D0991614

Blood Banking and Transfusion Medicine

Blood Banking and Transfusion Medicine

Basic Principles & Practice

Second Edition

Christopher D. Hillyer, MD
Director, Transfusion Medicine Program
Professor, Department of Pathology and Laboratory Medicine and the Division of Hematology/Oncology, Winship Cancer Institute
Emory University School of Medicine
Atlanta, Georgia

Leslie E. Silberstein, MD
Director, Joint Program in Transfusion Medicine
Children's Hospital Boston, Dana-Farber Cancer Institute, and Brigham and Women's Hospital
Professor of Pathology (Pediatrics)
Harvard Medical School
Boston, Massachusetts

Paul M. Ness, MD
Director, Transfusion Medicine Division, Johns Hopkins Medical Institutions
Professor, Pathology, Medicine, and Oncology, Johns Hopkins University School of Medicine
Baltimore, Maryland

Kenneth C. Anderson, MD
Chief, Division Hematologic Neoplasia
Director, Jerome Lipper Multiple Myeloma Center
Dana-Farber Cancer Institute
Kraft Family Professor of Medicine
Joint Program in Transfusion Medicine
Harvard Medical School
Boston, Massachusetts

John D. Roback, MD, PhD
Co-Director, Transfusion Medicine Program
Associate Professor, Department of Pathology and Laboratory Medicine
Emory University School of Medicine
Atlanta, Georgia

CHURCHILL LIVINGSTONE

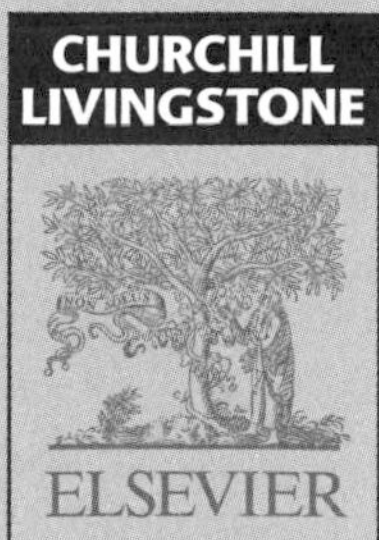

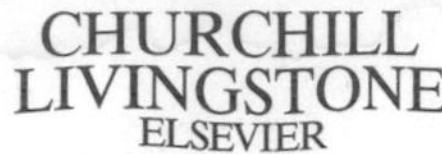

1600 John F. Kennedy Blvd.
Ste 1800
Philadelphia, PA 19103-2899

BLOOD BANKING AND TRANSFUSION MEDICINE, Second Edition

ISBN-13: 978-0-443-06981-9
ISBN-10: 0-443-06981-6

Notice

Knowledge and best practice in this field are constantly changing. As new research and experience broaden our knowledge, changes in practice, treatment and drug therapy may become necessary or appropriate. Readers are advised to check the most current information provided (i) on procedures featured or (ii) by the manufacturer of each product to be administered, to verify the recommended dose or formula, the method and duration of administration, and contraindications. It is the responsibility of the practitioner, relying on their own experience and knowledge of the patient, to make diagnoses, to determine dosages and the best treatment for each individual patient, and to take all appropriate safety precautions. To the fullest extent of the law, neither the Publisher nor the Editors assume any liability for any injury and/or damage to persons or property arising out or related to any use of the material contained in this book.

The Publisher

Library of Congress Cataloging-in-Publication Data
Blood banking and transfusion medicine: basic principles & practice /
Christopher D. Hillyer … [et al.].—2nd ed.
p. cm.
Includes bibliographical references and index.
ISBN 0-443-06981-6
1. Blood—Transfusion. 2. Blood banks. I. Hillyer, Christopher D. II. Title.
RM171.B583 2007
615′.39—dc22 2006048955

Acquisitions Editor: Dolores Meloni
Developmental Editor: Kristina Oberle/Kim DePaul
Project Manager: Bryan Hayward
Design Direction: Steven Stave

Printed in United States of America

Last digit is the print number: 9 8 7 6 5 4 3 2 1

About the Editors

Dr. Hillyer is a tenured professor in the Departments of Pathology and Pediatrics, as well as the Division of Hematology/Oncology, Winship Cancer Institute, Emory University School of Medicine. He serves as director of the Transfusion Medicine Program at Emory and oversees the Emory University Hospital Blood Bank, the blood and tissue banks of Children's Healthcare of Atlanta, and the Emory Center for the Advancement of International Transfusion Safety. He is an editor of three textbooks on transfusion medicine and an author of more than 120 articles and chapters pertaining to transfusion, HIV, cytokines, and herpesviruses (most notably CMV). Nationally recognized as an expert in hematology and blood transfusion, Dr. Hillyer is President of AABB (2006–2007) and is a Trustee of the National Blood Foundation (NBF). He has been awarded research funding from the NIH, CDC, NBF, and other agencies. He currently serves as principal investigator of a program project grant, several R-series awards, the Emory site of the NHLBI's Transfusion Medicine/Hemostasis Clinical Trial Network, and REDS-II. He also is a co-principal investigator of AABB's contract with HHS to provide technical assistance to six developing nations under the President's Emergency Plan for AIDS Relief (PEPFAR). Dr. Hillyer is an associate editor of *Transfusion* and part-time medical director of the American Red Cross Southern Region. Dr. Hillyer is board certified in Transfusion Medicine, Hematology, Medical Oncology, and Internal Medicine. He received his BS from Trinity College and his MD from the University of Rochester School of Medicine, with postgraduate training and fellowships in hematology-oncology, transfusion medicine, and bone marrow transplantation at Tufts–New England Medical Center in Boston.

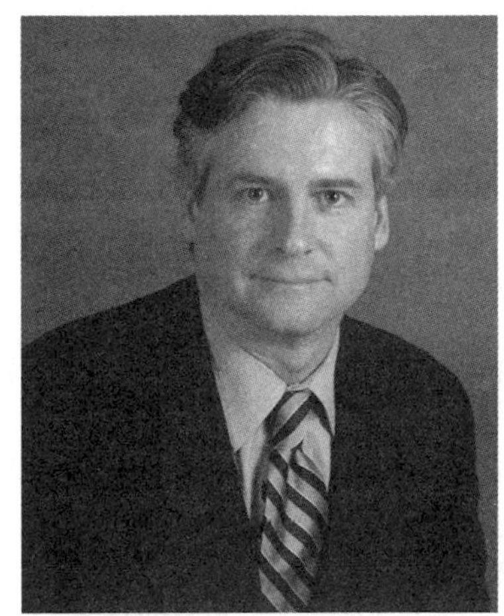

Dr. Silberstein is a tenured professor in the Department of Pathology, Harvard Medical School, and a Senior Investigator at the CBR Institute for Blood Research. He serves as director of the Joint Program in Transfusion Medicine, with responsibility for the blood and tissue programs at Boston Children's Hospital, the Brigham and Women's Hospitals, and the Dana-Farber Cancer Institute. Dr. Silberstein has recently created the Center for Human Cell Therapy at Harvard Medical School. The goal of this innovative center related to transfusion medicine is to facilitate the translation of proof-of-principle discoveries to clinical applications. Dr. Silberstein is editor of several texts, including *Hematology* and the *Handbook of Transfusion Medicine.* He is a member of the editorial boards of *Blood* and *Transfusion.* Dr. Silberstein is a highly respected physician-scientist well known for his mentorship; he has trained more than 45 fellows with PhD and MD backgrounds in transfusion medicine-related research. A leader and expert in transfusion medicine and hematology, Dr. Silberstein's research has focused on the immunology of B-cells and hematopoiesis, leading to the publication of more than 75 papers and numerous book chapters and reviews. Dr. Silberstein is board certified in Transfusion Medicine, Hematology, and Internal Medicine. He received his Baccalaureate and MD degrees from the University of Leiden, the Netherlands, and accomplished postgraduate training in Hematology/Oncology and Transfusion Medicine at Tufts–New England Medical Center in Boston.

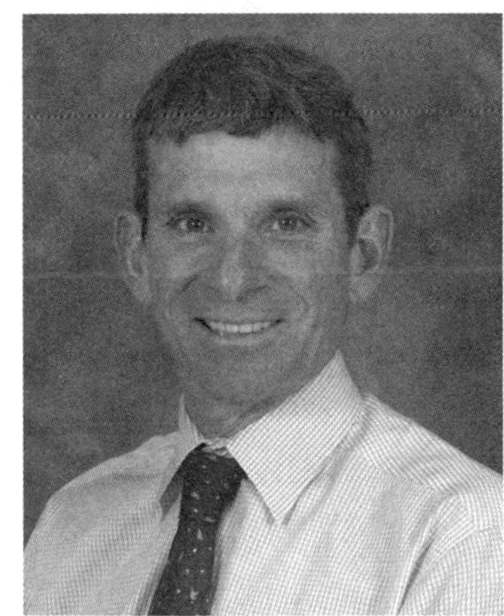

Dr. Ness is director of the Transfusion Medicine Division at The Johns Hopkins Hospital and professor of Pathology, Medicine, and Oncology at The Johns Hopkins University School of Medicine. For many years he also acted as CEO and medical director of the Greater Chesapeake and Potomac Region of the American Red Cross Blood Services. Dr. Ness has served the AABB for a number of years and was President in 1999. He served on the editorial board of *Transfusion* until named Editor in 2003. Dr. Ness has been a member of the American Society of Clinical Pathologists Board of Registry Blood Bank examination committee, and the FDA Blood Products Advisory Committee, and he consults for many commercial and nonprofit organizations. He is the editor of several textbooks on transfusion medicine and has published more than 150 articles. Dr. Ness' research focuses on transfusion-related complications and has been funded by the NIH and CDC. He was involved in the initial REDS program and now acts as consultant to REDS-II. He serves as principal investigator for the Johns Hopkins site of the Transfusion Medicine/Hemostasis Clinical Trial Network, funded by NHLBI. Dr. Ness is co-principal investigator of a project funded by the REDS-II program to study donor virus epidemiology issues in China. He has worked extensively in international blood safety initiatives in China, Thailand, Vietnam, Botswana, and Nigeria. Dr. Ness received his undergraduate education at the Massachusetts Institute of Technology and his MD degree from the State University of New York at Buffalo. His postgraduate work includes residency in internal medicine at Johns Hopkins, fellowship training in hematology-oncology at the University of California, San Francisco, and a transfusion medicine fellowship at Irwin Memorial Blood Bank in San Francisco.

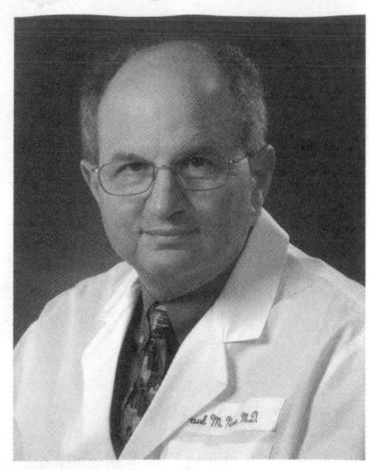

Dr. Anderson is the Kraft Family Professor of Medicine at Harvard Medical School and serves as chief of the Division of Hematologic Neoplasia, director of the Jerome Lipper Multiple Myeloma Center, and vice chair of the Joint Program in Transfusion Medicine at Dana-Farber Cancer Institute. Currently, Dr. Anderson is chair of the NCCN Multiple Myeloma Clinical Practice Guidelines Committee, is a Cancer and Leukemia Group B Principal Investigator, and is on the Board of Scientific Advisors of the International Myeloma Foundation. He has published more than 300 original articles and 200 book chapters, and has edited multiple textbooks on multiple myeloma and transfusion medicine. He is a Doris Duke Distinguished Clinical Research Scientist and has had long-term RO1, PO1, and SPORE funding from the NIH and other agencies. Dr. Anderson has received numerous awards, including the 2001 Charles C. Lund Award of the American Red Cross Blood Services, the 2003 Waldenstrom's award for research in plasma cell dyscrasias, the 2004 Johnson & Johnson Focused Giving Award for Setting New Directions in Science and Technology, and the 2005 Robert A. Kyle Lifetime Achievement Award. Dr. Anderson graduated from Johns Hopkins Medical School, trained in internal medicine at Johns Hopkins Hospital, and completed hematology, medical oncology, and tumor immunology fellowships at the Dana-Farber Cancer Institute.

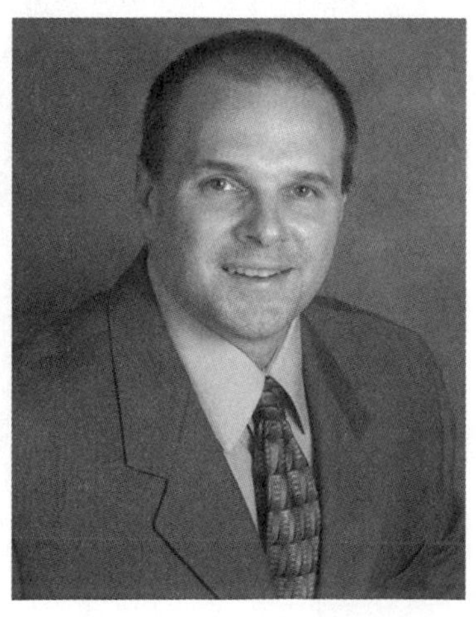

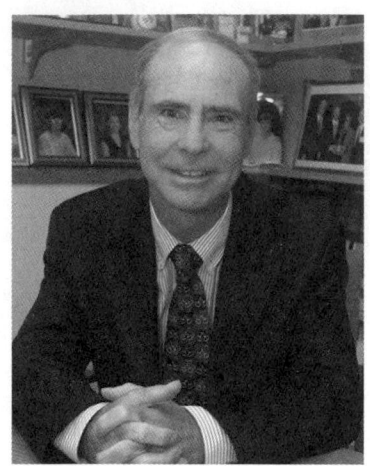

Dr. Roback is a tenured associate professor in the Department of Pathology and Laboratory Medicine at Emory University, associate director of the Emory Transfusion Medicine Program, and co-director of the Emory University Hospital Blood Bank and Stem Cell Processing Laboratory. Dr. Roback's research focuses on human and animal models of CMV infection, emphasizing approaches to accelerate and improve the antiviral immune response following hematopoietic stem cell transplantation. He also is inventor or co-inventor of a number of novel devices and methodologies for rapid pretransfusion blood testing. Dr. Roback's investigations have been funded by the NIH, CDC, NBF, and DOD. He is a co-principal investigator of the Emory site for REDS-II. Dr. Roback has authored 40 peer-reviewed publications and invited reviews, as well as 16 book chapters. He teaches medical, residency, and graduate school courses and was recognized for excellent clinical pathology teaching with the Golden Apple Award. An active member of a number of AABB committees, Dr. Roback is editor-in-chief of the 16th edition of the AABB's Technical Manual, member of the editorial board for the journal *Transfusion*, and co-chair of the NHLBI's Global Blood Safety and Availability task force on future transfusion medicine research initiatives. He is a Diplomate of the American Board of Pathology in Clinical Pathology and Blood Banking and Transfusion Medicine. Dr. Roback received his Baccalaureate degree from Johns Hopkins University and was awarded a PhD in experimental pathology and an MD from the University of Chicago. He completed a postdoctoral research fellowship and anatomic pathology residency training at Albert Einstein College of Medicine and subsequently completed clinical pathology and transfusion medicine training at Emory University.

Contributors

Sharon Adams, MT, CHS (ABHI)
Supervisor, HLA Laboratory
Department of Transfusion Medicine
Warren G. Magnuson Clinical Center
National Institutes of Health
Bethesda, Maryland, USA

Barbara Alving, MD, MACP
Professor of Medicine
Uniformed Services University of the Health Sciences
Bethesda, Maryland, USA

Kenneth C. Anderson, MD
Chief, Division Hematologic Neoplasia
Director, Jerome Lipper Multiple Myeloma Center
Dana-Farber Cancer Institute
Kraft Family Professor of Medicine
Harvard Medical School
Boston, Massachusetts

James P. AuBuchon, MD
E. Elizabeth French Professor and Chair of Pathology
Dartmouth-Hitchcock Medical Center
Lebanon, New Hampshire, USA

Nicholas Bandarenko, MD
Associate Professor of Pathology and Laboratory Medicine
Transfusion Medicine Service
University of North Carolina, Chapel Hill
Chapel Hill, North Carolina, USA

Jon Barrett, MBBCh, FRCOG, MD, FRCSC
Associate Professor, Department of Obstetrics and Gynecology, University of Toronto
Senior Investigator Maternal and Infant Research Unit of Center for Research in Women's Health
Chief of Maternal Fetal Medicine, Sunnybrook and Women's College Health Sciences Center
Toronto, Ontario, Canada

Richard J. Benjamin, MS, MBChB, PhD
Chief Medical Officer
American Red Cross Biomedical Services
National Headquarters, Washington, D.C.
Assistant Professor of Pathology
Joint Program in Transfusion Medicine
Harvard Medical School
Boston, Massachusetts, USA

Howard Benn, MD
Chief Fellow, Department of Hematology/Oncology
Seton Hall University School of Graduate Medical Education
South Orange, New Jersey, USA

Ginine M. Beyer, MD
Department of Pathology
University of Maryland School of Medicine
Baltimore, Maryland, USA

Morris A. Blajchman, MD, FRCP
Professor, Pathology and Molecular Medicine
Head, Transfusion Medicine Services, Hamilton Regional Laboratory
Medical Director, Canadian Blood Services
Hamilton, Ontario, Canada

Neil Blumberg, MD
Director, Clinical Laboratories
Director, Transfusion Medicine
Professor of Pathology and Laboratory Medicine, University of Rochester School of Medicine
Rochester, New York, USA

Mark E. Brecher, MD
Professor, Department of Pathology and Laboratory Medicine
Director, Clinical Pathology
University of North Carolina
Chapel Hill, North Carolina, USA

Hal E. Broxmeyer, PhD
Distinguished Professor, Chairman and Mary Margaret Walther Professor of Microbiology and Immunology
Professor of Medicine
Scientific Director of the Walther Oncology Center
Indiana University School of Medicine
Indianapolis, Indiana, USA

Michael P. Busch, MD, PhD
Vice President, Research, Blood Systems, Inc., Scottsdale, Arizona
Director, Blood Systems Research Institute, San Francisco, California
Adjunct Professor, Department of Laboratory Medicine
University of California,
San Francisco, California, USA

Jeannie L. Callum, BA, MD, FRCPC
Assistant Professor, Department of Laboratory Medicine and Pathobiology
University of Toronto
Director, Blood and Tissue Banks
Sunnybrook and Women's College Health Sciences Center
Toronto, Ontario, Canada

Sally A. Campbell-Lee, MD
Assistant Professor, Department of Pathology
Associate Medical Director, Division of Transfusion Medicine
Medical Director, Johns Hopkins Bayview Transfusion Medicine Service
Baltimore, Maryland, USA

Jeffrey L. Carson, MD
Richard C. Reynolds Professor of Medicine
Chief, Division of General Internal Medicine
University of Medicine and Dentistry, New Jersey
Robert Wood Johnson Medical School
New Brunswick, New Jersey, USA

Kenneth A. Clark, MD, MPH
Head, International Blood Safety
Global AIDS Program
Centers for Disease Control and Prevention
Atlanta, Georgia, USA

Laurence Corash, MD
Professor, Laboratory Medicine, University of California, San Francisco
Attending Physician, Laboratory Medicine and Medicine-Hematology Division
The Medical Center at the University of California, San Francisco
Chief Medical Officer and Vice President, Research and Medical Affairs
Cerus Corporation
Concord, California, USA

Robert L. Crookes, MBChB
Medical Director
South African National Blood Service
Johannesburg, South Africa

Elizabeth E. Culler, MD
Medical Director
Blood Assurance, Inc.
Chattanooga, Tennessee, USA

Melody J. Cunningham, MD
Assistant Professor of Pediatrics
Harvard Medical School
Children's Hospital Boston
Boston, Massachusetts, USA

Richard J. Davey, MD
Director, Transfusion Service
The Methodist Hospital
Houston, Texas, USA

Dana V. Devine, PhD
Professor of Pathology and Laboratory Medicine
Centre for Blood Research
University of British Columbia
Executive Director, Research and Development
Canadian Blood Services
Vancouver, British Columbia, Canada

Roger Y. Dodd, PhD
Vice President, Research and Development
Director, Holland Laboratory
American Red Cross, Biomedical Services
Rockville, Maryland, USA

Alexander Duncan, MD
Assistant Professor, Department of Pathology and Laboratory Medicine
Emory University School of Medicine
Director, Coagulation Laboratories
Atlanta, Georgia, USA

Walter H. Dzik, MD
Co-Director, Blood Transfusion Service
Massachusetts General Hospital
Associate Professor of Pathology
Harvard Medical School
Boston, Massachusetts, USA

James R. Eckman, MD
Director, Georgia Comprehensive Sickle Cell Center
Grady Health System
Professor of Hematology/Oncology and Medicine
Winship Cancer Institute
Emory University School of Medicine
Atlanta, Georgia, USA

A. Bradley Eisenbrey, MD, PhD
Chief, Transfusion Medicine Services
William Beaumont Hospital, Royal Oak, Michigan
HLA Laboratory Associate Director
Gift of Life of Michigan, Ann Arbor, Michigan
Assistant Professor of Pathology
Wayne State University School of Medicine
Detroit, Michigan, USA

Eberhard W. Fiebig, MD
Associate Professor, Department of Laboratory Medicine
Chief, Divisions of Hematology and Transfusion Medicine
University of California
San Francisco, California, USA

John M. Fisk, MD
Clinical Instructor, Laboratory Medicine
SUNY Upstate Medical University College of Medicine
Assistant Director, Transfusion Medicine
University Hospital of the State University of New York
Syracuse, New York, USA

Terrence L. Geiger, MD, PhD
Assistant Professor, Department of Pathology
St. Jude Children's Research Hospital
Memphis, Tennessee, USA

Mindy Goldman, MD, FRCP(C)
Executive Medical Director
Donor and Transplantation Services
Canadian Blood Services
Ottawa, Ontario, Canada

Shealynn B. Harris, MD
Assistant Medical Director
American Red Cross Blood Services, Southern Region
Atlanta, Georgia, USA

Joanna M. Heal, MRCP, MBBS
Associate Medical Director, American Red Cross Blood Services, New York-Penn Region
Associate Clinical Professor of Medicine, Hematology-Oncology Unit
University of Rochester School of Medicine
Rochester, New York, USA

Paul C. Hébert, MD, FRCPC, MHSc(Epid)
Vice-Chair, Department of Medicine
Professor of Medicine and Epidemiology
Chair in Transfusion and Critical Care Research
Ottawa Health Research Institute and the University of Ottawa
Ottawa, Ontario, Canada

Nancy Heddle, MSc, FCSMLS(D)
Director, McMaster Transfusion Research Program
Associate Professor, Department of Medicine
McMaster University
Hamilton, Ontario, Canada

John R. Hess, MD, MPH
Professor of Pathology and Medicine
University of Maryland School of Medicine
Baltimore, Maryland, USA

Christopher D. Hillyer, MD
Director, Transfusion Medicine Program
Professor, Department of Pathology and Laboratory Medicine and the Division of Hematology/Oncology, Winship Cancer Institute
Emory University School of Medicine
Atlanta, Georgia, USA

Krista L. Hillyer, MD
Chief Medical Officer, American Red Cross Blood Services, Southern Region
Assistant Professor, Department of Pathology and Laboratory Medicine
Emory University School of Medicine
Atlanta, Georgia, USA

Paul V. Holland, MD
Clinical Professor of Medicine and Pathology
UC Davis Medical Center, Sacramento, California
Scientific Director, Delta Blood Bank
Stockton, California, USA

Kim A. Janatpour, MD
Assistant Professor, University of California Davis School of Medicine, Department of Pathology and Laboratory Medicine
Davis Medical Center
Sacramento, California, USA

Viviana V. Johnson, MD
Transfusion Medicine Fellow
Department of Pathology
Georgetown University Hospital
Washington, D.C., USA

Cassandra D. Josephson, MD
Assistant Professor, Departments of Pathology and Pediatrics
Emory University School of Medicine
Assistant Director, Blood Banks and Transfusion Services
Attending Pediatric Hematologist/Oncologist, Department of Pediatrics
Children's Healthcare of Atlanta
Atlanta, Georgia, USA

Richard M. Kaufman, MD
Medical Director, Adult Transfusion Service, Brigham and Women's Hospital
Assistant Professor of Pathology, Harvard Medical School
Boston, Massachusetts, USA

Thomas S. Kickler, MD
Professor of Medicine and Pathology
Johns Hopkins University School of Medicine
Baltimore, Maryland, USA

Diane Killion, JD
Staff Counsel
AABB
Bethesda, Maryland, USA

Karen E. King, MD
Associate Medical Director
Transfusion Medicine Division
Johns Hopkins University School of Medicine
Baltimore, Maryland, USA

Steven H. Kleinman, MD
Kleinman Biomedical Research
Victoria, British Columbia, Canada
University of British Columbia
Vancouver, British Columbia, Canada

Thomas J. Kunicki, PhD
Associate Professor
Division of Experimental Hemostasis and Thrombosis
Department of Molecular and Experimental Medicine
The Scripps Research Institute
La Jolla, California, USA

Tzong-Hae Lee, MD, PhD
Director, Molecular Biology
Blood Systems Research Institute
San Francisco, California, USA

Karen Shoos Lipton, JD
Chief Executive Officer
AABB
Bethesda, Maryland, USA

Lennart E. Lögdberg, MD, PhD
Associate Professor, Department of Pathology and Laboratory Medicine
Director, Crawford W. Long Hospital Transfusion Services
Emory University School of Medicine
Atlanta, Georgia, USA

Naomi L. C. Luban, MD
Interim Executive Director, Center for Cancer and Blood Disorders
Chair, Laboratory Medicine and Pathology
Director, Transfusion Medicine/The Edward J. Miller Donor Center
Vice Chair for Academic Affairs, Department of Pediatrics
Children's National Medical Center
Professor, Pediatrics and Pathology
The George Washington University Medical Center
Washington, D.C., USA

Catherine S. Manno, MD
Professor and Associate Chair for Clinical Affairs
Department of Pediatrics
Children's Hospital of Philadelphia
University of Pennsylvania School of Medicine
Philadelphia, Pennsylvania, USA

Simon Mantha, MD
Department of Laboratory Medicine
Yale University School of Medicine
Yale–New Haven Hospital
New Haven, Connecticut, USA

Francesco M. Marincola, MD
Director, HLA and Immunogenetics Research Laboratory
Department of Transfusion Medicine
Warren G. Magnuson Clinical Center
National Institutes of Health
Bethesda, Maryland, USA

Bruce C. McLeod, MD
Professor of Medicine and Pathology
Director, Blood Center
Rush University Medical Center
Chicago, Illinois, USA

Jay E. Menitove, MD
Clinical Professor, Internal Medicine
University of Kansas School of Medicine
Kansas City, Kansas; Executive Director and Medical Director, Community Blood Center of Greater Kansas City
Kansas City, Missouri, USA

Peter A. Millward, MD
Assistant Professor, Clinical Pathology
Milton S. Hershey Medical Center
Pennsylvania State University
Hershey, Pennsylvania, USA

Edward L. Murphy, MD, MPH
Professor, Laboratory Medicine and Epidemiology/Biostatistics
University of California, San Francisco
San Francisco, California, USA

Paul M. Ness, MD
Director, Transfusion Medicine Division
Johns Hopkins Medical Institutions
Professor, Pathology, Medicine, and Oncology
Johns Hopkins University School of Medicine
Baltimore, Maryland, USA

Diane J. Nugent, MD
Assistant Professor
David Geffen School of Medicine at UCLA
University of California, Los Angeles
Director, Division of Hematology
Children's Hospital of Orange County
General Pediatrics, Irvine Medical Center
Los Angeles, California, USA

Peter L. Perrotta, MD
Associate Professor of Pathology
West Virginia University
Morgantown, West Virginia, USA

Patricia T. Pisciotto, MD
Professor, Laboratory Medicine
University of Connecticut Health Sciences Center
Director, Blood Bank, John Dempsey Hospital
Farmington, Connecticut, USA

Thomas H. Price, MD
Executive Vice-President, Medical Division
Medical Director, Puget Sound Blood Center
Professor of Medicine, University of Washington
Seattle, Washington, USA

Jayashree Ramasethu, MD
Associate Professor of Clinical Pediatrics
Division of Neonatology
Department of Pediatrics
Georgetown University Hospital
Washington, D.C., USA

Sandra M. Ramirez-Arcos, MSc, PhD
Associate Scientist, Canadian Blood Services
Adjunct Professor, University of Ottawa
Research and Development, Infectious Diseases
Ottawa, Ontario, Canada

William Reed, MD
Assistant Medical Director, Research
Blood Systems Research Institute
Clinical Associate Professor
Department of Laboratory Medicine
Medical Director, Human Islet and Cellular Therapy Laboratory
University of California
San Francisco, California, USA

Marion E. Reid, PhD
Director, Immunohematology
New York Blood Center
New York, New York, USA

John D. Roback, MD, PhD
Co-Director, Transfusion Medicine Program
Associate Professor, Department of Pathology and Laboratory Medicine
Emory University School of Medicine
Atlanta, Georgia, USA

Scott D. Rowley, MD, FACP
Chief, Adult Blood and Marrow Transplantation Program
Hackensack University Medical Center
Hackensack, New Jersey, USA

S. Gerald Sandler, MD
Professor of Medicine and Pathology
Georgetown University School of Medicine
Director, Transfusion Medicine
Department of Laboratory Medicine
Georgetown University Hospital
Washington, D.C., USA

Audrey N. Schuetz, MD
Department of Pathology and Laboratory Medicine
Emory University School of Medicine
Atlanta, Georgia, USA

Eileen Selogie, MT(ASCP)SBB
Consultant Compliance Officer
Department of Pathology, Blood Donor Services
Presbyterian Intercommunity Hospital
Whittier, California, USA

Beth Shaz, MD
Assistant Professor, Emory University School of Medicine
Department of Pathology and Laboratory Medicine
Director, Grady Memorial Hospital Blood Bank
Atlanta, Georgia, USA

R. Sue Shirey, MD, MT(ASCP) SBB
Technical Specialist, Transfusion Medicine Division,
Johns Hopkins Hospital
Baltimore, Maryland, USA

Ira A. Shulman, MD
Director of Transfusion Medicine
Professor and Vice Chair of Pathology
Keck School of Medicine of the University of Southern California
Director of Laboratories and Pathology, LAC + USC Medical Center
Los Angeles, California, USA

Suzanne Shusterman, MD
Instructor, Harvard Medical School
Department of Pediatric Oncology
Dana-Farber Cancer Institute
Children's Hospital Boston
Boston, Massachusetts, USA

Leslie E. Silberstein, MD
Director, Joint Program in Transfusion Medicine
Children's Hospital Boston, Dana-Farber Cancer Institute, Brigham and Women's Hospital
Professor of Pathology, Harvard Medical School
Boston, Massachusetts, USA

Steven R. Sloan, MD, PhD
Assistant Professor of Pathology Pediatrics
Joint Program in Transfusion Medicine
Harvard Medical School
Boston, Massachusetts, USA

Edward L. Snyder, MD
Professor, Laboratory Medicine
Yale University School of Medicine
Director, Blood Bank, Yale–New Haven Hospital
New Haven, Connecticut, USA

Ronald G. Strauss, MD
Professor of Pathology and Pediatrics
University of Iowa College of Medicine
Iowa City, Iowa, USA

David F. Stroncek, MD
Chief, Laboratory Services Section
Department of Transfusion Medicine
Warren G. Magnuson Clinical Center
National Institutes of Health
Bethesda, Maryland, USA

D. Michael Strong, PhD, BCLD(ABB)
Executive Vice President, COO
Puget Sound Blood Center
Research Professor
Department of Orthopaedics and Sports Medicine
Department of Surgery
University of Washington School of Medicine
Seattle, Washington, USA

Leon L. Su, MD
Associate Medical Director
Blood Systems, Inc.
Assistant Medical Director
United Blood Services, Arizona
Scottsdale, Arizona, USA

Zbigniew M. Szczepiorkowski, MD, PhD
Associate Professor of Pathology and Medicine
Director, Transfusion Medicine Service
Dartmouth-Hitchcock Medical Center
Lebanon, New Hampshire, USA

Gary E. Tegtmeier, PhD
Scientific Director
Community Blood Center of Greater Kansas City
Kansas City, Missouri, USA

Alan Tinmouth, MD, FRCPC, MSc
Director, Adult Hemophilia and Bleeding Disorders Comprehensive Care Program
Assistant Professor of Medicine
Associate Scientist, Center for Transfusion Research
Ottawa Health Research Institute and the University of Ottawa
Ottawa, Ontario, Canada

Ena Wang, MD
Staff Scientist, Immunogenetics Research Laboratory
Department of Transfusion Medicine
Warren G. Magnuson Clinical Center
National Institutes of Health
Bethesda, Maryland, USA

Kathryn E. Webert, MD, FRCPC
Assistant Professor, Department of Medicine
McMaster University
Medical Consultant, Canadian Blood Services
Hamilton, Ontario, Canada

Connie M. Westhoff, SBB, PhD
Scientific Director, Molecular Blood Group and Platelet Antigen Testing Laboratory
American Red Cross
Adjunct Assistant Professor, University of Pennsylvania Department of Pathology and Laboratory Medicine
Philadelphia, Pennsylvania, USA

Robert M. Winslow, MD
President, Chairman and CEO, Sangart, Inc.
Adjunct Professor, Department of Bioengineering
University of California, San Diego
San Diego, California, USA

Edward C. C. Wong, MD
Assistant Professor of Pediatrics and Pathology
Department of Laboratory Medicine
George Washington School of Medicine
Director of Hematology, Associate Director of Transfusion Medicine
Children's National Medical Center
Washington, D.C., USA

Gary Zeger, MD
Associate Professor, Keck USC School of Medicine
Co-Medical Director, USC University Hospital Clinical Laboratories
Medical Director, Blood Bank, USC University Hospital
Medical Director, USC Blood Donor Center
Los Angeles, California, USA

James C. Zimring, MD, PhD
Assistant Professor, Transfusion Medicine Program
Department of Pathology and Laboratory Medicine
Emory University School of Medicine
Atlanta, Georgia, USA

Preface to the Second Edition

The editors are pleased to introduce the Second Edition of *Blood Banking and Transfusion Medicine.* Substantial modifications and additions have been made to the text, reflecting advancements in a number of areas, including cellular therapy, component preparation, infectious disease testing, and the underlying biology of transfusion therapy. In addition, we have continued to integrate elements of Anderson and Ness's excellent textbook *The Scientific Basis of Transfusion Medicine*, which can be noted by the reader as a number of new chapters entitled "Principles of . . . ." We are grateful for the many suggestions offered by readers of the First Edition that led to additional improvements in the text. We have made a concerted effort to ensure that each chapter includes the most up-to-date scientific underpinnings of transfusion biology as well as detailed information that can be applied to clinical transfusion practice. It is our goal that this textbook remain the definitive source of blood banking and transfusion medicine biology, technology, and practice for physicians, technologists, nurses, and administrative personnel, and we sincerely welcome readers' observations, criticisms, and suggestions so that we can continue to work to improve this book. Finally, we thank you for your support of this text, the field of transfusion medicine, and the patients we serve.

C. D. Hillyer

L. E. Silberstein

P. M. Ness

K. C. Anderson

J. D. Roback

Acknowledgments

We, the editors, would like to acknowledge the outstanding technical and professional support of Sue Rollins and the expertise, guidance, and friendship of Dolores Meloni. We would also like to thank our friends and families for their unconditional love and support, without which this edition could not have come to fruition. We thank especially Krista, Whitney, Peter, Margot, Jackson, and James Hillyer; the family and friends of Les Silberstein; Barbara, Jennie, Steven, and Molly Ness; Cynthia, Emily, David, and Peter Anderson; and Linda, Evan, and Ethan Roback. Finally, we would like to acknowledge and thank the many mentors, physicians, and patients who have served as inspiration, colleagues, and friends.

Contents

B. Complications of Transfusion, 584

i. Infectious Complications, 584

ii. Noninfectious Complications, 668

C. Therapeutic Apheresis, 727

D. Cellular Therapies and Tissue Banking, 780

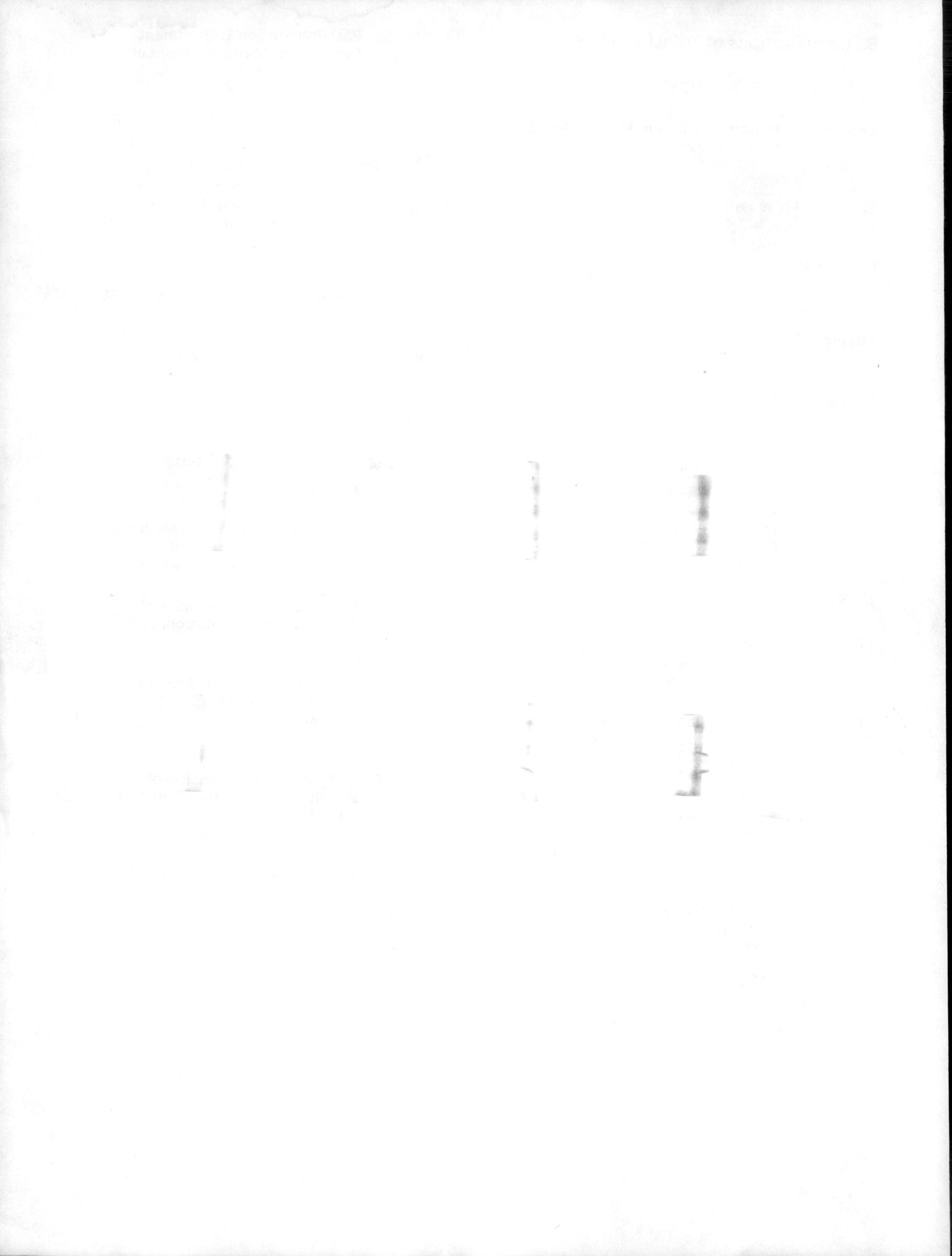

D. Specific Blood Components, 250

E. Special Processes and Products, 359

Section III
TRANSFUSION MEDICINE, 443

A. Transfusion in Specific Clinical Settings, 445

Section I

History

Chapter 1

A Brief History of Blood Transfusion

Kim A. Janatpour • Paul V. Holland

EARLY HISTORY

Since the beginning of human history, blood has been recognized as a vital force, the essence of life. Prehistoric man created cave drawings showing individuals bleeding from traumatic wounds. In the Bible, Leviticus states "the life of the flesh is in the blood." The Chinese Huang Di Nei Ching (770–221 BC) held that blood contained the soul. Blood played a central theme in ancient rituals. Egyptians and Romans took blood baths for physical and spiritual restoration,[1] and Romans even drank the blood of fallen gladiators in the belief that the blood could transmit the gladiator's vitality. Precolumbian North American Indians bled the body "of its greatest power" as self-punishment. In the Middle Ages, the drinking of blood was advocated as a tonic for rejuvenation and for the treatment of various diseases.[2] Pope Innocent VIII drank the blood from three young boys in 1492. Unfortunately, the boys and the Pope died.[2] The idea that infusion of blood could be beneficial did not emerge until the 17th century.

From the time of Hippocrates (c. 450 BC), disease was believed to be caused by an imbalance of the four humours—blood, phlegm, yellow bile, and black bile. Of these, blood was the most important (Galen [130–201 AD] really advanced the humoural theory). The most popular treatment for most ailments, even as late as the 18th century, was blood letting (Fig. 1–1). Without the correct understanding of blood circulation, intravenous blood infusion could not even be imagined. This changed in 1628 with William Harvey's description of the circulatory system. Harvey's identification of separate yet connected arterial and venous systems in his *De Motu Cordis* paved the way for an entirely new arena of blood investigation.[3]

In 1656, Christopher Wren used a quill with an attached bladder to demonstrate that the intravenous injection of substances into animals had systemic effects.[1,2] In 1666, Richard Lower successfully transfused blood from one dog to another, which led Samuel Pepys to speculate on the potential benefits of human transfusion, stating that "bad blood" might be mended by "borrowing" blood "from a better body."[3]

THE FIRST ANIMAL-TO-HUMAN TRANSFUSIONS

The first published animal-to-human transfusion was performed June 15, 1667, by Jean Baptiste Denis, a physician to Louis XIV, on a 16-year-old boy who had been "tormented with a contumacious and violent fever." The boy had been treated with multiple bleeds, following which "his wit seemed wholly sunk, his memory perfectly soft, and his body so heavy and drowsie that he was not fit for any thing." Denis attributed these symptoms to the bloodletting he had received. As treatment, Denis exchanged 3 ounces of the boy's blood for 9 ounces of lamb's blood. Denis chose animal blood because he believed it purer than that of humans due to man's "debauchery and irregularities in eating and drinking" and reasoned that if man could use animal milk as nutrient, animal blood would be safe. Following the infusion of lamb's blood, the patient complained about "a great heat along his arm," but otherwise suffered no ill effects. Denis subsequently performed such transfusions on three more patients, the last of which resulted in the first malpractice suit for blood transfusion.[4] Antoine Mauroy was a 34-year-old madman who was brought to Denis after he was found wandering the streets of Paris in the winter of 1667. Mauroy had suffered for years from severe "phrensies," during which he would beat his wife, strip off his clothes, and run through the streets, setting house fires. At this time, blood was believed to affect one's temperament and character; therefore, it was reasoned that blood transfusion could be used to treat mental ailments. Denis's patron, Monsieur de Montmort, proposed transfusing Mauroy to allay the "heat of his blood."[5] Denis transfused Mauroy with calf's blood, hoping that the calf's docile nature would be imparted to Mauroy. Although the patient complained of heat moving up his arm, he tolerated the transfusion well. A few days later, a second, larger transfusion was performed. This time, however, the patient complained "of great pains in his kidneys, and that he was not well in his stomack, that he was ready to [choak] unless they gave him his liberty."[6] The transfusion was quickly discontinued, after which the patient vomited and passed urine "black as soot." Miraculously, the patient not only survived this hemolytic transfusion reaction, but also appeared to be cured, showing "a surprising calmness, and a great presence of mind ... and a general lassitude in all his limbs." In fact, upon seeing his wife a few days later, Mauroy greeted her tenderly, relating "with great presence of mind all that had befallen him." Denis was astonished—the man who "used to do nothing but swear and beat his wife" had dramatically, almost magically, been cured.[7]

Also, later in 1667, Richard Lower successfully transfused a Cambridge University student described as "cracked a little in the head" with sheep's blood.[3,4] A bitter debate followed between Denis and Lower as to who could claim to have discovered blood transfusion.[4]

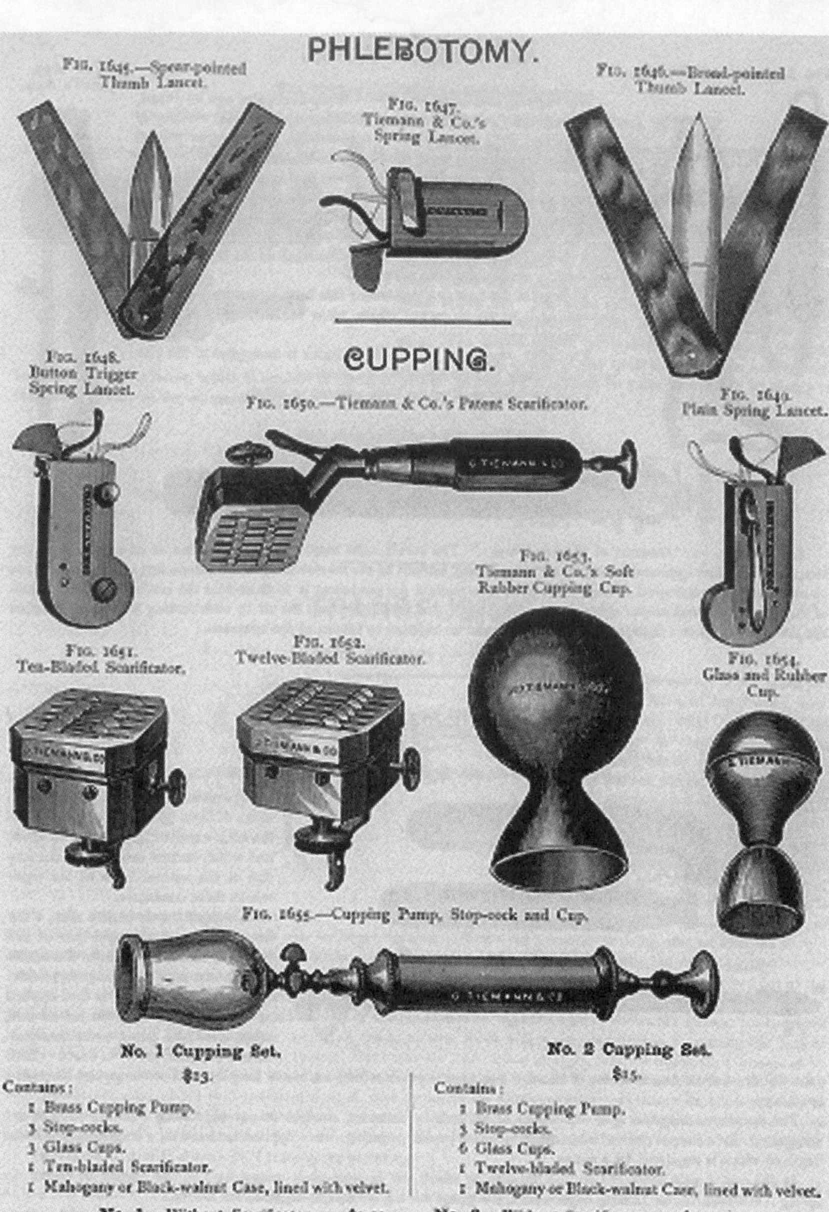

Figure 1–1 A collection of bloodletting instruments. (From Star D. Blood. An epic history of medicine and commerce. New York, HarperCollins Publishers, 2002. With permission.)

Although a select group of scientists was excited about the concept of transfusion, others were adamantly opposed to the practice. Denis, in particular, suffered harsh criticism from his peers. With this intense debate and criticism as the backdrop, Mauroy suffered a relapse; his wife begged Denis to transfuse her husband again. Denis found the patient to be very ill, so was hesitant to perform the transfusion, but reluctantly agreed. Before the transfusion began, however, Mauroy died and his widow refused to allow Denis to examine the body. The widow had been offered money from Denis's rivals to charge him with murder; she offered to drop the matter if Denis would agree to support her financially. Denis refused, and the case went to court. Denis was exonerated when it was discovered that Mauroy had been poisoned with arsenic by his wife. Nonetheless, although Denis was acquitted of malpractice, the general opposition to transfusion ultimately led the French and English courts, and much of the rest of Europe, to ban all human transfusions.[1,4,5,7,8]

FIRST HUMAN-TO-HUMAN TRANSFUSION

After being banned for more than 150 years, the use of blood transfusion was revived during the late 18th century. A footnote in an American journal indicates that the first human-to-human transfusion had been performed by Philip Syng Physick, the "Father of American Surgery," in 1795, although this has never been confirmed.[5,9] In 1816, John Henry Leacock, a Barbados physician, presented his dissertation "On the Transfusion of Blood in Extreme Cases of Haemorrhage." Leacock subsequently performed and published a set of animal experiments that proved that the donor and recipient must be of the same species.[10]

Although Leacock apparently went no further with the experiments, his work inspired James Blundell, an obstetrician and physiologist at Guy's Hospital in London, to carry out additional investigations. At the time, obstetricians could only stand by and watch helplessly as patients exsanguinated postpartum. Blundell was convinced that blood transfusion could save patients' lives. His extensive experimentation confirmed Leacock's findings that blood could be used to treat hemorrhagic shock, but only blood from the same species could be used. Recognizing the potentially serious risks of transfusion, Blundell began attempting human-to-human transfusion in cases that were otherwise hopeless. Over a decade, he performed 10 such transfusions, all without success. However, in August 1825, Blundell successfully transfused a woman dying from postpartum hemorrhage with blood from her husband. Other successes followed, including three cases of postpartum hemorrhage, and a young boy who was hypovolemic following amputation of his leg.[11] Subsequently, other reports of transfusion followed from Europe and then the United States, where it was reported that transfusion was used by the Union Army during the American Civil War.[5,9]

Significant progress in understanding the basis for the incompatibility between species was made by Emil Ponfick and Leonard Landois in the late 1800s.[8] The first revelation came from Ponfick, who observed red cell lysis in the blood of a woman who died after receiving a transfusion of sheep blood. From animal experiments, Ponfick found that incompatible transfusions were associated with hemorrhage and "congestion" of the kidneys, lungs, and liver. He also recognized that the red urine that transfused animals excreted was caused by hemoglobinuria, not hematuria. Landois's observation that human red cells would lyse when mixed in vitro with the sera of other animals set the stage for the study of the immunologic basis of blood incompatibility.[8]

DISCOVERY OF ABO BLOOD GROUPS

Before 1901, the prevailing belief was that all human blood was the same. However, this changed in 1901 with Karl Landsteiner's landmark discovery of ABO blood groups.[12] Landsteiner, an Austrian immunologist, noticed that human blood mixed in test tubes with other specimens of human blood sometimes resulted in agglutination. By incubating red cells from some individuals with serum from others, he identified agglutination patterns, leading to the initial identification of three blood groups, A, B, and C (C was later renamed O).[3,13] In 1902, Alfred Decastello and Adriano Sturli, two of Landsteiner's former students, found the fourth blood group, AB.[3] Landsteiner also contributed to forensic science by developing a method for blood typing of dried blood specimens.[14]

Interestingly, the importance of the blood groups was not immediately recognized; blood group typing did not become part of routine practice for several years. Richard Weil, a pathologist at the German Hospital in New York, was the first to perform ABO typing and began compatibility testing in 1907; he was also the first to suggest inheritance of ABO types.[5] Also in 1907 and 1910, respectively, Jan Jansky of Czechoslovakia and Moss of the United States independently identified four human blood groups.[3] However, the Roman numeral systems that Jansky and Moss each used for designating the four blood groups were completely reversed. Tremendous confusion ensued with the three different nomenclatures. Finally, in 1927, the American Association of Immunologists adopted a new classification scheme proposed by Landsteiner, the current ABO terminology.[3]

The discovery of blood groups led Ludvig Hektoen of Chicago to advocate selecting donors by blood group and crossmatching.[8] In 1913, Reuben Ottenberg conclusively demonstrated the importance of compatibility testing in his report of 128 cases of transfusion.[15] However, even as recently as 1937, some suggested that crossmatching was unnecessary if the selection of donors was restricted to individuals of the same blood group.[5]

The inheritance pattern of blood groups was finally proved by Felix Bernstein in 1924.[3] Sadly, differences in race distribution of blood groups were manipulated and misused in Germany during World War I (WWI) and World War II (WWII), during which time blood group B was deemed a marker for Slavic or Jewish race, and blood group A was considered associated with intelligence and industry. In the 1950s in Louisiana, it was a misdemeanor for a physician to give blood from a black donor to a white person without consent. In the United States, segregation of blood by race existed until the 1960s.[3]

DISCOVERY OF RH BLOOD GROUPS

Although a major discovery in transfusion medicine, ABO blood group typing was not sufficient to prevent many fatal hemolytic transfusion reactions. In 1939 Philip Levine published a case report of post-transfusion hemolysis in a blood group O patient who received blood from her blood group O husband. Levine found that incubation of the patient's serum with her husband's red cells resulted in agglutination. Additionally, the woman's serum was found to agglutinate 80 of 104 other samples of ABO-compatible blood. The name of the offending antibody came from parallel experiments conducted by Landsteiner and Alex Wiener in which antibodies produced by immunization of rabbits and guinea pigs with blood from rhesus monkeys caused red cell agglutination of 85% of humans tested. Those individuals whose red cells were agglutinated by these antibodies were classified as rhesus (Rh) positive.[3] Levine was able to show that Rh antibodies were the main cause of serious hemolytic disease of the newborn (erythroblastosis fetalis).[16] Later, it was appreciated that the Rh system is composed of numerous alleles. The current system of nomenclature—c, C, d, D, e, E—was proposed in 1944 by Cambridge geneticist Sir Ronald Fisher. Subsequent development of Rh immune globulin (RhIG) for prevention of hemolytic disease of the newborn was a major advance. The use of the antiglobulin test, first described by Carlo Moreschi in 1908 and rediscovered in 1945 by Robin Coombs, Rob Race, and Arthur Mourant, allowed the identification of many other blood group antigens in the decades that followed.[3,17]

BLOOD COAGULATION, PRESERVATION, AND STORAGE

Despite some successes by Blundell and contemporaries, transfusions often failed to save lives, and remained a rarity until the early 20th century. Clotting remained a significant problem. A variety of devices, involving valves, syringes, and tubing, were invented to facilitate the collection and infusion of blood from one individual to another, including two invented by Blundell—the "Gravitator" and the "Impellor." The impellor consisted of a double-walled funnel in which

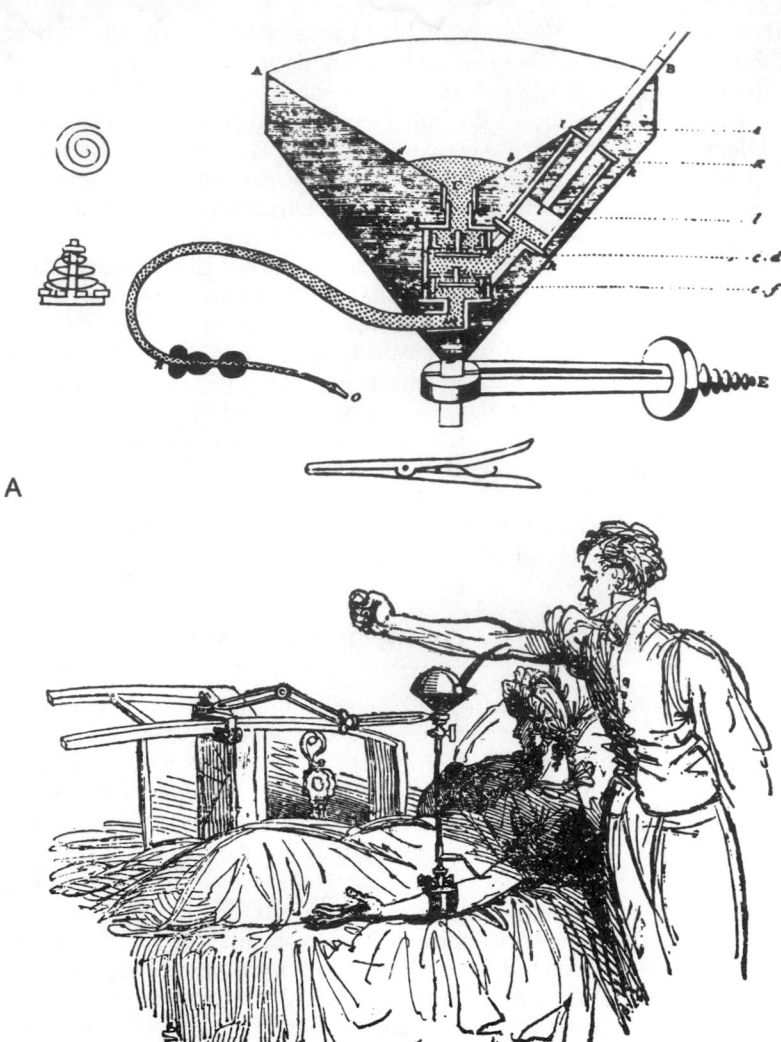

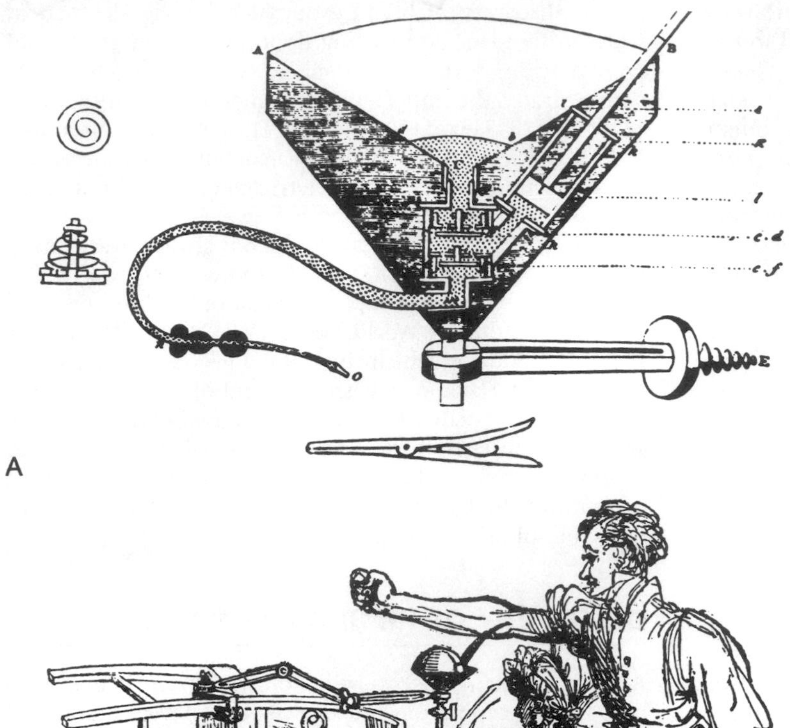

Figure 1–2 A. Blundell's "impellor." (Modified from Jones HW, Mackmull G. The influence of James Blundell on the development of blood transfusion. Ann Med Hist 1928;10:242.) B, Sketch of Blundell's gravitator. (Modified from Blundell J. Observations on transfusion of blood. Lancet 1828;2:321.)

the outer compartment was filled with warm water. The donor blood flowed into the funnel, was sucked into a syringe, and was forced along tubing into a cannula inserted into the patient's vein by means of two oppositely acting spring valves below the funnel[8] (Fig. 1–2). Gesellius used an equally complex device, in which the donor's back was lanced multiple times and capillary blood extracted using suction cups[5,8] (Fig. 1–3). James Aveling used a simpler method for direct blood transfusion from a donor using two silver cannulae, inserted into the recipient and donor, and connected by rubber tubing with a compressible bulb in the middle to promote and sustain flow.[11] The Aveling device is featured in the first known photograph of an actual blood transfusion, taken at Bellevue Hospital in New York City in the 1870s[9] (Fig. 1–4). In 1908, Alexis Carrel, a French researcher working at the Rockefeller Institute for Medical Research in New York, perfected a surgical technique for the direct anastomosis of donor artery to recipient vein.[3] Although highly effective at providing blood to the patient without clotting, performance of this technique required tremendous skill. Further, it required donors willing to undergo the painful procedure. It was also impossible to accurately estimate the amount of blood passed from donor to recipient; donors often became hypotensive or recipients developed circulatory overload.[3]

CITRATE ANTICOAGULATION

A chemical approach to anticoagulation was first attempted by Braxton Hicks, a 19th-century obstetrician, who experimented with phosphate of soda. Unfortunately, none of the four patients in whom it was used survived.[8] Other substances used in anticoagulation attempts included sodium bicarbonate, ammonium oxalate, arsphenamine, sodium iodide, sodium sulfate, and hirudin.[8] Surprisingly, these initial attempts did not include sodium citrate, which had long been used in laboratories as an anticoagulant.[8] The 1% concentration of citrate commonly used in the laboratory, however, was toxic to humans.[3] Nonetheless, in 1914 Albert Hustin reported the first human transfusion using citrated blood.[8] In 1915, Richard Lewisohn of the Mount Sinai Hospital in New York proved that a 0.2% sodium citrate solution was effective as an anticoagulant for blood, while having no toxicity even when as much as 2500 mL of citrated blood were transfused.[3] Also in 1915, Richard Weil, an American pathologist, found that citrated blood could be refrigerated for several days before use.[18] Lewinsohn and Weil, as well as Rous and Turner, found that addition of dextrose to citrate would preserve blood for up to 2 weeks[1,5] (Fig. 1–5). This permitted the first transfusion of stored blood in WWI by an American army physician, Oswald Robertson,

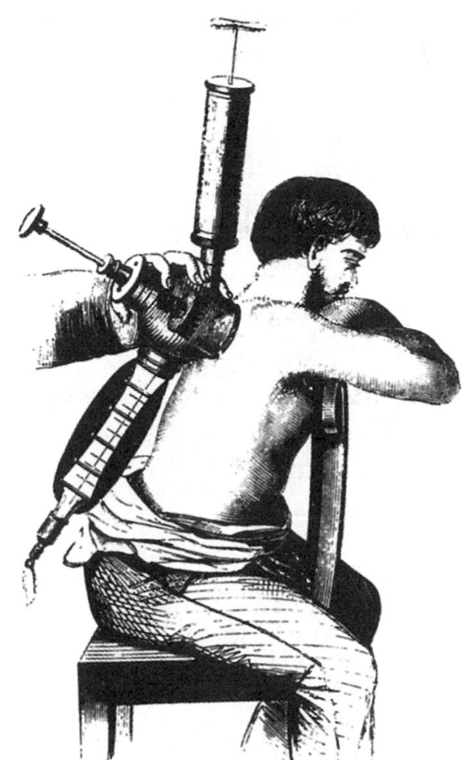

Figure 1–3 Collection and transfusion of capillary blood by the method of Gesellius. (Modified from Gesellius F: Die Transfusion des Blutes. Leipzig, E. Hoppe, 1873.)

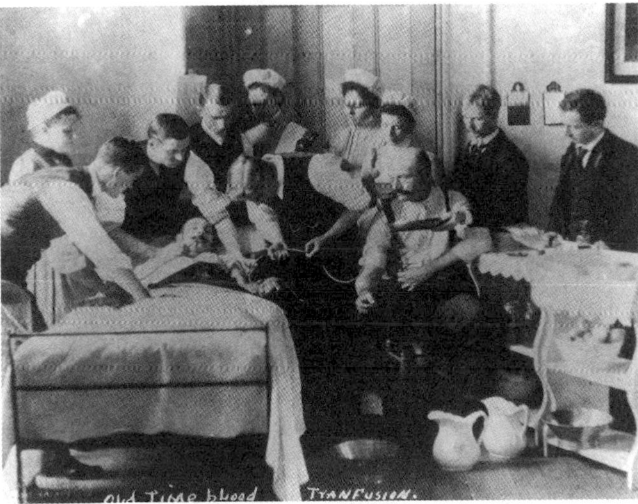

Figure 1–4 Medical and nursing staff administering transfusion, Bellevue Hospital, 1876. Note that the Bellevue staff has placed both needles in the wrong orientation. (From Schmidt PJ. The first photograph of blood transfusion. Transfusion 2001;41:968–969.)

who transfused 20 casualties on 22 occasions during the battle of Cambrai in November 1917. Nine of the 20 recipients lived.[19] The primary disadvantages of the Rous-Turner solution were that it was difficult to prepare and required a large volume of preservative solution in relation to the amount of blood. However, it remained the only anticoagulant–preservative solution available through most of WWII.[5] Acid citrate dextrose (ACD), developed in 1943 by Loutit and Mollison, allowed for blood to be stored for up to 3 to 4 weeks,[20] could be autoclaved, and had the advantage of being easier to prepare,

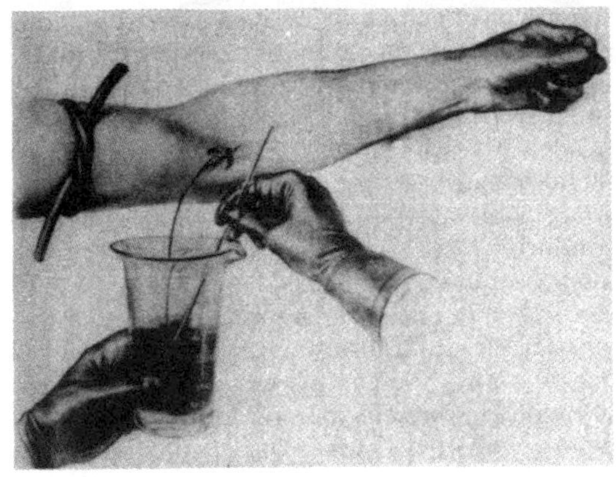

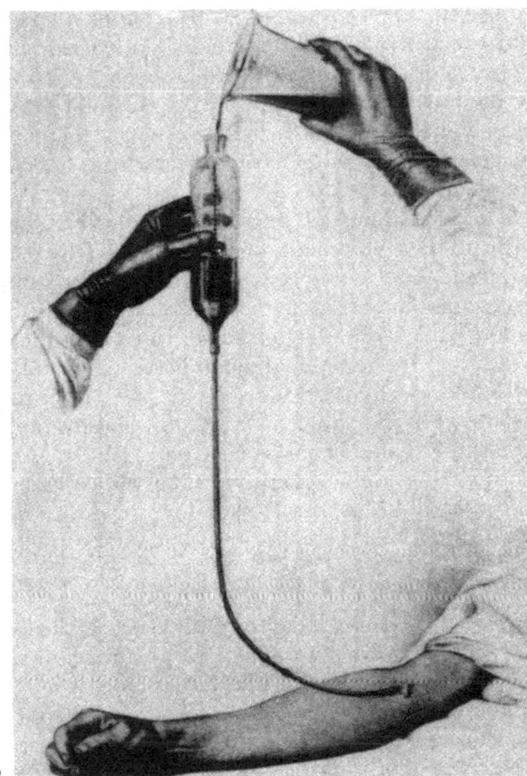

Figure 1–5 Lewisohn's method of transfusion of citrated blood. Blood is collected in a graduated flask (**A**) and is promptly transfused to the patient (**B**). (Modified from Lewisohn R: The citrate method of blood transfusion after ten years. Boston Med Surg J 1924;190:733.)

while requiring a smaller volume of solution relative to the amount of blood. Citrate phosphate dextrose (CPD) solution was subsequently adopted after studies showed blood could be stored for up to 28 days with better red cell survival than ACD.[3,21] Long-term red cell preservation by freezing began in 1950, when Smith and colleagues showed that glycerol could prevent freeze–thaw damage.[22]

ADVENT OF BLOOD BANKS

The first blood donor service was established in 1921 by Percy Oliver, Secretary of the Camberwell Division of the British Red Cross.[3] At this time, donors generally came from an unreliable supply; most from the patient's family and friends, or from indigents. Sometimes, no compatible donor could be found. On one such occasion, Oliver was contacted by a hospital with an urgent request for blood. Oliver and his coworkers rushed to the hospital to see if they could help. Blood from one individual in the group, a nurse, was found to be compatible with the patient. This experience gave Oliver the idea to create a stable supply of potential blood donors. In the program he developed, each potential blood donor underwent a physical examination, blood typing, and testing for syphilis before placement on the volunteer list. Because many physicians were still reluctant to use anticoagulation, the volunteer would go to the hospital and provide direct donation via venous cutdown (rendering the vein useless for subsequent donations). The service was supported entirely by donations, and the services were provided free. In 1922, the donor list consisted of 20 volunteers whose services were requested 13 times. By 1925, the number of requests had risen to 428, and it doubled the following year.[3,7] The increasing demand ultimately led to establishment of a new organization, the Greater London Red Cross Blood Transfusion Service.[7]

The first true predecessor to the modern blood bank was established in 1935 at the Mayo Clinic.[23] Others credit the first blood bank to Bernard Fantus, who established a blood bank at Cook County Hospital in Chicago in 1937.[24] In this latter facility, blood was collected into glass flasks containing sodium citrate, sealed, and stored refrigerated. Pilot tubes were prepared for typing and serology testing. Fantus was the first to coin the phrase "blood bank" for the operation because blood could be stored and saved for future use.[24] During the Spanish Civil War (1936–1939), Federico Duran-Jorda organized a highly successful mobile blood bank that could be transported wherever needed. Every donor was assessed with a questionnaire, physical examination, syphilis testing, and testing for blood type and red cell concentration. Only universal type O blood was collected. Using an entirely closed system of his own design, Duran-Jorda collected the blood into glass bottles containing a citrate and glucose solution.[7,25] Blood was then transported to front-line hospitals in vehicles fitted with refrigerators.[26] At the height of fighting, Duran-Jorda's blood center in Barcelona was processing up to 75 blood donations per hour.[7] When it became evident that the Nationalists would win the war, Duran-Jorda left Spain for England, where he assisted Janet Vaughan in establishing a blood bank at Hammersmith Hospital in 1938. Because war with Germany was imminent, the Medical Research Council supported Vaughan's proposal to establish four blood depots in London. In 1938, the War Office also created the army blood supply depot under the control of Lionel Whitby.[3] The Army's policy, to supply blood group O red cells at the battlefronts with blood that had been collected centrally rather than collected at the front from troops, proved to be highly successful.[3]

TRANSFUSION IN WWII

Beginning in September 1940, London was relentlessly assaulted for months by nightly German bombs that caused tens of thousands of deaths and injuries. The efficient organization of the blood depots provided for rapid transfusion of the wounded. Through experience, it became clear that blood transfusion could be used to treat injuries other than hemorrhage, including traumatic shock, crush injuries, fractures, and burns, creating a need for an even greater blood supply than could be provided by Britain alone. Americans were eager to help, but knew that whole blood could not survive the long transatlantic journey.[7]

Use of Plasma

John Elliott, laboratory chief at Rowan Hospital in North Carolina, had been experimenting with methods of separating plasma from blood when a patient who had been stabbed in the heart presented at the emergency room. Because there was no time to obtain a blood sample for type and crossmatching, Elliott decided to try transfusing the patient with the plasma he had in the laboratory. The patient survived. Elliott found that, in addition to having many of the beneficial properties of whole blood transfusion, plasma retained its usefulness for months. He was convinced that plasma could be the best transfusion liquid available and became a relentless advocate for its widespread transfusion.[7] Elliott's campaign efforts were successful. In August 1940, the Americans launched the Plasma for Britain program, headed by Charles Drew (Fig. 1–6). Drew was an African American surgeon whose 1938 doctoral thesis, "Banked Blood," was considered the most authoritative work on the science of blood storage at the time.[27] Under Drew's directorship, the Plasma for Britain program was a tremendous success, collecting blood from nearly 15,000 people, which produced 5500 vials of plasma (Fig. 1–7). Drew's contribution, however, extended beyond the sheer number of units collected. He was said to be the first to develop and implement strict procedures for blood collection and testing on a large, "industrial" scale.[7] In 1941, Drew was appointed director of the first American Red Cross Blood Bank, in charge of blood for use by the U.S. Army and Navy. In 1942, however, he resigned his official posts following the armed forces' decision that the blood of African Americans would be accepted but would have to be stored separately from that of whites.[7,27]

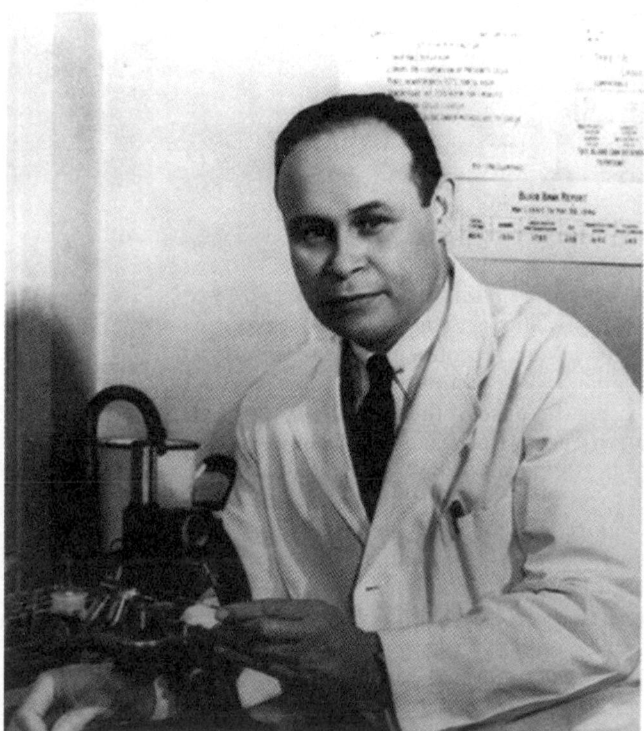

Figure 1–6 Dr. Charles Drew. (From Star D. Blood. An epic history of medicine and commerce. New York, HarperCollins Publishers, 2002.)

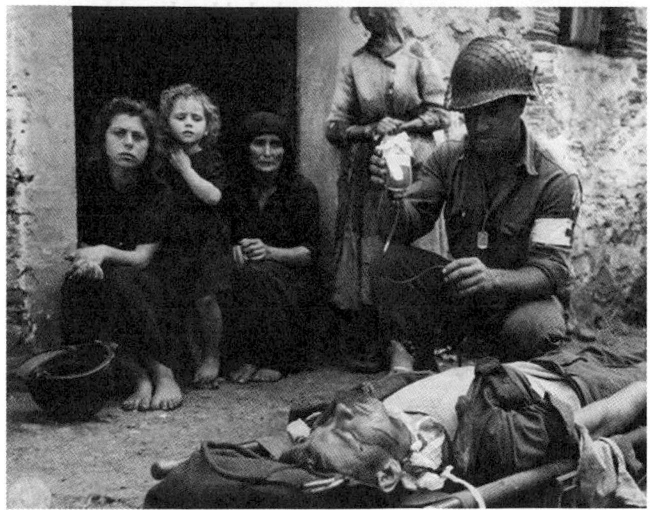

Figure 1–7 An American medic administers plasma to a wounded soldier in Sicily. (From Star D. Blood. An epic history of medicine and commerce. New York, HarperCollins Publishers, 2002.)

Eleanor Roosevelt took over his position. Drew became a professor of surgery at Howard University and trained numerous black surgeons. He died in an automobile accident in the late 1950s. It was widely alleged he didn't receive blood, because no "black blood" was available. This canard, however, is simply not true. Drew was transfused appropriately, but died as a result of injuries to his great vessels and his heart.[28]

Blood Fractionation

The benefits of plasma for treatment of injuries during WWII were evident, but like whole blood, plasma had its limitations. The protein-rich solution was highly prone to bacterial contamination. Freeze-dried plasma circumvented this problem, but was cumbersome and awkward to use on the battlefield. In 1940, Edwin Cohn, a Harvard chemist, isolated various fractions of plasma. Fraction V was found to be composed of albumin, which, in limited clinical studies of volunteers and accident victims, was found to restore circulatory collapse. Professor I. S. Ravdin at the University of Pennsylvania established albumin's efficacy following the bombing of Pearl Harbor in 1942, where albumin was used to treat injuries of 87 patients.[7] Most of these patients showed some clinical improvement, and only four suffered minor reactions.[3] Based on this success, the U.S. military added albumin production to efforts to produce plasma on a large scale.[7] Albumin had a number of advantages over plasma. Because of the method of production, cold ethanol precipitation/fractionation, albumin is free of bacteria. In addition, because albumin is highly concentrated, it could be transported in small vials easily on the battlefield. However, production of a single unit of albumin required pooling of multiple blood donations, and, like plasma, production of albumin was difficult. During WWII, both plasma and albumin were produced in vast amounts. By the end of 1943, over 2.5 million packages of dried plasma and nearly 125,000 units of albumin had been sent to the U.S. military.[7]

Cohn's fractionation of plasma yielded numerous benefits beyond the purification of albumin. Fraction I was found to contain fibrinogen; fractions II and III contained immunoglobulins that proved effective in the temporary prevention of a variety of infectious diseases, including infectious hepatitis (hepatitis A), rubella, and measles, and in the treatment of hypogammaglobulinemia.[16] Of particular significance, the isolation of Rh antibodies paved the way for discovery of methods to prevent most severe cases of hemolytic disease of the fetus and newborn.

IMMUNOGLOBULIN IN THE PREVENTION OF RH-HEMOLYTIC DISEASE OF THE FETUS AND NEWBORN

The first major advance, following Levine's discovery that maternal Rh antibodies were the cause of erythroblastosis fetalis, was the development of a practical procedure for umbilical vein exchange transfusion by a Boston pediatrician, Louis Diamond, in 1947. However, it took another 20 years before a treatment to prevent hemolytic disease of the newborn was discovered.[3] Initial experiments by Stern and colleagues in 1961 showed that passively administered "incomplete" anti-Rh antibody could interfere with primary Rh immunization.[16,29,30] Because immunoglobulin M (IgM) antibodies would not cross the placenta, investigators initially attempted to use "complete" or IgM anti-Rh antibody to block Rh immunization in Rh-negative males, but found that antibody formation was enhanced rather than suppressed.[31] Subsequently, suppression of Rh immunization by "incomplete" IgG anti-Rh antibody was demonstrated by Clarke and coworkers[30,31] and Freda and coworkers,[32,33] who were the first to use an immunoglobulin concentrate of IgG anti-Rh antibody given intramuscularly. Shortly afterward, it was realized that transplacental hemorrhage occurred chiefly at the time of delivery, and both groups showed that anti-Rh antibody given soon after delivery would suppress Rh immunization.[16,34,35]

BLOOD COMPONENTS

Another advance in transfusion was development of the first cell separator in 1951 by Edwin Cohn; the cell separator allowed blood to be separated into red cells, white cells, platelets, and plasma. Although in principle it was possible to harvest any particular component of the blood, in practice, satisfactory yields of only red cells or plasma could be obtained.[16]

Cohn's cell separator paved the way for component therapy, but the development of plastic containers made modern component therapy possible. Up until the 1950s, blood was collected through steel needles and rubber tubing into glass, rubber-stoppered bottles, which were reused following washing and sterilization.[1] Pyrogenic reactions and air embolism were known risks to blood collected using these materials. In 1952, Carl Walter, a researcher under Harvey Cushing, and William Murphy described a system in which the blood was collected into a collapsible bag of polyvinyl resin.[1,36] Plastic had the flexibility to permit the removal of plasma following sedimentation or centrifugation, techniques that became the foundations for component production.[1,37]

FACTOR VIII CONCENTRATES

The ability to separate blood into components resulted in major advances for the treatment of hemophilia. Initially, hemophiliacs were treated with fresh frozen plasma; however, massive volumes were required to replenish the deficient factor VIII in these patients. A more concentrated form of the required factor VIII was found in the cryoprecipitated portion of plasma by Judith Pool in 1965.[38] In 1968 Brinkhous and Shanbrom produced concentrated factor VIII by pooling hundreds to thousands of units of plasma. These factor concentrates could be carried by the patient and administered by self-injection at the earliest sign of bleeding.[7,39] Factor VIII concentrates were a major advance in the treatment of hemophilia A, but they came with a very high risk of infectious disease transmission, first with hepatitis and later with human immunodeficiency virus (HIV).

INFECTIOUS DISEASE TRANSMISSION

The first hint that hepatitis could be caused by blood transfusion came during WWII following administration of yellow fever vaccines produced using human serum as a stabilizer.[1] This was followed by a report in 1943 of a series of seven cases of jaundice following transfusion of whole blood or plasma.[40] At the time, serum hepatitis (or hepatitis B) was assumed to be the major cause of transfusion-associated hepatitis. This began the awareness that blood transfusion could transmit potentially deadly viral diseases. In 1962, the connection between paying for units and an increased risk of post-transfusion hepatitis was made by J. Garrett Allen, a Stanford surgeon[41]; however, it wasn't until a decade later that the National Blood Policy mandated a voluntary (unpaid) donation system in the United States.[1] Subsequently, in 1975 transfusion-associated hepatitis was shown to be primarily due to non-A, non-B hepatitis, or what became identified later as hepatitis C.[42] Despite the risk of hepatitis transmission, blood utilization continued to increase. In the United States, for example, blood utilization doubled between 1971 and 1980.[1] However, the emergence of acquired immunodeficiency syndrome (AIDS) changed this trend.

The first case of AIDS was reported in 1981. This mysterious disease initially occurred only in gay men. However, within a few years, it became clear that AIDS was caused by a blood-borne virus. The first reported case of transfusion-associated AIDS occurred in a 20-month-old infant who had received multiple transfusions for hemolytic disease of the newborn.[43] Hemophiliacs, dependent on lifelong infusions of factor VIII concentrates, were particularly devastated by the disease. In 1985, the first serologic test to detect HIV was implemented by blood banks to protect the blood supply. However, the possibility that other, as yet unknown, pathogens could also be transmitted by blood transfusion resulted in a new awareness that blood should be used judiciously. Multiple serologic tests are now routinely employed on every blood component for a variety of infectious agents, including hepatitis B, hepatitis C, HIV, cytomegalovirus (CMV), syphilis, and human T-lymphotropic virus (HTLV). Despite the improvement in blood safety that serologic testing provides, the risk of infectious disease transmission is not completely eradicated from the blood supply due to the window period in which donors are infectious, but have not yet developed detectable antibody. The development of nucleic acid amplification technology (NAT) has limited the risk of infectious disease transmission even more by allowing the direct detection of even small quantities of pathogen. Currently, NAT testing is widely employed for HIV and hepatitis C detection, and is used, in certain areas, for detection of hepatitis B virus and West Nile virus. Some type of pathogen inactivation applied to blood components might obviate the need for yet more testing of known and unknown pathogens that might be transfusion-transmissible.

NONINFECTIOUS COMPLICATIONS OF TRANSFUSION

In addition to infectious diseases, other risks of transfusion became apparent as transfusions increased. Transfused leukocytes were found to have a number of undesirable effects (e.g., graft-versus-host disease [GVHD] and febrile reactions).[8] In 1970, Graw and colleagues demonstrated that GVHD could be prevented by the irradiation of blood components.[44] In 1962, the first-generation leukocyte filter was shown to be effective in the prevention of febrile transfusion reactions.[45] The additional benefits of leukoreduction, including reduction of leukotropic viruses, such as HTLV 1/2 and CMV, and minimization of the risk of human leukocyte antigen (HLA) sensitization, have resulted in the widespread adoption of leukoreduction of cellular blood components.

THE MODERN ERA

Transfusion medicine continues to evolve in the modern era. New, problematic infectious agents emerge, such as West Nile virus, which is usually transmitted to humans by mosquitoes. West Nile virus was first reported to be transmitted by transfusion and organ transplantation in 2002.

As detection and prevention of transfusion-transmitted viral infections has improved, bacterial contamination has evolved into one of the most significant causes of transfusion-transmitted infectious disease. Bacterial detection systems are being used on platelet components with some success. Fortunately, new methodologies designed to inactivate bacteria have been developed and are undergoing evaluation.[46]

Alternatives to human blood for transfusion, so called "blood substitutes," continue to be actively investigated but have thus far had limited success. Current "blood substitutes" are limited to substances designed to carry oxygen. Unfortunately, these substances have limited application and are associated with a unique set of risks and potential complications.[47]

The history of transfusion medicine parallels mankind's understanding of physiology, immunology, chemistry, infectious diseases, and advances in technology. What began as a belief that blood carries important healing properties has been validated by science. However, despite numerous advances over the centuries, blood remains an indispensable, life-giving force. Interestingly, some of the more important advances in blood banking/transfusion medicine have occurred as the result of wars.

SUMMARY REMARKS

Blood transfusions today are an indispensable part of many medical and surgical therapies. The use of blood and its components temporarily replaces what may be lost or not produced before, during, or after a disease process and/or its treatment. The benefits of transfusion today far outweigh their minute (yet real) risks with all the current safeguards to select donors, test blood, and ensure that compatible blood is transfused to the correct patient. Transfusion medicine has come a long way due to multiple pathfinders, adventurous physicians, and courageous donors and patients, especially in the last half century. We owe much to these pioneers.

Acknowledgments

The authors wish to acknowledge Drs. Leo McCarthy and Paul Schmidt for their generous contributions of photos, information, and review of this chapter.

REFERENCES

1. Rossi E, Simon T, Moss G (eds). Principles of Transfusion Medicine. Baltimore, Williams & Wilkins, 1991.
2. Zmijewski CM. Immunohematology, 3rd ed. New York, Appleton-Century-Crofts, 1978.
3. Giangrande PL. The history of blood transfusion. Br J Haematol 2000;110:758–767.
4. Myhre BA. The first recorded blood transfusions: 1656 to 1668. Transfusion 1990;30:358–362.
5. Petz L, Swisher S, Kleinman S, Spence R (eds). Clinical Practice of Transfusion Medicine, 3rd ed. New York, Churchill Livingstone, 1996.
6. Denis J. A letter concerning a new way of curing sundry diseases by transfusion of blood. Philos Trans R Soc Lond [Biol] 1667;2:489.
7. Star D. Blood. An epic history of medicine and commerce. New York, HarperCollins Publishers, 2002.
8. Greenwalt TJ. A short history of transfusion medicine. Transfusion 1997;37:550–563.
9. Schmidt PJ. The first photograph of blood transfusion. Transfusion 2001;41:968–969.
10. Schmidt PJ, Leacock AG. Forgotten transfusion history: John Leacock of Barbados. BMJ 2002;325:1485–1487.
11. Baskett TF. James Blundell: the first transfusion of human blood. Resuscitation 2002;52:229–233.
12. Landsteiner K. Uber Agglunationserscheinungen normalen menschlichen Blutes. Wein Klin Wschr 1901;14:1132–1134.
13. Watkins WM. The ABO blood group system: historical background. Transfus Med 2001;11:243–265.
14. Levine P. A review of Landsteiner's contributions to human blood groups. Transfusion 1961;1:45–52.
15. Ottenberg R, Kaliski DJ. Accidents in transfusion: their prevention by preliminary blood examination: based on an experience of 128 transfusions. JAMA 1913;61:2138–2140.
16. Mollison PL. Blood Transfusion in Clinical Medicine, 7th ed. Oxford, Blackwell Scientific Publications, 1983.
17. Moreschi C. Neue Tatsachen Uber die Blutkorperchen-agglutination. Zentralbl Bakteriol Parasitenkd Infektkr 1908;1 Originale 46:49–51.
18. Weil R. Sodium citrate in the transfusion of blood. JAMA 1915;64: 425–426.
19. Hess JR, Schmidt PJ. The first blood banker: Oswald Hope Robertson. Transfusion 2000;40:110–113.
20. Loutit JF, Mollison PL. Advantages of a disodium-citrate-glucose mixture as a blood preservative. BMJ 1943;2:744–745.
21. Gibson JG, Gregory CB, Button LN. Citrate-phosphate-dextrose solution for preservation of human blood: a further report. Transfusion 1961;1:280–287.
22. Smith AU. Prevention of haemolysis during freezing and thawing of red blood cells. Lancet 1950;2:910–911.
23. Moore SB. A brief history of the early years of blood transfusion at the Mayo Clinic: the first blood bank in the United States (1935). Transfus Med Rev 2005;19:241–245.
24. Telischi M. Evolution of Cook County Hospital blood bank. Transfusion 1974;14:623–628.
25. Jorda FD. The Barcelona blood transfusion service. Lancet 1939;1:773–776.
26. www.pbs.org/wnet/redgold
27. www.cdrewu.edu
28. Schmidt PJ. Charles Drew, a legend in our time. Transfusion 1997;37:234–236.
29. Stern K, Goodman HS, Berger M. Experimental isoimmunization to hemoantigens in man. J Immunol 1961;87:189–198.
30. Clarke CA, Donohoe WT, McConnell RB, et al. Further experimental studies on the prevention of Rh haemolytic disease. BMJ 1963;5336:979–984.
31. Clarke CA, McConnell RB. Prevention of Rh-hemolytic disease. Springfield, Ill., Charles C Thomas, 1972.
32. Freda VJ, Gorman JG, Pollack W. Successful prevention of experimental Rh sensitization in man with an anti-Rh gamma$_2$globulin antibody preparation: A preliminary report. Transfusion 1964;77:26–32.
33. Freda VJ, Gorman JG, Pollack W. Rh factor; prevention of immunization and clinical trial on mothers. Science 1966;151:828–830.
34. [No authors listed]. Prevention of Rh-haemolytic disease: results of the clinical trial. A combined study from centres in England and Baltimore. BMJ 1966;2:907–914.
35. Pollack W, Gorman JG, Freda VJ, et al: Results of clinical trials of RhoGAM in women. Transfusion 1968;8:151–153.
36. Walter CW, Murphy WP. A closed gravity technique for the preservation of whole blood in ACD solution utilizing plastic equipment. Surg Gynecol Obstet 1952;95:113–119.
37. Sack T, Gibson JG, Buckley ES. The preservation of whole ACD blood collected stored and transfused in plastic equipment. Surg Gynecol Obstet 1952;95:113–119.
38. Pool JG, Shannon AE. Production of high-potency concentrates of antihemophilic globulin in a closed-bag system. N Engl J Med 1965;273:1443–1447.
39. Brinkhous KM, Shanbrom E, Roberts HR, et al. A new high-potency glycine-precipitated antihemophilic factor (AHF) concentrate. Treatment of classical hemophilia and hemophilia with inhibitors. JAMA 1968;205:613–617.
40. Beeson PB. Jaundice occurring one to four months after transfusion of blood or plasma. JAMA 1943;121:1332–1334.
41. Allen JG, Sayman WA. Serum hepatitis from transfusion of blood. JAMA 1962;180:1079–1085.
42. Feinstone SM, Kapikian AZ, Purcell RH, et al. Transfusion associated hepatitis not due to viral hepatitis type A or B. N Engl J Med 1975;292:767–770.
43. Ammann AJ, Cowan MJ, Wara DW, et al. Acquired immunodeficiency in an infant: possible transmission by means of blood products. Lancet 1983;1:956–958.
44. Graw RG Jr, Buckner CD, Whang-Peng J, et al. Complication of bone-marrow transplantation. Graft-versus-host disease resulting from chronic-myelogenous-leukaemia leucocyte transfusions. Lancet 1970;2:338–341.
45. Greenwalt TJ, Gajewski M, McKenna JL. A new method for preparing buffy coat-poor blood. Transfusion 1962;2:221–229.
46. Lin L, Hanson CV, Alter HJ, et al. Inactivation of viruses in platelet concentrates by photochemical treatment with amotosalen and long-wavelength ultraviolet light. Transfusion 2005;45:580–590.
47. Klein HG. Blood substitutes: how close to a solution? Dev Biol (Basel) 2005;120:45–52.

Section II

Blood Banking

A. Immunohematology

i. Basic Principles

Chapter 2

Principles of the Immune System Central to Transfusion Medicine

Terrence L. Geiger

INTRODUCTION

The histories of immunology and transfusion medicine intertwine, and efforts in each field have revealed fundamental truths about the other. One of the early leaders in both areas was Paul Ehrlich.[1,2] At the turn of the 19th century, Ehrlich observed that goats were able to produce an immune substance—antibodies—which could destroy red blood cells (RBCs) derived from other goats. Interestingly this substance did not affect a goat's own RBCs. From these findings Ehrlich developed the concept of *horror autotoxicus,* that in order to avoid "autotoxicity," or self-harm, immune responses are directed against foreign and not self compounds. Karl Landsteiner expanded on Ehrlich's work.[3] He demonstrated that anti-red cell agglutinins found in human serum, as in goats, were never directed against self, or autologous, RBCs. However, he also observed that some serum specimens were able to agglutinate samples of homologous RBCs, while other serum specimens could not. He categorized these agglutinins in analyses that led to the description of the ABO blood group system and thereby formed a scientific basis for modern transfusion medicine.

One hundred years after the pioneering studies of Ehrlich and Landsteiner, we still struggle to understand the immune mechanisms they described. The human immune system, functioning as a barrier against pathogen attack, can prevent the transfusion of cells and proteins and the transplantation of tissues. These cells and tissues, which are foreign to our bodies, contain antigens, or chemical structures recognized by the immune system. As Ehrlich observed, our immune system generally does not respond to self-antigens, antigens that are intrinsic to our bodies. In contrast, it can and often will respond against foreign antigens. In the case of transfusion, these foreign antigens result from differences between the structures of proteins and sugars present in transfused blood and those native to the recipient.

The recognition of antigens within transfused blood by the immune system may have several consequences. It may lead to the destruction of transfused cells and the neutralization of transfused proteins. This can occur through the generation of specific antibodies or less frequently through the activation of cellular immunity. Immune engagement may also inactivate the immune system. This is called *immune tolerance.* If tolerance develops against antigens on transfused or transplanted cells, the immune system will not respond when it encounters the same antigens again, even if they are present on different cells or tissues. Finally, the immune system may neither elaborate an effective response against an antigen nor become tolerant of it, an event sometimes called *immune ignorance.*[4,5] In each of these circumstances a transfusion is not passively witnessed by the immune system. Whether or not we observe a clinical consequence of immune engagement after a transfusion, the immune system is continuously active, identifying antigens and determining whether and how to respond.

The immune system consists of two lines of defense. The first, termed the *innate immune response,* is triggered by substances common to many pathogens, such as bacterial lipopolysaccharide or viral nucleic acid. These substances indicate potential danger to a host. Innate immunity is immediate. It is found in most multicellular organisms, even those with very short life spans, and it rapidly neutralizes the offending agent. A second, more complex immune response may follow the innate response. This response, which specifically targets antigens present in the immunizing substance, is called the *adaptive immune response.* Adaptive immunity requires days to weeks to develop and is only found in complex organisms. It is characterized by the development of antigen-specific antibody and T-cell responses.

THE INNATE IMMUNE SYSTEM

The innate immune system includes an amalgamation of interacting pathways that use invariant proteins to protect our bodies from specific types of assault. It continuously monitors our internal environment for the presence of pathogens and other hazards. It also defines the type of danger present, initiates a protective response, and establishes an environment conducive to the formation of effective adaptive immunity.[6]

The innate immune system includes dedicated cell types that lack antigen-specific receptors yet are able to recognize and neutralize pathogens and infected cells. These cells can destroy pathogens through phagocytosis, or ingestion, or through the production of cytocidal compounds such as reactive oxygen species and nitric oxide. They can also sound an alarm, recruiting other inflammatory cells to sites of infection and initiating inflammatory reactions. Examples of innate immune cells include macrophages, mast cells, neutrophils, eosinophils, and natural killer (NK) cells.

Innate immunity is, however, not limited to specific cell types. Elements of innate immunity are present in and around virtually all cells in our body. Some of these elements are produced within our cells, such as the cytoplasmic antiviral proteins that are produced in response to viral infections. Others, such as secreted antimicrobial peptides called *defensins* and *cathelicidins*, are exclusively extracellular.[7]

Activation of innate immunity begins with the recognition of pathogen motifs by specific receptors.[8] These motifs tend to be conserved within a class of organisms. An example is gram-negative bacteria, whose double membrane contains endotoxin, a unique complex of lipid and polysaccharide also called *lipopolysaccharide* (LPS). LPS binds to an LPS-specific receptor present on innate immune cells called *Toll-like receptor 4* (Tlr4).[9] Tlr4 is one of a group of similar receptors that are expressed on the cell surface or in endosomes (internalization vacuoles) and signal when danger is present.[10] Other Toll-like receptors recognize motifs specific to gram-positive bacteria, viruses, or other pathogens (Table 2–1).

When a Toll-like receptor is activated, it induces signaling molecules that coordinate the early response against an offending pathogen. These signaling molecules are called *biological response modifiers* (BRMs). BRMs include lipids, such as leukotrienes, and other small signaling molecules, such as histamine and serotonin. They also include a group of messenger proteins called *cytokines* that are critical in orchestrating the innate immune response (Table 2–2). There are several classes of cytokines with distinct roles in innate immunity. The interaction of viral DNA or RNA with specific Toll-like receptors induces the synthesis of Type I interferons (IFNs), a class of cytokines that binds IFN receptors on cells and promotes the formation of proteins that block virus replication. Another class of cytokines is called chemokines. The word *chemokine* is a conjunction of chemotactic, the promotion of migration along a chemical gradient, and cytokine. As chemokines diffuse from their site of production, they form a gradient along which immune cells migrate. An example is interleukin-8 (IL-8), which recruits inflammatory cells to the site of an infection.[11,12] Other released cytokines promote inflammation. For example, tumor necrosis factor (TNF) activates endothelial cells, aiding in the diapedesis of reactive cells into tissue, and increases the production of pathogen-neutralizing effector molecules such as reactive oxygen species and nitric oxide.[13] Yet other cytokines, such as IL-12, primarily link innate and adptive immunity. IL-12 promotes T-lymphocyte differentiation into helper T cells (Th1 cells) capable of recruiting and activating macrophages that destroy pathogens.[14] Cumulatively, the cytokines and other BRMs released during the innate immune response form a communication network between cells that identifies the pathogen class and severity of the infection and establishes an initial response to it.

Table 2–1 Recognition of Pathogen-Specific Motifs by Toll-like Receptors

Receptor	Recognition Motif	Pathogen
Tlr1 (associates with Tlr2)	Triacyl lipoproteins	Gram-negative bacteria
Tlr2	Peptidoglycan, lipoproteins, lipopeptides	Gram-positive and other bacteria, parasites, fungi
Tlr3	Double-stranded RNA	Viruses
Tlr4	Lipopolysaccharide	Gram-negative bacteria
Tlr5	Flagellin	Bacteria
Tlr6 (associates with Tlr2)	Diacetylated lipoproteins	Mycobacteria
Tlr7	Viral single-stranded RNA; imidazoquinalines and other guanosine nucleotide-related synthetic compounds	Viruses; synthetic agents
Tlr8	Viral single-stranded RNA	Viruses
Tlr9	Unmethylated CpG DNA	DNA viruses, prokaryotes

Table 2–2 Some Important Cytokines and Their Functions

Cytokine	Function
IL-1	T-cell and APC stimulatory, fever
IL-2	T-cell expansion and apoptosis sensitivity
IL-4	B-cell stimulation, IgE production, Th2 differentiation
IL-5	Eosinophil expansion and development
IL-10	Suppression of macrophage and DC function
IL-12	Th1 differentiation, NK activation
IL-15	NK cell and T-cell expansion and survival
IFN-γ	Macrophage activation, enhancement of antigen presentation, promotion of IL-12 production
IFN-α, β	Antiviral
TNF-α	Inflammation, sepsis
TGF-β	Anti-inflammatory, T-cell inhibition, IgA production

Although critical for innate immune pathogen detection, Toll-like receptors are not exclusive in this ability. Other proteins have complementary functions.[15] A cytoplasmic protein called *retinoic acid inducible gene 1* binds viral RNA and induces production of IFN-α and IFN-β. Other proteins that include nucleotide-binding oligomerization domains have been found to recognize intracellular bacteria. Mannose-binding lectins in the extracellular fluid bind the surfaces of pathogens and then activate complement. Recent data have also documented a completely new manner through which our bodies can recognize pathogens. Very short RNA sequences, microRNAs, are able to specifically recognize viral genetic material and in so doing inhibit viral replication within a cell.[16] Our ability to withstand the onslaught of potential invaders surrounding us is critical to our survival, and our bodies invest heavily in our innate immune system as a first line of defense.

The activation of innate immunity through pathogen-specific receptors may seem irrelevant to immune responses to blood transfusions, which to the best of our abilities lack contaminating pathogens. However, the innate immune system establishes a basal inflammatory state. Transfused RBC or plasma antigens are presented to the adaptive immune system in the context of this state, which may influence the immune response to them. Although a direct link between a specific type of inflammatory response and the type of response generated against transfused allogeneic blood products has not been demonstrated, associations between infection and other alloimmune responses, particularly graft rejection, have been documented.[17,18] Furthermore, specific immune reactivity against "bystander" antigens during responses against pathogens has been described in other circumstances and is therefore likely present in the context of transfusion.[19–21] Indeed, establishing such a bystander response forms the scientific rationale for the adjuvants present in modern vaccines. Adjuvants, by stimulating specific innate immune receptors, influence the magnitude and quality of the adaptive immune response against co-administered antigens.[22] Thus, the innate immune context in which a transfusion is administered may have a significant effect on the immunologic outcome of that transfusion.

THE ADAPTIVE IMMUNE SYSTEM

The adaptive immune system selectively neutralizes pathogens and nonpathogenic foreign antigens. It recognizes these through specific antigen receptors. Whereas receptors of the innate immune system detect just a handful of pathogen-specific chemical motifs, antigen receptors of the adaptive immune system are able to selectively identify billions of distinct antigenic structures. The 3 billion base pair long human genome would be insufficient to encode adequate numbers of proteins to accomplish this feat if each receptor was a separate gene, as is the case for Toll-like receptors. To circumvent this problem, antigen receptors are built up from modules that allow the incorporation of variability as they form (Fig. 2–1).[23] Each polypeptide of an antigen receptor is composed of three or four fragments of DNA. These fragments are called variable (V), diversity (D), junctional (J), and constant (C) fragments. More than a single piece of DNA can encode for each of these fragments, and their arbitrary linkage results in combinatorial variation. For example, if an organism has 20 V regions, 2 D regions, 10 J regions, and 1 C region for a receptor in its genome, random recombination would allow the formation of 20×2×10×1 or 400 unique receptors from the 20+2+10+1, or 33, gene segments.

Two additional features promote variation. As the receptor fragments recombine, enzymes randomly insert or remove nucleotides at the recombination sites. The sites where these alterations are made correspond to parts of the receptor that directly contact antigen and are called *hypervariable regions.*[24]

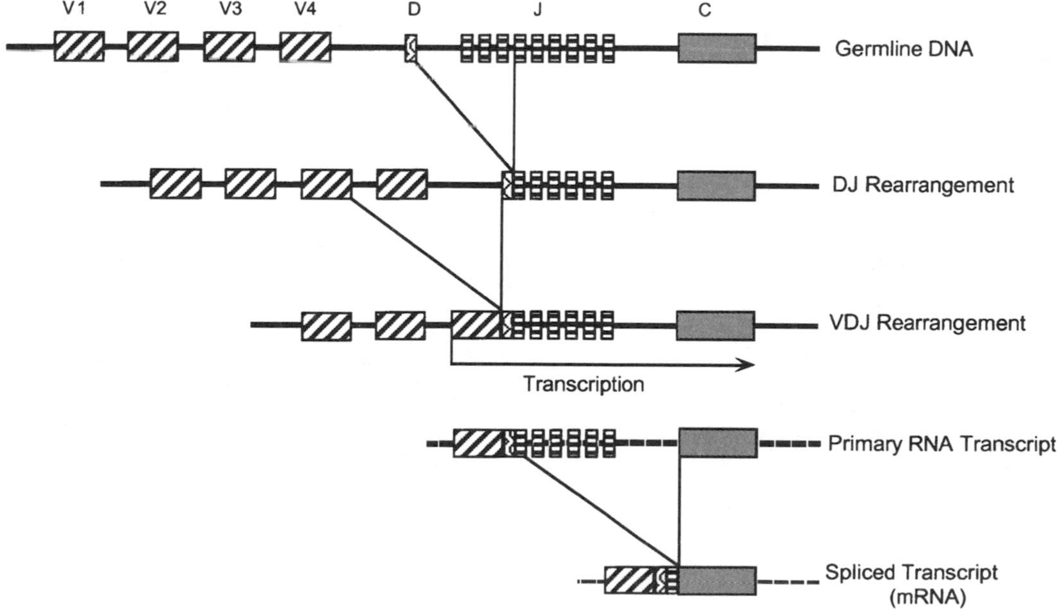

Figure 2–1 Antigen receptor gene rearrangement. The germline genetic sequence consists of multiple variable (V), diversity (D), and junctional (J) segments. Rearrangement of a D and J segment with excision of intervening DNA sequence is followed by that of the DJ sequence to a V region. Completion of rearrangement juxtaposes sequences necessary for RNA transcription. The RNA transcript is spliced to create an mRNA that is translated into an antigen receptor chain. The diagram is illustrative and does not indicate the full complexity of the T-cell receptor or B-cell receptor loci.

Thus antigen receptors are most variable at critical antigen-binding sites. Further, antigen receptors are heterodimers composed of two polypeptides, a V-D-J-C chain, and a V-D-J chain. Each of these receptor components uses an independent set of V, D, J, and C fragments. The chains recombine independently but recognize antigen together. Thus billions of distinct antigen receptors may form from a relatively small number of gene fragments.

Antigen receptors are expressed on only two classes of cells, B lymphocytes and T lymphocytes. On B cells they form the B-cell receptor (BCR), which is a cell surface form of immunoglobulin. On T cells they form the T-cell receptor (TCR). Each T cell or B cell expresses only a single (or in some rare cases two) immune receptors on their cell surface.[25] Therefore, each T cell or B cell is essentially a clone recognizing a distinct piece of an antigen, called an *epitope.* Because of the diversity of immune receptors, the frequency of T cells or B cells able to respond to any single antigenic protein is extremely low, typically ranging from 1/10,000 to 1/100,000 cells.[26] Receptor engagement activates a lymphocyte and may lead to the selection and rapid outgrowth of rare antigen-specific clones. Cell activation by antigen may also induce differentiation into effector lymphocyte forms designed to participate in distinct types of immune responses, such as allergic responses or delayed type hypersensitivity responses.

The Trail of Antigen

Foreign antigens can enter the body through different routes. In the case of infection, entry is generally through the skin or mucosal tissues. In the case of transfusion, direct intravenous inoculation occurs. In both situations, antigens make their way to lymphoid tissue. Antigens in the skin are picked up by specialized resident skin dendritic cells called *Langerhans cells* and are then carried to draining lymph nodes.[27] Antigens in the blood are picked up by cells in the spleen. Antigens in the gut are taken up by cells in the gut-associated lymphoid tissue.[28] They are then presented to T lymphocytes and B lymphocytes by specialized antigen-presenting cells (APCs), also called *professional APCs,* in the lymphoid tissues. The lymphoid tissues are specifically designed to facilitate the interaction between rare antigen-specific T cells and B cells and APCs bearing their cognate antigen (Fig. 2–2).

The cell carrying antigen to lymphoid tissue may transfer that antigen to professional APCs within that tissue.[27] Alternatively the courier cell, often a resident tissue dendritic cell, may serve as the APC within the lymphoid tissue, directly presenting antigen to lymphocytes. Conversion of such courier cells to effective professional APCs requires their maturation under the influence of cytokines or Toll-like receptor signals that are present in the context of inflammation and innate immune activation. These stimuli induce the formation of signaling molecules on the surface of the APC that can bind and activate lymphocyte receptors. They also induce the secretion of cytokines and other BRMs by the APCs.[29,30] Such supplemental, or costimulatory, signals can both modify and augment the signal received by a lymphocyte through its antigen receptor. In the presence of costimulatory signaling, a lymphocyte may become more fully activated, permitting its expansion and differentiation into an effector cell. In contrast, the absence of costimulatory signals indicates to a lymphocyte that antigen is not being presented in the context of inflammation or host danger. Signals through antigen receptor in this circumstance lead to incomplete stimulation that may promote the development of immune tolerance, sometimes through the death of the responding antigen-specific lymphocyte.[31,32] As self-derived antigens will tend not to be presented in the context of inflammation, this form of tolerance is one route through which the immune system rids itself of self-reactive lymphocytes that may cause autoimmunity.

Antigen Presentation to T Cells

The TCR is a complex that includes six different polypeptides, most commonly α, β, γ, δ, ε, and ζ (Fig. 2–3).[33,34] The α and β chains, which include recombined VJC and VDJC regions, respectively, are directly involved in antigen recognition. The remaining polypeptides do not recognize antigen but transmit signals into T cells after antigen engagement occurs. The γ, δ, and ε signaling chains are collectively referred to as the CD3 complex.

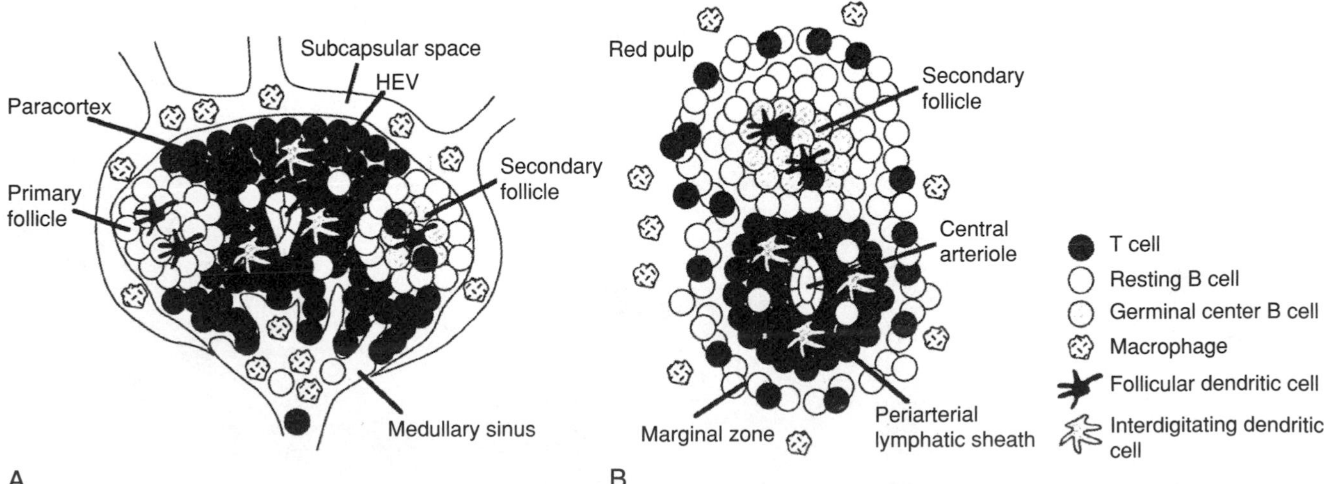

Figure 2–2 Schematic depiction of the structure of a lymph node (**A**) and an area of the splenic white pulp (**B**). Lymphocytes enter through the high endothelial venule (HEV) or central arteriole and then migrate to T- or B-rich areas where they may interact with antigen-presenting cells. T cells and B cells may also engage each other, often at the interface between the B- and T-cell zones of the spleen or lymph node. (From Mondino A, Khoruts A, Jenkins MK. The anatomy of T cell activation. Proc Natl Acad Sci USA 1996;93:2246.)

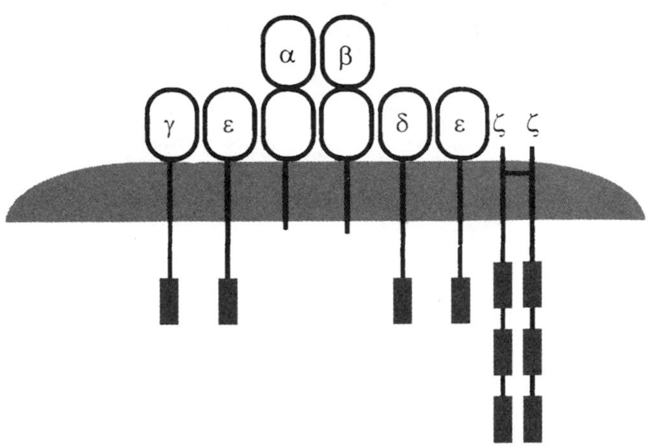

Figure 2–3 The TCR–CD3 complex consists of eight polypeptide chains. Specificity is determined by the αβ chains or, in some T cells, by analogous γδ TCR chains. Expression of the CD3 γ, δ, and ε chains, as well as ζ or its splice variants, are necessary for surface expression and signaling.

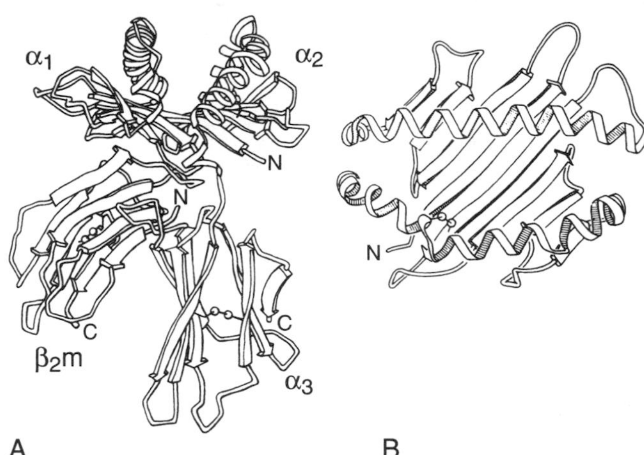

Figure 2–4 Structure of a class I MHC molecule. **A,** Three-dimensional ribbon model of the extracellular portion of the molecule. The peptide-binding groove lies between the helices at the top of the molecule. **B,** Top view. (From Bjorkman PJ et al Structure of the human class I histocompatability antigen, HLA-A2. Nature 1987;329:506.)

T cells do not see antigen alone through their TCR. They see it only in the context of major histocompatibility complex, or MHC, proteins. The significance of the MHC, also called the human leukocyte antigen (HLA) complex in humans, was first recognized through the work of Peter Gorer and George Snell in the 1930s.[2] Gorer and Snell were studying tumor graft rejection and determined that this genetic locus was absolutely critical in determining whether grafted cells were rejected. We now know that the MHC serves as a window through which T cells see the world around them. T lymphocytes recognize antigen only in the context of MHC molecules. Recognition is remarkably specific. Even subtle allelic variations in a single MHC molecule are sufficient to abrogate T-cell recognition.[35]

MHC proteins fall into two categories, class I and class II molecules.[36] Class I MHC molecules are heterodimers consisting of a larger α or "heavy" chain, which is membrane bound, and a smaller soluble protein called *β_2-microglobulin.* Class II MHC molecules are heterodimers of two membrane-bound polypeptides, an α chain and a β chain of roughly equal size. How the MHC presents antigen to T cells was not clear until the late 1980s when x-ray crystallographic structures of MHC molecules were solved (Fig. 2–4).[37–39] Although the amino acid sequences of class I and class II molecules are distinct, they form similar three-dimensional structures. The upper surface of the MHC molecule forms a platter, called a *β sheet,* on top of which lie two parallel tubular coils of peptide, called *α helices.* Between the α helices lies a groove into which various protein fragments, or peptides, may bind. These peptides, presented together with their restricting MHC molecules, are the antigenic structures recognized by T lymphocytes.

Class I MHC molecules bind peptides approximately 8 to 10 amino acids in length, whereas class II MHC molecules bind longer peptides, approximately 13 to 24 amino acids. Only a few interactions between peptide amino acids and the MHC are needed to stabilize binding.[40,41] This allows for the formation of large numbers of different peptide–MHC complexes. A typical antigenic protein will have one or more peptides able to bind any specific MHC molecule. The MHC therefore serves as a platform that displays the antigenic universe to T cells. The T cells view these peptides through their TCR, which recognize and bind the peptide–MHC complex.

It could be imagined that a pathogen may readily evade the immune system by simply designing proteins that do not contain MHC-binding motifs. However, this is not possible for two reasons. First, we express several different class I and class II MHC molecules, three of each for the major, or classical, MHC forms on each chromosome. These are called HLA-A, -B, and -C for the human class I locus, and HLA-DR, -DQ, and -DP for the class II locus. Therefore, an individual heterozygous for each locus may have a total of six different class I molecules, and, because the α and β chains of the class II molecule encoded on each chromosome may heterodimerize either in cis or in trans, an even larger number of distinct class II MHC molecules. If a pathogen's proteins failed to bind one HLA protein, it would likely bind one of the others. More importantly, the MHC genes are remarkable among all genes for their polymorphism, or allelic variability. Because of this variability, most of us have different sets of MHC genes. Indeed, no other human genetic locus is as polymorphic as the MHC.[42] Sequence variation of the allelic variants is particularly prominent at the peptide-binding groove, and different alleles of even a single MHC gene therefore often have distinct peptide-binding and antigen-presentation properties. MHC polymorphism ensures that a pathogen that attempted to evade the immune system of one individual would not be able to do so for others, thereby protecting the population as a whole.

The polymorphism and polygenicity of the MHC also presents a problem in transfusion and transplantation. T lymphocytes respond particularly vigorously against allogeneic (allelically distinct) MHC molecules. Each of these allogeneic MHC molecules can bind thousands of different peptides. Peptides derived from self-antigens, to which a person's immune system is normally tolerant, when combined with allogeneic MHC molecules, form complexes that are foreign to the host immune system.[43] It is estimated that roughly 1% to 10% of a person's T cells will respond to another person's allogeneic MHC combined with the array of self-peptides that may bind in its groove. For stem cell transplant recipients, this recognition may be manifested by the development of graft-versus-host disease (GVHD) or graft rejection. In the case of transfusion, it may be made apparent by the development of immune responses resulting in transfusion-associated GVHD or platelet refractoriness.

Specialized Functions of Class I and Class II MHC Molecules

Despite their similar structures, class I and class II MHC molecules have distinct roles. Key to this distinction is the repertoire of peptides that each MHC molecule binds. Class I MHC binds peptides derived from within a cell and thus displays a cell's intracellular milieu. Class II MHC displays antigens acquired from the extracellular space. Thus, each set of MHC proteins is telling T cells a different tale. In the event of a viral infection, presentation of viral antigens on a cell's class I MHC would indicate to a T cell that the cell is infected. Presentation on class II MHC molecules would instead indicate that virus is present in the environment, but not necessarily within that cell.

The distinct presentation capabilities of class I and class II MHC results from the different mechanisms through which each protein acquires its peptides. Within the cytoplasm of the cell proteins are continuously being degraded by a large proteolytic complex called the *proteasome.*[44] The peptide fragments formed by the proteasome are perfectly sized for binding class I MHC molecules. The production of antigenic peptides may be enhanced and the sites of proteolysis modified by cytokines produced during an immune response, most notably interferon-γ.[45] As class I MHC molecules are synthesized, they are extruded into a membranous compartment within the cell called the *endoplasmic reticulum.* Appropriately sized, proteasomally derived peptide fragments are continuously transported into the endoplasmic reticulum by a special peptide transporter, called *transporter of antigenic peptides,* or TAP1/2.[46,47] The transported peptides can then bind to the nascent class I MHC molecules (Fig. 2–5).[48] MHC molecules bound to peptide are then transported to the cell surface.

Class II MHC molecules take a different route to the cell surface. They are also extruded into the endoplasmic reticulum. However, unlike class I MHC molecules, they bind to a protein called the *invariant chain* as they are synthesized (Fig. 2–6). A peptide segment of the invariant chain folds into the peptide-binding groove of the class II molecule, blocking any other peptides from binding. Rather than going directly to the cell surface like class I MHC molecules, the class II molecules are first diverted to specialized vesicles, or membrane-contained compartments, within the cell where they meet up with extracellularly derived antigens.[49–51]

Cells may take up external antigens through a variety of processes, including phagocytosis, or wholesale consumption of cells or particles; pinocytosis, or internalization of small

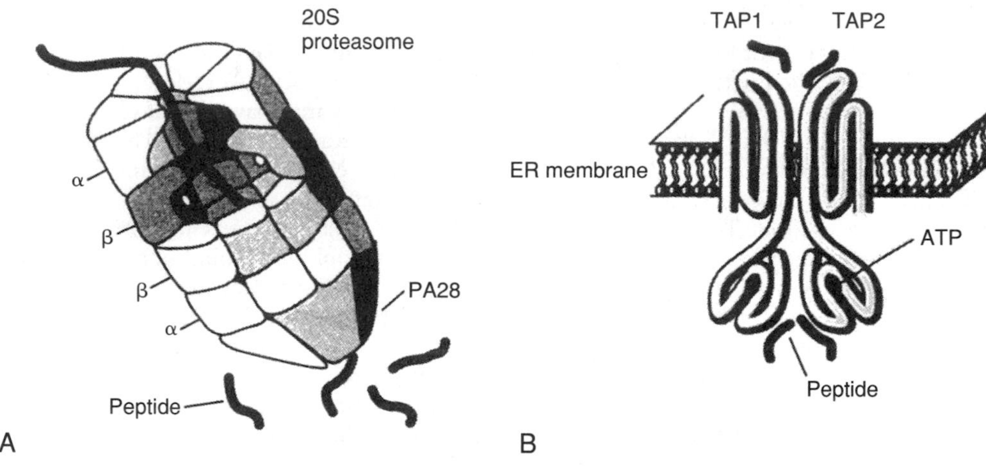

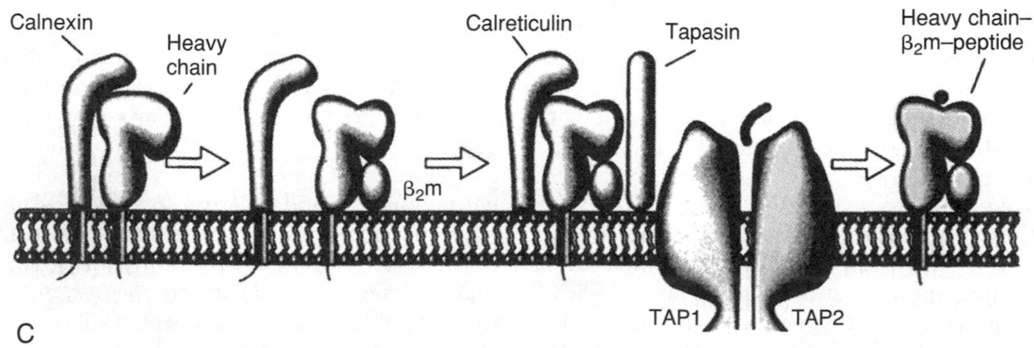

Figure 2–5 **A,** Schematic drawing of a cut-open 20S proteasome generating peptide fragments from an unfolded polypeptide chain threaded into the narrow entry formed by an outer ring of β-type subunits. Cleavage occurs in the central cavity formed by two seven-membered rings of β-type subunits. A PA28 regulator complex, inducible by IFN-γ is bound at the bottom of the cylinder. **B,** Hypothetical cross-section of TAP1/TAP2 heterodimer embedded into the endoplasmic reticulum membrane. The adenosine triphosphate (ATP)-binding domain, which extends into the cytoplasm, is shown. ATP cleavage provides energy for peptide translocation. **C,** Maturation of class I molecules in the endoplasmic reticulum. Nascent class I heavy chains initially associate with calnexin. On binding of β_2-microglobulin, the heterodimer dissociates from calnexin and forms a complex with calreticulin, tapasin, and TAP1/2. After peptide binding, the heavy-chain β_2-microglobulin complexes are released and exit to the cell surface. (From Koopman JO, Hammerling GJ, Momburg F. Generation, intracellular transport, and loading of peptides associated with MHC class I molecules. Curr Opin Immunol 1997;9:81.)

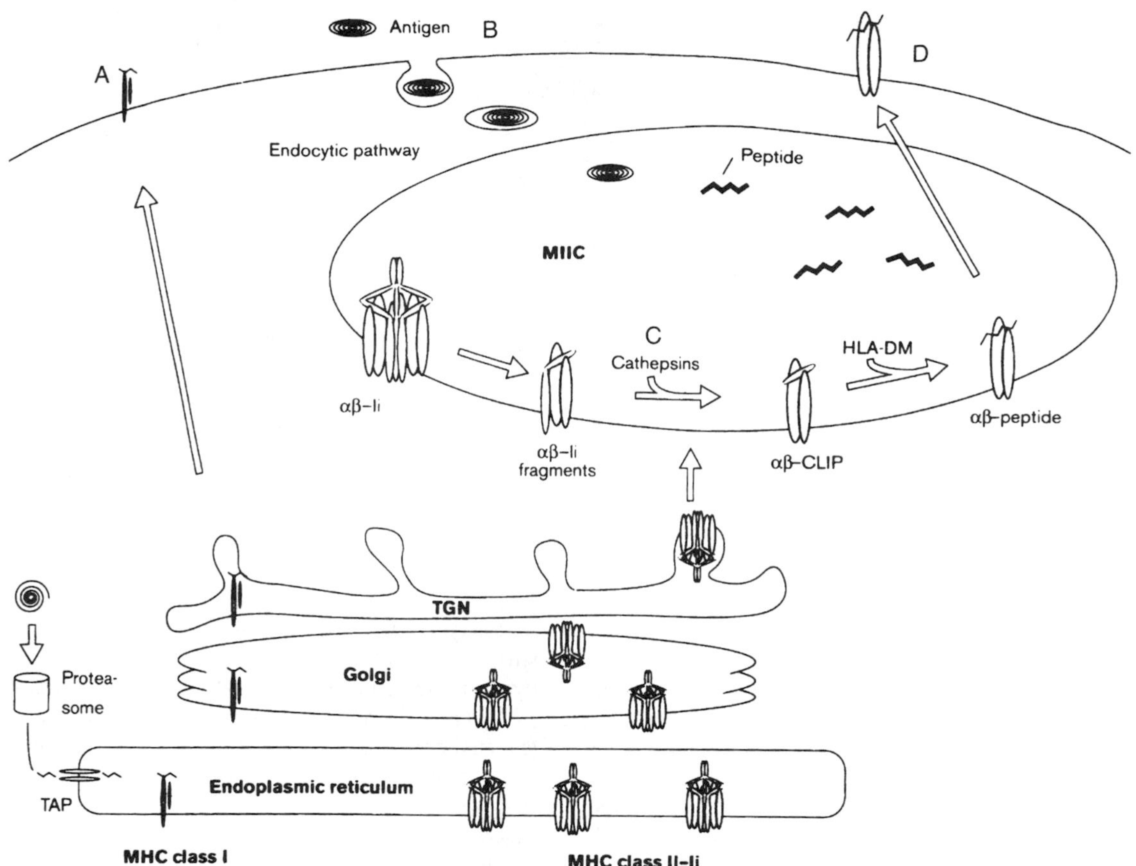

Figure 2–6 Intracellular pathways of class I and class II MHC molecules. Class I MHC molecules acquire antigenic peptides, generated by the proteasome in the cytosol, that are translocated into the endoplasmic reticulum by the TAP molecules (bottom of figure). The class I MHC–peptide complex is transported through the Golgi complex directly to the cell surface for presentation to CD8 T cells (**A**). In contrast, class II MHC molecules acquire antigenic peptides derived from antigens that are internalized in the endocytic pathways (**B**). Class II MHC heterodimers associate in the endoplasmic reticulum (bottom of figure) with invariant chains to form nonameric αβ–Ii complexes. At the trans-Golgi network (TGN), these complexes are targeted to class II MHC compartments (MIIC) in the endocytic pathway as a result of targeting signals within the Ii cytoplasmic tail (not shown). There the class II MHC-associated Ii is degraded in distinct steps, at least partially by cathepsin proteases (**C**), leaving a peptide from Ii in the class II MHC–peptide-binding groove. This peptide is exchanged for antigenic peptides in a process catalyzed by HLA-DM molecules. Peptide-loaded class II MHC complexes are then transported to the plasma membrane for presentation to CD4 T cells (**D**). (From Pieters J. MHC class II restricted antigen presentation. Curr Opin Immunol 1997;9:91.)

amounts of the extracellular fluid; and receptor-mediated internalization, which may occur through bound immunoglobulin or sugar-binding receptors such as the mannose receptor.[52–54] This material is broken down by enzymes within the endocytic, or internalization, pathway. Vesicles containing endocytosed and degraded material merge with the class II MHC containing vesicles. The invariant chain is degraded by proteases at this point, and vesicular peptides can then bind within the class II MHC-binding groove. The class II MHC, with externally derived bound peptide, then makes its way to the cell surface.

T-Cell Co-receptors and the Recognition of Class I and Class II MHC Molecules

MHC molecules present the antigenic universe to T lymphocytes. Considering the different types of antigens presented by class I and class II MHC, intracellular versus extracellular, it is not surprising that these molecules will engage different types of T cells and that this engagement will result in different types of responses. To understand how this occurs requires some background in how T cells recognize antigen.

The variable α and β chains of the TCR recognize peptide–MHC complexes. However, their affinity for peptide–MHC is poor, approximately 100- to 1000-fold lower than the binding affinity, or interaction strength, of antibodies for their target antigens.[55,56] For most TCRs, this interaction is too weak and too transient to generate a signal capable of fully activating a T cell. The TCR is able to signal because it also receives assistance from co-receptors called CD4 and CD8. CD4 binds to class II MHC molecules and CD8 binds to class I MHC molecules. When the TCR engages cognate peptide–MHC, CD4 or CD8 co-associates.

CD4 and CD8 are transmembrane proteins that perform two tasks.[57] First, because they both associate with the TCR and bind MHC at a site different from where the TCR binds peptide–MHC, they increase the binding affinity of the TCR complex for peptide–MHC. Second, and more importantly, they carry bound to their intracellular domain an enzyme of the src family, called lck (Fig. 2–7).[58] Lck is a type of enzyme called a *tyrosine kinase*. It adds phosphates to certain tyrosine residues present in proteins. Tyrosine phosphorylation of the γ, δ, ε, and ζ chains of the TCR is the first step in generating a signal once a TCR recognizes antigen. The complex of CD4 or CD8 co-receptor with the TCR and peptide–MHC aligns the lck kinase with specific conserved tyrosines present within the signaling chains of the TCR called *immunoreceptor tyrosine-based activation motifs,* or ITAMs.[59] Once phosphorylated, these ITAMs

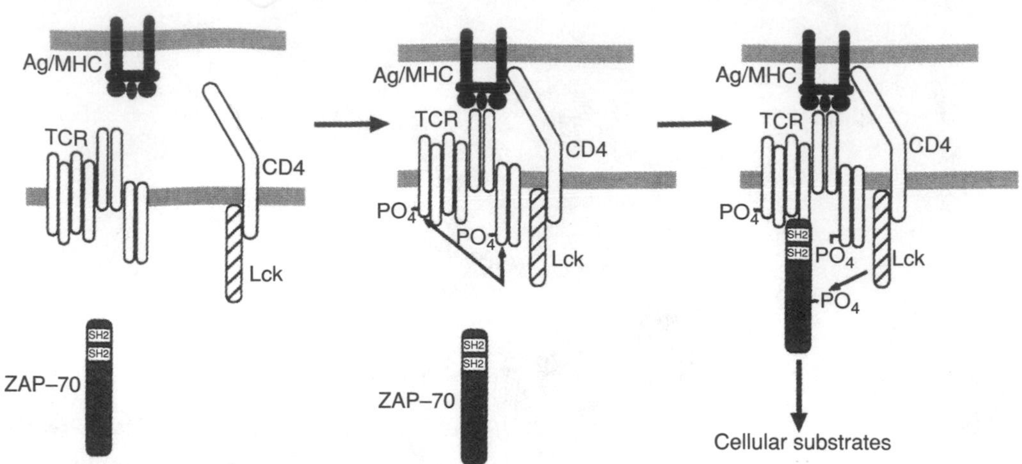

Figure 2–7 Model of TCR, Lck and ζ-associated protein (ZAP)-70 interactions during antigen recognition by a CD4 T cell. The phosphorylation of tyrosine residues of the immunoreceptor tyrosine-based activation motifs within the ζ and CD3 chains has been simplified. (From Weiss A. T-cell antigen receptor signal transduction: A tale of tails and cytoplasmic protein kinases. Cell 1993;73:211.)

serve as docking sites for additional proteins, particularly ZAP-70, another tyrosine kinase that is in turn phosphorylated and activated by lck. This triggers a cascade of signaling inside the cell as additional proteins are recruited to these phosphorylated molecules. In a manner analogous to how the coagulation cascade may be triggered by single event, such as exposure to tissue factor, a low amplitude signal that initially results from TCR–MHC engagement is enzymatically amplified within a T cell. The impact of CD4 and CD8 is dramatic, and it has been estimated that these molecules enhance signaling through the TCR by a factor of 100.[57] Through its sophisticated signaling apparatus, T cells may be discriminately stimulated by 100 or fewer antigen–MHC complexes on the surface of an APC.[60]

Mature T cells express either CD4 or CD8 and do not co-express both of these. This contrasts with their progenitors that develop in the thymus, which co-express CD4 and CD8. During development, these $CD4^+D8^+$ thymocytes are tested.[61] Cells that interact strongly with self-antigen–MHC complexes in the thymus are deleted in a process termed *negative selection.* Negative selection is a major mechanism through which the adaptive immune repertoire is depleted of self-antigen–specific T cells. Cells that do not interact with MHC present in the thymus do not receive necessary survival signals and undergo death through neglect. In contrast, in a process termed *positive selection,* cells with receptors that interact loosely with class I MHC molecules receive survival signals, downmodulate CD4, and are left expressing only CD8. Thymocytes that interact with class II MHC downmodulate CD8 and become CD4-expressing T cells. Thus, T cells can be divided into two major groups based on their interaction with either class I or class II MHC molecules, and these groups can be identified by the alternative expression of CD4 or CD8. Further, CD4 and CD8 define classes of T cells with distinct functional potentials.

Cells That Present Antigen

Because class I MHC presents antigens derived from intracellular pathogens, like viruses, or that result from intrinsic abnormalities, such as malignant transformation, it is important that all cells capable of self-propagation express class I MHC. $CD8^+$ T cells recognizing class I MHC-derived antigens may eliminate these aberrant or infected cells. The majority of nucleated cells indeed express class I MHC constitutively, though class I MHC expression can be enhanced by cytokines, such as in the setting of inflammation.[62]

Not all cells need to express class II MHC, which presents external antigens. Class II MHC expression is limited to specialized cells that provide T cells with environmental information. These include professional APCs, dendritic cells, macrophages, B cells, and endothelial cells, though other cell types may be induced to express class II MHC in the context of inflammation.

Of the professional APCs that present antigen to T cells on class II MHC, dendritic cells are particularly efficient. They reside in tissues in a quiescent state. When activated by any of a large variety of inflammatory stimuli, such as cytokines or Toll-like receptor signals, they sample antigens from their environment, which they present on cell surface class II MHC molecules.[30] After accumulating large quantities of antigen, the dendritic cells cease internalizing antigen and migrate to lymphoid tissues, particularly lymph nodes, where they present antigen to lymphocytes.

There are several types of dendritic cells.[63] Some, the follicular dendritic cells, are particularly adept at presenting whole antigen to B lymphocytes.[64] This is important because B cells recognize whole antigens or large pieces of antigens through their immunoglobulin receptors. In contrast, most dendritic cells, including myeloid, lymphoid, and plasmacytoid dendritic cells, digest antigens into small fragments and present these to T lymphocytes. Because of the scarcity of lymphocytes specific for any single antigen, presentation in specialized lymphoid tissue is essential. The professional APCs structure themselves into a reticular network through which lymphocytes continuously and rapidly percolate.[65] After a dendritic cell is stimulated through its Toll-like receptor or other receptors, it may secrete chemokines that will attract T lymphocytes to it and costimulatory molecules that can activate them. The lymphocytes scan these dendritic cells with their antigen receptor for the presence of cognate antigen. With recognition through their antigen and costimulatory receptors, the lymphocytes pause, alter their metabolism, and modulate gene expression. They may then expand and differentiate into effector forms.

Other professional APCs are macrophages and B lymphocytes. Macrophages are potent phagocytic cells when activated and may internalize a variety of different pathogens as well as dead and dying cells. Macrophages may present the antigen acquired at the site of tissue injury or within lymphoid organs and are important in guiding some types of T-cell responses. B cells primarily internalize antigens through their BCR, surface immunoglobulin. The high affinity of the BCR for specific antigens allows them to focus small quantities of antigen present in the environment and to display this to cognate antigen-specific T cells.

Functionally and Phenotypically Distinct Classes of T Cells

T cells are categorized into discrete groups based on their phenotype, function, and differentiation potential. The broadest categorization relates to the type of TCR expressed. The large majority of T cells express the αβ TCR described above, though a small number of cells express an alternative receptor composed of a parallel heterodimer of chains called γ and δ. These γ and δ chains recognize antigen–MHC complexes and are distinct from the signaling γ and δ chains that are part of the CD3 complex. Indeed, γδ TCR associate with the CD3 and ζ signaling chains, forming a signaling complex identical to that of αβ receptors. The function of γδ T cells is unclear. Some of these cells reside in lymphoid tissue and have a highly diverse receptor repertoire. Other γδ T cells reside in intraepithelial spaces. These cells have limited receptor diversity within a specific location. This suggests that they recognize relatively invariant molecules, either pathogen or host derived.[66] Indeed, some γδ T cells recognize nonclassical, nonpolymorphic class I MHC molecules called class Ib MHC.[67] Recent data indicates that they may also efficiently present antigen to αβ T cells and may promote the rapid induction of αβ T-cell responses after they are activated.[68] Therefore, these cells may act more as facilitators and regulators rather than mediators of adaptive immunity.

The more common αβ class of T cells is typically divided into helper and effector classes. Helper T cells integrate the environmental cues they receive and then signal to other cells, effector cells, orchestrating their response. Helper T-cell signals may include the release of cytokines, such as IL-2, IL-4, and IFN-γ. They also may signal by interacting with other cells through cell surface receptors. Helper T cells fall largely in the CD4 class of T cells. As a consequence, often the terms helper T cell and CD4 T cell are used interchangeably. On a biological level, this is inaccurate and should be avoided. CD4 T cells in some circumstances have effector functions and CD8 T cells may have helper activities. Nevertheless, it should not be surprising that CD4 T cells tend to be dominantly helper cells by nature. CD4 T cells probe the antigenic environment through class II MHC. Their response to environmental cues that may suggest danger should not be directed against the APC, which is merely a messenger carrying antigen to the T cell. They must choreograph a broader response that will directly target harmful antigens.

When a freshly formed CD4 T cell exits the thymus it is "naive," never having seen its cognate antigen. The cell will home to lymphoid tissues, occasionally circulating through the bloodstream to a different lymphoid location.[69] As it does this, it searches for antigen able to stimulate its TCR, which is delivered to it by APCs present within lymphoid tissue. Once stimulated this T cell may differentiate into one of a variety of forms. Two of the best studied types of CD4 T cells are Th1 and Th2 cells.[70,71] Cytokines secreted by Th1 cells, such as IFN-γ and TNF-β, are responsible for delayed-type hypersensitivity (DTH) reactions.[72,73] Th2 cells, which secrete IL-4, IL-5, IL-10, and IL-13, are responsible for allergic responses.[71,74]

In the DTH response, Th1 T cells stimulate B cells to produce specific antibodies that efficiently activate complement after antigen binding. The Th1 cells also migrate to sites of antigen presentation in tissues. Once there, they secrete cytokines, such as IFN-γ and TNF, and chemokines that promote the recruitment and activation of macrophages, additional lymphocytes, and other inflammatory cells.[75,76] Activation of endothelial cells leads to a loss of vascular integrity and the development of induration, a hallmark of the DTH response. The activated macrophages locally present antigen and amplify the immune response. Macrophages also serve as primary effector cells, ingesting and eliminating pathogens, and producing reactive oxygen species that can kill microorganisms. If this response is unable to clear the inciting agent, granuloma formation and scarring may wall it off.

In Th2 responses, CD4 T cells stimulate the production of antibodies that may be neutralizing or promote antibody-dependent cell-mediated cytotoxicity. Cytokines produced by the Th2 cells activate and promote the expansion of eosinophils and other cell types. Th2 T cells prominently support the production of IgE, which binds specific high-affinity receptors on mast cells and basophils.[77] Antigen crosslinks these antibodies, thereby activating the mast cells and basophils. This induces the release of histamine and other BRMs that are associated with allergic or anaphylactic symptoms, such as vascular dilatation, mucus production, urticaria, and diarrhea. We commonly associate these symptoms with pathologic responses to allergens and not with the clearance of infections. However, Th2 responses appear to be important for the clearance of some parasitic infections.[78,79]

The final form a naïve T cell differentiates into is determined by its microenvironment after antigen stimulation.[80,81] Th1 cell differentiation is promoted by the presence of IL-12 and IFN-γ. Th2 cell differentiation is promoted by the presence of IL-4 and prostaglandin E_2. These stimuli may be produced after innate immune signaling in cells. IL-4 is produced by activated mast cells and basophils.[82–84] Activated dendritic cells may produce IL-12 and the closely related IL-23.[82,85] NK cells may produce IFN-γ.[86] These differentiation cytokines may also be produced by T cells themselves. Th1 cells produce IFN-γ, which further promotes Th1 differentiation and inhibits Th2 differentiation. Th2 cells produce IL-4, which promotes Th2 and inhibits Th1 development. Thus Th1 or Th2 antigen-specific T cells that developed in prior immune responses or in an earlier phase of an active immune response may polarize a nascent immune response, promoting the development and expansion of T cells of their own class while inhibiting those of other classes. This ensures an unadulterated response to a particular pathogen type, DTH or allergic in the case of Th1 and Th2 cells, respectively.

CD8 T cells are typically effector in nature. When activated they differentiate into a class of cells called *cytotoxic T lymphocytes* (CTLs). In many circumstances this differentiation depends on signals provided by CD4 helper T cells.[87,88] One manner by which stimulated CD4 T cells do this is through the upregulation of a TNF-family protein, CD40L, on their cell surface.[89] CD40L interacts with CD40 on the surface of APCs, signaling into the APC. This signal is important to "license" the APC, that is, induce in the APC production of cytokines and signaling molecules that are needed to adequately stimulate the CD8 T cell. If a CD8 T cell does not receive these supplemental signals, it will not appropriately expand and differentiate in response to antigen and may die after antigen encounter.

When a CTL's TCR encounters and engages its target MHC–antigen complex on a cell, it extrudes preformed granules that contain lytic proteins.[90] These proteins include perforin, which forms pores in the membranes of the target cells, and granzymes, enzymes that kill targets through a preprogrammed cell death pathway called *apoptosis.* They also include a protein called fasL, which binds to a receptor called fas on many cell types, also inducing apoptosis. The absence of adequate lytic activity can have severe consequences. Patients with mutations in perforin develop a disease called *hemophagocytic lymphohistiocytosis.*[91,92] Failure to control infections results in an unrestrained activation of the immune system that is most often fatal.

Regulation of T-Cell Responses

The effector responses that T cells coordinate can cause substantial bystander damage to host tissues if unrestricted. Because of this, homeostatic mechanisms that limit immune responses are essential. There are several such mechanisms.

One mechanism is the apoptosis, or programmed cell death, of lymphocytes. After immune activation, T cells proliferate profusely. This is physically manifested by the splenomegaly and adenopathy commonly identified with infection. Failure to eliminate this expanded cell population would result in a plethora of activated immune effector cells. Most of these cells, however, die through apoptosis.[93–95] Members of the TNF family of proteins are particularly important for this. For example, in many circumstances activated T cells will express a pair of TNF family molecules, fas and fasL. When fasL engages fas, it stimulates the fas receptor. This activates a set of cellular proteases called *caspases* that can cause a loss of mitochondrial and ultimately cellular integrity. In the absence of molecules that inhibit apoptosis, caspase activation ultimately leads to cell death. Dysfunctional apoptosis mechanisms in lymphocytes can lead to autoimmunity by allowing the persistence of self-reactive T cells that normally would be eliminated. Indeed, patients with mutations in fas or apoptotic signaling develop a disease called *autoimmune lymphoproliferative syndrome.*[96]

Cytokines and other BRMs may also restrict immune responses. Many cytokines have dual properties, both enhancing and suppressing immune effector mechanisms even within a single type of immune response. For example, IFN-γ activates macrophages and other effector cells and promotes Th1-cell differentiation. It also inhibits proliferation and may in some circumstances promote apoptosis.[86] A good example of the dual effects of IFN-γ is observed in an experimental murine model of multiple sclerosis, an autoimmune disease that is predominantly Th1 in nature. IFN-γ produced early in the pathologic response promotes the induction of Th1-polarized T cells and therefore disease development. Later in the disease course, IFN-γ is protective, and its neutralization exacerbates disease.[97,98]

Although many cytokines have mixed pro- and anti-inflammatory effects, some cytokines have dominantly inhibitory roles.[99–101] For example, transforming growth factor-β (TGF-β) strongly suppresses T-cell activity. Mice genetically modified so that their T cells are unable to respond to this cytokine develop a spontaneous lethal autoinflammatory condition. IL-10, while able to activate B cells, is also a critical downregulatory cytokine for activated macrophages. Mice lacking IL-10 develop spontaneous inflammatory bowel disease.[102]

Negative signaling is not limited to cytokines but can also occur through cell associated proteins. As mentioned above, professional APCs provide T cells with access to costimulatory proteins. These generally promote signaling in the context of TCR activation.[29] The proteins B7.1 and B7.2 are prime examples.[103] These are upregulated on APC after exposure to Tlr signaling or CD40L, and bind to CD28 on T cells. In the absence of adequate costimulatory signaling a T cell will become unresponsive to its cognate antigen, a condition called anergy, or may die.[31] The B7 proteins are only one of a large group of essential costimulatory molecules expressed on APC.

However, costimulatory molecules need not transduce a positive signal into a T cell. Examples include PD-1L and B7h3, which when expressed on an APC downmodulate T-cell signaling and T-cell responses.[104,105] T cells may also express variant ligands for a single costimulatory molecule. Thus CD28 transduces a strong growth and survival signal when it engages B7 ligand. But a similar molecule, CTLA-4, when expressed on T cells, binds the same B7 ligands but downmodulates T-cell activation.[106,107] Mice that lack CTLA-4 develop uncontrolled lymphoproliferation. Temporal regulation of CD28 and CTLA-4 on a T cell may specify the magnitude of the T-cell response. Whereas most T cells express CD28 constitutively, they only express CTLA-4 after activation. Thus initial antigen exposure provides a strong signal to T cells. This signal is downmodulated by CTLA-4 if the exposure persists.

Not all T cells are involved in choreographing and mediating immune effector functions. The dominant role of several classes of T cells is the suppression of immune responses. These antagonize the pro-inflammatory activities of effector T cells. One important category of regulatory T cells co-expresses CD4 and the high-affinity receptor for IL-2, CD25.[108,109] Development of these cells is defined by the expression of a DNA-binding protein, or transcription factor, called FoxP3. Patients with the IPEX syndrome (immune polyendocrinopathy, X-linked) have mutations in this transcription factor and lack these regulatory T cells.[110] Overwhelming multiorgan autoimmunity develops early in life. When stimulated by antigen, FoxP3-expressing regulatory T cells inhibit T-cell responses both through direct cell–cell contact effects and through the production of cytokines, particularly IL-10 and TGF-β. Other classes of regulatory cells, which have been given different names by investigators, including Th3 and Tr1 cells, primarily inhibit immune responses through the production of regulatory cytokines.[99,101,111] Again, TGF-β and IL-10 seem to be critical.

The complexity to immune regulation parallels the complexity of immune activation. At any point in time the integration of many different signals, some promoting activation and others signaling restraint, will define the ultimate direction taken.

B-Lymphocyte Responses

B lymphocytes are critical effector cells for immune protection. They act through the production of immunoglobulin, or antibodies. Antibodies specifically bind to target antigens. By so doing, they may sterically block the function of some antigens, such as toxins, enzymes, and receptors. Antibody binding may promote complement fixation and thereby the lysis or phagocytosis of cells. Antibody–antigen complexes may crosslink immunoglobulin receptors, Fc receptors, on the surface of effector cell types, such as NK cells, neutrophils, macrophages, and mast cells.[112,113] If the Fc receptor is an activating form of the receptor, it will stimulate functions capable of clearing or neutralizing the antigen through a variety of mechanisms, including phagocytosis, antibody-dependent cell-mediated cytotoxicity (ADCC), cytotoxic granule release, and the generation of reactive oxygen and other cytocidal compounds. The antibody, or humoral, immune response is therefore essential to host defense. In its absence, there is a dramatic increase in the susceptibility to and severity of infections.[114]

Like the T-cell repertoire, the B-cell repertoire is richly diverse, with billions of possible unique receptors. Like T cells, B cells only express a single receptor on their surface. And like T cells, B cells are not constitutively activated, secreting random immunoglobulins. Rather, they produce soluble immunoglobulins only after being activated through their antigen receptor. Unlike T cells, B cells do not recognize antigen complexed with MHC; they recognize whole antigens.

B cells can differentiate to secrete antibodies in the absence of T cells. These responses are called *T-independent* or *helper-independent responses.*[115,116] There are two types of T-independent humoral immune responses. In T-independent-1 responses, the antigen is able to simultaneously stimulate the B lymphocyte through the BCR and other activating receptors. For example, B cells specific for LPS will receive stimulatory signals both through their antigen receptor and through their LPS-specific Toll-like receptor. This may occur in the setting of a gram-negative bacterial infection. Whereas high concentrations of LPS will polyclonally stimulate all B cells through Tlr4, low doses will only simulate those T-independent-1 B cells that are able to concentrate the LPS with their BCR. The combined Toll-like receptor/BCR signal promotes antibody secretion. In T-independent-2 responses, the antigen is not intrinsically stimulatory, but acts by cross-linking a threshold number of BCRs on the B lymphocyte. Too strong a BCR stimulus can turn off a B lymphocyte, and too small a stimulus will not adequately activate a B cell. However, intermediate levels of stimulus may be sufficient to activate subgroups of B lymphocytes, most prominently B cells that express the CD5 antigen (B-1 B cells) and marginal zone B cells.

Often the immune response to T-independent antigens is directed against polysaccharides and other polyvalent structures present in the cell walls of pathogens. The T-independent response may allow an early antibody response against these antigens. This antibody may promote internalization of infecting organisms by phagocytes and antigen presentation to T lymphocytes. Activation of the T-cell response may then further drive the B-cell response through the provision of T-cell help in the form of cytokines and other signaling molecules. Patients with Wiskott-Aldrich syndrome fail to produce T-independent responses to bactetrial antigens and consequentially are at great risk for infection with encapsulated bacteria.[117] T-independent immunoglobulin responses are primarily of the IgM class of antibodies (described in the following section). Further differentiation of the B cell is required to produce other types of antibody, and T-cell help must be provided for this.

Generally, T-cell help is available to promote B-cell responses. As B cells enter the spleen or lymph node from the circulation, they initially enter T-cell rich areas. If the B cell has encountered its antigen, either in the circulation or in the lymphatic tissue, it will internalize the BCR–antigen complex. This will be degraded and presented by the B cell on the surface of its class II MHC molecules. Because B cells internalize antigens almost exclusively through their BCR, they are able to selectively capture and concentrate their specific antigens from the extracellular environment. If a T cell that has been stimulated by its cognate antigen on a dendritic cell or other APC then discovers the same antigen on a B cell, the cells will transiently join together and stimulate each other.[118] The B lymphocyte along with the T lymphocyte will proliferate, expanding typically at the interface between the T and B regions of the lymph node.

The epitope recognized by a B lymphocyte's antigen receptor need not be the same as that recognized by the TCR of the T cell that stimulates it. When the BCR binds to and endocytoses antigen, it may internalize whole proteins; complexes containing multiple proteins, DNA, lipids, and polysaccharides; or even whole organisms. All of this will be digested and presented to T cells on the B cell's class II MHC. The antigenic epitope recognized by the T cell therefore does not need to be identical to that recognized by the B cell, but it must be co-internalized and therefore linked to it. The help provided to B cells by T cells is thus often termed *linked recognition.*[119]

Stimulated B cells that secrete antibodies are called *plasma cells.* These cells functionally transform themselves, upregulating protein synthetic machinery so as to be able to produce large quantities of antibodies. They localize to the medulla, or central core of the lymph nodes, or specific regions of the spleen or bone marrow, where they secrete copious amounts of specific antibodies.[120,121]

Some stimulated B cells will migrate into the B-cell rich follicles of the lymph node or spleen and form what is called a *germinal center.*[122] Germinal centers consist of large numbers of proliferating and differentiating antigen-specific B cells accompanied by smaller numbers of supporting T lymphocytes. Within the germinal centers the B cells are continuously stimulated by antigen presented by follicular dendritic cells. They receive further help from T cells, which promotes their survival, growth, and differentiation. Under the influence of these signals, the B cells may isotype switch, or replace the constant region of their immunoglobulin receptor to allow production of antibody isotypes other than IgM. Isotype switching involves the excision of DNA sequence encoding upstream antibody constant domains, placing the rearranged VDJ region in proximity with a different C region. It is fostered by the expression of CD40L on activated T cells, which binds CD40 on B cells. Cytokines, such as IL-4 and IL-6, also promote B-cell differentiation and isotype switching. B cells from patients lacking CD40L or an enzyme required for DNA rearrangement, activation-induced cytidine deaminase, fail to isotype switch and exclusively produce IgM.[123,124]

B lymphocytes are capable of an additional trick unavailable to T cells. B cells in the germinal center can actually mutate their BCR, a process termed *somatic hypermutation.*[125,126] The mutations are focused in the antigen-binding region of the receptor. Within the germinal center a process of selection occurs for B cells based on their affinity for antigen. As antigen recedes, the rare B cells in which immunoglobulin mutations have increased their affinity for antigen will survive best, whereas B cells that less effectively bind, internalize, and concentrate antigen will fail to receive necessary survival signals and will perish. Due to somatic hypermutation, B cells may acquire mutated antibodies that have 100-fold or higher affinity for antigen than their antecedent antibodies. Affinity-matured B cells may then form plasma cells, secreting high-affinity antibody. Alternatively, high-affinity B cells may become quiescent, forming what is called a *memory B cell.* Memory cells are long-lived formerly activated lymphocytes, either T or B, capable of rapid response on restimulation.[127] Because of the presence of memory cells, the antibody response on secondary stimulation is of a higher magnitude and affinity than the primary response that develops after initial exposure to antigen.

Antibodies

Antibodies come in several forms, each of which has the same basic structure, consisting of two linked dimers of a heavy and light chain. Each of the chains includes tandem globular domains called *immunoglobulin domains* that are conserved within the immunoglobulin superfamily of proteins (Fig. 2–8).[128] The heavy chain is composed of a variable region encompassing the V, D, and J segments, and a C region with three or four immunoglobulin domains depending on the antibody isotype. This heavy chain is linked through a disulfide bond (two cysteines bound together through their sulfur moiety) to a light chain. The light chain consists of V and J segments linked to a constant region with a single immunoglobulin domain. Two identical heavy-light chain dimers are fastened by disulfide linkages between the two heavy chain genes adjacent to the second immunoglobulin domain. Each heavy and light chain pair may independently bind antigen, and a single immunoglobulin monomer thus has a valency for antigen of 2.

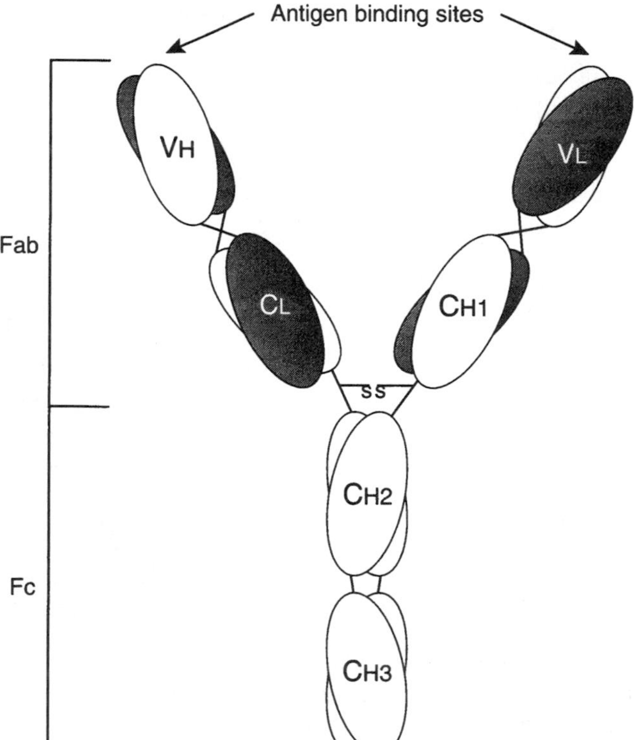

Figure 2–8 Structure of a prototypical, monomeric, secreted antibody molecule. Ovals represent immunoglobulin domains. Heavy chains are indicated by white fill, light chains by gray fill. Polypeptide linkages are indicated by lines. A single representative disulfide linkage between the hinge regions of the heavy chain is indicated; other interchain and intrachain disulfide bonds are not shown.

Different functional regions are encoded within immunoglobulin molecules. The Fv consists of the paired heavy and light chain variable domains. Fv are not independently stable when separated from the rest of the immunoglobin molecule; however, engineered single chain Fv in which the heavy and light variable domains are genetically linked have been created and are capable of binding antigen. These engineered scFv may become increasingly common as the use of engineered antibodies for therapy and diagnostics becomes more routine.[129–131]

The addition of the first constant region domain to the Fv domain incorporates a disulfide linkage between the heavy and light chains and stabilizes the Fv. These Fab (fraction antibody binding) retain the antigen-binding properties of the parent immunoglobulin. Fab fragments may be released from immunoglobulin molecules by protease digestion.

The final two or three constant regions of the heavy chain form the Fc domain. Where the Fab domains connect to the Fc stalk, there is a flexible hinge that allows each Fab domain to independently bend. This helps the antibody bind to multivalent antigens, where the spacing between individual epitopes may vary. The Fc binds to immunoglobulin-binding receptors on cells, Fc receptors, and is therefore responsible for ADCC and other cell-mediated activities. The Fc also binds complement and participates in the activation of this effector pathway. Fab and Fv antibody fragments lack the Fc domain and therefore lack these activities.

Immunoglobulin heavy chains come in five basic varieties—μ, γ, δ, ε, and α. When linked to either of the two varieties of light chain—κ or λ—these form IgM, IgG, IgD, IgE, and IgA, respectively, the different isotypes of immunoglobulin. Each of the immunoglobulin isotypes come in a membrane-bound form expressed on the surface of B cells. A transmembrane domain pierces the cell membrane, attaching the immunoglobulin to the cell surface. Transmembrane forms of immunoglobulin associate with cell membrane proteins, called Igα and Igβ, which allow BCR signaling in a manner analogous to the CD3 chains of the TCR. All isotypes except IgD may also be secreted, in which case the antibody protein is synthesized without the transmembrane anchor. The role of IgD is poorly characterized. Cells expressing IgD also express an IgM version of the same antibody.

The secreted forms of different antibodies differ structurally. Secreted IgM consists of five immunoglobulin molecules that are linked together by a junctional chain, forming a pentamer with 10 antigen-binding sites. IgA may be secreted as a single immunoglobulin, and this is its most common form in plasma. However, IgA produced by plasma cells underlying epithelia in the gut, respiratory, or reproductive tracts typically is dimeric, and therefore antibodies secreted into these locations have four antigen-binding sites.[132] The remaining immunoglobulin isotypes are only produced as monomers with two antigen-binding sites.

Soluble antibody can bind cognate antigen in solution. The binding affinity an antibody has for its antigen is related to the chemical energy of binding of the Fv domain with its antigen. When an antigen is polyvalent, however, the ability of immunoglobulin to multimerize with its respective antigen will significantly increase its ability to bind the antigen. In this circumstance dissociation of the antibody from antigen would not simply require the dissociation of a single interaction, but would require all Fv regions to simultaneously disconnect from the antigenic particle. This increases net binding capacity, or avidity, of immunoglobulin molecules.

Table 2–3 Properties of Immunoglobulin Classes[138]

Ig Class	Conc (mg/dL)	No. of Ab	% Intra-vascular	Half-life (d)	Complement Fixation (– to ++++)	Agglutination Capacity	Placental Transport	Epithelial Transport
IgM	120–400	5	41	5–6	++++	++++	–	+
IgG	800–1600	1	48	18–23		+/–	+	–
IgG1		1			+++			
IgG2		1			+/–			
IgG3		1			+++			
IgG4		1			–			
IgA	40–220	1–2	76	5–6.5	+/–	++	–	++++
IgE	17–450 ng/mL	1	51	2.3	–	–	–	–

Increased avidity is particularly important for IgM. IgM is formed early in the course of an immune response, and because it will not have undergone somatic hypermutation, is typically of low affinity. This is compensated for by its high valency and thereby enhanced avidity.

As described, naive B cells secrete IgM when stimulated to produce antibody. A minimal requirement for B cells to switch isotypes is the engagement of cell surface CD40 by CD40L on T cells. The isotype the B cell converts to depends on the inflammatory environment at the time of isotype switching. Cytokines are particularly important. IFN-γ will promote formation of subclasses of IgG that efficiently bind complement. IL-4 will promote IgE formation. TGF-β promotes the formation of IgA.[133–135] These different antibody isotypes and even subclasses within isotypes have distinct functional properties, including complement fixation, Fc-receptor binding, and transport across epithelial barriers or the placenta. Some of these properties are listed in Table 2–3.

All antibodies are not equivalent, and the properties an antibody possesses will define its functional capabilities. These properties include the antibody isotype and valency, affinity for antigen, temperature dependence in binding, and titer. For instance, IgM cold agglutinins generally bind poorly at physiologic temperatures and require high titers for clinically significant effects. Some antibody isotypes are most efficient at fixing complement, and anti-RBC alloantibodies of these isotypes are of most concern for intravascular hemolytic reactions. Only IgG isotype anti-RBC antibodies pass the placenta and cause hemolytic disease of the newborn. IgE antibodies bind to specific IgE receptors on mast cells and when crosslinked activate the mast cells to secrete histamine and other BRMs that generate allergic symptoms. Sometimes we can take advantage of the properties of an antibody. For example, the rate of IgM diffusion into the extravascular space is low compared with IgG. This facilitates IgM removal by plasmapheresis.

CONCLUSION

The immune system is a dynamic web of interacting cells and molecules that protect our bodies from harm. In the practice of transfusion medicine, we may only become aware of the immune system when our patients manifest symptoms, such as when they become alloimmunized or develop allergic reactions. However, underlying these responses are not only end-effector molecules, cytokines, or antibodies, but also complex pathways of innate and adaptive immunity involving many cell types and continuous intercellular dialogue. This dialogue occurs even when we fail to clinically observe an immunologic consequence of transfusion. It even occurs within stored blood components, which respond to their storage conditions by producing cytokines and other BRMs that are then infused into patients.[136,137] The complexity of the immune response leads to unpredictability in the effects of a transfusion. We still cannot predict who will or will not have an adverse outcome to a specific transfusion event. Nevertheless, a continuous conscientiousness toward the nature of the immune response, how the immune response may perturb the intended outcomes of our transfusions, and how transfusion may perturb the immune system itself, can only help inform the clinical decisions we make.

REFERENCES

1. Silverstein AM. Autoimmunity versus horror autotoxicus: the struggle for recognition. Nat Immunol 2001;2:279–281.
2. Silverstein AM. The History of immunology. In Paul WE (ed). Fundamental Immunology. New York, Raven Press, 1989, pp 21–38.
3. Owen R. Karl Landsteiner and the first human marker locus. Genetics 2000;155:995–998.
4. Ohashi PS, Oehen S, Buerki K, et al. Ablation of tolerance and induction of diabetes by virus infection in viral antigen transgenic mice. Cell 1991;65:305–317.
5. Soldavila G, Geiger T, Flavell R. Breaking immunologic ignorance to an antigenic peptide of simian virus 40 large T antigen. J Immunol 1995; 155:5590–5600.
6. Krutzik SR, Modlin RL. The role of Toll-like receptors in combating mycobacteria. Semin Immunol 2004;16:35–41.
7. Selsted ME, Ouellette AJ. Mammalian defensins in the antimicrobial immune response. Nat Immunol 2005;6:551–557.
8. Janeway CA Jr, Medzhitov R. Innate immune recognition. Annu Rev Immunol 2002;20:197–216.
9. Miller SI, Ernst RK, Bader MW. LPS, TLR4 and infectious disease diversity. Annu Rev Immunol 2005;3:36–46.
10. Iwasaki A, Medzhitov R. Toll-like receptor control of the adaptive immune responses. Nat Immunol 2004;5:987–995.
11. Murphy PM. The molecular biology of leukocyte chemoattractant receptors. Annu Rev Immunol 1994;12:593–633.
12. Hedrick JA, Zlotnik A. Chemokines and lymphocyte biology. Curr Opin Immunol 1996;8:343–347.
13. Munoz-Fernandez MA, Fernandez MA, Fresno M. Synergism between tumor necrosis factor-α and interferon-γ on macrophage activation for the killing of intracellular *Trypanosoma cruzi* through a nitric oxide-dependent mechanism. Eur J Immunol 1992;22:301–307.
14. Trinchieri G. Interleukin-12 and the regulation of innate resistance and adaptive immunity. Nat Rev Immunol 2003;3:133–146.
15. Takeda K, Akira S. Toll-like receptors in innate immunity. Int Immunol 2005;17:1–14.
16. Lecellier CH, Dunoyer P, Arar K, et al. A cellular microRNA mediates antiviral defense in human cells. Science 2005;308:557–560.
17. Gao LH, Zheng SS. Cytomegalovirus and chronic allograft rejection in liver transplantation. World J Gastroenterol 2004;10:1857–1861.

18. Cainelli F, Vento S. Infections and solid organ transplant rejection: a cause-and-effect relationship? Lancet Infect Dis 2002;2:539–549.
19. Falcone M, Bloom BR. A T helper cell 2 (Th2) immune response against non-self antigens modifies the cytokine profile of autoimmune T cells and protects against experimental allergic encephalomyelitis. J Exp Med 1997;185:901–907.
20. Stohlman SA, Pei L, Cua DJ, et al. Activation of regulatory cells suppresses experimental allergic encephalomyelitis via secretion of IL-10. J Immunol 1999;163:6338–6344.
21. Aharoni R, Teitelbaum D, Sela M, Arnon R. Bystander suppression of experimental autoimmune encephalomyelitis by T cell lines and clones of the Th2 type induced by copolymer 1. J Neuroimmunol 1998;91:135–146.
22. Marciani DJ. Vaccine adjuvants: Role and mechanisms of action in vaccine immunogenicity. Drug Discov Today 2003;8:934–943.
23. Toyonaga B, Mak T. Genes of the T-cell antigen receptor in normal and malignant T cells. Annu Rev Immunol 1987;5:585–620.
24. Chothia C, Boswell DR, Lesk AM. The outline structure of the T cell αβ receptor. EMBO 1988;7:3745–3755.
25. Malissen M, Trucy J, Jouvin-Marche E, et al. Regulation of TCR alpha and beta gene allelic exclusion during T-cell development. Immunol Today 1992;13:315–322.
26. Tse H, Schwarz R, Paul W. Cell–cell interactions in the T cell proliferative response. J Immunol 1980;125:401.
27. Carbone FR, Belz GT, Heath WR. Transfer of antigen between migrating and lymph node-resident DCs in peripheral T-cell tolerance and immunity. Trends Immunol 2004;25:655–658.
28. Man AL, Prieto-Garcia ME, Nicoletti C. Improving M cell mediated transport across mucosal barriers: do certain bacteria hold the keys? Immunology 2004;113:15–22.
29. Frauwirth KA, Thompson CB. Activation and inhibition of lymphocytes by costimulation. J Clin Invest 2002;109:295–299.
30. Guermonprez P, Valladeau J, Zitvogel L, et al. Antigen presentation and T cell stimulation by dendritic cells. Annu Rev Immunol 2002;20:621–667.
31. Schwartz RH. T cell anergy. Annu Rev Immunol 2003;21:305–334.
32. Heath WR, Carbone FR. Cross-presentation, dendritic cells, tolerance and immunity. Annu Rev Immunol 2001;19:47–64.
33. Malissen B, Ardouin L, Lin SY, et al. Function of the CD3 subunits of the pre-TCR and TCR complexes during T cell development. Adv Immunol 1999;72:103–148.
34. Davis MM, Bjorkman PJ. T-cell antigen receptor genes and T-cell recognition. Nature 1988;334:395–402.
35. Sprent J. T lymphocytes and the thymus. In Paul W (ed). Fundamental Immunology. New York, Raven Press, 1989, pp 69–93.
36. Campbell R, Trowsdale J. Map of the human MHC. Immunol Today 1993;14:349–352.
37. Bjorkman PJ, Saper MA, Samraoui B, et al. The foreign antigen binding site and T cell recognition regions of class I histocompatibility antigens. Nature 1987;329:512–518.
38. Bjorkman PJ, Saper MA, Samraoui B, et al. Structure of the human class I histocompatibility antigen, HLA-A2. Nature 1987;329:506–512.
39. Fremont D, Hendrikson W, Marrack P, Kappler J. Structures of an MHC class II molecule with covalently bound single peptide. Science 1996;272:1001–1004.
40. Falk K, Rotzsche O, Stevanovic S, Jung G, Rammensee H. Allele specific motifs revealed by sequencing of self peptides eluted from MHC molecules. Nature 1991;351:290–296.
41. Hunt D, Henderson R, Shabanowitz J, et al. Characterization of peptides bound to the class I molecule HLA-A2.1 by mass spectrometry. Science 1992;255:1261–1263.
42. Parham P, Ohta T. Population biology of antigen presentation by MHC class I molecules. Science 1996;272:67–74.
43. Sherman LA, Chattopadhyay S. The molecular basis of allorecognition. Annu Rev Immunol 1993;11:385–402.
44. Groettrup M, Soza A, Kuckelkorn U, Kloetzel P. Peptide antigen production by the proteasome: complexity provides efficiency. Immunol Today 1996;17:429–435.
45. Groettrup M, Khan S, Schwarz K, Schmidtke G. Interferon-gamma inducible exchanges of 20S proteasome active site subunits: why? Biochimie 2001;83:367–372.
46. Lehner P, Cresswell P. Processing and delivery of peptides presented by MHC class I molecules. Curr Opin Immunol 1996;8:59–67.
47. Koopmann J, Post M, Neefjes J, et al. Translocation of long peptides by transporters associated with antigen processing (TAP). Eur J Immunol 1996;26:1720–1728.
48. Sadasivan B, Lehner P, Ortmann B, et al. Roles for calreticulin and a novel glycoprotein, tapasin, in the interaction of class I MHC molecules with TAP. Immunity 1996;5:103–114.
49. Bakke O, Doberstein B. MHC class II associated invariant chain contains a sorting signal for endosomal compartments. Cell 1990;63:707–716.
50. Amigorena S, Drake J, Webster P, Mellman I. Transient accumulation of new MHC molecules in a novel endocytic compartment in B lymphocytes. Nature 1994;369:113–120.
51. Castellino F, Germain R. Extensive trafficking of MHC class II invariant chain complexes in the endocytic pathway and appearance of peptide loaded class II in multiple compartments. Immunity 1995;2:73–88.
52. Sallusto F, Sella M, Danieli C, Lanzavecchia A. Dendritic cells use macropinocytosis and the mannose receptor to concentrate macromolecules in the major histocompatibility complex class II compartment: downregulation by cytokines and bacterial products. J Exp Med 1995;182:389–400.
53. Bonnerot C, Lankar D, Hanau D, et al. Role of B cell receptor Ig α and β subunits in MHC class II-restricted antigen presentation. Immunity 1995;3:335–347.
54. Lanzavecchia A. Mechanisms of antigen uptake for presentation. Curr Opin Immunol 1996;8:348–354.
55. Sykulev Y, Brunmark A, Jackson M, et al. Kinetics and affinity of reactions between an antigen-specific TCR and peptide–MHC complexes. Immunity 1994;1:15–22.
56. Matsui K, Boniface J, Steffner P, et al. Kinetics of T cell receptor binding to peptide/IEk complexes: correlation of the dissociation rate with T-cell responsiveness. Proc Natl Acad Sci USA 1994;91:12862–12866.
57. Janeway CA Jr. The T cell receptor as a multicomponent signalling machine: CD4/CD8 coreceptors and CD45 in T cell activation. Annu Rev Immunol 1992;10:645–674.
58. Li QJ, Dinner AR, Qi S, et al. CD4 enhances T cell sensitivity to antigen by coordinating Lck accumulation at the immunological synapse. Nat Immunol 2004;5:791–799.
59. Weiss A, Littman D. Signal transduction by lymphocyte antigen receptors. Cell 1994;76:263–274.
60. Demotz S, Grey HM, Sette A. The minimal number of class II MHC–antigen complexes needed for T cell activation. Science 1990;249: 1028–1030.
61. Starr TK, Jameson SC, Hogquist KA. Positive and negative selection of T cells. Annu Rev Immunol 2003;21:139–176.
62. Boehm U, Klamp T, Groot M, Howard JC. Cellular responses to interferon-γ. Annu Rev Immunol 1997;15:749–795.
63. Wilson HL, O'Neill HC. Murine dendritic cell development: difficulties associated with subset analysis. Immunol Cell Biol 2003;81:239–246.
64. Park CS, Choi YS. How do follicular dendritic cells interact intimately with B cells in the germinal centre? Immunology 2005;114:2–10.
65. Huang AY, Qi H, Germain RN. Illuminating the landscape of in vivo immunity: insights from dynamic in situ imaging of secondary lymphoid tissues. Immunity 2004;21:331–339.
66. Kabelitz D, Holtmeier W. γδ T cells link innate and adaptive immune responses. Chem Immunol Allergy 2005;86:151–183.
67. Shin S, El-Diwany R, Schaffert S, et al. Antigen recognition determinants of γδ T cell receptors. Science 2005;308:252–255.
68. Brandes M, Willimann K, Moser B. Professional antigen-presentation function by human γδT cells. Science 2005;309:264–268.
69. Mackay CR. Migration pathways and immunologic memory among T lymphocytes. Semin Immunol 1992;4:51–8.
70. Mossman T, Coffman R. Th1 and Th2 cells: different patterns of lymphokine secretion lead to different functional properties. Annu Rev Immunol 1989;7:145–173.
71. Abbas A, Murphy M, Sher A. Functional diversity of helper T lymphocytes. Nature 1996;383:787–793.
72. Romagnani S. Type 1 T helper and type 2 T helper cells: functions, regulation and role in protection and disease. Int J Clin Lab Res 1991;21:152–158.
73. Cher D, Mossman T. Two types of murine helper T cell clone. II. Delayed type hypersensitivity is mediated by Th1 clones. J Immunol 1987;138:3688–3694.
74. Coffman R, Seymour B, Lebman D, et al. The role of helper T cell products in mouse B cell differentiation and isotype regulation. J Immunol 1988;102:5–28.
75. Bernhagen J, Bacher M, Calandra T, et al. An essential role for macrophage migration inhibitory factor in the tuberculin delayed-type hypersensitivity reaction. J Exp Med 1996;183:277–282.
76. Grabbe S, Schwarz T. Immunoregulatory mechanisms involved in elicitation of allergic contact hypersensitivity. Immunol Today 1998; 19:37–44.
77. Siraganian RP. Mast cell signal transduction from the high-affinity IgE receptor. Curr Opin Immunol 2003;15:639–46.
78. Capron A, Dessaint JP. Immunologic aspects of schistosomiasis. Annu Rev Med 1992;43:209–218.

79. Grencis RK. Th2-mediated host protective immunity to intestinal nematode infections. Philos Trans R Soc Lond B Biol Sci 1997;352:1377–1384.
80. Kamogawa Y, Minasi L, Carding S, et al. The relationship of IL-4 and IFN gamma producing T cells studied by lineage ablation of IL-4 producing cells. Cell 1993;75:985–995.
81. Constant S, Bottomly K. Induction of Th1 and Th2 responses: the alternative approaches. Annu Rev Immunol 1997;15:297–322.
82. Dvorak AM. New aspects of mast cell biology. Int Arch Allergy Immunol 1997;114:1–9.
83. Yoshimoto T, Paul W. CD4pos, NK1.1pos T cells promptly produce interleukin 4 in response to in vivo challenge with anti-CD3. J Exp Med 1994;179:1285–1295.
84. MacDonald HR. Development and selection of NKT cells. Curr Opin Immunol 2002;14:250–254.
85. Langrish CL, McKenzie BS, Wilson NJ, et al. IL-12 and IL-23: master regulators of innate and adaptive immunity. Immunol Rev 2004; 202:96–105.
86. Billiau A, Heremans H, Vermeire K, Matthys P. Immunomodulatory properties of interferon-γ. An update. Ann NY Acad Sci 1998;856: 22–32.
87. Smith CM, Wilson NS, Waithman J, et al. Cognate CD4+ T cell licensing of dendritic cells in CD8+ T cell immunity. Nat Immunol 2004;5:1143–1148.
88. Behrens G, Li M, Smith CM. Helper T cells, dendritic cells and CTL immunity. Immunol Cell Biol 2004;82:84–90.
89. van KC, Banchereau J. CD40-CD40 ligand. J Leukoc Biol 2000;67:2–17.
90. Berke G. The CTL's kiss of death. Cell 1995;81:9–12.
91. Ueda I, Morimoto A, Inaba T. Characteristic perforin gene mutations of haemophagocytic lymphohistiocytosis patients in Japan. Br J Haematol 2003;121:503–510.
92. Grunebaum E, Roifman CM. Gene abnormalities in patients with hemophagocytic lymphohistiocytosis. Isr Med Assoc J 2002;4:366–369.
93. Russell JH. Activation-induced death of mature T cells in the regulation of immune responses. Curr Opin Immunol 1995;7:382–388.
94. de Alborán, IM, Robles MS, Bras A, et al. Cell death during lymphocyte development and activation. Semin Immunol 2003;15:125–133.
95. Green DR, Droin N, Pinkoski M. Activation-induced cell death in T cells. Immunol Rev 2003;193:70–81.
96. Lenardo M, Chan KM, Hornung F, et al. Mature T lymphocyte apoptosis—immune regulation in a dynamic and unpredictable antigenic environment. Annu Rev Immunol 1999;17:221–253.
97. Ferber IA, Brocke S, Taylor-Edwards C, et al. Mice with a disrupted IFN-γ gene are susceptible to the induction of experimental autoimmune encephalomyelitis (EAE). J Immunol 1996;156:5–7.
98. Willenborg DO, Fordham SA, Staykova MA, IFN-γ is critical to the control of murine autoimmune encephalomyelitis and regulates both in the periphery and in the target tissue: a possible role for nitric oxide. J Immunol 1999;163:5278–5286.
99. Battaglia M, Gianfrani C, Gregori S, Roncarolo MG. IL-10-producing T regulatory type 1 cells and oral tolerance. Ann NY Acad Sci 2004;1029:142–153.
100. Grutz G. New insights into the molecular mechanism of interleukin-10-mediated immunosuppression. J Leukoc Biol 2005;77:3–15.
101. O'Garra A, Vieira P. Regulatory T cells and mechanisms of immune system control. Nat Med 2004;10:801–805.
102. Rennick DM, Fort MM. Lessons from genetically engineered animal models. XII. IL-10-deficient (IL-10(-/-) mice and intestinal inflammation. Am J Physiol Gastrointest Liver Physiol 2000;278:G829–G833.
103. Lenschow DJ, Walunas TL, Bluestone JA. CD28/B7 system of T cell costimulation. Annu Rev Immunol 1996;14:233–258.
104. Loke P, Allison JP. Emerging mechanisms of immune regulation: the extended B7 family and regulatory T cells. Arthritis Res Ther 2004;6:208–214.
105. Greenwald RJ, Freeman GJ, Sharpe AH. The B7 family revisited. Annu Rev Immunol 2005;23:515–548.
106. Nakaseko C, Miyatake S, Iida T, et al. Cytotoxic T lymphocyte antigen 4 (CTLA-4) engagement delivers an inhibitory signal through the membrane-proximal region in the absence of the tyrosine motif in the cytoplasmic tail. J Exp Med 1999;190:765–774.
107. Oosterwegel MA, Greenwald RJ, Mandelbrot DA, et al. CTLA-4 and T cell activation. Curr Opin Immunol 1999;11:294–300.
108. Fontenot JD, Rudensky AY. A well adapted regulatory contrivance: regulatory T cell development and the forkhead family transcription factor Foxp3. Nat Immunol 2005;6:331–337.
109. Wraith DC, Nicolson KS, Whitley NT. Regulatory CD4+ T cells and the control of autoimmune disease. Curr Opin Immunol 2004;16: 695–701.
110. Bennett CL, Christie J, Ramsdell F, et al. The immune dysregulation, polyendocrinopathy, enteropathy, X-linked syndrome (IPEX) is caused by mutations of FOXP3. Nat Genet 2001;27:20–21.
111. Roncarolo MG, Bacchetta R, Bordignon C, et al. Type 1 T regulatory cells. Immunol Rev 2001;182:68–79.
112. Ravetch JV, Bolland S. IgG Fc receptors. Annu Rev Immunol 2001; 19:275–290.
113. Ravetch JV. Fc receptors. Curr Opin Immunol 1997;9:121–125.
114. Conley ME. Early defects in B-cell development. Curr Opin Allergy Clin Immunol 2002;2:517–522.
115. Fagarasan S, Honjo T. T-Independent immune response: new aspects of B cell biology. Science 2000;290:89–92.
116. Mond JJ, Lees A, Snapper CM. T cell-independent antigens type 2. Annu Rev Immunol 1995;13:655–692.
117. Rijkers GT, Sanders LA, Zegers BJ. Anti-capsular polysaccharide antibody deficiency states. Immunodeficiency 1993;5:1–21.
118. Heyzer-Williams LJ, Heyzer-Williams MG. Antigen-specific memory B cell development. Annu Rev Immunol 2005;23:487–513.
119. Parker DC. T cell-dependent B cell activation. Annu Rev Immunol 1993;11:331–360.
120. Cyster JG. Homing of antibody secreting cells. Immunol Rev 2003; 194:48–60.
121. Kunkel EJ, Butcher EC. Plasma-cell homing. Nat Rev Immunol 2003; 3:822–829.
122. Cozine CL, Wolniak KL, Waldschmidt TJ. The primary germinal center response in mice. Curr Opin Immunol 2005;17:298–302.
123. Durandy A, Revy P, Imai K, Fischer A. Hyper-immunoglobulin M syndromes caused by intrinsic B-lymphocyte defects. Immunol Rev 2005;203:67–79.
124. Fuleihan RL. The X-linked hyperimmunoglobulin M syndrome. Semin Hematol 1998;35:321–331.
125. Maizels N. Immunoglobulin gene diversification. Annu Rev Genet 2004;39:22–46.
126. Wu X, Feng J, Komori A, et al. Immunoglobulin somatic hypermutation: double-strand DNA breaks, AID and error-prone DNA repair. J Clin Immunol 2003;23:235–246.
127. Gourley TS, Wherry EJ, Masopust D, Ahmed R. Generation and maintenance of immunological memory. Semin Immunol 2004;16: 323–333.
128. Williams AF, Barclay AN. The immunoglobulin superfamily—domains for cell surface recognition. Annu Rev Immunol 1988;6:381–405.
129. Bilbao G, Contreras JL, Curiel DT. Genetically engineered intracellular single-chain antibodies in gene therapy. Mol Biotechnol 2002;22: 191–211.
130. Hombach A, Heuser C, Abken H. The recombinant T cell receptor strategy: insights into structure and function of recombinant immunoreceptors on the way towards an optimal receptor design for cellular immunotherapy. Curr Gene Ther 2002;2:211–226.
131. Adams GP, Schier R. Generating improved single-chain Fv molecules for tumor targeting. J Immunol Methods 1999;231:249–260.
132. Mestecky J, Lue C, Russell MW. Selective transport of IgA. Cellular and molecular aspects. Gastroenterol Clin North Am 1991;20:441–471.
133. Oettgen HC. Regulation of the IgE isotype switch: new insights on cytokine signals and the functions of epsilon germline transcripts. Curr Opin Immunol 2000;12:618–623.
134. Purkerson J, Isakson P. A two-signal model for regulation of immunoglobulin isotype switching. FASEB J 1992;6:3245–3252.
135. Lebman DA, Edmiston JS. The role of TGF-β in growth, differentiation, and maturation of B lymphocytes. Microbes Infect 1999; 1:1297–1304.
136. Stack G, Baril L, Napychank P, Snyder EL. Cytokine generation in stored, white cell-reduced, and bacterially contaminated units of red cells. Transfusion 1995;35:199–203.
137. Stack G, Snyder EL. Cytokine generation in stored platelet concentrates. Transfusion 1994;34:20–25.
138. Bawa N, Tomar RH. Laboratory evaluation of immunoglobulin function and humoral immunity. In Henry JB (ed). Clinical Diagnosis and Management by Laboratory Methods. Philadelphia, W.B. Saunders, 1996, pp 913–927.

Chapter 3

Principles of the Complement System Central to Transfusion Medicine

Dana V. Devine

The existence of the complement system has great impact on the practice of transfusion medicine. In its normal immune activities, complement functions to kill pathogens, mediate inflammation, maintain the solubility of immune complexes, promote a normal adaptive immune response, and opsonize particles for phagocytosis. However, complement can also mediate pathogenic processes, including anaphylaxis, intravascular hemolysis of transfused blood cells, leukocyte mobilization in transfusion-related acute lung injury (TRALI), and activation of platelets.

The group of proteins known to constitute the complement system was first recognized in the 1880s as the labile bactericidal activity in serum.[1] Paul Ehrlich coined the term for the phenomenon by proposing a model of antibody-mediated cytotoxicity in which a serum factor *complements* the bactericidal activity of antibody. A detailed understanding of the biochemistry of the complement system required the development of techniques that would permit the isolation of individual complement proteins; this technology finally appeared in the 1960s. With the explosion of research activity in the complement field in the 1970s came the recognition that this system was much more complex than had been imagined. This complexity is amply demonstrated by the fact that at least 25 complement proteins are involved in the activation and regulation of that activity known to Ehrlich simply as *complement.*

The understanding of the complement system is made easier by setting a proper context. Like coagulation, the complement system is an activated enzyme cascade. In such cascades, proteins normally circulate in an inactive form, the zymogen. When the pathway is initiated, the first protein in the sequence is converted from a zymogen to an activated enzyme, which acts on the next protein zymogen in the cascade. Such pathways are amplifying, because each enzyme molecule generated can act on multiple substrate molecules. Activated enzyme pathways are also characterized by the presence of regulatory proteins, both humoral and cellular, that prevent the activated enzymes from converting all available substrate.

The nuances of the complement system have long struck fear into the hearts of basic scientist and clinician alike. Clinical aspects of complement biology in the pathophysiology of disease have been reviewed by Morgan[2] and more recently by others.[3,4] This chapter describes the central role of complement in many physiologic processes, including those associated with the use of blood components.

BASIC BIOCHEMISTRY OF THE COMPLEMENT SYSTEM

Classical Pathway Activation

Activation of the complement system occurs via two pathways; with the activation of C3 (the third component of complement), these pathways join to form a common pathway that completes the cascade (Fig. 3–1). The primary function of both pathways is the generation of enzyme complexes that activate C3 by cleaving it to C3b. The antibody-mediated activation of complement occurs by the *classical pathway,* so called because it was the first pathway recognized. Activators of the classical pathway include not only antibody molecules, but also several nonimmunoglobulin proteins (Table 3–1). Only immunoglobulins (Ig) of the M and G isotypes activate complement by the classical pathway. In humans, IgG3 and IgG1 are strong complement activators, but IgG2 is a poor activator, and IgG4 does not activate complement. These differences result fro m variation in the ability of the different IgG subclasses to bind the first component of complement, C1. The ability of an antibody to activate complement, with the accompanying opsonization and perhaps lysis of the cell, parallels the opsonic potential of the IgGs themselves. The varying risk of phagocytic destruction by crystallizable fragment (Fc) receptor-mediated recognition of IgG is an important feature in distinguishing clinically significant antibodies from those with less destructive potential.

C1 is a multisubunit complex that contains the initial antibody-binding subunits, C1q, as well as two types of zymogen subunits, C1r and C1s, that acquire serine protease activity on activation of the complex. Each molecule of C1 contains six C1q subunits, and two each of the C1r and C1s subunits. The fixation of a C1 molecule to the surface of the cell by the C1q subunits requires a minimum of one molecule of IgM or at least two molecules of IgG for efficient activation. C1q itself contains six identical subunits composed of a triple helical region with homology to collagen and a globular domain at the distal end. The proximal end of C1q is associated with the other subunits of the C1 complex, C1r and C1s, in a calcium-dependent manner. Two of the six C1q subunits must be bound by antibody to effect activation. Although a single molecule of IgM is capable of activating complement, it must be bound to antigen, where it assumes a staple-shaped conformation. Fluid-phase or planar IgM does not activate complement, inasmuch as the C1q-binding sites are exposed only in the staple form.[5]

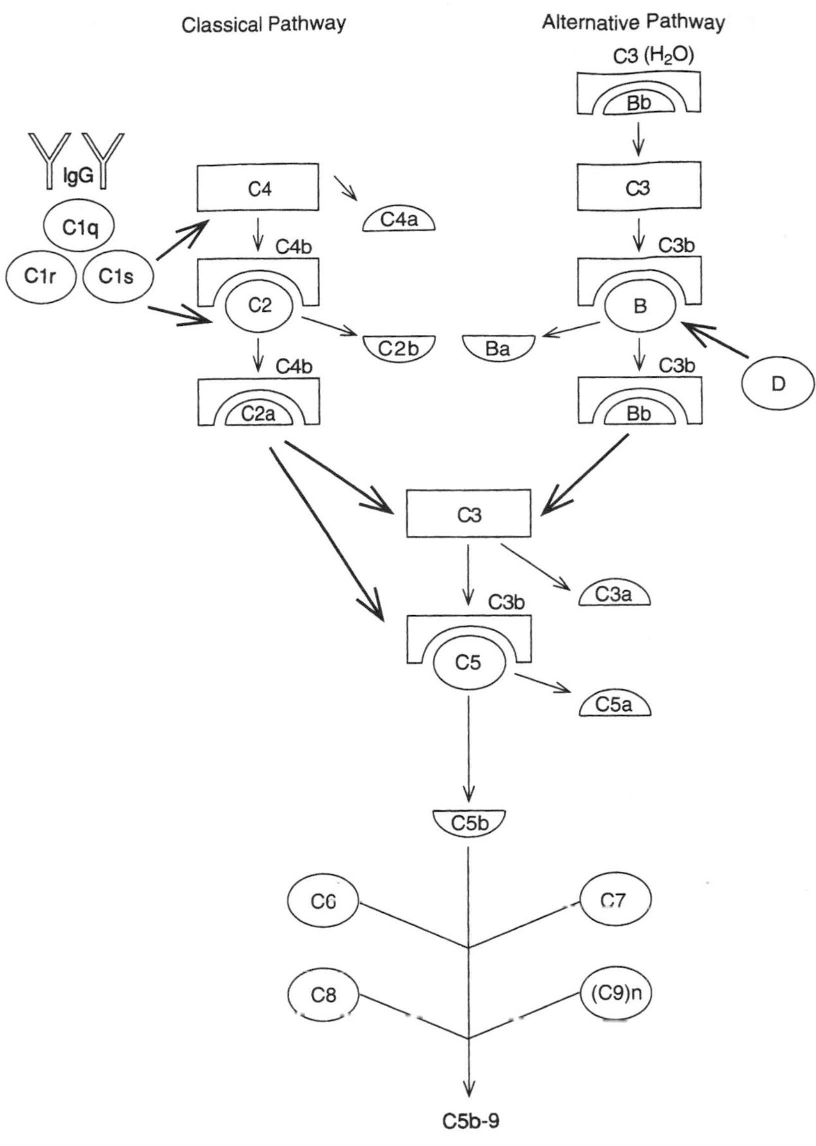

Figure 3–1 The activation pathway of complement. The activation of complement may proceed by the classical pathway or the alternative pathway. Inactive (zymogen) forms of complement proteins are cleaved by activated proteins that have serine protease activity (*heavy arrows*). Once cleaved, a substrate acquires enzymatic activity and acts on the next substrate in the pathway. The membrane attack complex forms by the assembly of the individual components in an enzyme-independent manner. (From Anderson KC, Ness PM. Scientific Basis of Transfusion Medicine, 2nd ed. Philadelphia, Saunders, 2000.)

Once two subunits of C1q are bound to antibody, the molecular conformation changes, in that the angle between the subunits is greatly reduced; the resulting stress on the molecule facilitates the autocatalysis of the C1r subunits.[6] On autoactivation, C1r acquires serine protease activity, which is directed against the C1s subunits. Once C1s is cleaved by activated C1r, it also acquires serine protease activity. This activated C1 complex is the initiation complex of the classical pathway.

Although the majority of classical pathway activation is antibody mediated, antibody-independent activation of the classical pathway has been described in several situations (see Table 3–1). Such activation may involve the direct binding of C1q to a surface, or it may be mediated by other plasma

Table 3–1 Complement Activators

Lectin Pathway	Classical Pathway	Alternative Pathway
Surfaces containing *N*-acetylglucosamine and mannose	IgG_1 and IgG_3; IgG_2 weakly; IgM Some negatively charged surfaces Crystalline cholesterol	Some dialysis membranes, especially cuprophane Desialated erythrocytes Surfaces that promote the binding of factor B IgA complexes Protein aggregates Microbial pathogens Tumor cells

proteins, such as C-reactive protein (CRP) or mannose-binding lectin. Activated C1s has the next two proteins in the pathway, C4 and C2, as its substrates. The C4 molecule is cleaved by C1s to C4a and C4b. Some of the C4b molecules bind covalently to the cell surface through a reactive thiol ester bond that is exposed when the C4a fragment is removed; most C4b molecules are inactivated by hydrolysis and never bind to a cell surface. In a magnesium-dependent reaction, a C2 molecule binds to a molecule of C4b; the C2 is then also cleaved by C1s. This cleavage results in the generation of the active serine protease, C2a, which remains associated with C4b. Clearly, the cleavage of both C4 and C2 by the same molecule of C1s is sensitive to the local geometry; deposition of the C4b molecule far from the activated C1 molecule results in the termination of the activation pathway.

The bimolecular complex, C4b2a, is the C3-converting complex of the classical pathway. The cleavage of C3 by C4b2a results in the formation of two fragments, C3a and C3b. C3b, like C4b, contains a reactive thiol ester bond that enables it to bind covalently to the cell surface. The intramolecular thiol ester present within C3 is formed by a transacylation reaction between the thiol group of ^{988}Cys and the gamma amide group of ^{991}Gln.[7] The exposure of this reactive center results in the interaction with cell surface moieties through the formation of an ester or an amide bond.

As indicated earlier, the activation of the classical pathway does not require immunoglobulin. The most recent developments in complement biochemistry have included an appreciation for the role of molecules of the pentraxin and lectin families in the activation of complement. Pentraxins, a family of molecules named for their cyclic pentameric subunit structure, include two proteins that have been implicated in complement activation: CRP and serum amyloid P.[8–10] Both proteins bind C1q, thereby initiating the classical pathway without a requirement for antibody.

Lectin Pathway Activation

The carbohydrate-binding properties of plant-derived lectins are well known in the field of blood banking, in which they are useful phenotyping reagents. Lectins or lectin-like proteins are also found in mammals. One of the C-type animal lectins, mannose-binding lectin (MBL), belongs to a group of soluble pattern recognition receptors. These molecules and their membrane-bound cousins the Toll-like receptors, recognize pathogen-associated molecular patterns located on infectious organisms. MBL recognizes mannose-containing carbohydrates and also binds *N*-acetylglucosamine. MBL binding to its substrates has been reported to mediate complement activation.[11] The hexameric form of MBL is structurally similar to C1q and will bind the $C1r_2s_2$ complex. MBL is found in association with one of three forms of a serine protease, MBL-associated protease (MASP1, MASP2, or MASP3). Complement activation may be mediated by either $C1r_2s_2$ or by the direct action of MASPs. The relative biological significance of the pentraxin and lectin pathways is not fully understood.[12] However, both CRP and MBL are acute-phase reactants and may reach significant serum concentration during infection or inflammation.

Alternative Pathway Activation

A different C3-converting complex is generated by the activation of the alternative pathway of complement. The term *alternative* arises from the fact that this mechanism of C3 cleavage was discovered many decades after the classical pathway. It should in no way be considered a secondary pathway of complement activation, because it is the only pathway of complement that can respond to microorganisms in the absence of specific antibody. It is, therefore, a front-line host defense. Activators of the alternative pathway include a broad spectrum of substances, from renal dialysis membranes to immune complexes to microorganisms (Table 3–2). The initial step in the activation of the alternative pathway is the generation of a partially activated molecule of C3, which has been described as C3b-like.[13] This molecule is presumably generated by the low-grade, spontaneous hydrolysis of C3 that occurs in the body and is not the result of the presence of the activator substance per se. $C3(H_2O)$ has the important characteristic of being able to interact in the fluid phase with the complement protein factor B in a magnesium-dependent manner. Once factor B has associated with $C3(H_2O)$, it is cleaved by factor D, a circulating serine protease that has specificity for factor B bound to $C3(H_2O)$. This cleavage results in the formation of two fragments, Ba and Bb. The Bb fragment has serine protease activity and remains associated with $C3(H_2O)$. The bimolecular complex $C3(H_2O)Bb$ has C3 as its substrate. The $C3(H_2O)Bb$ complex cleaves C3 in the same way as C4b2a, and the resulting C3b molecules can bind covalently to the cell surface. If C3b binds to an activator surface, factor B associates with it and is cleaved by factor D. This results in the formation of an alternative pathway C3-converting complex on the surface of the activator. Because this complex has C3 as its substrate, it produces a feedback amplification loop for the deposition of C3b onto the activator.

The binding of a C3b molecule in the immediate vicinity of a C4b2a or C3bBb enzyme complex produces a trimolecular complex that is capable of cleaving C5. The C3b molecule has a binding site for C5; if the geometry is appropriate, C5 is presented to the enzyme complex, where it is cleaved by C2a or Bb serine proteases. The cleavage produces the fragments C5a and C5b. Although there is a great deal of homology among C3, C4, and C5, there is no reactive thiol ester in the C5 molecule. Therefore, the cleavage of C5 does not generate a fragment capable of binding covalently to a cell surface. The C5b molecule remains briefly associated with C3b before its association with the terminal proteins of the complement pathway.

Formation of the Membrane Attack Complex

Membrane attack complex of complement refers to the association of the complement proteins C5, C6, C7, C8, and C9 to form a potentially cytolytic complex. When C5 is activated in either the classical or alternative pathway, the resulting C5b molecule contains binding sites for the next components in the pathway. This part of the complement pathway is still a cascade, but the activation of a component results in the exposure of binding sites for other terminal complement proteins rather than in the acquisition of enzymatic activity. C5b, but not C5, contains a binding site for C6, which becomes bound while the C5b molecule is associated with its C3b tether. The C5b6 complex may be released from C3b, or it may remain anchored until it binds a molecule of C7. Once C7 is attached, the trimolecular complex undergoes a transition in which the normal hydrophilic character of the

Table 3–2 Characteristics of the Proteins of Complement

Pathway	Protein	Molecular Weight (kDa)	Structure	Average Serum Concentration (mg/mL)
Activation complex classical pathway	C1q	Subunit A: 27 Subunit B: 27 Subunit C: 27 Complex: 465	6 each of subunits A, B, and C	80
	C1r	83	If full complex, C1q + 2 C1r + 2 C1; if no C1q, then 2 C1r + 2 C1s	50
	C1s	83		50
	C4	Subunit a: 97 Subunit b: 75 Subunit c: 33 Complex: 205	One each of subunits a, b, and c synthesized from a single precursor	600
Activation complex alternative pathway	Factor B	92	Single chain	210
Common pathway	Factor D	24	Single chain	<2
	C3	Subunit a: 110 Subunit b: 75 Complex: 185	One each of subunits a and b synthesized from a single precursor	1300
	C5	Subunit a: 115 Subunit b: 75 Complex: 190	One each of subunits a and b synthesized from a single precursor	70
	C6	120	Single chain	65
	C7	110	Single chain	56
	C8	Subunit a: 64 Subunit b: 64 Subunit c: 22 Complex: 150	One each of subunits a, b, and c	55
	C9	70	Single chain	60

individual members of the complex is lost and a transient hydrophobic character is acquired. At this time, C5b-7 may associate with a membrane through the hydrophobic region; if it fails to interact with a membrane, the complex inactivates by self-aggregation or by interaction with the inhibitors described later.

Once C5b-7 is membrane associated, a binding site for C8 is exposed in C5b. The binding of C8 causes the complex to insert more deeply into the membrane. C9 binds to C8 and undergoes significant conformational changes. Not only does it acquire considerable hydrophobic character, pushing the membrane attack complex deeper into the membrane, but it also gains affinity for other molecules of C9, which polymerize into the complex. Electron microscopic studies suggest that the C5b-$9_{(n)}$ complex resembles a hollow cylinder. This cylinder is formed by the polymerized C9 molecules, which number between 12 and 18 in each complex. The C5b-8 is thought to play little active role in the structure of the cylindrical pore; it is, however, the essential catalyst for the pore's formation. The biochemical characteristics of the complement proteins are given in Table 3–2.

The Regulation of Complement Activation

Plasma Proteins

As discussed previously, the activation of the complement system is expressed as the activation of several enzymes of the serine protease group. As with any zymogen-to-enzyme conversion, there must be a way of regulating the activity of the enzyme, or else it will cleave all available substrate molecules. With the complement proteins, this regulation is achieved by multiple mechanisms. The geometric arrangement of the proteins is the simplest of these, inasmuch as several of the key enzymes function only when surface associated. The continuing activation of the complement pathway is highly dependent on the spatial arrangement of the enzyme and substrate molecules. For example, a C2 molecule associated with a C4b molecule that has been deposited more than 60 nm from the activated C1 will not be activated. Also, the enzymatic proteins of complement all occur in multisubunit or multimolecular complexes, each of which has a divalent cation requirement. The reduction of divalent cation concentration, as well as the inherent dissociation constant of the protein–protein interaction, means that the complement enzyme complexes simply fall apart.

An important way in which the body controls complement activation is through the action of specific protein inhibitors of the complement proteins. These proteins are of two sorts: plasma proteins and cellular membrane proteins (Table 3–3). Cells that are constantly exposed to the plasma milieu have evolved their own defense mechanisms against complement activation. Selective pressure to evolve defense proteins is present because the complement system does not distinguish between "good" and "bad" targets. A variety of proteins that are involved in complement regulation on cell surfaces have been described.[14]

The plasma proteins that inhibit complement work at all steps of complement activation. The only known inhibitor of activated C1 is the C1 inhibitor protein, which is also an inhibitor of kallikrein, plasmin, factor XIa, and factor XIIa. C1 inhibitor inactivates C1 by binding to the active sites of the C1r and C1s subunits with very high affinity; this binding has been suggested to be covalent. Because the C1 complex is composed of two subunits each of C1r and C1s, the inactivation of the complex requires the binding of two molecules

Table 3–3 Characteristics of the Complement Regulatory Proteins

Pathway	Protein	Molecular Weight (kDa)	Structure	Average Serum Concentration (mg/mL)
Activation complex classical pathway	C1 inhibitor	110	Single chain	200
	C4BP	Subunit: 70 Complex: 500	Complex of 7 subunits	250
	Factor I	Subunit a: 50 Subunit b: 38 Complex: 80	One each of subunits a and b	35
	Decay accelerating factor (DAF)	70	Single chain; phosphatidylinositol membrane anchor	N/A
	Membrane cofactor protein (MCP)	45–70	Single chain	N/A
Activation complex alternative pathway	Factor H	150	Single chain	500
	CR1	160–250	Single chain	N/A
Terminal complex	S-protein (vitronectin)	83	Single chain	500
	Sp-40,40	Subunit: 40 Complex: 75	Two subunits in complex	50
	CD59	20	Single chain; phosphatidylinositol membrane anchor	N/A

N/A, not applicable.

of C1 inhibitor. Inhibition of enzymatic activity of C1 by C1 inhibitor does not modulate the ability of the C1q subunits to bind either to immunoglobulin or to specific cellular receptors for C1q.

The critical role of C1 inhibitor in the control of the complement pathway can be illustrated by the disease hereditary angioedema (HAE).[15] Approximately 80% of patients with type I HAE are shown, by both immunologic and functional assays, to have less than 50% normal levels of C1 inhibitor. The remaining 20% of patients have a normal level of a dysfunctional protein. Patients with both types of HAE are subjected to periodic attacks of acute edema that may be life threatening if there is laryngeal involvement. HAE attacks are thought to arise from minor trauma that produces localized complement activation. The ineffective regulation of C1, caused by the depletion of C1 inhibitor, results in the generation of activation peptides that induce edema. Although the exact nature of the mediators is yet to be determined, both kinin and bradykinin are candidate molecules. The levels of C2 and C4 in patients suffering HAE attacks are greatly reduced, which reflects the requirement for rapid inactivation of activated C1 to prevent substrate depletion. A similar clinical picture also arises in patients who have acquired angioedema as a result of the presence of an autoantibody reactive with C1 inhibitor. These antibodies can cause accelerated clearance of C1 inhibitor or may functionally interfere with the protein.

The other plasma proteins that regulate the classical pathway all act on the C4b2a complex. Two plasma proteins that bind C4b have been described. C4-binding protein is a multisubunit protein that circulates complexed with protein S of the coagulation system.[16] Bound protein S does not affect the complement inhibitory activity of C4-binding protein. C4-binding protein accelerates the decay of the C4b2a complex, as well as acting as a cofactor for the degradation of C4b by factor I. The other C4-binding plasma protein is a sialoglycoprotein called SGP120.[17] This molecule copurifies with C2 during C4b-sepharose affinity chromatography. It apparently is a competitive inhibitor for the C2-binding site on C4b. The precise biological role of SGP120 remains to be determined.

The plasma proteins that regulate the alternative pathway are molecules that are either inhibitory or stabilizing for the C3bBb complex. As described previously, the alternative pathway begins in the fluid phase. It is the fate of the C3b molecules deposited on the surface that distinguishes an activator from a nonactivator. The major plasma protein that regulates complement activation is factor H. The interplay between factor B and factor H, in their competition for C3b, actually determines whether a surface is "activating." On some surfaces, the binding of factor B is promoted over the binding of factor H; these surfaces are said to be activators of the alternative pathway because the C3bBb complex readily forms. If the binding of factor H is favored, the surface does not activate complement. Factor H has cofactor activity for factor I, the C3b inactivator. Factor I is a circulating serine protease that has C4b and C3b as its substrates. The degradation of C3b by factor I results in the formation of biologically important fragments of C3 that interact with specific cellular receptors. The importance of C3bBb regulation by factor H is highlighted by the manifestation of atypical hemolytic uremic syndrome in patients with diminished factor H due to congenital deficiency or the presence of autoantibody against factor H.

Although the plasma regulatory proteins just described act to downregulate the activation of complement, one protein of the alternative pathway, properdin, modulates the activity of the pathway by stabilizing the C3bBb complex. Properdin circulates in an inactive form, which becomes activated on association with C3b. Although properdin apparently binds to a site on C3b, the binding affinity increases considerably if C3b is complexed to Bb.[18]

The terminal complex of complement is regulated by two plasma proteins: vitronectin and clusterin (or Sp-40,40).

Vitronectin, the major plasma regulator of the membrane attack complex, was initially called *S-protein* by investigators in the complement field; current literature may still use this designation. This molecule is not the same as protein S of the coagulation system. Vitronectin regulates the membrane attack complex at the C5b-7 stage. When C5b-7 is formed, several molecules of vitronectin bind to the hydrophobic regions of the complex, increasing its water solubility. Inactivated C5b-7, known as SC5b-7, is capable of binding C8 and C9, but C9 polymerization is blocked. Sp-40,40 was described as an inhibitor of the membrane attack complex, which appears to act at the C5-6 level.[19,20] The protein is a disulfide-linked heterodimer; each subunit has a molecular weight of approximately 40 kDa. Sp-40,40 co-localizes with vitronectin and membrane attack complexes in tissue sections. There is some in vitro evidence to suggest that Sp-40,40 may be complexed in plasma with vitronectin. Sp-40,40 most likely shares identity with the protein clusterin, a cell-agglutinating protein that circulates in plasma complexed to apolipoprotein A-I.[21] The relative functions of this molecule in complement regulation, cholesterol transport, and cell–cell interaction remain to be determined.

Cell Membrane Proteins

Cells that come into contact with activated complement have evolved additional mechanisms to protect themselves from opsonization or cytolysis. One such adaptation is to evolve proteins that inactivate complement at the membrane surface. The analysis of such proteins has been the focus of much of the activity in complement biology since their discovery in the early 1980s.

The first such molecule described was *decay accelerating factor* (DAF; CD55), which was discovered simultaneously by two groups.[22,23] As its name suggests, DAF functions by accelerating the decay of the C3bBb or C4b2a enzyme complexes. In the alternative pathway, DAF binds to C3b, thereby disrupting the C3bBb complex. The mode of action of DAF on C4b2a is not completely clear; published studies have demonstrated the binding of DAF to both C2a and C4b.[24,25] DAF is expressed on a wide variety of tissues other than blood cells, including endothelial cells and kidney glomerular epithelial cells. The number of molecules of DAF per cell varies from 10^3 to 10^4, depending on the cell type; in addition, DAF expression in some cells can be modulated in response to mitogens and cytokines.[26] DAF has no cofactor activity for factor I inactivation of either C3b or C4b.

Membrane cofactor protein (MCP; CD46) is an integral membrane protein that regulates the C3bBb and C4b2a complexes by binding to C3b or C4b and acting as a cofactor for factor I inactivation.[27] The molecule has no decay accelerating activity. MCP acts only on C3b and C4b bound to the cell that contains the MCP; that is, it acts to regulate complement only at a very local level. The affinity of MCP for C3b is much greater than for C4b; hence its cofactor function is greater for C3b inactivation.

The third membrane protein capable of regulating complement activation at the C3 step is the complement receptor CR1 (CD35). The ligand for this receptor is C3b or C4b that is present on an exogenous cell—that is, not on the cell that bears the CR1 molecule. CR1 is an integral membrane protein with a wide tissue distribution; as discussed later, it is crucially important in the clearance of C3b-containing immune complexes from the circulation.

The plethora of proteins that have been identified as regulators of the C3/C5-converting enzymes seems at first to suggest redundancy in the complement system. However, these proteins, both plasma and membrane, act in concert to regulate complement activation in all situations in which it may arise. In the fluid phase of plasma, C4-binding protein, SGP120, and factor I control the activation of the classical pathway; factor H and factor I control the alternative pathway. The membrane proteins DAF and MCP regulate the activation of complement on autologous cell surfaces, whereas CR1 acts to regulate exogenous complement activation, particularly in immune complexes. The evolution of proteins to specifically control all activation scenarios prevents the negative physiologic sequelae of unregulated complement enzymes.

Two membrane proteins that regulate the membrane attack complex of complement by preventing the complete assembly of $C5b\text{-}9_{(n)}$ have been described.[28,29] These proteins are important in controlling the formation of membrane attack complex on cells that bear C5-converting enzyme complexes. They are also essential for protecting the cell from *reactive lysis* or *bystander lysis,* whereby the cell picks up C5b-7 from the surrounding medium even though it may not bear the C5-converting enzymes that generated the C5b-7 complex. C8-binding protein, also known as *homologous restriction factor,* is a 65-kDa protein first identified in the red blood cell membrane. It binds to C8 and prohibits the polymerization of C9 into the membrane attack complex. This protein has the characteristic of homologous restriction; that is, human C8-binding protein works best on human membrane attack complex and less efficiently or not at all with complement proteins from other species. Such species selectivity has been noted for other proteins in the complement pathway. In 1988 and 1989, four separate groups found another membrane protein that regulates the activity of the membrane attack complex.[30–33] This molecule, now known as CD59, was also called 1F5 antigen, P-18, MEM-43, homologous restriction factor 20, H-19, membrane inhibitor of reactive lysis, and MAC inhibitory factor. CD59 contains binding sites for C8 and C9 and thus appears to regulate at both C5b-8 and C5b-9.[34,35]

The regulatory proteins DAF, CD59, and C8-binding protein all belong to an unusual group of proteins that are attached to the cell membrane by a phosphatidylinositol anchor, rather than by cytoplasmic and transmembrane stretches of amino acids.[36] This anchor structure, which is synthesized in the endoplasmic reticulum, involves the attachment of a protein moiety to the phospholipid through a series of carbohydrate residues. Abnormalities in genes encoding enzymes responsible for the addition of carbohydrates to the anchor structure are associated with the development of the acquired myelodysplastic condition paroxysmal nocturnal hemoglobinuria (PNH).[36] Gene defects in PNH are clustered in the so-called *PIG-A* gene, a putative glycosyltransferase with specificity for *N*-acetylglucosamine; abnormalities often result in the complete lack of protein product. The defects in *PIG-A* gene in PNH are expressed phenotypically as the complete or near-complete absence of phosphatidylinositol-anchored proteins from the cell membrane. The lack of CD55, CD59, and C8-binding protein from PNH cells is associated with accelerated complement-mediated intravascular hemolysis and gives rise to the hemoglobinuria that is a hallmark of the disease.

Two sets of observations in other conditions suggest that it is the deficiency of membrane attack complex regulatory proteins that is responsible for the hemolytic anemia of PNH. First, it was determined by two groups of investigators that erythrocytes lacking the blood group antigens of the Cromer complex (the Inab phenotype) are deficient in DAF, the molecule that carries the Cromer antigen system.[37,38] Affected persons demonstrate no intravascular hemolysis. The second observation is a description of one patient who has a genetic deficiency of CD59.[39] This condition is associated, in this patient, with a mild hemolytic anemia and cerebrovascular thrombosis; thrombosis is the major cause of mortality in PNH. Together, these observations suggest that the regulators of the terminal complex are the most important in protecting cells from destruction by complement. The relative importance of CD59 and C8-binding protein in vivo remains to be determined.

These factors—molecular geometry, complex instability, and regulatory proteins—contribute to the marked inefficiency of the complement system. Circulating erythrocytes from a patient with cold agglutinin disease can carry over 100,000 molecules of C3 per cell; normal erythrocytes can defend themselves against as many as 20,000 membrane attack complexes. Even given the inherent inefficiency of complement, the presence of multiple regulatory mechanisms at each step of the complement pathway attests to the importance of regulating the activity of this system.

The Ontogeny and Phylogeny of Complement Proteins

The application of molecular biology to the complement system has demonstrated heretofore unidentified relationships among the proteins of complement. Many structural homologies exist within the complement system. As might be expected, structure and function are closely aligned in the complement proteins (Table 3–4). Four distinct "families" of complement proteins can be identified. The first of these is the serine protease family, which contains C1r, C1s, C2, factor B, factor D, and factor I. These proteins are related to the well-studied serine proteases trypsin and chymotrypsin. All of these proteins contain a 25-kDa protease domain at the carboxyl terminus of the protein. Because 25 kDa is the approximate molecular weight of factor D, this activator of factor B can be considered the quintessential serine protease. C1r and C1s are identical in size and contain very similar molecular features, including a set of 60–amino acid short consensus repeats (SCRs) and a type III cysteine-rich domain similar to that in epidermal growth factor. The genes encoding these two proteins are closely linked on chromosome 12 and presumably arose by gene duplication.

As indicated previously, the serine proteases of the early classical and alternative pathways are both C3/C5-converting enzymes. In addition to this functional similarity, C2 and factor B have considerable structural homology. They are similarly sized proteins composed of a single polypeptide chain; they contain similar SCRs, similar serine protease domains (shared by all serine proteases), and a region shared only by these two. The genes for both C2 and factor B lie in the class III region of the major histocompatibility complex (MHC) on chromosome 6, a region that also contains the genes for C4.

C3, C4, and C5 are highly homologous proteins. As discussed, each protein is activated by the cleavage of a small "a" fragment from the α chain of the native molecule. C3 and C4 share the feature of the reactive thiol ester bond in the α chain; this bond is lacking in C5. All three proteins are synthesized as single proproteins that undergo modification before release into the plasma to generate the two chains of C3 and C5 and the three chains of C4. Interestingly, despite the high degree of overall homology of amino acids in these proteins (about 25%), the genes for the three proteins are located on three different chromosomes: the C3 gene is on chromosome 19, the C4 genes are in the MHC on chromosome 6, and the C5 gene is on chromosome 9. Although both C3 and C5 are encoded by single genes, two genes encode C4. These genes, known as C4A and C4B, give rise to the isotypic variants of the C4 protein. On the basis of the structure of C3-like proteins in other organisms, it has been postulated that C3 arose first and C4 and C5 arose later as gene duplication products.

The terminal complement proteins (C6 to C9) also exhibit a considerable degree of homology. Each of the terminal proteins exhibits an overall amino acid homology of 18% to 33% with the other proteins. If an analysis is made considering conservative substitutions, the homology increases to more than 50%. The predominant characteristic of the terminal complement proteins is the presence of

Table 3–4 Structural/Functional Homologies within the Complement System

Proteins	Homology
C1r, C1s	Serine proteases with similar subunit structure Genes linked
C2, factor B	Similar size, activation Highly homologous by structure Linked in major histocompatibility complex locus
C3, C4, C5	Activation by cleavage from α chain C3 and C4 contain reactive thiol ester Amino acid sequences show >20% overall identity
C6, C7, C8, C9	Share overall homology to one another ranging from 16% to 33% C6 and C7 share greatest homology All undergo amphipathic conversion to acquire membrane-binding character
CR1, CR2, factor H, DAF, MCP, C4 binding protein	All function to regulate complement activation All have multiple (60–70) amino acid short consensus repeats

DAF, delay accelerating factor; MCP, membrane cofactor protein.

cysteine-rich regions. From the amino terminus, using the nomenclature of Morgan,[2] the four types of cysteine-rich domains are known as type I, type II, type III, and the SCR (Fig. 3–2). The terminal complement proteins all contain type I cysteine-rich domains of approximately 60 amino acids, as well as other cysteine-rich domains of approximately 40 amino acids that share sequence homology to those in the low-density lipoprotein receptor (types II and III). These cysteine-rich domains, which greatly contribute to the tertiary structure of the protein, are clearly important for function. The SCRs are present in at least 12 of the complement proteins, and 8 proteins contain the other types of cysteine-rich domains. C6, C7, and C9 are single-polypeptide chains encoded by single genes; C8 is composed of three polypeptide chains, each of which is encoded by its own gene. The C8 α and β proteins are highly homologous, but the C8 γ chain shows no homology to any complement protein; it shows homology to α_1-microglobulin.

The proteins involved in the regulation of complement activation are also structurally related. In addition, the genes encoding the proteins that modulate C3 and C4 activation are grouped in one region of the long arm of chromosome 6 known as the *regulators of complement activation* (RCA) cluster.[40] The RCA group includes factor H, C4-binding protein, DAF, MCP, and the complement receptors CR1 and CR2. These proteins contain a variable number of SCRs of 60 to 70 amino acids. The chromosomal assignments of the complement proteins are given in Table 3–5.

Molecular biology has also proved invaluable in the identification of polymorphisms of complement proteins that had previously been noted as variants in electrophoretic mobility or antigenicity. Polymorphisms have been described for most of the complement proteins.[41,42] Some of the complement protein polymorphisms are associated with a loss or decrease of complement activity. Others demonstrate some degree of disease association; however, no disease associations have been established for any polymorphisms of the terminal complex proteins.

THE PHYSIOLOGIC RESPONSE TO COMPLEMENT ACTIVATION

Anaphylatoxins

The cleavage of C3, C4, or C5 by the enzyme complexes of the alternative or classical pathways results in the formation of two fragments. The fate of the C3b, C4b, and C5b fragments was discussed previously. The other fragments, C3a, C4a, and C5a, are known as the *anaphylatoxic fragments of complement.* These very small fragments of complement can produce a very large and potentially life-threatening physiologic response. The C3bBb and C4b2a enzyme complexes recognize an Arg-X sequence near the amino terminus of C3, C4, and C5. Cleavage of this bond results in the formation of a small N-terminal peptide of 77 amino acids for C3a and C4a and a small N-terminal peptide of 74 amino acids for C5a, each with a C-terminal arginine residue.

Although these peptides are very similar in structure, their potency in mediating cellular responses varies considerably. C5a is the most potent of the complement-derived anaphylatoxins, and C3a is the least potent. These complement fragments exert their anaphylatoxic effects by interacting with specific cellular receptors present on the surface of mast cells and basophils. The occupation of the receptor triggers the release of histamine and serotonin from intracellular granules. These two soluble factors cause contraction of smooth muscle cells and increased vascular permeability of blood vessels. Neutrophils, monocytes, macrophages, and platelets also bind anaphylatoxic fragments of complement; the occupation of these receptors activates the cell and, in the case of neutrophils, induces chemotaxis toward the site of complement activation.

Although the anaphylatoxic fragments of C3, C4, and C5 are potent biological response modifiers, they are rapidly inactivated in plasma by the action of a pair of carboxypeptidases. The best known, serum carboxypeptidase N, removes the C-terminal arginine residue from the peptide. Another

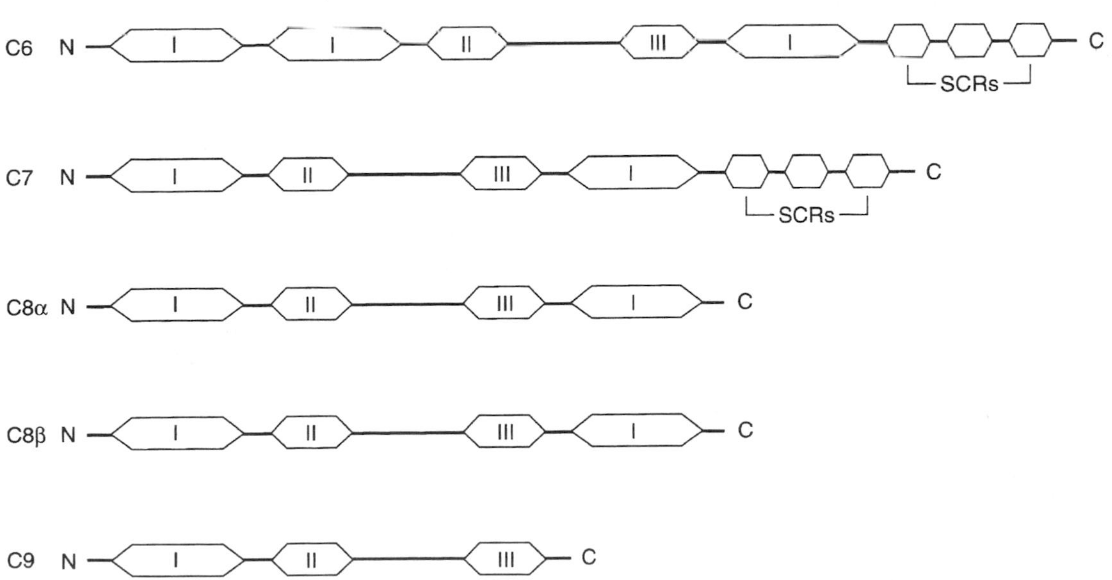

Figure 3–2 The domain structure of the terminal complex proteins. This figure illustrates the relative homologies among the proteins of the membrane attack complex. The highly homologous regions are found within cysteine-rich domains types I, II, and III (according to Morgan[2]). In addition, C6 and C7 contain cysteine-rich short consensus repeats (SCRs). (From Anderson KC, Ness PM. Scientific Basis of Transfusion Medicine, 2nd ed. Philadelphia, Saunders, 2000.)

Table 3–5 Chromosomal Assignments of the Complement Proteins

Protein(s)	Chromosomal Assignment
C1q	A, B and C chains on 1
C1r/C1s	Closely linked on 12
C2, C4A, C4B, factor B	In MHC locus on 6
C1 inhibitor, CD59	11
C4-binding protein, factor H, CR1, CR2, MCP, DAF	In RCA cluster on 1
Factor D	19
Factor I	4
Properdin	X
C3	19
C5	9
C6/C7	Closely linked on 5
C8	α and β chains on 1; γ chain on 9
C9	5

DAF, delay accelerating factor; MCP, membrane cofactor protein; MHC, major histocompatibility complex; RCA, regulators of complement activation.

enzyme, carboxypeptidase R, has been identified as the primary inactivator of kinin as well as anaphylatoxin peptides.[43] Unlike carboxypeptidase N, carboxypeptidase R is itself rapidly inactivated under normal purification conditions. After removal of the arginine, the peptide acquires the designation "des arg." C3a and C4a are rapidly and completely inactivated by the two carboxypeptidases; C5a is somewhat more resistant to inactivation. In addition, neutrophils can still respond to C5a des arg, albeit with some 10^3 weaker affinity; the removal of arginine from C3a and C4a results in complete loss of biological activity.

The relative resistance to carboxypeptidases and retention of bioactivity make C5a the most physiologically important of the anaphylactic complement peptides. Generation of C5a causes many of the effects seen in inflammation that are mediated by neutrophils. After activation by the binding of C5a into specific receptors, neutrophils bind to the capillary endothelium and migrate through the vessel wall, after the concentration gradient of the C5a. Once they are in contact with the higher concentrations of C5a present at the site of complement activation, neutrophils release granule contents and reactive metabolites, including lysozyme, reactive oxygen species, and eicosanoids. Although this is part of the normal mechanism of response to tissue injury or infection, the generation of large amounts of C5a or its presence in inappropriate locations can cause significant damage to uninvolved tissues.

Other Complement Activation Peptides

Other peptides generated during the course of complement activation have been identified as inducing cell activation or chemotaxis. Factor Ba, the peptide cleaved from factor B by factor D, is a weak chemotactic factor. The cleavage products of factor B—Ba and Bb—have been reported to inhibit and stimulate B-cell proliferation, respectively. Peptides with functions similar to those of C3a and C5a can be generated by the action of noncomplement enzymes, particularly plasmin, on C3 and C5. These C3a-like and C5a-like peptides may play a role in the activation of both platelets and white cells under existing blood storage protocols. The use of negatively charged leukoreduction filters may significantly affect the levels of various contact activation peptides in blood products.[44] In general, negatively charged artificial membrane surfaces promote complement activation; however, some types of filters appear to remove C3a that is generated during processing and storage.[45]

The membrane attack complex itself causes significant activation in a wide variety of cell types. Because most studies of the C5b-9 complex have focused on its lytic effect on erythrocytes, the functional effect on nucleated cells and platelets has lately gained appreciation. Although there are some reports in the literature that C5b-7 has chemotactic activity for neutrophils, it is the fully formed C5b-9 that has the greatest effect on these cells. In comparison with erythrocytes, nucleated cells are very resistant to C5b-9 lysis. In response to C5b-9, nucleated cells and platelets coalesce the C5b-9 complexes and bud them off in vesicles of plasma membrane. In nucleated cells, especially neutrophils, this process is accompanied by the activation of the cell and the release of enzymes, leukotrienes, prostaglandins, thromboxanes, and reactive oxygen metabolites from the cell.[46]

Platelets interact with the activated proteins of the complement system at several levels.[47] Specific platelet receptors for C1q have been identified.[48–50] Although the precise role of C1q receptors remains to be determined, one such receptor has been reported to play a role in phagocytosis in other cell types.[51] The exposure of human platelets to C3a alters the response to physiologic agonists but does not induce platelet aggregation. The effect of C5a on human platelets has not been investigated. Membrane attack complex can also affect platelet function.[52] C5b-9 can induce the formation of platelet membrane vesicles (or microparticles), increase the procoagulant activity of the platelet, and cause some degree of arachidonic acid generation.[53] Studies of the effects of C5b-9 on platelets have been carried out in purified protein systems; the significance of these observations for the whole plasma system remains to be determined. The platelet may modify the effects of activated complement fragments through the action of its surface regulatory proteins, DAF, MCP, C8-binding protein, and CD59. Platelets also contain internal pools of vitronectin, which may contribute to the local modulation of complement. The significant effects of activated complement fragments on the physiologic processes of platelets must be considered in the setting of platelet concentrate storage. Complement is activated under storage conditions,[54] with or without prestorage leukoreduction. Activated complement fragments as well as C5b-9 may contribute to the platelet storage lesion.[55]

EFFECTS OF COMPLEMENT ACTIVATION ON CELL SURVIVAL

Cytotoxic Effects

In the transfusion medicine setting, the effects of complement activation are graphically illustrated by the acute intravascular transfusion reaction. The generation of C3a and C5a produces bronchospasm and hypotension. C5a can also stimulate the production of interleukin-1 from macrophages, thereby causing fever.[56] The recruitment of large numbers of neutrophils to the lung by C5a generation produces ventilation–perfusion abnormalities. This effect may have devastating consequences for the recipients of transfusion products who develop TRALI subsequent to the fixation of complement by anti-HLA antibodies. Two other hallmarks of the acute intravascular transfusion reaction, hemoglobinemia and hemoglobinuria, result from the activation of complement on the red cell surface in sufficient amounts to overwhelm the cellular and plasma control proteins, thereby lysing the cell. The generation of activated complement proteins affects more than red cell survival. The activation of cells with the concomitant release of enzymes contributes to the activation of the coagulation system, as does the action of complement proteins on coagulation substrates and endothelial cells. In vitro studies suggest that these processes may trigger the disseminated intravascular coagulation seen in severe cases of hemolytic transfusion reaction. Evidence for the direct cytolysis of platelets or granulocytes during transfusion is not abundant, perhaps because of the difficulty in constructing an adequate study design. However, complement activation may be directly linked to platelet destruction in the setting of paroxysmal nocturnal hemoglobinuria, sepsis, and thrombotic thrombocytopenic purpura/hemolytic uremia syndrome. Each of these conditions is associated with complement activation and platelet dysfunction. The complement-mediated destruction of antibody-coated platelets can be experimentally induced. Antibody to the human platelet antigen $P1^{A1}$ (HPA-1) fixes sufficient complement to lyse target platelets.[57] In vitro platelet lysis can also be induced by cold agglutinin anti-I antibodies[58]; antibodies of this specificity have been proposed to mediate the thrombocytopenia associated with Epstein-Barr virus infection.

Opsonic Effects

The opsonic effects of complement activation result in the accelerated clearance of particles or cells that bear C3 as well as IgG. Although complement activation is the primary mechanism of cell destruction in the acute hemolytic transfusion reaction, the extravascular destruction of erythrocytes does not have the absolute requirement of complement activation. The primary clearance mechanism is through the phagocyte Fc receptor with recognition of the IgG present on the cell surface.[59] Opsonization of cells by complement, rather than through lysis, means that the cell has been able to regulate complement effectively to prevent the assembly of cytolytic membrane attack complexes. This regulation may reflect the titer, avidity, affinity, or thermal amplitude of the antibody in its interaction with the cell target.

In addition, as described previously, only IgG1 and IgG3 are efficient complement activators. The presence of C3b (or its degradation products) on the cell target in addition to antibody accelerates the clearance by the reticuloendothelial system. If a macrophage is already activated, it will bind and ingest cells that bear only C3b. Normal, resting macrophages require that IgG also be present on the erythrocyte surface. This experimental result is supported by the in vivo observation that the erythrocytes of patients with cold agglutinin disease circulate through the spleen bearing C3b but no IgG and are not sequestered. That is not to say that C3 has no in vivo role in clearance. Bacteria coated with C3 only are efficiently phagocytized by macrophages, resting or activated, even in the absence of IgG. Macrophages in the liver (Kupffer cells) are capable of clearing erythrocytes coated with C3b only. In addition, persons who are genetically deficient in one of the components of the early classical pathway are unable to bind C3 to anti-D-coated erythrocytes; those target cells are cleared from the circulation much more slowly than in persons with intact complement systems.[60]

The opsonic and cytotoxic effects of complement are important in the ex vivo setting of blood storage. Many types of bacteria that have been implicated in transfusion-mediated sepsis are either lysed or opsonized by the complement proteins in the blood unit. These bacteria are then engulfed by phagocytes also present in the bag. The removal of phagocytes by leukodepletion within 24 hours of collection results in the removal of contaminating bacteria as well. Leukodepletion more than 24 hours after collection may fail to sterilize the unit, because white cell breakdown may result in the release of viable bacteria from phagolysosomes.

The Role of Complement Receptors in Cell Clearance and in Maintenance of the Immune Response

The removal of complement-coated target cells is mediated by specific receptors for C3 and its activation and degradation fragments. As previously discussed, the activation of C3 produces two fragments, C3a, the anaphylatoxin, and C3b, which is covalently bound to the cell surface. In the presence of factor H, MCP, or the complement receptor CR1, C3b is rapidly cleaved by factor I to an inactivated form, iC3b (Fig. 3–3). This cleavage is estimated to occur in vivo within 5 minutes of the generation of C3b. Inactivated C3b undergoes another, slower interaction with factor I that results in a second cleavage on the opposite side of the thiol ester bond from the initial cleavage. This second cleavage occurs within 30 minutes of generation of C3b and results in the generation of the C3c fragment, which is no longer tethered to the cell, and the C3dg fragment, which contains the thiol ester bond and remains bound to the cell surface. Under laboratory conditions, the C3dg fragment can be further cleaved by trypsin to leave the C3d fragment on the cell surface; the frequency of generation of this fragment in vivo is uncertain.

Several complement receptors have been identified to date. They have overlapping cell distribution (Table 3–6). The specificity of these receptors for individual fragments of C3 is reflected in the biological response to receptor occupation. The central function of the complement receptor CR1 is clearance of immune complexes from the circulation through its interaction with C3b contained in the complex.[61] The bulk of the total CR1 in the circulation is present on red cells, because they provide the greatest mass of cells in the peripheral blood. The erythrocyte is therefore essential in transporting immune complexes from the plasma to the resident macrophages in the spleen.

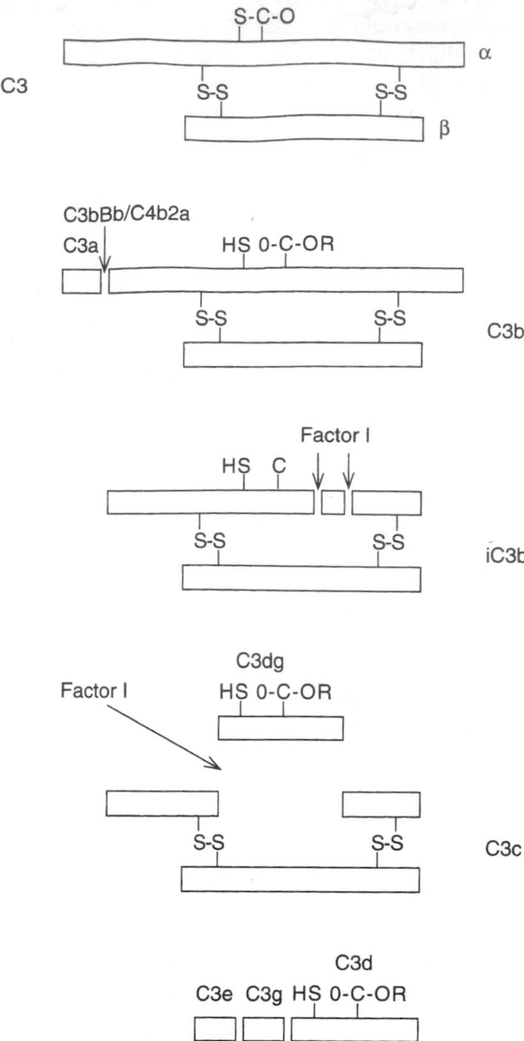

Figure 3–3 Degradation fragments of C3. Native C3 is cleaved by C4b2a or C3bBb, resulting in the exposure of a reactive thiol ester in the α chain of C3 and the generation of two fragments, C3a and C3b. C3b is inactivated by factor I in the presence of factor H or CR1 to iC3b, which remains bound to the surface by the thiol ester. A further cleavage by factor I on the other side of the covalent bond from the first cleavage results in the release of the C3c fragment; the C3dg fragment remains surface bound. In vitro, the C3dg fragment may be further degraded to C3d, C3e, and C3g. The C3d fragment, a terminal breakdown product of C3, remains covalently bound to the surface. (From Anderson KC, Ness PM. Scientific Basis of Transfusion Medicine, 2nd ed. Philadelphia, Saunders, 2000.)

The further processing of C3b to iC3b enables the complement fragment to interact with the complement receptor CR3, also known as CD11b/CD18. This receptor, with its distribution on monocytes, macrophages, and neutrophils, plays a major role in immune-mediated phagocytosis. CR3 belongs to a family of related receptor molecules that have the β chain CD18. The pairing of the CD11a α chain to CD18 defines the leukocyte function-associated antigen 1, which is important in mediating killing by T lymphocytes. CD18 may also pair with the α chain CD11c, forming the complex known as p150,95. This molecule has been unofficially designated CR4 in recognition of its binding affinity for iC3b.

The importance of the complement receptors CR3 and CR4 is indicated by the severity of the deficiency state, in which patients have defective phagocytic function and are susceptible to recurrent infections.[62] The degradation of iC3b by factor I produces C3dg, the principal ligand for the receptor CR2. The expression of CR2 is restricted to B lymphocytes, on which the binding of C3dg triggers B-cell activation and proliferation. In addition to its role as a C3dg-binding protein, CR2 is the cellular receptor through which the Epstein-Barr virus gains entry to B lymphocytes. The identification and characterization of the complement receptors has led to the development of new therapeutic modalities. For example, a recombinant CR1 has been engineered with the transmembrane region missing. This molecule retains the complement-regulatory ability of CR1 but is soluble in plasma. In animal models, this protein, sCR1, has proved efficacious in reducing the complement activation seen during thrombolytic therapy.[63]

Fragments of C3 are important in maintaining the immune response.[64] Animals with an experimental depletion of C3 fail to mount a normal IgG response to secondary immunization. This observation suggests that C3 is important in the development of immunologic memory, but such a role for C3 has not been confirmed in humans. It has also been established that the complement receptors CD21 and CD35 are important in the regulation of B-cell immunity while the complement regulatory proteins CD46 and CD55 have an additional role in T-cell function through the regulation of cytokine production.[65,66]

Therapeutic Complement Inhibition

The great advances in our understanding of both complement system biochemistry and the role of complement in

Table 3–6 Structure and Distribution of Complement Receptors

Receptor	Molecular Structure	Cellular Distribution
C1q	65 kDa, single chain	Platelets, monocytes, macrophages, B lymphocytes, endothelial cells
C3a	Single chain protein predicted to have 7 transmembrane regions	Mast cells, monocytes, macrophages, neutrophils, basophils, T cells
C5a	45 kDa, single chain	Monocytes, macrophages, neutrophils, mast cells
CR1 (CD35)	Four allotypes ranging from 160 to 250 kDa	Erythrocytes, monocytes, neutrophils, B lymphocytes
CR2 (CD21)	145 kDa, single chain	B cells, follicular dendritic cells
CR3 (CD11b/CD18)	Two chains, 165 kDa and 95 kDa	Neutrophils, monocytes, macrophages, follicular dendritic cells, natural killer cells
CD11c/CD18 (CR4)*	Two chains, 150 kDa and 95 kDa	Neutrophils, monocytes, macrophages, natural killer cells
(CR5)*	Unknown	Neutrophils, platelets

*CR designation is unofficial.

pathophysiology have led to the creation of strategies to control complement activation in order to minimize its deleterious effects.[67] Several promising compounds are in preclinical development; one monoclonal antibody against C5 has been used successfully in a clinical trial in the treatment of PNH to reduce ongoing hemolysis.[68] Although complement inhibitors have been proposed for use in acute hemolytic transfusion reactions, no clinical studies have yet been performed.[69]

LABORATORY ANALYSIS OF COMPLEMENT

Measurement of Cell-Associated Complement

The methods available for the measurement of cell-associated immunoglobulins are readily adaptable to the detection of cell-bound complement. Traditionally, the presence of cell-associated C3b and its cleavage products is *detected* by means of an aggregating anti-C3d antibody (C3 Coombs' test). The presence of small amounts of C4d antigen on the erythrocyte is identified in the blood bank as the Chido-Rodgers blood group antigen system. The antigenic difference is actually determined by the C4A and C4B alleles, with Rodgers specificity found in the C4A isotypes and Chido specificity found in the C4B isotypes. Techniques developed to measure cell-associated immunoglobulin can all be adapted to measure cell-bound complement, especially C3. These methods include fluorescence flow cytometry, radioimmunoassay, and enzyme-linked immunosorbent assay (ELISA).[70,71] In addition, the development of monoclonal antibodies that can distinguish among the various fragments of C3 may prove useful in laboratory diagnosis.

Measurement of Complement Activation or Deficiency States

Until the mid-1980s, there were no readily accessible tests of complement activation. The activation of complement was implied by a decrease in the level of an individual component, most often C4, in a clinical setting in which activation was suspected. Although this approach may be of some utility in the outpatient setting, it is of little use in the investigation of very sick patients, especially those receiving blood products. The problem with this diagnostic approach is twofold. First, reduction in the C4 level can occur from decreased synthesis of the protein in the liver rather than from consumption. Second, because of the presence of null genes for C4, the normal range for C4 is very wide; a person with a C4 level that usually is at the high end of the normal range may activate more than 50% of C4 before the measured level exceeds the normal range. Only laboratories with specialized complement expertise had methods permitting the detection of activation peptides of complement, generally by gel electrophoresis techniques or by radioimmunoassay of small complement fragments remaining in solution after precipitation of native protein and large fragments.

With the advent of monoclonal antibody technology, antibodies have been made that are capable of recognizing neoantigens expressed in the activation peptides of complement. These antibodies have been used in the formulation of commercial ELISA kits. ELISA tests that detect the activation peptides of either the classical (C4d) or alternative (factor Bb) pathway or both (C3a, C5a, iC3b, and C5b-9) are currently available. In addition, descriptions of many other monoclonal antibody-based activation peptide assays can now be found in the literature. These activation-dependent assays enable definite differentiation between patients with complement activation and those with decreased production of complement proteins.

Until recently, the assessment of patients with suspected complement deficiencies has relied on somewhat cumbersome gel methods. However, a new ELISA-based procedure has been developed for detection of complement deficiencies, including those due to a loss of proteins in the lectin pathway.[72] The continuing improvement of testing methods should make these assays more accessible to nonspecialists.

In summary, the burgeoning of research activity on the complement system has produced a clearer understanding of the biochemistry of these important proteins. This knowledge has led to the development of better diagnostic tools, to an increased clarity around the role of complement in disease pathophysiology, as well as to the invention of therapeutic modalities to control unwanted complement activation.

REFERENCES

1. Ross GD. Immunobiology of the Complement System. Orlando, Fla., Academic Press, 1986, pp 1–19.
2. Morgan BP. Complement: Clinical Aspects and Relevance to Disease. New York, Academic Press, 1990.
3. Sjoholm AG, Jonsson G, Braconier JH, et al. Complement deficiency and diseases: an update. Mol Immunol 2006;43:78–85.
4. Thiel S, Frederiksen PD, Jensenius JC. Clinical manifestations of mannan-binding lectin deficiency. Mol Immunol 2006;43:86–96.
5. Sim RB, Reid KBM. C1: Molecular interactions with activating systems. Immunol Today 1991;12:307–311.
6. Perkins SJ, Nealis AS. Solution structure of human and mouse immunoglobulin M by synchrotron X-ray scattering and molecular graphics modelling. J Mol Biol 1991;221:1345–1366.
7. Levine RP, Dodds AW. The thiolester bond of C3. Curr Top Microbiol Immunol 1989;153:73–82.
8. Szalai AJ, Briles DE, Volanakis JE. Role of complement in C-reactive protein-mediated protection of mice from *Streptococcus pneumoniae*. Infect Immunol 1996;64:4850–4853.
9. Bristow CL, Boackle RJ. Evidence for the binding of human serum amyloid P component to C1q and Fab. Mol Immunol 1986;23:1045–1052.
10. Pepys MB, Blatz ML. Acute phase proteins with special reference to C-reactive protein and related proteins (pentraxins) and serum amyloid A protein. Adv Immunol 1983;34:141–212.
11. Lu JH, Thiel S, Wiedemann H, et al. Binding of the pentamer/hexamer forms of mannan-binding protein to zymosan activates the proenzyme C1rC1s2 complex of the classical pathway of complement, without involvement of C1q. J Immunol 1990;144:2287–2294.
12. Fujita T, Matushita M, Endo Y. The lectin-complement pathway—its role in innate immunity and evolution. Immunol Rev 2004;198:195–202.
13. Lachmann PJ, Hughes-Jones NC. Initiation of complement activation. Springer Semin Immunopathol 1984;7:143–162.
14. Devine DV. The regulation of complement on cell surfaces. Trans Med Rev 1991;5:123–131.
15. Donaldson VH, Bissler JJ. C1 inhibitors and their genes: an update. J Clin Lab Med 1992;119:330–222.
16. Hillarp A, Dahlback B. The protein S-binding site localized to the central core of C4b-binding protein. J Biol Chem 1987;262:11300–11307.
17. Hammer CH, Jacobs RM, Frank MM. Isolation and characterization of a novel plasma protein which binds to activated C4 of the classical complement pathway. J Biol Chem 1989;264:2283–2291.
18. Farries TC, Lachmann PJ, Harrison RA. Analysis of the interaction between properdin and factor B, components of the alternative pathway C3 convertase of complement. Biochem J 1988;253:667–675.
19. Murphy BF, Kirszbaum L, Walker ID, et al. SP-40,40, a newly identified normal human serum protein found in the SC5b-9 complex of complement and in the immune deposits in glomerulonephritis. J Clin Invest 1988;81:1858–1864.

20. Choi NH, Mazda T, Tomita M. A serum protein Sp-40,40 modulates the formation of membrane attack complex of complement on erythrocytes. Mol Immunol 1989;26:835–840.
21. Jenne DE, Lowin B, Peitsch MC, et al. Clusterin (complement lysis inhibitor) forms a high density lipoprotein complex with apolipoprotein A-I in human plasma. J Biol Chem 1991;266:11030–11036.
22. Nicholson-Weller A, Burge J, Fearon DT, et al. Isolation of a human erythrocyte membrane glycoprotein with decay accelerating activity for C3 convertases of the complement system. J Immunol 1982;129:184–189.
23. Medof ME, Kinoshita T, Nussenzweig V. Inhibition of complement activation on the surface of cells after incorporation of decay-accelerating factor (DAF) into their membranes. J Exp Med 1984;160:1558–1578.
24. Pangburn MK. Differences between the binding sites of the complement regulatory proteins DAF, CR1, and factor H on C3 convertases. J Immunol 1986;136:2216–2221.
25. Kinoshita T, Medof ME, Nussenzweig V. Endogenous association of decay-accelerating factor (DAF) with C4b and C3b on cell membranes. J Immunol 1986;136:3390–3395.
26. Berger M, Medof ME. Increased expression of complement decay accelerating factor during activation of human neutrophils. J Clin Invest 1987;79:214–220.
27. Seya T, Atkinson JP. Functional properties of membrane cofactor protein of complement. Biochem J 1989;264:581–588.
28. Schoermark S, Rauterberg, EW, Shin ML, et al. Homologous species restriction in lysis of human erythrocytes: a membrane-derived protein with C8-binding capacity functions as an inhibitor. J Immunol 1986;136:1772–1776.
29. Zalman LS, Wood LM, Muller-Eberhard JH. Isolation of a human erythrocyte membrane protein capable of inhibiting expression of homologous complement transmembrane channels. Proc Nat Acad Sci USA 1986;83:6975–6979.
30. Holguin MH, Frederick LR, Bernshaw NJ, et al. Isolation and characterization of a membrane protein from normal human erythrocytes that inhibits reactive lysis of the erythrocytes of paroxysmal nocturnal hemoglobinuria. J Clin Invest 1989;84:7–17.
31. Sugita Y, Nakamo Y, Tomita M. Isolation from human erythrocytes of a new membrane protein which inhibits the formation of complement transmembrane channels. J Biochem (Tokyo) 1988;104:633–637.
32. Okada N, Harada R, Fujita T, et al. A novel membrane glycoprotein capable of inhibiting membrane attach by homologous complement. Int Immunol 1989;1:205–208.
33. Stefanova I, Hilgert I, Kirstofova H, et al. Characterization of a broadly expressed human leukocyte antigen MEM-43 anchored in membrane through phosphatidylinositol. Mol Immunol 1989;26:153–161.
34. Lockert DH, Kaufman KM, Chang CP, et al. Identity of the segment of human complement C8 recognized by complement regulatory protein CD59. J Biol Chem 1995;270:19723–19728.
35. Husler T, Lockert DH, Kaufman KM, et al. Chimeras of human complement C9 reveal the site recognized by complement regulatory protein CD59. J Biol Chem 1995;270:3483–3486.
36. Parker CJ, Omine M, Richards S, et al. Diagnosis and management of paroxysmal nocturnal hemoglobinuria. Blood 2005;106:3699–3709.
37. Telen MJ, Green AM. The Inab phenotype: characterization of the membrane protein and complement regulatory defect. Blood 1989;74: 437–441.
38. Merry AH, Rawlinson VI, Uchikawa M, et al. Studies on the sensitivity to complement-mediated lysis of erythrocytes (Inab phenotype) with a deficiency of DAF (decay accelerating factor). Br J Haematol 1989;73:248–253.
39. Yamashina M, Ueda E, Kinoshita T, et al. Inherited complete deficiency of 20-kilodalton homologous restriction factor (CD59) as a cause of paroxysmal nocturnal hemoglobinuria. N Engl J Med 1990;323:1184–1189.
40. Farries TC, Atkinson JP. Evolution of the complement system. Immunol Today 1991;12:295–300.
41. Marcus D, Alper CA. Methods for allotyping complement proteins. In Rose N, Manual of Clinical Immunology. Washington, D.C., American Society for Microbiology, 1986, pp 185–196.
42. Winkelstein JA, Colten HR. Genetically determined disorders of the complement system. In The Metabolic Basis of Disease. St. Louis, McGraw-Hill, 1987, pp 2711–2737.
43. Campbell W, Okada H. An arginine specific carboxypeptidase generated in blood during coagulation or inflammation which is unrelated to carboxypeptidase N or its subunits. Biochem Biophys Res Comm 1989;162:933–939.
44. Shiba M, Tadokoro K, Sawanobori M, et al. Activation of the contact system by filtration of platelet concentrates with a negatively charged white cell-removal filter and measurement of venous blood bradykinin level in patients who received filtered platelets. Transfusion 1997;37:457–462.
45. Snyder EL, Mechanic S, Baril L, et al. Removal of soluble biologic response modifiers (complement and chemokines) by a bedside white cell-reduction filter. Transfusion 1996;36:707–713.
46. Morgan BP. Complement membrane attack on nucleated cells: Resistance, recovery and non-lethal effects. Biochem J 1989;264:1–14.
47. Devine DV. The effects of complement activation on platelets. Curr Top Microbiol Immunol 1992;178:101–113.
48. Peerschke EIB, Ghebrehiwet B. Human blood platelets possess specific binding sites for C1q. J Immunol 1987;138:1537–1541.
49. Nepomuceno RR, Henschen-Edman AH, Burgess WH, et al. cDNA cloning and primary structure analysis of C1qR(P), the human C1q/MBL/SPA receptor that mediates enhanced phagocytosis in vitro. Immunity 1997;6:119–129.
50. Nepomuceno RR, Tenner AJ. C1qRP, the C1q receptor that enhances phagocytosis, is detected specifically in human cells of myeloid lineage, endothelial cells, and platelets. J Immunol 1998;160:1929–1935.
51. Butko P, Nicholson-Weller A, Wessels MR. Role of complement and complement receptor C1qR in the antibody-independent killing of group B streptococcus. Adv Exp Med Biol 1997;418:941–943.
52. Sims PJ, Wiedmer T. The response of human platelets to activated components of the complement system. Immunol Today 1991;12:338–342.
53. Wiedmer T, Esmon CT, Sims PJ. Complement proteins C5b-9 stimulate procoagulant activity through platelet prothrombinase. Blood 1986; 68:875–880.
54. Bode AP, Miller DT, Newman SL, et al. Plasmin activity and complement activation during storage of citrated platelet concentrates. J Lab Clin Med 1989;113:94–102.
55. Gyongyossy-Issa MIC, McLeod E, Devine DV. Complement activation in platelet concentrates is surface-dependent and modulated by the platelets. J Lab Clin Med 1994;123:859–868.
56. Dalmasso AP. Complement in the pathophysiology and diagnosis of human disease. CRC Crit Rev Clin Lab Sci 1986;24:123–283.
57. Cines DB, Schreiber RD. Effect of anti-P1^{A1} antibody on human platelets: I. The role of complement. Blood 1979;53:567–577.
58. Dixon RH, Rosse WF. Mechanisms of complement-mediated activation of human blood platelets in vitro: comparison of normal and paroxysmal nocturnal hemoglobinuria platelets. J Clin Invest 1977;59: 360–368.
59. Lutz HU. Innate immune and non-immune mediators of erythrocyte clearance. Cell Mol Biol 2004;50:107–116.
60. Schreiber AD. An experimental model of immune hemolytic anemia. Ann Intern Med 1977;87:211–217.
61. Schifferli JA, Ng YC, Peters DK. The role of complement and its receptor in the elimination of immune complexes. N Engl J Med 1986;315:488–495.
62. Anderson DC, Springer TA. Leukocyte adhesion deficiency: an inherited defect in the MAC-1, LFA-1, and p150,95 glycoproteins. Annu Rev Med 1987;38:175–194.
63. Weisman HF, Bartow T, Leppo MK, et al. Soluble complement receptor type 1: in vivo inhibitor of complement suppressing post-ischemic myocardial inflammation and necrosis. Science 1990;249:146–151.
64. Erdei A, Fust G, Gergely J. The role of C3 in the immune response. Immunol Today 1991;12:332–337.
65. Liu J, Miwa T, Hilliard B, et al. The complement inhibitory protein DAF (CD55) suppresses T cell immunity in vivo. J Exp Med 2005;201: 567–577.
66. Wagner C, Hansch GM. Receptors for complement C3 on T-lymphocytes: relics of evolution or functional molecules? Mol Immunol 2006;43:22–30.
67. Mollnes TE, Kirschfink M. Strategies of therapeutic complement inhibition. Mol Immunol 2006;43:107–121.
68. Hill A, Hillmen P, Richards SJ, et al. Sustained response and long-term safety of eculizumab in paroxysmal nocturnal hemoglobinuria. Blood 2005;106:2559–2265.
69. Yazdanbakhsh K, Kang S, Tamasauskas D, et al. Complement receptor 1 inhibitors for prevention of immune-mediated red cell destruction: Ppotential use in transfusion therapy. Blood 2003;15:5046–5052.
70. Garratty G. The significance of IgG on the red cell surface. Trans Med Rev 1987;1:47–57.
71. Schwartz KA. Platelet antibody: review of detection methods. Am J Hematol 1988;29:106–14.
72. Seelen MA, Roos A, Wieslander J, et al. Functional analysis of the classical, alternative and MBL pathways of the complement system: standardization and validation of a simple ELISA. J Immunol Meth 2005;296:187–198.

Chapter 4

Principles of Red Blood Cell Allo- and Autoantibody Formation and Function

James C. Zimring

INTRODUCTION

Humoral immunity represents the main barrier to transfusion of red blood cells (RBCs) in humans. Crossmatching units of RBCs for the naturally occurring antibodies against the ABO carbohydrate antigens is an absolute requirement to avoid acute hemolysis. However, the majority of immunohematology focuses on the identification of acquired antibodies to RBC antigens, which are typically generated after previous exposure to foreign RBCs. Several hundred different RBC antigens have now been described (see Chapters 5, 6, 7, and 8). These antigens can consist of carbohydrates, linear peptides, and tertiary confirmations dependent on proper folding and membrane insertion. Different blood group antigens have distinct immunogenicities, because RBC antigens vary in their likelihood of inducing an antibody response. In addition, antibodies to some blood group antigens frequently cause hemolysis (clinically significant), whereas others cause no deleterious effect (clinically insignificant). The current understanding of the basic science regarding immunogenicity of transfused RBCs and the immune-mediated mechanisms of RBC destruction are detailed in this chapter.

BASIC SCIENCE OF ALLOANTIBODY FORMATION

Most anti-RBC antibodies detected in the practice of transfusion medicine are humoral responses to alloantigens encountered during previous exposures to foreign RBCs, typically via transfusion or pregnancy. A great deal is now understood about the general mechanics of humoral immunization to soluble and particulate antigens (see Chapter 2). However, although sheep red blood cells have been used as a model antigen for many years, the current paradigms of immunology have been largely developed outside the context of immunization by RBC transfusion. Transfused RBCs appear to be only weakly immunogenic, and it is currently unclear if immune responses to RBC transfusion are qualitatively different from general mechanisms of immune response to foreign antigen. However, it is safe to say that there are several notable differences between traditional microbial or protein immunogens and transfusion of sterile blood, including route of immunization, potential absence of inflammation and danger signals, dose and kinetics of antigenic exposure, type of antigen-presenting cell involved, and the molecular nature of the antigen. The exact role and importance of these variables in RBC transfusion is currently unknown, but the theoretical potential for their importance is discussed in the following sections.

Frequency of Alloimmunization to RBC Transfusion: Immunity and Tolerance

Despite there being numerous foreign epitopes on essentially all transfusions of nonautologous RBCs, transfusion is not a highly immunogenic stimulus. Even in response to multiple transfusions, alloimmunization to alloantigens on transfused RBCs has an overall frequency of approximately 2% to 6%.[1–3] However, it has been hypothesized that frequency of alloimmunization may vary with the underlying pathophysiology of the transfused patient. One study revealed alloimmunization rates as follows, based on underlying disease: lymphocytic leukemia 0%, gastrointestinal bleed 11%, aplastic anemia 11%, renal failure 14%, myelogenous leukemia 16%, and hemoglobinopathy 29%.[4] These findings indicated a trend, with a clear decrease in lymphocytic leukemia, presumably due to immunosuppression. There is also an apparent increase in other disease states, but these differences were not found to be statistically significant.

It has been proposed that alloimmunization is unusually high in some disease states, such as sickle cell anemia, myelodysplastic anemia, and autoimmune hemolytic anemia. However, rates of alloimmunization can vary widely from study to study. For example, the range of alloimmunization in adult sickle cell patients ranges from 18.6%[5] to 47%,[6] depending on the study, with an average rate of 25%.[7] The presence of alloantibodies in patients with autoimmune hemolytic anemia, when excluding autoantibodies that mimicked alloantibodies, ranges from 12%[8] to 40%,[9] with an average frequency of 32%.[10] Likewise, two different groups reported alloimmunization rates in patients with myelodysplastic syndrome as 21% and 58.6%, respectively.[11,12]

Analysis of the above literature demonstrates considerable variation in the rates of alloimmunization reported by different groups. A number of factors may lead to varying results, including differences in patient demographics, differences in diagnostic criteria or subclasses of disease, and differences in methodology of alloantibody detection. In addition, it has been reported that up to 40% of alloantibodies subsequently become undetectable,[13,14] raising the possibility that the time after transfusion that specimens are collected may influence outcome. It has also been reported that leukoreduction may decrease immunogenicity of transfused RBCs.[15] Since use of leukoreduced blood varied in the above studies, this may be a relevant issue. A further complicating factor is that most studies are retrospective and do not compare pretransfusion specimens to post-transfusion specimens and it is unclear if the presence of an alloantibody is necessarily the result of an antecedent transfusion.

The precise mechanism by which different patient populations may differ in their alloimmunization rates is unclear. However, a number of potential factors may be involved. First, the volume and frequency of transfusion are important variables, because they reflect the magnitude and kinetics of antigen dose. Second, the extent to which donor units differ phenotypically from recipient RBCs will always be an important factor. Thus, one must consider the genetic similarity of the donor and recipient populations. A third variable is the extent to which the underlying pathophysiology of the condition necessitating transfusion may perturb immune function. For example, systemic immunosuppression linked to the pathophysiology likely contributes to a low rate of seroconversion in patients with lymphocytic leukemia.[4] In contrast, the pathophysiology of other disease states may lead to immune dysregulation resulting in increased alloimmunization.

Given that only a small percentage of individuals make detectable alloantibodies, despite multiple transfusion, it appears as though RBCs may represent a fairly weak immunogen. Of course, this notion is biased by the fact that RBCs are typically matched a priori for the most immunogenic antigens (i.e., Rh_0D). Immunization rates to Rh_0D have been estimated at 30% to 90%,[16–23] depending on the study. Still, even for the Rh_0D antigen, up to 20% of Rh-negative individuals do not mount an anti-Rh response, despite repeated exposure to Rh-positive blood. The nonresponse of such individuals may in part be due to Rh actually being self in the case of recipients who are weak D and do not type D+ by routine methods. In addition, nonresponders may have genetic factors such that they lack the ability to respond to the Rh antigen. However, this pattern is also consistent with initial exposure to Rh-positive RBCs inducing a state of active tolerance against Rh antigens, although such has not been demonstrated. Thus, overall, transfused RBCs are strongly immunogenic in some recipients, only weakly immunogenic or nonimmunogenic in other patients, and the theoretical potential for tolerance exists.

VARIABLES ASSOCIATED WITH RBCs AS AN IMMUNOGEN

The context in which the immune system encounters antigens on transfused RBCs is associated with a number of characteristics that may contribute to the relatively weak immunogenicity of RBCs in some settings.

Route of Immunization

Unlike subcutaneous and intramuscular routes, which are generally immunogenic, intravenous administration is among the most tolerogenic methods of antigen administration.[24–26] Because transfusion of a sterile unit of RBCs involves introduction of intravenous antigen, one might predict that no immune response should occur to RBC antigens. However, the induction of tolerance to intravenous antigen has typically been described with soluble proteins, and aggregated protein complexes are typically immunogenic. Although blood group antigens are polymeric as a result of being in a membrane, the molecules that carry blood group antigens are neither free-floating soluble proteins nor are they insoluble protein aggregates. Thus, it is unclear how this molecular form fits into the paradigm of soluble versus aggregate. It is worth noting that although intraperitoneal injection of soluble protein is not immunogenic, injection of the same protein chemically coupled to autologous RBCs results in an antibody response equivalent to immunization with the antigen in Freund's complete adjuvant, which is among the strongest known methods for immunization.[27,28] The same observation has recently been made regarding both humoral and cellular immunity using the intravenous route.[29,30] Thus, the intravenous route through which blood is given may influence the immunogenicity of antigens on RBCs, but the particulars of this are unclear given the form in which the immune system encounters RBC antigens.

Absence of a Danger Signal

It has been argued that without an inflammatory stimulus (also called a *danger signal*), immunity will not typically occur.[31,32] Danger signals are not present on healthy self-tissues and typically need to be introduced by microbial infections or inflammation.[33–37] In support of this concept, even a subcutaneous injection into the footpad of mice, which is typically the best route to induce humoral immunity, can induce tolerance when performed in the absence of an inflammatory adjuvant.[24] Properly processed units of RBCs should not contain any microbial products. However, it is possible that processing and transfusion of blood introduces danger signals from nonmicrobial sources. It is also possible that the danger signal is provided by ongoing inflammation in the transfusion recipient. Thus, the role of inflammation and/or danger signals during RBC transfusion is unclear. However, whereas danger signals would be typically present during infection and immunization, they may be altered or absent during transfusion, which could influence the nature of anti-RBC immune responses.

Dose of Antigen

Another important difference between an RBC transfusion and other immune stimuli is the amount of antigen present. The dose of foreign antigen received during the early stages of an infection can be quite low, especially when the infection begins as a small inoculum. As the infection proceeds, levels of antigen will rise rapidly and then decline within several weeks in the case of adequate clearance. Alternatively, in a chronic infection, the antigen will often still decline, but will persist at some level long term. In contrast, transfusion of blood results in a sudden burst of high-level antigen that persists for a moderate period of time (several months).

In the case of fresh blood, transfused RBCs have a life span of approximately 120 days. Starting with a transfusion of a single 200-mL unit of packed RBCs, approximately 1.67 mL of packed RBCs are consumed per day, which translates to consumption of about 12.8 million RBCs per minute. Because these cells are removed by macrophages of the reticuloendothelial system, RBC transfusion essentially represents a selective targeting of large doses of foreign antigen to professional antigen-presenting cells (APCs). Transfusion of a stored unit of blood will result in a slightly different pattern of consumption, because RBCs continue to senesce during storage of blood products.[38] Transfusion of a 200-mL bag of blood that has been stored for 4 weeks may result in more rapid removal of packed RBCs due to senescence of stored blood.[38] Thus, in contrast to the patterns seen with infectious pathogens, transfusion of RBCs results in a sudden introduction of large amounts of antigen (or very large amounts in the case of stored blood), followed by persistence of the antigen for several months. In the case of chronically transfused patients, exposure to common blood group antigens may be extended to a considerably longer period of time, depending on the frequency of transfusion.

Dose alterations can profoundly affect immune responses. It has been known for decades that moderate doses of antigen generally promote immune responses, whereas both low levels and very high levels of antigen lead to tolerance.[39] Duration of antigen persistence also has a significant effect on the nature of the immune response. Although CD4+ T cells expand and differentiate into helper T (Th) cells on initial exposure to antigen, extended exposure to antigens during chronic infection results in the inactivation and downregulation of viral antigen-specific CD4+ T cells.[40,41] Moreover, the level of antigen present during chronic exposure can regulate immunity versus tolerance at the level of CD4+ Th cells.[42]

Antigen-Presenting Cells Involved in Processing and Presenting RBC Antigens

In order for a primary immune response to occur, a professional APC (typically a macrophage or dendritic cell) must process and present the antigen. Although macrophages are not required for immune responses to antigens in tissues,[43–45] evidence suggests that they are necessary for generating immune responses to transfused RBCs.[43–45] Thus, the type of APC required for a primary immune response to transfused RBCs may differ from the APC required for responses to other better-studied antigens.

Evidence also suggests that the lymphatic compartment, and thus the immunologic microenvironment, varies for antigens injected into tissues and transfused RBCs. Tissue-injected antigens are consumed by resident dendritic cells, which then migrate to draining lymph nodes and accumulate in areas of naive T-cell activation, whereas macrophages are excluded from these areas.[44] Likewise, lessons can be learned from solid tissue transplantation, where immune responses can be generated via two mechanisms. The direct pathway involves donor dendritic cells migrating to recipient lymph nodes and priming recipient T cells. In the indirect pathway, however, recipient dendritic cells enter the transplanted tissues, consume donor antigens, and return to recipient lymph nodes to prime T cells with donor antigens on recipient MHC. In both cases, the predominant APC is a dendritic cell in the specialized microenvironment of a lymph node. In contrast, the majority of transfused RBCs are consumed by macrophages in the spleen and liver, and there is no discrete tissue parenchyma where recipient dendritic cells can enter.

Polymeric Nature of Antigens on RBCs

Erythrocyte surface antigens are physically linked via their mutual association with the cellular membrane and are thus polymeric in nature. As a group, polymeric antigens tend to be T-cell independent antigens that directly activate B cells[46] to secrete immunoglobulin M (IgM) without the requirement of T-cell help. However, responses to T-cell independent antigens typically fail to class switch to high-affinity IgG. Thus, it is possible that transfused RBCs activate T-cell independent pathways of humoral immunization. In support of this notion, it has been shown that initial anti-RBC IgM responses can be T-cell independent.[46] However, in animal models, subsequent class switching to anti-RBC IgG depends on T-cell help.[46] In addition, human patients with defective helper T-cell function secondary to infection with human immunodeficiency virus have significantly decreased rates of alloimmunization to transfused RBCs.[47] Thus, as an immunogen, RBCs appear to have a unique combination of early T-cell independence for IgM synthesis followed by T-cell dependence for class switching and memory.

BASIC SCIENCE OF ANTI-RBC AUTOANTIBODY FORMATION

Loss of immunologic tolerance to self-tissues can result in autoimmune processes targeted against specific organs or broadly reactive with self-tissues. Among the known autoimmune pathologies is the generation of autoantibodies against self-RBC antigens. This process can result in a clinically silent autoagglutinin that is detected incidentally by a positive direct antiglobulin test (DAT) during alloantibody screening. However, if the autoantibodies promote erythrocyte destruction, the clinical manifestation of autoimmune hemolytic anemia (AIHA) can result. AIHA can range in severity from a transient mild clinical course to massive lethal hemolysis. Although the exact etiology of AIHA is unclear, it can occur either spontaneously or in close temporal association to transfusion of RBCs. Because the basic processes that lead to AIHA in these two settings are likely different, they are considered separately in the following discussion.

AIHA Not Associated with a Transfusion (Spontaneous AIHA)

Although the loss of tolerance to self-tissues is a general feature of all AIHA, it is unlikely that a single mechanism accounts for the process by which anti-RBC autoantibodies are generated. In the general field of autoimmune pathophysiology, a number of mechanisms may explain how loss of self-tolerance occurs. Because there is evidence for several of these mechanisms playing a potential role in the generation of AIHA in different settings, each will be considered here.

Central and Peripheral Tolerance to Blood Group Antigens

The fine-tuning of the immune system such that it can respond to a wide variety of microbial antigens without recognizing self-tissues is essential to both maintaining immune competence and avoiding autoimmunity. The process begins when T-cell receptors and B-cell receptors recombine randomly and generate a highly diverse repertoire of specificities. Then, in a process referred to as *central tolerance*, immature autoreactive T cells are deleted in the thymus, and autoreactive B cells either become anergic or are deleted, first in the bone marrow and then in the periphery. Such deletion events depend on the exposure of these lymphocytes to self-antigens during development. Although a great variety of antigens are expressed in the thymus, and the majority of autoreactive T cells are deleted, some autoreactive T cells escape this thymic education.

If RBC-specific T cells and B cells survive deletion, AIHA could develop. This theory has been formally demonstrated in an animal model. In the NZB mouse, which spontaneously develops AIHA, $CD4^+$ helper T cells specific for peptides from RBC autoantigens survive thymic education, whereas in other strains that do not develop AIHA, the cells are deleted.[48] Moreover, it has recently been shown that autoreactive T cells specific for peptides from Rh antigens are detectable in human patients with measurable anti-Rh autoantibodies.[49] It thus seems likely that escape of some autoreactive $CD4^+$ T cells may be involved in generation of AIHA. However, it has also been reported that γ/δ T cells, which are not specific for RBC antigens, can provide help to anti-RBC autoreactive B cells.[50] Thus, it is also possible that T cells of other specificities can give bystander help to anti-RBC B cells. In addition, T cells specific for cryptic epitopes may also be involved. Thus, it appears that although T cells are likely involved in helping autoreactive B cells differentiate into plasma cells, the exact nature of such help may vary.

The activation of autoreactive B cells specific for RBC antigens is an absolute requirement for the generation of AIHA. Like thymic education of T cells, education of autoreactive B cells requires that immature B cells encounter the self-antigen, which results in either deletion or the induction of anergy.[51] Although deletion of autoreactive B cells can occur in the periphery,[52] B cells that encounter the antigen, recognized by their rearranged immunoglobulin gene, while still in the bone marrow undergo arrested development and death.[53] In addition, B cells are more easily tolerized to membrane-bound surface antigens than to soluble antigens.[52] Because erythroid development occurs in the bone marrow where immature B cells appear to first undergo education, and because blood group antigens are membrane-bound proteins, it seems likely that deletion of autoreactive B cells that recognize RBC antigens is a highly efficient process. Nonetheless, it has been demonstrated that while autoreactive B cells specific for RBC antigens are mostly deleted or rendered anergic, there is sufficient survival of autoreactive B cells to cause AIHA in some settings.[54,55] The autoreactive B cells that survive in this setting appear to reside predominantly in gut tissues, and their activation can be significantly influenced by the presence of enteric pathogens or inflammation.[55]

If autoreactive cells manage to escape central tolerance, they can still be deleted or inhibited via peripheral tolerance, a second process that prevents autoreactive cells from differentiating into mature effector cells that may cause autoimmunity. The distinction between central and peripheral tolerance, which is clear for T cells (thymic versus extrathymic), is less well defined for B cells. Mechanisms of peripheral tolerance include induction of apoptosis, anergy, and active inhibition by suppressor/regulatory T cells. This combination of central tolerance, which eliminates most autoreactive cells, and peripheral tolerance, which inhibits those few autoreactive cells that escape, is generally effective; AIHA is a relatively rare event. However, the presence of autoreactive lymphocytes essentially constitutes a pre-existing risk factor for AIHA if the normal factors that keep autoreactive lymphocytes at bay are sufficiently perturbed.

Several events can lead to the inappropriate activation of peripheral autoreactive cells. Infection with a pathogen that carries epitopes similar to blood group antigens *(molecular mimicry)* can provide sufficient stimulation of autoreactive cells in an inflammatory environment such that peripheral tolerance is overcome. Alternatively, general immune dysregulation and polyclonal activation of lymphocytes may nonspecifically activate T and/or B cells that happen to be specific for RBC antigens. In support of this concept, development of AIHA is associated with chronic inflammation and lymphoproliferative disorders in both human and animal models[56,57] and is also associated with a variety of infections, including *Mycoplasma pneumoniae*, Epstein-Barr virus, cytomegalovirus, and rubella.[58] Cytokine dysregulation may also play a role, as a polarization to a Th2-type profile in AIHA has been observed in both humans and in the NZB/W murine model of AIHA.[59,60] Additional mechanisms include a loss of regulatory T cells, as CD4+ CD25+ T reg levels appear to be decreased in AIHA.[61] Thus, the breakdown of peripheral tolerance by a variety of mechanisms may allow the few autoreactive lymphocytes that escape central tolerance to differentiate into mature effectors that ultimately result in the formation of plasma cells that secrete antibodies specific for blood group antigens.

An additional mechanism of loss of tolerance involves the generation of cryptic peptide epitopes. For any given protein, only a limited number of peptides are normally presented by MHC molecules. The repertoire of peptides presented by each individual is largely a function of their HLA type, because peptides differ in their affinities for the grooves of different MHC variants. The range of peptides presented is also a function of how a protein is processed and broken down by a system of protease complexes called the *proteosome.* It has been demonstrated that a given protein may contain peptide sequences that fit well into an MHC molecule but are not typically presented on MHC because that particular peptide fragment is not generated by proteolysis of the protein in question. Such a peptide is called a *cryptic epitope.*

Because cryptic epitopes will not be processed and presented by normal thymic tissues, T cells that recognize cryptic epitopes will not be deleted in the thymus. Such T cells are technically not autoreactive, because the cryptic epitopes are also not presented on peripheral tissues and thus do not constitute a self-antigen. However, abnormal processing of self-proteins can result in presentation of cryptic epitopes on self-tissues. For example, ongoing inflammation and microbial infection leads to the release of microbial proteases and a large-scale breakdown of self-proteins by inflammatory proteases released from leukocytes. Infection of APCs by microbes may also change the processing of self-antigens. Furthermore, cryptic epitopes may be generated by exposure to caustic stimuli that denature or destroy proteins, such as burns or chemicals. The generation of such peptides may lead to activation of T cells specific for the cryptic epitope, which would then be capable of providing T-cell help to a B cell presenting the same cryptic epitope. Once a B cell has differentiated into an antibody-secreting plasma cell, it no longer requires immune stimulation to produce antibodies. Thus, in theory, a sustained autoantibody response can be generated during a transient exposure to cryptic epitopes. Direct experimental evidence demonstrates that cryptic epitopes of Rh antigens are recognized by T cells in patients with AIHA of anti-Rh specificity.[62–65]

Transfusion-Associated AIHA

A considerable percentage of AIHA patients develop an anti-RBC autoantibody subsequent to transfusion with allogeneic RBCs. Several studies have examined the association between transfusion and the development of anti-RBC autoantibodies. The phenomenon has been observed with considerable frequency in patients with sickle cell anemia. For example, one study reported that 8% of pediatric patients and 9.7% of adults with sickle cell anemia who received transfusions developed anti-RBC autoantibodies. In a separate retrospective study, of 2618 patients with a positive DAT or indirect antiglobulin test, 121 (4.6%) were reported to also have autoantibodies. Of the patients with autoantibodies, 10% also had an identifiable alloantibody and generated both the alloantibody and autoantibody subsequent to transfusion.[66] Due to the inability to obtain transfusion records on all patients, this frequency of autoimmunization secondary to transfusion may be an underestimate.

Although the generation of new anti-RBC autoantibodies can have a strong temporal association to antecedent RBC transfusion, such observations constitute only a correlation and do not establish causality. Moreover, as transfusion recipients clearly have an underlying pathology that necessitates the transfusion in the first place, it is practically impossible to isolate the transfusion as the only variable. However, several settings do allow independent investigation of the role of transfusions on autoantibody development. For example, normal Rh-negative volunteers can be transfused with Rh-positive blood to generate a source of anti-Rh immunoglobulin.[17] In one study involving 34 volunteers, two participants developed a positive DAT on their own RBCs during the immunization protocol.[17] No clinical hemolysis was observed in these two individuals, but RBC survival studies that could detect low-level hemolysis were not carried out. Additionally, in an animal model of transfusion-induced AIHA, repeated transfusion of xenogeneic RBCs (rat into mouse) results in the generation of autoantibodies.[67] Taken together, these observations indicate that generation of autoantibodies can be a direct sequelae of transfusion of RBCs.

Mechanisms of Autoimmunization by Transfusion

The mechanisms by which allogeneic RBC transfusion induces an anti-RBC autoantibody are undetermined. However, as with the development of spontaneous autoantibodies, it is likely that several mechanisms are involved. First, any of the aforementioned immunologic perturbations involving loss of tolerance, which may contribute to the spontaneous generation of AIHA, may also contribute to transfusion-associated AIHA. However, in addition to the general breakdown of immune tolerance, several mechanisms unique to transfusion-induced AIHA require special mention here.

Linked Recognition of Foreign T-Cell Epitopes and Self B-Cell Epitopes

One detriment of the human immune system's use of linked recognition of T-cell and B-cell epitopes is that slightly altered self-antigens run a considerable risk for inducing humoral autoimmunity. For example, there are cases in which, although thymic education is complete, some B cells with immunoglobulins that recognize self-antigens persist. This appears to be the case for B cells specific for RBC antigens.[54,55] When these autoreactive B cells encounter the antigen recognized by their rearranged immunoglobulins, the antigen is phagocytosed and peptides from that antigen are presented on class II MHC molecules of the B cell. In this scenario, because all T cells that are capable of recognizing such peptide–MHC complexes have been deleted in the thymus, humoral tolerance is maintained. However, this mechanism of tolerance fails if the self-protein recognized by an autoreactive B cell has a foreign T-cell epitope attached to it. In this setting, the B cell now presents a foreign peptide–class II MHC epitope and receives the help required to differentiate into an antibody-secreting plasma cell. Thus, the linkage of a foreign T-cell epitope to a self B-cell epitope may result in humoral autoimmunity.

For such a mechanism to have physiologic relevance, one must ask in what situations would the immune system encounter a self B-cell epitope linked to a foreign T-cell epitope. One scenario is the exposure to foreign human tissues during transfusion. Many genes have numerous allelic variants throughout the human population. This is perhaps best demonstrated in the extensive catalog of human blood group antigens that have now been described. Although the described allelic variations of blood group antigens have been predominantly detected serologically, and are thus best known as B-cell epitopes, they can also serve as T-cell epitopes if the HLA of a given individual can present peptides containing the amino acid variation. Moreover, there may be a considerable number of polymorphisms that do not alter B-cell epitopes and have thus not been detected serologically, but can still constitute a variant of a T-cell epitope presented by class II MHC molecules. For example, a donor and recipient may both be positive for the Rh D epitope. However, the donor may have an amino acid difference in an internal portion of the Rh molecule. If the peptide containing this variation can be presented by the recipient HLA, then this constitutes the linkage of a foreign T-cell epitope to a self B-cell epitope. This is precisely the situation in which T-cell tolerance would be circumvented. This mechanism is hypothetical in the context of RBC transfusion and has not been formally tested. However, it is consistent with well-established experimental immunology in which linkage of foreign T-cell epitopes to self B-cell epitopes can lead to autoantibodies.[68]

"Autoantibodies" of Donor Origin: RBC-Specific Humoral Graft-versus-Host Disease

When an individual's immune system generates antibodies against their own tissue, it is generally assumed that their own B cells are the origin of the antibody. However, transfusion of blood results in the introduction of foreign B cells into the recipient. Because transfused leukocytes have the capacity to proliferate, transfusion of very few cells can be sufficient to generate a chimeric state. Indeed, it has been reported that even in the case of leukoreduced blood, sufficient leukocytes are transfused to cause microchimerism in some patients.[69] Thus, transfusion of RBCs introduces donor lymphocytes into the recipient immune system.

Aside from special populations at risk for transfusion-associated graft-versus-host disease (GVHD), including immunosuppressed patients and related individuals, the clinical consequences of transfusing foreign leukocytes are seldom significant. Transfusion of nonleukoreduced blood is routinely performed without any observable negative consequences. However, there are exceptions. It has been reported that in one patient transfusion-associated anti-RBC "autoantibodies" had immunoglobulin allotypes that were not part of the patient's genome.[70] Although one cannot rule out the possibility of spontaneous mutation of a patient's allotypes, the most likely explanation is that the antibodies were produced by B cells from a transfusion donor. A certain number of transfusion-associated anti-RBC autoantibodies may therefore not actually be "autoantibodies," but instead may be alloantibodies synthesized in situ by donor B cells, thus actually representing humoral GVHD.

Typically, transfused leukocytes are rejected by the recipient immune system as foreign. It is thus unclear why a transfused B cell would survive and differentiate into a plasma cell. In addition, it seems very unlikely that alloreactive B cells would be transfused, because the precursor frequency of donor B cells specific for recipient RBC antigens is expected to be low and relatively few B cells are transfused even in nonleukoreduced blood. However, it has been pointed out that up to 10% of transfusion donors were previously transfusion recipients.[71] In addition, any female who has carried a child may be alloimmunized to paternal RBC antigens. Given these facts, donor precursor frequencies of anti-RBC B cells may be higher than expected. Because these RBC-specific B cells would likely be memory cells, their activation requirements would be lower, which may make engraftment and antibody production more likely. The frequency by which this phenomenon occurs is undetermined.

CELLULAR IMMUNIZATION IN RESPONSE TO RBC TRANSFUSION

Typically and traditionally, clinical monitoring of immunization to RBCs is carried out by screening for antibodies that are detected by an agglutination reaction. This process of mounting an antibody response to transfused RBCs is known to involve activation and differentiation of $CD4^+$ helper T cells that recognize peptides from RBC antigens presented on class II MHC molecules of the recipient's APCs. The activated helper T cells then give the required signals to antigen-specific B cells to allow differentiation into antibody-secreting plasma cells.

However, in addition to helper T cells, it has also been appreciated that transfusion of blood products can result in the generation of class I MHC-restricted $CD8^+$ T cells with lytic activity. Except in exceptionally rare cases of autoimmunity, cellular immunity is not known to be capable of contributing to hemolysis of transfused RBCs.[72] Nonetheless, to the extent that multiply transfused patients ultimately receive bone marrow or organ transplants, the generation of cellular immunity is relevant in that it can contribute to subsequent transplant rejection.

Traditionally, units of packed RBCs have not been stringently leukoreduced. This results in the transfusion of a small but significant number of leukocytes of donor origin. Because leukocytes express class I MHC and can also serve as APCs, direct alloimmunization to donor MHC molecules results in activation of recipient T cells specific for donor human leukocyte antigens (HLAs). This can contribute to rejection of donor organs and bone marrow if they share the same HLA.

The widespread implementation of leukoreduction filters for units of RBCs has significantly limited the exposure of transfusion recipients to donor leukocytes. Because human RBCs do not express MHC (with the possible exception of the Bg blood group), direct alloimmunization of recipient T cells is highly unlikely. However, it has been reported that minor histocompatibility antigens on donor RBCs are efficiently crosspresented into the class I MHC of recipient APCs.[30] This results in expansion of recipient $CD8^+$ T cells specific for the minor histocompatibility antigen. In the context of transplantation of HLA-matched tissues, this immunization to minor histocompatibility antigens may contribute to rejection if the organ donor and transfusion donor have the same minor histocompatibility antigens. Thus, although leukoreduction of blood products may significantly decrease rates of alloimmunization to major histocompatibility antigens, transfusion of RBCs themselves has the potential to immunize against minor histocompatibility antigens. As previously discussed, this has little relevance to transfusion, because cellular responses do not typically lyse RBCs. However, it is relevant in the setting of the patient receiving transfusions as support prior to transplantation.

BASIC SCIENCE OF RBC DESTRUCTION

Nonimmunologic Mechanisms of Hemolysis

Hemolysis of transfused RBCs is the major sequelae prevented by crossmatching blood prior to transfusion. Despite this precaution, occasionally one observes the hemolysis of crossmatch-compatible blood. In some cases, hemolysis of crossmatch-compatible blood is an immune-mediated mechanism that involves undetected antibodies. However, mechanisms exist by which transfused RBCs can be hemolyzed in the absence of an alloantibody.

To begin with, nonimmune-based physical factors can lead to hemolysis. For example, erythrocytes are highly sensitive to osmotic damage. Thus, if RBCs are transfused through an intravenous line that is simultaneously delivering hypotonic saline, direct lysis can occur. This can lead to massive hemolysis that presents clinically as an acute hemolytic transfusion reaction. Alternatively, RBC hemolysis can occur in the recipient due to nonantibody-based factors. For example, it has been reported that transfusion of RBCs from donors deficient in glucose-6-phosphate dehydrogenase can result in considerable hemolysis, especially in infants.[73–76]

There are also antibody-dependent mechanisms of RBC destruction that do not require antibody binding to the RBCs. For example, large-scale complement activation by immune complexes not associated with RBCs can lead to complement sensitization of nearby RBCs that leads to "bystander hemolysis" of RBCs not coated with antibodies.[77] In addition, cellular immunity can lead to hemolysis in rare settings, and it has been reported that natural killer cells can lyse RBCs in DAT-negative AIHA.[72]

Despite these nonimmunologic mechanisms of RBC destruction, one must take care not to mistakenly exclude antibody-mediated hemolysis on the basis of a negative antibody screen. Although an anti-RBC antibody is usually detectable with immune-mediated destruction of transfused RBCs, there are exceptions. It has been observed that Rh-positive RBCs have a decreased life span in Rh-negative individuals previously exposed to Rh-positive blood, even if no anti-Rh is detectable.[78] Such individuals typically proceed to generate detectable anti-Rh antibodies on subsequent transfusion with Rh-positive blood. Thus, there appears to be a level of anti-RBC antibody that is capable of causing hemolysis but is below the threshold of detection by agglutination-based assays. In addition, not all antibodies that bind RBCs in vivo are detected in vitro. Also, anamnestic responses may result in an initial negative screen followed by a delayed hemolysis and conversion to a positive screen.

Antibody-Mediated Hemolysis

Although certain antibodies, such as anti-A and anti-B IgM, cause rapid intravascular hemolysis through complement fixation, the majority of clinically significant anti-RBC antibodies lead to delayed hemolytic transfusion reactions, in which hemolysis occurs over a matter of days to weeks. In this process, RBCs are opsonized by IgG, which can be augmented by complement proteins and results in removal of the RBCs by cells of the reticuloendothelial system. This occurs in the extravascular space and is mediated predominantly by tissue macrophages in the spleen and liver. In addition to hemolysis as a result of RBC phagocytosis, RBCs can also be lysed by the direct release of lysosomal proteases.[77] However, in either case, the process is facilitated by anti-RBC immunoglobulin.

There has been considerable investigation into the isotype and subclass of antibodies involved in hemolysis of RBCs. The majority of this work has been performed in the setting of AIHA, but likely applies to hemolysis of incompatible transfusions as well. The predominant antibody involved in delayed hemolytic transfusion reaction is of the IgG type. The presence of IgG on the RBC surface effectively opsonizes the RBC through interaction with Fc receptors on phagocytic macrophages predominantly in the spleen and liver. Although anti-RBC IgM typically results in complement-mediated intravascular hemolysis, IgM has been reported to promote a delayed hemolytic reaction in some settings.[77] This likely occurs through deposition of complement proteins on the RBC surface, which opsonizes RBCs via complement receptors on macrophages, because macrophages do not express IgM-binding Fc receptors. In support of this notion, it has been reported that IgM-coated RBCs have a normal life span in humans with complement deficiencies.[77] Although very uncommon, isolated anti-RBC IgA molecules have also been reported in patients with hemolysis.[77] However, the conclusion that the IgA is responsible for hemolysis in this setting is predicated on the assumption that no IgG was present. As it has been shown that the level of IgG necessary to induce hemolysis can be below the level of detection by standard anti-RBC IgG assays, the legitimacy of this assumption is unclear.

The potential of different IgG subclasses to induce hemolysis has been studied in both humans and mice. Several groups have performed large-scale analysis of DAT-positive patients with or without clinically evident AIHA in an attempt to identify the IgG subclass dependence of hemolysis.[79–82] Garratty performed an in-depth comparison of IgG subclasses involved in DAT-positive individuals with or without AIHA.[82] This analysis of 78 patients showed IgG1 to be the sole IgG subclass present in the majority of AIHA cases. However, IgG1 was also found on 72% of patients without clinical AIHA, and the presence of IgG1 does not predict whether a DAT-positive individual will experience hemolysis. In an analysis of 304 patients, Sokol and colleagues reported similar findings, with anti-RBC IgG1 present in 98% of cases and IgG1 as the sole subclass in 64% of cases.[80] A smaller analysis of 34 patients also had similar findings concerning the predominance of IgG1.[80] Garratty's analysis also demonstrated that some patients had IgG2 alone or IgG3 alone, but that neither was more prevalent in patients with AIHA compared with patients with no hemolysis. Isolated IgG4 was found only in five normal blood donors and none of the AIHA patients analyzed.

The above findings demonstrate that although IgG1 is the most common anti-RBC IgG subclass, isolated IgG1, IgG2, and IgG3 can lead to hemolysis. However, the detection of an isolated IgG subclass does not predict the likelihood of hemolysis. In contrast, the presence of multiple simultaneous subclasses clearly shows an increased risk for hemolysis.[82] Although this could represent a cooperativity of subclass, the presence of multiple IgG subclasses resulted in a larger amount of overall IgG on the RBC surface.[80] Indeed, it has been reported that the overall quantity of IgG on the RBC surface predicts the likelihood of hemolysis in vivo.[77,79,80,83–87]

Considerable evidence exists suggesting that additional genetic and environmental factors may play a role in the question of IgG subclass and hemolysis. For instance, in contrast to the above conclusions, it has been reported that IgG3 is more potent than other subclasses at promoting RBC phagocytosis by monocytes,[88] and it has also been reported that AIHA with IgG3 involvement may be less responsive to treatment.[89] However, a direct comparison in the clearance of Rh-positive cells from Rh-negative volunteers given monoclonal anti-Rh of the IgG1 or IgG3 type showed that RBCs were cleared from IgG1 recipients at a significantly higher rate than in IgG3 recipients.[90] Interestingly, volunteers receiving IgG3 had a wide distribution of responses, with rapid clearance in some individuals and slow clearance in others. Subsequent studies by Kumpel and colleagues demonstrated that naturally occurring allelic variants in the FcγRIIIa receptor alter the efficiency with which IgG3-coated RBCs are cleared.[91] In addition, an animal model of IgG-induced hemolytic anemia demonstrated that concurrent viral infection significantly enhances disease with a hemolytic IgG2a antibody but not with a hemolytic IgG1 antibody due to an increase in erythrophagocytic capacity of macrophages.[92] Thus, genetic variation in accessory molecules other than IgG may alter the IgG subclass dependence of AIHA in different patient populations. Likewise, environmental factors and patient-specific pathology that leads to inflammation and macrophage activation may significantly affect hemolysis by RBC-binding antibodies.

Although animal models are biologically distinct from human physiology, they represent a setting in which highly controlled studies can be carried out on genetically identical subjects in a controlled environment. Izui and colleagues and others have made extensive use of a murine model of AIHA to dissect out the biology of IgG-mediated RBC hemolysis.[92–98] In this model system, both high-affinity and low-affinity monoclonal antibodies against the RBC autoantigen have been isolated. Similar to human IgG-mediated hemolysis, complement does not appear to be required for RBC removal in the murine model, because hemolytic anemia still occurs in mice lacking C5 or C3.[93] However, both Fc receptor-dependent phagocytosis (mostly in the liver) and RBC sequestration of RBCs (mostly in the spleen) contribute to decreased hematocrit in response to autoantibodies.[93]

To control for intrinsic differences in the epitope specificity and affinity of different monoclonal antibodies, recombinant genetics have been employed to create artificial monoclonal antibodies of each murine IgG subclass that have precisely the same epitope-binding domains. IgG1, IgG2a, and IgG2b were each hemolytic, whereas IgG3 did not promote significant hemolysis.[96] IgG2a was 20 to 100 times more potent in inducing hemolysis than IgG1 or IgG2b. Gene deletion studies demonstrated that the FcγRIII receptor was responsible for hemolysis by IgG1, whereas both FcγRI and FcγRIII were involved in hemolysis by IgG2a and IgG2b. FcγRIIB did not appear to contribute to hemolysis, consistent with its generally understood role as an inhibitory molecule. Recently, a new FcγR has been identified (FcγRIV), which binds both IgG2a and IgG2b and can contribute to antibody-mediated thrombocytopenia.[99] The role of FcγRIV has not yet been formally tested in antibody-mediated hemolysis.

Antibody-Induced Antigen Loss/Suppression

Although many anti-RBC antibodies can result in either intravascular or extravascular hemolysis of the RBCs that they bind, hemolysis is not the inevitable result of antibody binding. There are certainly a considerable number of individuals who have strongly positive DATs without hemolysis. Moreover, numerous antibodies have been described against "clinically insignificant" blood group antigens for which crossmatch-incompatible blood can be transfused without ill effect. Additionally, there is a somewhat obscure (but well described) phenomenon in which the RBC phenotype will convert from positive to negative for a given antigen after encountering immunoglobulins that bind to the antigen. This phenomenon has been referred to as weakened antigenicity, antigen reduction, antigen suppression, or acquired loss and has been reported to occur for many blood group antigens, including Rh (D and e), Kell, Kidd, Duffy, Lutheran, LW, Co, Ge, En(a), AnWj, and Sc1.[77,100–112]

Although the mechanisms of antigen loss have not been fully elucidated, publications documenting the phenomenon have proposed a number of possible explanations. It has been suggested that the antibodies to a given RBC antigen are toxic to newly formed RBCs and that the presence of such antibodies alters hematopoiesis such that only antigen-negative RBCs escape the marrow intact.[102,105] However, this proposed mechanism cannot account for the observation that antigen loss can also be seen in the setting of transfusion of crossmatch-incompatible RBCs, which have already synthesized the antigen being recognized.[101,107] It has also been suggested that antigens might be lost due to factors other than immunoglobulins, such as destruction by microbial enzymes. However, suppression of antigen correlates more with the presence of antibody and, in most cases, antigen suppression does not involve a documented infection. Nonetheless, the presence of subclinical infections cannot be ruled out. It has also been suggested that antibody binding results in the shedding of antigen from mature erythrocytes through formation of antigen–antibody immune complexes.[102]

Insights into the mechanisms of antibody-induced antigen loss have been gained from an animal model of this phenomenon. It has been reported that presynthesized antigen is shed from transfused RBCs while leaving the RBC intact and without decreasing circulatory life span.[113] This process requires the presence of both IgG and FcγRIII, but it occurs normally in splenectomized animals. Thus, in this animal model, antigen loss involves neither bone marrow suppression of RBC antigen synthesis nor microbial destruction. In contrast, antigen appears to be lost through interactions between RBCs coated with IgG and FcγRIII-bearing cells. However, the exact mechanism in humans remains to be determined, and antigen loss may occur as a result of distinct mechanisms in different settings.

It is unclear why mechanisms that result in antibody-induced antigen loss may evolve. In this context, it is worth noting that biological mechanisms have been described by which RBCs shed whole antigens as part of normal RBC biology. CD35, which is also known as the CR1 complement receptor and the Knops blood group antigen, is a receptor for the C3b fragment of complement.[114] In what has been termed the *immune-adherence phenomenon,* circulating immune complexes or antibody-bound bacteria bind to RBCs via interactions of CD35 on RBC and C3b on the immune complex.[115,116] When a RBC encounters hepatic macrophages, the immune complex is transferred to the phagocyte. Like antibody-induced antigen loss, RBCs delivering immune complexes to macrophages lose their CD35 surface antigen but are not destroyed.[117–119] Because this process appears to depend on the Fc portion of the antibodies, interactions with Fc receptors may also be involved.[120] Furthermore, because immune complex transfer occurs in the liver,[120,121] an intact spleen is presumably not required. Whether loss of CD35 is due to complete removal of the molecule or due to proteolytic fragmentation by Fc-bearing cells is unresolved. However, it has been demonstrated that no residual cytoplasmic domain of CD35 remains after loss of CD35 from podocytes during immune complex–based pathophysiology of lupus, a situation that resembles CD35 loss from RBC delivering immune complexes to phagocytes.[122] Thus, despite the fact that CD35 is a transmembrane protein, complete extrusion of the CD35 molecule seems a distinct possibility. Overall, the natural process of RBC-mediated delivery of immune complexes to the liver resembles antibody-mediated antigen loss in several regards and suggests that antibody-induced antigen loss may be functioning through existing pathways that evolved to deliver immune complexes to hepatic macrophages.

REFERENCES

1. Heddle NM, Soutar RL, O'Hoski PL, et al. A prospective study to determine the frequency and clinical significance of alloimmunization post-transfusion. Br J Haematol 1995;91:1000–1005.
2. Hoeltge GA Domen RE, Rybicki LA, Schaffer PA. Multiple red cell transfusions and alloimmunization. Experience with 6996 antibodies detected in a total of 159,262 patients from 1985 to 1993. Arch Pathol Lab Med 1995;119:42–45.
3. Seyfried H, Walewska I. Analysis of immune response to red blood cell antigens in multitransfused patients with different diseases. Materia Medica Polona 1990;22:21–25.
4. Blumberg N Peck K, Ross K, Avila E. Immune response to chronic red blood cell transfusion. Vox Sang 1983;44:212–217.
5. Rosse WF. Gallagher D, Kinney TR, et al. Transfusion and alloimmunization in sickle cell disease. The Cooperative Study of Sickle Cell Disease. Blood 1990;76:1431–1437.
6. Aygun B, Padmanabhan S, Paley C, Chandrasekaran V. Clinical significance of RBC alloantibodies and autoantibodies in sickle cell patients who received transfusions. Transfusion 2002;42:37–43.
7. Garratty G. Severe reactions associated with transfusion of patients with sickle cell disease. Transfusion 1997;37:357–361.
8. Issitt PD, Combs MR, Bumgarner DJ, et al. Studies of antibodies in the sera of patients who have made red cell autoantibodies. Transfusion 1996;36:481–486.
9. Leger RM, Garratty G. Evaluation of methods for detecting alloantibodies underlying warm autoantibodies. Transfusion 1999;39:11–16.
10. Branch DR Petz LD. Detecting alloantibodies in patients with autoantibodies.. Transfusion 1999;39:6–10.
11. Stiegler G, Sperr W, Lorber C, et al. Red cell antibodies in frequently transfused patients with myelodysplastic syndrome. Ann Hematol 2001;80:330–333.
12. Novaretti MC, Sopelete CR, Velloso ER, et al. Immunohematological findings in myelodysplastic syndrome. Acta Haematol 2001;105:1–6.

13. Lostumbo MM, Holland PV, Schmidt PJ. Isoimmunization after multiple transfusions. N Engl J Med 1966;275:141–144.
14. Schonewille H, Haak HL, van Zijl AM. Alloimmunization after blood transfusion in patients with hematologic and oncologic diseases. Transfusion 1999;39:763–771.
15. Blumberg N, Heal JM,Gettings KF. WBC reduction of RBC transfusions is associated with a decreased incidence of RBC alloimmunization. Transfusion 2003;43:945–952.
16. Frohn C, Dumbgen L, Brand JM, et al. Probability of anti-D development in D– patients receiving D+ RBCs. Transfusion 2003;43:893–898.
17. Cook IA. Primary rhesus immunization of male volunteers. Br J Haematol 1971;20:369–375.
18. Freda VJ, Gorman JG, Pollack W, et al. Prevention of Rh isoimmunization. Progress report of the clinical trial in mothers. JAMA 1967;199:390–394.
19. Gunson HH, Stratton F, Cooper DG, Rawlinson VI. Primary immunization of Rh-negative volunteers. BMJ 1970;1:593–595.
20. Hattersley P. Two popular fallacies regarding Rh. J Lab Clin Med 1947;32:423.
21. Waller RK. Intentional isoimmunizations against the antigen D(Rh_0). J of Lab Clin Med 1949;34:270.
22. Wiener AS. Further observations on isosensitization to the Rh factor. Proc Soc Exper Biol Med 1949;70:576.
23. Clarke CA, Donohoe WT, Mc C R, et al. Further experimental studies on the prevention of Rh haemolytic disease. BMJ 1963;5336:979.
24. Azar MM, Wyche AA. Route of antigen administration for tolerance production. Life Sciences 1974;14:2151–2157.
25. Endres RO, Grey HM. Antigen recognition by T cells. II. Intravenous administration of native or denatured ovalbumin results in tolerance to both forms of the antigen. J Immunol 1980;125:1521–1525.
26. Weigle WO. Immunological unresponsiveness. Adv Immunol 1973; 16:61–122.
27. Magnani M, Chiarantini L, Vittoria E, et al. Red blood cells as an antigen-delivery system. Biotech Appl Biochem 1992;16:188–194.
28. Dominici S, Laguardia ME, Serafini G, et al. Red blood cell-mediated delivery of recombinant HIV-1 Tat protein in mice induces anti-Tat neutralizing antibodies and CTL. Vaccine 2003;21:2073–2081.
29. Zimring JC, Hair GA, Anderson KM, et al. Use of red blood cells as a vaccine vector to induce humoral and cellular immunity. Transfusion 2005;45S:24A.
30. Zimring JC, Hair GA, Deshpande SS, Horan JT. Immunization to minor histocompatibility antigens on transfused RBC through crosspriming into recipient MHC class I pathways. Blood 2005;107:187–189.
31. Matzinger P. The danger model: a renewed sense of self. Science 2002;296:301–305.
32. Matzinger P. Tolerance, danger, and the extended family. Annu Rev Immunol 1994;12:991–1045.
33. Akira S, Takeda K. Toll-like receptor signalling. Nature Rev Immunol 2004;4:499–511.
34. Takeda K, Kaisho T, Akira S. Toll-like receptors. Annu Rev Immunol 2003;21:335–376.
35. Imler JL, Hoffmann JA. Toll and Toll-like proteins: An ancient family of receptors signaling infection. Rev Immunogenetics 2000;2:294–304.
36. Murillo LS, Morre SA, Pena AS. Toll-like receptors and NOD/CARD proteins: Pattern recognition receptors are key elements in the regulation of immune response. Drug Today 2003;39:415–438.
37. Modlin RL. Mammalian Toll-like receptors. Ann Allergy Asthma Immunol 2002;88:543–547.
38. Mollinson PL, Engelfriet CP, Contreras M. Blood Transfusion in Clinical Medicine. Oxford, Blackwell Science, 1997, pp 288–291.
39. Mitchison NA. Induction of immunological paralysis in two zones of dosage. Proc R Soc Lond B Biol Sci 1964;161:275–292.
40. Ciurea A, Hunziker L, Klenerman P, et al. Impairment of $CD4^+$ T cell responses during chronic virus infection prevents neutralizing antibody responses against virus escape mutants. J Experiment Med 2001;193:297–305.
41. Fuller MJ, Zajac AJ. Ablation of CD8 and CD4 T cell responses by high viral loads. J Immunol 2003;170:477–486.
42. Singh NJ, Schwartz RH. The strength of persistent antigenic stimulation modulates adaptive tolerance in peripheral CD4+ T cells. J Experiment Med 2003;198:1107–1117.
43. Delemarre FG, Kors N, van Rooijen N. Elimination of spleen and of lymph node macrophages and its difference in the effect on the immune response to particulate antigens. Immunobiol 1990;182:70–78.
44. Trombetta ES, Mellman I. Cell biology of antigen processing in vitro and in vivo. Annu Rev Immunol 2005;23:975–1028.
45. Guermonprez P, Valladeau J, Zitvogel L, et al. Antigen presentation and T cell stimulation by dendritic cells. Annu Rev Immunol 2002;20:621–667.
46. Mond JJ, Lees A, Snapper CM. T cell-independent antigens type 2. Annu Rev Immunol 1995;13:655–692.
47. Boctor FN, Ali NM, Mohandas K, Uehlinger J. Absence of D-alloimmunization in AIDS patients receiving D-mismatched RBCs. Transfusion 2003;43:173–176.
48. Perry FE, Barker RN, Mazza G, et al. Autoreactive T cell specificity in autoimmune hemolytic anemia of the NZB mouse. Eur J Immunol 1996;26:136–141.
49. Hall AM, Vickers MA, McLeod E, Barker RN. Rh autoantigen presentation to helper T cells in chronic lymphocytic leukemia by malignant B cells. Blood 2005;105:2007–2015.
50. Watanabe N, Ikuta K, Fagarasan S, et al. Migration and differentiation of autoreactive B-1 cells induced by activated γ/δ T cells in antierythrocyte immunoglobulin transgenic mice. J Experiment Med 2000;192:1577–1586.
51. Goodnow CC, Crosbie J, Adelstein S, et al. Altered immunoglobulin expression and functional silencing of self-reactive B lymphocytes in transgenic mice. Nature 1988;334:676–682.
52. Hartley SB, Crosbie J, Brink R, et al. Elimination from peripheral lymphoid tissues of self-reactive B lymphocytes recognizing membrane-bound antigens. Nature 1991;353:765–769.
53. Hartley SB, Cooke MP, Fulcher DA, et al. Elimination of self-reactive B lymphocytes proceeds in two stages: Arrested development and cell death. Cell 1993;72:325–335.
54. Okamoto M, Murakami M, Shimizu A, et al. A transgenic model of autoimmune hemolytic anemia. J Experiment Med 1992;175:71–79.
55. Murakami M, Nakajima K, Yamazaki K, et al. Effects of breeding environments on generation and activation of autoreactive B-1 cells in anti-red blood cell autoantibody transgenic mice. J Experiment Med 1997;185:791–794.
56. Stellrecht KA, Vella AT. Evidence for polyclonal B cell activation as the mechanism for LCMV-induced autoimmune hemolytic anemia. Immunol Lett 1992;31:273–277.
57. De Rossi G, Granati L, Girelli G, et al. Incidence and prognostic significance of autoantibodies against erythrocytes and platelets in chronic lymphocytic leukemia (CLL). Nouv Rev Franc Hematol 1988;30:403–406.
58. Roelcke D. Cold agglutination. Transfus Med Rev 1989;3:140–166.
59. Fagiolo E. Immunological tolerance loss vs. erythrocyte self antigens and cytokine network disregulation in autoimmune hemolytic anaemia. Autoimmunity Rev 2004;3:53–59.
60. Toriani-Terenzi C, Fagiolo E. Th2 cytokine role in autoimmune haemolytic anaemia (AIHA) pathogenesis. Panminerva Medica 2001;43:1–5.
61. Mqadmi A, Zheng X, Yazdanbakhsh K. CD4+CD25+ regulatory T cells control induction of autoimmune hemolytic anemia. Blood 2005;105:3746–3748.
62. Barker RN, Elson CJ. Multiple self epitopes on the Rhesus polypeptides stimulate immunologically ignorant human T cells in vitro. Eur J Immunol 1994;24:1578–1582.
63. Fagiolo E, Toriani-Terenzi C. Mechanisms of immunological tolerance loss versus erythrocyte self-antigens and autoimmune hemolytic anemia. Autoimmunity 2003;36:199–204.
64. Barker RN, Hall AM, Standen GR, et al. Identification of T-cell epitopes on the Rhesus polypeptides in autoimmune hemolytic anemia. Blood 1997;90:2701–2715.
65. Elson CJ, Barker RN, Thompson SJ, Williams NA. Immunologically ignorant autoreactive T cells, epitope spreading and repertoire limitation. Immunol Today 1995;16:71–76.
66. Young PP, Uzieblo A, Trulock E, et al. Autoantibody formation after alloimmunization: Are blood transfusions a risk factor for autoimmune hemolytic anemia? [see comment]. Transfusion 2004;44:67–72.
67. Cox KO, Keast D. Erythrocyte autoantibodies induced in mice immunized with rat erythrocytes. Immunol 1973;25:531–539.
68. Dalum I, Jensen MR, Hindersson P, et al. Breaking of B cell tolerance toward a highly conserved self protein. J Immunol 1996;157:4796–4804.
69. Lee TH, Paglieroni T, Utter GH, et al. High-level long-term white blood cell microchimerism after transfusion of leukoreduced blood components to patients resuscitated after severe traumatic injury. Transfusion 2005;45:1280–1290.
70. Ishikura H, Endo J, Saito Y, et al. Graft-versus-host antibody reaction causing a delayed hemolytic anemia after blood transfusion. Blood 1993;82:3222–3223.
71. Garratty G. Autoantibodies induced by blood transfusion [comment]. Transfusion 2004;44:5–9.
72. Gilsanz F, De La Serna J, Molto L, Alvarez-Mon M. Hemolytic anemia in chronic large granular lymphocytic leukemia of natural killer cells: Cytotoxicity of natural killer cells against autologous red cells is associated with hemolysis. Transfusion 1996;36:463–466.

73. Kumar P, Sarkar S, Narang A. Acute intravascular haemolysis following exchange transfusion with G-6-PD deficient blood. Eur J Pediatr 1994;153:98–99.
74. Mimouni F, Shohat S, Reisner SH. G6PD-deficient donor blood as a cause of hemolysis in two preterm infants. Isr J Medical Sci 1986;22:120–122.
75. Gulati S, Singh S, Narang A, Bhakoo ON. Exchange transfusion with G-6-PD deficient donor blood causes exaggeration of neonatal hyperbilirubinemia. Ind Pediatr 1989;26:499–501.
76. Shalev O, Bogomolski-Yahalom V, Sharon R. Hemolysis following transfusion of erythrocytes from a donor with G6PD deficiency and beta-thalassemia minor. Isr J Medical Sci 1993;29:214–216.
77. Petz LD, Garratty G. Immune Hemolytic Anemias. Philadelphia, Churchill Livingstone, 2004.
78. Petz LD, Swisher SN, Kleinman S, et al. Clinical Practice of Transfusion Medicine. New York, Churchill Livingstone, 1996, p 42.
79. Dubarry M, Charron C, Habibi B, et al. Quantitation of immunoglobulin classes and subclasses of autoantibodies bound to red cells in patients with and without hemolysis. Transfusion 1993;33:466–471.
80. Sokol RJ, Hewitt S, Booker DJ, Bailey A. Erythrocyte autoantibodies, subclasses of IgG and autoimmune haemolysis. Autoimmunity 1990;6:99–104.
81. Sokol RJ, Hewitt S, Booker DJ, Bailey A. Red cell autoantibodies, multiple immunoglobulin classes, and autoimmune hemolysis. Transfusion 1990;30:714–717.
82. Garratty G. Factors affecting the pathogenicity of red cell auto- and alloantibodies: immune destruction of red blood cells. Arlington, Va., American Association of Blood Banks, 1989.
83. Lynen R, Neuhaus R, Schwarz DW. Flow cytometric analyses of the subclasses of red cell IgG antibodies. Vox Sang 1995;69:126–130.
84. Garratty G, Nance SJ. Correlation between in vivo hemolysis and the amount of red cell-bound IgG measured by flow cytometry. Transfusion 1990;30:617–621.
85. Merry AH, Thomson EE, Rawlinson VI, Stratton F. Quantitation of IgG on erythrocytes: Correlation of number of IgG molecules per cell with the strength of the direct and indirect antiglobulin tests. Vox Sang 1984;47:73–81.
86. Merry AH, Thomson EE, Rawlinson VI, Stratton F. A quantitative antiglobulin test for IgG for use in blood transfusion serology. Clin Lab Haematol 1982;4:393–402.
87. van der Meulen FW, de Bruin HG, Goosen PC, et al. Quantitative aspects of the destruction of red cells sensitized with IgG1 autoantibodies: an application of flow cytofluorometry. Br J Haematol 1980;46:47–56.
88. Zupanska B, Brojer E, Thomson EE, et al. Monocyte–erythrocyte interaction in autoimmune haemolytic anaemia in relation to the number of erythrocyte-bound IgG molecules and subclass specificity of autoantibodies. Vox Sang 1987;52:212–218.
89. Li Z, Shao Z, Xu Y, et al. Subclasses of warm autoantibody IgG in patients with autoimmune hemolytic anemia and their clinical implications. Chin Medical J 1999;112:805–808.
90. Kumpel BM, Goodrick MJ, Pamphilon DH, et al. Human Rh D monoclonal antibodies (BRAD-3 and BRAD-5) cause accelerated clearance of Rh D+ red blood cells and suppression of Rh D immunization in Rh D− volunteers. Blood 1995;86:1701–1709.
91. Kumpel BM, De Haas M, Koene HR, et al. Clearance of red cells by monoclonal IgG3 anti-D in vivo is affected by the VF polymorphism of Fcγ RIIIa (CD16). Clin Exper Immunol 2003;132:81–86.
92. Meite M, Leonard S, Idrissi ME, et al. Exacerbation of autoantibody-mediated hemolytic anemia by viral infection. J Virol 2000;74:6045–6049.
93. Shibata T, Berney T, Reininger L, et al. Monoclonal anti-erythrocyte autoantibodies derived from NZB mice cause autoimmune hemolytic anemia by two distinct pathogenic mechanisms. Int Immunol 1990;2:1133–1141.
94. Azeredo da Silveira S, Kikuchi S, Fossati-Jimack L, et al. Complement activation selectively potentiates the pathogenicity of the IgG2b and IgG3 isotypes of a high affinity anti-erythrocyte autoantibody. J Exper Med 2002;195:665–672.
95. Fossati-Jimack L, Reininger L, Chicheportiche Y, et al. High pathogenic potential of low-affinity autoantibodies in experimental autoimmune hemolytic anemia. J Exper Med 1999;190:1689–1696.
96. Fossati-Jimack L, Ioan-Facsinay A, Reininger L, et al. Markedly different pathogenicity of four immunoglobulin G isotype-switch variants of an antierythrocyte autoantibody is based on their capacity to interact in vivo with the low-affinity Fcγ receptor III. J Experiment Med 2000;191:1293–1302.
97. Izui S, Fossati-Jimack L, da Silveira SA, Moll T. Isotype-dependent pathogenicity of autoantibodies: analysis in experimental autoimmune hemolytic anemia. Springer Semin Immunopathol 2001;23:433–445.
98. Meyer D, Schiller C, Westermann J, et al. FcγRIII (CD16)-deficient mice show IgG isotype-dependent protection to experimental autoimmune hemolytic anemia. Blood 1998;92:3997–4002.
99. Nimmerjahn F, Bruhns P, Horiuchi K, Ravetch JV. FcγRIV: A novel FcR with distinct IgG subclass specificity. Immunity 2005;23:41–45.
100. Beck ML, Marsh WL, Pierce SR, et al. Auto anti-Kpb associated with weakened antigenicity in the Kell blood group system: A second example. Transfusion 1979;19:197–202.
101. Brendel WL, Issitt PD, Moore RE, et al. Temporary reduction of red cell Kell system antigen expression and transient production of anti-Kpb in a surgical patient. Biotest Bull 1985;2:201–206.
102. Williamson LM, Poole J, Redman C, et al. Transient loss of proteins carrying Kell and Lutheran red cell antigens during consecutive relapses of autoimmune thrombocytopenia. Br J Haematol 1994;87:805–812.
103. Seyfried H, Gorska B, Maj S, et al. Apparent depression of antigens of the Kell blood group system associated with autoimmune acquired haemolytic anaemia. Vox Sang 1972;23:528–536.
104. Puig N, Carbonell F, Marty ML. Another example of mimicking anti-Kpb in a Kp(a+b−) patient. Vox Sang 1986;51:57–59.
105. Marsh WL, Oyen R, Alicea E, et al. Autoimmune hemolytic anemia and the Kell blood groups. Am J Hematol 1979;7:155–162.
106. Manny N, Levene C, Sela R, et al. Autoimmunity and the Kell blood groups: Auto-anti-Kpb in a Kp(a+b-) patient. Vox Sang 1983;45:252–256.
107. Vengelen-Tyler V, Gonzalez B, Garratty G, et al. Acquired loss of red cell Kell antigens. Br J Haematol 1987;65:231–234.
108. Koscielak J. Session on blood group substances and red cell membrane receptors. Vox Sang 1980;39:289.
109. Issitt PD, Gruppo RA, Wilkinson SL, Issitt CH. Atypical presentation of acute phase, antibody-induced haemolytic anaemia in an infant. Br J Haematol 1982;52:537–543.
110. Ganly PS, Laffan MA, Owen I, Hows JM. Auto-anti-Jka in Evans' syndrome with negative direct antiglobulin test. Br J Haematol 1988; 69:537–539.
111. Issitt PD, Obarski G, Hartnett PL, et al. Temporary suppression of Kidd system antigen expression accompanied by transient production of anti-Jk3. Transfusion 1990;30:46–50.
112. Garratty G. Target antigens for red-cell-bound autoantibodies. In Nance SJ (ed). Clinical and Basic Science Aspects of Immunohematology. Arlington, Va., American Association of Blood Banks, 1991, p 33–72.
113. Zimring JC, Hair GA, Chadwick TE, et al. Nonhemolytic antibody-induced loss of erythrocyte surface antigen. Blood 2005;106:1105–1112.
114. Fearon DT. Identification of the membrane glycoprotein that is the C3b receptor of the human erythrocyte, polymorphonuclear leukocyte, B lymphocyte, and monocyte. J Exper Med 1980;152:20–30.
115. Nelson RA Jr. The immune-adherence phenomenon: a hypothetical role of erythrocytes in defence against bacteria and viruses. Proc Royal Soc Med 1956;49:55–58.
116. Nelson RA Jr. The immune-adherence phenomenon: an immunologically specific reaction between microorganisms and erythrocytes leading to enhanced phagocytosis. Science 1953;118:733–737.
117. Cosio FG, Shen XP, Birmingham DJ, et al. Evaluation of the mechanisms responsible for the reduction in erythrocyte complement receptors when immune complexes form in vivo in primates. J Immunol 1990;145:4198–4206.
118. Cornacoff JB, Hebert LA, Smead WL, et al. Primate erythrocyte-immune complex-clearing mechanism. J Clin Invest 1983;71:236–247.
119. Davies KA, Hird V, Stewart S, et al. A study of in vivo immune complex formation and clearance in man. J Immunol 1990;144:4613–4626.
120. Nardin A, Lindorfer MA, Taylor RP. How are immune complexes bound to the primate erythrocyte complement receptor transferred to acceptor phagocytic cells? Molec Immunol 1999;36:827–835.
121. Nardin A, Schlimgen R, Holers VM, Taylor RP. A prototype pathogen bound ex vivo to human erythrocyte complement receptor 1 via bispecific monoclonal antibody complexes is cleared to the liver in a mouse model. Eur J Immunol 1999;29:1581–1586.
122. Moll S, Miot S, Sadallah S, et al. No complement receptor 1 stumps on podocytes in human glomerulopathies. Kidney Int 2001;59:160–168.

ii. Red Blood Cell, Platelet, and Leukocyte Antigens and Antibodies

Chapter 5

Membrane Blood Group Antigens and Antibodies

Marion E. Reid • Connie M. Westhoff

Erythrocyte blood group antigens are polymorphic, inherited carbohydrate or protein structures located on the outside surface of the red blood cell (RBC) membrane. Our ability to detect and identify blood group antigens and antibodies has contributed significantly to the current safe, supportive blood transfusion practice and to the appropriate management of pregnancies at risk for hemolytic disease of the fetus and newborn (HDN). Exposure to erythrocytes carrying an antigen lacking on the RBCs of the recipient can elicit an immune response in some individuals. Thus, blood group antigens are clinically important in allogeneic blood transfusions, maternofetal blood group incompatibility, and organ transplantation.

By virtue of their relative ease of detection and generally straightforward mode of inheritance, blood group antigens have been used in genetic, forensic, and anthropologic investigations. The polymorphisms of blood groups have been exploited as a tool to monitor in vivo survival of transfused RBCs, to monitor engraftment of bone marrow transplants, and to monitor for blood doping by allogeneic transfusion in sports and athletics. Antigen profiles have been used to predict inheritance of diseases encoded by a gene in close proximity to the gene encoding the blood group antigen (e.g., the association of gene deletions causing chronic granulomatous disease with the loss of expression of Kell). Blood group antigens have also contributed to our understanding of cell membrane structure. The lack of Kell/Kx expression is associated with acanthocytes, Rh-deficient RBCs are stomatocytic, and mild elliptocytosis occurs in RBCs lacking Gerbich glycophorin C (GPC) and/or glycophorin D (GPD).

More recently, in the postgenomic era, knowledge about the molecular basis associated with blood group antigens and phenotypes is being applied to the detection of single nucleotide polymorphisms (SNPs) associated with blood group antigens. Microarray and microchip technologies hold promise for transfusion medicine testing.

This chapter reviews the scientific basis of molecules that express RBC blood group antigens and their relevance and application to the practice of transfusion medicine. One of the most important clinical concerns in contemporary transfusion medicine occurs with the discovery that a patient requiring transfusion has an unexpected blood group antibody. Although the laboratory can characterize an antibody in terms of specificity, immunoglobulin class, and in vitro characteristics, it cannot always predict the antibody's clinical significance. Therefore, when a blood group antibody is detected, an important, although often overlooked, first step is to review all available pertinent patient information (Table 5–1). One can then assess the potential for adverse effects by correlating the serologic information with the patient history and also with historical clinical experience in other patients. A patient who has not been exposed to RBCs by transfusion or pregnancy is unlikely to have a clinically significant alloantibody.

ERYTHROCYTE MEMBRANE

The erythrocyte membrane consists of lipids, proteins, and carbohydrates, which interact to form a dynamic and fluid structure. By dry weight, the ratio of protein-to-lipid-to-carbohydrate in the RBC membrane is 49:43:8. The RBC membrane behaves as a semisolid, with elastic and viscous properties that are not observed with simple lipid vesicles. These properties are critical for the RBC to survive in the circulation for approximately 120 days during numerous cycles (approximately 75,000) and passages through narrow veins and sinusoids in the spleen. The RBC accomplishes this goal without intracellular machinery to repair damage. The multiple connections between the membrane skeleton and the lipid bilayer cause the bilayer to follow the contours of the membrane skeleton. Together, the membrane skeleton and lipid bilayer give the erythrocyte shape and resilience.[1,2]

Lipids

The lipids in the RBC membrane form a bilayer, with the hydrophobic tails on the inside and the hydrophilic polar head groups to either the outside (extracellular) or the inside (cytoplasmic) surface (Fig. 5–1). The following three types of lipids occur in the RBC membrane: phospholipid (50%), cholesterol (40%), and glycolipids (10%). The arrangement

Table 5–1 Information for Problem-Solving in Immunohematology

Available Information	Considerations
Patient demographics	Diagnosis, age, sex, ethnicity, transfusion and/or pregnancy history, drugs, intravenous fluids (lactated Ringer's solution, IVIgG, antilymphocyte globulin), infections, malignancies, hemoglobinopathies, stem cell transplantation
Initial serologic results	ABO, Rh, direct antiglobulin test, phenotype, antibody detection, autologous control, crossmatch
Hematology/chemistry values	Hemoglobin, hematocrit, bilirubin, lactate dehydrogenase, reticulocyte count, haptoglobin, hemoglobinuria, albumin:globulin ratio, red blood cell (RBC) morphology
Sample characteristics	Site and technique of collection, age of sample, anticoagulant, hemolysis, lipemic, color of serum/plasma, agglutinates/aggregates in the sample
Other	Check records in current and previous institutions for antibodies to blood group antigens
Antibody identification	Autologous control, phase of reactivity, potentiator (saline, albumin, low-ionic-strength solution, polyethylene glycol), reaction strength, effect of chemicals on antigen (proteases, thiol reagents), pattern of reactivity (single antibody or mixture of antibodies), characteristics of reactivity (mixed field, rouleaux), hemolysis, preservatives/antibiotics in reagents, use of washed RBCs

of phospholipids in the bilayer is asymmetrical. The outer leaflet predominantly contains the neutral phospholipids (phosphatidylcholine and sphingomyelin), and the inner leaflet predominantly contains the aminophospholipids (phosphatidylethanolamine and phosphatidylserine). The presence of phosphatidylserine, which is negatively charged, on the inner monolayer results in a significant difference in charge between the two sides of the bilayer. The lipid molecules can diffuse rapidly within their own monolayer, but they rarely "flip-flop," maintaining membrane "sidedness."[1]

Proteins

Peripheral proteins form a meshwork under the lipid bilayer that is called the *membrane skeleton.* This name implies a relatively rigid structure; however, the meshwork is actually fluid and flexible. The RBC membrane skeleton is associated with the lipid bilayer through specific interactions with transmembrane proteins.

Specific protein components of the RBC membrane skeleton, which is associated with the inner leaflet of the lipid bilayer, interact with the cytoplasmic domains of some antigen-carrying transmembrane proteins.[3–5] Two major and well-defined interactions are ankyrin, which binds to spectrin in the membrane skeleton and the cytoplasmic domain of the multipass transmembrane protein, band 3 (anion exchanger, AE1),[6–14] and protein 4.1, which provides a link between spectrin, actin, and p55 in the membrane skeleton to the single-pass transmembrane proteins GPC and GPD.[15–22] Some integral transmembrane proteins interact with other transmembrane proteins, forming either small or large macromolecular complexes (e.g., glycophorin A (GPA) with glycophorin B (GPB)[2]; band 3 with GPA[23–27]; Kell with Kx[28,29]; RhD, RhCE, RhAG,

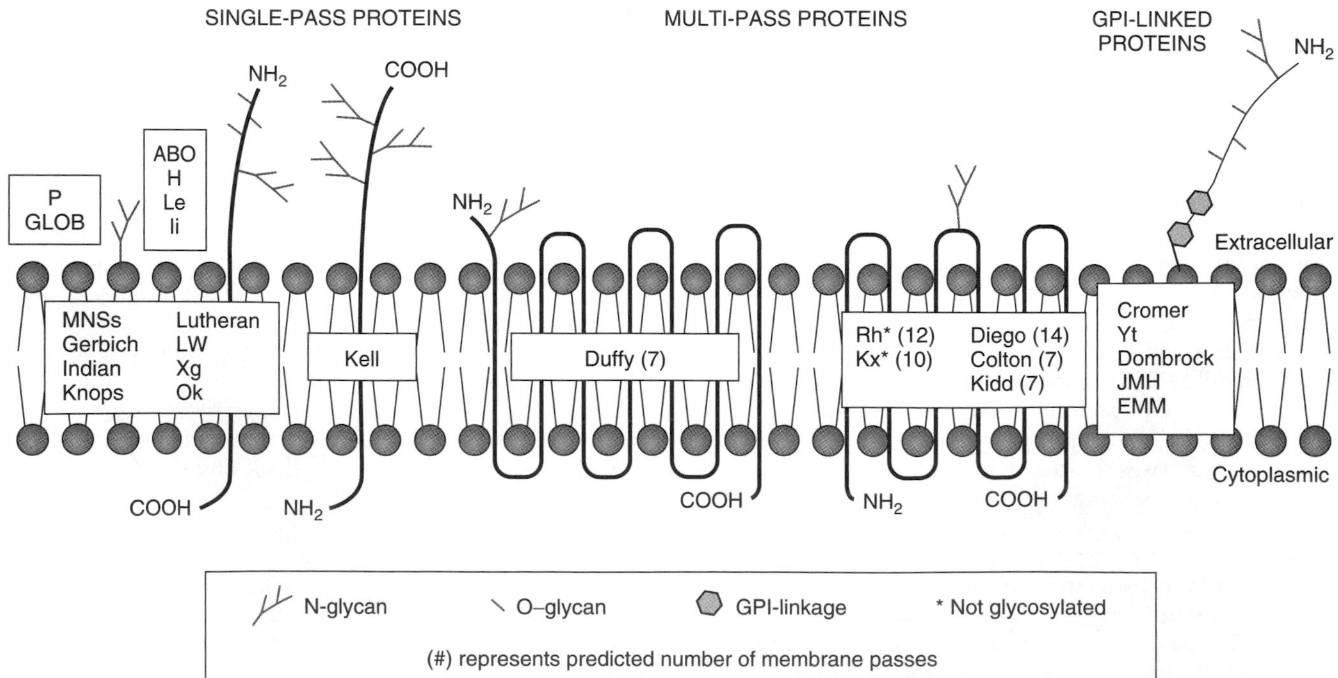

Figure 5–1 Diagram of a cross-section of the red blood cell membrane lipid bilayer and various membrane components that carry blood group antigens. GPI, glycosylphosphatidylinositol.

LW (ICAM4), CD47, and GPB).[4,30] The recent discovery that the Rh–RhAG complex interacts with cytoskeletal ankyrin[31] suggests that there are additional attachment sites between integral membrane proteins and the membrane skeleton and provides an possible explanation for the stomatocytosis associated with Rh-null erythrocytes.

Many blood group antigens are carried on transmembrane proteins or glycoproteins; however, a few antigens are carried on glycosylphosphatidylinositol (GPI)-linked proteins (see Fig. 5–1). Antigens in two blood group systems (Lewis and Chido-Rodgers) are carried on proteins that are adsorbed onto RBCs from the plasma.

Carbohydrates

Carbohydrates are essentially restricted to the extracellular surface of the RBC membrane, where they collectively form a negatively charged environment that is largely responsible for keeping the RBCs from adhering to one another and to the endothelium. The majority of carbohydrates are attached to lipids on ceramide and to proteins by attachment to asparagine (N-linked) or to serine or threonine (O-linked) during passage through the lumen of the Golgi.[32] Some blood group antigens are determined by the terminal carbohydrate residue (e.g., A and B) whereas others require the presence of a chain of carbohydrate residues (e.g., Le^b and I).

The carbohydrates form the *glycocalyx,* a negatively charged barrier approximately 10 Å thick around the outside of the RBC membrane. This barrier can keep immunoglobulin G (IgG) antibodies, particularly those recognizing antigens that reside close to the lipid bilayer, from readily interacting with the corresponding antigen. Thus, the glycocalyx affects the ability of an IgG antibody to cause direct agglutination.

RBC BLOOD GROUP ANTIGENS

Figure 5–1 depicts the membrane components that are known to carry blood group antigens. Some antigens are carbohydrates attached to lipids or to proteins, some are protein, and some require both protein and carbohydrates. Although the blood group antigens do not themselves have a function, the molecules on which they are carried do. The function of proteins carrying blood group antigens has been determined through observation of the morphology of RBCs that lack the protein (Table 5–2), direct experimentation, or comparison of the predicted protein sequence with protein databases to identify similar proteins whose function is known, even if in other tissues or organisms.

Recognition of a blood group antigen begins with discovery of an antibody. When an individual whose RBCs lack an antigen is exposed to RBCs that possess that antigen, the person may mount an immune response and produce an antibody that reacts with the antigen. Depending on the immunoglobulin class of the antibody and, to some extent, on the number and topology of antigens on the RBC membrane, the interaction between antibody and antigen may be detected by agglutination or hemolysis or may require an antiglobulin reagent. In human blood grouping, most tests involve agglutination, in which clumping of the RBCs serves as the detectable end point.[33] The polymorphic erythrocyte marker is given a blood group antigen name after genetic and family studies.

Terminology

A working party on terminology for RBC surface antigens, sanctioned by the International Society for Blood Transfusion (ISBT), has categorized the blood group antigens into four classifications[34]: the genetically discrete blood group systems (Table 5–3 summarizes the name, ISBT system number, chromosome location, gene name, associated antigens, component name, and possible functions for each system); blood group collections that consist of serologically, biochemically, or genetically related antigens; 700 series of low-incidence antigens; and 901 series of high-incidence antigens (Table 5–4 contains the ISBT name, number, and associated antigens. The chromosome location for these antigens has not yet been determined).

As RBC antigens were discovered, notations were devised to describe them. The terminology used is inconsistent: a single letter (e.g., A, D, K), a symbol with a superscript (e.g., Fy^a, Jk^b, Lu^a), or a numerical notation (e.g., Fy3, Lu4, K12) is used. Even within the same blood group system, antigens have been named with different schemes, resulting in a cumbersome terminology for describing phenotypes. The use of the same symbol with a different superscript letter (e.g., Fy^a and Fy^b) indicates products of alleles (antithetical antigens).[34] Some confusing terminology persists; for example, the P1 antigen is the sole antigen in the P blood group system, and the P antigen is the only antigen in the GLOB system. There is also a GLOB collection, with Pk and LKE antigens. In clinical practice, the traditional terminology is still extensively used; this is the terminology that will be used throughout this chapter for the discussion of red cell antigens.

Collectively, there are over 260 antigens recognized by the ISBT. We restrict discussion to the more commonly encountered antibodies and antigens.

Inheritance

Most blood group antigens are encoded by genes on autosomes.[35] Most are codominant (e.g., M/N, E/e, K/k, Fy^a/Fy^b),

Table 5–2 Red Blood Cell Morphology and Associated Phenotype

Shape	Clinical Manifestation	Protein	Phenotype
Stomatocyte	Mild hemolytic anemia	Absent Rh or RhAG (Rh50)	Rh-null, Rh-mod
Elliptocyte	Slightly reduced red blood cell survival	Absent GPC and GPD	Ge2, Ge3, Ge4 (Leach)
Acanthocyte	Elevated creatinine phosphokinase, muscular choreiform movements, neurologic defects, reduced RBC survival	Absent Kx	McLeod

Table 5–3 Genetically Discrete Blood Group Systems

Name	ISBT Number	Chromosome Location	Gene Name ISBT	Gene Name ISGN	Associated Antigens	Component Name	Possible Function
ABO	001	9q34.2	*ABO*	*ABO*	A, B, A,B, A_1	Carbohydrate	
MNS	002	4q28.2–q31.1	*MNS*	*GYPA, GYPB*	M, N, S, s, U, He Mi^a, Vw +35 more	GPA; GPB	Carrier of sialic acid
P	003	22q11.2-qter	*P1*	*P1*	P1	Carbohydrate	
Rh	004	1p36.13-p34.3	*RH*	*RHD, RHCE*	D, C, E, c, e, f, C^w and more	RhCE; RhD	Structural/Transport
Lutheran	005	19q13.2	*LU*	*LU*	Lu^a, Lu^b, Lu3, Lu4 and more	Lutheran	
Kell	006	7q33	*KEL*	*KEL*	K, k, Kp^a, Kp^b, Ku, Js^a and more	Kell glycoprotein	Enzymatic
Lewis	007	19p13.3	*LE*	*FUT3*	Le^a, Le^b, Le^{ab}, Le^{bh} and more	Carbohydrate	
Duffy	008	1q22–q23	*FY*	*DARC*	Fy^a, Fy^b, Fy3, Fy4 and more	Fy glycoprotein	Chemokine receptor
Kidd	009	18q11-q12	*JK*	*SLC14A1*	Jk^a, Jk^b, Jk3	Kidd glycoprotein	Urea transport
Diego	010	17q21-q22	*DI*	*SLC4A1*	Di^a, Di^b, Wr^a, Wr^b, Wd^a and more	Band 3	Anion transport
Yt	011	7q22	*YT*	*ACHE*	Yt^a, Yt^b	Acetylcholinesterase	Enzymatic
Xg	012	Xp22.32	*XG*	*XG*	Xg^a	Xg^a glycoprotein	Adhesion
Scianna	013	1p35-p32	SC	*SC*	Sc1, Sc2, Sc3	Sc glycoprotein	
Dombrock	014	12p13.2–p12.1	*DO*	*DO*	Do^a, Do^b, Gy^a, Hy, Jo^a	Do glycoprotein CD297	Enzymatic
Colton	015	7p14	*CO*	*AQP1*	Co^a, Co^b, Co3	Channel-forming	Water transport
Landsteiner-Wiener	016	19p13.3	*LW*	*LW*	LW^a, LW^{ab}, LW^b	LW glycoprotein	Adhesion
Chido-Rodgers	017	6p21.3	*CH/RG*	*C4A, C4B*	Ch1, Ch2, Rg1 and more	C4A; C4B	Complement
Hh	018	19q13.3	*H*	*FUT1*	H	Carbohydrate	
Kx	019	Xp21.1	*XK*	*XK*	Kx	Kx glycoprotein	Transport
Gerbich	020	2q14–q21	*GE*	*GYPC*	Ge2, Ge3, Ge4, Wb and more	GPC; GPD	Interacts with protein 4.1 and p55
Cromer	021	1q32	*CROM*	*DAF*	Cr^a, Tc^a, Tc^b, Tc^c and more	CD55 (DAF)	Complement
Knops	022	1q32	*KN*	*CR1*	Kn^a, Kn^b, McC^a, Sl^a, Yk^a	CD35 (CR1)	Complement
Indian	023	11p13	*IN*	*CD44*	In^a, In^b	CD44	Adhesion
Ok	024	19pter-p13.2	*OK*	*CD147*	OK^a	CD147	Adhesion
Raph	025	11p15.5	*MER2*	*MER2*	MER2	Tetraspanin (CD151)	Adhesion
JMH	026	15p22.3–q23	*JMH*	*CD108*	JMH	CD108	Adhesion
I	027	6p24.2	*IGNT*	*IGNT*	I	*N*-Acetylglucosaminyltransferase A	Glycocalyx
Globoside	028	3q26.1	*βGalNAcT1*	*β3GALT*	P	*N*-Acetylgalactosaminyltransferase	Glycocalyx
GIL	029	9p13.1	*GIL*	*AQP3*	GIL	AQP3	Glycerol/water/urea transport

B-CAM, cell adhesion molecule; GP, glycophorin; ISBT, International Society of Blood Transfusion; ISGN, International Society for Gene Nomenclature.

Table 5–4 Other Blood Groups Whose Chromosome Locations Have Not Yet Been Determined

Name	International Society of Blood Transfusion Number	Associated Antigens
Collections		
Cost	205	Cs^a, Cs^b
i	207	i
Er	208	Er^a, Er^b
Globoside	209	P, P^k, LKE
Unnamed	210	Le^c, Le^d
Series		
Low-incidence antigens	700	By, Chr^a, Bi, Bx^a, Rd, Pt^a + 15 more
High-incidence antigens	901	Vel, Lan, At^a, Jr^a, JMH, Emm, AnWj, Sd^a, Duclos, PEL, ABTI, MAM

but some appear to be dominant if an antibody to the presumed antithetical antigen has not been discovered (e.g., Ul[a], Cr[a]). Some rare phenotypes appear to be inherited in a dominant manner, for example, dominant type Lu(a–b–), or in a recessive manner, for example, recessive type Lu(a–b–). Xg[a] and Kx are encoded by genes on the X chromosome and are inherited in a classic X-linked manner. See Table 5–3 for the chromosomal location of genes encoding blood groups.

Expression

Some blood group antigens are also found on nonerythroid cells. Some examples are A, B, H, Kn[a] (CD35), In[a] (CD44), Ok[a] (CD147), and Cromer-related antigens (CD55), which have a wide tissue distribution.[36,37]

The ability to culture stem cells and sort erythroid lineages and the availability of monoclonal antibodies have enabled the estimation of the timing of expression of blood group antigens during in vitro erythroid maturation. The blood group antigens appear in the following order: GPC, Kell, RhAG, LW, RhCE, GPA, band 3, RhD, Lutheran, and Duffy.[38,39]

Maturation

Several blood group antigens are not expressed or are only weakly expressed on fetal RBCs and do not reach adult levels until a person is approximately age 2. Cord RBCs do not express Le[a], Sd[a], Ch, Rg, or AnWj antigens. Antibodies to these antigens are unlikely to cause HDN, because RBC expression is a prerequisite for HDN. Expression of A, B, H, P1, I, Le[b], Lu[a], Lu[b], Yt[a], Vel, Do[a], Do[b], Gy[a], Hy, Jo[a], Xg[a], Kn, and Bg is greatly reduced on RBCs from cord blood compared to adult RBCs. In contrast, the i and LW antigens are more strongly expressed on RBCs from cord blood than on RBCs from adults. Furthermore, although adults express more LW on D-positive RBCs than on D-negative RBCs, cord RBCs express LW antigens equally regardless of D type. This information makes the testing of cord RBCs useful in antibody identification studies.

Molecular Genetic Basis

Of the 29 genes (or gene families) that encode blood group antigens, 28 have been cloned and sequenced (only the gene encoding P remains to be clarified),[40–44] and the genetic basis of many blood group antigens has been determined.[45–48] This knowledge is being applied to transfusion medicine and is discussed later in the chapter. Relevant details about blood groups and molecular knowledge are given in Chapters 6 through 8. Information concerning the genetic basis of blood group antigens can also be obtained from the Blood Group Antigen Mutation Database: www.bioc.aecom.yu.edu/bgmut/index.php.

Evolution

It has been known for many years from agglutination with human sera that blood group antigens have homologues in anthropoid apes.[49] The availability of monoclonal antibodies and molecular analysis of the gene homologues from nonhuman primates have contributed to defining the epitopes of human blood group antigens.[26,49–52] Additionally, because of the conserved nature of proteins, protein sequence comparisons are contributing to predictions about the function of human proteins (see Table 5–3). The sequencing of the genomes of many model organisms has allowed researchers to make testable inferences about protein function. The understanding of blood groups has benefited from this revolution.

Natural Knockouts

The detection of an alloantibody to a high prevalence antigen during compatibility testing or prenatal testing has led to the discovery of RBCs with null phenotypes. Such RBCs lack the specific carbohydrate or carrier protein and therefore, all blood group antigens within that system. Thus, these RBCs serve as natural knockout models and these null phenotypes have provided insights into the function of the carrier proteins.

Function

In general, the polymorphisms that we recognize as blood group antigens and that have significance in transfusion medicine do not appear to alter the function of the carrier molecule. The predicted functions are often based on the function of closely related proteins in other tissues; however, their role in the mature RBC may not be the same as in other cells, altered forms may function as recognition signals in senescent RBCs, or they may have an important role during earlier stages of erythroid development.[5]

The possible functions of the various components carrying blood group antigens can be divided into the following broad categories: contributors to membrane structural integrity, transport proteins, receptors for extracellular ligands, adhesion proteins, extracellular enzymes, complement regulatory proteins, and maintainers of surface charge in the glycocalyx (see Table 5–3).[4,45,46,53–55] Specific details can be found in the chapters that follow.

BLOOD GROUP ANTIBODIES

An *antigen* can be defined as a substance that will induce the production of antibodies, although there are certain properties of a molecule, such as foreignness, size, and chemical complexity, that are associated with increased immunogenicity. Proteins usually induce the most vigorous immune responses, followed by carbohydrates, whereas lipids and nucleic acids are usually not strong immunogens, although clinically significant antibodies specific for these types of molecules do exist (e.g., antiphospholipid antibodies and anti-DNA antibodies found in some autoimmune diseases). Most antigens require helper activity, usually in the form of cytokines, from helper T cells to induce strong antibody responses, and this helper activity is required for production of antibody classes other than IgM. Some antigens, usually carbohydrate in nature, can induce antibodies in the absence of helper T-cell activity, but these responses are primarily IgM, with little, if any, antibodies of other classes produced.

Antibodies are produced by B lymphocytes, also known as B cells. The basic antibody molecule consists of four polypeptide chains—two heavy chains of 50 to 70 kilodaltons, depending on the antibody class, and two light chains of approximately 25 kilodaltons. The two heavy chains produced by a B cell are identical, as are the two light chains. In each polypeptide chain, whether it is a heavy chain or a light chain, approximately the first 100 amino acids are known as the *variable region,* and the remainder of the polypeptide chain constitutes the *constant region,* which is identical in all antibodies of the same class. The antigen-binding site is formed by association of the variable regions of one heavy chain and one light chain, which means that each four-chain unit has two identical antigen-binding sites. However, in most immune responses, a large number of B cells are stimulated by an antigen, and each antigen-specific B cell will produce a unique antibody, resulting in a heterogeneous response consisting of many different antibody molecules directed toward multiple sites on the antigen.

Immunogenicity

Several factors influence the ability to stimulate antibody production, including antigen size, complexity, and dose as well as host human leukocyte antigen genotype and other, as yet unidentified, susceptibility factors. Most carbohydrate-based RBC antigens are T independent and therefore tend to elicit an IgM response. The protein-based antigens usually are T dependent and induce an IgM primary response that progresses to IgG.[56] Antigen exposure usually occurs by transfusion of products containing RBCs or during pregnancy (immune antibodies) or by exposure to microbes (apparently, naturally occurring antibodies). Table 5–5 summarizes the usual type of immunoglobulin response and the potential clinical significance, in transfusion or in HDN, of selected blood group antibodies, which are listed in order of clinical significance.[36]

Clinical Significance

Antibodies recognizing antigens in the ABO blood group system are by far the most clinically significant. This is because they occur naturally in people whose RBCs lack the corresponding antigen. Other clinically significant antibodies occur in the following order, from the most commonly to the least commonly encountered in transfusion practice: anti-D, anti-K, anti-E, anti-c, anti-Fy^a, anti-C, anti-Jk^a, anti-S, anti-Jk^b. All other clinically significant antibodies occur with an incidence of less than 1% of immunized patients.[57–59] Antibodies that are considered clinically insignificant unless the antibody reacts in tests performed strictly at 37°C are anti-P1, anti-M, anti-N, anti-Lu^a, anti-Le^a, anti-Le^b, and anti-Sd^a. Other clinically insignificant antibodies that react at 37°C in the indirect antiglobulin test (IAT) are those of the Knops and Chido-Rodgers systems and anti-JMH (Table 5–6).

The incidence of a blood group antibody depends on both the prevalence in the population and the immunogenicity of the antigen. Immunized patients frequently produce multiple antibodies, and the more antibodies present, the more difficult they are to identify.

Detection and Identification

Compatibility testing (testing patient's serum against donor's RBCs) still uses techniques that were described 100 years ago for direct agglutination and 50 years ago for indirect agglutination. Even today, with our detailed understanding of blood group antigens, we have no single technical procedure able to detect all known blood group antibodies. The hemagglutination technique is simple and inexpensive, does not require sophisticated equipment, and when done correctly is sensitive and specific in terms of clinical relevance. Agglutination should be graded according to the strength of reaction, and an evaluation of the reaction strength can aid in identification of antibodies, especially when multiple antibodies are present in a serum.[33]

The first blood group antigens to be identified were those that could be agglutinated by the alloantibodies when antigen-positive RBCs were suspended in a saline medium (direct agglutination). This direct agglutination reflects the fact that these antibodies are usually IgM and detect carbohydrate antigens (ABO, P1, Le, and H antigens). Although

Table 5–5 Characteristics of Some Blood Group Alloantibodies

			Clinical	
Antibody Specificity	**IgM (Direct)**	**IgG (Indirect)**	**Transfusion Reaction**	**HDN**
ABO	Most	Some	Immediate; mild to severe	Common; mild to moderate
Rh	Some	Most	Immediate/delayed; mild to severe	Common; mild to severe
Kell	Some	Most	Immediate/delayed; mild to severe	Sometimes; mild to severe
Kidd	Few	Most	Immediate/delayed; mild to severe	Rare; mild
Duffy	Rare	Most	Immediate/delayed; mild to severe	Rare; mild
M	Some	Most	Delayed (rare)	Rare; mild
N	Most	Rare	None	None
S	Some	Most	Delayed; mild	Rare; mild to severe
s	Rare	Most	Delayed; mild	Rare; mild to severe
U	Rare	Most	Immediate/delayed; mild to severe	Rare; severe
P1	Most	Rare	None (rare)	None
Lutheran	Some	Most	Delayed	Rare; mild
Le^a	Most	Few	Immediate (rare)	None
Le^b	Most	Few	None	None
Diego	Some	Most	Delayed; none to severe	Mild to severe
Colton	Rare	Most	Delayed; mild	Rare; mild to severe
Dombrock	Rare	Most	Immediate/delayed; mild to severe	Rare; mild
LW	Rare	Most	Delayed; none to mild	Rare; mild
Yt^a	Rare	Most	Delayed (rare); mild	None
I	Most	Rare	None	None
Chido-Rodgers	Rare	Most	Anaphylactic (several cases)	None
JMH	Rare	Most	Delayed (rare)	None
Knops	Rare	Most	None	None
Xg^a	Rare	Most	None	None

Clinically Significant?	Alloantibodies
Always	A and B H in O_h Rh Kell Duffy Kidd Diego S, s, U P, PP1, P^k Vel
Sometimes	At^a Colton Cromer Dombrock Gerbich Indian Jr^a JMH Lan LW Scianna Yt
Not unless reactive at 37°C	A_1 H Le^a Lutheran M, N P1 Sd^a
Not usually	Chido-Rodgers Cost Knops Le^b Xg^a

Table 5–6 **Clinical Significances of Some Alloantibodies to Blood Group Antigens**

anti-A and anti-B are highly clinically significant, antibodies to the other carbohydrate antigens generally are not.

Most of the other antigens (e.g., Rh, Kell, Duffy, and Kidd) are proteins and are detected by antibodies that react in the IAT. This test detects IgG antibodies, complement attached to RBCs, or both. The sensitized RBCs are washed to remove unattached immunoglobulin (which would inhibit the antiglobulin reagent), and anti-human immunoglobulin is added. The specimen is centrifuged and examined for agglutination. The antiglobulin test can be direct or indirect. The direct antiglobulin test is used to detect RBCs sensitized in vivo, such as alloantibodies causing transfusion reactions or HDN and autoantibodies in autoimmune hemolytic anemia or cold agglutinin disease. The IAT is used to detect RBCs sensitized in vitro; for instance, antigen typing, antibody detection and identification, and compatibility testing.

To identify antibodies, serum is tested against RBCs of known phenotype by various techniques. It is sometimes helpful to treat antigen-positive test RBCs with proteolytic enzymes and chemical agents and to compare the antibody reactivity in tests against treated and untreated RBCs to aid antibody identification (Table 5–7).[47] Brief, but informative, descriptions of the technical and clinical aspects of most blood group antibodies can be found elsewhere.[33,60]

Locating Antigen-Negative Blood

Once a patient is actively immunized to an RBC antigen and produces a clinically significant alloantibody, the patient is considered immunized for life and must be transfused with antigen-negative RBCs, even if the antibody is no longer detectable. Patients with passively acquired antibody (e.g., neonates and recipients of plasma products, Rh immune globulin, or IVIgG) are not actively immunized and may be transfused with antigen-negative RBCs only while the passive antibody is still present. Selection of blood for transfusion of a patient with blood group alloantibodies is the joint responsibility of the staff at the transfusion service, the donor center, and the patient's physician. Thus, it is very important that there be communication regarding the number of units of RBC products required and the time frame involved. Figure 5–2 is a flow chart that outlines the process for locating blood. Table 5–8 lists the prevalence of donors whose RBCs lack selected antigens.

To locate antigen-negative blood for transfusion, it is not necessary to identify an antibody to a low-prevalence antigen detected in the recipient's blood during compatibility testing, because another unit of donor blood is highly unlikely to be positive for the same uncommon antigen. In contrast, if an antibody to a low-prevalence antigen is detected in the serum of a pregnant woman, identification of the antibody or determination of its reactivity with paternal RBCs is required to predict the likelihood and severity of HDN in the baby. Locating blood for exchange transfusion is not difficult, for the reason previously described.

If a patient's serum contains alloantibodies to a high-prevalence antigen, blood for transfusion may be very difficult to locate. Whether the investigation is for transfusion purposes or for prediction of HDN, the antibody should be identified. The identification aids in both the assessment of its clinical significance and the location of appropriate blood for transfusion. Family members, in particular siblings, are

Table 5–7 **Reactivity of Antigen-Positive Red Blood Cells after Treatment with Ficin/Papain or DTT**

Ficin/Papain	Dithiothreitol (200 mM)	Possible, Antibody Specificity
Negative	Positive	M,N,S,s†; Fy^a,Fy^b; Ge2,Ge4; Xg^a; Ch/Rg
Negative	Negative	Indian; JMH
Positive	Weak	Cromer; Knops (weak in ficin), Lutheran; Dombrock; AnWj; MER2
Variable	Negative	Yt^a
Positive	Negative	Kell; LW; Scianna
Positive	Positive	A, B; H; P1; Rh; Lewis; Kidd; Fy3; Diego; Co; Ge3; Ok^a, I, i; P, LKE; At^a; Cs^a; Emm; Er^a; Jr^a; Lan; Vel, Sd^a, PEL
Positive	Enhanced	Kx

†variable with ficin/papain.

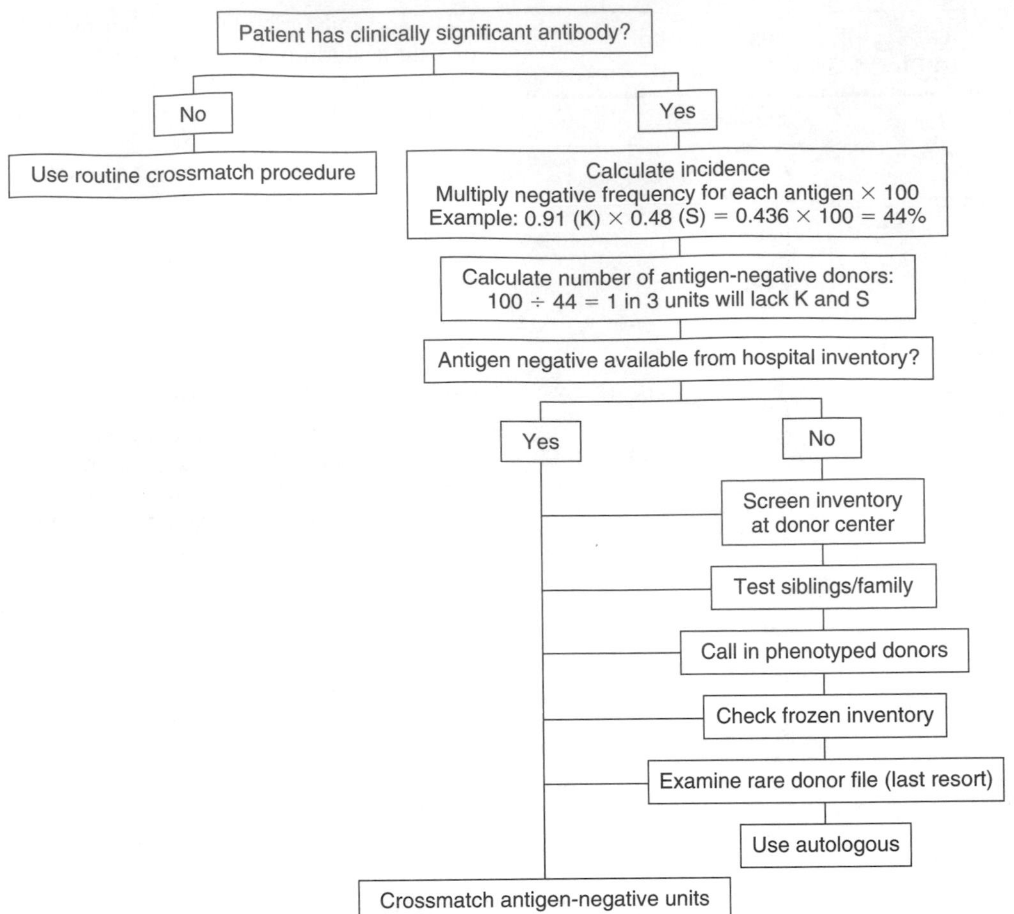

Figure 5–2 Flow chart for locating antigen-negative blood.

the first source to investigate for antigen-negative units. Most national blood donor centers can often assess national and international Rare Donor Registries and can help provide the appropriate antigen-negative blood.

COMPATIBILITY PROCEDURES

Most laboratories follow recommendations made by the American Association of Blood Banks,[61] and all must comply with regulations of state and federal agencies. Routine approaches to compatibility testing involve testing a blood sample from a prospective recipient for ABO and D blood groups and for the presence of blood group antibodies. In most cases, no unexpected antibodies are detected, and donor RBCs of appropriate ABO and D blood type are selected for transfusion. A sample of the donor's RBCs may be tested (crossmatched) with the patient's serum by means of either an immediate spin procedure or the IAT. Alternatively, the blood can be issued without direct cross-testing if a computer check is performed.[33] Any blood typing problems should be resolved, and when antibodies are detected, they should be identified. Knowing the specificity of an antibody helps establish whether it is likely to be clinically significant and determine the approach necessary to provide an adequate supply of compatible blood. Once an antibody has been identified, antigen-negative RBC products selected for transfusion should be tested with the patient's serum by the IAT to ensure compatibility.

It is important not to delay surgery or transfusion unnecessarily by attempting to obtain antigen-negative RBCs for patients with clinically insignificant antibodies. Also, in hemolytic anemia due to warm-reactive autoantibodies, compatibility may be difficult to demonstrate. The important issue is to be sure that there are no underlying, clinically significant alloantibodies. This fact can be determined with autologous or homologous autoabsorptions,[33] which require extra time and, possibly, the services of an immunohematology reference laboratory. It is helpful to remember that patients without a history of immunization (transfusion or pregnancy) are unlikely to have underlying alloantibodies. Unfortunately, a patient's transfusion history is not always reliable, because many patients are unaware or forget that they have received transfusions.[62]

CHOICE OF ANTIGEN-NEGATIVE BLOOD FOR DISEASES REQUIRING LONG-TERM TRANSFUSION THERAPY

Transfusion management of patients who require long-term transfusion therapy, in particular patients with sickle cell anemia, has been the subject of controversy and debate.[63,64] There is still no consensus as to the best and most practical approach, although the goal is to provide blood with maximal survival. In addition to the traditional practice of providing antigen-negative blood only after the patient has made an antibody, approaches that have been adopted

Table 5–8 **Antigen-Negative Incidence—Common Polymorphic Antigens***

System	Antigen	Incidence of Antigen Negativity	
		White	Black
Rh	D	0.15	0.08
	C	0.32	0.73
	E	0.71	0.78
	c	0.20	0.04
	e	0.02	0.02
	f	0.35	0.08
	C^w	0.98	0.99
	V	>0.99	0.70
	VS	>0.99	0.73
	CE	<0.01	<0.01
	cE	0.72	0.78
	Ce	0.32	0.73
MNS	M	0.22	0.26
	N	0.30	0.25
	S	0.48	0.69
	s	0.11	0.06
	M,S	0.15	0.19
	M,s	0.01	0.02
	N,S	0.1	0.16
	N,s	0.06	0.02
P	P1	0.21	0.06
Lewis	Le^a	0.78	0.77
	Le^b	0.28	0.45
Lutheran	Lu^a	0.92	0.95
	Lu^b	<0.01	<0.01
Kell	K	0.91	0.98
	k	0.002	<0.01
	Kp^a	0.98	>0.99
	Kp^b	<0.01	<0.01
	Js^a	>0.99	0.80
	Js^b	<0.001	0.01
Duffy	Fy^a	0.34	0.90
	Fy^b	0.17	0.77
Kidd	Jk^a	0.23	0.08
	Jk^b	0.26	0.51
Dombrock	Do^a	0.33	0.45
	Do^b	0.18	0.11
Colton	Co^a	<0.01	
	Co^b	0.90	

*To calculate the incidence of compatible donors, multiply the incidence of antigen-negative donors for each antibody, e.g., the incidence of K, S, and Jk^a negative donors in the general donor pool is (0.91) × (0.48) × (0.23) = 0.10 in 100, or 1 in 1000.

include providing phenotype-matched blood after the first antibody is made; providing blood matched for D, C, E, and K antigens; providing fully antigen-matched blood (i.e., matched for D, C, E, c, e, K, Fy^a, Fy^b, Jk^a, and Jk^b antigens); and providing blood based on ethnic background combined with antigen matching for D, C, E, and K.[65–70]

Clearly, if the objective is to prevent immunization to blood group antigens, initial phenotype matching is the logical approach; however, this approach does not prevent the production of antibodies to high-prevalence antigens, such as U, Js^b, Cr^a, hr^S, and hr^B. The decision as to whether the blood donor community can support this approach lies with the directors of the transfusion service and of the donor center that supplies the blood. Providing phenotypically matched RBC products is logistically difficult and expensive. Although from the patient's perspective it is desirable to be transfused only with phenotype-matched blood, the community may not be able to support that approach. Indeed, in some regions, it is a challenge to provide antigen-negative blood to patients who have already made the antibodies. Extensive screening for antigen-negative donors may be realized with the advent of microarray technology.

COMPLICATIONS OF TRANSFUSION

As previously described, physicians in some locations may choose to provide phenotype-matched blood for patients with sickle cell anemia who undergo long-term transfusion therapy. Because the incidences of antigens differ in various ethnic groups, blood for these patients is most likely to be found among African American donors, whose RBCs more commonly lack C, E, K, S, Fy^a, Fy^b, and Jk^b antigens than the RBCs of white donors.[70] However, it is worth noting that RBCs from African American donors are more likely (approximately 1 in 5) to express antigens for which we do not routinely test, such as VS, Js^a, Go^a, and DAK.[71] Thus, because all these antigens are immunogenic but are not present on screening cells, it is recommended in this group of patients that blood be crossmatched using the IAT in preference to performing a computer match. This crossmatching approach would prevent a potential transfusion reaction due to antibodies such as anti-VS, anti-Js^a, anti-Go^a, and anti-DAK.

Although current pretransfusion practice has drastically reduced the incidence of hemolytic transfusion reactions, they still occur. The single most common cause of a hemolytic transfusion reaction is clerical error. It should be noted that several conditions mimic hemolytic transfusion reactions; they are summarized in Table 5–9. Additional details can be found in the review by Beauregard and Blajchman.[72]

HEMAGGLUTINATION AS AN AID IN DIAGNOSIS

Hemagglutination can be used to diagnose syndromes that are caused by the absence of a component carrying blood group antigens (null phenotypes). For example, an absence of the Rh proteins causes stomatocytosis and compensated hemolytic anemia (Rh syndrome),[30,73,74] and an absence of Xk protein causes the McLeod syndrome.[28,75–77] These individuals can be identified with a simple test of their RBCs with antibody to common Rh antigens and to Kx antigen, respectively. RBCs and white blood cells (WBCs) from patients with leukocyte adhesion deficiency II (also known as congenital disorder of glycosylation) lack antigens that are dependent on fucose. Thus, the RBCs have a Bombay, Le(a−b−) phenotype. Their WBCs lack sialyLe^x, which explains the high WBC count and infections in these patients.[78,79]

APPLICATIONS OF DNA-BASED ASSAYS IN TRANSFUSION MEDICINE

The astounding pace of growth in the field of molecular biology and in the understanding of the genetic changes associated with most blood group antigens and phenotypes enables us to consider identification of blood group antigens and antibodies using nucleic acid-based approaches. Indeed, the knowledge is already being applied to help resolve some long-standing clinical problems that cannot be resolved by classical hemagglutination.

Table 5–9 Causes of Apparent in Vivo Hemolysis

Immune Causes	Microbial
ABO incompatibility	Sepsis
Clinically significant alloantibody	Malaria
Anamnestic alloantibody response	Contamination of donor blood
Autoimmune hemolytic anemia	**Chemical**
Cold agglutinin disease	Inappropriate solutions infused
Hemolytic disease of the newborn	Drugs infused
Drug-induced hemolytic anemia	Serum phosphorus <0.2 mg/dL
Polyagglutination (sepsis T-active plasma)	Water irrigation of bladder
Paroxysmal cold hemoglobinuria	Azulfidine
Thrombotic thrombocytopenic hemolytic uremia syndrome (a microangiopathic process)	Dimethyl sulfoxide
Nonimmune Causes	Venom (snake, bee, brown recluse spider)
Mechanical	Certain herbal preparations, teas, enemas
Poor sample collection	**Inherent Red Blood Cell Abnormalities**
Small-bore needle used for infusion	Paroxysmal nocturnal hemoglobinuria
Excessive pressure during infusion	Sickle cell anemia
Malfunctioning blood warmer	Spherocytosis
Donor blood exposed to excessive heat or cold	Hemoglobin H
Urinary catheter	Glucose-6-phosphate dehydrogenase deficiency
Crush trauma	
Prosthetic heart valves	
Aortic stenosis	
March hemoglobinuria	

Although direct and indirect hemagglutination tests have served the transfusion community well for more than 100 and more than 50 years, respectively, in some aspects, hemagglutination has limitations. For example, it gives only an indirect measure of the potential complications in an at-risk pregnancy, it cannot indicate *RHD* zygosity in D-positive people, it cannot be relied on to type some recently transfused patients, and it requires the availability of specific reliable antisera. The characterization of genes and determination of the molecular basis of antigens and phenotypes has made it possible to use the polymerase chain reaction[80,81] to amplify regions of DNA of interest to detect alleles encoding blood groups. The knowledge can also be applied to express antigens in heterologous systems as a first step to detect and identify blood group antibodies in a single, objective, automated assay.

DNA Basis of Blood Group Antigens

Once a gene is shown to encode a protein that carries a blood group, focused analysis of people with known serologically defined antigen profiles is used to determine the molecular basis of variant forms of the gene. This approach has been extremely powerful because antisera-based definitions of blood groups readily distinguish variants within each blood group system. The molecular basis associated with many blood group antigens has been determined over a relatively short period.[30,46,54,73,82–99] The available wealth of serologically defined variants has contributed to the rapid rate with which the genetic diversity of blood group genes has been revealed. Initially, molecular information associated with each variant was obtained from only a small number of samples and applied to analysis with the hopeful assumption that the molecular analysis would always correlate with RBC antigen typing. With the gathering of more information it became obvious that several molecular events can result in discrepant genotype and RBC phenotype (some are listed in Table 5–10). Furthermore, analyses of the null phenotypes have demonstrated that multiple, diverse genetic events can give rise to the null phenotype, for example, for Rh,[30,73] Kell,[100] and Jk systems,[101] and the p phenotype.[102]

Antigen Identification by DNA Testing

Although there are many molecular events that give rise to blood group antigens and phenotypes, the majority of genetically defined blood group antigens are the consequence of an SNP. Thus, simple DNA-based assays can be used to identify defined SNPs in genes encoding blood groups. Innumerable DNA-based assays have been described to detect specific blood group SNPs. They include polymerase chain reaction (PCR)-restriction fragment length polymorphism (RFLP), allele-specific (AS)-PCR, sequence-specific (SS)-PCR as single or multiplex assays, real-time quantitative PCR (Q-PCR; RQ-PCR), a single nucleotide dye terminator extension method, and high throughput microarray technology. The PCR-RFLP, AS-PCR, and SS-PCR assays can be visualized in a gel or by electropherogram printouts. Semi-automated methods that use a specific tag attached to the primers, which can then be analyzed in a digital readable format by a mass-spectrometer or pyrosequencer, have tremendous potential in the clinical laboratory. Another exciting opportunity is the use of microchip technology for the purpose of antigen identification.[103,104] The process uses a "chip," which is composed of spots of DNA from many genes attached to a solid surface in a gridlike array. The fluorescent-labeled cDNA or DNA with a sequence that matches the sequence of one of the gene fragments adheres and can be detected. The system is most frequently used for studying genes involved in regulation and expression.[105] However, it is now also being used to analyze specific blood group genes. Some clinical applications of DNA analysis for blood groups are listed in Table 5–11.

In the Transfusion Setting

FOR TRANSFUSION-DEPENDENT PATIENTS

Certain medical conditions, such as sickle cell disease, thalassemia, autoimmune hemolytic anemia, and aplastic

Table 5–10 Examples of Events That Confound Analysis of Genotype and Phenotype

Event	Mechanism	Blood Group Phenotype
Promoter mutation	Nucleotide change in GATA box	Fy(b–)
Alternative splicing	Nucleotide change in splice site: partial/complete skipping of exon	S–s–; Gy(a–)
	Deletion of nucleotides	Dr(a–) Cromer weak
Premature stop codon	Deletion of nucleotide(s) → frameshift	Fy(a–b–); D–; Rh null; Ge2, Ge3, Ge4; Gy(a–); K_0; McLeod
	Insertion of nucleotide(s) → frameshift	D–; Co(a–b–)
	Nucleotide change	Fy(a–b–); r′; Gy(a–); K_0; McLeod
Amino acid change	Missense mutation	D–; Rh null; K_0; McLeod
Reduced amount of protein	Missense mutation	Fy^X; Co(a–b–)
Hybrid genes	Crossover	GP.Vw; GP.Hil; GP.TSEN
	Gene conversion	GP.Mur; GP.Hop; D– –; R_0^{Har}
Interacting protein	Absence of RhAG	Rh null
	Absence of Kx	Weak expression of Kell antigen
	Absence of amino acids 59 to 76 of GPA	Wr(b–)
	Absence of protein 4.1	Weak expression of Ge antigens
Modifying gene	*In(LU)*	Lu(a–b–)
	In(Jk)	Jk(a–b–)

anemia, often require chronic blood transfusion. In this situation or when a patient receives a massive transfusion, the presence of donor RBCs in the patient's peripheral blood makes RBC phenotyping by conventional hemagglutination techniques complex, time-consuming, and possibly inaccurate. Indeed the interpretation of RBC typing results of multitransfused patients, based on such parameters as number of units transfused, length of time between transfusion and sample collection, and size of patient (the "best guess"), is often incorrect.[106] It is desirable to determine the blood type of a patient as part of the antibody identification process, and molecular DNA approaches are being used to type patients to overcome this limitation of hemagglutination. Interference or false results from transfused donor WBCs surviving in the recipient's circulation depends on the design of the assay used.[107] PCR assays designed for transfusion medicine testing do not detect post-transfusion DNA chimerism, and blood group determinations can reliably be made using DNA prepared from a blood sample collected after the patient has received recent chronic or even massive transfusions.[108–111] Determination of a patient's blood type by analysis of DNA is particularly useful when a patient who is transfusion-dependent has produced alloantibodies. This is because identification of the patient's probable phenotype allows the laboratory to determine to which antigens the patient can and cannot respond to make alloantibodies.

Table 5–11 Clinical Applications of DNA Analysis for Blood Group Antigens

To type patients who have been recently transfused
To type patients whose RBCs are coated with immunoglobulin
To identify a fetus at risk for hemolytic disease of the newborn
To determine which phenotypically antigen-negative patients can receive antigen-positive RBCs
To type donors for antibody identification panels
To type patients who have an antigen that is expressed weakly on RBCs
To determine *RHD* zygosity
To mass screen for antigen-negative donors
To resolve blood group A, B, and D discrepancies
To determine the origin of engrafted leukocytes in a stem cell recipient
To determine the origin of lymphocytes in a patient with graft-versus-host disease
For tissue typing
For paternity and immigration testing
For forensic testing

For Patients Whose RBCs Have a Positive DAT. DNA-based antigen typing of patients with autoimmune hemolytic anemia, whose RBCs are coated with immunoglobulin, is valuable when available diagnostic antibodies require the IAT and IgG removal techniques (e.g., EDTA-acid-glycine, chloroquine diphosphate) are not effective at removing bound immunoglobulin, or when these techniques destroy the antigen of interest.

For Donors. DNA-based assays can be used to antigen-type donor blood both for transfusion and for antibody identification reagent panels. This is particularly useful when antibodies are not available or are weakly reactive. A good example is the Dombrock blood group polymorphism, where DNA-based assays[112–114] are used to type patients and donors for Do^a and Do^b to overcome the problem of not having reliable typing reagents. Furthermore, the newer DNA technologies have the potential for screening pools of DNA for rare blood types and thereby increasing the number of donors that can be tested. As automated procedures attain higher and faster throughput at lower cost, typing of blood donors by DNA-based assays is likely to become more widespread, revolutionizing the provision of antigen-negative blood to patients.

With donor DNA-based typing, the presence of a grossly normal gene whose product is not expressed on the RBC surface would lead to the donor being falsely typed as antigen-positive, and although this would mean loss of an antigen-negative donor, it would not jeopardize the safety of the patient in blood transfusion practice.

IN THE PRENATAL SETTING

Hemagglutination titers give only an indirect indication of the risk and severity in HDN. Thus, antigen typing by DNA-based assays has particular value in the prenatal setting to determine whether the fetus has inherited the paternal antigen of clinical relevance. If the fetus is predicted to be antigen-negative, the fetus is not at risk for HDN and the mother need not be aggressively monitored.

Specific criteria should be met before initiating fetal DNA testing. The mother's serum contains an IgG antibody of potential clinical significance and the father is heterozygous for the gene encoding the antigen of interest (or paternity is in doubt). It is helpful to know the ethnic origin and to genotype both mother and father concurrently with the fetus to confirm the inheritance and to identify potential variants that could influence interpretation of the test results.

Fetal DNA can be isolated from cells obtained by invasive procedures such as amniocentesis or chorionic villus sampling and by noninvasive procedures from trophoblasts collected by transcervical sampling[115–117] and from fetal erythroblasts isolated from the maternal circulation.[118] Remarkably, cell-free fetal-derived DNA can be extracted from maternal serum or plasma[119–122] and *RHD* typing is possible.[120,123–129] Use of cell-free fetal DNA from maternal plasma has overcome concerns that fetal lymphocytes from previous pregnancies can persist in maternal blood[130] or skin[131] for years. This is not a problem with cell-free fetal DNA because it clears the maternal circulation within 3 days of termination of the pregnancy.[120,121] Fetal DNA obtained from maternal plasma appears to be less stable and reports vary regarding optimal sample storage.[120,129] Large-scale trials and standardization of protocols are still needed; however, it is likely that determination of fetal *RHD* using this noninvasive procedure will become routine clinical practice. *RHD* testing for D expression is the prime target because, at least in the majority of white individuals, the D-negative mother has a complete deletion of *RHD*, thereby permitting detection of the paternally derived fetal *RHD* gene. For analysis of the inheritance of blood group antigens determined by SNPs (e.g., K/k) rather than by the presence or absence of the gene, a sample source that contains primarily fetal DNA (e.g., amniocytes) is preferred. When isolating fetal DNA from maternal plasma, proper positive controls that test for the presence of fetal DNA are critical. Y chromosome markers are useful when the fetus is a male, but polymorphic paternal markers are needed in the case of a female.

DNA analysis for the prediction of fetal D phenotype is based on detecting the presence or absence of portions of *RHD*. A prerequisite to the accurate interpretation of DNA analysis in clinical applications is the extensive molecular characterization of apparently identical phenotypes in mother and fetus. The Rh blood group system is complex, and many hybrid genes have been described. For example, in Europeans, the molecular basis of the D-negative phenotype was, with few exceptions, associated with deletion of the entire *RHD*, until a study of serologically D-negative samples revealed nine novel *RHD* gene-positive haplotypes.[95,132] Approximately one third of Japanese D-negative people have an intact but inactive *RHD*. The majority of D-negative Africans and approximately one quarter of D-negative African Americans have an inactive *RHD* pseudogene (*RHDΨ*), and many others have hybrid *RHD-CE-D* genes.[133] These hybrid genes complicate DNA testing and can lead to false results if they are not understood by the investigator.[30,74]

When recommendations for clinical practice are based on molecular analyses, it is important to remember that, in rare situations, a genotype determination will not correlate with antigen expression on the RBC (see Table 5–10).[48,95–97,133–138] If a patient has a grossly normal gene that is not expressed (usually a null phenotype), he or she could produce an antibody if transfused with antigen-positive blood. When feasible, the appropriate assay to detect a mutation that silences a gene should be part of the DNA-based testing (e.g., GATA box analysis with *FY* typing,[137] presence of *RHD* pseudogene with *RHD* typing,[133] and exon 5 analysis with *GYPB(S)* typing).[139] Also, it is important to obtain an accurate medical history for the patient because with certain medical treatments, such as stem cell transplantation and kidney transplants, typing results in tests using DNA from different sources (such as WBCs, buccal smears, or urine sediment) may differ. Thus, thought should be given as to the purpose of the testing when establishing standard operating procedures for use in the clinical laboratory.

Before interpreting the results of DNA testing, it is important to obtain an accurate medical history and to establish if the study subject is a surrogate mother, if she has been impregnated with nonspousal sperm, or if she has received a stem cell transplant. This information, although critical, is often not provided. For prenatal diagnosis of a fetus at risk of HDN, the approach to genotyping should err on the side of caution.

When performing any blood group DNA analysis in the prenatal setting, determining the *RHD* status of the fetus, in addition to the test being ordered, can be important. If the fetus has a normal *RHD*, there is no need to provide Rh-negative blood for intrauterine transfusions. This is especially true if the mother has anti-c and fetal DNA is being typed for *RHc*.

Antibody Identification

In addition to the value of typing donors for antibody identification panels when appropriate antibodies are not available, DNA analyses are being used to aid in the identification of Dombrock (anti-Hy, anti-Jo^a), Knops (anti-Kn^a, anti-Sl^a, and anti-McC^a), and Rh (anti-hr^S, anti-hr^B) antibodies. Determination of the phenotype of the patient allows more accurate classification in Dombrock and Knops blood group systems.

DNA can be transfected into cells and grown in tissue culture to express blood group antigens. Indeed, single-pass (Kell) and multipass (Duffy) proteins have been expressed in high levels in mouse erythroleukemic cells or 293T cells and detected by human polyclonal antibodies.[140] Similar experiments have been performed on Lutheran antigens.[141] Thus, it is theoretically possible to produce a panel of cell lines expressing individual proteins for development of an automated, objective, single-step antibody detection and identification procedure. Such an approach would eliminate the need for antigen-matched, short-dated, potentially biohazardous RBC screening and panel products derived from humans. However, although promising, some major hurdles are yet to be overcome; for example, antigens from all blood group systems must be expressed at levels that are at least equivalent to those on RBCs and the detection system should have low background levels of reactivity. The highly clinically significant Rh antigens are proving difficult to express in adequate levels.

Recombinant cells expressing blood group antigens can be used for adsorption of specific antibodies as part of antibody detection and identification procedures, or prior to crossmatching if the antibody is clinically insignificant. In addition, genes can be engineered to express soluble forms of antigens for use in antibody inhibition, again as part of antibody detection and identification procedures, or prior to crossmatching.[142–144] Concentrated forms of recombinant CR1 (CD35) would be valuable to inhibit clinically insignificant antibodies in the Knops system, thereby allowing a compatible crossmatch. So far it has proven difficult to prepare the recombinant material in sufficient quantity to be of practical use.

General Considerations

The quality of DNA may be compromised in clinical samples that are not stored correctly, but this is often overcome by restricting the size of the amplified PCR product.[145] To maximize the value of DNA analysis in transfusion medicine, several areas of expertise are desirable when using molecular approaches to identify blood groups: an expertise in antibody identification, a knowledge of and ability to troubleshoot techniques, a knowledge of the genes encoding blood group antigens and their variant forms, an expertise in interpretation of the PCR-based assays used, and knowledge about the clinical significance of blood group alloantibodies.

Hemagglutination has identified many phenotypic variants encoded by *RHD*, *RHCE*, or hybrids of the two, and molecular analysis has revealed remarkable variation within the variants. Of clinical concern is the distinction, difficult to make serologically, between weak partial D and weak D phenotypes because the former may make alloantibodies to D, whereas the latter are unlikely to do so. Numerous partial D and weak D phenotypes have been defined at the molecular level,[30,73,132,138,146] and it is anticipated that this information, together with clinical (and serologic) data, will be used to guide transfusion and testing policy for patients and donors.[74]

Molecular analysis of samples with aberrant e and E antigen expression have highlighted the complexity of polymorphisms. In whites, variant e antigen expression was associated with the presence of a 48G>C nucleotide change in *RHCE*.[147] Depressed e antigen expression in black persons, which is often associated with the loss of hr^S antigen, results from different molecular backgrounds, many which have a Met238Val substitution in the Rhce protein.[148,149] To identify serologically, with certainty, that a person is truly hr^S-negative and to screen for compatible donors has always been challenging due to the lack of suitable reagents. Thus, the possibility of using a molecular approach to fulfill the transfusion requirements of such patients will quickly have a positive impact by providing the means to identify those patients at risk of making anti-e-like antibodies and a valuable screening tool for donors.

Many new *ABO* alleles have been defined,[82–84] and *ABO* genotyping is a useful clinical tool for the resolution of typing discrepancies and is especially valuable for distinguishing acquired variant phenotypes from inherited ones. DNA analysis makes it possible to define a person's ABO genotype without laborious family studies. However, improvements in testing and population studies are needed to ensure detection of the multitude of *ABO* alleles now known. DNA-based analyses will be useful to explain apparent discrepancies in typing blood donors for certain ABO subgroups that may otherwise be reportable to the FDA. In summary, the multitude of ABO and Rh alleles indicates that a large number of people from a variety of ethnic backgrounds need to be studied to determine the occurrence of particular genotypes and to establish more firmly the correlation between blood group genotype and phenotype.

Our growing understanding of the molecular basis underlying blood group polymorphisms can be used to develop automated systems for antigen typing and for antibody detection and identification. Development of DNA microarray technology continues at a rapid rate. Thus, it should soon be possible to analyze major and many minor blood group alleles on a single synthetic chip that is smaller than the head of a pin.

Currently, DNA-based assays provide a valuable adjunct to the classic hemagglutination assays. Molecular analyses have the advantage that genomic DNA is readily available from peripheral blood leukocytes, buccal epithelial cells, and even cells in urine, and it is remarkably stable. The current disadvantage is that the genotype determined on DNA may not, in some instances, reflect the RBC phenotype.

The next three chapters provide details about specific blood group antigens. Chapter 6 focuses on the ABO system and other carbohydrate antigens. Chapter 7 concentrates on the Rh, Kell, Duffy, and Kidd systems, in which the corresponding antibodies are potentially highly clinically significant. Chapter 8 describes aspects of the other blood groups.

Many websites have useful information about blood group systems. Some URL addresses that may be of interest to the reader are as follows:

1. http://www.ncbi.nlm.nih.gov/projects/mhc/xslcgi.fcgi?cmd=bgmut/home
   The website of the Blood Group Antigen Mutation Database, a mutation database of gene loci encoding common and rare blood group antigens. This site provides links to many other relevant sites.
2. www.iccbba.com
   The website of the International Society for Blood Transfusion, with links to information about topics such as ISBT128.
3. www.iccbba.com/page25.htm
   The website for the ISBT Working Party on Terminology for Red Cell Surface Antigens.
4. www.aabb.org
   The website of the American Association for Blood Banks.
5. www.bbts.org.uk
   The website of the British Blood Transfusion Society.

REFERENCES

1. Alberts B, Bray D, Lewis J, et al. Molecular Biology of the Cell, 3rd ed. New York, Garland Publishing, 1994.
2. Hoffman R, Benz EJ, Shattil SJ, et al. (eds). Hematology: Basic Principles and Practice, 2nd ed. New York, Churchill Livingstone, 1995.
3. Telen MJ. Erythrocyte blood group antigens: Not so simple after all. Blood 1995;85:299–306.
4. Cartron JP, Colin Y. Structural and functional diversity of blood group antigens. Transfus Clin Biol 2001;8:163–199.
5. Reid ME, Mohandas N. Red blood cell blood group antigens: structure and function. Semin Hematol 2004;41:93–117.
6. Tanner MJA. The structure and function of band 3 (AE1): recent developments. Mol Membr Biol 1997;14:155–165.
7. Jennings ML. Structure and function of the red blood cell anion transport protein. Annu Rev Biophys Biophys Chem 1989;18:397–430.
8. Vince JW, Reithmeier RA. Carbonic anhydrase II binds to the carboxyl terminus of human band 3, the erythrocyte C1-/HCO_3^- exchanger. J Biol Chem 1998;273:28430–28437.
9. Lux SE, Palek J. Disorders of the red cell membrane. In Handin RI, Lux SE, Stossel TP (eds). Blood: Principles and Practice. Philadelphia, J.B. Lippincott, 1995, pp 1701–1817.
10. Bruce LJ, Tanner MJA. Structure-function relationships of band 3 variants. Cell Mol Biol 1996;42:953–973.

11. Delaunay J, Alloisio N, Morle L, et al. Molecular genetics of hereditary elliptocytosis and hereditary spherocytosis. Ann Genet 1996;39: 209–221.
12. Hassoun H, Palek J. Hereditary spherocytosis: a review of the clinical and molecular aspects of the disease. Blood Rev 1996;10:129–147.
13. Wang DN, Kuhlbrandt W, Sarabia VE, Reithmeier RA. Two-dimensional structure of the membrane domain of human band 3, the anion transport protein of the erythrocyte membrane. EMBO J 1993;12:2233–2239.
14. Low PS. Structure and function of the cytoplasmic domain of band 3: center of erythrocyte membrane–peripheral protein interactions. Biochim Biophys Acta 1986;864:145–167.
15. Hemming NJ, Anstee DJ, Mawby WJ, et al. Localisation of the protein 4.1-binding site on human erythrocyte glycophorins C and D [published erratum appears in Biochem J 1994;300(Pt 3):920]. Biochem J 1994;299:191–196.
16. Nunomura W, Takakuwa Y, Parra M, et al. Regulation of protein 4.1R, p55, and glycophorin C ternary complex in human erythrocyte membrane. J Biol Chem 2000;275:24540–24546.
17. Reid ME, Chasis JA, Mohandas N. Identification of a functional role for human erythrocyte sialoglycoproteins beta and gamma. Blood 1987;69:1068–1072.
18. Reid ME, Takakuwa Y, Conboy J, et al. Glycophorin C content of human erythrocyte membrane is regulated by protein 4.1. Blood 1990;75:2229–2234.
19. Alloisio N, Dalla Venezia N, Rana A, et al. Evidence that red blood cell protein p55 may participate in the skeleton-membrane linkage that involves protein 4.1 and glycophorin C. Blood 1993;82:1323–1327.
20. Workman RF, Low PS. Biochemical analysis of potential sites for protein 4.1-mediated anchoring of the spectrin-actin skeleton to the erythrocyte membrane. J Biol Chem 1998;273:6171–6176.
21. Hemming NJ, Anstee DJ, Staricoff MA, et al. Identification of the membrane attachment sites for protein 4.1 in the human erythrocyte. J Biol Chem 1995;270:5360–5366.
22. Marfatia SM, Morais-Cabral JH, Kim AC, et al. The PDZ domain of human erythrocyte p55 mediates its binding to the cytoplasmic carboxyl terminus of glycophorin C—Analysis of the binding interface by in vitro mutagenesis. J Biol Chem 1997;272:24191–24197.
23. Bruce LJ, Ring SM, Anstee DJ, et al. Changes in the blood group Wright antigens are associated with a mutation at amino acid 658 in human erythrocyte band 3: a site of interaction between band 3 and glycophorin A under certain conditions. Blood 1995;85:541–547.
24. Hassoun H, Hanada T, Lutchman M, et al. Complete deficiency of glycophorin A in red blood cells from mice with targeted inactivation of the band 3 (AE1) gene. Blood 1998;91:2146–2151.
25. Peters LL, Shivdasani RA, Liu SC, et al. Anion exchanger 1 (band 3) is required to prevent erythrocyte membrane surface loss but not to form the membrane skeleton. Cell 1996;86:917–927.
26. Xie SS, Huang C-H, Reid ME, et al. The glycophorin A gene family in gorillas: structure, expression, and comparison with the human and chimpanzee homologues. Biochem Genet 1997;35:59–76.
27. Tanphaichitr VS, Sumboonnanonda A, Ideguchi H, et al. Novel AE1 mutations in recessive distal renal tubular acidosis—Loss-of-function is rescued by glycophorin A. J Clin Invest 1998;102:2173–2179.
28. Russo D, Redman C, Lee S. Association of XK and Kell blood group proteins. J Biol Chem 1998;273:13950–13956.
29. Jung HH, Russo D, Redman C, Brandner S. Kell and XK immunohistochemistry in McLeod myopathy. Muscle Nerve 2001;24:1346–1351.
30. Avent ND, Reid ME. The Rh blood group system: a review. Blood 2000;95:375–387.
31. Nicolas V, Kim CL, Gane P, et al. Rh-RhAG/ankyrin-R, a new interaction site between the membrane bilayer and the red cell skeleton, is impaired by Rh-null-associated mutation. J Biol Chem 2003;278:25526–25533.
32. Paulson JC, Colley KJ. Glycosyltransferases. Structure, localization, and control of cell type-specific glycosylation. J Biol Chem 1989;264: 17615–17618.
33. Brecher M (ed). Technical Manual, 15th ed. Bethesda, Md., American Association of Blood Banks, 2005.
34. Garratty G, Dzik WH, Issitt PD, et al. Terminology for blood group antigens and genes: Historical origins and guidelines in the new millennium. Transfusion 2000;40:477–489.
35. Reid ME, McManus K, Zelinski T. Chromosome location of genes encoding human blood groups. Transf Med Rev 1998;12:151–161.
36. Mollison PL, Engelfriet CP, Contreras M. Blood Transfusion in Clinical Medicine, 10th ed. Oxford, Blackwell Science, 1997.
37. Anstee DJ, Spring FA. Red cell membrane glycoproteins with a broad tissue distribution. Transf Med Rev 1989;3:13–23.
38. Southcott MJG, Tanner MJ, Anstee DJ. The expression of human blood group antigens during erythropoiesis in a cell culture system. Blood 1999;93:4425–4435.
39. Green CA, Daniels GL. Development of erythroid cell surface markers during in vitro erythropoiesis: a comparison of two methods (abstract). Transf Med 1999;9(Suppl 1):9.
40. Lögdberg L, Reid ME, Miller JL. Cloning and genetic characterization of blood group carrier molecules and antigens. Transf Med Rev 2002; 16:1–10.
41. Crew VK, Burton N, Kagan A, et al. CD151, the first member of the tetraspanin (TM4) superfamily detected on erythrocytes, is essential for the correct assembly of human basement membranes in kidney and skin. Blood 2004;104:2217–2223.
42. Wagner FF, Poole J, Flegel WA. The Scianna antigens including Rd are expressed by ERMAP. Blood 2003;101:752–757.
43. Yu LC, Twu YC, Chou ML, et al. The molecular genetics of the human I locus and molecular background explaining the partial association of the adult i phenotype with congenital cataracts. Blood 2003;101: 2081–2087.
44. Hellberg A, Poole J, Olsson ML. Molecular basis of the Globside-deficient P^k blood group phenotype. identification of four inactivating mutations in the UDP-*N*-acetylgalactosamine: Globotriaosylceramide 3-beta-*N*-acetylgalactosaminyltransferase gene. J Biol Chem 2002;277:29455–29459.
45. Avent ND. Human erythrocyte antigen expression: its molecular bases. Br J Biomed Sci 1997;54:16–37.
46. Issitt PD, Anstee DJ. Applied Blood Group Serology, 4th ed. Durham, N.C., Montgomery Scientific, 1998.
47. Reid ME, Lomas-Francis C. Blood Group Antigen FactsBook, 2nd ed. San Diego, Academic Press, 2003.
48. Reid ME, Yazdanbakhsh K. Molecular insights into blood groups and implications for blood transfusions. Curr Opin Hematol 1998;5: 93–102.
49. Blancher A, Reid ME, Socha WW. Cross-reactivity of antibodies to human and primate red cell antigens. Transf Med Rev 2000;14: 161–179.
50. Salvignol I, Calvas P, Socha WW, et al. Structural analysis of the RH-like blood group gene products in nonhuman primates. Immunogenetics 1995;41:271–281.
51. Huang C-H, Xie S-S, Socha WW, Blumenfeld OO. Sequence diversification and exon inactivation in glycophorin A gene family from chimpanzee to human. J Mol Evol 1995;41:478–486.
52. Westhoff CM, Silberstein LE, Wylie DE. Evidence supporting the requirement for two proline residues for expression of the "c" antigen. Transfusion 2000;40:321–324.
53. Daniels G. Human Blood Groups, 2nd ed. Oxford, Blackwell Science, 2002.
54. Cartron JP. Molecular basis of red cell protein antigen deficiencies. Vox Sang 2000;78:7–23.
55. Minetti G, Low PS. Erythrocyte signal transduction pathways and their possible functions. Curr Opin Hematol 1997;4:116–121.
56. Roitt I, Brostoff J, Male D. Immunology, 4th ed. London, Mosby, 1996.
57. Giblett ER. A critique of the theoretical hazard of inter vs. intra-racial transfusion. Transfusion 1961;1:233–238.
58. Giblett ER. Blood group alloantibodies: an assessment of some laboratory practices. Transfusion 1977;4:299–308.
59. Hoeltge GA, Domen RE, Rybicki LA, Schaffer PA. Multiple red cell transfusions and alloimmunization: experience with 6996 antibodies detected in a total of 159,262 patients from 1985 to 1993. Arch Pathol Lab Med 1995;119:42–45.
60. Reid ME, Øyen R, Marsh WL. Summary of the clinical significance of blood group alloantibodies. Semin Hematol 2000;37:197–216.
61. Standards Committee of American Association of Blood Banks. Standards for Blood Banks and Transfusion Services, 23rd ed. Bethesda, Md., American Association of Blood Banks, 2004.
62. Regan F, Hewitt P, Vincent B, Nolan A. Do patients know they have been transfused? Vox Sang 1999;76:248–249.
63. Wayne AS, Kevy SV, Nathan DG. Transfusion management of sickle cell disease. Blood 1993;81:1109–1123.
64. Ness PM. To match or not to match: the question for chronically transfused patients with sickle cell anemia. Transfusion 1994;34:558–560.
65. Rosse WF, Gallagher D, Kinney TR, et al. Cooperative Study of Sickle Cell Disease. Transfusion and alloimmunization in sickle cell disease. Blood 1990;76:1431–1437.
66. Pegelow CH, Adams RJ, McKie V, et al. Risk of recurrent stroke in patients with sickle cell disease treated with erythrocyte transfusions. J Pediatr 1995;126:896–899.

67. Adams RJ, McKie VC, Brambilla D, et al. Stroke prevention trial in sickle cell anemia. Control Clin Trials 1998;19:110–129.
68. Adams RJ, McKie VC, Hsu L, et al. Prevention of a first stroke by transfusions in children with sickle cell anemia and abnormal results on transcranial Doppler ultrasonography. N Engl J Med 1998;339:5–11.
69. Fullerton HJ, Adams RJ, Zhao S, Johnston SC. Declining stroke rates in Californian children with sickle cell disease. Blood 2004;104:336–339.
70. Sosler SD, Jilly BJ, Saporito C, Koshy M. A simple, practical model for reducing alloimmunization in patients with sickle cell disease. Am J Hematol 1993;43:103–106.
71. Sausais L, Øyen R, Rios M, et al. DAK, a low incidence antigen shared by D^{IIIA} and R^{N} (abstract). Transfusion 1999;39(Suppl 1):79S.
72. Beauregard P, Blajchman MA. Hemolytic and pseudo-hemolytic transfusion reactions: an overview of the hemolytic transfusion reactions and the clinical conditions that mimic them. Transf Med Rev 1994;8:184–199.
73. Huang C-H, Liu PZ, Cheng JG. Molecular biology and genetics of the Rh blood group system. Semin Hematol 2000;37:150–165.
74. Westhoff CM. The Rh blood group system in review: a new face for the next decade. Transfusion 2004;44:1663–1673.
75. Redman CM, Russo D, Pu J, Lee S. Kell blood group protein: Its relation to XK and its function as an endothelin-3 converting enzyme. In Danek A(ed.). Neuroacanthocytosis Syndromes: New Perspectives for the Study of Basal Ganglia Degeneration. Berlin, Springer-Verlag, 2004, pp 197–203.
76. Russo DCW, Lee S, Reid ME, Redman CM. Point mutations causing the McLeod phenotype. Transfusion 2002;42:287–293.
77. Danek A, Rubio JP, Rampoldi L, et al. McLeod neuroacanthocytosis: Genotype and phenotype. Ann Neurol 2001;50:755–764.
78. Hirschberg CB. Golgi nucleotide sugar transport and leukocyte adhesion deficiency II. J Clin Invest 2001;108:3–6.
79. Luhn K, Wild MK, Eckhardt M, et al. The gene defective in leukocyte adhesion deficiency II encodes a putative GDP-fucose transporter. Nat Genet 2001;28:69–72.
80. Mullis KB, Faloona FA. Specific synthesis of DNA in vitro via a polymerase-catalyzed chain reaction. Methods Enzymol 1987;155: 335–350.
81. Mullis KB. The unusual origin of the polymerase chain reaction. Sci Am 1990;262:56–65.
82. Chester MA, Olsson ML. The ABO blood group gene: a locus of considerable genetic diversity. Transfus Med Rev 2001;15:177–200.
83. Yamamoto F. Cloning and regulation of the *ABO* genes. Transf Med 2001;11:281–294.
84. Olsson ML, Irshaid NM, Hosseini-Maaf B, et al. Genomic analysis of clinical samples with serologic ABO blood grouping discrepancies: identification of 15 novel A and B subgroup alleles. Blood 2001;98:1585–1593.
85. Yamamoto F. Molecular genetics of ABO. Vox Sang 2000;78(Suppl 2): 91–103.
86. Reid ME, Rios M, Yazdanbakhsh K. Applications of molecular biology techniques to transfusion medicine. Semin Hematol 2000;37: 166–176.
87. Lee S, Russo D, Redman CM. The Kell blood group system: Kell and XK membrane proteins. Semin Hematol 2000;37:113–121.
88. Pogo AO, Chaudhuri A. The Duffy protein: a malarial and chemokine receptor. Semin Hematol 2000;37:122–129.
89. Schenkel-Brunner H. Human Blood Groups: Chemical and Biochemical Basis of Antigen Specificity, 2nd ed. New York, Springer-Verlag Wien, 2000.
90. Reid ME, Lomas-Francis C. The Blood Group Antigen FactsBook. San Diego, Academic Press, 1996.
91. Daniels G. Human Blood Groups. Oxford, Blackwell Science, 1995.
92. Oriol R, Candelier JJ, Mollicone R. Molecular genetics of H. Vox Sang 2000;78:105–108.
93. Reid ME, Storry JR. Low-incidence MNS antigens associated with single amino acid changes and their susceptibility to enzyme treatment. Immunohematology 2001;17:76–81.
94. Wagner T, Vadon M, Staudacher E, et al. A new *h* allele detected in Europe has a missense mutation in $\alpha^{1,2}$-fucosyltransferase motif II. Transfusion 2001;41:31–38.
95. Wagner FF, Frohmajer A, Flegel WA. *RHD* positive haplotypes in D-negative Europeans. BMC Genetics 2001;2:10
96. Flegel WA, Wagner FF. Molecular genetics of *RH*. Vox Sang 2000;78: 109–115.
97. Huang C-H, Blumenfeld OO. MNSs blood groups and major glycophorins: Molecular basis for allelic variation. In Cartron J-P, Rouger P (eds). Molecular Basis of Human Blood Group Antigens. New York, Plenum Press, 1995, pp 153–188.
98. Poole J. Red cell antigens on band 3 and glycophorin A. Blood Rev 2000;14:31–43.
99. Zelinski T. Erythrocyte band 3 antigens and the Diego blood group system. Transf Med Rev 1998;12:36–45.
100. Lee S, Russo DCW, Reiner AP, et al. Molecular defects underlying the Kell null phenotype. J Biol Chem 2001;276:27281–27289.
101. Lucien N, Sidoux-Walter F, Olivès B, et al. Characterization of the gene encoding the human Kidd blood group/urea transporter protein: evidence for splice site mutations in Jknull individuals. J Biol Chem 1998;273:12973–12980.
102. Furukawa K, Iwamura K, Uchikawa M, et al. Molecular basis for the p phenotype. Identification of distinct and multiple mutations in the α 1,4-galactosyltransferase gene in Swedish and Japanese individuals. J Biol Chem 2000;275:37752–37756.
103. Cuzin M. DNA chips: A new tool for genetic analysis. Transfus Clin Biol 2001;8:291–296.
104. Petrik J. Microarray technology: The future of blood testing? Vox Sang 2001;80:1–11.
105. Miyazato A, Ueno S, Ohmine K, et al. Identification of myelodysplastic syndrome-specific genes by DNA microarray analysis with purified hematopoietic stem cell fraction. Blood 2001;98:422–427.
106. Reid ME, Oyen R, Storry J, et al. Interpretation of RBC typing in multi-transfused patients can be unreliable (abstract). Transfusion 2000;40 (Suppl):123S.
107. Reed WF, Lee TH, Trachtenberg E, et al. Detection of microchimerism by PCR is a function of amplification strategy. Transfusion 2001;41: 39–44.
108. Wenk RE, Chiafari FA. DNA typing of recipient blood after massive transfusion. Transfusion 1997;37:1108–1110.
109. Legler TJ, Eber SW, Lakomek M, et al. Application of RHD and RHCE genotyping for correct blood group determination in chronically transfused patients. Transfusion 1999;39:852–855.
110. Reid ME, Rios M, Powell VI, et al. DNA from blood samples can be used to genotype patients who have recently received a transfusion. Transfusion 2000;40:48–53.
111. Rozman P, Dovc T, Gassner C. Differentiation of autologous *ABO*, *RHD*, *RHCE*, *KEL*, *JK*, and *FY* blood group genotypes by analysis of peripheral blood samples of patients who have recently received multiple transfusions. Transfusion 2000;40:936–942.
112. Rios M, Hue-Roye K, Lee AH, et al. DNA analysis for the Dombrock polymorphism. Transfusion 2001;41:1143–1146.
113. Wu G-G, Jin Z-H, Deng Z-H, Zhao T-M. Polymerase chain reaction with sequence-specific primers-based genotyping of the human Dombrock blood group *DO1* and *DO2* alleles and the *DO* gene frequencies in Chinese blood donors. Vox Sang 2001;81:49–51.
114. Storry JR, Westhoff CM, Charles-Pierre D, et al. DNA analysis for donor screening of Dombrock blood group antigens. Immunohematology 2003;19:73–76.
115. Adinolfi M, Sherlock J, Kemp T, et al. Prenatal detection of fetal RhD DNA sequences in transcervical samples. Lancet 1995;345:318–319.
116. Bennett PR, Overton TG, Lighten AD, Fisk NM. Rhesus D typing. Lancet 1995;345:661–662.
117. Kingdom J, Sherlock J, Rodeck C, Adinolfi M. Detection of trophoblast cells in transcervical samples collected by lavage or cytobrush. Obstet Gynecol 1995;86:283–288.
118. Cheung M-C, Goldberg JD, Kan WK. Prenatal diagnosis of sickle cell anemia and thalassaemia by analysis of fetal cells in maternal blood. Nature Genet 1997;14:264–268.
119. Lo YMD, Corbetta N, Chamberlain PF, et al. Presence of fetal DNA in maternal plasma and serum. Lancet 1997;350:485–487.
120. Nelson M, Eagle C, Langshaw M, et al. Genotyping fetal DNA by non-invasive means: extraction from maternal plasma. Vox Sang 2001;80:112–116.
121. Lo YM, Tein MS, Lau TK, et al. Quantitative analysis of fetal DNA in maternal plasma and serum: implications for noninvasive prenatal diagnosis. Am J Hum Genet 1998;62:768–775.
122. Lo YMD. Fetal DNA in maternal plasma: application to non-invasive blood group genotyping of the fetus. Transfus Clin Biol 2001;8:306–310.
123. Avent ND, Finning KM, Martin PG, Soothill PW. Prenatal determination of fetal blood group status. Vox Sang 2000;78:155–162.
124. Lo YMD, Hjelm NM, Fidler C, et al. Prenatal diagnosis of fetal RhD status by molecular analysis of maternal plasma. NEJM 1998;339:1734–1738.
125. Lo YM. Fetal DNA in maternal plasma. Ann NY Acad Sci 2000;906: 141–147.
126. Hahn S, Zhong XY, Burk MR, et al. Multiplex and real-time quantitative PCR on fetal DNA in maternal plasma. A comparison with fetal cells isolated from maternal blood. Ann NY Acad Sci 2000;906: 148–152.

127. Faas BH, Beuling EA, Christiaens GC, et al. Detection of fetal RHD-specific sequences in maternal plasma. Lancet 1998;352:1196.
128. Bischoff FZ, Nguyen DD, Marquez-Do D, et al. Noninvasive determination of fetal RhD status using fetal DNA in maternal serum and PCR. J Soc Gynecol Invest 1999;6:64–69.
129. Brojer E, Zupanska B, Guz K, et al. Noninvasive determination of fetal RHD status by examination of cell-free DNA in maternal plasma. Transfusion 2005;45:1473–1480.
130. Bianchi DW, Zickwolf GK, Weil GJ, et al. Male fetal progenitor cells persist in maternal blood for as long as 27 years postpartum. Proc Natl Acad Sci USA 1996;93:705–708.
131. Artlett CM, Smith JB, Jimenez SA. Identification of fetal DNA and cells in skin lesions from women with systemic sclerosis. NEJM 1998;338: 1186–1191.
132. Wagner FF, Frohmajer A, Ladewig B, et al. Weak D alleles express distinct phenotypes. Blood 2000;95:2699–2708.
133. Singleton BK, Green CA, Avent ND, et al. The presence of an *RHD* pseudogene containing a 37 base pair duplication and a nonsense mutation in Africans with the Rh D-negative blood group phenotype. Blood 2000;95:12–18.
134. Cartron JP, Bailly P, Le Van Kim C, et al. Insights into the structure and function of membrane polypeptides carrying blood group antigens. Vox Sang 1998;74(Suppl 2):29–64.
135. Huang C-H. Molecular insights into the Rh protein family and associated antigens. Curr Opin Hematol 1997;4:94–103.
136. Reid ME. Molecular basis for blood groups and function of carrier proteins. In Silberstein LE (ed). Molecular and Functional Aspects of Blood Group Antigens. Arlington, Va., American Association of Blood Banks, 1995, pp 75–125.
137. Tournamille C, Colin Y, Cartron JP, Le Van Kim C. Disruption of a GATA motif in the *Duffy* gene promoter abolishes erythroid gene expression in Duffy-negative individuals. Nature Genet 1995;10: 224–228.
138. Müller TH, Wagner FF, Trockenbacher A, et al. PCR screening for common weak D types shows different distributions in three Central European populations. Transfusion 2001;41:45–52.
139. Storry JR, Reid ME, Fetics S, Huang CH. Mutations in GYPB exon 5 drive the S-s-U+(var) phenotype in persons of African descent: implications for transfusion Transfusion 2003;43:1738–1747.
140. Yazdanbakhsh K, Øyen R, Yu Q, et al. High level, stable expression of blood group antigens in a heterologous system. Am J Hematol 2000;63:114–124.
141. Ridgwell K, Dixey J, Parsons SF, et al. Screening human sera for anti-Lu antibodies using soluble recombinant Lu antigens (abstract). Transf Med 2001;11(Suppl 1):P25.
142. Moulds JM, Brai M, Cohen J, et al. Reference typing report for complement receptor 1 (CR1). Exper Clin Immunogenetics 1998;15: 291–294.
143. Daniels GL, Green CA, Powell RM, Ward T. Hemagglutination inhibition of Cromer blood group antibodies with soluble recombinant decay-accelerating factor. Transfusion 1998;38:332–336.
144. Lee S, Lin M, Mele A, et al. Proteolytic processing of big endothelin-3 by the Kell blood group protein. Blood 1999;94:1440–1450.
145. Reid ME, Rios M. Applications of molecular genotyping to immunohaematology. Br J Biomed Sci 1999;56:145–152.
146. Wagner FF, Gassner C, Müller TH, et al. Molecular basis of weak D phenotypes. Blood 1999;93:385–393.
147. Westhoff CM, Silberstein LE, Wylie DE, et al. 16Cys encoded by the *RHce* gene is associated with altered expression of the e antigen and is frequent in the R_0 haplotype. Br J Haematol 2001;113:666–671.
148. Noizat-Pirenne F, Mouro I, Le Pennec PY, et al. Two new alleles of the *RHCE* gene in Black individuals: the *RHce* allele *ceMO* and the *RHcE* allele *cEMI*. Br J Haematol 2001;113:672–679.
149. Noizat-Pirenne F, Lee K, Le Pennec P-Y, et al. Rare RHCE phenotypes in black individuals of Afro-Caribbean origin: identification and transfusion safety. Blood 2002;100:4223–4231.

Chapter 6

ABO and Related Antigens and Antibodies

Connie M. Westhoff • Marion E. Reid

This chapter summarizes current knowledge of the blood groups composed of terminal carbohydrate moieties, the ABO, H, Lewis, Ii, and P systems (International Society of Blood Transfusion [ISBT] system or collection numbers given in parentheses). The antigens are the products of the action of glycosyltransferase enzymes, and they share biochemical synthesis pathways and precursor framework oligosaccharide molecules. The antigens are carried on large oligosaccharide chains covalently linked to proteins (glycoproteins), lipids (glycolipids), or both on the red blood cell (RBC). In addition, some are expressed on tissues, and soluble forms can be found in various secretions and excretions.

ABO AND Hh SYSTEMS (ISBT SYSTEMS 001 AND 018)

History

ABO was the first blood group system to be discovered. In 1900, Landsteiner mixed sera and RBCs from his colleagues and observed agglutination.[1] On the basis of the agglutination pattern, he named the first two blood group antigens A and B, using the first two letters of the alphabet. RBCs not agglutinated by either sera were first called type C but became known as "ohne A" and "ohne B" (*ohne* is German for "without") and finally O. Landsteiner received the Nobel Prize in 1930, 30 years after the discovery of the ABO blood groups.

Unfortunately, administering transfusions based on agglutination reactions was largely ignored, and surgeons continued performing direct donor-to-patient blood transfusions. This practice provided many opportunities to observe symptoms of severe and fatal hemolytic transfusion reactions. Not until methods were developed to store and preserve blood (1914–1917) did blood transfusion move to the blood bank environment, and World War I saw the first large-scale transfusions based on serologic ABO selection of donors.[2]

Antigens

The ABO antigens were biochemically characterized in the 1950s and 1960s (reviewed in Yamamoto[3]) as carbohydrate structures on glycoproteins and glycolipids. The ABO system consists of four antigens with ISBT numbers—A, B, A,B, and A_1—but there are additional subgroups (e.g., A_2, A_3, A_X, A_{el}, B_3), and Hh is a separate system.[4] The antigens are synthesized in a stepwise fashion by glycosyltransferase enzymes that sequentially add specific monosaccharide sugars in specific linkages to a growing oligosaccharide precursor chain. The terminal sugar determines antigen specificity: an *N*-acetylgalactosamine residue results in expression of the A antigen, and a terminal galactose residue is responsible for the B antigen. These structures are similar, differing only in that A antigen has a substituted amino group on carbon 2 (Fig. 6–1). The precursor substrate for A and B antigens is the H antigen (Fig. 6–2). The terminal fucose in $\alpha(1,2)$ linkage to galactose is responsible for H antigen specificity, and large amounts of H are present on group O RBCs, because H is not converted to A or B. Some H antigen precursor also remains on A and B RBCs, listed as follows in descending order of frequency: A_2, B, A_2B, A_1, A_1B.

RBC membrane proteins carry well over 2×10^6 A, B, and H antigens (ABH) combined per RBC, and most (80%) are located on the major integral membrane protein, band 3 (anion exchanger 1, or AE1), which is the RBC $Cl^-HCO_3^-$ anion exchanger. In addition, the glucose transporter, Rh-associated glycoprotein (RhAG), and aquaporin-1 (Colton) also carry A, B, and H, but in smaller amounts (reviewed in Lowe[5]). A, B, and H antigens are also found in lesser amounts as lipid-linked glycoconjugates associated with the RBC membrane via a ceramide moiety.

After their discovery on RBCs, the ABH antigens were also found on many tissues. Large amounts are expressed on endothelial and epithelial cells of the lung and gut and on the epithelial cells of the urinary and reproductive tracts; hence, they are called *histo-blood group antigens*. ABH antigens are also found in secretions (particularly saliva) and fluids (milk and urine) of 80% of the population who have the secretor (Se) phenotype.[6]

ABH antigens are also found on platelets. The amount of A or B antigen on platelets varies between individuals, with approximately 8% of blood group A and 10% of B donors reported to have "high" level expression.[7] Thus, ABO incompatibility can compromise the outcome in platelet transfusions. Recent studies have refocused attention on the interesting observation that platelets from donors with an A_2 phenotype lack both A and H antigens.[8,9] The biochemical basis for the lack of A antigen is not yet known, but this observation has implications for transfusion practice in that approximately 20% of group A platelets would be from A_2 donors (see incidence of A_2 phenotype). These platelets would be appropriate for "universal" use, and platelets from A_2 donors may also be a superior product for patients undergoing A/O major mismatch allogeneic progenitor cell transplantation.[9]

As tissue antigens, ABH are important in solid organ transplantation. Recipient antibodies react with antigens on the transplanted organ, and complement activation at the surface of endothelial cells results in rapid destruction and

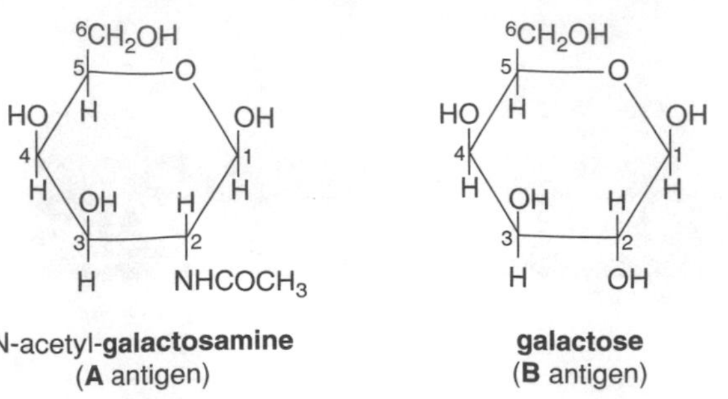

Figure 6–1 Terminal carbohydrates that define the A and B antigens. The terminal galactose residues differ only in that the A antigen has a substituted amino-acetyl group on carbon number 2.

acute rejection.[10] However, successful transplantation across ABO barriers is possible, particularly with blood group A_2 to O, and combined with current immunosuppressive and pretreatment regimens (reviewed by Rydberg[11]). As observed for platelets, the absence of A antigen on tissues of group A_2 indicates significant lack of A_2-transferase activity in nonerythroid tissues.[12,13]

The incidence of ABO blood groups differs in populations (Table 6–1).[14] Group B is found twice as frequently in African Americans and Asians as in white persons. Group A subgroups are more common than group B subgroups, and A_2 has an average incidence of 20% of group A patients.[15] Subgroup A_2 is rare in Asians.

Inherited and Acquired ABH Antigen Variants

Subgroups of A and B have weaker expression of the respective antigens. The difference between A_1 and A_2 is quantitative, because the number of A antigens is reduced on A_2. The difference is also qualitative, because there are structural differences in the branching of the oligosaccharide chains. The structural difference explains why A-subgroup individuals often make anti-A_1. The reagent *Dolichos biflorus* lectin distinguishes A_1 from A_2 and other A subgroups.

Acquired B antigen results from the action of bacterial deacetylase, an enzyme that can remove an acetyl group from the A-terminal sugar, *N*-acetylgalactosamine. Galactosamine is similar to galactose, the B-specific terminal residue, and anti-B reagents can cross-react with the deacetylated structure.[16] Acquired B usually occurs in individuals suffering from colon or rectal carcinoma, intestinal obstruction, or infections involving gram-negative bacteria from the gut. It is transient and, because the acquired B develops at the expense of A antigen, the phenotype is found only in group A patients. There is a report of a transfusion fatality in a group A patient mistyped as AB because of acquired B who was transfused with group AB blood.[17]

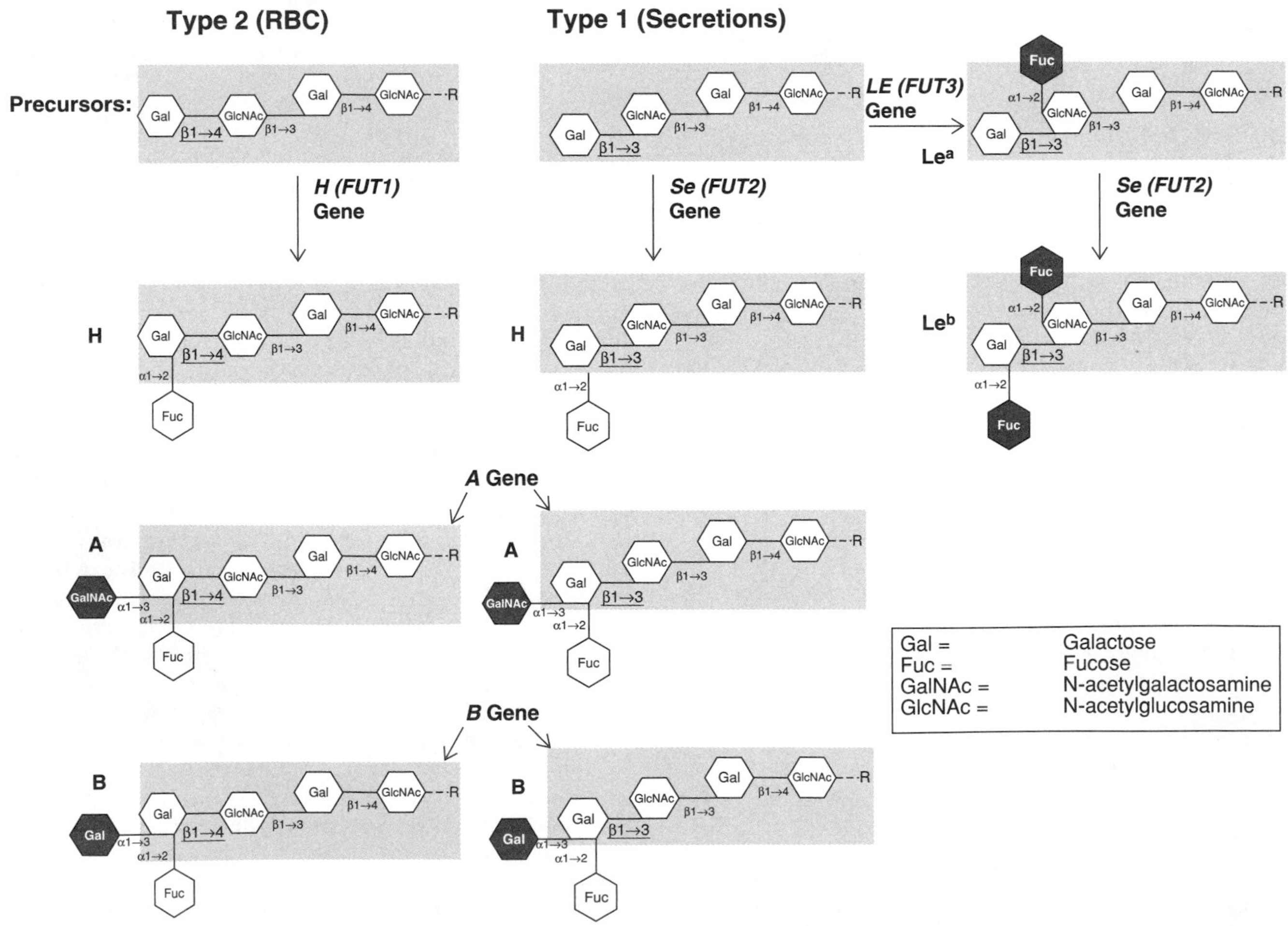

Gal =	Galactose
Fuc =	Fucose
GalNAc =	N-acetylgalactosamine
GlcNAc =	N-acetylglucosamine

Figure 6–2 Synthesis of A, B, and H, and Lewis antigens. Oligosaccharide precursor core type 1 and type 2 structures differ only in the linkage between the terminal galactose (Gal) and the *N*-acetylglucosamine (GlcNAc), shown underscored. Terminal carbohydrates that define the antigens are shown in black.

Table 6–1 ABO Blood Groups and Incidence

Phenotype	Incidence (%)		
	White	African American	Asian
A_1	34	19	27
A_2	10	8	Rare
B	9	19	25
A_1B	3	3	5
A_2B	1	1	Rare
O	44	49	43

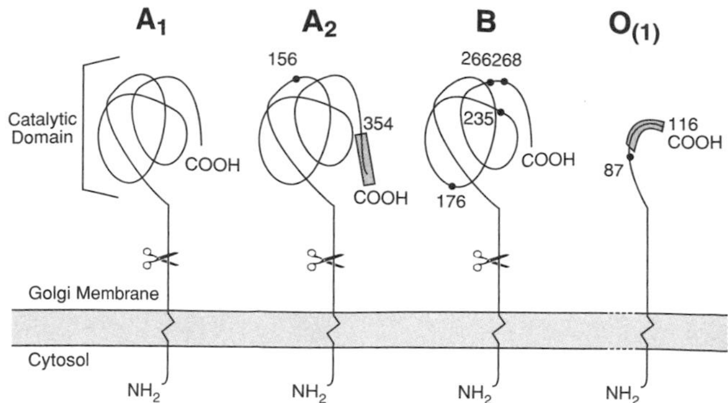

Figure 6–3 Model of the glycosyltransferases and their location in the lumen of the Golgi. Proteolytic cleavage, shown as *scissors*, generates the soluble enzyme found in body fluids and plasma. The *boxed areas* on the A_2 and O_1 glycosyltransferases indicate the altered protein sequence that results from the frameshift gene mutations. (The O truncated enzyme probably does not reach the Golgi membrane.)

A or B antigen expression can weaken in patients with acute leukemia or stress hematopoiesis. Chromosomal deletions and lesions that involve the ABO locus can result in the loss of transferase expression in the leukemic cell population. A decrease in A or B antigen expression, when found without a hematologic disorder, can be prognostic of a preleukemic state. In stress hematopoiesis, the higher turnover and early release from the bone marrow results in reduced branching of the carbohydrate chains, causing weakened expression.[18]

Rare Bombay phenotype RBCs (first reported in Bombay, India) lack H antigen; consequently, without H precursor, they also lack A and B antigens. These RBCs type routinely as group O, designated O_h, and the serum contains potent anti-H in addition to anti-A and anti-B.[18,19]

ABO Genes

In 1959, Watkins and Morgan[20] correctly suggested that the genes for the carbohydrate ABO determinants actually encoded enzymes responsible for the assembly of the subunits. The ABO locus encodes the A and B glycosyltransferases, which were mapped by linkage analysis to chromosome 9q34.[21] Researchers cloned the A-glycosyltransferase in 1990 by exploiting the fact that some tumors have increased expression of ABH antigens and the corresponding glycosyltransferase. Soluble enzyme was isolated from lung tissue for amino acid sequencing,[22] and complementary DNA libraries from gastric carcinoma and colon adenocarcinoma cell lines from individuals with different ABO phenotypes were screened and sequenced to determine the molecular differences among the transferases.[23,24]

The ABO glycosyltransferase gene contains seven exons and spans approximately 18 to 20 kb.[25] It encodes a 354-amino acid, 41-kD transferase that has a short N-terminal region, a hydrophobic transmembrane segment for retention in the Golgi membrane, and a large C-terminal, catalytically active domain (Fig. 6–3). The glycosyltransferase enzymes are membrane-bound in the lumen of the Golgi,[26] and glycosylation of membrane proteins takes place during transit through the Golgi. Some soluble enzyme is also found in body fluids and plasma and is derived from the membrane-bound enzyme through proteolysis that cleaves the catalytic domain from the membrane-spanning domain.[27]

A and B transferases

The A and B transferase enzymes differ by only 4 of 354 amino acids, Arg176Gly, Gly235Ser, Leu266Met, and Gly268Ala. The last two, residues 266 and 268, are primarily responsible for the substrate specificity (see Fig. 6–3).[24] Mutations in A or B transferase genes can result in weak expression (subgroup phenotypes) or in nonfunctional O alleles. A and B subgroups result from a large variety of mutations that cause reduced activity of the glycosyltransferase. To date, DNA studies reveal the presence of 41 different A subgroup alleles and 18 B subgroup alleles in various populations.[28] The less common B(A) phenotype results from B-transferase-catalyzed addition of small amounts of A antigen on RBCs that is only detected with highly potent anti-A monoclonal reagents. (Individuals have anti-A in their serum). In cisAB phenotypes, A and B are inherited together from a single locus. Both of these phenotypes, B(A) and cisAB, result from variant glycosyltransferases that, at critical substrate selective positions, have a combination of A- and B-specific residues. For example, in the cisAB shown (Fig. 6–4), the first substitution is identical to that described for the A_2 transferase (Leu156), and the second is that found in the B transferase (Ala268).[29] Five different cisAB and five B(A) backgrounds have now been reported.[28]

Nonfunctional O transferases

The group O phenotype results from any mutation in an A or B transferase gene that causes loss of glycosyltransferase activity and a nonfunctional enzyme. Consequently, there are numerous group O genetic backgrounds. The most common group O (designated O^1 or O_{01}) results from a single nucleotide deletion early in the gene near the N terminus. This allele is referred to as 261delG. The deletion causes a frameshift and a truncated product with no enzyme activity that probably does not reach the Golgi membrane (see Fig. 6–3). Another common O allele (designated O^{1var} or O_{02}) has the same 261delG with nine additional point mutations. Alleles with 261delG are referred to as "deletion phenotypes" to distinguish them from O alleles that result from point mutations or splice site mutations. This distinction has become important with the finding that some "nondeletion" O alleles may retain low levels of glycosyltransferase activity and are often associated with ABO typing discrepancies.[30–32] Although approximately 61 different O alleles have been reported, the two O alleles, O^1 and O^{1var}, are common in all populations examined.[33]

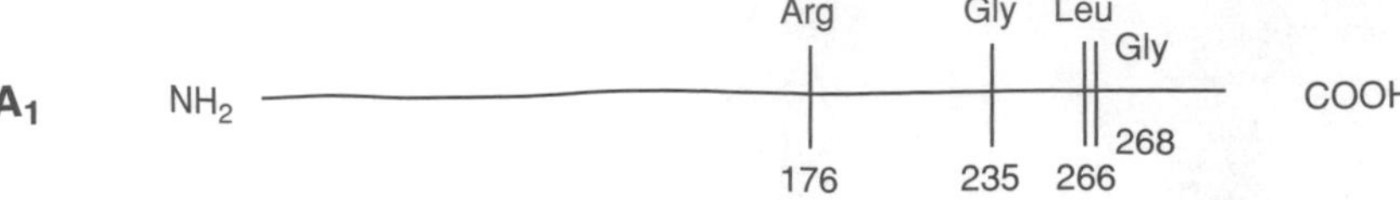

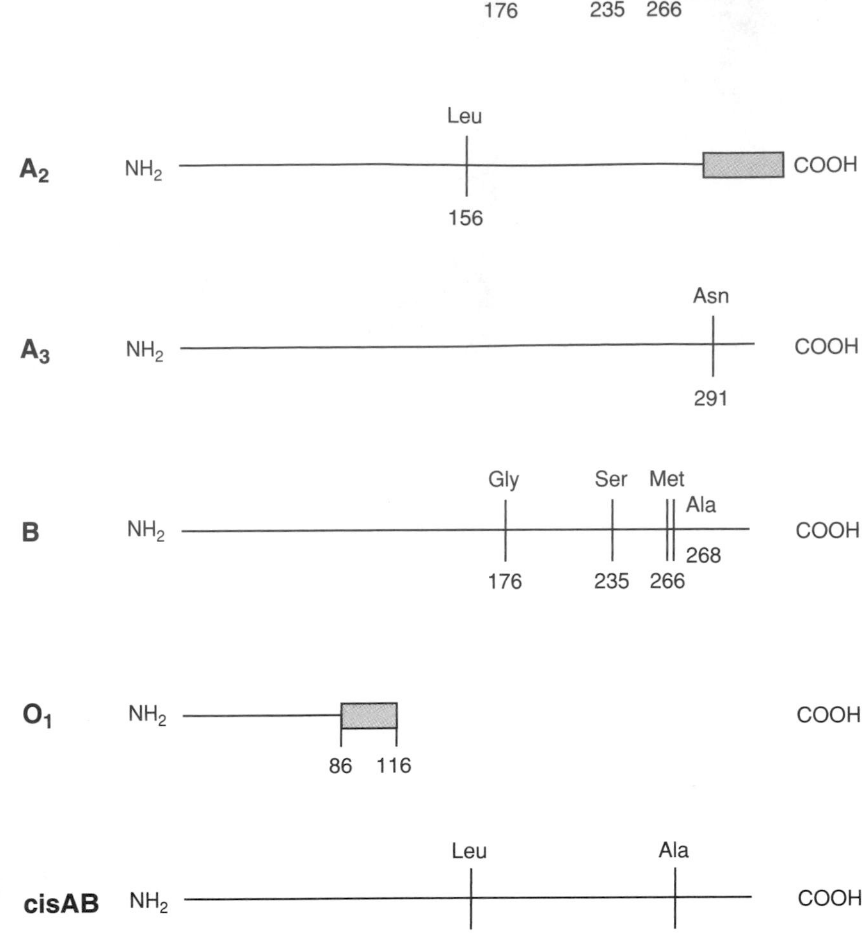

Figure 6–4 Representation of the amino acid sequence differences in the ABO glycosyltransferases. The grey boxes on the A_2 and O_1 glycosyltransferases indicate the altered protein sequence that results from the frameshift gene mutations.

Information regarding the ABO system alleles is maintained and updated on the Blood Group Antigen Mutation Database website (www.ncbi.nlm.nih.gov/projects/mhc/xslcgi.fcgi?cmd=bgmut/home), and can also be found in an issue of *Transfusion Medicine* that is dedicated to the ABO system.[34]

DNA genotyping

A polymerase chain reaction restriction fragment length polymorphism assay can be used to discriminate the common ABO genotypes.[35] This assay will not correctly assign subgroups of A (other than A_2) or subgroups of B, B(A), or cisAB phenotypes, and gene sequencing is often required. Determination of the ABO type with DNA-based approaches is complicated by the number of different subgroup and variant alleles present in populations. Serologic methods also have limitations when testing RBCs from ABO subgroups, but the hope would be that DNA genotyping would be a superior methodology. The observation that the same genotype can give rise to different phenotypes even within families, possibly due to genetic or somatic recombination events,[32] has added an additional layer of complexity to the ABO system. Although uncommon, these samples present challenges for development of DNA-based testing methods for ABO.

H (FUT1) and Secretor *(FUT2)* Genes

The biosynthesis of H antigen found on RBCs and epidermis and that found in secretions involves two different α1,2-fucosyltransferase enzymes encoded by two closely linked genes on chromosome 19q13.3,[36] *FUT1* and *FUT2*. These genes are also referred to as the *H* gene and the *Se* (secretor) gene. Both encode enzymes that add an H-specific fucose sugar to a precursor oligosaccharide core structure, but they act on different precursor structures. Four different core structures, all tetrasaccharides (four sugars) with terminal galactose residues, are found in human cells, and these core structures differ among tissues.[5] Type 1 precursors are found in the acinar cells of salivary glands and the epithelial lining of the pulmonary, gastrointestinal, urinary, and reproductive tracts. Type 2 precursors are expressed by RBCs and other tissues.[5] These precursors are identical except for the terminal galactose linkage (see Fig. 6–2). H antigen is synthesized in RBCs when the *H* (*FUT1*) gene-encoded fucosyltransferase attaches a fucose via an α1,2 linkage to the terminal galactose of type 2 precursor chains. H antigen in secretions is synthesized when the *Se* (Secretor, *FUT2*) gene-encoded fucosyltransferase attaches a fucose via an α1,2 linkage to the terminal galactose on type 1 precursor chains in secretory tissues. The A and B glycosyltransferases do not discriminate type 1 or type 2 chains and add *N*-acetylgalactosamine (A) or galactose (B) sugars to H antigens on both (i.e., in secretions and on RBCs) (see Fig. 6–2).

H (*FUT1*) encodes a 365-amino acid type II transmembrane protein, and *Se* (*FUT2*) encodes either a 332- or a 343-amino acid (there are two potential initiator codons) type II transmembrane protein. These genes are similar to A and B transferases in structure. They share 68% identity in a region of 292 amino acids and are clearly homologous. *H (FUT1)* is only 9 kb, and the coding region is contained in a single 1.1-kb exon.[37,38]

Homozygosity for defective *Se (FUT2)* is responsible for the nonsecretor (sese) phenotype, which has an incidence of approximately 20%. Numerous mutations cause loss of enzyme activity,[39] and these differ among populations. In white persons, a nonsense mutation at nucleotide G428A (se428) is found, whereas a mutation at se571 is common in Asians, and se849 is often found in Taiwanese. In addition, a normally functioning variant, designated Se^{l}, and a variant with reduced enzyme activity, *Se(W)*, are found in Asians. (The reduced activity of the *Se(W)* fucosyltransferase is responsible for the rare Le(a+b+) phenotype in Asians).

The majority of nonsecretors have functional *H (FUT1)* with synthesis of H antigen on RBCs. The exceptions, who are homozygous for null alleles at both *H (FUT1)* and *Se (FUT2)* loci, have the rare Bombay phenotype. They lack H antigen both in secretions and on RBCs; therefore, they make potent anti-H and must be transfused with RBCs from other Bombay people. In contrast, para-Bombay individuals are homozygous for null alleles at *H (FUT1)* but have at least one functional *Se (FUT2)* allele; they lack H antigen on their RBCs, but have H antigen in secretions (Table 6–2).[5] Those with a para-Bombay phenotype who are nonsecretors have clinically significant anti-H in their serum. More than 20 different mutations in *H (FUT1)* have been associated with Bombay and para-Bombay phenotypes (summarized by Costache and associates[40]).

Expression

ABO antigens are not fully developed at birth. Cord and infant RBCs have linear oligosaccharide structures with single termini to which the A, B, and H sugars can be added. Not until a person is approximately age 2 to 4 do complex branching oligosaccharide structures appear on the RBCs, which create additional termini. The antigens are then fully developed (and can accurately be tested for A_1 status) and remain fairly constant throughout life.[41–43] ABO-related hemolytic disease of the newborn (ABO-HDN) is usually mild because of the weaker RBC expression of A and B antigens and also because tissue expression provides additional antigen targets for maternal antibodies. Tissue expression of the ABO antigens varies during fetal development, but they are expressed on endothelial and epithelial cells of most organs and RBCs in 5- to 6-week-old embryos.[44]

A, B, and H antigens may be detected on lymphocytes of people with a secretor *(Se)* gene as a result of adsorption from the plasma as glycolipids. In contrast, platelets contain A-, B-, and H-transferases, making A, B, and H antigens intrinsic on platelet glycoproteins.[45]

Evolution

The ABH antigens appear earlier on epithelial cells than on blood cells,[46] so they may have or may have had functions in early development. ABO antigens are present on the RBCs of nonhuman primates—chimpanzee, gorilla, orangutan, gibbon, baboon, and several species of Old and New World monkeys.[47] Therefore, the ABO polymorphism has been maintained from species to species for more than 37 million years,[48] suggesting that there must be some importance to maintaining variation in ABO types. Primate studies reveal that the oldest common ancestral gene is A and that B alleles have arisen from the ancestral A alleles on at least three independent occasions.[49] However, the nonfunctional O allele has become one of the most common alleles and is even fixed in some South American populations. Nonfunctional or null alleles are expected to remain rare, unless they confer a selective advantage. Why the null allele evolved can only be speculated upon at present, but the presence in group O individuals of natural antibodies against A and B determinants may have offered important protection against bacteria and parasites[49] or even smallpox.[50]

Antibodies

Anti-A and anti-B are found in the sera of individuals who lack the corresponding antigens. They are produced in response to environmental stimulants, such as bacteria, and have therefore been termed *natural antibodies*.[51–53] Antibody production begins after birth, reaching a peak at age 5 to 10 and declining with increasing age. The antibodies formed to carbohydrate antigens are mostly immunoglobulin M (IgM). IgM antibodies activate complement, which, in conjunction with the high density of ABO antigen sites on RBCs, is responsible for the severe, life-threatening transfusion reactions that may be caused by ABO-incompatible transfusions.

Table 6–2 Comparison of H Antigen in Bombay, Para-Bombay, and Normal Phenotypes

	H Antigen			
Phenotype	**Blood Cells**	**Secretion**	**Predicted Genotype**	**Antibody**
Common				
Secretor	H+	Yes	*HH, Hh, SeSe, Sese*	
Nonsecretor	H+	No	*HH, Hh, sese*	
H-Deficient				
Bombay	H-	No	*hh, sese*	Anti-H
Para-Bombay	H weak	No	*(H), sese*	Anti-H
Para-Bombay	H weak	Yes	*(H), SeSe, Sese*	Anti-HI

Hemolytic disease of the newborn caused by ABO antibodies is usually mild, for the following reasons: placental transfer is limited to the fraction of IgG anti-A and anti-B found in maternal serum, fetal ABO antigens are not fully developed,[54] and ABO tissue antigens provide additional targets for the antibodies. ABO-HDN is most often seen in non-group O infants of group O mothers, because anti-A, anti-B, and anti-A,B of group O mothers often has a significant IgG component.

Potent anti-H (along with anti-A and anti-B) found in O_h (Bombay) or para-Bombay nonsecretors destroys transfused RBCs of any ABO group, so these individuals must be transfused only with blood of the Bombay phenotype.[55] In contrast, anti-H in non-Bombay individuals is usually IgM and clinically insignificant. Anti-IH is not uncommonly found in patient sera and is usually IgM; compatible blood is easily found among donors of identical ABO type.[15,56]

Enzyme-Converted O Cells (ECO)

Blood group O is considered the *universal donor* because it can be transfused to patients of all ABO types. Therefore, enzymes that remove terminal carbohydrates from the nonreducing end of carbohydrate chains could be used to remove terminal A and B sugars to convert the blood supply to all universal group O units. An enzyme from coffee beans, α-galactosidase, has been the most successful at removing galactose to convert blood group B to group O. RBCs treated in this manner have normal survival when transfused to group B, A, or O recipients.[57] Removal of *N*-acetylgalactosamine to convert group A to group O has been much more problematic, owing to the inaccessibility of the carbohydrates on internal branching chains, especially those found on A_1 cells. The procedures required to convert B to O, which include exposure to low pH followed by numerous washings, make them impractical for general use. This is an active area of research and alternative enzymes and improved methodologies are under investigation.[58,59]

THE LEWIS SYSTEM (ISBT SYSTEM 007)

History

The Lewis system, first reported in 1946 by Mourant,[60] was named after the first patient to make the antibody. What was thought at the time to be the antithetical antigen was found in 1948, and the designations Le^a and Le^b were applied at a later time.[19] We now know that these antigens are not antithetical, because they are not products of alternative forms of a single gene. Rather, they result from the sequential action of two fucosyltransferases encoded at independent loci (*LE-FUT3* and *Se-FUT2*).

Antigens

Lewis antigens, unlike antigens of all other blood group systems except Chido-Rodgers, are not intrinsic to the RBC but are synthesized in the intestinal epithelial cells. Lewis antigens circulate in plasma while bound to glycosphingolipids and are passively adsorbed onto RBCs.[61,62]

There are four Lewis phenotypes—Le(a+b−), Le(a−b+), Le(a−b−), and the rare Le(a+b+). African Americans have a higher incidence of the Le(a−b−) phenotype, and Le(a+b+) is very rare in white persons and African Americans but not uncommon in Asians (Table 6–3).

Le^a and Le^b are synthesized in a stepwise manner by two transferase enzymes that add fucose residues only to type 1 chains, which are found in secretions but not in RBCs (see Fig. 6–2). The nature and substrate specificity of the enzymes have been elucidated only recently. The α1,4-fucosyltransferase encoded by *LE (FUT3)* catalyzes the addition of a fucose to carbon 4 of the subterminal *N*-acetylglucosamine (GlcNAc) residue of the type 1 precursor chains, creating the Le^a structure (see Fig. 6–2). (Note that this transferase cannot act similarly on the type 2 chains found on RBCs, because they already have Gal on carbon 4 of the subterminal GlcNAc, which blocks the acceptor site; this fact explains why the Lewis antigens are not synthesized in RBCs.)

Table 6–3 Lewis Blood Group Phenotypes and Incidence

Phenotype	Incidence (%) White	African	Asian
Le(a−b+)	72	55	72
Le(a+b−)	22	23	22
Le(a−b−)	6	22	6
Le(a+b+)	Rare	Rare	3

The Le^a structure remains unchanged, resulting in the Le(a+b−) phenotype, unless the individual is a secretor *(Se-FUT2)*. In the presence of the α1,2-fucosyltransferase encoded by the secretor locus, the Le^a structure is converted to Le^b by the addition of a fucose residue to carbon 2 of the terminal galactose residue on the same chain. Le^b antigen is synthesized at the expense of Le^a antigen, resulting in the Le (a−b+) phenotype. This finding explains early observations that individuals with RBCs that typed as Le(b+) were secretors of ABH substance, those with Le(a+) RBCs were nonsecretors, and individuals with Le(a−b−) RBCs could be either secretors or nonsecretors of ABH. Ninety percent of white persons inherit normal *LE (FUT3)*, and 80% carry a functional *Se (FUT2)*, accounting for the prevalence of the Le(a−b+) phenotype in the white population (see Table 6–3).[5,50]

Le(a−b−) arises from homozygous defects in *LE (FUT3)*, regardless of the *Se (FUT2)*. Le(a+b+) individuals have weak expression of both Le^a and Le^b and are sometimes called *partial secretors.* They have significantly reduced α1,2-fucosyltransferase activity, and this uncommon phenotype is principally found in Taiwanese.

Genes

The gene responsible for Lewis carbohydrates, *LE (FUT3)*, located on chromosome 19 (19p13.3), encodes a 361-amino acid, type II membrane-bound enzyme.[63] It is one of the series of genes located on chromosome 19 that encode fucosyltransferases. Chromosome 19 is also the location for both the secretor gene *Se (FUT2)*—which not only determines ABH secretor status but also interacts with *LE* (*FUT3*) to synthesize Le^b antigens—and the *H* gene (*FUT1*)—which is responsible for H antigen on RBCs.

Le(a−b+) individuals have a least one functional *LE (FUT3)* and *Se (FUT2)*, and are secretors of ABH antigens. Le(a+b−) individuals have at least one functional *LE (FUT3)*, but this phenotype identifies the 20% of individuals with defective *Se (FUT2)* (see discussion of the ABO system). Le(a+b+), found in relatively high prevalence in Taiwan, results from inheritance of *Se(w)*, which encodes an amino acid change in the catalytic domain resulting in reduced activity of the enzyme encoded by *Se (FUT2)*. Le(a−b−) individuals have point mutations in the *LE (FUT3)* gene *(le/le)*. Many different defective alleles (le^1-le^6) have been reported, and mutations at nucleotides 508, 1067, and 202 severely reduce or inactivate the fucosyltransferase.[39] A mutation at nucleotide 59 results in an amino acid change in the transmembrane domain, which does not affect the enzyme activity but may affect the Golgi localization. This mutation is responsible for the paradoxical Le(a−b−) RBC phenotype in people with Lewis antigens in their saliva.[64]

Expression

Lewis antigens are not expressed on cord RBCs. Lewis antigen levels on RBCs are often diminished during pregnancy, possibly due to pregnancy-associated changes in plasma lipoproteins.[65] Lewis antigens are also found on lymphocytes and platelets (secondarily adsorbed from the plasma); on other tissues, including pancreas, stomach, intestine, skeletal muscle, renal cortex, and adrenal glands; and in soluble form in saliva as glycoproteins. Lewis antigens may be of some consequence in renal allografts. Graft survival has been reported to be reduced in patients who lack Lewis antigens, but this issue is controversial.[18] The Le^b antigen may be a receptor for *Helicobacter pylori,* a feature that could explain the association of gastric ulcers and secretor status.[66,67]

Antibodies

Lewis antibodies are primarily IgM and are usually not clinically significant. Lewis antibodies often complicate antibody identification when multiple antibodies are present, but they are easy to inhibit with saliva (made isotonic) from secretors or with commercially prepared Lewis substance. Lewis antibodies occur in the sera of Le(a−b−) persons and may be naturally occurring.[15]

Rare hemolytic transfusion reactions, due to transfusion of Le(a+) RBCs to recipients with anti-Le^a, have been reported.[68] Because Le(a−) RBCs are found in almost 80% of donors, it is easy to select Le(a−) RBCs for transfusion to recipients with anti-Le^a when the antibody is reactive at 37°C.[69] Because Lewis antigens are not intrinsic to the RBC membrane and are present in plasma, selection of Le(b−) RBCs is unnecessary for recipients with anti-Le^b, because Lewis antigens in donor plasma readily neutralize Lewis antibodies in transfusion recipients.[61]

The intimate relationship between Lewis and ABH antigens is revealed by antibodies such as anti-Le^{bH}, which reacts best with O Le(b+) cells. Crossmatching ABO-identical RBCs (rather than O) usually provides compatible blood. Anti-Le^{bA} reacts best with A Le(b+) cells. These antibodies are IgM and not clinically significant.

Anti-Le^a and anti-Le^b are not known to cause HDN, because they are usually IgM, and because fetal RBCs type as Le(a−b−).[15]

THE Ii BLOOD GROUP COLLECTION (ISBT COLLECTION 207)

History

In 1956, Wiener and colleagues[70] described the I antigen after making an intense study of a particularly severe case of hemolysis, or cold agglutinin disease, due to anti-I. They used the symbol I to emphasize the high degree of *I*ndividuality of RBCs failing to react with the patient's serum at room temperature. Because the patient's serum was only weakly reactive in vitro with bovine RBCs, she was transfused with a small volume of bovine RBCs, but an anaphylactic-type reaction discouraged Wiener and colleagues[70] from further attempts to transfuse bovine RBCs.

Antigens

I and i antigens on RBCs are subterminal portions of the same carbohydrate chains that carry ABH antigens.[18] I and i are not allelic; rather, they differ in their branching structure. The i antigen, found predominantly on fetal and infant RBCs, is characterized by disaccharide units (Gal-GlcNAc) linked in a straight chain.[71] During the first 2 years of life, many of these linear chains are modified into branched chains,[41] resulting in the appearance of I antigens found on adult RBCs. I specificity develops at the expense of i antigens when the branched structures appear.

Gene

The gene responsible for I antigen synthesis on RBCs and in tissues, called *IGnT* (GCNT2), consists of three exons and is located on chromosome 6p24.[72] The gene encodes β1,6-*N*-acetylglucosaminyltransferase, a type II membrane protein similar in structure to other glycosyltransferases.[73] This enzyme is responsible for the branching synthesis of I antigen and so is probably developmentally regulated. The gene has three forms of exon 1 that are differentially spliced to give three transcripts—IGnTA, IGnTB, or IGnTC—each responsible for synthesis of I antigen in various tissues (Fig. 6–5).[72,74,75] For example, I antigen on RBCs is encoded by IGnTC, and expression of I antigen in lens epithelium is encoded by IGnTB.

The I-negative phenotype (adult i) in Taiwanese and in Japanese is associated with three different mutant alleles; all have a Gly348Glu change encoded in exon 3, with or without Arg383His (exon 3) or Gly334Arg (exon 2), or a large gene deletion encompassing exons 1B, 1C, and exons 2 and 3.[72] In whites, an Ala169Thr change, with or without Arg228Gln, encoded by IGnTC exon 1C causes adult i. In Japanese, the adult i phenotype has been associated with congenital cataracts,[76,77] but this has not been observed in whites.[78] The different genetic backgrounds explains these observations, because the white mutation in exon 1C affects RBC expression of the I antigen, but normal I antigen is expressed in lens epithelium. In contrast, mutations in exon 3 of *IGnT* found in Taiwanese and Japanese persons result in lack of transferase

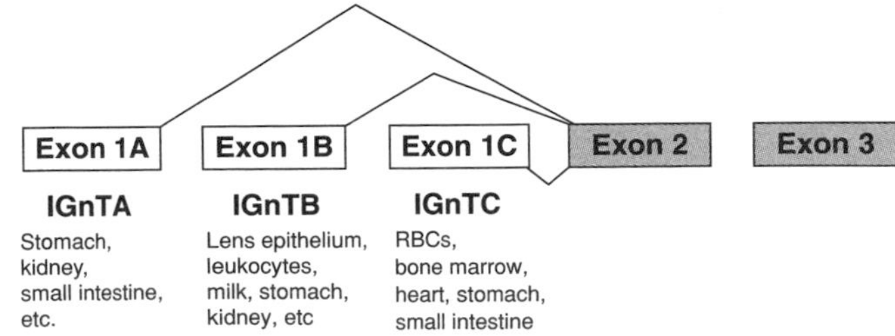

Figure 6–5 Representation of the *IGnT* gene. Altenative splicing generates three different transcripts responsible for I antigen synthesis in the tissues indicated.

activity on RBCs and lens epithelium. The human *IGnT* gene appears to have some role in maintaining lens transparency (reviewed in Reid[79]).

Expression

Adult RBCs express predominantly I antigens and little or no i antigen, whereas newborn infant RBCs have strong expression of i antigens and small amounts of I antigen.[80] Adult RBCs vary in the amount of I antigen. I and i can also be found on lymphocytes and platelets. The I and i antigens are referred to by some as *histo-blood group antigens* because, like ABH antigens, they are not restricted to RBCs but are found on most cells and in various body fluids.[18] Many conditions that result in stress hematopoiesis result in altered I and i antigen expression; typically, I expression is weakened but i expression is enhanced. For example, decreased expression of I antigen with concomitant increase in i antigen expression are associated with leukemia, Tk polyagglutination, thalassemia, sickle cell disease, hereditary erythroblastic multinuclearity with positive acidified serum, congenital hypoplastic anemia, myeloblastic erythropoiesis, and sideroblastic erythropoiesis.[81]

Antibodies

The sera of all individuals contain anti-I as a common autoantibody that is reactive at or below room temperature and is usually benign. These autoantibodies are commonly referred to as *cold agglutinins.* If the autoantibody is reactive at room temperature, problems in compatibility testing may result, but prewarming components and testing at 37°C easily circumvents them.[82] Even in patients undergoing hypothermia during surgical procedures, there are no reports of anti-I causing RBC destruction. Alloantibody to I made by the rare i adult phenotype is clinically significant and causes destruction of transfused I+ RBCs.

In contrast, cold agglutinin disease is characterized by high titers of monoclonal anti-I antibodies, which cause in vivo hemolysis and hemolytic anemia. These pathologic autoantibodies often react at 30°C in albumin and can fix complement.[83] The autologous circulating RBCs of a patient with cold agglutinin disease are often strongly coated with complement component C3d, making them relatively resistant to destruction. In contrast, when donor RBCs are transfused to a patient with cold agglutinin disease, they may be rapidly destroyed by circulating antibody. If transfusion cannot be avoided, donor RBCs should be transfused through a blood warmer.[15]

The titer and thermal range of anti-I are often increased after infection with *Mycoplasma pneumoniae.*[16] Approximately 50% of patients with infectious mononucleosis may have transient anti-i in their sera, but less than 1% have hemolysis.[84] Transient autoantibody to i can occur in patients with lymphoproliferative disorders (e.g., Hodgkin's disease).

THE P SYSTEM (ISBT SYSTEM 003) AND GLOB COLLECTION (ISBT COLLECTION 209)

History

The P blood group system was first discovered by Landsteiner and Levine[85] in 1927 after they injected rabbits with human RBCs. The first antigen discovered in this system appeared to be present on all human RBCs. It was named the P antigen because this was the first letter after M, N, and O, which had already been used. This antigen, present in 79% of white people, was renamed P_1; according to current ISBT terminology, however, the name is now written as P1, whereas P_1 denotes the P1+ phenotype.[4,19] This chapter uses the more familiar P_1 terminology. Other related antigens P, P^k, and LKE have been assigned to the GLOB collection because, although they are related biochemically to the P_1 antigen, their genetic association is still unclear.

Antigens

The P_1, P, and P^k blood group antigens are defined by sugars added to precursor glycosphingolipids and are not found on glycoproteins. Biosynthesis occurs by the sequential addition of monosaccharides to a precursor substrate catalyzed by glycosyltransferases. Two pathways are involved in the production of these antigens from a common precursor, galactose β1,4-glucose-ceramide, also called *lactosylceramide* (Fig. 6–6). In one pathway, lactosylceramide is converted to P^k (also called CD77), an antigen of very high incidence that is the precursor structure for synthesis of P. P is produced by the action of a second enzyme, and P antigen is found on all RBCs except the rare p and P^k phenotypes.

The P antigen is a cellular receptor for the B19 parvovirus, which causes erythema infectosum (fifth disease), a common childhood illness, and occasionally can cause more severe disorders of erythropoiesis. The virus causes both transient aplastic crises in patients with underlying hemolysis and anemia in immunocompromised patients.[86] Individuals with the p phenotype lack both P and P^k and are naturally resistant to parvovirus B19 infection. P^k (CD77) is present on epithelial cells and immature B cells in the germinal center and is a receptor molecule for Shiga-like toxins from *Escherichia coli* 0157.[87] LKE antigen is formed when two additional carbohydrate residues (galactose and sialic acid) are added to P (see Fig. 6–6).

In the second pathway, lactosylceramide is converted to P_1 antigen. The biochemical pathway is not completely established, and whether the same α1,4-galactosyltransferase gene is responsible for synthesis of both P^k and P_1 antigens is debated. P_1 antigen is a receptor for uropathogenic strains of *E. coli,* and it has been suggested that P_1 on urinary tract tissue allows the bacteria to bind to and ascend the urinary tract more easily.[50]

The RBC phenotypes that carry various combinations of these antigens are shown in Table 6–4. The nomenclature can be confusing, but five phenotypes, depending on the presence or absence of the three antigens—P_1, P, and P^k—are known. The presence of all three antigens results in the P_1 phenotype. The absence of P_1 results in the P_2 phenotype. P_1 and P_2 phenotypes are common. Among white persons, 21% are P_1 negative, but the incidence of P_1 negative people is greater in Southeast Asian populations; 80% of Cambodians and Vietnamese are P_1 negative. The absence of all three antigens is associated with the "null" p phenotype.

Genes

Two genes code for the P^K and P synthesizing enzymes, 4-α-galactosyltransferase (α4Gal-T, Gb3)[88] and 3-β-*N*-acetylgalactosaminyltransferase (β3GalNAcT, Gb4)[89] (see Fig. 6–6).

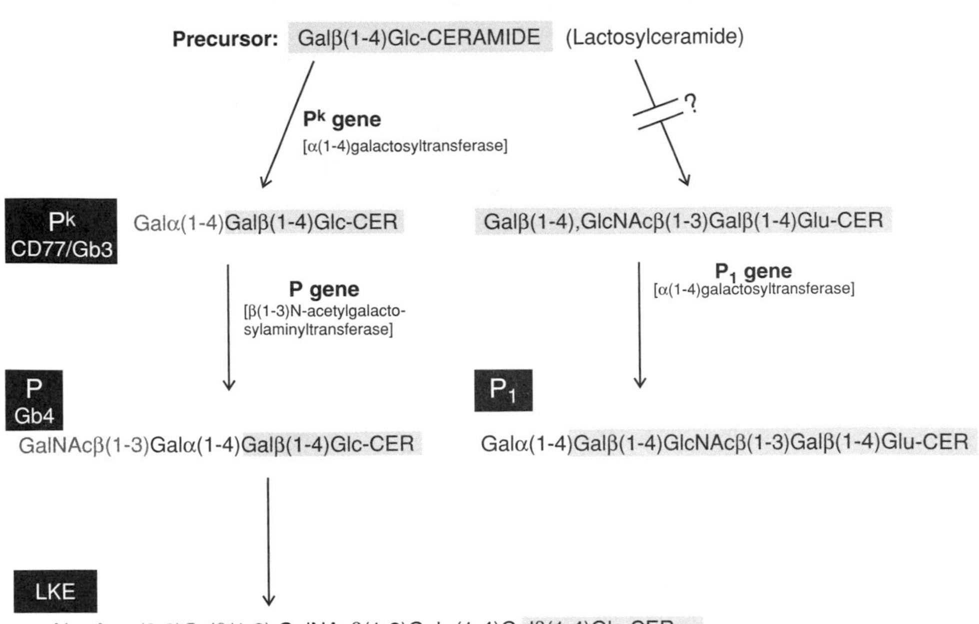

Figure 6–6 Biosynthesis of the P_1, P^k, P, and LKE antigens. Glu, glucose; CER, ceramide.

Table 6–4 P Blood Group System Phenotypes and Incidence

	Incidence (%)		
Phenotypes	Whites	African Americans	Antigens
P_1	79	94	P_1, P, P^{k*}
P_2	21	6	P, P^{k*}
P_1^k	Very rare	Very rare	P^1, P^k
P_2^k	Very rare	Very rare	P^k
p	Very rare	Very rare	None

*P^k is difficult to detect on these cells because it is converted to P.

The p "null" phenotype is due to alterations and mutations in the *α4Gal T* transferase gene, which acts on the precursor lactosylceramide.[90] Eleven different P^k-null (p phenotype) alleles have been reported from donors with different geographic backgrounds (summarized in Hellberg et al.[91]). Mutations in the gene for β3GalNAcT, Gb4 lead to the P_1^k and P_2^k phenotypes[92] (see Fig. 6–6). The genetic background for the P_1 antigen remains unknown, and why the P_2 and p phenotypes are associated with the absence of P_1 antigen has not been established.

Expression

P_1 antigen is considerably weaker in children than in adults, and its expression does not reach adult level until age 7. However, P_1 antigen is more strongly expressed on fetal RBCs than on neonatal RBCs, and P_1 expression weakens as the fetus ages. RBCs from different people show variation in the strength of the P_1 antigen, which can be seen during analysis of panel results in the identification of anti-P_1. P_1 and P are also expressed on lymphocytes, granulocytes, and monocytes.[18]

P_1 antigens are expressed in a wide variety of organisms, including bacteria, nematodes, earthworms, liver flukes, pigeons, and tapeworms.[18]

Antibodies

P_1-negative individuals frequently produce anti-P_1. This cold-reactive IgM antibody does not cross the placenta and has rarely been reported to cause hemolysis in vivo.[93] Like Lewis antibodies, anti-P_1 can often complicate antibody identification when multiple antibodies are present. However, anti-P_1 antibodies are easily neutralized with commercially prepared P_1 substance. Hydatid cyst fluid, *Echinococcus* cyst fluid, or pigeon egg white may be used. Anti-P^k is also neutralized by these substances.

Persons with the very rare p phenotype lack P_1, P, and P^k antigens and may produce anti-P,P_1,P^k (anti-Tj^a), a potent hemolytic IgM antibody that can cause immediate hemolytic transfusion reactions.[15,19] In women with the p, P_1^k, or P_2^k phenotypes, cytotoxic IgM and IgG3 antibodies directed against P antigens, P^k antigens, or both, are associated with a higher than normal rate of spontaneous abortions.[18,94]

Autoantibody to P, the Donath-Landsteiner autoantibody, is found in patients with paroxysmal cold hemoglobinuria and in some patients with acquired immune hemolytic anemia.[95] The autoantibody, complement-fixing IgG, is a biphasic hemolysin that binds to RBCs in the cold and then hemolyzes them when warmed. Thus, the patient's serum causes hemolysis of RBCs that have been first incubated in melting ice and then incubated at 37°C.[96] This antibody should be considered when the patient has hemoglobinuria and C3 alone is present on the RBCs. Transfusion is seldom required in paroxysmal cold hemoglobinuria, because the anemia is usually transient. P-negative blood is rare, and P-positive blood has been used successfully for transfusion in patients with severe anemia.[15]

SUMMARY

Despite the clinical relevance, especially of the ABO blood groups, the physiologic function of the carbohydrate antigens is unclear. The fact that some microbes and parasites use the carbohydrate blood group determinants as receptors certainly may contribute to their variation but does not shed light on their function. Specific interactions between cells might involve the blood group portions of cell surface glycoconjugates. Certainly, the carbohydrate structures on RBCs are important to impart the net negative charge on the membrane, keeping RBCs from adhering to one another and to the extracellular matrix. However, at present, the specific function of these carbohydrate molecules is unknown.

REFERENCES

1. Landsteiner K. Zur Kenntnis der antifermentativen, lytischen und agglutinierenden Wirkungen des Blutserums und der Lymphe. Zbl Bakt 1900;27:357
2. Hess JR, Schmidt PJ. The first blood banker: Oswald Hope Robertson. Transfusion 2000;40:110–113.
3. Yamamoto F. Molecular genetics of the ABO histo-blood group system. Vox Sang 1995;69:1–7.
4. Daniels GL, Anstee DJ, Cartron J-P, et al. Blood group terminology 1995. ISBT working party on terminology for red cell surface antigens. Vox Sang 1995;69:265–279.
5. Lowe JB. The blood group-specific human glycosyltransferases. Baillieres Clin Haematol 1993;6:465–492.
6. Clausen H, Hakomori S. ABH and related histo-blood group antigens: immunochemical differences in carrier isotypes and their distribution. Vox Sang 1989;56:1–20.
7. Curtis BR, Edwards JT, Hessner MJ, et al. Blood group A and B antigens are strongly expressed on platelets of some individuals. Blood 2000;96:1574–1581.
8. Skogen B, Rossebo Hansen B, Husebekk A, et al. Minimal expression of blood group A antigen on thrombocytes from A2 individuals. Transfusion 1988;28:456–459.
9. Cooling LL, Kelly K, Barton J, et al. Determinants of ABH expression on human blood platelets. Blood 2005;105:3356–3364.
10. Platt JL, Bach FH. The barrier to xenotransplantation. Transplantation 1991;52:937–947.
11. Rydberg L. ABO-incompatibility in solid organ transplantation. Transf Med 2001;11:325–342.
12. Fishbein TM, Emre S, Guy SR, et al. Safe transplantation of blood type A2 livers to blood type O recipients. Transplantation 1999;67:1071–1073.
13. Nelson PW, Helling TS, Shield CF, et al. Current experience with renal transplantation across the ABO barrier. Am J Surg 1992;164:541–544.
14. Wallace ME, Gibbs FL (eds). Blood Group Systems: ABH and Lewis. Arlington, Va., American Association of Blood Banks, 1986.
15. Mollison PL, Engelfriet CP, Contreras M. Blood Transfusion in Clinical Medicine, 10th ed. Oxford, Blackwell Science, 1997.
16. Gerbal A, Maslet C, Salmon C. Immunological aspects of the acquired B antigen. Vox Sang 1975;28:398–403.
17. Garratty G, Arndt P, Co A, et al. Fatal hemolytic transfusion reaction resulting from ABO mistyping of a patient with acquired B antigen detectable only by some monoclonal anti-B reagents. Transfusion 1996;36:351–357.
18. Daniels G. Human Blood Groups, 2nd ed. Oxford, Blackwell Science, 2002.
19. Race RR, Sanger R. Blood Groups in Man, 6th ed. Oxford, Blackwell Scientific, 1975.
20. Watkins WM, Morgan WTJ. Possible genetical pathways for the biosynthesis of blood group mucopolysaccharides. Vox Sang 1959;4:97–119.
21. Ferguson-Smith MA, Aitken DA, Turleau C, de Grouchy J. Localisation of the human ABO: Np-1: AK-1 linkage group by regional assignment of AK-1 to 9q34. Hum Genet 1976;34:35–43.
22. Clausen H, White T, Takio K, et al. Isolation to homogeneity and partial characterization of a histo-blood group A defined Fucα1→2Galα1→3-*N*-acetylgalactosaminyltransferase from human lung tissue. J Biol Chem 1990;265:1139–1145.
23. Yamamoto F, Clausen H, White T, et al. Molecular genetic basis of the histo-blood group ABO system. Nature 1990;345:229–235.
24. Yamamoto F, Hakomori S. Sugar-nucleotide donor specificity of histo-blood group A and B transferases is based on amino acid substitutions. J Biol Chem 1990;265:19257–19262.
25. Yamamoto F, McNeill PD, Hakomori S. Genomic organization of human histo-blood group ABO genes. Glycobiology 1995;5:51–58.
26. Paulson JC, Colley KJ. Glycosyltransferases. Structure, localization, and control of cell type-specific glycosylation. J Biol Chem 1989;264: 17615–17618.
27. Watkins WM. Biochemistry and genetics of the ABO, Lewis, and P blood group systems. Adv Hum Genetics 1980;10:1–136.
28. Human Genome Variation Society. Blood Group Antigen Gene Mutation Database. New York, Albert Einstein College of Medicine, Yeshiva University 2004 (Abstract).
29. Yamamoto F-I. Review: Recent progress in the molecular genetic study of the histo-blood group ABO system. Immunohematology 1994;10:1–7.
30. Wagner FF, Blasczyk R, Seltsam A. Nondeletional ABO*O alleles frequently cause blood donor typing problems. Transfusion 2005;45:1331–1334.
31. Seltsam A, Das GC, Wagner FF, Blasczyk R. Nondeletional *ABO*O* alleles express weak blood group A phenotypes. Transfusion 2005;45:359–365.
32. Hosseini-Maaf B, Irshaid NM, Hellberg A, et al. New and unusual O alleles at the ABO locus are implicated in unexpected blood group phenotypes. Transfusion 2005;45:70–81.
33. Olsson ML, Irshaid NM, Hosseini-Maaf B, et al. Genomic analysis of clinical samples with serologic ABO blood grouping discrepancies: identification of 15 novel A and B subgroup alleles. Blood 2001;98:1585–1593.
34. Commemoration of the centenary of the discovery of the ABO blood group system. Transfu Med 2001;11(4) (entire issue).
35. Olsson ML, Chester MA. A rapid and simple ABO genotype screening method using a novel B/O^2 versus A/O^2 discriminating nucleotide substitution at the ABO locus. Vox Sang 1995;69:242–247.
36. Ball SP, Tongue N, Gibaud A, et al. The human chromosome 19 linkage group *FUT1 (H), FUT2 (SE), LE, LU, PEPD, C3, APOC2, D19S7* and *D19S9*. Ann Hum Genet 1991;55:225–233.
37. Kelly RJ, Rouquier S, Giorgi D, et al. Sequence and expression of a candidate for the human *secretor* blood group (α1,2-fucosyltransferase) gene (*FUT2*). J Biol Chem 1995;270:4640–4649.
38. Larsen RD, Ernst LK, Nair RP, Lowe JB. Molecular cloning, sequence, and expression of a human GDP-L fucose:β-D-galactoside 2-α-L-fucosyltransferase cDNA that can form the H blood group antigen. Proc Natl Acad Sci USA 1990;87:6674–6678.
39. Spitalnik PF, Spitalnik SL. Human blood group antigens and antibodies. Part 1: Carbohydrate determinants. In Hoffman R, Benz EJ, Shattil SJ, et al. (eds). Hematology: Basic Principles and Practice. Philadelphia, Churchill Livingstone, 2000, pp 2188–2196.
40. Costache M, Cailleau A, Fernandez-Mateos P, et al. Advances in molecular genetics of α-2- and α-3/4-fucosyltransferases. Transfus Clin Biol 1997;4:367–382.
41. Hakomori S. Blood group ABH and Ii antigens of human erythrocytes: Chemistry, polymorphism, and their developmental change. Semin Hematol 1981;18:39–62.
42. Witebsky E, Engasser LM. Blood groups and subgroups of the newborn. I. The A factor of the newborn. J Immunol 1949;61:171.
43. Watanabe K, Hakomori S. Status of blood group carbohydrate chains in ontogenesis and oncogenesis. J Exp Med 1976;144:644–653.
44. Szulman AE. The histological distribution of the blood group substances in man as disclosed by immunofluorescence. IV. The ABH antigens in embryos at the fifth week post fertilization. Hum Pathol 1971;2:575–585.
45. Cartron J-P, Mulet C, Bauvois B, et al. ABH and Lewis glycosyltransferases in human red cells, lymphocytes and platelets. Rev Franc Transf 1980;23:271–282.
46. Hakomori S, Kobata EA. Blood group antigens. In Sela M (ed). The Antigens, Vol. 2. San Diego, Academic Press, 1975, pp 79–140.
47. Moor-Jankowski J, Wiener AS, Rogers CR. Human blood group factors in non-human primates. Nature 1964;202:663–665.
48. Martinko JM, Vincek V, Klein D, Klein J. Primate ABO glycosyltransferases: Evidence for trans-species evolution. Immunogenetics 1993;37:274–278.
49. Saitou N, Yamamoto F. Evolution of primate ABO blood group genes and their homologous genes. Mol Biol Evol 1997;14:399–411.

50. Issitt PD, Anstee DJ. Applied Blood Group Serology, 4th ed. Durham, N.C., Montgomery Scientific Publications, 1998.
51. Springer GF, Horton RE, Forbes M. Origin of anti-human blood group B agglutinins in white leghorn chicks. J Exp Med 1959;110:221–224.
52. Thomsen O. Immunisierung von Menschen mit Antigenem Gruppenfremden Blute. Z Rassenphysiol 1930;2:105.
53. Baumgarten A, Kruchok AH, Weirich F. High frequency of IgG anti-A and -B antibody in old age. Vox Sang 1976;30:253–260.
54. Romans DG, Tilley CA, Dorrington KJ. Monogamous bivalency of IgG antibodies. I. Deficiency of branches ABHI-active oligosaccharide chains on red cells of infants causes the weak antiglobulin reactions in hemolytic disease of the newborn due to ABO incompatibility. J Immunol 1980;124:2807–2811.
55. Davey RJ, Tourault MA, Holland PV. The clinical significance of anti-H in an individual with the O_h (Bombay) phenotype. Transfusion 1978;18: 738–742.
56. Brecher M (ed). Technical Manual, 15th ed. Bethesda, Md., American Association of Blood Banks, 2005.
57. Goldstein J, Siviglia G, Hurst R, et al. Group B erythrocytes enzymatically converted to group O survice normally in A, B, and O individuals. Science 1982;215:168–170.
58. Lenny LL, Hurst R, Goldstein J, Galbraith RA. Transfusions to group O subjects of 2 units of red cells enzymatically converted from group B to group O. Transfusion 1994;34:209–214.
59. Lenny LL, Hurst R, Zhu A, et al. Multiple-unit and second transfusions of red cells enzymatically converted from group B to group O: Report on the end of Phase 1 trials. Transfusion 1995;35:899–902.
60. Mourant AE. A "new" human blood group antigen of frequent occurence. Nature 1946;158:237–238.
61. Sneath JS, Sneath PHA. Transformation of the *Lewis* groups of human red cells. Nature 1955;176:172.
62. Marcus DM, Cass LE. Glycosphingolipids with Lewis blood group activity: uptake by human erythrocytes. Science 1969;164:553–555.
63. Kukowska-Latallo JF, Larsen RD, Nair RP, Lowe JB. A cloned human cDNA determines expression of a mouse state-specific embryonic antigen and the Lewis blood group α(1,3/1,4)-fucosyltransferase. Genes Devel 1990;4:1288–1303.
64. Mollicone R, Reguigne I, Kelly RJ, et al. Molecular basis for Lewis α(1,3/1,4)-fucosyltransferase gene deficiency *(FUT3)* found in Lewis-negative Indonesian pedigrees. J Biol Chem 1994;269:20987–20994.
65. Hammar L, Mansson S, Rohr T, et al. Lewis phenotype of erythrocytes and Le^b-active glycolipid in serum of pregnant women. Vox Sang 1981;40:27–33.
66. Boren T, Falk P, Roth KA, et al. Attachment of *Helicobacter pylori* to human gastric epithelium mediated by blood group antigens. Science 1993;262:1892–1895.
67. Clyne M, Drumm B. Absence of effect of Lewis A and Lewis B expression on adherence of *Helicobacter pylori* to human gastric cells. Gastroenterology 1997;113:72–80.
68. Waheed A, Kennedy MS, Gerhan S, Senhauser DA. Transfusion significance of Lewis system antibodies. Am J Clin Pathol 1981;76:294–298.
69. Issitt PD. Antibodies reactive at 30°C, room temperature and below. In American Association of Blood Banks (ed). Clinically Significant and Insignificant Antibodies. Washington, D.C., American Association of Blood Banks, 1979, pp 13–28.
70. Wiener AS, Unger LJ, Cohen L, Feldman J. Type-specific cold auto-antibodies as a cause of acquired hemolytic anemia and hemolytic transfusion reactions: biologic test with bovine red cells. Ann Intern Med 1956;44:221–240.
71. Feizi T. The blood group Ii system: A carbohydrate antigen system defined by naturally monoclonal or oligoclonal autoantibodies of man. Immunol Commun 1981;10:127–156.
72. Yu L-C, Twu Y-C, Chang C-Y, Lin M. Molecular basis of the adult i phenotype and the gene responsible for the expression of the human blood group I antigen. Blood 2001;98:3840–3845.
73. Bierhuizen MF, Mattei MG, Fukuda M. Expression of the developmental I antigen by a cloned human cDNA encoding a member of a β-1,6-*N*-acetylglucosaminyltransferase gene family. Genes Dev 1993;7:468–478.
74. Yu LC, Twu YC, Chou ML, et al. The molecular genetics of the human I locus and molecular background explaining the partial association of the adult i phenotype with congenital cataracts. Blood 2003;101:2081–2087.
75. Inaba N, Hiruma T, Togayachi A, et al. A novel I-branching βb-1,6-*N*-acetylglucosaminyltransferase involved in human blood group I antigen expression. Blood 2003;101:2870–2876.
76. Yamaguchi H, Okubo Y, Tanaka M. A note on possible close linkage between the Ii blood group and congenital cataract locus. Proc Jpn Acad 1972;48:625–628.
77. Ogata H, Okubo Y, Akabane T. Phenotype i associated with congenital cataract in Japanese. Transfusion 1979;19:166–168.
78. Page PL, Langevin S, Petersen RA, Kruskall MS. Reduced association between the Ii blood group and congenital cataracts in white patients. Am J Clin Pathol 1987;87:101–102.
79. Reid ME. The gene encoding the I blood group antigen: review of an I or an eye. Immunohematology 2004;20:249–252.
80. Marsh WL. Anti-i: A cold antibody defining the Ii relationship in human red cells. Br J Haematol 1961;7:200–208.
81. Hillman RS, Giblett ER. Red cell membrane alteration associated with 'marrow stress'. J Clin Invest 1965;44:1730–1736.
82. Issitt PD, Jackson VA. Useful modifications and variations of technics in work on I system antibodies. Vox Sang 1968;15:152–153.
83. Garratty G, Petz LD, Hoops JK. The correlation of cold agglutinin titrations in saline and albumin with haemolytic anaemia. Br J Haematol 1977;35:587–595.
84. Worlledge SM, Dacie JV. Haemolytic and other anaemias in infectious mononucleosis. In Carter RL, Penman HG (eds). Infectious Mononucleosis. Oxford, Blackwell Scientific, 1969, pp 82–89.
85. Landsteiner K, Levine P. Further observations on individual differences of human blood. Proc Soc Exp Biol Med 1927;24:941.
86. Luban NL. Human parvoviruses: Implications for transfusion medicine. [Review]. Transfusion 1994;34:821–827.
87. Karmali MA. Infection by verocytotoxin-producing *Escherichia coli.* Clin Microbiol Rev 1989;2:15–38.
88. Steffensen R, Carlier K, Wiels J, et al. Cloning and expression of the histo-blood group P^k UDP-galactose: Galb-4Glcbl-cer α1,4-galactosyltransferase. Molecular genetic basis of the p phenotype. J Biol Chem 2000;275:16723–16729.
89. Okajima T, Nakamura Y, Uchikawa M, et al. Expression cloning of human globoside synthase cDNAs. Identification of β 3Gal-T3 as UDP-*N*-acetylgalactosamine:globotriaosylceramide β 1,3-*N*-acetylgalactosaminyltransferase. J Biol Chem 2000;275:40498–40503.
90. Furukawa K, Iwamura K, Uchikawa M, et al. Molecular basis for the p phenotype. Identification of distinct and multiple mutations in the α1,4-galactosyltransferase gene in Swedish and Japanese individuals. J Biol Chem 2000;275:37752–37756.
91. Hellberg Å, Steffensen R, Yahalom V, et al. Additional molecular bases of the clinically important p blood group phenotype. Transfusion 2003;43:899–907.
92. Hellberg A, Poole J, Olsson ML. Molecular basis of the Globoside-deficient P^k blood group phenotype. Identification of four inactivating mutations in the UDP-N-acetylgalactosamine: globotriaosylceramide 3-β-*N*-acetylgalactosaminyltransferase gene. J Biol Chem 2002;277:29455–29459.
93. Chandeysson PL, Flye MW, Simpkins SM, Holland PV. Delayed hemolytic transfusion reaction caused by anti-P_1 antibody. Transfusion 1981;21:77–82.
94. Levine P. Comments on hemolytic disease of newborn due to anti-PP_1P(k) (anti-Tj(a)). Transfusion 1977;17:573–578.
95. Levine P, Celano MJ, Falkowski F. The specificity of the antibody in proxysmal cold hemoglobinuria. Transfusion 1963;3:278–280.
96. Petz LD, Garratty G. Acquired Immune Hemolytic Anemias. New York, Churchill Livingstone, 1980.

Chapter 7

Rh, Kell, Duffy, and Kidd Antigens and Antibodies

Connie M. Westhoff • Marion E. Reid

This chapter summarizes four clinically significant blood group systems that are defined by protein polymorphisms. The proteins that carry these blood group antigens were difficult to isolate because they are integral membrane proteins present as minor components of the total red blood cell (RBC) protein. Biochemical techniques developed in the 1970s and 1980s enabled their purification and partial amino acid sequencing. In the 1990s, the protein sequence data were used to construct nucleic acid probes for amplification and screening of bone marrow cDNA libraries to isolate the genes. In the past decade, there has been a considerable increase in the amount of information about these blood group antigens; principally, the development and use of the polymerase chain reaction (PCR) has resulted in the rapid elucidation of the molecular basis for the antigens and phenotypes. In addition, the structure and function of these membrane proteins is an active area of investigation.

Rh BLOOD GROUP SYSTEM

History

The Rh system is second only to the ABO system in importance in transfusion medicine. Rh antigens, especially D, are highly immunogenic and can cause hemolytic disease of the newborn (HDN) and severe transfusion reactions. HDN was first described by a French midwife in 1609 in a set of twins, of whom one was hydropic and stillborn, and the other was jaundiced and died of kernicterus.[1,2] In 1939, Levine and Stetson[3] described a woman who delivered a stillborn fetus and suffered a severe hemolytic reaction when transfused with blood from her husband. Her serum agglutinated the RBCs of her husband and 80 of 104 ABO-compatible donors. Subsequently, in 1941, Levine and colleagues[4] correctly concluded that the mother had been immunized by the fetus, which carried an antigen inherited from the father, and suggested that the cause of the *erythroblastosis fetalis* was maternal antibody in the fetal circulation. Attempts to immunize rabbits against this new antigen were not successful.[1] Levine and colleagues did not name the antigen.[5]

Meanwhile, Landsteiner and Wiener, in an effort to discover additional blood groups, injected rabbits and guinea pigs with rhesus monkey RBCs. The antiserum agglutinated not only rhesus cells but also the RBCs of 85% of a group of white subjects from New York, whom the researchers called *Rh positive;* the remaining 15% were *Rh negative.*[1] Because the *anti-Rhesus* appeared to have reactivity indistinguishable from the maternal antibody reported by Levine and Stetson, the antigen responsible for HDN was named *Rh.* Later it was realized that the rabbit antiserum was not recognizing the same antigen but was detecting an antigen found in greater amounts on Rh-positive than on Rh-negative RBCs.[6] This antigen was named LW for Landsteiner and Wiener,[1] and the original human specificity became known as anti-D.

As early as 1941, it was obvious that Rh was not a simple single antigen system. Fisher named the C and c antigens (A and B had been used for ABO) on the basis of the reactivity of two antibodies that recognized antithetical antigens, and used the next letters of the alphabet, D and E, to define antigens recognized by two additional antibodies.[1] Anti-e, which recognized the e antigen, was identified in 1945.[7]

Nomenclature

The Rh system has long been acknowledged as one of the most complex blood group systems because of its large number of antigens (45) and the heterogeneity of its antibodies. The introduction of two different Rh nomenclatures reflected the differences in opinion concerning the number of genes that encoded these antigens. The Fisher-Race nomenclature was based on the premise that three closely linked genes — C/c, E/e, and D — were responsible, whereas the Wiener nomenclature (Rh-Hr) was based on the belief that a single gene encoded one *agglutinogen* that carried several blood group factors.

Even though neither theory was correct (there are two genes, *RHD* and *RHCE*, correctly proposed by Tippett[8]), the Fisher-Race designation (CDE) for haplotypes is often preferred for written communication, and a modified version of Wiener's nomenclature (the original form is nearly obsolete) is preferred for spoken communication (Table 7–1). A capital "R" indicates that D is present, and a lowercase "r" (or "little r") indicates that it is not. The C or c and E or e Rh antigens carried with D are represented by subscripts: 1 for Ce (R_1), 2 for cE (R_2), 0 for ce (R_0), and Z for CE (R_z). The CcEe antigens present without D (r) are represented by superscript symbols: "prime" for Ce (r'), "double-prime" for cE (r") and "y" for CE (r^y) (see Table 7–1). The "R" versus "r" terminology allows one to convey the common Rh antigens present on one chromosome in a single term (a phenotype). Dashes are used to represent missing antigens of the rare deletion (or CE-depleted) phenotypes; for example, D– – (referred to as D dash, dash) lacks C/c and E/e antigens.

In 1962, Rosenfield and associates[9] introduced numerical designations for the Rh antigens to more accurately represent

Table 7–1 Nomenclature and Prevalence for Rh Haplotypes				
		Prevalence (%)		
Haplotype Based on Antigens Present	Shorthand for Haplotype	White	African American	Asian
DCe	R_1	42	17	70
DcE	R_2	14	11	21
Dce	R_0	4	44	3
DCE	R_Z	<0.01	<0.01	1
ce	r	37	26	3
Ce	r′	2	2	2
cE	r″	1	<0.01	<0.01
CE	r^y	<0.01	<0.01	<0.01

the serologic data, to be free of genetic interpretation, and to be more compatible for computer use (Table 7–2). However, this numerical nomenclature, with a few exceptions (Rh17, Rh32, Rh33), is not widely used in the clinical laboratory.

Terminology

Current Rh terminology distinguishes the genes and the proteins from the antigens, which are referred to by the letter designations, D, C, c, E, e, and so on. To indicate the RH genes, capital letters, with or without italics, are used (i.e., RHD, RHCE, and RHAG). The different alleles of the *RHCE* gene are designated *RHce, RHCe, RHcE,* according to which antigens they encode. In contrast, the proteins are designated RhD, RhCE (or according to the specific antigens they carry, Rhce, RhCe, or RhcE), and RhAG. RH haplotypes are designated Dce, DCe, DcE, etc., or ce, Ce, cE when referring to a specific CE haplotype.

Proteins

Despite the clinical importance of the Rh blood groups, the RBC membrane proteins that carry them were identified only in the late 1980s.[10,11] The extremely hydrophobic nature of these multipass transmembrane proteins made the biochemical isolation difficult and limited progress in their characterization until the genes were cloned.

The Rh proteins, designated RhD and RhCE, are 417-amino acid, nonglycosylated proteins; one carries the D antigen, and the other carries various combinations of the CE antigens (ce, cE, Ce, or CE).[12–14] RhD differs from RhCE by 32 to 35 amino acids (depending on which form of RhCE is present), and both are predicted to span the membrane 12 times. They migrate in SDS-PAGE (sodium dodecyl sulfate–polyacrylamide gel electrophoresis) gels with an approximate molecular weight ratio (M_r) of 30,000 to 32,000, and hence are sometimes referred to as the *Rh30 proteins.* They are covalently linked to fatty acids (palmitate) in the lipid bilayer.[15]

A 409-amino acid glycosylated protein that coprecipitates with RhD and RhCE proteins and migrates with an approximate M_r of 40,000 to 100,000 is called RhAG (*Rh-a*ssociated *g*lycoprotein) or Rh50 glycoprotein to reflect its apparent molecular weight.[16] RhAG (Rh50) shares 37% amino acid identity with the RhD and RhCE proteins and has the same predicted membrane topology. RhAG is not polymorphic and does not carry Rh antigens. It is important for targeting the RhD and RhCE to the membrane, because mutations in, or lack of expression of, RhAG results in a lack of Rh antigen expression (Rh-null) or a marked reduction of Rh antigen expression (Rh-mod).[17] RhAG has one N-glycan chain that also carries ABO and Ii specificities (Fig. 7–1).

Rh-null and the Rh-Core Complex

Rh-null erythrocytes, which lack expression of Rh antigens, are stomatocytic and spherocytic, and affected individuals have variable degrees of anemia.[18,19] The phenotype is rare, occurring on two different genetic backgrounds; the *regulator* type, caused by mutations in the *RHAG* gene, and the *amorph* type, which maps to the *RH* locus. The amorph Rh-null results from mutations in *RHCE* on a deleted *RHD* background.[20] Regulator RBCs express no Rh and RhAG proteins, whereas amorph type RBCs have no Rh proteins but have reduced (20% of normal) RhAG.

Rh and RhAG proteins are associated in the membrane, possibly as a tetramer consisting of two molecules of each as a core complex,[21] although the precise configuration is not yet known. Evidence that other proteins interact with this Rh-core complex comes from observations that Rh-null RBCs have reduced expression of CD47 (an integrin-associated protein) and of glycophorin B (a sialoglycoprotein that carries S or s and U antigens). Rh-null RBCs also lack LW (ICAM-4), a glycoprotein of approximate M_r 42,000 that belongs to the family of intercellular adhesion molecules. Band 3 (the red cell anion exchanger AE1) may also be associated with the Rh complex.[22] The Rh complex is linked to the membrane skeleton via Rh/RhAG–ankyrin interaction[23] and CD47–protein 4.2 association.[24] Some mutations underlying Rh-null disease involve potential contact sites between RhAG and RhCE/RhD and cytoskeleton ankyrin, which may explain the morphologic defect in these erythrocytes.[23]

Genes

Two genes, designated *RHD* and *RHCE*, encode the Rh proteins. Rh-positive individuals have both genes, whereas most Rh-negative white people have only the *RHCE* gene.[25] The genes are 97% identical. Each gene has 10 exons and is the result of a gene duplication on chromosome 1p34–p36.[26] A comprehensive diagram of the intron–exon structure of *RHD* and *RHCE* can be found in the review by Avent and Reid.[27]

The single gene, *RHAG*, located at chromosome 6p11–p21.1 encodes RhAG. *RHAG* is 47% identical to the *RH* genes and also has 10 exons.[16,28]

Table 7–2 Rosenfield Numerical Terminology for Rh Antigens

Numerical Term	ISBT Symbol
Rh1	D
Rh2	C
Rh3	E
Rh4	c
Rh5	e
Rh6	ce or f
Rh7	Ce
Rh8	C^W
Rh9	C^X
Rh10	V
Rh11	E^W
Rh12*	G
Rh17	Hr_0†
Rh18	Hr
Rh19	hr^s
Rh20	VS
Rh21	C^G
Rh22	CE
Rh23*	D^W
Rh26	c-like
Rh27	cE
Rh28	hr^H
Rh29	Rh29
Rh30	Go^a
Rh31	hr^B
Rh32	Rh32‡
Rh33	Rh33§
Rh34	Hr^B
Rh35	Rh35‖
Rh36	Be^a
Rh37	Evans
Rh39	Rh39
Rh40	Tar
Rh41	Rh41
Rh42	Rh42
Rh43	Crawford
Rh44	Nou
Rh45	Riv
Rh46	Sec
Rh47	Dav
Rh48	JAL
Rh49	STEM
Rh50	FPTT
Rh51	MAR
Rh52	BARC
Rh53	JAHK
Rh54	DAK
Rh55	LOCR
Rh56	CENR

*Rh13 through Rh16, Rh24, and Rh25 are obsolete.

†High-incidence antigen; the antibody is made by D– –/D– and similar phenotypes.

‡Low-incidence antigen expressed by $\bar{\bar{R}}^N$ and DBT phenotypes.

§Originally described on R_0^{Har} phenotype, but also found on $\bar{\bar{R}}^N$ and D^{VIa} (C)–, R_0^{JOH}, and R_1^{Lisa}.

‖Low-incidence antigen on D(C)(e) cells.

ISBT, International Society for Blood Transfusion.

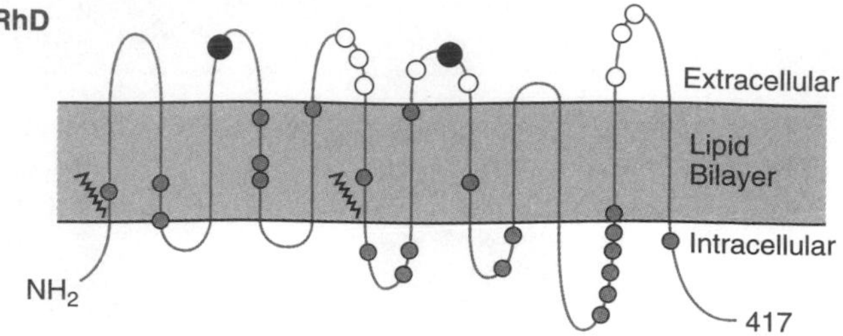

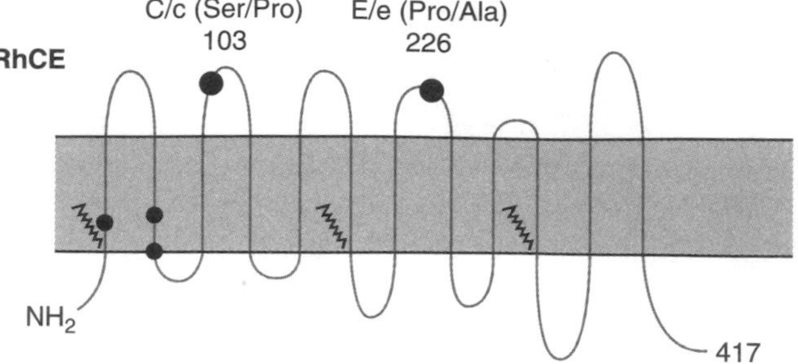

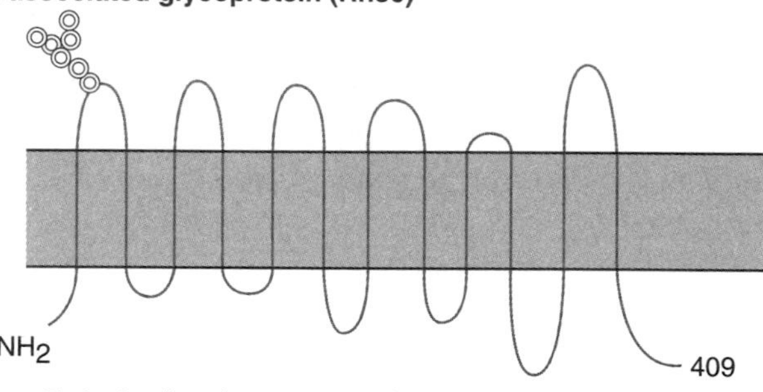

Figure 7–1 Predicted 12-transmembrane domain model of the RhD, RhCE, and RhAG proteins in the red blood cell membrane. The amino acid differences between RhD and RhCE are shown as symbols. The eight extracellular differences between RhD and RhCE are indicated as *open circles*. The *zigzag lines* represent the location of possible palmitoylation sites. Positions 103 and 226 in RhCE that are critical for C/c and E/e expression, respectively, are indicated as *black circles*. The N-glycan on the first extracellular loop of the Rh-associated glycoprotein is indicated by the *branched structure*.

Antigens

As previously described, the major Rh antigens are D, C, c, E, and e. The many other Rh antigens (see Table 7–2) define compound antigens in *cis* (e.g., f (ce), Ce, and CE), low-incidence antigens arising from partial D hybrid proteins (e.g., D^w, Go^a, BARC), high-incidence antigens, and other variant antigens. The molecular bases of most Rh antigens have been determined.

Studies to estimate the number of D, C/c, and E/e antigen sites on RBCs found differences between Rh phenotypes. The number of D antigens ranges from 10,000 on Dce/ce RBCs to 33,000 on DcE/DcE. The number of C, c, and e antigens per RBC varies from 8500 to 85,000.[6] Because C or c and E or e are carried on the same protein, their numbers should be equivalent. The equivalency was not always demonstrated in these studies, reflecting the inherent difficulty in the use of radiolabeled polyclonal antiserum to estimate antigen numbers. Results of tests with monoclonal antibodies to high-incidence Rh antigens suggest that the total number of Rh proteins (RhD and RhCE) per RBC is 100,000 to 200,000. The number of RhAG is also estimated to be 100,000 to 200,000,[29] consistent with predictions that Rh and RhAG may be present in the membrane as a tetramer of two molecules of each.[21]

D Antigen

Rh positive and *Rh negative* refer to the presence and absence, respectively, of the D antigen, which is the most immunogenic of the Rh antigens. The Rh-negative (D-negative) phenotype occurs in 15% to 17% of white persons but is not common in other ethnic populations. The absence of D in people of European descent is primarily the result of deletion of the entire *RHD* gene and occurred on a Dce (R_0) haplotype because the allele most often carried with the deletion is ce. However, rare D-negative white persons carry an *RHD* gene that is not expressed because of a premature stop codon,[30] a 4-base pair (bp) insertion at the intron 3/exon 4 junction,[31] point mutations, or *RHD/CE* hybrids.[32,33] Most of these are associated with the uncommon Ce (r′) or cE (r″) haplotypes.

D-negative phenotypes in Asian or African persons, however, are most often caused by inactive or silent *RHD* rather than a complete gene deletion. Asian D-negative individuals occur with a frequency of less than 1%, and most carry mutant *RHD* genes associated with *Ce*,[34] indicating that the gene mutations probably originated on a DCe (R_1) haplotype. Only 3% to 7% of South African black persons are D negative, but 66% of this group have *RHD* genes that contain a 37-bp internal duplication,[35] which results in a premature stop codon. The 37-bp insert *RHD*-pseudogene was also found in 24% of D-negative African Americans. In addition, 15% of the D-negative phenotypes in Africans result from a hybrid *RHD-CE-D*^{s} gene characterized by expression of VS, weak C and e, and no D antigen.[35] Only 18% of D-negative Africans and 54% of D-negative African Americans completely lack *RHD*.

WEAK D (FORMERLY D^u)

An estimated 0.2% to 1% of white persons (and a greater number of African Americans) have reduced expression of the D antigen, which is characterized serologically as failure of the RBCs to agglutinate directly with anti-D typing reagents and requires the use of the indirect antiglobulin test (IAT) for detection. The number of samples classified as *weak D* depends on the characteristics of the typing reagent. These weak D antigens were previously referred to as *D*^{u}, a term that has been abolished. The molecular basis of weak D expression is heterogeneous. In a large study of samples from Germany,[36] expression of weak D was found to be associated with the presence of point mutations in *RHD*. More than 70% of the samples had a Val270Gly amino acid change, but a total of 16 different mutations were found in the initial study. Since then, a large number of different mutations have been associated with the weak D phenotype (42 to date).[37] Collectively, the weak D phenotypes have amino acid changes predicted to be intracellular or in the transmembrane regions of the RhD protein and not on the outer surface of the RBC,[36] suggesting that the mutations affect the efficiency of insertion and, therefore, the quantity of RhD protein in the membrane but do not affect D epitopes.

The majority of individuals with a weak D phenotype can safely receive D-positive blood and do not make anti-D. However, two weak D types (type 4.2.2 and type 15) have been reported to make anti-D.[38] These weak D individuals would more accurately be classified as partial-D. The serologic differentiation of weak D from partial D is not unequivocal. Importantly, donor center typing procedures must detect and label weak D RBC components as *D-positive*.

A very weak form of D, designated D_{el}, detected by absorption and *el*ution of anti-D, has a high incidence in Hong Kong Chinese and Japanese persons. The D_{el} phenotype most often results from a splice site mutation or deletion that results in the absence of amino acids encoded by exon 9 of *RHD*[39] in Asians or a M295I mutation in whites. These RBCs type as D negative (even when tested using the IAT), and they are usually only recognized if they stimulate production of anti-D in a D-negative recipient.[40,41]

PARTIAL D ANTIGENS (D CATEGORIES OR D MOSAICS)

The D antigen has long been described as a *mosaic* on the basis of the observation that some Rh-positive individuals make alloanti-D when exposed to normal D antigen. It was hypothesized that the RBCs of these individuals lack some part of RhD and that they can produce antibodies to the missing portion. Molecular analysis has shown that this hypothesis is correct, but what was not predicted is that the missing portions of *RHD* are replaced by corresponding portions of *RHCE* (Fig. 7–2).[27,42] Some replacements involve entire exons, and the novel sequence of amino acids generates new antigens (e.g., D^w, BARC, Rh32) (Table 7–3). In addition, several exon rearrangements can give rise to the same partial D category (e.g., D^{VI} can result from type I, II, or III rearrangements; see Fig. 7–2). Other partial D antigens result from multiple amino acid conversions between *RHCE* and *RHD*, and some are the result of single point mutations in *RHD* (D^{VI}, DMH, DFW; see Table 7–3). These point mutations are predicted to be located on an extracellular loop or portion of the RhD protein, in contrast to the weak D antigens already described, which are predicted to have mutations located in cytoplasmic or transmembrane regions. Individuals with partial D antigens can make anti-D and therefore ideally should receive D-negative donor blood. In practice, however, most are typed as D positive and are recognized only after they have made anti-D.

ELEVATED D

Several phenotypes, including D– –, Dc–, and DC^W–, have an elevated expression of D antigen and no, weak, and variant CE antigens, respectively.[6] They are caused by replacement of portions of *RHCE* by *RHD*,[27,42] analogous to the partial D rearrangements already described. The additional *RHD* sequences in *RHCE* along with a normal *RHD* may explain the enhanced D and accounts for the reduced or missing CE antigens. Immunized people with these CE-depleted phenotypes make anti-Rh17.

D EPITOPES EXPRESSED ON RHCE PROTEINS (R_0HAR, ceCF, ceRT)

Some Rhce proteins carry D-specific amino acids that react with some monoclonal anti-D reagents, adding further complexity to D antigen typing. Two examples, R_0^{Har} (D^{HAR}), found in individuals of German ancestry,[43] and Crawford (ceCF, Rh43), found in individuals of African ancestry, deserve attention because of their strong reactivity (3+-4+) with some FDA-licensed monoclonal reagents and lack of reactivity with others (including the weak D test) (Table 7–4). Individuals with R_0^{Har} do not have a *RHD* gene, but exon 5 of the *RHCE* gene is from *RHD* (see Fig. 7–2). Those that carry a Crawford allele, ceCF, also do not have a *RHD* gene, but have a Rhce protein with three amino acid changes, Trp16Cys, Leu245Val, and Gln233Glu. The latter two are D-specific residues responsible for reactivity with a monoclonal anti-D (see Table 7–4 and Fig. 7–2).[44,45] Individuals with R_0^{Har} or Crawford phenotypes make anti-D when stimulated[46] (our unpublished observations), and should be considered Rh negative for transfusion and Rh immune globulin prophylaxis.

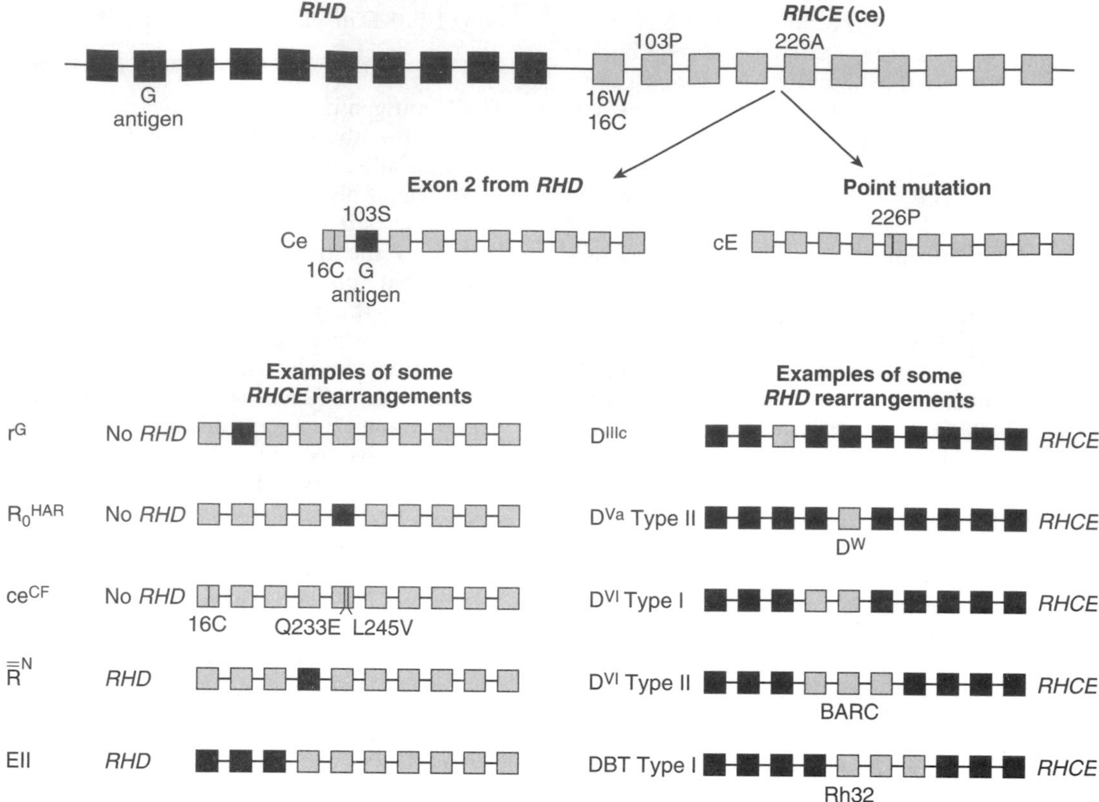

Figure 7–2 *Top panel,* Diagram of the *RHD* and *RHCE* genes, indicating the changes that resulted in the common RhCE polymorphisms. The shared exon 2 of *RHD* and *RHCE* (shown as a *black box*) explains the expression of G antigen on RhCe and RhD proteins. *Bottom panel,* Examples of some *RHCE* and *RHD* rearrangements.

Table 7–3 Molecular Basis of Some Rh Antigens, Partial D, and Unusual Phenotypes

Molecular Basis	Gene	Phenotype/Antigen/Genotype
Single point mutations	*RHD*	Partial D: DMH, D^{VII}, D+G–, DFW, DHR, D^{Va}, D^{HMi}, DNU, D^{II}, DNB, DHO Weak D (previously called D^{u})
	RHCE	C^{X}, C^{W}, Rh–26, E type I, IV, V+,VS+
Multiple mutations (gene conversions)	RHD RHCE	Partial D: D^{IIIa}, D^{IVa}, D^{Va}, DFR type I E type III, IV, V+VS+
Rearranged gene(s) *RHD*	RHD-CE-D	Partial D: D^{IIIb}, D^{IIIc}, D^{IVb}, D^{Va}, D^{VI}, DFR type II, DBT r''^{G}, (Ce)Ce, (C)ce^{s} VS+V–
RHCE	*RHCE-D-CE* *RHD-CE*	D^{Har}, r^{G}, $\bar{\bar{R}}^{N}$ E type II
RHD: RHCE	*RHD-CE: RHCE-D* *RHD: RHCE-D-CE* *RHD: RHD-CE* *RHCE-D: RHD-CE*	DC^{W}– D– –, D••, Dc– D•• D••

Table 7–4 Composition (IgM and IgG Clones) and Reactivity of FDA-Licensed Anti-D Reagents with Some Rh Variant RBCs That Can Result in D Typing Discrepancies

Reagent	IgM Monoclonal	IgG	DVI	DBT	DHAR (Whites)	Crawford (Blacks)
Gammaclone	GAMA401	F8D8 monoclonal	Neg/Pos*	Pos	Pos	Pos
Immucor Series 4	MS201	MS26 monoclonal	Neg/Pos	Pos	Pos	Neg
Immucor Series 5	Th28	MS26 monoclonal	Neg/Pos	Pos	Vary/Pos	Neg
Ortho BioClone	MAD2	Polyclonal	Neg/Pos	Neg/Pos	Neg/Neg	Neg
Ortho Gel (ID-MTS)	MS201		Neg	Pos	Pos	Neg
Polyclonal			Neg/Pos	Neg/Pos	Neg/Neg	Neg/Neg

* Result following slash denotes anti-D test result by the IAT, as permitted by the manufacturer.

Lastly, an Rhce protein with an R154T mutation, designated ceRT, demonstrates weak reactivity with some anti-D monoclonal reagents, and the reactivity is enhanced at lower temperatures. Interestingly, this variant does not carry any D-specific amino acid but mimics a D-epitope (epD6) structure.[47]

C/c and E/e Antigens

There are four major allelic forms of *RHCE*: ce, Ce, cE, and CE.[14] C and c differ by four amino acids: Cys16Trp (cysteine at residue 16 replaced by tryptophan) encoded by exon 1, and Ile60Leu, Ser68Asn, and Ser103Pro encoded by exon 2. Only residue 103 is predicted to be extracellular; it is located on the second loop of RhCE (see Fig. 7–1). The amino acids encoded by exon 2 of *RHC* are identical to those encoded by exon 2 of *RHD*. At the genomic level, *RHCe* appears to have arisen from transfer of exon 2 from *RHD* into *RHce* (see Fig. 7–2). The shared exon 2 explains the expression of the G antigen on both RhD and RhC proteins.

E and e differ by one amino acid, Pro226Ala. This polymorphism, predicted to reside on the fourth extracellular loop of the protein (see Fig. 7–1), is encoded by exon 5. A single point mutation in *RHce* resulted in *RHcE* (see Fig. 7–2).[14,48]

C^W and C^X antigens result from single amino acid changes, encoded by exon 1, which are predicted to be located on the first extracellular loop of the RhCE protein.[49]

The antigens V and VS are expressed on RBCs of more than 30% of black persons. They are the result of a Leu245Val substitution located in the predicted eighth transmembrane segment of Rhce.[50] The close location of the e antigen, Ala226 on the fourth extracellular loop, suggests that Leu245Val causes a local conformation change responsible for the weakened expression of e antigen in many black persons who are V and VS positive. The V−VS+ phenotype results from a Gly336Cys change on the 245Val background,[51] and these alleles are referred to as ce^S (Fig. 7–3). Loss of VS expression (the V+VS− phenotype) is associated with additional amino acid changes and is characteristic of the ceAR haplotype (see Fig. 7–3).

Other modifications of *RHCE*, which are uncommon, are the hybrids r^G, R^N, and several E/e variants (see Fig. 7–2). R^N RBCs are found in people of African origin and type as e-weak (or negative) with polyclonal reagents, but are indistinguishable from "normal" e-positive RBCs with some monoclonal anti-e. The E variants—EI, EII, and EIII—result either from a point mutation (EI) or from gene conversion events that lead to replacement of several extracellular RhcE amino acids with RhD residues (EII and EIII) and loss of some E epitope expression.[52] Category EIV RBCs, which have an amino acid substitution in an intracellular domain, do not lack E epitopes but have reduced E expression.[53] The very rare RH:-26 results from a Gly96Ser transmembrane amino acid change that abolishes Rh26 and weakens c expression.[54]

VARIATION IN e EXPRESSION AND SICKLE CELL PATIENTS

Variation in expression of the e antigen is not uncommon and can result from several different mutations. Deletion of the codon for Arg229, which is close to the Ala226 residue found in normal e expression,[55] and substitution of a Cys residue for Trp at position 16 in the Rhce protein[56] weaken expression of the antigen. Individuals of African ancestry often have *RHce* genes that encode variant e antigens. The RBCs type as e positive, but they often make alloantibodies with e-like specificities. The antibodies, designated anti-hr^S, -hr^B, -RH18, and -RH34, are difficult to identify serologically, are clinically significant, and have caused transfusion fatalities.[57] The prevalence of e variants in this population, together with the incidence of sickle cell disease requiring transfusion support often provided by white donors with conventional *RHce*, make the occurrence of alloanti-e in these patients not uncommon. Some of the *RH* genetic backgrounds have now been defined[58] and include the *RHCE* haplotypes shown in Figure 7–3. All encode the Trp16Cys difference in exon 1, and have additional changes, primarily localized to exon 5. The ce^S allele is associated with RBCs that are hr^B−, whereas individuals homozygous for ceAR, ceMO, ceEK, and ceBI alleles lack

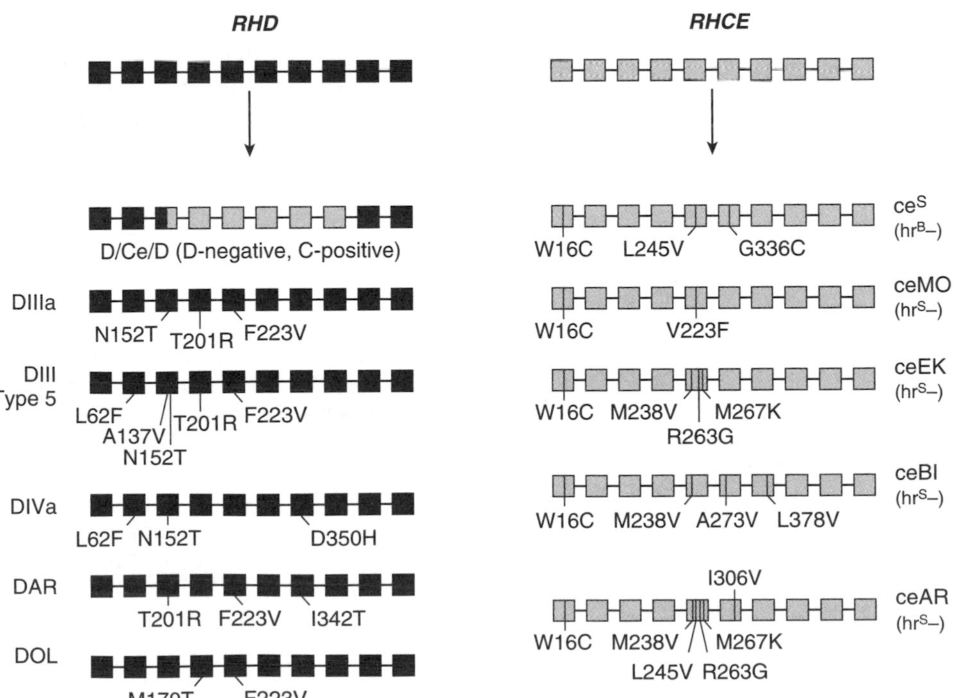

Figure 7–3 Diagram of the *RHD* and *RHCE* genes indicating changes often found in African backgrounds that complicate transfusion in sickle cell patients.

the high-incidence hr^S antigen (see Fig. 7–3). Importantly, because of the multiple molecular backgrounds responsible for the hr^B– and hr^S– phenotypes, some of which are not yet elucidated, the antibodies produced are not all serologically compatible. This explains why it is difficult to find compatible blood for patients with these antibodies, and often only rare deleted D– – RBCs appear compatible. As an additional complication, these variant *RHce* can often be inherited with an altered *RHD* (e.g., DAR, DAU, or DIIIA), so they can also make anti-D (see Fig. 7–3).

Rh Genotyping

RH genotyping is a useful means to determine the Rh phenotype of patients who have been recently transfused or whose RBCs are coated with IgG. RH genotyping in the prenatal setting can be used to determine paternal *RHD* zygosity and to predict fetal D status to prevent invasive and expensive monitoring for the possibility of HDN. The ethnic background of the parents is important to the design of the assay, because the different molecular events responsible for D-negative phenotypes must be considered. Testing of samples from the parents limits the possibility of misinterpretation.

RH genotyping can aid resolution of D typing discrepancies. These often are the result of differences in manufacturers' reagents, but in the donor setting they can be FDA reportable. Genotyping can determine a specific weak D type, partial D category, or the presence of D_{el}.

Genotyping to detect the inheritance of altered or variant e alleles, which are often linked to variant *RHD,* aids resolution of antibody specificities and is helpful to determine alloantibody versus autoantibody specificity. This can be of significance, especially in sensitized sickle cell patients. Molecular genotyping can aid in the selection of compatible blood for transfusion and ultimately improve long-term transfusion support. Currently, these investigations can sometimes be cumbersome, often requiring complete gene sequencing. The development of automated, high-throughput platforms that sample many regions of both *RHD* and *RHCE,* along with detailed algorithms for accurate interpretation, are needed.

Antibodies

Most Rh antibodies are IgG, subclasses IgG1 and IgG3 (IgG2 and IgG4 have also been detected), and some sera have an IgM component.[59] Rh antibodies do not activate complement, although two rare exceptions have been reported. The lack of complement activation by Rh antibodies is thought to be due to the distance between antigens, but is probably due to a lack of mobility.[6] Reactivity of Rh antibodies is enhanced by enzyme treatment of the test RBCs, and most react optimally at 37°C.

Anti-D can cause severe transfusion reactions and severe HDN. Approximately 80% to 85% of D-negative persons make anti-D after exposure to D-positive RBCs. The lack of response in 15% may be due to antigen dose, recipient HLA-DR alleles, and other as yet unknown genetic factors. Anti-D was the most common Rh antibody, but its incidence has greatly diminished with the prophylactic use of Rh immune globulin for prevention of HDN. ABO incompatibility between the mother and the fetus has a partial protective effect against immunization to D; this finding suggested the rationale for development of Rh immune globulin.[59]

Anti-c, clinically the most important Rh antibody after anti-D, may cause severe HDN. Anti-C, anti-E, and anti-e do not often cause HDN, and when they do, it is usually mild.[6,59]

Autoantibodies to high-incidence Rh antigens often occur in the sera of patients with warm autoimmune hemolytic anemia and in some cases of drug-induced autoimmune hemolytic anemia. These autoantibodies are nonreactive with Rh-null cells.[60]

Anti-D reagents

A large number of IgM, direct-agglutinating, anti-D monoclonals have been generated by immortalizing human B lymphocytes in vitro with Epstein-Barr virus. D-typing reagents licensed for use in the United States are a blend of monoclonal IgM reactive at room temperature along with monoclonal or polyclonal IgG reactive by the IAT for the determination of weak D. Four different FDA-licensed reagents are available for tube testing and one for gel (see Table 7–4). All but two contain different IgM clones. The reactivity of each with variant D antigens may result in D typing discrepancies. Importantly, the *IgM* anti-D component of these reagents has been selected to not react with D^{VI} RBCs (see Table 7–4). D^{VI} is the most common partial D found in white populations, and these individuals often make anti-D when exposed to conventional D. Most agree that they should be classified as Rh-negative for transfusion or Rh immune globulin. The *IgG* component in these reagents reacts with D^{VI} RBCs in the IAT phase (see Table 7–4). D^{VI} RBCs can stimulate production of anti-D in an Rh-negative recipient and must be typed as Rh-positive as donors. The composition of current FDA-licensed reagents has prompted the movement away from weak D testing in the hospital and prenatal setting to classify individuals with D^{VI} RBCs, or some of the other partial D phenotypes (see Table 7–4), as Rh negative.

Monoclonal anti-D has not yet been tested clinically for its ability to prevent immunization after pregnancy but has been shown to suppress D immunization in D-negative male volunteers.[61]

Expression

Northern blot analysis indicated that Rh and RhAG messenger RNA (mRNA) are restricted to cells of erythroid and myeloid lineage, but reverse transcriptase-PCR (RT-PCR) found Rh mRNA splicing isoforms in B and T lymphocytes and monocytes.[62] The significance of this observation is not yet known. During erythropoiesis, RhAG appears early (on $CD34^+$ progenitors), but the Rh proteins appear later—RhCE first, followed by RhD.[63]

Evolution

The *RHD* and *RHCE* genes arose from an early duplication of the erythrocyte *RHAG* gene. *RH* and *RHAG* have been investigated in nonhuman primates[64,65] and rodents,[66–68] and most, with the exception of gorillas and chimpanzees, have a *RHAG* and only one *RH* gene. The *RH* gene duplicated in some common ancestor of gorillas, chimpanzees, and humans, leading to *RHCE* and *RHD.* Chimpanzees and some gorillas have three *RH* genes, indicating that a third duplication has taken place in these species.

Function

The predicted membrane structures of Rh and RhAG suggest that they are transport proteins, and the analysis of their amino acid sequence reveals distant similarity to ammonium transporters in bacteria, fungi, and plants.[69] Evidence for ammonia transport by RhAG comes from yeast complementation experiments,[70,71] expression studies in *Xenopus* oocytes,[72] and direct evidence in RBCs.[73] Rh and RhAG homologues have been found in many organisms, including the sponge *(Geodia)*, the slime mold *(Dictyostelium)*, the fruit fly *(Drosophila)*, and the frog *(Xenopus)*,[74] indicating that they are conserved throughout evolution.

Nonerythroid homologues, designated RhCG and RhBG, are found in the kidney,[75] liver,[76,77] testis, brain, gastrointestinal tract,[78] and skin[79,80] and are localized to regions where ammonium production and elimination are critical in mammalian tissues, strongly suggesting a role for these proteins in ammonia/ammonium homeostasis. When expressed in *Xenopus* oocytes, RhBG and RhCG also mediate transport of ammonia.[81] In the kidney ammonium ions act as expendable cations that facilitate excretion of acids, and renal ammonium metabolism and transport are critical for acid-base balance. In the collecting segment and collecting duct, where large amounts of ammonia are excreted, RhBG and RhCG are found on the basolateral and apical membranes, respectively, of the intercalated cells.[76] These localization studies suggest that RhBG and RhCG are ideally situated to mediate transepithelial movement of ammonium from the interstitium to the lumen of the collecting duct. In support, mouse collecting duct (mIMCD-3) cells, which show polarized expression of these proteins, demonstrate transporter-mediated movement of ammonia.[82]

The function of RhCE and RhD has not been determined. Co-expression of RhCE/RhAG did not influence the rate or total substrate accumulated in oocytes compared to that seen with expression of RhAG alone.[83] Although further studies are necessary to determine if RhCE/D are involved in membrane transport, RhCE/D may have lost transport function and may have a structural role in the RBC membrane.

Summary

The molecular basis of many of the Rh antigens has now been elucidated. The revelation that RhD and RhCE proteins differ by 35 amino acids explains why D antigen is so immunogenic. In addition, exchanges between *RHD* and *RHCE*, mainly by gene conversion, have generated many Rh polymorphisms. The proximity of the two genes on the same chromosome probably affords greater opportunity for exchange. This finding finally explains the myriad of antigens observed in the Rh blood group system and gives interesting insight into the evolutionary history of duplicated genes and the interactions that can take place between them. The complexity hampers molecular genotyping, and additional Rh variants are still being discovered. The challenge is to develop automated platforms that sample several regions of the genes for unequivocal interpretation.

The discovery that members of the Rh family of proteins, RhAG, RhBG, and RhCG, are involved in ammonia/ammonium transport and are ideally positioned in key tissues essential for ammonium elimination is a significant finding because it was long assumed that the high membrane permeability of ammonia would obviate the need for specific transport pathways in mammalian cells.

RBC membrane protein–cytoskeleton and protein–protein interactions are an active area of investigation. Although the major attachment sites between the erythrocyte cytoskeleton and the lipid bilayer are understood to be through glycophorin C and band 3, an additional attachment site mediated by the Rh complex explains the Rh-null defect. Additional studies are needed to determine the protein–protein associations and the dynamics of the assembly of the Rh-membrane complex.

THE KELL AND Kx SYSTEM

History

The Kell blood group system was discovered in 1946, just a few weeks after the introduction of the antiglobulin test. The RBCs from a newborn baby who was thought to be suffering from HDN gave a positive reaction in the direct antiglobulin test.[84] The serum of the mother reacted with RBCs from her husband, her older child, and 9% of random donors. The system was named from Kelleher, the mother's surname, and the antigen is referred to as K (synonyms: Kell, K1). Three years later, the more common antigen, k (synonyms: Cellano, K2), which has a high incidence in all populations, was identified through the typing of large numbers of RBC samples with an antibody that had also caused a mild case of HDN.[85] The Kell system remained a simple two-antigen system until 1957, when the antithetical Kp^a and Kp^b antigens were reported, as was the K_0 (Kell-null) phenotype.[6] Subsequently, the number of Kell antigens has grown to 25, making Kell one of the most polymorphic blood group systems known.

Proteins

The Kell protein is a type II glycoprotein with an approximate M_r of 93,000. It has a 665-amino acid carboxyl terminal extracellular domain, a single 20-amino acid transmembrane domain, and a 47-amino acid N-terminal cytoplasmic domain.[86] The protein has five N-glycosylation sites and 15 extracellular cysteine residues that cause folding through the formation of multiple intrachain disulfide bonds (Fig. 7–4). This explains why Kell blood group antigens are inactivated when RBCs are treated with reducing agents, such as dithiothreitol and aminoethylisothiouronium bromide, which disrupt disulfide bonds.[87] All Kell system antigens are carried on this glycoprotein, which is present at 3500 to 17,000 copies per RBC.[88,89] All but two (Js^a and Js^b) of the Kell antigens are localized in the N-terminal half of the protein before residue 550, strongly suggesting that the C-terminal domain does not tolerate change and is functionally important. Indeed, the Kell glycoprotein is a zinc endopeptidase, and the C terminus contains a zinc-binding domain that is the catalytic site.[90,91]

Kx is a 444-amino acid, 37-kD protein that is linked by a disulfide bond to the Kell protein.[17] Kx is predicted to span the membrane 10 times (see Fig. 7–4), is not glycosylated, and may be a membrane transport protein. RBCs lacking Kx have the McLeod phenotype, which is characterized by a marked reduction of Kell antigens, acanthocytosis, and reduced in vivo RBC survival.

Genes

The *KEL* gene has been localized on chromosome 7q33. It consists of 19 exons spanning approximately 21.5 kb.[92,93] The Kell antigens result from nucleotide mutations that cause

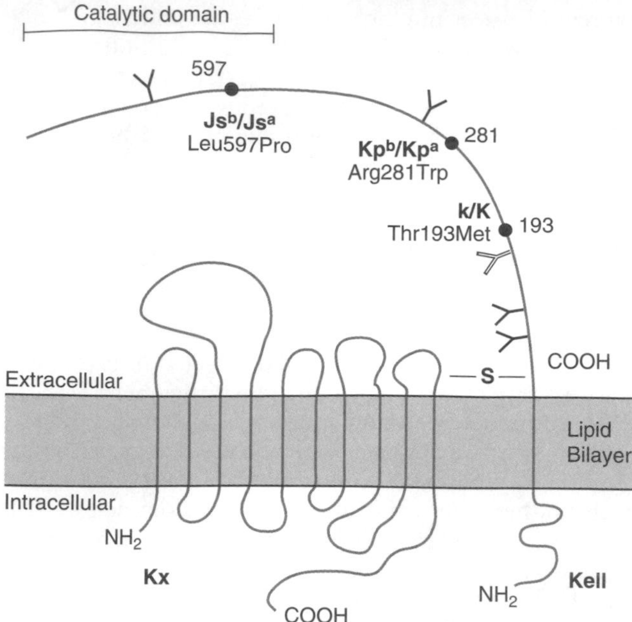

Figure 7–4 Kell and Kx proteins. Kell is a single-pass protein, but Kx is predicted to span the red blood cell membrane 10 times. Kell and Kx are linked by a disulfide bond, shown as -S—. The amino acids that are responsible for the more common Kell antigens are shown. The N-glycosylation sites are shown as *Y*. The *hollow Y* represents the N-glycosylation site that is not present on the K (K1) protein.

single amino acid substitutions in the protein (Table 7–5). The lack of Kell antigens, K_0, is caused by several different molecular defects, including nucleotide deletion, defective splicing, premature stop codons, and amino acid substitutions.[91,94,95]

The *XK* gene is on the short arm of the X chromosome at Xp21.[96] *XK* has three exons, and mutations cause the McLeod syndrome, which, because the gene is X linked, affects males. Carrier females, because of X-chromosome inactivation, have two populations of RBCs (one of the McLeod phenotype and one normal), and the proportion varies from 5% McLeod:95% normal to 85% McLeod:15% normal.[97,98]

McLeod Syndrome

When testing medical students in 1961, Allen and coworkers[99] found that one of the students, Mr. McLeod, had RBCs with very weak expression of Kell antigens. It is now evident that he lacked Kx, which is important for expression of Kell, and that lack of Kx is the basis for the McLeod syndrome. Males with the McLeod syndrome have muscular and neurologic defects, including skeletal muscle wasting, elevated serum creatine phosphokinase, psychopathology, seizures with basal ganglia degeneration, and cardiomyopathy.[90,100] Most symptoms develop after the fourth decade of life. The syndrome is very rare. Approximately 60 males have been identified, and all but 2 have been white; however, because of the plethora of symptoms, the syndrome is probably underdiagnosed.

Fifteen different mutations in the *XK* gene were found in a study of 17 families; these mutations involve major and minor deletions, point mutations, and splice site or frameshift mutations that result in the absence or truncation of Kx protein.[17,100] At one time, chronic granulomatous disease (CGD) was thought to be related to the McLeod syndrome, but the gene controlling CGD is near the *XK* gene on the X chromosome, and the small minority of patients with CGD who have the McLeod phenotype have X-chromosome deletions encompassing both genes.[6,101]

Table 7–5 Molecular Basis of Antigens in the Kell Blood Group System

Antigen	Amino Acid	Position
k(K2)	Threonine	193
K(K1)	Methionine	
Kp^a(K3)	Tryptophan	281
Kp^b(K4)	Arginine	
Kp^c(K21)	Glutamine	
Js^a(K6)	Proline	597
Js^b(K7)	Leucine	
K11	Valine	302
K17	Alanine	
K14	Arginine	180
K24	Proline	
Ul^a	Glutamic acid→Valine	494

Antigens

The Kell system consists of five sets of high-incidence and low-incidence antigens, as follows (the names of the high-incidence antigens appear in **boldface**):

- K and **k**
- Kp^a, **Kp^b**, and Kp^c
- Js^a and **Js^b**
- **K11** and K17
- **K14** and K24

In addition, 14 independently expressed antigens, 3 low-incidence (Ul^a, K23, VLAN), and 11 high-incidence (Ku, Km, K12, K13, K16, K18, K19, K22, Tou, KALT, KTIM), have been identified. The null phenotype, K_0, lacks Kell antigens, and Kell-mod phenotypes have a weak expression of Kell antigens.

Kell antigens show population variations (Table 7–6). K has an incidence of 9% in white persons but is much less common in people of other ethnic backgrounds.[1,58] Kp^a and K17 are also mainly found in white persons. Js^a is almost exclusively found in African Americans, with an incidence of 20%. Ul^a is found in Finnish and Japanese persons.[1,58]

The molecular basis of most of the Kell antigens has been determined (see Table 7–5).[91,102] The K methionine substitution disrupts a glycosylation consensus sequence so that K has one less N-glycan than k.[103] Js^a and Js^b are located within a cluster of cysteine residues,[104] a finding that explains why they are more susceptible than other Kell antigens to treatment with reducing agents.[105] No Kell haplotype has been found to express more than one low-incidence Kell antigen, not because of structural constraints, but because multiple expression would require more than one mutation encoding a recognized Kell system antigen to occur in the same gene.[106]

Weaker expression of Kell antigens is found when RBCs carry Kp^a in *cis*.[107–109] Weak expression of Kell antigens can be inherited or can be acquired and transient. Inherited weak expression occurs when the Kell-associated Kx protein is absent (McLeod phenotype), when glycophorins C and D are absent (Leach phenotype), or when a portion of the extracellular domain of glycophorin C and D, specifically exon 3, is

Table 7–6 Kell Phenotypes and Prevalence

Phenotype	Prevalence (%) White	African American
K−k+	91	98
K+k+	8.8	2
K+k−	0.2	Rare
Kp(a+b−)	Rare	0
Kp(a−b+)	97.7	100
Kp(a+b+)	2.3	Rare
Kp(a−b−c+)	0.32 Japanese	0
Js(a+b−)	0	1
Js(a−b+)	100	80
Js(a+b+)	Rare	19
K11	High incidence	
K17	Low incidence	
K14	High incidence	
K24	Low incidence	
Ul^a	Low incidence (2.6% in Finns, 0.46% in Japanese)	

deleted (some Gerbich-negative phenotypes).[109,110] Transient depression of Kell system antigens has been associated with the presence of autoantibodies mimicking alloantibodies in autoimmune hemolytic anemia and with microbial infections. Kell expression was reduced in two cases of idiopathic thrombocytopenic purpura but returned to normal after remission.[6]

Antibodies

Kell antigens are highly immunogenic, and anti K is common. However, because more than 90% of donors are K negative, it is not difficult to find compatible blood for patients with anti-K. The other Kell system antibodies are less common but are also usually IgG, and they have caused transfusion reactions and HDN or neonatal anemia. In HDN due to Kell antibodies, neither maternal antibody titers nor amniotic bilirubin levels are good predictors of the severity of the disease. Reports demonstrate that Kell antigens are expressed very early during erythropoiesis[63] and that Kell antibodies can cause suppression of erythropoiesis in vitro.[111] This finding suggests that the low level of bilirubin observed, in the presence of neonatal anemia, is due to Kell antibodies that bind to erythroid progenitors and exert effects before hemoglobinization.

Anti-Ku is the antibody made by immunized K_0 individuals, and Ku represents the high-incidence or "total-Kell" antigen. McLeod males with CGD make anti-Kx+Km; this antibody reacts strongly with K_0 cells, weaker with RBCs of common Kell phenotype, and not at all with McLeod phenotype RBCs. Anti-Km, made by McLeod persons who do not have CGD, reacts with RBCs of common Kell phenotypes but not with K_0 or McLeod RBCs, suggesting that it detects one or more epitopes requiring both the Kell and Kx proteins. One case has been reported of a McLeod male without CGD who made an apparent anti-Kx without the presence of anti-Km.[101]

Expression

Kell system antigens appear to be erythroid specific and are expressed very early during erythropoiesis.[63] Kx mRNA is found in muscle, heart, brain, and hematopoietic tissue.[17]

Evolution

Primate RBCs express the k antigen but not the K antigen, indicating that the K mutation appeared in human lineage. Chimpanzees are Js(a+b−),[112] and Js^a is also present on RBCs from Old World monkeys,[113] suggesting that Js^b also arose after human speciation. Kell protein is not found on immunoblots of RBCs from sheep, goat, cattle, rabbit, horse, mouse, donkey, cat, dog, or rat.[114]

Function

The Kell glycoprotein is a member of the M13 or neprilysin family of zinc endopeptidases that cleave a variety of physiologically active peptides. One member of this family, endothelin converting enzyme 1 (ECE-1), is a membrane-bound metalloprotease that catalyzes the proteolytic activation of big endothelin-1 (big ET-1).[115] Like ECE-1, Kell protein can proteolytically cleave endothelins, specifically big ET-3 to generate ET-3, which is a potent vasoconstrictor.[116] ET-3 is also involved in the development of the enteric nervous system and in migration of neural crest-derived cells. The biologic role of the endothelins is not yet completely elucidated, but they act on two G protein–coupled receptors, ET_A and ET_B, which are found on many cells. Kell-null individuals, who lack Kell protein, do not have any obvious defect, so they do not immediately give insight into the biologic function of the Kell protein. This lack of defect in Kell-null people may be because other enzymes probably also cleave ET-3,[116] and determining whether Kell-null individuals have abnormal levels of plasma endothelins is an active area of investigation.

DUFFY (Fy) BLOOD GROUP SYSTEM

History

The Duffy (Fy^a) blood group antigen was first reported in 1950 by Cutbush and associates,[117] who described the reactivity of an antibody found in a hemophiliac male who had received multiple transfusions. This blood group system bears the patient's surname, Duffy, the last two letters of which provide the abbreviated nomenclature (Fy). Fy^b was found 1 year later.[118] In 1975, Fy was identified as the receptor for the malarial parasite *Plasmodium vivax*.[119] This discovery explained the predominance of the Fy(a−b−) (Fy-null) phenotype, which confers resistance to malarial invasion, in persons originating from West Africa.

Proteins

The Fy protein is a transmembrane glycoprotein of 35 to 43 kD consisting of a glycosylated amino terminal region, which protrudes from the membrane and has seven transmembrane-spanning domains (Fig. 7–5).[120,121] In 1993, it was realized that Fy was the erythrocyte chemokine receptor that could bind interleukin-8 and monocyte chemotactic peptide-1 (MCP-1).[122] The cloning of the *FY* gene[123] confirmed that it belongs to the conserved family of chemokine receptors.

Gene

The *FY* gene is located on the long arm of chromosome 1q22–q23[124] and spans 1.5 kb. The gene, which has only two

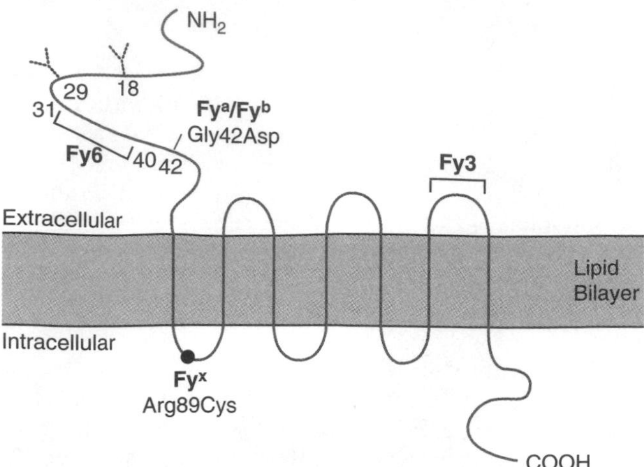

Figure 7–5 The predicted seven-transmembrane domain structure of the Duffy protein. The amino acid change responsible for the Fy^a/Fy^b polymorphism, the mutation responsible for Fy^x glycosylation sites, and the regions where Fy3 and Fy6 map are indicated.

exons, contains two ATG codons. The upstream exon contains the major start site.[125,126] The same two-exon organization is also found in genes for other chemokine receptors.[127]

Antigens

The Fy^a and Fy^b antigens are encoded by two allelic forms of the gene, designated *FYA* and *FYB*, and are responsible for the Fy(a+b−), Fy(a−b+), and Fy(a+b+) phenotypes.[126] They differ by a single amino acid located on the extracellular domain (see Fig. 7–5).

Fy^x, which is a weak expression of Fy^b, is found in white persons and is due to a single mutation in the *FYB* gene.[128,129] The amino acid change, which is located in the first intracellular cytoplasmic loop, is associated with a decrease in the amount of protein in the membrane and results in diminished expression of Fy^b, Fy3, and Fy6 antigens as well as reduced binding of chemokine.[127,130,131]

Fy3, as determined with one monoclonal anti-Fy3, is located on the third extracellular loop,[132] whereas Fy6 maps to the amino terminal loop of the protein. The aspartic acid at amino acid 25 and glutamic acid at 26 are critical for anti-Fy6 binding.[133]

The Fy(a−b−) phenotype found in African Americans is caused by a mutation in the promoter region of *FYB* (T>C at position −46), which disrupts a binding site for the erythroid transcription factor GATA-1 and results in the loss of Fy expression on RBCs.[134,135] The Fy protein has also been found on endothelial cells. Because the erythroid promoter controls expression only in erythroid cells, expression of Fy proteins on endothelium is normal in these Fy(a−b−). All African persons with a mutated GATA sequence to date have been shown to carry *FYB;* therefore, Fy^b is expressed on their nonerythroid tissues. This finding explains why Fy(a−b−) individuals make anti-Fy^a but not anti-Fy^b.[136] It also is relevant in the selection of antigen-matched units for Fy(a−b−) patients with sickle cell disease, because they would not be expected to make anti-Fy^b. Rare Fy(a−b−) who do make anti-Fy^b should be investigated at the genetic level, because the molecular basis for this observation has not yet been explained. Lastly, a *FYA* allele with a mutated GATA sequence has been found in Papua New Guinea.[137]

Table 7–7 Duffy Phenotypes and Prevalence

Phenotype	Prevalence (%)				
	Caucasians	Blacks	Chinese	Japanese	Thai
Fy(a+b−)	17	9	90.8	81.5	69
Fy(a−b+)	34	22	0.3	0.9	3
Fy(a+b+)	49	1	8.9	17.6	28
Fy(a−b−)*	Rare	68	0	0	0
Fy^X	1.4	0	0	0	0

*Fy(a−b−), incidence in Israeli Arabs 25%; Israeli Jews, 4%

The Fy(a−b−) phenotype in white persons is very rare (Table 7–7).[1] One propositus, an Australian (AZ) woman, appears to be homozygous for a 14-bp deletion in *FYA*, which introduces a stop codon in the protein[138]; a Cree Indian female (Ye), a white female (NE), and a Lebanese Jewish male (AA) carry different Trp to stop codon mutations.[139] Because these mutations would result in a truncated protein, these people would not be expected to express endothelial or erythroid Fy protein. All four people made anti-Fy3.

There are 13,000 to 14,000 Fy antigen sites per RBC,[140] and Fy^a, Fy^b, and Fy6 antigens are sensitive to proteolytic enzyme treatment of antigen-positive RBCs, although Fy3 is resistant.

Antibodies

Fy antigens are estimated to be 40 times less immunogenic than K antigens, and most Fy antibodies arise from stimulation by blood transfusion. They are mostly IgG, subclass IgG1, and only rarely are IgM. Anti-Fy^b is less common than anti-Fy^a, and Fy antibodies are often found in sera with other antibodies. Anti-Fy3 is made by rare white Fy(a−b−) individuals.[6] Anti-Fy6 is a mouse monoclonal antibody.[127]

Expression

Duffy mRNA is present in kidney, spleen, heart, lung, muscle, duodenum, pancreas, placenta, and brain.[123,127] Cells responsible for Fy expression in these tissues are the endothelial cells lining postcapillary venules,[141–143] except in the brain, where expression is localized to the Purkinje cell neurons.[144,145] The same polypeptide is expressed in endothelial cells and RBCs, but in brain, a larger, 8.5-kb mRNA is present. The function of Fy on neurons is an area of active investigation.

In the fetus, Fy antigens can be detected at 6 to 7 weeks' gestation and are well developed at birth.[1] The expression of these antigens was found to occur late during erythropoiesis and RBC maturation.[63]

Evolution

RBCs of monkeys and apes react with anti-Fy^b, and the conserved GT repeat sequences in the 3 flanking region of the gene both suggest that *FYB* was the ancestral gene.[146,147] The first human divergence occurred when a mutation in the erythroid promoter region of *FYB* resulted in the loss of Fy^b expression on RBCs. This mutation conferred resistance to malaria infection in regions where *P. vivax* was endemic and selected for the high proportion of Fy(a−b−) in populations of African ancestry. Later, a single nucleotide change in the *FYB* gene caused the *FYA* polymorphism in people of European and Asian ancestry. Fy has been cloned from several nonhuman primates, including chimpanzees, squirrel monkeys, and rhesus monkeys, and from cows, pigs, rabbits, and mice.[127]

Function

The importance of Fy as a receptor for the malarial parasite *P. vivax* is well established, but its biologic role as a chemokine receptor on RBCs, endothelial cells, and brain is not yet clear. The chemokine receptors are a family of proteins that are receptors on target cells for the binding of chemokines. Chemokines are so named because they are *cytokines* that are *chemotactic* (cause cell migration), and their receptors are an active area of investigation.[148] Chemokine receptors have been found principally on lymphocytes, where they are coupled to G proteins and activate intracellular signaling pathways that regulate cell migration into tissues. Unlike other chemokine receptors, Fy does not have a conserved amino acid DRY-motif in the second extracellular loop, and cells transfected with Fy and stimulation with chemokines do not mobilize free calcium.[120] Also, Fy can bind chemokines from both the CXC (IL-8, MGSA) and the CC (RANTES, MCP-1, MIP-1) classes of chemokines.[127] These features have led investigators to hypothesize that it may act as a scavenger or sink for excess chemokine release into the circulation.[149,150] If the function of Fy on RBCs is to scavenge excess chemokine, it may be that Fy(a−b−) individuals would be more susceptible to septic shock[143] or to cardiac damage after infarction. Renal allografts have been reported to have shorter survival in African American Fy(a−b−) recipients,[151] and Fy has been shown to be upregulated in the kidney during renal injury.[152]

Abundant expression of Fy on high endothelial venules and sinusoids in the spleen,[143] which is a site central to chemokine-induced leukocyte trafficking, suggests a role in leukocyte migration into the tissues. Fy is also similar to the receptor for endothelins (ET_B), vasoactive proteins that strongly influence vascular biology and that may also be mitogenic.[127]

THE KIDD BLOOD GROUP SYSTEM

History

The Kidd blood group system was discovered in 1951, when a "new" antibody in the serum of Mrs. Kidd (who also had anti-K) caused HDN in her sixth child. Jk came from the initials of the baby (John Kidd), because K had been used previously for Kell.[153] Anti-Jk^b was found 2 years later in the serum of a woman who had a transfusion reaction (she also had anti-Fy^a).[154] Kidd system antibodies are characteristically found in sera with other blood group antibodies, suggesting that Kidd antigens are not particularly immunogenic. However, Kidd antibodies induce a rapid and robust anamnestic response that is responsible for their reputation for causing severe delayed hemolytic transfusion reactions.

Proteins

The Kidd glycoprotein has an approximate M_r of 46,000 to 60,000 and is predicted to span the membrane 10 times. The

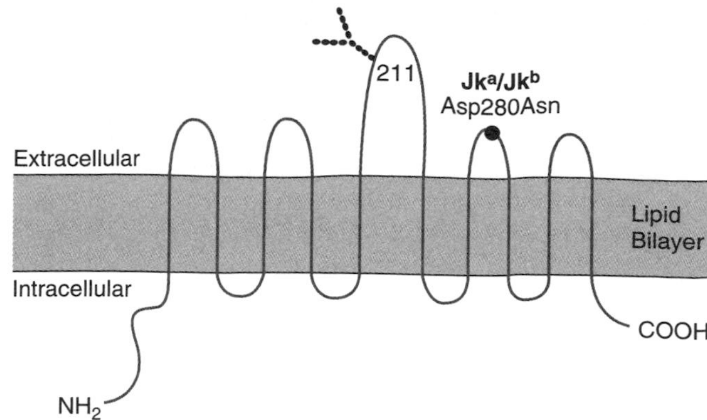

Figure 7–6 Predicted 10-transmembrane domain structure of the Kidd/urea transporter. The polymorphism responsible for the Kidd antigens and the site for the N-glycan are indicated.

third extracellular loop is large and carries an N-glycan at Asn211 (Fig. 7–6). The protein has 10 cysteine residues, but only 1 is predicted to be extracellular, a fact that explains why the antigens are not sensitive to disulfide reagents. There is internal homology between the N-terminal and C-terminal halves of the protein, with each containing an LP box (LPXXTXPF) characteristic of urea transporters.[155] Isolation of the Kidd protein from RBCs was elusive, and cloning of the Kidd gene was accomplished with primers complementary to the rabbit kidney urea transporter. A clone isolated from a human bone marrow library with the PCR product was confirmed by in vitro transcription–translation to encode a protein that carried Kidd blood group antigens.[156]

Gene

The Kidd blood group gene (*HUT11* or *SLC14A1*) is located at chromosome 18q11–q12.[157,158] The *HUT11* gene has 11 exons and spans approximately 30 kb. Two alternative polyadenylation sites generate transcripts of 4.4 and 2.0 kb, which appear to be used equally. Exons 4 to 11 encode the mature protein.[17,159]

Antigens

Two antigens, Jk^a and Jk^b, are responsible for the three common phenotypes—Jk(a+b−), Jk(a−b+), and Jk(a+b+). The two antigens are found with similar frequency in white persons but show large differences in other ethnic groups (Table 7–8).[1] The Jk(a−b−) phenotype is rare but occurs with greater incidence in Asian and Polynesian people.

Table 7–8 Kidd Phenotypes and Prevalence

	Prevalence(%)		
Phenotype	White	African	Asian
Jk(a+b−)	26.3	51.5	23.2
Jk(a−b+)	23.4	8.1	26.8
Jk(a+b+)	50.3	40.8	49.1
Jk(a−b−)	Rare	Rare	0.9 (Polynesian)

The Jk^a and Jk^b polymorphism is located on the fourth extracellular loop and is caused by a single amino acid substitution (see Fig. 7–6).[160] The null phenotype has been reported to arise on the following two genetic backgrounds: homozygous inheritance of a silent allele and inheritance of a dominant inhibitor gene, *In(Jk)*, which is unlinked to *JK (HUT11)*.[1] The silent alleles were found to have acceptor or donor splice site mutations that cause skipping of exon 6 or exon 7.[159,161] In Finnish persons, a single point mutation (Ser291Pro) was the only change associated with silencing of the expression of Jk^b.[161] The unlinked dominant inhibitor gene has not yet been identified.

The Jk3 antigen ("total Jk") is found on RBCs that are positive for Jk^a, Jk^b, or both, but the specific amino acid residues responsible for Jk3 are unknown. There are approximately 14,000 Jk^a antigen sites on Jk(a+b−) RBCs.[140]

Antibodies

Neither anti-Jk^a nor anti-Jk^b is common, and anti-Jk^b is found less often than anti-Jk^a. Once a Kidd antibody is identified, compatible blood is not difficult to find, because 25% of donors are negative for each antigen. Unfortunately, Kidd antibodies are often found in sera that contain other alloantibodies, so the situation is often more complicated. In addition, the antibodies are known to cause delayed hemolytic transfusion reactions and are responsible for at least one third of all cases of delayed hemolytic transfusion reactions.[59] The antibodies often decrease in titer, react only with cells that are from persons homozygous for the antigen (the dosage phenomenon), or may escape detection altogether in the sensitized patient's serum before transfusion. If the patient is transfused with antigen-positive RBCs, an anamnestic response results, with an increase in the antibody titer and hemolysis of the transfused RBCs.[59]

Because Kidd antibodies are mainly IgG, it was assumed that they must activate complement to cause such prompt RBC destruction. Kidd antibodies can be partially IgM, however, and the minor IgM component may be responsible for the pattern of destruction of incompatible RBCs in delayed hemolytic transfusion reactions. This theory is based on evidence that serum fractions containing only IgG anti-Jk^a do not bind complement.[162] Kidd antibodies only rarely cause HDN; if they do, it is typically not severe. Anti-Jk^a has occasionally been found as an autoantibody, and the concurrent, temporary suppression of antigen expression has also been reported.[59] Anti-Jk3, sometimes referred to as anti-Jk^{ab}, is produced by Jk(a−b−) individuals and reacts with RBCs that are positive for Jk^a, Jk^b, or both.[163]

Expression

In the fetus, Kidd antigens can be detected at 11 weeks' gestation and are well developed at birth.[6] Immunohistochemical and in situ hybridization have shown that Kidd/HUT11 is also expressed on endothelial cells of vasa recta in the medulla of the human kidney.[17]

Evolution

Expression of RBC Kidd antigens has not been investigated in nonhuman primates, but the human RBC Kidd protein is clearly a member of a family of urea transporters, which have homologues in the human kidney and in nonhuman primates.

Function

A first clue to the function of Kidd came from the observation in 1982 that the RBCs of a male of Samoan descent were resistant to lysis in 2M urea, which was being used to lyse RBCs for platelet counting.[164] His RBCs were Jk(a−b−), and subsequent investigations revealed that movement of urea into Jk(a−b−) RBCs was equivalent to passive diffusion, in contrast to RBCs with normal Kidd antigens, with rapid urea influx. Fast urea transport in human RBCs is thought to be advantageous for RBC osmotic stability in the kidney, especially during transit through the vasa recta from the papilla to the isoosmotic renal cortex.[165] Urea transport in the kidney contributes to urine concentration and water preservation. Two types of urea transporters have now been characterized, vasopressin-sensitive transporters and constitutive transporters. The Kidd/HUT11 in RBCs and kidney medulla is a constitutive transporter. A vasopressin-sensitive transporter, HUT2, which is expressed in the collecting ducts of the kidney, has 62% sequence identity with Kidd/HUT11. *HUT2* is also located on chromosome 18q12, suggesting that both transporters evolved from an ancestral gene duplication.[166] Jk-null individuals do not suffer a clinical syndrome except for a reduced capacity to concentrate urine,[167] suggesting that other mechanisms or other gene family members, such as *HUT2*, can compensate for the missing Kidd/HUT11 protein.

Summary

The last decade has witnessed the rapid elucidation of the molecular basis for the various blood group antigens and phenotypes. In the next decade, research focus is turned to determination of the structure and function of the proteins carrying these blood group antigens. Null individuals *(natural knockouts)*, persons who lack the antigens and the proteins that carry them, exist for all four of these blood group systems. Reminiscent of what is being found in many genetically engineered knockout mice, most of the individuals with null phenotypes do not have serious or any obvious defects. This observation is consistent with growing evidence that many genes have evolved as members of larger gene families, which appear to have overlapping abilities to substitute for the disrupted gene family member. Evidence is accumulating that genes encoding blood group proteins are also members of larger gene families. The mouse homologues of some of these blood group genes have been cloned, and knockout mice are being generated to study them. This process may aid in the further elucidation of the structure and function of the molecules carrying blood group antigens.

REFERENCES

1. Race RR, Sanger R. Blood Groups in Man, 6th ed. Oxford, Blackwell Scientific, 1975.
2. Bowman JM. RhD hemolytic disease of the newborn [editorial; comment]. NEJM 1998;339:1775–1777.
3. Levine P, Stetson RE. An unusual case of intragroup agglutination. JAMA 1939;113:126–127.
4. Levine P, Burnham L, Katzin EM, Vogel P. The role of iso-immunization in the pathogenesis of erythroblastosis fetalis. AJOG 1941;42:925–937.

5. Rosenfield RE. Who discovered Rh? A personal glimpse of the Levine-Wiener argument. Transfusion 1989;29:355–357.
6. Daniels G. Human Blood Groups, 2nd ed. Oxford, Blackwell Science, 2002.
7. Mourant AE. A new rhesus antibody. Nature 1945;155:542.
8. Tippett P. A speculative model for the Rh blood groups. Ann Hum Genet 1986;50:241–247.
9. Rosenfield RE, Alen FHJr, Swisher SN, Kochwa S.A review of Rh Serology and presentation of a new terminology. Transfusion 1962;2:287–312.
10. Agre P, Saboori AM, Asimos A, Smith BL. Purification and partial characterization of the M_r 30,000 integral membrane protein associated with the erythrocyte Rh(D) antigen. J Biol Chem 1987;262:17497–17503.
11. Bloy C, Blanchard D, Dahr W, et al. Determination of the N-terminal sequence of human red cell Rh(D) polypeptide and demonstration that the Rh(D), (c), and (E) antigens are carried by distinct polypeptide chains. Blood 1988;72:661–666.
12. Arce MA, Thompson ES, Wagner S, et al. Molecular cloning of RhD cDNA derived from a gene present in RhD-positive, but not RhD-negative individuals. Blood 1993;82:651–655.
13. Chérif-Zahar B, Bloy C, Le Van Kim C, et al. Molecular cloning and protein structure of a human blood group Rh polypeptide. Proc Natl Acad Sci USA 1990;87:6243–6247.
14. Simsek S, de Jong CA, Cuijpers HT, et al. Sequence analysis of cDNA derived from reticulocyte mRNAs coding for Rh polypeptides and demonstration of of E/e and C/c polymorphisms. Vox Sang 1994;67:203–209.
15. Hartel-Schenk S, Agre P. Mammalian red cell membrane Rh polypeptides are selectively palmitoylated subunits of a macromolecular complex. J Biol Chem 1992;267:5569–5574.
16. Ridgwell K, Spurr NK, Laguda B, et al. Isolation of cDNA clones for a 50 kDa glycoprotein of the human erythrocyte membrane associated with Rh (rhesus) blood-group antigen expression. Biochem J 1992;287:223–228.
17. Cartron JP, Bailly P, Le Van Kim C, et al. Insights into the structure and function of membrane polypeptides carrying blood group antigens. Vox Sang 1998;74(Suppl 2):29–64.
18. Ballas SK, Clark MR, Mohandas N, et al. Red cell membrane and cation deficiency in Rh null syndrome. Blood 1989;63:1046–1055.
19. Sturgeon P. Hematological observations on the anemia associated with blood type Rhnull. Blood 1970;36:310–320.
20. Huang C-H, Chen Y, Reid ME, Seidl C. Rh_{null} disease: The amorph type results from a novel double mutation in RhCe gene on D-negative background. Blood 1998;92:664–671.
21. Eyers SA, Ridgwell K, Mawby WJ, Tanner MJ. Topology and organization of human Rh (rhesus) blood group-related polypeptides. J Biol Chem 1994;269:6417–6423.
22. Beckmann R, Smythe JS, Anstee DJ, Tanner MJA. Functional cell surface expression of band 3, the human red blood cell anion exchange protein (AE1), in K562 erythroleukemia cells: Band 3 enhances the cell surface reactivity of Rh antigens. Blood 1998;92:4428–4438.
23. Nicolas V, Kim CL, Gane P, et al. Rh-RhAG/ankyrin-R, a new interaction site between the membrane bilayer and the red cell skeleton, is impaired by Rh_{null}-associated mutation. J Biol Chem 2003;278:25526–25533.
24. Dahl KN, Parthasarathy R, Westhoff CM, et al. Protein 4.2 is critical to CD47-membrane skeleton attachment in human red cells. Blood 2004;103:1131–1136.
25. Colin Y, Chérif-Zahar B, Le Van Kim C, et al. Genetic basis of the RhD-positive and RhD-negative blood group polymorphism as determined by Southern analysis. Blood 1991;78:2747–2752.
26. Chérif-Zahar B, Mattei MG, Le Van Kim C, et al. Localization of the human Rh blood group gene structure to chromosome region 1p34.3–1p36.1 by in situ hybridization. Hum Genet 1991;86:398–400.
27. Avent ND, Reid ME. The Rh blood group system: a review. Blood 2000;95:375–387.
28. Huang C-H. The human Rh50 glycoprotein gene—Structural organization and associated splicing defect resulting in Rh_{null} disease. J Biol Chem 1998;273:2207–2213.
29. Chérif-Zahar B, Raynal V, Gane P, et al. Candidate gene acting as a suppressor of the *RH* locus in most cases of Rh-deficiency. Nature Genet 1996;12:168–173.
30. Avent ND, Martin PG, Armstrong-Fisher SS, et al. Evidence of genetic diversity underlying Rh $D,^-$ weak D (D^u), and partial D phenotypes as determined by multiplex polymerase chain reaction analysis of the *RHD* gene. Blood 1997;89:2568–2577.
31. Andrews KT, Wolter LC, Saul A, Hyland CA. The RhD− trait in a white patient with the RhCCee phenotype attributed to a four-nucleotide deletion in the *RHD* gene. Blood 1998;92:1839–1840.
32. Huang C-H. Alteration of *RH* gene structure and expression in human dCCee and DC^W-red blood cells: phenotypic homozygosity versus genotypic heterozygosity. Blood 1996;88:2326–2333.
33. Wagner FF, Frohmajer A, Flegel WA. *RHD* positive haplotypes in D negative Europeans. BMC Genetics 2001;2:10
34. Okuda H, Kawano M, Iwamoto S, et al. The *RHD* gene is highly detectable in RhD-negative Japanese donors. J Clin Invest 1997;100:373–379.
35. Singleton BK, Green CA, Avent ND, et al. The presence of an *RHD* pseudogene containing a 37-base pair duplication and a nonsense mutation in Africans with the Rh D-negative blood group phenotype. Blood 2000;95:12–18.
36. Wagner FF, Gassner C, Müller TH, et al. Molecular basis of weak D phenotypes. Blood 1999;93:385–393.
37. Blumenfeld OO, Patnaik SK. Allelic genes of blood group antigens: a source of human mutations and cSNPs docmented in the Blood Group Antigen Mutation Database. Hum Mutat 2004;23:8–16. Available at www.ncbi.nlm.nih.gov/projects/mhc/xslcgi.fcgi?cmd=bgumt/home.
38. Wagner FF, Frohmajer A, Ladewig B, et al. Weak D alleles express distinct phenotypes. Blood 2000;95:2699–2708.
39. Chang JG, Wang JC, Yang TY, et al. Human RhD_{el} is caused by a deletion of 1,013 bp between introns 8 and 9 including exon 9 of RHD gene. Blood 1998;92:2602–2604.
40. Yasuda H, Ohto H, Sakuma S, Ishikawa Y. Secondary anti-D immunization by Del red blood cells. Transfusion 2005;45:1581–1584.
41. Wagner T, Kormoczi GF, Buchta C, et al. Anti-D immunization by DEL red blood cells. Transfusion 2005;45:520–526.
42. Huang C-H. Molecular insights into the Rh protein family and associated antigens. Curr Opin Hematol 1997;4:94–103.
43. Wallace M, Lomas-Francis C, Tippett P. The D antigen characteristic of R_0^{Har} is a partial D antigen. Vox Sang 1996;70:169–172.
44. Schlanser G, Moulds MK, Flegel WA, Wagner FF. Crawford (Rh43), a low-incidence antigen, is associated with a novel RHCE variant RHce allele (abstract). Transfusion 2003;43(Suppl):34A–35A.
45. Westhoff CM, Vege S, Nance S, et al. Determination of the molecular background of the Crawford antigen occurring with a weak C antigen (abstract). Vox Sang 2004;87(Suppl 3):42.
46. Beckers EAM, Porcelijn L, Ligthart P, et al. The R_0^{Har} antigenic complex is associated with a limited number of D epitopes and alloanti-D production: A study of three unrelated persons and their families. Transfusion 1996;36:104–108.
47. Wagner FF, Ladewig B, Flegel WA. The RHCE allele ceRT: D epitope 6 expression does not require D-specific amino acids. Transfusion 2003;43:1248–1254.
48. Mouro I, Colin Y, Chérif-Zahar B, et al. Molecular genetic basis of the human Rhesus blood group system. Nature Genet 1993;5:62–65.
49. Mouro I, Colin Y, Sistonen P, et al. Molecular basis of the RhC^W (Rh8) and RhC^X (Rh9) blood group specificities. Blood 1995;86:1196–1201.
50. Faas BHW, Beckers EAM, Wildoer P, et al. Molecular background of VS and weak C expression in blacks. Transfusion 1997;37:38–44.
51. Daniels GL, Faas BHW, Green CA, et al. The VS and V blood group polymorphisms in Africans: a serological and molecular analysis. Transfusion 1998;38:951–958.
52. Noizat-Pirenne F, Mouro I, Gane P, et al. Heterogeneity of blood group RhE variants revealed by serological analysis and molecular alteration of the *RHCE* gene and transcript. Br J Haematol 1998;103:429–436.
53. Noizat-Pirenne F, Mouro I, Roussel M, et al. The molecular basis of a D(C)(E) complex probably associated with the RH35 low frequency antigen (abstract). Transfusion 1999;39(Suppl):103S.
54. Faas BHW, Ligthart PC, Lomas-Francis C, et al. Involvement of Gly96 in the formation of the Rh26 epitope. Transfusion 1997;37:1123–1130.
55. Huang C-H, Reid ME, Chen Y, Novaretti M. Deletion of Arg229 in RhCE polypeptide alters expression of RhE and CE-associated Rh6 (abstract). Blood 1997;90(Suppl 1):272a.
56. Westhoff CM, Silberstein LE, Wylie DE, et al. 16Cys encoded by the *RHce* gene is associated with altered expression of the e antigen and is frequent in the R_0 haplotype. Br J Haematol 2001;113:666–671.
57. Noizat-Pirenne F, Lee K, Le Pennec P-Y, et al. Rare RHCE phenotypes in black individuals of Afro-Caribbean origin: identification and transfusion safety. Blood 2002;100:4223–4231.
58. Reid ME, Lomas-Francis C. Blood Group Antigen FactsBook, 2nd ed., San Diego, Academic Press, 2003.
59. Mollison PL, Engelfriet CP, Contreras M. Blood Transfusion in Clinical Medicine, 10th ed., Oxford, Blackwell Science, 1997.
60. Petz LD, Garratty G. Acquired Immune Hemolytic Anemias. New York, Churchill Livingstone, 1980.
61. Kumpel BM, Goodrick MJ, et al. Human Rh D monoclonal antibodies (BRAD-3 and BRAD-5) cause accelerated clearance of Rh D^+ red blood cells and suppression of Rh D immunization in Rh D^- volunteers. Blood 1995;86:1701–1709.

62. Kajii E, Umenishi F, Nakauchi H, Ikemoto S. Expression of Rh blood group gene transcripts in human leukocytes. Biochem Biophys Res Comm 1994;202:1497–1504.
63. Southcott MJG, Tanner MJ, Anstee DJ. The expression of human blood group antigens during erythropoiesis in a cell culture system. Blood 1999;93:4425–4435.
64. Westhoff CM, Wylie DE. Investigation of the human Rh blood group system in nonhuman primates and other species with serologic and Southern blot analysis. J Mol Evol 1994;39:87–92.
65. Salvignol I, Calvas P, Socha WW, et al. Structural analysis of the RH-like blood group gene products in nonhuman primates. Immunogenetics 1995;41:271–281.
66. Westhoff CM, Schultze A, From A, et al. Characterization of the mouse RH blood group gene. Genomics 1999;57:451–454.
67. Blancher A, Klein J, Socha WW (eds). Molecular Biology and Evolution of Blood Group and MHC Antigens in Primates. Berlin, Springer-Verlag, 1997.
68. Kitano T, Sumiyama K, Shiroishi T, Saitou N. Conserved evolution of the Rh50 gene compared to its homologous Rh blood group gene. Biochem Biophys Res Commun 1998;249:78–85.
69. Marini AM, Urrestarazu A, Beauwens R, André B. The Rh (rhesus) blood group polypeptides are related to NH_4^+ transporters. Trends Biochem Sci 1997;22:460–461.
70. Marini AM, Matassi G, Raynal V, et al. The human rhesus-associated RhAG protein and a kidney homologue promote ammonium transport in yeast. Nature Genet 2000;26:341–344.
71. Westhoff CM, Siegel DL, Burd CG, Foskett JK. Mechanism of genetic complementation of ammonium transport in yeast by human erythrocyte Rh-associated glycoprotein. J Biol Chem 2004;279:17443–17448.
72. Westhoff CM, Ferreri-Jacobia M, Mak D-OD, Foskett JK. Identification of the erythrocyte Rh blood group glycoprotein as a mammalian ammonium transporter. J Biol Chem 2002;277:12499–12502.
73. Ripoche P, Bertrand O, Gane P, et al. Human Rhesus-associated glycoprotein mediates facilitated transport of NH_3 into red blood cells. Proc Natl Acad Sci USA 2004;101:17222–17227.
74. Huang C-H, Liu PZ, Cheng JG. Molecular biology and genetics of the Rh blood group system. Semin Hematol 2000;37:150–165.
75. Eladari D, Cheval E, Quentin F, et al. Expression of RhCG, a new putative NH3/NH4+ transporter, along the rat nephron. J Amer Soc Nephrology 2002;13:1999–2008.
76. Weiner ID, Miller RT, Verlander JW. Localization of the ammonium transporters, Rh B glycoprotein and Rh C glycoprotein, in the mouse liver. Gastroenterology 2003;124:1432–1440.
77. Weiner ID, Verlander JW. Renal and hepatic expression of the ammonium transporter proteins, Rh B glycoprotein and Rh C glycoprotein. Acta Physiol Scand 2003;179:331–338.
78. Handlogten ME, Hong SP, Zhang L, et al. Expression of the ammonia transporter proteins Rh B glycoprotein and Rh C glycoprotein in the intestinal tract. Am J Physiol Gastrointest Liver Physiol 2005;288: G1036–G1047.
79. Liu Z, Peng J, Mo R, et al. Rh type B glycoprotein is a new member of the Rh superfamily and a putative ammonia transporter in mammals. J Biol Chem 2001;276:1424–1433.
80. Liu Z, Chen Y, Mo R, Hui C, Cheng J-F, Mohandas N, Huang C-H. Characterization of human RhCG and mouse RhCG as novel nonerythroid Rh glycoprotein homologues predominantly expressed in kidney and testis. J Biol Chem 2000;275:25641–25651.
81. Mak DO, Dang B, Weiner ID, et al. Characterization of ammonia transport by the kidney Rh glycoproteins, RhBG and RhCG. Am J Physiol Renal Physiol 2006;290:F297–F305.
82. Handlogten ME, Hong SP, Westhoff CM, Weiner ID. Apical ammonia transport by the mouse inner medullary collecting duct cell (mIMCD-3). Am J Physiol Renal Physiol 2005;289:F347–F358.
83. Westhoff CM. The Rh blood group system in review: a new face for the next decade. Transfusion 2004;44:1663–1673.
84. Coombs RRA, Mourant AE, Race RR. In vivo isosensitisation of red cells in babies with haemolytic disease. Lancet 1946;i:264–266.
85. Levine P, Backer M, Wigod M, Ponder R. A new human hereditary blood property (Cellano) present in 99.8% of all bloods. Science 1949;109:464–466.
86. Lee S, Zambas ED, Marsh WL, Redman CM. Molecular cloning and primary structure of Kell blood group protein. Proc Natl Acad Sci USA 1991;88:6353–6357.
87. Advani H, Zamor J, Judd WJ, Johnson CL, Marsh WL. Inactivation of Kell blood group antigens by 2-aminoethylisothiouronium bromide. Br J Haematol 1982;51:107–115.
88. Hughes-Jones NC, Gardner B. The Kell system: studies with radiolabeled anti-K. Vox Sang 1971;21:154–158.
89. Masouredis SP, Sudora E, Mohan LC, Victoria EJ. Immunoelectron microscopy of Kell and Cellano antigens on red cell ghosts. Haematologia 1980;13:59–64.
90. Marsh WL, Redman CM. The Kell blood group system: a review. Transfusion 1990;30:158–167.
91. Lee S. Molecular basis of Kell blood group phenotypes. Vox Sang 1997;73:1–11.
92. Lee S, Zambas ED, Marsh WL, Redman CM. The human Kell blood group gene maps to chromosome 7q33 and its expression is restricted to erythroid cells. Blood 1993;81:2804–2809.
93. Lee S, Zambas E, Green ED, Redman C. Organization of the gene encoding the human Kell blood group protein. Blood 1995;85:1364–1370.
94. Lee S, Russo DCW, Reiner AP, et al. Molecular defects underlying the Kell null phenotype. J Biol Chem 2001;276:27281–27289.
95. Yu LC, Twu YC, Chang CY, Lin M. Molecular basis of the Kell-null phenotype: a mutation at the splice site of human KEL gene abolishes the expression of Kell blood group antigens. J Biol Chem 2001;276: 10247–10252.
96. Bertelson CJ, Pogo AO, Chaudhuri A, et al. Localization of the McLeod locus *(XK)* within Xp21 by deletion analysis. Am J Hum Genet 1988; 42:703–711.
97. Marsh WL, Redman CM. Recent developments in the Kell blood group system. Transf Med Rev 1987;1:4–20.
98. Øyen R, Reid ME, Rubinstein P, Ralph H. A method to detect McLeod phenotype red blood cells. Immunohematology 1996;12:160–163.
99. Allen FH, Krabbe SMR, Corcoran PA. A new phenotype (McLeod) in the Kell blood group system. Vox Sang 1961;6:555–560.
100. Danek A, Rubio JP, Rampoldi L, et al. McLeod neuroacanthocytosis: genotype and phenotype. Ann Neurol 2001;50:755–764.
101. Oyen R, Powell VI, Reid ME, et al. The first non-CGD McLeod phenotype male to make anti-Kx: definition of the molecular basis (abstract). Transfusion 1999;39(Suppl 1):90S.
102. Lee S, Wu X, Son S, et al. Point mutations characterize *KEL10*, the *KEL3*, *KEL4*, and *KEL21* alleles, and the *KEL17* and *KEL11* alleles. Transfusion 1996;36:490–494.
103. Lee S, Wu X, Reid ME, Zelinski T, Redman C. Molecular basis of the Kell (K1) phenotype. Blood 1995;85:912–916.
104. Lee S, Wu X, Reid ME, Redman C. Molecular basis of the K:6,-7 [Js(a+b−)] phenotype in the Kell blood group system. Transfusion 1995;35:822–825.
105. Branch DR, Muensch HA, Sy Siok Hian AL, Petz LD. Disulfide bonds are a requirement for Kell and Cartwright (Yt^a) blood group antigen integrity. Br J Haematol 1983;54:573–578.
106. Yazdanbakhsh K, Lee S, Yu Q, Reid ME. Identification of a defect in the intracellular trafficking of a Kell blood group variant. Blood 1999;94:310–318.
107. Allen FH Jr, Lewis SJ, Fudenberg H. Studies of anti-Kp^b, a new antibody in the Kell blood group system. Vox Sang 1958;3:1–13.
108. Allen FH, Lewis SJ. Kp^a (Penney), a new antigen in the Kell blood group system. Vox Sang 1957;2:81–87.
109. Øyen R, Halverson GR, Reid ME. Review: Conditions causing weak expression of Kell system antigens. Immunohematology 1997;13:75–79.
110. Anstee DJ. Blood group-active surface molecules of the human red blood cell. Vox Sang 1990;58:1–20.
111. Vaughan JI, Warwick R, Letsky E, et al. Erythropoietic suppression in fetal anemia because of Kell alloimmunization. AJOG 1994;171:247–252.
112. Redman CM, Lee S, ten Huinink D, et al. Comparison of human and chimpanzee Kell blood group systems. Transfusion 1989;29:486–490.
113. Blancher A, Reid ME, Socha WW. Cross-reactivity of antibodies to human and primate red cell antigens. Transf Med Rev 2000;14:161–179.
114. Jaber A, Loirat MJ, Willem C, et al. Characterization of murine monoclonal antibodies directed against the Kell blood group glycoprotein. Br J Haematol 1991;79:311–315.
115. Xu D, Emoto N, Giaid A, et al. ECE-1: A membrane-bound metalloprotease that catalyzes the proteolytic activation of big endothelin-1. Cell 1994;78:473–485.
116. Lee S, Lin M, Mele A, et al. Proteolytic processing of big endothelin-3 by the Kell blood group protein. Blood 1999;94:1440–1450.
117. Cutbush M, Mollison PI, Parkin DM. A new human blood group. Nature 1950;165:188.
118. Ikin EW, Mourant AE, Pettenkofer HJ, Blumenthal G. Discovery of the expected haemagglutinin anti-Fy^b. Nature 1951;168:1077–1078.
119. Miller LH, Mason SJ, Dvorak JA, et al. Erythrocyte receptors for *(Plasmodium knowlesi)* malaria: Duffy blood group determinants. Science 1975;189:561–563.
120. Neote K, Mak JY, Kolakowski LF Jr, Schall TJ. Functional and biochemical analysis of the cloned Duffy antigen: identity with the red blood cell chemokine receptor. Blood 1994;84:44–52.

121. Chaudhuri A, Zbrzezna V, Johnson C, et al. Purification and characterization of an erythrocyte membrane protein complex carrying Duffy blood group antigenicity. Possible receptor for *Plasmodium vivax* and *Plasmodium knowlesi* malaria parasite. J Biol Chem 1989; 264:13770–13774.
122. Horuk R, Colby TJ, Darbonne WC, et al. The human erythrocyte inflammatory peptide (chemokine) receptor. Biochemical characterization, solubilization, and development of a binding assay for the soluble receptor. Biochemistry 1993;32:5733–5738.
123. Chaudhuri A, Polyakova J, Zbrzezna V, et al. Cloning of glycoprotein D cDNA, which encodes the major subunit of the Duffy blood group system and the receptor for the *Plasmodium vivax* malaria parasite. Proc Natl Acad Sci USA 1993;90:10793–10797.
124. Mathew S, Chaudhuri A, Murty VV, Pogo AO. Confirmation of Duffy blood group antigen locus (FY) at 1q22→23 by fluorescence in situ hybridization. Cytogenet Cell Genet 1994;67:68.
125. Iwamoto S, Li J, Omi T, et al. Identification of a novel exon and spliced form of Duffy mRNA that is the predominant transcript in both erythroid and postcapillary venule endothelium. Blood 1996;87:378–385.
126. Iwamoto S, Omi T, Kajii E, Ikemoto S. Genomic organization of the glycophorin D gene: Duffy blood group Fy^a/Fy^b alloantigen system is associated with a polymorphism at the 44-amino acid residue. Blood 1995;85:622–626.
127. Hadley TJ, Peiper SC. From malaria to chemokine receptor: the emerging physiologic role of the Duffy blood group antigen. Blood 1997;89:3077–3091.
128. Parasol N, Reid M, Rios M, et al. A novel mutation in the coding sequence of the FY*B allele of the Duffy chemokine receptor gene is associated with an altered erythrocyte phenotype. Blood 1998;92:2237–2243.
129. Olsson ML, Smythe JS, Hansson C, et al. The Fy^x phenotype is associated with a missense mutation in the Fy^b allele predicting Arg89Cys in the Duffy glycoprotein. Br J Haematol 1998;103:1184–1191.
130. Tournamille C, Le Van Kim C, Gane P, et al. Arg89Cys substitution results in very low membrane expression of the Duffy antigen/receptor for chemokines in Fy^x individuals (erratum in 95:2753). Blood 1998;92:2147–2156.
131. Yazdanbakhsh K, Øyen R, Yu Q, et al. High level, stable expression of blood group antigens in a heterologous system. Am J Hematol 2000;63:114–124.
132. Lu ZH, Wang ZX, Horuk R, et al. The promiscuous chemokine binding profile of the Duffy antigen/receptor for chemokines is primarily localized to sequences in the amino-terminal domain. J Biol Chem 1995;270:26239–26245.
133. Wasniowska K, Blanchard D, Janvier D, et al. Identification of the Fy6 epitope recognized by two monoclonal antibodies in the N-terminal extracellular portion of the Duffy antigen receptor for chemokines. Mol Immunol 1996;33:917–923.
134. Tournamille C, Colin Y, Cartron JP, Le Van Kim C. Disruption of a GATA motif in the *Duffy* gene promoter abolishes erythroid gene expression in Duffy-negative individuals. Nature Genet 1995;10:224–228.
135. Iwamoto S, Li J, Sugimoto N, et al. Characterization of the Duffy gene promoter: evidence for tissue-specific abolishment of expression in Fy(a−b−) of black individuals. Biochem Biophys Res Commun 1996; 222:852–859.
136. Le Pennec PY, Rouger P, Klein MT, et al. Study of anti-Fy^a in five black Fy(a−b−) patients. Vox Sang 1987;52:246–249.
137. Zimmerman PA, Woolley I, Masinde GL, et al. Emergence of *FY* A*-null in a *Plasmodium vivax*-endemic region of Papua New Guinea. Proc Natl Acad Sci USA 1999;96:13973–13977.
138. Mallinson G, Soo KS, Schall TJ, et al. Mutations in the erythrocyte chemokine receptor (Duffy) gene: The molecular basis of the Fy^a/Fy^b antigens and identification of a deletion in the Duffy gene of an apparently healthy individual with the Fy(a−b−) phenotype. Br J Haematol 1995;90:823–829.
139. Rios M, Chaudhuri A, Mallinson G, et al. New genotypes in Fy(a−b−) individuals: Nonsense mutations (Trp to stop) in the coding sequence of either *FY A* or *FY B*. Br J Haematol 2000;108:448–454.
140. Masouredis SP, Sudora E, Mahan L, Victoria EJ. Quantitative immunoferritin microscopy of Fy^a, Fy^b, Jk^a, U, and Di^b antigen site numbers on human red cells. Blood 1980;56:969–977.
141. Hadley TJ, Lu ZH, Wasniowska K, et al. Postcapillary venule endothelial cells in kidney express a multispecific chemokine receptor that is structurally and functionally identical to the erythroid isoform, which is the Duffy blood group antigen. J Clin Invest 1994;94:985–991.
142. Peiper SC, Wang ZX, Neote K, et al. The Duffy antigen/receptor for chemokines (DARC) is expressed in endothelial cells of Duffy negative individuals who lack the erythrocyte receptor. J Exp Med 1995;181:1311–1317.
143. Chaudhuri A, Nielsen S, Elkjaer ML, et al. Detection of Duffy antigen in the plasma membranes and caveolae of vascular endothelial and epithelial cells of nonerythroid organs. Blood 1997;89:701–712.
144. Horuk R, Martin A, Hesselgesser J, et al. The Duffy antigen receptor for chemokines: Structural analysis and expression in the brain. J Leukocyte Biol 1996;59:29–38.
145. Horuk R, Martin AW, Wang Z, et al. Expression of chemokine receptors by subsets of neurons in the central nervous system. J Immunol 1997;158:2882–2890.
146. Li J, Iwamoto S, Sugimoto N, et al. Dinucleotide repeat in the 3 flanking region provides a clue to the molecular evolution of the Duffy gene. Hum Genet 1997;99:573–577.
147. Chaudhuri A, Polyakova J, Zbrzezna V, Pogo O. The coding sequence of Duffy blood group gene in humans and simians: restriction fragment length polymorphism, antibody and malarial parasite specificities, and expression in nonerythroid tissues in Duffy-negative individuals. Blood 1995;85:615–621.
148. Luster AD. Chemokines—Chemotactic cytokines that mediate inflammation. NEJM 1998;338:436–445.
149. Tilg H, Shapiro L, Atkins MB, et al. Induction of circulating and erythrocyte-bound IL-8 by IL-2 immunotherapy and suppression of its *in vitro* production by IL-1 receptor antagonist and soluble tumor necrosis factor receptor (p75) chimera. J Immunol 1993;151: 3299–3307.
150. de Winter RJ, Manten A, de Jong YP, et al. Interleukin 8 released after acute myocardial infarction is mainly bound to erythrocytes. Heart 1997;78:598–602.
151. Danoff TM, Hallows KR, Burns JE, et al. Influence of the Duffy blood group on renal allograft survival in African-Americans (abstract). J Amer Soc Nephrology 1998;9:670A.
152. Liu X-H, Hadley TJ, Xu L, et al. Up-regulation of Duffy antigen receptor expression in children with renal disease. Kidney Int 1999;55:1491–1500.
153. Allen FH, Diamond LK, Niedziela B. A new blood-group antigen. Nature 1951;167:482.
154. Plaut G, Ikin EW, Mourant AE, et al. A new blood-group antibody, anti-Jk^b. Nature 1953;171:431.
155. Rousselet G, Ripoche P, Bailly P. Tandem sequence repeats in urea transporters: identification of an urea transporter signature sequence. Am J Physiol 1996;270:F554–F555.
156. Olivès B, Neau P, Bailly P, et al. Cloning and functional expression of a urea transporter from human bone marrow cells. J Biol Chem 1994;269:31649–31652.
157. Geitvik GA, Hoyheim B, Gedde-Dahl T, et al. The Kidd (*JK*) blood group locus assigned to chromosome 18 by close linkage to a DNA-RFLP. Hum Genet 1987;77:205–209.
158. Leppert M, Ferrell R, Kambok MI, et al. Linkage of the polymorphic protein markers *F13B, CIS, CIR* and blood group antigen Kidd in CEPH reference families (abstract). Cytogenet Cell Genet 1987;46:647.
159. Lucien N, Sidoux-Walter F, Olivès B, et al. Characterization of the gene encoding the human Kidd blood group/urea transporter protein: Evidence for splice site mutations in Jk_{null} individuals. J Biol Chem 1998;273:12973–12980.
160. Olivès B, Merriman M, Bailly P, et al. The molecular basis of the Kidd blood group polymorphism and its lack of association with type 1 diabetes susceptibility. Hum Mol Genet 1997;6:1017–1020.
161. Irshaid NM, Henry SM, Olsson ML. Genomic characterization of the Kidd blood group gene: different molecular basis of the Jk(a−b−) phenotype in Polynesians and Finns. Transfusion 2000;40:69–74.
162. Yates J, Howell P, Overfield J, et al. IgG anti-Jk^a/Jk^b antibodies are unlikely to fix complement. Transf Med 1998;8:133–140.
163. Pinkerton FJ, Mermod LE, Liles BA, Jack JA, Noades J. The phenotype Jk(a−b−) in the Kidd blood group system. Vox Sang 1959;4:155–160.
164. Heaton DC, McLoughlin K. Jk(a−b−) red blood cells resist urea lysis. Transfusion 1982;22:70–71.
165. Macey RI, Yousef LW. Osmotic stability of red cells in renal circulation requires rapid urea transport. Am J Physiol 1988;254:C669–C674.
166. Martial S, Olivès B, Abrami L, et al. Functional differentiation of the human red blood cell and kidney urea transporters. Am J Physiol Renal Fluid Electrolyte Physiol 1996;271:F1264–F1268.
167. Sands JM, Gargus JJ, Frohlich O, et al. Urinary concentrating ability in patients with Jk(a−b−) blood type who lack carrier-mediated urea transport. J Amer Soc Nephrol 1992;2:1689–1696.

Chapter 8

Other Blood Group Antigens and Antibodies

Marion E. Reid • Connie M. Westhoff

This chapter provides information for the 16 blood group systems not covered in Chapters 6 and 7. The systems are discussed here in the order of their International Society of Blood Transfusion (ISBT) numbers (see Table 5–3). Antibodies to antigens in these systems are less common than those described in the preceding chapters, and information regarding their general clinical significance, when known, is summarized in Tables 5–5 and 5–6. The red blood cell (RBC) membrane components carrying the antigens of the systems described in this chapter are depicted in Figure 8–1. The antigens of the Chido-Rodgers system are adsorbed onto the RBC and are not integral membrane components; thus, they are not included in Figure 8–1.

THE MNS SYSTEM (ISBT SYSTEM 002)

History

The MNS system, discovered in 1927, was the second blood group system to be recognized. The first two antigens, M and N, were named from the second and fifth letters of the word *immune*, because the corresponding antibodies were produced through immunization of rabbits with human RBCs, and it was thought that the first letter, I, might be confused with the number 1.[1,2] The S antigen, the next to be identified, was named from the city (Sydney) where the first anti-S was discovered.[3] When the antithetical antigen was identified, the logical name s was used. The name for the high-incidence antigen U was derived from the "almost *universal* distribution of the new blood factor."[4] Many of the other antigens were named after the original family in which an antigen-positive neonate suffered from hemolytic disease of the newborn (HDN).

Gene, Protein, and Antigens

MNS antigens are carried on glycophorin A (GPA) and GPB, which are encoded by homologous genes (*GYPA* and *GYPB*, respectively) on chromosome 4q28–q31.[5] *GYPA* has seven exons, and *GYPB* has five exons and one pseudo-exon. A third homologous gene, *GYPE*, completes this glycophorin gene family, but it is not clear whether the product of *GYPE* is expressed on the RBC membrane. The glycophorin gene cluster encompasses approximately 330 kb in the following order: *GYPA*, *GYPB*, *GYPE*.[6]

Glycophorin A and GPB are single-pass membrane sialoglycoproteins oriented with their N termini to the exterior of the RBC. GPA has 15 potential sites for O-glycans, one N-glycan, and an approximate M_r of 43,000 on sodium dodecyl sulfate polyacrylamide gel electrophoresis (SDS-PAGE); there are approximately 1million copies of GPA per RBC. GPB has 11 potential sites for O-glycans, no N-glycan, an approximate M_r of 25,000 on SDS-PAGE, and there are approximately 200,000 copies per RBC.[7,8]

M and N antigens are carried on alternative forms of GPA and are the result of amino acid substitutions at residues 1 and 5. The M antigen has Ser at position 1 and Gly at position 5, whereas the N antigen has Leu at position 1 and Glu at position 5. The first 26 amino acids of the N form of GPA are identical to those of GPB. Anti-N reagents prepared for use in the clinical setting are formulated to detect the N antigen on GPA but not the N on GPB (N).[9–13] Using these reagents, human RBCs type as M+N−, M−N+, or M+N+.

S and s antigens are carried on alternative forms of GPB. At amino acid residue 29, Met is critical for the S antigen and Thr for the s antigen. Both antigens also involve the amino acids at residues 25, 28, 34, and 35.[14] Persons who are S−s−, usually blacks, may be negative for the high-incidence antigen U owing to a deletion of or an altered form of *GYPB*.[15–17] Because M/N and S/s are on homologous proteins that are encoded by adjacent genes, they are inherited en bloc, accounting for linkage dysequilibrium between the antigens (Table 8–1).

The MNS blood group system is highly polymorphic, with 43 antigens.[7] Many of the antigens are uncommon, resulting from an amino acid substitution or multiple rearrangements between *GYPA* and *GYPB* (Table 8–2).[7,15] Low-incidence antigens in the MNS blood group system are as follows, in alphabetical order: Cl^a, DANE, Dantu, ERIK, Far, HAG, He, Hil, Hop, Hut, MARS, M^e, M^g, Mi^a, MINY, Mit, Mt^a, Mur, MUT, M^v, Nob, Ny^a, Or, Os^a, Ri^a, s^D, SAT, St^a, TSEN, Vr, Vw.[7] The rare null phenotypes of this system—En(a−), which lacks MN antigens; U−, which lacks S_s−antigens; and M^k M^k, which lacks both MN and Ss antigens—most often result from gene deletions.[7,18] Some antigens that are associated with the MNS system but are not numbered by the ISBT Working Party on Terminology for Red Cell Surface Antigens are a consequence of altered glycosylation at residues 2, 3, and 4 of GPA. They include Tm, Sj, M_1, Can, Sext, and Hu.[19]

Antibodies

Anti-M and anti-N antibodies are usually cold-reactive, clinically insignificant antibodies that are naturally occurring; that is, present in persons who have not been previously transfused

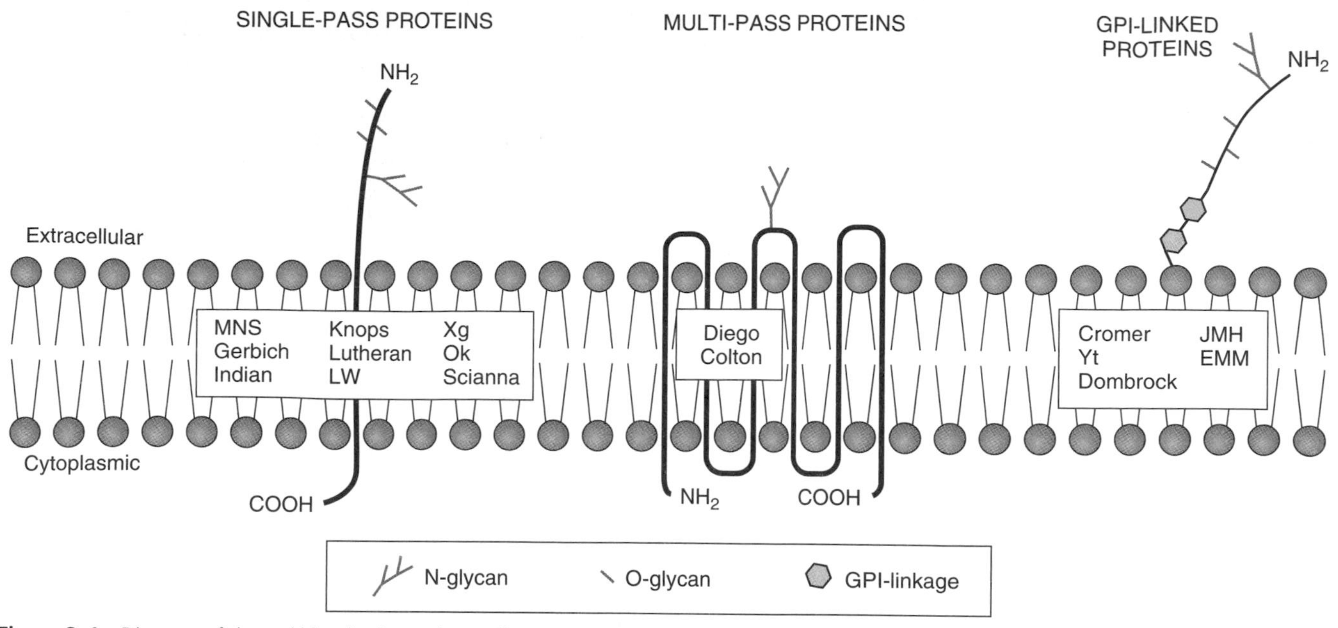

Figure 8–1 Diagram of the red blood cell membrane illustrates the type of membrane components that carry the blood group antigens described herein. The figure does not show components carrying Chido/Rodgers antigens, because they are not integral membrane components, or most of the components carrying the blood group collections, and high- and low-incidence antigens, because their structure is unknown.

Table 8–1 Incidence of Various MNS Phenotypes

	Percentage	
Phenotype	**Whites**	**Blacks**
M+N–S+s–	6	2
M+N–S+s+	14	7
M+N–S–s+	10	16
M+N+S+s–	4	2
M+N+S+s+	22	13
M+N+S–s+	23	33
M–N+S+s–	1	2
M–N+S+s+	6	5
M–N+S–s+	15	19
M+N–S–s–	0	0.4
M+N+S–s–	0	0.4
M–N+S–s–	0	0.7

or pregnant. Anti-M can be immunoglobulin M (IgM) or IgG (mostly cold-reactive), but anti-N are mostly IgM and rarely IgG. Reactivity of anti-M is often enhanced by acidification of the serum, whereas anti-N are more specific at alkaline pH. Technical problems with these antibodies can usually be avoided if the test is performed strictly at 37°C.

Anti-M is more common than anti-N. Anti-M is common in antenatal patients (even when the fetus is M-negative); however, there are few reports of potent IgG anti-M that is active at 37°C and causes HDN. If a rare example of anti-M, reactive at 37°C, is identified, the patient should be transfused with M-negative blood as a precaution. Anti-N is not known to cause hemolytic transfusion reactions or HDN; therefore, selection of N-negative blood for transfusion of patients with the antibody is not necessary. It should be noted, however, that rare examples of anti-N, which are compatible only with N–U–RBCs, may be clinically significant.[20]

In contrast, antibodies to S, s, and U usually occur after stimulation and are capable of causing hemolytic transfusion reactions and HDN.[21] Antigen-negative blood should be selected for transfusion of persons with these antibodies. Most anti-S and anti-s are IgG antibodies shown to be reactive on the indirect antiglobulin test (IAT). However, IgM anti-S exist and are more common than IgM anti-s. Anti-U is IgG, reacts on the IAT, and can cause severe transfusion reactions or severe HDN.

Human sera often contain antibodies against one or more of the MNS system antigens, particularly antibodies directed at the low-incidence antigens, but the source of the stimulation is usually unknown.[21] These antibody specificities are often not separable by absorption or elution, and they recognize amino acid sequences common to more than one antigenic determinant. Antibodies to low-incidence antigens in the MNS system may be IgG or IgM. The corresponding antigens are well-developed on RBCs from newborn babies, and the antibodies may cause HDN. Almost all random donors are compatible, and there is no difficulty in finding blood for transfusion.

Anti-En^a is an umbrella term for immune antibodies that react with high-incidence determinants along GPA. The reactivity of anti-En^a in serologic tests using protease-treated RBCs depends on the location of the specific antigen on GPA. En^a antibodies are usually IgG, react on the IAT, and may cause transfusion reactions or HDN.[7,20] It is difficult, if not impossible, to find compatible donor blood for patients with these antibodies. Siblings of such patients should be tested for compatibility, and patients should be urged to donate blood for long-term cryogenic storage when their clinical state permits.

Expression

Antigens in the MNS system are expressed on RBCs from newborns. GPA and GPB are expressed in renal endothelium and epithelium.[22,23] Expression of GPA and GPB in erythroid

Table 8–2 Hybrid Glycophorin Molecules, Phenotype Symbol, and Associated Low-Incidence Antigens

Molecular Basis	Glycophorin	Phenotype Symbol	Associated Novel Antigens
GYP(A-B)	GP(A-B)	(GP.MEP(En[a–]UK) GP.Hil(Mi.V) GP.JL(Mi.XI) GP.TK	None known Hil, MINY TSEN, MINY SAT
GYP(B-A)	GP(B-A)	GP.Sch(M^r) GP.Dantu	St^a Dantu
GYP(A-ψB-A)	GP(A-B-A)	GP.Vw(Mi.I) GP.Hut(Mi.II) GP.Nob(Mi.VII) GP.Joh(Mi.VIII) GP.Dane(Mi.IX)	Vw Hut, MUT Nob Nob, Hop Mur, DANE
*GYP(A-ψB-A)**	Gp(A-A)	GP.Zan(M^z)	St^a
GYP(A-ψB-A-B)	Gp(B-A-B)	GP.Mur(Mi.III) GP.Bun(Mi.VI) GP.HF(Mi.X) GP.Hop(Mi.IV)	Mur, MUT, Hil, MINY Mur, MUT, Hop, Hil, MINY MUT, Hil, MINY Mur, MUT, Hop, TSEN, MINY
GYPA nucleotide substitution	GPA (t1) GP(A-A) (t2)	GP.EBH GP.EBH	ERIK St^a

*Genes that result in more than 1 transcript (t).

tissues occurs early in erythroid differentiation, but the associated antigens are detectable only later in erythroid development.[8,24]

Evolution

Glycophorin A and the MN antigens are found on RBCs of all anthropoid apes (chimpanzee, gorillas, orangutan, and gibbon) and Old World monkeys, but GPB has been found only in humans and the anthropoid apes. Only humans have S and s antigens. The glycophorin gene duplication that generated GPA and GPB is not present in gibbons or orangutans and probably occurred in a common ancestor of anthropoid apes.[25]

Function

Glycophorin A (also known as *membrane inhibitor of reactive lysis type II*, MIRL II) may function as a complement regulator[26] and is a receptor for bacteria, viruses, and *Plasmodium falciparum* malaria parasites.[9,27,28] It is a chaperone for band 3 transport to the RBC membrane and is the major component contributing to the negatively charged RBC glycocalyx,[8,29] which may contribute antiadhesion properties.[30–32] As single-pass membrane proteins, the glycophorins have been considered candidate mediators of transmembrane signaling in RBCs.[33] Rare GPA and GPB null phenotypes—En(a−), U−, and M^{k}M^k—have RBCs that survive normally; people with these rare phenotypes have no apparent health defects.[8]

THE LUTHERAN SYSTEM (ISBT SYSTEM 005)

History

Anti-Lu^a was first found in 1946 in the serum of a patient who had received multiple transfusions, and it agglutinated 8% of random samples.[34] The system should have been named *Lutteran*, after the name of the donor of the Lu(a+) RBCs; however, the handwritten label on the blood sample from the original donor was misread.

Gene, Protein, and Antigens

Lutheran (LU), along with *Secretor*, provided the first example of autosomal linkage in humans, the first example of autosomal crossing over, and the first indication that crossing over in humans is more common in females than in males.[35,36]

The *LU* gene, located on chromosome 19q13.2–q13.3, consists of 15 exons distributed over approximately 12 kb of DNA. *LU* encodes the Lutheran (Lu) glycoprotein and a spliced form of the glycoprotein, basal cell adhesion molecule (B-CAM). Lu glycoprotein passes through the RBC membrane once with the N terminus oriented to the extracellular surface, and the cytoplasmic region of Lutheran glycoprotein interacts with the membrane cytoskeleton.[37] The protein is predicted to have five disulfide-bonded, extracellular, Ig superfamily (IgSF) domains (two variable-region and three constant-region sets).[38] The Lu glycoprotein has five sites for N-glycans and is O-glycosylated and has an approximate M_r of 85,000 on SDS-PAGE; there are 1500 to 4000 copies per RBC.[39,40] The minor isoform (B-CAM) has an approximate M_r of 78,000, because it lacks the cytoplasmic tail and has an increased expression on epithelial cancer cells.[38,41]

The Lutheran system consists of four pairs of antigens (Lu^a/Lu^b, Lu6/Lu9, Lu8/Lu14, Au^a/Au^b) and 10 independent antigens. The Lu^a antigen is present in 5% of blacks and 8% of whites, and the antithetical antigen, Lu^b, is present in more than 99% of random blood samples.[7] Only Lu9 and Lu14 are low-incidence antigens; the others are either polymorphic (Lu^a, Au^a, and Au^b) or of high incidence (Lu^b, Lu3, Lu4, Lu5, Lu6, Lu7, Lu8, Lu11, Lu12, Lu13, Lu16, Lu17, and Lu20). The molecular basis of Lu^a/Lu^b is His77Arg, and that of Au^a/Au^b is Thr539Ala.[42,43]

The Lu^a and Lu^b antigens, and most of the other Lutheran antigens, are resistant to treatment by papain, ficin, sialidase, and low concentrations (50 mM) of dithiothreitol (DTT), and are sensitive to treatment by trypsin and α-chymotrypsin.[7]

Lutheran-null phenotypes have three genetic backgrounds: homozygozity for a recessive gene mutation *Lu*, a dominant suppressor gene *In(Lu)* (inhibitor of Lutheran), and an X-linked recessive gene *XS*[44] (Table 8–3). Only the autosomal recessive Lu(a−b−) is a true null phenotype;

Table 8–3 Characteristics of Lu(a–b–) Phenotypes

Lu(a–b–) Phenotype	Lutheran Antigens	Make Anti-Lu3	CD44	CDw75	I/i Antigen
Recessive	Absent	Yes	Normal	Normal	Normal/normal
Dominant	Weak	No	Weak (25%–39% of normal)	Strong	Normal/weak
X-linked	Weak	No	Normal	Absent	Weak/strong

weak expression of Lutheran antigens are found on RBCs of the two other types. The original Lu(a–b–) phenotype was discovered by the proposita herself when her own RBCs were not agglutinated by anti-Lu^a or anti-Lu^b.[44] Later, it was shown that these RBCs had weak expression of Lutheran antigens and that the phenotype was inherited in a dominant manner and unlinked to *LU*.[44] The presence of an inhibitor gene, *In(Lu)*,[45] was proposed. *In(Lu)* is also associated with reduced expression of CD44,[46,47] and weak expression of P_1, AnWj, In^b, i, and MER2 blood group antigens.[48]

Antibodies

Antibodies in this system are rarely encountered because the antigens are not highly immunogenic (see Table 5–5).[21] Anti-Lu^a are usually IgG and reactive on the IAT, but they may be IgM and may directly agglutinate Lu(a+) RBCs, giving characteristic stringy agglutinates surrounded by unagglutinated RBCs. Anti-Lu^a has not been implicated in transfusion reactions and has rarely caused mild HDN. Anti-Au^a and anti-Au^b are rare, usually found in sera that contain other antibodies. They are IgG, react on the IAT, and can cause mild transfusion reactions, but neither has caused HDN.

Several Lutheran antibodies are directed at antigens of high incidence; the one most frequently encountered is anti-Lu^b. Anti-Lu^b are IgG and react by the IAT but can occasionally be IgM. Anti-Lu^b can cause mild transfusion reactions and has rarely caused mild HDN. Lu(b–) blood should be used for transfusion, but only about 1 in 500 donors are Lu(b–). Anti-Lu3 is found only in the serum of immunized people of the rare recessive Lu(a–b–) phenotype. The antibody is usually IgG, is reactive on the IAT, and may cause a delayed transfusion reaction or HDN. Blood with the Lu(a–b–) phenotype should be used for transfusion of patients with these antibodies.

Antibodies to other high-incidence Lutheran antigens, usually weak IgG antibodies, have not been reported to cause HDN. With the exception of one example of anti-Lu6, which was shown to destroy transfused Lu6 RBCs, these specificities have not caused transfusion reactions. If a patient has formed a Lutheran antibody directed at a high-incidence antigen, it is important to test for compatible siblings and encourage the patient to donate blood for long-term storage when clinical status permits. Anti-Lu9 and anti-Lu14 define low-incidence antigens that have not been reported to cause transfusion reactions or HDN.[7] Most randomly collected blood is antigen negative and compatible.

Expression

Lutheran antigens are expressed weakly on cord RBCs. The antigens are present in various tissues, including brain, heart, kidney, liver, lung, pancreas, placenta, and skeletal muscle.[38]

Lutheran glycoprotein is expressed late during erythroid differentiation and may play a role in mediating erythroblast–extracellular matrix interactions in the marrow and reticulocyte release into the circulation.[33]

Function

Lutheran blood group protein and B-CAM bind laminin, a major component of basement membranes.[49] The cytoplasmic domain interacts with the erythroid skeleton through spectrin binding,[37,50] and the nature of the extracellular and cytoplasmic domains suggests receptor and signal transduction functions. On RBCs, Lutheran glycoprotein may be involved in the adherence of RBCs to vascular endothelial cells and in the vaso-occlusion that is characteristic of sickle cell disease.[51] RBCs from patients with sickle cell disease express approximately 1½ times more Lutheran glycoprotein than do normal RBCs, and have a proportional increase in binding to laminin.[52] Lutheran is phosphorylated in sickle cells, and phosphorylation has been shown to regulate the adhesion to laminin.[53] Although the function of the Lutheran glycoprotein is not fully defined, its involvement in cell-to-cell and cell-to-substrate adhesion is probable.

DIEGO SYSTEM (ISBT SYSTEM 010)

History

The Diego blood group system was named after the producer of the first example of anti-Di^a. The antibody, which had caused HDN in a Venezuelan baby, was reported in detail in 1955. Anti-Di^b was described in 1967, and for many years, the system consisted of two antithetical antigens, Di^a and Di^b.[20] The finding that Di^a and Di^b are carried on band 3, the anion exchanger (AE1),[54,55] was the beginning of the expansion of the Diego system. In 1995, Bruce and colleagues[55,56] located the Wr^a and Wr^b antigens on band 3. Since then, many low-incidence antigens have been assigned to this system, which now consists of 18 antigens.[57–59]

Gene, Protein, and Antigens

The gene encoding band 3 and the Diego antigens, *SLC4A1* (solute carrier family 4, anion exchanger member 1; *DI*; *AE1*; *EPB-3*), consists of 20 exons distributed over 18 kb of DNA and is located on chromosome 17q12–q21.[60,61] There are more than 1 million copies of band 3 in the RBC membrane, making it the most abundant integral RBC protein. The glycoprotein passes through the RBC membrane multiple times and has both the N terminus and the C terminus oriented to the cytoplasm. Band 3 has one large N-glycan, on the fourth extracellular loop, with repeating lactosaminyl groups that accounts for the broad banding pattern of approximate M_r 95,000 to 105,000 on SDS-PAGE. The N-glycan of band 3 carries over half of the red cell A, B, H, I, and i blood group activity.[62]

The Di^a/Di^b polymorphism is located on the last extracellular loop and is defined by Pro854 (Di^b) or Leu854 (Di^a).[55] The Di^a antigen is rare in most populations but is polymorphic in people of Mongoloid ancestry. The incidence in South American Indians may be as high as 54%, and 10% to 12% of Native Americans are Di(a+).[63] The incidence of Di^b is generally greater than 99.9%; however, the incidence of Di^b among Native Americans is reduced to 96% and is likely to be lower in those populations with a high incidence of Di^a. The Wr^a/Wr^b polymorphism is located on the fourth extracellular loop, close to the insertion into the RBC membrane, and is defined by Lys658 (Wr^b) or Glu658 (Wr^a); however, for expression, the Wr^b antigen also requires the presence of normal GPA.[56,64,65]

The other antigens in the Diego system—Wd^a, Rb^a, WARR, ELO, Wu, Bp^a, Mo^a, Hg^a, Vg^a, Sw^a, BOW, NFLD, Jn^a, and KREP[57]—are of low incidence and are each associated with a single point mutation.[58,59] The antigens are resistant to treatment of RBCs by proteolytic enzymes, sialidase, DTT, chloroquine, and acid.[7]

Antibodies

Diego antibodies are usually IgG that react on the IAT and do not bind complement. These antibodies have caused transfusion reactions (usually delayed) and HDN.[7,66]

Expression

Diego antigens are expressed on RBCs of newborns. Band 3, in addition to its presence on RBCs, is present in the intercalated cells of the distal and collecting tubules of the kidney and on granulocytes.[62]

Evolution

A variant form of band 3, Memphis I (56Glu), has a faster migration on SDS-PAGE than the more common form (56Lys). Evidence suggests that the primordial gene encodes 56Glu and that 56Lys is the result of a more recent mutation.[67]

Function

Band 3 is the major anion $HCO_3^-Cl^-$ exchanger in RBC membrane. This function is critical for RBC CO_2 uptake from the tissues and release of CO_2 in the lungs. In addition, band 3 has an important structural role in the RBC membrane through the interaction of its N-terminal domain with ankyrin, band 4.2, and band 4.1 in the membrane skeleton.[61,62] An altered form of band 3, with a deletion of amino acid residues 400 through 408, is present in ovalocytes of Southeast Asian people and causes the RBCs to be rigid.[68–70] Numerous mutations exist in the predicted cytoplasmic or transmembrane domains of band 3 and give rise to hereditary spherocytosis, congenital acanthocytosis, and distal renal tubular acidosis.[59,71]

Yt BLOOD GROUP SYSTEM (ISBT SYSTEM 011)

History

The Yt system was named in 1956,[72] the last letter of the antibody producer's name, Cartwright, being used because the other letters of the name were already in use. The logic was that if all the other letters had been used, "Why not t?," or "Why t?" (Yt) (M. Pickles, personal communication, 1999).

Gene, Protein, and Antigens

ACHE encodes acetylcholinesterase (AChE), a glycosylphosphatidylinositol-linked (GPI-linked) glycoprotein that exists as a dimer in the RBC membrane.[73] The gene is located on chromosome 7q22 and consists of six exons.[7,74,75] Alternative splicing results in different domains at the C terminus of AChE. AChE glycoprotein has N-glycans and O-glycans and an approximate M_r of 160,000 (72,000 monomer) on SDS-PAGE; there are 10,000 copies per RBC.[7,73]

Yt^a and Yt^b antigens are antithetical and a consequence of an amino acid substitution on AChE, His353Asn (originally numbered 322).[76] Yt^a occurs with an incidence of more than 99% in random blood samples. Yt^b has an incidence of 8% in most populations, but of 20% or higher in Israelis.[77]

The antigens are sensitive to treatment of RBCs by papain, ficin, α-chymotrypsin, and DTT but resistant to treatment by trypsin, sialidase, chloroquine, and acid.[7]

Antibodies

Yt antibodies usually are IgG, are reactive on IAT, and do not bind complement. These antibodies have caused delayed transfusion reactions but not HDN.

Expression

Acetylcholinesterase is expressed on hematopoietic and innervated tissue (including brain and muscle).[78,79] The antigens are expressed weakly on RBCs of newborns and are absent from RBCs of people with paroxysmal nocturnal hemoglobinuria (PNH) III.[80]

Evolution

A form of AChE has been found in the electric fish *Torpedo californica.*[81]

Function

Acetylcholinesterase is a well-characterized enzyme that hydrolyzes acetylcholine and is an essential component of cholinergic neurotransmission.[78] The role of AChE in RBCs is unknown,[82] but the molecule is enzymatically active.[73]

Xg BLOOD GROUP SYSTEM (ISBT SYSTEM 012)

History

Anti-Xg^a, discovered in 1962, detects an antigen encoded by a locus on the X chromosome. The "X" was used because of the association with the X chromosome, and the g stood for Grand Rapids, Michigan, the home of the male patient who had received multiple transfusions and who made the first anti-Xg^a.[83] Xg^a has been useful in linkage studies involving the X chromosome and in sex chromosome aneuploidy, in which an abnormal number of X chromosomes occurs.[63]

Gene, Protein, and Antigens

The gene encoding Xg^a^ is located at Xp22.32; it is not subject to X inactivation due to the expression of a duplicate gene, *MIC2,* located telomeric and in the pseudoautosomal region of the X chromosome. The first three of the ten exons of *XG* are in the pseudoautosomal region of the X chromosome; exons 4 through 10 are X-specific; hence the alternative name *PBDX* (pseudoautosomal boundary divided on X) for *XG.*[84]

The Xg glycoprotein passes through the membrane once with the amino terminus to the outside of the RBC. N-glycans are not present, but there are 16 potential sites for O-glycans, and the protein has numerous proline residues. On SDS-PAGE, Xg has a M_r of 22,000 to 29,000, and there are approximately 9000 copies per RBC.[7] The difference between Xg(a+) and Xg(a−) is the level of Xg^a antigen on the RBC, rather than a different gene product.[33,85] Xg glycoprotein has 48% identity with the CD99 glycoprotein.[84] Because an altered form of CD99 in a person with alloanti-CD99 has been described, the ISBT Working Party assigned CD99 the number XG2 (012.002).[86]

The incidence of Xg^a differs in males (65.6%) and females (88.7%), and there is a phenotypic association between the expression of Xg^a and CD99 (formerly known as 12E7 antigen) (Table 8–4). The Xg^a antigen is sensitive to treatment of RBCs by proteolytic enzymes but resistant to treatment by sialidase and DTT.[7]

Antibodies

Anti-Xg^a is usually IgG that is reactive on the IAT and may bind complement. Some anti-Xg^a are apparently naturally occurring. These antibodies have not caused transfusion reactions or HDN.[7]

Expression

The antigen is expressed weakly on RBCs of newborns. Xg is expressed on fibroblasts as well as on fetal liver, spleen, thymus, and adrenal glands and on adult bone marrow.[84]

Evolution

Xg^a is on the RBCs of some gibbons *(Hylobates lar).* RBCs of other great apes, various monkeys (including baboons), mice, and dogs are Xg(a−).[63]

Function

The role of the protein carrying Xg^a in RBCs is unknown, but it is thought to be important in hematopoietic cell differentiation. Xg is homologous with CD99.[87] CD99 has been implicated in cell-to-cell adhesion events,[85,88] activates a caspase-independent apoptosis pathway in T cells,[89] and is expressed on human RBCs, all leukocyte lineages, and all other human tissue tested.

Table 8–4 Phenotype Relationship of Xg^a and 12E7[CD99] Antigens

Sex	Xg^a	CD99 Expression
Male	Positive	High
	Negative	High or low
Female	Positive	High
	Weak positive	High
	Negative	Low

SCIANNA BLOOD GROUP SYSTEM (ISBT SYSTEM 013)

History

The Scianna system was named after the first antibody producer. The first example of anti-Sc1 (initially called anti-Sm) was reported in 1962. The antithetical antigen, Sc2, was originally called Bu^a.[63] In 1974 the relationship of these antigens was recognized and they were renamed Scianna.[90]

Gene, Protein, and Antigens

Scianna is the last of the blood group systems carried on a membrane protein to be elucidated. The gene encoding Sc antigens was known to be located on chromosome 1p36.2–p22.1, but only recently was it shown that the antigens are expressed by the red cell adhesion protein, erythrocyte membrane-associated protein (ERMAP).[91,92] The ERMAP glycoprotein has at least one N-glycan, one or more disulfide bonds, and an approximate M_r of 60,000 to 68,000 on SDS-PAGE.[93] The glycoprotein is predicted to have one extracellular transmembrane immunoglobulin-like domain.

The high-incidence antigen Sc1 (incidence ≈99.9%) is antithetical to the low-incidence antigen Sc2 (1%). Sc1, Sc2, and the high-incidence antigen Sc3 are lacking on RBCs of the very rare null phenotype Sc:−1,−2,−3. The low frequency antigen Rd (Radin) is also carried on the ERMAP protein and is part of the Scianna blood group system.[92] The antigens are resistant to treatment of RBCs by papain, ficin, trypsin, α-chymotrypsin, sialidase, acid, and 50 mM of DTT, but sensitive to treatment of RBCs with 200 mM of DTT.[7]

Antibodies

Scianna antibodies are usually IgG reactive on the IAT, and some bind complement. These antibodies have not caused transfusion reactions, but have caused a positive direct antiglobulin test (DAT) requiring transfusion support in a newborn.[94] Several examples of autoanti-Sc1 have been reported, some reactive in tests using patient serum but not plasma. Autoanti-Sc3-like antibodies have been described in one patient with lymphoma and in one patient with Hodgkin's disease whose RBCs had suppressed Sc antigens.[7]

Expression

The Sc antigens are erythrocyte specific and are expressed on RBCs of newborns.[94] ERMAP is expressed throughout erythropoiesis.[91]

Function

The function of ERMAP is not known. In addition to an extracellular transmembrane immunoglobulin-like domain, the intracellular region has multiple kinase-dependent phosphorylation consensus motifs, suggesting it may be a receptor/signal transduction molecule.[95] Individuals with the Sc:−1,−2 null phenotype appear to be healthy.

DOMBROCK BLOOD GROUP SYSTEM (ISBT SYSTEM 014)

History

The first antibody of the Dombrock system, anti-Do^a, was identified in 1965 in the serum of Mrs. Dombrock. Anti-Do^b was found in 1973. In 1995, it was realized that the Gregory-negative phenotype was the null of the Dombrock system.[96]

Gene, Protein, and Antigens

The Dombrock antigens are carried on a mono-ADP-ribosyltransferase (ART4), encoded by the *DO* gene.[97] The gene, located at chromosome 12p13.2–p12.1,[98] is composed of three exons distributed over 14 kb.[97,99,100]

The glycoprotein has an approximate M_r of 47,000 to 58,000 on SDS-PAGE and is attached to the RBC membrane via a GPI anchor.[80] The number of copies per RBC is not known.

The incidence of each Dombrock phenotype and the association of Gregory (Gy^a), Holley (Hy), and Joseph (Jo^a) phenotypes with Do^a and Do^b are summarized in Table 8–5. Although three nucleotide substitutions are associated with the various *DO* alleles, the amino acid substitutions associated with expression of the antigens are as follows: Do^a/Do^b, Asn265Asp;[97] Hy+/Hy–, Gly108Val; and Jo(a+)/Jo(a–), Thr117Ile.[101] The Gy(a–) phenotype arises from different molecular backgrounds—donor and acceptor splice site mutations, nonsense mutation, and deletion of eight nucleotides.[102–104] The antigens are resistant to treatment of RBCs by ficin, papain, sialidase, 50 mM of DTT, and acid, weakened by treatment with α-chymotrypsin, and sensitive to treatment by trypsin and 200 mM of DTT.[7]

Antibodies

Do^a and Do^b antigens are poor immunogens, and anti-Do^a and anti-Do^b are rarely found as single specificities. In contrast, Gy^a is immunogenic. Antibodies in the Do system are usually IgG reactive on the IAT and do not bind complement. These antibodies have caused delayed transfusion reactions and a positive DAT result, but no clinical HDN. Anti-Do^a and anti-Do^b are notorious for disappearing in vivo.[66]

Expression

The Dombrock antigens are expressed on RBCs of newborns. They are absent from PNH III RBCs.[80]

Function

The function of Dombrock glycoprotein is not known. Although the enzyme ART4 acts as a regulator of protein function through post-translational modification by addition of adenosine diphosphate (ADP)-ribose to a target molecule, the Dombrock glycoprotein has not been shown to have enzymatic activity.[33]

COLTON BLOOD GROUP SYSTEM (ISBT SYSTEM 015)

History

The Colton system, named after the first producer of anti-Co^a, was reported in 1967. The association of this blood group system with a 28-kDa integral membrane protein (CHIP-28) led to the discovery of the first water channel protein.

Gene, Protein, and Antigens

The Colton blood group antigens are carried on the water transport protein, known as *channel-forming integral protein* (CHIP-1) or *aquaporin 1* (AQP-1).[105] The gene (*AQP1* or *CO*) encoding the Colton glycoprotein is on chromosome 7q14 and comprises four exons distributed over 17 kb.

The glycoprotein passes through the RBC membrane multiple times, has cytoplasmic N and C termini, and is N-glycosylated. The N-glycan carries A, B, H, I, and i blood group activity. On SDS-PAGE, the Colton glycoprotein has an approximate M_r of 28,000 in the unglycosylated form and 40,000 to 60,000 in the glycosylated form.[105] There are 120,000 to 160,000 molecules of AQP-1 arranged in tetramers on the RBC membrane.[7]

The Colton blood group system consists of three antigens: Co^a, Co^b, and Co3. Co^a has an incidence of 99.9%, its antithetical antigen Co^b has an incidence of 10%, and Co3 is present on all RBCs except those of the very rare null phenotype Co(a–b–). Only four Co(a–b–) propositi are reported, all of which were found because of the presence of anti-Co3 in their sera. The Co(a–b–) phenotype arises from various molecular backgrounds, including exon deletion, missense mutations, and a single nucleotide insertion.[106–108]

The amino acid substitution responsible for the Co^a/Co^b polymorphism is on the first extracellular loop of AQP-1 and results from an Ala45Val substitution.[109] The antigens are resistant to treatment of RBCs by proteases, sialidase, DTT, and acid.[7]

Antibodies

Antibodies in the Co system are usually IgG reactive on the IAT, and some bind complement. The antibodies have caused delayed transfusion reactions and HDN.[66]

Table 8–5 Dombrock Phenotypes and Their Incidences (in Percentage)

Phenotype	Do^a	Do^b	Gy^a	Hy	Jo^a	Whites	Blacks
Do(a+b–)	+	0	+	+	+	18	11
Do(a+b+)	+	+	+	+	+	49	44
Do(a–b+)	0	+	+	+	+	33	45
Gy(a–)	0	0	0	0	0	Rare	0
Hy–	0	Weak	Weak	0	0	0	Rare
Jo(a–)	Weak	0/Weak	+	Weak	0	0	Rare

Expression

The Co antigens are expressed on RBCs of newborns. AQP-1 is strongly expressed in the kidney on the apical surface of proximal tubules, the basolateral membrane subpopulation of collecting ducts in the cortex, and the descending tubules in the medulla, as well as on liver bile ducts, gallbladder, brain, lung, eye epithelium, cornea, lens, choroid plexus, hepatobiliary epithelia, and capillary endothelium.[105,110]

Evolution

AQP-1 is a member of a large family of proteins that are involved in water transport and are found in all domains of life.[111]

Function

The function of AQP-1 is to transport water, and it accounts for 80% of water reabsorption in kidneys. Defective urine-concentrating ability[112] and decreased pulmonary vascular permeability[113] are seen with complete AQP-1 deficiency. The function of AQP-1 in RBCs may be to rehydrate rapidly after shrinking in the hypertonic environment of the renal medulla.[114] Apparently healthy propositi with the Co(a−b−) phenotype and AQP-1 deficiency have RBCs with an 80% reduction in the ability to transport water.[96] The residual water transport in these RBCs may be through another member of the water channel protein family, AQP-3, which transports water, glycerol, and urea[115] and carries the blood group antigen GIL.[116]

LW BLOOD GROUP SYSTEM (ISBT SYSTEM 016)

History

In 1940, Landsteiner and Wiener[117] produced an antibody by injecting rabbits and guinea pigs with RBCs from rhesus monkeys; they named the antibody Rh after rhesus monkey. A few years later, it was shown that the animal anti-Rh were different from the human Rh antibody (i.e., anti-D); thus, the animal anti-Rh was renamed anti-LW in honor of Landsteiner and Wiener.

The historical terminology LW_1, LW_2, LW_3, and LW_4 to describe phenotypes was changed when the antithetical relationship of the antigen defined by anti-Ne^a (now called anti-LW^b) and that defined by anti-LW made by LW_3 people (now called anti-LW^a) was recognized.[7,118]

Gene, Protein, and Antigens

The LW glycoprotein, also called *intracellular adhesion molecule 4* (ICAM-4), is a member of the IgSF.[119] The gene *(LW)* encoding the LW glycoprotein consists of three exons distributed over 2.65 kb of DNA on chromosome 19.

The LW glycoprotein passes through the RBC membrane once, and the N-terminal extracellular region is organized into two IgSF domains.[119] LW glycoprotein has an approximate M_r of 37,000 to 43,000 on SDS-PAGE, has three pairs of cysteine residues and four potential N-glycan sites, and is O-glycosylated.

LW^a is a common antigen, whereas LW^b has an incidence of less than 1% in most Europeans (but is found in 6% of Finns and in 8% of Estonians). RBCs with the Rh-null phenotype lack LW antigens and type LW(a−b−). The LW^{ab} antigen was originally defined by the alloantibody made by the only genetically LW(a−b−) person. There is a phenotypic relationship between LW and the D antigen of the Rh system; D-positive RBCs have stronger expression of LW antigen than D-negative RBCs, and the expression of LW is stronger on cord RBCs than on RBCs from adults.[120]

The LW^a/LW^b polymorphism is due to the amino acid substitution Gln70Arg.[121] LW antigens require intramolecular disulfide bonds and the presence of divalent cations, notably Mg^{2+}, for expression.[122] The antigens are resistant to treatment of RBCs by ficin, papain, trypsin, α-chymotrypsin (but may be weakened), sialidase, and acid; they are sensitive to treatment of RBCs by pronase and DTT. These features are helpful in the differentiation of anti-LW from anti-D, because the D antigen is resistant to pronase and DTT treatment.[7]

The LW gene of the only genetic LW(a−b−) person has a 10-deletion and a premature stop codon in the first exon.[123]

Transient loss of LW antigens from the RBC has been described in pregnancy and in patients with diseases, particularly Hodgkin's disease, lymphoma, leukemia, sarcoma, and other forms of malignancy. Such loss of LW antigens is usually associated with the production of LW antibodies.[124]

Antibodies

Antibodies in the LW system are IgM and IgG that are reactive at room temperature or on the IAT and do not bind complement. They have occasionally caused mild delayed transfusion reactions and mild HDN. Autoanti-LW are common in patients with transient depression of LW antigens and can appear to be alloantibodies.[66]

Expression

The LW antigens are expressed on RBCs of newborns in equal amounts regardless of D type. In contrast, D-positive RBCs of adults express more LW than D-negative RBCs. LW glycoprotein appears early in erythropoiesis, before GPA.

Evolution

LW antigen has been detected on RBCs of all primate species tested, including chimpanzee, gorilla, orangutan, and a variety of monkey species.

Function

LW glycoprotein has homology to ICAMs, and interacts with integrins LFA1 (CD11/CD18),[125] α4β1, and αV[126] and also binds platelet-specific integrin, αIIbβ3.[127] The significance of these observations is not yet known, but LW glycoprotein may function in erythroblast–macrophage interactions in erythroblastic islands.[128] The proband and her brother who have the rare inherited LW-null phenotype do not have an apparent hematologic defect.

CHIDO-RODGERS BLOOD GROUP SYSTEM (ISBT SYSTEM 017)

History

Antigens in the Chido-Rodgers system were named after the first antibody producers, Ch for *Ch*ido and Rg for *R*od*g*ers.

Anti-Ch was first described in 1967, and when anti-Rg was reported in 1976, there were obvious similarities between them. Although the Ch and Rg antigens are readily detected on RBCs and were given blood group system status, later work revealed that Ch and Rg antigens are located on the fourth component of complement (C4), which becomes bound to RBCs from the plasma.

Gene, Protein, and Antigens

In complement activation through the classical pathway, C4 becomes bound to the RBC membrane and undergoes further cleavage; ultimately, a tryptic fragment, C4d, remains on the RBC. This C4d glycoprotein carries the Chido-Rodgers blood group antigens. Electrophoresis identified the following two isoforms of C4: C4B, the slower-migrating molecule, expresses Ch antigens, and C4A, the faster molecule, expresses Rg antigens.[129] C4A and C4B are not the products of alleles, but are encoded by genes at two very closely linked loci located at chromosome 6p21.3. Silent alleles are relatively common at each locus. *C4A* and *C4B* have been cloned, and each consists of 41 exons and is 22 kb long, although a shorter form of *C4B* exists. C4A and C4B glycoproteins are 99% identical in their amino acid sequences.

The Chido-Rodgers blood group system contains nine antigens. Some or all of the antigens may be expressed by a particular phenotype. Ch1 to Ch6, Rg1, and Rg2 have frequencies greater than 90%. The WH antigen has an incidence of about 15%. The various antigens are associated with amino acid differences in eight residues.[130,131] The antigens are stable in stored serum or plasma, and the phenotypes of this system are most accurately defined in plasma by hemagglutination inhibition tests.[7]

The antigens are sensitive to treatment of RBCs by proteases and resistant to treatment by sialidase, DTT, and acid. RBCs coated with C4 (+C3) through the use of low-ionic strength 10% sucrose solution give enhanced reactivity with anti-Ch and anti-Rg; this feature has been used to aid identification of antibodies.[7]

Antibodies

Antibodies in the Chido-Rodgers system are usually IgG reacting by the IAT, do not activate complement, and are considered benign and nebulous. There can be considerable variation in the reaction strength obtained with different RBC samples. Although these antibodies do not generally cause transfusion reactions, they have caused anaphylactic reactions.[132] The antibodies have not caused HDN. Anti-Ch and anti-Rg are neutralized in the test tube or in the circulation by plasma from Ch-positive and Rg-positive persons, respectively.

Expression

Chido-Rodgers antigens are absent or weakly expressed on RBCs of newborns. They are weakly expressed on RBCs of some people with the dominant Lu(a−b−) phenotype and on GPA-deficient (i.e., sialidase-deficient) RBCs. Indeed, it is not possible to coat sialidase-deficient RBCs with C4 in vitro through the 10% sucrose technique.[133]

Function

C4A binds preferentially to proteins and C4B to carbohydrates. C4B binds more effectively to the RBC surface (through sialic acid) and thus is more effective at promoting hemolysis. A single amino acid substitution, Asp1106His, converts the functional activity of C4B to C4A, whereas Cys1102Ser affects hemolytic activity and IgG binding.[134]

Inherited low levels of C4 may be a predisposing factor for diseases such as insulin-dependent diabetes and autoimmune chronic active hepatitis. Specific C4 allotypes and null genes have been associated with numerous autoimmune disorders, including Graves' disease and rheumatoid arthritis. Lack of C4B (Ch−) bestows greater susceptibility to bacterial meningitis on children. Lack of C4A (Rg−) results in a predisposition for systemic lupus erythematosus (SLE).[134]

GERBICH BLOOD GROUP SYSTEM (ISBT SYSTEM 020)

History

The Gerbich system was named in 1960 after Mrs. Gerbich, the first antibody producer.

Gene, Protein, and Antigens

The three high-incidence antigens (Ge2, Ge3, and Ge4) and four low-incidence antigens (Wb, Ls^a, An^a, and Dh^a) of the Gerbich blood group system are carried on GPC, GPD, or both. The two glycoproteins are products of the *GYPC* gene.[135] The gene, located at chromosome 2q14–q21, consists of four exons. The smaller GPD polypeptide is generated by the use of alternative translation initiation sites. On SDS-PAGE, GPC has an approximate M_r of 40,000; it has one N-glycan and 13 sites for O-glycans. GPD has an approximate M_r of 30,000, no N-glycan, and 8 sites for O-glycans. There are approximately 135,000 copies of GPC and 50,000 copies of GPD per RBC. GPC and GPD pass through the RBC membrane once with their N terminus oriented to the outside of the membrane.

Ge2 is located on the N terminus of GPD, Ge3 is located between amino acid residues 40 and 50 on GPC and between residues 19 and 28 on GPD, and Ge4 is located at the N terminus of GPC. Of the four low-incidence antigens, three (Wb, An^a, Dh^a) are the result of an amino acid substitution, and one (Ls^a) is created by a novel amino acid sequence derived from a duplication of exon 3 and encoded by nucleotides at the exon 3 to exon 3 junction.[135]

Except in Papua New Guinea, Gerbich-negative RBCs are seldom found. The three Gerbich-negative phenotypes are as follows: Ge:−2,3,4 (the Yus phenotype), Ge:−2,−3,4 (the Gerbich phenotype), and Ge:−2,−3,−4 (the Leach phenotype). The Leach phenotype is the null of the Gerbich system. The PL type (the original propositus) arises from a deletion of exons 3 and 4 of *GYPC*. The LN type is caused by a deletion of nucleotide 134, changing Pro45Arg of GPC, a frameshift mutation, and a premature stop codon. The Gerbich phenotype is due to a deletion of exon 3, and the Yus phenotype is due to a deletion of exon 2 of *GYPC*.[135–139] The Yus and Gerbich phenotypes have been found in diverse populations, but in the Melanesians of Papua New Guinea only the

Gerbich type has been found.[135] The Leach phenotype has been restricted to people of Northern European extraction.

Ge2 and Ge4 are sensitive to treatment of RBCs by ficin, papain, and trypsin; Ge3 is sensitive to trypsin but resistant to ficin and papain; and all antigens are resistant to treatment of RBCs with α-chymotrypsin, DTT, and acid.[7]

Antibodies

The antibodies may be immune or naturally occurring. Most are IgG and are reactive on the IAT, and some of these bind complement; some antibodies may be IgM. Although some antibodies have caused delayed transfusion reactions, others have been benign. Clinical HDN due to these antibodies has not been reported, but the antibodies have been eluted from cord RBCs that tested positive on DAT. Antibodies to the high-incidence Gerbich antigens are rare; the least rare specificity is anti-Ge2, which can be produced by any of the three Gerbich-negative phenotypes. Clinically significant auto-anti-Ge have been reported. Because Ge-negative donors are rare, it is important to test siblings of Ge-negative patients for compatibility, and to urge such patients to donate blood for long-term storage.[66]

Antibodies to low-incidence antigens in the Ge blood group system are rare, and RBCs from almost all random donors are compatible; there is no difficulty in finding blood for transfusion of patients with these antibodies. One brief report implicated anti-Ls^a in HDN,[140] but there are no reports of HDN due to anti-Wb, anti-An^a, or anti-Dh^a.

Expression

Ge antigens are expressed on RBCs of newborns. Gerbich antigens are weak on protein 4.1-deficient RBCs because the membranes of such cells have reduced levels of GPC and GPD. The majority of RBC samples with Leach or Gerbich phenotypes have a weak expression of Kell blood group system antigens. GPC and GPD are expressed on erythroblasts and fetal liver and in several nonerythroid tissues, including kidney, brain cerebellum, and ileum.[7]

Function

Glycophorin C and GPD are possibly involved in RBC membrane integrity via interaction with protein 4.1. Both glycophorins are markedly reduced in protein 4.1-deficient RBCs.[141]

CROMER BLOOD GROUP SYSTEM (ISBT SYSTEM 021)

History

The Cromer system was named after the first antibody producer, Mrs. Cromer. When the antibody was first identified in 1965, it was believed to be anti-Go^b; later, however, it was recognized as a new specificity, and in 1975, it was renamed anti-Cr^a.

Gene, Protein, and Antigens

Blood group antigens in the Cromer system are carried on the complement regulatory protein, decay accelerating factor (DAF, CD55). The *DAF* gene, located at chromosome 1q32, is one of a group of genes known as the regulators of complement activation (RCA) cluster. The gene spans approximately 40 kb and comprises 11 exons.[142] The DAF glycoprotein is arranged into four extracellular short consensus repeat domains, each with about 60 amino acid residues, and is attached to the RBC membrane through GPI linkage. On SDS-PAGE, DAF has an approximate M_r of 64,000 to 73,000 (reduced) and 60,000 to 70,000 (nonreduced). One N-glycan and 15 O-glycans are present on each glycoprotein, and there are 20,000 copies of DAF per RBC.[143]

Cromer is a system of 11 antigens with two sets of antithetical antigens, Tc^a/Tc^b/Tc^c and WES^a/ WES^b. Eight of the antigens (Cr^a, Tc^a, Dr^a, Es^a, IFC, WES^b, UMC, and GUTI) are of high incidence, and three (Tc^b, Tc^c , and WES^a) are of low incidence. These antigens are lacking from the Cromer null phenotype, the Inab phenotype. The amino acids required for expression of all the antigens have been determined; with the exception of Dr^a, all are due to a single amino acid change.[144,145] In the Dr(a−) phenotype, the level of expression of DAF, and therefore of all Cromer system antigens, is greatly reduced. The Cr(a−) phenotype is the least rare of the negative phenotypes, and with the exception of one Spanish-American woman, all people with Cr(a−) RBCs are black. Most of the other phenotypes are exceedingly rare.

Cromer antigens are resistant to treatment of RBCs by ficin, papain, trypsin, 50 mM of DTT, sialidase, and acid, are sensitive to α-chymotrypsin, and are weakened by 200 mM of DTT.[7]

Antibodies

Antibodies in the Cromer system are usually IgG, are reactive on the IAT, and do not bind complement. The antibodies have caused mild delayed transfusion reactions but not HDN. When a patient's antibody is directed at a high-incidence antigen, it is important to test siblings in the quest for compatible blood and to urge the patient to donate blood for long-term storage when clinical status permits.[66]

Expression

The Cromer antigens are expressed on RBCs of newborns. DAF is preferentially expressed on the apical surface of trophoblasts and may protect the conceptus from antibody-mediated hemolysis.[146] DAF is not expressed on RBCs from patients with PNH III. Dr(a−) variant RBCs express inherited Cromer antigens very weakly.

Cromer antigens are present in the plasma and urine of people with the corresponding antigen on their RBCs. This soluble form of the antigens can be used for hemagglutination inhibition tests, although the urine requires prior concentration.[147]

Function

Decay accelerating factor prevents assembly and accelerates the decay of C3 and C5 convertases, decreasing the deposition of C3 on the RBC surface and thereby reducing complement-mediated hemolysis.[143]

Five of the six known people with the Inab phenotype, the null of the system, do not have significant complement-induced lysis in vivo.[148] Protein-losing intestinal disorders have been reported to be associated with Inab, but there is not a clear disease association.[33] Dr^a is the receptor for uropathogenic *Escherichia coli*.[7]

KNOPS BLOOD GROUP SYSTEM (ISBT SYSTEM 022)

History

The antigens Kn^a, Kn^b, McC^a, Sl^a, and Yk^a had long been grouped together for serologic reasons. In 1991, the Knops blood group system was established when these antigens were shown to be on complement receptor 1 (CR1). The system was named after Mrs. Knops, the first antibody producer.

Gene, Protein, and Antigens

Knops antigens are encoded by various forms of *CR1*.[149] Like *DAF*, the *CR1* gene is located within the RCA cluster on chromosome 1q32. *CR1* has four allotypes: A, B, C, and D. The most common allotypes are A (82%) and B (18%); the other two are rare.

CR1 (CD35) is an unusual protein with 30 short consensus repeat domains. SDS-PAGE reveals the approximate M_r of the CR1 allotypes as follows: 190,000 (C allotype), 220,000 (A allotype), 250,000 (B allotype), and 280,000 (D allotype). Of 20 potential N-glycan sites, only 6 to 8 are usually occupied; there are four cysteine residues. Each RBC contains 20 to 1500 copies of CR1. The CR1 glycoprotein passes through the RBC membrane once with its N terminus toward the extracellular surface. The molecular basis of the McC^a/McC^b polymorphism is associated with a Lys1590Glu missense mutation, and the Sl^a/Vil polymorphism with an Arg1601Gly missense mutation.[150] The antigens are weakened by treatment of RBCs with ficin and papain, are sensitive to treatment by trypsin, α-chymotrypsin, and 200 mM of DTT, and are resistant to sialidase, 50 mM of DTT, and acid.[7]

With the exception of the low-incidence antigen Kn^b, the antigens in this system are fairly common and have a similar prevalence (>90%) in different populations; however, Sl^a is present on RBCs of 98% of whites but on only 60% of blacks.

Typing for Knops system antigens can be challenging because of the low level of expression on the RBCs of some people as well as the lack of potent antisera. Disease processes causing CR1 deficiency and, therefore, weak expression of Knops system antigens can lead to false-negative results. Furthermore, the low level of expression can lead to variable results in tests on different samples from the same patient.

Antibodies

Antibodies in the Knops system are usually IgG and reactive on the IAT, and they do not bind complement. The antibodies do not cause transfusion reactions or HDN; once identified, they can be ignored for clinical purposes. Identification may be complicated by the fluctuation of antigen expression on RBCs. Anti-Kn^a is the most common antibody in white persons, and anti-Sl^a is the most common in black persons.[20]

Expression

The Knops antigens are weakly expressed on RBCs of newborns, RBCs with the dominant Lu(a−b−) phenotype, and RBCs of patients with autoimmune diseases. CR1 is present on B cells, a subset of T cells, monocytes, macrophages, neutrophils, eosinophils, glomerular podocytes, and splenic follicular dendritic cells.[151]

Function

CR1 has an inhibitory effect on complement activation by both the classical and alternative pathways. CR1 binds C3b and C4b, thereby mediating phagocytosis by neutrophils and monocytes. RBC CR1 is important in the processing of immune complexes, binding them for transport to the liver and spleen for removal from the circulation. The presence of CR1 on other blood cells and tissues suggests that it has multiple functions.[149] The CR1 copy number per RBC (and thus antigen strength) is reduced in SLE, cold agglutinin disease, PNH, hemolytic anemia, insulin-dependent diabetes mellitus, acquired immunodeficiency syndrome, some malignant tumors, and any condition associated with increased clearance of immune complexes.

CR1, and the Sl^a antigen in particular, may act as a receptor for the malarial parasite *Plasmodium falciparum*, and thus, the Sl(a−) phenotype may provide selective advantage.[152]

INDIAN BLOOD GROUP SYSTEM (ISBT SYSTEM 023)

History

The In^a antigen, reported in 1973, is on RBCs from 4% of Indians from Bombay. This blood group system was named because of its association with India.

Gene, Protein, and Antigens

In^a and In^b, the antigens of the Indian system, are carried on CD44 (synonyms: In(Lu)-related p80; HUTCH-1; H-CAM; GP90(HERMES), Pgp-1; ECRMIII; Ly-24; p85).[153] The *CD44* gene is located at chromosome 11p13 and consists of at least 19 exons, 10 of which are variably spliced. The CD44 glycoprotein passes through the RBC membrane once, and the extracellular N terminus has six cysteine residues, six N-glycan sites, four chondroitin sulfate sites, and potential sites for O-glycans. There are 2000 to 5000 copies of CD44 per RBC. SDS-PAGE shows that CD44 has an approximate M_r of 80,000 when reduced. The In^a/In^b polymorphism is due to Pro46Arg on CD44.[154] In^b is a common antigen, and In^a is rare in white persons but has an incidence of 4% in Indians, 10% in Iranians, and nearly 12% in Arabs. The antigens are sensitive to treatment of RBCs by proteases and DTT but resistant to treatment with sialidase and acid.[7]

The In(a−b−) phenotype was described in a patient with a novel form of congenital dyserythropoietic anemia (CDA) and CD44 deficiency,[155] but it was not possible to ascertain whether the phenotype was genetically determined or related to the patient's hematologic disorder. The RBCs of the patient also typed AnWj− and Co(a−b−) and had a reduced level of LW^{ab} expression.

Antibodies

Antibodies in the Indian system are usually IgG and reactive on the IAT, and they do not bind complement. Some antibodies may directly agglutinate RBCs, but the reactivity is greatly enhanced by the IAT. These antibodies have caused decreased RBC survival and a positive DAT result in the neonate but not HDN. A severe, delayed, hemolytic transfusion reaction due to anti-In^b has been reported.[156]

Expression

Indian antigens are weakly expressed on cord RBCs as well as on RBCs from people with the dominant Lu(a−b−) phenotype and from pregnant women. CD44 is expressed on neutrophils, lymphocytes, monocytes, brain, breast, colon epithelium, gastric tissue, heart, kidney, liver, lung, placenta, skin, spleen, thymus, and fibroblasts.

Joint fluid from patients with inflammatory synovitis has higher than normal levels of soluble CD44.[155] The serum CD44 value is elevated in some patients with lymphoma.

Function

CD44 has a diverse range of biologic functions involving cell–cell and cell–matrix interactions in cells other than RBCs.[153] It is an adhesion molecule in lymphocytes, monocytes, and some tumor cells. CD44 binds to hyaluronate and other components of the extracellular matrix and is also involved in immune stimulation as well as signaling between cells.[157]

OK BLOOD GROUP SYSTEM (ISBT SYSTEM 024)

History

Anti-Ok^a was first identified in 1979 in the serum of a Japanese woman (Mrs. Okbutso) who had received a transfusion, and was therefore named after her. After the identification of the gene encoding the Ok protein, the Ok^a antigen attained system status in 1999.[57]

Gene, Protein, and Antigens

The Ok^a blood group antigen is carried on CD147 and is encoded by the *OK* gene at 19pter-p13.2. CD147 (also known as *extracellular matrix metalloproteinase inducer* [EMMPRIN]), M6, OX-47, CE9, basigin, gp42, neurothelin, HT7, 5A11) is an N-glycosylated glycoprotein that passes through the RBC membrane once with its N terminus to the extracellular surface. It is also a member of the IgSF. On SDS-PAGE, CD147 is shown to have an approximate M_r of 35,000 to 69,000. The Ok^a polymorphism is due to an amino acid substitution at residue 92 [Glu for Ok(a+) and Lys for Ok(a−)].[158,159] Ok^a is resistant to treatment of RBCs by proteases, sialidase, DTT, and acid.[7] The eight known Ok(a−) probands are Japanese.

Antibodies

The original example of anti-Ok^a is IgG and is reactive on the IAT; it does not bind complement. This antibody caused reduced cell survival but not HDN. Only one other example of human anti-Ok^a is known.

Expression

The Ok^a antigen on RBCs is well-developed at birth. CD147 has a broad expression pattern in both hematopoietic and nonhematopoietic tissues and is upregulated on activated lymphocytes and monocytes.[160,161]

Evolution

The Ok^a antigen is on RBCs from gorillas and chimpanzees but not on RBCs from rhesus monkeys, baboons, and marmosets.[158] Homologues of the Ok^a glycoprotein have been found in the rat (OX-47 or CE9), mouse (basigin), rabbit, and chicken (neurothelin or HT7).[160]

Function

Human CD147 on tumor cells is thought to bind an unknown ligand on fibroblasts, which stimulates their production of collagenase and other extracellular matrix metalloproteinases, thus enhancing tumor cell invasion and metastasis.[162] In studies with CD147 knockout mice, RBCs were apparently not compromised. CD147 may be involved in the function of the blood-brain barrier[163] and lymphocyte inactivation.[164]

RAPH BLOOD GROUP SYSTEM (ISBT SYSTEM 025)

History

A new polymorphism on RBCs was originally defined by monoclonal antibodies (1D12, 2F7) and called MER2 (M for monoclonal; ER for Eleanor Roosevelt, the name of the laboratory producing the antibodies). Later, the polymorphism was also recognized by human polyclonal antibodies, and when the MER2 antigen attained system status in 1999, the system was named RAPH after the first patient to make the specificity.

Gene, Protein, and Antigens

The MER2 antigen is encoded by a gene located on chromosome 11p15, but it has not been cloned, and the molecular basis of the antigen is not known. Ninety-two percent of English blood donors are MER2 positive, and 8% are MER2-negative. The antigen strength varies among different RBC samples. The antigen is resistant to treatment of RBCs by papain, ficin, and sialidase but sensitive to treatment by trypsin, α-chymotrypsin, and DTT.[7]

Antibodies

The three examples of human anti-MER2 (anti-RAPH) are IgG and reactive on the IAT, and two of the three antibodies bind complement. These antibodies have not caused HDN nor transfusion reactions; indeed, two siblings with the antibody have received numerous crossmatch-incompatible RBC transfusions without problems. The three antibody producers were Indian Jews.[165]

Expression

The antigen is expressed on RBCs of newborns. MER2 is expressed on fibroblasts, and its expression may be reduced on Lu(a−b−) RBCs of persons with the *In(Lu)* gene.

Function

All three people (two probands) with anti-MER2 (anti-RAPH) had renal failure requiring dialysis. It is possible that the protein carrying the MER2 antigen is required for normal kidney function.[165]

OTHER ANTIGENS

Table 5–4 lists antigens that are not included in blood group systems. Three of the blood group collections are carbohydrate antigens (Ii, GLOB, Unnamed). Antigens of the Ii and GLOB collections are discussed in Chapter 6. The other two (Cost, Er) are presumed to be protein antigens, and the antibodies to antigens in these systems are generally not clinically significant. Antigens in the 700 series of low-incidence antigens occur in less than 1% of most populations and have no known alleles. Antibodies to many of these low-incidence antigens have caused HDN.[7] Antigens in the 901 series of high-incidence antigens occur in more than 90% of people, have no known alleles, and cannot be placed in a blood group system or collection. Antibodies to Vel, Lan, At^a, Jr^a, AnWj, PEL, ABTI, and MAM can cause HDN and transfusion reactions.[7,57] Finding blood for patients with any of the antibodies to these antigens can be difficult, and the patient should be encouraged to predeposit autologous units for long-term frozen storage. JMH and EMM are carried on GPI-linked proteins, and antibodies to these antigens are of little clinical concern.

REFERENCES

1. Landsteiner K, Levine P. A new agglutinable factor differentiating human blood. Proc Soc Exp Biol Med 1927;24:600–603.
2. Levine P. A review of Landsteiner's contributions to human blood groups. Transfusion 1961;1:45–52.
3. Garratty G, Dzik WH, Issitt PD, et al. Terminology for blood group antigens and genes: historical origins and guidelines in the new millennium. Transfusion 2000;40:477–489.
4. Wiener AS, Unger LF, Gordon EG. Fatal hemolytic transfusion reaction caused by sensitization to a new blood factor U. JAMA 1953;153: 1444–1446.
5. Rahuel C, London J, d'Auriol L, et al. Characterization of cDNA clones for human glycophorin A. Use for gene localization and for analysis of normal or glycophorin-A-deficient (Finnish type) genomic DNA. Eur J Biochem 1988;172:147–153.
6. Vignal A, London J, Rahuel C, Cartron J-P. Promoter sequence and chromosomal organization of the genes encoding glycophorins A, B and E. Gene 1990;95:289–293.
7. Reid ME, Lomas-Francis C. Blood Group Antigen FactsBook, 2nd ed. San Diego, Academic Press, 2003.
8. Chasis JA, Mohandas N. Red blood cell glycophorins. Blood 1992;80: 1869–1879.
9. Dahr W. Immunochemistry of sialoglycoproteins in human red blood cell membranes. In Vengelen-Tyler V, Judd WJ (eds). Recent Advances in Blood Group Biochemistry. Arlington, Va., American Association of Blood Banks, 1986, pp 23–65.
10. Fukuda M. Molecular genetics of the glycophorin A gene cluster. Semin Hematol 1993;30:138–151.
11. Anstee DJ, Spring FA, Parsons SF, et al. Molecular background of human blood group antigens. In Hackel E, Tippett P (eds). Human Genetics 1994: A Revolution in Full Swing. Bethesda, Md., American Association of Blood Banks, 1994, pp 1–52.
12. Blanchard D. Human red cell glycophorins: biochemical and antigenic properties. Transf Med Rev 1990;4:170–186.
13. Reid ME. Some concepts relating to the molecular genetic basis of certain MNS blood group antigens. Transf Med 1994;4:99–111.
14. Dahr W, Gielen W, Beyreuther K, Krüger J. Structure of the Ss blood group antigens. I. Isolation of Ss-active glycopeptides and differentiation of the antigens by modification of methionine. Hoppe-Seylers Z Physiol Chem 1980;361:145–152.
15. Huang C-H, Blumenfeld OO. MNSs blood groups and major glycophorins: Molecular basis for allelic variation. In Cartron J-P, Rouger P (eds). Molecular Basis of Human Blood Group Antigens. New York, Plenum Press, 1995, pp 153–188.
16. Storry JR, Reid ME. Characterization of antibodies produced by S–s– individuals. Transfusion 1996;36:512–516.
17. Greenwalt TJ, Sasaki T, Sanger R, et al. An allele of the S(s) blood group genes. Proc Natl Acad Sci USA 1954;40:1126–1129.
18. Daniels G. Human Blood Groups, 2nd ed. Oxford, Blackwell Science, 2002.
19. Dahr W, Knuppertz G, Beyreuther K, et al. Studies on the structures of the Tm, Sj, M1, Can, Sext and Hu blood group antigens. Biol Chem Hoppe-Seyler 1991;372:573–584.
20. Issitt PD, Anstee DJ. Applied Blood Group Serology, 4th ed. Durham, N.C., Montgomery Scientific Publications, 1998.
21. Mollison PL, Engelfriet CP, Contreras M. Blood Transfusion in Clinical Medicine, 10th ed. Oxford, Blackwell Science, 1997.
22. Harvey J, Parsons SF, Anstee DJ, Bradley BA. Evidence for the occurrence of human erythrocyte membrane sialoglycoproteins in human kidney endothelial cells. Vox Sang 1988;55:104–108.
23. Anstee DJ, Holmes CH, Judson PA, Tanner MJA. The use of monoclonal antibodies to determine the distribution of red cell surface proteins on cells and tissues. In Agre PC, Cartron J-P (eds). Protein Blood Group Antigens of the Human Red Cell: Structure, Function, and Clinical Significance. Baltimore, Johns Hopkins University Press, 1992, pp 170–181.
24. Southcott MJG, Tanner MJ, Anstee DJ. The expression of human blood group antigens during erythropoiesis in a cell culture system. Blood 1999;93:4425–4435.
25. Blancher A, Reid ME, Socha WW. Cross-reactivity of antibodies to human and primate red cell antigens. Transf Med Rev 2000;14:161–179.
26. Tomita A, Radike EL, Parker CJ. Isolation of erythrocyte membrane inhibitor of reactive lysis type II. Identification as glycophorin A. J Immunol 1993;151:3308–3323.
27. Hadley TJ, Miller LH, Haynes JD. Recognition of red cells by malaria parasites: the role of erythrocyte-binding proteins. Transf Med Rev 1991;5:108–113.
28. Miller LH. Impact of malaria on genetic polymorphism and genetic diseases in Africans and African Americans. Proc Natl Acad Sci USA 1994;91:2415–2419.
29. Jentoft N. Why are proteins *O*-glycosylated? Trends Biochem Sci 1990;15:291–294.
30. Groves JD, Tanner MJ. The effects of glycophorin A on the expression of the human red cell anion transporter (band 3) in *Xenopus* oocytes. J Membr Biol 1994;140:81–88.
31. Groves JD, Tanner MJ. Role of N-glycosylation in the expression of human band 3-mediated anion transport. Mol Membr Biol 1994;11:31–38.
32. Groves JD, Tanner MJ. Glycophorin A facilitates the expression of human band 3-mediated anion transport in *Xenopus* oocytes. J Biol Chem 1992;267:22163–22170.
33. Reid ME, Mohandas N. Red blood cell blood group antigens: Structure and function. Semin Hematol 2004;41:93–117.
34. Callender STE, Race RR. A serological and genetical study of multiple antibodies formed in response to blood transfusion by a patient with lupus erythematosus diffusus. Ann Eugen 1946;13:102.
35. Cook PJL. The Lutheran-secretor recombination fraction in man: a possible sex-difference. Ann Hum Genet 1965;28:393–401.
36. Mohr J. A search for linkage between the Lutheran blood group and other hereditary characters. Acta Path Microbiol Scand 1951;28:80–96.
37. Parsons SF, Lee G, Spring FA, et al. Lutheran blood group glycoprotein and its newly characterized mouse homologue specifically bind α5 chain-containing human laminin with high affinity. Blood 2001;97: 312–320.
38. Parsons SF, Mallinson G, Holmes CH, et al. The Lutheran blood group glycoprotein, another member of the immunoglobulin superfamily, is widely expressed in human tissues and is developmentally regulated in human liver. Proc Natl Acad Sci USA 1995;92:5496–5500.
39. Parsons SF, Mallinson G, Judson PA, et al. Evidence that the Lu^b blood group antigen is located on red cell membrane glycoproteins of 85 and 78 kd. Transfusion 1987;27:61–63.
40. Anstee DJ. Blood group-active surface molecules of the human red blood cell. Vox Sang 1990;58:1–20.
41. Rahuel C, Kim CL, Mattei MG, et al. A unique gene encodes spliceoforms of the B-cell adhesion molecule cell surface glycoprotein of epithelial cancer and of the Lutheran blood group glycoprotein. Blood 1996;88:1865–1872.

42. El Nemer W, Rahuel C, Colin Y, et al. Organization of the human LU gene and molecular basis of the Lu[a]/Lu[b] blood group polymorphism. Blood 1997;89:4608–4616.
43. Parsons SF, Mallinson G, Daniels GL, et al. Use of domain-deletion mutants to locate Lutheran blood group antigens to each of the five immunoglobulin superfamily domains of the Lutheran glycoprotein: Elucidation of the molecular basis of the Lu[a]/Lu[b] and the Au[a]/Au[b] polymorphisms. Blood 1997;89:4219–4225.
44. Crawford MN. The Lutheran blood group system: Serology and genetics. In Pierce SR, Macpherson CR (eds). Blood Group Systems: Duffy, Kidd and Lutheran. Arlington, Va., American Association of Blood Banks, 1988, pp 93–117.
45. Taliano V, Guevin RM, Tippett P. The genetics of a dominant inhibitor of the Lutheran antigens. Vox Sang 1973;24:42–47.
46. Telen MJ, Eisenbarth GS, Haynes BF. Human erythrocyte antigens. Regulation of expression of a novel erythrocyte surface antigen by the inhibitor Lutheran In(Lu) gene. J Clin Invest 1983;71:1878–1886.
47. Spring FA, Dalchau R, Daniels GL, et al. The In[a] and In[b] blood group antigens are located on a glycoprotein of 80,000 MW (the CDw44 glycoprotein) whose expression is influenced by the *In(Lu)* gene. Immunology 1988;64:37–43.
48. Poole J. Review: The Lutheran blood group system—1991. Immunohematology 1992;8:1–8.
49. El Nemer W, Gane P, Colin Y, et al. The Lutheran blood group glycoproteins, the erythroid receptors for laminin, are adhesion molecules. J Biol Chem 1998;273:16686–16693.
50. Kroviarski Y, El NW, Gane P, et al. Direct interaction between the Lu/B-CAM adhesion glycoproteins and erythroid spectrin. Br J Haematol 2004;126:255–264.
51. Udani M, Zen Q, Cottman M, et al. Basal cell adhesion molecule Lutheran protein—The receptor critical for sickle cell adhesion to laminin. J Clin Invest 1998;101:2550–2558.
52. Hines PC, Zen Q, Burney SN, et al. Novel epinephrine and cyclic AMP-mediated activation of BCAM/Lu-dependent sickle (SS) RBC adhesion. Blood 2003;101:3281–3287.
53. Gauthier E, Rahuel C, Wautier MP, et al. Protein kinase A-dependent phosphorylation of Lutheran/basal cell adhesion molecule glycoprotein regulates cell adhesion to laminin α5. J Biol Chem 2005;280: 30055–30062.
54. Spring FA, Bruce LJ, Anstee DJ, Tanner MJ. A red cell band 3 variant with altered stilbene disulphonate binding is associated with the Diego (Di[a]) blood group antigen. Biochem J 1992;288:713–716.
55. Bruce LJ, Anstee DJ, Spring FA, Tanner MJ. Band 3 Memphis variant II. Altered stilbene disulfonate binding and the Diego (Di[a]) blood group antigen are associated with the human erythrocyte band 3 mutation Pro^{854}→Leu. J Biol Chem 1994;269:16155–16158.
56. Bruce LJ, Ring SM, Anstee DJ, et al. Changes in the blood group Wright antigens are associated with a mutation at amino acid 658 in human erythrocyte band 3: a site of interaction between band 3 and glycophorin A under certain conditions. Blood 1995;85:541–547.
57. Daniels GL, Anstee DJ, Cartron JP, et al. Terminology for red cell surface antigens Oslo report. Vox Sang 1999;77:52–57.
58. Zelinski T. Erythrocyte band 3 antigens and the Diego blood group system. Transf Med Rev 1998;12:36–45.
59. Jarolim P, Rubin HL, Zakova D, et al. Characterization of seven low incidence blood group antigens carried by erythrocyte band 3 protein. Blood 1998;92:4836–4843.
60. Zelinski T, Coghlan G, White L, Philipps S. The Diego blood group locus is located on chromosome 17q. Genomics 1993;17:665–666.
61. Tanner MJ. Molecular and cellular biology of the erythrocyte anion exchanger (AE1). Semin Hematol 1993;30:34–57.
62. Tanner MJA. The structure and function of band 3 (AE1): recent developments. Mol Membr Biol 1997;14:155–165.
63. Race RR, Sanger R. Blood Groups in Man, 6th ed. Oxford, Blackwell Scientific, 1975.
64. Blumenfeld OO, Huang C-H, Xie SS, Blancher A. The MNSs blood group system: molecular biology of glycophorins in humans and nonhuman primates. In Blancher A, Klein J, Socha WW (eds). Molecular Biology and Evolution of Blood Group and MHC Antigens in Primates. Berlin, Springer-Verlag, 1997, pp 113–146.
65. Reid ME. Contribution of MNS to the study of glycophorin A and glycophorin B. Immunohematology 1999;15:5–9.
66. Reid ME, Øyen R, Marsh WL. Summary of the clinical significance of blood group alloantibodies. Semin Hematol 2000;37:197–216.
67. Palatnik M, Simoes ML, Alves ZM, Laranjeira NS. The 60 and 63 kda proteolytic peptides of the red cell membrane band-3 protein: their prevalence in human and nonhuman primates. Hum Genet 1990;86:126–130.
68. Jarolim P, Palek J, Amato D, et al. Deletion in erythrocyte band 3 gene in malaria-resistant Southeast Asian ovalocytosis. Proc Natl Acad Sci USA 1991;88:11022–11026.
69. Tanner MJ, Bruce L, Martin PG, et al. Melanesian hereditary ovalocytes have a deletion in red cell band 3. Blood 1991;78:2785–2786.
70. Schofield AE, Reardon DM, Tanner MJ. Defective anion transport activity of the abnormal band 3 in hereditary ovalocytic red blood cells. Nature 1992;355:836–838.
71. Jarolim P, Shayakul C, Prabakaran D, et al. Autosomal dominant distal renal tubular acidosis is associated in three families with heterozygosity for the R589H mutation in the AE1 (band 3) Cl^-–HCO_3^- exchanger. J Biol Chem 1998;273:6380–6388.
72. Eaton BR, Morton JA, Pickles MM, White KE. A new antibody, anti-Yt[a], characterizing a blood group of high incidence. Br J Haematol 1956;2:333–341.
73. Spring FA, Gardner B, Anstee DJ. Evidence that the antigens of the Yt blood group system are located on human erythrocyte acetylcholinesterase. Blood 1992;80:2136–2141.
74. Coghlan G, Kaita H, Belcher E, et al. Evidence for genetic linkage between the *KEL* and *YT* blood group loci. Vox Sang 1989;57:88–89.
75. Getman DK, Eubanks JH, Camp S, et al. The human gene encoding acetylcholinesterase is located on the long arm of chromosome 7. Am J Hum Genet 1992;51:170–177.
76. Bartels CF, Zelinski T, Lockridge O. Mutation at codon 322 in the human acetylcholinesterase *(ACHE)* gene accounts for YT blood group polymorphism. Am J Hum Genet 1993;52:928–936.
77. Levene C, Bar-Shany S, Manny N, et al. The Yt blood groups in Israeli Jews, Arabs, and Druse. Transfusion 1987;27:471–474.
78. Taylor P. The cholinesterases. J Biol Chem 1991;266:4025–4028.
79. Li Y, Camp S, Rachinsky TL, et al. Gene structure of mammalian acetylcholinesterase: Alternative exons dictate tissue-specific expression. J Biol Chem 1991;266:23083–23090.
80. Telen MJ, Rosse WF, Parker CJ, et al. Evidence that several high-frequency human blood group antigens reside on phosphatidylinositol-linked erythrocyte membrane proteins. Blood 1990;75:1404–1407.
81. Sussman JL, Harel M, Frolow F, et al. Atomic structure of acetylcholinesterase from *Torpedo californica:* a prototypic acetylcholine-binding protein. Science 1991;253:872–879.
82. Lawson AA, Barr RD. Acetylcholinesterase in red blood cells. Am J Hematol 1987;26:101–111.
83. Mann JD, Cahan A, Gelb AG, et al. A sex-linked blood group. Lancet 1962;1:8–10.
84. Ellis NA, Tippett P, Petty A, et al. *PBDX* is the *XG* blood group gene. Nature Genet 1994;8:285–290.
85. Tippett P, Ellis NA. The Xg blood group system: A review. Transf Med Rev 1998;12:233–257.
86. Daniels GL, Anstee DJ, Cartron JP, et al. International Society of Blood Transfusion working party on terminology for red cell surface antigens: Vienna report. Vox Sang 2001;80:193–197.
87. Schlossman SF, Bounsell L, Gilks W, et al. CD antigens 1993. Blood 1994;83:879–880.
88. Gelin C, Aubrit F, Phalipon A, et al. The E2 antigen, a 32 kd glycoprotein involved in T-cell adhesion processes, is the MIC2 gene product. EMBO J 1989;8:3253–3259.
89. Bernard G, Breittmayer JP, de Matteis M, et al. Apoptosis of immature thymocytes mediated by E2/CD99. J Immunol 1997;158:2543–2550.
90. Lewis M, Kaita H, Chown B. Scianna blood group system. Vox Sang 1974;27:261–264.
91. Xu H, Foltz L, Sha Y, et al. Cloning and characterization of human erythroid membrane-associated protein, human ERMAP. Genomics 2001;76:2–4.
92. Wagner FF, Poole J, Flegel WA. The Scianna antigens including Rd are expressed by ERMAP. Blood 2003;101:752–757.
93. Spring FA, Herron R, Rowe G. An erythrocyte glycoprotein of apparent M_r 60,000 expresses the Sc1 and Sc2 antigens. Vox Sang 1990; 58:122–125.
94. DeMarco M, Uhl L, Fields L, et al. Hemolytic disease of the newborn due to the Scianna antibody, anti-Sc2. Transfusion 1995;35:58–60.
95. Su YY, Gordon CT, Ye TZ, et al. Human ERMAP: An erythroid adhesion/receptor transmembrane protein. Blood Cells Mol Dis 2001;27:938–949.
96. Banks JA, Hemming N, Poole J. Evidence that the Gy[a], Hy and Jo[a] antigens belong to the Dombrock blood group system. Vox Sang 1995;68:177–182.
97. Gubin AN, Njoroge JM, Wojda U, et al. Identification of the Dombrock blood group glycoprotein as a polymorphic member of the ADP-ribosyltransferase gene family. Blood 2000;96:2621–2627.
98. Eiberg H, Mohr J. Dombrock blood group (*DO*): assignment to chromosome 12p. Hum Genet 1996;98:518–521.

99. Koch-Nolte F, Haag F, Braren R, et al. Two novel human members of an emerging mammalian gene family related to mono-ADP-ribosylating bacterial toxins. Genomics 1997;39:370–376.
100. Koch-Nolte F, Haag F, Braren R, et al. Erratum (to Koch-Nolte et al. Genomics 1997;39:370–376). Genomics 1999;55:130.
101. Rios M, Hue-Roye K, Øyen R, et al. Insights into the Holley-negative and Joseph-negative phenotypes. Transfusion 2002;42:52–58.
102. Rios M, Hue-Roye K, Lee AH, et al. DNA analysis for the Dombrock polymorphism. Transfusion 2001;41:1143–1146.
103. Lucien N, Celton J-L, Le Pennec P-Y, et al. A short deletion within the blood group Dombrock locus causing a Do-null phenotype. Blood 2002;100:1063–1064.
104. Rios M, Storry JR, Hue-Roye K, et al. Two new molecular bases for the Dombrock null phenotype. Br J Haematol 2002;117:765–767.
105. Preston GM, Agre P. Isolation of the cDNA for erythrocyte integral membrane protein of 28 kilodaltons: Member of an ancient channel family. Proc Natl Acad Sci USA 1991;88:11110–11114.
106. Preston GM, Smith BL, Zeidel ML, et al. Mutations in *aquaporin-1* in phenotypically normal humans without functional CHIP water channels. Science 1994;265:1585–1587.
107. Chretien S, Catron JP. A single mutation inside the NPA motif of aquaporin-1 found in a Colton-null phenotype [letter]. Blood 1999;93:4021–4023.
108. Joshi SR, Wagner FF, Vasantha K, et al. An *AQP1* null allele in an Indian woman with Co (a−b−) phenotype and high-titer anti-Co3 associated with mild HDN. Transfusion 2001;41:1273–1278.
109. Smith BL, Preston GM, Spring FA, et al. Human red cell aquaporin CHIP. I. Molecular characterization of ABH and Colton blood group antigens. J Clin Invest 1994;94:1043–1049.
110. King LS, Agre P. Pathophysiology of the aquaporin water channels. Ann Rev Physiol 1996;58:619–648.
111. King LS, Kozono D, Agre P. From structure to disease: the evolving tale of aquaporin biology. Nat Rev Mol Cell Biol 2004;5:687–698.
112. King LS, Choi M, Fernandez PC, et al. Defective urinary-concentrating ability due to a complete deficiency of aquaporin-1. NEJM 2001;345:175–179.
113. King LS, Nielsen S, Agre P, Brown RH. Decreased pulmonary vascular permeability in aquaporin-1-null humans. Proc Natl Acad Sci USA 2002;99:1059–1063.
114. Smith BL, Baumgarten R, Nielsen S, et al. Concurrent expression of erythroid and renal aquaporin CHIP and appearance of water channel activity in perinatal rats. J Clin Invest 1993;92:2035–2041.
115. Roudier N, Verbavatz JM, Maurel C, et al. Evidence for the presence of aquaporin-3 in human red blood cells. J Biol Chem 1998;273:8407–8412.
116. Roudier N, Ripoche P, Gane P, et al. AQP3 deficiency in humans and the molecular basis of a novel blood group system, GIL. J Biol Chem 2002;277:45854–45859.
117. Landsteiner K, Wiener AS. An agglutinable factor in human blood recognized by immune sera for rhesus blood. Proc Soc Exp Biol Med 1940;43:223.
118. Sistonen P, Tippett P. A "new" allele giving further insight into the LW blood group system. Vox Sang 1982;42:252–255.
119. Bailly P, Hermand P, Callebaut I, et al. The LW blood group glycoprotein is homologous to intercellular adhesion molecules. Proc Natl Acad Sci USA 1994;91:5306–5310.
120. Mallinson G, Martin PG, Anstee DJ, et al. Identification and partial characterization of the human erythrocyte membrane component(s) that express the antigens of the LW blood-group system. Biochem J 1986;234:649–652.
121. Hermand P, Gane P, Mattei MG, et al. Molecular basis and expression of the LW^a/LW^b blood group polymorphism. Blood 1995;86:1590–1594.
122. Bloy C, Hermand P, Blanchard D, et al. Surface orientation and antigen properties of Rh and LW polypeptides of the human erythrocyte membrane. J Biol Chem 1990;265:21482–21487.
123. Hermand P, Le Pennec PY, Rouger P, et al. Characterization of the gene encoding the human LW blood group protein in LW^+ and LW^- phenotypes. Blood 1996;87:2962–2967.
124. Giles CM. The LW blood group: a review. Immunol Commun 1980;9:225–242.
125. Bailly P, Tontti E, Hermand P, et al. The red cell LW blood group protein is an intercellular adhesion molecule which binds to CD11/CD18 leukocyte integrins. Eur J Immunol 1995;25:3316–3320.
126. Spring FA, Parsons SF, Ortlepp S, et al. Intercellular adhesion molecule-4 binds $\alpha_4 b_1$ and α_V-family integrins through novel integrin-binding mechanisms. Blood 2001;98:458–466.
127. Hermand P, Gane P, Huet M, et al. Red cell ICAM-4 is a novel ligand for platelet-activated $\alpha_{IIb}\beta_3$ integrin. J Biol Chem 2003;278:4892–4898.
128. Lee G, Spring FA, Parsons SF, et al. Novel secreted isoform of adhesion molecule ICAM-4: potential regulator of membrane-associated ICAM-4 interactions. Blood 2003;101:1790–1797.
129. O'Neill GJ, Yang SY, Tegoli J, et al. Chido and Rodgers blood groups are distinct antigenic components of human complement C4. Nature 1978;273:668–670.
130. Yu CY, Campbell RD, Porter RR. A structural model for the location of the Rodgers and the Chido antigenic determinants and their correlation with the human complement component C4A/C4B isotypes. Immunogenetics 1988;27:399–405.
131. Giles CM, Jones JW. A new antigenic determinant for C4 of relatively low frequency. Immunogenetics 1987;26:392–394.
132. Westhoff CM, Sipherd BD, Wylie DE, Toalson LD. Severe anaphylactic reactions following transfusions of platelets to a patient with anti-Ch. Transfusion 1992;32:576–579.
133. Tippett P, Storry JR, Walker PS, et al. Glycophorin A-deficient red cells may have a weak expression of C4-bound Ch and Rg antigens. Immunohematology 1996;12:4–7.
134. Moulds JM. Association of blood group antigens with immunologically important proteins. In Garratty G (ed). Immunobiology of Transfusion Medicine. New York, Marcel Dekker, 1994, pp 273–297.
135. Reid ME, Spring FA. Molecular basis of glycophorin C variants and their associated blood group antigens. Transf Med 1994;4:139–149.
136. Colin Y, Rahuel C, London J, et al. Isolation of cDNA clones and complete amino acid sequence of human erythrocyte glycophorin C. J Biol Chem 1986;261:229–233.
137. Chang S, Reid ME, Conboy J, et al. Molecular characterization of erythrocyte glycophorin C variants. Blood 1991;77:644–648.
138. Telen MJ, Le Van Kim C, Chung A, et al. Molecular basis for elliptocytosis associated with glycophorin C and D deficiency in the Leach phenotype. Blood 1991;78:1603–1606.
139. Winardi R, Reid M, Conboy J, Mohandas N. Molecular analysis of glycophorin C deficiency in human erythrocytes. Blood 1993;81:2799–2803.
140. Sistonen P. Some notions on clinical significance of anti-Ls^a and independence of *Ls* from Colton, Kell, and Lewis blood group loci (abstract). XIX Congress of the International Society of Blood Transfusion 1986;652.
141. Alloisio N, Morle L, Bachir D, et al. Red cell membrane sialoglycoprotein b in homozygous and heterozygous 4.1(−) hereditary elliptocytosis. Biochim Biophys Acta 1985;816:57–62.
142. Post TW, Arce MA, Liszewski MK, et al. Structure of the gene for human complement protein decay accelerating factor. J Immunol 1990;144:740–744.
143. Lublin DM, Atkinson JP. Decay-accelerating factor: Biochemistry, molecular biology and function. Ann Rev Immunol 1989;7:35–58.
144. Telen MJ, Rao N, Udani M, et al. Molecular mapping of the cromer blood group Cr^a and Tc^a epitopes of decay accelerating factor: toward the use of recombinant antigens in immunohematology. Blood 1994;84:3205–3211.
145. Lublin DM, Kompelli S, Storry JR, Reid ME. Molecular basis of Cromer blood group antigens. Transfusion 2000;40:208–213.
146. Holmes CH, Simpson KL, Wainwright SD, et al. Preferential expression of the complement regulatory protein decay accelerating factor at the fetomaternal interface during human pregnancy. J Immunol 1990;144:3099–3105.
147. Daniels GL, Okubo Y, Yamaguchi H, et al. UMC, another Cromer-related blood group antigen. Transfusion 1989;29:794–797.
148. Telen MJ, Green AM. The Inab phenotype: Characterization of the membrane protein and complement regulatory defect. Blood 1989;74:437–441.
149. Ahearn JM, Fearon DT. Structure and function of the complement receptors, CR1 (CD35) and CR2 (CD21). Adv Immunol 1989;46:183–219.
150. Moulds JM, Zimmerman PA, Doumbo OK, et al. Molecular identification of Knops blood group polymorphisms found in long homologous region D of complement receptor 1. Blood 2001;97:2879–2885.
151. Rao N, Ferguson DJ, Lee SF, Telen MJ. Identification of human erythrocyte blood group antigens on the C3b/C4b receptor. J Immunol 1991;146:3502–3507.
152. Rowe JA, Moulds JM, Newbold CI, Miller LH. *P. falciparum* rosetting mediated by a parasite-variant erythrocyte membrane protein and complement-receptor 1. Nature 1997;388:292–295.
153. Telen MJ, Ferguson DJ. Relationship of Inb antigen to other antigens on In(Lu)-related p80. Vox Sang 1990;58:118–121.
154. Telen MJ, Udani M, Washington MK, et al. A blood group-related polymorphism of CD44 abolishes a hyaluronan-binding consensus sequence without preventing hyaluronan binding. J Biol Chem 1996;271:7147–7153.

155. Parsons SF, Jones J, Anstee DJ, et al. A novel form of congenital dyserythropoietic anemia associated with deficiency of erythroid CD44 and a unique blood group phenotype [In(a−b−), Co(a−b−)]. Blood 1994;83:860–868.
156. Joshi SR. Immediate haemolytic transfusion reaction due to anti-In^{b}. Vox Sang 1992;63:232–233.
157. Goldstein LA, Zhou DFH, Picker LJ, et al. A human lymphocyte homing receptor, the Hermes antigen, is related to cartilage proteoglycan core and link proteins. Cell 1989;56:1063–1072.
158. Williams BP, Daniels GL, et al. Biochemical and genetic analysis of the OK^{a} blood group antigen. Immunogenetics 1988;27:322–329.
159. Spring FA, Holmes CH, Simpson KL, et al. The Ok^{a} blood group antigen is a marker for the M6 leukocyte activation antigen, the human homolog of OX-47 antigen, basigin and neurothelin, an immunoglobulin superfamily molecule that is widely expressed in human cells and tissues. Eur J Immunol 1997;27:891–897.
160. Kasinrerk W, Fiebiger E, Stefanova I, et al. Human leukocyte activation antigen M6, a member of the Ig superfamily, is the species homologue of rat OX-47, mouse basigin, and chicken HT7 molecule. J Immunol 1992;149:847–854.
161. Anstee DJ, Spring FA. Red cell membrane glycoproteins with a broad tissue distribution. Transf Med Rev 1989;3:13–23.
162. Biswas C, Zhang Y, DeCastro R, et al. The human tumor cell-derived collagenase stimulatory factor (renamed EMMPRIN) is a member of the immunoglobulin superfamily. Cancer Res 1995;55:434–439.
163. Seulberger H, Unger CM, Risau W. HT7, neurothelin, basigin, gp42 and OX-47—many names for one developmentally regulated immunoglobulin-like surface glycoprotein on blood-brain barrier endothelium, epithelial tissue barriers and neurons. Neurosci Lett 1992;140:93–97.
164. Ghebrehiwet B, Lu PD, Zhang W, et al. Identification of functional domains on gC1Q-R, a cell surface protein that binds to the globular "heads" of C1Q, using monoclonal antibodies and synthetic peptides. Hybridoma 1996;15:333–342.
165. Daniels GL, Levene C, Berrebi A, et al. Human alloantibodies detecting a red cell antigen apparently identical to MER2. Vox Sang 1988;55:161–164.

Chapter 9

Human Platelet Antigens

Thomas J. Kunicki • Diane J. Nugent

INTRODUCTION

Platelet Membrane Glycoproteins

Among the variety of glycoproteins on the human platelet surface, there are several that contribute to the immunogenic makeup of the platelet (Table 9–1).

Integrins

The integrins are membrane glycoprotein heterodimers, each consisting of noncovalently associated α and β subunits.[1] The specificity of an integrin is dictated in large part by the identity of its α subunit, even though ligand binding per se may occur with a significant portion of the β subunit. These ubiquitous receptors mediate a wide range of cell adhesion events that are important to every fundamental area of human biology, including embryonal development, immunocompetence, wound healing, and hemostasis. Two platelet integrins figure prominently in the antigenic profile of platelets, the cohesion receptor $\alpha_{IIb}\beta_3$ and the collagen receptor $\alpha_2\beta_1$.

THE PLATELET COHESION RECEPTOR, INTEGRIN $\alpha_{IIb}\beta_3$

The numerically predominant platelet integrin $\alpha_{IIb}\beta_3$ (initially designated *glycoprotein [GP] IIb/IIIa*) mediates the common cohesive pathway that follows platelet activation in vivo (i.e., platelet aggregation supported by the binding of adhesive proteins, such as fibrinogen and von Willebrand factor ([vWF]). The α subunit of this integrin, α_{IIb}, is synthesized exclusively by megakaryocytes. Consequently, $\alpha_{IIb}\beta_3$ is a unique marker for platelets or cell lines with a megakaryocytic lineage. Glanzmann thrombasthenia is an inherited disorder of platelet function characterized by an inability of platelets to bind fibrinogen and undergo agonist-induced aggregation.[2] The molecular defect in this disease involves either a quantitative or a qualitative abnormality of $\alpha_{IIb}\beta_3$.

THE PLATELET COLLAGEN RECEPTOR, INTEGRIN $\alpha_2\beta_1$

Another integrin that contributes significantly to platelet function is the collagen receptor $\alpha_2\beta_1$ (GPIa/IIa). A high-affinity interaction of platelet $\alpha_2\beta_1$ with collagen anchors the platelet more firmly to the matrix, permitting the formation of an activated, procoagulant platelet monolayer.[3] Platelet adhesion in flowing blood mediated by $\alpha_2\beta_1$ is supported by several collagen types, including types I, III, IV, and VI, and the rate of platelet monolayer formation is directly proportional to platelet $\alpha_2\beta_1$ density.[4] Signal transduction is mediated by both $\alpha_2\beta_1$ and the platelet-specific collagen receptor, glycoprotein VI (GPVI) facilitating and likely accelerating platelet activation, leading to aggregate formation.[5,6]

Unlike α_{IIb}, the α_2 subunit is a single-chain molecule and, like several other integrin α subunits, contains an additional 129–amino acid segment known as the I-domain.[1] Inherited platelet deficiencies of the α_2 subunit have been described, and patients with these deficiencies exhibit chronic mucocutaneous bleeding and prolonged bleeding times.[7,8] The expression of $\alpha_2\beta_1$ on platelets differs markedly between normal subjects, depending on the inheritance of α_2 gene (*ITGA2*) haplotypes.[4]

Regulation of $\alpha_2\beta_1$ expression could certainly modulate the antigenicity of this membrane receptor. It is also possible that similar factors influence expression of other platelet integrins, including $\alpha_{IIb}\beta_3$, but the extent to which that occurs remains to be determined. Two other integrins, the fibronectin receptor $\alpha_5\beta_1$,[9] and the laminin receptor $\alpha_6\beta_1$,[10] are expressed by platelets, but neither has yet been shown to contribute significantly to platelet immunogenicity.

The Receptor Complex Glycoprotein Ib-IX-V

The functional GPIb complex is a heptamer composed of one molecule of glycoprotein V associated with two molecules each of three other gene products, glycoproteins Ibα, Ibβ, and IX [(2) Ibα:(2)Ibβ:(2)IX:(1)V].[11] With blood flow conditions ranging from low ($\leq$300 sec^{-1}) to high shear ($\geq$1500 sec^{-1}), the initial *transient* arrest of platelets on collagen requires vWF acting as a bridge between collagen and the GPIb complex.[12] The vWF binding site on the complex is located within the amino-terminal domain of glycoprotein Ibα.[13] The Bernard-Soulier syndrome (BSS) is an inherited disorder of platelet function characterized by defective platelet adhesion to subendothelium and a quantitative or qualitative defect in the GPIb complex caused by mutations in genes encoding either the GPIbα, Ibβ, or IX components.[2,14]

ALLOANTIGENS

The proliferation of serologically defined alloantigens on platelet glycoproteins has led to the development of a consensus nomenclature, in which each of the alloantigens is prefixed as human platelet antigen (HPA-).[15] These designations as well as alternate and/or original names are depicted in Table 9–2. The HPA- nomenclature does not take into consideration linkage disequilibrium between these polymorphisms.

Two clinically significant syndromes are the direct result of sensitization to platelet-specific alloantigens: neonatal alloimmune thrombocytopenia (NAIT) and post-transfusion purpura (PTP).

Table 9–1 Functional Properties of Selected Membrane Glycoprotein (GP) Complexes

GP	Alternate Names	Receptor Function	Protein Ligands
Ib-IX-V	GPIb complex	Adhesion	vWF
VI-FcγR	p62	Adhesion	Collagen
$\alpha_{IIb}\beta_3$	GPIIb/IIIa, CD41/CD61	Adhesion	Fibrinogen
		Cohesion	Fibrinogen
			Fibronectin
			Vitronectin
			vWF
$\alpha_2\beta_1$	GPIa/IIa, VLA-2, CD49b/CD29	Adhesion	Collagen
$\alpha_5\beta_1$	GPIc/IIa, VLA-5, CD49e/CD29	Adhesion	Fibronectin
$\alpha_6\beta_1$	GPIc /IIa, VLA-6, CD49f/CD29	Adhesion	Laminin

FcγR, Fc receptor γ chain; vWF, von Willebrand factor; VLA, very late activation (antigen); CD, cell differentiation (antigen).

Table 9–2 Human Platelet Alloantigens

Antigen	Synonym	Glycoprotein	Nucleotide Substitution	Amino Acid Substitution	Reference
HPA-1a	Pl^{A1}, Zw^a	Integrin β_3	T_{196}	Leu^{33}	173
HPA-1b	Pl^{A2}, Zw^b		C_{196}	Pro^{33}	
HPA-2a	Ko^b	GPIbα	C_{524}	Thr^{145}	35
HPA-2b	Ko^a, Sib^a		T_{524}	Met^{145}	
HPA-3a	Bak^a, Lek^a	Integrin α_{IIb}	T_{2622}	Ile^{843}	37
HPA-3b	Bak^b		G_{2622}	Ser^{843}	
HPA-4a	Yuk^b, Pen^a	Integrin β_3	G_{526}	Arg^{143}	174
HPA-4b	Yuk^a, Pen^b		A_{526}	Gln^{143}	
HPA-5a	Br^b, Zav^b	Integrin α_2	G_{1648}	Glu^{505}	175
HPA-5b	Br^a, Zav^a, Hc^a		A_{1648}	Lys^{505}	
HPA-6bW	Ca^a, Tu^a	Integrin β_3	A_{1564}	Gln^{489}	176
			G_{1564}	Arg^{489}	
HPA-7bW	Mo^a	Integrin β_3	G_{1317}	Ala^{407}	177
			C_{1317}	Pro^{407}	
HPA-8bW	Sr^a	Integrin β_3	T_{2004}	Cys^{636}	178
			C_{2004}	Arg^{636}	
HPA-9bW	Max^a	Integrin α_{IIb}	A_{2603}	Met^{837}	179
			G_{2603}	Val^{837}	
HPA-10bW	La^a	Integrin β_3	A_{281}	Gln^{62}	180
			G_{281}	Arg^{62}	
HPA-11bW	Gro^a	Integrin β_3	A_{1996}	His^{633}	181
			G_{1996}	Arg^{633}	
HPA-12bW	Iy^a	GPIbβ	A_{141}	$Glu^{15}Gly^{15}$	182
			G_{141}	Gly^{15}	
HPA-13bW	Sit^a	Integrin α_2	T_{2531}	Met^{799}	183
			C_{2531}	Thr^{799}	
HPA-14bW	Oe^a	Integrin β_3	$\Delta\ AAG_{1929-31}$	ΔLys^{611}	184
			$AAG_{1929-31}$	Lys^{611}	
HPA-15a	Gov^b	CD109	C_{2108}	Ser^{703}	43
HPA-15b	Gov^a		A_{2108}	Tyr^{703}	
HPA-16bW	Duv^a	Integrin β_3	T_{517}	Ile^{140}	185
			C_{517}	Thr^{140}	
	Va^a	Integrin β_3			186
	Pe^a	GPIbα			187

Neonatal Alloimmune Thrombocytopenia

Neonatal alloimmune thrombocytopenia occurs in neonates and is caused by transplacental transfer of maternal alloantibodies produced by sensitization to paternal alloantigens on fetal platelets (Table 9–3). A correct diagnosis of NAIT must first eliminate other causes of thrombocytopenia that may occur during pregnancy. When severe, NAIT may result in intracerebral hemorrhage leading to hydrocephalus and fetal death. Fetal hydrocephalus, unexplained fetal thrombocytopenia with or without anemia, or recurrent miscarriages should be considered as indicators of possible NAIT.[16] Multiparous women with a history of at least one incident of NAIT should be monitored carefully for subsequent episodes. Postnatal management involves transfusion of compatible platelets, and washed maternal platelets are often used. Antenatal management is controversial but can include a combination of maternal intravenous immune globulin (IVIG) administration, intrauterine platelet transfusions, and corticosteroid therapy, while monitoring fetal platelet counts closely throughout the pregnancy.[16]

Table 9–3 Alloimmune Thrombocytopenias

NAIT

Incidence: 1 per 3000 in a retrospective study, 1 per 2200 births in one prospective study.
Maternal antibodies produced against paternal antigens on fetal platelets.
Similar to erythroblastosis fetalis, except that 50% of cases occur during first pregnancy.
Most frequently implicated antigens are HPA-1a and HPA-5b (United States/Europe).
In the case of responsiveness to HPA-1a, there is a high-risk association with HLA-DRB3*0101or DQB1*02.
In the case of responsiveness to HPA-6b, there is an increased association with HLA-DRB1*1501, DQA1*0102 or-DQB1*0602.

PTP

Nearly all of the reported patients have been females previously sensitized by pregnancy or transfusion (<5% were males).
Thrombocytopenia usually occurs 1 week after transfusion.
Homozygous HPA-1b individuals account for a majority (>60%) of cases.
High-risk association with HLA DRB3*0101or DQB1*02.
Enigmatically, the recipient's antigen-negative platelets are destroyed by autologous antibody.

The laboratory diagnosis is normally made by a comparison of maternal and paternal genotypes and a serologic search for antibodies in maternal plasma or serum that react with paternal platelets.

Only a fraction of those mothers negative for the platelet antigen in question deliver infants affected with NAIT. For example, in the western world, responsiveness to HPA-1a is most commonly the cause of NAIT, with severe thrombocytopenia due to maternal alloantibodies occurring in 1 per 1200 pregnancies, yet the frequency of homozygous HPA-1b mothers among white non-Hispanics is much higher (2%). A key to understanding this discrepancy lies in the finding that responsiveness to HPA-1a shows a human leukocyte antigen (HLA) restriction.[17] Individuals who are homozygous for Pro_{33} (homozygous HPA-1b) and responsive to the predominant HPA-1a antigen are almost exclusively HLA DRB3*0101[17] or DQB1*02.[18] In the case of DRB3*0101, the calculated risk factor is 141, a risk level equivalent to that of the hallmark of HLA restriction in autoimmune disease, ankylosing spondylitis and HLA-B27.[19] In contrast, responsiveness of homozygous HPA-1a individuals to the HPA-1b allele is not linked to HLA.[19,20] T cells are the likely candidates for providing HLA restriction in this case, and Maslanka and coworkers[19] provided elegant evidence that in one case of NAIT, T cells that share CDR3 motifs are stimulated by peptides that contain the same Leu_{33} polymorphism that is recognized by anti-HPA-1a alloantibodies.

In five cases of alloimmunization against the less frequent antigen, HPA-6b, there was a clear association between responsiveness and the major histocompatibility complex (MHC) haplotype DRB1*1501, DQA1*0102, DQB1*0602.[21] This alloimmunization likely involves different HLA class II molecules than those involved in immunization against HPA-1a.

Responsiveness to HPA-1a is not the sole cause of NAIT. In a large study of 348 cases of clinically suspected NAIT,[22] 78% of serologically confirmed cases were due to anti-HPA-1a and 19% to anti-HPA-5b. All other specificities accounted for no more than 5% of cases. In reports from other laboratories, the association of NAIT with other alloantigens, such as HPA-3a, HPA-3b, HPA-1b, and HPA-2b, has been noted, but is rare.[23] Obviously, differences in haplotype frequencies between racial or ethnic populations will have an important impact on the frequency of responsiveness to a particular alloantigen.

Haplotype Frequencies in Different Racial/Ethnic Groups

A substantial amount of information has been accumulated with respect to the relative frequency of the major alloantigen haplotypes among different racial and ethnic populations (see Figs. 9–1 through 9–4). The data for four of the most clinically prominent alloantigen haplotypes are depicted, namely, HPA-1b, HPA-2b, HPA-3b, and HPA-5b (*ITGA*2 haplotype 3). Each of these alloantigens represent one of a diallelic system. Consequently, the frequencies of the immunogenic (less common alleles) are depicted, and those of the more common alleles can be deduced.

HPA-1b has a relatively higher frequency among North Africans (0.26), whites of European background (0.15), and black Americans (0.1), and is much rarer among Asians (0.009), Aboriginals (0.008), and Native North Americans (<0.001) (Fig. 9–1). Not surprisingly, the most frequent antigen target in NAIT in white populations is HPA-1a (estimated at 78%).[22] However, among Asians, anti-HPA-1a has never been shown to be involved in NAIT.[24]

HPA-2b has the highest frequencies among Central Africans (0.3), North Africans (0.19), black Americans (0.17), and Native North Americans (0.12) (Fig. 9–2). A somewhat lower frequency is found among whites (0.09), native South Americans (Amerindians) (0.07), Asians (0.05), and Southeast

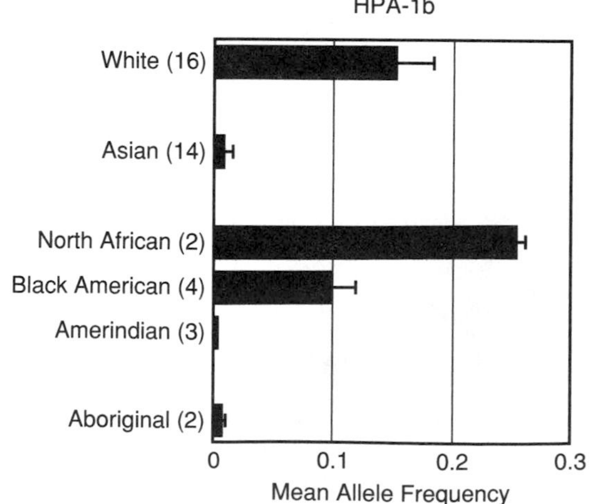

Figure 9–1 HPA-1b frequencies among selected racial/ethnic populations. The frequencies of HPA-1b (abscissa) among the populations listed on the ordinate are depicted. Each data entry (bar) represents the mean and standard deviation for the number of studies indicated in parentheses. References: White,[188–202] Asian,[190,203–215] North African,[216,217] black American,[188–190,203] Amerindian,[188,189,218] and Aboriginal.[202,219]

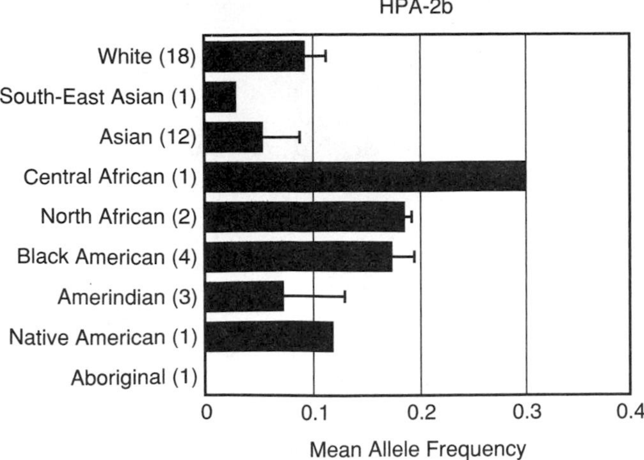

Figure 9–2 HPA-2b frequencies among selected racial/ethnic populations. The frequencies of HPA-2b (abscissa) among the populations listed on the ordinate are depicted. Each data entry (bar) represents the mean and standard deviation for the number of studies indicated in parentheses. References: White,[36,188–203] Southeast Asian,[36] Asian,[36,190,204,205,207–213,215] Central African,[36] North African,[36,216] black American,[188–190,203] Amerindian,[188,189,218] Native American,[220] and Aboriginal.[202]

Asians (0.03), and it is essentially nonexistent among Aboriginals (<0.001). The reports of HPA-2b frequency among Asians have provided disparate values ranging from 0 to 0.1 (mean = 0.05). HPA-2a has been implicated in NAIT among both whites and Asians,[23,25–27] but is much more common among whites.

HPA-3b appears at a very low frequency (0.05) uniquely among Aboriginals. Otherwise, HPA-3b seems to be prominently represented among all other races tested: Asians (0.47), whites (0.4), Amerindians (0.36), black Americans (0.34), and North Africans (0.32) (Fig. 9–3). HPA-3a is a frequent target for alloimmunization in NAIT and PTP among whites.

The highest frequencies of HPA-5b are found among Central Africans (0.25), Aboriginals (0.2), North Africans (0.18), and black Americans (0.17) (Fig. 9–4). Lower frequencies are found among whites (0.09) and Southeast Asians (0.09), and the lowest frequencies occur among Asians (0.03), Amerindians (0.02), and Native North Americans (0.02).

Post-transfusion Purpura

Post-transfusion purpura follows 7 to 10 days after an immunogenic blood (platelet) transfusion (see Table 9–3). It most often affects previously nontransfused, multiparous women. As with NAIT, there is an increased risk to develop PTP among HLA-DR3–positive individuals, and HPA-1a is the antigen most often implicated (in European white populations).[28,29]

Immunochemistry of Platelet Alloantigens

By convention, the designation human platelet antigen has been assigned to alloantigen systems in which the precise polymorphism that accounts for the serologic difference between alleles has been identified. Of 16 HPA systems defined to date (see Table 9-2), 9 are expressed by the integrin β_3 subunit (HPA-1, HPA-4, HPA-6, HPA-7, HPA-8, HPA-10W, HPA-11W, HPA-14W, and HPA-16W), 2 are localized on the integrin α_{IIb} subunit (HPA-3 and HPA-9W), 2 are found on the integrin α_2 subunit (HPA-5 and HPA-13W), 1 is expressed by the GPIbα (HPA-2), 1 by GPIbβ (HPA-12W), and the last is located on the CD109 (HPA-15).

The vast majority of clinical episodes following alloimmunization involve five of these systems: HPA-1, HPA-2, HPA-3, HPA-5, and HPA-15.

HPA-1

The HPA-1 alloantigen system is defined by the Leu_{33}/Pro_{33} polymorphism that is enclosed within a small 13–amino acid loop formed by the pairing of Cys_{26} with Cys_{38}. This region of the molecule is held proximal to the distal cysteine-rich region in the middle of β_3 by a long-range disulfide bond linking Cys_5 and Cys_{435}.[30] The complex structure of the β_3 molecule and the sensitivity of the determinants to this structure is the likely explanation for observed heterogeneity in binding properties of anti-HPA-1a alloantibodies.[31] Although all alloantibodies would bind to the denatured molecule or to recombinant amino-terminal segments of the molecule expressed in *Escherichia coli*,[32] a subset of antibodies appear to require presentation of the antigenic loop within a more native environment (e.g., the nondenatured molecule).[31] Anti-HPA-1a antibodies inhibit clot retraction and platelet aggregation; in the latter case, presumably because they block the binding of fibrinogen.[33]

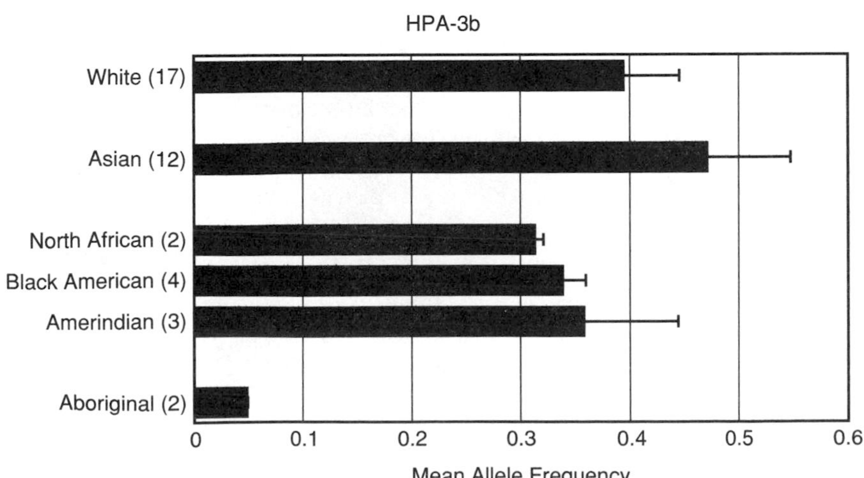

Figure 9–3 HPA-3b frequencies among selected racial/ethnic populations. The frequencies of HPA-3b (abscissa) among the populations listed on the ordinate are depicted. Each data entry (bar) represents the mean and standard deviation for the number of studies indicated in parentheses. References: White,[36,188–202] Asian,[36,189,190,204,207–213,215] North African,[36,216] black American,[188–190,203] Amerindian,[188,189,218] and Aboriginal.[202,219]

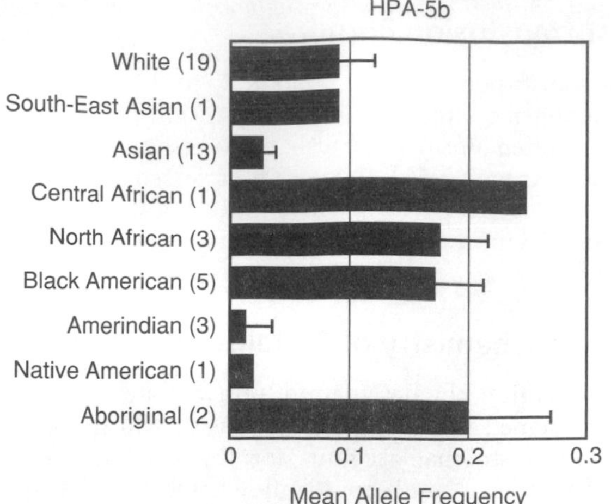

Figure 9–4 HPA-5b frequencies among selected racial/ethnic populations. The frequencies of HPA-5b (abscissa) among the populations listed on the ordinate are depicted. Each data entry (bar) represents the mean and standard deviation for the number of studies indicated in parentheses. References: White,[36,188–203,220] Southeast Asian,[36] Asian,[36,189,190,204,205,207–213,215] Central African,[36] North African,[36,216,217] black American,[188–190,203,220] Amerindian,[188,189,218] Native American,[220] and Aboriginal.[202,219]

Other cells that express β_3, as the β subunit of the vitronectin receptor, including endothelial cells, fibroblasts, and smooth muscle cells, also express HPA-1 epitopes.[34] This could contribute to the complexity of the clinical symptoms in alloimmune-mediated thrombocytopenia. At this time, little, if anything, is known about the involvement of tissues other than platelets in these conditions.

HPA-2

Two previously described polymorphisms of the GP Ib-IX-V complex, termed Ko and Sib, are now known to be reflections of two linked polymorphisms, one of which defines the diallelic system, HPA-2.[35] In the GPIbα sequence, a Thr/Met polymorphism at residue 145 is associated with HPA-2a and HPA-2b epitopes, respectively.

There are several major GPIbα gene *(GP1BA)* haplotypes that can be defined by linkage disequilibrium between the alleles at positions –5 (Kozak), 1018 (Thr145Met; HPA-2), and 1285 (variable number of tandem repeats [VNTR] A, B, C, and D).[36]

HPA-3

The HPA-3 system is associated with an Ile_{843}/Ser_{843} polymorphism of α_{IIb}.[37]

HPA-5

The HPA-5 system is located on the integrin subunit α_2.[38] The detection of this system was facilitated by the development of a highly sensitive murine monoclonal antibody-based monoclonal antibody immobilization of platelet antigen assay.[39] Like the preceding alloantigenic systems, the HPA-5 system is diallelic. Roughly 500 to 2000 copies of α_2 are present on the surface of normal platelets, and each α_2 molecule expresses a single HPA-5 epitope.[38] The integrin α_2 is distributed on a wide variety of cells, but nothing is currently known about the antigenicity of the HPA-5 determinants on receptors expressed by cell types other than platelets.

The density of the $\alpha_2\beta_1$ integrin is known to correlate with the α_2 single-nucleotide polymorphism (SNP) C807T. However, in a study of 79 HPA-5(a/a) mothers giving birth to HPA-5(a/b) offspring, Panzer and colleagues[40] determined that there was no increased risk of maternal-fetal HPA-5 incompatibility among mothers whose genotype is 807T.

There are at least 6 major haplotypes of the integrin α_2 gene *(ITGA2)* that are defined by linkage disequilibrium between alleles at position –52 (C/T), 807 (C/T), and 1643 (A/G; HPA-5).[36]

HPA-15

Kelton and coworkers[41] initially described the Gov system, which is now known to be carried by the 175-kDa glycosyl phosphatidylinositol-anchored glycoprotein CD109 and has been designated HPA-15. Alloantibodies defining each of the two alleles have been detected in patients who had received multiple platelet transfusions[41] as well as in patients who developed NAIT.[42] An A2108C SNP of the CD109 gene results in a Tyr703Ser substitution that defines the HPA-15 alloantigen system.[43] The detection of antibodies against HPA-15 is complicated by variation in expression and instability of CD109 during preparation and storage.[44] Nonetheless, relative to all detected HPA-specific antibodies, HPA-15 was found to account for roughly 6% of alloimmunization in a white population.[44]

ISOANTIGENS

Isoantibodies are produced against an epitope that is expressed by all normal individuals and is not polymorphic. In the area of human platelet immunology, a classic example of isoimmunization occurs when a patient with an inherited deficiency of a membrane glycoprotein has been subjected to multiple platelet transfusions to correct a bleeding diathesis. Glanzmann thrombasthenia and BSS are such inherited disorders, wherein the individual either lacks or expresses an altered form of $\alpha_{IIb}\beta_3$ (Glanzmann thrombasthenia) or GP Ib-IX-V (BSS), respectively. Isoantibodies developed by transfused patients do not distinguish any of the allelic forms of the glycoproteins (such as HPA-3 or HPA-1 alloantigens on $\alpha_{IIb}\beta_3$) but react with the platelets of all normal persons tested. Because the propositus does not express the platelet glycoprotein that carries the epitope in question, these antibodies do not bind to their own platelets.

Isoantibodies in Glanzmann Thrombasthenia

Several cases have been documented in which patients with Glanzmann thrombasthenia have produced antibodies specific for α_{IIb}, β_3, or the $\alpha_{IIb}\beta_3$ complex. Recently, we defined an idiotype (OG) that is associated at high frequency with isoantibodies specific for integrin subunit β_3 generated by Glanzmann thrombasthenia patients.[45,46] Patient OG suffered from persistent often-serious bleeding episodes as a result of both his Glanzmann thrombasthenia phenotype and the fact that he had generated a very high-titered, IgG isoantibody inhibitor of platelet cohesion.[46]

Isoantibodies in Bernard-Soulier Syndrome

Because BSS is less frequently encountered than Glanzmann thrombasthenia, it follows that isoantibodies produced in conjunction with this syndrome are also less frequently encountered. In the only clearcut case of such an isoantibody,[47] the isolated IgG impaired both normal platelet adhesion to subendothelial elements and in vitro aggregation in response to ristocetin and bovine factor VIII.

CD36

The frequency of platelet CD36 (GPIV) deficiency, which occurs most often in Asians and blacks, is approximately 4%, and a subset of these individuals is at risk for immunization against CD36.[48] In five cases of neonatal thrombocytopenia, isoantibodies reactive with CD36 were identified in the mothers of the affected infants. Two black mothers were homozygous for a T1264G substitution in the CD36 gene, and a European white mother was homozygous for a novel deletion of exons 1 through 3. These findings and the results of prior reports indicate that isoimmunization against CD36 can cause neonatal *isoimmune* thrombocytopenia, refractoriness to platelet transfusions, and PTP.[48]

AUTOANTIGENS AND IDIOPATHIC THROMBOCYTOPENIC PURPURA

Autoimmune (or idiopathic) thrombocytopenic purpura (ITP) is the most frequently encountered form of immune thrombocytopenia.[49] This disorder can be classified as acute or chronic on the basis of the duration of the thrombocytopenia, the chronic form persisting longer than 6 months. The acute, self-limiting form occurs predominantly in children, often following a viral illness or immunization, and affects males and females with equal frequency. Although 10% to 15% of childhood ITP lasts longer than 6 months, the chronic form of immune thrombocytopenia is mainly an adult illness and affects twice as many females as males. Life-threatening bleeding occurs in up to 1% of patients with ITP. The reason that some patients sustain severe hemorrhagic complications and others do not remains unexplained, but because of differences seen in the clinical expression of chronic and acute ITP, it has been theorized that the mechanisms of disease for each form stem from different etiologies.[50] Although most autoantibodies apparently induce thrombocytopenia, a minority can induce platelet dysfunction with or without an increase in platelet clearance.[51,52] The proportion of the two types of autoantibody, that which leads to platelet clearance and that which blocks platelet function, may be a very important factor controlling the unpredictable clinical severity of ITP.

It had been hoped that the antigenic targets in acute and chronic forms of ITP might be distinct, so that antigen identity might one day be used as an early indicator of clinical outcome. Subsequent studies have shed more light on this issue and have demonstrated that autoantibody specificity in chronic versus acute ITP is quite similar, particularly in children.[53,54] Nonetheless, a distinction between antigen specificity and an acute versus chronic course in ITP may yet be found in the early stages of the autoimmune response, particularly if additional risk factors such as cytokine response and predisposing high-risk polymorphisms in immune response genes are included in the evaluation.[55–57]

Suppression of Megakaryocyte Production and Maturation

One area where both autoantigen and age may play a role in predicting chronicity in ITP is megakaryocyte expansion and thrombopoiesis.[58–64] Initial studies by McMillan and coworkers[58] showed that immunoglobulin G (IgG) produced in vitro by splenic cells from ITP patients would bind to megakaryocytes but IgG produced by normal splenic cells or purified normal sera IgG would not, thus suggesting that autoantibody might directly interfere with platelet production. Later studies examining the effect of ITP plasma on megakaryocytic growth in culture confirmed that those plasmas containing antiplatelet antibodies resulted in a direct suppression of replication. Of note, these studies once again suggested that there might be significant differences in the etiology of megakaryocytic suppression by plasma from children versus adults with ITP. In addition, autoantigen specificity, especially those antibodies directed against GPIb/IX complex in pediatric patients, may have a profound effect on thrombopoiesis.

In childhood ITP, the mean yield of megakaryocytic cells in culture was significantly reduced in the presence of patient plasmas containing either antiplatelet GPIb autoantibodies alone (p<0.001) or antibodies against both GPIb and $\alpha_{IIb}\beta_3$(p<0.001), as compared to control plasmas.[61] There was no significant difference between the mean megakaryocytic yield in cultures containing control plasmas or patient plasmas with either no autoantibodies or autoantibodies specific solely for $\alpha_{IIb}\beta_3$. The ploidy distribution of megakaryocytic precursors in cultures containing either control or ITP plasma was not significantly different. The importance of autoantibodies in the suppression of megakaryocyte production was demonstrated by platelet adsorption studies. Platelet absorption of anti-GPIb autoantibodies in ITP plasmas resulted in a doubling of megakaryocyte production compared to that in the presence of the same plasmas without absorption. On the other hand, platelet absorption of normal control plasma had no effect on megakaryocyte yield.

Studies with plasmas from adult ITP patients demonstrated similar suppression of megakaryocytic production, with one striking difference: The ploidy distribution of megakaryocytic precursors in cultures containing either control or ITP plasma was also significantly different. ITP plasmas that suppressed in vitro megakaryocyte production clearly reduced the percentages of 4N, 8N, and 16N megakaryocytes as well.[63] Houwerzijl and colleagues[64] showed that megakaryocytes in bone marrow aspirates of adult ITP patients exhibit morphologic alterations characteristic of para-apoptosis: mitochondrial swelling with cytoplasmic vacuolization, distention of the demarcation membranes, and chromatin condensation within the nucleus. Importantly, they found that similar para-apoptotic changes could be induced in normal CD34+ cells differentiated to megakaryocytes in the presence of ITP plasma. These authors suggested that the binding of antiplatelet autoantibodies to megakaryocytes may play an important role in initiating the cascade of programmed cell death.[64] These ploidy and para-apoptotic changes were not observed in cultures co-incubated with pediatric ITP plasmas despite their ability to suppress megakaryopoiesis.[61] In addition, when megakaryocytes cultured with ITP plasma were also treated with FMK, a general caspase inhibitor, the differential effect of adult and pediatric ITP plasmas remained. This result would rule out a difference in caspase-mediated apoptotic mechanisms between adults and children as the cause of these findings.[61–64]

It is more likely that a difference in autoantigen epitopes or the intensity of autoantibody binding to certain platelet receptors accounts for the difference in apoptotic changes seen in adult megakaryocytes that is absent in pediatric studies. In addition, since the immune system is still maturing in patients younger than age 5, one would expect to observe increased variability in antibody specificity, affinity, and isotypes among children, with an increased suppression of megakaryocytopoiesis compared to adults.[61,62] Adolescent ITP patients are much more likely to have autoantibodies specific for the GPIb/IX complex and a clinical course similar to that of adult ITP.[57] Autoantibody binding to the GPIb/IX complex at a certain stage of megakaryocyte development may trigger signaling pathways that predispose to apoptotic changes, resulting in a more profound and lasting suppression of megakaryopoiesis and concomitant thrombocytopenia.

Glycoproteins as Platelet Autoantigens

An extensive characterization of platelet target autoantigens has been accomplished within the past decade. It is now evident that both T and B cells mediate self-reactivity in immune thrombocytopenia. Under normal circumstances, immune recognition may serve to clear damaged or senescent cells, but in ITP patients, these processes result in the pathologic destruction of platelets. In normal individuals, the network of autoreactive T and B cells remains tightly regulated, allowing the effective maintenance of platelet production and integrity. In autoimmune states, following infection or environmental triggers, pathologic platelet autoreactivity results from an imbalance in T-cell signaling and regulation. This state allows the clonal expansion and somatic mutation of B cells through epitope spreading, resulting in pathologic autoantibodies. An understanding of the role of autoantigens in promoting and perpetuating this response has been assisted by an extensive characterization of platelet glycoproteins and glycolipids.[65,66]

Integrin $\alpha_{IIb}\beta_3$

Integrin $\alpha_{IIb}\beta_3$ was the first platelet membrane component to be identified as a dominant antigen in chronic ITP,[67] and subsequent studies from several laboratories have confirmed the important contribution of this receptor to the autoantigenic makeup of the human platelet.[49] An excellent review of the specific assays used to identify serum antiplatelet antibodies and their autoantigen targets has recently been published for readers interested in a detailed description of the technology and use of these assays in the diagnosis of ITP.[68]

Integrin Subunit β_3

Initially, attempts to further localize autoepitopes on either integrin subunit were more successful with regard to β_3. Early on, Kekomaki and coworkers[69] defined a prominent autoantigenic region as the 33-kDa chymotryptic fragment of β_3 located within the cysteine-rich region of β_3, which was bound by both plasma autoantibodies and autoantibody eluted from patients' platelets. Using recombinant fusion proteins containing the extracellular disulfide-rich region of β_3, Beardsley and coworkers[70] more recently confirmed that a disulfide-rich segment of β_3 (residues 468–691) immediately external to the proposed membrane spanning domain (residues 693–721) contains peptide target antigens for autoantibodies from ITP patients.

Fujisawa and colleagues[71] also determined that plasma autoantibodies in 5 of 13 patients with chronic ITP bound to peptides representing β_3 residues 721–744 or 742–762, namely, the carboxy-terminal region of β_3, which is presumed to be located in the cytoplasm of the platelet. Their role in the pathogenesis of immune thrombocytopenia is unclear because this portion of the β_3 molecule is located within the cytoplasm, rather than on the surface, of the resting platelet. However, internal autoantigens are the hallmark of many immune-mediated diseases, such as polymyositis and systemic lupus erythematosus (SLE).[72] As in those diseases, one can postulate that certain autoantigens are normally internal but, at some point, are expressed on the surface of the platelet, perhaps as a result of activation or senescence, at which time the autoantibodies can bind and trigger the removal of platelets from the circulation.

The report by Fujisawa and colleagues[71] is one of many suggesting that autoantibodies to $\alpha_{IIb}\beta_3$ may bind to cryptic epitopes or neoantigens that are expressed on platelet activation or senescence.[73] Platelets normally accumulate IgG on the membrane surface as they age over 7 to 10 days in the circulation and/or become activated, and then they are cleared by reticuloendothelial cells in the spleen.[74] Using a Fab′2 fraction of IgG, it has been shown that normal individuals have autoantibodies in their sera that specifically bind to senescent antigens on red cells and platelets and can mediate clearance of spent or dysfunctional cells.[75,76] The role of these naturally occurring autoantibodies in pathologic immune destruction of cells is unclear. Animal studies suggest that the initial binding of the pathogenic antiplatelet autoantibody may trigger the expression of senescent or cryptic antigens on the platelet membrane, resulting in a second wave of immunoglobulin binding and clearance by naturally occurring autoantibodies.[77]

More recently, additional autoantigenic epitopes have been identified on the β_3 subunit. Nardi and coworkers[78] identified the peptide β_3^{49-66} as a site that is bound by a majority of affinity-purified antibodies isolated from serum immune complexes of human immunodeficiency virus-1–infected patients with immune thrombocytopenia. This is not a peptide region that is bound by serum IgG antibodies from control subjects or patients with the classic form of ITP.

Identification of autoimmune epitopes has been aided by the development of the phage-display peptide library. Bowditch and coworkers[79] used a filamentous phage library that displayed random linear hexapeptides to identify peptide sequences recognized by platelet-specific autoantibodies. Plasma antibody eluates from ITP patients were used to select for phage-displaying autoantibody-reactive peptides. They identified anti-$\alpha_{IIb}\beta_3$ antibody-specific phage encoding the hexapeptide sequences Arg-Glu-Lys-Ala-Lys-Trp (REKAKW), Pro-Val-Val-Trp-Lys-Asn (PVVWKN), and Arg-Glu-Leu-Leu-Lys-Met (RELLKM). Each phage showed saturable dose-dependent binding to immobilized autoantibody, and binding could be blocked with purified $\alpha_{IIb}\beta_3$. The binding of plasma autoantibody to the phage encoding REKAKW could be blocked with a synthetic peptide derived from the β_3 cytoplasmic tail; however, binding to the PVVWKN-bearing phage was not inhibited. Using sequential overlapping peptides from the β_3 cytoplasmic region, an epitope was localized to the sequence Arg-Ala-Arg-Ala-Lys-Trp (β_3 734–739).

Using a similar phage peptide display approach, Gevorkian and coworkers[80] identified other mimotopes of platelet autoantigens recognized by autoantibodies in sera from 20 ITP patients. These mimotopes exhibited potential homology with sequences on both β_3 and GPIb, although a specific sequence identity was not proposed.

Integrin Subunit α_{IIb}

In a growing body of literature, it now appears that the α_{IIb} molecule may be the dominant target in the adult form of chronic ITP.[81] Autoantibodies reactive with α_{IIb} were identified in two patients with chronic ITP,[82,83] and in one of these patients, the antibody was subsequently shown to react with a chymotryptic, 65-kDa, COOH-terminal fragment of the α_{IIb} heavy chain.[83] Ethylenediaminetet-raacetic acid (EDTA)-dependent autoantibodies represent a special category that are adsorbed by autologous platelets when whole blood is drawn in EDTA. In one such case of EDTA-dependent "pseudothrombocytopenia," an IgM antibody was shown to bind to α_{IIb} by immunoblot assay and crossed immunoelectrophoresis.[84]

In subsequent studies, Gevorkian and colleagues[80,85] used phage display to map an autoepitope on α_{IIb}. A filamentous phage library was employed that displays random peptides, 11 amino acids in length, flanked on each side by a cysteine to identify peptide sequences recognized by antiplatelet autoantibodies previously determined to block fibrinogen binding to $\alpha_{IIb}\beta_3$. Phage expressing the sequence CTGRVPLGFEDLC exhibited saturable dose-dependent binding to the immobilized autoantibody that could be blocked with purified $\alpha_{IIb}\beta_3$ or α_{IIb}, but not β_3. This amino acid sequence exhibits partial identity with amino acid residues 4–10 and 31–35 on α_{IIb}. These results suggest that the autoantibodies in question bind to a combinatorial epitope within the amino-terminal 35 amino acids of α_{IIb}.

Other critical autoantigen epitopes have been identified on α_{IIb} in recent years. Using a combination of lysates from platelets with known protein mutations, Kosugi and colleagues[86] demonstrated that one third of patients with chronic ITP produced anti-$\alpha_{IIb}\beta_3$ autoantibodies with a unique specificity. The binding of these autoantibodies is inhibited by the single amino acid substitution (D163A) and a 2-amino acid insertion in the W3 4–1 loop of α_{IIb}.

Autoantigenic epitopes may be conformational, thereby dependent on the tertiary configuration of the molecule. Given the fluid nature of the platelet membrane and the remarkable morphologic changes that can occur on adhesion and activation, it is not surprising that conformational epitopes might be dynamically expressed. In one of the first descriptions of this kind, Shadle and Barondes[87] described a neoantigen on α_{IIb}, which is only revealed following the normal binding of fibrinogen to its receptor, the $\alpha_{IIb}\beta_3$ complex. In addition, serum autoantibodies have been described that demonstrate increased binding to platelets in the presence of calcium chelators, such as EDTA, heparin, or other drugs.[84] Some of this autoantibody specificity may be directed to neoantigens and thus is enhanced following changes in membrane glycoproteins induced by agents such as EDTA or heparin.

Human Monoclonal Autoantibodies

One important question that needs to be resolved is the extent of the autoepitope repertoire on a given platelet glycoprotein antigen. The answer will have an impact on the feasibility of developing therapeutic and diagnostic measures based on epitope specificity. Because the autoantibodies that react with a given epitope are likely to share idiotypes, one can approach this question from two directions, analyzing the epitope repertoire or the idiotype repertoire.

Two studies have addressed the extent of the autoantigen repertoire on $\alpha_{IIb}\beta_3$ by analyzing the competitive binding between human autoantibodies and murine monoclonal antibodies.[88,89] However, the limited number of studies that have used this approach have generated conflicting results, and insufficient data are available to judge the size of the autoepitope repertoire on $\alpha_{IIb}\beta_3$. Additional analyses aimed at epitope localization will be necessary, and perhaps novel approaches will expedite this task. One such novel approach is the development of human monoclonal autoantibodies specific for $\alpha_{IIb}\beta_3$ and other platelet glycoproteins.

Human monoclonal antibodies are an alternative tool in the search for glycoprotein epitopes that are autoimmunogenic in humans. The first human monoclonal antibody against a platelet glycoprotein was derived from an ITP individual producing an antibody against β_3.[72] This human monoclonal antibody detects a neoantigen associated with β_3 that is expressed only on stored or thrombin-activated platelets. A number of human monoclonal autoantibodies specific for the heavy chain of GPIb were generated from the lymphocytes of an ITP patient with serum autoantibody specific for GPIb.[90] The heavy-chain variable region genes of four of these antibodies have been sequenced and found to be markedly homologous to human immunoglobulin, germline, heavy-chain variable region genes.[90] Another human monoclonal autoantibody was produced that is specific for the heavy chain of α_{IIb}.[73] The epitope recognized by this antibody (2E7) has been identified as a contiguous amino acid sequence with residues 231–238 with an immunodominant tryptophan residue at position 235.[91] This was the first time that the precise epitope on α_{IIb} or β_3 recognized by a human antibody had been identified.

The $\alpha_{IIb}\beta_3$ molecule is a member of the greater family of adhesion molecules or integrins, and α_{IIb} has significant homology with other integrin α chains. A comparison of the 220–238 sequences of α_{IIb} and seven other integrin α subunits revealed significant homology between α_{IIb} and other α integrin chains, yet 2E7 did not bind to the other cell types that express these related integrin family members, such as endothelial cells, lymphocytes, monocytes, or neutrophils. In the highly homologous region spanning residues 234–238, α_{IIb} differs from the other α chains only in position 235 (W→L). Ironically, this tryptophan plays a critical role in determining the immunogenic epitope recognized by 2E7.

From the foregoing analysis, it is clear that further studies are required to determine the extent to which the production of human autoantibodies to platelet glycoproteins is clonally restricted. Given a selected number of idiotypes related to autoimmunity to $\alpha_{IIb}\beta_3$, one could potentially use the anti-idiotype (anti-Id) to modulate immunization to $\alpha_{IIb}\beta_3$. Along these lines, it has been reported that IVIG, which is routinely used to reverse acute thrombocytopenia in ITP, may contain anti-Id directed to idiotypes of autoantibody but not alloantibodies that recognize $\alpha_{IIb}\beta_3$.[92] Other investigators have defined a DM idiotype that is characteristic of human autoantibodies that are specific for the GPIb heavy chain.[93] The latter study clearly suggests that the repertoire of idiotypes expressed by human autoantibodies specific for membrane glycoproteins, such as those of the human platelet, will be narrowly defined and, thus, amenable to study.

The production of human monoclonal autoantibodies or recombinant Fab fragments from patients with immune thrombocytopenia provides researchers with specific antibody probes to map target antigens. Human monoclonal antibodies have an advantage over serum antibodies in that they are monoclonal and circumvent problems associated with using a polyclonal serum where many different, low titer autoantibodies may be found with reactivity against a variety of epitopes.

GPIb/IX Complex

Unlike the $\alpha_{IIb}\beta_3$ complex, autoantibodies directed against GPIb are almost universally associated with pathologic immune destruction of platelets. Thus far, no one has described naturally occurring antibodies reacting with GPIb in either resting or activated platelets. Although only 15% to 30% of ITP patients have autoantibodies that bind to GPIb, there is no background binding of antibodies in normal plasma so the characterization of this antigen is much more straightforward. Autoantibodies to components of the GPIb complex are also frequently encountered in adult chronic ITP.

He and colleagues[94] have made progress in the localization of selected autoantigenic epitopes on the GPIb molecule. Epitopes were most frequently found on a recombinant fragment of Ibα corresponding to residues 240–485, and next most often on a fragment representing residues 1–247. In the case of those antibodies reactive with the former sequence, further epitope mapping identified the dominant determinant as the 9-amino acid sequence TKEQTTFPP (residues 333–341).[94] In some cases in which autoantibody to GPIb/IX was detected, the clinical presentation proved to be particularly severe and refractory to therapy.[93] One case of "pseudo-Bernard-Soulier syndrome" (dysfunction of the Ib-IX-V receptor complex) was reported to be caused by an autoantibody to GPIb.[95] Finally, in a subset of childhood ITP, that associated with *Varicella zoster* infection, the GPV component of this receptor was found to be the dominant target of serum autoantibodies that do not crossreact with viral antigens.[96] At the same time, in another group of children with this disease, it was found that serum antibodies specific for viral antigens can crossreact with normal platelet antigens and may thus contribute to platelet clearance.[97]

The GPIbα heavy chain is a large molecule and contains leucine-rich repeats and a region in the middle of the glycoprotein that is heavily glycosylated. The NH2-terminal region of GPIb is responsible for binding to von Willebrand antigen, mediating platelet adhesion. Theoretically, there could be a variety of antigenic sites on this molecule. However, using anti-Id reagents, it appears that the repertoire of idiotypes expressed by anti-GPIb antibodies from patients with ITP is very narrowly defined.[93]

GPV

In the mid-1980s, when screening for antigen-specific autoantibodies became available, many researchers hoped that the patterns of target antigen reactivity might be predictive of the clinical course of ITP (i.e., acute versus chronic). In fact, an initial report looking at eight children with acute ITP using immunoblot technique failed to demonstrate anti-β_3 antibody even though this was the dominant antigenic target recognized by autoantibodies from patients with chronic ITP.[98] This was followed by a report from the same laboratory[99] demonstrating serum antibody reactivity to Glycoprotein V (GPV) in four pediatric patients with thrombocytopenia associated with varicella (chickenpox) infection. GPV is a thrombin-sensitive, 85-kDa glycoprotein of unknown function on the platelet surface. There was no evidence of immune complexes in these patients or varicella antigens adsorbed to the surface of their platelets. As all of the children with varicella-related ITP and acute childhood form of ITP resolved their thrombocytopenia within 6 months, there was some hope that GPV reactivity would be a marker for mild disease and these patients could escape aggressive immunosuppressive therapy.

Integrin $\alpha_2\beta_1$

Platelet integrin $\alpha_2\beta_1$ is an important collagen receptor on the platelet membrane. Although present in a much lower concentration than $\alpha_{IIb}\beta_3$ or the GPIb complex, this receptor has also been shown to be a target autoantigen in 10% to 20% of chronic ITP patients.[100] Moreover, serum IgG autoantibodies specific for integrin subunit α_2 were identified in a unique case of autoimmune platelet dysfunction following myasthenia gravis.[100] This autoantibody inhibited aggregation of normal platelets induced by collagen or wheat germ agglutinin. This was the first case wherein autoantibodies to α_2 were associated with a chronic hemorrhagic disorder.

Efforts to map the specific epitope on this receptor have been unsuccessful even though a number of groups have suggested that the binding of these antibodies, since they impair function, might be near the binding site of collagen. Deckmyn and colleagues describe a plasma autoantibody directed against a protein comigrating with α_2 and recognized by the patient's antibody when affinity-purified $\alpha_2\beta_1$ was used as antigen.[100] The $\alpha_2\beta_1$ complex was immunoprecipitated from a platelet lysate by the patient's plasma, and purified platelet specific IgG from this patient inhibited aggregation of normal platelets induced by collagen or by wheat germ agglutinin. Dromigny and coworkers[101] described a 48-year-old woman in whom they found increased bleeding times, impaired collagen-induced platelet aggregation, and the presence of autoantibodies directed against $\alpha_2\beta_1$ and the GPIb complex.

GPVI

Sugiyama and coworkers[102] and Moroi and coworkers[103] were the first to identify and characterize autoantibodies from an ITP patient specific for GPVI, a 62-kDa membrane glycoprotein present on both human and murine platelets noncovalently associated with a coreceptor FcγR chain.

More recently, Boylan and colleagues[104] described a patient with a mild bleeding disorder and a moderately reduced platelet count whose platelets were nonresponsive to collagen, although no abnormalities were found in the genomic DNA sequence of *GP6* and the level of platelet *GP6* mRNA was normal. The plasma of this patient was found to contain an autoantibody that binds specifically to GPVI. Because shedding of GPVI on mouse platelets in vivo by infusion of specific anti-GPVI antibody had already been described,[105] it was proposed that in this patient the GPVI/FcγR complex is cleared from the platelet by this autoantibody, resulting in a chronic "acquired" deficiency of platelet GPVI.

This case represents a unique effect of platelet-specific autoantibodies and emphasizes that acquired defects in platelet function can also be a pathologic outcome of autoimmunity to platelets.

Glycolipids as Autoantigens

A number of reports have implicated cardiolipin, lactosylceramide, and other glycosphingolipids (GSL) as autoantigenic targets (Table 9–4).[106,107] Van Vliet and colleagues[107] analyzed the binding of serum IgG/IgM antibodies from 30 ITP patients to platelet glycosphingolipids separated by high-performance thin-layer chromatography. Acidic GSL, namely sulfatides and gangliosides, were identified as the major targets of serum autoantibodies. Thirteen of the 30 sera, five with anticardiolipin antibodies, had antibodies that bound to

Table 9–4 Glycolipid Antigens of Platelets
Cardiolipin
Lactosylceramide
Glycosphingolipids (GSL)
Acidic: sulfatides/gangliosides
Monogalactosyl sulfatide (16/6 idiotype)
Neutral: globotriosyl ceramide
Globotetraosyl ceramide

sulfatides; four sera showed antibody binding to gangliosides. Koerner and colleagues[106] employed a more efficient phase partition separation of acidic GSL from neutral GSL and were able to demonstrate that serum antibodies specific for neutral GSL were more characteristic of ITP. Two classes of GSL autoantigens were defined: those associated with general autoimmunity and detected in the sera of patients with either SLE or ITP, and those peculiar to platelet-specific autoimmunity and detected only in the sera of ITP patients. Two GSL forms belong to the platelet-specific group, but they are present at minute levels, and further characterization awaits large-scale purification. One half (6/12) of patients with ITP had serum IgG or IgM antibodies that bound these platelet-specific GSL. Sera from none of 10 patients with nonimmune thrombocytopenia, none of 10 patients with SLE, and only 1 of 18 normal subjects gave positive reactions with the platelet-specific GSL group. The general GSL antigen group includes globotriaosyl ceramide, globotetraosyl ceramide, and a third unidentified neutral GSL. Antigens in the general group were bound by IgG or IgM antibodies in the sera of 10 of 10 patients with SLE, 8 of 12 patients with ITP, and none of 10 patients with nonimmune thrombocytopenia or 18 control subjects. These findings provide compelling support for a role of neutral GSL as antigenic targets in selected cases of ITP.

Animal Models of ITP

Many investigators have searched in animals for clinical correlates of human ITP. These attempts have been largely unsuccessful, but an exception may have recently evolved from concerted studies in dogs. As pointed out in a recent series of reports by Lewis and Meyers,[108] there is now substantial evidence that ITP in dogs and ITP in humans are clinically analogous syndromes. In 32 cases of canine ITP, increased platelet-bound IgG was detected in a majority of the animals (30 of 32), and immunoglobulin eluted from the platelets of 11 of 19 affected dogs bound to homologous normal canine platelets.[108] Furthermore, immunoglobulin specific for integrin subunits α_{IIb} and/or β_3 was detected in sera of 4 of 17 dogs tested. They have concluded that, in canine ITP, immunoglobulin bound to the surface of platelets is directed against host antigens and that the target antigen is frequently $\alpha_{IIb}\beta_3$. Given the similarities between these findings and the cumulative experience with human ITP, the canine model may prove to be a valuable tool to further understand the pathogenesis of the autoimmune response to platelet antigens.

Recent attempts to create a murine model of ITP have produced initial results that are promising for researchers interested in studying the pathophysiology of immune-mediated thrombocytopenias. Monoclonal antibodies of different IgG subclasses directed against mouse $\alpha_{IIb}\beta_3$, β_3, GPIba, GPIb/IX, GPV, and CD31 were generated. When injected into mice, monoclonal antibodies against GPIb/IX, GPV, CD31, and linear epitopes on β_3 had mild and transient effects on platelet counts and induced no spontaneous bleeding. On the other hand, anti-GPIba monoclonal antibodies induced profound irreversible thrombocytopenia (to <3% of normal) by an Fc-independent mechanism.[65]

Immunologic Abnormalities in ITP

Increasing insights into the etiology and pathophysiology of ITP have stimulated an examination of immune abnormalities that distinguishes adult from childhood immune thrombocytopenia. Given the elegant and extensive regulatory network inherent in the immune system that optimizes our response to external organisms and safeguards us against autoimmune disease, one wonders why antibodies to platelet antigens appear to be preserved in our repertoire of immunoglobulins.

Kazatchkine and coworkers[109] were among the first to demonstrate the presence of antiplatelet antibodies in normal human serum and anti-Id antibodies in IVIG, suggesting that immunoglobulin reactive with common platelet antigens, such as the GPIb/IX complex and $\alpha_{IIb}\beta_3$, are critical components of the naturally occurring autoantibody repertoire.[109–115] These observations, along with a growing body of evidence, suggest that antiplatelet antibodies are produced as a result of epitope shift[116,117] after exposure to certain infectious organisms or external antigens. This response must be tightly controlled with a network of regulatory cells and plasma factors, such the anti-Id antibodies found in IVIG.[115,118,119] In childhood ITP, which is seasonal and transient in nature, the regulatory network can usually restore itself to proper order within 6 months following the acute insult in a majority of patients.[57]

In animal models, loss of peripheral tolerance to self-antigens is emerging as a possible mechanism for autoimmune disease, with particular focus on the regulatory CD4+25+ T-lymphocyte subset.[120–122] These cells prevent autoimmune disease by modulating self-reactive T cells and secretion of suppressor cytokines, such as interleukin-10 (IL-10) and transforming growth factor beta (TGF-β).[123,124] As summarized in the following section, the finding of inherent T-cell abnormalities and alterations in the expression of accessory molecules on autoreactive T cells provides a novel avenue for the development of immunotherapy in ITP.[119,125]

T Lymphocytes

As in other autoimmune diseases, elevated numbers of T-cell receptor (TCR) γ/δ-positive T lymphocytes have been noted in both acute and chronic ITP patients, as initially described by Ware and Howard.[126] Analysis of the nucleotide sequences used by these TCR γ/δ T cells demonstrated a diverse set of VDJC gene rearrangements, characteristic of a superantigen response. Further evidence for T-cell reactivity in ITP came from the observations that isolated T-cell clones showed in vitro proliferation against allogeneic platelets, the numbers of Vβ8+ T cells were elevated, and platelet stimulation resulted in measurable IL-2 secretion.[126] These results provided the first evidence that patients with ITP have platelet-reactive T lymphocytes identifiable at the clonal level.

T-cell proliferative responses to platelet membrane glycoproteins were examined in 21 patients with chronic ITP or SLE, with or without thrombocytopenia, and 10 healthy donors.[127] T cells from all subjects failed to respond to detergent-soluble native glycoproteins, but tryptic peptides of integrin $\alpha_{IIb}\beta_3$ stimulated T cells from nearly all subjects, including the normal individuals. Similar T-cell proliferation in healthy individuals in response to $\alpha_{IIb}\beta_3$ had been described previously by Filion and colleagues.[128] These findings implied that some autoreactive T cells, directed against membrane antigens present on platelets, were not necessarily eliminated by intrathymic deletion but are present in a suppressed state in normal individuals. In the ITP patients, the T-cell response was restricted by HLA-DR, the responding T cells had a CD4+ phenotype, and the proliferation was accelerated relative to normal subjects, suggesting in vivo T-cell activation.[128] None of the peripheral blood mononuclear cell culture supernatants from healthy donors contained a significant amount of IgG anti-$\alpha_{IIb}\beta_3$ antibody, but all showed trypsin-digested $\alpha_{IIb}\beta_3$-induced T-cell proliferation. These findings led to the conclusion that CD4+ HLA-DR-restricted T cells reactive with $\alpha_{IIb}\beta_3$ epitopes are involved in production of antiplatelet autoantibody and are implicated in the pathogenesis of chronic ITP.

T-cell activation, proliferation, and T-B cell cognate recognition in response to specific autoantigens require signaling through a variety of membrane immune receptors. The MHC and TCR were recognized as major receptors for many years, but it is now understood that there are accessory molecules that facilitate or modulate the response and that these are potential therapeutic targets in treating ITP.[119,125,129] Antigen-presenting cells, which include B cells as well as macrophages, require specific recognition and signaling through the receptors B7, LFA-3, and ICAM-1, whereas the T cell employs the receptors CD28, LFA-1, and CD2.[125,130] Increased expression of CD40L on platelets may be a normal response of platelets activated by infection or other inflammatory mediators. However, this increase in CD40L has the potential to drive B-cell production of platelet autoantibody. Two research groups reported that administration of a humanized anti-CD40L antibody resulted in increased T-cell tolerance in patients with ITP, suggesting that blockade of CD40L may prove to be a useful therapeutic approach.[125,131] Likewise, Zimmerman and colleagues[132] reported that IVIG and dexamethasone induced an alteration of T-lymphocyte subsets and suppression of T-lymphocyte proliferation in vitro in ITP patients. Although equally effective in the treatment of ITP in children, they found that high-titer anti-D immunoglobulin caused significantly less inhibition than IVIG or dexamethasone in children with chronic ITP, and anti-D did not affect T-lymphocyte subsets.

Cytokines

Considerable work has been focused on the measurement of cytokines in ITP in an effort to further characterize the influence of T-helper subsets (Th0, Th1, and Th2) in the autoimmune etiology of this disease.[130,133] Unfortunately, the majority of these studies draw conclusions based on a single cytokine profile determination. Because cytokine signaling is dynamic and may fluctuate rapidly, it is difficult to draw valid conclusions from a single assay. In addition, the presence of soluble cytokine receptors may confound the results if these are not measured directly in parallel with cytokines. To distinguish a normal versus pathologic immune response in both acute and chronic ITP, multiple samples must be obtained over time, with attention paid to both the cytokines and their soluble receptors. The referenced studies have incorporated multiple samples and controls in the overall analysis. Nonetheless, a degree of disparity remains between the results obtained in children[57] versus those found in adults,[134,135] which likely reflects a difference in the primary pathophysiology of the thrombocytopenia.

In pediatric ITP patients, a Th1 type of cytokine response is the customary finding, characterized by very low IL-4 and IL-6, but elevated levels of IL-2, interferon-γ, and TNF-β.[136] In adults with chronic ITP, malignancy associated with ITP, or the autoimmune lymphoproliferation syndrome associated with defects in the Fas apoptosis pathway, there are elevated levels of IL-10, IL-11, IL-6, and IL-13.[137–140] One would expect that successful therapy might be associated with favorable changes in cytokine profiles. Although many treatment regimens have been efficacious in ITP, in only a few instances has there been documentation of cytokine profile changes following therapeutic intervention with the most common drugs, IVIG and anti-D immunoglobulin.[57,132,141]

Bussel and coworkers[141] compared the changes in IL-6, IL-10, MCP-1, and TNF-α cytokine levels after treatment with IVIG and anti-D in thrombocytopenic adults. There was an increase in all but TNF-α within 2 hours after administration of anti-D. After IVIG, there was a significant increase in IL-10 levels within 4 hours (but not 2 hours) post-therapy. It was concluded that the early increase in these macrophage-synthesized cytokines following anti-D administration reflects the substantial interaction of antibody-coated erythrocytes with macrophages.[132] Mouzaki and coworkers measured a panel of Th0-, Th1-, and Th2-related cytokines over 0.5 to 5 years following the onset of ITP and found that patients who did not convert from a Th1- to Th2-dominant cytokine profile were more likely to have a chronic or relapsing course of thrombocytopenia.[57] Interestingly, the same group of researchers found that adults with ITP were likely to have a striking polarization toward Th1 phenotype, but this profile did not change in response to disease status over time or with treatment.[135] This is in contrast to another group who found an association between improved platelet count and disease outcome in adults with a lower Th1/Th2 ratio.[134] Again, these differences may arise from disparities in population, differences in timing and technology of assays, and differences in treatment regimens, which vary greatly between centers. A better understanding of the relevance of Th1/Th2 ratio and cytokine profiles will emerge with the establishment of coordinated clinical trials and the incorporation into such trials of the newly recognized components of the cellular immune response, such as CD4+25+ (Treg) cells and the antigen-specific idiotypic network.

DRUG-INDUCED IMMUNE THROMBOCYTOPENIA (QUININE/ QUINIDINE PURPURA)

Although drug-induced immune thrombocytopenia (DITP) may be a complication of therapy employing a variety of drugs, it is most frequently seen in the United States with the administration of quinine and quinidine.[142] It has been proposed that the following criteria be met before an individual can be considered to have DITP: the patient is not thrombocytopenic before administration of the drug; thrombocytopenia follows drug ingestion and begins to reverse shortly after cessation of drug; thrombocytopenia does not recur after cessation of drug treatment; and all other causes of thrombocytopenia are ruled out.[143]

Cumulative evidence now favors a mechanism whereby the drug induces the expression of a neoantigen on the platelet surface[144] that is recognized by circulating antibodies only in the presence of the drug. The observation that platelets from BSS patients (lacking Ib-IX-V) failed to lyse in the presence of drug-dependent antibody, specific drug, and complement, was the first indication that a specific platelet antigen is recognized by such antibodies.[145] This finding led other laboratories to confirm that purified GPIb/IX would compete for drug plus antibody and was therefore likely to contain the antigenic epitope in question. Evidence of direct binding of such antibodies to GPIb/IX was first provided by Chong and coworkers,[146] and Berndt and coworkers[147] established that the complex of both Ib and IX is likely required for maximum antigen expression.

Chong and coworkers[148] showed that one quinine-dependent antibody binds to an epitope on the amino-terminal portion of Ibα, and five other quinine-dependent antibodies recognize a complex-specific epitope proximal to the membrane-associated region of GPIb/IX. Each of six quinidine-dependent antibodies contained two specificities, one for the same Ib/IX complex epitope described above, the other for IX alone. Additional observations were that antibodies reactive with GPIb/IX are more predominant (12/12 patients) than those that bind $\alpha_{IIb}\beta_3$ (3/12 patients), and antibodies specific for Ib-IX-V are present in titers 8- to 32-fold higher than the corresponding antibodies that bind to $\alpha_{IIb}\beta_3$ in the same patient samples. In each case, those antibodies that bound to Ib-IX-V were distinct from those that recognized $\alpha_{IIb}\beta_3$. The specificity of quinine- and quinidine-dependent antibodies for a conformation-sensitive epitope(s) on the GPIX component of the complex was confirmed by Lopez and colleagues[149] using monoclonal antibody inhibition assays. Rifampicin-dependent antibodies bind to a similar or identical epitope on GPIX as that recognized by quinine-dependent antibodies.[150]

Regions of $\alpha_{IIb}\beta_3$ that bind to quinine- or quinidine-dependent antibodies have also been further localized by Visentin and colleagues.[151] Of 13 patient sera containing such antibodies, 10 were reactive with both GPIb-IX and $\alpha_{IIb}\beta_3$, 2 reacted with Ib-IX alone, and 1 reacted with $\alpha_{IIb}\beta_3$ alone. Again, in those sera where both specificities were identified, the anti-Ib-IX-V antibodies were distinct from those that bound to $\alpha_{IIb}\beta_3$. Seven sera containing anti-$\alpha_{IIb}\beta_3$ antibodies were further characterized: Three bound only to the $\alpha_{IIb}\beta_3$ complex, one bound to α_{IIb} alone, and three bound to β_3 alone. On β_3, a 17-amino acid sequence in the "hybrid" and PSI homology domains of β_3 is a dominant epitope.[144] In the case of sulfonamide-induced immune thrombocytopenia,[152] the causative antibodies are almost exclusively specific for calcium-dependent (complex-specific) epitopes on the integrin $\alpha_{IIb}\beta_3$.

In addition, sera from 20 patients with quinine-induced thrombocytopenia and 5 patients with DITP following intake of carbimazole were found to have drug-dependent antibodies specific for PECAM-1.[153] Thus, integrin $\alpha_{IIb}\beta_3$ and the GPIb-IX-V complex are not the only antigenic targets in DITP.

One additional intriguing aspect of certain cases of DITP is worthy of mention, because it may have an important bearing on our understanding of the autoimmune response to platelets in general. Based on anecdotal evidence, it has been suspected that some cases of chronic ITP[154] are initiated in clinical situations that, from all appearances, could be classified as DITP. The only difference is that selected autoantibodies persist long after exposure to the insulting drug. Direct evidence to support this contention was obtained by Nieminen and Kekomäki.[155] In that report, it was found that the DITP patients with GPIb/IX-specific antibodies, despite a very intense and acute thrombocytopenia, recovered promptly after drug removal. On the other hand, DITP patients with more prolonged thrombocytopenia and persistently elevated platelet immunoglobulins, more than 1 month after drug removal, had antibodies that reacted with additional target antigens, including integrin $\alpha_{IIb}\beta_3$. To better understand the pathogenesis of both DITP and classic ITP, in the future it may become important to distinguish the acute but readily reversible clinical situation that we accept as DITP from the more complex disease situation that may be initiated by drug exposure but evolves into a more classic form of ITP.

Compounds that inhibit the binding of fibrinogen to the platelet receptor $\alpha_{IIb}\beta_3$ are a novel group of antithrombotics that are being used more frequently to inhibit acute episodes of thrombosis or restenosis in patients with cardiovascular disease.[156] Thrombocytopenia has been observed within hours of the initiation of treatment with such inhibitors and has become a recognized side effect of this drug therapy. Accumulated evidence argues that drug-dependent antibodies may be responsible for platelet destruction in a substantial portion of the affected recipients. Because these antibodies are often detected in persons not previously exposed to the inhibitor drug, there is a high likelihood that thrombocytopenia is caused by naturally occurring or pre-existing antibodies. This complication of antithrombotic therapy warrants further investigation.

HEPARIN-ASSOCIATED IMMUNE THROMBOCYTOPENIA

Heparin-induced thrombocytopenia (HIT) is a life-threatening condition that occurs in 1% to 5% of patients treated with unfractionated high-molecular-weight heparin. In these patients, use of high-molecular-weight heparin results in thrombocytopenia and can be associated with life-threatening thrombotic complications. Unlike quinine- or quinidine-dependent antibodies, the actual binding of heparin-dependent antibodies to the platelet surface appears to be of very low affinity, and was difficult to demonstrate in earlier studies, until the report of Lynch and Howe.[157] It was also determined that heparin-dependent antibodies differ from other forms of drug-dependent antibodies in that they can often be *activating*, causing not only thrombocytopenia, but also heparin-dependent platelet aggregation, thromboxane synthesis, and granule release that can be quantitated by preloading platelets with [^{14}C]serotonin. The consequences of HIT therefore are multiplied by often serious thrombotic complications. Approximately 30% of these patients die, with an additional 20% developing vascular occlusions that result in gangrene and subsequent amputation.[158]

Although the precise mechanism of heparin-dependent antibodies binding to platelets eluded investigators for many years, it was generally accepted that the activating properties of heparin-dependent antibodies must be mediated by Fc-dependent binding to platelets. In this regard, Kelton and colleagues[159] showed that the platelet release reaction induced by heparin-dependent antibodies could be blocked by pretreating platelets with human or goat IgG Fc fragments, Adelman and colleagues showed that the Fab regions of heparin-dependent antibodies alone are not sufficient to cause platelet activation,[160] Chong and colleagues[161] showed that purified rabbit IgG and its Fc, but not Fab, fragments markedly inhibited platelet aggregation induced by heparin-dependent antibodies, and a number of groups observed that the monoclonal anti-Fc receptor antibody, IV.3, could block platelet activation by HDA.[159,162]

It is now accepted that HIT is caused by antibody specific for a complex of heparin (H) and platelet factor 4 (PF4). H–PF4 complexes, which are detected in 85% of patients with HIT,[163] can bind to the membrane of platelets[164–166] or endothelial cells,[164] leading directly to thrombocytopenia in the former case. In those cases in which the heparin-dependent antibodies are IgG, the Fc portion can crosslink to the platelet FcγRIIA receptor, inducing platelet activation, release, aggregation, and thrombosis.[164,167,168] However, HIT can also be associated with antibodies of IgM and IgA isotypes,[169] in which case the Fc(μ)R of lymphocytes or the Fc(α)R of monocytes and neutrophils, as well as complement activation, may play a role in the pathology of this disorder.

Poncz[170] has proposed that this disease is probably initiated by an excessive release of platelet PF4, which then binds to the platelet membrane or other vascular cell membranes and initiates HIT by three mechanisms that are not mutually exclusive. First, the infused heparin could neutralize a proportion of membrane surface PF4, thus enhancing local thrombosis. Second, the excess PF4 could be mobilized into H–PF4 complexes that stimulate HIT antibody production. Third, the remaining PF4 that has been complexed with heparin on the vascular surfaces could be bound by HIT antibodies and through an FcγRII-mediated reaction, lead to additional platelet activation, thrombosis, and inflammation. When present at equimolar concentrations, unfractionated heparin and tetrameric PF4 can form ultralarge (>670 kDa) complexes that are particularly more reactive with respect to binding to HIT antibodies and capacity to promote FcγRII-dependent platelet activation.[171] These processes would stimulate further PF4 release, exacerbating the clinical manifestations.

Alternative protein targets may be involved in selected cases of HIT. For example, in 9 of 15 patients with HIT that lacked detectable antibodies to H–PF4 complexes, Amiral and coworkers[172] found evidence of autoantibodies specific for the chemokines neutrophil-activating peptide 2 (NAP2) and IL-8. PF4 is about 60% homologous to NAP2 and 40% homologous to IL-8, leading to the proposal that HIT involving these proteins could proceed along a mechanism similar to that invoked for PF4.

REFERENCES

1. Hynes RO. Integrins: Bidirectional, allosteric signaling machines. Cell 2002;110:673–687.
2. Nurden AT, Nurden P. Inherited defects of platelet function. Rev Clin Exp Hematol 2001;5:314–334.
3. Kunicki TJ. The influence of platelet collagen receptor polymorphisms in hemostasis and thrombotic disease. Arterioscler Thromb Vasc Biol 2002;22:14–20.
4. Kritzik M, Savage B, Nugent DJ, et al. Nucleotide polymorphisms in the α2 gene define multiple alleles which are associated with differences in platelet α2β1. Blood 1998;92:2382–2388.
5. Moroi M, Jung SM, Shinmyozu K, et al. Analysis of platelet adhesion to a collagen-coated surface under flow cond itions: the involvement of glycoprotein VI in the platelet adhesion. Blood 1996;88:2081–2092.
6. Kehrel B, Wierwille S, Clemetson KJ, et al. Glycoprotein VI is a major collagen receptor for platelet activation: it recognizes the platelet-activating quaternary structure of collagen, whereas CD36, glycoprotein IIb/IIIa, and von Willebrand factor do not. Blood 1998;91:491–499.
7. Nieuwenhuis HK, Akkerman JWN, Houdijk WPM, Sixma JJ. Human blood platelets showing no response to collagen fail to express surface glycoprotein Ia. Nature 1985;318:470–472.
8. Kehrel B, Balleisen L, Kokott R, et al. Deficiency of intact thrombospondin and membrane glycoprotein Ia in platelets with defective collagen-induced aggregation and spontaneous loss of disorder. Blood 1988;71:1074–1078.
9. Piotrowicz RS, Orchekowski RP, Nugent DJ, et al. Glycoprotein Ic-IIa functions as an activation-independent fibronectin receptor on human platelets. J Cell Biol 1988;106:1359–1364.
10. Sonnenberg A, Modderman PW, Hogervorst F. Laminin receptor on platelets is the integrin VLA-6. Nature 1988;336:487–489.
11. Modderman PW, Admiraal LG, Sonnenberg A, Von dem Borne AEGK. Glycoproteins V and Ib-IX form a noncovalent complex in the platelet membrane. J Biol Chem 1992;267:364–369.
12. Savage B, Almus-Jacobs F, Ruggeri ZM. Specific synergy of multiple substrate–receptor interactions in platelet thrombus formation under flow. Cell 1998;94:657–666.
13. Vicente V, Houghten RA, Ruggeri ZM. Identification of a site in the α chain of platelet glycoprotein Ib that participates in von Willebrand factor binding. J Biol Chem 1990;265:274–280.
14. Liang HP, Morel-Kopp MC, Clemetson JM, et al. A common ancestral glycoprotein (GP) 9 1828A<G (Asn45Ser) gene mutation occurring in European families from Australia and Northern Europe with Bernard-Soulier syndrome (BSS). Thromb Haemost 2005;94:599–605.
15. von dem Borne AEGKr. Nomenclature of platelet antigen systems. Br J Haematol 1990;74:239–240.
16. Kaplan C. Alloimmune thrombocytopenia of the fetus and the newborn. Blood Rev 2002;16:69–72.
17. Valentin N, Vergracht A, Bignon JD, et al. HLA-Drw52a is involved in alloimmunization against PL-A1 antigen. Human Immunol 1990;27:73–79.
18. L'Abbé D, Tremblay L, Filion M, et al. Alloimmunization to platelet antigen HPA-1a (PI[A1]) is strongly associated with both HLA-DRB3*0101 and HLA-DQB1*0201. Hum Immunol 1992;34:107–114.
19. Maslanka K, Yassai M, Gorski J. Molecular identification of T cells that respond in a primary buk culture to a peptide derived from a platelet glycoprotein implicated in neonatal alloimmune thrombocytopenia. J Clin Invest 1996;98:1802–1808.
20. Kuijpers RWAM, von dem Borne AE, Kifel V, et al. Leucine 33-Proline 33 substitution in human platelet glycoprotein IIIa determines HLA-DRw52a (Dw24) association of the immune response against HPA-1a (Zw[a]/PI[A1]) and HPA-1b (Zw[b]/PI[A2]). Hum Immunol 1992;34:253–256.
21. Westman P, Hashemi-Tavoularis S, Blanchette V, et al. Material DRB1*1501, DQA1*0102,DQB1*0602 haplotype in fetomaternal alloimmunization against human platelet alloantigen HPA-6b (GPIIIa-Gln489). Tissue Antigens 1997;50:113–118.
22. Mueller-Eckhardt C, Kiefel V, Grubert A, et al. 348 cases of suspected neonatal alloimmune thrombocytopenia. Lancet 1989;1:363–366.
23. McGrath K, Minchinton R, Cunningham I, Ayberk H. Platelet anti-Bak[b] antibody associated with neonatal alloimmune thrombocytopenia. Vox Sang 1989;57:182–184.
24. Shibata Y, Matsuda I, Miyaji T, Ichikawa Y. Yuk[a], a new platelet antigen involved in two cases of neonatal alloimmune thrombocytopenia. Vox Sang 1986;50:177–180.
25. von dem Borne A, von Riesz E, Verheugt F, et al. Bak[a], a new platelet-specific antigen involved in neonatal Alloimmune thrombocytopenia. Vox Sang 1980;39:113–120.
26. Mueller-Eckhardt C, Becker T, Weishet M, et al. Neonatal alloimmune thrombocytopenia due to fetomaternal Zw[b] incompatability. Vox Sang 1986;50:94–96.
27. Grenet P, Dausset J, Dugas M, et al. Purpura thrombopenique neonatal avec isoimmunisation foeto-maternelle anti-Ko[a]. Arch Fr Pediatr 1965;22:1165–1174.
28. Reznikoff-Etievant MF, Dangu C, Lobet R. HLA-B8 antigen and anti-P1[A1] alloimmunization. Tissue Antigens 1981;18:66–68.
29. Mueller-Eckhardt C. HLA-B8 antigen and anti-P1[A1] alloimmunization. Tissue Antigens 1982;19:154–158.
30. Beer J, Coller BS. Evidence that platelet glycoprotein IIIa has a large disulfide- bonded loop that is susceptible to proteolytic cleavage. J Biol Chem 1989;264:17564–17573.
31. Honda S, Honda Y, Ruan C, Kunicki TJ. The impact of three-dimensional structure on the expression of PI[A1] alloantigens on human integrin β3. Blood 1995;86:234–242.
32. Bowditch RD, Tani P, McMillan R. Reactivity of autoantibodies from chronic ITP patients with recombinant glycoprotein IIIa peptides. Br J Haematol 1995;91:178–184.
33. Furihata K, Nugent DJ, Bissonette A, et al. On the association of the platelet-specific alloantigen, Pen[a], with glycoprotein IIIa. Evidence for heterogeneity of glycoprotein IIIa. J Clin Invest 1987;80:1624–1630.
34. Newman PJ, Kawai Y, Montgomery RR, Kunicki TJ. Synthesis by cultured human umbilical vein endothelial cells of two proteins structurally and immunologically related to platelet membrane glycoproteins IIb and IIIa. J Cell Biol 1986;103:81–86.
35. Kuijpers RWAM, Faber NM, Cuypers HTM, et al. NH2-terminal globular domain of human platelet glycoprotein Iba hs a Methionine145T hreonine145 amino acid polymorphism, which is associated with the HPA-2 (Ko) alloantigens. J Clin Invest 1992;89:381–384.
36. Di Paola J, Jugessur A, Goldman T, et al. Platelet glycoprotein Ibα and integrin αβ polymorphisms: gene frequencies and linkage disequilibrium in a population diversity panel. J Thromb Haemost 2005; 3:1511–1521.
37. Lyman S, Aster RH, Visentin GP, Newman PJ. Polymorphism of human platelet membrane glycoprotein IIb associated with the Bak[a]/Bak[b] alloantigen system. Blood 1990;75:2343–2348.
38. Kiefel V, Santoso S, Katzmann B, Mueller-Eckhart C. The Br[a]/Br[b] alloantigen system on human platelets. Blood 1989;73:2219–2223.

39. Kiefel V, Santoso S, Weisheit M, Mueller-Eckhardt C. Monoclonal antibody-specific immobilization of platelet antigens (MAIPA): a new tool for the identification of platelet-reactive antibodies. Blood 1987;70:1732–1733.
40. Panzer S, Janisiw M, Fischer G, Jilma B. The platelet α2-Integrin (GPIa) nucleotide-807 polymorphism is not associated with a risk for maternal-fetal human platelet antigen-5 incompatibility. Ann Hematol 2000;79:296–298.
41. Kelton JG, Smith JW, Horsewood P, et al. Gov$^{a/b}$ alloantigen system on human platelets. Blood 1990;75:2172–2176.
42. Bordin JO, Kelton JG, Warner MN, et al. Maternal immunization to Gov system alloantigens on human platelets. Transfusion 1997;37: 823–828.
43. Schuh AC, Watkins NA, Nguyen Q, et al. A Tyrosine703Serine polymorphism of CD109 defines the Gov platelet alloantigens. Blood 2002;99:1692–1698.
44. Ertel K, Al Tawil M, Santoso S, Kroll H. Relevance of the HPA-15 (Gov) polymorphism on CD109 in alloimmune thrombocytopenic syndromes. Transfusion 2005;45:366–373.
45. Gruel Y, Brojer E, Nugent DJ, Kunicki TJ. Further characterization of the thrombasthenia-related idiotype OG. Anti-idiotype defines a novel epitope(s) shared by fibrinogen B β chain, vitronectin and von Willebrand factor and required for binding to β3. J Exp Med 1995;180:2259–2267.
46. Ishida F, Gruel Y, Brojer E, et al. Repertoire cloning of a human IgG inhibitor of $\alpha_{IIb}\beta_3$ function. The OG idiotype. Mol Immunol 1995;32:613–622.
47. Tobelem G, Levy-Toledano S, Bredoux R, et al. New approach to determination of specific functions of platelet membrane sites. Nature 1976;263:427–429.
48. Curtis BR, Ali S, Glazier AM, et al. Isoimmunization against CD36 (glycoprotein IV): description of four cases of neonatal isoimmune thrombocytopenia and brief review of the literature. Transfusion 2002;42:1173–1179.
49. Beardsley DS. Pathophysiology of immune thrombocytopenic purpura. Blood Rev 2002;16:13–14.
50. Cines DB, Blanchette VS. Immune thrombocytopenic purpura. NEJM 2002;346:995–1008.
51. Niessner H, Clemetson KJ, Panzer S, et al. Acquired thrombasthenia due to GPIIb/IIIa-specific platelet autoantibodies. Blood 1986;68:571–576.
52. Balduini C, Grignani G, Sinigaglia F, et al. Severe platelet dysfunction in a patient with autoantibodies against membrane glycoproteins IIb/IIIa. Haemostasis 1987;7:98–104.
53. Berchtold P, McMillan R, Tani P, et al. Autoantibodies against platelet membrane glycoproteins in children with acute and chronic immune thrombocytopenic purpura. Blood 1989;74:1600–1602.
54. Winiarski J. IgG and IgM antibodies to platelet membrane glycoprotein antigens in acute childhood idiopathic thrombocytopenic purpura. Br J Haematol 1989;73:88–92.
55. Yang R, Han ZC. Pathogenesis and management of chronic idiopathic thrombocytopenic purpura: an update. Int J Hematol 2000;71:18–24.
56. Semple JW. Immune pathophysiology of autoimmune thrombocytopenic purpura. Blood Rev 2002;16:9–12.
57. Mouzaki A, Theodoropoulou M, Gianakopoulos I, et al. Expression patterns of Th1 and Th2 cytokine genes in childhood Idiopathic Thrombocytopenic Purpura (ITP) at Presentation and their Modulation by intravenous immunoglobulin G (IVIg) treatment: their role in prognosis. Blood 2002;100:1774–1779.
58. McMillan R, Luiken GA, Levy R, et al. Antibody against megakaryocytes in idiopathic thrombocytopenic purpura. JAMA 1978;239:2460–2462.
59. Ballem PJ, Segal GM, Stratton JR, et al. Mechanisms of thrombocytopenia in chronic autoimmune thrombocytopenic purpura. Evidence of both impaired platelet production and increased platelet clearance. J Clin Invest 1987;80:33–40.
60. Abgrall JF, Berthou C, Sensebe L, et al. Decreased in vitro megakaryocyte colony formation in chronic idiopathic thrombocytopenic purpura. Br J Haematol 1993;85:803–804.
61. Chang M, Nakagawa PA, Williams SA, et al. Immune thrombocytopenic purpura (ITP) plasma and purified ITP monoclonal autoantibodies inhibit megakaryocytopoiesis in vitro. Blood 2003;102:887–895.
62. Takahashi R, Sekine N, Nakatake T. Influence of monoclonal antiplatelet glycoprotein antibodies on in vitro human megakaryocyte colony formation and proplatelet formation. Blood 1999;93:1951–1958.
63. McMillan R, Wang L, Tomer A, et al. Suppression of in vitro megakaryocyte production by antiplatelet autoantibodies from adult patients with chronic ITP. Blood 2004;103:1364–1369.
64. Houwerzijl EJ, Blom NR, van der Want JJ, et al. Ultrastructural study shows morphologic features of apoptosis and para-apoptosis in megakaryocytes from patients with idiopathic thrombocytopenic purpura. Blood 2004;103:500–506.
65. Nieswandt B, Bergmeier W, Rackebrandt K, et al. Identification of critical antigen-specific mechanisms in the development of immune thrombocytopenic purpura in mice. Blood 2000;96:2520–2527.
66. McMillan R. Autoantibodies and autoantigens in chronic immune thrombocytopenic purpura. Semin Hematol 2000;37:239–248.
67. Van Leeuwen EF, van der Ven JTM, Engelfriet CP, von dem Borne AEGKr. Specificity of autoantibodies in autoimmune thrombocytopenia. Blood 1982;59:23–29.
68. McMillan R. The role of antiplatelet autoantibody assays in the diagnosis of immune thrombocytopenic purpura. Curr Hematol Rep 2005;4:160–165.
69. Kekomaki R, Dawson B, McFarland J, Kunicki TJ. Localization of human platelet autoantigens to the cysteine-rich region of glycoprotein IIIa. J Clin Invest 1991;88:847–854.
70. Beardsley DJ, Tang C, Chen BG, et al. The disulfide-rich region of platelet glycoprotein (GP) IIIa contains hydrophilic peptide sequences that bind anti-GPIIIa autoantibodies from patients with immune thrombocytopenic purpura (ITP). Biophys Chem 2003;105:503–515.
71. Fujisawa K, Tani P, McMillan R. Platelet-associated antibody to glycoprotein IIb/IIIa from chronic immune thrombocytopenic purpura patients often binds to divalent cation-dependent antigens. Blood 1993;81:1284–1289.
72. Nugent DJ, Kunicki TJ, Berglund C, Bernstein ID. A human monoclonal autoantibody recognizes a neoantigen on glycoprotein IIIA expressed on stored and activated platelets. Blood 1987;70:16–22.
73. Kunicki TJ, Furihata K, Kekomaki R, et al. A human monoclonal autoantibody specific for human platelet glycoprotein IIb (integrin α_{IIb}) heavy chain. Hum Antibodies Hybridomas 1990;1:83–95.
74. Kelton JG, Carter CJ, Rodger C, et al. The relationship among platelet-associated IgG, platelet lifespan, and reticuloendothelial cell function. Blood 1984;63:1434–1438.
75. Kay MM. Appearance of a terminal differentiation antigen on senescent and damaged cells and its implications for physiologic autoantibodies. Biomembranes 1983;11:119–150.
76. Khansari N, Fudenberg HH. Immune elimination of autologous senescent erythrocytes by Kupffer Cells in vivo. Cell Immunol 1983;80: 426–430.
77. Sinha TK, Horsewood P, Koltan JG. Nonimmune and immune binding of IgG to platelets in an animal model of immune thrombocytopenia. Blood 1991;78:344a.
78. Nardi MA, Liu LX, Karpatkin S. GPIIIa-49–66 is a major pathophysiologically relevant antigenic determinant for anti-platelet GPIIIa of HIV-1-related immunologic thrombocytopenia. Proc Natl Acad Sci USA 1997;94:7589–7594.
79. Bowditch RD, Tani P, Fong KC, McMillan R. Characterization of autoantigenic epitopes on platelet glycoprotein IIb/IIIa using random peptide libraries. Blood 1996;12:4579–4584.
80. Gevorkian G, Manoutcharian K, Govezensky T, et al. Identification of mimotopes of platelet autoantigens associated with autoimmune thrombocytopenic purpura. J Autoimmun 2000;15:33–40.
81. McMillan R, Lopez-Dee J, Loftus JC. Autoantibodies to $\alpha_{IIb}\beta_3$ in patients with chronic immune thrombocytopenic purpura bind primarily to epitopes on α_{IIb}. Blood 2001;97:2171–2172.
82. Tomiyama Y, Kurata Y, Mizutani H, et al. Platelet glycoprotein IIb as a target antigen in two patients with chronic idiopathic thrombycytopenic purpura. Br J Haematol 1987;66:535–538.
83. Tomiyama Y, Kurata Y, Shibata Y, et al. Immunochemical characterization of an autoantigen on platelet glycoprotein IIb in chronic ITP: Comparison with the Bak^a alloantigen. Br J Haematol 1989;71:76–83.
84. van Vliet H, Kappers-Klunne M, Abels J. Pseudothrombocytopenia: A cold antibody against platelet glycoprotein GPIIb. Br J Haematol 1986;62:501–511.
85. Gevorkian G, Manoutcharian K, Almagro JC, et al. Identification of autoimmune thrombocytopenic purpura-related epitopes using phage-display peptide library. Clin Immunol Immunopathol 1998;86: 305–309.
86. Kosugi S, Tomiyama Y, Honda S, et al. Platelet-associated anti-GPIIb-IIIa autoantibodies in chronic immune thrombocytopenic purpura recognizing epitopes close to the ligand-binding site of glycoprotein (GP) IIb. Blood 2001;98:1819–1827.
87. Shadle PJ, Barondes SH. Platelet–collagen adhesion: Evidence for participation of antigenically distinct entities. J Cell Biol 1984;99:2048–2055.
88. Varon D, Karpatkin S. A monoclonal antiplatelet antibody with decreased reactivity for autoimmune thrombocytopenic platelets. Proc Natl Acad Sci USA 1983;80:6992–6995.
89. Tsubakio T, Tani P, Woods VL, McMillan R. Autoantibodies against platelet GPIIb/IIIa in chronic ITP react with different epitopes. Br J Haematol 1987;67:345–348.

90. Hiraiwa A, Nugent DJ, Milner EB. Sequence analysis of monoclonal antibodies derived from a patient with idiopathic thrombocytopenic purpura. Autoimmunity 1990;8:107–113.
91. Kunicki TJ, Plow EF, Kekomaki R, Nugent DJ. A human monoclonal autoantibody 2E7 is specific for a peptide sequence of platelet glycoprotein IIb: Localization of the epitope to IIb231–238 with an immunodominant Trp-235. J Autoimmun 1991;4:415–431.
92. Berchtold P, Dale GL, Tani P, McMillan R. Inhibition of autoantibody binding to platelet glycoprotein IIb/IIIa by anti-idiotypic antibodies in intravenous immunoglobulin. Blood 1989;74:2414–2417.
93. Nugent DJ. Human monoclonal antibodies in the characterization of platelet antigens. In Kunicki TJ, George JN (eds). Platelet Immunobiology: Molecular and Clinical Aspects. Philadelphia, J.B. Lippincott, 1989, pp 123–148.
94. He R, Reid DM, Jones CE, Shulman NR. Extracellular epitopes of platelet glycoprotein Iba reactive with serum antibodies from patients with chronic idiopathic thrombocytopenic purpura. Blood 1995;86:3789–3796.
95. Devine DV, Curie MS, Rosse WF, Greenberg CS. Pseudo-Bernard-Soulier syndrome: Thrombocytopenia caused by autoantibody to platelet glycoprotein Ib. Blood 1987;70:428–431.
96. Mayer JL, Beardsley DS. Varicella-associated thrombocytopenia: Autoantibodies against platelet surface glycoprotein V. Pediatr Res 1996;40:615–619.
97. Wright JF, Blanchette VS, Wang H, et al. Characterization of platelet-reactive antibodies in children with varicella-associated acute immune thrombocytopenic purpura (ITP). Br J Haematol 1996;95:145–152.
98. Beardsley DS, Spiegel JE, Jacobs MM, et al. Platelet membrane glycoprotein IIIa contains target antigens that bind anti-platelet antibodies in immune thrombocytopenias. J Clin Invest 1984;74:1701–1707.
99. Beardsley DJS, Ho J, Beyer EC. Varicella-associated thrombocytopenia: Antibodies against an 85-kDa thrombin-sensitive protein (?GPV). Blood 1985;66(Suppl 1):1030.
100. Deckmyn H, Chew SL, Vermylen L. Lack of platelet response to collagen associated with an autoantibody against glycoprotein Ia: a novel cause of acquired qualitative platelet dysfunction. Thromb Haemost 1990;64:74–79.
101. Dromigny A, Triadou P, Lesavre P, et al. Lack of platelet response to collagen associated with autoantibodies against glycoprotein (GP) Ia/IIa and Ib/IX leading to the discovery of SLE. Hematol Cell Ther 1996;38:355–357.
102. Sugiyama T, Ishibashi T, Okuma M. Functional role of the antigen recognized by an antiplatelet antibody specific for a putative collagen receptor in platelet–collagen interaction. Int J Hematol 1993;58:99–104.
103. Moroi M, Jung SM, Okuma M, Shinmyozu K. A patient with platelets deficient in glycoprotein VI that lack both collagen-induced aggregation and adhesion. J Clin Invest 1989;84:1440.
104. Boylan B, Chen H, Rathore V, et al. Anti-GPVI-associated ITP: An acquired platelet disorder caused by autoantibody-mediated clearance of the GPVI/FcRγ-chain complex from the human platelet surface. Blood 2004;104:1350–1355.
105. Nieswandt B, Schulte V, Bergmeier W, et al. Long-term antithrombotic protection by in vivo depletion of platelet glycoprotein VI in mice. J Exp Med 2001;193:459–470.
106. Koerner TAW, Weinfeld HM, Bullard LSB, Williams LCJ. Antibodies against platelet glycosphingolipids: detection in serum by quantitative HPTLC-autoradiography and association with autoimmune and alloimmune processes. Blood 1989;74:274–284.
107. Van Vliet HHDM, Kappers-Klunne MC, van der Hel JWB, Abels J. Antibodies against glycosphingolipids in sera of patients with idiopathic thrombocytopenic purpura. Br J Haematol 1987;67:103–108.
108. Lewis DC, Meyers KM. Studies of platelet-bound and serum platelet-bindable immunoglobulins in dogs with idiopathic thrombocytopenic purpura. Exp Hematol 1996;24(6):696–701.
109. Kazatchkine MD, Dietrich G, Hurez V, et al. V region-mediated selection of autoreactive repertoires by intravenous immunoglobulin (IVIg). Immunol Rev 1994;139:79–107.
110. Rossi F, Kazatchkine MD. Antiidiotypes against autoantibodies in pooled normal human polyspecific Ig. J Immunol 1989;143:4104–4109.
111. Dietrich G, Kaveri SV, Kazatchkine MD. A V region-connected autoreactive subfraction of normal human serum immunoglobulin G. Eur J Immunol 1992;22:1701–1706.
112. Hurez V, Kaveri SV, Kazatchkine MD. Expression and control of the natural autoreactive IgG repertoire in normal human serum. Eur J Immunol 1993;23:783–789.
113. Hurez V, Dietrich G, Kaveri SV, Kazatchkine MD. Polyreactivity is a property of natural and disease-associated human autoantibodies. Scand J Immunol 1993;38:190–196.
114. Mouthon L, Haury M, Lacroix-Desmazes S, et al. Analysis of the normal human IgG antibody repertoire. Evidence that IgG autoantibodies of healthy adults recognize a limited and conserved set of protein antigens in homologous tissues. J Immunol 1995;154:5769–5778.
115. Coutinho A, Kazatchkine MD, Avrameas S. Natural autoantibodies. Curr Opin Immunol 1995;7:812–818.
116. Roark JH, Bussel JB, Cines DB, Siegel DL. Genetic analysis of autoantibodies in idiopathic thrombocytopenic purpura reveals evidence of clonal expansion and somatic mutation. Blood 2002;100:1388–1398.
117. Oldstone MB. Molecular mimicry and immune-mediated diseases. FASEB J 1998;12:1255–1265.
118. Ephrem A, Misra N, Hassan G, et al. Immunomodulation of autoimmune and inflammatory diseases with intravenous immunoglobulin. Clin Exp Med 2005;5:135–140.
119. Andersson PO, Wadenvik H. Chronic idiopathic thrombocytopenic purpura (ITP): molecular mechanisms and implications for therapy. Expert Rev Mol Med 2004;6:1–17.
120. Seddon B, Mason D. Peripheral autoantigen induces regulatory T cells that prevent autoimmunity. J Exp Med 1999;189:877–882.
121. Walker LS, Abbas AK. The enemy within: keeping self-reactive T cells at bay in the periphery. Nat Rev Immunol 2002;2:11–19.
122. Sarween N, Chodos A, Raykundalia C, et al. CD4+CD25+ cells controlling a pathogenic CD4 response inhibit cytokine differentiation, CXCR-3 expression, and tissue invasion. J Immunol 2004;173:2942–2951.
123. Shevach EM. Regulatory/suppressor T cells in health and disease. Arthritis Rheum 2004;50:2721–2724.
124. Shevach EM. CD4+ CD25+ suppressor T cells: More questions than answers. Nat Rev Immunol 2002;2:389–400.
125. Kuwana M, Kawakami Y, Ikeda Y. Suppression of autoreactive T-cell response to glycoprotein IIb/IIIa by blockade of CD40/CD154 interaction: implications for treatment of immune thrombocytopenic purpura. Blood 2003;101:621–623.
126. Ware RE, Howard TA. Phenotypic and clonal analysis of T lymphocytes in childhood immune thrombocytopenic purpura. Blood 1993;82(7):2137–2142.
127. Kuwana M, Kaburaki J, Ikeda Y. Autoreactive T cells to platelet GPIb-IIIa in immune thrombocytopenic purpura. Role in production of anti-platelet autoantibody. J Clin Invest 1998;102:1393–1402.
128. Filion MC, Proulx C, Bradley AJ, et al. Presence in peripheral blood of healthy individuals of autoreactive T cells to a membrane antigen present on bone marrow-derived cells. Blood 1996;88:2144–2150.
129. Peng,J, Liu C, Liu D, et al. Effects of B7-blocking agent and/or CsA on induction of platelet-specific T-cell anergy in chronic autoimmune thrombocytopenic purpura. Blood 2003;101:2721–2726.
130. Semple JW. T cell and cytokine abnormalities in patients with autoimmune thrombocytopenic purpura. Transfus Apher Sci 2003;28:237–242.
131. Nomura S, Kuwana M, Ikeda Y. Induction of T-cell tolerance in a patient with idiopathic thrombocytopenic purpura by single injection of humanized monoclonal antibody to CD40 ligand. Autoimmunity 2003;36:317–319.
132. Zimmerman SA, Malinoski FJ, Ware RE. Immunologic effects of anti-D (WinRho-SD) in children with immune thrombocytopenic purpura. Am J Hematol 1998;57:131–138.
133. Andersson J. Cytokines in idiopathic thrombocytopenic purpura (ITP). Acta Paediatr 1998;(Suppl):61–64.
134. Ogawara H, Handa H, Morita K, et al. High Th1/Th2 ratio in patients with chronic idiopathic thrombocytopenic purpura. Eur J Haematol 2003;71:283–288.
135. Panitsas FP, Theodoropoulou M, Kouraklis A, et al. Adult chronic idiopathic thrombocytopenic purpura (ITP) is the manifestation of a type-1 polarized immune response. Blood 2004;103:2645–2647.
136. Garcia-Suarez J, Prieto A, Reyes E, et al. Abnormal γIFN and αTNF secretion in purified CD2+ cells from autoimmune thrombocytopenic purpura (ATP) patients: their implication in clinical course of the disease. Am J Hematol 1995;49:271–276.
137. Dianzani U, Bragardo M, DiFranco D, et al. Deficiency of the Fasapoptosis pathway without Fas gene mutations in pediatric patients with autoimmunity/lymphoproliferation. Blood 1997;89(8):2871–2879.
138. Crossley AR, Dickinson AM, Proctor SJ, Dalvert JE. Effects of interferon-α therapy on immune parameters in immune thrombocytopenic purpura. Autoimmunity 1996;24:81–100.
139. Lazarus AH, Joy T, Crow AR. Analysis of transmembrane signaling and T cell defects associated with idiopathic thrombocytopenic purpura ITP. Acta Paediatr 1998;(Suppl):21–25.
140. Erduran E, Aslan Y, Aliyazicioglu Y, et al. Plasma soluble interleukin-2 receptor levels in patients with idiopathic thrombocytopenic purpura. Am J Hematol 1998;57:119–123.

141. Bussel J, Heddle N, Richards C, Woloski M. MCP-1, IL-10, IL-6 and TNF-αlevels in patients with ITP before and after IV anti-D and IVIG treatments. Blood 1999;94:15a.
142. Shulman NR. Immunoreactions involving platelets: I. A steric and kinetic model for formation of a complex from a human antibody, quinidine as a haptene, and platelets; and for fixation of complement by the complex. J Exp Med 1975;107:665–690.
143. Hackett T, Kelton JG, Powers, P. Drug-induced platelet destruction. Semin Thromb Hemost 1982;8:116–137.
144. Peterson JA, Nyree CE, Newman PJ, Aster RH. A site involving the "hybrid" and PSI homology domains of GPIIIa (β 3-integrin subunit) is a common target for antibodies associated with quinine-induced immune thrombocytopenia. Blood 2003;101:937–942.
145. Kunicki TJ, Johnson MM, Aster RH. Absence of the platelet receptor for drug-dependent antibodies in the Bernard-Soulier syndrome. J Clin Invest 1978;62:716–719.
146. Chong BH, Berndt MC, Koutts J, Castaldi PA. Quinidine-induced thrombocytopenia and leukopenia: demonstration and characterization of distinct antiplatelet and antileukocyte antibodies. Blood 1983;62:1218–1223.
147. Berndt MC, Chong BH, Bull HA. Molecular characterization of quinine/quinidine drug-dependent antibody platelet interaction using monoclonal antibodies. Blood 1985;66:1292–1301.
148. Chong BH, Du X, Berndt MC, et al. Characterization of the binding domains on platelet glycoproteins Ib-IX and IIb-IIIa complexes for the quinine/quinidine-dependent antibodies. Blood 1991;77: 2190–2199.
149. Lopez JA, Li CQ, Weisman S, Chambers M. The glycoprotein Ib-IX complex-specific monoclonal antibody SZ1 binds to a conformation-sensitive epitope on glycoprotein IX: implications for the target antigen of quinine/quinidine-dependent autoantibodies. Blood 1995;85:1254–1258.
150. Burgess JK, Lopez JA, Gaudry LE, Chong BH. Rifampicin-dependent antibodies bind a similar or identical epitope to glycoprotein IX-specific quinine-dependent antibodies. Blood 2000;95:1988–1992.
151. Visentin GP, Newman PJ, Aster RH. Characteristics of quinine- and quinidine-induced antibodies specific for platelet glycoproteins IIb and IIIa. Blood 1991;77:2668–2676.
152. Curtis BR, McFarland JG, Wu GG, et al. Antibodies in sulfonamide-induced immune thrombocytopenia recognize calcium-dependent epitopes on the glycoprotein IIb/IIIa complex. Blood 1994;84:176–183.
153. Kroll H, Sun QH, Santoso S. Platelet endothelial cell adhesion molecule-1 (PECAM-1) is a target glycoprotein in drug-induced thrombocytopenia. Blood 2000;96:1409–1414.
154. Szatkowski NS, Kunicki TJ, Aster RH. Identification of glycoprotein Ib as a target for autoantibody in idiopathic (autoimmune) thrombocytopenic purpura. Blood 1986;67:310–315.
155. Nieminen U, Kekomäki R. Quinidine-induced thrombocytopenic purpura: Clinical presentation in relation to drug-dependent and drug-independent platelet antibodies. Br J Haematol 1992;80:77–82.
156. Aster RH, Curtis BR, Bougie DW. Thrombocytopenia resulting from sensitivity to GPIIb-IIIa inhibitors. Semin Thromb Hemost 2004;30:569–577.
157. Lynch DM, Howe SE. Heparin-associated thrombocytopenia: Antibody binding specificity to platelet antigens. Blood 1985;66:1176.
158. Berndt MC, Chong BH, Andrews RK. Biochemistry of drug-dependent platelet autoantigens. In Kunicki TJ, George JN (eds). Immunobiology. Philadelphia, J.B. Lippincott, 1989, pp 78–93.
159. Kelton JG, Sheridan D, Santos A, et al. Heparin-induced thrombocytopenia: Laboratory studies. Blood 1988;72:925–930.
160. Adelman B, Sobel M, Fujimura Y, et al. Heparin-associated thrombocytopenia: Observations on the mechanism of platelet aggregation. J Lab Clin Med 1989;113:204–210.
161. Chong BH, Castaldi PA, Berndt MC. Heparin-induced thrombocytopenia: Effects of rabbit IgG and its Fab and Fc fragments on antibody-heparin-platelet interaction. Thromb Res 1989;55:291–295.
162. Chong BH, Fawaz I, Chesterman CN, Berndt MC. Heparin-induced thrombocytopenia: Mechanism of interaction of the heparin-dependent antibody with platelets. Br J Haematol 1989;73:235–240.
163. Greinacher A, Amiral J, Dummel V, et al. Laboratory diagnosis of heparin-associated thrombocytopenia and comparison of platelet aggregation test, heparin-induced platelet activation test, and platelet factor 4/heparin enzyme-linked immunosorbent assay. Transfusion 1994;34:381–385.
164. Visentin GP, Ford SE, Scott JP, Aster RH. Antibodies from patients with heparin-induced thrombocytopenia/thrombosis are specific for platelet factor 4 complexed with heparin or bound to endothelial cells. J Clin Invest 1994;93:81–88.
165. Arepaly G, Reynolds C, Tomaski A, et al. Comparison of PF4/heparin ELISA assay with 14C-serotonin release assay in the diagnosis of heparin induced thrombocytopenia. Am J Clin Pathol 1995;104:648.
166. Greinacher A, Michels I, Liebenhoff U, et al. Heparin associated thrombocytopenia: Immune complexes are attached to the platelet membrane by the negative charge of highly sulphated oligosaccharides. Br J Haematol 1993;84:711–716.
167. Kelton JG, Smith JW, Warkentin TE, et al. Immunoglobulin G from patients with heparin-induced thrombocytopenia binds to a complex of heparin and platelet factor 4. Blood 1994;83:3232–3239.
168. Amiral J, Bridey F, Wolf M, et al. Antibodies to macromolecular platelet factor 4–heparin complexes in heparin-induced thrombocytopenia: a study of 44 cases. Thromb Haemost 1995;73:21–28.
169. Amiral J, Wolf M, Fischer AM, et al. Pathogenicity of IgA and/or IgM antibodies to heparin–PF4 complexes in patients with heparin-induced thrombocytopenia. Br J Haematol 1996;92:954–959.
170. Poncz M. Mechanistic basis of heparin-induced thrombocytopenia. Semin Thorac Cardiovasc Surg 2005;17:73–79.
171. Rauova L, Poncz M, McKenzie SE, et al. Ultralarge complexes of PF4 and heparin are central to the pathogenesis of heparin-induced thrombocytopenia. Blood 2005;105:131–138.
172. Amiral J, Marfaing-Koka M, Wolf M, et al. Presence of autoantibodies to interleukin-8 or neutrophil-activating peptide-2 in patients with heparin-associated thrombocytopenia. Blood 1996;88:410–416.
173. Newman PJ, Derbes RS, Aster RH. The human platelet alloantigens, PLA1 and PLA2, are associated with a Leucine33/Proline33 amino acid polymorphism in membrane glycoprotein IIIa, and are distinguishable by DNA typing. J Clin Invest 1989;83:1778–1781.
174. Wang R, Furihata K, McFarland JG, et al. An amino acid polymorphism within the RGD binding domain of platelet membrane glycoprotein IIIa is responsible for the formation of the Pen^a/Pen^b alloantigen system. J Clin Invest 1992;90:2038–2043.
175. Santoso S, Kalb R, Walka V, et al.The human platelet alloantigens Br^a and Br^b are associated with a single amino acid polymorphism on glycoprotein Ia (integrin subunit α2). J Clin Invest 1993;92:2427–2432.
176. Wang R, McFarland JG, Kekomaki R, Newman PJ. Amino acid 489 is encoded by a mutational "hot spot" on the β3 integrin chain: the CA/TU human platelet alloantigen system. Blood 1993;82(11):3386–3391.
177. Kuijpers RWAM, Simsek S, Faber NM, et al. Single point mutation in human glycoprotein IIIa is associated with a new platelet-specific alloantigen (Mo) involved in neonatal alloimmune thrombocytopenia. Blood 1993;81:70–76.
178. Santoso S, Kalb R, Kiefel V, et al. A point mutation leads to an unpaired cysteine residue and a molecular weight polymorphism of a functional platelet β3 integrin subunit. The Sra alloantigen system of GPIIIa. J Biol Chem 1994;269:8439–8444.
179. Noris P, Simsek S, De Bruijne-Admiraal LG, et al. Max^a, a new low-frequency platelet-specific antigen localized on glycoprotein IIb, is associated with neonatal alloimmune thrombocytopenia. Blood 1995;86:1019–1026.
180. Peyruchaud O, Bourre F, Morel-Kopp M-C, et al. HPA-10wb (Laa): Genetic determination of a new platelet-specific alloantigen on glycoprotein IIIa and its expression in COS-7 cells. Blood 1997;89:2422–2428.
181. Simsek S, Folman C, Van der Schoot CE, Von dem Borne AEGK. The Arg633His substitution responsible for the platelet antigen Gro^a unravelled by SSCP analysis and direct sequencing. Br J Haematol 1997;97:330–335.
182. Sachs UJH, Kiefel V, Bohringer M, et al. Single amino acid substitution in human platelet glycoprotein Ib β Is responsible for the formation of the platelet-specific alloantigen Iy^a. Blood 2000;95:1849–1855.
183. Santoso S, Amrhein J, Hofmann HA, et al. A point mutation (Thr799et) on the α2 integrin leads to the formation of new human platelet alloantigen Sit(a) and affects collagen-induced aggregation. Blood 1999;94:4103–4111.
184. Santoso S, Kiefel V, Richter IG, et al. A functional platelet fibrinogen receptor with a deletion in the cysteine-rich repeat region of the β3 Integrin: the Oe^a alloantigen in neonatal alloimmune thrombocytopenia. Blood 2002;99:1205–1214.
185. Jallu V, Meunier M, Brement M, Kaplan C. A new platelet polymorphism Duva+, localized within the RGD binding domain of glycoprotein IIIa, is associated with neonatal thrombocytopenia. Blood 2002;99:4449–4456.
186. Kekomaki R, Raivio P, Kero P. A new low-frequency platelet alloantigen, Va(a), on glycoprotein IIb/IIIa associated with neonatal alloimmune thrombocytopenia. Transf Med 1992;2:27–33.
187. Kekomaki R, Partanen J, Pitkanen S, et al. Glycoprotein Ib/IX-specific alloimmunization in an HPA 2b-homozygous mother in association with neonatal thrombocytopenia. Thromb Haemost 1993;69:99.

188. Covas DT, Delgado M, Zeitune MM, et al. Gene frequencies of the HPA-1 and HPA-2 platelet antigen alleles among the Amerindians. Vox Sang 1997;73:182–184.
189. Covas DT, Biscaro TA, Nasciutti DC, et al. Gene frequencies of the HPA-3 and HPA-5 platelet antigen alleles among the Amerindians. Eur J Haematol 2000;65:128–131.
190. Castro V, Origa AF, Annichino-Bizzacchi JM, et al. Frequencies of platelet-specific alloantigen systems 1–5 in three distinct ethnic groups in Brazil. Eur J Immunogenet 1999;26:355–360.
191. Holensteiner A, Walchshofer S, Adler A, et al. Human platelet antigen gene frequencies in the Austrian population. Haemostasis 1995;25: 133–136.
192. Steffensen R, Kaczan E, Varming K, Jersild C. Frequency of platelet-specific alloantigens in a Danish population. Tissue Antigens 1996;48:93–96.
193. Simsek S, Faber NM, Bleeker PM, et al. Determination of human platelet antigen frequencies in the Dutch population by immunophenotyping and DNA (allele-specific restriction enzyme) analysis. Blood 1993;81:835–840.
194. Kekomaki S, Partanen J, Kekomaki R. Platelet alloantigens HPA-1, -2, -3, -5 and -6b in Finns. Transfus Med 1995;5:193–198.
195. Merieux Y, Debost M, Bernaud J, et al. Human platelet antigen frequencies of platelet donors in the French population determined by polymerase chain reaction with sequence-specific primers. Pathol Biol (Paris) 1997;45:697–700.
196. Chen DF, Pastucha LT, Chen HY, et al. Simultaneous genotyping of human platelet antigens by hot start sequence-specific polymerase chain reaction with DNA polymerase AmpliTaq Gold. Vox Sang 1997;72:192–196.
197. Kunicki TJ, Federici AB, Salomon DR, et al. An association of candidate gene haplotypes and bleeding severity in von Willebrand disease (VWD) Type 1 pedigrees. Blood 2004;104:2359–2367.
198. Drzewek K, Brojer E, Zupanska B. The frequency of human platelet antigen (HPA) genotypes in the Polish population. Transfus Med 1998;8:339–342.
199. Rozman P, Drabbels J, Schipper RF, Genotyping for human platelet-specific antigens HPA-1, -2, -3, -4 and -5 in the Slovenian population reveals a slightly increased frequency of HPA-1b and HPA-2b as compared to other European populations. Eur J Immunogenet 1999;26:265–269.
200. Nogues N, Subirana L, Garcia Manzano a, et al. Human platelet alloantigens in a Mexican population: a comparative gene frequency study. Vox Sang 2000;78:P060.
201. Sellers J, Thompson J, Guttridge MG, Darke C. Human platelet antigens: Typing by PCR using sequence-specific primers and their distribution in blood donors resident in Wales. Eur J Immunogenet 1999;26:393–397.
202. Bennett JA, Palmer LJ, Musk AW, Erber WN. Gene frequencies of human platelet antigens 1–5 in indigenous Australians in Western Australia. Transfus Med 2002;12:199–203.
203. Kim HO, Jin Y, Kickler TS, et al. Gene frequencies of the five major human platlet antigens in African American, white and Korean populations. Transfusion 1995;35:863–867.
204. Seo DH, Park SS, Kim DW, et al. Gene frequencies of eight human platelet-specific antigens in Koreans. Transfus Med 1998;8:129–132.
205. Legler TJ, Kohler M, Mayr WR, et al. Genotyping of the human platelet antigen systems 1 through 5 by multiplex polymerase chain reaction and ligation-based typing. Transfusion 1996;36:426–431.
206. Tanaka S, Ohnoki S, Shibata H, et al. Gene frequencies of human platlet antigens on glycoprotein IIIa in Japanese. Transfusion 1996;36: 813–817.
207. Romphruk AV, Akahat J, Srivanichrak P, et al. Genotyping of human platelet antigens in ethnic northeastern Thais by the polymerase chain reaction-sequence specific primer technique. J Med Assoc Thai 2000;83:1333–1339.
208. Shih MC, Liu TC, Lin IL, et al. Gene frequencies of the HPA-1 to HPA-13, Oe and Gov platelet antigen alleles in Taiwanese, Indonesian, Filipino and Thai populations. Int J Mol Med 2003;12:609–614.
209. Liu TC, Shih MC, Lin CL, et al. Gene frequencies of the HPA-1 to HPA-8w platelet antigen alleles in Taiwanese, Indonesian, and Thai. Ann Hematol 2002;81:244–248.
210. Chang YW, Mytilineos J, Opelz G, Hawkins BR. Distribution of human platelet antigens in a Chinese population. Tissue Antigens 1998;51:391–393.
211. Dazhuang L, Zhenyu L, Yuqin B, et al. Genotyping of human platelet antigens (HPA) and investigation of their gene frequencies. Chin J Blood Transfus 2001;14:177–192.
212. Tsao KC, Sun CF, Lai NC. The phenotype and gene frequencies of human platelet specific antigens among Chinese in Taiwan. Zhonghua Min Guo. Wei Sheng Wu Ji. Mian. Yi. Xue. Za Zhi. 1992;25:48–55.
213. Chu CC, Lee HL, Chu TW, Lin M. The use of genotyping to predict the phenotypes of human platelet antigens 1 through 5 and of neutrophil antigens in Taiwan. Transfusion 2001;41:1553–1558.
214. Santoso S, Kiefel V, Masri R, Mueller-Eckhardt C. Frequency of platelet-specific antigens among Indonesians. Transfusion 1993;33:739–741.
215. Halle L, Bach KH, Martageix C, et al. Eleven human platelet systems studied in the Vietnamese and Ma'Ohis Polynesian populations. Tissue Antigens 2004;63:34–40.
216. Ferrer G, Muniz-Diaz E, Aluja MP, et al. Analysis of human platelet antigen systems in a Moroccan Berber population. Transfus Med 2002;12:49–54.
217. Mojaat N, Halle L, Proulle V, et al. Gene frequencies of human platelet antigens in the Tunisian population. Tissue Antigens 1999;54:201–204.
218. Chiba AK, Bordin JO, Kuwano ST, et al. Platelet alloantigen frequencies in Amazon Indians and Brazilian blood donors. Transfus Med 2000;10:207–212.
219. Chen Z, Lester S, Boettcher B, McCluskey J. Platelet antigen allele frequencies in Australian Aboriginal and Caucasian populations. Pathology 1997;29:392–398.
220. Reiner AP, Aramaki KM, Teramura G, Gaur L. Analysis of platelet glycoprotein Ia (α_2 Integrin) allele frequencies in three North American populations reveals genetic association between nucleotide 807C/T and amino acid 505 Glu/Lys (HPA-5) dimorphisms. Thromb Haemost 1998;80:449–456.

Chapter 10

Human Leukocyte and Granulocyte Antigens and Antibodies: The HLA and HNA Systems

Ena Wang • Sharon Adams • Francesco M. Marincola • David F. Stroncek

INTRODUCTION

The structure, function, and nomenclature of the human leukocyte antigen (HLA) and human neutrophil antigen (HNA) systems and their relevance in transfusion medicine are reviewed in this chapter. Analysis of HLA gene products is applied in several settings, including the selection of compatible donor–recipient pairs for hematopoietic stem cell transplantation, selection of HLA-compatible platelet components for transfusion to thrombocytopenic patients refractory to platelet transfusions, and screening of genetic factors that may contribute to the prevalence of diseases. In addition, we discuss new applications that have broadened the relevance of HLA in immune pathology. HLA phenotypes are being used to determine the eligibility of patients for epitope-specific immunization to treat cancer or viral infections. Tetrameric HLA–epitope complexes (tHLA) are being used to enumerate antigen-specific T-cell responses. Furthermore, the molecular identification of T-cell epitopes associated with distinct diseases and characterization of the communication between immune effector cells through HLA–HLA ligand interactions has extended the relevance of the HLA antigen system to several biologic fields, which encompass natural killer (NK) and cytotoxic T-cell function, and antigen recognition in the context of infection, autoimmunity, graft-versus-neoplasia effect, and autologous cancer rejection.

Neutrophil antigens are a group of immunogenetic molecules expressed by neutrophils but few if any other blood cells. The antigens are located on a number of different and otherwise unrelated molecules. A few of these polymorphisms affect neutrophil function, but the importance of these antigen systems is primarily due to clinical problems caused by antibodies directed to these antigens, including alloimmune neonatal neutropenia, autoimmune neutropenia of childhood, and transfusion-related acute lung injury (TRALI).

HUMAN LEUKOCYTE ANTIGENS

Genes of the Major Histocompatibility Complex

Human leukocyte antigens are a family of genes clustered in the short arm of chromosome 6 and are the human version of the major histocompatibility complex (MHC). MHC was initially identified in mice as the antigen responsible for graft rejection between genetically unrelated strains (transplantation antigens).[1] HLA genes comprise a group of coding sequences that regulate the expression of molecules with similar but not identical function as the mouse MHC.

The HLA genes reside in a region that spans approximately 4000 kilobases (kb) of chromosome 6 band p21.3[2] (Fig. 10–1). This region contains a number of genes and pseudogenes characterized by sequence homology and functional similarity. Of them, 47 are officially recognized by the World Health Organization (WHO) nomenclature committee.[3] The HLA genes are separated into classical and nonclassical categories. Classical HLA genes have been well characterized and are clearly associated with presentation of antigen to immune cells. The classical genes include HLA class I (HLA-A, HLA-B, and HLA-C) and class II (HLA-DR, HLA-DQ, and HLA-DP). The nonclassical HLA genes include HLA-E, HLA-F, HLA-G, HLA-DM, and HLA-DO.

Human leukocyte antigens and HLA-associated genes can be grouped into three subregions according to chromosomal location. On the centromeric end of the MHC region is the HLA class II region, comprising genes encoding the α- and β-chains of HLA-DR, HLA-DQ, HLA-DP, HLA-DM, and HLA-DO as well as transporter associated with antigen processing (TAP) and psmB genes. The class I region is most telomeric and includes HLA-A, HLA-B, and HLA-Cw loci; the nonclassical HLA-E, HLA-F, and HLA-G loci; and several pseudogenes. Located between the class I and class II region is the class III region, which encodes several genes that are not functionally related to the HLA genes, such as complement components, heat shock proteins, and tumor necrosis factor. The functional basis for the genetic link of the genes in the class III region to those in the class I and II region is unknown, although the immunologic function of the genes in the class III region and their inclusion in the MHC seems more than coincidental.

Genetics, Structure, and Function of HLA molecules

Genetics of HLA Molecules

In general, HLA class I and II genes have a very similar structure and function.[4–6] Both class I and class II molecules

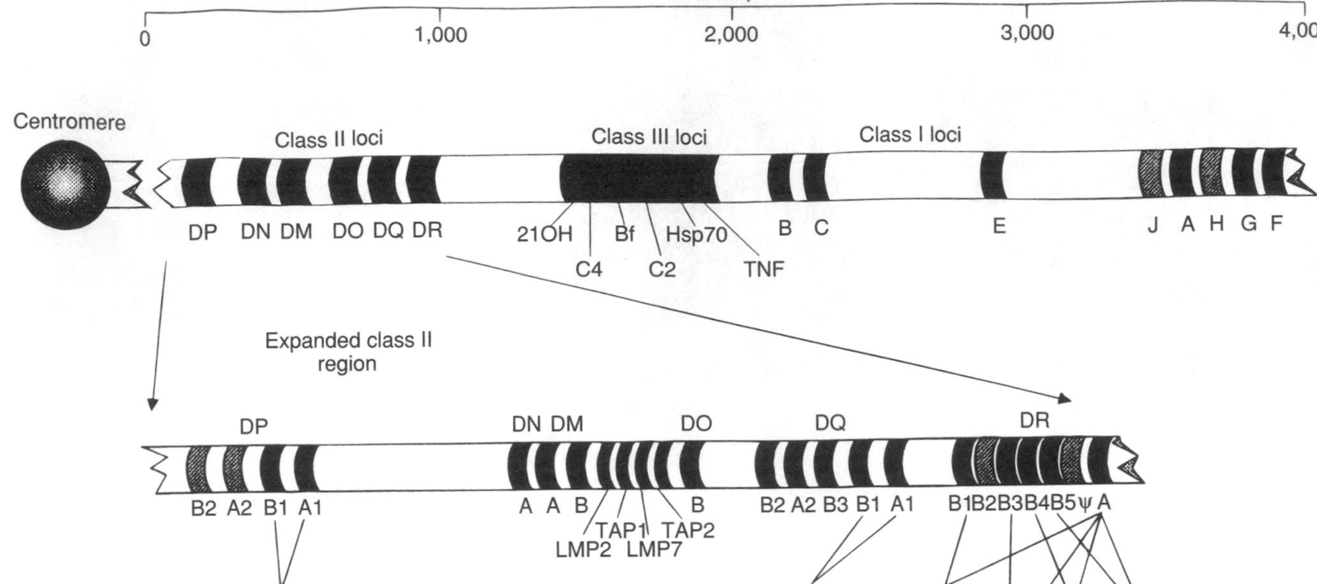

Figure 10–1 Physical map of the HLA genetic complex, illustrating the clusters of genes according to the class of encoded gene products. The symbol ψ represents four DRB pseudogenes, designated 7, 8, and 9. Other pseudogenes are shown in gray. (From Hoffman R, et al. Hematology: Basic Principles and Practice, 4th ed. Philadelphia, Churchill Livingstone, 2005.)

are made up of a heavy and light chain. The genes encoding the HLA class I heavy chain and both the HLA class II heavy and light chains are located in the MHC region. All HLA class I molecules share the same light chain, β_2-microglobulin, which is encoded outside the MHC on chromosome 15.[7]

Three separate genes encode the class I HLA-A, HLA-B, and HLA-C heavy chains, *HLA-A*, *HLA-B*, and *HLA-C*, and the three have a similar structure. Each contains eight exons encoding for the α_1, α_2, and α_3 extracytoplasmic domains, a transmembrane domain, and a cytoplasmic tail (Fig. 10–2). The first exon of the class I α chain encodes a leader sequence. Exons 2 through 4 are highly polymorphic and encode extracellular domains, α_1, α_2, and α_3, that are responsible for peptide binding and T-cell receptor (TCR) engagement. Exon 5 encodes the transmembrane region, exons 6 and 7 the cytoplasmic tail, and exon 8 the 3′ untranslated region.

The HLA class II molecules are heterodimers composed of an α and β chain of approximately the same size. The genes encoding the class II α and β chains have a similar structure, but the α chain has 5 exons and the β chain has 6 exons. For both the α and β chain genes exon 1 encodes the leader peptide, and exons 2 and 3 encode the two extracellular domains. For the β chain gene exon 4 encodes the transmembrane domain, exon 5 the ctyoplasmic tail, and exon 6 the 3′ untranslated region. For the gene encoding the α chain exon 4 encodes the transmembrane domain and the cytoplasmic tail and exon 5 encodes the 3′ untranslated region.

Class I

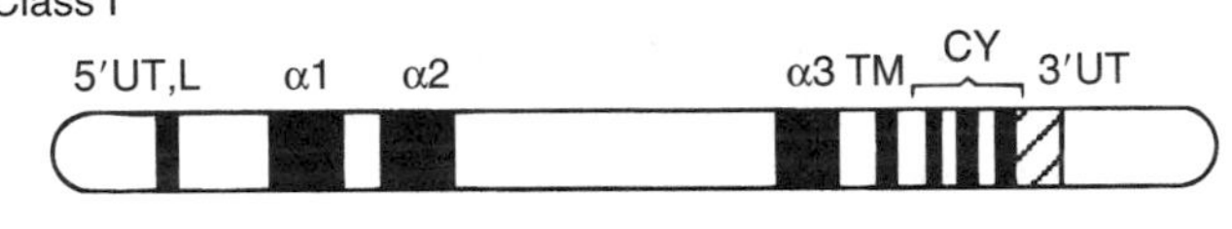

Class II

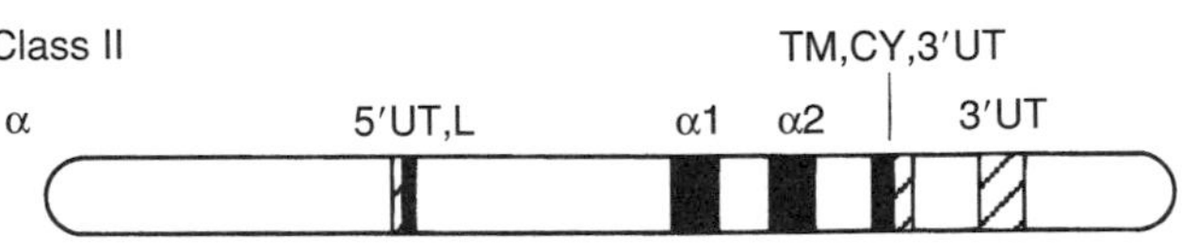

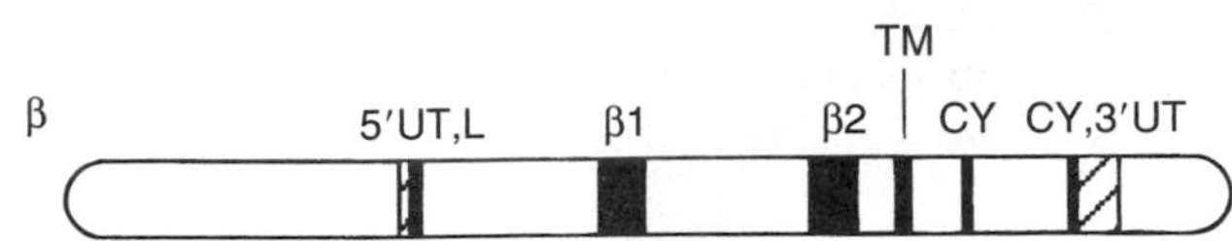

Figure 10–2 The organization of class I and II MHC genes. 5′UT and 3′UT are the untranslated regions in the 5′ and 3′ ends of the gene. L is the leader sequence, TM the exons encoding the transmembrane domains, and CY the exons encoding the cytoplasmic tails. (From Germain RN, Malissen B. Analysis of the expression and function of class-II major histocompatibility complex-encoded molecules by DNA-mediated gene transfer. Annu Rev Immunol 1986;4:281–315.)

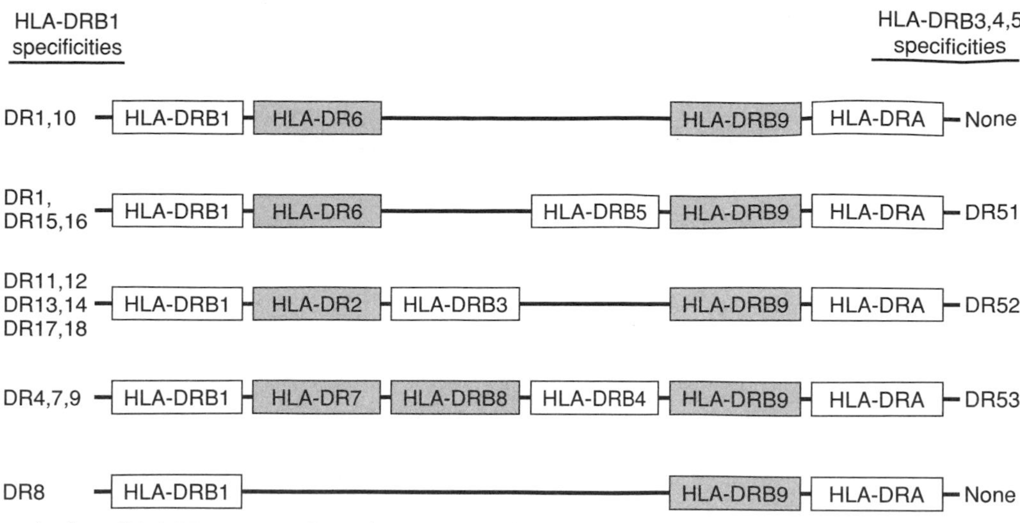

Figure 10–3 Organization of HLA-DRB genes and pseudogenes in DRB haplotypes. The *white boxes* represent expressed HLA-DRB gene and the *gray boxes* pseudogenes.

There are 5 isotypes of the class II molecules, which are designated as HLA-DM, HLA-DO, HLA-DP, HLA-DQ, and HLA-DR. Within the class II region of the MHC, the α and β genes encoding most of the isotypes are organized as pairs of α and β chains that contribute to the same isotype. The genes encoding the α chains are designated as A and those encoding the β chain B. The HLA-DM molecules are the product of HLA-DMA and HLA-DMB, HLA-DO of HLA-DOA and HLA-DOB, HLA-DP of HLA-DPA1 and HLA-DPB1, and HLA-DQ of DQA1 and DQB1 genes, respectively.

There are several HLA class II pseudogenes that are not expressed. There is one HLA-DPA pseudogene, HLA DPA2, and one HLA-DPB pseudogene, HLA-DPB2. There is also one HLA-DQA pseudogene, HLA-DQA2, and two HLA-DQB pseudogenes, HLA-DQB2 and HLA-DQB3.

The expression of HLA-DR molecules is more complicated than the expression of the other HLA class II molecules. All HLA-DR α chains are encoded by the same DRA gene, HLA-DRA1. However, there are several functional HLA-DRB genes that encode the HLA-DR β chains and several HLA-DRB pseudogenes. In addition, the number of HLA-DRB genes and pseudogenes present varies among individuals. The different combinations of HLA-DRB genes are known as *DRB haplotypes;* several different haplotypes have been described. The HLA-DR molecules can use alleles coded by the DRB1, DRB3, DRB4, or DRB5 genes for β chains. HLA-DRB2, HLA-DRB6, HLA-DRB7, HLA-DRB8, and HLA-DRB9 are pseudogenes. The HLA-DRB1 gene and HLA-DRB9 pseudogene loci are expressed in all HLA haplotypes. At most one other HLA-DRB gene is present in each of the five haplotypes. Some haplotypes have no functional DRB genes other than DRB1 (DR8 and DR10 haplotypes). The other haplotypes have DRB1 plus one of the other three functional DRB genes: DRB3, DRB4, or DRB5 (Fig. 10–3).[2]

HLA Gene Inheritance and Linkage Disequilibrium

Because of their proximity within a short chromosomal distance, HLA genes are inherited en bloc from each parent unless a recombinant event occurs. Thus, each HLA haplotype behaves as a unit and is transmitted through generations according to mendelian principles. Because each individual inherits two of four possible haplotypes (two from each parent), there are four possible genotypes for each individual and the probability of genotypic identity between two siblings is 25% (Fig. 10–4). Because HLA genes are inherited as haplotypes, most HLA phenotypically identical siblings are also HLA genotypically identical. In 2% of cases, recombinant HLA haplotypes (a set of genes derived partially from two chromosomes through recombination) yield genotypes that deviate from this rule.

In large populations gene frequencies achieve equilibrium within a few generations unless selective pressure influences individuals' survival and mating capacity (Hardy-Weinberg law). In equilibrium, gene prevalence is maintained based solely on its frequency. However, within specific populations the presence of specific combinations of HLA antigens occurs with a higher frequency than expected from the prevalence of

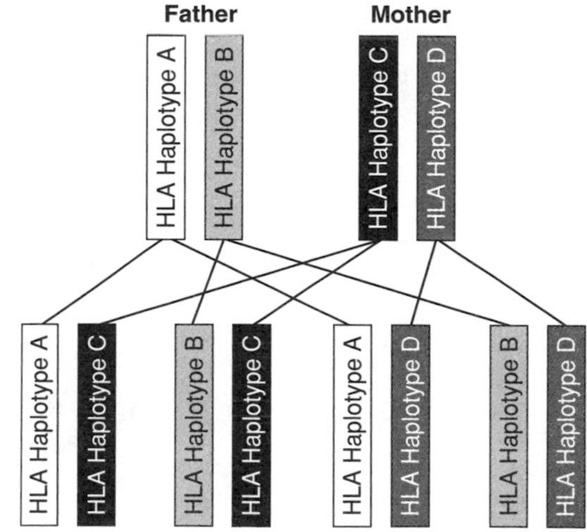

Figure 10–4 Potential HLA haplotypes inherited from two parents. Because four different haplotype combinations are possible, the chances that any two siblings will inherit the same HLA haplotyes and be an HLA "identical" match are 1 in 4.

individual alleles within the same population. This association of specific antigens as HLA haplotypes is called *linkage disequilibrium* and is due to the close proximity of class I and class II on chromosome 6.

Assuming that there were 414, 728, and 210 alleles for the HLA-A, HLA-B, and HLA-C loci, respectively (number of alleles known when this example was described[8]), then theoretically $414 \times 728 \times 210 = 63{,}292{,}320$ HLA class I allelic combinations or haplotypes would be possible. The addition of HLA class II genes to these calculations yields an astronomical number of combinations, making unlikely the identification of two HLA-matched individuals. However, some individual alleles occur with high frequency and are predominant in certain populations (i.e., HLA-A2 in whites and HLA-A24 or HLA-A11 in Asians).[9] Because predominant alleles are often associated with other high-frequency alleles in related haplotypes, the chances of identifying matched individuals are much higher than theoretically possible.

Structure of HLA Class I and II Molecules

Although the genetics of the HLA class I and II molecules differ, the HLA class I and class II protein products are structurally similar. The structure of HLA molecules and their relationship with their natural ligand, the TCR, has been well characterized by crystallography.[10–12] HLA molecules are heterodimer glycoproteins belonging to the immunoglobulin superfamily. Several features are common to all HLA molecules (Fig. 10–5), including two α-helical domains protruding toward the extracellular milieu. Class I molecules consist of two chains: a heavy or α chain and a light chain, β_2-microglobulin. The α chain has a transmembrane portion, but β_2-microglobulin does not. The extracellular portion of the α chain contains three α-helical domains and that of β_2-microglobulin a single α-helical domain (Fig. 10–6). Class II molecules consist of two chains, α and β, both of which consists of two α-helical domains and a transmembrane portion (see Fig. 10–6).

The two outer α–helical domains of both HLA class I and class II form the peptide-binding groove, and they contain the regions with the most amino acid variability. Between the two outer α–helical domains lies a flat surface formed by β-sheet structures that contributes to the formation of a groove that accommodates peptides generated from intracellular (HLA class I) or extracellular proteins (HLA class II) (Fig. 10–7). After a peptide binds to this groove, the helixes–peptide complex is exposed for TCR recognition and receptor activation.

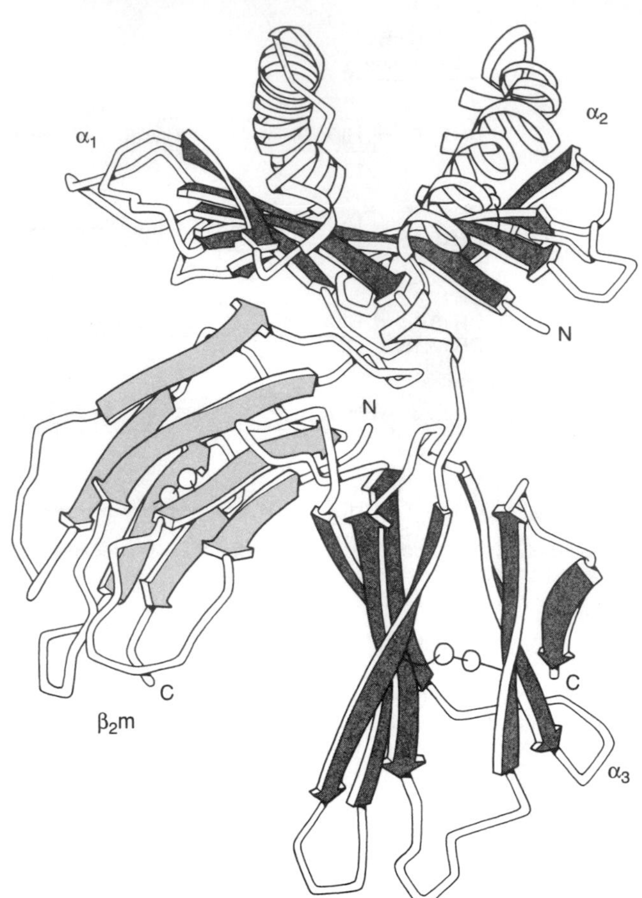

Figure 10–5 Three-dimensional configuration of HLA-A2, modeled from x-ray crystallographic studies. (From Bjorkman PJ, Saper MA, Samraoui B, et al. Structure of the human class I histocompatibility antigen, HLA-A2. Nature 1987;329:506–512.)

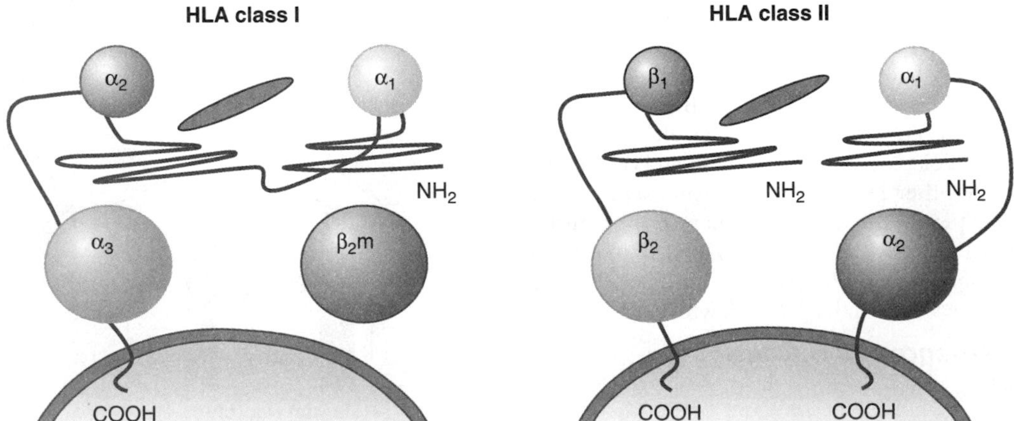

Figure 10–6 Schematic diagram of HLA class I and class II molecules, pointing to their structural similarity. In both HLA classes two immunoglobulin-type domains reside close to the cell membrane (α_3 and β_2 for class I and α_2 and β_2 for class II). The other two domains project toward the extracellular milieu with α-helices (α_1 and α_2 for class I and α_1 and β_1 for class II) and a platform of parallel β-sheets that form a peptide-binding groove. (From Hoffman R, et al. Hematology: Basic Principles and Practice, 4th ed. Philadelphia, Churchill Livingstone, 2005.)

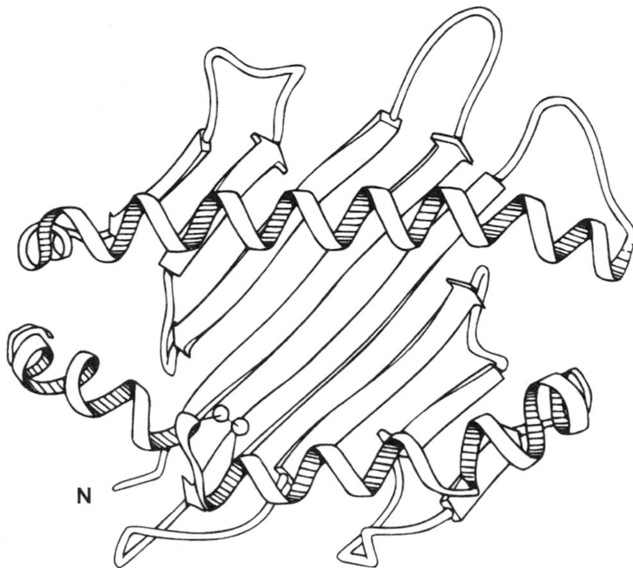

Figure 10–7 Scheme of the peptide groove of an HLA class I molecule, formed by the α_1 and α_2 domains at the side and the β-sheets at the bottom. The view is looking down on the vertically oriented molecule, the T-cell receptor point of view. (From Bjorkman PJ, Saper MA, Samraoui B, et al. Structure of the human class I histocompatibility antigen, HLA-A2. Nature 1987;329:506–512.)

T-cell activation requires the interaction of the TCR with a compatible peptide–HLA molecule complex. The nature of the TCR interaction with the HLA molecule required for productive engagement of the TCR with the HLA–peptide complex spans a surface that includes the peptide and portions of the α and β helixes of the HLA molecule.[12–15] This double requirement of interaction of peptides with both the TCR and HLA complex represents the structural basis for HLA restriction. Because HLA polymorphism is clustered within the α-helices and β-sheet domains that form the peptide-binding groove, specific peptides display a highly variable affinity for distinct HLA alleles.[16,17]

It has been proposed that a given peptide can bind to closely related HLA alleles and as a result HLA superfamilies with similar binding characteristics exist.[18–20] However, peptide binding to related but distinct HLA alleles is associated with conformational dissimilarity due to differential interaction with variant residues in the binding groove.[21] Degenerate and promiscuous TCR recognition of peptides presented by distinct HLA alleles within the same superfamily has also been described.[22] Although the concept of HLA superfamilies holds in general, several exceptions can be expected because single amino acid variants in the HLA molecule may disallow binding of a peptide[23] or may not be permissive to TCR engagement.[24,25]

The binding affinity of a given peptide for an HLA allele can be predicted through computer algorithms that compile available information to identify amino acid residues that fit the distinct pockets of the HLA groove.[16,26] Many of these algorithms supplement this information with experimental testing that analyzes the refolding capability of HLA heavy chains exposed to known peptide sequences in the presence of β_2-microglobulin and/or their dissociation rates (http://bimas.dcrt.nih.gov or http://www.uni-tuebingen.de/uni/kxi). These algorithms are based on the principle that the binding of a peptide to a specific HLA class I molecule promotes stability of the noncovalent assembly of the heavy chain with β_2-microglobulin.[16,27] In addition to using algorithms to predict affinity of specific peptides to a specific HLA molecule, peptide binding can be evaluated directly by elution of peptides from purified HLA heavy chains.[17,28]

In addition to the component of the HLA molecule that is interactive with the TCR, other HLA domains act as coreceptors for the TCR. The association of the CD8+ cytotoxic T cells to the TCR is enhanced by the binding of the CD8 molecule to the α_3 domain of HLA class I, and the association of CD4+ T cells with the TCR is enhanced by the binding of the CD4 molecule to the β_2 domain of HLA class II. Although the coreceptor–TCR interaction is not an absolute requirement, in most cases it determines the HLA class I or II restriction of the individual T cells.[29]

The HLA class I molecules are unique in that the heavy chain and β_2-microglobulin can only be assembled when they are stabilized by a high-affinity peptide derived from the cleavage of intracellular proteins (endogenous pathway of antigen presentation).[6] Most of these intracellular peptides are derived from degradation of self-proteins in the cytosol by proteasomes (psmB) and other proteases.[30] After the proteins are degraded they are assembled into a heavy chain/β_2-microglobulin–peptide complex. To assemble this complex, soluble peptides 9 to 10 amino acids in length are chaperoned into the endosomal compartment by transporter molecules associated with antigen processing (TAP1 and TAP2). While the peptides are in this compartment, they bind to heavy chains according to their amino acid sequence and the individual's HLA type. The binding and stability of the HLA–peptide complex is dependent on the affinity of each peptide for a particular allele. If the stability is sufficient, the peptide-loaded HLA molecule migrates to the cell surface.

In addition to self-peptides, intracellular pathogens produce proteins that are degraded by proteasomes into peptides that compete with the self-peptides for HLA class I molecule-binding sites. Thus, the function of the endogenous pathway of antigen presentation is to provide information to the extracellular compartment of intracellular events. In physiologic conditions, only self-peptides are presented and, therefore, minimal interactions occur with circulating T cells. During infection, pathogen-derived peptides are presented and signal cellular infection to T cells, but antibodies that cannot cross the cell membrane remain insensitive to intracellular pathogens.

Several pathogens such as cytomegalovirus (CMV) can interfere with peptide processing by reducing the density of HLA–/peptide complexes on the cell surface and, consequently, diminish T-cell recognition.[31,32] This escape mechanism can be counteracted by the host through increased susceptibility of virally infected cells to NK cell-mediated cytolysis.[33] Reciprocally, viruses can evade NK cells and escape the recognition by modulating HLA expression.[34–36]

HLA class II molecules bind longer peptides derived from the metabolism of molecules endocytosed from the extracellular compartment. This is known as the *exogenous pathway of antigen presentation.*[6] This is a specialized process used by professional antigen-presenting cells such as macrophages and dendritic cells. HLA class II molecules are assembled within the endosomal compartment, where they are composed of a heterotrimer, including the α and β chains plus a short invariant chain that stabilizes the molecule by occupying its groove while chaperoning its migration to the endosomal compartment (MHC class II peptide-loading compartment, MIIC) where exogenous antigens are processed.

On entering the MIIC, the pre-HLA class II complex is degraded and antigenic peptides are loaded with the help of the nonclassical HLA-DM molecule.[37] On uptake of an exogenous antigen by the HLA class II molecule the antigen peptide undergoes limited proteolysis in the membrane-bound acidic endosomal compartment.

Expression of HLA Molecules

Although there are genetic and structural differences between HLA class I and class II molecules, there are striking functional differences between these two molecules because their expression varies greatly. HLA class I molecules are expressed by most nucleated cells with the exception of germinal cells; HLA class II molecules are expressed mainly by specialized antigen-presenting cells.[38,39] HLA class I molecules are also expressed by platelets[40] and are responsible for refractoriness after multiple transfusion.[41–44] HLA class I molecules are also expressed weakly, though significantly, by reticulocytes and can be the targets of alloantibodies during hemolytic transfusion reactions.[45,46] HLA class II proteins are expressed constitutively by cells associated with the initiation of the immune response, such as monocytes, macrophages, and B cells,[46] and by immune cells activated by cytokines during inflammation. HLA class II molecules initiate immune responses by taking up pathogen components and presenting them to CD4+ helper T cells that in turn initiate humoral immune responses and facilitate cellular immune responses.

The expression of HLA alleles is sensitive to environmental conditions and can be modulated by cytokines, especially interferons.[47] This is particularly important for HLA-B and HLA-C molecules, which are normally expressed at a lower density than HLA-A.[48,49] In addition, HLA class II molecules can be expressed by most cells following cytokine stimulation.[50,51] This might explain why chronic inflammation induced by alloreactions during graft-versus-host disease (GVHD) may facilitate the presentation of tumor-specific antigens by tumor cells with consequent development of graft-versus-neoplasia (GVN) effect. In addition, it might explain how systemic administration of pro-inflammatory cytokines such as interleukin-2 (IL-2) may stimulate immune responses by increasing the antigen-presenting ability of cells within the tumor microenvironment.[52]

HLA Polymorphism and Its Clinical Significance

A striking characteristic of the HLA system is its extreme polymorphism. By chance, most individuals are heterozygous and therefore carry two different alleles for each HLA gene that, being codominant, are equally expressed on the cell surface. As everybody carries three HLA class I (-A, -B, and -C) and three HLA class II (-DR, -DQ, and -DP) genes, most individuals (with the exception of homozygotes) express six different HLA class I and six different HLA class II molecules on the surface of their cells. This has important functional implications because HLA polymorphism is clustered in domains of the HLA molecule that are associated with peptide binding and interactions with the TCR. Thus, most individuals have a broad repertoire of molecules capable of presenting different pathogen components to immune cells. It is, therefore, believed that HLA polymorphism improves a given species' chances of surviving infectious agents.[53] This paradigm is difficult to demonstrate in human pathology, in which the natural history of infectious diseases rarely correlates with HLA phenotype. An exception is the strong association between HLA-B*5701 and lack of progression to AIDS of HIV-infected individuals.[54] Associations have been observed between HLA phenotype and predisposition for Epstein-Barr virus (EBV)-associated nasopharyngeal carcinoma.[55,56] This is of particular interest because nasopharyngeal carcinoma is a virally induced cancer against which T cells may mediate immune surveillance. HLA associations have also been described with less consistency for other virally driven tumors such as cervical carcinoma[57] or immunogenic tumors such as melanoma.[58,59]

HLA polymorphism is at the basis of alloimmunization because most individuals are likely to have different HLA molecules on the surface of their cells. Hundreds of HLA alleles have been identified through high-resolution typing, making the chances that two individuals have identical HLA phenotypes extremely low. The complete and partial mismatches that exist between almost all individuals are at the basis of hyperacute, acute, and chronic rejection of transplanted organs and tissues. Hyperacute rejection is due to preformed antibodies that are directed against donor HLA alleles and usually a result of presensitization of the transplant recipient by multiple transfusions.[60] Acute and chronic rejection result from a combination of humoral and cellular immune reactivity toward donor HLA alleles.[61,62] In addition to allosensitization, HLA alleles can mediate GVHD, whereby hematopoietic cells derived from the grafted organs recognize and reject the host tissues by identifying polymorphisms of intracellular proteins of the host (minor histocompatiblity antigens) presented in association with donor–recipient-matched HLA alleles.

Nonclassical MHC and MHC Class I and Class II Related Molecules

In addition to the genes that encode the α chains of the class I HLA-A, HLA-B, and HLA-C molecules, the class I region of the MHC also encodes the nonclassical HLA-E, HLA-F, and HLA-G molecules. These selectively expressed class I genes are also known as MHC-1b.[63,64] These molecules are characterized by unique patterns of transcription, protein structure, and immunologic function.[65]

The class I MHC region also includes two other genes that are structurely but not functionally related to the HLA genes: MIC and HFE. Several other genes have a structure that is related to the class I genes but are encoded outsided the MHC region. These include the CD1 gene family and MR1(HALs) on chromosome 1, the FCGRT gene on chromosome 19, and zince α_2-glycoprotein on chromosome 7. In addition to the classical HLA-DP, HLA-DQ, and HLA-DR molecules, the class II MHC region encodes the nonclassical HLA-DM and HLA-DO molecules.

HLA-E, HLA-F, and HLA-G

HLA-G is characterized by low polymorphism, and its expression differs from the expression of the classical class I molecules. "Aberrant" cytokine-responsive regulatory sequences[66,67] may be responsible for low levels of HLA-G expression in a variety of human tissues[68] and for the predominant expression of HLA-G by trophoblasts that, in turn, do not express other HLA molecules.[69] Lack of responsiveness of expression to common immune stimulatory pathways (NF-*k*B, interferon-γ, or CIITA) is most pronounced for HLA-G molecules, although this characteristic is shared by other nonclassical MHC such as HLA-E.[70] HLA-G is also expressed in a variety of cancers. The importance of HLA-G expression by specific cell types is not known because HLA-G can be expressed in various membrane-bound or soluble isoforms with distinct functional characteristics. Functional HLA-G isoforms that include the α_1 and α_2 domains bind and present peptides derived from cytoplasmic proteins.[71] Because of the minimal polymorphism of HLA-G, the repertoire of peptides presented by HLA-G is likely to be limited, suggesting that peptide binding is necessary to stabilize the HLA-G molecule rather than being involved in antigen presentation.

Functionally, HLA-G is thought to modulate the function of NK cells through interactions with their inhibitory receptors.[72] In addition, the HLA-G leader sequence contains a peptide that can bind and stabilize the expression of HLA-E, which also inhibits NK cells.[73] Because the HLA-G derived leader peptide has the strongest affinity for HLA-E among all HLA class I molecules, it is likely that HLA-G is a powerful direct and indirect inhibitor of NK cells that is capable of reducing the risk of cardiac rejection or inducing immune escape of cancer cells.[74] Although much has been published about the immune regulatory role of HLA-G, its true function remains uncertain, principally due to discordant findings reported by various groups.[66]

HLA-E is minimally polymorphic,[3] binds hydrophobic peptides from other HLA class I leader sequences, and interacts with CD94/NKG2 lectin-like receptors present predominantly on NK cells and partially on CD8+ T cells.[75–78] The binding of peptides derived from leader sequences is highly specific and stabilizes the HLA-E molecule, allowing its migration to the cell surface. Thus, the surface density of HLA-E is an indirect reflection of the number of HLA class I alleles expressed by a cell.[79] The interaction of HLA-E with CD94/NKG2 protects HLA-E expressing cells from NK cell killing. Cells damaged by viral infection or neoplastic degeneration may lose HLA class I expression. As a backup mechanism of host protection, reduced HLA class I expression leads to decreased expression of HLA-E, leading to vulnerability to NK cells.[80] Interestingly, some viruses express mimic peptides that bind and stabilize HLA-E so that, while classical MHC molecules are downregulated, HLA-E expression is maintained, allowing the pathogen to simultaneously escape CD8+ T-cell and NK cell killing.[81]

The function of HLA-F remains enigmatic. Its transcriptional regulation is closest to classical HLA molecules because it can be induced by NF-*k*B, interferon regulatory factor-1, and class II transactivator.[82] However, contrary to the classical HLA molecules HLA-F is predominantly empty, mostly intracellular, and has a restricted pattern of expression.[83] Its tissue distribution appears to be limited to B cells; therefore, it is mostly found in lymphatic organs.[83] Structural studies suggest that HLA-F is a peptide-binding molecule, and it may reach the cell surface under favorable conditions when a suitable peptide is present.[84] Once on the cell surface, HLA-F may interact with the effector cell receptors ILT2 and ILT4 as suggested by HLA-F tetrameric complex-binding studies.[84] Thus, it is possible that in specific yet unknown conditions, HLA-F may modulate the function of immune effector cells similarly to HLA-E and HLA-G.

Other Class I and Class II MHC–Related Genes

The class I MHC–related chain genes MIC-A and MIC-B are located within the MHC region and are characterized by high polymorphism (more than 50 alleles so far identified). The molecules encoded by these genes do not appear to bind peptides nor to associate with β_2-microglobulin. Their polymorphic variants are not concentrated around the peptide-binding groove, yet they seem to have functional significance because most of the mutations are nonsynonymous, suggesting selective pressure as driving force. Their tissue distribution is restricted to epithelial cells, endothelial cells, and fibroblasts. It appears that MIC genes modulate the function of NK and CD8+ T cells by binding the NKG2D-stimulating receptor.[85] MIC has also been implicated in transplant rejection; alloantibodies against them are often found in transplant recipients. The alloantibodies may exert complement-mediated cytotoxicity against endothelial cells from the graft.

Other "unusual" MHC-like molecules are present in the genome and have disparate functions, including presentation of lipid antigens (CD1), transport of immunoglobulins (Fc receptor), and regulation of iron metabolism (hemochromatosis gene product).[86] Contrary to classical class I MHC genes, which are constitutively expressed, nonclassical MHC and MIC gene expression depends on stimulation by pro-inflammatory cytokines.[87]

In addition, two nonclassical class II MHC proteins (HLA-DM and HLA-DO) have been described that function as mediators of peptide exchange by stabilizing empty class II MHC molecules.[37] Finally, it is possible that several nonclassical MHC molecules whose function is to present peptides to lymphocytes may be present throughout the genome. Because of their limited polymorphism, however, these genes may have evolved to serve specialized presentation functions.[88]

Non-HLA Polymorphism and Its Clinical Significance

This chapter would be incomplete without mentioning polymorphisms of several other important immune modulators. The significance of these non-HLA polymorphisms is evidenced by the development of GVHD in the presence of HLA identical matching among relatives. Three general areas of polymorphism being investigated are NK cell receptor genes, minor histocompatibility antigens, and cytokines.

During the past decade much progress has been made in identifying the mechanisms of action of NK cells. A major breakthrough was the discovery of HLA class I–specific inhibitory receptors and the role that they play in the regulation of NK function, with consequent effects on the eradication of hematologic malignancies and on prevention of graft rejection and the induction of GVHD.[89] NK cells recognize HLA molecules via killer cell immunoglobulin-like receptors (KIRs), and as a consequence they kill target cells that have lost HLA molecule expression. KIRs are glycoproteins encoded by a compact family of at least 17 different genes located on chromosome 19q13.4 in the lymophocyte receptor complex.[90] All human KIR genes derive from a gene encoding three immunoglobulin (Ig)-like domains (D0, D1, and D2) and a long cytoplasmic tail. However, the KIR genes are diverse and may encode either two or three Ig-like domains and either a long or short cytoplasmic tail (Table 10–1). The long cytoplasmic tails contain one or two immunoreceptor tyrosine-based inhibition motifs (ITIM).[91] KIR molecules with long cytoplasmic tails inhibit NK cytotoxicity; those with short tails do not. The names given to KIR genes are based on the molecule that they encode. The

Table 10–1 **Structural Features and HLA Class I Alleles Recognized by Different Killer Immunoglobulin-like Receptors (KIR)**

KIR	Type of Ig-like Domain	Type of Intracellular Chain	Ligand
KIR2DL1	D1, D2	Long with 2 ITIMs	HLA-C^{Lys80}
KIR2DL2,3	D1, D2	Long with 2 ITIMs	HLA-C^{Asn80}
KIR2DS1	D1, D2	Short	HLA-C^{Lys80}
KIR2DS2	D1, D2	Short	HLA-C^{Asn80}
KIR2DS3,5	D1, D2	Short	Unknown
KIR2DS4	D1, D2	Short	Unknown
KIR2DL4	D0, D2	Long with 1 ITIM	HLA-G
KIR2DL5A/B	D0, D2	Long with 1 ITIM	Unknown
KIR3DL1	D0, D1, D2	Long with 2 ITIMs	HLA-B^{Bw4}
KIR3DL2	D0, D1, D2	Long with 2 ITIMs	HLA-A
KIR3DL3	D0, D1, D2	Long with 2 ITIMs	
KIR3DS1	D0, D1, D2	Short	Unknown

ITIM, immunoreceptor tyrosine inhibitory motif.

first digit corresponds to the number of Ig-like domains in the molecule and a "D" denotes *domain.* The D is followed by either an "L" for *long* cytoplasmic tail, S for *short* cytoplasmic tail, or "p" for a *pseudogene.* The last digit indicates the number of the KIR gene.[92]

Expression of KIR in individual NK cells is complex because NK cells may express several members of the KIR family. The number of KIR genes in each haplotype varies among individuals. The most common haplotype, known as group A, is made up of 6 genes (2DL1, 2DL2 or 2DL3, 3DL1, 3DL2, 2DS4, and 2DL4). Various KIR genes can recognize different HLA-A, HLA-B, and HLA-C molecules. HLA-C antigens can be divided into two groups based on polymorphisms at amino acid positions 77 and 80 of their class I heavy chains. One group has asparagine (Asn) at position 77 and lysine (Lys) at 80; the other has serine (Ser) at 77 and Asn at 80. Some KIRs recognize HLA-C antigens with Asn77 and Lys80; other KIRs recognize HLA-C antigens with Ser77 and Lys80. The polymorphism at position 80 is most important. Another group of KIRs reacts with HLA-B antigens that carry specific combinations of amino acids at positions 77 and 83 of the heavy chain that form HLA-Bw4. KIR recognition of HLA class I molecules is degenerate because a single KIR can interact with multiple HLA class I alleles. Another NK inhibitory receptor (CD94-NKG2A) recognizes the nonclassical HLA-E molecule. In addition, each of the KIR genes is extensively polymorphic.

Because the genes for KIR, HLA, and CD94-NKG2A are located in separate chromosomes, they segregate independently; consequently, individuals may carry genes for KIRs for which there is no correspondent HLA ligand.[93] Because HLA-E is expressed in all individuals, NK cells that bear the CD94-NKG2A receptor are not alloreactive. Because the specificity of KIRs for their ligands is broad and each individual carries several KIRs, it is likely that in the majority of cases all NK cells of a given person express at least one KIR that is specific for a self-HLA class I allele. Thus, in autologous settings NK cells kill only aberrant cells that have lost HLA class I expression. In contrast, NK cells can kill allogeneic cells that do not express HLA class I alleles recognized by their KIR. Thus, by knowing the KIR repertoire of a given transplant recipient and the HLA type of the donor, it is theoretically possible to predict the likelihood of an NK-mediated alloreaction. Importantly, it appears that "alloreactive" NK cells undergo proliferation on exposure to stimulatory cells; therefore, they can preferentially expand in the presence of allogeneic tissue.

NK cells also express activating receptors that are responsible for their lytic activity. These activating receptors include KIRs with short cytoplasmic tails. Although the ligands for these activating receptors have not been identified, it is possible that they are expressed primarily by activated or proliferating cells. It is, therefore, possible that during the inflammatory process induced in allogeneic conditions, normal cells may become activated by cytokines and express ligands responsible for NK activation in the absence of HLA class I molecules reactive with the inhibitory receptors.[89]

The relevance of KIR in haploidentical hematopoietic transplantation has been well studied. In haploidentical transplants several KIR–HLA class I allele combinations are possible, including NK cells from the graft that express KIR but do not interact with the donor's HLA molecules (graft-versus-host alloreactivity) and NK cells from the donor that do not interact with the host's HLA molecules (graft rejection alloreactivity). The presence of graft-versus-host reactive NK cells due to incompatibilities between donor and recipient (especially HLA-Cw families) has favorable effects in the outcome of acute myeloid leukemia.[94] Alternatively, a good match may be present between graft NK cells and host's HLA and between host's NK cells and graft HLA. In such a case no alloreactivity will occur. If the stem cell donor is incompatible with the host's NK cell repertoire, the host's reactivity may lead to graft rejection. Interestingly, alloreactive grafted NK cells seem to prevent GVHD while inducing GVN.[89]

Like HLA, KIR genes are polymorphic, and their variability is clustered in positions likely to impact the overall structure of the molecule. The relevance of KIR gene polymorphism in the outcome of bone marrow transplantation (BMT) is unclear. It appears that the risk of GVHD is highest in the context of unrelated BMT when the recipient KIR genotype is "included" in the donor KIR genotype.[95] These results show that compatibility between KIR genotypes themselves may influence the outcome of BMT.

Minor histocompatibility antigens (mHA) are polymorphic molecules whose peptides contain variant sequences that are presented by HLA alleles. They have been shown to be targets of cytotoxic T lymphocytes that can lyse leukemia cells.[96] In addition, some mHA are selectively expressed by neoplastic cells.[97] At present little is known about the identity of mHA epitopes in the context of various HLA types and their significance in the development of GVHD and GVN.

Cytokines are another large family of molecules associated with antigen recognition, graft rejection, and GVHD. Their polymorphism is becoming an important area of investigation in the context of transplantation, autoimmunity, and cancer. Generally, polymorphic sites of cytokines reside in regulatory regions so that genetic variants are associated with high or low production of a given cytokine rather than differences in its function. Information about cytokine polymorphism is being compiled on a website (http://www.bris.ac.uk/Depts/PathAndMicro/services/GAT/cytokinet.htm). Although no consensus has been achieved yet, several studies have shown associations between various cytokine genotypes and propensity to disease or transplant outcome. Interestingly, a strong association has recently been noted between a low IL-10 production genotype and a tendency to develop melanoma and prostate cancer.[98,99]

HLA Nomenclature

The HLA system nomenclature[100] began as HL-A for human leukocyte locus A. With the recognition that HLA molecules are encoded by more than one locus, the A came to represent *antigen* and a locus designation was added after HLA (i.e., HLA-A, HLA-B, HLA-C, HLA-D).[8] The WHO has taken responsibility for updating the nomenclature; the most recent update was in 2004 following the 14th International Histocompatibility Workshop.[3] At present, two nomenclature systems are used. An immunologically defined nomenclature is based on the identification of HLA antigens on the surface of leukocytes. HLA phenotypes described by immunologic methods are, therefore, conventionally called *HLA antigens.*[101] The second system is based on the molecular identification of nucleotide sequences in genomic DNA; the results are conventionally referred to as *HLA alleles.* Because molecular typing has higher resolution, this nomenclature has gained widespread acceptance.

Immunologically Defined HLA Nomenclature

Immunologically defined nomenclature follows this convention: HLA is separated by a hyphen from a capital letter identifying the locus encoding distinct HLA class I (-A, -B, -C) or class II (-DR, -DQ, -DP) antigens. The letter is followed by a number that identifies a serologic family of alleles sharing epitopes recognized by alloantibodies or alloreactive cytotoxic T cells. With improved understanding of the molecular genetics of the HLA region, various appendages have been removed from the HLA nomenclature. For instance, the letter *w* was used to indicate a provisional assignment; this has been discontinued, although it is occasionally added to HLA-C antigen nomenclature to distinguish it from complement genes. HLA-DP and HLA-DW also maintained this letter to reinforce the dependency of their immune identification predominantly through cellular techniques. Finally, HLA-Bw4 and HLA-Bw6 retain the *w* to emphasize that these public epitopes are shared by several HLA-B and some HLA antigens.

Sequence-defined Allelic Nomenclature

Recently, a bridge between immunologic and molecular nomenclature has been proposed whereby HLA antigens that encompass a single gene product can be attributed a two-digit numeric extension corresponding to the molecular nomenclature for that allele.[102] The 10th International Histocompatibility Workshop recommended a sequence-based nomenclature in 1987[102] to describe alleles not distinguishable by immunologic methods. Since then, the number of HLA alleles has rapidly increased. A total of 422 new alleles were named between the previous report in 2003 and December 2004[3]: 349 designations were given to HLA-A, 627 to HLA-B, and 182 to HLA-Cw alleles (1180 named HLA class I alleles). Assignments for HLA class II included 394 HLA-DRB1, 61 HLA-DQB1, and 116 HLA-DPB1 alleles. Other designations are summarized in Table 10–2. In this nomenclature system HLA designates molecules belonging to the human MHC followed by the locus (i.e., -A, -B). Alleles are then identified after an asterisk (*). A four-digit number is used in which the first two digits refer to the original serologic family (i.e., HLA-A2 serologic would be HLA-A*02). The last two digits designate alleles sequentially identified within that family. Often numbers are missing because an original assignment was revoked (this is why there is no HLA-A*2401 allele). When silent mutations are identified (variations in nucleotide sequences that do not translate into changes in amino acid sequence), the name of the allele remains identical, but another two digits are added to designate that it is a variant that has no functional significance. When new sequences are identified they are submitted to EMBL (www.ebi.ac.uk/Submissions/index.html) GeneBank (www.ncbi.nlm.nih.gov/Genbank/index.html), or DDBJ (http://www.ddbj.nig.ac.jp/sub-e.html).

The requirements for new allele naming were described by Marsh and colleagues.[103] The WHO committee also made recommendations about the naming of alleles with aberrant expression, such as HLA-G isoforms and KIRs. Some alleles are identifiable at the genomic level, but they are not translated into protein (pseudogenes) and are indicated by the addition of an N (for *null*) following the numerical designation of the allele. Mutations inducing a reduction of expression are marked by L (for *low expression*). An "S" denotes alleles expressed as *soluble* or *secreted* molecules; such molecules, such as HLA-B*4402010S, are characterized by an intronic variant that disallows the expression of the transmembrane domain of the HLA molecule and therefore only exists in a soluble form. Differential splicing of HLA-G leads to production of membrane-bound and soluble forms, which are denoted by a lowercase "m" or "s," respectively, before HLA. Limited cytoplasmic expression is denoted by "C," and aberrant expression by "A." Finally, KIR polymorphism will be classified by a new system that is in preparation.[93,103,104] A nomenclature system for cytokine polymorphism has not been developed yet.[105]

HLA Typing in Transfusion Medicine and Determination of Compatibility

HLA Typing

Originally, HLA phenotyping was used to support transplantation and transfusion needs with the purpose of identifying the best match between donors and recipients. Allosensitization of recipients previously exposed to heterologous cell products was tested by identifying alloreactive antibodies in serum. Crossmatch procedures involving serum from alloimmunized patients and cells from donors were performed to grade compatibility of candidate donor–recipient pairs.

Table 10–2 Name of Genes in the HLA Region Considered by the WHO Nomenclature Committee and Numbers of Named Alleles[3]

Name	Previous Equivalents	Molecular Characteristics	No. of Alleles (Dec. 2004)
HLA-A	—	Class I α-chain	349
HLA-B	—	Class I α-chain	627
HLA-B	—	Class I α-chain	182
HLA-E	E, '6.2'	Associated with class I 6.2-kB Hind III fragment	5
HLA-F	F, '5.4'	Associated with class I 5.4-kB Hind III fragment	2
HLA-G	G, '6.0'	Associated with class I 6.0-kB Hind III fragment	15
HLA-H	H, AR, '12.4', HLA-54	Pseudogene assoc. with class I 5.4-kb Hind III fragment	
HLA-J	cda 12, HLA-59	Pseudogene assoc. with class I 5.9-kb Hind III fragment	
HLA-K	HLA-70	Pseudogene assoc. with class I 7.0-kb Hind III fragment	
HLA-L	HLA-92	Pseudogene assoc. with class I 9.2-kb Hind III fragment	
HLA-N	HLA-30	Pseudogene assoc. with class I 1.7-kb Hind III fragment	
HLA-S	HLA-17	Pseudogene assoc. with class I 3.0-kb Hind III fragment	
HLA-X	—	Class I gene fragment	
HLA-Z	HLA-Z1	Class I gene fragment located in HLA class II region	
HLA-DRA	DRα	DR α chain	3
HLA-DRB1	DRβI, DR1B	DR β1 determining specificity for DR1, DR2, DR3, etc.	394
HLA-DRB2	DRβII2	Pseudogene with DRβ-like sequence	1
HLA-DRB3	DRβIII, DR3B	DR β3 determining DR52, Dw24, w25, –26 specificity	41
HLA-DRB4	DRβIV, DR4B	DR β4 determining DR53 specificity	13
HLA-DRB5	DRβV, DR5B	DR β5 determining DR52, Dw24, w25, –26 specificity	18
HLA-DRB6	DRBX, DRBσ	Pseudogene found in DR1, DR2, and DR10 haplotypes	3
HLA-DRB7	DRBψ1	Pseudogene found in DR4, DR7, and DR9 haplotypes	2
HLA-DRB8	DRBψ2	Pseudogene found in DR4, DR7, and DR9 haplotypes	1
HLA-DRB9	M 4.2 β exon	Pseudogene isolated fragment	1
HLA-DQA1	DQα1, DQ1A	DQ α chain as expressed	28
HLA-DQB1	DQβ1, DQ1B	DQ β chain as expressed	61
HLA-DQA2	DXα, DQ2A	DQ α-related chain, not known to be expressed	
HLA-DQB2	DXβ, DQ2B	DQ β-related chain, not known to be expressed	
HLA-DQB3	DVβ, DQB3	DQ β-related chain, not known to be expressed	
HLA-DOA	DNA, DZα, DOα	DO α chain	8
HLA-DOB	DOβ	DO β chain	9
HLA-DMA	RING 6	DM α chain	4
HLA-DMB	RING 7	DM β chain	7
HLA-DPA1	DPα1, DP1A	DP α chain as expressed	22
HLA-DPB1	DPβ1, DP1B	DQ β chain as expressed	116
HLA-DPA2	DPα2, DP2A	DP α chain-related pseudogene	
HLA-DPA3	DPA 3	DP α chain-related pseudogene	
HLA-DPB2	DPβ2, DP2B	DP β chain-related pseudogene	
TAP1	ABCB2, RING4	ABC (ATP-binding cassette) transporter	7
TAP2	ABCB3, RING 11	ABC (ATP-binding cassette) transporter	4
PSMB9	LMP2, RING 12	Proteasome-related sequence	
PSMB8	LMP7, RING 10	Proteasome-related sequence	
MICA	PERB 11.1	Class I chain-related gene	57
MICB	PERB 11.2	Class I chain-related gene	18
MICC	PERB 11.3	Class I chain-related gene	
MICD	PERB 11.4	Class I chain-related gene	
MICE	PERB 11.5	Class I chain-related gene	

HLA phenotyping has also been applied to identify links between a given disease and the genetic makeup of its carriers.[106] Strong associations are exemplified by birdshot uveitis, a disease occurring exclusively in HLA-A29 individuals[107]; type I diabetes and other autoimmune diseases[108–110]; or long-term survival of HIV-infected individuals.[54] These studies evaluated the role that genetic background may have contributed over environmental factors.[106,111] HLA associations are thought to be due to differential ability of distinct alleles to present immunogenic epitopes[107,108] or to the close linkage of HLA class I and II antigens to the HLA class III region where potent immune modulators such as TNF-α are located.[112]

HLA phenotype associations have also been suggested as predictors of immune responsiveness of cancer to immune therapy.[59] However, such associations have remained difficult to reproduce. Most recently, patient HLA typing is being required before enrollment into immunization protocols[25] because the response to the vaccine may be HLA-restricted. Analysis of specific HLA–epitope combinations for immunization protocols requires high-resolution typing because allelic variations may affect antigen presentation and the immune response to vaccination.[23,113]

Traditional serologic assessment of HLA antibodies and antigens takes advantage of fetomaternal sensitization. In mammals, the progeny carries a full haplotype of paternal origin, and pregnant women may develop antibodies against antigens expressed by the paternal haplotype. Maternal sera are collected at term and characterized by testing their ability to kill HLA-bearing cell lines of known phenotype in the presence of complement (complement-dependent cytotoxicity, or CDC).[114] CDC is then used for HLA typing by exposing circulating cells expressing HLA class I (most cells) and class II (predominantly B cells) antigens from the individual to be typed to previously characterized alloantisera or monoclonal antibodies.[115]

Traditionally, when sera from sensitized patients are screened for antibodies directed to HLA antigens, a HLA-phenotyped repository of cell lines are used in a CDC assay to identify alloantibodies. The fraction of cell lines killed by the sera serves as a rough grade or indicator of the intensity of allosensitization and is referred to as *panel-reactive antibody (PRA) reactivity.*

Some antibodies activate complement and kill with poor efficiency: the cytotoxicity-negative-absorption-positive (CYNAP) phenomenon.[116] CYNAP may cause the underestimated allosensitization judged by cytotoxicity testing. By modifying CDC with the addition of antihuman antibodies capable of activating complement, CYNAP can be circumvented (augmented CDC). However, with this assay relatively innocuous antibodies may cause overestimation of clinically relevant allosensitization.[117]

Other methods identify alloantibodies, including the immobilization of HLA molecules on solid surface to capture soluble antibodies[118–120] and a flow cytometry method that uses a spectrum of microbeads coated with HLA molecules of known type.[121,122] An interlaboratory comparison of serum screening for HLA antibody determination suggested that enzyme-linked immunosorbent assay (ELISA) and flow cytometry yield higher PRA activity values compared with CDC or augmented CDC.[119] However, the study suggested a lack of consistency among participant laboratories, leaving unsolved which method most accurately defines clinically relevant allosensitization; a panel of various methods may be most informative.

The CDC phenotyping assay is declining in interest in the United States because most laboratories are switching to easier-to-handle and higher-resolution molecular methods. However, cellular immunologic methods remain valuable to characterize functional aspects of HLA molecules because molecular genotyping methods cannot define whether an HLA allele is expressed.[123] Thus, it is likely that immunologic methods will continue to complement molecular methods in the future.[123]

The usefulness of conventional serologic typing has been limited by the availability of allele-specific sera. Most importantly, because antibodies identify structural differences on the surface of HLA molecules, variations caused by nucleotide polymorphism in areas that are not exposed, such as the peptide-binding groove of the HLA heavy chain, are not detectable. However, the differences that are located in the peptide-binding groove are of functional significance because they determine the specificity and affinity of peptide binding[124,125] and T-cell recognition of self and allogeneic target cells.[24,126]

DNA-based typing methods directly determine the sequence of HLA molecules.[127] Various polymerase chain reaction (PCR)-based methods have been described, among which sequence-specific primer (SSP)[127,128] and sequence-specific oligonucleotide probe (SSOP)-based methods[129] are the most universally used. The resolution of SSP and SSOP assays is limited only by the number of allele-specific primers or probes used to identify an ever growing number of alleles (http://www.anthonynolan.com/HIG/index.htm). The realization of the richness of HLA polymorphism has led to a proportional increase in the complexity of the assays utilized to cover all possible alleles. As a consequence, accurate HLA typing for donor and recipient matching in transplantation has become increasingly complex and burdensome. In addition, due to the important role that HLA molecules play in antigen presentation and the stringency of the relationship between epitope and associated HLA allele, high-resolution typing is increasingly requested for appropriate enrollment of patients into immunization protocols aimed at the enhancement of T-cell responses. Therefore, high-resolution HLA typing is increasingly in demand in clinical and experimental settings.

Although oligonucleotide-based methods could theoretically discriminate any known polymorphic site, they have two major limitations. First, they require a specific PCR for each allele investigated. Because each individual has only two alleles for each locus a disproportionately large number of PCRs need to be performed to cover all possible polymorphisms in order to identify the two alleles in the individual tested. In addition, because both oligonucleotide-based methods are based on specific interactions with known oligonucleotide sequences unique to a particular allele, they cannot identify unknown polymorphisms unless, by chance, the variation occurs within the region spanned by one of the oligonucleotide primers or pairs used in the assay. Because of these limitations interest is growing for definitive typing methods that yield conclusive information about the identity of the alleles typed. The most comprehensive method is sequence-based typing (SBT), however, its utilization has been limited by cost of equipment and reagents and by the high level of expertise and time required for the interpretation of each typing. In addition, some of the alleles and allele combinations are difficult to resolve even with SBT.[130] More recently, high-throughput robotic SBT has been developed that allows sequencing of hundreds of genomic fragments each day.[131] Finally, new methods based on high-density array technology are being developed that may allow extensive typing of known and unknown polymorphisms on microchips.[132]

High-resolution HLA genotyping methods yield high-resolution information of an individual's HLA type. The wealth of information is, however, counterbalanced by increased difficulty in identifying suitable HLA alleles during donor–recipient pairing or accrual into immunization protocols restricted to specific HLA–epitope combinations. Thus, at present clinicians are faced with the daunting task of applying high-resolution typing results of unclear relevance to clinical settings.[133]

TESTING FOR ALLOSENSITIZATION AND DETERMINATION OF COMPATIBLE RECIPIENT–DONOR PAIRS

Ideally, any cell containing a human product transfused or transplanted between different individuals should be HLA compatible. Yet, in most cases histocompatibility is not prospectively sought. Thus, patients who have received long-term therapies often become reactive to various antigens, including HLA. Transfusion of leukocyte-depleted products has decreased the incidence of allosensitization, yet organ transplant candidates often develop alloreactivity before the transplant. To prevent rejection in organ transplant recipients alloreactivity must be documented before transplantation. Alloreactive patients can still receive a transplant if the documentation provided states that the donor organ has no mismatched HLA antigens reactive with the patient's antibodies. Similarly, patients who have received repeated platelet transfusions may become allosensitized and consequently refractory to further transfusions unless platelets from HLA-compatible donors are used.

Obviously, the best compatibility among organ, hematopoietic progenitor cell, and platelet donors and recipients is identical matching. However, particularly in the case of rare HLA types, it is often impossible to identify a perfectly matched unrelated donor. Thus, other strategies have been adopted to identify the best possible match or "compatible mismatch." Selection of compatible unrelated donor–recipient pairs is carried out through typing with serologic, cellular, and molecular methods.[134] With the increasing resolution of these typing methods, the chances of identifying compatible donors based on full or partial HLA matching has become increasingly low.[133] To broaden compatibility-matching criteria for donor–recipient pairs, matching systems have been developed based on shared public epitopes assigned to crossreacting groups (CREGs)[135] or shared amino acid polymorphisms defined through sequence information.[136] Pre-existing alloantibodies further restrict the availability of compatible donors. Highly sensitized recipients with PRA reactivity exceeding 85% of tested specificities represent a particularly challenging group.[137] An alternative approach to the exclusion of alloreactive determinants is the inclusion of "acceptable" antigen mismatches expressed in a panel of cells that give negative reactions with the recipient sera,[138] thereby extending the repertoire of possible donors. Unfortunately, even these tools for the identification of unrelated, partially matched donor–recipient pairs often fail to identify a suitable match.

Recently Duquesnoy[137] described a molecularly based algorithm to identify histocompatible donor–recipient pairs called HLAMatchmaker. This method focuses on the structural basis of HLA class I polymorphism so that compatible HLA mismatches can be identified without extensive serum screening. This algorithm is based on the principle that short amino acid sequences, triplets, characterizing polymorphic sites of the HLA molecules, are the critical components of allosensitizing epitopes. Such amino acids reside in the α-helices and β-loops of the heavy chain. Because each HLA molecule expresses a characteristic string of these determinants, it is possible to characterize each molecule according to the linear sequence of amino acid triplets present on its surface. Based on the reasonable assumption that none of the triplets present in the HLA repertoire of the recipient are self-immunogenic, it is possible through a process of "electronic recombination" to identify donors with HLA alleles different from the recipient's but containing exclusively shared triplets. The selected HLA alleles will be compatible because they do not contain any epitope absent in the recipient.

In theory, a large number of triplets could occur if polymorphisms were randomly distributed. However, most HLA molecules span conserved domains and only a total of 142 different polymorphic triplets designate serologically defined HLA-A, HLA-B, and HLA-C antigens.[137] Triplet polymorphism can occur in 30 locations on HLA-A, 27 in HLA-B, and 19 in HLA-C chains. Because the HLAMatchmaker algorithm includes interlocus comparison, it is possible to accumulate the information into a single database. Among the 142 polymorphic triplets, 29 are polymorphic for one class I locus but monomorphic for another. Such polymorphic triplets cannot be immunogenic because they are always present on the patient's own HLA antigens, whereas the remaining 113 triplets have immunogenic potential. With this algorithm it is possible to significantly broaden the number of "molecularly matched" HLA alleles and therefore significantly increase the chances of identifying a compatible donor, particularly in those cases when the recipient has a rare HLA phenotype.

In addition, if information on the specificity of HLA antibodies in the recipient is known, HLAMatchmaker considers triplets that are present in the panel of screening cells that give negative reactions with the recipient's serum. These negative panel cells can be expected to share antigens with the patients; however, other HLA antigens may be present and contain mismatched triplets that apparently are not immunogenic for that recipient. Such triplets are therefore acceptable and can be added to the algorithm for the identification of possible donors.

Thus, HLAMatchmaker assesses HLA compatibility at a molecular level by determining whether or not a triplet in a given position of a mismatched HLA antigen is also found in the same position in any of the recipient's own HLA-A, HLA-B, and HLA-C molecules. A shared triplet in the same position on a mismatched HLA antigen cannot elicit a specific antibody response in that patient. This hypothesis needs future testing as this strategy might represent a revolutionary tool for the identification of potential donors. Preliminary verification of the algorithm in a series of high PRA renal patients suggested that this is a proper strategy, at least in highly sensitized renal transplant candidates waiting for kidneys from unrelated donors.[139] HLAMatchmaker is also effective at selecting the best HLA-typed platelet component to transfuse to alloimmunized thrombocytopenic patients.[140]

The HLA Molecules as Antigens and HLA Alloimmunization

Because of their high density on the surface of cells HLA molecules can become immunogenic when cells from one individual are exposed to another's immune system. The mechanism(s) leading to HLA allosensitization are believed to follow two pathways. The first pathway is followed during most immune reactions and involves donor antigen uptake by donor antigen-presenting cells and presentation to recipient lymphocytes (indirect pathway). In this case, the donor's HLA molecules are processed into peptides through the exogenous pathway of antigen presentation and presented to recipient T cells as linear peptides.[141,142] This pathway is believed to be responsible for the development of alloantibodies as well as helper T-cell responses, but its role in the development of cytotoxic T-cell responses remains unclear. Because this pathway depends on the presentation of donor HLA molecules by the recipient's HLA alleles, it may explain why the humoral response to HLA class I allodeterminants correlates with the HLA phenotype of the recipient.[143] The indirect pathway of HLA allorecognition has been associated with allograft rejection.[144]

Because the function of HLA molecules is to present antigenic determinants to T cells, it could be easily envisioned how minor changes in their structure could be misinterpreted as antigenic epitopes. Thus, intact HLA molecules residing on the surface of donor cells are a perfect target for T cell–mediated allorecognition (direct pathway) by recipient cells either through direct cytotoxic effect of T cells against target cells or by the activation of helper T cells, through HLA class II engagement, which leads to stimulation of antibody-mediated immune responses.[145]

Humoral alloresponses mediated most frequently by immunoglobulin M (IgM) are predominant when sensitization involves infrequent allogeneic exposure because they require smaller amounts of antigenic material. T-cell responses become more predominant in the context of transplantation where the persistence of the continuous allogeneic stimulation allows the expansion and sustenance of alloreactive cytotoxic T cells.

Because antibodies and TCR have different requirements for engagement, epitopes recognized by T cells and antibodies are different. Antibodies require interaction with a small structure, including a limited number of amino acids; thus, any amino acid sequence combination on the surface of an HLA allele not present in the individual exposed to the alloreaction may represent an epitope. The TCR has a much lower binding affinity for their ligand and binding requires the complete interaction of the TCR with the antigenic peptide as well as the α– and β–helices of the HLA class I heavy chain.[12] Thus, although several B-cell epitopes recognized by antibodies can be identified in a given HLA molecule, generally the whole HLA molecule is necessary for T cell–dependent allorecognition.

Two types of antibody-defined epitopes can be identified according to their frequency among HLA alleles. Private epitopes are almost, but not totally, unique for each single serologically defined HLA antigen, and antibodies directed to private epitopes are used for phenotyping. Private epitopes are generally shared by all molecularly defined alleles in a given family; for this reason fine differences among alleles within a general family cannot be distinguished serologically. Public epitopes are more widely distributed among serologically defined antigens and have been used to cluster distinct serologic families into groups. Public epitopes have an immune dominant character. Immune sera that identify public epitopes have been considered to be predictive of major CREGs. When donors and recipients belong to the same CREG, alloreactivity is thought to be less likely to develop (Table 10–3). The predictive value of CREG matching of donor–recipient pairs on transplant outcome or platelet transfusion results, however, remains to be demonstrated.

Not all subjects that have been exposed to HLA alloantigens develop alloantibodies and, in fact, exposure to low doses of donor-specific HLA antigens through donor-specific blood transfusions may have a beneficial effect on the survival of organ allografts.[146] Several hypotheses have been proposed for the capriciousness of allosensitization, including presence of regulatory immune responses or cytokine-mediated immune suppression. However, the mechanisms that modulate the quality and quantity of alloimmunity remain elusive; different aspects of this algorithm are discussed ad hoc in this chapter with particular attention to molecularly defined algorithms for the prediction of histocompatibility.[123,137,147,148]

HLA matching enhances the outcome of some types of organ transplants. An analysis of more than 150,000 renal transplant recipients performed by centers participating in the Collaborative Transplant Study showed that a complete mismatch (6 HLA-A+B+DR) had a 17% lower survival expectation than no mismatch ($p<0.0001$),[149] and matching was particularly beneficial in patients with highly reactive preformed alloantibodies. The same study suggested that high-resolution matching based on molecular typing improved graft survival. Similar results were observed in cardiac transplantation where HLA matching yielded significantly ($p< 0.0001$) better results. This is particularly important because in most centers donor hearts are currently not allocated according to HLA match. HLA matching was not beneficial in liver transplantation.[150]

The induction of donor-specific hyporesponsiveness has been particularly well documented in the context of renal allotransplantation and may limit the need for immune suppression. A recent randomized study suggested that pretransplant donor transfusions improved the survival of cadaver kidney grafts in patients receiving modern immune

Table 10–3 Population Frequencies of Major Cross-Reactive Groups or Determinants Present on HLA-A and HLA-B Gene Products

Major Cross-Reactive Group	Public Epitope	Associated Private Epitopes	Approximate Epitope Frequency (%)
1C	1p	A1, 3, 9 (23, 24), 11, 29, 30, 31, 36, 80	79
	10p	A10 (25, 26, 34, 43, 66), 11, 28 (68, 69), 32, 33, 74	
2C	28p	A2, 28 (68, 69), 9, 17	70
	9p	A2, 28 (68, 69), 9 (23, 24)	
	17p	A2, B17 (57,58)	
5C	5p	B5 (51, 52), 18, 35, 53, 78	50
	21p	B5 (51,52), 15 (62, 63, 75, 76, 77), 17 (57, 58), 21 (49, 50), 35, 53, 70 (71, 72), 73, 74, 78	
7C	7p	B7, 8, 41, 42, 48, 81	54
	22p	B7, 22 (54, 55, 56), 27, 42, 46	
	27p	B7, 13, 27, 40 (60, 61), 47	
8C	8p	B8, 14 (64, 65), 16 (38, 39), 18	38
12C	12p	B12 (44, 45), 13, 21 (49,50), 40 (60, 61), 41	44
Bw4	Bw4	B13, 27, 37, 38, 47, 49, 51, 52, 53, 57, 58, 59, 63, 77, A24, 25, 32	79
Bw6	Bw6	B7, 8, 18, 35, 39, 41, 42, 45, 46, 48, 50, 54, 55, 56, 60, 61, 62, 64, 65, 67, 71, 72, 73, 75, 76, 78, 81	87

*North American white populations of European origin.

suppressive regimens, although the mechanism remains unclear.[151,152] Thus, although most centers presently do not implement deliberate blood transfusions, the usefulness of this approach needs to be further investigated.

Patients who have been previously exposed to HLA class I expressing heterologous cells and who have produced HLA antibodies often require platelet transfusions. Such patients are refractory to random donor platelets and must be given HLA-matched or "semi-matched" apheresis components.[41–44] However, the provision of HLA-matched platelets does not always improve platelet recovery and survival. Possibly, the ineffectiveness of some "HLA-matched" platelet transfusions is due, at least, in part to unrecognized HLA mismatches between the donor and recipient resulting from low-resolution methods used for typing the donor and recipients. Higher-resolution typing methods have been advocated, but it remains controversial whether molecularly based HLA typing confers an advantage over serologic typing; this principle was recently questioned in the context of hematopoietic cell transplantation.[153,154]

HLA as a Functional Mediator of Graft-versus-Host Disease and/or Graft-versus-Neoplasia Effect

Allogeneic or syngeneic hematopoietic progenitor cell (HPC) transplantation is used to treat hematologic malignancies[155,157]; hematologic disorders such as aplastic anemia,[158] thalassemia,[159] or myelodysplastic syndrome[160]; immune difficiency states; and some types of cancers.[161] The objective of HCP transplantation in malignancies is to cure the patient by eradicating the neoplastic cells with high-dose myeloablative chemotherapy followed by restoration of hematopoiesis through the transplantation of normal hematopoietic stem cells derived from HLA-compatible normal donors. This strategy, however, is characterized by the reaction by the transplanted (donor's) immune system toward the host's normal cells, GVHD.[162,164] The development of GVHD is often associated with an immune reaction that preferentially targets neoplastic cells (the GVN effect).[161,165,171] GVHD and the GVN effect can occur in the presence of a complete HLA match, suggesting that the HLA molecules themselves are not the targets of the allosensitization reaction responsible for GVHD or the GVN effect. Instead cells involved with GVHD and the GVN effect are induced by polymorphic molecules presented by the HLA molecules and expressed by the recipient's cells and recognized by the grafted immune cells.

Graft-versus-Host Disease

Graft-versus-host disease represents the alloimmune reaction of donor lymphocytes against normal cells of the recipient. GVHD occurs predominantly in association with HPC transplantation because HPC transplantation also replaces the host humoral and cellular immune systems. GVHD is a major complication of HPC transplantation but for a successful transplant a fine balance must be maintained between GVHD and graft rejection by modulating the level of post-transplant immune suppression.[169] In addition, other major events associated with HPC transplantaion, such as post-transplant infection, leukemic or tumor relapse, and other regimen-related mortalities, are strongly influenced by the methods use to treat GVHD.

T-cell depletion has been advocated as a means of preventing GVHD by decreasing the probability of cellular and humoral alloresponses.[172,173] This strategy decreases the occurrence of GVHD but is associated with an increased risk of graft rejection and tumor/leukemia relapse.[174] In fact, Weiden and colleagues[175] observed that survivors of severe acute GVHD had a significantly lower incidence of tumor relapse compared with patients who did not experience GVHD. This association appeared mandatory and it was felt that the beneficial GVN effect was inseparable from GVHD.

The risk of GVHD increases with genetic distancing between donor and recipient. Recipients of HPC transplantation from identical siblings have a lower chance of developing GVHD compared with recipients of HPC transplants from HLA-matched unrelated donors and partial HLA-matched realated donors.[176,177] However, although the genetic closeness between donor and recipient appears to decrease the risk of GVHD, it also decreases the therapeutic benefit of the GVN effect and increases the chances of tumor relapse.

Graft-versus-Neoplasia Effect

It was first recognized that a beneficial collateral effect of GVHD was the rejection of neoplastic cells by the donor immune system in the context of hematologic malignancies (graft-versus-leukemia effect).[165] It was rapidly recognized that the graft-versus-leukemia effect could play a powerful therapeutic role in the treatment of refractory malignant disorders, including some solid tumors (graft-versus-tumor effect).[161] Because the biology and clinical principles underlining the two effects are likely similar, for simplicity, in this chapter we coin a unifying term: graft-versus-neoplasia effect.

It is believed that the GVN reaction is the most potent form of tumor immunotherapy currently in clinical use. However, the mechanism(s) responsible for the GVN effect are still poorly understood. T cells definitely play a fundamental role in the initiation and maintenance of the alloreaction toward neoplastic cells.[178] In fact a sevenfold increase in the chance of disease relapse was noted in patients with chronic myelogenous leukemia who received a T cell–depleted HPC transplant compared with a subset of patients who had received a T cell–replete HPC transplant but did not develop GVHD.[172,173] This result suggests that GVHD is a biologic entity different from the GVN effect. In addition, on relapse of chronic myelogenous leukemia, the administration of lymphocytes from the transplant donor can re-induce clinical remission.[179] Finally, leukemia-specific CD8+ T cells have been identified among circulating lymphocytes at the time of leukemia regression.[180] NK cells also play a role in mediating this phenomenon; clinical data suggests that mismatch of NK receptor and ligands during allogeneic BMT may be used to enhance the GVN effect.[89,181]

Appreciation of the GVN effect has led to the development of nonmyeloablative stem cell transplants designed to immune suppress the host only to a level sufficient to permit engraftment of the donor immune cells to generate the GVN effect without inducing the serious complications associated with myeloablation.[174] With nonmyeloablative HPC transplantation, GVHD and the GVN effect are being used as the primary antitumor therapy rather than high-dose chemotherapy. The use of nonmyeloablative HCP transplants and their associated GVN effect has gained popularity in the last decade to the point that this allogeneic-based immunotherapeutic approach has been advocated for several nonhematologic malignancies.[174] The rationale is largely based on the assumption that the immune cell repertoire capable of recognizing cancer cells in the allogeneic context is broader than that in the autologous system. Donor T cells may target not only tumor-specific antigens, but also allelic variants of antigens expressed by the tumor such as mHA and, in the case of HLA-mismatched transplants, HLA antigens disparate from the donor.[182–184] Although there are several theories about how GVN effect occurs, it remains unclear why allo-T cells have a better chance of targeting tumor cells compared with the natural antitumor immunity described in patients with several type of solid tumors.

HLA and T Cell–Directed Immunization

The past decade has witnessed remarkable progress in the identification and mapping of T-cell epitopes for various infectious diseases and cancers. In particular, progress has been made in mapping HLA-associated epitopes for HIV, CMV, and EBV.[185–188] In addition, the molecular identification of tumor-associated antigens has yielded a large number of epitopes that could be used to immunize against neoplasia.[189] A comprehensive discussion of these topics is beyond the scope of this chapter, but we address a few points framing the relevance of HLA in the context of T cell–directed immunization.

The identification of T-cell epitopes led to two major areas of clinical investigation: active-specific immunization to prevent or treat ongoing infections or cancer and the harvest and in vitro expansion of immunization-induced T cells for adoptive transfer. In general, active immunization has proven successful in inducing epitope-specific T cells easily detectable among circulating lymphocytes.[113,190–192] However, in most cases, the immunization-induced enhancement of T-cell function is not associated with clinical improvement. Although the reason for the clinical ineffectiveness of immunization-induced T cells is unclear, it has been postulated that they may be quantitatively[191] or qualitatively[193] inadequate for eradicating disease. Therefore, a second strategy is being pursued, whereby the number of antigen-specific T cells is amplified in vitro for autologous or donor-derived adoptive transfer. This second strategy has met some promising success in the context of ganciclovir-resistant CMV infection,[194] EBV-induced post-transplant lymphoproliferative disorders,[195] and metastatic melanoma.[196]

Whether delivered as a primary form of therapy or to prime in vivo T cells for further ex vivo expansion, epitope-specific vaccination is limited by the stringent requirement for HLA allelic association or HLA restriction. Although superfamilies of HLA alleles may share epitopes,[18,19] in practical terms, clinically relevant HLA–epitope associations are restricted to a few peptide–allele combinations for a given protein.[23] Thus, patients considered for enrollment in immunization protocols are best served by high-resolution HLA typing to exclude subtypes with unproven immunogenic potential for a given epitope.

To overcome the stringent HLA requirements for successful epitope-specific vaccination, some protocols have used entire peptides, based on the assumption that the epitope repertoire of a protein can be adjusted to specific HLA phenotypes by a cellular process of self-selection that naturally couples peptides to HLA molecules according to their binding affinity. The peptide(s) within the protein with the greatest binding affinity are bound by the molecules. Although theoretically sound, in practice the truth of this assumption depends on the efficiency with which individual molecules are processed and presented in association with distinct HLA alleles. Even in clinical settings where this method of vaccination or sensitization is used, high-resolution typing is desirable because it allows accurate interpretation of immunization results by allowing a comparison between the detailed genetic makeup of the individual receiving the vaccine and his or her antigen-specific immune response. Thus, it is likely that in the future HLA laboratories will increasingly be required to provide high-resolution, definitive typing for enrollment of patients into vaccination protocols and for subsequent interpretation of immune responses.

Monitoring Immune Responses with Tetrameric HLA–Peptide Complexes

The growing understanding of the molecular immunology of T-cell interactions with HLA–epitope complexes in the context of infectious disease, virally induced malignancies, and spontaneous tumors and interest in their treatment with T cell–directed vaccines has sparked an interest in accurate methods to quantify ex vivo the extent of antigen-specific immune responses.[197] The most widely used assays for the enumeration of antigen-specific T cells include tetrameric HLA–peptide complexes (tHLA), intracellular flow cytometry staining for cytokines expressed on cognate peptide stimulation, detection of cytokine release by ELISPOT, and quantitative real-time PCR.[198]

Tetrameric HLA–peptide are complexes of four HLA molecules combined with a specific peptide and bound to a fluorochrome[199] (Fig. 10–8). These complexes bind to the complementary TCR and therefore identify antigen-specific T cells.[200] These tHLA can measure cellular responses against specific epitopes with sensitivity as low as 1/5000 CD8+ T cells. To synthesize tHLA molecules, soluble HLA heavy chain containing a biotinylation site and recombinant β_2-microglobulin are synthesized and purified. They are then refolded in the presence of the specific epitope and the monomer is isolated by gel filtration and biotinylated. Fluorescent streptavidin is added to induce tetramerization. An aliquot of tetramer is added to the peripheral blood mononuclear cells together with other antibodies for a more detailed characterization of antigen-specific T cells.[193] Analysis is performed using a flow cytometer. Due to the specificity of vaccines, the HLA type of the patient and the specific peptide must be identified and synthesized to provide the adequate tetramer.

Analysis of tHLA offers many potential advantages over other T-cell assays. This method is quantitative and enables an estimation of the avidity between TCR and peptide-loaded HLA class I molecules. In addition, tHLA staining does not kill the labeled cells, allowing sorting of subpopulations by flow cytometry for additional analysis or expansion for adoptive transfer. With tHLA, specific T cells can be analyzed from blood samples without the prerequisite of in vitro culture, and all specific cytotoxic T lymphocytes are detected, regardless of their functional status.[191,193]

Summary

The relevance of HLA in clinical pathology has broadened from a predictor of allosensitization to a mediator of GVHD and the GVN effect. In addition, understanding of the mechanism of action of various nonclassical HLA genes as well as KIRs has opened a new field involving the study of the innate immune response in the context of transplantation.

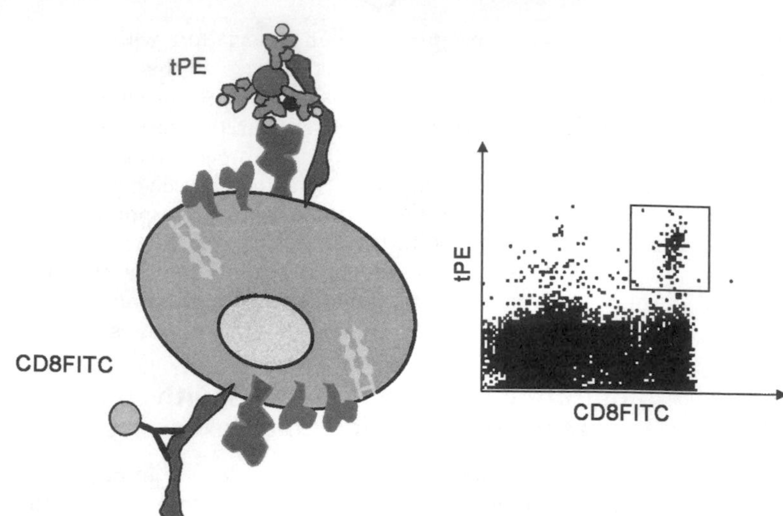

Figure 10–8 Schematic representation of the mechanism of binding of tetrameric peptide–HLA complexes (tHLA) to antigen-specific T cells. *A,* Binding of tHLA to TCR. The tHLA consists of four HLA–peptide complexes identical to the ones recognized by the T cell on the surface of live cells. Each HLA molecule is modified to contain one biotin molecule that serves as a bridge for binding to tetravalent strepavidin molecules fluorescently labeled. *B,* Actual FAC analysis result of CD8+, tHLA-positive T cells. (Modified with permission from Monsurro V, Nagorsen D. Immunotracking of specific cancer vaccine CD8+ lymphocytes. ASHI Quarterly 2003;26:100–102.)

Table 10–4 International Society of Blood Transfusion (ISBT) Human Neutrophil Antigen Nomenclature

Antigen System	Antigens	Location	Former Name	Alleles
HNA-1	HNA-1a	FcγRIIIb	NA1	*FCGR3B*1*
	HNA-1b	FcγRIIIb	NA2	*FCGR3B*2*
	HNA-1c	FcγRIIIb	SH	*FCGR3B*3*
HNA-2	HNA-2a	CD177 (NB1 gp)	NB1	*CD177*1*
HNA-3	HNA-3a	70–95 kD gp	5b	Not defined
HNA-4	HNA-4a	CD11b (CR3 or Mac-1)	Mart[a]	*CD11B*1*
HNA-5	HNA-5a	CD11a (LFA-1)	Ond[a]	*CD11A*1*

CR3, C3bi receptor; gp, Glycoprotein; ISBT, International Society of Blood Transfusion; LFA-1, leukocyte functional antigen-1.

Together with HLA, the study of immunogenetics is experiencing rapid growth that is driven by the realization that polymorphism in molecules such as mHA, KIR, cytokines, and their receptors is an important hallmark of human immune pathology. Modern histocompatibility and immunogenetics laboratories must be able to adopt high-throughput systems for the parallel assessment of all these variables when addressing the genetic makeup of an individual in correlation with the natural or therapeutic history of his or her disease. The comparison of donor and recipient protein profiling and cytokine polymorphism may offer new insights on the mechanism of rejection, GVHD, and GVN in transplant recipients. Finally, the increased utilization of T cell–directed immunization protocols is driving an increase in demand for high-resolution typing of HLA molecules to allow a more accurate interpretation of clinical and immunologic results.

HUMAN NEUTROPHIL ANTIGENS AND THEIR CLINICAL SIGNIFICANCE

Introduction

Lalezari and colleagues described the first neutrophil-specific antigens. These antigens were designated "N" for *neutrophil.* Each antigen system was described alphabetically and each allele was described numerically in order of discovery. They identified human neutrophil antigen 1a (HNA-1a) or NA1 in 1966; its allele, HNA-1b or NA2 in 1972[201,202]; and HNA-2a or NB1 in 1971.[203] Reports of several other granulocyte antigens followed.

The current neutrophil antigen nomenclature was established in 1998 by an International Society of Blood Transfusion (ISBT) Working Party[204] (Table 10–4). In this nomenclature antigen systems are referred to as human neutrophil antigens, or HNA. The antigen systems are indicated by integers, and specific antigens within each system are designated alphabetically by date of publication. Alleles of the coding genes are named according to the Guidelines for Human Gene Nomenclature. Five neutrophil antigen systems have been described: HNA-1, HNA-2, HNA-3, HNA-4, and HNA-5.

Genetics, Structure, and Function of Neutrophil Antigens

Genetics

HNA-1 antigens, which are located on the neutrophil low-affinity Fc receptor, Fc-γ receptor IIIb (FcγRIIIb), are encoded by the Fc-γ receptor gene, *FCGR3B,* which is located on chromosome 1q23.[205–208] This area of chromosome 1 contains a cluster of two families of FcγR genes, *FCGR2* and *FCGR3.* The *FCGR3* family is made up of *FCGR3A* and *FCGR3B,* which are located adjacent to each other on chromosome 1q23. *FCGR3B* is highly homologous to *FCGR3A,* which encodes FcγRIIIa (Table 10–5). The most important difference between the two genes is a C to T change at position 733nt in *FCGR3B* that

Table 10–5 Nucleotide Differences among the Genes Encoding the FcγRIIIa and the HNA-1a, HNA-1b, and HNA-1c Antigens of FcγRIIIb

Molecule	Gene	Base Pair Position										
		141	147	227	266	277	349	473	505	559	641	733
FcγRIIIb HNA-1a	FCGR3B*1	AGG	CTC	A**A**C	GCT	GAC	**G**TC	GAC	CAC	GTT	TCT	TGA*
FcγRIIIb HNA-1b	FCGR3B*2	AG**C**	CT**T**	AGC	GCT	**A**AC	ATC	GAC	CAC	GTT	TCT	TGA*
FcγRIIIb HNA-1c	FCGR3B*3	AG**C**	CT**T**	AGC	G**A**T	**A**AC	ATC	GAC	CAC	GTT	TCT	TGA*
FcγRIIIa	FCGR3A	AGG	CTC	AGC	GCT	GAC	ATC	G**G**C	**T**AC	**T**TT	T**T**T	**C**GA

* Stop codon.
Differences among genes are in bold.

creates a stop codon. As a result *FCGR3A* has 21 more amino acids than *FCGR3B*.

The HNA-2a antigen is encoded by the gene *CD177*, which is located on chromosome 19q13.2. *CD177* belongs to the *Ly6* gene superfamily.[209–211] The coding region of *CD177* consists of 1311 bp that code for a protein of 416 and a signal peptide of 21 amino acids.[209] The predicted protein has two cysteine-rich domains, three potential N-linked glycosylation sites, and a potential ω-site for attachment of the glycosylphosphatidylinositol (GPI) anchor.[209]

The *Ly6* gene superfamily is also known as the urokinase-type plasminogen activator receptor (uPAR) or snake toxin family. This superfamily is characterized by conserved cysteine-rich domains. Typically these domains contain 70 to 100 amino acids, including 8 to 10 cysteine residues spaced at conserved distances. The *Ly6* superfamily includes two subfamilies, one encodes GPI-anchored glycoproteins and the other encodes secretory proteins without a GPI anchor. In general, the GPI-anchored *Ly6* proteins have domains with 10 cysteines and the secretory proteins have 8. The protein encoded by *CD177*, NB1 gp, is an exception in that it is GPI anchored, but it has only six cysteine residues in its cysteine-rich domains.[209] Most *Ly6* proteins have one cysteine-rich domain. Two exceptions are uPAR, which has three cysteine-rich domains and NB1 gp, which has two.[212] Members of this family tend to have little homology. At most, 20% to 30% of amino acids are conserved among members. The functions of these proteins are diverse, but not well understood.

Genes in the *Ly6* superfamily were first described in mice and are widely used as markers of murine hematopoietic stem cells and T-cell differentiation. *Ly6A/E* (stem cell antigen 1, or Sca-1) is used as a marker of murine hematopoietic precursor cells. Among the *Ly6* superfamily genes found in humans, CD59 or membrane inhibitor of reactive lysis and CD87 or uPAR are best described. *CD177* is most similar to *uPAR*; however, *CD177* and *uPAR* are only approximately 30% homologous.[209,210]

The gene encoding HNA-3a has not yet been identified. HNA-4a and HNA-5a are encoded by genes belonging to the integrin family of leukocyte cell adhesion molecules. This family is made up of three members sharing a common integrin β chain, β_2, but a different α chain. The leukocyte function-associated antigen (LFA-1) is a heterodimer made up of α_L or CD11a and β_2 or CD18 and is expressed on all leukocytes. The second member of this group, complement receptor 3 (CR3) or Mac-1, is made up of α_M or CD11b and β_2. The other member, CD11c/CD18, is made up of α_x (CD11c) and β_2. Mac-1 and CD11c/CD18 are expressed by granulocytes, monocytes, and NK cells. The HNA-4a antigen is located on CD11b and is encoded by *CD11B*1*; HNA-5a antigen is located on CD11a and is encoded by *CD11A*1*.[213]

Structure and Function of Neutrophil Antigens

The HNA-1a antigens are located on FcγRIIIb or CD16. This glycoprotein has 233 amino acids and is GPI-anchored.[205,208] The molecular weight of this heavily glycosylated protein ranges from 50 to 80 kD; differences in N-glycosylation account for the differences in molecular mass. FcγRIIIb has N-linked carbohydrate side chains, and the number of side chains differs between the HNA-1a and HNA-1b forms of the glycoprotein. The HNA-1a form of FcγRIIIb has 4 N-link side chains and it ranges in size from 50 to 65 kD; the HNA-1b form of FcγRIIIb has 6 N-linked side chains and is 65 to 80 kD.

FcγRIIIb is a low-affinity Fc receptor. It is the most abundant neutrophil low-affinity Fc-γ receptor. The low-affinity Fc-γ receptors link humoral immunity to cellular immune function; specifically, Fcγ receptors on effector cells recognize cytotoxic IgG molecules and immune complexes containing IgG molecules.

HNA-2a antigen is on NB1 gp, which is located on neutrophil plasma membranes and secondary granules[214,215] and is linked to the plasma membrane via a GPI anchor.[215,216] The molecular weight of NB1 gp is 58 to 64 kD and it contains N-linked carbohydrate side chains.[214,215] NB1 gp has been well characterized, but its function is not known.

HNA-3 antigens are located on a 70 to 95 kD glycoprotein that has not yet been fully characterized.[217] The function of this glycoprotein is not known. The HNA-4a and HNA-5 antigens are located on the $\alpha_M\beta_2$ or CR3 and $\alpha_L\beta_2$ or LFA-1 integrin molecules, which are important leukocyte adhesion molecules. The integrin $\alpha_M\beta_2$ also serves as a receptor for complement component C3bi.

Expression of Neutrophil Antigens

FcγRIIIb and HNA-1 antigens are expressed only on neutrophils. FcγRIIIb, HNA-1a, and HNA-1b antigens are expressed on all segmented neutrophils, about one half of neutrophilic metamyelocytes, and about 10% of neutrophilic myelocytes.[218] Soluble FcγRIIIb is found in plasma and both the HNA-1a and HNA-1b forms of the glycoprotein can be found in plasma.[219,220] Neutrophils release FcγRIIIb when they are stimulated in vitro or in vivo. Soluble FcγRIIIb levels are increased when neutrophils are stimulated or granulopoiesis is increased.[221] In healthy subjects given granulocyte colony-stimulating factor (G-CSF), FcγRIIIb expression by neutrophils is reduced and levels of soluble FcγRIIIb are increased.

HNA-2a is a neutrophil-specific antigen. It is expressed only on neutrophils, neutrophilic metamyelocytes, and myelocytes.[218,222] Although some GPI-anchored proteins, such as FcγRIIIb, are shed by stimulated neutrophils, NB1 gp is not, nor is soluble NB1 gp present in plasma.[215] HNA-2a is unique in that it is expressed on subpopulations of neutrophils. The mean size of the HNA-2a-positive subpopulation of neutrophils is 45% to 65%.[215,223,224] The expression of HNA-2a is greater on neutrophils from women than men.[224,225] The size of the HNA-2a-positive subpopulation of neutrophils from women is approximately 60% to 70% compared to approximately 50% to 60% for men. The expression of HNA-2a falls with age in women, but remains constant in men.[224] Neutrophil expression of HNA-2a is greater in pregnant women than in healthy female blood donors.[226,227]

The surface expression of HNA-2a is slightly upregulated by treatment with the chemotactic peptide f-Met-Leu-Phe.[215,216] The administration of G-CSF to healthy subjects for several days increases the proportion of neutrophils expressing HNA-2a to near 90%.[228] Patients with polycythemia vera have markedly increased levels of *CD177* mRNA, but the levels of NB1 gp expressed by neutrophils from patients with polycythemia vera have been reported to be normal.[229] However, NB1 gp expression has not been studied thoroughly in patients with polycythemia vera.

Unlike the HNA-1 and HNA-2 antigens, the other neutrophil antigens HNA-3, HNA-4, and HNA-5 are expressed by several other cell types. HNA-3a is expressed by neutrophils, lymphocytes, platelets, endothelial cells, and kidney, spleen, and placental cells.[217] HNA-4a is expressed on granulocytes, monocytes, and NK cells; HNA-5a is expressed on all leukocytes.

Neutrophil Antigen Polymorphisms and Clinical Significance

Neutrophil Antigen Polymorphisms

The neutrophil-specific HNA-1 antigen system is made up of the three alleles HNA-1a, HNA-1b, and HNA-1c[230,231] (see Table 10–4). The gene frequencies of the three alleles vary widely among different racial groups. Among whites the frequency of the gene encoding HNA-1a, *FCGR3B*1*, is between 0.30 and 0.37 and the frequency of the gene encoding HNA-1b, *FCGR3B*2*, is from 0.63 to 0.70.[231–236] In contrast, among Asian populations the *FCGR3B*2* gene is more common. In Japanese and Chinese populations the *FCGR3B*1* gene frequency ranges from 0.60 to 0.66 and the *FCGR3B*2* gene frequency from 0.30 to 0.33.[233,235–237] The gene frequency of the gene encoding HNA-1c, *FCGR3B*3*, also varies among racial groups. *FCGR3B*3* is expressed by neutrophils from 4% to 5% of Caucasians and 25% to 38% of African Americans.[231]

The structures of *FCGR3B*1*, *FCGR3B*2*, and *FCGR3B*3* alleles are very similar. The *FCGR3B*1* gene differs from the *FCGR3B*2* gene by only five nucleotides in the coding region, at positions 141, 147, 227, 277, and 349[205–208] (see Table 10-5). Four of the nucleotide changes result in changes in amino acid sequence between the HNA-1a and HNA-1b forms of the glycoprotein. The fifth polymorphism at 147 is silent. The glycosylation pattern of the protein differs between the two antigens because of two nucleotide changes at bases 227 and 277. The HNA-1b form has six N-linked glycosylation sites and the HNA-1a form has four glycosylation sites.

The gene encoding the HNA-1c form FcγRIIIb, *FCGR3B*3*, is identical to *FCGR3B*2* except for a C to A substitution at nucleotide 266. The nucleotide substitution results in an Alanine to Aspartate change at amino acid 78 of FcγRIIIb[230] (see Table 10–5). In many cases *FCGR3B*3* exists on the same chromosome with a second or duplicate *FCGR3B* gene.[238] One group has found that in Danish people, *FCGR3B*3* always exists as a duplicate gene in association with *FCGR3B*1*.[239] However, in other populations duplicate *FCGR3B*3* genes were associated with both *FCGR3B*1* and *FCGR3B*2*.

Several other sequence variations in *FCGR3B* have been described.[234,237] These chimeric alleles have single-base substitutions involving one of the five single nucleotide polymorphisms that distinguish *FCGR3B*1* and *FCGR3B*2*. *FCGR3B* alleles that more closely resembled *FCGR3B*2* were found more often in African Americans than in whites or Japanese.[237]

Neutrophils from some people do not express any HNA antigens.[240–242] Blood cells from patients with paroxysmal nocturnal hemoglobinuria (PNH) lack GPI-linked glycoproteins and their granulocytes express reduced amounts of FcγRIIIb and the HNA-1 antigens. In addition, genetic deficiencies of granulocyte FcγRIIIb and HNA-1 antigens have also been reported. With inherited deficiency of FcγRIIIb, the *FCGR3B* gene is deleted along with an adjacent gene, *FCGR2C*.[242] Among whites the incidence of individuals homozygous for the *FCGR3B* gene deletion is about 0.1%.[243,244] However, among Africans and African Americans the incidence is much higher; in one study 3 of 126 Africans were found to have homozygous *FCGR3B* deletions[231] and in another 1 of 53 were found to have homozygous *FCGR3B* deletions.[237]

HNA-2a is expressed on neutrophils by approximately 97% of whites, 95% of African Americans, and 89% to 99% of Japanese.[224,225,245] HNA-2a has been reported to have an allele, *NB2*, but the product of this gene cannot be reliably identified with alloantisera and no monoclonal antibody specific for NB2 has been identified.[246] Several *CD177* polymorphisms have been described. Two different groups sequenced *CD177* independently. One group sequenced it as the gene encoding HNA-2a and called the gene *NB1*[209]; the other group sequenced it as a gene overexpressed in granulocytes from people with polycythemia rubra vera and called the gene *PRV-1*.[210] The *NB1* and *PRV-1* alleles differ at only four nucelotides.[209] Bettinotti and colleagues used Human Genomic Project databases to characterize the structure of the *PRV-1* and *NB1* genes.[211] They described the intron and exon structure of *NB1;* however, they found only one gene, *CD177*, homologous to both *PRV-1* and *NB1*, suggesting that they are alleles of the same gene. In addition, they described a pseudogene homologous to exons 4 through 9 of *CD177* and adjacent to *CD177* on 19q13.2.[211]

One of the four single nucleotide substitutions that distinguish the *NB1* and *PRV-1* alleles of *CD177* affects the size of the neutrophil population that expresses HNA-2a, but these single nucleotide polymorphisms are not responsible for the HNA-2a-negative phenotype.[247,248] Instead, the HNA-2a-negative neutrophil phenotype is due to a *CD177* transcription defect.[249] HNA-2a genes from two women with HNA-2a-negative neutrophils who produced HNA-2a-specific alloantibodies have been studied, and abnormal *CD177* mDNA sequences of variable lengths were detected in both women.[249] Their neutrophil mRNA had both exons and accessory sequences that were considered to be introns. Some cDNA containing the entire *CD177* coding sequence was identified, but all cDNA had some accessory sequences.[249]

HNA-3a has a gene frequency of 0.66, but the molecular basis of this antigen is not known.[217] HNA-4a has a phenotype frequency of 99.1% in whites and is due to a single nucleotide substitution of G to A at position 302 of *CD11B*.[213] This substitution results in an Arg to His polymorphism at amino acid 61 of the α chain of CR3, α_M. A second polymorphism of the β_2 integrins, HNA-5a, was first described as Ond[a]. A chronically transfused male with aplastic anemia became alloimmunized to HNA-5a. HNA-5a is due to a G to C single nucleotide substitution at position 2446 of *CD11A*. This change leads to an amino acid change of Arg to Thr at amino acid 766 of the α chain of LFA-1, α_L.[213]

Clinical Significance of Neutrophil Antigens

Polymorphisms of HNA-1 have been found to have only a few clinical consequences. The deletion of the entire *FCGR3B* gene does not have major clinical consequences, and most people with FcγRIIIb deficiency are healthy. However, too few patients have been studied to identify a slight increase in susceptibility to infection or autoimmune disease due to FcγRIIIb deficiency. In a study of 21 people with FcγRIIIb deficiency, 2 people were found to have autoimmune thyroiditis and 4 had multiple episodes of bacterial infections.[242] Other smaller studies and case reports have found that despite their FcγRIIIb deficiency, all individuals, except for the one person with systemic lupus erythematosus, were healthy, had no circulating immune complexes, and showed no increased susceptibility to infections.

Despite the lack of serious illness in people with FcγRIIIb deficiencies, HNA-1 polymorphisms have some effect on neutrophil function. Neutrophils that are homozygous for HNA-1b have a lower affinity for IgG3 than granulocytes homozygous for HNA-1a.[250] Neutrophils from people who are homozygous for HNA-1b phagocytize erythrocytes sensitized with IgG1 and IgG3 anti-Rh monoclonal antibodies[251] as well as bacteria opsonized with IgG1 at a lower level than granulocytes homozygous for HNA-1a.[251,252]

Several studies suggest that *FCGR3B* polymorphisms affect the incidence and outcomes of some autoimmune and inflammatory diseases, but the results of some of these studies seem contradictory. However, because *FCGR3B* is clustered with *FCGR3A* and *FCGR2* on chromosome 1q22, it is possible that some of these findings may be due in part to linkage disequilibrium among Fc receptors. Children with chronic immune thrombocytopenia purpura are more likely to be *FCGR3B**1* homozygous than controls,[253] but Spanish patients with systemic lupus erythematosus are more likely to be *FCGR3B**2* homozygous.[254] Myasthenia gravis is more severe in *FCGR3B**1* homozygous patients,[255] but multiple sclerosis is more benign in *FCGR3B**1* homozygous patients.[256] Patients with chronic granulomatous disease who are *FCGR3B**1* homozygous are less likely to develop major gastrointestinal or genital urinary tract infectious complications compared to those with chronic granulomatous disease who are heterozygous and *FCGR3B**2* homozygous.[257]

The role of NB1gp in neutrophil function is unknown. The rare women who produce HNA-2a specific alloantibodies and who lack NB1 gp are healthy. The expression of HNA-2a is reduced on neutrophils from people with PNH and chronic myelogenous leukemia.[218] It is not known if the lack of expression of HNA-2a on neutrophils from patients with PNH or chronic myelogenous leukemia has any clinical significance.

CD177 has become an important biomarker for polycythemia vera. The diagnosis of polycythemia vera can be difficult because several other clinical conditions are associated with increased hemoglobin levels. Hemoglobin levels can be increased as a secondary response to reduced arterial oxygen levels, increased erythropoietin levels, and the presence of high-oxygen affinity hemoglobin. It is important to distinguish patients with secondary erythrocytosis from those with polycythemia vera, because if not treated, patients with polycythemia vera can suffer serious thrombotic and hemorrhagic complications.

The measurement of neutrophil *CD177* mRNA is being used along with other assays by many centers to distinguish patients with increased hemoglobin levels due to secondary erythrocytosis from those with polycythemia vera.[258,259] Quantitative real-time PCR is being used to measure neutrophil *CD177* mRNA levels, and several studies have found that neutrophil levels of *CD177* mRNA are increased in polycythemia vera patients. Overall, 91% to 100% of patients with polycythemia vera have increased *CD177* mRNA levels.[258–260] In contrast, none of the patients with secondary erythrocytosis have increased *CD177* mRNA levels.[258,259]

Neutrophil *CD177* mRNA levels are also increased in some patients with myeloproliferative disorders related to polycythemia vera.[259] Neutrophil *CD177* mRNA is overexpressed in 30% to 60% of patients with essential thrombocythemia and in approximately 60% of patients with idiopathic myelofibrosis. In patients with essential thrombocythemia the overexpression of *CD177* may affect the course of their disease. Essential thrombocythemia patients with increased neutrophil *CD177* mRNA levels have an increased incidence of thrombosis and bleeding.[261]

CD177 mRNA overexpression in myeloproliferative disorders is likely secondary to a point mutation in the Janus kinase 2 (JAK2). Approximately 75% to 95% of patients with polycythemia vera have a G to T substitution in *JAK2,* which causes a Phenylalanine to be substituted for Valine at position 617 of JAK2 (V617F).[262–265] JAK2 is involved with signaling of a number of hematopoietic growth factors, including G-CSF. The JAK2 V617F gain of function mutation and the stimulation of neutrophils by physiologic G-CSF likely leads to increased JAK2 activation, increased expression of secondary signaling molecules such as the transcription factor STAT3, and increased *CD177* mRNA transcription. Interestingly, *CD177* mRNA is also overexpressed by neutrophils from healthy subjects given G-CSF.[248]

Testing for Neutrophil Antibodies and Neutrophil Antigen Typing

Many barriers surround neutrophil antibody testing and antigen typing, including limited availability of reagents, lack of commercially available test kits, and the need to use fresh neutrophils. However, neutrophil antibodies remain clinically important, and many laboratories test for these antibodies. As a result of the reduced risk of transmitting infectious diseases via blood component transfusion, attention has focused on TRALI. TRALI is now one of the most frequent causes of transfusion-associated mortality. Neutrophil antibody testing, phenotyping, and crossmatching are an important part of evaluation of patients and donors.

Neutrophil Antibody Testing

Screening for neutrophil antibodies remains technically challenging. Antibodies to some neutrophil antigens can be detected using solid phase assays; however, the clinically important antibodies to HNA-1 antigens cannot. As a result, intact neutrophils must be used for antibody screening assays. Unfortunately, neutrophils have a short life span so fresh neutrophils must be prepared daily for testing. Neutrophils are prepared from fresh whole blood using density gradient separation. Patient sera are tested in one of several assays against panels of neutrophils prepared from several donors with known phenotypes to distinguish antibodies with different specificities. The presence of HLA antibodies with broad specificities can make the detection of neutrophil antibodies difficult because neutrophils express class I antigens. HLA-specific antibodies can be separated from neutrophil-specific antibodies by absorbing serum with platelets. Alternatively, monoclonal antibody capture assays can be used to test for antibodies specific to neutrophil membrane glycoproteins.

Granulocyte Agglutination

In this assay antibodies cause neutrophils to actively agglutinate. Cells and serum are incubated for 4 to 6 hours at 30°C. When antibodies are present, neutrophils will clump. The granulocyte agglutination assay is very reliable but less sensitive than other assays. It can detect antibodies to HNA-1, HNA-2, HNA-3, HNA-4, and HNA-5 antigens and it is the only assay that can identify antibodies specific for HNA-3a.

Granulocyte Immunofluorescence and Flow Cytometry

In the granulocyte immunofluorescence assay, antigen–antibody reactions are detected using fluorescence-conjugated secondary antibodies and a fluorescent microscope. Before incubation with sera, neutrophils are treated with 1% paraformaldehyde for 5 minutes at 20°C to 24°C to help prevent nonspecific binding of antibodies to neutrophil Fc receptors and to stabilize the cell membranes. Treated neutrophils and patient sera are then incubated for 30 minutes at 37°C. Binding of antibody to the neutrophils is detected with a fluorochrome conjugated secondary antibody. To prevent nonspecific binding of the secondary antibody to neutrophil Fc receptors, $F(ab')_2$ secondary antibodies are used. The binding of antibodies in the test serum results in a uniform staining of the outside of the neutrophils. Strong reactions are readily distinguished, but considerable training is required to distinguish weak reactions from background staining.

Testing for neutrophil antibodies with flow cytometry is technically similar to the granulocyte immunofluorescence assay except that neutrophils are evaluated with a flow cytometer rather than a fluorescent microscope. The flow cytometer can more readily compare the reactions of test sera with positive and negative control sera than the fluorescent microscope.

Mixed Passive Agglutination

The mixed passive agglutination assay uses a granulocyte antigen preparation for antibody screening. This assay allows granulocyte testing trays to be prepared in large batches and frozen until testing. Antigens are extracted from isolated neutrophils using 3% sucrose.[266] The neutrophil extract is used to coat U-bottom Terasaki plates. Sera to be tested is incubated with neutrophil extract in wells for 3 hours at 22°C. Antibody binding is detected using sheep erythrocytes coated with antihuman IgG. The antigen-coated plates can be prepared and stored for at least 1 year at −80°C. The assay has been shown to detect antibodies specific for HNA-1a, HNA-1b, HNA-2a, and HNA-3a. Although results of this assay look promising, it has yet to be compared extensively with other assays or tested in international workshops.

Monoclonal Antibody Capture Assays

The monoclonal antibody capture, or monoclonal antibody immobilization of neutrophil antigens (MAINA), assay allows the detection of antibodies to specific neutrophil membrane glycoproteins. In this assay, neutrophils are incubated with test sera, washed, incubated with a murine monoclonal antibody to a specific neutrophil glycoprotein, and washed again. The neutrophils are then dissolved in a mild detergent. The soluble glycoprotein–monoclonal antibody complex is "captured" in a well with an antibody specific to mouse IgG fixed to the well bottom. An antibody specific to human IgG conjugated to alkaline phosphatase is added followed by a substrate, and the reaction is detected with a spectrophotometer.

The MAINA assay can be used to detect antibodies to FcγRIIIb (CD16), NB1 gp (CD177), LFA-1 (CD11a), and CR3 (CD11b). This assay will detect antibodies to HNA-1, HNA-2, HNA-4, and HNA-5. The use of neutrophils from panels of donors with known HNA-1 phenotypes allows the identification of antibodies specific to HNA-1a and HNA-1b. In addition, antibodies are sometimes detected that are directed to FcγRIIIb but are not specific to HNA-1a, HNA-1b, or HNA-1c. The MAINA assay permits the recognition of antibodies to specific neutrophil glycoproteins even when antibodies to HLA antigens are present.

Strategy for Antibody Detection

Most laboratories screen serum for neutrophil antibodies by granulocyte agglutination and granulocyte immunofluorescence or flow cytometry. The serum reactive with neutrophils must also be screened in an assay that can detect HLA antibodies. If the serum is reactive with neutrophils and HLA antibodies are present, then the MAINA or a similar assay is used to determine if both HLA antibodies and antibodies to neutrophil-specific antigens are present. Because the monoclonal antibody capture assays sometimes identify antibodies that cannot be detected in other assays, some laboratories test all serum samples in MAINA assays.

Phenotyping and Genotyping of Neutrophil Antigens

Phenotyping

Traditionally, neutrophil antigen phenotyping has been performed using human alloantibodies in the granulocyte agglutination or granulocyte immunofluorescence assays. However, alloantisera are difficult to obtain. Monoclonal antibodies specific to HNA-1a, HNA-1b, and HNA-2a have been described, are commercially available, and have been used to phenotype neutrophils using flow cytometry. Phenotyping with monoclonal antibodies and flow cytometry is faster and easier than phenotyping with alloantibodies because phenotyping with monoclonal antibodies can be done with whole blood instead of isolated neutrophils.

Genotyping

Because alloantibodies are difficult to obtain and monoclonal antibodies are not available for all neutrophil antigens, genotyping assays have become important. The characterization of the genes encoding the HNA-1 antigens has allowed for the development of genotyping assays for these antigens. Genotyping of HNA-1 antigens is especially important because alloantisera to HNA-1c are rare and monoclonal antibodies specific to HNA-1c do not exist. Distinguishing single nucleotide polymorphisms is usually straightforward, but genotyping for *FCGR3B* alleles is complicated by the high degree of homology between *FCGR3B* and the gene that encodes FcγRIIIa, *FCGR3A*. As a result, most laboratories use PCR-SSP to distinguish *FCGR3B* alleles.[231,233] A unique set of primers is used to amplify each of the three alleles.

Unfortunately, HNA-2a genotyping methods are not available. Because the HNA-2a-negative phenotype is due to *CD177* mRNA splicing defects,[249] SSP have been used to determine HNA-4a[267] and HNA-5a[268] genotypes. These assays are less complex than genotyping for HNA-1 antigens because these polymorphisms are due to single nucleotide polymorphisms.

Clinical Significance of Antibodies to Neutrophil Antigens

Alloimmune Neonatal Neutropenia

During pregnancy mothers can become alloimmunized to neutrophil antigens. Maternal IgG directed to neutrophils can cross the placenta and destroy the neonate's neutrophils. Maternal alloimmunization to neutrophil antigens can occur in utero and affect the first child. Most neonates experience isolated neutropenia, but the cytopenias are self-limiting and resolve as the antibody is cleared. The alloimmunized mothers produce and carry the antibodies, but the antibodies do not react with the mother's blood cells or tissues, and they have normal neutrophil counts. Antibodies to neutrophil-specific antigens HNA-1a, HNA-1b, and HNA-2a most commonly cause neonatal alloimmune neutropenia.[269] Rarely antibodies to HNA-1c and HNA-3a cause alloimmune neonatal neutropenia. Mothers with FcγRIIIb deficiency have produced FcγRIIIb-specific antibodies that caused neonatal neutropenia.[240,241,244,245] In addition, mothers without FcγRIIIb deficiency have produced antibodies specific for a high incidence FcγRIIIb antigen that have resulted in alloimmune neonatal neutropenia.[270] Neutrophil autoantibodies can cross the placenta and cause neonatal neutropenia.[271]

Newborns with alloimmune neutropenia are usually asymptomatic. Most often the neutropenia is detected in the first week of life when the neonate becomes febrile or develops an infection and a neutrophil count is done. Typically the counts are 0.1 to 0.2 × 10^9/L. Some neonates have normal neutrophil counts the first day of life, but they become neutropenic on their second day.[269] White blood cell count, platelet count, and hemoglobin are usually normal, but eosinophilia or monocytosis may be present. If a bone marrow biopsy is performed, it often shows normal numbers of erythroid progenitors and megakarocytes with hyperplasia of myeloid progenitors.

The clinical course is quite variable. An occasional infant is asymptomatic, but most affected children have an infection. The most common infections are umbilicus infections, skin infections, abscesses, and respiratory tract infections. Less commonly infants experience otitis media, urinary tract infections, and gastroenteritis. Serious infections such as sepsis, pneumonia, and meningitis can occur. The duration of the neutropenia may be as short as a few days or as long as 28 weeks.[269] The mean duration of neutropenia is about 11 weeks.[269]

For an asymptomatic child no immediate treatment may be required. Prompt and aggressive antibiotic treatment of children with fevers or other signs of infections is indicated. Intravenous immunoglobulin (IVIG) has a limited role in the treatment of neonatal alloimmune neutropenia. Approximately half the patients treated have a transient increase in count lasting only a few days. The use of G-CSF to treat alloimmune neutropenia has also had mixed results, elevating the neutrophil count in some but not all neonates.[269]

Autoimmune Neutropenia of Childhood

Autoimmune neutropenia has been well described in children.[272–275] Typically, the onset of autoimmune neutropenia of childhood begins at age 8 months, but children between ages 1 and 36 months can be affected. Most studies found that neutrophil counts recover spontaneously by age 5 years, with a median of 13 to 20 months of neutropenia.[269,272–275]

In most cases, children presented with severe neutropenia, having neutrophil counts less than 0.5 × 10^9/L. Monocytosis has been reported to occur in up to 38% of patients. Bone marrow biopsies in infected patients usually show normal to hypercellular marrow with a decreased number of mature granulocytes. Febrile episodes and infections, including bacterial skin infections, otitis media, respiratory tract infections, and urinary tract infections, are common. Life-threatening complications are rare.

Antibodies to neutrophils can be detected in up to 98% of affected patients. If an antibody specificity is identified, the antibodies are almost always specific to epitopes located on FcγRIIIb. The antibodies are directed to HNA-1a in 10% to 46% of patients, to HNA-1b in 2% to 3% of patients, and rarely to FcγRIIIb eptitopes expressed by granulocytes from all donors.[273,274]

Autoimmune neutropenia has been treated with corticosteroids, IVIG, and G-CSF. Approximately half the patients responded to IVIG, but neutrophil counts remained elevated for only 1 week. Almost all of the patients responded to G-CSF and 75% to corticosteroids; neutrophil counts remained elevated as long as the drugs were given.

Transfusion Reactions

Prior to the widespread transfusion of leukocyte-reduced blood components, approximately 0.5% of transfusions were associated with febrile nonhemolytic transfusion reactions. These febrile reactions are due to the interaction of leukocyte antibodies in the transfusion recipient with leukocytes contained in the transfused blood components. These reactions can be prevented by the use of components that have been filtered to remove leukocytes.

A more serious type of transfusion reaction associated with leukocyte antibodies is acute noncardiac pulmonary edema, or TRALI. It has been known for more than 45 years that the transfusion of leukocyte antibodies can cause pulmonary distress.[276] Evidence for the role of neutrophils in lung injury was provided in 1977 by Craddock and colleagues, who found that activated neutrophils can cause acute lung injury and respiratory distress.[277] They found that some hemodialysis membranes activated complement, which resulted in transient neutropenia and respiratory distress.[278] In addition, they found that activated complement caused neutrophils to aggregate and resulted in pulmonary vessel leukostasis and interstitial edema.[277,278] In 1983 Popovsky and coworkers found that the transfusion of blood components containing leukocyte antibodies was sometimes associated with acute respiratory distress, which they called TRALI.[279] TRALI is characterized by acute respiratory distress occurring within 4 to 6 hours after a transfusion, characterized by dyspnea, hypoxia, and bilateral pulmonary infiltrates on chest x-ray without cardiomegaly or pulmonary vascular congestion. The mortality associated with TRALI is approximately 5%.[279] Eighty percent of patients with TRALI have rapid resolution of pulmonary infiltrates and return of arterial blood gas values to normal within 96 hours after the initial respiratory insult. However, pulmonary infiltrates have persisted for at least 7 days after the transfusion reaction in 17% of TRALI patients.

Leukocyte antibodies have also been found to cause lung injury in animal models. The infusion of alloanti-HNA-3a in an isolated rabbit lung perfused with human neutrophils caused lung injury 3 to 6 hours after the transfusion of anti-HNA-3a.[280] In this model, lung injury was dependent on the presence of complement.

Initially, TRALI was defined as only occurring when leukocyte antibodies were present in the implicated blood component.[279] However, TRALI can occur after transfusion of blood components that do not contain leukocyte antibodies. In these cases TRALI is thought to be due to the transfusion of biologically active lipids that accumulate in blood components during storage, which primes neutrophils and potentiates the toxic effects of activated neutrophils in the transfusion recipient.[281] Other studies suggest that the activation of monocytes may cause TRALI.[282] As a result a consensus group developed a definition of TRALI that was not dependent on leukocyte antibodies in the blood component.[283] TRALI was defined as acute lung injury occurring within 6 hours of a transfusion in a patient without pre-existing acute lung injury or alternative acute lung injury risk factors.[283] Acute lung injury is the acute onset of lung injury with pulmonary artery occlusion pressure $\leq$ 18 mmHg or without clinical evidence of left atrial hypertension, bilateral infiltrates on chest x-ray, and hypoxemia with a ratio of $PaO_2/FIO_2 \leq 300$ mmHg or oxygen saturation of $\leq$ 90% on room air.[283]

Transfusion-related acute lung injury has been associated with transfusion of blood components containing both neutrophil and HLA antibodies. Antibodies specific to HNA-1a, HNA-1b, HNA-3a, and HLA class I have been reported to cause TRALI.[284] Recently HLA class II antibodies have also been implicated in TRALI.[285] Antibodies specific to HNA-3a seem to be particularly potent in causing TRALI.[286–288] Three fatal cases of TRALI following the transfusion of platelet or fresh frozen plasma components containing HNA-3a specific antibodies have recently been reported. Two of the three donors with anti-HNA-3a were regular blood donors. A review of the transfusion of 25 previous donations from one of the donors found that no transfusion reactions were reported.[287] However, a review of 36 transfusions from the other donor found 15 transfusion reactions, 8 of which were severe and included respiratory symptoms.[288]

Granulocyte Transfusions

Granulocyte transfusion recipients sometimes produce antibodies specific to HNA-1a, HNA-1b, and HNA-2a.[289,290] The transfusion of granulocytes to patients with these antibodies can result in febrile transfusion reactions and pulmonary transfusion reactions.[290] Hematopoietic progenitor cell transplant recipients who produce HNA-2a antibodies as a result of granulocyte transfusions have experienced marrow graft failure.[289]

Summary

Four neutrophil antigen systems—HNA-1, HNA-2, HNA-4, and HNA-5—have been well described and the other—HNA-3—described in part. HNA-1 antigens are located on FcγRIIIb, and antibodies to these antigens are frequently implicated in autoimmune and alloimmune neutropenia. HNA-2a is located on NB1 gp, and antibodies to HNA-2a are found in patients with alloimmune and autoimmune neutropenia. This protein is overexpressed by neutrophils in patients with polycythemia rubra vera. The significance of the overexpression of the *CD177* gene is not certain, but measurement of *CD177* levels is being used to help diagnose polycythemia rubra vera. Antibodies to HNA-3a are rare, but they appear to be more likely than other neutrophil antibodies to cause TRALI. The significance, if any, to HNA-4a and HNA-5a antibodies is not certain.

REFERENCES

1. Gorer PA. The detection of antigenic differences in mouse erythrocytes by employment of immune sera. Br J Exper Pathol 1938;17:42–49.
2. Trowsdale J, Ragoussis J, Campbell RD. Map of the human MHC. Immunol Today 1991;12:443–446.
3. Marsh SG, Albert ED, Bodmer WF, et al. Nomenclature for factors of the HLA system, 2004. Hum Immunol 2005;66:571–636.
4. Malissen M, Malissen B, Jordan BR. Exon/intron organization and complete nucleotide sequence of an HLA gene. Proc Natl Acad Sci USA 1982;79:893–897.
5. Germain RN, Malissen B. Analysis of the expression and function of class-II major histocompatibility complex-encoded molecules by DNA-mediated gene transfer. Annu Rev Immunol 1986;4:281–315.
6. Yewdell JW, Bennink JR. The binary logic of antigen processing and presentation to T cells. Cell 1990;62:203–206.
7. Goodfellow PN, Jones EA, Van HV, et al. The β_2-microglobulin gene is on chromosome 15 and not in the HL-A region. Nature 1975;254:267–269.
8. Klein J. Natural History of the Major Histocompatibility Complex. New York, John Wiley & Sons, 1986.
9. Terasaki IP, Gjertson DW. HLA. Los Angeles, UCLA Tissue Typing Laboratory, 1997.
10. Bjorkman PJ, Saper MA, Samraoui B, et al. Structure of the human class I histocompatibility antigen, HLA-A2. Nature 1987;329:506–512.
11. Brown JH, Jardetzky TS, Gorga JC, et al. Three-dimensional structure of the human class II histocompatibility antigen HLA-DR1. Nature 1993;364:33–39.
12. Garboczi DN, Ghosh P, Utz U, et al. Structure of the complex between human T-cell receptor, viral peptide and HLA-A2. Nature 1996;384:134–141.
13. Hennecke J, Wiley DC. Structure of a complex of the human α/βT cell receptor (TCR) HA1.7, influenza hemagglutinin peptide, and major histocompatibility complex class II molecule, HLA-DR4 (DRA*0101 and DRB1*0401): insight into TCR cross-restriction and alloreactivity. J Exp Med 2002;195:571–581.
14. Hennecke J, Wiley DC. T cell receptor–MHC interactions up close. Cell 2001;104:1–4.
15. Hennecke J, Carfi A, Wiley DC. Structure of a covalently stabilized complex of a human αβ T-cell receptor, influenza HA peptide and MHC class II molecule, HLA-DR1. EMBO J 2000;19:5611–5624.
16. Ruppert J, Sidney J, Celis E, et al. Prominent role of secondary anchor residues in peptide binding to HLA-A2.1 molecules. Cell 1993;74:929–937.
17. Falk K, Rotzschke O, Stevanovic S, et al. Allele-specific motifs revealed by sequencing of self-peptides eluted from MHC molecules. Nature 1991;351:290–296.
18. del Guercio MF, Sidney J, Hermanson G, et al. Binding of a peptide antigen to multiple HLA alleles allows definition of an A2-like supertype. J Immunol 1995;154:685–693.

19. Sidney J, Grey HM, Southwood S, et al. Definition of an HLA-A3-like supermotif demonstrates the overlapping peptide-binding repertoires of common HLA molecules. Hum Immunol 1996;45:79–93.
20. Sidney J, del Guercio MF, Southwood S, et al. The HLA molecules DQA1*0501/B1*0201 and DQA1*0301/B1*0302 share an extensive overlap in peptide binding specificity. J Immunol 2002;169:5098–5108.
21. Madden DR, Garboczi DN, Wiley DC. The antigenic identity of peptide–MHC complexes: a comparison of the conformations of five viral peptides presented by HLA-A2. Cell 1993;75:693–708.
22. Threlkeld SC, Wentworth PA, Kalams SA, et al. Degenerate and promiscuous recognition by CTL of peptides presented by the MHC class I A3-like superfamily: implications for vaccine development. J Immunol 1997;159:1648–1657.
23. Bettinotti MP, Kim CJ, Lee KH, et al. Stringent allele/epitope requirements for MART-1/Melan A immunodominance: implications for peptide-based immunotherapy. J Immunol 1998;161:877–889.
24. Rivoltini L, Loftus DJ, Barracchini K, et al. Binding and presentation of peptides derived from melanoma antigens MART-1 and glycoprotein-100 by HLA-A2 subtypes. Implications for peptide-based immunotherapy. J Immunol 1996;156:3882–3891.
25. Kim CJ, Parkinson DR, Marincola F. Immunodominance across HLA polymorphism: implications for cancer immunotherapy. J Immunother 1998;21:1–16.
26. Parker KC, Bednarek MA, Coligan JE. Scheme for ranking potential HLA-A2 binding peptides based on independent binding of individual peptide side-chains. J Immunol 1994;152:163–175.
27. Parker KC, DiBrino M, Hull L, et al. The β_2-microglobulin dissociation rate is an accurate measure of the stability of MHC class I heterotrimers and depends on which peptide is bound. J Immunol 1992;149:1896–1904.
28. Hunt DF, Henderson RA, Shabanowitz J, et al. Characterization of peptides bound to the class I MHC molecule HLA-A2.1 by mass spectrometry. Science 1992;255:1261–1263.
29. Lanzavecchia A, Lezzi G, Viola A. From TCR engagement to T cell activation: a kinetic view of T cell behavior. Cell 1999;96:1–4.
30. Pamer E, Cresswell P. Mechanisms of MHC class I–restricted antigen processing. Annu Rev Immunol 1998;16:323–358.
31. Wiertz EJ, Jones TR, Sun L, et al. The human cytomegalovirus US11 gene product dislocates MHC class I heavy chains from the endoplasmic reticulum to the cytosol. Cell 1996;84:769–779.
32. Wiertz EJ, Mukherjee S, Ploegh HL. Viruses use stealth technology to escape from the host immune system. Mol Med Today 1997;3:116–123.
33. Falk CS, Mach M, Schendel DJ, et al. NK cell activity during human cytomegalovirus infection is dominated by US2-11-mediated HLA class I down-regulation. J Immunol 2002;169:3257–3266.
34. Lopez-Botet M, Llano M, Ortega M. Human cytomegalovirus and natural killer-mediated surveillance of HLA class I expression: a paradigm of host-pathogen adaptation. Immunol Rev 2001;181:193–202.
35. Ulbrecht M, Martinozzi S, Grzeschik M, et al. Cutting edge: The human cytomegalovirus UL40 gene product contains a ligand for HLA-E and prevents NK cell-mediated lysis. J Immunol 2000;164:5019–5022.
36. Chen Y, Rocha V, Bittencourt H, et al. Relationship between HLA alleles and cytomegalovirus infection after allogenic hematopoietic stem cell transplant. Blood 2001;98:500–501.
37. Kropshofer H, Hammerling GJ, Vogt AB. The impact of the non-classical MHC proteins HLA-DM and HLA-DO on loading of MHC class II molecules. Immunol Rev 1999;172:267–278.
38. Daar AS, Fuggle SV, Fabre JW, et al. The detailed distribution of HLA-A, B, C antigens in normal human organs. Transplantation 1984;38:287–292.
39. Kowalik I, Kurpisz M, Jakubowiak A, et al. Evaluation of HLA expression on gametogenic cells isolated from human testis. Andrologia 1989;21:237–243.
40. Datema G, Stein S, Eijsink C, et al. HLA-C expression on platelets: studies with an HLA-Cw1-specific human monoclonal antibody. Vox Sang 2000;79:108–111.
41. Ornstein DL, Mortara KL, Smith MB, et al. Treatment of severe thrombocytopenia in alloimmunized, transfusion-refractory patients. Mil Med 2001;166:269–274.
42. Petz LD, Garratty G, Calhoun L, et al. Selecting donors of platelets for refractory patients on the basis of HLA antibody specificity. Transfusion 2000;40:1446–1456.
43. Kekomaki S, Volin L, Koistinen P, et al. Successful treatment of platelet transfusion refractoriness: the use of platelet transfusions matched for both human leucocyte antigens (HLA) and human platelet alloantigens (HPA) in alloimmunized patients with leukaemia. Eur J Haematol 1998;60:112–118.
44. Gelb AB, Leavitt AD. Crossmatch-compatible platelets improve corrected count increments in patients who are refractory to randomly selected platelets. Transfusion 1997;37:624–630.
45. Panzer S, Puchler K, Mayr WR, et al. Haemolytic transfusion reactions due to HLA antibodies. A prospective study combining red-cell serology with investigations of chromium-51-labelled red-cell kinetics. Lancet 1987;1:474–478.
46. Daar AS, Fuggle SV, Fabre JW, et al. The detailed distribution of MHC Class II antigens in normal human organs. Transplantation 1984;38:293–298.
47. Skoskiewicz MJ, Colvin RB, Schneeberger EE, et al. Widespread and selective induction of major histocompatibility complex-determined antigens in vivo by gamma interferon. J Exp Med 1985;162:1645–1664.
48. Hakem R, Le Bouteiller P, Jezo-Bremond A, et al. Differential regulation of HLA-A3 and HLA-B7 MHC class I genes by IFN is due to two nucleotide differences in their IFN response sequences. J Immunol 1991;147:2384–2390.
49. Hakem R, Jezo-Bremond A, Le Bouteiller P, et al. Differential transcription inducibility by interferon of the HLA-A3 and HLA-B7 class-I genes. Int J Cancer Suppl 1991;6:2–9.
50. Marincola FM, Shamamian P, Alexander RB, et al. Loss of HLA haplotype and B locus down-regulation in melanoma cell lines. J Immunol 1994;153:1225–1237.
51. Marincola FM, Shamamian P, Simonis TB, et al. Locus-specific analysis of human leukocyte antigen class I expression in melanoma cell lines. J Immunother Emphasis Tumor Immunol 1994;16:13–23.
52. Panelli MC, Wang E, Phan G, et al. Gene-expression profiling of the response of peripheral blood mononuclear cells and melanoma metastases to systemic IL-2 administration. Genome Biol 2002;3: RESEARCH0035.
53. Kaufman J, Volk H, Wallny HJ. A "minimal essential MHC" and an "unrecognized MHC": two extremes in selection for polymorphism. Immunol Rev 1995;143:63–88.
54. Migueles SA, Sabbaghian MS, Shupert WL, et al. HLA B*5701 is highly associated with restriction of virus replication in a subgroup of HIV-infected long term nonprogressors. Proc Natl Acad Sci USA 2000;97:2709–2714.
55. Hildesheim A, Apple RJ, Chen CJ, et al. Association of HLA class I and II alleles and extended haplotypes with nasopharyngeal carcinoma in Taiwan. J Natl Cancer Inst 2002;94:1780–1789.
56. Goldsmith DB, West TM, Morton R. HLA associations with nasopharyngeal carcinoma in Southern Chinese: a meta-analysis. Clin Otolaryngol Allied Sci 2002;27:61–67.
57. Wank R, Thomssen C. High risk of squamous cell carcinoma of the cervix for women with HLA-DQw3. Nature 1991;352:723–725.
58. Lee JE, Reveille JD, Ross MI, et al. HLA-DQB1*0301 association with increased cutaneous melanoma risk. Int J Cancer 1994;59:510–513.
59. Marincola FM, Shamamian P, Rivoltini L, et al. HLA associations in the antitumor response against malignant melanoma. J Immunother Emphasis Tumor Immunol 1995;18:242–252.
60. Braun WE. Update on kidney transplantation: increasing clinical success, expanding waiting lists. Cleve Clin J Med 2002;69:501–504.
61. Shirwan H. Chronic allograft rejection. Do the Th2 cells preferentially induced by indirect alloantigen recognition play a dominant role? Transplantation 1999;68:715–726.
62. Ponticelli C, Tarantino A, Vegeto A. Renal transplantation, past, present and future. J Nephrol 1999;12(Suppl 2):S105–S110.
63. Adams EJ, Parham P. Species-specific evolution of MHC class I genes in the higher primates. Immunol Rev 2001;183:41–64.
64. Natarajan K, Li H, Mariuzza RA, et al. MHC class I molecules, structure and function. Rev Immunogenet 1999;1:32–46.
65. Paul P, Rouas-Freiss N, Moreau P, et al. HLA-G, -E, -F preworkshop: tools and protocols for analysis of non-classical class I genes transcription and protein expression. Hum Immunol 2000;61:1177–1195.
66. Bainbridge D, Ellis S, Le Bouteiller P, et al. HLA-G remains a mystery. Trends Immunol 2001;22:548–552.
67. Gobin SJ, van den Elsen PJ. The regulation of HLA class I expression: is HLA-G the odd one out? Semin Cancer Biol 1999;9:55–59.
68. Onno M, Guillaudeux T, Amiot L, et al. The HLA-G gene is expressed at a low mRNA level in different human cells and tissues. Hum Immunol 1994;41:79–86.
69. Ellis SA, Palmer MS, McMichael AJ. Human trophoblast and the choriocarcinoma cell line BeWo express a truncated HLA Class I molecule. J Immunol 1990;144:731–735.
70. Gobin SJ, van den Elsen PJ. Transcriptional regulation of the MHC class Ib genes HLA-E, HLA-F, and HLA-G. Hum Immunol 2000;61:1102–1107.
71. Lee N, Malacko AR, Ishitani A, et al. The membrane-bound and soluble forms of HLA-G bind identical sets of endogenous peptides but differ with respect to TAP association. Immunity 1995;3:591–600.
72. Lopez-Botet M, Llano M, Navarro F, et al. NK cell recognition of non-classical HLA class I molecules. Semin Immunol 2000;12:109–119.

73. Lee N, Goodlett DR, Ishitani A, et al. HLA-E surface expression depends on binding of TAP-dependent peptides derived from certain HLA class I signal sequences. J Immunol 1998;160:4951–4960.
74. Lila N, Amrein C, Guillemain R, et al. Human leukocyte antigen-G expression after heart transplantation is associated with a reduced incidence of rejection. Circulation 2002;105:1949–1954.
75. Braud VM, Allan DS, O'Callaghan CA, et al. HLA-E binds to natural killer cell receptors CD94/NKG2A, B and C. Nature 1998;391:795–799.
76. Lee N, Llano M, Carretero M, et al. HLA-E is a major ligand for the natural killer inhibitory receptor CD94/NKG2A. Proc Natl Acad Sci USA 1998;95:5199–5204.
77. Borrego F, Ulbrecht M, Weiss EH, et al. Recognition of human histocompatibility leukocyte antigen (HLA)-E complexed with HLA class I signal sequence-derived peptides by CD94/NKG2 confers protection from natural killer cell-mediated lysis. J Exp Med 1998;187: 813–818.
78. Garcia P, Llano M, de Heredia AB, et al. Human T cell receptor-mediated recognition of HLA-E. Eur J Immunol 2002;32:936–944.
79. Maier S, Grzeschik M, Weiss EH, et al. Implications of HLA-E allele expression and different HLA-E ligand diversity for the regulation of NK cells. Hum Immunol 2000;61:1059–1065.
80. O'Callaghan CA. Molecular basis of human natural killer cell recognition of HLA-E (human leucocyte antigen-E) and its relevance to clearance of pathogen-infected and tumour cells. Clin Sci (Lond) 2000;99:9–17.
81. Tomasec P, Braud VM, Rickards C, et al. Surface expression of HLA-E, an inhibitor of natural killer cells, enhanced by human cytomegalovirus gpUL40. Science 2000;287:1031.
82. Carosella ED, Paul P, Moreau P, et al. HLA-G and HLA-E: Fundamental and pathophysiological aspects. Immunol Today 2000;21:532–534.
83. Wainwright SD, Biro PA, Holmes CH. HLA-F is a predominantly empty, intracellular, TAP-associated MHC class Ib protein with a restricted expression pattern. J Immunol 2000;164:319–328.
84. Lepin EJ, Bastin JM, Allan DS, et al. Functional characterization of HLA-F and binding of HLA-F tetramers to ILT2 and ILT4 receptors. Eur J Immunol 2000;30:3552–3561.
85. Cerwenka A, Lanier LL. Ligands for natural killer cell receptors: Redundancy or specificity. Immunol Rev 2001;181:158–169.
86. Wilson IA, Bjorkman PJ. Unusual MHC-like molecules: CD1, Fc receptor, the hemochromatosis gene product, and viral homologs. Curr Opin Immunol 1998;10:67–73.
87. Daser A, Mitchison H, Mitchison A, et al. Non-classical-MHC genetics of immunological disease in man and mouse. The key role of pro-inflammatory cytokine genes. Cytokine 1996;8:593–597.
88. Fischer LK. Peptide antigen presentation by non-classical MHC class I molecules. Semin Immunol 1993;5:117–126.
89. Velardi A, Ruggeri L, Alessandro M, et al. NK cells: a lesson from mismatched hematopoietic transplantation. Trends Immunol 2002;23: 438–444.
90. Trowsdale J, Barten R, Haude A, et al. The genomic context of natural killer receptor extended gene families. Immunol Rev 2001;181:20–38.
91. Moretta L, Moretta A. Killer immunoglobulin-like receptors. Curr Opin Immunol 2004;16:626–633.
92. Middleton D, Williams F, Halfpenny IA. KIR genes. Transpl Immunol 2005;14:135–142.
93. Vilches C, Parham P. KIR: Diverse, rapidly evolving receptors of innate and adaptive immunity. Annu Rev Immunol 2002;20:217–251.
94. Ruggeri L, Capanni M, Urbani E, et al. Effectiveness of donor natural killer cell alloreactivity in mismatched hematopoietic transplants. Science 2002;295:2097–2100.
95. Gagne K, Brizard G, Gueglio B, et al. Relevance of KIR gene polymorphisms in bone marrow transplantation outcome. Hum Immunol 2002;63:271–280.
96. Falkenburg JH, Marijt WA, Heemskerk MH, et al. Minor histocompatibility antigens as targets of graft-versus-leukemia reactions. Curr Opin Hematol 2002;9:497–502.
97. Klein CA, Wilke M, Pool J, et al. The hematopoietic system-specific minor histocompatibility antigen HA-1 shows aberrant expression in epithelial cancer cells. J Exp Med 2002;196:359–368.
98. Howell WM, Turner SJ, Bateman AC, et al. IL-10 promoter polymorphisms influence tumour development in cutaneous malignant melanoma. Genes Immun 2001;2:25–31.
99. McCarron SL, Edwards S, Evans PR, et al. Influence of cytokine gene polymorphisms on the development of prostate cancer. Cancer Res 2002;62:3369–3372.
100. Bodmer WF. HLA: What's in a name? A commentary on HLA nomenclature development over the years. Tissue Antigens 1997;49:293–296.
101. Tiercy JM, Marsh SG, Schreuder GM, et al. Guidelines for nomenclature usage in HLA reports: ambiguities and conversion to serotypes. Eur J Immunogenet 2002;29:273–274.
102. Dupont B. Nomenclature for factors of the HLA system, 1987. Decisions of the Nomenclature Committee on Leukocyte Antigens, which met in New York on November 21–23, 1987. Hum Immunol 1989;26:3–14.
103. Marsh SG, Albert ED, Bodmer WF, et al. Nomenclature for factors of the HLA system, 2002. Eur J Immunogenet 2002;29:463–515.
104. Shilling HG, Guethlein LA, Cheng NW, et al. Allelic polymorphism synergizes with variable gene content to individualize human KIR genotype. J Immunol 2002;168:2307–2315.
105. Turner D, Choudhury F, Reynard M, et al. Typing of multiple single nucleotide polymorphisms in cytokine and receptor genes using SNaPshot. Hum Immunol 2002;63:508–513.
106. Svejgaard A, Ryder LP. HLA and disease associations: Detecting the strongest association. Tissue Antigens 1994;43:18–27.
107. Boisgerault F, Khalil I, Tieng V, et al. Definition of the HLA-A29 peptide ligand motif allows prediction of potential T-cell epitopes from the retinal soluble antigen, a candidate autoantigen in birdshot retinopathy. Proc Natl Acad Sci USA 1996;93:3466–3470.
108. Friday RP, Trucco M, Pietropaolo M. Genetics of Type 1 diabetes mellitus. Diabetes Nutr Metab 1999;12:3–26.
109. Luppi P, Alexander A, Bertera S, et al. The same HLA-DQ alleles determine either susceptibility or resistance to different coxsackievirus-mediated autoimmune diseases. J Biol Regul Homeost Agents 1999;13:14–26.
110. Cope AP, Patel SD, Hall F, et al. T cell responses to a human cartilage autoantigen in the context of rheumatoid arthritis-associated and nonassociated HLA-DR4 alleles. Arthritis Rheum 1999;42:1497–1507.
111. Luppi P, Rossiello MR, Faas S, et al. Genetic background and environment contribute synergistically to the onset of autoimmune diseases. J Mol Med 1995;73:381–393.
112. Jongeneel CV, Briant L, Udalova IA, et al. Extensive genetic polymorphism in the human tumor necrosis factor region and relation to extended HLA haplotypes. Proc Natl Acad Sci USA 1991;88:9717–9721.
113. Cormier JN, Salgaller ML, Prevette T, et al. Enhancement of cellular immunity in melanoma patients immunized with a peptide from MART-1/Melan A. Cancer J Sci Am 1997;3:37–44.
114. Hopkins KA, van Leeuwen A, Tardiff GN, Lefor WM. Lymphocytoxocity testing. In Zachary AA, Teresi GA (eds). ASHI Laboratory Manual, 2nd ed. Lenexa, Kan., American Society for Histocompatibility and Immunogenetics, 1990, pp 195–199.
115. Sakaguchi K, Ono R, Tsujisaki M, et al. Anti-HLA-B7, B27, Bw42, Bw54, Bw55, Bw56, Bw67, Bw73 monoclonal antibodies: specificity, idiotypes, and application for a double determinant immunoassay. Hum Immunol 1988;21:193–207.
116. Yunis EJ, Ward EE, Amos DB. Observation of the CYNAP phenomenon. In Terasaki IP (ed). Histocompatibility 1970. Copenhagen, Munksgaard, 1970, p 351.
117. Scornik JC, Brunson ME, Schaub B, et al. The crossmatch in renal transplantation. Evaluation of flow cytometry as a replacement for standard cytotoxicity. Transplantation 1994;57:621–625.
118. Christiaans MH, Nieman F, van Hooff JP, et al. Detection of HLA class I and II antibodies by ELISA and complement-dependent cytotoxicity before and after transplantation. Transplantation 2000;69:917–927.
119. Duquesnoy RJ, Marrari M. Multilaboratory evaluation of serum analysis for HLA antibody and crossmatch reactivity by lymphocytotoxicity methods. Arch Pathol Lab Med 2003;127:149–156.
120. Buelow R, Chiang TR, Monteiro F, et al. Soluble HLA antigens and ELISA—a new technology for crossmatch testing. Transplantation 1995;60:1594–1599.
121. Pei R, Lee J, Chen T, et al. Flow cytometric detection of HLA antibodies using a spectrum of microbeads. Hum Immunol 1999;60:1293–1302.
122. Moses LA, Stroncek DF, Cipolone KM, et al. Detection of HLA antibodies by using flow cytometry and latex beads coated with HLA antigens. Transfusion 2000;40:861–866.
123. Duquesnoy RJ, Marrari M. HLAMatchmaker: A molecularly based algorithm for histocompatibility determination. II. Verification of the algorithm and determination of the relative immunogenicity of amino acid triplet-defined epitopes. Hum Immunol 2002;63:353–363.
124. Parker KC, Bednarek MA, Hull LK, et al. Sequence motifs important for peptide binding to the human MHC class I molecule, HLA-A2. J Immunol 1992;149:3580–3587.
125. Rotzschke O, Falk K, Stevanovic S, et al. Peptide motifs of closely related HLA class I molecules encompass substantial differences. Eur J Immunol 1992;22:2453–2456.

126. Sette A, Vitiello A, Reherman B, et al. The relationship between class I binding affinity and immunogenicity of potential cytotoxic T cell epitopes. J Immunol 1994;153:5586–5592.
127. Bunce M, O'Neill CM, Barnardo MC, et al. Phototyping: Comprehensive DNA typing for HLA-A, B, C, DRB1, DRB3, DRB4, DRB5 & DQB1 by PCR with 144 primer mixes utilizing sequence-specific primers (PCR-SSP). Tissue Antigens 1995;46:355–367.
128. Krausa P, Browning MJ. A comprehensive PCR-SSP typing system for identification of HLA-A locus alleles. Tissue Antigens 1996;47:237–244.
129. Ng J, Hurley CK, Carter C, et al. Large-scale DRB and DQB1 oligonucleotide typing for the NMDP registry: Progress report from year 2. Tissue Antigens 1996;47:21–26.
130. Adams SD, Barracchini KC, Chen D, et al. Ambiguous allele combinations in HLA Class I and Class II sequence-based typing: when precise nucleotide sequencing leads to imprecise allele identification. J Transpl Med 2004;2:30.
131. Adams SD, Barracchini KC, Simonis TB, et al. High throughput HLA sequence-based typing (SBT) utilizing the ABI Prism 3700 DNA Analyzer. Tumori 2001;87:S40–S43.
132. Wang E, Adams S, Zhao Y, et al. A strategy for detection of known and unknown SNP using a minimum number of oligonucleotides applicable in the clinical settings. J Transpl Med 2003;1:4.
133. Tiercy JM, Bujan-Lose M, Chapuis B, et al. Bone marrow transplantation with unrelated donors: What is the probability of identifying an HLA-A/B/Cw/DRB1/ B3/B5/DQB1-matched donor? Bone Marrow Transplant 2000;26:437–441.
134. Tiercy JM, Villard J, Roosnek E. Selection of unrelated bone marrow donors by serology, molecular typing and cellular assays. Transpl Immunol 2002;10:215–221.
135. Duquesnoy RJ, White LT, Fierst JW, et al. Multiscreen serum analysis of highly sensitized renal dialysis patients for antibodies toward public and private class I HLA determinants. Implications for computer-predicted acceptable and unacceptable donor mismatches in kidney transplantation. Transplantation 1990;50:427–437.
136. Duquesnoy RJ, Marrari M. Determination of HLA-A,B residue mismatch acceptability for kidneys transplanted into highly sensitized patients: a report of a collaborative study conducted during the 12th International Histocompatibility Workshop. Transplantation 1997;63:1743–1751.
137. Duquesnoy RJ. HLAMatchmaker: a molecularly based algorithm for histocompatibility determination. I. Description of the algorithm. Hum Immunol 2002;63:339–352.
138. Claas FH, De Meester J, Witvliet MD, et al. Acceptable HLA mismatches for highly immunized patients. Rev Immunogenet 1999;1:351–358.
139. Lobashevsky AL, Senkbeil RW, Shoaf JL, et al. The number of amino acid residues mismatches correlates with flow cytometry crossmatching results in high PRA renal patients. Hum Immunol 2002;63:364–374.
140. Nambia A, Duquesnoy RJ, Adams S, et al. HLAMatchmaker-driven analysis of responses to HLA-typed platelet transfusions in alloimmunized thrombocytopenic patients. Blood 2006;107:1680–1687.
141. Shoskes DA, Wood KJ. Indirect presentation of MHC antigens in transplantation. Immunol Today 1994;15:32–38.
142. Semple JW, Freedman J. Recipient antigen-processing pathways of allogeneic platelet antigens: Essential mediators of immunity. Transfusion 2002;42:958–961.
143. Fuller TC, Fuller A. The humoral immune response against an HLA class I allodeterminant correlates with the HLA-DR phenotype of the responder. Transplantation 1999;68:173–182.
144. Liu Z, Colovai AI, Tugulea S, et al. Indirect recognition of donor HLA-DR peptides in organ allograft rejection. J Clin Invest 1996;98:1150–1157.
145. Benichou G, Valujskikh A, Heeger PS. Contributions of direct and indirect T cell alloreactivity during allograft rejection in mice. J Immunol 1999;162:352–358.
146. Salvatierra O Jr, Melzer J, Potter D, et al. A seven-year experience with donor-specific blood transfusions. Results and considerations for maximum efficacy. Transplantation 1985;40:654–659.
147. Hardy S, Lee SH, Terasaki PI. Sensitization 2001. Clin Transpl 2001;271–278.
148. Clark BD, Geer LI, Park MS, et al. Association of high sensitization to the structure of HLA class I alleles. Clin Transpl 1991;347–362.
149. Opelz G, Wujciak T, Dohler B, et al. HLA compatibility and organ transplant survival. Collaborative Transplant Study. Rev Immunogenet 1999;1:334–342.
150. Matzinger P. An innate sense of danger. Semin Immunol 1998;10: 399–415.
151. Terasaki PI. The beneficial transfusion effect on kidney graft survival attributed to clonal deletion. Transplantation 1984;37:119–125.
152. Opelz G, Vanrenterghem Y, Kirste G, et al. Prospective evaluation of pretransplant blood transfusions in cadaver kidney recipients. Transplantation 1997;63:964–967.
153. Petersdorf EW, Hansen JA, Martin PJ, et al. Major-histocompatibility-complex class I alleles and antigens in hematopoietic-cell transplantation. NEJM 2001;345:1794–1800.
154. Rubinstein P. HLA matching for bone marrow transplantation—how much is enough? NEJM 2001;345:1842–1844.
155. Champlin RE, Goldman JM, Gale RP. Bone marrow transplantation in chronic myelogenous leukemia. Semin Hematol 1988;25:74–80.
156. Hansen JA, Gooley TA, Martin PJ, et al. Bone marrow transplants from unrelated donors for patients with chronic myeloid leukemia. NEJM 1998;338:962–968.
157. Clift RA, Buckner CD. Marrow transplantation for acute myeloid leukemia. Cancer Invest 1998;16:53–61.
158. Storb R, Leisenring W, Anasetti C, et al. Long-term follow-up of allogeneic marrow transplants in patients with aplastic anemia conditioned by cyclophosphamide combined with antithymocyte globulin. Blood 1997;89:3890–3891.
159. Gaziev D, Galimberti M, Lucarelli G, et al. Bone marrow transplantation from alternative donors for thalassemia: HLA-phenotypically identical relative and HLA-nonidentical sibling or parent transplants. Bone Marrow Transplant 2000;25:815–821.
160. Jurado M, Deeg HJ, Storer B, et al. Hematopoietic stem cell transplantation for advanced myelodysplastic syndrome after conditioning with busulfan and fractionated total body irradiation is associated with low relapse rate but considerable nonrelapse mortality. Biol Blood Marrow Transplant 2002;8:161–169.
161. Childs RW, Barrett J. Nonmyeloablative allogeneic immunotherapy for solid tumors. Annu Rev Med 2004;55:459–475.
162. Teshima T, Ferrara JL. Understanding the alloresponse: New approaches to graft-versus-host disease prevention. Semin Hematol 2002;39:15–22.
163. Ratanatharathorn V, Ayash L, Lazarus HM, et al. Chronic graft-versus-host disease: Clinical manifestation and therapy. Bone Marrow Transplant 2001;28:121–129.
164. Flowers ME, Kansu E, Sullivan KM. Pathophysiology and treatment of graft-versus-host disease. Hematol Oncol Clin North Am 1999;13: 1091–1099.
165. Michallet M. Graft-versus-host disease and graft-versus-leukemia. Hematol Cell Ther 1996;38:459–460.
166. Mavroudis D, Barrett J. The graft-versus-leukemia effect. Curr Opin Hematol 1996;3:423–429.
167. Porter DL, Antin JH. The graft-versus-leukemia effects of allogeneic cell therapy. Annu Rev Med 1999;50:369–386.
168. Shimoni A, Giralt S, Khouri I, et al. Allogeneic hematopoietic transplantation for acute and chronic myeloid leukemia: non-myeloablative preparative regimens and induction of the graft-versus-leukemia effect. Curr Oncol Rep 2000;2:132–139.
169. Srinivasan R, Barrett J, Childs R. Allogeneic stem cell transplantation as immunotherapy for nonhematological cancers. Semin Oncol 2004;31:47–55.
170. Feinstein L, Sandmaier B, Maloney D, et al. Nonmyeloablative hematopoietic cell transplantation. Replacing high-dose cytotoxic therapy by the graft-versus-tumor effect. Ann NY Acad Sci 2001; 938:328–337.
171. Barrett J, Childs R. The benefits of an alloresponse: Graft-versus-tumor. J Hematother Stem Cell Res 2000;9:347–354.
172. Horowitz MM, Gale RP, Sondel PM, et al. Graft-versus-leukemia reactions after bone marrow transplantation. Blood 1990;75:555–562.
173. Marmont AM, Horowitz MM, Gale RP, et al. T-cell depletion of HLA-identical transplants in leukemia. Blood 1991;78:2120–2130.
174. Barrett J, Childs R. New directions in allogeneic stem cell transplantation. Semin Hematol 2002;39:1–2.
175. Weiden PL, Flournoy N, Thomas ED, et al. Antileukemic effect of graft-versus-host disease in human recipients of allogeneic-marrow grafts. NEJM 1979;300:1068–1073.
176. Sasazuki T, Juji T, Morishima Y, et al. Effect of matching of class I HLA alleles on clinical outcome after transplantation of hematopoietic stem cells from an unrelated donor. Japan Marrow Donor Program. NEJM 1998;339:1177–1185.
177. Hansen JA, Yamamoto K, Petersdorf E, et al. The role of HLA matching in hematopoietic cell transplantation. Rev Immunogenet 1999;1:359–373.
178. Barrett AJ. Mechanisms of the graft-versus-leukemia reaction. Stem Cells 1997;15:248–258.
179. Kolb HJ, Mittermuller J, Clemm C, et al. Donor leukocyte transfusions for treatment of recurrent chronic myelogenous leukemia in marrow transplant patients. Blood 1990;76:2462–2465.

180. Barrett AJ, Malkovska V. Graft-versus-leukaemia: understanding and using the alloimmune response to treat haematological malignancies. Br J Haematol 1996;93:754–761.
181. Farag SS, Fehniger TA, Ruggeri L, et al. Natural killer cell receptors: New biology and insights into the graft-versus-leukemia effect. Blood 2002;100:1935–1947.
182. de Bueger M, Bakker A, Van Rood JJ, et al. Tissue distribution of human minor histocompatibility antigens. Ubiquitous versus restricted tissue distribution indicates heterogeneity among human cytotoxic T lymphocyte-defined non-MHC antigens. J Immunol 1992;149:1788–1794.
183. Goulmy E. Human minor histocompatibility antigens. Curr Opin Immunol 1996;8:75–81.
184. Warren EH, Greenberg PD, Riddell SR. Cytotoxic T-lymphocyte-defined human minor histocompatibility antigens with a restricted tissue distribution. Blood 1998;91:2197–2207.
185. Frahm N, Korber BT, Adams CM, et al. Consistent cytotoxic T-lymphocyte targeting of immunodominant regions in human immunodeficiency virus across multiple ethnicities. J Virol 2004;78:2187–2200.
186. Solache A, Morgan CL, Dodi AI, et al. Identification of three HLA-A*0201-restricted cytotoxic T cell epitopes in the cytomegalovirus protein pp65 that are conserved between eight strains of the virus. J Immunol 1999;163:5512–5518.
187. Provenzano M, Mocellin S, Bettinotti M, et al. Identification of immune dominant cytomegalovirus epitopes using quantitative real-time polymerase chain reactions to measure interferon-γ production by peptide-stimulated peripheral blood mononuclear cells. J Immunother 2002;25:342–351.
188. Meij P, Leen A, Rickinson AB, et al. Identification and prevalence of $CD8^+$ T-cell responses directed against Epstein-Barr virus-encoded latent membrane protein 1 and latent membrane protein 2. Int J Cancer 2002;99:93–99.
189. Rosenberg SA. Progress in human tumour immunology and immunotherapy. Nature 2001;411:380–384.
190. Lin CL, Lo WF, Lee TH, et al. Immunization with Epstein-Barr virus (EBV) peptide-pulsed dendritic cells induces functional CD8+ T-cell immunity and may lead to tumor regression in patients with EBV-positive nasopharyngeal carcinoma. Cancer Res 2002;62:6952–6958.
191. Lee KH, Wang E, Nielsen MB, et al. Increased vaccine-specific T cell frequency after peptide-based vaccination correlates with increased susceptibility to in vitro stimulation but does not lead to tumor regression. J Immunol 1999;163:6292–6300.
192. Parmiani G, Castelli C, Dalerba P, et al. Cancer immunotherapy with peptide-based vaccines: What have we achieved? Where are we going? J Natl Cancer Inst 2002;94:805–818.
193. Monsurro V, Nagorsen D, Wang E, et al. Functional heterogeneity of vaccine-induced $CD8^+$ T cells. J Immunol 2002;168:5933–5942.
194. Einsele H, Roosnek E, Rufer N, et al. Infusion of cytomegalovirus (CMV)-specific T cells for the treatment of CMV infection not responding to antiviral chemotherapy. Blood 2002;99:3916–3922.
195. Bollard CM, Savoldo B, Rooney CM, et al. Adoptive T-cell therapy for EBV-associated post-transplant lymphoproliferative disease. Acta Haematol 2003;110:139–148.
196. Dudley ME, Wunderlich JR, Robbins PF, et al. Cancer regression and autoimmunity in patients after clonal repopulation with antitumor lymphocytes. Science 2002;298:850–854.
197. Nagorsen D, Marincola FM. How to analyze ex vivo T-cell responses in cancer patients. In Vivo 2002;16:519–525.
198. Keilholz U, Weber J, Finke JH, et al. Immunologic monitoring of cancer vaccine therapy: results of a workshop sponsored by the Society for Biological Therapy. J Immunother 2002;25:97–138.
199. Monsurro V, Nagorsen D. Immunotracking of specific cancer vaccine CD8+ lymphocytes. ASHI Quarterly 2003;26:100–102.
200. Altman JD, Moss PA, Goulder PJ, et al. Phenotypic analysis of antigen-specific T lymphocytes. Science 1996;274:94–96.
201. Lalezari P, Bernard GE. An isologous antigen–antibody reaction with human neutrophiles, related to neonatal neutropenia. J Clin Invest 1966;45:1741–1750.
202. Boxer LA, Yokoyama M, Lalezari P. Isoimmune neonatal neutropenia. J Pediatr 1972;80:783–787.
203. Lalezari P, Murphy GB, Allen FH Jr. NB1, a new neutrophil-specific antigen involved in the pathogenesis of neonatal neutropenia. J Clin Invest 1971;50:1108–1115.
204. Bux J. Nomenclature of granulocyte alloantigens. ISBT Working Party on Platelet and Granulocyte Serology, Granulocyte Antigen Working Party. International Society of Blood Transfusion. Transfusion 1999;39:662–663.
205. Trounstine ML, Peltz GA, Yssel H, et al. Reactivity of cloned, expressed human FcγRIII isoforms with monoclonal antibodies which distinguish cell-type-specific and allelic forms of FcγRIII. Int Immunol 1990;2:303–310.
206. Ravetch JV, Perussia B. Alternative membrane forms of FcγRIII (CD16) on human natural killer cells and neutrophils. Cell type-specific expression of two genes that differ in single nucleotide substitutions. J Exp Med 1989;170:481–497.
207. Ory PA, Clark MR, Kwoh EE, et al. Sequences of complementary DNAs that encode the NA1 and NA2 forms of Fc receptor III on human neutrophils. J Clin Invest 1989;84:1688–1691.
208. Huizinga TW, Kleijer M, Tetteroo PA, et al. Biallelic neutrophil Na-antigen system is associated with a polymorphism on the phospho-inositol-linked Fc γ receptor III (CD16). Blood 1990;75:213–217.
209. Kissel K, Santoso S, Hofmann C, et al. Molecular basis of the neutrophil glycoprotein NB1 (CD177) involved in the pathogenesis of immune neutropenias and transfusion reactions. Eur J Immunol 2001;31:1301–1309.
210. Temerinac S, Klippel S, Strunck E, et al. Cloning of PRV-1, a novel member of the uPAR receptor superfamily, which is overexpressed in polycythemia rubra vera. Blood 2000;95:2569–2576.
211. Bettinotti MP, Olsen A, Stroncek D. The use of bioinformatics to identify the genomic structure of the gene that encodes neutrophil antigen NB1, CD177. Clin Immunol 2002;102:138–144.
212. Plesner T, Behrendt N, Ploug M. Structure, function and expression on blood and bone marrow cells of the urokinase-type plasminogen activator receptor, uPAR. Stem Cells 1997;15:398–408.
213. Simsek S, van der Schoot CE, Daams M, et al. Molecular characterization of antigenic polymorphisms (Ond[a] and Mart[a]) of the β_2 family recognized by human leukocyte alloantisera. Blood 1996;88: 1350–1358.
214. Stroncek DF, Skubitz KM, McCullough JJ. Biochemical characterization of the neutrophil-specific antigen NB1. Blood 1990;75:744–755.
215. Goldschmeding R, van Dalen CM, Faber N, et al. Further characterization of the NB 1 antigen as a variably expressed 56–62 kD GPI-linked glycoprotein of plasma membranes and specific granules of neutrophils. Br J Haematol 1992;81:336–345.
216. Skubitz KM, Stroncek DF, Sun B. Neutrophil-specific antigen NB1 is anchored via a glycosyl-phosphatidylinositol linkage. J Leukoc Biol 1991;49:163–171.
217. de Haas M, Muniz-Diaz E, Alonso LG, et al. Neutrophil antigen 5b is carried by a protein, migrating from 70 to 95 kDa, and may be involved in neonatal alloimmune neutropenia. Transfusion 2000;40:222–227.
218. Stroncek DF, Shankar R, Litz C, et al. The expression of the NB1 antigen on myeloid precursors and neutrophils from children and umbilical cords. Transfus Med 1998;8:119–123.
219. Huizinga TW, de Haas M, Kleijer M, et al. Soluble Fcγ receptor III in human plasma originates from release by neutrophils. J Clin Invest 1990;86:416–423.
220. Koene HR, de Haas M, Kleijer M, et al. NA-phenotype-dependent differences in neutrophil FcγRIIIb expression cause differences in plasma levels of soluble FcγRIII. Br J Haematol 1996;93:235–241.
221. Huizinga TW, de Haas M, van Oers MH, et al. The plasma concentration of soluble Fc-γ RIII is related to production of neutrophils. Br J Haematol 1994;87:459–463.
222. Clement LT, Lehmeyer JE, Gartland GL. Identification of neutrophil subpopulations with monoclonal antibodies. Blood 1983;61:326–332.
223. Stroncek DF, Shankar RA, Noren PA, et al. Analysis of the expression of NB1 antigen using two monoclonal antibodies. Transfusion 1996;36:168–174.
224. Matsuo K, Lin A, Procter JL, et al. Variations in the expression of granulocyte antigen NB1. Transfusion 2000;40:654–662.
225. Taniguchi K, Kobayashi M, Harada H, et al. Human neutrophil antigen-2a expression on neutrophils from healthy adults in western Japan. Transfusion 2002;42:651–657.
226. Caruccio L, Bettinotti M, Matsuo K, et al. Expression of human neutrophil antigen-2a (NB1) is increased in pregnancy. Transfusion 2003;43:357–363.
227. Taniguchi K, Nagata H, Katsuki T, et al. Significance of human neutrophil antigen-2a (NB1) expression and neutrophil number in pregnancy. Transfusion 2004;44:581–585.
228. Stroncek DF, Jaszcz W, Herr GP, et al. Expression of neutrophil antigens after 10 days of granulocyte-colony-stimulating factor. Transfusion 1998;38:663–668.
229. Klippel S, Strunck E, Busse CE, et al. Biochemical characterization of PRV-1, a novel hematopoietic cell surface receptor, which is overexpressed in polycythemia rubra vera. Blood 2002;100:2441–2448.
230. Bux J, Stein EL, Bierling P, et al. Characterization of a new alloantigen (SH) on the human neutrophil Fc γ receptor IIIb. Blood 1997;89: 1027–1034.

231. Kissel K, Hofmann C, Gittinger FS, et al. HNA-1a, HNA-1b, and HNA-1c (NA1, NA2, SH) frequencies in African and American Blacks and in Chinese. Tissue Antigens 2000;56:143–148.
232. Bux J, Stein EL, Santoso S, et al. NA gene frequencies in the German population, determined by polymerase chain reaction with sequence-specific primers. Transfusion 1995;35:54–57.
233. Hessner MJ, Curtis BR, Endean DJ, et al. Determination of neutrophil antigen gene frequencies in five ethnic groups by polymerase chain reaction with sequence-specific primers. Transfusion 1996;36:895–899.
234. Matsuo K, Procter JL, Chanock S, et al. The expression of NA antigens in people with unusual Fcγ receptor III genotypes. Transfusion 2001;41:775–782.
235. Lin M, Chen CC, Wang CL, et al. Frequencies of neutrophil-specific antigens among Chinese in Taiwan. Vox Sang 1994;66:247.
236. Ohto H, Matsuo Y. Neutrophil-specific antigens and gene frequencies in Japanese. Transfusion 1989;29:654.
237. Matsuo K, Procter J, Stroncek D. Variations in genes encoding neutrophil antigens NA1 and NA2. Transfusion 2000;40:645–653.
238. Koene HR, Kleijer M, Roos D, et al. FcγRIIIB gene duplication: Evidence for presence and expression of three distinct FcγRIIIB genes in $NA^{1+,2+}SH^{+}$ individuals. Blood 1998;91:673–679.
239. Steffensen R, Gulen T, Varming K, et al. FcγRIIIB polymorphism: Evidence that NA1/NA2 and SH are located in two closely linked loci and that the SH allele is linked to the NA1 allele in the Danish population. Transfusion 1999;39:593–598.
240. Huizinga TW, Kuijpers RW, Kleijer M, et al. Maternal genomic neutrophil FcRIII deficiency leading to neonatal isoimmune neutropenia. Blood 1990;76:1927–3192.
241. Stroncek DF, Skubitz KM, Plachta LB, et al. Alloimmune neonatal neutropenia due to an antibody to the neutrophil Fc-γ receptor III with maternal deficiency of CD16 antigen. Blood 1991;77:1572–1580.
242. de Haas M, Kleijer M, van Zwieten R, et al. Neutrophil Fc γa RIIIb deficiency, nature, and clinical consequences: a study of 21 individuals from 14 families. Blood 1995;86:2403–2413.
243. Muniz-Diaz E, Madoz P, de la Calle MO, et al. The polymorphonuclear neutrophil Fc γ RIIIb deficiency is more frequent than hitherto assumed. Blood 1995;86:3999.
244. Fromont P, Bettaieb A, Skouri H, et al. Frequency of the polymorphonuclear neutrophil Fc γ receptor III deficiency in the French population and its involvement in the development of neonatal alloimmune neutropenia. Blood 1992;79:2131–2134.
245. Bierling P, Poulet E, Fromont P, et al. Neutrophil-specific antigen and gene frequencies in the French population. Transfusion 1990; 30:848–849.
246. Stroncek DF, Shankar RA, Plachta LB, et al. Polyclonal antibodies against the NB1-bearing 58- to 64-kDa glycoprotein of human neutrophils do not identify an NB2-bearing molecule. Transfusion 1993;33:399–404.
247. Caruccio L, Walkovich K, Bettinotti M, et al. CD177 polymorphisms: Correlation between high-frequency single nucleotide polymorphisms and neutrophil surface protein expression. Transfusion 2004;44:77–82.
248. Wolff J, Brendel C, Fink L, et al. Lack of NB1 GP (CD177/HNA-2a) gene transcription in NB1 GP-neutrophils from NB1 GP-expressing individuals and association of low expression with NB1 gene polymorphisms. Blood 2003;102:731–733.
249. Kissel K, Scheffler S, Kerowgan M, et al. Molecular basis of NB1 (HNA-2a, CD177) deficiency. Blood 2002;99:4231–4233.
250. Nagarajan S, Chesla S, Cobern L, et al. Ligand binding and phagocytosis by CD16 (Fc γ receptor III) isoforms. Phagocytic signaling by associated zeta and gamma subunits in Chinese hamster ovary cells. J Biol Chem 1995;270:25762–25770.
251. Bredius RG, Fijen CA, de Haas M, et al. Role of neutrophil FcγRIIa (CD32) and FcγRIIIb (CD16) polymorphic forms in phagocytosis of human IgG1- and IgG3-opsonized bacteria and erythrocytes. Immunology 1994;83:624–630.
252. Salmon JE, Edberg JC, Kimberly RP. Fc γ receptor III on human neutrophils. Allelic variants have functionally distinct capacities. J Clin Invest 1990;85:1287–1295.
253. Foster CB, Zhu S, Erichsen HC, et al. Polymorphisms in inflammatory cytokines and Fcγreceptors in childhood chronic immune thrombocytopenic purpura: A pilot study. Br J Haematol 2001;113:596–599.
254. Gonzalez-Escribano MF, Aguilar F, Sanchez-Roman J, et al. FcγRIIA, FcγRIIIA and FcγRIIIB polymorphisms in Spanish patients with systemic lupus erythematosus. Eur J Immunogenet 2002;29:301–306.
255. Raknes G, Skeie GO, Gilhus NE, et al. FcγRIIA and FcγRIIIB polymorphisms in myasthenia gravis. J Neuroimmunol 1998;81:173–176.
256. Myhr KM, Raknes G, Nyland H, et al. Immunoglobulin G Fc-receptor (FcγR) IIA and IIIB polymorphisms related to disability in MS. Neurology 1999;52:1771–1776.
257. Foster CB, Lehrnbecher T, Mol F, et al. Host defense molecule polymorphisms influence the risk for immune-mediated complications in chronic granulomatous disease. J Clin Invest 1998;102:2146–2155.
258. Klippel S, Strunck E, Temerinac S, et al. Quantification of PRV-1 mRNA distinguishes polycythemia vera from secondary erythrocytosis. Blood 2003;102:3569–3574.
259. Tefferi A, Lasho TL, Wolanskyj AP, et al. Neutrophil PRV-1 expression across the chronic myeloproliferative disorders and in secondary or spurious polycythemia. Blood 2004;103:3547–3548.
260. Kralovics R, Buser AS, Teo SS, et al. Comparison of molecular markers in a cohort of patients with chronic myeloproliferative disorders. Blood 2003;102:1869–1871.
261. Griesshammer M, Klippel S, Strunck E, et al. PRV-1 mRNA expression discriminates two types of essential thrombocythemia. Ann Hematol 2004;83:364–370.
262. Kralovics R, Passamonti F, Buser AS, et al. A gain-of-function mutation of JAK2 in myeloproliferative disorders. NEJM 2005;352:1779–1790.
263. Levine RL, Wadleigh M, Cools J, et al. Activating mutation in the tyrosine kinase JAK2 in polycythemia vera, essential thrombocythemia, and myeloid metaplasia with myelofibrosis. Cancer Cell 2005;7:387–397.
264. Baxter EJ, Scott LM, Campbell PJ, et al. Acquired mutation of the tyrosine kinase JAK2 in human myeloproliferative disorders. Lancet 2005;365:1054–1061.
265. James C, Ugo V, Le Couedic JP, et al. A unique clonal JAK2 mutation leading to constitutive signalling causes polycythaemia vera. Nature 2005;434:1144–1148.
266. Araki N, Nose Y, Kohsaki M, et al. Anti-granulocyte antibody screening with extracted granulocyte antigens by a micro-mixed passive hemagglutination method. Vox Sang 1999;77:44–51.
267. Clague HD, Fung YL, Minchinton RM. Human neutrophil antigen-4a gene frequencies in an Australian population, determined by a new polymerase chain reaction method using sequence-specific primers. Transfus Med 2003;13:149–152.
268. Sachs UJ, Reil A, Bauer C, et al. Genotyping of human neutrophil antigen-5a (Ond). Transfus Med 2005;15:115–117.
269. Bux J, Jung KD, Kauth T, et al. Serological and clinical aspects of granulocyte antibodies leading to alloimmune neonatal neutropenia. Transfus Med 1992;2:143–149.
270. Bux J, Hartmann C, Mueller-Eckhardt C. Alloimmune neonatal neutropenia resulting from immunization to a high-frequency antigen on the granulocyte Fc γ receptor III. Transfusion 1994;34:608–611.
271. Fung YL, Pitcher LA, Taylor K, et al. Managing passively acquired autoimmune neonatal neutropenia: a case study. Transfus Med 2005; 15:151–155.
272. Bux J, Behrens G, Jaeger G, et al. Diagnosis and clinical course of autoimmune neutropenia in infancy: analysis of 240 cases. Blood 1998;91:181–186.
273. Bruin MC, dem Borne AE, Tamminga RY, et al. Neutrophil antibody specificity in different types of childhood autoimmune neutropenia. Blood 1999;94:1797–1802.
274. Lalezari P, Khorshidi M, Petrosova M. Autoimmune neutropenia of infancy. J Pediatr 1986;109:764–769.
275. Conway LT, Clay ME, Kline WE, et al. Natural history of primary autoimmune neutropenia in infancy. Pediatrics 1987;79:728–733.
276. Brittingham TE. Immunologic studies on leukocytes. Vox Sang 1957;2:242–248.
277. Craddock PR, Fehr J, Brigham KL, et al. Complement and leukocyte-mediated pulmonary dysfunction in hemodialysis. NEJM 1977;296:769–774.
278. Craddock PR, Fehr J, Dalmasso AP, et al. Hemodialysis leukopenia. Pulmonary vascular leukostasis resulting from complement activation by dialyzer cellophane membranes. J Clin Invest 1977;59:879–888.
279. Popovsky MA, Abel MD, Moore SB. Transfusion-related acute lung injury associated with passive transfer of antileukocyte antibodies. Am Rev Respir Dis 1983;128:185–189.
280. Seeger W, Schneider U, Kreusler B, et al. Reproduction of transfusion-related acute lung injury in an ex vivo lung model. Blood 1990;76:1438–1444.
281. Silliman CC, Boshkov LK, Mehdizadehkashi Z, et al. Transfusion-related acute lung injury: epidemiology and a prospective analysis of etiologic factors. Blood 2003;101:454–462.
282. Kopko PM, Paglieroni TG, Popovsky MA, et al. TRALI: correlation of antigen-antibody and monocyte activation in donor-recipient pairs. Transfusion 2003;43:177–184.
283. Toy P, Popovsky MA, Abraham E, et al. Transfusion-related acute lung injury: definition and review. Crit Care Med 2005;33:721–726.
284. Bux J. Transfusion-related acute lung injury (TRALI): a serious adverse event of blood transfusion. Vox Sang 2005;89:1–10.

285. Kopko PM, Popovsky MA, MacKenzie MR, et al. HLA class II antibodies in transfusion-related acute lung injury. Transfusion 2001;41:1244–1248.

286. Nordhagen R, Conradi M, Dromtorp SM. Pulmonary reaction associated with transfusion of plasma containing anti-5b. Vox Sang 1986;51:102–107.

287. Davoren A, Curtis BR, Shulman IA, et al. TRALI due to granulocyte-agglutinating human neutrophil antigen-3a (5b) alloantibodies in donor plasma: a report of 2 fatalities. Transfusion 2003;43:641–645.

288. Kopko PM, Marshall CS, MacKenzie MR, et al. Transfusion-related acute lung injury: report of a clinical look-back investigation. JAMA 2002;287:1968–1971.

289. Stroncek DF, Shapiro RS, Filipovich AH, et al. Prolonged neutropenia resulting from antibodies to neutrophil-specific antigen NB1 following marrow transplantation. Transfusion 1993;33:158–163.

290. Stroncek DF, Leonard K, Eiber G, et al. Alloimmunization after granulocyte transfusions. Transfusion 1996;36:1009–1015.

B. Blood Donation

Chapter 11
Blood Donation and Collection

Gary Zeger • Eileen Selogie • Ira A. Shulman

Blood donation is critical to all of transfusion therapy, as it provides the starting product. In the United States and many other economically developed nations, all of the blood is given by volunteer, nonremunerated donors. Donated whole blood is then made into transfusable components, which include but are not limited to packed red blood cells (RBCs), platelets, and frozen plasma or cryoprecipitate. Other lesser utilized blood components, such as granulocytes and cryoprecipitate-depleted plasma, also have important therapeutic value. Individual plasma proteins, such as factor VIII, have been manufactured using recombinant methods for years; however, there is no commercial product, single or combined, with the clinical properties of frozen plasma. Each of these components make possible an extraordinary number of traditional and state-of-the-art medical therapies, including trauma surgery, organ transplantation, and cancer chemotherapy. At the time of this writing, there are no clinically effective or available substitutes for RBCs, platelets, or plasma in the United States.

In 2001, the National Blood Donor Resource Center estimated that 8 million volunteer U.S. blood donors contributed approximately 15 million whole blood donations per year, the majority of which were manufactured into separate components, such as RBCs, fresh frozen plasma, and platelets.[1] These components allowed transfusion of 29 million blood components in the United States. Thus, in the United States, the average volunteer blood donor gives blood about 1.6 times a year. Of that total, almost 2% represent donations indicated for a specific recipient other than the donor. These are generally referred to as *directed* or *designated donations.* In addition, approximately 3% of blood donations are *autologous:* blood that is donated by an individual for his or her own use, usually for a prescheduled elective surgery.[2–4] Although it is estimated that 60% of the adult population in the United States is eligible to donate blood, at present it is believed that less than 5% of the eligible population donates within any given year.[5,6] The various reasons that some people give blood readily and others do not have been studied for several decades, but the blood donation process and applicable statistics during this time have changed little, if at all.

THE PROCESS OF BLOOD DONATION

Blood donation can be divided into five processes that are directly related to the donor: recruitment, screening, physical examination, collection, and post-donation care.

Recruitment of blood donors is a specialized task. It is often performed by telerecruiters, and the message delivered must be convincing and compelling to result in a scheduled appointment to donate blood.

Once a donor has been recruited, the screening process is carried out to make sure that the donation process will be safe for the donor and that the collected blood will be safe for the recipient. The prospective donor is initially given information about criteria for eligibility for blood donation and about the process itself. The screening process consists of a questionnaire that seeks to find medical conditions and behaviors that might make donation unsafe for the donor or recipient. Critical information is confirmed by direct verbal questioning to ensure that the answers are accurate. If no disqualifying information is uncovered during the screening process, a brief physical examination follows, which includes examination of antecubital veins, followed by measurement of body temperature, donor hematocrit or hemoglobin, and heart rate.

After the venipuncture is performed, blood is collected, labeled, and temporarily stored until it can be transferred to a manufacturing center for further processing and distribution. Specimen tubes are drawn at the time of collection for infectious disease testing; these tubes are sent for testing immediately after collection.

After the donation, donors receive oral fluids and remain under observation for a period of time so that any post-donation reactions may be treated appropriately. Post-donation instructions are given to help the donor avoid untoward side effects. The donor is instructed to call the blood center with any post-donation information, such as the development of worrisome physical symptoms or information remembered that would change the answers given during the screening process.

Donor Recruitment

Maintaining an adequate blood supply is an ongoing challenge. Attrition of blood donors due to older age and illness, implementation of new regulations resulting in deferrals, or other reasons makes it difficult for blood collection centers to keep pace with the increasing demand for blood. Thus, the recruitment of new blood donors must be ongoing and vigorous. New exclusionary criteria and serologic testing make this task increasingly difficult, as does the fact that newly recruited blood donors are nearly twice as likely to have disqualifying medical conditions as are established blood donors.[7]

It is unacceptable to provide volunteer blood donors with monetary compensation (i.e., cash or cash equivalents), so the act of blood donation in the United States is voluntary. Thus, without paying donors for their time and blood, the formidable challenges of encouraging volunteer blood donation begin at the first step of the blood collection process: donor recruitment.

Sources of Donor Motivation

The most successful approach to recruitment of volunteer blood donors has been an appeal to community responsibility. Individuals often first learn about the need for donation during blood shortages via public service announcements and appeals for blood from newspapers, radio, and television. Other donors become aware of the importance of blood donation when transfusions are needed for family and friends (or themselves).

Appeals after disasters tend to bring out community spirit in Americans. This was particularly evident after the September 11, 2001, terrorist attack on the New York World Trade Center and the Pentagon in Washington, D.C. In both instances, blood donations vastly exceeded the local demand, due to the motivation of the entire community to contribute to their fellow Americans in need.

Donating blood for a friend or relative (directed donation) has proven to be an excellent motivator and has brought many first-time blood donors into the system. Donating for one's own use (autologous donation) has also been an effective motivator.

For whatever reason each donor is motivated to give blood, he or she must be convinced that donation is truly necessary and will be appreciated. For this reason, appeals for blood should only be made when there is a significant shortage. Once the donor has been motivated to donate, making his or her blood donation a convenient and pleasant experience is critical to retaining that donor for subsequent donations. Excellent customer service is the key to retaining blood donors.

A Note about Minority Donors

Latino Americans, particularly immigrants from Mexico, are the largest growing demographic group in the United States.[8] Adequate donor recruitment and collection among this minority group is especially important because of the high percentage of blood group O among Latinos. Because group O individuals can only receive group O RBCs, a higher percentage of group O blood is necessary in areas with large Latino populations. Specialized recruiting programs are important to attract and maintain these essential donors. Appeals in Spanish to Latino organizations and in the media are of key importance. In areas with large Latino populations, an effort should be made to provide Spanish versions of all donor materials. It is also advisable to have staff members who are conversant in Spanish or to have translators readily available.

With the exception of Chagas disease, the incidence of infectious disease markers among whole blood donors in areas with large Latino populations is similar to that of other repeat whole blood donors.[9] However, the seroprevalence of Chagas disease among whole blood donors in Los Angeles is 1 in 7200, versus 1 in 93,000 among plateletpheresis donors.[10] The significant difference in this seroprevalence is due to the fact that very few Latino individuals donate apheresis platelets in Los Angeles.

African American donors are currently the second largest minority population in the United States.[9] Recruitment and donation by African Americans is particularly important, due to many factors: they make up a large percentage of the general eligible blood donor population in certain communities; the high prevalence of blood group B in the African American population; and the higher prevalence of African Americans with specific blood types (e.g., antigen-negativity for a variety of RBC antigens to which antibodies are frequently made in highly transfused populations, such as patients with sickle cell disease) that may be used for patients who have made antibodies to these antigens.

Few publications adequately address the reasons why certain minority populations do not donate blood at the same percentages as the white population. Much research is necessary to understand the needs and wants of these important donors, so that these minority donors can be successfully recruited into the blood donor system.

Paid Donors

Aside from paid plasma donors at centers that manufacture fractionated, licensed plasma products, it is not acceptable to provide monetary compensation (cash or cash equivalents) to blood donors in the United States. In the early days of blood banking, paying for blood donors was a commonplace and accepted practice. These donors were often motivated by a lack of funds to maintain drug or alcohol habits; subsequently, paid donors had a higher incidence of transfusion-transmissible diseases, particularly hepatitis, which infected many early blood recipients. In the 1970s, growing recognition of this problem[11] led the Food and Drug Administration (FDA), in its Code of Federal Regulations (CFR), to require blood from paid donors to be labeled as such.[12] As these "paid donor"-labeled units were considered to be undesirable by clinicians and hospitals, the practice of paid whole blood donations effectively died out.

In some states, however, the shortage of single donor platelet concentrates collected by apheresis technology prompted exceptions for these donations. Until January 1, 2003,[13] a few U.S. blood collection facilities continued to pay apheresis donors. Due to the previous stigma attached to paid blood donation, these centers employed screening procedures that met or exceeded those of "all-volunteer" centers. Despite studies demonstrating that these donors had infectious disease marker frequencies similar to, or better than, those of volunteer donors, these centers were eventually forced to cease paying plateletpheresis donors.[14]

Paid donation, however, is regularly utilized for the recruitment of donors in the United States for commercial source plasma. This plasma is collected by apheresis and sent for further manufacture into various plasma-derived products. Because the pooled plasma from these donations is effectively "sterilized" during the fractionation and manufacturing process, there is less concern about the potentially increased risk for infectious disease transmission by using paid donors for "source plasma." Most countries with all-volunteer commercial plasma programs have struggled, usually unsuccessfully, to meet their population's plasma derivative needs.[15]

Health Benefits of Whole Blood Donation

The proven health benefit to blood donors is the free mini-physical examination and the infectious disease screening testing performed at the time of donation. Many donors might not have otherwise become aware of diseases such as hypertension, anemia, cardiac arrhythmia, hepatitis, or human immunodeficiency virus (HIV) infection. This information alerts the donor to seek further appropriate medical diagnosis and treatment, and may limit the transmission of infectious disease to others. Aside from these benefits, a controversial hypothesis that depletion of iron stores through whole blood donation can improve cardiovascular status[16,17] has been proposed; more research needs to be performed prior to making any claims regarding cardiac health benefits from blood donations.

Donor Incentives

Improved screening and infectious disease testing methods used for donor blood have made widespread infectious disease transmission by transfusion, as occurred in the early days of paid blood donors, a thing of the past. All-volunteer donor programs have become the base of the blood collection establishment. Although blood donor incentives such as t-shirts, gift certificates, and paid time off are acceptable gifts, rewards that can easily be converted to cash (or cash itself) are not. The issue of donor motivation caused by incentives continues to be an area of concern to the FDA and the American Association of Blood Banks (AABB). The CFR, in its definition of paid and volunteer donors, states that "Benefits, such as time off from work, membership in blood assurance programs, and cancellation of nonreplacement fees that are not readily convertible to cash, do not constitute payment within the meaning of this paragraph." The AABB[18] and FDA[19] have provided some guidance on donor incentives (Table 11–1). There is still a concern that a potential donor might be untruthful about high-risk behaviors for infectious disease to receive a gift being offered at a blood collection site. For this reason, incentives should be provided for simply attending a blood drive and attempting to donate, rather than the gift being given based on the condition of the actual donation.

Blood Credit Programs

Blood credit programs, which in the past were more popular entities, are difficult to manage logistically and practically. The implication that a blood donor will receive a credit that can eventually be cashed in for "free" blood in the future is almost always misleading. The credits are often symbolic "credits to the blood supply" and have no direct application to the donor, monetarily or otherwise. The logistics of a true crediting program are generally prohibitive, because the time and place that the credits will be redeemed is unknown, and the involved health care providers may not be party to the program.

Patients are sometimes encouraged to have friends and relatives donate blood to "replace" any that they might use. This appears to be a reasonable recruitment strategy, as long as the patient is not made to feel stressed and anxious about finding replacement donors. It is most important for the patient to understand that he or she will never be denied blood because of inability to replace blood that has been, or might be, used. Poor communication, however, might cause the patient to put blood donation pressure on family, friends, and acquaintances who may have valid reasons for not donating, thus potentially endangering the blood supply.

Motivation by Free Testing

A serious concern throughout the blood industry following the discovery of HIV in the early 1980s (and the subsequent knowledge that HIV was transmissible through transfusions), was that high-risk individuals would donate blood to obtain a free confidential HIV test. The concern that people might now donate blood to receive free blood tests (a magnet effect) has been shown to be generally unfounded, at least for HIV p24 antigen testing.[20] Nevertheless, donor centers generally make available a list of testing sites where confidential or anonymous HIV blood testing is available, to discourage a potential high-risk individual from donating.

Factors for Success

Any donor's internal motivation will only provide a finite amount of impetus for continued participation in the blood donation process. It is the job of the entire blood collection team to make the donation process as pleasant as possible. If they are successful, a hesitant first-time donor may be converted into a regular repeat blood donor. This is a worthwhile goal: regular, repeat blood donors are more reliable and have less risk of infectious disease.

Making blood donation as convenient as possible is of prime importance. After a national disaster, blood donors have stood in long lines for hours to donate blood for anonymous victims. In such times, the truly heroic nature of the motivated blood donor is evident. Under more routine circumstances, inhospitable conditions and/or poor customer service may almost certainly discourage a blood donor from making a donation. A safe and convenient location is critical to attract and retain repeat blood donors. Parking should be easily available and free. The waiting area should be clean and pleasant. Excessive waits are to be avoided, and donors should be given an accurate wait-time whenever possible. Blood center staff should be professional, knowledgeable, and courteous. Of particular importance is making sure

Table 11–1 Examples of Donor Incentives.

Items Considered "Paid" Incentives	Items That May Qualify as "Nonpayment"
Cash payment or cash equivalent	Tokens or prizes of nominal value (e.g., coffee cups, t-shirts, pins)
Tickets to concerts or sporting events where market for resale exists	Employee paid time off
Music media not associated with product promotions where market for resale exists	Raffle tickets, regardless of value of prize. Prize must not be transferable or readily convertible to cash
Transferable product discounts or coupons convertible to cash	Membership in blood assurance program
Vouchers for free medical tests	Medical tests performed at the time of donation
Scholarships paid directly to students	Scholarships transferred directly to academic institution
	Gift cards and gift certificates that are nontransferable, not redeemable for cash, and bear the donor's name

From Compliance Policy Guide for FDA Staff and Industry, Chapter 2, Section 230.150. Issued May 7, 2002, revised November 22, 2005. Available at http://www.fda.gov/ora/compliance_ref/cpg/cpgbio/cpg230=150final.htm. Last modified December 12, 2005. Accessed June 3, 2006.

that a new donor understands the donation process and fully knows what to expect. Donors appreciate honesty, and unpleasant or painful surprises often provoke bad feelings.

Blood Collection Sites: Fixed and Mobile

Fixed site is a widely used term for a permanent or freestanding blood collection center. The fixed site may be located in a hospital-based donor room or in a community blood center building. The site should be clean and pleasant and must meet standards of current Good Manufacturing Practices (GMP)[21] for cleanliness, ventilation, space, and temperature. Donor confidentiality must be maintained, and there must be compliance with the Health Insurance Portability and Accountability Act of 1996. Compliance with these regulations requires a screening area that provides the donor with privacy to discuss the many personal questions on the donor-screening questionnaire. There must be adequate room in the collection area for the phlebotomists to function freely, and there must be a "canteen," or refreshment area, where the donor can be orally rehydrated and observed for post-donation reactions. Properly monitored storage areas must be available for storage of blood products and equipment.

Most autologous and directed donations are performed at fixed sites. Donations that require apheresis technology, such as plateletpheresis and granulocyte collections, are also typically performed at fixed sites, although new automated blood collection technology has allowed for the collection of multiple blood products by apheresis at mobile sites as well.

Fixed sites are generally less convenient for donors than are mobile sites, as they often require additional travel, parking, and time. For this reason, a friendly, attractive, and professional staff is important. Most regular blood donors look forward to their visits and, in a sense, become part of the blood collection "family." Intensive telephone recruitment of repeat blood donors is usually necessary for a fixed site to be successful.

Plateletpheresis donations are most often collected at fixed sites. Regular plateletpheresis donors tend to differ from whole blood donors in their levels of motivation and willingness to endure longer and more uncomfortable procedures to donate their blood platelets. These donors have their blood processed by a machine for as long as 2 hours, compared to the 7 or 8 minutes needed to complete a whole blood donation. Plateletpheresis donors are able to donate more frequently (up to 24 times per year) than are whole blood donors (regular whole blood donors may only donate every 56 days). For these reasons, positive relationships between platelet donors and blood center staff appear to play a more important role in plateletpheresis donor retention. These donors are generally recruited from the ranks of repeat whole blood donors and tend to be quite steadfast and reliable.

Mobile blood drives are the ultimate in convenience for the blood donor. The donor room is essentially transported to the donor. The mobile blood collection team generally arranges mobile blood drives with a sponsoring organization, often a business, school, hospital, public service organization, religious group, or military installation. Although it is generally easier and more cost effective to run a fixed site, the convenience of a mobile drive brings many otherwise "unavailable" blood donors into the system. Once these mobile site donors have had a positive and successful blood donation experience, it is often possible to bring them to a fixed site for further donations, with effective and continuous recruitment techniques.

An adequate area must be provided by the sponsoring organization for the mobile team to set up. An experienced, well-trained collections staff is important, because everything necessary for the blood drive must be properly set up and organized on site. Essential equipment and supplies are brought by the mobile collection team, and any omission may result in cancellation of the drive or unacceptable delays. Delays and cancellations of mobile blood drives can lead to ill will between the sponsor and the blood collection center, which may dampen the likelihood of another blood drive being sponsored by that group in the future.

An alternative to using space within a school or business for a mobile blood drive is a self-contained mobile unit, usually a specially adapted bus, typically of four- to six-bed capacity. These buses are most often used for small blood drives.

Mobile blood drives should be set up along the same basic principles as fixed sites, although a certain amount of flexibility is often in order. Donor confidentiality concerns must be adhered to as best as possible, often by use of portable modular components to maintain privacy.

Recruiting for mobile blood drives requires an entirely different approach than recruiting blood donors for a fixed site. An individual from the sponsor group is often asked to organize the blood drive, by providing a personal message of support, hosting employee rallies, and designating organizers to work with a blood center representative to produce a plan for a productive and well-run blood drive. Sponsor organizers work on a personal level to recruit donors, who sign up to donate on a particular day and time. A good sponsor organizer will also do whatever is necessary to make certain each donor arrives at the appointed time. A successful drive is often followed by a recognition ceremony for all involved.

After a first successful mobile blood drive with a sponsor, future drives are generally easier to organize and run. Setting up a first-time blood drive, however, requires a blood collection center donor recruiter with excellent interpersonal and organizational skills, because it is often not a simple process to convince a sponsor to commit to a blood drive in the workplace, because of disruptions of work due to employees' taking time away from their jobs to donate blood.

Special Donations

Autologous Donation

Autologous blood donation is blood donated for the donor's own use, usually in preparation for an upcoming elective surgery. The major impetus for autologous donation is the donor's perception of eliminating the risk of transfusion-transmitted viral disease, particularly HIV and hepatitis. Recognition of transfusion-transmitted HIV in the mid-1980s greatly increased the utilization of autologous donation, which was used less frequently before that time. Another benefit of autologous donation is minimization of exposure to allogeneic red cells and leukocyte antigens that may stimulate alloantibody formation and create future transfusion compatibility problems. Some literature also suggests that allogeneic blood transfusion can lead to modulation of the recipient's immune system.[22–27]

Because the autologous donor is also the patient who will receive the donated product, deferral criteria are less stringent than for allogeneic blood donation. For example, the autologous donor can donate every 72 hours (and typically no less than 72 hours before surgery), rather than at an interval of at least 56 days. Similarly, the minimum hemoglobin level is lowered from 12.5 to 11 g/dL for autologous donors. When multiple autologous units are requested, it is best to begin donation a few weeks in advance of the upcoming surgery. In some cases, the donor is given supplemental iron or erythropoietin injections to maintain hemoglobin levels during the autologous donation process.[28]

Collections staff who evaluate and draw autologous blood donors must have more extensive training than those who handle only routine donations. This is in part due to the fact that autologous donors tend to be older than allogeneic donors, resulting in more age-related health problems (which may thus increase the incidence of serious adverse reactions at the time of donation). The frequency of severe donor reactions requiring hospitalization, although quite low for all donors, is significantly higher among autologous donors than allogeneic donors (1 in 17,000 versus 1 in 200,000).[29] Blood center staff must also take into consideration the disease processes that made the elective surgeries necessary in the first place. Cardiac patients, for example, may have arrhythmias or symptoms of vascular disease. Orthopedic patients often have mobility problems that would adversely affect their donation experience. Blood collection staff screeners should be especially mindful of identifying those autologous donors who are at risk for ischemic heart disease, cerebrovascular disease,[30] and seizures.

The donor history form is typically abbreviated for autologous donation, insofar as risk factors for infectious disease transmission are concerned. Acceptability criteria for autologous donation often differ from routine allogeneic donation: there is a far broader list of health problems that make a donor acceptable for autologous donation that would necessitate deferral for allogeneic or routine directed donation.

Bacterial contamination of the blood product remains a risk, even for the autologous donor. Individuals with evidence of bacterial infection should be deferred from donation until the condition is resolved. Blood collection staff screeners should question the autologous donor regarding signs or symptoms of infection (e.g., fever and antibiotic use), indwelling catheters, and open wounds. Donors who have had recent procedures that could lead to a transient bacteremia, such as recent dental work or colonoscopy, are typically deferred for at least 24 hours.

Improved screening and infectious disease testing have significantly minimized the infectious disease risks of allogeneic transfusion. However, many donors and physicians continue to request autologous donation as a transfusion option. Autologous donations require more complicated donor screening and collection procedures, associated logistical problems, and associated higher costs. The autologous unit must be specifically labeled for the designated patient, and systems must be in place in both the blood center and the hospital that will guarantee that the blood arrives at the proper place, in the right condition, and in time for surgery. Occasionally, autologous blood is not available for use, due to surgery being delayed beyond the expiration of the donated blood components or due to failure of proper communication between the collection center and the hospital staff. Positive infectious disease testing or clerical errors may also delay availability of autologous blood. At the hospital, care must be taken to transfuse autologous blood before allogeneic or directed donor blood. If an adverse effect is attributed to an allogeneic or directed unit that, arguably, would never have been transfused had the autologous unit been available for use and transfused first, medicolegal consequences may ensue.

Autologous transfusion is not risk-free, so autologous units should never be transfused simply because they are available. However, individual clinicians' thresholds for transfusion of autologous blood may be somewhat lower than for allogeneic blood transfusions.[31,32] Bacterial contamination remains a risk with autologous units, and clerical errors may cause an autologous unit with positive infectious disease markers to be transfused to an unintended recipient.[33]

Excessive wastage of unused autologous blood is often an issue, because unused units are very rarely, if ever, given to other patients (i.e., "crossed over"). These units are allowed to expire at the hospital and must be discarded. "Cross-over" has been discouraged, in part, because, as a group, autologous donors have a higher frequency of infectious disease markers than regular allogeneic donors.[34] They may also have underlying disease conditions that would make them unacceptable as donors for allogeneic blood transfusion. Another factor making autologous units less desirable for allogeneic transfusion is the lower hematocrit acceptable for autologous donation, which does not meet allogeneic criteria and may provide a substandard (less potent) red cell product.

Because modern screening and testing methodologies reduce the risk of transfusion-transmitted disease, the primary medical indications for autologous donations have been reduced; however, these donations are still often medically indicated, particularly for patients who have a rare blood type. Autologous donation is also beneficial as a means of supplementing the blood supply and does provide a degree of psychological benefit to patients who fear transfusion-transmitted disease. Autologous donation may also introduce repeat donors into the system; however, the process tends not to be cost effective, as measured by traditional cost-benefit estimations.[35] Autologous donations will likely continue to decrease in popularity, unless a frightening new transfusion-transmitted pathogen, such as HIV, is discovered in the blood supply in the future.

Infectious disease testing of autologous blood and transfusion of units with positive infectious disease markers is controversial. If the blood is collected in a hospital-based donor room for use in that hospital only, infectious disease testing is not mandated. Autologous blood drawn at a community blood center, however, must be fully tested (as for allogeneic units). Autologous units positive for infectious disease must be labeled with biohazard stickers.[36,37] The AABB Standards require that if an autologus unit is to be shipped to another facility and the unit tests positive for any marker of transfusion-transmitted disease, the shipping facility shall notify the receiving trasfusion service.[38] It is the prerogative of the hospital transfusion service whether to accept autologous blood components that are positive for infectious disease(s).

Some transfusion services agree to store and transfuse autologous units that are confirmed positive for HIV, or hepatitis B or C (HBV, HCV). Evidence presented by the College of American Pathologists (CAP) indicates that many transfusion services either do not test autologous blood for infectious disease markers or knowingly collect, store, and transfuse infectious units.[39] Although transfusion of these infected units may not present an obvious risk to the donor/patient, accidental needle-sticks and splatters do put blood handlers at risk. Accidental transfusion of an infected autologous unit to the wrong recipient is possible. Storage of infectious blood components in hospital blood banks also presents some risk to other patients, considering that at least 1 in every 25,000 blood products is transfused to the "wrong" individual.[40] In 1992, the CAP conducted a survey of 3852 hospital transfusion services and found that 34 (0.9%) had issued one or more autologous blood products to the wrong patient during the previous year, and that 20 of these units were actually transfused.[40] An analysis of 256 licensed transfusion services by The New York State Department of Health, from 1990 through 1998, indicated that 1 in 19,000 RBC units where transfused to the wrong patient or were of incorrect ABO group or Rh type.[41] In addition, preliminary data indicate the frequency of infectious disease markers among autologous donors is significantly higher than that of allogeneic donors (Table 11–2). This data, along with the decreasing benefits of autologous transfusion due to improved infectious disease testing of allogeneic blood, make the practice of storing and transfusing infected units less attractive to hospital transfusion services.

One possible reason why many transfusion services permit storage of infectious autologous units is for fear of legal action based on the Americans with Disabilities Act, which affords to asymptomatic individuals infected with HIV a protected class status.[42–46] There is a concern that not offering autologous services to these donor/patients might be interpreted as a violation of this act.[47]

Directed Donations

A directed donation is a blood donation made specifically for use by a designated patient. Directed donations are usually made by friends and family members of the patient. These donations are typically manufactured into RBCs; however, directed plateletpheresis donations are not uncommon. Using new apheresis technology, a combination of red cells and platelets (or plasma) can be donated in one sitting.

Directed donation was initially discouraged by most blood centers, for fear that the practice would institute an inequitable two-tiered blood system in which well-connected patients would have access to a safe and adequate blood supply while less fortunate patients might have none. However, the discovery of HIV in the blood supply in the early 1980s created so much demand that today directed donations have become a routine part of blood donation.

There were two schools of thought in the early days of directed donations. One suggested that individuals, under pressure to donate by friends and family members, might not be truthful about risk factors for infectious disease. These donors would, therefore, present an increased risk of infectious disease transmission to the recipient. The other way of thinking suggested that individuals would be more careful about admitting potential risk factors when making such donations. Eventually it became evident that directed donations are likely to be as safe as most first-time blood donations, but not as safe as donations from repeat donors who have a history of safe donations.[48] Although there is no evidence that directed donations are safer than routine volunteer donations, the practice often does provide a psychological sense of well-being for the patient and may alleviate the feelings of helplessness that occur when a loved one is suffering from health care problems.

Blood from directed donors is collected and tested in accordance with the same criteria that is in place for allogeneic donations and hence can be "crossed-over" and used by other patients when not required by the original intended recipient. It is the choice of the hospital transfusion service whether to utilize the practice of "crossing over." This option, however, is important to recognize, because the blood types of the donor and/or intended recipients are often not known at the time of donation; thus, incompatible directed donations are not uncommon. These units can be transfused to other patients, improving the overall blood supply. The practice of directed donation is also a valuable means of getting donors into the system, because a sizable number of these donors go on to become repeat allogeneic donors. Rather than creating a two-tiered system, as was initially feared, directed donations tend to increase the amount of blood available for all patients.

Directed donation presents a series of logistical problems not present in allogeneic donation. A physician's order must be in place indicating the number and type (e.g., platelets, RBCs) of directed units required. The blood types of the directed donors and intended recipients are often incompatible. Additionally, directed units may not be available at the time of need, because the intended directed donor was unable to donate due to fear, time constraints, or exclusionary health conditions. Fully screened and motivated donors may be unable to donate due to inadequate venous access or technical errors. Directed donations testing positive for infectious disease are discarded. For these reasons and perhaps others, directed donations may not be available for use as expected by the patient.

Communication among donors, patients, clinicians, the blood center, and the hospital transfusion service is critical

Table 11–2 Prevalence of Donors Confirmed Positive for Transfusion-Transmitted Disease (per 10,000 donors)

Confirmed Infection	Autologous*	Allogeneic†
HIV	3.38	0.38
HCV	110.08	8.32
HBV	13.64	3.62

HBV, hepatitis B virus; HCV, hepatitis C virus; HIV, human immunodeficiency virus.

*Systemwide collection data from American Red Cross for calendar year 2004. Personal communication from Edward P. Notari IV, M.P.H, American Red Cross, Jerome H. Holland Laboratory, ARCNET Data Center.

†Wang B, Schreiber GB, Glynn SA, et al. Retrovirus Epidemiology Donor Study: Does prevalence of transfusion-transmissible viral infection reflect corresponding incidence in United States blood donors? Transfusion 2005;45:1089–1096.

for a successful directed donation program. A system must be in place to allow the patient and attending physician to know how many directed donor units are available for transfusion, so that more donors can be recruited if necessary. Good communication and successful procedures for directed donation programs avoid last-minute misunderstandings, in circumstances in which the anticipated number of directed units is not available when needed.

Medically Indicated Directed Donations

Directed donations are not safer than allogeneic donations, but they do increase the blood supply and provide a sense of security to the recipients. Most directed donations are not clinically necessary. However, circumstances do exist that require directed donations or in which a directed donation offers medical benefit. Using the same directed donor to provide small volumes of blood at regular intervals to neonates should reduce the risk of transfusion-transmitted diseases that would presumably be present with the use of multiple donors.[49] Similarly, one can use a small group of donors for chronically transfused patients (e.g., patients with sickle cell anemia or thalassemia).[50] Patients requiring rare blood types also benefit from specific directed donations, often from a blood relative. With proper authorization, the frequency of these medically indicated donations can be increased beyond that which would be acceptable for routine donation. In these instances, the slight potential donor risk is offset by the benefit to the recipient.

HLA-Matched Platelet Donors

Some blood collection centers test their plateletpheresis donors for human leukocyte antigen (HLA) type and store the data in a computerized database to have a readily available pool of donors to treat patients who have developed anti-HLA alloantibodies and require HLA-compatible platelets. The advent of platelet crossmatching techniques and the reduced frequency of alloimmunization, possibly due to leukoreduced blood products, have made the availability of a large HLA-typed donor pool less necessary than in previous years. However, orders for HLA-matched plateletpheresis products are still made, and most blood centers still offer this option to their hospital customers.

Donors with Hemochromatosis

Therapeutic phlebotomy is an accepted modality for preventing iron overload and subsequent organ damage for patients with hereditary hemochromatosis. Some blood collection centers, in the United States and elsewhere, have used units collected from individuals with hemochromatosis for allogeneic transfusion. These donors must meet all other allogeneic criteria. Recently the FDA has sanctioned this process by allowing variances for blood centers to collect blood from these individuals, provided certain donor follow-up and other stringent criteria are met.[51]

Donor Screening

Blood donors are carefully screened to minimize the risk of adverse consequences to the donor and to the recipient of the transfused blood. The screening process is made up of two distinct steps. The first is the donor history questionnaire (DHQ), a series of questions designed to expose potential health problems that might lead to adverse effects to the donor or blood recipient. The second step is an abbreviated physical evaluation of donor blood pressure, pulse, temperature, and venous access. The donor's hematocrit or hemoglobin levels are also evaluated at this time.

Donor screening and blood collection must be conducted under specific rules found in the CFR, as well as in applicable FDA guidelines and memoranda. In addition, the AABB, the preeminent nongovernmental organization involved with transfusion medicine in the United States, issues a publication, the *Standards for Blood Banks and Transfusion Services* (*Standards*),[52] which is adhered to by the majority of American blood centers and has been adopted into law, in varying degrees, by many states. The AABB *Standards* are upgraded regularly, to keep pace with current trends in transfusion medicine and the most recent federal regulations. Websites for the AABB (www.aabb.org) and the FDA (www.fda.gov/cber) are good sources for the most up-to-date transfusion-related regulations and information. Additionally, state and local regulations regarding blood collection practices often apply. Qualifying donor requirements, as stipulated in the most recent edition of the AABB *Standards,* are listed in Table 11–3.

Donor Identification and the Deferred Donor Registry (DDR)

Proper identification, often photographic, is required to confirm the donor's identity before donation.[53] This information is important if it becomes necessary to track down and notify the donor of any positive infectious disease test results. Proper identification is also required to perform a "lookback" study, to investigate whether a donor may have transmitted an infectious disease, unknown at the time of donation, to a blood recipient. Donors are asked if they have ever donated under any other name, possibly a maiden name or nickname, which would make it difficult to confirm previous donations. Correct personal identifiers are also necessary to calculate if adequate time has passed between donations.

Computers are becoming a mainstay of donor screening and tracking, but they can only work properly if supplied with accurate information. As an added precaution, the donor's name is compared against a database of individuals, the deferred donor registry (DDR), who have been disqualified from donating in the past, usually due to a positive infectious disease marker.[54] This database can be maintained with computers or by using manual methods such as microfiche.

During the early days of the HIV epidemic in the early and mid-1980s, the DDR was instituted as a precaution against individuals falsifying information to donate blood to obtain a free HIV test. The use of the DDR is still in effect today.

The Donor History Questionnaire (DHQ)

The donor history questionnaire is an extensive series of questions, often quite personal, designed to minimize the chance of adverse consequences to the blood donor and ensure a safe and potent blood product for the recipient. Questions are typically phrased in a "yes-no" format, other than the few open-ended questions regarding health care problems. The questionnaire must comply with requirements of the CFR and *Standards.* The AABB has developed a questionnaire that fulfills these requirements, which has been adopted, to some extent, by most blood centers in the United States (Table 11–4).[55]

A blood collection staff screener is required to answer any of the donor's questions and makes sure the forms are accurate and complete. It is crucial that the DHQ be completed properly: a false

Table 11–3 AABB Standards Requirements for Donor Qualification*

Item	Category	Criteria
1	Age	≥17 years or applicable state law
2	Whole Blood Volume Collected	Maximum of 10.5 mL/kg of donor weight, including samples; blood collection container shall be cleared for volume collected
3	Donation Interval	8 weeks after whole blood donation (Standard 5.6.7.1 applies) 16 weeks after 2-unit red cell collection 4 weeks after infrequent plasmapheresis ≥2 days after plasma-, platelet-, or leukapheresis (see exceptions in Standard 5.5)
4	Blood Pressure	≤180 mm Hg systolic ≤100 mm Hg diastolic
5	Pulse	50–100 beats per minute, without pathologic irregularities; <50 beats per minute acceptable if an otherwise healthy athlete
6	Temperature	≤37.5°C (99.5°F) if measured orally, or equivalent if measured by another method
7	Hemoglobin/ Hematocrit	≥12.5 g/dL/≥38%; blood obtained by earlobe puncture shall not be used for this determination
8	Drug Therapy	Medication evaluation: Finasteride (Proscar, Propecia), isotretinoin (Accutane)—defer 1 month after last dose Dutasteride (Avodart)—defer for 6 months after last dose Acitretin (Soriatane)—defer for 3 years after last dose Etretinate (Tegison)—defer indefinitely Bovine insulin manufactured in UK—defer indefinitely Medications that irreversibly inhibit platelet function preclude use of the donor as sole source of platelets: Defer for 36 hours after ingestion of aspirin Defer for other medications as defined by the facility's medical director
9	Medical History	
	General health	The prospective donor shall appear to be in good health and shall be free of major organ disease (e.g., heart, liver, lungs), cancer, or abnormal bleeding tendency, unless determined eligible by the medical director. The venipuncture site shall be evaluated for lesions on the skin. Family history of Creutzfeldt-Jakob disease (CJD)—defer indefinitely†
	Pregnancy	Defer if pregnant in the last 6 weeks
	Receipt of blood, component, or other human tissue	Receipt of dura mater or pituitary growth hormone of human origin—defer indefinitely Receipt of blood, components, human tissue, or plasma-derived clotting factor concentrates—defer for 12 months
	Immunizations and vaccinations	Receipt of toxoids or synthetic or killed viral, bacterial, or rickettsial vaccines if donor is symptom-free and afebrile—no deferral [anthrax, cholera, diphtheria, hepatitis A, hepatitis B, influenza, Lyme disease, paratyphoid, pertussis, plague, pneumococcal polysaccharide, polio (Salk/injection), Rocky Mountain spotted fever, tetanus, typhoid (by injection)] Receipt of live attenuated viral and bacterial vaccines—defer for 2 weeks [measles (rubeola), mumps, polio (Sabin/oral), typhoid (oral), yellow fever] Receipt of live attenuated viral and bacterial vaccines—defer 4 weeks [German measles (rubella), chickenpox (varicella zoster)] Smallpox (refer to FDA Guidance) Receipt of other vaccines, including unlicensed vaccines—defer for 12 months unless otherwise indicated by medical director‡
	Infectious diseases	Defer indefinitely: History of viral hepatitis after 11th birthday Confirmed positive test for HBsAg Repeatedly reactive test for anti-HBc on more than one occasion Present or past clinical or laboratory evidence of infection with HCV, HTLV, or HIV or as excluded by current FDA regulations and recommendations for the prevention of HIV transmission by blood and components Donated the only unit of blood or component that resulted in the apparent transmission of hepatitis, HIV, or HTLV A history of babesiosis or Chagas disease Evidence or obvious stigmata of parenteral drug use Use of a needle to administer nonprescription drugs Donors recommended for indefinite deferral for risk of vCJD, as defined in most recent FDA Guidance 12-month deferral from the time of: Mucous membrane exposure to blood

*Reference Standard 5.4.1A- Requirements for Allogeneic Donor Qualification.

†FDA Guidance for Industry, January 9, 2002. Revised Preventative to Reduce the Possible Risk of Transmission of Creutzfeldt-Jakob disease (CJD) and variant Creutzfeldt-Jakob disease (vCJD) by Blood and Blood Products.

‡AABB Association Bulletin 05–11. Interim Standard for *Standards for Blood Banks and Transfusion Services* (23rd edition). Sept. 30, 2005.

Table 11–3 **AABB Standards Requirements for Donor Qualification—Continued**

Item	Category	Criteria
		Nonsterile skin penetration with instruments or equipment contaminated with blood or body fluids other than the donor's own. Includes tattoos or permanent makeup unless applied by a state-regulated entity with sterile needles and ink that is not re-used. Sexual contact with an individual with a confirmed positive test for HBsAg Sexual contact with an individual who is symptomatic (clinical evidence or diagnosis) for any viral hepatitis Sexual contact with an HCV-positive individual who has had clinically apparent hepatitis within the past 12 months Sexual contact with an individual with HIV infection or at high risk of HIV infection[§, ‖] Incarceration in a correctional institution (including juvenile detention, lockup, jail, or prison) for more than 72 consecutive hours Completion of therapy for treatment of syphilis or gonorrhea or a reactive screening test for syphilis in the absence of a negative confirmatory test History of syphilis or gonorrhea Other: West Nile virus—defer in accordance with FDA Guidance[#]
	Malaria	Prospective donors who have had a diagnosis of malaria or who have traveled or lived in an area where malaria is endemic and have had unexplained symptoms suggestive of malaria, shall be deferred for 3 years after becoming asymptomatic. Individual(s) who have lived for at least 5 consecutive years in areas where malaria is considered endemic by the Malarial Branch, Centers for Disease Control and Prevention, U.S. Department of Health and Human Services, shall be deferred for 3 years after departure from that area(s). Individuals who have traveled to an area where malaria is endemic shall be deferred for 12 months after departing that area.[**]
10	Travel	The prospective donor's travel history shall be evaluated for potential risks.[††]

§FDA Memorandum, April 23, 1992, Revised Recommendation for the Prevention of Human Immunodeficiency Virus (HIV) Transmission by Blood and Blood Products.

‖FDA Memorandum, December 11, 1996. Interim Recommendations for Deferral of Donors at Increased Risk for HIV-1 Group O Infection.

#FDA Guidance for Industry, June 2005, Assessing Donor Suitability and Blood and Blood Product Safety in Cases of Known of Suspected West Nile Virus.

**The Department of Defense has recommended a 24-month deferral. Department of Defense Memorandum, October 14, 1999, "Deferral of Service Members Stationed in Possible Malaria Areas in the Republic of Korea," and February 28, 2001 update.

†† http://www.cdc.gov/travel

or missing entry must be corrected before the blood is released for transfusion. For additional clarity, screeners may be required to confirm certain critical questions verbally.[56] For autologous donors, who may have special health problems, it is often wise to have a well-trained registered nurse participate in the screening.

Other than the "yes" or "no" questions, the DHQ uses "capture questions" that cover a variety of broad topics. When an affirmative answer is given to a particular question, additional follow-up questions are asked by the screener to obtain additional information. For example, the question "Have you ever had any type of cancer, including leukemia?" often serves as a capture question that would elicit further information.

Additionally, to ensure that donors who self-administer a paper DHQ maintain focus, several "attention" questions are included. They serve to indicate if a donor is actually paying attention to the DHQ questions. The following is an example of one of the attention questions:

In the past 6 weeks, have you been pregnant or are you pregnant now? (Males check "I am male.")

An inappropriate answer to the question would be a male answering "yes" or "no." Each blood center must define the action of the screener when a donor inappropriately answers the attention questions. Attention questions may not be necessary when using other techniques to assure donor focus, such as an audiovisual computer-assisted self-interviewing system. In recent years, methods of computerized data entry have become more common.[57]

Several blood centers have investigated the use of an abbreviated donor history questionnaire (aDHQ) for repeat donors. The aDHQ eliminates nonrepeatable event questions; identifies recent changes in health, travel, or behavior; and retains questions about risk-associated activities that might have changed since the last donation. Data presented to the FDA Blood Products Advisory Committee on March 18, 2005, showed that a significant number of donors desire faster processing with a less complicated interview. This data demonstrated no indication that the abbreviated questionnaire increases blood safety risk.[58] At this time, the FDA has not accepted the aDHQ and has requested that the AABB Donor History Task Force develop a pre-implementation study of the aDHQ (currently in progress).

The minimum age for blood donation is typically age 17, but laws vary from state to state. Collections teams must follow local regulations and make certain proper consent is obtained. In some states, parental notification and/or consent may also be necessary.

Donor History Questionnaire and Donor Safety

For the majority of blood donors, the blood volume lost at donation is restored within 48 to 72 hours. With normal vascular elasticity, blood pressure is maintained and adverse reactions are kept at a minimum. Experienced screeners are more conservative with individuals who have a history of hypertension, diabetes, atherosclerosis, or other vascular diseases that can interfere with the normal physiologic response to acute blood loss, which might precipitate a hypotensive vasovagal reaction. Although rare, an acute drop in blood pressure could precipitate symptoms of otherwise occult coronary artery or cerebrovascular disease. The incidence of these disorders increases with age, so it is wise to be cautious with elderly donors or smaller donors with lesser blood volumes, for whom the acute loss of a pint of blood provides relatively more severe strain to the circulatory system.

Open-ended questions about a donor's general state of health, medications, previous surgeries, or current health care

Table 11–4 **AABB Full-Length Donor History Questionnaire, Version 1.1, June 2005***

	Yes	No	
Are you			
1. Feeling healthy and well today?	❒	❒	
2. Currently taking an antibiotic?	❒	❒	
3. Currently taking any other medication for an infection?	❒	❒	
Please read the Medication Deferral List.			
4. Are you now taking or have you ever taken any medications on the Medication Deferral List?	❒	❒	
5. Have you read the educational materials?	❒	❒	
In the past 48 hours			
6. Have you taken aspirin or anything that has aspirin in it?	❒	❒	
In the past 6 weeks			
7. Female donors: Have you been pregnant or are you pregnant now? (Males: check "I am male.")	❒	❒	❒ I am male
In the past 8 weeks have you			
8. Donated blood, platelets, or plasma?	❒	❒	
9. Had any vaccinations or other shots?	❒	❒	
10. Had contact with someone who had a smallpox vaccination?	❒	❒	
In the past 16 weeks			
11. Have you donated a double unit of red cells using an apheresis machine?	❒	❒	
In the past 12 months have you			
12. Had a blood transfusion?	❒	❒	
13. Had a transplant such as organ, tissue, or bone marrow?	❒	❒	
14. Had a graft such as bone or skin?	❒	❒	
15. Come into contact with someone else's blood?	❒	❒	
16. Had an accidental needle-stick?	❒	❒	
17. Had sexual contact with anyone who has HIV/AIDS or has had a positive test for the HIV/AIDS virus?	❒	❒	
18. Had sexual contact with a prostitute or anyone else who takes money or drugs or other payment for sex?	❒	❒	
19. Had sexual contact with anyone who has ever used needles to take drugs or steroids, or anything *not* prescribed by their doctor?	❒	❒	
20. Had sexual contact with anyone who has hemophilia or has used clotting factor concentrates?	❒	❒	
21. Female donors: Had sexual contact with a male who has ever had sexual contact with another male? (Males: check "I am male.")	❒	❒	❒ I am male
22. Had sexual contact with a person who has hepatitis?	❒	❒	
23. Lived with a person who has hepatitis?	❒	❒	
24. Had a tattoo?	❒	❒	
25. Had ear or body piercing?	❒	❒	
26. Had or been treated for syphilis or gonorrhea?	❒	❒	
27. Been in juvenile detention, lockup, jail, or prison for more than 72 hours?	❒	❒	
In the past three years have you			
28. Been outside the United States or Canada?	❒	❒	
From 1980 through 1996,			
29. Did you spend time that adds up to three (3) months or more in the United Kingdom? (Review list of countries in the UK)	❒	❒	
30. Were you a member of the U.S. military, a civilian military employee, or a dependent of a member of the U.S. military?	❒	❒	
From 1980 to the present, did you			
31. Spend time that adds up to five (5) years or more in Europe? (Review list of countries in Europe.)	❒	❒	
32. Receive a blood transfusion in the United Kingdom? (Review list of countries in the UK.)	❒	❒	
From 1977 to the present, have you			
33. Received money, drugs, or other payment for sex?	❒	❒	
34. Male donors: had sexual contact with another male, even once? (Females: check "I am female.")	❒	❒	❒ I am female
Have you EVER			
35. Had a positive test for the HIV/AIDS virus?	❒	❒	
36. Used needles to take drugs, steroids, or anything *not* prescribed by your doctor?	❒	❒	
37. Used clotting factor concentrates?	❒	❒	
38. Had hepatitis?	❒	❒	
39. Had malaria?	❒	❒	
40. Had Chagas disease?	❒	❒	

*Final Guidance from FDA not yet released on this version. Current version is 1.0 from April 23, 2004.

Table 11–4 AABB Full-Length Donor History Questionnaire, Version 1.1, June 2005—Continued

	Yes	No
Have you EVER—cont'd		
41. Had babesiosis?	❒	❒
42. Received a dura mater (or brain covering) graft?	❒	❒
43. Had any type of cancer, including leukemia?	❒	❒
44. Had any problems with your heart or lungs?	❒	❒
45. Had a bleeding condition or a blood disease?	❒	❒
46. Had sexual contact with anyone who was born in or lived in Africa?	❒	❒
47. Been in Africa?	❒	❒
48. Have any of your relatives had Creutzfeldt-Jakob disease?	❒	❒

problems serve to elicit potential risk factors that require careful evaluation prior to donation. Additional questions target specific medical conditions such as cardiac, lung, liver, and blood diseases; pregnancy; and cancer. A detailed discussion of the many disease states that would affect donation is beyond the scope of this chapter; however, cardiovascular disease, cerebrovascular disease, and seizure disorders are some of the primary reasons for which deferral may be indicated. Many properly controlled medical problems, such as thyroid disease, hypertension, mild seizure disorders, diabetes, and certain heart conditions, such as mitral valve prolapse, may not interfere with blood donation. It is good policy to refer difficult cases to the blood center's medical director for a final decision as to whether it is safe for the donor to donate blood. If it is not clear whether an individual meets criteria for donation, it is generally wise to err on the side of donor safety and defer the donor.

Medications are rarely of significance from the aspect of donor safety. Although angiotensin-converting enzyme inhibitors have fostered concern about potential hypotensive episodes, medications often serve to alert the screener to health problems that otherwise may have been inadvertently left out of the donor history. Use of a coronary artery dilator, for example, would indicate a history of ischemic heart disease, which might have gone unmentioned. Experienced screeners are often impressed by the lack of information that many individuals have about their own health history. Some pre-existing disease states are not mentioned by donors when completing the DHQ, as are medications and the reasons for which the medications are being taken. This may be a matter of denial or may be symptomatic of a language problem. The latter is of increasing significance as our donor population becomes more diverse.

Donor History Questionnaire and Recipient Safety

Most significantly, the DHQ exists to protect the transfusion recipient. The driving force for much of the DHQ involves screening for transfusion-transmissible infectious diseases. The greatest danger exists for diseases in which an undetected, asymptomatic carrier state exists at the time of donation. Often there are geographic or behavioral indicators that place a donor at increased risk for transmitting these diseases. The DHQ seeks to identify these risk factors to reduce the chance of disease transmission.

Viral diseases are the most tested for transfusion-transmitted pathogens. Most notorious among these is HIV, which devastated the blood supply in the early to mid 1980s. HBV and HCV (once called *non-A, non-B hepatitis*) have also caused significant morbidity and mortality in transfusion recipients. Although sophisticated infectious disease testing methodologies have significantly reduced the rate of transfusion-transmitted viral disease, the *window period* (the time during which a recently infected donor is infectious but tests negative for infectious disease markers) contributes to a low-level risk. The introduction of sensitive nucleic acid amplification technology (NAT) has shortened the window period for HCV and HIV, when compared to previous HCV and HIV antibody or HIV p24 antigen testing. However, no matter how small the risk, it is unlikely that testing will ever detect every infected blood donor, so reliance on screening cannot diminish.

Some behaviors, which have been associated with increased risk for HIV or hepatitis infection, result in indefinite deferral. These include intravenous drug use and prostitution. Male homosexual or bisexual activity, often defined as "men having sex with other men, even once, since 1977," is also considered high-risk behavior and results in indefinite deferral from allogeneic donation. Other behaviors, such as having sexual contact with a prostitute or an intravenous drug user, require a 12-month deferral from the last contact.

The DHQ is the first line of defense against such pathogens as malaria and the agents responsible for Chagas disease and Creutzfeldt-Jakob disease (CJD), for which no practical screening tests are now available in the United States.[59,60]

Donor centers should have information to indicate areas where malaria is endemic.[61] Potential donors who have traveled to an endemic area are deferred for 12 months from the date of return. Donors with a history of malaria are deferred for 3 years if symptoms do not recur.

Transmission of variant CJD (vCJD) through blood transfusion has been a controversial topic in recent years.[62,63] There has been documented disease transmission of classic CJD through dura mater grafts, pituitary-derived human growth hormone, and ineffectively sterilized electroencephalogram electrodes. Animal studies and a few reported cases in humans suggest strongly that vCJD can be transmitted by blood transfusion. Although the risk seems to be very low, the magnitude is unknown, due to the long (e.g., 30-year) incubation period. Those stricken with vCJD by eating contaminated meat products during the 1990s became symptomatic and died in just a few years.

To deal with this difficult problem, geographical screening is now in place to exclude donors who have spent time in countries where cases of vCJD have been known to occur, including the United Kingdom (UK) and much of Europe. Potential donors are indefinitely deferred who have spent a cumulative 3 months in the United Kingdom between 1980 and 1996, the period when unsafe cattle feeding practices led to an outbreak of bovine spongiform encephalopathy, or "mad cow" disease. Ingestion of infected beef at that time is believed to responsible for a number of cases of human vCJD.[64] Also indefinitely deferred are those who spent a cumulative 6 months on European military bases or a cumulative 5 years in certain European countries other than the UK, as are those who received a blood transfusion in the UK from 1980 to the present.[65] Recipients of pituitary-derived growth hormone are deferred as are individuals with known exposure to vCJD or CJD. Until practical mass serological screening becomes available, geographical exclusions may stay in place and thousands of otherwise eligible donors will be excluded.

Exclusionary criteria are changed and updated regularly based on new threats to the blood supply. Deferral criteria may change based on improved serologic testing, and better understanding of the disease processes involved. Criteria to avoid severe acute respiratory syndrome[66] were in effect at one time, and Gulf War veterans were deferred from blood donation from 1991 to 1993 to avoid the transmission of leishmaniasis.[67–70] Donors with a history of blood-borne parasites such as babesiosis and Chagas disease are permanently deferred.

Diseases that present with severe clinical symptoms, such as hepatitis A, tend not to require special screening, because the victims are generally too sick to donate. Standards allow prospective donors who have a history of hepatitis before age 11 to be eligible for donation, provided no other cause for deferral exists.

A number of DHQ questions deal with hematologic disease, leukemia, and previous use of clotting factors. These conditions may cause abnormalities in RBCs, platelets, or plasma proteins that may lead to substandard blood products being produced.

Exposure, or even potential exposure, to another individual's blood requires a 12-month deferral. The rationale for the 12-month deferral period is that the vast majority of transfusion-transmitted infectious diseases would manifest positive serologic markers within 1 year's time. Besides blood transfusion and accidental needle-sticks, other sources of blood exposure include human bites and acupuncture, tattoos, and piercings performed with nonsterile instruments. Nonsterile body piercing (including ears) has become increasingly problematic in recent years due to the increase in popularity of piercings and tattoos. The screener should ask if the procedure was done using sterile techniques.

Vaccinations provide another area of concern for donor screening. This is particularly true for live-attenuated viral vaccines, which could theoretically infect immunocompromised individuals. Recipients of rubella and varicella zoster vaccines are deferred for 4 weeks. A 2-week deferral is required of recipients of rubeola (measles), polio (Sabin/oral), mumps, typhoid (oral), and yellow fever vaccines. Individuals vaccinated for exposure to HBV or rabies are deferred for 12 months to avoid the remote possibility of disease transmission. The American Red Cross requires a 7-day deferral period for routine (not exposure-related) HBV vaccination; the deferral time varies among different organizations. Vaccination with nonviable agents such as toxoids and nonviable antigenic material requires no deferral. Donors who are vaccinated with experimental vaccines should be carefully evaluated and deferred for at least 12 months if there is any doubt as to the safety of the agent.[71]

The September 11, 2001, terrorist attacks on the United States and subsequent attacks of anthrax, real or hoax, through the postal system created concern about bioterrorism. The United States' vulnerability to a smallpox attack resulted in plans for mass vaccinations that have caused concern in the blood banking community. Vaccination with the vaccinia virus requires a minimum of a 21-day deferral; complicated additional criteria have been established related to vaccine-related complications and whether the scab separates spontaneously. There are also deferrals for individuals who may have come in contact with a vaccine recipient. For more information, see FDA Guidance (http://www.fda.gov/cber/gdlns/smpoxdefquar.htm#iv).

Medications taken by potential donors present a significant concern for the donor screeners. Medication deferrals fall into three major categories: those that might have adverse effects on the blood recipient, those that are taken for a medical condition that might make donation unacceptable, and those that would reduce the effectiveness of a blood product.

Some drugs are teratogenic and could cause birth defects if transfused to pregnant women. These medications include finasteride (Proscar, Propecia) and isotretinoin (Accutane), each of which requires a 1-month deferral after the last dose. Leflunomide (Arava) and dutasteride (Avodart) require 3-month and 6-month deferrals, respectively. Etretinate (Tegison) requires an indefinite deferral. Drugs that might transmit infections, such as human pituitary-derived growth hormone, which is associated with CJD, are cause for indefinite deferral. In the 1980s, prior to improved screening and purification processes, hemophiliac recipients of pooled clotting factor concentrates were at very high risk for transmitting HIV and hepatitis.

Antibiotic use may indicate an active bacterial infection. Associated subclinical bacteremia may result in a contaminated blood product, which could cause serious, even fatal, consequences to the recipient.

Medications may interfere with the quality of certain blood products. This is especially true of medications that inhibit platelet function, such as aspirin. Platelet donors must have not taken aspirin within 36 hours of donation. Other medications interfering with platelet function include clopidogrel (Plavix) and ticlopidine (Ticlid).

The CFR and AABB *Standards* provide some specific guidelines with which blood collections facilities must adhere, but it is impossible to attempt to provide specific guidance for all situations. This most often becomes an issue when evaluating donors with underlying health care problems. Not only might a particular condition require medical director consideration, but often the degree of clinical severity of that condition must also be considered.[72] For example, an active case of rheumatoid arthritis may require deferral, whereas a history of rheumatoid arthritis may not. In these instances, a collection center must develop its own procedures and criteria. Although not every circumstance can be dealt with in a comprehensive manner, some centers have developed comprehensive procedures to standardize this as best as possible.[73] It is occasionally necessary, however, particularly for autologous donations, to have a properly credentialed medical director review ambiguous situations and make informed decisions on a case-by-case basis. The medical director may also be needed to resolve issues about medications, potential risk factors, and any other circumstance where a medical doctor's decision is needed.

Donor Consent and Additional Information

It is necessary to obtain informed consent prior to donation. To help ensure that the prospective donor is properly informed, educational material about the donation process is distributed, including information about screening, phlebotomy, and potential donation-related complications. The goal of this material is for the donor to understand the reasons for self-deferral and the importance of self-deferral when appropriate. The notification process for positive serologic tests may be explained as well as donor confidentiality issues. AABB *Standards* requires review of information about the symptoms of AIDS, and the possibility of infectious disease transmission through blood transfusion. This reading material should be in language simple enough that every donor can comprehend it.[74] When local demographics demand, it may be wise to accommodate donors with materials written in a language that they can understand; otherwise, translators may be necessary. The donor must acknowledge that these materials were read and that all questions were answered.

Donor Physical Examination and Hematocrit

A brief physical examination is performed to help ensure the donor's suitability for blood donation. The physical examination consists of evaluation of the donor's pulse, blood pressure, temperature, and weight. There is also an inspection of antecubital fossae as sites of venous access.

Generally, a donor must weigh at least 110 pounds to undergo routine donation. *Standards* allows donation of 10.5 mL of whole blood for every kilogram of donor weight, but most centers purchase blood bags with a premeasured amount of anticoagulant/preservative. These have a specified minimum and maximum amount of blood that can be collected for the anticoagulant and preservatives to function according to manufacturer's specifications. For this reason, the volume of whole blood donated is fairly constant: approximately 1 pint. Assuring that the donor is of the minimum weight is important because a smaller donor, with a smaller blood volume, will suffer greater relative stress to the circulatory system. This will increase the likelihood of an adverse reaction, possibly loss of consciousness or seizures. Underweight donors are particularly likely among younger individuals, who also have a higher incidence of adverse donation reactions than older individuals.[75,76] Although the weight is generally noted from the history, it is wise to actually weigh those donors who appear to be underweight. There is no maximum weight for blood donation, but the donor's weight should not exceed the maximum capacity of the center's collection equipment.

The donor's pulse must be regular and between 50 and 100 beats per minute. A lower pulse is sometimes acceptable in athletic donors, although a medical director's approval may be necessary. A physician should also evaluate first-time donors with an irregular pulse. Allogeneic donors should be deferred if there is any question about the potential donor's cardiovascular fitness. For autologous donors with irregular heartbeats, consultation or written permission from the patient's physician may be necessary.

The donor's blood pressure must be less than 180/100 mmHg on the day of donation. First-time donors may present with elevated blood pressure due to donation-related anxiety. Allowing them a few moments' rest may lower the blood pressure to acceptable levels. Screeners should also be wary of low blood pressure in donors of small stature, advanced age, or with vascular disease, such as diabetes or atherosclerosis. These individuals may not tolerate acute blood loss as well as a normotensive donor. Blood pressure medications are acceptable if the blood pressure is controlled and the donor otherwise meets donation criteria.

The prospective donor's temperature should be less than 99.6°F. An elevated temperature may indicate a disease process that might affect the blood recipient (i.e., bacterial contamination of the product) and may require medical attention for the donor.

The potential donor's antecubital fossae are evaluated for acceptable venous access. The skin is checked for rashes, scars, or other lesions that would make phlebotomy unacceptable. The presence of "tracks" indicative of intravenous drug abuse also leads to deferral.

Determination of hemoglobin/hematocrit level is an essential part of the donation process. Whole blood collection from an anemic donor jeopardizes the donor and provides a substandard product for the transfusion recipient. *Standards* and the CFR require that donors have a minimum hemoglobin of 12.5 g/dL or hematocrit of 38% or greater.

Venous blood or finger pricks are common methods for obtaining blood for hemoglobin/hematocrit determination. Earlobe sampling, once a commonly used method, has been proven inaccurate and is not longer acceptable according to *Standards*.[77–79] Hematocrit determinations are often done using the manual microcapillary tube method or a portable point of care technology. Some facilities use the copper sulfate method, which relies on the specific gravity of blood relative to copper sulfate, to determine whether a blood sample has an adequate hemoglobin level.

Confidential Unit Exclusion

Blood donors with unacceptable risk factors for transfusion-transmitted disease might be coerced into blood donation. This situation may arise at an institutional blood drive or with directed donations for a friend or family member. The donor may deny risk factors, such as homosexuality or drug abuse, for fear that a breach of confidentiality might allow this behavior to become widely known. The confidential unit exclusion (CUE) provides the opportunity for a donor to request, with confidentiality guaranteed, that unacceptable donated blood not be used for transfusion. This procedure is accomplished by affording the donor a CUE card containing the unit number and a means of indicating, if necessary, that the unit not be used for transfusion. The CUE is then placed in a locked box to be reviewed at a later time, at which time excluded units are earmarked for destruction. In addition, centers can provide a designated telephone number so that a donor can call back with additional information, when necessary, that would exclude a unit for transfusion. When first used, the infectious disease marker frequency of units designated for nonuse by CUE was significantly higher than other units: as many as 20% of anti-HIV positive units would have been diverted from transfusion due to the CUE.[80] Improved donor education, infectious disease testing, and screening techniques have made the CUE a less valuable tool.[81–83] Many CUEs are the result of donors misunderstanding the CUE directions and inadvertently checking the wrong box.[84,85] For this reason, after investigation, some centers will destroy an excluded unit but will continue to allow the donor to donate blood.[86]

Infectious Disease Testing

Although donor screening plays an undeniable role in maintaining a safe blood supply, infectious disease testing remains the gold standard. As of 2005, blood is routinely screened for the following disease markers:

Hepatitis B surface antigen (HBsAg)
Hepatitis B core antibody (anti-HBc)
Hepatitis C virus antibody (anti-HCV)
HIV-1 and HIV-2 antibody (anti-HIV-1 and anti-HIV-2)
HTLV-I and HTLV-II antibody (anti-HTLV-I and anti-HTLV-II)
Nucleic acid amplification testing (NAT) for HIV-1 and HCV
NAT for West Nile virus (WNV)
Serologic test for syphilis

Although hepatitis plagued the blood supply for many years, it was not until the mid-1980s and the discovery that HIV was transmitted through blood transfusion that blood safety became a national obsession. Currently, the risk of transfusion-transmitted HIV may be as low as 1 in 2 million units.[87] Despite this, HIV is the most feared transfusion-transmitted disease.

Risk of HBV contamination may be as low as 1 in 100,000. NAT testing for HBV is still not in widespread use, although it is under consideration.[88,89] The debate, in part, consists of whether it is more cost effective to spend public funds on HBV vaccination programs or for NAT testing of the blood supply, and whether NAT testing would be more sensitive for "window period" detection of donors who have lost HBV antigenemia.[90,91]

The anti-HBc test is somewhat controversial.[92] It was once considered a surrogate marker for HIV, but improved serologic testing for HIV would seem to make anti-HBc unnecessary. The high false-positive rate for this marker further limits its usefulness. However, its proponents suggest that anti-HBc detects those donors who remain infectious of HBV who have lost HBsAg positivity.

Hepatitis C virus was once considered responsible for a transfusion-transmitted hepatitis rate of up to 10%. Current estimates of HCV transmission may be as low as 1 in 2 million units.

The test for antibodies to HTLV is also controversial.[93] Early on, HTLV-II was considered a possible etiologic agent of hairy-cell leukemia. This has been proven not to be the case, and HTLV-II is currently not associated with any disease process. HTLV-I is associated with adult T-cell leukemia/lymphoma in Japan and HTLV-associated myelopathy and tropical spastic paraparesis, chronic demyelinating diseases found in the Caribbean. The confirmatory test for HTLV is often time consuming and expensive. Many screening test results are not confirmed, however; the donated blood is destroyed and the donor is alarmed for no apparent reason.[94] Because HTLV-associated diseases are highly unusual in the United States, the necessity of HTLV as a screening test is unclear.

The most recent threat to the blood supply is West Nile virus. WNV is a mosquito-borne pathogen known to cause meningoencephalitis. Once it was recognized as a threat to the blood supply in 2003, NAT became available in fairly short order. In 2005, WNV seems to be an increasing threat, but the highly successful screening program has reduced its transmission by transfusion significantly.

Serologic testing for syphilis is another somewhat controversial test because transfusion-related transmission of this disease has been documented only recently. Some consider it to have value as an indicator of lifestyle problems that might make blood donation undesirable.

Collection

Prevenipuncture Procedures

The collection process begins with accurate identification of the blood donor. This is especially important in large centers where screening and phlebotomy are done in separate areas and by different staff. A unique identification number is placed on the collection bags, paperwork, and the pilot tubes collected for serologic testing. The phlebotomist applies mild pressure over the upper arm, usually with a blood pressure cuff or tourniquet. The increased venous pressure engorges the veins in the anticubital fossa, making them easier to detect for phlebotomy. Once a vein is selected, the skin is thoroughly disinfected, often using a two-step procedure utilizing soap and iodine solutions.[95] After the skin has been disinfected, the phlebotomist performs the venipuncture and the collection begins.

Whole Blood Collection

Whole blood is collected by means of venous pressure and gravity. Usually, the phlebotomy needle comes attached to a preconfigured bag system containing a premeasured amount of anticoagulant and preservative. A number of different anticoagulant/preservative preparations are available. The maximum liquid storage time for any RBC unit is currently 42 days. The number of bags in the collection set depends on intentions for further manufacture: whole blood, packed cells and plasma, or packed cells, plasma, and platelets. Multiple small bags can be attached if the blood is designated for pediatric transfusion. It is possible, through a sterile docking device, to add additional bags to a set. It is also possible to manually adjust the amount of anticoagulant in a collection bag for an underweight donor, but this requires significant time and expertise and is not done in most centers.

The collection bag is often placed on a trip-scale, which impedes further blood flow once the desired amount (usually 450 or 500 mL) has been drawn. The blood is agitated during collection, either manually or with an automated device, to ensure adequate mixing with the anticoagulant-preservative mixture in the bag. Many facilities choose to utilize a blood collection system that diverts the initial aliquot of donor blood into an integrally connected pouch. This diversion reduces the possibility that a skin plug or core cut with the needle during phlebotomy, possibly harboring bacteria, will contaminate the collection bag. Blood in the diversion pouch can be used for blood typing and viral marker testing without increasing blood loss associated with donation. This technique (diversion pouch) may reduce bacterial contamination rates in blood components overall by about 40%, with the highest reduction observed for common skin contaminants.[96,97]

Apheresis Platelet Collections

Plateletpheresis is a sophisticated technology by which blood is processed by an apheresis machine that uses centrifugation to remove a selected component of the blood and returns the rest to the donor. The most common use of this technology is for collection of apheresis platelets. Platelet donors are usually recruited from the ranks of whole blood donors. The minimum platelet count required to donate apheresis platelets is 150,000/μL. Apheresis platelet donors can donate more frequently than whole blood donors: AABB *Standards* limits apheresis platelet donations to no more than twice in a 7-day period and no more than 24 times per year. The apheresis procedure is more rigorous than whole blood collection because the donor must remain connected to the apheresis machine for an extended period, often 1 to 2 hours. Another difficulty is the high incidence of hypocalcemic reactions, due to the calcium-binding anticoagulant used to keep blood from clotting in the machine.

Platelets collected through apheresis technology have some advantages over random donor platelets (RDPs, collected by centrifugation from individual whole blood units) because 1 apheresis platelet unit is the equivalent of 6 to 10 RDPs. This decreases the risk of transfusion-transmitted disease and allergic transfusion reactions. If an apheresis donor's platelet count (and patience) is sufficient, a double or even triple product can be collected at one sitting. Many apheresis platelet technologies provide a leukocyte-reduced product.

Granulocytapheresis

Granulocytapheresis produces a product of concentrated neutrophils using apheresis technology. Granulocytes are used to treat neutropenic patients with infections that are not responding to antibiotics. Donors are placed on an apheresis machine with granulocytapheresis capabilities. Not all machines can perform granulocytapheresis: many of the newer machines are specialized for collection of platelets or plasma. The machine must be properly programmed and the operator specially trained for granulocyte collections.

A significant challenge to granulocytapheresis therapy is collecting enough granulocytes to produce a therapeutic response. Granulocytapheresis donors are premedicated with corticosteroids and/or granulocyte-colony stimulating factor (G-CSF) before collection, to maximize granulocyte yield. These medications cause release of marginated granulocytes from the spleen and major blood vessels, markedly increasing the peripheral blood granulocyte count before donation.[98] Higher peripheral granulocyte blood counts result in larger granulocyte collections.

Regimens for premedication vary. An example dosage is 5 to 10 μg/kg administered subcutaneously, 12 hours before the collection procedure. It is recommended that one consult the manufacturer's package insert for specific dosage guidelines.[99–101] Corticosteroids are usually given as prednisone or dexamethasone. The latter is given as a dose of 8 to 12 mg, depending on the donor's weight, at intervals of 4 and 12 hours before the collection procedure. A uniform dose of 450 μg of G-CSF coupled with 8 mg of dexamethasone, both given 12 hours before collection, has been shown to be as effective as larger combined doses.[102]

Producing a granulocytapheresis product that is not heavily contaminated with RBCs has also been a challenge. The density of granulocytes is only slightly lower than that of RBCs, which makes it difficult to produce a clean separation. RBCs in the granulocyte product must be compatible with the recipient to avoid the possibility of an acute hemolytic transfusion reaction. To help remedy the problem of red cell contamination, differential sedimentation is enhanced by use of rouleaux-inducing agents. Both hetastarch and pentastarch are employed for this purpose, although hetastarch is more widely used for its higher granulocyte yields.[103] Hetastarch, however, is less rapidly cleared from the body and accumulates more readily in the extravascular space, which can lead to localized edema, headache, and fluid retention in repeat donors, often family members, who donate regularly over a period of several days. It may be wise to use reduced dosages for frequent donors to help avoid these effects. These adverse effects tend to be less of a problem for infrequent donors and with collections using pentastarch. Although traces of hetastarch may be detected in the donor for years, there has been no demonstrated clinical significance. Combined premedication with G-CSF, dexamethasone, and collection with the use of hetastarch have been reported to provide a product with a granulocyte yield of 4.1 to 10.8×10^{10} compared to 2.1 to 2.6×10^{10} using dexamethasone alone.[104]

Granulocytapheresis products should be administered at least daily to an adult patient to achieve a physiologic dose, and this must be repeated for a number days. This requirement creates serious logistical problems and is one reason why (along with the cost) granulocytapheresis is not more frequently utilized. Improved antibiotic therapy and the high incidence of adverse effects in the recipients of granulocytapheresis products, including pulmonary reactions and leukocyte alloimmunization, have further decreased the functionality of this therapy.[105,106]

Hematopoietic Progenitor Cells, Apheresis

Collection of hematopoietic progenitor cells by apheresis (HPC-A), often referred to as *peripheral blood stem cells* or *stem cells,* has become increasingly prevalent over the past decade. The main advantage of HPC-A over hematopoietic progenitor cells, marrow (HPC-M) is that adequate HPC-A can be collected to support several courses of high-dose chemotherapy. Furthermore, transplantation of autologous HPC-A results in a more rapid hematopoietic recovery compared to autologous HPC-M. HPCs are mobilized into the donor's peripheral blood from the bone marrow with the use of recombinant colony-stimulating factors, either G-CSF, granulocyte-macrophage colony-stimulating factor, or a combination of the two.

Autologous HPC-A collections may be performed following, without, or in conjunction with chemotherapy. Apheresis is performed for several days as necessary, until an adequate stem cell dose is achieved. The adequacy is determined by the CD34+ dose (the number of CD34+ cells per kilogram of recipient body weight). It is generally agreed that a minimum dose of 2.5×10^6/kg CD34+ cells is necessary for successful engraftment.[107] In most autologous collections, venous access is obtained through a dual- or triple-lumen catheter.

Collection of allogeneic HPC-A from HLA-matched relatives is primarily performed using G-CSF mobilization. Clinical trials have suggested that a dose of 2.0×10^6/kg CD34+ cells is a minimum threshold for transplantation.[108]

Collections of HPC-A can be stored unmodified or can be processed further with the intent of improving outcomes. These include purging of cancer cells utilizing monoclonal antibodies,[109] CD34+ selection techniques,[110] and ex vivo expansion[111] (i.e., culture techniques).

Plasmapheresis

Most plasma for transfusion is produced by centrifugation of a unit of whole blood, which produces a unit of platelet-rich plasma and a unit of RBCs. Plasma can also be obtained using apheresis technology. Apheresis plasma is usually collected from group AB donors, which is of particular value because it can be transfused to patients with any blood type, although several investigators have raised concerns regarding the impact of ABO nonidentical blood product transfusions on patient outcomes.[112] The advantage of apheresis plasma technology is the ability to collect larger units, often called *jumbo plasma.* Larger units are desirable because fewer units are required per dose, which lessens the chance of infectious disease transmission and allergic reactions per recipient. For blood centers collecting blood for transfusion, plasma collections usually occur at an interval of 4 weeks or greater and must be compliant with FDA guidelines for "infrequent plasmapheresis."[113] These donors must meet whole blood criteria and are limited to an annual maximum of 12 L of plasma (14.4 L if at least 80 kg).

"Source" plasma is collected in large quantities by commercial firms for fractionation into plasma derivatives used to produce reagents and other plasma products. Source plasma is not for direct human transfusion. Because source plasma donors are often paid and tend to be aggressively recruited, specific regulatory requirements have been designed to protect the frequent plasmapheresis donor. These donors can donate a maximum of twice in a 7-day period, with at least 2 days between donations. Frequent donors require periodic physical examination by a physician and periodic determination of serum protein levels.

Multiple Apheresis Products

New apheresis technologies now make possible the collection of multiple products in a single donation when appropriate donor criteria are met. A double red cell product can be collected every 16 weeks if the donor meets the specified weight and hematocrit criteria. Some donors appreciate the convenience of donating less frequently. The collection of multiple products from a single donation helps to maintain an adequate blood supply and is often more cost efficient for the collection facility.

Adverse Donor Reactions and Injuries

The vasovagal reaction is the most common systemic donor reaction, occurring in 2% to 3% of donors.[114–117] These reactions often present as loss of consciousness due to a drop in blood pressure without a normal compensatory increase in heart rate. Vasovagal reactions are 5 to 10 times more frequent in younger donors (8% to 11%),[118] making careful observation especially important at high school and college blood drives. Other predisposing factors include first-time donor status,[119] low weight,[120] and a history of a previous donation reaction.[121,122] An anxiety-related psychosomatic component appears to be present because vasovagal reactions have occurred before donation and epidemic fainting is known to occur.

Vasovagal reactions often occur with short warning, during or immediately or after phlebotomy. Experienced phlebotomists know to look for lightheadedness, weakness, pallor, nausea, and diaphoresis. Excessive anxiety, often manifested by nervous talkativeness and hyperventilation, can precipitate a vasovagal reaction. Hyperventilation can result in respiratory alkalosis and hypocalcemia, which can help precipitate a vasovagal reaction.[123] In these instances, having the donor breathe into a paper bag may increase carbon dioxide levels, reversing the alkalosis and hypocalcemia. A calm, assuring demeanor by the phlebotomist will also do much to alleviate anxiety.

Approximately 5% of vasovagal reactions are syncopal and progress to loss of consciousness in about 0.08% to 0.34% of donors.[124] Syncopal reactions tend to occur after phlebotomy—about 60% occur at the refreshment table and 12% occur after the donor has left the collection site. This underscores the importance of closely observing donors even after the donation has been completed without incident. From 30% to 45% of the syncopal reactions include involuntary tetany or tonic-clonic convulsive movements.[125] These usually last less than 30 seconds; however, 20% may last longer, up to a minute or two. These can also progress to full-blown tonic-clonic seizures with associated urine incontinence. Prolonged hyperventilation can rarely lead to tetany without syncope as a result of hypocapnea leading to hypocalcemia. Severe vasovagal reactions may resemble shock clinically, except that the pulse is slow rather than fast. When the blood pressure becomes extremely low the donor often becomes pale and even cyanotic.

Mild vasovagal reactions are treated by elevating the donor's legs above his or her heart, helping to improve blood flow to the brain. Ammonium salts, cold neck compresses, and reassurance are often all that is necessary, and the donation can proceed. Treatment with intravenous fluids or medications is usually unnecessary if the donor does not have an underlying medical condition such as coronary artery or cerebrovascular disease. Experienced staff can help avoid a severe vasovagal reaction by recognizing and treating a reaction in the early stages.[126,127] Treatment of more severe vasovagal reactions, which may proceed to loss of consciousness and seizure activity, require that the donation be stopped and the needle be withdrawn to prevent local tissue injury from convulsive movements. The main risk associated with syncopal vasovagal reaction is trauma, particularly head trauma. Fractures and other significant injuries have been reported.[114] Some centers keep tongue protectors available, but damage to the tongue from convulsive movements is rare. The typical time for recovery from a vasovagal reaction is 5 to 30 minutes.

On occasion, a particularly severe reaction may require additional resources. Hospital-based donor rooms may have access to an emergency response team with a crash cart to deal with these situations. For remote centers without an on-site emergency response team, it may be prudent to call paramedics and have the donor transferred to a local emergency room if necessary. Maintaining a crash cart in the donor center with emergency life support equipment and medications is controversial. Centers that rarely see a severe reaction may have little or no actual experience with advanced life support procedures despite formal accreditation and may be unfamiliar with the available emergency equipment when needed. It may be better to have an emergency backup system, often calling 911, than to have an crash cart and not know how to use it.

Vasovagal reactions may recur within the next several hours and so donors who have had one should be advised to use caution when driving or operating heavy machinery. Donors with severe or multiple reactions should be discouraged from attempting to give blood again in the near future. Even donors who have had severe vasovagal reactions tend to recover spontaneously. No reports of deaths caused by blood donation-related vasovagal reaction appear in the medical literature, although there are reports of cardiac arrest in patients after venipuncture for blood sample collection.[128,129]

The sudden drop in blood pressure caused by a vasovagal reaction may evoke an ischemic event in donors with occlusive atherosclerotic vascular disease. These reactions tend to be rare, likely due to successful donor screening techniques.[114] The risk, of course, is higher for individuals with pre-existing disease, so these donors should be accepted only if their disease is stable and even then with caution. Some degree of risk may be acceptable for autologous donation, which is commonplace for elective cardiac bypass surgery (if the patient does not have unstable angina).[30,130] Taking chances with a routine allogeneic donor is unacceptable, and if there is any real uncertainty, the donor should be deferred.

Cerebrovascular disease presents a special problem because loss of consciousness and mild seizure activity may be manifestations of both a vasovagal reaction and cerebrovascular ischemia. For a donor with a known history of cerebrovascular disease, distinguishing a donation reaction from a stroke or transient ischemic attack may be difficult. For the same reasons, it is generally a good idea to be cautious about accepting a donor with a poorly controlled seizure disorder.

Minor local tissue injury at the venipuncture site is a well-known complication of any venipuncuture. Postphlebotomy bruising is the most common adverse donor event. Two studies of outpatient phlebotomy suggest that the incidence of bruising may range from 9% to 16%.[131,132] Hematomas occur less commonly: approximately 0.3% at the time of donation and an additional 0.05% reported by the donor later. Hematomas, bruising, and soreness can usually be treated with compresses and acetaminophen. These hematomas generally resolve within 2 weeks.

Accidental arterial punctures are rare.[125] They may present as an unusually rapid phlebotomy with bright red blood and a pulsating needle. On recognition, the phlebotomy should be stopped and pressure should be applied for at least 10 minutes. The donor should be closely observed for an extended period. If there is any question about effective hemostasis, competent medical consultation should be obtained. Brachial artery pseudoaneurysm,[133,134] arteriovenous fistula,[135] and compartment syndrome[136] are possible sequelae of arterial puncture. All three complications are rare but do require surgical repair.

Nerve damage due to a hematoma or direct trauma is an unusual event. Reports suggestive of nerve damage occur in approximately 1 of every 6000 blood donors.[137,138] Symptoms may include pain and paresthesias at the venipuncture site extending into the donor's hand, fingers, or shoulder area. A hematoma is present in approximately 25% of cases. Approximately 40% recover in a few days and 70% recover completely within 30 days. The remaining 30% take as long as 9 months to recover. A few donors have a small area of persistent numbness even after 9 months. Rarely, significant permanent neurologic damage occurs.

Bactericidal skin cleansing solutions and adhesive tape can cause local allergic reactions and irritation despite extensive prerelease testing and FDA approval. For iodine-sensitive donors, alternative solutions can be used. Post-donation hemostasis can be attained with pressure dressings rather than adhesive tape.

A common adverse effect of apheresis donation is hypocalcemia, due to the calcium-binding citrate anticoagulant used to keep blood from clotting in the apheresis machine tubing. Return of citrated blood to the donor may cause lightheadedness and perioral and peripheral paresthesias. These are readily treated by ingestion of calcium-containing antacid tablets. On machines that allow more extensive operator control, the rate of citrate infusion can be lowered to help diminish these reactions.

Apheresis removes a limited amount of blood from the donor at any given time, so vasovagal reactions and other adverse effects precipitated by acute volume loss are less pronounced. The two-needle continuous flow technology draws blood from one vein at the same rate as processed blood is returned in the other. Intermittent single-needle technology removes and replaces blood in very small increments. The decreased rate of vasovagal reactions among apheresis donors may also be due to the fact that these donors tend to be older and more experienced with the donation process. As with whole blood donation, the frequency of adverse reactions is higher in first-time apheresis donors. Vasovagal reactions, for instance, range from 2.0% in first-time to 0.5% in repeat donations.

Other than mild citrate reactions, adverse events are seen with an overall frequency of 2.18% (428 of 19,611 donations from 17 centers).[139] The most common adverse events are related to the venipuncture, with a frequency of 1.30%. Palpable hematoma accounted for 88% of these events. The risk of a hematoma is higher for a plateletpheresis procedure than for a whole blood donation (0.3% for the latter; Table 11-5). This may be due to the extended time frame that the needle is in place compared with the 10 to 15 minutes for a whole blood collection.

Other adverse effects of apheresis include RBC hemolysis, air emboli, clots, and leaks. These have been reported but are extremely rare with improved apheresis technology and better-trained operators. The incidence of adverse apheresis reactions varies among institutions, which may be due to donor selection, operator training, or even record keeping. One program has reported an overall 0.81% frequency of adverse events; of 19,736 procedures, 47 (0.24%) were rated as serious.[140] Seven of these 47 donors required transfer to an emergency department.

A single unit plateletpheresis procedure will cause a drop in the donor's platelet count of approximately 30,000 to 50,000 platelets/μL, although a return to prepheresis levels will usually occur in a few days.[141,142] In some donors, frequent plateletpheresis may cause a gradual drop in platelets, such that collections must be discontinued, or possibly donations can be scheduled with longer intervals between donations.[143] The platelet count usually recovers in these donors over several months without treatment. Donors with persistent thrombocytopenia are deferred from platelet donation.

Lymphocytes, which have a density similar to platelets, are often lost during a plateletpheresis procedure. In theory, frequent plateletpheresis could remove enough lymphocytes, especially long-lived T lymphocytes, to cause immune dysfunction. At this time, however, no adverse clinical effects have been observed in healthy donors.[144]

The same adverse effects of plateletpheresis are also be seen with granulocytapheresis. In addition, the sedimenting agents used to effectively remove granulocytes and the medications used to stimulate the donors' granulocyte counts have additional side effects. Small doses of corticocosteroids have been reported to cause insomnia in up to 25% of donors.[145] Frequent granulocyte donors should be free of peptic ulcers, diabetes mellitus, hypertension, glaucoma, and other diseases exacerbated by prolonged use of corticosteroids. A combined dose of G-CSF and dexamethasone may cause side effects in as many as 72% of donors; these are commonly insomnia (30%), mild bone pain (41%), and headaches (30%). The latter two are readily relieved by analgesics.[146] Sedimentation agents, usually hetastarch, may cause fluid retention and allergic reactions.

Table 11–5 The Incidence of Whole-Blood Donor Complications and of outside Medical Care

Variable	Incidence: Observation/ Donor Complaints†,%	Incidence: Observation and Postdonation Interview‡, %	Outside Medical Care Reported to American Red Cross in 2003§ (cases per 10,000)
Arm injuries			
Bruise	NA	22.7	See hematoma
Sore arm	NA	10.0	Unknown
Hematoma	0.35	1.7	0.57 (1/17,500)
Nerve irritation	0.02	0.9	0.46 (1/21,700)
Local allergy	0.5 (estimate)	NA	Unknown
Arterial puncture	0.01	NA	0.07 (1/142,900)
Thrombophlebitis	0.002 (estimate)	NA	0.01 (1/75,000)
Thrombosis	Very rare	NA	<0.001
Local infection	0.002 (estimate)	NA	<0.01 (1/225,000)
Systemic			
Fatigue	NA	7.8	Unknown
Vasovagal reaction	2.5	7.0	1.08 (1/9300)
Syncope	0.08–0.34	NA	See above
Syncope with injury	0.01–0.05	NA	See above
Nausea, vomiting	NA	0.4	Unknown
MI, stroke, etc.	Very rare	Very rare	Unknown
Total (donors)	3.5	37	2.94 (1/3400)‖

‖MI, myocardial infarction; NA, not applicable.

From Newman BH. Blood donor complications after whole-blood donation. Curr Opin Hematol 2004;Sep;11(5):339–345.

† Newman BH. Donor reactions and injuries from whole-blood donation. Transfusion Med Rev 1997;11:64–75.

‡Newman BH, Pichette S, Pichette D, et al. Adverse effect in blood donors after whole-blood donation: a study of 1,000 blood donors interviewed 3 weeks after whole-blood donation. Transfusion 2003;43:598–603.

§Newman B, Crooks N, Zhou L, et al. Whole-blood donor complications leading to outside medical care: National overview and a detailed review at one blood center [abstract]. Transfusion 2004;44(Suppl):77A.

‖Includes an unlisted category of "other."

Post-Donation Procedures

When the collection is complete, the tubing between the donor and the collection bag is clamped to stop the blood flow. Typically, pilot tubes for serologic testing are filled according to procedure, and the needle is removed. A pressure dressing is applied to the venipuncture site to achieve hemostasis. When the bleeding is stopped, a bandage is generally applied and the donor is escorted to a refreshment area.

Blood remaining in the collection tubing is "stripped" into the collection bag to ensure adequate mixing with the anticoagulant/preservative solution. Refilled tubing is sealed into individual attached segments to be used for compatibility testing at a later time. The unit is then documented, stored, and transported to its next stop according to procedure.

The donor must remain in the canteen area under observation for approximately 15 minutes to ensure that the staff can quickly react should a reaction occur. Liquids are given to help replace those removed during the donation procedure.

The donor should receive a post-donation packet that includes information about caring for the venipuncture site, drinking liquids, and describes appropriate post-donation activity levels. A telephone number is provided to call if the donor has an adverse reaction or wishes to modify the health history information. Once stable, the donor can be released and possibly scheduled for the next donation.

Safety Concerns

Safety is always a concern when working with biohazardous materials. Safety issues have come under increasing regulatory surveillance, and there is particular concern about accidental exposure through used needles, lancets, and microhematocrit tubes.[147] Retractable needle covers to avoid accidental needle-sticks have become mandatory in some states. Safety devices are also available for filling pilot tubes. Disposable lancets and glass microhematocrit tubes can puncture skin if not handled properly. Proper disposal of used needles, lancets, and microcapillary hematocrit tubes in specialized "sharps" containers is mandatory. A properly designed and enforced Exposure Control Plan is a key element in preventing occupational blood exposures and transmission of blood-borne pathogens.

Although volunteer blood donors have a low prevalence of transfusion-transmitted disease,[148] use of disposable gloves should be encouraged, especially for staff with open wounds on exposed skin.[149] If a staff member is exposed, the employee should be counseled immediately and offered postexposure testing and prophylaxis for HIV infection.[150] Postexposure prophylaxis (PEP) should begin within 2 hours of exposure, so it may not be possible to delay treatment until infectious disease testing results on the donor are available. Although PEP for potential HIV transmission should be offered, its use is not justified for exposures that pose a negligible risk.[151,152] PEP, if taken, should be discontinued if the source is later determined to be HIV negative. Rapid testing of HIV of source donors or patients can facilitate making timely decisions regarding the use of HIV PEP.

Treatment for exposure to other transfusion-transmitted diseases is less time sensitive and can usually wait until testing of the donor in complete. If the donor is found to be HBsAg positive, a nonimmune staff member should be offered hepatitis B immune globulin within 7 days of exposure and HBV vaccine.[153] It is recommended that staff receive the HBV vaccine on initial employment, unless one is prohibited from receiving the vaccine for medical reasons or is otherwise already immune.

Table 11–6 Example of Causes for Lookback Notification

Item	Lookback Initiated If
HBsAg	Repeatedly reactive HBsAg confirmed positive by neutralization (or neutralization not done) is found in a subsequent donation whose prior test results were nonreactive **OR** Repeatedly reactive HBsAg, negative neutralization AND repeatedly reactive HBcore is found in a subsequent donation whose prior test results were nonreactive
HBcore	Repeatedly reactive anti-HBcore, and the test result of the second test method is reactive in a subsequent donation whose prior test results were nonreactive **OR** Repeatedly reactive anti-HBcore and repeatedly reactive HBsAg in a subsequent donation whose prior test results were nonreactive
HTLV-I/II	Repeatedly reactive anti-HTLV-I/II and the second test result is repeatedly reactive or not performed is found in a subsequent donation, whose prior test results were nonreactive or not previously tested
Anti-HIV-1,2	Repeatedly reactive anti-HIV-1,2 confirmed positive HIV-1 Western Blot **OR** HIV-2 EIA reactive found in a subsequent donation not previously tested or whose prior test results were nonreactive
HIV-1 NAT	NAT reactive AND HIV-1 Western Blot (or IFA) indeterminate positive or HIV-2 EIA reactive is found in a subsequent donation whose prior test results were nonreactive or prior donation was not tested
Anti-HCV	Repeatedly reactive anti-HCV with a supplemental test result of positive, indeterminate OR no supplemental test performed found in a subsequent donation whose prior donation was not previously tested with the currently licensed test, or whose prior test results were nonreactive
HCV NAT	NAT reactive with a supplemental test result of positive, indeterminate OR no supplemental test performed found in a subsequent donation whose prior donation was not previously tested, or whose prior test results were nonreactive
WNV	Current donation sample has a reactive WNV NAT. Relevant collections include those occurring between 120 days prior to the date of the reactive test and 120 days after the date of the reactive test. Donor reports a diagnosis of West Nile virus occurring between 14 days prior to the onset of illness and up to and including 120 days subsequent to the onset of illness or diagnosis, whichever is the later date. Donor reports unexplained febrile illness with headache or symptoms suggestive of WNV infection between June 1 and November 30, and Medical Director has determined this represents likely infection by WNV. A report is received regarding possible transmission of WNV by a blood component received within the 120 days prior to the onset of symptoms, or a WNV- fatality in a transfused recipient. Prompt quarantine and retrieval for in-date components collected from the donor of suspect donation in the period between 120 days before the suspect donation and up to and including 120 days after the suspect donation must be performed.
CJD or vCJD Risk factors	Subsequent to donation, the donor: is diagnosed with Creutzfeldt-Jakob disease indicates a family history of Creutzfeldt-Jakob disease acknowledges receipt of human pituitary-derived growth hormone (HGH) acknowledges receipt of a dura mater transplant indicates having spent a total time of 3 months or more in the United Kingdom from 1980 through 1996 indicates receipt of injectable products from cattle in BSE-endemic countries acknowledges spending a total time of 5 years or more in Europe, including time spent in the UK If a member of the U.S. military, a civilian military employee or a dependent of a member of the US military and spent a total of 6 months or more associated with a military base in any of the following countries: From 1980 through 1990 in Belgium, the Netherlands, or Germany From 1980 through 1996 in Spain, Portugal, Turkey, Italy, or Greece
AIDS-related	If a donor implicated in the investigation of transfusion-associated AIDS has a reactive test result for anti-HIV-1, 2 and/or HIV-1 antigen. If information is received that a patient with AIDS has previously donated blood.
High-risk behavior (e.g., travel, vaccination malaria, tattoo, blood exposure)	Post-donation information becomes available regarding a donor who would have been deferred had the information been known at the time of donation.

Compliance Issues

The management of unexpected events may often be referred to as *error* or *deviation management*. Because humans are fallible, limiting the incidence of errors to absolute zero can never be achieved.[154, 155] Well-prepared organizations approach error management from a systems level, anticipating that errors and deviations will occur, and prepare system defenses for dealing with their inevitable occurrence rather than focusing on blaming individuals for forgetfulness or inattention.[154]

Lookbacks

Being human, blood donors themselves represent a source of deviation. With the incubation time between exposure and onset of disease, some individuals are unaware that they may be infectious to others. To identify these individuals, a donor center must develop procedures to notify the recipients of blood or components of previous donations when a donor becomes confirmed positive for an infectious disease marker, or when a statement of high-risk information dis closed at a subsequent time determines that the donor was actually ineligible at the time of their donation. Identification of persons who may have received blood or components from such donors is referred to as *lookback*. Examples of causes for lookback may be seen in Table 11–6.

On identification of a unit meeting lookback criteria, a facility must search records for prior donations by the same individual. A sample worksheet may be seen in Figure 11–1. The highest priority should be placed on the most recently donated units. This should be done within 72 hours, so that any unit(s) remaining in inventory may be immediately quarantined. Policies must include consignee notification, so that any components shipped to other facilities may be immediately quarantined and returned. A sample notification letter and product disposition record may be seen in Figures 11–2 and 11–3.

If the implicated donor has donated on many occasions, lookback notification should be started with the most recent recipients. Reasonable and timely attempts must be made to notify transfusion recipients, particularly if a lookback is due to HIV[156] or HCV,[157] so that recipients may obtain testing, counseling, and medical referral as needed.

Recalls and Market Withdrawals

Errors can also result from improper testing, incorrect labeling of components, improperly interpreting test results, improperly using equipment, or failure to follow the manufacturers' directions or facility procedures. These kinds of errors may result in recalls or market withdrawals.

Recalls are defined as actions taken by a facility to remove a product from the market.[158,159] Recalls may be conducted

Somewhere Donor Center
Anywhere, State, Zip

LOOKBACK WORKSHEET **Case Number:** ______________

Unit Number		Unit # of
Date/Time Initiated		By:
Unit collected by (facitlity name)		
Notified by (name, date, time)		

Components prepared/received (✓)	Unit status (INV, QU, TF, DS, or SHIP)	**If in Inventory,** Quarantined Date/Time	**If Shipped** Date Shipped	Consignee Name	Consignee Notified Date/Time/By	Consignee Contact Name	**If Transfused** Patient Name	Medical Record Number	Patient Status
❑ Whole Blood									
❑ Red Cells									
❑ Fresh Frozen Plasma									
❑ Platelets									
❑ Recovered Plasma									
❑ Cryoprecipitate									
❑									
❑									
❑									

FOR USE BY COMPLIANCE:

Other information (Patient primary physician notifications, final outcomes, response from consignees). List by component. Use other side as necessary and attach all related documents.

Unit Status Legend: INV = Inventory; QU = Quarantined; TF = Transfused; DS = Destroyed; SHIP = Shipped

SOP # attachment #
Effective date

Figure 11–1 Sample lookback worksheet.

Date: December 1, 2005

John Doe, MD
Director, Blood Bank
General Hospital
Anywhere, CA 90000

This confirms our telephone notification that your hospital received a blood component from a donor that was subsequently found to be confirmed positive for HIV-1. All test results from prior donations were nonreactive, including those for the blood component shipped to your facility.

On November 30, 2005, at 11:25am, we telephoned your facility and spoke to Jane Doe and conveyed the following information:

UNIT NUMBER	Z987654321
TYPE OF COMPONENT	Whole Blood
ABO/RH:	O negative
EXPIRATION DATE:	12/6/2005
SHIPMENT DATE	11/25/2005

Your transfusion service reported the unit to be **transfused.**

Please complete and return the enclosed *Lookback Product Disposition Record.* Maintain a copy of the record for your files.

If you have any questions concerning this matter, please contact the Somewhere Donor Center at (555) 123-4567 x891.

Sincerely,

Name & credentials
Authorized Somewhere Donor Center contact

Figure 11–2 Sample confirmation letter.

on a facility's own initiative, by FDA request, or by FDA order under statutory authority. FDA guidelines categorize all recalls into one of three classes according to the level of hazard involved.

A Class I recall is a situation in which there is a reasonable probability that the use of or exposure to a violative product will cause serious adverse health consequences or death. An example of products in this category would be a unit issued that was found to be HIV positive.

A Class II recall is a situation in which use of or exposure to a violative product may cause temporary or medically reversible adverse health consequences or where the probability of serious adverse health consequences is remote. An example of products in this category would be a unit later found to be collected from a donor whose hemoglobin did not meet the minimum criteria.

A Class III recall is a situation in which use of or exposure to a violative product is not likely to cause adverse health consequences. Examples of products in this category might be those that do not meet FDA labeling regulations.

Somewhere Donor Center
123 Main Street
Anywhere, State, Zip
(555) 123-4567 extension 891

Section A: *To be completed by Somewhere Donor Center*

Case ID: ______________________

Consignee: ______________________ Contact Person: ______________________

Street Address: ______________________ Phone: ______________________

City/State/Zip: ______________________ Email: ______________________

Re: (Unit number) __________ ABO/Rh: __________ Component: __________

Date Shipped: __________ Expiration Date: __________ Date Notified: __________

Reason for Notification: ______________________

Form Completed by: ______________________ Date: ______________________

Section B: *To be completed by Consignee*

Final Disposition of Component: __________ Date of final disposition: __________

❑ Transfused

❑ Returned

❑ Discarded (Reason) ______________________

❑ Transferred to another facility (Please complete the information on the receiving facility below)

Name ______________________

Street Address ______________________

City/State/Zip ______________________

Phone (   ) ______________________

Informed ❑ No ❑ Yes If Yes, Date notified __________

For Manufacturers only: ❑ Put into production ❑ Quarantined ❑ Discarded

Form Completed by: ______________________ Date ______________________

Title ______________________

Figure 11–3 Sample lookback product disposition record.

A market withdrawal occurs when a product has a minor violation that would not be subject to FDA legal action. The firm removes the product from the market or corrects the violation. For example, a product removed from the market due to tampering, without evidence of manufacturing or distribution problems, would be a market withdrawal.

Biological Product Deviation Reporting

On November 7, 2000, the FDA published a final rule[160] to amend the requirements of reporting errors and accidents in manufacturing of products. This rule was issued as part of a program to improve the effectiveness of the FDA's regulatory program. FDA replaced the term *error and accident* with the term *biological product deviation* (BPD).

Licensed blood establishments, unlicensed blood establishments, registered blood establishments, and transfusion services are required to report to the FDA all BPDs. BPDs are defined as any event associated with manufacturing of blood or blood components that EITHER:

1. Represent a deviation from current GMPs, applicable regulations, or established specifications that may

affect the safety, purity, or potency of that product OR

2. Represent an unexpected or unforeseeable event that may affect the safety, purity, or potency of that product AND
   - Occurs in your facility or a facility under contract to you AND
   - Involves a distributed blood or blood component.

Post-donation information is considered reportable to the FDA as a BPD if the donor should have been deferred had the information been known at the time of donation and the safety, purity, or potency of the product could be affected. Post-donation information also includes information that a blood center obtains when it adds new donor history questions.

In many cases blood establishments cannot control post-donation information. For example, a donor may call after donating to report a post-donation illness, or information obtained post-donation about exposure to a disease or a sex partner at high risk. Reports of post-donation information continue to represent the largest percentage of BPDs submitted by blood and plasma establishments (71%). In 88% of the reports the donor was aware of the information at the time they were interviewed, but failed to provide the information during the interview. Most often (91%), the donor center staff is made aware during a subsequent donation interview.[161]

CONCLUSION

The products of blood donation—RBCs, platelets, and plasma—are a vital resource making possible modern medicine. At this time, there are no comparable substitutes. A debt of gratitude is owed to those blood donors who give their blood, for no monetary compensation, to anonymously help save the lives of others.

At one time, all that was needed to collect blood was a collection set and a donor with suitable veins. Since then, thousands of transfusion medicine professionals have transformed the early donor rooms to a multibillion dollar industry collecting tens of millions of blood products per year. Their ceaseless efforts to improve transfusion safety have had remarkable success on the well-being of the blood recipient, donor, and even the collections staff. Unremitting efforts to improve donor screening and serologic testing for infectious disease are needed to keep ahead of potential threats to the blood supply.

For these reasons, change occurs very rapidly in the world of blood banking, and all decision-making processes require checking for the latest information available, which can be obtained through the AABB or FDA websites.

REFERENCES

1. American Association of Blood Banks. Available at http://www.aabb.org/content/All_Blood/Facts_About_Blood_and_Blood_Banking/aabb_ faqs.htm. Last modified April12, 2006.
2. Sullivan MT, Wallace EL, Umana WO, Schreiber GB. Trends in the collection and transfusion of blood in the United States, 1987–1997 [abstract]. Transfusion 1999;39(Suppl):1S.
3. Brecher ME, Goodnough LT. The rise and fall of preoperative autologous blood donation (editorial). Transfusion 2001;41:1459–1462.
4. Goodnough LT, Brecher ME, Kanter MH, AuBuchon JP. Transfusion medicine. First of two parts—blood transfusion. NEJM1999;340:438–447.
5. Canadian Blood Services News Release. Ipsos-Reid poll: over half of Canadians say they or their family have needed blood. Less than four percent of eligible population donated blood last year. Available at http://www.bloodservices.ca/Centreps/Internet/UW_V502_MainEngine.nsf/page/E_NR2005-09-07_IpsosReid_Touched+by+system?OpenDocument. Accessed September 8, 2005.
6. Newman BH. Whole-blood donation: blood donor suitability and adverse events. Curr Hematol Rep 2004;3:437–443.
7. U.S. General Accounting Office. blood Supply: Availability of Blood (GAO/HEHS-99-187R). Washington, D.C., U.S. General Accounting Office, September 20, 1999.
8. U.S. Department of State. Hispanics Replace African Americans as Largest U.S. Minority Group. January 23, 2003. Available at http://usinfo.state.gov/usa/diversity/a012303.htm.
9. Glynn SA, Schreiber GB, Busch MP, et al. Demographic characteristics, unreported risk behaviors, and the prevalence and incidence of viral infections: a comparison of apheresis and whole blood donation. Transfusion 1998;38:350–358.
10. Leiby DA, Herron RM Jr, Read EJ, et al. *Trypanosoma cruzi* in Los Angeles and Miami blood donors: impact of evolving donor demographics on seroprevalence and implications for transfusion transmission. Transfusion 2002;42:549–555.
11. Eastlund T. Monetary blood donation incentives and the risk of transfusion-transmitted infection. Transfusion 1998;38:874–882.
12. Code of Federal Regulations. 21 CFR 606.121(c)(5). Washington, D.C., U.S. Government Printing Office, April 1, 2005.
13. California Health and Safety Code. 1626(d). Available at http://www.leginfo.ca.gov.
14. Strauss RG. Blood donations, safety, and incentives. Transfusion 2001;41:165–167.
15. Barker LF, Westphal RG. Voluntary, nonremunerated blood donation: still a world health goal? Transfusion 1998;38:803–806.
16. Sullivan JL. Iron and the sex differences in heart disease risk. Lancet 1981;1:1293–1294.
17. Meyers DG. The iron hypothesis: does iron play a role in atherosclerosis? Transfusion 2000;40:1023–1029.
18. Wallas CH, Lipton KS. Donor Incentives—A Report of the AABB Board of Directors (Association Bulletin 94-6). Bethesda, Md., American Association of Blood Banks, October14, 1994.
19. U.S. Food and Drug Administration. Compliance Policy Guidance for FDA Staff and Industry, Chapter 2, Section 230.150. Issued May 7, 2002, revised November 22, 2005. Available at http://www.fda.gov/ora/compliance—ref/cpg/cpgbio/cpg230=150final.htm. Last modified December 12, 2005.
20. Busch M, Stramer S. The efficiency of HIV p24 antigen screening of US blood donors: projections versus reality. Infus Ther Transfus Med 1998;25:194–197.
21. Code of Federal Regulations. 21 CFR 606.40. Washington, D.C., U.S. Government Printing Office, April 1, 2005.
22. Dellinger EP, Anaya DA. Infectious and immunologic consequences of blood transfusion. Crit Care (London) 2004;8(Suppl 2):S18–S23.
23. Blumberg N. Deleterious clinical effects of transfusion immunomodulation: proven beyond a reasonable doubt. Transfusion 2005;45 (2 Suppl):33S–39S.
24. Raghavan M, Marik PE. Anemia, allogenic blood transfusion, and immunomodulation in the critically ill. Chest 2005;127:295–307.
25. Blajchman MA. Immunomodulation and blood transfusion. Am J Therap 2002;9:389–395.
26. Vamvakas EC. Blajchman MA. Deleterious clinical effects of transfusion-associated immunomodulation: fact or fiction? Blood 2001;97: 1180–1195.
27. Rouger P. Transfusion induced immunomodulation: myth or reality? Transfus Clin Biol 2004;11:115–116.
28. Goodnough LT, Monk TG, Andriole GL. Erythropoietin therapy. NEJM 1997;336:933–938.
29. Popovsky MA, Whitaker B, Arnold N. Severe outcomes to allogeneic and autologous blood donation: frequency and characterization. Transfusion 1995;35:734–737.
30. Kiyama H, Ohshima N, Imazeki T. Safety and efficacy of blood donation prior to elective cardiac surgery in anemic patients. Japan J Thorac Cardiovasc Surg 2000;48:101–105.
31. From California Blood Bank Society. Available at http://www.cbbsweb.org/enf/2001/adtxtrigger.html. Last revised March 1, 2001.
32. Dupuis JY, Bart B, Bryson G, Robblee J. Transfusion practices among patients who did and did not predonate autologous blood before elective cardiac surgery. Can Med Assoc J 1999;160:97–1002.
33. From California Blood Bank Society. Available at http://www.cbbsweb.org/enf/2004/ad_positivetests.html. Last modified August 5, 2005.
34. Grossman BJ, Stewart NC, Grindon AJ. Increased risk of a positive test for antibody to hepatitis B core antigen (anti-HBc) in autologous blood donors. Transfusion 1988;28:283–285.

35. Etchason J, Petz L, Keeler E, et al. The cost-effectiveness of preoperative autologous blood donations. NEJM 1995;332:719–724.
36. Code of Federal Regulations. 21 CFR 610.40(d). Washington, D.C., U.S. Government Printing Office, April 1, 2005.
37. Code of Federal Regulations. 21 CFR 606.121. Washington, D.C., U.S. Government Printing Office, April 1, 2005.
38. Silva MA (ed). Standards for Blood Banks and Transfusion Services, 23rd ed. Bethesda, Md., American Association of Blood Banks, 2004. Standard 5.8.5.1.2.
39. Shulman IA, Osby M. Storage and transfusion of infected autologous blood or components. Arch Pathol Lab Med 2005;129:981–983.
40. Shulman IA. 1992 CAP Surveys. Comprehensive Transfusion Medicine Survey, 1992 Set J-C. Interlaboratory Comparison Program. Northfield, Ill., College of American Pathologists, 1992.
41. Linden JV, Wagner K, Voytovich AE, Sheehan J. Transfusion errors in New York State: an analysis of 10 years' experience. Transfusion 2000;40:1207–1213.
42. Pub. Law No. 101–336, 104 Stat. 327 (1990). Codified at 42 U.S.C. §12101–12213.
43. Rothstein RF. Bragdon v. Abbott—Supreme Court Decision Addresses Application of Americans with Disabilities Act to Individuals with HIV. Houston, Tex., University of Houston Health Law & Policy Institute, June 26, 1998.
44. Bragdon v. Abbott et al. (97-156). Cornell Law School Legal Information Institute Supreme Court Selection. Available at http://supct.law.cornell.edu/supct/html/97-156.ZS.html. Accessed June 3, 2006.
45. Mintz PD. Participation of HIV-infected patients in autologous blood programs. JAMA 1993;269:2892–2894.
46. Yomtovian R, Kelly C, Bracey AW, et al. Procurement and transfusion of human immunodeficiency virus-positive or untested autologous blood units: issues and concerns: A report prepared by the Autologous Transfusion Committee of the American Association of Blood Banks. Transfusion 1995;35:353–361.
47. The ADA, HIV, and autologous blood donation. Association Bulletin 98–5. Bethesda, Md., American Association of Blood Banks, 1998.
48. Williams AE, Wu Y, Kleinman SH. The declining use and comparative seroprevalence of directed whole blood donations [abstract]. Transfusion 2000;40(Suppl):5S.
49. Strauss RG, Barnes A, Blanchette VS, et al. Directed and limited-exposure blood donations for infants and children. Transfusion 1990; 30:68–72.
50. Hare VW, Liles BA, Crandall LW, Nufer CN. "Partners for Life"—a safer therapy for chronically transfused children [abstract]. Transfusion 1994;34(Suppl):92S.
51. U.S. Food and Drug Administration. Guidance for industry: variances for blood collection from individuals with hereditary hemochromatosis. FDA Docket No. 00D-1618. Federal Register August 23, 2001;66(164).
52. Silva MA (ed). Standards for Blood Banks and Transfusion Services, 23rd ed. Bethesda, Md, American Association of Blood Banks, 2004.
53. From California Blood Bank Society. Available at http://www.cbbsweb.org/enf/2003/donor_id.html. Last modified July 5, 2003.
54. Grindon AJ, Norrell S, Robertson WR, et al. Predonation determination of donor eligibility [abstract]. Transfusion 1995;35(Suppl):72S.
55. From U.S. Food and Drug Administration. Available at http://www.fda.gov/cber/gdlns/donorhistques.htm. Accessed July 5, 2006.
56. Silvergleid AJ, Leparc GF, Schmidt PJ. Impact of explicit questions about high-risk activities on donor attitudes and donor deferral patterns: results in two community blood centers. Transfusion 1989;29:362–364.
57. Zuck TF, Cumming PD, Wallace EL. Computer-assisted audiovisual health history self-interviewing. Results of the pilot study of the Hoxworth Quality Donor System. Transfusion 2001;41:1469–1474.
58. From U.S. Food and Drug Administration. Available at http://www.fda.gov/ohrms/dockets/ac/05/slides/2005-4096S2_03.ppt. Accessed July 5, 2006.
59. Brown P, Cervenakova L. The modern landscape of transfusion-related iatrogenic Creutzfeldt-Jakob disease and blood screening tests. Curr Opin Hematol 2004;11:351–356.
60. McCullough J, Anderson D, Brookie D, et al. Consensus conference on vCJD screening of blood donors: report of the panel. Transfusion 2004;44:675–683.
61. National Center for Infectious Diseases. Available at http://www2.ncid.cdc.gov/travel/yb/utils/ybGet.asp?section=dis&obj=index.htm&cssNav=browseoyb. Accessed July 5, 2006.
62. Dodd RY. Bovine spongiform encephalopathy, variant CJD, and blood transfusion: beefer madness? Transfusion 2004;44:628–630.
63. Ironside JW, Head MW. Variant Creutzfeldt-Jakob disease: risk of transmission by blood and blood products. Haemophilia 2004;10(Suppl 4): 64–69.
64. Boulton F. The impact of variant CJD on transfusion practices in the UK. Transf Apheresis Sci 2003;28:107–116.
65. U.S. Department of HHS, Food and Drug Administration, Center for Biologics Evaluation and Research. Guidance for Industry: Revised Preventive Measures to Reduce the Possible Risk of Transmission of Creutzfeldt-Jakob Disease (CJD) and Variant Creutzfeldt-Jakob Disease (vCJD) by Blood and Blood Products. Federal Register Docket No. 97D-0318. Washington, D. C., Government Printing Office, January 16, 2002.
66. Schmidt M, Brixner V, Ruster B, et al. NAT screening of blood donors for severe acute respiratory syndrome coronavirus can potentially prevent transfusion associated transmissions. Transfusion 2004;44:470–475.
67. le Fichoux Y, Quaranta JF, Aufeuvre JP, et al. Occurrence of *Leishmania infantum* parasitemia in asymptomatic blood donors living in an area of endemicity in southern France. J Clin Microbiol 1999;37:1953–1957.
68. Eastman RT, Barrett LK, Dupuis K, et al. Leishmania inactivation in human pheresis platelets by a psoralen (amotosalen HCl) and long-wavelength ultraviolet irradiation. Transfusion 2005;45:1459–1463.
69. Pomper GJ, Wu Y, Snyder EL. Risks of transfusion-transmitted infections: 2003. Curr Opin Hematol 2003;10:412–418.
70. Busch MP, Kleinman SH, Nemo GJ. Current and emerging infectious risks of blood transfusions. JAMA 2003;289:959–962.
71. Mintz PD, Liption KS. Interim Standard for Standards for Blood Banks and Transfusion Services, 23rd ed. AABB Association Bulletin #05–07. Bethesda, Md., American Association of Blood Banks, September 30, 2005.
72. Newman B. Blood donor suitability and allogeneic whole blood donation. Transfus Med Rev 2001;15:234–244.
73. Department of Defense. Available at http://www.militaryblood.dod. mil/library/policies/downloads/conditions_list.doc. Revised July 5, 2005.
74. Mayo DJ, Rose AM, Matchett SE, et al. Screening potential blood donors at risk for human immunodeficiency virus. Transfusion 1991; 31:466–474.
75. Newmand BH. Vasovagal reactions in high school students: findings relative to race, risk factor synergism, female sex, and non-high school participants. Transfusion 2002;42:1557–1560.
76. Trouern-Trend JJ, Cable RG, Badon SJ, et al. A case-controlled multicenter study of vasovagal reaction in blood donors: influence of sex, age, donation status, weight, blood pressure, and pulse. Transfusion 1999;39:316–320.
77. Coburn TJ, Miller WV, Parrill WD. Unacceptable variability of hemoglobin estimation on samples obtained from ear punctures. Transfusion 1977;17:265–268.
78. Avoy DR, Canuel ML, Otton BM, et al. Hemoglobin screening in prospective blood donors: a comparison of methods. Transfusion 1977;17:261–264.
79. Newman B. Very anemic donors pass copper sulfate screening test [letter]. Transfusion 1997;37:670–671.
80. Nusbacher J, Chiavetta J, Naiman R, et al. Evaluation of a confidential method of excluding blood donors exposed to human immunodeficiency virus. Transfusion 1986;26:539–541.
81. Peterson LR, Lackritz E, Lewis WF, et al. The effectiveness of the confidential unit exclusion option. Transfusion 1994;34:865–869.
82. Korelitz JJ, Williams AE, Busch MP, et al. Demographic characteristics and prevalence of serologic markers among donors who use the confidential unit exclusion process: The Retrovirus Epidemiology Donor Study. Transfusion 1994;34:870–876.
83. Zou S, Notari EP, Musavi F, Dodd RY. Current impact of the confidential unit exclusion option. Transfusion 2004;44651–44657.
84. Kean CA, Hsueh Y, Querrin JJ, et al. A study of confidential unit exclusion. Transfusion 1990;30:707–709.
85. Kessler D, Valinsky JE, Bianco C. Sensitivity and specificity of confidential unit exclusion (CUE)-does it work? [abstract] Transfusion 1993;33(Suppl):35S.
86. From California Blood Bank Society. Available at http://www.cbbsweb.org/enf//2003/donor_cue_deferral.html. Last modified April 14, 2003.
87. Goodnough LT, Shander A, Brecher ME. Transfusion medicine: looking to the future. Lancet 2003;361:161–169.
88. Kleinman SH, Strong DM, Tegtmeier GG, et al. Hepatitis B virus (HBV) DNA screening of blood donations in minipools with the COBAS AmpliScreen HBV test. Transfusion 2005;45:1247–1257.
89. Busch MP. Should HBV DNA NAT replace HBsAg and/or anti-HBc screening of blood donors? Transfus Clin Biol 2004;11:26–32.
90. Ringwald J, Mertz I, Zimmermann R, et al. Hepatitis B virus vaccination of blood donors—what costs may be expected? Transfus Med 2005;15:83–92.
91. Marshall DA, Kleinman SH, Wong JB, et al. Cost-effectiveness of nucleic acid test screening of volunteer blood donations for hepatitis B, hepatitis C and human immunodeficiency virus in the United States. Vox Sang 2004;86:28–40.
92. Muhlbacher A, Zdunek D, Melchior W, Michl U. Is infective blood donation missed without screening for antibody to hepatitis B core antigen and/or hepatitis B virus DNA? Vox Sang 2001;81:139.

93. Witt D, Kuramoto K, Kemper M, Holland P. Utility of prospective study of donors deferred as HTLV indeterminate. [Letter] Vox Sang 2000;78:130–131.
94. False-positive serologic tests for human T-cell lymphotropic virus type I among blood donors following influenza vaccination, 1992. MMWR 1993;42:173–175.
95. Brecher M (ed). Technical Manual, 15th ed. Bethesda, Md., American Association of Blood Banks, 2005, pp 800–801.
96. de Korte D, Marcelis JH, Verhoeven AJ, Soeterboek AM. Diversion of first blood volume results in a reduction of bacterial contamination for whole-blood collections. Vox Sang 2002;83:13–16.
97. U.S. Department of Health and Human Services, Advisory Committee on Blood Safety and Availability. April 2004 Presentations. Available at http://www.hhs.gov/bloodsafety/presentations/Jaroslav.pdf. April 7–8, 2004.
98. Lord LI, Bronchud MH, Owens S, et al. The kinetics of human granulopoiesis following treatment with granulocyte colony-stimulating factor in vivo. Proc Natl Acad Sci USA 1989;86:9499–9503.
99. Neupogen (filgrastim) prescribing information. Amgen, Inc. Thousand Oaks, Calif., Issued December 20, 2004.
100. Neulasta (pegfilgrastim) prescribing information Amgen, Inc. Thousand Oaks, Calif., Issued December 20, 2004.
101. Granocyte (lenograstim) patient information leaflet. Chugai Pharma UK Limited, Tokyo, Japan. Revision November 2001.
102. Liles WC, Rodger E, Dale DC. Combined administration of G-CSF and dexamethasone for the mobilization of granulocytes in normal donors: optimization of dosing. Transfusion 2000;40:643–644.
103. Lee J-H, Leitman SF, Klein HG. A controlled comparison of the efficacy of hetastarch and pentastarch in granulocyte collections by centrifugal leukapheresis. Blood 1995;86:4662–4666.
104. Burgstaler EA. Blood component collection by apheresis. D01-10.1002/jca.20043.
105. Robinson SP, Marks DI. Granulocyte transfusions in the G-CSF era. Where do we stand? Bone Marrow Transplant 2004;34:839–846.
106. Stanworth S, Massey E, Hyde C, et al. Granulocyte transfusions for treating infections in patients with neutropenia or neutrophil dysfunction. Cochrane Database Syst Rev 2005;D005339.
107. Jillella AP, Ustun C. What is the optimum number of C34+ peripheral blood stem cells for an autologous transplant? Stem Cells Dev 2004;13:597–606.
108. Singhal S, Powles R, Treleaven J, et al. A low CD34+ cell dose results in higher mortality and poorer survival after blood or marrow stem cell transplantation from HLA-identical siblings: should 2×10^6 CD34+ cells/kg be considered the minimum threshold? Bone Marrow Transplant 2000;26:489–496.
109. Feller N, van der Pol MA, Waaijman T, et al. Immunologic purging of autologous peripheral blood stem cell products based on CD34 and CD133 expression can be effectively and safely applied in half of the acute myeloid leukemia patients. Clin Cancer Res 2005;11:4793–4801.
110. Kawabata Y, Hirokawa M, Komatsuda A, Sawada K. Clinical applications of CD34+ cell-selected peripheral blood stem cells. Ther Apher Dial 2003;7:298–304.
111. Ziegler BL, Kanz L. Expansion of stem and progenitor cells. Curr Opin Hematol 1998;5:434–440.
112. Heal JM, Liesveld JL, Phillips GL, Blumberg N. What would Karl Landsteiner do? The ABO blood group and stem cell transplantation. Bone Marrow Transplant 2005;36:747–755.
113. FDA Memorandum: Revision of FDA Memorandum of August 27, 1982: Requirements for Infrequent Plasmapheresis Donors. Bethesda, Md., Food and Drug Administration, 1995.
114. Boynton MH, Taylor ES. Complications arising in donors in a mass blood procurement project. Am J Med Sci 1945;209:421–436.
115. Fainting in blood donors. A report to the Medical Research Council prepared by a subcommittee of the Blood Transfusion Research Committee. BMJ 1944;1:279–283.
116. Tomasulo PA, Anderson AJ, Paluso MB, et al. A study of criteria for blood donor deferral. Transfusion 1980;20:511–518.
117. Kasprisin DO, Glynn SH, Taylor F, et al. Moderate and severe reactions in blood donors. Transfusion 1992;32:23–26.
118. Khan W, Newman B. Comparison of donor reaction rates in high-school, college, and general blood drives [abstract]. Transfusion 1999;39(Suppl):31S.
119. Trouern-Trend J, Cable R, Badon S, et al. Vasovagal reaction in blood donors: Influence of gender, age, donation status, weight, blood pressure, and pulse. A case-controlled multicenter study. Transfusion 1999;39:316–320.
120. Poles FC, Boycott M. Syncope in blood donors. Lancet 1942;2:531–535.
121. Maloney WC, Lonnergan LR, McClintock JK, et al. Syncope in blood donors. NEJM 1946;234:114–118.
122. Brown H, McCormack P. An analysis of vasomotor phenomena (faints) occurring in blood donors. BMJ 1942;1:1–5.
123. McHenry LC, Fazekas JF, Sullivan JF. Cerebral hemodynamics of syncope. Am J Med Sci 1961;241:173.
124. Williams GE. Syncopal reactions in blood donors. BMJ 1942;1:783–786.
125. Newman B. Donor reactions and injuries from whole blood donations. Transfus Med Rev 1997;11:64–75.
126. Williams GE. Syncopal reactions in blood donors. BMJ 1942;1:783–786.
127. Ogata H, Iinuma N, Nagashima K, et al. Vasovagal reactions in blood donors. Transfusion 1980;20:679–683.
128. Engel GL. Psychologic stress, vasodepressor (vasovagal) syncope, and sudden death. Ann Intern Med 1978;89:403–412.
129. Tizes R. Cardiac arrest following routine venipuncture. JAMA 1976;236:1846–1847.
130. Yoda M, Nonoyama M, Shimakura T. Autologous blood donation before elective off-pump coronary artery bypass grafting. Surgery Today 2004;34:21–23.
131. Galena HJ. Complications occurring from diagnostic venipuncture. J Fam Pract 1992;34:582–584.
132. Howanitz PJ, Cembrowski GS, Bachner P. Laboratory phlebotomy. College of American Pathology Q-probe study of patient satisfaction and complication in 23,783 patients. Arch Pathol Lab Med 1991;115: 867–872.
133. Newman B. Arterial punctures in whole blood donors. Transfusion 2001;41:1390–1392.
134. Kumar S, Agnihotri SK, Khanna SK. Brachial artery pseudoaneurysm following blood donation. Transfusion 1995;35:791.
135. Lung J, Wilson S. Development of arteriovenous fistula following blood donation. Transfusion 1971;11:145–146.
136. Gibble J, Ness P, Anderson G, Conry-Cantilena C. Compartment syndrome and hand amputation after whole blood phlebotomy: report of a case [abstract]. Transfusion 1999;39(Suppl):30S.
137. Newman BH, Waxman DA. Blood donation-related neurologic needle injury: evaluation of 2 years' worth of data from a large blood center. Transfusion 1996;36:213–215.
138. Berry PR, Wallis WE. Venipuncture nerve injuries. Lancet 1977;1: 1236–1237.
139. McLeod BC, Price TH, Owen H, et al. Frequency of immediate adverse effects associated with apheresis donation. Transfusion 1998; 38:938–943.
140. Despotis GJ, Goodnough LT, Dynis M, et al. Adverse events in platelet apheresis donors: a multivariate analysis in a hospital-based program. Vox Sang 1999;77:24–32.
141. Katz AJ, Genco PV, Blumberg N, et al. Platelet collection and transfusion using the Fenwal CS-3000 cell separator. Transfusion 1981;21:560–563.
142. Simon TL, Sierra ER, Ferdinando B, et al. Collection of platelets with a new cell separator and their storage in a citrate-plasticized container. Transfusion 1991;31:335–339.
143. Lazarus EF, Browning J, Norman J, et al. Sustained decreases in platelet count associated with multiple, regular plateletpheresis donations. Transfusion 2001;41:756–761.
144. McCullough J. Introduction to apheresis donations including history and general principles. In McLeod BC, Price TH, Drew MJ (eds). Apheresis: Principles and Practice. Bethesda, Md., American Association of Blood Banks, 1997, p 40.
145. Leitman SF, Oblitas JM. Optimization of granulocytapheresis mobilization regimens using granulocyte colony stimulating factor (G-CSF) and dexamethasone [abstract]. Transfusion 197;37(Suppl):67S.
146. Price TH, Bowden RA, Boeckh M, et al. Phase I/II trial of neutrophil transfusions from donors stimulated with G-CSF and dexamethasone for treatment of patients with infections in hematopoietic stem cell transplantation. Blood 2000;95:3302–3309.
147. Occupational Safety and Health Administration. Occupational exposure to bloodborne pathogens: needlesticks and other sharps injuries: Final rule. Fed Register 2001;66:5317–5325.
148. Page PL. Risk of hepatitis B exposure in regional blood services. Transfusion 1987;27:242–244.
149. From California Blood Bank Society. Available at http://www.cbbsweb.org/enf/2001/gloves.html, last modified November 27, 2001 and http://www.cbbsweb.org/enf/2005/gloves2.html, last modified August1, 2005.
150. Code of Federal Regulations. 29 CFR 1910.1030. Washington, D.C., U.S. Government Printing Office, July 1, 2003.
151. Grindon AJ, Keelan LT, Lenes BA. HIV post-exposure prophylaxis for blood center healthcare workers [abstract]. Transfusion 1998;38(Suppl):109S.
152. Updated U.S. Public Health Service guidelines for the management of occupational exposure to HIV and recommendations for postexposure prophylaxis. MMWR 2005;54(RR09):1–17.

153. Updated U.S. Public Health Service guidelines for the management of occupational exposures to HBV, HCV, and HIV and recommendations for postexposure prophylaxis. MMWR 2001;50(RR11):1–52.
154. Reason J. Human error: Models and management. BMJ 2000;320: 768–770.
155. Reason J. Beyond the organisational accident: The need for "error wisdom" on the frontline. Qual Saf Health Care 2004;13:28–33.
156. U.S. Food and Drung Administation, FDA 21 CFR 610, 46 and 47 Medicare and Medicaid programs: hospital standard for potentially HIV infectious blood and blood products. Washington, D.C., Government Printing Office, September 9, 1996, revised April 1, 2005.
157. U.S. Department of Health and Human Services, U.S. Food and Drug Administration, Center for Biologics Evaluation and Research Guidance for Industry. Current good manufacturing practice for blood and blood components: (1) Quarantine and disposition of units from prior collections from donors with repeatedly reactive screening tests for antibody to Hepatitis C Virus (anti-HCV);(2) Supplemental testing, and the notification of consignees and blood recipients of donor test results for anti-HCV. Federal Register Docket No. 98D-0143. Washington, D.C., Government Printing Office, September 23, 1998.
158. Nordenberg T. Recalls: FDA, industry cooperate to protect consumers. FDA Consumer Magazine 1995;29:24–27.
159. U.S. Food and Drug Administration, Center for Food Safety and Applied Nutrition. FDA recall policies. Industry Affairs Staff Brochure, June 2002. Avaiable at http://www.cfsan.fda.gov/~Ird/recall2.html. Accessed June 4, 2006.
160. U.S. Department of Health and Human Services. U.S. Food and Drug Administration. Final Rule: Reporting of Biological Product Deviations in Manufacturing. Federal Register Docket No. 97N-0242. Washington D.C. Government Printing Office, November 7, 2000.
161. U.S. Food and Drug Administation, Center for Biologics and Research. Biological Product Devitation Reports—Annual Summary for Fiscal Year 2004. Avilable at http://www.fda.gov/cber/biodev/bpdrfy04.htm. Last modified April 28, 2005.

Chapter 12

Blood Manufacturing: Component Preparation, Storage, and Transportation

Shealynn B. Harris • Christopher D. Hillyer

Modern transfusion medicine in highly developed nations is based on the use of components, including cellular and plasma components, prepared or manufactured from whole blood collected from a volunteer donor. This is often called *component therapy* and offers both therapeutic and economic advantages, including the provision of concentrated products for specific and targeted transfusion management and the cost-effective and efficient use of this valuable and often limited resource. Along with the benefits of component therapy, however, there are also challenges posed by the complex manufacturing process required for component production.

In this chapter, the essentials of the blood manufacturing process will be discussed, with an emphasis placed on blood collection, component preparation, labeling, and storage. Although they are mentioned in this chapter, the areas of regulation, donor eligibility, quality control, infectious disease testing, and clinical use of components are addressed in greater detail in dedicated chapters elsewhere in this textbook.

BLOOD COLLECTION

Donor Preparation and Care

Essentially, the manufacturing of components can be thought of as beginning with the collection of blood from an eligible volunteer donor by whole blood phlebotomy or automated apheresis. Indeed, the process of blood collection is regulated under the CFR and is subject to AABB Standards. Accordingly, establishments that collect blood for transfusion or "for further manufacture" need to have adequate and appropriate standard operating procedures (SOPs), training, and equipment validation for donor collection. An effective donor selection, preparation, and collection process serves several purposes: it ensures the quality of the final products and components; it minimizes risks to both the donor and transfusion recipient; and it enhances donor satisfaction, which increases the likelihood of repeat donations.

Prior to collection, all allogeneic blood donors must be accurately identified, provide informed consent, and be evaluated for general suitability requirements, which include criteria for age, weight, donation interval, medical and pregnancy history, infectious diseases and related risk behavior, hemoglobin level, temperature, pulse, and blood pressure. If a donor is accepted for collection, the donor's identity must be effectively linked to all resulting components and test samples by a unique alphanumeric identifier.

Skin Antisepsis

Bacterial contamination of blood products is a leading cause of transfusion-related morbidity and mortality.[1] Because the donor is most often the source of bacterial contamination, either through bacteremia or skin flora, methods to reduce the risk of contamination begin with proper donor screening, arm inspection, and skin antisepsis.[2] For all types of collection procedures, donor preparation starts with the inspection of both arms for signs of intravenous drug use or skin lesions that pose an infectious disease risk.[3] This is followed by the appropriate application of one of the FDA approved skin disinfection methods for blood collection.[4] Most methods specify use of an iodine disinfectant, either povidone iodine or tincture of iodine. Because iodine can result in skin reactions in sensitive individuals, the FDA-approved 2% chlorhexidine gluconate in 70% isopropyl alcohol method is recommended by the AABB for iodine-allergic donors.[5] The use of green soap and 70% isopropyl alcohol for iodine-allergic donors is no longer recommended by the AABB, based on data that show significantly more residual skin flora after cleaning as compared to the other currently approved skin antisepsis methods listed previously.[6]

Donor Care and Complications

Care of the donor is essential to a safe and effective donation process. Because the collection staff serve as the primary interface between donors and the blood community, it is imperative that staff act in a courteous, professional manner to help promote donor satisfaction and repeat donations. In addition, to ensure donor safety, collection staff must also be aware of potential donor reactions and must be trained in collection facility procedures for reaction management.

Venipuncture, intravascular volume shifts, and apheresis-specific citrate use present risks for donation complications.[7,8] For apheresis donation, the overall frequency of complications is approximately 2%, with the majority related to mild hypocalcemia from the citrate anticoagulant.[9] In contrast, for whole blood donation, the overall frequency of complications is at least 10 times greater (20% to 40%), with bruising, arm discomfort, fatigue, vasovagal events, and nerve irritation, listed in order of decreasing frequency, as the complications most often reported.[7]

In general, for the common complications just listed, donors typically do not require significant medical intervention and readily recover without lasting sequelae. However, for donors with phlebotomy-related cutaneous nerve irritation or injury (incidence, 0.02%–0.9%), a study by Newman and Waxman[10] showed that approximately 30% will experience symptoms, typically mild numbness, lasting 1 month or longer, and the majority of these donors will request a physician consultation. In the same study, approximately 25% of nerve injury cases were associated with a hematoma, indicating improper phlebotomy technique as a contributing factor. However, in another report by Newman,[11] approximately 40% of nerve injuries occurred after an uncomplicated phlebotomy, which suggests that phlebotomy-related nerve injury may not be completely preventable. Furthermore, an anatomical study by Horowitz[12] of the cutaneous nerve-superficial vein relationships at common venipuncture sites suggests that cutaneous nerves often overlie superficial veins, which increases the likelihood for mild nerve injury, even with proper phlebotomy technique.

Rarely, phlebotomy-related nerve injury is more severe, resulting in a chronic, disabling neuropathic pain syndrome, Complex Regional Pain Syndrome Type 2 (CRPS-II), which is characterized by shooting, burning, or electrical pain often associated with motor dysfunction.[13] In contrast to donors with mild nerve injury, 80% of donors with CRPS-II report traumatic phlebotomy with multiple attempts or hematoma formation.[13]

Although the vast majority of donor complications do not require emergency intervention or hospitalization, very serious events, defined by the need for hospitalization, do occur and are more likely with apheresis donation (1 in 20,000)[14] than with whole blood donation (1 in 200,000).[15] Because serious adverse events can take place during or immediately after donation, a plan for managing these events must be in place at the collection facility. Collection staff should be familiar with signs and symptoms of donation complications and should closely monitor donors throughout the donation process.[16]

As complications can occur or be noted after the donor leaves the collection facility, donors should be provided with postphlebotomy information,[17] which includes care of the venipuncture site, limits on strenuous physical activity, discussion of the need for increased fluid consumption, and contact instructions in the event of an adverse reaction.

Donor Test Samples

Current standards require that donors be tested for multiple infectious disease markers, ABO and Rh type, and if previously transfused or pregnant, red cell alloantibodies.[18] These testing requirements necessitate the collection of several vacuum tubes of blood from the donor. To eliminate the need for a second donor venipuncture, most collection and storage kits include a convenient method for donor sampling, either a diversion pouch or an in-line sampling system. Once test samples are obtained, the tubes must be properly labeled with the donor identifier to ensure effective traceability and proper result reporting.

Collection and Storage Kits

In addition to donor-derived bacteria, environmental pathogens, such as *Serratia marcecsens*, encountered during blood manufacturing and transport serve as a potential contamination source.[2,19] A closed manufacturing system helps to ensure that all surfaces in direct contact with the blood remain sterile and pyrogen free throughout blood manufacturing and storage. Closed collection, processing, and storage kits (also known as *disposables*) have been developed as an effective means of preventing the introduction of environmental pathogens.

Whole blood collection and storage kits incorporate, at a minimum, a 16-gauge phlebotomy needle, tubing, and a primary collection bag with an anticoagulant-preservative solution. For routine donations, a collection kit that contains a 450-mL or 500-mL primary bag is used to accommodate the standard whole blood collection. In addition, 250-mL and 450-mL bags can be used for special collections, such as autologous donations and low-volume units. In the United States, 250-mL collection kits are not licensed for volunteer or directed donation and must be reserved for autologous donors. Depending on the kit manufacturer and processing requirements, the integrated system may include one or more of the following: a diversion pouch, satellite bags for component preparation (i.e., double, triple, or quad packs), a bag with additive solution for red blood cell (RBC) storage, and an in-line leukoreduction filter.

Some collection kit accessories are provided separately and can be attached to the primary collection kit through a sterile connection device (SCD), which applies a sterile weld between two pieces of compatible tubing. To effectively maintain the integrity of the closed system, SCDs must be used as recommended, and the sterile weld must be checked for defects. If there is a defective connection, the system is considered open, and the product expiration is affected.[20] Guidelines for the proper use of SCDs are provided by the FDA in a guidance document.[21]

Manufacturers of apheresis equipment supply customized apheresis collection and storage kits that meet the unique specifications of each apheresis instrument and type of component collection. In general, apheresis disposables incorporate a specialized, integrated system of tubing and bags that allows for closed, sterile collection. Similar to whole blood collection kits, the type of blood bags in an apheresis kit depends on the type of component collected and the component's storage requirements.

Diversion Pouches

Diversion pouches have been recently introduced as a means to help further reduce bacterial contamination from donor skin flora. Even with proper skin antisepsis during donor preparation, residual deep-seated bacteria can be introduced into the collected blood through coring of the skin during venipuncture.[22] Several studies have shown that the collection of the initial volume of blood into an in-line diversion pouch can provide an additional safeguard against skin flora contamination. By using an in vitro model with the common skin contaminant *Staphylococcus aureus*, Wagner and colleagues[23] demonstrated that the diversion of the first 21 mL to 42 mL of blood flow results in a 95% to 98% reduction of bacteria in the final collection volume. Another study by de Korte and associated[24] showed a significant overall decrease in *Staphylococcus* species in whole blood collections (0.14% to 0.03%, $p = 0.015$) with the use of a 10-mL diversion system. Several manufacturers offer an FDA-approved, in-line diversion pouch as part of a blood collection kit. In addition to reducing bacterial contamination, these pouches have been designed to accommodate sufficient volume for donor sampling for required and standard infectious disease and serological testing.

Blood Bag Plastics: Polymers and Plasticizers

All blood collection and storage systems are made of disposable plastic. There are many types of plastics available; however, only a few plastic materials meet the specifications for blood processing and storage. The fundamental structure of a plastic is the polymer, which is a repeatedly linked chain of a simple base chemical called a *monomer*.[25] To be functional, polymers require additives, such as plasticizers, to increase flexibility and stability. In general, the unique properties of each type of plastic are determined by the monomer, chain length, and additives.

Plastic materials for blood bags must have particular qualities. These qualities include, depending on the bag's intended use, adequate flexibility and strength to withstand centrifugation and handling; temperature resistance for both steam sterilization and freezing; limited toxicity to the transfusion recipient; compatibility with cells and plasma to reduce component adulteration; selective permeability for cellular gas exchange; water and pathogen impermeability; and transparency for effective product visualization.[25] Of all available polymers, polyvinylchloride (PVC) has been shown to be the most compatible with component manufacturing. During the past 50 years, most innovations in blood bag materials have focused on improvements in PVC with the incorporation of different plasticizers. The two most common plasticizers in current use for PVC blood bags are di-2-ethylhexylphthalate (DEHP) and tri-2-ethylhexyl trimellitate (TEHTM).[25] In addition to increasing PVC flexibility, plasticizers act to improve gas exchange across the bag barrier and help to stabilize the RBC membrane during storage.

Effective gas exchange is especially important for maintaining platelet viability during storage. Platelets are particularly sensitive to an acidic environment, with major shape changes and cell death occurring at a pH less than 6.0.[26] In a gas-impermeable container, the high metabolic rate of room-temperature platelets causes the pH to drop rapidly as lactic acid accumulates with oxygen consumption and compensatory anaerobic metabolism.[27] To meet the need for enhanced platelet viability and longer storage, platelet storage bags in current use ("second-generation bags") are made with selectively permeable plastics, thinner walls, and increased surface area for better gas exchange.[28–31] In addition to PVC-based bags, a polyolefin-based bag has been shown to effectively maintain platelet viability and is approved by the FDA for platelet storage.[28]

For RBCs, in addition to the benefit of improved gas exchange, plastic containers also appear to improve RBC stability during storage. This property was initially suggested by early work that showed significantly reduced hemolysis and osmotic fragility of blood stored in plastic bags compared to blood stored in glass containers.[32] It was later shown that RBCs stored in the presence of the plasticizer DEHP have improved in vitro survival,[33] decreased microvesicle formation,[34] and better post-transfusion survival[35] compared to RBCs stored in the absence of DEHP. Additional studies have shown that DEHP, a highly lipophilic compound, leaches out of PVC-DEHP containers and into the RBC membrane during storage,[36,37] thus stabilizing the RBC membrane and prolonging RBC survival. Given the superior quality of RBCs stored in DEHP and the lack of a commercially available alternative, PVC-DEHP is currently the only plastic used for RBC storage.[25]

The use of DEHP is not without concern, and the relative safety of PVC-DEHP has been questioned for the past 20 years.[38] Early work by Jacobson and colleagues,[39] using a rhesus monkey chronic platelet transfusion model, suggested that the chronic transfusion of DEHP-stored platelets is associated with an increased rate of hepatic dysfunction and liver histopathology compared to chronic transfusion with non–DEHP-stored platelets. A postmortem study by Hillman and coworkers[40] also showed accumulation of DEHP in the tissues of critically ill human neonates who had received blood products. Further studies of DEHP toxicity in rodents have suggested the potential for developmental and reproductive effects in humans, although human toxicity has not been conclusively proven.[41] The National Toxicology Program's Center for Risks to Human Reproduction provides a recent extensive review of DEHP toxicity studies and suggests the need for additional evidence to conclusively prove DEHP's toxic effects.[41] As stated in the report, the primary concern is the effect of DEHP in neonates and children who are chronically transfused or undergo blood volume exchange and are exposed to a high cumulative dose of DEHP. For example, with a single-procedure double-volume exchange in a neonate, the dose of DEHP is approximately 1800 μg/kg bw/day; and for a neonate treated with replacement transfusions, the average dose is 300 μg/kg bw/day. For comparison, the current maximum allowable occupational inhalational exposure to DEHP in an adult is 700 μg/kg bw/day. At this time, the potential toxicity of DEHP is still unclear, and currently, DEHP remains the most common plasticizer used for blood bags.

Anticoagulant and Preservative Solutions

Under storage conditions, RBCs show predictable, time-dependent adverse changes, which together are known as the *red cell storage lesion* (Table 12–1). Key consequences of the storage lesion are a reduction in post-transfusion RBC survival and impairment of oxygen transport, which are effects that lead to an overall decrease in transfusion efficacy.[42] Although the cellular and molecular events that lead to the storage lesion have not been completely elucidated, certain principles are known. RBCs are anucleate, and thus, they lack the synthetic machinery to renew structural proteins and enzymes. Without replacement of structural proteins and enzymes to maintain the RBC membrane and metabolic machinery, RBCs undergo senescence during storage. RBCs are also devoid of mitochondria, the organelle required for oxidative phosphorylation. To produce ATP for cellular energy, RBCs rely on anaerobic metabolism (the Embden-Meyerhof pathway), which requires a continuous supply of glucose and adenine and produces large quantities of lactic acid and hydrogen ions.[43] With acid accumulation and decreasing pH, enzymes and structural proteins undergo changes that compromise cell metabolism and stability.

In addition to these structural and metabolic changes, RBC function is affected with storage. To effectively deliver oxygen, RBCs require sufficient levels of 2,3-diphosphoglycerate (2,3-DPG). By competing with oxygen for hemoglobin binding sites, 2,3-DPG acts to displace oxygen from hemoglobin, thus making the oxygen more readily available for tissue uptake. During storage, the concentration of 2,3-DPG in RBCs declines. With low levels of 2,3-DPG, hemoglobin binds oxygen more avidly, and the oxygen delivery function of the stored RBCs is reduced. Within approximately 3 weeks of storage, RBC 2,3-DPG concentration falls to below 10%.[44] This effect is reversed after transfusion, however, because the transfused RBCs replenish 2,3-DPG within 24 to 48 hours in circulation.[45,46]

Two important methods for RBC preservation are refrigeration and the use of supplemental anticoagulant-preservative solutions. With refrigeration (1°C–6°C), the metabolic rate of RBCs is reduced significantly, and senescence is delayed.[47] However, to effectively extend red cell storage beyond 5 days, a preservative solution is necessary.[48] The efficacy of a preservative in maintaining stored red cells is

Table 12–1 Biochemical Changes of Stored Red Blood Cells (RBC Storage Lesion)

	CPD		CPDA-1				AS-1*	AS-3†	AS-5*
Variable	**Whole Blood**		**Whole Blood**	**Red Blood Cells**	**Whole Blood**	**Red Blood Cells**	**Red Blood Cells**	**Red Blood Cells**	**Red Blood Cells**
Days of storage	0	21	0	0	35	35	42	42	42
No. of viable cells (24 hours post-transfusion)	100	80	100	100	79	71	76(64–85)	84	80
pH (measured at 37°C)	7.20	6.84	7.60	7.55	6.98	6.71	6.6	6.5	6.5
ATP (% of initial value)	100	86	100	100	56(±16)	45(±12)	60	59	68.5
2,3-DPG (% of initial value)	100	44	100	100	<10	<10	<5	<10	<5
Plasma K^+ (mmol/L)	3.9	21	4.20	5.10	27.30	78.50‡	50	46	45.6
Plasma hemoglobin (mg/L)	17	191	82	78	461	658.0‡	N/A	386	N/A
% Hemolysis	N/A	N/A	N/A	N/A	N/A	N/A	0.5	0.9	0.6

*Based on information supplied by the manufacturer.
†Simon TL, Hunt WC, Garry PJ. Iron supplementation for menstruating female blood donors. Transfusion 1984;24:469–472.
‡Values for plasma hemoglobin and potassium concentrations may appear somewhat high in 35-day stored RBC units; the total plasma in these units is only about 70 mL. From American Association of Blood Banks. Technical Manual, 14th ed. Bethesda, MD, AABB, 2002.

determined by assessing the preservative-stored RBC viability post-transfusion. Specifically, in order to meet established regulations and standards, 75% of the stored RBCs must remain in circulation at 24 hours after transfusion,[42] as measured by an in vivo ^{51}Cr red cell radiolabeling and transfusion method.[49]

The common anticoagulant-preservative solutions used in transfusion practice are acid citrate dextrose (ACD-A), citrate phosphate dextrose (CPD and CP2D), and citrate phosphate dextrose adenine CPDA-1. RBCs suspended in these solutions are stored at a hematocrit (Hct) between 70% and 80%. As seen in Table 12–2, anticoagulant-preservative solutions vary in content and the approved length of RBC storage, with the RBC storage limit for CPD and CP2D at 21 days and CPDA-1 at 35 days. Additive solutions (AS-1, AS-3, AS-5), discussed in the following section, are approved for RBC storage up to 42 days.

Each component of the preservative solution has a specific metabolic support function. Dextrose and adenine serve as substrates for ATP production, and phosphate acts as a pH buffer and substrate for 2,3-DPG formation. For a whole blood collection kit, the volume of the anticoagulant-preservative solution is specific for the collection volume. For a 450-mL primary collection bag, the anticoagulant-preservative solution is 63 mL, and for a 500-mL primary collection bag, the solution volume is 70 mL. If the whole blood collection is less than 300 mL, the volume of anticoagulant-preservative solution must be adjusted to maintain an approximate anticoagulant-to-blood ratio of 1.4:10.

To extend the expiration time to 42 days, RBCs are suspended in an additive solution (100 mL) that is transferred to the primary bag after the plasma is expressed from the whole blood collection. Additive solutions decrease in vitro hemolysis by stabilizing the RBC membrane, either through the action of mannitol or citrate.[42] With an approximate hematocrit of 60% for additive-stored RBCs, these solutions also act to enhance transfusion flow and reduce product administration time by decreasing the viscosity of packed RBCs. Listed in Table 12–3, the currently approved additive solutions include the saline-adenine-glucose-mannitol (SAGM) formulations, AS-1 (Adsol) and AS-5 (Optisol), and a non–mannitol-based solution, AS-3 (Nutricel). AS-1 and AS-5 can be coupled with any of the anticoagulant-preservative solutions in a whole blood collection system; however, AS-3 requires supplemental glucose and must be paired with CP2D for a whole blood collection kit.[43]

Current efforts to develop media that prolong RBC storage beyond 6 weeks have led to a new generation of experimental additive solutions (EASs) that are under investigation.[50-52] Although most EASs increase storage to between 7 and 10 weeks, reports by Meryman and associates[53] and Hess and associates[54] provide evidence for effective liquid RBC storage

Table 12–2 Content of Anticoagulant-Preservative Solutions (g/L)

Component	ACD-A	CPD	CP2D	CPDA-1
Trisodium citrate	22.00	26.30	26.30	26.30
Citric acid	8.00	3.27	3.27	3.27
Dextrose	24.50	25.50	51.10	31.90
Monobasic sodium phosphate		2.22	2.22	2.22
Adenine				0.275

ACD, acid citrate dextrose; CPD, citrate phosphate dextrose; CPDA-1, citrate phosphate dextrose adenine.

Table 12–3 **Content of Additive Solutions (mM)**

Component	AS-1 (Optisol)	AS-3 (Nutricel)	AS-5 (Adsol)
Dextrose	111.00	55.50	45.50
Adenine	2.00	2.22	2.22
Monobasic sodium phosphate	0.00	23.00	0.00
Mannitol	41.20	0.00	45.40
Sodium chloride	154.00	70.00	150.00

for up to 12 weeks. The potential benefits of prolonged storage with EASs include reduction of allogeneic RBC outdate rates; decreased donor exposure for premature infants who require repeat, small-volume maintenance transfusions; and an increased collection window for autologous donors. The primary limitation of these new solutions is the inability to adequately preserve 2,3-DPG levels. Because most RBC transfusions are given between 12 and 21 days of storage, the value of extended RBC storage for routine transfusion practice is debatable; however, extended storage may be of benefit in rural outposts and military settings.[54]

As previously mentioned, although 2,3-DPG levels replenish within 48 hours of transfusion, stored RBCs older than 2 weeks have reduced oxygen transport function immediately after transfusion. This property of "older" RBCs may have implications for effective resuscitation of certain patients with more urgent or greater oxygen delivery needs, such as those in cardiac surgery, trauma, massive transfusion, and critical care settings.[55-59] Thus, research efforts for improving additive solutions continue to focus on methods for improving 2,3-DPG preservation. A recent report by Högman and colleagues[60] provides promising data for a modified EAS, Erythro-Sol 2, which maintains RBC 2,3-DPG levels at a normal level over a 2-week storage period. Another study by Kurup and coworkers[61] compared the RBC storage properties of SAGM and a modified SAGM solution. Although the SAGM showed a 99% decrease in 2,3-DPG levels by day 28, the modified SAGM maintained day 28 RBC 2,3-DPG levels near baseline, with an overall decrease of less than 1%. Although EASs have received approval in Europe,[62] an extended storage solution is not currently approved in the United States.

Whole Blood Collection

Donor Requirements

In addition to enhancing transfusion recipient safety, some of the donor eligibility requirements for allogeneic and directed whole blood donation are established for the purpose of enhancing donor safety and include limits for donor volume deficit, weight, hemoglobin, and donation frequency. Studies of controlled blood loss in normal, healthy adult volunteers indicate that up to 15% of a donor's blood volume (BV) can be safely removed without significant physiologic signs or symptoms.[63,64] Thus, the maximum allowable intravascular volume deficit for a single donation is 10.5 mL/kg (15% BV), which includes the volume for test samples and in residual tubing.[65] In the United States, the standard volume for a whole blood donation is 450 mL to 500 mL ± 10%. With test samples, the entire collected blood volume for a typical donation is approximately 525 mL. Therefore, the standard minimum donor weight for routine whole blood donation is 50 kg or 110 lb (10.5 mL/kg × 50 kg = 525 mL). To prevent overcollection, a practical method for monitoring volume during donation is to weigh the whole blood unit. For a normal donor hematocrit, the specific gravity of whole blood is 1.053,[66] so a commonly used conversion factor to calculate the collected volume (mL) from the unit weight (g) is 1.06 g/mL.

Another physiologic consequence of blood donation is the temporary reduction of donor RBC mass. Because most of the body's iron is carried in RBCs, loss of RBC mass after repeated donations can lead to anemia, especially in premenopausal females.[67] To reduce the risk of anemia, an allogeneic donor is required to have a hemoglobin level of greater than or equal to 12.5 g/dL (Hct 38%) and is limited to donating once every 8 weeks, unless examined and cleared by a physician to donate more frequently, which in practice occurs only in unusual situations with directed donors.

Donors with Hereditary Hemochromatosis

Whole blood collected for the purpose of therapeutic phlebotomy must be labeled with the donor's disease if the blood is used for transfusion.[68] Although therapeutic collections from otherwise healthy individuals with hereditary hemochromatosis are considered safe for allogeneic transfusion, these units are often rejected by hospital transfusion services due to the required disease label.[69] Recently, however, the FDA introduced the option for a variance that allows collection facilities to exclude the disease designation from whole blood units obtained by therapeutic phlebotomy from individuals with hereditary hemochromatosis.[70] Under the variance, the donor must meet the standard allogeneic donor suitability requirements, and the collection facility must not charge a fee for the collection. In addition, to collect from a donor more frequently than every 8 weeks, a physician prescription for therapeutic phlebotomy or a physical exam and physician's certification of good health is required.

Collection Procedure

Phlebotomy is performed using the integral donor needle supplied with the sterile collection and storage kit. Immediately prior to phlebotomy, a tourniquet or blood pressure cuff is applied and is kept in position throughout collection. To limit trauma to subcutaneous tissue, a single venipuncture is performed, and the needle is secured to prevent movement or displacement. If signs of an arterial puncture are present, such as rapid filling of the blood bag (<4 minutes) and bright red, pulsating blood flow, the procedure should be immediately discontinued, the needle removed, and extended pressure applied.[7]

Because the internal surface of the collection tubing is not filled with an anticoagulant, adequate blood flow must be maintained to prevent coagulation factor activation and clotting prior to the blood entering the primary collection bag. As the blood enters the primary container, it should be mixed frequently with the anticoagulant to avoid clot formation. With sufficient flow, the duration of a whole blood collection is approximately 10 minutes. The effect of donation time on whole blood–derived plasma and platelets does not appear to be significant until the donation exceeds 15 minutes.[71,72] For whole blood collections that exceed 15 minutes, data suggest increased thrombin generation in the plasma and decreased platelet counts in the platelet concentrates. Although there is no FDA regulation for maximum collection time, based on these data, it is recommended that whole blood collections that exceed 15 minutes be restricted to red cell production and not be used for platelet concentrates or plasma components for transfusion.[73]

Automated Apheresis Collection

Apheresis is the process by which a desired component of whole blood is separated and collected, and the unselected constituents of whole blood are returned to the donor. The types of blood components collected by apheresis of volunteer donors include plasma (plasmapheresis), platelets (plateletpheresis), RBCs (erythrocytapheresis), and leukocytes (leukapheresis). Although manual apheresis methods are available, automated apheresis is more convenient and provides better product safety and quality. Hence, manual apheresis is not routinely employed for component collection.

Donation Requirements

In addition to meeting the standard eligibility requirements for allogeneic blood donation, routine apheresis donors must also meet criteria specific for the type of apheresis procedure and frequency of donation. For all apheresis collections, a donor is not eligible if a whole blood donation or equivalent apheresis RBC loss (>200 mL) occurred within the previous 8 weeks, unless the extracorporeal RBC volume during the current apheresis procedure is less than 100 mL.[74–76] If the RBC loss for a single procedure is greater than 300 mL, the donor is deferred for 16 weeks.[76] The collection facility must monitor total annual donor RBC loss from all apheresis and whole blood donations to ensure that the RBC volume does not exceed that allowed for cumulative yearly whole blood donation.[77] Regardless of standard requirements, when a specific component is deemed to be of particular value to a specific recipient (e.g., human leukocyte antigen [HLA]-matched platelets), an otherwise ineligible donor may donate if approved by the medical director.[78]

For automated plasmapheresis, in addition to the routine donor test samples, the FDA requires the collection of a blood sample on the day of the first physical exam for donation or on the day of the first plasmapheresis procedure.[79] Tests on the sample include a total protein quantification and plasma or serum immunoglobulin composition (e.g., serum protein electrophoresis). Additional donor qualifications are defined by donation interval. "Infrequent" plasmapheresis is performed every 4 weeks or less frequently, and "frequent" plasmapheresis is performed at an interval of 4 weeks, or more frequently.[75] For frequent donors, a serum or plasma protein study is required prior to each donation, and the cumulative results must be evaluated by a qualified, licensed physician within 21 days of the sample draw to determine donor acceptability for subsequent plasmapheresis collections. If the total protein level is less than 6 g/dL or the immunoglobulin composition is abnormal, the donor is ineligible until the values normalize. Frequent donors can donate a maximum of 2 times in a week, as long as the collections occur at least 2 days apart. The FDA-approved volume limits for a single, automated plasma collection are specific for each apheresis instrument and provided by the instrument manufacturer.[80] The annual limits for maximum donated plasma volume are 12 liters (110 to 175 lb) and 14.4 liters (>175 lb).[75]

For plateletpheresis, a platelet count is not required for the first collection and is only required for subsequent collections if the donation interval is more frequent than every 4 weeks.[81] If the platelet count drops below 150,000/μL, the donor usually is temporarily deferred until the count rises above 150,000/μL. Regardless of platelet count, a donor who has ingested aspirin or aspirin-containing medications within 36 hours prior to collection is ineligible for plateletpheresis donation, because aspirin irreversibly inhibits platelet function. The frequency limits for plateletpheresis are two collections in a 7-day period with at least a 48-hour interval between collections, and a maximum of 24 collections performed in a year.[74] The total volume limits (excluding anticoagulant) for a single, automated plateletpheresis collection are 500 mL (110 to 175 lb) and 600 mL (>175 lb). As with automated plasma collection, the annual volume limits for automated plateletpheresis are 12 liters (110 to175 lb) and 14.4 liters (>175 lb).

At the time of this writing, the FDA has posted a draft guidance document for automated platelet collection, and if accepted for implementation, it will replace previous guidelines.[82] Proposed changes to the previous guidelines include additional eligibility criteria for platelet-inhibiting medications, such as Clopidogrel, Ticlopidine, and NSAIDs, and an extension of the aspirin deferral from 3 days to 5 days post-ingestion. In addition, because modern apheresis instruments are capable of more than one platelet collection, new recommendations for double and triple platelet donors have been proposed.

Automated RBC apheresis donor requirements, including height, weight, and hemoglobin/hematocrit, are defined for each FDA-approved instrument and provided by the manufacturer. In addition to instrument-specific criteria, there are general donor suitability requirements for automated RBC collections.[76] For single apheresis collections (RBC volume of 200 mL to 300 mL), the requirements are similar to whole blood donation (e.g., limited to 8-week intervals). However, the criteria for double RBC collections (RBC volume > 300 mL) are somewhat different. A donor hemoglobin or hematocrit level is required prior to each donation, as measured by a quantitative method and not by the copper sulfate (CuSO4) method. This preprocedure value, along with the donor's height, weight, and gender, is used to determine a predicted postprocedure hemoglobin or hematocrit for donor eligibility.[76] If a drop in hemoglobin of <10g/dL or in hematocrit of <30% is predicted, the donor should not be considered for a double RBC collection. Instrument manufacturers provide device-specific nomograms and formulae to assist collection facilities with this determination. If a double RBC collection is performed, the donor is deferred from whole blood or apheresis collection for 16 weeks.

Several apheresis devices are capable of collecting multiple concurrent components (see Table 12–4). For multicomponent collection, the donor must meet eligibility and donation frequency criteria for each collected component. In

Table 12–4 Components That Can Be Collected from Various Instruments

	Gran	Plt	cRBC	2-RBC	Plasma	cPlasma
Fenwal CS3000	×	×				×
Fenwal CS3000 +	×	×				×
Baxter Amicus		×	×			×
Fenwal Autopheresis C					×	
COBE Spectra	×	×				×
Gambro Trima V4		×	×	×		×
Gambro Trima Accel		×	×	×		×
Haemonetics LN9000	×	×				×
Haemonetics MCS + LN8150			×	×		×
Haemonetics PCS-2					×	
Baxter Alyx				×		
Fresenius AS104	×					

cPlasma, concurrent plasma; concurrent, more than one component can be collected; cRBC, concurrent 1 unit red blood cells; Gran, granulocytes; PH, plateletapheresis (single, double, triple); 2-RBC, double unit RBC; V4, software version 4.
From Burgstaler EA. Blood component collection by apheresis. J Clin Apher, May 6, 2005 [Epub ahead of print].

addition, the combined donor plasma and RBC losses must be determined and must not exceed the device-specific limits approved by the FDA.[83]

Granulocyte collection is a more involved process compared to other automated apheresis donations and necessitates special donor preparation. To obtain sufficient granulocyte dose ($>1.0 \times 10^{10}$), donors are treated with leukocyte mobilizing agents, such as corticosteroids and granulocyte colony-stimulating factor (G-CSF), prior to granulocyte collection (see Chapter 24).[84] Although there are limited data on the long-term effects of mobilization in healthy donors, several studies indicate that in the short-term there is minimal risk, even after repeat donations.[85–87] However, donors often experience side effects, such as headache, bone pain, myalgias, and arthralgias after mobilization, particularly with G-CSF administration. These symptoms are generally transient (<24 hours) and well tolerated by donors.[88] In addition to precollection leukocyte mobilization, an erythrocyte sedimenting agent, such as hydroxyethyl starch (HES), is added during granulocyte apheresis for more effective granulocyte–red cell separation. The addition of HES improves granulocyte yield and reduces donor RBC loss during the procedure.[89] For donors, the disadvantages of HES include the immediate side effects of intravascular volume expansion, such as headache and pulmonary edema, and the potential cumulative toxic side effects, such as severe pruritus and coagulopathy.[90] Because HES persists for weeks to years in circulation,[91,92] the additive volume of HES for a repeat donor must be routinely determined and monitored for cumulative toxic dose.[93] As part of the eligibility assessment for granulocyte donation, donors should be evaluated for medical conditions that may be exacerbated by HES and leukocyte-mobilizing drugs. In addition, donors should receive information about the potential side effects of these drugs as part of the informed consent process. As with other apheresis collections, the standard allogeneic donor eligibility criteria and infectious disease testing requirements apply to granulocyte collection, though the release of collected granulocytes to the transfusing facility often occurs before all test results have been obtained, as these cells lose viability quickly, within 8 to 24 hours of collection. In addition, the automated platelet collection frequency limits and cumulative RBC loss limits apply to granulocyte collection.

Collection Procedure

For automated apheresis, the donor is connected by intravenous access to a programmable device that draws, processes, collects, and returns blood to the donor all in a single donation session. To separate a component, most automated devices employ differential centrifugation, which separates by specific gravity. Instruments that collect by centrifugation are designed to process blood by continuous flow centrifugation (CFC), with an uninterrupted separation and return circuit, or by intermittent flow centrifugation (IFC), with alternating separation and return cycles. The process of cell separation during centrifugation isolates leukocytes for "process leukoreduction" during the apheresis collection. In addition, depending on the manufacturer, the apheresis disposable kit may include an in-line filter for leukoreduction. Leukoreduction can also be performed off-line with a sterile-docked leukoreduction filter. Automated apheresis instruments also differ in terms of required intravenous access (single- or double-arm) and collection capability (single- or multiple-component collection). See Table 12–4 for a summary of current available instruments and collection capabilities. Because each apheresis instrument has a unique design and function, a disposable collection kit that meets the specifications of an individual instrument and type of collection is required.

As with whole blood donation, the maximum extracorporeal blood volume allowed at any time during apheresis is 10.5 mL/kg. Most instruments are equipped with a control panel for the apheresis operator to input donor and collection data, calculate donor blood volume, and monitor fluids and flow rate during the procedure. To maintain relatively constant volume during apheresis, normal saline is often used both to prime the circuit and to balance fluid shifts. A citrate-based anticoagulant, such as ACD-A, is also added to prevent clotting and to maintain extracorporeal flow during apheresis. Citrate, which chelates calcium, can cause symptomatic hypocalcemia, which can result in seizures, hypotension, and fatal arrhythmias if left untreated.[8] In practice, these severe reactions are unusual, because early signs of hypocalcemia, such as perioral tingling, are monitored in donors. If signs and symptoms of hypocalcemia are noted, temporary cessation of the procedure and reduction of apheresis flow rate are usually effective.[8] If symptoms persist, oral calcium supplementation may be given, or with more severe symptoms, an intravenous calcium solution is administered.

Quality control criteria for apheresis component collections are established to ensure consistent and adequate product dose. For apheresis RBCs, the method employed should result in a mean hemoglobin of 60 g in the final product, and at least 95% of the units tested should have a hemoglobin of 50 g.[94] For leukoreduced, apheresis red cells, the procedure should result in a mean hemoglobin of 51 g, with fewer than 5×10^6 residual white cells in the final component, and 95% of the units tested should have a hemoglobin of 42.5 g.[95] For plateletpheresis quality control, the method should result in a final platelet count of 3×10^{11} in at least 90% of the units tested, and a residual white cell count of fewer than 5×10^6 in 95% of the units tested.[95]

COMPONENT PREPARATION AND STORAGE

Components are prepared from the processing of a whole blood donation or via automated apheresis collection methods, as just described. Component preparation from whole blood entails distinct manufacturing steps for collection, transportation, and separation, each of which involves unique logistical issues. With automated apheresis, the whole blood collection and component separation steps are integrated into a single process, as described in the previous section.

After collection and separation, individual components can be further modified by leukoreduction, irradiation, or washing to reduce the likelihood of certain transfusion-related complications. Each component and modified component has specific processing, transportation, and storage requirements, established to optimize product quality, safety, and therapeutic efficacy. Table 12–5 provides a summary of components, modified components, and manufacturing requirements.

In the following sections, component preparation, modification, and storage are discussed. The clinical and therapeutic aspects of blood transfusion are presented in greater detail in the dedicated chapters of this textbook.

Whole Blood Processing

With the advent of component therapy, the use of whole blood for transfusion in the United States has become uncommon. Whole blood is still reported to be a replacement for massive blood loss, such as in trauma and transplant cases.[96] In practice, however, intravenous fluids and blood components serve as the standard therapy for massive resuscitation, and whole blood is rarely used for this purpose. The primary exception is autologous blood, which, for simplicity, is often transfused as whole blood. Currently, the primary purpose of whole blood is as source material for blood component preparation.

For collection facilities, the logistics of whole blood processing depend on the components that are planned to be produced from the whole blood unit. If the whole blood unit is to be processed into plasma and RBCs only, the unit is transported on ice; however, if the whole blood unit is intended for platelet production, then the unit is maintained at room temperature until after separation of the platelet-rich plasma from the RBCs.

For plasma and RBC production, the unit is immediately stored at 1°C to 6°C or transported in a refrigerated system that cools the unit toward the range of 1°C to 10°C to maintain the optimal storage temperature for RBCs. If fresh frozen plasma (FFP) is to be produced, the plasma is separated from the whole blood unit within 8 hours of collection and stored in a freezer at −18°C or colder. A whole blood unit intended for *plasma frozen within 24 hours of phlebotomy* (FP24) is processed and frozen between 8 and 24 hours after collection.

In the case of platelet production, refrigeration leads to changes in the platelet membrane that result in poor in vivo platelet recovery after transfusion.[97–99] Thus, if the whole blood unit is intended for production of a platelet concentrate, then the unit is transported in a container capable of maintaining a temperature as close as possible to the optimal temperature range for platelet viability, 22°C to 24°C.[98] At the component preparation laboratory, the whole blood unit is processed to form a platelet concentrate within 8 hours of collection, and the remaining RBCs are then immediately refrigerated.

In addition to whole blood transport and storage, collection facilities must take into account the whole blood separation method to be employed when planning for component preparation. Whole blood is separated by differential centrifugation based on the specific gravity (relative density) of the blood constituents. The relative density of blood constituents ranges from most dense to least dense, as follows: RBCs, white blood cells (WBCs), platelets, and plasma. The degree of separation and component yield depend primarily on the centrifuge rotor size, speed (*g*- force or rpm), and spin time.[100] A temperature-controlled centrifuge is required to maintain the proper temperature range for the specific type of component being prepared.

The following general methods are used in the United States for whole blood separation. If a whole blood unit is intended for platelet production, the centrifuge temperature is set at 20°C, and a *soft spin* (low *g*- force) is used to separate the whole blood into platelet-rich plasma (PRP) and RBCs. The PRP is then manually expressed with a spring-loaded plasma expresser, through a top port of the primary bag into a satellite bag. The remaining RBCs in the primary bag are refrigerated at 1°C to 6°C. The PRP is further processed at 20°C by a *hard spin* (high *g*- force) to separate the plasma from the platelets. This method of platelet concentrate production is often referred to as the *PRP method*, as opposed to the *buffy coat method* used in European countries.

If the whole blood is not intended for platelet production, the unit is centrifuged at 4°C with a hard spin to separate the whole blood into a platelet-poor plasma (PPP) layer, a buffy coat layer containing platelets and WBCs, and a packed RBC layer. The PPP is then expressed into a satellite bag, leaving the majority of the platelets and WBCs with the RBCs in the primary bag. The RBCs are then immediately refrigerated at 1°C to 6°C.

Pooled Buffy Coat Method

In most European countries and Canada, the buffy coat method is applied to the processing of whole blood for platelet production. With this method, a specialized primary collection bag with ports on the bottom and top, referred to as the *bottom-and-top system* (BAT), is used. A whole blood unit is first centrifuged to produce a buffy coat (platelets and WBCs). With a semiautomated extractor, plasma is then

Table 12–5 **Requirements for Storage, Transportation, and Expiration**

Item No.	Components	Storage	Transport	Expiration*	Additional Criteria
1	Whole Blood	1–6°C, unless for room temperature components, then 1–6°C within 8 hours	Cooling toward 1–10°C	ACD/CPD/CP2D: 21 days	
			If intended for room temperature components, approaching (as close as possible to) 20–24°C	CPDA-1: 35 days	
2	Whole Blood Irradiated	1–6°C	1–10°C	Original expiration or 28 days from date of irradiation, whichever is sooner	
3	Red Blood Cells	1–6°C	1–10°C	ACD/CPD/CP2D: 21 days CPDA-1: 35 days Additive solution: 42 days Open system: 24 hours	
4	RBCs Deglycerolized	1–6°C	1–10°C	24 hours	
5	RBCs Frozen		Maintain frozen state	10 years (A policy shall be developed if rare frozen units are to be retained beyond this time.)	Frozen within 6 days of collection without an additive.
	40% Glycerol	≤–65°C if 40% Glycerol			Prior to red blood cell expiration if with an additive.
	20% Glycerol	≤–120°C if 20% Glycerol			
6	RBCs Irradiated	1–6°C	1–10°C	Original expiration or 28 days from date of irradiation, whichever is sooner	
7	RBCs Leukocytes Reduced	1–6°C	1–10°C	ACD/CPD/CP2D: 21 days CPDA-1: 35 days Open system: 24 hours Additive solution: 42 days	
8	RBCs Rejuvenated	1–6°C	1–10°C	24 hours	
9	RBCs Rejuvenated Deglycerolized	1–6°C	1–10°C	24 hours	
10	RBCs Rejuvenated Frozen	≤–65°C	Maintain frozen state	10 years AS1: 3 years (A policy shall be developed if rare frozen units are to be retained beyond this time.)	
11	RBCs Washed	1–6°C	1–10°C	24 hours	
12	Platelets	20–24°C with continuous gentle agitation	20–24°C (as close as possible to)	24 hours to 5 days, depending on collection system	Maximum time without agitation 24 hours
13	Platelets Irradiated	20–24°C with continuous gentle agitation	20–24°C (as close as possible to)	No change from original expiration date	Maximum time without agitation 24 hours

Table continued on following page

Table 12–5 Requirements for Storage, Transportation, and Expiration (Continued)

Item No.	Components	Storage	Transport	Expiration*	Additional Criteria
14	Platelets Leukocytes Reduced	20–24°C with continuous gentle agitation	20–24°C (as close as possible to)	Open system: 4 hours Closed system: No change in expiration	Maximum time without agitation 24 hours
15	Platelets Pooled or Open System	20–24°C with continuous gentle agitation	20–24°C (as close as possible to)	4 hours	
16	Platelets Pheresis	20–24°C with continuous gentle agitation	20–24°C (as close as possible to)	24 hours to 5 days, depending on collection system	Maximum time without agitation 24 hours
17	Platelets Pheresis Irradiated	20–24°C with continuous gentle agitation	20–24°C (as close as possible to)	No change from original expiration date	Maximum time without agitation 24 hours
18	Platelets Pheresis Leukocytes Reduced	20–24°C with continuous gentle agitation	20–24°C (as close as possible to)	No change from original expiration date	Maximum time without agitation 24 hours
19	Granulocytes	20–24°C	20–24°C (as close as possible to)	24 hours	Transfuse as soon as possible
20	Granulocytes Irradiated	20–24°C	20–24°C (as close as possible to)	No change from original expiration date	Transfuse as soon as possible
21	Cryoprecipitated AHF	≤–18°C	Maintain frozen state	12 months from original collection	Thaw the FFP at 1–6°C Refreeze cryoprecipitate within 1 hour
22	Cryoprecipitated AHF Thawed	20–24°C	20–24°C (as close as possible to) Single unit: 6 hours	Open system or pooled: 4 hours	Thaw at 30–37°C
23	Fresh Frozen Plasma (FFP) (including donor retested FFP)	≤–18°C or ≤–65°C	Maintain frozen state	≤–18°C: 12 months	Placed in freezer within 8 hours of collection in CPD, CP2D, CPDA-1 or within 6 hours of collection in ACD or as FDA-cleared.

				≤−65°C: 7 years	
24	FFP Thawed	1–6°C	1–10°C	24 hours	Thaw at 30–37°C or using an FDA-cleared device
25	Plasma Cryoprecipitate Reduced	≤−18°C	Maintain frozen state	12 months from original collection	
26	Plasma Cryoprecipitate Reduced Thawed	1–6°C	1–10°C	24 hours	
27	Plasma Frozen within 24 Hours of Collection	≤−18°C	Maintain frozen state	12 months from original collection	Placed in freezer within 24 hours of collection
28	Plasma, Frozen within 24 Hours, Thawed	1–6°C	1–10°C	24 hours	Thaw at 30–37°C or using an FDA-cleared device
29	Liquid Plasma	1–6°C	1–10°C	5 days after expiration of RBCs	
30	Thawed Plasma	1–6°C	1–10°C	5 days	Closed system
31	Solvent/Detergent-Treated Pooled Plasma	≤−18°C	Maintain frozen state	24 months from manufacture; manufacturer will state expiration date on label	
32	Solvent/Detergent-Treated Pooled Plasma Thawed	20–24°C	20–24°C (as close as possible to)	24 hours	Thaw at 30–37°C or using an FDA-cleared device
33	Recovered Plasma	≤−18°C	≤−18°C	Must be shipped for further manufacture within 12 months	Requires a short supply agreement.†
34	Tissue	Conform to source facility's written instructions	Conform to source facility's written instructions		

*If the seal is broken during processing, components stored at 1–6°C shall have an expiration time of 24 hours, and components stored at 20–24°C shall have an expiration time of 4 hours, unless otherwise indicated.

†21 CFR 601.22.

From American Association of Blood Banks. Standards for Blood Banks and Transfusion Services, 21st ed. Bethesda, MD, AABB, 2002.

expressed out of the top port, and the RBCs are expressed out of the bottom port.[101] The buffy coat platelet concentrate (BC-PC) remaining in the primary bag contains the majority of platelets and WBCs, along with approximately 30 mL of plasma and 30 mL of the RBCs. A pool of BC-PCs is prepared by suspending 4 to 6 units in a platelet additive solution. The BC-PC pool is centrifuged, and the platelet-rich supernatant is passed through a leukoreduction filter and stored.[102] With a pool of 6 BC-PC units, this method will result in more than 3×10^{11} platelets in the final product greater than 75% of the time.[103] Compared to the PRP method, advantages of the BC-PC method include greater plasma volume for plasma components, the ability to perform bacterial testing on stored pools (likely increasing the effective and allowed utilization of these components to 6 or 7 days), and improved metabolic stability of the platelets.[102] The disadvantage of this method is the increased RBC loss (10% to 15% loss) that occurs during processing.[102] An automated method for BC-PC processing is now available that results in increased efficiency, more consistent product volume, and better platelet yield than the manual BC-PC method.[104]

Red Blood Cells

The primary indication for RBC transfusion is the restoration of oxygen-carrying capacity in such conditions as blood loss, anemia, or hemoglobinopathy. RBCs are prepared either by whole blood processing (red blood cells) or by automated erythrocytapheresis (apheresis red blood cells). Often, RBCs are further modified by leukoreduction to reduce the risk of cytomegalovirus (CMV) transmission, alloimmunization, and febrile nonhemolytic transfusion reactions. For special circumstances, RBCs can be irradiated to prevent graft-versus-host disease (GVHD) or washed to prevent severe allergic reactions. For routine storage, RBCs are refrigerated between 1°C and 6°C and stored for 21 days (CPD, CP2D), 35 days (CPDA-1), or 42 days (AS-1, AS-3, AS-5). RBCs that have passed the expiration by up to 3 days can be rejuvenated for immediate transfusion or frozen storage.

Rejuvenated Red Blood Cells

Within the first 2 weeks of refrigerated storage, RBC ATP and 2,3-DPG are depleted.[43] To increase intracellular ATP and 2,3-DPG to normal or above-normal levels, refrigerated RBCs can be *rejuvenated* through a treatment process with the FDA-approved solution Rejuvesol (enCyte Systems, Braintree, Mass.). This rejuvenating solution contains the substrates inosine, adenine, phosphate, and pyruvate for RBC ATP and 2,3-DPG biosynthesis. CPD and CPDA-1 RBCs are approved for rejuvenation up to 3 days after expiration. After rejuvenation, CPD and CPDA-1 RBCs can be stored in the frozen state for up to 10 years, or they can be transfused within 24 hours of rejuvenation. CPD/AS-1 (Adsol) RBCs are approved for rejuvenation and cryopreservation within the 42-day storage period and may be stored in the frozen state for up to 3 years. As opposed to CPD and CPDA-1 units, CPD/AS-1 units are not approved for rejuvenation after expiration or for same-day transfusion after rejuvenation. In addition, the rejuvenation of RBCs stored in an additive system other than CPD/AS-1 (i.e., AS-3 or AS-5) is not currently approved by the FDA. Because rejuvenation early in storage results in excessive 2,3-DPG levels that can potentially impair the oxygen delivery function of the transfused cells in vivo,[105] it is not recommended to rejuvenate RBCs that have been in refrigerated storage less than 6 days.[106]

For rejuvenation of a single unit of stored RBCs, a 50-mL vial of rejuvenating solution is added through a sterile, disposable, Y-type connection and transfer set supplied by the rejuvenating solution manufacturer. Once suspended in the rejuvenating solution, the unit is sealed in a waterproof, double plastic bag overwrap and incubated in a 37 °C water bath for 60 minutes. After rejuvenation, the RBCs are prepared for same-day transfusion (CPD and CPDA-1 units) or processed for frozen storage (CPD, CPDA-1, and CPD/AS-1 units).

For same-day transfusion, the rejuvenated unit is immediately washed with an unbuffered saline solution in an approved cell washer to remove the residual metabolites hypoxanthine, uric acid, inosine, and inorganic phosphates prior to transfusion.[107] Outdated, rejuvenated, washed RBCs that are stored at 4 °C for up to 3 days have been shown to have an approximate in vitro RBC recovery of 95% and a 24-hour, post-transfusion survival rate of greater than 75%.[107] Despite these favorable data, the open washing procedure, which has the potential for pathogen contamination of the product, limits the approved storage of refrigerated, washed, rejuvenated RBCs to 24 hours.

For cryopreservation by freezing, the rejuvenated RBCs in the primary collection bag are not immediately washed, but they are instead further processed for frozen storage. The RBCs are centrifuged to separate the rejuvenating solution, which is then expressed into a transfer bag and discarded. Following separation, the RBCs are immediately prepared with a 40% glycerol solution and stored at −80 °C. Prior to transfusion, these rejuvenated, frozen RBCs are deglycerolized and washed. The freeze–thaw–wash cycle results in an approximate in vitro RBC recovery of 90% and a 24-hour post-transfusion survival rate of greater than 75%. As for RBC function, the rejuvenated, frozen, washed units have normal or above-normal 2,3-DPG levels and adequate or improved oxygen delivery.[108,109]

Frozen and Deglycerolized Red Blood Cells

Cryopreservation by freezing slows or suspends most metabolic functions and thus limits cellular deterioration during prolonged storage. When processed correctly, studies of stored, frozen RBCs have shown acceptable post-thaw in vitro viability and function after several decades of storage.[110–113] The major limitation to cryopreservation for RBC storage is the cryoinjury effect that can occur during the freeze–thaw process.[114] To minimize the effects of cryoinjury, a permeable or nonpermeable cryoprotective agent is added to the cell solution prior to cryopreservation. Glycerol, a permeable cryoprotectant, is the recommended cryopreservative for transfusable RBCs, because it is considered to be nontoxic to humans and has proven efficacy.

There are two general methods employed for the preparation of frozen RBCs, the low glycerol/rapid cooling technique and the high glycerol/slow cooling technique. Because glycerolized RBCs are hypertonic and hemolyze on contact with plasma, both freezing methods require a specialized post-thaw–wash procedure to remove excess glycerol (deglycerolization) prior to transfusion.

With the low glyercol/rapid cooling method, which is primarily used by European blood manufacturers, RBCs are suspended in a 15% to 20% weight/volume (wt/vol) solution of glycerol, cooled at a rate of greater than −100 °C/min by immersion in −197 °C liquid nitrogen, and stored at temperatures below −150 °C in liquid nitrogen or nitrogen vapor.[115,116] To prepare for transfusion, the frozen RBCs are rapidly thawed in a 42 °C to 45 °C water bath and deglycerolized. Due to the required extreme storage conditions, RBCs frozen with low glycerol are not as amenable to transportation, and thus, they are typically thawed at the storage facility and shipped to the transfusing facility in the liquid state.[117]

In the United States, RBCs that have been in refrigerated storage for 6 days or less or have been rejuvenated are approved for glycerolization and frozen storage. For the high glycerol/slow cooling process, RBCs are prepared with a 40% wt/vol glycerol solution, slowly cooled at a rate of approximately −1°C/min, and stored at −80 °C in metal or cardboard containers in a mechanical freezer. There are two process variations for the 40% glycerol method: the Meryman-Hornblower technique and the Valeri or Naval Blood Research Laboratory (NBRL) technique.[112,118] With the traditional Meryman-Hornblower method, the excess glycerol solution is not removed from the RBCs prior to freezing, so the post-thaw deglycerolization step requires a large-volume wash to remove the excess glycerol. With the Valeri or NBRL variation for glycerolization, the glycerolized unit is centrifuged, and the supernatant glycerol is discarded prior to freezing. Thus, after thawing, there is a smaller volume of glycerol to remove and a less-extensive deglycerolization process compared to the Meryman-Hornblower method.

For transfusion, the frozen RBC unit is initially thawed in a 37°C water bath or dry warmer and then deglycerolized. With the traditional, open method of deglycerolization, the unit is diluted with hypertonic saline, and then washed with approximately 2 liters of 1.6% saline solution. After adequate washing, the RBCs are suspended in isotonic saline for transfusion. Frozen RBCs that have been deglycerolized in an open system are approved for transfusion within 24 hours. The 24-hour expiration of deglycerolized units and the tedious, semiautomated deglycerolization process have presented both logistic and work-flow challenges for the routine use of frozen units.[117] Recently, however, a more efficient, automated, closed glycerolization-deglycerolization system (ACP 215, Haemonetics, Braintree, Mass.) has been approved by the FDA.[119,120] This system utilizes a disposable processing set, sterile connector device, and an in-line 0.22 μ filter to prevent bacterial contamination during processing. After deglycerolization, the processed RBCs are resuspended in AS-3, instead of isotonic saline, and are approved for refrigerated storage up to 14 days.[121] Frozen RBCs glycerolized by the Meryman-Hornblower method cannot be deglycerolized on the ACP 215, because the system in unable to process the larger volume of supernatant glycerol in these units.

Unlike low-glycerol frozen RBCs, RBCs frozen in 40% glycerol are better suited for transport, because these units are more tolerant of temperature fluctuations and can be effectively transported on dry ice.[122] One factor that complicates the transportation of frozen units is the increased fragility of blood bags that occurs at approximately −78 °C, which makes the units prone to breakage.[123] Traditionally, RBCs have been stored in polyolefin bags inside metal containers (Meryman-Hornblower method). With transport, frozen units stored in this manner have an incidence of breakage of greater than 30%.[124] An alternative, improved method for storage and transport, developed at the NBRL, uses specialized PVC-based freezer bags protected in corrugated cardboard holders, which reduces the rate of transportation breakage to less than 3%.[124]

Platelets

Platelet transfusion is indicated for prophylactic or hemostatic therapy in individuals with acquired or congenital thrombocytopenia or thrombocytopathy. Platelet components are prepared from either whole-blood donation or apheresis collection. For whole blood–derived platelets (Platelets), the preparation method must yield at least 5.5×10^{10} platelets per unit in at least 75% of the units tested by the manufacturing facility. With whole blood–derived platelets, typically 4 to 6 units are pooled immediately prior to transfusion, for a dose comparable to a single apheresis-derived platelet unit. For apheresis-derived platelets (Platelets, Pheresis), the collection method must yield at least 3×10^{11} platelets per unit in at least 90% of the units tested by the manufacturing facility. Large-yield plateletpheresis collections can be divided into two separate apheresis-derived platelets units, also known as *splits*, as long as the platelet count in each unit is greater than or equal to 3×10^{11}. The platelet storage conditions, such as plasma volume, agitation, and temperature, must be optimized to maintain an adequate pH of greater than or equal to 6.2 in 90% of the units tested at the end of the approved storage period. As with RBCs, platelet components are often modified by leukoreduction, and for special conditions, platelets can be further modified by irradiation or washing. In addition, apheresis-derived platelets can be cross-matched or HLA-matched for alloimmunized individuals who exhibit poor platelet increments with random platelet transfusions.

Compared to other components, platelets are more sensitive to variable storage conditions. Although refrigerated or frozen storage would seem ideal for slowing cellular deterioration and retarding bacterial growth, cold storage of platelets results in significantly worse post-transfusion in vivo survival relative to room temperature–stored platelets.[97–99] Furthermore, platelets that remain undisturbed during storage are less efficacious than platelets that are agitated on a horizontal rocker, a process that helps ensure optimal gas exchange and maintenance of pH.[125] Thus, for optimum storage, platelets must be gently agitated and maintained at a temperature range from 20 °C to 24 °C. During transport, the period of time that platelets remain without gentle agitation should not exceed 24 hours, because interruption of agitation for greater than 1 day results in significant damage to the component.[126]

A major challenge with platelet storage is that the room temperature environment and nutrient-rich plasma favor bacterial proliferation.[127] To reduce the risk of significant bacterial burden, the approved storage period for platelets is limited to 5 days after collection,[128] even though platelets stored for longer periods show acceptable in vivo survival.[31,129] Even with 5-day storage, bacterial contamination of platelets with subsequent transfusion-related bacteremia or sepsis had been a leading cause of transfusion morbidity and mortality.[1] To address this issue, in the 23rd edition of the *Standard for Blood Banks and Transfusion Services*, AABB introduced a standard for blood establishments to have methods in place that limit and detect bacterial contamination of platelets.

Given the nonspecific nature of the standard, many methods are employed for bacterial testing, including Gram stain or bacterial culture, point-of-care testing by pH/glucose determination, and visualization of a lack of swirling, which is a sign of nonviable platelets.[1] A major limitation of the nonculture techniques is the lack of sensitivity (10^6 to 10^7 CFU/mL) compared to bacterial culture systems (10^2 to 10^3 CFU/mL or less).[130–133] Consequently, more false negatives should be expected with nonculture systems. Although more sensitive, the bacterial culture method has the limitations of a larger volume of sample required for testing and a longer wait for test results. In the case of the latter limitation, the platelet unit may be distributed and transfused prior to the reported culture result, so the bacterial status at the time or point of transfusion may be unknown. Typically, point-of-care methodologies are more commonly employed for whole blood–derived platelets, because the volume necessary for bacterial culture constitutes a more significant loss to this smaller-volume platelet product. Apheresis-derived platelets, as a larger-volume product, are more amenable to sampling for bacterial culture, and thus are more often tested by the bacterial culture method, using a sample obtained within 24 to 48 hours of storage. With all methodologies, if a true positive result is obtained, the facility is obligated to quarantine the product, identify the contaminating organism, and if already distributed, notify the customer and retrieve the product if not transfused. If the product has been transfused, the clinical service must be notified for proper assessment and treatment of the transfusion recipient.

Extended (7-Day) Platelet Storage

Room temperature platelets have been stored for up to 2 weeks with acceptable therapeutic efficacy.[102] Advantages of extended storage of platelets are improved logistics, increased inventory flexibility, and decreased cost associated with reduced outdate rates.[134] Although 7-day storage was previously approved by the FDA in the 1980s,[31] concern about the increased risk of transfusion-related sepsis with prolonged storage at room temperature led the FDA to limit platelet storage to 5 days. However, with the increased sensitivity of bacterial detection systems for platelet testing, extended storage of platelets has again become a possibility.[133,135] The FDA's position on 7-day platelet storage is currently in evolution. In 2003, the FDA approved, with restrictions, the use of specific plateletpheresis collection and storage systems for 7-day storage of platelets (COBE Spectra Apheresis System and Trima Automated Blood Collection System, Gambro BCT, Inc., Lakewood, Colo.). At this time, facilities cleared by the FDA for 7-day storage must comply with a specific protocol for bacterial testing, and approved facilities must participate in a postmarket surveillance study of the applied protocol.[136]

Prestorage Pooling of Platelets

Studies of prestorage pooled, whole blood–derived platelets show satisfactory in vitro and in vivo properties.[137–139] Although a common practice in Europe with buffy coat platelets, prestorage pooling of whole blood–derived platelet units has not been approved in the United States due to concerns about increased risk of bacterial growth in prestorage platelet pools.[140] With the introduction of required bacterial testing of platelets in the United States, it has become apparent that the most sensitive bacterial detection methods are based on automated bacterial culture. Given the relatively large sample volume required for bacterial culture and the increased number of units to test for a single transfusion, such methods are not routinely applied for bacterial testing of whole blood–derived platelets. Typically, due to these constraints, less sensitive methods are employed for bacterial testing of whole blood–derived versus apheresis–derived platelets. Prestorage pooling of whole blood–derived platelets provides sufficient sample volume for more sensitive automated bacterial culture methods, thus increasing the likelihood of bacterial detection and improving the safety of whole blood–derived platelets. Consequently, in the United States there is renewed interest in prestorage pooling of whole blood–derived platelets.[141–143] Recently, the FDA approved a system for prestorage leukoreduction and pooling of whole blood–derived platelets that contains an integrated bacterial culture system for automated bacterial detection (Acrodose PL, Pall Corporation, East Hills, NY). With improved technology, the availability and use of prestorage pooled platelets in the United States is likely to increase.

Plasma

Plasma components are obtained by separation from a centrifuged whole blood unit, from a plasmapheresis donation, or as a by-product of plateletpheresis. After collection, plasma can be processed as components for transfusion (FFP and PF24) or as source material for further manufacture (recovered plasma and source plasma) into injectable products (i.e., plasma derivatives) or noninjectable products (i.e., reagents). In general, plasma from a healthy blood donor contains normal levels of proteins, immunoglobulins, and coagulation factors. However, plasma units can vary somewhat in content and appearance based on the donor's diet, medication intake, and physiology. For example, plasma from female donors on estrogen-based contraceptives or hormone replacement therapy can appear green due to an estrogen-related elevation in ceruloplasmin levels.[144,145]

As a transfused product, plasma components primarily serve as a source of coagulation factors and are indicated in the management of coagulopathies associated with liver disease, warfarin therapy, disseminated intravascular coagulation, massive transfusion, and congenital factor deficiencies.[146,147] In addition, plasma components are used as replacement fluids during therapeutic plasma exchange.

Plasma Components for Transfusion: FFP and PF24

FFP and FP24 are indicated for the treatment of disorders of secondary hemostasis associated with multiple coagulation factor deficiencies. For most indications, FFP and FP24 are essentially comparable in therapeutic dose of coagulation factors, except that FFP has significantly higher factor VIII activity.[148] Because the activities of coagulation factors in stored plasma are dependent on temperature and length of storage, the processing and storage requirements for FFP and FP24 are established to optimize coagulation factor levels. In general, during refrigerated whole blood storage, coagulation factor levels remain relatively stable for up to 24 hours.[148] However, although remaining within the hemostatic range, factor VIII activity significantly decreases by 20% to 50% within 24 hours of whole blood storage.[149–151] Factor V exhibits variable stability during 24-hour whole blood storage, with some studies showing an insignificant decrease in activity[152] and others reporting a decrease in activity of greater than 10% from baseline.[148,153]

Due to the significant decrease in factor VIII activity between 8 and 24 hours of refrigerated storage, FFP collected in CPD, CP2D, and CPDA-1 is required to be frozen within

8 hours of collection. FFP collected in ACD is required to be frozen within 6 hours of phlebotomy. If maintained at −18 °C or colder, FFP is approved for storage for up to 1 year. If cleared by the FDA, facilities may store FFP for up to 7 years at −65 °C or colder. For plasma processed and frozen within 8 to 24 hours of collection, the component is designated as PF24. PF24 is approved for storage at −18 °C for up to 1 year after collection. During transport, FFP and PF24 are maintained in the frozen state by packaging with dry ice in an insulated container.

For transfusion, FFP and PF24 are thawed between 30 °C to 37 °C in a water bath for approximately 30 minutes or rapidly thawed in an FDA-approved microwave device for approximately 6 minutes.[154,155] Although less expensive than microwave devices, water baths contribute to a longer thaw time compared to microwave devices, which can impact the immediate provision of thawed plasma in situations that require urgent need, particularly in the trauma setting. In addition, although the frozen unit is placed in a waterproof plastic overwrap bag prior to immersion in the water bath, the baths contain nonsterile water, which may contaminate the entry ports of the unit if the unit is not sufficiently protected. Although microwave devices are more sterile and result in a more rapid turnaround time, these devices are relatively expensive. Furthermore, if not properly maintained, microwave devices have the potential to produce temperature "hot spots" in the unit during thawing, which can damage plasma proteins. Once thawed, FFP and PF24 are approved for storage at 1 °C to 6 °C for up to 24 hours. If prepared in a closed system and not transfused within 24 hours, thawed FFP and PF24 can be relabeled as "Thawed Plasma" and stored at 1 °C to 6 °C for up to 5 days. Although prolonged storage of refrigerated plasma is associated with cold activation of the coagulation system and decreased levels of some coagulation factors,[156,157] this has a clinically insignificant effect, as coagulation factor levels remain well within the acceptable range for adequate hemostasis.[150,158]

Plasma for Further Manufacture: Recovered Plasma and Source Plasma

Plasma that is separated from a unit of whole blood up to 5 days after the whole blood unit expiration is labeled as "Liquid Plasma" and stored between 1 °C and 6 °C. Plasma that is separated from a whole blood unit greater than 24 hours after collection and up to 5 days after the whole blood unit expiration is labeled "Plasma" and stored at −18 °C or colder. FFP that has exceeded the 12-month expiration can also be relabeled as "Plasma" and stored at −18 °C for an additional 4 years. Liquid plasma is approved for use up to 5 days after the expiration of the whole blood unit from which it was separated, and plasma is approved for storage up to 5 years from the whole blood collection date. Although liquid plasma and plasma are licensed for transfusion, these products are often relabeled as "Recovered Plasma" and designated for further manufacture. As an unlicensed product, recovered plasma can only be shipped to another manufacturer if the shipping facility has a "short supply agreement" with the receiving manufacturer.[159]

Source plasma is a licensed product that is collected by plasmapheresis for the purpose of fractionation into injectable or noninjectable plasma products. Donors of source plasma must meet the requirements for allogeneic plasmapheresis donors, including infectious disease testing, plasma protein evaluation, and donation interval limitations. The only exception is that donors of source plasma are not required to be tested for human T-lymphotropic virus (HTLV) 1 and 2.[160] In addition, in contrast to allogeneic donors, donors of source plasma are not required to have a negative result for antibody to hepatitis B core antigen (HBcAg).[160] Furthermore, donors that have a reactive serological test for syphilis can undergo plasmapheresis for source plasma only if the donor is being treated for syphilis and the plasma is specifically designated for further manufacture into control reagents for syphilis testing.[161]

Source plasma that is prepared for injectable products must be labeled "Caution: For Manufacturing Use Only." For noninjectable products, the source plasma product must be labeled "Caution: For Use in Manufacturing Noninjectable Products Only."[160] If intended for injectable products, source plasma is approved for storage at −20 °C or colder for up to 10 years.

Cryoprecipitate and Cryoprecipitate-Reduced Plasma

Cryoprecipitated antihemophilic factor (*cryoprecipitate AHF, cryoprecipitate, cryo*) is indicated for the treatment of coagulopathy associated with hypofibrinogenemia, dysfibrinogenemia, factor XIII deficiency, uremic thrombocytopathy, and tissue plasminogen activator (tPA) therapy.[162] Cryoprecipitate is also used in surgical settings as a source of fibrinogen, admixed with thrombin, for topically applied fibrin glue. In the past, prior to the development of pasteurized, purified plasma derivatives and recombinant factor concentrates, cryoprecipitate was a treatment for hemophilia A and von Willebrand disease (vWD). However, given the improved safety, purity, and efficacy of factor concentrates, cryoprecipitate is no longer a first-line therapy for hemophilia A or vWD when appropriate factor concentrates are available. *Cryoprecipitate-reduced plasma* (also called *cryo-poor supernatant*) is employed as a plasma replacement fluid in therapeutic plasma exchange for the treatment of TTP. Cryoprecipitate-reduced plasma is not an FDA-licensed product.

A unit of cryoprecipitate contains the following concentrated, cold, insoluble plasma proteins: fibrinogen (150 mg to 250 mg), factor VIII (80 IU to 120 IU), fibronectin (30 mg to 60 mg), factor XIII (40 IU to 60 IU), and von Willebrand factor (80 IU).[163] At a minimum, a cryoprecipitate unit is required to have a fibrinogen level of 150 mg and a factor VIII activity of 80 IU. To ensure an adequate concentration of plasma constituents, a unit of cryoprecipitate is prepared from an FFP unit that contains a volume of at least 200 mL. The unit of FFP is slowly thawed, in a refrigerator or water bath, to a range of 1 °C to 6 °C. At this temperature, a precipitate of cold, insoluble plasma proteins forms. After centrifugation at 4 °C to concentrate and pellet the insoluble proteins, the supernatant plasma, known as cryoprecipitate-reduced plasma, is expressed into a satellite bag, and approximately 15 mL is reserved for the cryoprecipitate unit. To maintain adequate factor VIII levels, cryoprecipitate must be refrozen within 1 hour of thawing of the FFP unit. For cryoprecipitate-reduced plasma, the unit is required to be refrozen with 24 hours of FFP thawing. Both cryoprecipitate and cryoprecipitate-reduced plasma are approved for storage at −18 °C or colder for up to 1 year from the original collection date.

For cryoprecipitate transfusion, approximately 8 units are thawed in a 30 °C to 37 °C water bath and then pooled into a single transfer bag. The pooled cryoprecipitate product is required to be stored at room temperature (20 °C to 24 °C) and is approved for administration within 4 hours of pooling. A single unit of thawed cryoprecipitate, stored at room temperature, is approved for use within 6 hours of thawing. Thawed cryoprecipitate-reduced plasma is approved for storage at 1 °C to 6 °C for up to 5 days.

Granulocytes

The general indication for granulocyte transfusion is treatment of a life-threatening fungal and bacterial infection in an individual with severe but reversible neutropenia, typically resulting from myeloablative chemotherapy that has not adequately responded to antibiotic therapy after 48 to 72 hours (see Chapter 24).[84] Granulocytes are collected by leukapheresis from an eligible donor who has received a leukocyte-mobilizing agent, such as corticosteroids and G-CSF, prior to the procedure. Although granulocytes for transfusion are not an FDA-licensed product, AABB requires that a minimum of 1.0×10^{10} granulocytes per unit are present in at least 75% of the products tested. In addition, because a granulocyte component contains greater than 2 mL of red blood cells, the donor and recipient ABO type and crossmatch must be compatible.

Starting immediately after collection, granulocyte function deteriorates rapidly; thus, a granulocyte component should be transfused as soon as possible after collection, usually within 8 to 24 hours.[164] Because granulocyte components contain viable T lymphocytes and are transfused to immunocompromised individuals, all granulocyte products should be irradiated to prevent GVHD. When transported or temporarily stored, the component should be kept at room temperature (20 °C to 24 °C) without agitation.[165] In addition, for obvious reasons, a granulocyte product should not be leukoreduced or transfused through a bedside leukoreduction filter. Although not an FDA-licensed product, granulocytes are considered a "product under development" under 21 CFR 601.21,[166] and thus are exempt from requirements for licensing for interstate transport and may be shipped from one state to another as long as the product is not "introduced into interstate commerce."

Modification Processes

Leukoreduction

Leukoreduction involves the removal of WBCs from cellular components to reduce the risk of HLA alloimmunization, CMV transmission, and febrile nonhemolytic transfusion reactions.[167] Leukoreduction can be performed by filtration prior to component storage (prestorage leukoreduction) or during the transfusion (bedside filtration). For apheresis-derived platelets, leukoreduction is often performed by cell separation during the apheresis collection. For whole blood, whole blood–derived platelets, and RBCs, leukoreduction is performed using third-generation leukoreduction filters, which are commercially available as an integral part of a whole blood collection kit or as a separate, sterilely docked device. This modification process is discussed in detail in Chapter 26.

Quality control standards for leukocyte-reduced components require that 95% of the units sampled contain fewer than 5×10^6 WBCs per unit for apheresis-derived platelets and RBCs and fewer than 8.3×10^5 WBCs per unit for whole blood–derived platelets.[168] In addition, for both apheresis-derived and whole blood–derived RBCs, the RBC loss from filtration must not exceed 15% of the original unit. The most common quality control method employed for white blood cell enumeration is light microscopy using a Nageotte chamber.[169] Although this manual method is relatively inexpensive, it is labor-intensive and results in a high degree of interindividual variation. Automated flow cytometry and microfluorometry hemocytometers provide a more accurate and precise method for WBC enumeration.[170] Although more expensive, automated devices offer greater convenience and are being increasingly employed by blood centers for leukofiltration quality control.

Washing

Washed cellular products are indicated for individuals who have a history of recurrent, severe allergic transfusion reactions.[171] In addition, for neonatal transfusion, washed maternal platelets are indicated for neonatal alloimmune thrombocytopenia (NAIT),[172] and washed RBCs, previously stored in additive solution, have been suggested as an option for neonatal massive transfusion.[173] Cell washing can be performed by manual or automated methods. Automated cell washing devices contain a specialized centrifugation device with fluid input and output channels that remove supernatant waste from the cells and add normal saline (0.9%) solution for cell resuspension. Manufacturers of cell-washing systems provide a customized, disposable processing kit that meets the specifications of the cell-washing device. With a 1-L to 2-L saline wash procedure, greater than 99% of the supernatant plasma is removed from the component, with approximately 90% recovery for washed platelets[174] and 80% to 85% recovery for washed RBCs.[173,175] This modification process is discussed in additional detail in Chapter 29.

Current cell-washing devices operate as an open system, so the expiration of the washed component is affected. For refrigerated, washed red blood cells, the expiration is 24 hours, and for room temperature, washed platelets, the expiration is to 4 hours. The shortened expiration time presents a logistic challenge for washed platelet transfusion, because an additional platelet "rest" step of approximately 1 hour is typically performed prior to release[172]; therefore, the actual allowable time to transfusion is between 2 and 3 hours. Finally, washed components are not FDA licensed, and thus they are not approved for interstate transport.

Irradiation

Irradiation of blood components is performed to prevent transfusion-associated graft-versus-host disease (TA-GVHD), a fatal transfusion complication. TA-GVHD occurs when donor T lymphocytes, present in cellular blood products, engraft, proliferate, and destroy the target organs in a susceptible transfusion recipient. Irradiation of cellular products, with either gamma rays or x-rays, prevents TA-GVHD by damaging donor T-lymphocyte DNA, with resultant inhibition of donor T-lymphocyte proliferation within the recipient.[176]

Blood component irradiation is considered a manufacturing process, so a facility that performs irradiation must be registered with the FDA. Free-standing irradiators used in blood manufacturing contain either a radioactive cesium (^{137}Cs) or cobalt (^{60}Co) source. Because the intensity of the radioactive source decays with time, the dose of radiation to which the blood product is exposed, measured in centiGray (1 cGy = 1 rad), is dependent on the source half-life. Thus, to obtain a predicted, fixed radiation dose, the radioisotope decay is calculated to determine radiation exposure time. In addition, the irradiator must be recalibrated periodically, semiannually for ^{60}Co irradiators and annually for ^{137}Cs irradiators, to ensure adequate delivered dose.[177] Although a dose of 1500 cGy significantly reduces T-lymphocyte proliferation, a dose of approximately 2500 cGy has been shown to completely inhibit T-lymphocyte proliferation, based on studies using the sensitive limiting dilution assay (LDA).[178,179] Accordingly, quality control standards require that the minimum radiation dose delivered to the component be 2500 cGy, with a minimum dose of 1500 cGy at any point in the blood product. This modification process is discussed in detail in Chapter 28.

Validation of the irradiation process is performed by a dose-mapping procedure, which measures the dose of radiation delivered to specific points over the entire area of a simulated blood product. For dose mapping, a phantom, composed of water or plastic and equipped with strategically placed dosimeters, is positioned inside the irradiation chamber. On irradiation, each dosimeter absorbs a specific dose of radiation, which is then measured and mapped. Available dose-mapping systems for blood irradiators employ one of the following: radiochromic film dosimeters, thermoluminescent dosimeters (TLD chips), or metal oxide semiconductor field effect transistors (MOSFET). Along with dose validation, a process for irradiation confirmation is necessary. This process is performed by affixing a label that contains radiosensitive film to the blood product prior to irradiation. On irradiation, the film changes from transparent to opaque, providing visual evidence that the product was irradiated.

With irradiation, the expiration date and time of granulocytes and platelets are unaffected. However, the shelf life of RBCs is shortened due to irradiation-induced acceleration of adverse storage effects, such as decreased in vivo survival[180,181] and increased potassium leakage.[182] For irradiated RBCs, the expiration date is 28 days from the day of irradiation or the original expiration date, whichever comes first.

LABELING

In 1985, due to concerns about potential transfusion errors related to inconsistent industry labeling practices, the FDA published the "Guidelines for the Uniform Labeling of Blood and Blood Components."[183] Along with specifications for label design, content, and product identifiers, these guidelines introduced to blood manufacturing a machine-readable bar code system, known as *ABC Codabar*, to better facilitate information transfer, product identification, traceability, and trackability. Although ABC Codabar enhanced blood manufacturing efficiency and decreased the likelihood of mistransfusion, the system was limited by the lack of controls for data substitution errors and an inadequate number of codes for newly developed products.[184] Thus, within a few years of ABC Codabar implementation, the need for an improved electronic data management process was recognized. To address this need, the International Society for Blood Transfusion (ISBT) proposed an alternative uniform product coding system, known as ISBT 128, to be managed by the International Council for Commonality in Blood Banking Automation (ICCBBA).

With its advanced coding system using discrete data structures, ISBT 128 is more amenable to automation, new product development, inventory control, global distribution, and future introduction of radio frequency identification (RFID) technology.[184] Both the FDA and AABB endorse the ICCBBA's "United States Industry Consensus Standard for the Uniform Labeling of Blood and Blood Components Using *ISBT 128*," and they have committed to a time line for ISBT 128 implementation by the U.S. blood industry.[185,186] Effective November 1, 2006, the 24th edition of the *AABB Standards for Blood Banks and Transfusion Services* will require accredited facilities to have a written plan for the transition to and implementation of ISBT 128; and effective May 1, 2008, the 25th edition will require accredited facilities to have fully implemented ISBT 128.[186] In addition to blood and blood products, ISBT 128 will be applied to labeling for cellular therapy products and tissues, with an effective implementation date of September 1, 2008.[186] In light of these developments, the following section will provide a general overview of the ISBT 128 labeling system, with reference to ABC Codabar for comparison purposes only. The reader is encouraged to visit the ICCBBA website (http://www.isbt128.org) and the AABB website (http://www.aabb.org) for additional resources on ISBT 128 implementation.

In general, the attributes of ISBT 128 include an enhanced unique donor identification system; an improved data structure for critical information (e.g., blood group, expiration date); an internationally recognized product description database; an eye-readable, machine-readable uniform labeling format; and a more accurate, flexible bar coding system.[187] In addition, unlike ABC Codabar, ISBT 128 supports concatenation, which is the ability to integrate data from paired bar codes into a single data message.[184] Furthermore, ISBT 128 contains check characters to further reduce scanning errors.[184] A sample ISBT 128 label is shown in Figure 12–1, which illustrates the standardized four-quadrant layout and the key label features of the ISBT 128 system.

Located in the upper left-hand corner is the unique donor identification code, which is a 13-character data set composed

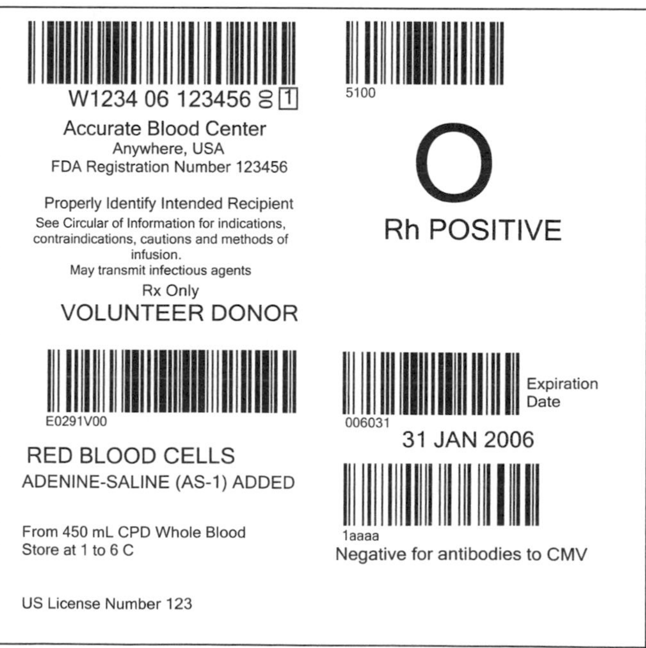

Figure 12–1 Sample ISBT 128 Label. (Used with permission of ICCBBA, Inc.)

of the collection facility identifier, the collection year, and a 6-digit donation sequence number. Adjacent to the unique donor identification code is an enclosed checksum digit to ensure accurate data entry if the number is entered manually by keyboard. Compared to the 7-digit donor identification number used by ABC Codabar that results in duplicate donor numbers, the ISBT 128 13-digit code provides more than sufficient characters to give each donation a unique identifier. The upper right-hand corner contains the ABO/Rh designation, which was previously required to be of a designated color. To accommodate the use of black-and-white, on-demand, in-house label printing, the FDA has proposed a regulatory change to the CFR that will allow for an alternative black-and-white color scheme with optional use of the traditional multicolor scheme.[188] The lower right-hand corner contains the section for product expiration and, if applicable, a space for a special testing label, such as for CMV-negative products. The lower left-hand quadrant contains the alphanumeric product code (up to eight characters), which includes information on the component class (e.g., red blood cells), modifier (e.g., washed), core conditions (anticoagulant, volume, and storage), attributes (e.g., irradiated), and intended use of the product. Currently, with all combinations of the component class, modifiers, and attributes, the ISBT 128 Product Code Database contains more than 5000 blood product codes that provide unique, specific product identification.

AABB has published the "ISBT Code 128 Implementation Plan," which provides specific information for the transition to ISBT 128 and a time line for implementation. ISBT 128 is not in the public domain, and all blood manufacturing facilities that plan to implement ISBT 128 must register with ICCBBA and pay an annual licensing fee based on the facility's annual product collections. For transfusion services that do not manufacture blood products, registration with ICCBBA is optional. In addition, at the time of this writing, the establishment must notify the FDA prior to conversion to ISBT 128.

A recent survey by AABB of blood facilities that have implemented ISBT 128 indicates that the typical time for complete implementation is less than 6 months. The most common logistic challenges encountered by the surveyed facilities were achieving compatibility between the new computer software and hardware and issues with label scanning, reading, and printing. Additional obstacles that were cited included coordination with facility customers and suppliers, validation of ISBT 128, and managing staffing for ISBT 128–associated activities while maintaining operations.[186]

SHIPPING

Shipping and receiving diagnostic specimens and blood products is an essential part of the blood manufacturing process. Regulations for the interstate transport of biological materials are established by the Department of Transportation (DOT) for ground transport, the International Air Transport Association (IATA) for air transport, and the United States Postal Service (USPS) for mail transport. Diagnostic specimens and components that have a high likelihood of containing an infectious agent must be packaged in compliance with 42 CFR 72 and shipped in accordance to the requirements set forth by the IATA, USPS, and the Centers for Disease Control and Prevention (CDC).[189] In general, the shipping requirements for clinical specimens and infectious materials include proper labeling formats to ensure clear recognition of the biohazardous contents and required packaging, such as use of leak-proof containers, shock-absorbent material, and liquid-absorbent material to reduce the risk of breakage and leakage of the transported contents. For diagnostic specimens, if damage or leakage does occur, only the shipper and receiver are to be notified. However, for infectious substances, if breakage or leakage occurs, the package must be appropriately isolated, and the CDC must be immediately notified by the contact information present on the required "Infectious Substance" shipping label.[189]

Blood products that have tested negative for infectious disease markers, or that are untested but have been obtained from screened, healthy donors, are not considered to be infectious; thus, they are not subject to all of the shipping requirements for diagnostic specimens or infectious materials. Blood products are required to be inspected for defects or abnormal appearance immediately prior to packaging and on receipt. In addition, for transport, a packaging system that protects the contents from damage and maintains the appropriate temperature range is necessary to ensure the safety and quality of the product.

With refrigerated whole blood and red blood cells, the required transport temperature range is 1 °C to 10 °C. To maintain this range, units are surrounded by bags of wet ice and encased in polyurethane insulation within a corrugated cardboard shipping container. On delivery, a procedure to confirm that the temperature remained within range during transport must be performed using one of the following methods: measurement with a thermometer at the time of delivery, use of a specialized "high-low" thermometer in the shipping container, or visual inspection of an "out-of-range" temperature indicator in the shipping container. For platelets, a room temperature platelet shipping system composed of a durable, insulated polyurethane container with gel-based temperature stabilizing (phase change) packs has been shown to maintain platelet temperature from 20 °C to 24 °C during transport, even in extreme conditions (−10 °C).[190] For frozen plasma products and RBCs, an insulated packaging system that uses dry ice is employed to maintain products in the frozen state during transport. Dry ice is considered a hazardous material, and its use requires special training, handling, packaging, and shipping procedures. Because dry ice can result in burns and asphyxiation if mishandled or improperly stored, individuals who handle or transport material containing dry ice must receive HAZMAT instruction on the use of personal protective equipment, effective packing and ventilation, and proper storage and disposal.

REFERENCES

1. Hillyer CD, Josephson CD, Blajchman MA, et al. Bacterial contamination of blood components: risks, strategies, and regulation: Joint ASH and AABB educational session in transfusion medicine. Hematology (Am Soc Hematol Educ Program) 2003:575–589.
2. Wagner SJ. Transfusion-transmitted bacterial infection: risks, sources and interventions. Vox Sang 2004;86:157–163.
3. Code of Federal Regulations, 21 CFR 604.3. U.S. Government Printing Office, Washington, D.C., 2005 (revised annually).
4. U.S. Food and Drug Administration (CBER). Options for Arm Preparation. Available at http://www.fda.gov/cber/blood/armpreprev.htm. Accessed October 30, 2005.
5. AABB Association Bulletin #03–07 and #03–10, August 2003.
6. Goldman M, Roy G, Frechette N, et al. Evaluation of donor skin disinfection methods. Transfusion 1997;37:309–312.

7. Newman BH. Blood donor complications after whole-blood donation. Curr Opin Hematol 2004;11:339–345.
8. Winters JL. Complications of donor apheresis. J Clin Apheresis 2005 (Epub ahead of print).
9. McLeod BC, Price TH, Owen H, et al. Frequency of immediate adverse effects associated with apheresis donation. Transfusion 1998; 38:938–943.
10. Newman BH, Waxman DA. Blood donation-related neurologic needle injury: evaluation of 2 years' worth of data from a large blood center. Transfusion 1996;36:213–215.
11. Newman B. Venipuncture nerve injuries after whole-blood donation. Transfusion 2001;41:571–572.
12. Horowitz SH. Venipuncture-induced causalgia: anatomic relations of upper extremity superficial veins and nerves, and clinical considerations. Transfusion 2000;40:1036–1040.
13. Horowitz SH. Venipuncture-induced neuropathic pain: the clinical syndrome, with comparisons to experimental nerve injury models. Pain 2001;94:225–229.
14. Despotis GJ, Goodnough LT, Dynis M, et al. Adverse events in platelet apheresis donors: a multivariate analysis in a hospital-based program. Vox Sang 1999;77:24–32.
15. Popovsky MA, Whitaker B, Arnold NL. Severe outcomes of allogeneic and autologous blood donation: frequency and characterization. Transfusion 1995;35:734–737.
16. Standard 5.3.2: Silva MA (ed). Standards for Blood Bank and Transfusion Services, 23rd Edition. Bethesda, MD: AABB, 2004.
17. Standard 5.3.3: Silva MA (ed). Standards for Blood Bank and Transfusion Services, 23rd Edition. Bethesda, MD: AABB, 2004.
18. Standard 5.8: Silva MA (ed). Standards for Blood Bank and Transfusion Services, 23rd Edition. Bethesda, MD: AABB, 2004.
19. Szewzyk U, Szewzyk R, Stenstrom TA. Growth and survival of Serratia marcescens under aerobic and anaerobic conditions in the presence of materials from blood bags. J Clin Microbiol 1993;31:1826–1830.
20. Standard 5.7.2: Silva MA (ed). Standards for Blood Bank and Transfusion Services, 23rd Edition. Bethesda, MD: AABB, 2004.
21. FDA Guidance for Industry. Use of sterile connecting devices in blood bank practices, November 2000. Available at http://www.fda.gov/cber/gdlns/bbconn.htm. Accessed October 30, 2005.
22. Blajchman MA. Bacterial contamination of cellular blood components: risks, sources and control. Vox Sang 2004;87(Suppl 1):98–103.
23. Wagner SJ, Robinette D, Friedman LI, et al. Diversion of initial blood flow to prevent whole-blood contamination by skin surface bacteria: an in vitro model. Transfusion 2000;40:335–338.
24. de Korte D, Marcelis JH, Verhoeven AJ, et al. Diversion of first blood volume results in a reduction of bacterial contamination for whole-blood collections. Vox Sang 2002;83:13–16.
25. Carmen R. The selection of plastic materials for blood bags. Transfus Med Rev 1993;7:1–10.
26. Murphy S, Sayar SN, Gardner FH. Storage of platelet concentrates at 22°C. Blood 1970;35:549–557.
27. Murphy S, Gardner FH. Platelet storage at 22°C: role of gas transport across plastic containers in maintenance of viability. Blood 1975;46:209–218.
28. Murphy S, Kahn RA, Holme S, et al. Improved storage of platelets for transfusion in a new container. Blood 1982;60:194–200.
29. Holme S, Heaton A, Momoda G. Evaluation of a new, more oxygen-permeable, polyvinylchloride container. Transfusion 1989;29:159–164.
30. Snyder EL, Pope C, Ferri PM, et al. The effect of mode of agitation and type of plastic bag on storage characteristics and in vivo kinetics of platelet concentrates. Transfusion 1986;26:125–130.
31. Hogge DE, Thompson BW, Schiffer CA. Platelet storage for 7 days in second-generation blood bags. Transfusion 1986;26:131–135.
32. Sasakawa S, Tokunaga E. Physical and chemical changes of ACD-preserved blood: a comparison of blood in glass bottles and plastic bags. Vox Sang 1976;31:199–210.
33. Horowitz B, Stryker MH, Waldman AA, et al. Stabilization of red blood cells by the plasticizer, diethylhexylphthalate. Vox Sang 1985; 48:150–155.
34. Estep TN, Pedersen RA, Miller TJ, et al. Characterization of erythrocyte quality during the refrigerated storage of whole blood containing di-(2-ethylhexyl) phthalate. Blood 1984;64:1270–1276.
35. AuBuchon JP, Estep TN, Davey RJ. The effect of the plasticizer di-2-ethylhexyl phthalate on the survival of stored RBCs. Blood 1988;71: 448–452.
36. Jaeger RJ, Rubin RJ. Contamination of blood stored in plastic packs. Lancet 1970;2:151.
37. Rock G, Tocchi M, Ganz PR, et al. Incorporation of plasticizer into red cells during storage. Transfusion 1984;24:493–498.
38. Rubin RJ, Ness PM. What price progress? An update on vinyl plastic bags. Transfusion 1989;29:358–361.
39. Jacobson MS, Kevy SV, Grand RJ. Effects of a plasticizer leached from polyvinyl chloride on the subhuman primate: a consequence of chronic transfusion therapy. J Lab Clin Med 1977;89:1066–1079.
40. Hillman LS, Goodwin SL, Sherman WR. Identification and measurement of plasticizer in neonatal tissues after umbilical catheters and blood products. N Engl J Med 1975;292:381–386.
41. Kavlock R, Boekelheide K, Chapin R, et al. NTP Center for the Evaluation of Risks to Human Reproduction: phthalates expert panel report on the reproductive and developmental toxicity of di(2-ethylhexyl) phthalate. Reprod Toxicol 2002;16:529–653.
42. Hess JR, Greenwalt TG. Storage of red blood cells: new approaches. Transfus Med Rev 2002;16:283–295.
43. Scott KL, Lecak J, Acker JP. Biopreservation of red blood cells: past, present, and future. Transfus Med Rev 2005;19:127–142.
44. Valeri CR, Collins FB. Physiologic effects of 2,3-DPG-depleted red cells with high affinity for oxygen. J Appl Physiol 1971;31:823–827.
45. Beutler E, Wood L. The in vivo regeneration of red cell 2,3 diphosphoglyceric acid (DPG) after transfusion of stored blood. J Lab Clin Med 1969;74:300–304.
46. Valeri CR, Hirsch NM. Restoration in vivo of erythrocyte adenosine triphosphate, 2,3-diphosphoglycerate, potassium ion, and sodium ion concentrations following the transfusion of acid-citrate-dextrose-stored human red blood cells. J Lab Clin Med 1969;73:722–733.
47. Högman CF. Preparation and preservation of red cells. Vox Sang 1998;74(Suppl 2):177–187.
48. Kendrick D. Chapter IX. Preservative Solutions Blood. Program in World War II. Washington, D.C. Office of the Surgeon General, Department of the Army, U.S. Government Printing Office, 1964.
49. Moroff G, Sohmer PR, Button LN. Proposed standardization of methods for determining the 24-hour survival of stored red cells. Transfusion 1984;24:109–114.
50. Högman CF, Eriksson L, Gong J, et al. Half-strength citrate CPD combined with a new additive solution for improved storage of red blood cells suitable for clinical use. Vox Sang 1993;65:271–278.
51. Hess JR, Rugg N, Knapp AD, et al. Successful storage of RBCs for 10 weeks in a new additive solution. Transfusion 2000;40:1012–1016.
52. Hess JR, Rugg N, Knapp AD, et al. Successful storage of RBCs for 9 weeks in a new additive solution. Transfusion 2000;40:1007–1011.
53. Meryman HT, Hornblower ML, Syring RL. Prolonged storage of red cells at 4 degrees C. Transfusion 1986;26:500–505.
54. Hess JR, Hill HR, Oliver CK, et al. Twelve-week RBC storage. Transfusion 2003;43:867–872.
55. Ho J, Sibbald WJ, Chin-Yee IH. Effects of storage on efficacy of red cell transfusion: when is it not safe? Crit Care Med 2003;31(12 Suppl): S687–S697.
56. Leal-Noval SR, Jara-Lopez I, Garcia-Garmendia JL, et al. Influence of erythrocyte concentrate storage time on postsurgical morbidity in cardiac surgery patients. Anesthesiology 2003;98:815–822.
57. Zallen G, Offner PJ, Moore EE, et al. Age of transfused blood is an independent risk factor for postinjury multiple organ failure. Am J Surg 1999;178:570–572.
58. Marik PE, Sibbald WJ. Effect of stored-blood transfusion on oxygen delivery in patients with sepsis. JAMA 1993;269:3024–3029.
59. Purdy FR, Tweeddale MG, Merrick PM. Association of mortality with age of blood transfused in septic ICU patients. Can J Anaesth 1997;44:1256–1261.
60. Hogman CF, Knutson F, Loof H, et al. Improved maintenance of 2,3 DPG and ATP in RBCs stored in a modified additive solution. Transfusion 2002;42:824–829.
61. Kurup PA, Arun P, Gayathri NS, et al. Modified formulation of CPDA for storage of whole blood, and of SAGM for storage of red blood cells, to maintain the concentration of 2,3-diphosphoglycerate. Vox Sang 2003;85:253–261.
62. Hogman CF, Eriksson L, Wallvik J, et al. Clinical and laboratory experience with erythrocyte and platelet preparations from a 0.5CPD Erythro-Sol opti system. Vox Sang 1997;73:212–219.
63. Ebert R, Stead EA, Gibson JG. Response of normal subjects to acute blood loss. Arch Intern Med. 1941;68:578.
64. Howarth S, Sharpey-Schafer EP. Low blood-pressure phases following haemorrhage. Lancet 1947;1:18.
65. Standard 5.6.6.1.3: Silva MA (ed): Standards for Blood Bank and Transfusion Services, 23rd Edition. Bethesda, MD: AABB, 2004.
66. Trudnowski RJ, Rico RC. Specific gravity of blood and plasma at 4 and 37°C. Clin Chem 1974;20:615–616.
67. Simon TL, Hunt WC, Garry PJ. Iron supplementation for menstruating female blood donors. Transfusion 1984;24:469–472.

68. Code of Federal Regulations, 21 CFR 640.3(d): U.S. Government Printing Office, Washington, D.C. (revised annually).
69. Jeffrey G, Adams PC: Blood from patients with hereditary hemochromatosis—a wasted resource. Transfusion 1999;39:549–550.
70. FDA Guidance for Industry: Variances for collections from individuals with hereditary hemochromatosis, August 2001. Available at http://www.fda.gov/cber/gdlns/hemchrom.pdf. Accessed October 30, 2005.
71. Huh YO, Lichtiger B, Giacco GG, et al. Effect of donation time on platelet concentrates and fresh-frozen plasma. An in vitro study. Vox Sang 1989;56:21–24.
72. Reiss RF, Katz AJ. Platelets and factor VIII as functions of blood collection time. Transfusion 1976;16:229–231.
73. Brecher M, ed. Technical Manual, 14th ed. Bethesda, MD: AABB, 2002.
74. U.S. Food and Drug Administration (CBER). Revised Guidelines for the Collection of Platelets, Pheresis. Memorandum, October 1988.
75. U.S. Food and Drug Administration (CBER). Revisions of FDA Memorandum of August 27, 1982: Requirements for Infrequent Plasmapheresis Donors. Memorandum, March 1995.
76. FDA Guidance for Industry. Recommendations for collecting red blood cells by automated apheresis methods, January 2001. Available at http://www.fda.gov/cber/gdlns/rbcautoph2.pdf. Accessed October 30, 2005.
77. Standard 5.5.3.4: Silva MA (ed). Standards for Blood Bank and Transfusion Services, 23rd Edition. Bethesda, MD: AABB, 2004.
78. Standard 5.5.1: Silva MA (ed). Standards for Blood Bank and Transfusion Services, 23rd Edition. Bethesda, MD: AABB, 2004.
79. Code of Federal Regulations, 21 CFR 640.65, U.S. Government Printing Office, Washington, D.C., 2005 (revised annually).
80. U.S. Food and Drug Administration (CBER). Volume Limits for Automated Collection of Source Plasma. Memorandum, November 1992.
81. Standard 5.5.3.5: Silva MA (ed). Standards for Blood Bank and Transfusion Services, 23rd Edition. Bethesda, MD: AABB, 2004.
82. FDA Draft Guidance for Industry. Collection of platelets by automated methods. September 2005. (http://www.fda.gov/cber/gdlns/plateletauto.pdf). Accessed November 18, 2005.
83. Standard 5.5.4: Silva MA (ed). Standards for Blood Bank and Transfusion Services, 23rd Edition. Bethesda, MD: AABB, 2004.
84. Briones MA, Josephson CD, Hillyer CD. Granulocyte transfusion: Revisited. Curr Hematol Rep 2003;2:522–527.
85. Stroncek DF, Clay ME, Herr G, et al. Blood counts in healthy donors 1 year after the collection of granulocyte-colony-stimulating factor-mobilized progenitor cells and the results of a second mobilization and collection. Transfusion 1997;3:304–308.
86. MacHida U, Tojo A, Takahashi S, et al. The effect of granulocyte colony-stimulating factor administration in healthy donors before bone marrow harvesting. Br J Haematol 2000;108:747–753.
87. Liles WC, Huang JE, Llewellyn C, et al. A comparative trial of granulocyte-colony-stimulating factor and dexamethasone, separately and in combination, for the mobilization of neutrophils in the peripheral blood of normal volunteers. Transfusion 1997;37:182–187.
88. Einsele H, Northoff H, Neumeister B. Granulocyte transfusion. Vox Sang 2004;87(Suppl 2):205–208.
89. Lee JH, Leitman SF, Klein HG. A controlled comparison of the efficacy of hetastarch and pentastarch in granulocyte collections by centrifugal leukapheresis. Blood 1995;86:4662–4666.
90. Strauss RG. Review of the effects of hydroxyethyl starch on the blood coagulation system. Transfusion 1981;21:299–302.
91. Trivedi SM, Humphrey RL, Braine HG, et al. Hydroxyethyl starch serum levels in leukapheresis donors measured by modified periodic acid-Schiff staining technique. Transfusion 1984;24:260–263.
92. Maguire LC, Strauss RG, Koepke JA, et al. The elimination of hydroxyethyl starch from the blood of donors experiencing single or multiple intermittent-flow centrifugation leukapheresis. Transfusion 1981;21:347–353.
93. Standard 5.6.6.1.2.1: Silva MA (ed). Standards for Blood Bank and Transfusion Services, 23rd Edition. Bethesda, MD: AABB, 2004.
94. Standard 5.7.5.8: Silva MA (ed). Standards for Blood Bank and Transfusion Services, 23rd Edition. Bethesda, MD: AABB, 2004.
95. Standard 5.7.5.8.1: Silva MA (ed). Standards for Blood Bank and Transfusion Services, 23rd Edition. Bethesda, MD: AABB, 2004.
96. Laine E, Steadman R, Calhoun L, et al. Comparison of RBCs and FFP with whole blood during liver transplant surgery. Transfusion 2003;43:322–327.
97. Murphy S, Gardner FH. Effect of storage temperature on maintenance of platelet viability—deleterious effect of refrigerated storage. N Engl J Med 1969;280:1094–1098.
98. Murphy S, Gardner FH. Platelet storage at 22°C; metabolic, morphologic, and functional studies. J Clin Invest 1971;50:370–377.
99. Slichter SJ, Harker LA. Preparation and storage of platelet concentrates. I. Factors influencing the harvest of viable platelets from whole blood. Br J Haematol 1976;34:395–402.
100. Kahn RA, Cossette I, Friedman LI. Optimum centrifugation conditions for the preparation of platelet and plasma products. Transfusion 1976;16:162–165.
101. Hogman CF, Eriksson L, Hedlund K, et al. The bottom and top system: a new technique for blood component preparation and storage. Vox Sang 1988;55:211–217.
102. Murphy S. Platelets from pooled buffy coats: an update. Transfusion 2005;45:634–639.
103. Murphy S, Heaton WA, Rebulla P. Platelet production in the Old World—and the New. Transfusion 1996;36:751–754.
104. Janetzko K, Kluter H, van Waeg G, et al. Fully automated processing of buffy-coat-derived pooled platelet concentrates. Transfusion 2004;44:1052–1058.
105. Valeri CR. Use of rejuvenation solutions in blood preservation. Crit Rev Clin Lab Sci 1982;17:299–374.
106. Package Insert. Rejuvesol. Braintree, Mass. enCyte Systems, 1997.
107. Valeri CR, Gray AD, Cassidy GP, et al. The 24-hour posttransfusion survival, oxygen transport function, and residual hemolysis of human outdated-rejuvenated red cell concentrates after washing and storage at 4°C for 24 to 72 hours. Transfusion 1984;24:323–326.
108. Szymanski IO, Teno RA, Lockwood WB, et al. Effect of rejuvenation and frozen storage on 42-day-old AS-1 RBCs. Transfusion 2001;41:550–555.
109. Valeri CR, Zaroulis CG, Vecchione JJ, et al. Therapeutic effectiveness and safety of outdated human red blood cells rejuvenated to restore oxygen transport function to normal, frozen for 3 to 4 years at –80°C, washed, and stored at 4°C for 24 hours prior to rapid infusion. Transfusion 1980;20:159–170.
110. Valeri CR, Ragno G, Pivacek LE, et al. An experiment with glycerol-frozen red blood cells stored at –80°C for up to 37 years. Vox Sang 2000;79:168–174.
111. Umlas J, Jacobson M, Kevy SV: Suitable survival and half-life of red cells after frozen storage in excess of 10 years. Transfusion 1991;31:648–649.
112. Valeri CR, Pivacek LE, Gray AD, et al. The safety and therapeutic effectiveness of human red cells stored at -80°C for as long as 21 years. Transfusion 1989;29:429–437.
113. Lecak J, Scott K, Young C, et al. Evaluation of red blood cells stored at -80°C in excess of 10 years. Transfusion 2004;44:1306–1313.
114. Mazur P. Freezing of living cells: mechanisms and implications. Am J Physiol 1984;247(3 Pt 1):C125–C142.
115. Rowe AW, Eyster E, Kellner A. Liquid nitrogen preservation of red blood cells for transfusion: a low glycerol-rapid freeze procedure. Cryobiology 1968;5:119–128.
116. Valeri CR. Simplification of the methods for adding and removing glycerol during freeze-preservation of human red blood cells with the high or low glycerol methods: biochemical modification prior to freezing. Transfusion 1975;15:195–218.
117. Hess JR. Red cell freezing and its impact on the supply chain. Transfus Med 2004;14:1–8.
118. Meryman HT, Hornblower M. A method for freezing and washing red blood cells using a high glycerol concentration. Transfusion 1972;12:145–156.
119. Valeri CR, Ragno G, Pivacek L, et al. In vivo survival of apheresis RBCs, frozen with 40-percent (wt/vol) glycerol, deglycerolized in the ACP 215, and stored at 4°C in AS-3 for up to 21 days. Transfusion 2001;41:928–932.
120. Valeri CR, Ragno G, Pivacek LE, et al. A multicenter study of in vitro and in vivo values in human RBCs frozen with 40-percent (wt/vol) glycerol and stored after deglycerolization for 15 days at 4°C in AS-3: assessment of RBC processing in the ACP 215. Transfusion 2001;41:933–939.
121. Valeri CR, Srey R, Tilahun D, et al. The in vitro quality of red blood cells frozen with 40 percent (wt/vol) glycerol at -80°C for 14 years, deglycerolized with the Haemonetics ACP 215, and stored at 4°C in additive solution-1 or additive solution-3 for up to 3 weeks. Transfusion 2004;44:990–995.
122. Valeri CR, Pivacek LE, Cassidy GP, et al. In vitro and in vivo measurements of human RBCs frozen with glycerol and subjected to various storage temperatures before deglycerolization and storage at 4°C for 3 days. Transfusion 2001;41:401–405.
123. Hmel PJ, Kennedy A, Quiles JG, et al. Physical and thermal properties of blood storage bags: implications for shipping frozen components on dry ice. Transfusion 2002;42:836–846.
124. Valeri CR, Lane JP, Srey R, et al. Incidence of breakage of human RBCs frozen with 40-percent wt/vol glycerol using two different methods for storage at -80°C. Transfusion 2003;43:411–414.

125. Bannai M, Mazda T, Sasakawa S. The effects of pH and agitation on platelet preservation. Transfusion 1985;25:57–59.
126. Hunter S, Nixon J, Murphy S. The effect of the interruption of agitation on platelet quality during storage for transfusion. Transfusion 2001;41:809–814.
127. Brecher ME, Holland PV, Pineda AA, et al. Growth of bacteria in inoculated platelets: implications for bacteria detection and the extension of platelet storage. Transfusion 2000;40:1308–1312.
128. Goldman M, Blajchman MA. Blood product-associated bacterial sepsis. Transfus Med Rev 1991;5:73–83.
129. Dumont LJ, AuBuchon JP, Whitley P, et al. Seven-day storage of single-donor platelets: recovery and survival in an autologous transfusion study. Transfusion 2002;42:847–854.
130. Wagner SJ, Robinette D. Evaluation of swirling, pH, and glucose tests for the detection of bacterial contamination in platelet concentrates. Transfusion 1996;36:989–993.
131. Chambers LA, Long KF, Wissel ME, et al. Multisite trial of a pH paper and a pH value of less than 7.0 to screen whole-blood-derived platelets: implications for bacterial detection. Transfusion 2004;44:1261–1263.
132. Hay SN, Brecher ME. Validation of pH and glucose determination for bacteria detection screening in platelet concentrates stored in the Terumo Teruflex XT612 platelet container. Transfusion 2004;44:1395.
133. Brecher ME, Means N, Jere CS, et al. Evaluation of an automated culture system for detecting bacterial contamination of platelets: an analysis with 15 contaminating organisms. Transfusion 2001;41:477–482.
134. Larsen CP, Ezligini F, Hermansen NO, et al. Six years' experience of using the BacT/ALERT system to screen all platelet concentrates, and additional testing of outdated platelet concentrates to estimate the frequency of false-negative results. Vox Sang 2005;88:93–97.
135. AuBuchon JP, Cooper LK, Leach MF, et al. Experience with universal bacterial culturing to detect contamination of apheresis platelet units in a hospital transfusion service. Transfusion 2002;42:855–861.
136. Vostal JG. FDA's current considerations for 7 day platelets and bacterial detection in single and pooled platelet products, January 25, 2005. Available at http://www.hhs.gov/bloodsafety/presentations/Vostal- FDA Positionfor7dayplatelets.pdf. Accessed October 30, 2005.
137. Moroff G, Holme S, Dabay MH, et al. Storage of pools of six and eight platelet concentrates. Transfusion 1993;33:374–378.
138. Snyder EL, Stack G, Napychank P, et al. Storage of pooled platelet concentrates. In vitro and in vivo analysis. Transfusion 1989;29:390–395.
139. Ferrer F, Rivera J, Corral J, et al. Evaluation of pooled platelet concentrates using prestorage versus poststorage WBC reduction: impact of filtration timing. Transfusion 2000;40:781–788.
140. Wagner SJ, Robinette D, Nazario M, et al. Bacteria levels in components prepared from deliberately inoculated whole blood held for 8 or 24 hours at 20 to 24 degrees C. Transfusion 1995;35:911–916.
141. Sweeney JD, Kouttab NM, Holme S, et al. Prestorage pooled whole-blood-derived leukoreduced platelets stored for seven days, preserve acceptable quality and do not show evidence of a mixed lymphocyte reaction. Transfusion 2004;44:1212–1219.
142. Heddle NM, Barty RL, Sigouin CS, et al. In vitro evaluation of prestorage pooled leukoreduced whole blood-derived platelets stored for up to 7 days. Transfusion 2005;45:904–910.
143. Heddle NM, Cook RJ, Blajchman MA, et al. Assessing the effectiveness of whole blood-derived platelets stored as a pool: a randomized block noninferiority trial. Transfusion 2005;45:896–903.
144. Tovey LA, Lathe GH. Caeruloplasmin and green plasma in women taking oral contraceptives, in pregnant women, and in patients with rheumatoid arthritis. Lancet 1968;2:596–600.
145. Wolf P, Enlander D, Dalziel J, et al. Green plasma in blood donors. N Engl J Med 1969;281:205.
146. American Society of Anesthesiologists Task Force on Blood Component Therapy. Practice guidelines for blood component therapy. Anesthesiology 1996;84:732–747.
147. O'Shaughnessy DF, Atterbury C, Bolton Maggs P, et al. Guidelines for the use of fresh-frozen plasma, cryoprecipitate and cryosupernatant. Br J Haematol 2004;126:11–28.
148. Cardigan R, Lawrie AS, Mackie IJ, et al. The quality of fresh-frozen plasma produced from whole blood stored at 4°C overnight. Transfusion 2005;45:1342–1348.
149. Weisert O, Jeremic M. Preservation of coagulation factors V and VIII during collection and subsequent storage of bank blood in ACD-A and CPD solutions. Vox Sang 1973;24:126–133.
150. Nilsson L, Hedner U, Nilsson IM, et al. Shelf-life of bank blood and stored plasma with special reference to coagulation factors. Transfusion 1983;23:377–381.
151. Kakaiya RM, Morse EE, Panek S. Labile coagulation factors in thawed fresh frozen plasma prepared by two methods. Vox Sang 1984;46:44–46.
152. O'Neill EM, Rowley J, Hansson-Wicher M, et al. Effect of 24-hour whole-blood storage on plasma clotting factors. Transfusion 1999;39:488–491.
153. Sohmer PR, Bolin RB, Scott RL, et al. Effect of delayed refrigeration on plasma factors in whole blood collected in CPDA-2. Transfusion 1982;22:488–490.
154. Churchill WH, Schmidt B, Lindsey J, et al. Thawing fresh frozen plasma in a microwave oven. A comparison with thawing in a 37°C waterbath. Am J Clin Pathol 1992;97:227–232.
155. Rock G, Tackaberry ES, Dunn JG, et al. Rapid controlled thawing of fresh-frozen plasma in a modified microwave oven. Transfusion 1984;24:60–65.
156. Suontaka AM, Silveira A, Soderstrom T, et al. Occurrence of cold activation of transfusion plasma during storage at +4°C. Vox Sang 2005;88:172–180.
157. Blomback M, Chmielewska J, Netre C, et al. Activation of blood coagulation, fibrinolytic and kallikrein systems during storage of plasma. Vox Sang 1984;47:355–342.
158. Buchta C, Felfernig M, Hocker P, et al. Stability of coagulation factors in thawed, solvent/detergent-treated plasma during storage at 4°C for 6 days. Vox Sang 2004;87:182–186.
159. Code of Federal Regulations, 21 CFR 601.22: U.S. Government Publishing Office, Washington, D.C. (revised annually).
160. Code of Federal Regulations 21 CFR 610.40: U.S. Government Printing Office, Washington, D.C. (revised annually).
161. Code of Federal Regulations, 21 CFR 640.65 2005: U.S. Government Printing Office, Washington, D.C. (revised annually).
162. Pantanowitz L, Kruskall MS, Uhl L. Cryoprecipitate. Patterns of use. Am J Clin Pathol 2003;119:874–881.
163. Hughes C, Thomas KB, Schiff P, et al. Effect of delayed blood processing on the yield of factor VIII in cryoprecipitate and factor VIII concentrate. Transfusion 1988;28:566–570.
164. McCullough J, Weiblen BJ, Fine D. Effects of storage of granulocytes on their fate in vivo. Transfusion 1983;23:20–24.
165. Glasser L, Lane TA, McCullough J, et al. Neutrophil concentrates: functional considerations, storage, and quality control. J Clin Apher 1983;1:179–184.
166. FDA Compliance Program Manual. Chapter 42: Blood and Blood Products: Inspection of Licensed and Unlicensed Blood Banks, Brokers, Reference Laboratories, and Contractors - 7342.001. FDA Office of Regulatory Affairs. Available at http://www.fda.gov/cber/7342001bld.htm. Accessed October 12, 2005.
167. Ratko TA, Cummings JP, Oberman HA, et al. Evidence-based recommendations for the use of WBC-reduced cellular blood components. Transfusion 2001;41:1310–1319.
168. Standard 5.7.4.1 Silva MA (ed). Standards for Blood Bank and Transfusion Services, 23rd Edition. Bethesda, Md, AABB, 2004.
169. Lutz P, Dzik WH. Large-volume hemocytometer chamber for accurate counting of white cells (WBCs) in WBC reduced platelets: Validation and application for quality control of WBC-reduced platelets prepared by apheresis and filtration. Transfusion 1993;33:409–412.
170. Dzik S, Moroff G, Dumont L. A multicenter study evaluating three methods for counting residual WBCs in WBC-reduced blood components: nageotte hemocytometry, flow cytometry, and microfluorometry. Transfusion 2000;40:513–520.
171. Buck SA, Kickler TS, McGuire M, et al. The utility of platelet washing using an automated procedure for severe platelet allergic reactions. Transfusion 1987;27:391–393.
172. Vesilind GW, Simpson MB, Shifman MA, et al. Evaluation of a centrifugal blood cell processor for washing platelet concentrates. Transfusion 1988;28:46–51.
173. Weisbach V, Riego W, Strasser E, et al. The in vitro quality of washed, prestorage leucocyte-depleted red blood cell concentrates. Vox Sang 2004;87:19–26.
174. Kalmin ND, Brown DJ. Platelet washing with a blood cell processor. Transfusion 1982;22:125–127.
175. Toth CB, Kramer J, Pinter J, et al. IgA content of washed red blood cell concentrates. Vox Sang 1998;74:13–14.
176. Orlin JB, Ellis MH. Transfusion-associated graft-versus-host disease. Curr Opin Hematol 1997;4:442–448.
177. FDA Guidance for Industry. Gamma irradiation of blood and blood components: a pilot program for licensing, February 2000. Available at http://www.fda.gov/cber/gdlns/gamma.pdf. Accessed November 18, 2005.
178. Pelszynski MM, Moroff G, Luban NL, et al. Effect of gamma irradiation of red blood cell units on T-cell inactivation as assessed by limiting dilution analysis: Implications for preventing transfusion-associated graft-versus-host disease. Blood 1994;83:1683–1689.

179. Luban NL, Drothler D, Moroff G, et al. Irradiation of platelet components: Inhibition of lymphocyte proliferation assessed by limiting-dilution analysis. Transfusion 2000;40:348–352.
180. Davey RJ, McCoy NC, Yu M, et al. The effect of prestorage irradiation on posttransfusion red cell survival. Transfusion 1992;32:525–528.
181. Mintz PD, Anderson G. Effect of gamma irradiation on the in vivo recovery of stored red blood cells. Ann Clin Lab Sci 1993;23:216–220.
182. Hillyer CD, Tiegerman KO, Berkman EM. Evaluation of the red cell storage lesion after irradiation in filtered packed red cell units. Transfusion 1991;31:497–499.
183. U.S. Food and Drug Administration (CBER). Guideline for the Uniform Labeling of Blood and Blood Components, August 1985. Available at http://www.fda.gov/cber/gdlns/unilabel.pdf. Accessed November 18, 2005.
184. Wallas CH. Closing the technology gap with supermarkets: implementation of ISBT 128. Transfusion 2005;45:1054–1055.
185. FDA Guidance for Industry. Recognition and use of a standard for the uniform labeling of blood and blood components, June 2000. Available at http://www.fda.gov/cber/gdlns/unilabbld.pdf. Accessed November 18, 2005.
186. AABB Association Bulletin #05–12, October 12, 2005.
187. Ashford P (ed). An Introduction to ISBT 128, 2nd Edition: ICCBBA, Inc, 2002.
188. Federal Register. 68 FR 146 July 30, 2003.
189. Federal Register. 67 FR 53118, August 14, 2002. Available at http://www.cdc.gov/od/ohs/pdffiles/DOTHazMat8-14-02.pdf. Accessed November 18, 2005.
190. George VM, Pringle TC, Kline L, et al. Development and evaluation of a shipping system for platelet components. Transfusion 1996;36:335–338.

Chapter 13

Red Blood Cell Metabolism during Storage: Basic Principles and Practical Aspects

John R. Hess • Ginine M. Beyer

INTRODUCTION

The mature human red blood cell (RBC), lacking nucleus and mitochondria, is released into the vascular space with a protein content that is 97% hemoglobin. Over its approximately 120-day life span, the RBC circulates, carrying oxygen nested in hemoglobin molecules and deriving nutrients from and excreting waste into the plasma. The demise of this apparently simple and monofunctional cell was historically assumed to be due to the slow breakdown of its metabolic machinery.

The RBC is now recognized to be more than just "a hapless sack of hemoglobin."[1] RBCs have a focused and sophisticated metabolism that supports biophysical responses to environmental changes and allows programmed cell death. RBC metabolism includes the glycolytic pathways producing both energy (as adenosine 5′- triphosphate, or *ATP*) and oxidation-reduction intermediates that support oxygen transport and membrane flexibility.[2] RBCs interact with their environment by changing shape in response to pH and by secreting ATP in response to sheer forces and nitric oxide in response to hypoxia.[3–5] At the end of their life span, RBCs undergo programmed cell death in two ways: by racemization of negatively charged membrane phospholipids in response to calcium or low concentrations of ATP, and by the active loss of membrane through microvesiculation.[6] Increasing knowledge of RBC metabolism and homeostasis has led to better understanding of the so-called red cell "storage lesion" and to improved methods of preserving viable RBCs for transfusion and as blood bank reagents.

The *storage lesion* is a blanket term used to encompass all of the "bad" things that happen to RBCs during storage.[7] These "bad" things include: decreased concentrations of ATP and 2,3-diphosphoglycerate (2,3-DPG), increased concentrations of extracellular potassium, changes in cell shape, loss of RBC viability, and hemolysis. Although elevated extracellular potassium concentrations in stored RBC units are not usually of clinical significance, they can, however, be fatal if RBC concentrates are infused in large volumes through central vascular catheters, as in neonatal exchange transfusions or when priming cardiopulmonary bypass machines.[8] Hemolysis results not only in a reduction of the relative number of stored RBCs that survive when returned to circulation, but also in the release of harmful breakdown products. Free hemoglobin causes vasoconstriction, endothelial cell activation, and renal tubular damage.[9] Free membrane phospholipids are procoagulant. The clinical consequences of the early forms of RBC shape change or reduced 2,3-DPG concentrations are much less clear. The loss of viability during storage reduces the effective transfused RBC dose, but the consequences of administering intact but nonviable cells are not known.[7]

The evolution of RBC storage solutions and storage systems has been driven historically by military need and funding for durable blood products, rather than by academic interests.[10,11] However, the addition of phosphate and adenine to blood storage solutions followed the recognition of the roles these compounds play in normal RBC metabolism.[12] The development of plastic bags and separate RBC additive solutions was a response to the need for sterile blood plasma for fractionation.[13] Leukoreduction of blood components was first undertaken as a safety measure, and only secondarily recognized to improve the quality of stored RBCs. Unfortunately, regulatory controversy and clinical inertia slowed the inclusion of these technical advances into routine clinical practice to about one per decade. In the past 10 years, however, the basic sciences of red cell metabolism and physiology have broken important new ground. These discoveries provide a basis for future advances in blood storage and product use that is at once broad, fertile, and reliable.

RBC METABOLIC PATHWAYS

RBCs use energy to pump ions and phospholipids, limit the effects of oxidation, and shed membrane.[14] RBC function depends on ion pumping and maintaining phospholipid asymmetry. If the cells do not pump out calcium and move the negatively charged phospholipid phosphatidylserine to the inner surface of their membrane, they are rapidly removed from circulation. The binding of oxygen to hemoglobin is not perfectly reversible.[15] In about 1% of binding events, the oxygen takes an electron from the hemoglobin iron, thus forming superoxide and methemoglobin. Methemoglobin is unstable and will not bind oxygen.[16] Without a methemoglobin reductase system, RBCs would function for only a few hours.[17] Some of the superoxide formed in hemoglobin oxidation goes on to damage membrane lipids.[18] RBCs have a mechanism to concentrate these damaged lipids and shed them in membrane microvesicles.[19]

RBC energy metabolism, in turn, uses four major biochemical pathways.[2] The Embden-Meyerhof glycolytic pathway allows glucose to be broken down to two molecules of lactate, with the net production of two molecules of ATP and two molecules of reduced nicotinamide-adenine dinucleotide (NADH). This pathway is the major source of biochemical energy for cellular processes and of reducing equivalents for methemoglobin reduction. The Rapoport-Leubering shunt diverts 1,3-diphosphoglycerate from the mainstream of glycolysis to allow the production of 2,3-DPG in a pH-regulated manner.[20] The hexose monophosphate shunt is an alternative pathway of glycolysis that produces reduced nicotinamide-adenine dinucleotide phosphate (NADPH) for glutathione reduction. This shunt can also accept ribose phosphate from inosine breakdown as an alternative energy source. Purine metabolic pathways provide adenine monophosphate (AMP) and adenine diphosphate (ADP) as substrates for ATP production. Enzymes involved in these energy pathways represent about 10% of the more than 300 proteins found in RBCs.

Embden-Meyerhof Pathway

Figure 13–1 shows the Embden-Meyerhof glycolytic pathway with the associated Rapoport-Leubering shunt.[2,21] In the first three steps of the glycolytic pathway, glucose is phosphorylated to glucose-6-phosphate, isomerized to fructose-6-phosphate, and phosphorylated again to fructose-1,6-diphosphate. Both the first and third steps require a molecule of ATP. Even in the presence of glucose, glycolysis stops if ATP is depleted. In the fourth step, the six carbon sugar fructose-1,6-diphosphate is broken down into two phosphorylated molecules of three carbons each. One of those molecules is glyceraldehyde-3-phosphate, and the other is dihydroxyacetone phosphate, which is then isomerized to glyceraldehyde-3-phosphate, as well. In the fifth step, the glyceraldehyde-3-phosphate is phosphorylated again to 1,3-diphosphoglycerate, with the energy provided by its dehydrogenation and with the simultaneous reduction of a molecule of NAD to NADH. In the final five steps of the pathway, 1,3-diphosphoglycerate gives up a phosphate to make a molecule of ATP and form 3-phosphoglyceric acid; 3-phosphoglyceric acid is mutated to 2-phosphoglyceric acid, which in turn is isomerized to phospho(enol)pyruvate; phospho(enol)pyruvate transfers its phosphate to ADP to make ATP and pyruvate; and pyruvate is oxidized to lactate, again reducing NAD to NADH. The result of this pathway is that one molecule of glucose is broken down to two molecules of lactate anion and two protons, with the net production of two molecules of ATP and two molecules of NADH.

The rates of glycolysis in the Embden-Meyerhof pathway are directly controlled by the availability of the substrates for its initial reactions, glucose and ATP, and by pH and PO_2.[22] Glucose can be replaced by fructose, both of which pass freely into human RBCs through a specific hexose transporter.[23] However, the initial energy-requiring steps of the pathway cannot be bypassed by providing the phosphorylated forms of the sugars, because these are not transported across the RBC membrane. As decreasing pH reduces the rate of glycolysis, a point is reached where ATP production does not keep up with ATP use. If glucose is removed and the RBC ATP concentrations are allowed to decrease, a point is reached where adding glucose back only rescues a fraction of the cells.

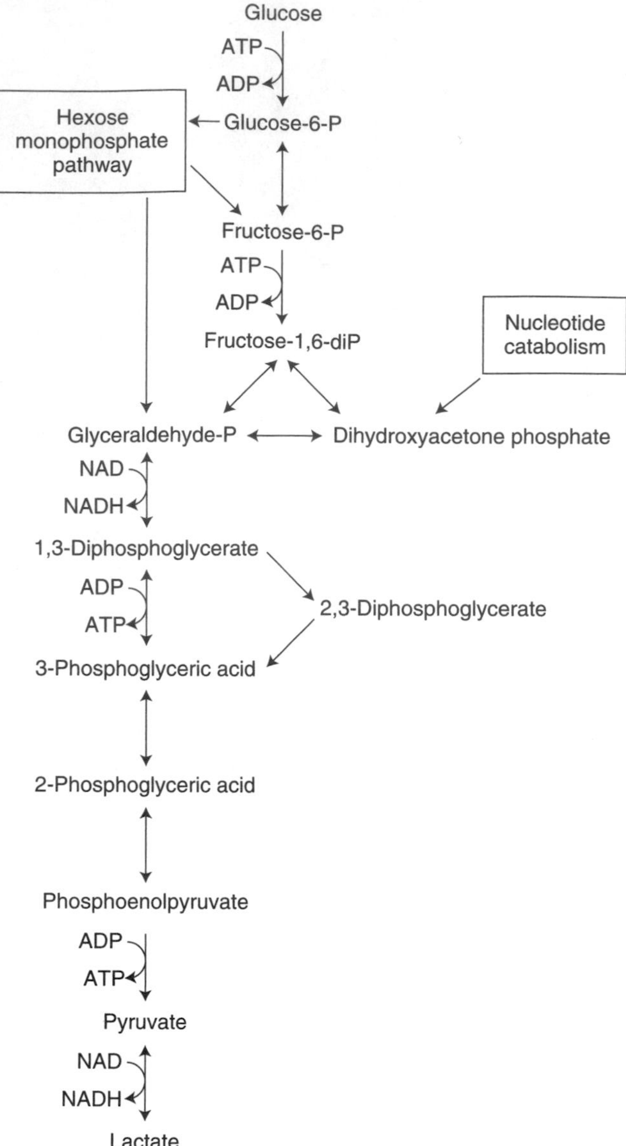

Figure 13–1 The Embden-Meyerhof glycolytic pathway along with the associated Rapoport-Leubering shunt. (From Beutler E. Red cell metabolism and storage. In Anderson KC, Ness PM, [eds]: Scientific Basis of Transfusion Medicine: Implications for Clinical Practice. Philadelphia, WB Saunders, 1994, pp 188–202.)

Rapoport-Leubering and Hexose Monophosphate Shunts

The Rapoport-Leubering shunt, also shown in Figure 13–1, allows 1,3-diphosphoglycerate to be mutated into 2,3-DPG. At an intracellular pH greater than 7.2, large amounts of 2,3-DPG are produced.[20] In the cell, 2,3-DPG serves as a steric effector of hemoglobin, stabilizing deoxyhemoglobin and thereby shifting the hemoglobin oxygen equilibrium curve to the right (reducing oxygen affinity). 2,3-DPG is broken down by phosphatase activity to 3-phosphoglyceric acid. The Rapoport-Leubering shunt thus makes 2,3-DPG at the expense of bypassing the ATP-making step in glycolysis from 1,3-diphosphoglycerate to 3-phosphoglyceric acid. If all of the three-carbon glycerate phosphates made from glucose went through the Rapoport-Leubering shunt, there would be no net ATP production from glycolysis.

The hexose monophosphate or pentose shunt also branches from and feeds back into the Embden-Meyerhof pathway, again shown as a block in Figure 13–1. In the first three steps, glucose-6-phosphate is dehydrogenated twice, making two molecules of NADPH for glutathione synthesis and reduction, at the cost of a carbon lost as CO_2, and leaving a pentose phosphate. In the remainder of the pathway, the pentose phosphates are variously isomerized, and pairs of them are mutated into 4- and 6- and 3- and 7-carbon phosphated sugars. The 3- and 6-carbon phosphated sugars, glyceraldehyde-3-phosphate and fructose-6-phosphate, respectively, can return to the Embden-Meyerhof pathway. Moreover, the pentose phosphate pool can be fed with ribose-1-phosphate from the breakdown of inosine monophosphate (IMP), providing a pathway for the manufacture of ATP and NADH in the distal Embden-Meyerhof pathway that is independent of both glucose and initial stores of ATP. The flux of sugars through the upper end of the hexose monophosphate shunt is regulated by the availability of NADP (i.e., the level of redox stress on the RBC) and the lower half by the availability of pentose phosphates.

RBC Nucleotide Metabolism

Nucleotide metabolism is necessary to maintain substrates that support the formation of the high-energy intermediate ATP and guanosine triphosphate (GTP). In the RBC, adenine and phosphoribosylpyrophosphate are converted to AMP, and adenosine can be activated to AMP by ATP. AMP, in turn, can also be activated to ADP by ATP. ATP is made from ADP and phosphate by specific enzymes in the lower limb of the Embden-Meyerhof pathway. ATP and AMP can also be made from two ADP, because the ADP activating reaction is reversible. AMP is slowly and irreversibly deaminated to form IMP, which is further broken down to hypoxanthine and pentose phosphate.

A similar set of enzymes supports the maintenance of GTP. GTP does not appear to have a role as an energy intermediate in RBCs, but instead it serves as a concentration-dependent inhibitor of the enzyme transglutaminase that crosslinks proteins in a primitive coagulation process.[24] Thus, maintaining normal concentrations of GTP appears to be necessary to prevent transglutaminase from randomly cross-linking RBC proteins, thereby damaging protein function and membrane flexibility.

THE STORAGE LESION

When RBCs are stored in liquid suspension in the cold, metabolism slows, metabolic byproducts and cellular breakdown products accumulate in the suspending fluid in the closed container, and the RBCs change shape, lose viability, and finally rupture.[7] The slowing of metabolism is the desired result of cooling, in that it allows RBCs to be stored for longer periods than is possible at room or body temperature. However, during storage, potassium and hemoglobin increase in concentration in the suspending plasma, and the pH falls. At the same time, the cells develop bumps, followed by spicules from which microvesicles bleb, and the cells finally fall apart. Overall, a decreasing fraction of RBCs survives after being returned to the circulation. These changes are collectively known as the *storage lesion.*

RBC glycolysis slows threefold for each 10°C decrease in temperature.[25] Thus, a conventional unit of RBCs can be stored about a day at 37°C, 3 to 4 days at room temperature, and 5 to 6 weeks at 1°C to 6°C. With each of those times and temperatures, sufficient glucose is metabolized to produce enough protons to reduce the pH to the point where further metabolism is inhibited; ATP concentrations then fall to levels that do not support cell viability.

However, the thermal coefficients of all of the individual enzymes and pumps in the RBC are not the same. This is most readily seen for the Na-K ATPase that pumps potassium into, and sodium out of, the RBC. At 4°C, the pump's activity is well below the small ion conductance of the membrane, leading to a decrease in cytosolic potassium concentration and a corresponding increase in extracellular potassium of about 1 mEq/L/day. The resulting high suspending fluid potassium concentrations are occasionally clinically important, causing arrhythmias when old RBC concentrates are infused at high volume into the central circulation, but the ion loss does not seem to have any direct effect on RBC viability.

The decreasing pH of metabolically active stored RBC inhibits the production of 2,3-DPG. Normal venous blood typically has a pH of about 7.35. When acidic storage solutions are added, the pH is reduced to below 7.2, and the Rapoport-Leubering shunt is largely bypassed during glycolysis. The concentrations of 2,3-DPG then fall over the first 10 days of storage.

During storage, RBCs change shape.[26] The biconcave disks first develop a knobbled appearance, which progresses into blunt echinocytic projections, and then into sharp spicules from which microvesicles are shed. The early stages in this process are reversible with warming, but the shedding of membrane cannot be undone. Membrane loss makes RBCs smaller and more rigid as they become spherical and finally rupture. The shape change progression can be measured by RBC morphology scoring systems, whereas the loss of membrane is seen as increasing osmotic fragility or shed microvesicle mass. However, the relationship between RBC membrane loss and reduced cell viability when returned to the circulation is not known.

The functional viability of RBCs during storage is measured by their ability to persist when returned to the circulation. Differential agglutination, radioactive labeling, and biotin labeling with flow cytometry have all been used to measure the persisting infused cell fraction. Most recent experience has depended on chromium-51 labeling of stored RBCs, and standard methods for the measurement have been published.[27] In most such studies, stored RBCs are labeled and returned to the circulation of the donor who initially provided them. Performed correctly, this practice prevents the transmission of disease to study subjects and avoids alloimmune removal of the cells that would invalidate the measurements.

A portion of the infused labeled and stored RBCs is cleared rapidly from the circulation, so the standard measurement for comparing storage systems is the fraction of infused cells that remains in the circulation 24 hours after infusion. Determining this fraction from the concentration of cells circulating at 24 hours requires a reasonable estimate of the number of cells circulating immediately after infusion. This number can be determined by statistical regression of a series of early measures made between 5 and 15 minutes after infusion back to the time of infusion, or by labeling fresh cells with a second isotope, such as technicium-99m, to obtain an independent measure of the whole body RBC volume. When the fraction of infused stored RBCs surviving for 24 hours (the *recovery*) is greater than 80%, the rapidly cleared fraction tends to be small, and the two estimates are usually close. Double-label recovery measures are useful for understanding poor recovery, but single-label measures are often sufficient when recoveries are high. Fifty years of storage studies using chromium-51 recovery measures have consistently shown that RBCs that persist in the circulation for 24 hours survive normally and have a 50-day half-life.

An important insight into the meaning of the early loss of RBCs in recovery measurements comes from work by Hogman and his colleagues in a study of the effect of metabolic rejuvenation.[28] RBCs stored for 6 weeks had a mean recovery of 77%. When RBCs from the same units were metabolically rejuvenated by warming and replenishing glycolytic intermediates with pyruvate, adenine, inosine, and phosphate for two hours, the recovery rose to 89%. Thus, more than half of the stored RBCs removed from the circulation in the first 24 hours were not dead.

It is now clear that stored RBCs do not just run out of metabolic energy. Rather, they are undergoing a program of cell death.[29] The program includes the racemization of negatively charged membrane phospholipids and the loss of membrane by microvesiculation. These activities are also components of the apoptotic process in nucleated cells. Both of these processes are inhibited by normal concentrations of ATP in RBCs, and the racemization of phospholipids is reversible with the restoration of ATP concentrations in the metabolic rejuvenation process just described. The relative contributions of senescent RBC death and programmed RBC death can be estimated in the ratio of microvesicular hemoglobin to free hemoglobin in the suspending fluid of stored RBCs.

RBC STORAGE IN LIQUID MEDIA

History

Lee described the use of citrate as an anticoagulant for human blood in 1913, and Rous and Turner showed that glucose delayed the hemolysis of RBC suspended in saline in 1915.[30] Rous and Turner went on to make the first RBC storage solution of citrate and glucose and showed that rabbit RBCs could be stored for 4 weeks with minimal hemolysis.[31] When the stored RBCs were returned to the rabbit donors, the hematocrit increased without significant bilirubinuria.[32] Robertson, who worked with Lee at Harvard and then with Rous and Turner at the Rockefeller, used their storage solution to collect group O whole blood in bottles and then demonstrated the utility of this stored blood as a resuscitation fluid on the battlefields of France in World War I.[33] Mollison has eloquently described the importance of the combination of citrate and glucose, saying that citrate allows the donor and the recipient to be separated in space, whereas glucose allows them to be separated in time. These and more sophisticated storage solutions are the basis for modern RBC banking.[34]

A problem with the original Rous-Turner solution was that the RBCs were stored in very dilute suspensions, 70% solution to 30% blood for a storage hematocrit of about 12%. In the late 1930s, DeGowin reformulated the solution for 60:40 mixtures, and in the early 1940s, Alsever again modified the solutions for 50:50 ratios.[35,36] However, the major advance during World War II was Loutit and Mollison's acid citrate dextrose (ACD) solution, designed for use in a 1:4 ratio and later concentrated further for 1:7 mixing with whole blood.[37] Acidifying the solution to pH 5.5 allowed the citrate and glucose to be autoclaved together without caramelizing the sugar, so that blood collection sets could be manufactured and distributed with sterile vacuum bottles containing premixed anticoagulant. Concentrated whole blood, and later, packed RBCs, made resuscitation faster. Sterile ACD allowed RBCs to be stored with minimal hemolysis for 3 weeks.

In addition to reduced bacterial contamination, the new ACD solution improved in vivo RBC recovery despite the acid pH. It took a decade to determine that ACD solution had little buffer capacity, so that its acidity did not much reduce the initial pH of stored blood. At the same time, the lower volume of anticoagulant solution added to whole blood reduced the amount of phosphate that diffused from stored RBCs, leaving more intracellular phosphate as a substrate for ATP production.[38] This realization led to the addition of phosphate to ACD to make citrate phosphate dextrose (CPD) solution. The added phosphate did increase the anticoagulant solution buffer capacity, but the resulting lower initial pH of the stored blood was less important than the provision of the metabolic substrate. CPD was better than ACD in clinical testing, providing higher in vivo recoveries and reduced hemolysis. Based on these results, CPD was considered but never approved for 4-week storage of whole blood.

Subsequent advancements in RBC storage include plastic bags in the 1960s, adenine to make citrate phosphate dextrose adenine (CPDA-1) for 5-week RBC storage in the 1970s, separate RBC additive solutions for 6-week storage in the 1980s, and leukoreduction in the 1990s.[39] This slow developmental cycle meant that CPDA-1, a solution designed for whole blood storage, was finally licensed eleven years later in the era of blood components. However, when plasma was removed to make component plasma products and platelets, the in vivo recovery of the stored packed RBCs decreased due to insufficient glucose.[40,41] Additive solutions were developed to replace the volume and nutrients removed with plasma, resulting in RBC survival that was as good or better than in native plasma. Current leukoreduced RBC concentrates in additive solution can be stored for 6 weeks with an 82% mean recovery and about 0.4% hemolysis. Leukocyte reduction, by removing highly metabolically active cells that will decrease the pH of the storage solution, and by removing sources of proteases and phospholipases that damage RBCs, generally improves the measured recovery of current 6-week stored RBC by about 4%.

Current Liquid RBC Storage Systems

Two types of liquid RBC storage systems, combined anticoagulant-nutrient solutions and additive solution systems, are in general use in the United States. RBC units stored in additive solutions are much more common. CPDA-1 is the only anticoagulant and nutrient solution in regular use. To make such RBC units, whole blood is drawn directly into the solution at a 7:1 volume ratio (450 mL blood to 63 mL of CPDA-1) and the plasma separated to leave an RBC concentrate with a storage hematocrit of about 75%. Such units are licensed for 5-week storage, and the in vivo RBC recovery at the end of 5 weeks of storage is approximately 75%. With additive solution systems, whole blood is first drawn into a CPD-like solution, again at a 7:1 volume ratio. Plasma is then removed for component manufacture, and 100 mL to 110 mL of additive solution is added. RBCs in additive solutions typically have a lower storage hematocrit, 55% to 60%, and a higher in vivo recovery, averaging 78% to 84% after 6 weeks of storage.

For many years, the two kinds of stored RBCs have been maintained side-by-side in blood banks because pediatricians did not want small children exposed to the mannitol or extra citrate in the commercially available additive solutions, and trauma surgeons complained that the concentrated RBCs in CPDA-1 flowed too slowly for effective resuscitation of the injured.[42,43] Now that infants have been shown to tolerate infusions of 15 mL/kg of RBCs in the common additive solutions, collection of RBCs into CPDA-1 is decreasing.[44,45]

The additive solutions (AS) used in North America, AS-1, AS-3, and AS-5, appear to store RBCs equally well. Theoretical reasons to prefer one solution over another do not appear to correlate with clinical differences. However, the additive solutions work in slightly different ways. AS-1 and AS-5 contain saline, adenine, glucose, and mannitol. The added adenine replaces RBC adenine lost to adenine deaminase, and the mannitol suppresses membrane loss, probably by a combination of direct physical interactions and by trapping oxygen free radicals. AS-3 contains saline, adenine, glucose, phosphate, and citrate. The citrate, another sugar, serves as a membrane protectant in a manner similar to that of mannitol. Citrate has the advantage that it is readily metabolized when infused and the disadvantage that it can contribute, although minimally, to citrate toxicity. The phosphate serves to maintain intracellular phosphate concentrations, a function that can be important if RBC units are underdrawn or drawn from anemic individuals. Under these conditions, the volume ratio of AS to RBCs can be high, and intracellular phosphate can be lost.

In Europe, a single additive solution, saline adenine glucose mannitol (SAG-M), has been standard for several decades. Although SAG-M has the same ingredients and essentially the same composition as the AS-1 and AS-5 solutions used in the United States for 6-week storage, it is usually used for 5-week RBC storage.

Two other, newer additive solutions are available with 7-week storage times. Walker developed an additive solution of phosphate, adenine, glucose, guanine, saline, and mannitol (PAGGS-M).[46] Its development followed the long tradition of searching for extra nutrients that might extend RBC storage. The phosphate prevents stored RBCs from becoming phosphate depleted from slow diffusional loss across a concentration gradient from inside to outside of the cells. Guanine was added to support GTP concentrations before it was understood that low GTP concentrations are rare in stored RBCs. The solution was licensed for 7-week storage in 1993, when the German government wanted a long-term RBC storage solution to support its United Nations peacekeeping mission in Somalia.[47] The studies that were submitted for licensure showed 74.7% in vivo recovery, a value that would not pass the U.S. standard of 75%.

A second system for 7-week storage, 1/2CPD-ErythroSol (Baxter), was designed to maintain pH at a higher level longer.[48] In this system, one half the normal volume of acid CPD is used in the collection phase, to blunt the decrease in pH associated with mixing venous blood with citric acid and monosodium phosphate. The additive solution portion of the storage system contains sodium chloride, adenine, glucose, mannitol, and phosphate at pH 7.5, which is achieved by mixing monosodium and disodium phosphate and made autoclavable by storing the sugar and phosphate in different pouches. The combined additive solution components have a final volume of 150 mL. The system allowed in vivo RBC recoveries of 78% at 7 weeks, but there were occasional problems with coagulation during whole blood collection because of the reduced amounts of primary CPD anticoagulant. The increased additive solution volume led to a reduced storage hematocrit of about 50%, which might cause problems with excessive hemodilution in massive transfusion situations.

Currently available liquid RBC storage systems work well in urban clinical medicine. Liquid RBC concentrates are easy to manufacture and handle, and the cells are accordingly safe, available, effective, and inexpensive. RBCs last long enough that almost 95% of all RBC components are transfused, and the majority of recipients receive cells that are only a few weeks old. Such cells are expected to have excellent in vivo recovery and little loss of membrane. However, at the end of the supply lines in small, rural hospitals and remote overseas territories and military bases, the average age of blood increases while the efficiency of use goes down. The use rate for RBCs sent to the peacekeeping forces in Bosnia from 1995 to 2000 was 1.7%, and for troops in Iraq and Afghanistan from 2002 to 2004 it was 2%. Moreover, in some retrospective studies the use of older cells has been associated with increased multiple organ failure and death.[49] Thus, the military wants a longer shelf-life for liquid-stored RBCs, and there is a perception that generally better storage is needed, as well.

Designing Better RBC Storage Systems

In 1986, Meryman and his colleagues described storing RBCs for 14 weeks in an ammonia-containing liquid storage solution at 1° C to 6° C, with occasionally excellent in vivo recovery.[50] They went on in 1994 to show that RBCs could be stored in very dilute suspensions for 35 weeks.[51] Such demonstrations show that the 5- to 7-week limits of conventional liquid RBC storage are not a result of anything intrinsic to the RBCs themselves but are a consequence of currently employed methods.

The Meryman solution appeared to work by maintaining very high concentrations of RBC ATP, presumably because ammonium prevented feedback inhibition of glucose phosphorylation.[52–55] Because ammonia would need to be washed out of the RBC component before it could be transfused, this storage solution was not compatible with routine clinical use. However, the idea that maintaining high concentrations of RBC ATP improved storage was compatible with the observation that the RBC ATP concentration was the laboratory measure that best correlated with the in vivo recovery of stored cells.

In 1992, Greenwalt and his colleagues described 9-week storage of RBC in a dilute, alkaline, ammonia- and phosphate-containing solution.[56] Again, ammonia made the solution unsuitable for clinical use, but it also appeared to work by maintaining high concentrations of ATP in the RBCs. However, careful review of several of Greenwalt's prior studies raised the possibility that it was the alkaline phosphate and not the ammonia that was driving the increase in ATP.[57,58] Hess and his colleagues then showed that the addition of disodium phosphate to conventional saline, adenine, glucose, and mannitol created a simple additive solution that increased RBC ATP concentrations and reduced hemolysis with increasing dose.[59] A 200-mL version of this experimental additive solution (EAS) allowed RBCs to be stored for 9 weeks, with 77 ± 7% in vivo recovery and 0.35% hemolysis.[60] A 300-mL version, EAS-64, allowed RBCs to be stored for 10 weeks, with 84 ± 8% in vivo recovery and 0.43% hemolysis.[61] Moreover, the loss of membrane through microvesiculation was one fifth that of control RBCs stored for 6 weeks in AS-1.

The combined groups of Greenwalt and Hess then tested the roles of pH and tonicity; the concentrations of phosphate, mannitol, and sodium; and the effect of plastic bags on these storage systems.[62–65] They showed that pH had to be maintained between 7.2 and 6.4. Above pH 7.2, 2,3-DPG was made at the expense of ATP, and the cells did not recover. Below pH 6.4, glycolysis essentially stopped. Phosphate in the extracellular fluid prevented the net loss of the intracellular phosphate necessary for ATP production. Phosphate also served as a pH buffer, but there were clinical limits on its safe concentration. Mannitol inhibited hemolysis, but most of the benefit was seen below 30-mM concentrations. Low sodium concentrations reducing tonicity to 290 mOsm resulted in cell swelling and reduced hemolysis. Storage in polyvinyl chloride (PVC) bags plasticized with diethylhexyl phthalate (DEHP) reduced hemolysis fourfold compared to storage in polyolefin bags.

This same series of studies examined the flow of metabolic energy through RBC storage systems. In 5-week CPDA-1, a unit of RBCs consumed 3 mM of glucose, produced 6 mM of lactate and protons, and dropped the pH from 7.0 to 6.5.[25] The proton buffering capacity of the system came almost entirely from the lysines on hemoglobin in the RBC. Lactate production was twice as fast in the first week as in the last. ATP production was maintained only above pH 6.7. During 10 weeks of storage in EAS-64, the pH decreased from 7.25 to 6.5, buffering 9 mM of protons with hemoglobin and 1 mM with phosphate. The additional storage time and membrane quality was bought with greater energy use. Better RBC storage required more proton buffering capacity, which could only be obtained by increasing the volume of the storage solutions or increasing their intrinsic buffering capacity. Clinical considerations suggested that patients would not tolerate the additional volume.

Buffering RBC storage was originally proposed and developed by Beutler in a solution called BAGPM (bicarbonate, adenine, glucose, phosphate, and mannitol).[66] When the bicarbonate picks up a proton, carbonic anhydrase converts the resulting carbonic acid to water and CO_2, the CO_2 diffuses out through the plastic bag, and the system effectively loses a proton. Unfortunately, Beutler added so much bicarbonate to BAGPM that he increased its pH to 7.8, reduced ATP concentrations in the stored blood, and observed poor in vivo recoveries. The Greenwalt and Hess groups used lower concentrations of bicarbonate and balanced the solutions to have a maximum pH of 7.2 at the beginning of storage. With bicarbonate, the groups made EAS that allowed 11 to 12 weeks of storage in 300-mL versions and a candidate 100-mL solution that stored RBC with 87 ± 2% in vivo recovery after 8 weeks, with reduced hemolysis and membrane loss. It is likely that such solutions can be improved further.[67–69]

Thus, it is possible to make better RBC storage systems by changing additive solutions to maintain ATP concentrations in the physiologic range. This goal can be accomplished by optimizing pH, buffering the solutions with bicarbonate and phosphate, using membrane protectants such as mannitol, and reducing sodium and chloride content. Solutions made using this general plan can store RBCs longer and with less membrane loss. The best balance between length of storage and membrane loss is not known at this time.

The best approach to integrate these advances into practice is still unclear. Current liquid storage systems appear to maintain RBCs with very little loss of membrane or viability for several weeks, followed by a phase marked by decreasing recovery and increasing stiffness. The regulatory standard of 75% in vivo recovery is a compromise between what had been achieved with storage system development in the past and what is compatible with meeting the demands of a national blood system. Shorter time limits on RBC storage will improve quality. Longer storage improves logistic efficiency at a time when blood availability is a serious problem. The new storage technology appears good enough that simultaneous improvement in RBC quality and shelf-life are possible.

REFERENCES

1. Greenwalt TJ. The Ernest Witebsky memorial lecture. Red but not dead: not a hapless sac of hemoglobin. Immunol Invest 1995;24:3–21.
2. Beutler E. Red cell metabolism and storage. In Anderson KC, Ness PM, (eds): Scientific Basis of Transfusion Medicine: Implications for Clinical Practice. Philadelphia, WB Saunders, 1994, pp 188–202.
3. Weed RI, Chailley B. Calcium-pH interactions in the production of shape change in erythrocytes. In Bessis M, Weed RI, Leblond PF (eds): Red cell shape: physiology, pathology, ultrastructure. New York, Springer Verlag, 1973, pp 55–67.
4. Sprague RS, Ellsworth ML, Stephenson AH, Lonigro AJ. Participation of cAMP in a signal-transduction pathway relating erythrocyte deformation to ATP release. Am J Physiol-Cell Ph 2001;281:C1158–C1164.
5. Gladwin MT. Hemoglobin as a nitrite reductase regulating red cell dependent hypoxic vasodilation. Am J Resp Cell Mol 2005;32: 363–366.
6. Lang KS, Lang PA, Bauer C, et al. Mechanisms of suicidal erythrocyte death. Cell Physiol Biochem 2005;15:195–202.
7. Tinmouth A, Chin-Yee I. The clinical consequences of the red cell storage lesion. Transfus Med Rev 2001;15:91–107.
8. Hall TL, Barnes A, Miller JR, Bethencourt DM, Nestor L. Neonatal mortality following transfusion of red cells with high plasma potassium levels. Transfusion 1993;33:606–609.
9. Hess JR. Update on alternative oxygen carriers. Vox Sang 2004;87:(Suppl 2):132 135.
10. Kendrick DB. Blood Program in World War II. Washington, D.C. Office of the Surgeon General, Department of the Army, 1964, pp 217–232.
11. Hess JR, Thomas MJG. Blood use in war and disaster: Lessons from the last century. Transfusion 2003;43:1622–1633.
12. Donohue DM, Finch CA, Gabrio BW. Erythorcyte preservation. VI. The storage of blood with purine nucleosides. J Clin Invest 1956; 35:562–567.
13. Beutler E. Experimental blood preservatives for liquid storage. In Greenwalt TJ, Jamieson GA (eds): The Human Red Cell In Vitro. New York, Grune & Stratton, 1973, pp 189–216.
14. Messana I, Ferroni L, Misiti F, et al. Blood bank conditions and RBCs: The progressive loss of metabolic modulation. Transfusion 2000;40:353–360.
15. Rifkind JM, Nagababu E, Ramasamy S, Ravi LB. Hemoglobin redox reactions and oxidative stress. Redox Rep 2003;8:234–237.
16. Jarolim P, Lahav M, Liu SC, Palek J. Effect of hemoglobin oxidation products on the stability of red cell membrane skeletons and the associations of skeletal proteins: correlations with a release of hemin. Blood 1990;76:2125–2113.
17. Sivilotti ML. Oxidant stress and haemolysis of the human erythrocyte. Toxicol Rev 2004;23:169–188.
18. Tavazzi B, Di Pierro D, Amorini AM, et al. Energy metabolism and lipid peroxidation of human erythrocytes as a function of increased oxidative stress. Eur J Biochem 2000;267:684–689.
19. Lutz HU, Liu HC, Palek J. Release of spectrin-free vesicles from human erythrocytes during ATP depletion. J Cell Biol 1977;73:548–560.
20. Rose ZB. Enzymes controlling 2,3-diphosphoglycerate in human erythrocytes. Fed Proc 1970;29:1105–1111.

21. Van Wijk R, van Solinge WV. The energy-less red blood cell is lost—erythorcyte enzyme abnormalities in glycolysis. Blood 2005;106:4032–4042.
22. Campanella ME, Chu H, Low PS. Assembly and regulation of a glycolytic enzyme complex on the human erythrocyte membrane. Proc Nat Acad Sci USA 2005;102:2402–2407.
23. Moses SW, Bashon N. Fructose metabolism in the human red blood cell. Isr J Med Sci 1974;10:707–711.
24. Murthy SNP, Lorand L. Nucleotide binding by the erythrocyte transglutaminase/Gh protein, probed with fluorescent analogs of GTP and GDP. Proc Nat Acad Sci USA 2000;97:7744–7747.
25. Ruddell JP, Babcock JG, Lippert LE, Hess JR. Effect of 24 hours of storage at 25 C on the in vitro storage characteristics of CPDA-1 packed red blood cells. Transfusion 1998;38:424–428.
26. Shohet SB, Haley JE. Red cell membrane shape and stability: relation to cell lipid renewal pathways and cell ATP. In Bessis M, Weed RI, Leblond PF (eds): Red Cell Shape: Physiology, Pathology, Ultrastructure. New York, Springer Verlag, 1973, pp 41–48.
27. Moroff G, Sohmer PR, Button LN. Proposed standardization of methods for determining the 24-hour survival of stored red cells. Transfusion 1984;24:109–114.
28. Hogman CF, de Verdier CH, Ericson A, et al. Studies of the mechanism of human red cell loss of viability during storage at 4+°C in vitro. I. Cell shape and total adenylate concentration as determinant factors for post-transfusion survival. Vox Sang 1985;48:257–268.
29. Kamp D, Sieberg T, Haest CW. Inhibition and stimulation of phospholipid scrambling activity. Consequences for lipid asymmetry, echinocytosis, and microvesiculation of erythrocytes. Biochemistry 2001;40:9438–9446.
30. Stansbury LG, Hess JR. Roger I. Lee: the right man at the right time. Transfus Med Rev 2005 Jan;19:81–84.
31. Rous P, Turner JW. The preservation of living red blood cells in vitro. J Exp Med 1916;23:219–237.
32. Rous P, Turner JW. The transfusion of kept cells. J Exp Med 1916; 23:239–247.
33. Robertson OH. Transfusion with preserved red blood cells. BMJ 1918;1:691 695.
34. Mollison PL. The introduction of citrate as an anticoagulant and of glucose as a red cell preservative. Br J Haematol 2000;108:13–18.
35. DeGowin EL, Harris JE, Plass ED. Studies on preserved human blood. I. Various factors influencing hemolysis. J Amer Med Assoc 1940; 114:850–855.
36. DeGowin EL, Hardin RC, Alsever JB. Blood Transfusion. Philadelphia and London, WB Saunders, 1949.
37. Loutit JF, Mollison PL. Advantages of a disodium-citrate-glucose mixture as a blood preservative. BMJ 1943;2:744–745.
38. Gibson JG, Rees SB, McManus TJ, Scheitlin WA II. A citrate phosphate dextrose solution for the preservation of human blood. Am J Clin Pathol 1957;28:569–578.
39. Heaton WAL, Holme S, Smith K, et al. Effects of 3–5 log10 pre-storage leucocyte depletion on red cell storage and metabolism. Brit J Haemat 1994;87:363–368.
40. Zuck TF, Bensinger TA, Peck CC, et al. The in vivo survival of red blood cells stored in modified CPD with adenine: report of a multi-institutional cooperative effort. Transfusion 1977;17:374–382.
41. Beutler E, West C. The storage of hard-packed red blood cells in citrate-phosphate-dextrose (CPD) and CPD-adenine (CPDA-1). Blood 1979;54:280–284.
42. Luban NL, Strauss RG, Hume HA. Commentary on the safety of red cells preserved in extended-storage media for neonatal transfusions. Transfusion 1991;31:229–235.
43. Hogman CF, Hedland K, Zetterstroem H. Clinical usefulness of red cells preserved in protein-poor mediums. N Engl J Med 1978;2999: 1377–1382.
44. Strauss R, Burmeister LF, Johnson K, et al. AS-1 red cells for neonatal transfusions: a randomized trial assessing donor exposure and safety. Transfusion 1996;36:873–878.
45. Strauss R, Burmeister LF, Johnson K, et al. Feasibility and safety of AS-3 red cells for neonatal transfusions. J Pediatr 2000;136:215–219.
46. Walker WH, Netz M, Ganshirt KH. 49 day storage of erythrocyte concentrates in blood bags with the PAGGS-mannitol. Beitr Infusionsther 1990;26:55–59.
47. Hess J. Extended liquid storage of red cells. In Manning FJ, Sparacino L (eds): Blood Donors and the Supply of Blood and Blood Products. National Academy Press, Washington, D.C. 1996, pp 99–102.
48. Hogman CF, Erickson L, Wallvik J, et al. Clinical and laboratory experience with erythrocyte and platelet preparations for 0.5 CPD ErythroSol opti systems. Vox Sang 1997;73:212–219.
49. Zallen G, Offner PJ, Moore EE, et al. Age of transfused blood is an independent risk factor for postinjury multiple organ failure. Am J Surg 1999 Dec;178:570–572.
50. Meryman HT, Hornblower M, Syring RL. Prolonged storage of red cells at 4°C. Transfusion 1986;26:500–505.
51. Meryman HT, Hornblower M, Syring RL, et al. Extending the storage of red cells at 4°C. Transfus Sci 1994;15:105–115.
52. Kay A, Beutler E. The effect of ammonium, phosphate, potassium, and hypotonicity on stored red cells. Transfusion 1992;32:37–41.
53. Mazor D, Dvilansky A, Meyerstein N. Prolonged storage of red cells with ammonium chloride and mannitol. Transfusion 1990;30:150–153.
54. Greenwalt TJ, Dumaswala UJ, Dhingra N, et al. Studies in red blood cell preservation. 7. In vivo and in vitro studies with a modified phosphate-ammonium additive solution. Vox Sang 1993;65:87–94.
55. Mazor D, Dvilansky A, Meyerstein N. Prolonged storage of red cells: The effect of pH, adenine and phosphate. Vox Sang 1994;66:264–269.
56. Greenwalt TJ, Dumaswala UJ, Rugg N. Studies in red blood cell preservation: 10. 51Cr recovery of red cells after liquid storage in a glycerol-containing additive solution. Vox Sang 1996;70:6–10.
57. Greenwalt TJ, Dumaswala UJ, Dhingra N, et al. Studies in red blood cell preservation: 7. In vivo and in vitro studies with a modified phosphate-ammonium additive solution. Vox Sang 1993;65:87–94.
58. Greenwalt TJ, Dumaswala UJ, Rugg N. Studies in red blood cell preservation: 10. 51Cr recovery of red cells after liquid storage in a glycerol containing additive solution. Vox Sang 1996;70:6–10.
59. Hess JR, Lippert LE, Derse-Anthony CP, et al. The effects of phosphate, pH, and AS volume on RBCs stored in saline-adenine-glucose-mannitol solutions. Transfusion 2000;40:1000–1006.
60. Hess JR, Rugg N, Knapp AD, et al. Successful storage of RBCs for nine weeks in a new additive solution. Transfusion 2000;40:1007–1011.
61. Hess JR, Rugg N, Knapp AD, et al. Successful storage of RBCs for 10 weeks in a new additive solution. Transfusion 2000 Aug;40:1012–1016.
62. Hess JR, Rugg N, Knapp AD, et al. The role of electrolytes and pH in RBC additive solutions. Transfusion 2001;41:1045–1051.
63. Hess JR, Hill HR, Oliver CK, et al. The effect of two different additive solutions on the post-thaw storage of RBCs. Transfusion 2001;41:923–927.
64. Hess JR, Hill HR, Oliver CK, et al. Alkaline CPD and the preservation of red blood cell 2,3-DPG. Transfusion 2002;42:747–752.
65. Hill HR, Oliver CK, Lippert LE, et al. The effects of polyvinyl chloride and polyolefin bags on red blood cells stored in a new additive solution. Vox Sang 2001;81:161–166.
66. Beutler E, Wood LA. Preservation of red cell 2,3-DPG and viability in bicarbonate-containing medium: the effect of blood-bag permeability. J Lab Clin Med 1972;80:723–728.
67. Hess JR, Rugg N, Gormas JF, et al. Eleven week red blood cell storage. Transfusion 2001;41:1586–1590.
68. Hess JR, Hill HR, Oliver CK, et al. 12-week red blood cell storage. Transfusion 2003;43:867–872.
69. Hess JR, Rugg N, Joines AD, et al. Buffering and dilution in red blood cell storage. Transfusion 2005;46:50–54.

Chapter 14

Infectious Disease Testing: Basic Principles and Practical Aspects

Roger Y. Dodd

BRIEF HISTORICAL REVIEW

The risk of disease transmission by blood transfusion is extremely low, particularly in developed nations. This situation is a consequence of a number of interlocking safety measures, including the selection of safe populations from which donors are drawn, careful donor questioning, laboratory testing, record keeping, and the use of quality systems and good manufacturing practices. These approaches have evolved over the years, and perhaps the most change has been seen in the area of blood testing. Indeed, blood collectors have now added nucleic acid amplification techniques to the battery of tests directed toward the safety of the blood supply. However, although transmission of known agents has almost been eliminated, residual fear of the unknown, fueled by a continuing stream of newly emerging or newly recognized microbes, continues.

Although some form of blood transfusion has been used for well over a century, organized testing approaches did not really commence until the 1940s. At that time, the transmissibility of syphilis by this route was recognized, and testing (albeit using nonspecific methods) was implemented. However, viral hepatitis was the biggest unresolved concern from the 1940s to about 1970. Clinical hepatitis was recognized as an almost inevitable consequence of transfusion, but little could be done to prevent it. The greatest benefits during that time were derived from epidemiologic studies that established the increased infection risk attributable to commercial donors and prisoners. There were also a number of attempts to use liver function tests to screen blood donors for risk of hepatitis transmission, but none of the tests was broadly adopted.

In 1965, Blumberg and colleagues[1] described the Australia antigen, mistakenly identifying it as an allotypic protein.[2] Subsequently, the antigen was recognized as a component of the hepatitis B virus (HBV), fortuitously produced in considerable excess during both acute and chronic infection. This discovery underlies the entire history of specific serologic testing for transfusion-transmissible infections. Between 1969 and 1972, all blood-collecting establishments in the United States adopted some form of testing for hepatitis B surface antigen (HBsAg), using agar gel diffusion, counter-electrophoresis, or rheophoresis. Subsequently, Ling and Overby[3] reported on a radioimmunoassay for HBsAg, and this assay was rapidly adopted. Interestingly, the insensitive gel precipitation methods seemed to affect only about 20% of post-transfusion hepatitis, and the frequency of radioimmunoassay–positive samples was about fivefold greater. A brief period of hope that the transfusion hepatitis problem was solved rapidly terminated in disillusion when it was found that most of the additional reactive results were false positive and that post-transfusion hepatitis continued to occur. As a result of the observations on specificity of the radioimmunoassay, confirmatory testing was implemented. Subsequently, testing for antibodies to the hepatitis B core antigen (anti-HBc) was licensed as a means to further reduce HBV infectivity, although it was initially introduced as a surrogate test for other forms of hepatitis. In 2004 and 2005, clinical trials of nucleic acid amplification tests (NAT) for HBV DNA were completed, and one test had been licensed as of July 2005.

Recognition of the hepatitis A virus and development of diagnostic tests for infection with this virus led to the definition of most cases of residual post-transfusion hepatitis as non-A, non-B (NANB).[4] Extensive studies were performed to characterize the agent(s) of NANB hepatitis, but such studies were without any real success until 1989.[5] Many attempts were also made to identify donor characteristics that might be used for screening. As a result of two of these studies, recommendations were made to screen donors for elevated levels of alanine aminotransferase (ALT) in the serum, and a small number of institutions adopted this measure around 1982.[6,7] Continuing studies also implicated antibodies to the hepatitis B core antigen (anti-HBc) as another surrogate for NANB infectivity.[8,9]

Further measures to reduce the incidence of post-transfusion NANB hepatitis were largely set aside as a result of the emergence of acquired immunodeficiency syndrome (AIDS) and recognition of its transmissibility by blood components and plasma fractions between 1981 and 1984. Although the potential value of the anti-HBc test as a surrogate for AIDS infectivity was discussed, this approach was adopted in only a limited number of blood establishments. Recognition of the human immunodeficiency virus (HIV) as the infectious agent of AIDS by Gallo and Montagnier and their colleagues[10,11] led to the rapid development and introduction of screening tests for antibodies to the virus. Testing started in March 1985. Because of the persistent nature of HIV infection, the presence of antibodies to HIV was closely linked to infectivity, and it is now clear that the introduction of this test played a major role in the almost total elimination of transfusion-transmitted HIV and AIDS. A problem with the exclusive use of anti-HIV as a viral marker is the fact that, early in infection, infectious virus can circulate before the appearance of detectable levels of antibody. Thus, there has been a continuing process of improvement of antibody tests and implementation of additional tests in order to reduce the length of this infectious window period and reduce risk. Not only have antibody tests become much more sensitive, but also tests for HIV p24 antigen and now for HIV RNA have been introduced. On licensure of NAT, the p24 antigen test was shown to be superfluous and has been discontinued.

The first human retrovirus to be recognized was the human T-lymphotropic virus 1 (HTLV-1).[12] This virus is an oncovirus, and its epidemiology is characterized by extreme geographic clustering in Japan, the Caribbean, and parts of Africa. Clinical outcomes of infection with this virus are relatively uncommon but include the serious T-cell lymphoma/leukemia and a neurologic disease called HTLV-associated myelopathy, otherwise termed *tropical spastic paraparesis.* Subsequently, a closely related virus, HTLV-2, was characterized. Its epidemiology is less well defined, but it appears to be naturally endemic in certain indigenous populations in the Americas and also circulates among users of injected drugs. The first serologic tests to be developed were designed to detect antibodies to HTLV-1, but as a result of cross-reactivity, they also identified the majority of HTLV-2 infections. Epidemiologic studies in the U.S. donor population revealed a 0.025% prevalence of anti-HTLV,[13] and this figure, along with the potentially serious outcomes of infection (which had been shown to occur through transfusion), led to the implementation of donor testing in 1988.

During the same period, there was a reevaluation of the severity of long-term outcomes of NANB hepatitis. As a result of this reevaluation and of a heightened awareness of blood safety, blood establishments adopted testing for both elevated ALT levels and anti-HBc, in the expectation that these tests together might reduce the incidence of transfusion-transmitted NANB hepatitis by about 60%.[8,9] This projection turned out to be quite accurate.

However, the most important advance in management of NANB was the cloning of a portion of the genome of a virus termed *hepatitis C virus.* This advance permitted the development of a test for antibodies to the virus based on peptides expressed from the viral genome. Use of this test revealed that almost all NANB hepatitis was due to hepatitis C. The first-generation test was implemented for donor screening in 1989 and 1990. Subsequently, with the expression of additional peptides, versions 2.0 and 3.0 of the test were successively implemented, with consequent gains in sensitivity. Nevertheless, because of a significant infectious window period, NAT for HCV has also been implemented. As a result, and because none of the supposed non-A, non-B, non-C hepatitis viruses were shown to be pathogenic, testing for ALT has also been discontinued.

Unexpectedly, in 2002 it became apparent that West Nile virus (WNV), which had entered the United States for the first time in 1999, was readily transmissible by blood transfusion. Although infection with WNV is acute, the frequency of infection was so great that a significant number of blood donors did give blood in the brief viremic, asymptomatic phase. As a result of these observations, tests for WNV RNA were developed and implemented within a relatively short time (about 9 months). Well over 1000 viremic and potentially infectious donations were identified in the first 2 years of testing.[14]

APPROACH TO TESTING

In the United States, blood, blood components, and plasma products are classified as biologics. By extension, tests used in the preparation of blood are also classified as biologics and, as such, are regulated by the U.S. Food and Drug Administration (FDA). This licensure involves extensive clinical trials and stringent regulatory oversight. However, these procedures are somewhat cumbersome and involve considerable resource use by manufacturers and regulators. As a consequence, the selection of available tests in the United States may differ from that in other parts of the world. A listing of FDA-licensed tests may be found on the FDA website (http://www.fda.gov/cber/products/testkits.htm). It should be noted that some of these tests may no longer be available. Typical results from the use of these tests in a large voluntary donor population are presented in Table 14–1.

There is a broad commonality in the implementation of all tests used to ensure the safety of blood and blood components. Every donation is tested, and current requirements in the United States are that the test be performed on a sample drawn at the time of donation. With the exception of testing for viral nucleic acids, which is described later, there are three phases of the testing. Each sample is tested singly; nonreactive results are considered to be negative for the marker, and the corresponding blood unit (and its components) may be issued for transfusion. If the result is reactive, the sample is retested in duplicate. If both of the repeated test results are nonreactive, the sample is classified as negative, and the unit, or its components, is released. However, if one or both of the repeated results is reactive, the sample is classified as repeatedly reactive, and the blood unit cannot be issued for transfusion. This practice was initiated when it was recognized that radioimmunoassays (and subsequently enzyme immunoassays [EIAs]) were subject to

Table 14–1 Prevalence and Incidence of Transfusion-Transmissible Infections among American Red Cross Blood Donors over the Two-year Period 2000–2001

	Prevalence among First-time Donors (n = 3.055 million)		Incidence among Repeat Donors (4.182 million person-years)	
	Number Confirmed Positive	Rate per Hundred Thousand	Number Confirmed Positive	Rate per Hundred Thousand Person-years
HBsAg	2229	72.9	53	1.27
HCV	9420	308.3	79	1.90
HIV	313	10.2	65	1.55
HTLV	299	9.8	10	0.24

Adapted from Dodd RY, Notari EP, Stramer SL. Current prevalence and incidence of infectious disease markers and estimated window-period risk in the American Red Cross blood donor population. Transfusion 2002;42:975–979.

nonrepeatable reactive results related to minor contamination with the labeled conjugate.

The final phase of testing is the application of confirmatory or supplementary tests, largely intended to ensure that the donor is properly advised about the significance of the screening test results. Although imperfect, this phase of testing markedly improves the accuracy of donor notification and counseling. In certain circumstances, these additional tests may also be used to support reentry of donors whose screening test results are definitively false positive. In some countries, a second screening test is used in place of different technology. In the United States, it has proved effective to use this second EIA strategy to reduce the number of confirmatory tests that have to be performed.[15] The strategy requires that the two EIA tests have essentially the same sensitivity. Despite the use of supplementary or confirmatory testing, the general rule in the United States is that a donor is indefinitely deferred on the basis of a repeatedly reactive screening test result.

There are some exceptions to this generalized algorithm. For example, there is no supplementary or confirmatory test for antibodies to the HBc antigen. In this case, a donor is not permanently deferred until he or she is found to be repeatedly reactive on a second occasion. Recent data, however, suggest that this policy is of little value and will become even less so as the specificity of tests for anti-HBc improves. Somewhat similarly, a donor does not need to be deferred the first time a test for anti–HTLV-1 or -2 is repeatedly reactive, provided the supplementary test result is nonreactive or indeterminate.

Starting in 1999, blood collection establishments in the United States implemented NAT for HCV and HIV RNA in donor samples. This testing was performed on small (i.e., 16 or 24) pools of samples. In some cases, primary testing was performed using a multiplex system.[16] Consequently, the testing algorithms differ significantly from those outlined previously. A second round of testing is used to resolve pools, followed, in some cases, by another test to differentiate HIV from HCV. In addition, a second, different NAT procedure is used to confirm or support the results of the primary test. Initially, all NAT for donor blood in the United States was performed under Investigational New Drug (IND) protocols, but tests were licensed in 2002. Table 14–2 outlines the results of NAT for the U.S. blood donor population from March 2000 through April 2002.[16]

Infectious disease testing is not static; there is continuing improvement in four broad areas. First, individual tests are being modified to ensure improved sensitivity and specificity. This process is perhaps best exemplified by the rapid progression of anti-HCV tests from version 1.0 to version 3.0. Second, the formats of the tests and the nature of the automated instrument systems are also subject to change and improvement. In some cases, these changes improve the performance characteristics of the tests, but they also reduce the need for human intervention and improve adherence to the requirements of good manufacturing practice. Third, a better understanding of the early (window) phase of infection has led to the addition of new test methods for some agents. For example, the measures for HIV now include a test for antibodies to the virus, and a test for viral nucleic acids. In addition, a number of tests are supplemented to detect additional strains or subtypes of a given agent. Fourth, continuing concern about blood safety is likely to lead to the implementation of tests for other agents including imported diseases such as Chagas disease[17] and emerging infections such as babesiosis.

WINDOW PERIOD

At least until the late 1980s, the serologic tests in use were considered to have adequate sensitivity for detecting well-established, chronic infection. Comparison of detection rates among first-time and repeat donors generally revealed that about 50% of all confirmed positive test results were found among first-time donors, although they contributed only 20% of all donations. Concern about the continued occurrence of transfusion-transmitted HIV infection led to much closer evaluation of the risk of infectivity during the early phases of infection, particularly the viremic but antibody-negative window period. Indeed, in a study by Petersen and colleagues,[18] HIV infectivity was demonstrated in one in five seronegative donations collected from individuals who were HIV antibody positive at their next donation. Mathematic modeling showed that the period of such infectivity averaged 45 days as of 1990.[18]

Knowledge of the length of the window period and of the incidence of new infection in the donor population also permitted estimation of the residual risk of infection from transfusion. The availability of closely spaced, sequential samples from commercial plasma donors permitted careful characterization of the window period and of the impact of additional tests. These studies showed that as the sensitivity of antibody tests was increased, the HIV window period was reduced to about 22 days.[19] The impact of the addition of tests for the HIV-1 p24 antigen and HIV RNA was also estimated.[19] Similarly, the dynamics of early infection with HCV and HBV are now well defined.[20] Although data published in 2002 suggested that the benefits of NAT were consistent with projections,[21] this was not the case for HIV-1 p24 antigen, which was detected much less frequently than anticipated. It is possible that because the HIV antigen peak corresponds

Table 14–2 Results of NAT for HIV and HCV, USA March 1999–April 2002, and for WNV, 2002–2003

	Donations tested (millions)	Number Confirmed Positive	Rate per Million
HIV	35.87	11	0.31
HCV	36.97	156	4.22
WNV*	5.32	540	101.5

*Data represents collections only during the period that WNV was detected among donors.

Adapted from Stramer SL, Fang CT, Foster GA, et al. West Nile virus among blood donors in the United States, 2003 and 2004. N Engl J Med 2005;253:451–459; Stramer SL, Glynn SA, Kleinman SH, et al. Detection of HIV-1 and HCV infections among antibody-negative blood donors by nucleic acid-amplification testing. N Eng J Med 2004;351:760–768.

with the symptomatic phase of early acute HIV infection, the affected donors feel unwell and are less likely to present for donation.

SCIENTIFIC BASIS FOR TEST SELECTION

Determining a Need for Testing

There are a number of levels of decision making relative to testing for transfusion-transmissible infections. At the highest level is the determination to test for a given agent. Many factors are considered in this process, including the potential frequency of transmission of the disease, its severity, and the efficacy of treatment. This is perhaps the most difficult decision to make, and there is no clear guidance, methodology, or prioritization process in place. In fact, in the United States, there are no clear decision-making hierarchies for implementing a new test, although final authority for requiring a test rests with the FDA. During the history of blood testing, there have been examples of voluntary initiation of tests, either by a local decision in one or more blood establishments, or through professional bodies, such as the AABB. In the first of these categories, a number of individual blood establishments independently initiated early testing for ALT, anti-HBc, or HIV-1 p24 antigen. In the past, the AABB, through its standard-setting procedures, has called for testing for ALT and anti-HBc, and more recently, for methods of detecting bacteria in platelet concentrates. In addition, even if it is clear that a preventative measure is required for a given agent, there is no process to make sure that a test will be developed and made available. Conversely, it appears that the development of a test will not necessarily lead to its adoption, at least in the short term. However, the development and implementation of a test for WNV RNA appears to be a good example of a case in which the need was clear, and all stakeholders worked together to achieve an effective outcome.[14]

Although it would seem appropriate to base a decision about test implementation on science and cost-benefit analyses, there is now a much greater tendency to invoke a variant of the precautionary principle. In effect, this tendency translates to implementing some measure to reduce transfusion risk before data are available to define the efficacy of such a measure. The major constraint is that the measure should not have any deleterious effect. It has been argued that the use of this approach has been successful in the case of donor deferral policies for risk of vCJD.[22] However, in this case, the argument was that measures had been taken before the disease had clearly been shown to be transmissible by transfusion. The selected measures had not been shown to be efficacious, so the argument for success was based on the finding of transmission, rather than a demonstration that the measures actually prevented it. If the precautionary principle is used to promote the use of unproven methods, it is important to recognize that the principle is not absolute and that certain constraints should be considered before it is invoked.[23]

Selecting a Test Methodology

Of more scientific interest is the selection of an appropriate methodology to be used to test for any given agent. In the past, this selection was often based on the historic availability of a given technology and its linkage to the discovery or characterization of the agent in question. The classic examples of this approach are the use of nontreponemal tests for syphilis and the implementation of testing for HBsAg. In fact, both of these approaches turned out to be appropriate and successful, but we are now in a much better position to select methods on the basis of the properties of the infectious agent itself, and of its pathology and natural history. Broadly speaking, the approaches are to identify the infectious agent itself, or to focus on the body's reaction to infection with the agent.

Direct Identification of Infectious Agents

Direct detection of the agent itself may involve techniques as simple as visualization, or as complex as nucleic acid amplification. Obviously, direct visualization is unlikely to be sensitive enough to support current needs for blood safety, although it is used in some circumstances—for example, evaluation of donor malaria infection in parts of the developing world. Most current technologies in widespread use involve the immunologic detection of specific antigens and amplification of nucleic acids. Antigen testing has undoubtedly been of greatest use up to the present time and has demonstrated its greatest efficacy in the detection of infection with HBV. Its efficacy is directly attributable to an essentially unique property of HBV infection, which is the synthesis of a great excess of the viral surface antigen. This, in effect, is an amplification mechanism, because immunologically based tests can usually only detect analytes at levels well above the picogram-per-mL range. It is not to be expected that many other infectious agents will be as readily detected through their antigenic components. Nevertheless, HBV has been considered to be a model, and a great deal of effort has been expended on a search for detectable soluble antigens from other transfusion-transmissible viruses. In fact, methods to identify antigens of both HIV and HCV have been successfully developed and deployed. However, the antigenic levels have been low, and their sensitivity in detecting infectivity is greatly surpassed by nucleic acid testing. For example, the maximum sensitivity of a test for HCV core antigen is equivalent to about 30,000 to 50,000 genome copies of RNA, although this sensitivity can be increased by the use of immune complex dissociation techniques.[24] Another issue with antigen detection is that, in general, antigens cease to be readily detectable once a significant level of antibody has developed. Thus, in the absence of methods using immune complex dissociation, antigens are detectable only during the early acute phases of infection. (This is not the case for HBV, because the levels of antigen synthesized during chronic infection are enough to overwhelm the antibody response and lead to a situation of antigen excess.) Thus, with the exception of HBsAg, antigen detection methods are used to supplement other detection procedures by providing for earlier detection of infection and thus reducing the length of the infectious window period. A test for HIV p24 antigen was in use for this purpose for a number of years in the United States and some other countries, but at least in the United States it has been supplanted by the much more sensitive NAT. Some countries have adopted a test for HCV core antigen instead of implementing the more costly and complex NAT. An evolving trend is the development of so-called *combo assays*, which permit the detection of both the viral antigen and the antibody. Such tests offer operational advantages, but they are generally somewhat less sensitive than individual tests alone. In general, it should not be anticipated that blood product contamination by any emerging infection will be effectively prevented solely by testing for its antigens.

Nucleic acid amplification tests are extremely sensitive, with the theoretical possibility of detecting a single molecule of nucleic acid, although this level is rarely achieved in practice. Conceptually, NAT was introduced into donor testing as a way to increase safety by identifying individuals in the viremic window period. In large part, it appears to have fulfilled this expectation, reducing the estimated risk of transfusion-transmitted HCV from 1 per 200,000 units to 1 per 1,390,000 units, and that of HIV from 1 per 1,048,000 units to 1 per 1,525,000 units.[21,25] However, it is clear that NAT is insufficiently sensitive to identify every infectious blood unit, and it is currently seen as a supplement to conventional immunologic tests for antibodies to HIV and HCV. NAT for HBV DNA is now available and, at the time of writing, one test has been licensed for routine use, but such use is has not been mandated by the FDA. This is the case largely because there appears to be relatively little benefit to implementing this test on pooled samples, relative to the use of highly sensitive tests for HBsAg. Nevertheless, a continuing question is whether NAT could displace currently used serologic tests for any of these viruses. Certainly, it is clear that a proportion of donor samples may have confirmed positive test results for antibodies, but they may be negative for RNA or DNA. This result occurs among about 20% of anti-HCV–positive, and about 0.4% of anti-HIV–positive donors (SL Stramer, unpublished observations). In some, but not all, cases, these findings do represent resolution of infection and viral clearance. Overall, at the time of writing, it seems unlikely that conventional test methods will be eliminated.

The value of NAT for managing emerging transfusion-transmissible infections has been amply illustrated by the U.S. experience with WNV. NAT for this virus was developed by two manufacturers and implemented within 9 months of the recognition of need. It is certainly easier to develop a nucleic acid-based assay than an immunoassay, because it does not require the expression of antigens or the production of antibodies. However, NAT may not necessarily be the most effective solution for all emerging infections. It has been very successful in the case of WNV because the infection itself is acute, and it appears that the period of blood-borne infectivity is restricted to the earliest phases of infection, prior to the development of significant levels of antibodies. In fact, there do not appear to have been any well-documented cases of transfusion transmission of WNV from donors who had developed antibodies to WNV.[14]

Detection of Antibody and Other Responses to Infection

The other broad approach to testing for infectivity is by assessing the body's response to the agent. Most frequently, of course, this assessment is done by detecting antibodies, although other methods have been used or considered. The major benefit of testing for antibodies is that the immune response is a form of amplification: infection with, or exposure to, a modest titer of a microorganism generates levels of circulating antibodies that are readily detectable by relatively simple procedures. Antibody tests have been highly effective as a measure to control transfusion-transmitted infection with a number of agents, but this effectiveness is really confined to persistent infections, such as HCV, HIV, or Chagas disease. In contrast, as pointed out above, antibody testing does not offer any benefit for the prevention of acute infections, as exemplified by WNV, where it appears that infectivity diminishes or disappears as antibody becomes detectable. Clearly, in such circumstances, direct detection of the agent is the preferred approach. More broadly, the use of any given test approach for donor screening should be based on knowledge of the natural history of each particular infection, rather than on the availability of a test method per se.

At the time of writing, there is interest in an entirely different approach to the detection of infection, based on proteomics. Modern technology permits the characterization of actual or relative concentrations of a very large number of proteins (for example, in the plasma). Some of these protein levels may change as a result of infection with a particular organism, and conceptually, at least, it may be possible to identify an infection through a particular pattern of change in the levels or distribution of these proteins. Rapid, simultaneous screening of large numbers of proteins, along with intensive computational capabilities, makes this identification possible. However, this approach has yet to be shown to be appropriately sensitive and specific, or even simple enough, for routine use.

Selecting a Specific Test

The final level of test selection is the choice of which particular manufacturer's test to use. Although it may be argued that in many parts of the world tests must be approved by a regulatory authority, this requirement does not ensure that all approved tests have equivalent performance characteristics. This fact is clearly demonstrated by the differences in analytic sensitivity for licensed (and unlicensed) HBsAg tests reported by the FDA.[26] Consequently, a process of evaluation of test characteristics is desirable in order to inform purchase decisions, in addition to issues of cost and convenience.

For blood screening tests, the key performance parameters are sensitivity and specificity. In the case of most markers, analytic sensitivity directly impacts epidemiologic sensitivity. In other words, a more sensitive test will identify more infected donors. Perhaps the most important aspect of sensitivity is the ability to detect infection at the earliest time, because this detection reduces the length of the infectious window period and hence the risk of transmitting infection to recipients. Sensitivity for early infection is best evaluated against panels of samples taken during seroconversion. Such panels are commercially available and have usually been collected from donors of plasma for further manufacture. It should, however, be noted that in an environment where multiple tests are used for any given infectious agent, the sensitivity of the overall test system is most important. For example, use of NAT may compensate for an antibody test that may not be the most sensitive one available. Another aspect of sensitivity is the ability of a given test to detect different serotypes, genotypes, or mutants of the agents of concern. Most available tests have been designed to have optimal sensitivity for the strains of agent that predominate in the United States. Even though a particular strain or genotype is very rare, there may be benefits to using tests with broader sensitivity. For example, in the United States, potential donors must be deferred if they have a history of travel, residence, or sexual contact in certain African countries where HIV-1 type O is present, unless a test with FDA-validated claims for group O detection is used.

Test specificity is another critical parameter. Tests with poor specificity result in unnecessary loss of products and their donors, and they require performance of additional confirmatory tests. Furthermore, blot-based confirmatory tests frequently generate indeterminate results that are hard to interpret and which cause unnecessary alarm when donors are notified. The very low prevalence of some infections among blood donors magnifies the impact of poor test specificity. For example, the positive predictive value of a repeat reactive test result for HIV is currently around 5% in the U.S. donor population, even though current tests have good to excellent specificity. A test's specificity is best evaluated by testing many nonreactive samples, preferably from donor populations.

Ideally, assessments of sensitivity and specificity should be made in field conditions. However, doing so may be unrealistic, and decisions may have to be based on available information. Although comparative evaluations of test kits are occasionally published in the open literature, every kit approved in the United States includes a product insert with summary information of the results of the clinical trials that define the claimed performance characteristics for the test. Tests should be expected to meet these performance claims in routine use. Clinical trials for licensure of tests for donation screening require evaluations of test sensitivity and specificity in field conditions, along with evaluations of the impact of samples with interfering substances. Sensitivity evaluations include the use of a wide variety of positive samples representing different genotypes. In addition, a population of high-risk samples is usually tested. Specificity is assessed by testing 10,000 or more routine donor samples. Samples giving positive results must be further investigated and the donors evaluated by follow up.

TESTS BY AGENT

Hepatitis B Virus

Hepatitis B Immunoassays

The primary means for the detection of hepatitis B infectivity is the test for HBsAg. This antigen is the first serologic marker to appear during acute HBV infection, and it persists during active, chronic infection. It is produced in the cytoplasm of HBV-infected cells, and it is often present in the serum at high levels, even up to micrograms per milliliter. The HBsAg represents the viral coat and is found in the serum or plasma in the form of self-assembled spheres and tubules 22 nm in diameter. It is readily detected by simple, sandwich-type immunoassays using animal antibodies to HBsAg (anti-HBs) as a solid-phase capture reagent and a conjugated anti-HBs as a probe. Conventional assays use either a bead or a microplate well as the solid phase, but tests (particularly automated ones) are increasingly based on microparticle substrates. Similarly, enzyme conjugates and chromogenic detection methods are being replaced by chemiluminescent labels.

Currently available tests have an analytic sensitivity on the order of 0.5 ng/mL, with a range of 0.08 ng/mL to 0.7 ng/mL. The epidemiologic sensitivity and specificity of the test are high. Nevertheless, because the prevalence of positive HBsAg findings in the donor population is quite low, the positive predictive value of the test is also low. Thus, as with any other donor screening test, any repeatedly reactive finding should be confirmed before the donor is notified. Manufacturers of HBsAg test kits also provide confirmatory reagents consisting of specific antibodies to HBsAg. The test is repeated in the presence of the antibody, and a control test is also run using normal serum. If the added antibody inhibits the test signal by 50% or more relative to the control, the reactive result is considered to be confirmed as positive. There are some additional steps that are required in specified circumstances (such as a strong primary test result). It should be noted that very weak reactive signals may also give false-positive results in this confirmatory procedure.

As indicated earlier, testing for anti-HBc was uniformly introduced in the United States in 1986 and 1987. It was originally used to screen for NANB hepatitis infectivity as a result of some epidemiologic correlation between HBV and HCV infection, but this use is no longer considered valid or appropriate. In fact, anti-HBc testing was licensed by the FDA as an additional measure to improve safety with respect to HBV. The core antigen is actually the viral capsid, and antibodies appear early in infection, but after HBsAg. Originally, it was hypothesized that anti-HBc was the only marker detectable during a window period after the decline of HBsAg and before the appearance of the corresponding protective antibody (anti-HBs). Current test methods are so sensitive that this is probably no longer the case. Nonetheless, there are both old and contemporary data suggesting that a minority of donations with anti-HBc as the sole marker of HBV infection may be infectious.[27–30] However, the presence of significant levels of anti-HBs seems to negate the risk of any infectivity through the blood (although not from a transplanted liver).[31] Consequently, in Japan, a country with a high prevalence of HBV infection, donors are tested for HBsAg, anti-HBc, and anti-HBs. All units with detectable HBsAg are discarded, as are those with anti-HBc in the absence of anti-HBs. However, units with both antibodies are used for transfusion.[32]

There are two approaches to anti-HBc testing. The initial test that was developed was an inhibition immunoassay, which is still available. The solid phase has recombinant HBc antigen as a capture reagent, and the probe is a labeled, partially purified anti-HBc antibody. The presence of anti-HBc in the test sample inhibits the signal. Perhaps surprisingly, this test has rather poor specificity, in part because of reduction-sensitive interfering molecules in some samples.[33] Newer versions of the test incorporate reductants, which clearly increase the specificity of the test. However, the inhibition procedure is also quite dependent on good technique, and reproducibility is not optimal. A second test, a direct antiglobulin assay for anti-HBc, is also available; it appears to be more specific than the inhibition procedure. There is no formal confirmatory procedure for anti-HBc, but the use of two different tests may help to increase the predictive value of a reactive result.

Nucleic Acid Amplification Testing for Hepatitis B Virus

A number of NAT procedures for HBV DNA have been developed and, in some cases, put into routine use, particularly in Japan and parts of Germany.[34,35] In the United States, two commercial procedures have been developed and evaluated in clinical trials.[36] At the time of writing (2005), one of these procedures has been licensed by the FDA. However, the FDA did not specifically require its use. Clinical trials of the licensed test using minipool procedures did result in the detection of HBV DNA–positive, serology-negative donations at a frequency of about 1 per 340,000 donations. In general, minipool testing for HBV DNA is considered to have a sensitivity similar to that of the most sensitive tests for HBsAg, and there is considerable debate about the real safety benefits of minipool NAT for HBV in the United States. It must be remembered that anti-HBc testing of donors is in routine use in the United States, and studies have shown that fewer than 1% of anti-HBc-reactive donations have detectable HBV DNA. Consequently, minipool NAT for HBV may have more value in an environment where anti-HBc testing is not in use. It is considered likely that the use of individual donation testing for HBV DNA would offer some increased safety, because the increased sensitivity may decrease the length of the window period. Finally, HBV NAT of plasma for further manufacture has been implemented using relatively large pools of samples (i.e., 512 to 1200).

Other Hepatitis B Virus Tests

There are other tests for markers of HBV infection, but, in general, they have little current relevance to transfusion medicine, at least in the United States. As pointed out earlier, tests for anti-HBs are available, and a positive result usually (but not always) signifies a resolved infection and the absence of circulating virus.[32] Indeed, the presence of anti-HBs may not signify complete elimination of HBV, because the virus may still be present in the liver; transplanted organs from donors with anti-HBs can result in HBV infection in a susceptible recipient.[31] Nonetheless, anti-HBs testing may be used to identify anti-HBc–reactive donations that are safe for transfusion, as in Japan. There are commercially available tests for immunoglobulin M anti-HBc, and this test is useful for diagnosis of acute HBV infection. Tests for the hepatitis B e antigen are of some value in defining the severity of an infection, but the value of a test for the corresponding antibody (anti-HBe) is less clear.

Hepatitis C Virus

HCV Immunoassays

The primary screening and diagnostic test for HCV infection is an antiglobulin EIA for antibodies to the virus. As of the end of 2005, only two tests were available in the United States. Both use immobilized, recombinant viral antigens as the capture reagent and an anti-immunoglobulin conjugate as the probe. One test is defined as a version 2.0 test, and the other as a version 3.0. Both tests use antigens representing the core and NS3/NS4 regions of the viral genome, and the 3.0 version includes an NS5 peptide. In comparison, the first test to be licensed (termed 1.0) used only a single peptide in the capture reagent. This HCV 1.0 test, although a considerable advance on surrogate testing, lacked both sensitivity and specificity. Subsequent versions are much improved with respect to both of these characteristics.

One licensed supplementary test for anti-HCV is available in the United States. This test is an immunoassay consisting of a nitrocellulose paper strip bearing HCV peptides at specified locations. There are also controls to ensure that the test is performed properly and to identify reactions due to antibodies to superoxide dismutase (SOD), a carrier protein for expression of some of the peptides. The strip is exposed to a test sample, and any adherent antibodies are detected and visualized by use of an antiglobulin conjugate and a chromogenic substrate. The test is designed to complement the version 3.0 EIA and consequently uses essentially the same peptides. Clearly, the test was developed to dissect out and identify the presence of antibodies to different viral epitopes. In common with the Western blot, this approach has two deficiencies: (1) it is a subjective test, and (2) it does not generate outcomes with unequivocal interpretations. That is, results may be defined as nonreactive, positive, or indeterminate. A positive test is defined on the basis of at least two bands with a density greater than or equal to that of the low-positive control, but in the absence of an SOD band. A negative result is defined as one or more bands with a density less than that of the low-positive control. A result is defined as indeterminate if there is only one band with a density greater than or equal to that of the weak-positive control or if an SOD band is present, irrespective of other band patterns. An indeterminate result does not clearly establish the presence or absence of current or prior infection with HCV. In testing donors, about 20% of EIA repeat-reactive donations are found to be indeterminate, but only about 1% of these donations are positive for HCV RNA by polymerase chain reaction (PCR).[37,38]

Hepatitis C Virus Nucleic Acid Amplification Testing

At the time of writing, two commercially available NAT procedures are in use for testing donor blood for evidence of HCV infectivity.[16] One is a PCR procedure that is conducted on RNA extracted by standard chemical methods from pools of 24 plasma samples. The other approach uses a transcription-mediated amplification procedure on nucleic acid preparations made by a solid-phase, probe-capture method. Both approaches are successful in detecting HCV antibody–nonreactive, RNA-positive window–phase donations. Furthermore, both methods seem to have the same performance characteristics when the different sensitivities of the version 2.0 and 3.0 EIAs are accounted for. Following infection, HCV RNA levels increase rapidly and reach values of 10^5 to 10^7 copies/mL during the period about 40 to 50 days before the appearance of detectable HCV antibody. In a review of national experience with NAT, Stramer and colleagues[16] showed that the detection rate for HCV RNA was about 1 in every 230,000 seronegative donations.[16] Accepted testing algorithms for blood donor screening differ somewhat from those for diagnosis or screening of the general population, inasmuch as the NAT procedures have not been formally accepted as part of the confirmatory process for donors. This subject is discussed in more detail in Chapter 44.

Although not in widespread use, immunologic tests for the HCV core antigen have been developed, with a sensitivity that is approximately equivalent to the detection of 30,000 to 50,000 copies of HCV RNA. Although less sensitive than NAT for HCV RNA, core antigen tests nevertheless are capable of substantially reducing the infectious window period.

Human Immunodeficiency Virus

Immunoassays for Human Immunodeficiency Virus Antibodies

As a direct result of the discovery of HIV, the causative agent of AIDS, the first tests for antibodies to this virus were licensed for donor screening in early 1985. All of the initial tests were antiglobulin EIA procedures using viral lysate as the solid-phase capture reagent and enzyme-conjugated antiglobulins as the probe. Early results using one of these procedures nationwide revealed that the prevalence of seropositive donations was 0.038%.[39] Tests for antibodies to HIV have been continuously upgraded. During this process, there have been two major changes. First, in 1992 the FDA required that blood donor testing should include a means of detecting infection with HIV-2. This goal was achieved by the development of combination ("combo") tests designed to identify antibodies to both viruses in the same test. Second, and in some cases as a means of satisfying this requirement, some of the tests evolved to a direct test in which both the capture reagent and the labeled probe were viral peptides (usually prepared by recombinant techniques). These approaches led to much-increased sensitivity, cutting the seronegative window period by as much as 23 days.[40] As a result of careful and intensive approaches to donor selection and questioning and of continued testing, fewer than 1 in 25,000 donations are currently confirmed positive for anti-HIV.

Two tests are licensed for confirmatory or supplemental testing for anti-HIV. The one more commonly used is the Western blot, essentially a research test that was reported in the earliest publication on HIV antibody testing.[41] Also approved for use is an indirect immunofluorescence procedure. The Western blot is similar to the strip immunoassay already mentioned, in that it identifies the presence of antibodies to individual viral components. The blot procedure involves separation of viral components by electrophoresis on polyacrylamide gel, followed by transfer (blotting) to a nitrocellulose paper. A strip of the paper is exposed to a test sample, and adherent antibodies are detected and visualized by the use of an appropriate conjugated antiglobulin.

A number of attempts have been made to define an effective set of interpretive criteria for the HIV blot, but none has been fully effective.[42–47] The criterion in current use was developed by the Centers for Disease Control and Prevention and the Association of State and Territorial Public Health Laboratory Directors. A positive finding is defined as the presence of at least two of the following bands at an intensity equal to or greater than that of the weak-positive control: p24, gp41, and gp120/160. A blot with no visible bands is considered to be negative, and any other band pattern is interpreted as indeterminate (even if the bands are nonviral).[47] In fact, the current approved criterion may lead to false-positive outcomes in as many as 10% of donor samples with a positive blot interpretation.[46,48] Indeterminate outcomes are also frequent; in the American Red Cross system, only 4.8% of EIA repeatedly reactive samples are found to be positive on the blot, 44.2% are negative, and 51% are indeterminate. Essentially all of the reactions in the indeterminate group are unrelated to HIV infection, but current recommendations permit them to be resolved only on the basis of follow-up. A clear advantage of the immunofluorescence alternative method is the much lower frequency of indeterminate results. The interpretation of HIV antibody test results is complicated by the requirement to evaluate EIA repeatedly reactive samples for evidence of HIV-2 infection using a second test based on a viral lysate. There are no licensed supplemental tests for HIV-2, and some individuals may be inappropriately notified that they have been infected with HIV-2 despite its extreme rarity in the U.S. donor population.

Human Immunodeficiency Virus p24 Antigen Testing

The inability to detect HIV in the infectious window period has engendered considerable concern since 1985. As pointed out earlier, the sensitivity of antibody tests has been improved, so that the window period has been halved. Nevertheless, the risk is still unacceptable. Although it was known that the soluble HIV-1 p24 antigen could be detected during the window period, an extensive study published in 1990 did not suggest that implementation of the antigen test for screening would have any appreciable yield.[49] Subsequently, the issue was reevaluated, and antigen testing was implemented in 1996. Despite predictions that approximately 5 to 10 antigen-positive, antibody-negative donations would be identified each year, the actual detection frequency has been only 1 in 4 million to 9 million donations.

Human Immunodeficiency Virus Nucleic Acid Amplification Tests

As is the case for HCV, NAT has been implemented for the detection of HIV RNA. The procedures used are those described previously for HCV. Subsequently, NAT for HIV was licensed, and two tests are available for routine use. During the period of use of these tests under IND, it was shown that all p24 antigen-positive samples were also clearly reactive by NAT, and the use of the p24 test has now been discontinued. Reviews of national data have shown that 1 in 3.1 million donations are HIV RNA positive, but seronegative.[16] Studies have shown that HIV RNA levels increase quite rapidly and normally reach 10^4 to 10^6 copies/mL before the appearance of anti-HIV antibodies. Nevertheless, there have been a handful of cases in which transfusion transmission of HIV has occurred from NAT-nonreactive blood components.[50–52] Again, the results of NAT have not been formally approved as a supplement to the serologic test results, even though such information would be of clear relevance in notifying and counseling seropositive donors.

Human T-Lymphotropic Virus

Although HTLV-1 was the first human retrovirus to be identified, donor testing was not initiated until 1988. Seroprevalence studies indicated that approximately 0.025% of the donor population had evidence of infection with the virus.[13] In actuality, as a result of the strong sequence and antigenic homologies, the tests originally developed to detect antibodies to HTLV-1 were also able to detect many (perhaps most) infections with HTLV-2. Although the viruses differ epidemiologically, there are insufficient data to determine the extent to which their pathologic outcomes differ.

Tests for antibodies to HTLV-1 and HTLV-2 are generally similar to the earliest tests for HIV antibodies. That is, they rely on a viral lysate as the capture reagent, and adherent donor antibodies are identified with an antiglobulin conjugate. In 1998, the FDA required that blood donations be additionally evaluated for the presence of antibodies to HTLV-2 using a test formally approved for that purpose. This requirement necessitated the development of tests that included specific HTLV-2–derived antigens, and manufacturers developed combo tests for this purpose. Consequently, available tests are designed for the detection of HTLV-1/HTLV-2 antibodies.

There are no licensed confirmatory or supplemental tests for the EIA procedures. Western blot tests are commercially available for use under research or IND protocols, but their performance characteristics are far from optimal. In fact, in the American Red Cross system, only 9% of EIA repeatedly reactive samples are positive by blot, 19.3% are negative, and the remaining 71.7% are indeterminate.[38] Radioimmunoprecipitation has been used to supplement these procedures, but this technique is more complex and arduous than the Western blot. A final problem is that additional tests may be required to distinguish HTLV-1 and HTLV-2 infections. A specific viral peptide–supplemented blot is designed to differentiate these two infections, but it is not readily available to blood collectors. It is, however, reasonable to ask whether there is any clear medical benefit to distinguish between these viruses; notification policy does not differ greatly.[53] NAT is available experimentally, but it appears unlikely to be adopted for screening donations.

Syphilis

Although (or perhaps because) testing for syphilis was the first procedure to be implemented for blood safety, it is now the least understood and least justified test in use. The nature and properties of serologic tests for syphilis are described in much greater detail elsewhere.[54] Initially, donor testing was undertaken using nontreponemal tests, such as the rapid plasma reagin (RPR) test. Although these tests were markedly nonspecific, they had the advantage of identifying primarily active or recent infections. Over the past 10 to 15 years, most blood collection agencies have adopted treponemal tests, mainly because they are adaptable to use on automated instruments, including those routinely used for blood typing. Treponemal tests generally indicate current and distant infection, even after successful treatment. Repeatedly reactive screening test results are generally confirmed or supplemented by the use of fluorescent treponemal antibody tests, treponemal EIA tests, or nontreponemal assays. The frequency of reactive screening test results among Red Cross donations is about 0.18%. Of these results, about 46% are confirmed by a fluorescent treponemal antibody absorption (FTA-ABS) test. Among the confirmed samples, 23% are RPR reactive. Even so, only about 50% of donors with an FTA-ABS–confirmed positive result report a history of syphilis.

Evolving data suggest that few, if any, donors who test positive for syphilis antibodies have detectable *Treponema pallidum* DNA or RNA in their circulation.[55] In contrast, many individuals identified through sexually transmitted disease clinics are clearly bacteremic. The FDA has indicated its willingness to evaluate data with a view to reconsidering the need to continue routine syphilis testing for blood donors. It should be noted that, although a history of syphilis results in a 1-year deferral because of concerns that active syphilis might correlate with increased risk for HIV, there is no evidence that a positive test result for syphilis has any meaningful association with window-phase HIV infection.[56]

Cytomegalovirus

Cytomegalovirus (CMV) infection is usually relatively benign, but it can have profound and life-threatening effects on persons with a compromised immune response, including low-birth-weight infants. The virus is ubiquitous, and seroprevalence rates of 50% or more are common among adult populations. For many years, the use of CMV-seronegative blood components has been recommended for particular groups of patients at risk for serious CMV disease.[57,58] It has been suggested that the use of leukoreduced components may similarly protect these vulnerable groups. Nevertheless, CMV testing continues to be used.[59] Both particle agglutination and EIA tests are available. Seronegative products are labeled as such, but there is no corresponding labeling of seropositive products, which are freely used for recipients who are not considered to be at risk. There is no program for donor notification or deferral for reactive CMV antibody tests. The performance characteristics of tests may differ, and there is no definitive "gold standard." Even the use of nucleic acid amplification techniques has generated results that are not always readily interpreted, perhaps as a consequence of interlaboratory variation in testing.[60]

SURROGATE TESTS

The usual approach to testing blood for transfusion is to apply an assay that identifies a specific marker of the infectious agent concerned. Serologic tests depend on the detection of circulating antigens or antibodies, and NAT methods provide direct detection of the pathogen's RNA or DNA. However, NANB hepatitis and AIDS were recognized as transfusion-transmissible diseases before any specific markers had been identified. In these cases, surrogate tests were considered or implemented. In the case of NANB, key studies clearly documented an association between elevated ALT levels in donors and the development of NANB in the recipients of the donations. Somewhat surprisingly, subsequent analysis showed a similar but nonoverlapping relationship between donor anti-HBc and recipient NANB. Although it was widely recognized that these tests were neither specific nor sensitive for NANB, they were projected to reduce the incidence of such post-transfusion infection by up to 60%, and testing for both markers was introduced during 1986 and 1987. Such projections were subsequently validated when tests for anti-HCV came into use.[61]

During the early years of the AIDS epidemic, it was recognized that individuals with the disease were often reactive for anti-HBc. Although a relationship between anti-HBc in donors and transmission of AIDS to recipients was understandably not demonstrable, some blood centers, particularly in the San Francisco Bay area, implemented anti-HBc testing as a surrogate.[28,62] Further expansion of this measure was overtaken by the recognition of HIV and by the anticipated availability of a specific test. Other measures based on some of the clinical characteristics of AIDS, such as changed T-cell subset ratios, were also proposed as surrogates and implemented in at least one location.[63]

Surrogate tests are inevitably less than satisfactory, usually failing to demonstrate adequate sensitivity or specificity. However, it should be recognized that perceptions have changed materially over the past 2 decades, and there is little doubt that surrogate tests would be seriously considered in the future. One example is the potential use of surrogate markers as a means of identifying individuals in the early stages of disease attributable to transmissible spongiform encephalopathies.

Testing is a key aspect of blood safety. Consequently, blood components are managed very conservatively with respect to test results. As pointed out earlier, a blood donation is discarded when found to be repeatedly reactive in a test. For the majority of assays, there is also a requirement to identify, retrieve, and quarantine any in-date products from prior donations from the affected donor. This action must be taken within a 3-day time frame, but it is not necessary if negative confirmatory or supplementary test results are available within this time.

A confirmed positive test result for HIV or HCV in a repeat donor triggers *lookback*. This process is designed to identify the recipients of prior donations from an individual now found to be seropositive. Such donations may have been in the infectious window period, may have been tested by a less-sensitive version of the test, or may have been given before the implementation of the test in question. Lookback may also be triggered by a report that implicates a donor in post-transfusion disease.

Donors with repeatedly reactive test results must be deferred from all further donations, and records must be kept to ensure that they are deferred. Clearly, this process results in the loss of many uninfected donors. At the same time, there is little point in continuing to collect blood from an individual who continues to generate false-positive test results, because the donations could not be used. In some circumstances a test that yields a false-positive result is not repeated, and so-called "reentry algorithms" have been developed to permit continued donation. These algorithms generally apply only to donors with repeatedly reactive screening test results that are negative in a licensed confirmatory or supplemental test. After a suitable waiting period, the donor must test nonreactive on screening and supplemental or confirmatory tests before being permitted to give blood again. Acceptable reentry protocols are published and updated by the FDA.

REFERENCES

1. Blumberg BS, Alter HJ, Visnich S. A 'new' antigen in leukemia sera. JAMA 1965;191:541–546.
2. Blumberg BS, Gerstley BJS, Hungerford DA, et al. A serum antigen (Australia antigen) in Down's syndrome, leukemia and hepatitis. Ann Intern Med 1967;66:924–931.
3. Ling CM, Overby LR. Prevalence of hepatitis B virus antigen as revealed by direct radioimmune assay with 125-I-antibody. J Immunol 1972;109:834–841.
4. Feinstone SM, Kapikian AZ, Purcell RH, et al. Transfusion-associated hepatitis not due to viral hepatitis type A or B. N Engl J Med 1975;292:767–770.
5. Choo Q-L, Kuo G, Weiner AJ, et al. Isolation of a cDNA clone derived from a blood-borne non-A, non-B viral hepatitis genome. Science 1989;244:359–362.
6. Alter HJ, Purcell RH, Holland PV, et al. Donor transaminase and recipient hepatitis. Impact on blood transfusion services. JAMA 1981;246: 630–634.
7. Aach RD, Szmuness W, Mosley JW, et al. Serum alanine aminotransferase of donors in relation to the risk of non-A, non-B hepatitis in recipients. The Transfusion-Transmitted Viruses Study. N Engl J Med 1981;304:989–994.
8. Stevens CE, Aach RD, Hollinger FB, et al. Hepatitis B virus antibody in blood donors and the occurrence of non-A, non-B hepatitis in transfusion recipients. An analysis of the Transmission-Transmitted Viruses Study. Ann Intern Med 1984;101:733–738.
9. Koziol DE, Holland PV, Alling DW, et al. Antibody to hepatitis B core antigen as a paradoxical marker for non-A, non-B hepatitis agents in donated blood. Ann Intern Med 1986;104:488–495.
10. Barre-Sinoussi F, Chermann J-C, Rey F, et al. Isolation of a T-lymphotropic retrovirus from a patient at risk for acquired immune deficiency syndrome (AIDS). Science 1983;220:868–871.
11. Gallo RC, Salahuddin SZ, Popovic M, et al. Frequent detection and isolation of cytopathic retroviruses (HTLV-III) from patients with AIDS and at risk for AIDS. Science 1984;224:500–503.
12. Poiesz BJ, Ruscetti FW, Gazdar AF, et al. Detection and isolation of type C retrovirus particles from fresh and cultured lymphocytes of a patient with cutaneous T-cell lymphoma. Proc Natl Acad Sci USA 1980;77:7415–7419.
13. Williams AE, Fang CT, Slamon DJ, et al. Seroprevalence and epidemiological correlates of HTLV-1 infection in U.S. blood donors. Science 1988;240:643–646.
14. Stramer SL, Fang CT, Foster GA, et al. West Nile virus among blood donors in the United States, 2003 and 2004. N Engl J Med 2005;253: 451–459.
15. Stramer SL, Layug L, Trenbeath J, et al. Use of a second EIA in an HTLV-I/HTLV-II algorithm [abstract]. Transfusion 1998;38(Suppl):81S.
16. Stramer SL, Glynn SA, Kleinman SH, et al. Detection of HIV-1 and HCV infections among antibody-negative blood donors by nucleic acid-amplification testing. N Eng J Med 2004;351:760–768.
17. Leiby DA, Read EJ, Lenes BA, et al. Seroepidemiology of *Trypanosoma cruzi*, etiologic agent of Chagas' disease, in US blood donors. J Infect Dis 1997;176:1047–1052.
18. Petersen LR, Satten GA, Dodd R, et al. Duration of time from onset of human immunodeficiency virus type 1 infectiousness to development of detectable antibody. Transfusion 1994;34:283–289.
19. Schreiber GB, Busch MP, Kleinman SH, Korelitz JJ. The risk of transfusion-transmitted viral infections. N Engl J Med 1996;334:1685–1690.
20. Busch MP. HIV, HBV and HCV: new developments related to transfusion safety. Vox Sang 2000;78:253–256.
21. Dodd RY, Notari EP, Stramer SL. Current prevalence and incidence of infectious disease markers and estimated window-period risk in the American Red Cross blood donor population. Transfusion 2002;42: 975–979.
22. Wilson K, Ricketts MN. The success of precaution? Managing the risk of transfusion transmission of variant Creutzfeldt-Jakob disease. Transfusion 2004;44:1475–1478.
23. Foster KR, Vecchia P, Repacholi MH. Risk management. Science and the precautionary principle. Science 2000;288:979–981.
24. Tobler LH, Stramer SL, Lee SR, et al. Performance of ORTHO(R) HCV core antigen and trak-C assays for detection of viraemia in pre-seroconversion plasma and whole blood donors. Vox Sang 2005;89:201–207.
25. Dodd RY. Current safety of the blood supply in the United States. Int J Hematol 2004;80:301–305.
26. Biswas R, Tabor E, Hsia CC, et al. Comparative sensitivity of HBV NATs and HBsAg assays for detection of acute HBV infection. Transfusion 2003;43:788–798.
27. Huang YY, Yang SS, Wu CH, et al. Impact of screening blood donors for hepatitis C antibody on posttransfusion hepatitis: a prospective study with a second-generation anti-hepatitis C virus assay. Transfusion 1994;34:661–665.
28. Dodd RY, Popovsky MA. Antibodies to hepatitis B core antigen and the infectivity of the blood supply. Scientific Section Coordinating Committee. Transfusion 1991;31:443–449.
29. Caspari G, Gerlich WH. Virus safety of blood and plasma products in Germany—state of knowledge and open problems. Infusionsther Transfusionsmed 2000;27:286–295.
30. Allain JP, Hewitt PE, Tedder RS, Williamson LM. Evidence that anti-HBc but not HBV DNA testing may prevent some HBV transmission by transfusion. Br J Haematol 1999;107:186–195.
31. Dodson SF, Issa S, Araya V, et al. Infectivity of hepatic allografts with antibodies to hepatitis B virus. Transplantation 1997;64:1582–1584.
32. Marusawa H, Uemoto S, Hijikata M, et al. Latent hepatitis B virus infection in healthy individuals with antibodies to hepatitis B core antigen. Hepatology 2000;31:488–495.
33. Cheng Y, Dubovoy N, Hayes-Rogers ME, et al. Detection of IgM to hepatitis B core antigen in a reductant containing, chemiluminescence assay. J Immunol Methods 1999;230:29–35.
34. Cardoso MD, Koerner K, Kubanek B. PCR screening in the routine of blood banking of the German Red Cross Blood Transfusion Service of Baden-Wurttemberg. Infusionsther Transfusionsmed 1998;25: 116–120.
35. Roth WK, Weber M, Seifried E. Feasibility and efficacy of routine PCR screening of blood donations for hepatitis C virus, hepatitis B virus, and HIV-1 in a blood-bank setting. Lancet 1999;353:359–363.
36. Stramer SL. Pooled hepatitis B virus DNA testing by nucleic acid amplification: implementation or not. Transfusion 2005;45:1242–1246.

37. Dow BC, Buchanan I, Munro H, et al. Relevance of RIBA-3 supplementary test to HCV PCR positivity and genotypes for HCV confirmation of blood donors. J Med Virol 1996;49:132–136.
38. Dodd RY, Stramer SL. Indeterminate results in blood donor testing: what you don't know can hurt you. Transfus Med Rev 2000;14:151–160.
39. Schorr JB, Berkowitz A, Cumming PD, et al. Prevalence of HTLV-III antibody in American blood donors. N Engl J Med 1985;313:384–385.
40. Busch MP, Lee LLL, Satten GA, et al. Time course of detection of viral and serologic markers preceding human immunodeficiency virus type 1 seroconversion: implications for screening of blood and tissue donors. Transfusion 1995;35:91–97.
41. Sarngadharan MG, Popovic M, Bruch L, et al. Antibodies reactive with human T-lymphotropic retroviruses (HTLV-III) in the serum of patients with AIDS. Science 1984;224:506–508.
42. Dodd RY, Fang CT. The Western immunoblot procedure for HIV antibodies and its interpretation. Arch Pathol Lab Med 1990;114: 240–245.
43. Dock NL, Kleinman SH, Rayfield MA, et al. Human immunodeficiency virus infection and indeterminate Western blot patterns: prospective studies in a low prevalence population. Arch Intern Med 1991;151: 525–530.
44. Kleinman S, Busch MP, Hall L, et al. False-positive HIV-1 test results in a low-risk screening setting of voluntary blood donation. JAMA 1998;280:1080–1085.
45. Mortimer PP. The fallibility of HIV western blot. Lancet 1991;337: 286–287.
46. Sayre KR, Dodd RY, Tegtmeier G, et al. False-positive human immunodeficiency virus type 1 Western blot tests in noninfected blood donors. Transfusion 1996;36:45–52.
47. Interpretation and use of the Western blot assay for serodiagnosis of human immunodeficiency virus type 1 infections. MMWR Morb Mortal Wkly Rep 1989;38(Suppl 7):1–7.
48. Aberle-Grasse J, Dodd RY, Layug L. Impact on human immunodeficiency virus type 1 (HIV-1) seroprevalence of the change in HIV-1 Western blot criteria. Transfusion 1997;37:246–247.
49. Alter HJ, Epstein JS, Swenson SG, et al. Prevalence of human immunodeficiency virus type 1 p24 antigen in U.S. blood donors-an assessment of the efficacy of testing in donor screening. N Engl J Med 1990;323: 1312–1317.
50. Delwart EL, Kalmin ND, Jones TS, et al. First report of human immunodeficiency virus transmission via an RNA-screened blood donation. Vox Sang 2004;86:171–177.
51. Phelps R, Robbins K, Liberti T, et al. Window-period human immunodeficiency virus transmission to two recipients by an adolescent blood donor. Transfusion 2004;44:929–933.
52. Stramer SL, Chambers L, Page PL, et al. Third reported US case of breakthrough HIV transmission from NAT screened blood (Abstract). Transfusion 2003;43(Suppl.):40A.
53. Khabbaz RF, Fukuda K, Kaplan JE. Guidelines for counseling human T-lymphotropic virus type I (HTLV-I)- and HTLV type II-infected persons. Transfusion 1993;33:694.
54. Larsen SA, Steiner BM, Rudolph AH. Laboratory diagnosis and interpretation of tests for syphilis. Clin Microbiol Rev 1995;8:1–21.
55. Orton SL, Liu H, Dodd RY, et al. Prevalence of circulating *Treponema pallidum* DNA and RNA in blood donors with confirmed positive syphilis tests. Transfusion 2002;42:94–99.
56. Herrera GA, Lackritz EM, Janssen RS, et al. Serologic test for syphilis as a surrogate marker for human immunodeficiency virus infection among United States blood donors. Transfusion 1997;37:836–840.
57. Preiksaitis JK. Indications for the use of cytomegalovirus-seronegative blood products. Transfus Med Rev 1991;5:1–17.
58. Preiksaitis JK. The cytomegalovirus-"safe" blood product: is leukoreduction equivalent to antibody screening? Transfus Med Rev 2000;14:112–136.
59. Blajchman MA, Goldman M, Freedman JJ, Sher GD. Proceedings of a consensus conference: prevention of post-transfusion CMV in the era of universal leukoreduction. Transfus Med Rev 2001;15:1–20.
60. Roback JD, Hillyer CD, Drew WL, et al. Multicenter evaluation of PCR methods for detecting CMV DNA in blood donors. Transfusion 2001;41:1249–1257.
61. Donahue JG, Muñoz A, Ness PM, et al. The declining risk of post-transfusion hepatitis C virus infection. N Engl J Med 1992;327:369–373.
62. Busch MP, Dodd RY, Lackritz EM, et al. Value and cost-effectiveness of screening blood donors for antibody to hepatitis B core antigen as a way of detecting window-phase human immunodeficiency virus type 1 infections. Transfusion 1997;37:1003–1011.
63. Galel SA, Lifson JD, Engleman EG. Prevention of AIDS transmission through screening of the blood supply. Annu Rev Immunol 1995;13: 201–227.

C. Regulatory, Quality, and Legal Principles

Chapter 15

Regulatory Principles and Issues Central to Blood Banking and Transfusion Medicine

Shealynn B. Harris • Christopher D. Hillyer

INTRODUCTION

Regulation is a government's oversight and control of a nongovernment entity's operations and practices through the enactment and enforcement of laws (i.e., regulations). Compliance with these legal requirements is not voluntary, and the potential consequences for a failure to comply with regulations include civil and criminal penalties. In general, the impetus for enacting regulatory legislation is the protection and promotion of public welfare; thus, regulations focus primarily on the overall safety of commercial and manufacturing operations, along with some professional services that directly impact the public welfare.

In the United States, the authority for federal regulatory oversight and enforcement is designated to a government agency; this agency is typically within one of the departments of the executive branch that is directed by a secretary, an appointee of the president of the United States. There are some exceptions to this regulatory organizational structure; for example, the Nuclear Regulatory Commission (NRC) is independent of a department and is led by a group of five commissioners who are all appointed by the president.[1] Although regulation is often more apparent at the federal level, regulation also occurs at the state level. There are similarities and overlap between federal and state regulation, a situation that is apparent in the parallel organizational structure of federal and state regulatory agencies and in the general purpose of federal and state regulatory code. In addition, federal authorities often partner with states through cooperative agreements to perform specific regulatory functions. However, for some operations and practices, it is the state government, and not the federal government, that sets regulations and maintains sole regulatory authority; examples include medical licensing, and in the case of blood establishments, the lower age limit for volunteer blood donation. The key federal regulatory agencies that have jurisdiction within blood banking and transfusion medicine are listed in Table 15–1.

As seen in Table 15–1, the U.S. blood industry as a whole is accountable to a variety of regulatory agencies. However, for an individual blood establishment, the extent of each agency's regulatory oversight depends on the breadth of the regulated establishment's operations and processes. In general, all U.S. blood establishments are subject to regulatory oversight by the Food and Drug Administration (FDA) for blood manufacturing and by the Centers for Medicare and Medicaid Services (CMS) for clinical laboratory testing.

This chapter focuses primarily on the FDA and the CMS in terms of agency structure, regulatory code, compliance oversight, and enforcement practices that are specific to the blood industry. The specific regulatory activities of the Department of Transportation (DOT), Occupational Safety and Health Administration (OSHA), and NRC that relate directly to blood establishments, blood manufacturing, and blood components are summarized in Table 15–1 and are not further addressed in this chapter. Finally, this chapter does not address regulation of non-U.S. blood banks and transfusion services, which range from highly developed to virtually nonexistent, depending on the location, nor does this chapter address the practice of medicine including aspects of transfusion medicine practice, because these aspects are not regulated by the government.

Regulation is sometimes confused with, or used as synonymous with, accreditation. *Accreditation* is a mechanism by which an organization's or an industry's practices are surveyed and formally approved by a private accrediting agency that promotes standards of practice for a specific industry or profession. In contrast to regulation, the accreditation process is voluntary, and failure to comply is not grounds for civil or criminal action. These private agencies not only serve an important role to the regulated entities, but they can also serve as a check and balance structure for government regulators. A more detailed discussion of accreditation and quality is presented in Chapter 16.

Table 15–1 Federal Regulatory Agencies in Blood Banking and Transfusion Medicine

Agency	Key Legislation	Regulatory Code (Title of CFR)	Applicability of Regulation
Department of Health and Human Services (HHS)			
Food and Drug Administration (FDA)	Federal Food Drug and Cosmetic Act of 1938 (FDC) Public Health Services Act of 1944 (PHS)	Title 21	Blood and blood manufacturing
Centers for Medicare & Medicaid (CMS)	Clinical Laboratory Improvement Amendment of 1988 (CLIA)	Title 42	Clinical laboratory testing
Department of Labor (DOL)			
Occupational Safety & Health Administration (OSHA)	Occupational Safety and Health Act of 1970 (OSH)	Title 29	Personnel safety (e.g., biohazard information, personal protective equipment (PPE), postexposure prophylaxis)
Department of Transportation (DOT)			
Pipeline and Hazardous Materials Safety Administration (PHMSA)	Federal Hazardous Materials Transportation Law (HAZMAT)	Title 49	Packaging, labeling, transport of biohazardous materials
Federal Motor Carrier Safety Administration (FMCSA)	Motor Carrier Safety Improvement Act of 1999	Title 49	Commercial drivers
Nuclear Regulatory Commission (NRC)	Nuclear Regulatory Legislation (NUREG)	Title 10	Free-standing irradiators

BLOOD AND BLOOD MANUFACTURING: THE FDA

Background

The federal government has regulatory authority over drugs, biologics, and devices, as mandated by the Federal Food, Drug, and Cosmetic (FDC) Act of 1938 and the Public Health Services (PHS) Act of 1944.[2] The FDA, an official agency of the Department of Health and Human Services (HHS), is the responsible body for the regulatory oversight and compliance enforcement of its regulations for drugs, biologics, and devices. Along with its regulatory duties, the FDA also engages in scientific and research endeavors, and it serves as an information resource for industry, health care, and the public.

Regulatory Organization

The FDA is organized into *offices*, which manage and direct FDA operations, and specialized program *centers*, which oversee the specific products regulated by the FDA.[3] For all FDA-regulated products and industries, the Office for Regulatory Affairs (ORA) serves as the lead office for compliance assurance.[4,5] The ORA's principle duty is the management and coordination of FDA regulatory field operations. These operations include routine inspections of registered and licensed facilities and compliance enforcement activities, such as assistance with legal and criminal investigations.[6]

Each regulated product and industry is also assigned to a specialized program center that is dedicated to non–field-based compliance management, regulatory guidance, and research efforts. The Center for Biologics Evaluation and Research (CBER) is the specialized program center committed to regulatory oversight of all biological products, including blood, vaccines, cellular therapies, gene therapies, tissues, and related devices.[4,7] CBER's research operations are further divided into offices and divisions. The Office of Blood Research and Review (OBRR) conducts research activities related to blood and blood safety through two divisions, the Division of Hematology and the Division of Emerging and Transfusion Transmitted Diseases.[8]

Regulatory Code

Although considered a biological product from an FDA organizational standpoint, in terms of legislation, blood is viewed as both a drug and a biological product. Accordingly, the legal requirements for blood products and blood manufacturing are contained in the FDC Act, which applies to drugs and devices, and the PHS Act, which applies to biologics. The specific federal statutes and amendments that pertain to blood and blood manufacturing are codified in Title 21 of the CFR in Parts 210 and 211 (drugs) and 600 to 680 (biologics).[9]

The entities and processes subject to this regulatory code are broadly defined by the FDA within the CFR and more clearly described in related compliance documents. According to the FDA, a *blood establishment* is "a place of business under one management at one general physical location." The term includes among others, human blood and plasma "donor centers, blood banks, transfusion services, other blood manufacturers and independent laboratories that engage in quality control and testing for registered blood product establishments."[10] For the purposes of FDA registration and compliance oversight, the types of blood establishments, as listed in Table 15–2, are more specifically defined by the FDA in terms of the extent of an establishment's manufacturing processes and level of manufacturing complexity.

Table 15–2 FDA-Defined Blood Establishments and Registration Requirements

Establishment	Definition	FDA Registration Requirements
Blood Bank, Blood Center (foreign and domestic)	A facility, sometimes located within a hospital, that engages in the manufacture of blood and blood components including: collection; processing of blood components product; testing compatibility testing; storing; distributing of blood products to consignees	Required to register
Blood and Plasma Broker	Takes physical possession of blood products or engages in any manufacturing step. Arranges for the sale or shipment of product.	Required to register Exempt if activities restricted to the arrangement of sale or shipment of products
Component Preparation Facility	Prepares components from blood collected at a mobile or fixed collection site and operates under the control of a parent blood bank or blood center	Required to register through parent establishment
Contractor	Person or entity that performs part or all of the steps in the manufacture of a licensed product or that performs a service for a blood or blood component manufacturer	Required to register Manufacturer and contractor share responsibility for product quality, however the manufacturer is ultimately responsible
Distribution Center or Depot	Stores blood and blood components under specific, controlled conditions for redistribution (intrastate or interstate) to final users and operates under the control of a parent blood bank or blood center	Required to register through parent establishment
Donor (Collection) Center	Fixed location that collects blood from donors by manual or automated methods and operates under the control of a parent blood bank or blood center. May operate blood mobiles or mobile blood drives	Required to register through parent establishment
Hospital Transfusion Service	Performs compatibility testing of (cross matching) for blood and blood components, but does not: routinely collect allogeneic or autologous blood process whole blood into componentswash components, prepare plasma cryoprecipitate reduced or leukocyte reduced products, or irradiate blood products May perform: product pooling of platelets or cryoprecipitate; compatibility testing; transfusion product thawing; division of products; preparation of recovered plasma or red blood cells from whole blood collected by a blood bank	Not required to register if the parent hospital participates in the Medicare reimbursement program Inspection responsibility granted to the CMS through a 1980 MOU
Indian Health Service (IHS) Hospital	Blood establishments maintained within the IHS See Blood Bank and Hospital Transfusion Service	
Military Blood Bank and Transfusion Service	Blood establishments, foreign and domestic, maintained by the Department of Defense	All foreign and domestic establishments must register Inspections are NOT unannounced; inspectors must notify respective military contacts 30 days before initiating an inspection
Testing Laboratory	Perform testing for a blood bank which may include testing for: infectious diseases; donor suitability and donor reentry; product quality	Required to register No registration is required if only testing patient samples or performing syphilis confirmatory tests
Veterans Health Administration Medical Center (VHAMC)	Blood banks and hospital transfusion services maintained within the VHAMC	All VHAMC blood banks and hospital transfusion services must register
Other Blood Establishment	Nonhospital-affiliated establishments that collect blood or prepare blood cells, serum, or plasma for "further manufacture" into drugs or devices	Required to register

Adapted from FDA Compliance Program Manual. Chapter 42: Blood and Blood Products: Inspection of Licensed and Unlicensed Blood Banks, Brokers, Reference Laboratories, and Contractors - 7342.001. FDA Office of Regulatory Affairs. Available at http://www.fda.gov/cber/7342001bld.htm. Accessed Oct. 12, 2005.

In order to operate legally in the United States, a blood establishment must comply with the specific blood manufacturing regulations outlined in the CFR, which include general criteria for licensing, registration, product quality, and component production. In addition to the CFR, which is updated annually, the FDA announces changes to regulations in the *Federal Register*, an official, daily publication of the federal government in which finalized rules and regulations, proposed regulations, and notices of regulatory agencies are posted. The final rules and regulations that are published in the *Federal Register* are incorporated into the CFR with the annual update. Electronic copies of both the CFR and recent editions of the *Federal Register* are available on the FDA website (http://www.fda.gov).

The regulatory requirements in the CFR are stated in broad, general terms. To assist blood establishments with interpretation, standardization, and implementation of regulatory requirements, CBER publishes *guidance documents* that provide background, explanation, interpretation and recommendations for more specific industry procedures and processes. Although not technically legally binding, guidance documents are considered by many to be standards for the blood industry and current good manufacturing practice (cGMP). Guidance documents for the blood industry are available on the CBER website (http://www.fda.gov/cber/guidelines.htm).

Current Good Manufacturing Practice

With regard to blood and blood establishments, relevant sections of the CFR focus primarily on cGMP. In general, cGMP requirements are set forth to ensure the safety, quality, identity, potency, and purity of drugs and biological products, also referred to as *SQuIPP*, in the blood industry.[11,12] More specifically, cGMP regulations are established for key areas of the blood manufacturing process that affect SQuIPP (Table 15–3). If a blood establishment fails to comply with cGMP, the manufactured product may be considered adulterated, and the establishment is subject to regulatory action. To effectively oversee blood establishment compliance with cGMP, the FDA employs several controls, which include registration, licensing, adverse event investigations, and facility inspections.

Blood Establishment Registration and Licensure

Registration

Under the FDC Act, all blood establishments are required to register with the FDA and submit a list of all products commercially distributed within 5 days of initiating manufacturing operations (see Table 15–2).[13] Manufacturers can register by completing either a paper Form FD-2830 (Blood Establishment Registration and Product Listing) or the electronic blood establishment registration (eBER) form on the FDA website. Certain blood establishments and blood distributors are exempt from CBER registration; these are facilities that do not engage in FDA-defined manufacturing activities that require a higher level of technical complexity or proficiency.[14] Manufacturing steps that are considered exempt are routine compatibility testing, product pooling, product thawing, and transfusion. A blood establishment that does not collect blood and restricts its operations to the above activities (e.g., a hospital transfusion service) is deemed exempt if its parent hospital participates in the Medicare reimbursement program. However, if the blood establishment performs more complex steps, as above, including but not limited to washing, irradiation, or preparation of plasma cryoprecipitate–reduced or leukocyte-reduced products and is not affiliated with a hospital in the Medicare reimbursement program, it is required to register with CBER. Exempt establishments are surveyed by the Center for Medicare and Medicaid Services (CMS) for regulatory compliance and are not routinely inspected by the FDA[15] unless just cause requires FDA inspection (e.g., a transfusion-related fatality).

Licensure

In addition to being registered, if a blood establishment engages in interstate commerce of a blood product, under Section 351 of the PHS Act, it must obtain a biologics license.[16] In December 1999, in an effort to improve regulatory efficiency as mandated by the FDA Modernization Act of 1997 (FDAMA), the previously separate establishment license application (ELA) and product license application (PLA) were consolidated into a single biologics license application (BLA).[17] CBER oversees the BLA process, which requires submission of specified documents and a prelicense inspection of the blood establishment. Once an establishment is licensed, any intentional changes to the manufacturing process that may impact product safety, purity, and potency must be reported to the FDA through CBER. Manufacturing changes are categorized into major, moderate, and minor, according to the effect that the change will have on the product. The reporting action that the manufacturer takes is based on the category of change. CBER provides a guidance document to help blood establishments with the process for reporting a change to an approved BLA.[18]

Facility Inspections and Compliance Enforcement

All registered, unlicensed and registered, licensed blood establishments are required to submit to routine, unannounced FDA inspections,[19] which are performed at a minimum of every 2 years. The only exception to unannounced inspections is for military blood establishments, for which the FDA must give at least 30 days notice prior to the inspection.[15] The primary objective of the inspection is to ensure SQuIPP by evaluating compliance with cGMP and thus the appropriate sections of the CFR. To focus on critical areas of blood safety, the FDA has identified five "blood systems" and five "layers of safety" (listed below) on which their inspection strategy is based.[15] The five blood systems are Quality Assurance, Donor (Suitability) Eligibility, Product Testing, Quarantine/Inventory Management, and Production and Processing. The five layers of safety are Donor Screening,

Table 15–3 A Summary of the Key cGMP Areas Referred to in 21 CFR 210, 211, and 600

Organization and Personnel
Buildings and Facilities
Equipment
Components, Containers, and Closures
Production and Processing
Packaging and Labeling
Quarantine, Storage, and Distribution
Testing
Records and Reports
Returned and Salvaged Products

II

Donor Deferral, Product Testing, Quarantining, and Monitoring and Investigating Problems. The extent of the inspection is determined by the blood establishment's specific manufacturing activities and is categorized by levels. A Level I inspection is a comprehensive assessment and requires an evaluation of compliance with all five systems. A Level II inspection is a more streamlined process that involves a review of three of the five blood systems.

On arrival for inspection of a blood establishment, the ORA investigator must provide a Form 482 (Notice of Inspection) that identifies the facility, the inspector, and the legal statutes by which the inspection is authorized.[20] This form must be signed by a facility representative or employee, often an individual of fairly high rank, indicating his or her recognition of the official nature of the inspection. On completion of the inspection, the inspector submits Form 483 (Inspectional Observations), which is a list of any observations of possible compliance violations.[20] This form is also signed by a facility official and acknowledges receipt of Form 483. Form 483 is not a final document of noncompliance, and the manufacturer may submit any objection to the observed violations or a plan for corrective action. Then, in consultation with ORA regional (or national, if needed) leadership and after final review, a formal inspection report is issued. After this compliance evaluation is completed, and if the facility is found to be in violation, the ORA may then begin compliance enforcement. The ORA's enforcement activities include advisory, administrative, and/or judicial actions.[21–23] The primary advisory action is a warning letter, which specifies significant regulatory violations and the necessity for prompt and adequate corrective action. If appropriate action is not taken by the manufacturer, or the action does not satisfactorily correct the violation, the ORA can then proceed with administrative and/or judicial actions, which include citations, license revocation or suspension, product recall or destruction, civil penalties, seizures, court action, and criminal prosecution.

In addition to the above enforcement activities, if a blood establishment fails to comply with regulations after multiple enforcement actions, the FDA may file a "Consent Decree of Permanent Injunction" (also known as a "Consent Decree"), which is a court order approved by a judge. A Consent Decree is a legally binding agreement, overseen by the court, between the FDA and a blood establishment that contains specific requirements and timelines for corrective action of regulatory violations. The Consent Decree defines the way in which the establishment must conduct its business while under the Consent Decree and allows for more frequent and in-depth FDA inspections. In addition, the Consent Decree defines the penalties, such as fines, placed on the establishment while it is under the Consent Decree. If the establishment satisfactorily meets the requirements outlined in the Consent Decree, the establishment will be released from the Consent Decree and considered "in good standing" by the FDA. Because the Consent Decree is a court order, if the establishment fails to comply with the Consent Decree, it is considered "in contempt of court," which is a criminal offense.

LABORATORY TESTING: CLIA AND CMS

Background

With the passage of the Public Health Service (PHS) Act of 1944, the federal government established regulatory authority over clinical laboratory facilities and, more specifically, set forth the requirements for certification of such facilities to operate legally in the United States. Under Section 353 of the PHS Act, the federal government introduced the following key certification requirements: (1) submission of records for types of tests performed, methodologies, and personnel training and experience; (2) accreditation by a government-approved, nonprofit, private accreditation body; and (3) participation in a proficiency testing program through a government-approved, nonprofit, private organization.[24,25] Furthermore, the PHS Act granted authority to the Department of Health and Human Services (HHS) for the oversight of clinical laboratory certification, development and promulgation of quality standards for clinical laboratory test performance, and inspection of clinical laboratory facilities and records.

In 1988, Congress passed the Clinical Laboratory Improvement Amendments of 1988 (*CLIA* or *CLIA 88*) in an effort to ensure the continuous improvement of the quality of clinical laboratory test performance, with a primary focus on the enhancement of test accuracy, reliability, and result turnaround time.[26] Furthermore, CLIA established parameters for the applicability and extent of clinical laboratory regulations by categorizing tests into levels of complexity.

Regulatory Organization

The HHS is charged with overseeing and providing services that relate to public health and welfare. The responsibilities for specific regulatory oversight functions and public services are divided among the twelve agencies within the HHS, each of which has a designated focus area. With regard to regulation of clinical laboratory testing, the HHS has charged its Centers for Medicare and Medicaid Services (CMS), formerly the Health Care Financing Administration (HCFA), with the authority for general CLIA implementation and oversight.[26] In addition, the HHS has given specific CLIA responsibilities to its Food and Drug Administration (FDA) for test complexity categorization, and to its Centers for Disease Control and Prevention (CDC) for convening the Clinical Laboratory Improvement Advisory Committee (CLIAC), which provides technical and scientific advice that relates to CLIA.[26]

The responsibilities and functions of CMS are divided into four "programs," which, in addition to the CLIA program, include Medicare, Medicaid, and the State Children's Health Insurance Programs (SCHIP). CMS performs its field operations through regional offices, which also serve as the liaisons with state and local agencies.[27] Through its Center for Medicaid and State Operations (CMSO), CMS also partners with state and local governments to manage CMS programs. In terms of CLIA, this partnership is most evident in functions that relate to compliance oversight, in particular, the performance of clinical laboratory inspections or surveys by state survey agencies.[28] Individual states may apply to be deemed as "exempt" under CLIA. When exempted, the state takes on the burden of clinical laboratory regulation. At the time of this writing, there are only two CLIA exempt states: Washington and New York.

The Regulatory Code and Regulated Entities

The regulations that pertain to clinical laboratory testing are codified in Title 42 of the CFR. CLIA defines a laboratory as "any facility that performs laboratory testing on specimens for the diagnosis, prevention, treatment of disease, or impairment of, or assessment of health."[25] All laboratories that perform even a single test on human specimens for these purposes, even those entities that do not bill to Medicare, are subject to federal regulation under CLIA and must register with the CLIA program.[25] The primary exception is a laboratory that performs testing for research purposes only. Thus, all laboratories within blood banking and transfusion services, except research laboratories, are regulated under CLIA.

Test Complexity and CLIA Certification

The applicability of specific CLIA regulations and the extent of regulatory oversight are based on the complexity of the test(s) performed by the clinical laboratory. Based on the technical demands of a test and the expertise required for the performance of a test, a test method is placed into one of the following categories: waived complexity, moderate complexity, or high complexity.[26] For each moderate- and high-complexity test, CLIA outlines requirements for quality control, quality assurance, personnel qualifications, proficiency testing, and patient sample and result management. CLIA does not specify such requirements for waived tests, for example, a point-of-care rapid diagnostic test for influenza performed in a physician's office. Although required to register with the CLIA program, clinical laboratories that perform only waived tests, also known as "waived laboratories," are only obligated to follow the test manufacturer's instructions.[30] Furthermore, these waived laboratories are not subject to routine inspections under CLIA.[31]

All clinical laboratories, even those that perform only waived tests, are required to apply to CMS for CLIA certification by submitting the "CLIA Application of Certification" (Form CMS-116) to the CMS-affiliated state agency in the state in which the clinical laboratory resides.[32] The application review focuses on the assessment of the complexity of test(s) performed by the clinical laboratory, the determination of the type of certificate to be issued, and the establishment of fees to be collected. The types of CLIA certificates are listed in Table 15–4. As a "user fee–funded" government program, all costs that relate to CLIA compliance, including registration, certification, and inspection fees, are required to be covered by the regulated laboratory.

Compliance Oversight

To ensure compliance with CLIA regulations, clinical laboratories that perform moderate- and/or high-complexity tests are obligated to submit to routine performance surveys. CMS follows an "outcome-oriented survey process," which focuses on assessing the overall quality of laboratory performance and not on an in-depth evaluation of each specific regulatory requirement.[33] The survey is typically an on-site inspection of the clinical laboratory; however, if the laboratory has shown consistently good performance, the survey can be in the form of a self-assessment, known as an *Alternate Quality Assessment Survey* (AQAS),[34] which does not require an on site inspection. Surveys are performed by the survey agency in the state in which the clinical laboratory resides or, in some cases, by the CMS regional office.

If a clinical laboratory fails to comply with regulations, maintains operations that pose an immediate threat to public welfare, and/or fails to show improvement in test performance deficiencies, then CMS is obligated under CLIA to proceed with enforcement actions. These enforcement actions include, but are not limited to, on-site monitoring of the laboratory by the state, mandatory retraining and technical assistance, civil penalties (fines), suspension or revocation of CLIA certification, suspension of Medicare/Medicaid payments, cancellation of Medicare/Medicaid approval, and court order of injunction to refrain from violative operations or practices.[35]

SUMMARY

In summary, regulation is a government's authority over a nongovernment body's operations and processes for the general intention of protecting public health and welfare. Compliance with regulations, which are the legal requirements established through the enactment of legislation, is nonvoluntary, and failure to comply with regulations is justification for civil and/or criminal action. Blood banks and transfusion services in the United States are subject to regulatory oversight by a variety of government agencies, with specific regulatory influence from the FDA for blood and blood manufacturing and the CMS for clinical laboratory performance. Regulations are codified in the CFR and organized into Titles according to the specific regulatory agency. Given that regulatory code is continuously updated, to ensure compliance, regulated entities must remain up-to-date on regulations and changes to regulatory code. Lastly, because the area of regulation is closely linked to the areas of accreditation and quality standards (Chapter 16) and legal practices (Chapter 17), a review of these subjects provides a more comprehensive view of regulation in the context of blood banking and transfusion practice.

Table 15–4 Types of CLIA Certificates

Certificate of Waiver. This certificate is issued to a laboratory to perform only waived tests.

Certificate for Provider-Performed Microscopy Procedures (PPMP). This certificate is issued to a laboratory in which a physician, midlevel practitioner, or dentist performs no tests other than the microscopy procedures. This certificate permits the laboratory to also perform waived tests.

Certificate of Registration. This is a certificate issued to a laboratory that enables it to conduct moderate- or high-complexity laboratory testing, or both, until it is determined by survey to be in compliance with the CLIA regulations.

Certificate of Compliance. This certificate is issued to a laboratory after an inspection that finds the laboratory is in compliance with all applicable CLIA requirements.

Certificate of Accreditation. This is a certificate that is issued to a laboratory on the basis of the laboratory's accreditation by an accreditation organization approved by HCFA.

Adapted from http://www.cms.hhs.gov/CLIA/downloads/TYPES_OF_CLIA_CERTIFICATES.pdf.

REFERENCES

1. U.S. Nuclear Regulatory Commission. Who We Are: The Commission. Available at http://www.nrc.gov/who-we-are/organization/commfunc-desc.html. Accessed Dec. 20, 2005.
2. U.S. Food and Drug Administration. Laws Enforced by the FDA and Related Statutes. Available at http://www.fda.gov/opacom/laws. Accessed Oct. 12, 2005.
3. U.S. Food and Drug Administration. FDA Organization. Available at http://www.fda.gov/opacom/7org.html. Accessed Oct. 30, 2005.
4. A Tour of FDA. U.S. Food and Drug Administration Office of Regulatory Affairs and EduNeering, Inc. Available at http://web.eduneering.com/fda/courses/fdatour/welcome.html. Accessed Oct. 12, 2005.
5. FDA's Sentinel of Public Health: Field Staff Safeguards High Standards. U.S. Food and Drug Administration: Just the Facts. Available at http://www.fda.gov/opacom/factsheets/justthefacts/7ora.pdf. Accessed Oct. 12, 2005.
6. Regulatory Procedures Manual March 2004. Chapter 1: Regulatory Organization. U.S. Food and Drug Administration. Available at www.fda.gov/ora/compliance_ref/rpm. Accessed Oct. 12, 2005.
7. FDA's Center on the Frontline of the Biomedical Frontier. U.S. Food and Drug Administration: Just the Facts. Available at http://www.fda.gov/opacom/factsheets/justthefacts/4cber.pdf. Accessed Oct. 12, 2005.
8. U.S. Food and Drug Administration. Center for Biologics Evaluation and Research: CBER Research Divisions and Investigators. Available at http://www.fda.gov/cber/research/rschovr.htm. Accessed October 12, 2005.
9. Code of Federal Regulations, Title 21, FDA. U.S. Government Printing Office, Washington, D.C. (revised annually).
10. Code of Federal Regulations, 21 CFR 607.3 (c). U.S. Government Printing Office, Washington, D.C. (revised annually).
11. Code of Federal Regulations, 21 CFR 210 and 211. U.S. Government Printing Office, Washington, D.C. (revised annually).
12. Code of Federal Regulations, 21 CFR 606. U.S. Government Printing Office, Washington, D.C. (revised annually).
13. Code of Federal Regulations, 21 CFR 607. U.S. Government Printing Office, Washington, D.C. (revised annually).
14. Code of Federal Regulations, 21 CFR 607.65. U.S. Government Printing Office, Washington, D.C. (revised annually).
15. FDA Compliance Program Manual. Chapter 42: Blood and Blood Products: Inspection of Licensed and Unlicensed Blood Banks, Brokers, Reference Laboratories, and Contractors - 7342.001. FDA Office of Regulatory Affairs. Available at http://www.fda.gov/cber/7342001bld.htm. Accessed Oct. 12, 2005.
16. Code of Federal Regulations, 21 CFR 601. U.S. Government Printing Office, Washington, D. C. (revised annually).
17. Federal Register. 64 FR 56441, October 20, 1999.
18. FDA Guidance to Industry: Changes to an Approved Application: Biological Products: Human Blood and Blood Components Intended for Transfusion or for Further Manufacture, August 7, 2001. Available at http://www.fda.gov/cber/gdlns/bldchanges.htm. Accessed Oct. 12, 2005.
19. Code of Federal Regulations, 21 CFR 600.20. U.S. Government Printing Office, Washington, D.C. (revised annually).
20. Investigations Operations Manual 2005. Chapter 5: Establishment Inspection: Subchapter 501: Authority to Inspect and Enter. FDA Office of Regulatory Affairs. Available at http://www.fda.gov/ora/inspect_ref/iom. Accessed Oct. 12, 2005.
21. Regulatory Procedures Manual March 2004. Chapter 4: Advisory Actions. Available at http://www.fda.gov/ora/compliance_ref/rpm. Accessed Oct. 12, 2005.
22. Regulatory Procedures Manual March 2004. Chapter 5: Administrative Actions. U.S. Food and Drug Administration. Available at http://www.fda.gov/ora/compliance_ref/rpm. Accessed Oct. 12, 2005.
23. Regulatory Procedures Manual March 2004. Chapter 6: Judicial Actions. U.S. Food and Drug Administration. Available at http://www.fda.gov/ora/compliance_ref/rpm. Accessed Oct. 12, 2005.
24. Public Health Service Act. Certification of Laboratories. Title 42 United States Code, Chapter 6A, Part F, Section 263a (42USC263a). Available at http://www.fda.gov/opacom/laws/phsvcact/phsvcact.htm. Accessed Oct. 30, 2005.
25. Code of Federal Regulations, 42 CFR 493. U.S. Government Printing Office, Washington, D.C. (revised annually).
26. Centers for Medicare & Medicaid Services: Program Descriptions/Projects. Available at http://www.cms.hhs.gov/CLIA/07_Program_Descriptions_Projects. asp. Accessed Dec. 20, 2005.
27. Centers for Medicare & Medicaid Services: Regional Office Overview. Available at http://www.cms.hhs.gov/RegionalOffices. Accessed Dec. 20, 2005.
28. Centers for Medicare & Medicaid Services: Office of the Administrator: Center for Medicaid and State Operations. Available at http://new.cms.hhs.gov/CMSLeadership/Downloads/CMSO.pdf. Accessed Dec. 20, 2005.
29. Centers for Medicare & Medicaid Services. List of Exempt States under the Clinical Laboratory Improvement Amendments (CLIA). Available at http://www.cms.hhs.gov/CLIA/downloads/Exempt.States.List.pdf. Accessed Dec. 20, 2005.
30. Centers for Medicare & Medicaid Services: Waived/PPMP Laboratory Project. Available at http://www.cms.hhs.gov/CLIA/08_Waived_PPMP_Laboratory_Project.asp. Accessed Dec. 20, 2005.
31. Code of Federal Regulations, 42 CFR 493.1775. U.S. Government Printing Office, Washington, D.C. (revised annually).
32. Centers for Medicare & Medicaid Services: How to How to Apply for a CLIA Certificate, Including Foreign Laboratories. Available at http://www.cms.hhs.gov/CLIA/06_How_to_Apply_for_a_CLIA_Certificate,_Including_Foreign_Laboratories.asp. Accessed Dec. 20, 2005.
33. Centers for Medicare & Medicaid Services. Outcome Oriented Survey Process. Available at http://new.cms.hhs.gov/CLIA/downloads/OUTCOME_ORIENTED_SURVEY_PROCESS.pdf. Accessed Dec. 20, 2005.
34. Centers for Medicare & Medicaid Services. Alternate Quality Assessment Survey. Available at http://new.cms.hhs.gov/CLIA/downloads/ALTERNATE_QUALITY_ASSESSMENT_SURVEY. pdf. Accessed Dec. 20, 2005.
35. Code of Federal Regulations, 42 CFR 493 Subpart R-Enforcement Procedures. U.S. Government Printing Office, Washington, D.C. (revised annually).

Chapter 16

Quality Assurance, Control and Improvement, and Accreditation

Richard J. Benjamin

INTRODUCTION

Quality, "a degree of excellence" or "superiority of kind,"[1] is difficult to define objectively, and thus it is often viewed differently by patients, regulatory agencies, and accrediting bodies. Consequently, blood bank professionals are held to quality standards set by a variety of agencies that have different foci. For example, the Food and Drug Administration (FDA), as a federal regulatory body, concentrates on the quality of the end product and applies pharmaceutical industry–type standards to the collection, testing, and provision of safe blood. In contrast, the Joint Commission for Accreditation of Healthcare Organizations (JCAHO), an independent, not-for-profit accrediting body, focuses primarily on quality of patient care and examines aspects of the hospital transfusion service involved with ordering, processing, and transfusion of blood. These complementary and overlapping approaches to ensuring quality have led to the need for transfusion services to maintain sophisticated programs in order to comply with the variety of state, federal, and industry regulations and standards.

QUALITY OVERSIGHT: REGULATION AND ACCREDITATION

Background

The general purpose of blood establishment regulation and accreditation is to guarantee safe, effective blood products and to ensure high-quality care of patients. Although similar in the overall promotion of quality, *regulation* and *accreditation* are distinct in terms of the structure for quality oversight and compliance enforcement. *Regulation* implies the enactment and enforcement by the government of laws and rules for required industry practices. If a regulated entity fails to comply with a regulation or, in other words, breaks a law, the potential consequences are civil or criminal penalties. *Accreditation*, conversely, involves a process by which an establishment demonstrates compliance with standards set by a nongovernmental professional or industry-related body. If compliance is not demonstrated, accreditation may not be granted or may be revoked; however, legal penalties cannot be applied for noncompliance with standards of an accrediting agency. Although technically distinct, in practice, regulation and accreditation often overlap. For example, accrediting standards are often viewed as standards of practice and may be invoked in a court of law as evidence for compliance with or deviation from accepted practice. In addition, accrediting agencies often incorporate government regulations into industry standards, and accreditation may serve as support for quality compliance in a government assessment of a regulated establishment. Finally, accrediting agencies can have influence on regulatory legislation through associated political action committees, industry testimony, and scientific panels.

Regulation of Blood Establishments

From a federal regulatory standpoint, blood products are viewed as both drugs and biologics.[2] Under the provisions of the Federal Food Drug and Cosmetic Act (FDC) of 1938 and the Public Health Service (PHS) Act of 1944, blood establishments are subject to federal regulations for registration, licensing, and inspection.[3] In 1972, the FDA was granted responsibility for regulatory oversight and enforcement of the blood industry, with the authority to inspect both licensed and unlicensed blood establishments. To ensure uniform blood component production throughout the United States, in 1975, the FDA issued Current Good Manufacturing Practices (cGMPs) that specifically focus on the blood industry.[4]

As defined in the Title 21 of the Code of Federal Regulations (CFR) Part 607.3, a blood establishment "means a place of business under one management at one general physical location" and includes, but is not limited to, blood banks, human blood and plasma donor (collection) centers, component preparation facilities, and hospital transfusion services. A blood establishment that enters into human blood and blood component manufacturing, which includes collection, preparation, and processing, must register with and submit to the FDA a list of all products for commercial distribution within 5 days of initiating operations. In addition, once registered and engaged in manufacturing operations, the blood establishment is required to register annually and submit an updated list of manufactured products.[5] Prior to engaging in interstate transport of blood or blood components, under Section 351 of the PHS Act, a registered blood establishment is further required to file a biologics license application (BLA), which includes a prelicense inspection by the FDA's Center for Biologics Evaluation and Research (CBER). Prior to December 1999, blood establishments were required to submit a separate establishment license application (ELA) and a product license application (PLA); however, in accordance with the FDA Modernization Act of 1997 (FDAMA), the ELA and PLA are now consolidated into a single BLA. To ensure that manufactured blood or blood components are safe, effective, free of adulteration, and appropriately labeled, the FDA's Office of Regulatory Affairs (ORA) performs routine announced or unannounced inspections of registered and licensed blood establishments. In addition to blood and blood component manufacturers, the FDA has recently extended its regulatory oversight to facilities that manufacture cellular and tissue-based therapeutics, including hematopoietic stem cells derived from blood, umbilical cord blood, and bone marrow.[6]

A blood establishment is considered exempt from registration with the FDA if it does not collect autologous or allogeneic blood and does not perform procedures that the FDA considers consistent with whole blood or component processing. An exempt hospital blood establishment, referred to as a "hospital transfusion service," may perform unit crossmatch, pool cryoprecipitate or platelet units, thaw frozen units, prepare recovered plasma, or transfuse blood components without being required to register. If the blood establishment performs prestorage leukoreduction, cell washing, or irradiation of blood or blood components, then the establishment is required to register with the FDA. In 1980, in accordance with a Memorandum of Understanding (MOU), the FDA transferred the responsibility for inspection of exempt transfusion services in hospitals approved for Medicare reimbursement to the Health Care Financing Administration (now called the Center for Medicaid and Medicare Services [CMS]).[7] Although CMS performs routine surveys of exempt hospital transfusion services, the FDA reserves the right to inspect these blood establishments, if required. For more information about federal regulation of blood manufacturing, the reader is referred to Chapters 12 and 15.

In addition to FDA regulatory oversight of blood manufacturing operations, blood banks, and transfusion services that test blood (e.g., ABO and Rh typing, antibody screening and identification) are subject to the Clinical Laboratory Improvement Amendments of 1988 (CLIA 1988),[8,9] which set standards for good laboratory practices. Responsibility for ensuring compliance with CLIA is assigned to the CMS. This compliance monitoring is achieved during triennial inspections by JCAHO, an accrediting agency with deemed status from the CMS. Finally, in many states in the United States, blood banks and transfusion services are subject to state regulations, which may include requirements for registration and annual reporting of adverse transfusion events. Requirements for reporting and inspections vary from state to state.

Accreditation of Blood Establishments

Professional societies and accrediting bodies such as AABB,[10] the College of American Pathologists (CAP),[11] and the Foundation for Accreditation of Hematopoietic Cell Therapy (FACT)[12] publish lists of voluntary standards to which many institutions subscribe. Regular inspections are undertaken to ensure compliance. These voluntary standards are intended to allow the profession to inspect and regulate its own practices outside the punitive environment of federal and state regulation. Accreditation by these agencies has yet to preclude inspection by the FDA or JCAHO.

AABB accreditation is based on the demonstration, through regular inspections, that the service has a detailed quality system under executive management, with written policies, processes, and procedures to cover the following: personnel qualification, training, competence, and proficiency; equipment qualification and validation; supplier qualification and vetting; appropriate process controls; secure and retained documents and records; internal and external assessments and audits; investigation of deviations, nonconformances and adverse events; process improvement through corrective and preventive action; and safe and adequate facilities. Similarly, CAP publishes a checklist of requirements for accreditation of all clinical laboratories, including the transfusion service. CAP accreditation is frequently used by smaller, non-FDA–registered facilities to demonstrate quality and compliance.

QUALITY ASSURANCE IN THE HOSPITAL AND THE ROLE OF THE TRANSFUSION COMMITTEE

Hospital transfusion practice is one focus of the JCAHO regulatory effort to ensure the quality of care, services, and treatment provided to patients. JCAHO standards and surveys form not only the basis for triennial inspections but also provide a framework for continuous operational improvement as hospitals incorporate guidelines into everyday practice.[13] Hospitals are required to have in place systems to collect data and monitor their performance, with blood and blood product use specifically mentioned as key parameters. Hemolytic transfusion reactions, in particular, are identified as sentinel events that should be reported and that should be subject to root cause analysis and formulation of an action plan. These requirements may be met by instituting systems for reviewing blood use, including: (1) ordering; (2) distribution, handling, and dispensing; (3) administration; and (4) the effects of transfusion. Oversight of these reviews is the responsibility of a hospital transfusion committee, or its equivalent, composed of members from departments that use blood, clinical laboratories, blood bank, nursing, and administration.[14,15] In this view, transfusion is a cooperative effort that requires quality assessment and documented improvement exercises that are performed continuously and according to objective guidelines used to monitor performance. Specific aspects that may be subject to audit and review include the adequacy of the blood supply, the use and wastage of autologous blood, mislabeling of patient specimens, turnaround time for completing immediate and routine transfusion orders, and the documentation of patient identification and vital signs at the time of transfusion. Further important aspects are investigations of transfusion reactions, appropriateness of blood orders, use of intraoperative blood salvage equipment, and use and maintenance of blood warmers.

Transfusion practice guidelines and criteria for specific product use vary between institutions and are developed by the transfusion committee with reference to criteria published in peer-reviewed journals. Examples are shown in Table 16–1. Such practice guidelines are not intended to serve as medical indications for transfusion; rather, they set limits outside of which the ordering physician should be required

Table 16–1 Examples of Criteria for Blood Component Administration in Adults

Red Blood Cells
Symptomatic anemia in a normovolemic patient
Acute loss of >15% of blood volume or evidence of inadequate O_2 delivery
Hematocrit <24% in a chronically transfused patient
Hematocrit <27% in a patient with severe cardiac or pulmonary dysfunction
Platelets
Platelet count <10,000/μL in a stable patient without bleeding risk factors
Platelet count <20,000/μL in a stable patient with risk factors for bleeding
Platelet count <50,000/μL for impending surgery or invasive procedure
Bleeding in patient with qualitative platelet defect, regardless of cause
Fresh Frozen Plasma
PT and/or PTT >1.5 normal value in patient undergoing surgery, an invasive procedure, or active bleeding
To reverse coumadin overdose in a bleeding patient
Bleeding after transfusion of more than one blood volume or signs of disseminated intravascular coagulation
For plasma exchange in patients with thrombotic thrombocytopenic purpura
Cryoprecipitate
Prevention or treatment of bleeding in patients with dysfibrinogenemia
Prevention or treatment of bleeding in patients with fibrinogen <100 mg/dL

to provide additional justification. Review of appropriateness of blood use is an important function of the transfusion committee, and there is a requirement that 5% of all transfusions be audited on a quarterly basis. Review may take one of three forms:

1. *Prospective review* is the process by which a blood bank designee evaluates the indication for transfusion at the time of the transfusion order. If the criteria for appropriate component use are met, the components are released. If not, the physician is asked to provide further justification for the specific order. If transfusion is urgent, however, the blood product may be released and the follow-up information obtained retrospectively.
2. *Concurrent review* requires transfusions to be assessed within 24 hours of issue, typically while the patient is still in the hospital and the indications are still fresh in the memory of the ordering physician. Both concurrent and prospective reviews provide opportunities to educate medical staff with respect to appropriate use of transfusions.
3. *Retrospective review* is undertaken more than 24 hours after transfusion. This type of review may be less effective. Trends in transfusion practice may be documented, although less educational benefit may be gained.

Overall, the purpose of blood use review is to provide opportunities to identify areas that need quality improvement. The emphasis is as much on ensuring that blood is available and used when it is needed as it is on preventing waste of a limited resource and unnecessary exposure of patients to the risks of transfusion.

QUALITY ASSURANCE IN THE COLLECTION AND MANUFACTURE OF BLOOD PRODUCTS

Blood components are considered drugs by the FDA because their use is meant to produce therapeutic benefit for the patient.[16] Establishments that collect blood (even autologous products) are viewed as pharmaceutical manufacturers. This approach raises significant practical issues. The principles of cGMP for drugs, as described in 21 CFR Parts 210 and 211,[17] are based on the concepts of continuous process control and lot release of products. In this view, blood donors are analogous to sources of raw material, and donor testing is simply quality control of incoming supplies. Furthermore, each blood product is a unique lot and therefore requires individual lot release, whereas with drugs, a batch of drug may be released. With blood products, quality control of each lot is not usually feasible. For this reason, more emphasis is placed on quality assurance of overall processes rather than on testing each product for quality parameters, such as volume, weight, hematocrit, and leukocyte content. The FDA clearly recognizes the unique nature of blood products as both blood and biologics and has promulgated a second series of regulations in 21 CFR Parts 600 to 680 that are specific for blood[4] and complement those in 21 CFR 210 and 211. The underlying principle of regulatory control of blood products is that by enforcing strict quality assurance of manufacturing processes, the statutory agencies hope to ensure the quality of individual blood products. Nevertheless, the advances in the field of blood safety, including the development of new tests (e.g., nucleic acid testing) and processes (e.g., leukoreduction), outstrip the ability of the federal government to promulgate law. Consequently, the industry relies on a series of guidelines and notices from the FDA that supplement the CFR and create many standards for the industry.

The Principles of cGMP

The concept of cGMPs is founded on the need to demonstrate control of all aspects of a manufacturing process, with documentation of all variables. This control should allow any single product to be tracked from donor to recipient and all reagents, facilities, and personnel to be traced so that any deviations may be fully identified, investigated, and rectified. Tight control of the manufacturing process, combined with suitable in-process quality control procedures and regular quality assurance exercises, serve to ensure the potency, efficacy, and purity of the final product.

The statutes promulgated in 21 CFR 211[17] and 21 CFR 606[4] cover all aspects of manufacturing, including personnel; buildings and facilities; equipment; components and containers; packaging; labeling; storage; holding and distribution; records; production and process controls; and salvaged products. Central to this regulatory structure is the need to document all procedures in standards of practice (SOP) and to qualify all facilities, equipment, and components by validation before use. A key role is ascribed to the quality control unit, which has overall responsibility for the release of final products.

Continuous Quality Improvement

Continuous quality improvement (CQI) is based on the premise that, despite the utmost care, processes and systems

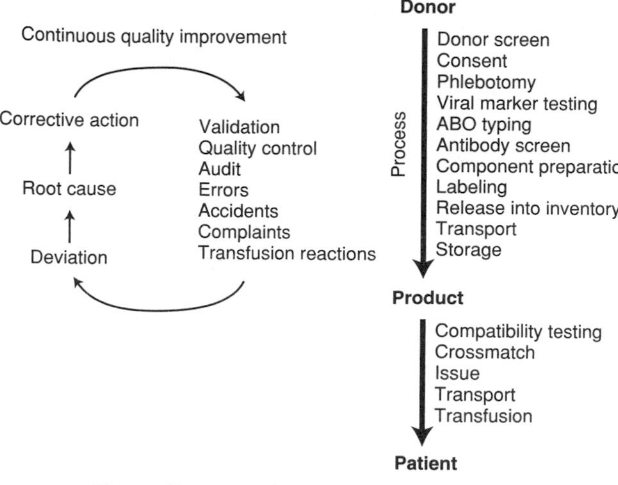

Figure 16–1 Continuous quality improvement.

cannot be designed to be perfect. It is therefore necessary to implement an evolutionary refining process to detect deviations and to put in place appropriate corrective actions (Fig. 16–1). The FDA requires that blood establishments have in place procedures for thoroughly searching for signs of deviations in processes. These deviations may become apparent during validation of a new process, during quality control (QC) and quality assurance (QA) audits, or through occurrences such as errors, accidents, complaints, and transfusion reactions. Establishments must have systems in place to investigate deviations, to determine their root cause, and to put in place corrective action. Central to this concept is the idea that staff and customers must be encouraged to report deviations; indeed, they should be encouraged to search actively for mistakes without fear of retribution. This view recognizes deviations as opportunities to improve and to provide better services. Well-designed processes performed by well-trained staff should ideally not allow deviations. When they occur, it is critical to thoroughly evaluate the problem and the involved processes to ensure systemic quality improvement.

The Role of the Quality Assurance Unit

Ensuring the safety of blood products requires the implementation of effective control over manufacturing processes and systems. In 1995 the FDA published guidelines that require blood establishments to develop written QA programs with an emphasis on error prevention rather than on retrospective detection.[18] QA is the sum of activities planned and performed to provide confidence that all systems and their elements that influence the quality of a product are functioning as expected and can be relied on. QA functions include QC procedures and audits, as well as ensuring that standards are in place for facilities, personnel, procedures, equipment, testing, and record keeping.

All blood establishments are required to have a QA function, either as a QA unit in large establishments or a single individual in small transfusion services. Whatever the size, the QA unit is required to be separate from the management of production and to report directly to the responsible head or the designated qualified person in charge of the operation. The QA unit has final responsibility for the quality of products released and must have the power to stop production and release of product if it deems necessary.

Major responsibilities of the QA unit include the following:

1. *Standard operating procedures.* Development of written procedures is a fundamental component of cGMP that promotes an environment with minimal variation. Ensuring that SOPs exist and that they accurately describe each procedure is a basic function of the QA unit. Each SOP must be reviewed, signed, and indexed in a master copy of the SOPs. SOPs must be available to employees who perform the tasks. SOPs must be updated promptly to reflect changes in processes, and these modifications must be appropriately documented. SOPs must exist for QA unit activities that define its role in reviewing, approving, and authorizing all SOPs.
2. *Training and education.* The QA unit should assist in developing, reviewing, and approving training and educational programs for all personnel. This responsibility includes new employee orientation; cGMP, SOP, and QA training; and technical, supervisory, managerial, and computer system training. The QA unit is ultimately responsible for ensuring that personnel are appropriately qualified and trained to perform their tasks. Written documentation of training must be on file.
3. *Competence evaluation.* The QA unit should implement a formal, regular competence evaluation program to ensure that staff maintain the skills to perform their tasks. This program should include direct observation of performance of routine and QC procedures, review of worksheets, preventive maintenance records, and written tests to assess theory and knowledge of SOPs. Remedial action and retraining should be documented in the personnel records.
4. *Proficiency testing.* The QA unit should review and monitor proficiency testing procedures and results to ensure adequate evaluation of test methods, equipment, and personnel competence. Proficiency testing should be performed by the same personnel who perform the tasks routinely and should include backup or alternative testing (e.g., manual procedures performed during computer downtime). There should also be a written plan for remedial action in the case of unsuccessful proficiency testing performance.
5. *Validation.* The QA unit is responsible for ensuring that validation protocols are designed prospectively, performed, and evaluated, and that written validation reports are prepared. Although validation of test methods is a standard practice in the clinical laboratory, the extension of these principles to manufacturing processes, computer systems, and facilities poses unique challenges. Validation requires documented evidence to demonstrate that the system is performing as designed and with the expected degree of accuracy and reproducibility. Complaints, errors, accidents, and problems at critical control points should be reviewed to determine the need for revalidation, according to the FDA's *Guideline on General Principles of Process Validation.*[19]
6. *Equipment and computers.* Equipment, in particular, should undergo installation qualification by the establishment (not the manufacturer). This is a form of validation that establishes "confidence that process equipment and ancillary systems are capable of consistently operating within established limits and tolerances." There should be written procedures for equipment qualification,

validation, maintenance, calibration, and monitoring. A major piece of equipment that is easily overlooked in the blood bank is the computer-based information system. The FDA has recognized that computers play a central role in practically all blood bank processes and that the risk of deviation caused by computer errors is high. For this reason, blood bank information systems are considered medical devices in their own right and are directly regulated by the Center for Biologics Evaluation and Research (CBER) at the FDA, requiring 510(k) approval before being marketed. This requirement places a unique burden on the manufacturers of blood bank software to demonstrate good software engineering practices and to document and validate all aspects of their systems.

Furthermore, blood establishments are required to validate all aspects of software on-site, an exhaustive process that was initially described in an FDA draft guidance, although a finalized guidance document had not yet been issued at the time of this writing.[20] As with other processes in the blood bank, there must be a system in place to document complaints and problems with computer software and hardware, with documented investigation, root cause analysis, and corrective actions. New versions of software require revalidation. Many institutions find that they require a dedicated computer person to perform these tasks despite the purchase of commercial software systems. The situation for homegrown computer programs has been less clear historically, as these programs are not for commercial sale. Homegrown systems may be used without preapproval, but the FDA has made it clear that they expect the same standards to apply to homegrown computer system design as to commercial vendors. Although FDA authorities do not routinely inspect the manufacturers of homegrown systems, they enforce the full weight of the law should major deficiencies in the computer system become apparent during routine blood bank inspection.

7. *Error/accident reports, complaints, and adverse reactions.* Licensed establishments are required to report to CBER all errors and accidents that affect the safety, quality, identity, potency, or purity ("SQuIPP") of a blood product. The FDA has announced that nonlicensed establishments, including hospital transfusion services, must report similar occurrences, now termed *biological product deviations* (BPDs), if the product has left the control of the establishment by the time the occurrence is detected.[21] It is the role of the QA unit to investigate all complaints, errors, and accidents to determine whether there is a need to report each occurrence. Similarly, all adverse reactions must be fully investigated and documented, and recalls and withdrawals must be handled according to established procedures. In particular, transfusion reactions must be fully investigated, and in cases of suspected bacterial contamination, a full review of manufacturing procedures must be undertaken. Fatalities that are related to either the donation process or the receipt of blood products are reportable within 24 hours to a special hotline at the FDA. This reporting must be followed within a week by a full written report describing the occurrence and its subsequent investigation. This written report, in turn, usually triggers a focused FDA inspection.

   As outlined earlier, an essential element of CQI is feedback into the QA system of knowledge acquired through investigation of complaints, errors, accidents, or adverse reactions. This is seen as a vital source of information on which continuous quality improvement efforts can be focused through a system of corrective actions and fine-tuning of existing processes.
8. *Records management.* The QA unit is responsible for ensuring that all records, including computer records, are adequately stored and held for the appropriate periods as defined by the FDA. Systems of storage, especially computerized systems, must be fully validated and reviewed as necessary to ensure completeness.
9. *Lot release procedures.* Each component released by a blood establishment represents one lot of product and bears a lot number, usually the unit number assigned at the time of collection. QA procedures must ensure that all records pertaining to manufacture are reviewed for accuracy, completeness, and compliance with existing standards before release. A second person should review the significant steps. Labeling procedures, especially, are considered critical control points and must be tightly controlled.
10. *QA audits.* A QA audit is one mechanism for evaluating the effectiveness of the total quality system. Comprehensive audits should be conducted periodically in accordance with written procedures and should consist of a review of a statistically significant number of records. On occasion, focused audits may be conducted when quality problems have been identified or to monitor a particular critical control point. Individuals conducting audits must have sufficient knowledge of and expertise in the process under review but must not be responsible for the processes being audited. There should be a written report documenting audit procedures and results; this written report should include a review by the responsible head or other designated qualified person to evaluate the results of the audit so that suitable corrective action can be implemented. QA audits should be constructed using a systems approach and may include review of donor suitability, blood collection, manufacturing, product testing, storage and distribution, lot release, and computers. QA audits should evaluate critical control points and key elements in each system, and each establishment should customize its audits for its own systems.

RECALLS AND WITHDRAWALS: PRACTICAL APPLICATION OF THE CONCEPT OF SQuIPP

Continuous quality improvement exercises aim to use all sources of information to identify BPDs, with a view to improving processes and systems. In the endeavor to identify deviations, problematic products may be identified that have been released from inventory or even transfused, requiring a consideration of the safety of the recipient. If the deviation from the standard was the result of an error in the collection or processing of the unit by the collecting facility, in violation of the laws overseen and enforced by the FDA, especially violations of cGMPs, "and against which the agency would initiate legal action,"[22] the process is called a *biologic recall.* Recalls may be conducted voluntarily on a firm's own initiative, by FDA request, or by FDA order under statutory authority.[23] All recalls must also be reported to the FDA, regardless of who initiated the action. The FDA subsequently classifies recalls as follows: A *Class I* recall is a situation in which there is a reasonable probability that the use of or exposure to a violative product will cause serious adverse health consequences or death. A *Class II* recall is a situation in which use of or exposure to a violative product may cause temporary or medically reversible adverse health consequences, or where the probability of serious adverse health consequences is remote. A *Class III* recall is a situation in which use of or exposure to a violative product is not likely to cause adverse health consequences.[22] These recalls are then reported publicly by the FDA several months later.[24] If large, multiunit recalls are excluded, the more common blood center recalls occur typically at an approximate rate of 1 in 5000 components distributed.[24]

A *market withdrawal* occurs when a product has a minor violation that would not be subject to FDA legal action (i.e., not an "actionable violation"). The firm removes the product from the market or corrects the violation. For example, a product removed from the market due to tampering, without evidence of manufacturing or distribution problems, would be a market withdrawal. For the blood center, withdrawals are most often triggered by information provided by a blood donor or a third party after donation that, if known at the time of donation, would have led to deferral of the donor. An example would be the withdrawal, in the late 1990s, of blood products that were obtained from donors at risk of Creutzfeldt-Jakob Disease (CJD), or variant CJD. The FDA became aware of a theoretical risk of transfusion transmission of these ailments and advised that previously collected, "in-date" products from donors at risk should be withdrawn. Likewise, in the fall of 2002, the discovery that West Nile virus could be transmitted by blood products led to the later, voluntary withdrawal of most frozen blood products from certain localities collected during the period of highest risk of transmission, on the grounds that they might be contaminated. These products met all the required standards of blood safety at the time of manufacture, but they were later considered unsafe and required withdrawal. Blood component–related market withdrawals occur with approximately the same frequency as recalls.[25]

In deciding whether postdistribution information warrants action on the part of a blood establishment, it is helpful to consider *SQuIPP* (Table 16–2). Any deviation from established procedures or deferral criteria that would lead to reduced *safety* in the product (i.e., greater potential for harmful effects) generally leads to withdrawal or recall. For instance, a presenting donor may state that he received a needlestick exposure to blood 4 months earlier, before a donation 3 months ago. Because donors with exposures to blood represent a group that may have a greater risk of carrying transfusion-transmissible disease, they are deferred. Had the center known of the blood exposure at the time of the earlier donation, the donor would have been deferred; therefore, components distributed from the donation 3 months ago must be withdrawn.

Quality represents conformance of a product or process with preestablished specifications or standards. If it is discovered after the release of a leukoreduced component that the leukoreduction quality control for that component failed, then the component must be recalled.

Identity indicates the need to ensure that the identification of the donor, the unit, and its components is certain throughout the collection, processing, and labeling steps. For instance, if a unit of red blood cells, acceptable in every other way, is stated on the label to be negative for Kell (K1) when it is not, the unit is "misbranded," and it could be harmful to a recipient whose serum contains anti-K1.

Purity deals with freedom from extraneous contaminating matter in a product. If, after a recipient febrile transfusion reaction, the residue from a unit of platelets is cultured and is found to contain microorganisms, the other components from that collection should be withdrawn, because they may also have been contaminated.

Potency represents the ability of a product to produce the desired effect. Here, loss of potency typically indicates a failure of quality control. The findings that fewer than 75% of platelets units have 5.5×10^{10} platelets and that red blood cell recovery after leukoreduction of red blood cells is less than the required amount represent a loss of potency. If these products had been distributed, discovery of their deficiencies would have led to a recall.

Table 16–2 SQuIPP

Use SQuIPP to help determine whether a product needs to be recalled or withdrawn
- Safety: does the product have a greater potential than usual for harmful effects?
- Quality: does the product conform to preestablished specifications or standards?
- Identity: is the identity of the final product and its labeling certain?
- Purity: is the product free of extraneous contaminating matter?
- Potency: can the product produce the desired effect?

Actions Taken by the Blood Center

When the collecting facility discovers that a product that does not meet SQuIPP criteria has been released, staff members must work rapidly to notify the receiving transfusion service. For in-date products that may still be in the hospital inventory, this notification is done typically by telephone, to allow immediate quarantine of the suspect product, followed by written notification. The center must also quarantine any in-date products in its inventory. Because the information is typically obtained at the time of a subsequent attempted donation, platelet and red blood cell components are usually outdated, but frozen plasma, frozen red blood cells, and cryoprecipitate may still be in the center or hospital inventory. The center in-date inventory must be identified and quarantined quickly. Hospitals must be notified of in-date components as soon as possible, with written notification following soon afterward. When the hospital returns suspect components, the center usually destroys them or corrects the underlying problem with appropriate documentation. If the postdonation information would lead to donor deferral in the future, the center must place the donor in the deferral registry and must notify the donor of this action, to prevent collection and distribution of any future donations. The center must document its actions and must seek from the consignee information regarding the final disposition of components.

Actions Taken by the Hospital Transfusion Service

When notified that products are being recalled or withdrawn, the hospital must act immediately to quarantine any such products in the inventory. The hospital must ensure that proper steps are taken and documented. When products have been transfused (75% of recalls in one hospital were found to be for components already transfused),[25] the hospital transfusion service must consider carefully the appropriate steps to take, in concert with hospital administration and risk management staff. For some recalls or withdrawals, no further action may be necessary. For instance, when a unit that was incorrectly labeled as K1 negative was subsequently transfused to a recipient who had no anti-K1, no clinician or patient notification would be needed, merely a note for the record of the facts. For other situations, the transfusion service may wish to notify the clinician but advise him or her that patient notification is probably unnecessary. For instance, red blood cells from a donor who had traveled to a malarial area and that were transfused 6 months earlier would have caused transfusion-induced malaria within 50 days of transfusion, and if no febrile disease developed, these red blood cells would represent no additional risk.[26] Finally, in some cases, the patient should be notified, particularly when there is some risk of infectious disease transmission, so that investigation, counseling, and treatment can be considered. Patient notification may be required, for instance, for possible transmission of human immunodeficiency virus (HIV) or hepatitis C virus (HCV).[27] In each case in which a component has been transfused, the transfusion service must balance the evidence that an infectious agent was transmitted through transfusion, the potential benefit to the recipient of receiving this information, and the potential harm to the recipient when no diagnostic test exists that can resolve whether such transmission has occurred.[28] If the transfusion service physician finds the information sent to be insufficient, sometimes more information can be obtained from the blood center. Fortunately, most recall and market withdrawal notifications have little clinical significance.[25,29]

LOOKBACK

When a donor unit is found to be positive for an infectious disease marker, several actions must be taken by the collecting blood center. Obviously, the implicated unit must be destroyed, and this disposition must be recorded. In addition, donor-related actions are required (notification, counseling, and placement in a donor deferral registry), and action may need to be taken to ensure that previous units donated by that donor have not transmitted disease. The latter process is termed *lookback.*

When determining the risk of transfusion transmission of disease, prevalence, measured for transfusion-transmitted diseases by an infectious disease marker, is usually of less concern than *incidence,* or the new acquisition and development of disease, because blood with a marker indicating prevalence is usually readily identified by testing and is discarded. For a newly acquired, incident viral agent, the concern is about transmission of disease during the *window period,* defined as the time between donor infection and the appearance of detectable markers of disease, a time in which current tests may not identify an infectious unit. The window period may be conveniently divided into two parts: an eclipse period, when the agent is undergoing proliferation in host tissue but is not present in sufficient numbers in the blood to be infectious,[30] and the subsequent infectious period, when circulating virus can be transmitted by the blood. The goal of test improvement has been to increase sensitivity to the extent that the infectious window period is reduced as much as possible. Because an infectious window period still exists, and may have been longer in the past, when a donor is found to have a newly acquired marker of an infectious disease, the more recent, previously seronegative donations of that donor must be regarded as suspect.[31] The risk of a previous donation's ability to transmit disease depends on the incidence of the disease and on the length of the infectious window period, the latter a function of the sensitivity of the test used. For HIV or HCV, using nucleic acid amplification testing, the infectious window period may be a few days, at most.[30] Notification of recipients of previously donated seronegative units is important, so that the recipients may be tested and, if they are positive for the agent, counseled and treated appropriately.

Actions by the Center and the Hospital

The blood center must identify previously donated units at risk from the implicated donor and must determine the components made from these units and the consignees to whom these components were shipped. The center must then notify the hospital of the situation and must obtain information about the final disposition of the components. If in-date components from such units may be available, the consignee should be notified as soon as possible after the detection of a repeat reactive screening test.

The specifics of the actions required vary by disease. For HIV and human T-cell leukemia/lymphoma virus (HTLV), the center searches for the first seronegative (or untested) unit previously donated and for all units donated for at least 1 year before that donation.[27] The center must identify all components made from the suspect units and must determine where they were sent. If any in-date components exist, these must be identified and quarantined if they are in the center. If these components have been distributed, the consignees of such components should be notified within a few days of the positive test result. The hospital, in turn, must ensure that the patient is notified (typically through the clinician, but if necessary, by the hospital directly) within a few weeks. For HIV, even if the patient is deceased, the patient's next of kin must be notified.[27] For HTLV, in contrast, the clinician can make the decision not to notify the patient or the recipient, if the decision is warranted clinically. Both the center and the hospital must document notification attempts.

For HCV lookback on a donor found to be seropositive, the same process is used. The center must identify units 12 months before the last seronegative unit, locate the consignees of components made from those units and shipped to the consignee, and notify the consignee within 45 days of the repeat reactive donation. The consignee must ensure that the patient is notified of the need for HCV testing and of the availability of testing and counseling. There must be documentation of three attempts to notify the recipient within 12 weeks of notification by the center.[32]

A massive retrospective HCV lookback of units donated between 1990 and 1999, on which lookback had not already been performed, was begun in 1999 and was completed by 2001. This *targeted* (identification of specific blood recipients) lookback process may not be very cost effective. One estimate is that of approximately 300,000 recipients to be notified, perhaps only 5000 to 10,000 will be living and will have newly recognized infections, and 1500 will benefit from therapy.[33] Interim data from the U.S. Centers for Disease Control and Prevention corroborate these numbers and indicate that approximately 0.5% of recipients will be found to have newly recognized infections.[34] Despite the inefficiency of the targeted lookback process, no compelling evidence indicates that general notification of all blood recipients would be effective[35]; indeed, many of those recipients identified by targeted lookback would not otherwise be identified and treated.

CONCLUSION

Quality management in transfusion medicine is a formalized process that is required by law. Over the past 2 decades, blood establishments have focused on regulatory compliance in order to meet the standards of accreditation set by multiple agencies. These regulatory pressures have engendered a change in mind-set that is now increasingly pervasive throughout the industry: Quality accepts only the best and works hard to improve, despite cost constraints, shortages in the skilled workforce, evolving technology, and a growing regulatory burden. Quality is the ultimate goal, and compliance is merely obeying the rules. It is now clear that, along with refinements in donor screening and viral marker testing, the implementation of Quality and cGMP principles and improved clinical practice are responsible for the safety revolution that continues in blood transfusion.

REFERENCES

1. Webster's 9th New Collegiate Dictionary. Springfield, Mass., Merriam-Webster, 1991.
2. Federal Food, Drug and Cosmetic Act. Title 21 USC Sec 201 (Amended by FDA Modernization Act of 1997).
3. Public Health Service Act, Biologic products. Title 42 USC Sec 262 (revised annually).
4. Code of Federal Regulations. Title 21 CFR 606. Washington, D.C., U.S. Government Printing Office, 2004 (revised annually).
5. Department of Health and Human Services, Food and Drug Administration, Office of Regulatory Affairs: FDA Compliance Policy Guide. Registration of Blood Banks and Other Firms Collecting, Manufacturing, Preparing and Processing Human Blood or Blood Products. Bethesda, Md., Food and Drug Administration, 2000, Sec 230.110.
6. Current good tissue practice for human cell, tissue, and cellular and tissue-based product establishments. Code of Federal Regulations. Title 21 CFR part 16, 1270 and 1271. Washington, D.C., US Government Printing Office, 2005.
7. Department of Health and Human Services, Food and Drug Administration: FDA Compliance Policy Guide. Memorandum of Understanding 1980: 7155e.03 Chapter 55e. Bethesda, Md., Food and Drug Administration, 1980.
8. Department of Health and Human Services: Medicare, Medicaid and CLIA programs: regulations implementing the Clinical Laboratory Improvement Amendments of 1988 (CLIA 1988). Fed Regist 1992;57:7002.
9. Code of Federal Regulations. Title 42 CFR 493.1. Washington, D.C., U.S. Government Printing Office, 2000 (revised annually).
10. Silva M (chair). Standards for Blood Banks and Transfusion Services, 23rd ed. Bethesda, Md., American Association of Blood Banks, 2005.
11. How to Inspect the Transfusion Medicine Laboratory. College of American Pathologists, Chicago, Ill., 1999.
12. FACT Standards for hematopoietic progenitor cell collection, processing and transfusion, 2nd edition. Foundation for Accreditation of Hematopoietic Cell Therapy. Omaha, Neb., 2003.
13. Comprehensive accreditation manual for hospitals: The official handbook. Joint Commission for Healthcare Organizations. Oakbrook Terrace, Ill., 2005.
14. Silberstein LE, Kruskall MS, Stehling LC, et al. Strategies for the review of transfusion practices. JAMA 1989;262:1993–1997.
15. Stehling L, Luban NLC, Anderson KC, et al. Guidelines for blood utilization review. Transfusion 1994;34:438–448.
16. Department of Health and Human Services, Food and Drug Administration, Office of Regulatory Affairs: FDA Compliance Policy Guide. Human Blood and Blood Products as Drugs (CPG 7134.02). Bethesda, Md., Food and Drug Administration, 1996, Sec 230.120.
17. Code of Federal Regulations. Title 21 CFR 211. Washington, D.C., U.S. Government Printing Office, 2004 (revised annually).
18. Department of Health and Human Services, Center for Biologics Evaluation and Research: Guideline for Quality Assurance in Blood Establishments (Docket no 91N-0450), 1995.
19. Department of Health and Human Services, Center for Drugs and Biologics, Center for Devices and Radiological Health: Guideline on General Principles of Process Validation. Rockville, Md., Division of Manufacturing and Product Quality, 1987.
20. Department of Health and Human Services, Center for Biologics Evaluation and Research: Draft Guideline for the Validation of Blood Establishment Computer Systems (Docket no 93N-0394). Office of Communication, Training and Manufacturers Assistance, 1993.
21. Department of Health and Human Services, Food and Drug Administration: Biological products: reporting of biological product deviations in manufacturing. Fed Regist 2000;65:66621.
22. Code of Federal Regulations. Title 21 CFR 7.1–7.59. Washington, D.C., U.S. Government Printing Office, 2005 (revised annually).
23. Bozzo T. Blood component recalls. Transfusion 39:439–441, 1999.
24. Ramsey G, Sherman L. Blood component recalls in the United States. Transfusion 1999;39:473–478.
25. Ramsey G, Fryxell LM, Russell DL, Sherman LA. Three-year hospital experience with a system for tracking blood supplier notifications about blood products. Transfusion 1998;38(Suppl):123S.
26. Guerrero IC, Weniger BC, Schultz MG. Transfusion malaria in the United States, 1972–1981. Ann Intern Med 1983;99:221–226.
27. United States Food and Drug Administration: Current good manufacturing practices for blood and blood components: Notification of consignees receiving blood and components at increased risk for transmitting HIV infection. Final rule: HHS docket No.91N-0152. Fed Regist 61:47413–47474, 1996.
28. Smith DM, Lipton KS. Association Bulletin 97–3: Consignee/Recipient Notification Guidelines. Bethesda, Md, American Association of Blood Banks, 1997.
29. Grindon AJ, Harris SL, Roback JD, et al. Low patient risk from market withdrawn (MW) blood components. Transfusion 1999;39(Suppl):125S.
30. Murthy KK, Henrard DR, Eichberg JW, et al. Redefining the HIV-infectious window period in the chimpanzee model: Evidence to suggest that viral nucleic acid testing can prevent blood-borne transmission. Transfusion 1999;39:688–693.
31. Ward JW, Holmberg SD, Allen JR, et al. Transmission of human immunodeficiency virus (HIV) by blood transfusion screened as negative for HIV antibody. N Engl J Med 1988;318:473–478.
32. United States Food and Drug Administration: Current good manufacturing practices for blood and blood components: Notification of consignees and transfusion recipients receiving blood and blood components at increased risk of transmitting HCV infection ("lookback"). Proposed rule. Fed Regist 65:69377–69416, 2000.
33. AuBuchon JP. Public health, public trust, and public decision making: making hepatitis C virus lookback work. Transfusion 1999;39:123–127.
34. Culver DH, Alter MJ, Mullan RJ, Margolis HS. Evaluation of the effectiveness of targeted lookback for HCV infection in the United States: Interim results. Transfusion 2000;40:1176–1181.
35. Zuck T. Cited in Busch MP: Let's look at human immunodeficiency virus look-back before leaping into hepatitis C look-back. Transfusion 1991;31:655–661.

Chapter 17

Legal Principles and Issues Central to Transfusion Medicine

Karen Shoos Lipton • Diane Killion

Today's transfusion medicine and cellular therapy professionals are challenged with striking an appropriate balance between optimizing and maintaining the safety of blood donors and recipients and effectively managing the legal risks inherent in the operation of blood-collection and blood-transfusion facilities. This chapter provides health care professionals with an overview of the growing number of legal issues that affect the transfusion medicine and cellular therapy communities and offers suggestions as to how to mitigate the associated risks in order to better serve donors and patients.

Because of the evolution of the law in these areas, more cases relate to the collection and transfusion of blood and blood components than to the collection, processing, storage, and administration of cellular therapy products. For this reason, this chapter focuses on cases relating to the transfusion of blood and blood components. As a practical matter, however, many of the legal issues that have affected transfusion medicine will similarly affect the cellular therapies field. Although the cases discussed in this chapter are intended to be illustrative of legal concepts, they are not intended to replace the advice of competent legal counsel.

LEGAL RISKS IN TRANSFUSION MEDICINE

Theories of Liability

A plaintiff complaining that he or she was wrongly injured by a transfusion typically looks to include the greatest number of defendants, based on as many causes of action as possible. For example, defendants may include clinician(s) who transfused blood and treated the patient, the hospital where the transfusion and treatment were provided, the blood center that collected the blood, and possibly the organization that set the applicable standards.

The claims may include failure properly to warn of the risks of treatment or surgery, failure adequately to discuss alternatives to transfusion such as autologous or directed donation, failure adequately to warn of the potential risks inherent in transfusion, negligent hiring and supervision of staff, failure adequately to test the donor for transfusion-transmitted disease, failure to develop or implement an appropriate "lookback" program for notifying recipients of infected blood, negligent standard setting, failure to transfuse at the proper rate, and negligently administering transfusions that were not medically necessary.

These causes of action are generally based on at least three different theories of liability: (1) negligence, (2) strict liability, and (3) breach of implied warranty. Appreciating the distinctions among the applicable theories is important to minimize the risk of liability.

NEGLIGENCE

Although the law of negligence varies significantly from state to state, the basic elements of a negligence claim are as follows: the defendant owed a duty of care to the plaintiff; the defendant breached the duty; the plaintiff's injury was directly or proximately caused by the breach; and the plaintiff suffered damages as a result.[1] In short, the theory of negligence holds that the provider of medical services is responsible for providing safe products and services that will not harm the patient and that are consistent with the prevailing standards of care.

Historically, negligence was grounded in fault-based liability: the negligent actions had to be proven to cause the injury. Beginning with the Restatement (Second) of Torts §402A (1964), a new basis for liability was widely adopted largely to hold manufacturers accountable for poorly designed products. This was termed *strict liability* or *liability without fault*.[2] To find a manufacturer strictly liable, one need prove only that the injury was due to the product's design, regardless of whether the manufacturer was at fault. The impetus for the adoption of the theory was to encourage manufacturers to make safer products by requiring them to absorb the real costs of the consequences of the unsafe product. However, recognizing that blood is a living tissue, inherently variable and incapable of being rendered uniform or completely safe, virtually every state has adopted special "Blood Shield Statutes" exempting blood from strict liability standards. Even in jurisdictions that have not yet adopted blood shield statutes, courts can decide that strict liability should not apply to blood collection and storage. A notable case is described in Box 17–1.

Elements of Negligence

Duty of Care

The first element in a successful negligence claim is establishing that the defendant owed a duty of care to the individual who is claiming harm. Traditionally, in cases involving the provision of health care services, a doctor-patient relationship between the defendant and plaintiff must be established

BOX 17–1 *Illustrative Case*

Nestor v. Hospital Pavia[3] involved a patient who was transfused during August 2001 and was later diagnosed with hepatitis C. The patient alleged that both the local blood bank and the hospital were negligent as they provided contaminated blood and therefore were strictly liable for marketing a defective product, despite the performance of the most sensitive, specific, licensed, and unlicensed tests available at that time. The court decided to follow the vast majority of states with blood-shield statutes and determined that, as a matter of law, strict liability should not apply to blood collection and storage.

before a duty of care may be attached, although courts are not unanimous in defining the parameters of the duty of care. Courts in a few states, including Arizona, Maryland, Mississippi, Ohio, and Washington, have broadened the duty of care between physicians and patients to situations in which no traditional doctor-patient relationship exists.

One of the most striking cases illustrating this trend is *Stanley v. McCarver*[4] detailed in Box 17–2. Citing cases in the District of Columbia,[5] Michigan,[6] and New Jersey,[7] the Arizona Supreme Court noted that "[t]he requirement of a formalized relationship between the parties has been quietly eroding in several jurisdictions."[4] The court held that, in deciding whether a duty exists with no formal doctor-patient relationship, it is appropriate to consider "whether the doctor was in a unique position to prevent harm, the burden of preventing harm, whether the plaintiff relied upon the doctor's diagnosis or interpretation, the closeness of the connection between the defendant's conduct and the injury suffered, the degree of certainty the plaintiff has suffered or will suffer harm, the skill or reputation of the actors, and public policy."[4]

In the blood-transfusion setting, some courts have recognized a duty in even more attenuated relationships, such as between the blood provider and the recipient of the blood. Examples of this duty arise in "lookback" cases, which involve the notification of recipients of components from donors who have previously tested positive for an infectious agent. Once a blood collector becomes aware that one of its donors has a disease transmissible by blood transfusion, the provider has a duty to develop and implement an appropriate program to notify the recipient of any component that might transmit the disease. An important example of this attenuated level of relationship is described in Box 17–3.

In *Snyder v. AABB*,[9] a New Jersey court went to great lengths in finding that a duty of care existed between a standard setting organization (American Association of Blood Banks; [AABB]) and a plaintiff who had contracted human immunodeficiency virus (HIV) from a transfusion, even though no direct relationship was found between the parties. The court concluded that AABB owed a duty of care to an individual treated by one of its voluntary members because the association had voluntarily assumed responsibility for the nation's blood supply by inviting blood banks, hospitals, physicians, and the public to rely on its Standards. At the time of this writing, this logic has been adopted in only one other jurisdiction.[10]

BOX 17–2 *Illustrative Case*

In *Stanley v. McCarver*,[4] a nursing home contracted with a radiologist to read chest radiographs of prospective employees of the nursing home to screen for tuberculosis. The radiologist never met with the plaintiff but noted a spot on her chest radiograph and, in his report to the nursing home, recommended further evaluation. Although the nursing home's procedures called for notifying a prospective employee of radiographic results within 72 hours of receiving the report, the plaintiff was never notified of the defendant's report. Relatively soon thereafter, she was diagnosed with lung cancer and ultimately died a few years later.

BOX 17–3 *Illustrative Case*

In *Smith v. American Red Cross*,[8] a blood-transfusion recipient who was infected by AIDS-contaminated blood in April 1984 and subsequently died, brought an action claiming, among other things, that the American Red Cross (Red Cross) did not promptly notify the recipient that the donor of the blood with which the recipient was transfused tested positive for human immunodeficiency virus (HIV). Rejecting a charge that Red Cross should have notified her immediately after the donor tested HIV positive in August 1985 instead of waiting until it developed its "lookback" program in July 1986, the court pointed out that the plaintiff had suffered no damages resulting from the delay because no allegation was made that the recipient spread the disease to anyone else, and, in 1985, no early-treatment protocols existed for those infected with HIV.

In general, the majority of courts require some greater connection or relationship between the health care provider and the recipient of health care services. One court, refusing to impose liability on AABB as a standard setting organization, specifically recognized that "adverse consequences to the public by chilling scientific and medical debate on important issues and leaving these matters to the often slow and cumbersome processes of governmental agencies" significantly weighed against finding AABB liable under the circumstances presented.[11]

Breach

Once a plaintiff establishes the existence of a legal duty, the plaintiff must prove that the defendant breached the standard of care. The breach may be a failure to diagnose, a delay in diagnosis, improper treatment, a negligent rate of infusion, failure to obtain informed consent, and/or inferior care, including substandard surgery or any number of other purported acts of malfeasance. A review of transfusion-related case law reveals that courts apply three distinct standards of care: medical negligence, ordinary negligence, and professional negligence. Subtle but important differences exist among these standards, and the outcome of an individual lawsuit is often based on which standard is applied.

Medical Negligence: The standard of care applicable in a medical negligence action requires that a physician exercise the degree of knowledge and care ordinarily possessed and exercised by other members of the profession acting under similar conditions and circumstances. Expert testimony is generally required to establish medical negligence.

Ordinary Negligence: Ordinary negligence is a standard of care that can be assessed by a "reasonable man of ordinary prudence."[12] Thus, ordinary negligence cases do not require expert testimony. In general, plaintiffs prefer to frame their cases as ordinary negligence actions rather than as medical negligence cases specifically to avoid the added burden of introducing expert testimony. This approach allows the defendant's actions to be judged by the finder of fact, often a jury, who measures the actions against what a reasonable person would do in similar circumstances. Very few cases involving donor screening or donor testing have been successfully asserted as a matter of simple negligence, although other blood center and transfusion service activities have been judged against the ordinary negligence standard.

Professional Negligence: In the blood banking and transfusion setting, most jurisdictions view the production and safeguarding of blood as a professional activity to be judged against the actions of a "reasonable professional" (the professional standard) as opposed to a reasonable person, as in ordinary negligence cases mentioned earlier. In its most traditional form, the professional standard requires that an expert offer testimony on the prevailing standard of care in the field. This evidence typically includes government regulations and applicable private standards and guidelines. Under this same standard, a single expert may not second-guess an entire profession.[13] Some courts, however, have broadened the evidence that can be introduced to establish the prevailing standard of care, including evidence about practices of other hospitals and transfusion services. This is most likely to occur in situations in which the standard of practice in the field is not settled. For most professional negligence cases, the less consensus that exists within the medical community concerning a specific course of action, the greater the opportunity for divergent outcomes in litigation.

Causation

The third element of negligence is establishing causation, in other words, determining that the defendant's breach of the duty of care was the actual or proximate cause of the plaintiff's injury.[14] In the transfusion setting, this means that the plaintiff must prove that it is more likely than not that the blood transfusion caused some form of injury, for example, HIV infection. Where the hospital, physician, or transfusion service can show that the plaintiff engaged in high-risk activities before the transfusion or that the particular morbidity or mortality could have been caused by a different source, it is more difficult to satisfy the element of causation.

When considering causation, the concept of foreseeability is relevant to determining whether certain actions or inactions constitute negligence. When the manner in which an injury occurs is so improbable or unpredictable that the defendant could not have "foreseen" it, the injury is not actionable. As cases discussed later in this chapter illustrate, the more foreseeable an untoward outcome is or was, the greater the potential exposure to liability.

Damages

The final element of negligence is proving that the plaintiff has suffered actual damages; a patient must have been injured as a result of the breach of the standard of care. The proper measure of damages is the amount that will compensate the plaintiff for the injury proximately caused by the defendant. These are called *compensatory damages* and are further subdivided into economic and noneconomic damages. Possible economic damages can include lost wages and medical expenses. Noneconomic damages are subjective and include pain and suffering, physical impairment, emotional harm, inconvenience, loss of society and companionship, and humiliation. In determining the amount of damages, it is appropriate to consider past, present, and future economic and noneconomic damages.

BOX 17–4 *Illustrative Case*

In 2003, a New Jersey court awarded $300,000 in damages to a patient who, after a blood test for human immunodeficiency virus (HIV), was incorrectly informed by a doctor that he was HIV positive.[17] The patient brought a medical malpractice action against the doctor and hospital where the patient was treated, claiming that, as a result of the misdiagnosis, he became depressed and suffered from physical and psychological injuries. The court found that, although the hospital was not negligent, the doctor had deviated from the standard of care by failing to give the plaintiff pretest and posttest counseling, by misinterpreting the test results, by incorrectly advising the plaintiff that he was HIV positive, and by giving the results over the telephone rather than informing the plaintiff in person.

Plaintiffs sometimes claim that their fear of contracting a disease is a compensable injury.[15] These types of cases arose originally in the asbestos context, and plaintiffs have had mixed success expanding this cause of action into the transfusion arena. Pennsylvania, for example, does not allow monetary damages for an asymptomatic plaintiff's fear of contracting acquired immunodeficiency syndrome (AIDS) in the absence of actual exposure to the disease.[16] The opposite occurred in New Jersey, as described in Box 17–4.

CONTRACTUAL CAUSES OF ACTION: IMPLIED WARRANTY

Some plaintiffs apply a broad approach to litigation and sue not only on negligence theories, but also on theories founded in contract. Typically, such claims allege that the physician promised certain results from procedures or treatments, the patient is unsatisfied with the results, and the physician's failure to produce the promised results gives rise to an action for breach of contract or breach of warranty.

In one such case, a blood bank that supplied the wrong type of blood, resulting in a patient's death, was held not liable under the doctrine of implied warranty, because the transfused blood was not in any way unwholesome or defective.[18] The court reasoned that the patient's death resulted from the negligence of an employee who recorded the wrong blood-type number on the decedent's card. In the court's opinion, supplying blood for a fee constitutes the provision of a service, rather than the sale of a product and, accordingly, breach of warranty did not apply.

The best way to prevent breach of contract or breach of warranty claims is to avoid promising specific results; managing patient expectations is not only sound practice, but also can help to protect against certain causes of action.

DONOR SCREENING, DONOR TESTING, AND COMPONENT PROCESSING

In the field of transfusion medicine, most legal cases brought against blood centers, hospitals, and physicians involve challenges to donor-screening and infectious disease–testing practices. Although blood center and transfusion medicine professionals regard donor screening and, in particular, donor questioning as relatively noninclusive and nonspecific for mitigating the risk of transfusion-transmitted disease, plaintiffs have often made this issue the focus of their complaints. In general, donor-screening complaints have centered around alleged "failures" in the donor-screening process, notably either the failure to ask a donor a specific question or a failure to rely on direct questioning to screen the donor for a particular risk.

Infectious disease–screening testing cases most often revolve around the failure to implement an available test, typically a test that is a "surrogate marker" for populations at risk for transmitting a specific agent but that does not directly identify the infectious agent. The period between the emergence of infectious disease and the development of a test for the agent responsible for transmission of the disease often presents the greatest risk of liability for a defendant. Additionally, in these same cases, the closer the injury is temporally to the implementation of testing for the agent, the greater the risk of liability. This concept is best illustrated by the early history of HIV and blood transfusion. The emergence of the first incidences of HIV related to blood transfusion occurred in 1981,[19] and the licensure of the first HIV test occurred on March 2, 1985.[20] This several-year period gave rise to a significant number of transfusion-transmitted (TT)-HIV cases aimed at standard-setting organizations, blood centers and hospitals, transfusion medicine professionals in both blood centers and hospitals, and clinicians involved in the patients' care. Courts have come to different conclusions about the liability of these parties for alleged deficiencies in donor screening and blood-donation testing to prevent the transmission of disease through blood transfusion.

In most jurisdictions, courts have applied the professional negligence standard and required only that the actions of blood-collection facilities be measured against the conduct of other members of the defendant's profession, through the testimony of expert witnesses. In those jurisdictions, blood collectors whose donor-screening and donation-testing procedures conformed to the standard of care in the profession and, in particular, the recommendations of standard-setting organizations such as AABB, the Food and Drug Administration (FDA), and the Centers for Disease Control and Prevention (CDC) have not been held responsible for transmission of a disease. In these cases, courts reject allegations of alleged failure to screen donors[13,21] and failure to implement tests not yet adopted by standard-setting organizations or mandated by government agencies.[22,23]

This articulation of the professional negligence standard was most recently applied in a case involving transfusion-related acute lung injury (TRALI). Although not an infectious disease risk, TRALI is, as of today, the most commonly reported cause of transfusion-related death in the United States, surpassing deaths caused by ABO incompatibility and bacterial contamination.[24] Unfortunately, because this clinical syndrome remains poorly defined and its pathophysiology is not understood, the medical community lacks consensus as to the appropriate way to prevent the syndrome. An interesting and illustrative case is presented in Box 17–5.

The court specifically noted that the plaintiff's malpractice contentions with respect to the blood center were that the blood products administered to the patient should have been screened for antibodies and that the entire blood-banking community was negligent for failing to follow this practice. The court dismissed the case, finding that the plaintiff had failed adequately to dispute the defendants' proof that the decedent's "treatment was consistent with good and acceptable medical practice."

BOX 17–5 *Illustrative Case*

In *Boland v. Montefiore*,[14] a patient diagnosed with myelogenous leukemia underwent a bone marrow transplant and was told by his treating physician that he required outpatient transfusions to increase his platelet count. The hospital blood bank director responsible for the management of outpatient transfusions performed in the blood center was present in the blood bank during the transfusions. The first two units were transfused without incident; however, during transfusion of the third unit, the patient experienced shortness of breath. Although all appropriate actions were taken, including stopping the transfusion and providing emergency care, the patient suffered cardiac arrest and died. The patient's estate filed suit against the blood center for negligent screening and testing of the units and failure to prepare properly the blood administered to the plaintiff. The treating and transfusing physicians, as well as the hospital, were sued for conscious pain and suffering, wrongful death, and failure to obtain informed consent.

In other jurisdictions, however, the question of a defendant's negligence concerning donor screening or testing has been judged under a different application of the professional negligence standard. Specifically, the highest state court in Colorado overturned a verdict rendered in favor of the blood center and held that a blood collector's compliance with governmental regulations and the standards and guidelines of a professional association was not conclusive proof that additional precautions were not required, because some other blood centers were using "additional precautionary measures."[25] When evidence concerning the appropriate standard of care is broadened to include not only the testimony of expert witnesses but also the practices of other individual blood centers, courts have determined that sufficient conflicting evidence exists about the standard to create a question of fact to be determined by a jury.

Even if a traditional professional negligence standard is applied, once the testimony of experts creates a question of material fact for the jury, the specific instruction to the jury on the standard becomes exquisitely important in determining the outcome of the case.

In *Ray v. American National Red Cross* (ANRC),[26] the plaintiff argued that the ANRC was obliged to act as a reasonable blood bank with the knowledge and skill level similar to that of the ANRC, whereas the ANRC contended that it had only to act according to industry standards. In applying the ordinary negligence standard, the appellate court reasoned that, "particularly where the Red Cross is in a position to substantially establish the industry standard, it may not use that standard as a safe harbor to insulate its activities from scrutiny if competent evidence demonstrates that it would have been reasonable for the Red Cross to adhere to a higher standard or a different practice."[26]

As a practical matter, the outcome of any case that challenges donor-screening or -testing practices will largely depend on the specific facts presented, including the specific time and circumstances of the harm or injury. The *Boland* case (see Box 17–5), which involved a patient who died of TRALI and allegations of a failure to screen donors in 1995, was successfully defended.[14] Whether that same case could be successfully defended today is uncertain, as several options for mitigating the risk of TRALI have recently been presented and discussed at a consensus conference.[27] Although the panel stopped short of recommending that any specific intervention practice be adopted, some major blood-transfusion systems, including the National Blood Service in the United Kingdom, have implemented practices to mitigate the risk of TRALI.[28] As practices in the profession change, so too does the standard of care against which facilities and individuals are judged.

A few of the changing standards of practice are discussed later.

CHANGING STANDARDS OF CARE IN TRANSFUSION MEDICINE–RELATED CASES

Bacterial Contamination

Prior to 1995, virtually no filed cases involved negligence in testing or screening to prevent transfusion-associated morbidity and mortality from bacterial contamination of platelet or red blood cell units. One of the few reported cases of bacterial contamination calls into question not the failure to test, but the failure to provide directed donations as an alternative to conventional transfusions. In 1995, a woman who received a transfusion of two units of packed red blood cells in the course of coronary bypass surgery developed sepsis and died the day after her surgery.[29] It was later determined that her death was caused by an extremely rare blood-borne bacterial infection. The woman's family claimed that the medical facility was negligent in refusing their request for directed donation of blood and that this refusal was the proximate cause of death. The judge awarded the woman's family $400,000; however, the medical facility appealed, and the finding was reversed. The appellate court specifically determined that the applicable standard of care should reflect the community standard of care, including FDA and/or AABB recommendations and standards, not just the hospital's internal policies.

Then, in 1997, the family of a man who died of transfusion-associated sepsis brought suit against a hospital in Providence, Rhode Island, and was awarded $5.6 million.[30] Although the plaintiff alleged that the hospital was negligent in failing to prevent transfusion of the contaminated unit, the jury appeared to base its award on the alleged failure of the hospital to recognize and treat the infection. With the implementation of AABB Standard 5.1.5.1,[31] requiring that blood collectors and transfusion services have in place a method both to limit and to detect bacterial contamination in platelet components, undoubtedly increased attention will be focused on adverse reactions in patients related to undetected bacterial contamination.

Given evolving technologies, ongoing determination of residual risk, and the lack of uniform methods for meeting AABB Standard 5.1.5.1, the possibility of exposure to a lawsuit for injuries relating to death or injury resulting from bacterial contamination is real. Bacterial contamination of platelets has been one of the greatest transfusion-transmitted infectious risks in the United States, and is now significantly higher than the risk of transfusion-transmitted viral infection.[32] Although lack of consensus appears to be present as to the best way to eradicate the risk, transfusion-medicine professionals clearly now have a duty to try to minimize the risk through available means.

What is not as clear is the effect of divergent practices on a defendant's ability to avoid a risk of litigation. The increasing trend toward the use of single-donor platelets, the debate over the necessity of testing for aerobic as well as anaerobic bacteria, and the discrepancies in the relative predictive value of available test methods[33] may constitute grounds for negligence claims. The true measure of potential legal exposure, however, will be the incidence and severity of the adverse reactions relating to the transfusion of bacterially contaminated units. Current anecdotal survey data and data from some larger facilities suggest that morbidity and mortality directly relating to failures to implement two-bottle culture systems, eliminate or reduce the use of pooled platelets, or substitute more sensitive and specific testing will be limited.

West Nile Virus and Variant Creutzfeldt-Jakob Disease

The transmission of West Nile virus (WNV) or variant Creutzfeldt-Jakob Disease (vCJD) through blood transfusion is often proffered as a source of potential liability for blood collectors, hospitals, and transfusing physicians. These two threats and the blood community response to each are illustrative of two separate approaches to mitigating transfusion risk. As a practical matter, however, the blood community's rapid and system-wide response to both of these threats mitigates the risk of liability for blood-transfusion professionals.

The management of the WNV threat to blood safety serves as a model for effective threat containment. Beginning with the first diagnosis of potential TT-WNV in 2002,[34] through the implementation of donor screening[35] and inventory management to reduce the risk of distribution of infected units[36,37] to the implementation of pooled[38] and then individual nucleic acid testing (NAT) in high-incidence locations,[39] the response of the government and the private sector was swift, coordinated, and evidence based.[40] Although a number of blood recipients were infected with WNV through transfusion, the broad-based development of national recommendations for donor screening and inventory management, as well as the rapid development and implementation of testing for the virus, established a clear national standard of practice against which blood-center and transfusion-service response could be measured.

The management of vCJD as a risk of blood transfusion has proven to be more difficult. The primary method for controlling the risk of vCJD has been the implementation of geographic and time-defined donor exclusions.[41] As a method for mitigating risk, these deferrals, which are based in part on scientific data and in part on the need to maintain public confidence in the safety of the blood supply, are neither sensitive nor specific. Yet, with the publication of FDA guidance on the issue[42] and the adoption of donor-exclusion criteria in other countries, it is unlikely that a plaintiff who contracted vCJD through blood collected and issued by a facility that followed these recommendations could successfully argue negligence.

The primary reason that a case alleging the negligent transmission of vCJD through blood transfusion is likely to fail is the difficulty of proving causation, and, specifically, associating transmission of the disease with a particular unit, as no specific test exists for the pathologic prion at the time of this writing. In addition, given the extremely low prevalence of vCJD in the human population, it is evident that only a small number of cases, if any, will occur.

Component Processing

In the blood-transfusion field, significant discussion has occurred over the potential for increased liability relating to the failure to adopt certain component-processing steps. As an example, increasing consensus is found that certain patients will benefit from receiving leukocyte-reduced red blood cells. The failure to prescribe leukocyte-reduced red cells for patients who have previously experienced febrile nonhemolytic transfusion reactions, those who need cytomegalovirus (CMV)-safe units, or those who need to have their risk of human leukocyte antigen (HLA) alloimmunization limited can create a potential risk of liability for a transfusing physician. Conversely, the obligation to provide leukoreduced units to every patient (universal leukoreduction) has not been clearly established. Conflicting, underpowered, and inconclusive studies,[43–46] as well as the very public and documented discussion over the cost/benefit ratio of leukoreduction,[47] suggest that similar debates over leukoreduction would be repeated in any litigation asserting the obligation to provide leukoreduced units to all patients. In addition, because many of the asserted benefits of leukoreduction are difficult to capture in a single episode (e.g., the prevention of immunomodulation or the transmission of viruses not invariably associated with symptomatic disease) and because many of the risks of not using leukocyte-reduced units can be masked or corrected through the administration of other drugs (e.g., acetaminophen for fever reduction), both causation and the specific injury to the plaintiff would likely to be difficult to establish.

The utility of irradiation of blood components is another area in which consensus has not yet developed. Most physicians recognize the utility of blood-component irradiation to prevent graft-versus-host disease (GVHD) in certain at-risk patients.[48] The literature strongly supports the conclusion that patients with hematologic malignancies, patients with congenital immunodeficiencies, patients who are receiving allogeneic bone marrow transplants, and patients who receive intrauterine or exchange transfusion should receive irradiated blood components (see Chapter 28). However, some documented medical cases exist in which the implementation of universal irradiation would have prevented the death of patients not known to be at risk.[49,50] Although some in the transfusion-medicine community have advocated the adoption of universal irradiation of blood components, others debate whether the high severity and low frequency of these adverse events warrant the implementation of universal irradiation. Nonetheless, facilities must keep abreast of the growing body of literature on patients who may benefit from receiving irradiated units.

Donor Injury

With an overall frequency of donor complications reported as approximating 20% on average and including severities of reactions from bruising to death, blood-collection facilities have policies and procedures in place to minimize the risk of both donor injury and litigation resulting from injury. Best practices require a facility to continually update the information in the consent for donation, to have a plan for adverse reactions at the donation site, and to provide donors with postdonation care and contact information. Most facilities also have adopted a policy of paying for immediate emergency care in the event an injury occurs.

Such preventive measures are critically important because, as previously noted, areas of activity in blood collection and transfusion services may be analyzed under principles of ordinary negligence, as opposed to the professional negligence standard. Instructive examples are described in Box 17–6.

Although it is difficult to predict which standard will be applied in all situations, a blood-collection facility will be best protected by an annual review of its policies and procedures against what a reasonable donor might understand and expect.

BOX 17–6 ***Illustrative Cases***

McDonnell v. American National Red Cross[51] revolved around a donor who fainted immediately after blood donation while walking unescorted from the donation table across a stone floor to the snack table and suffered a concussion and a postconcussion syndrome. The court, in an unpublished opinion, adopted ordinary negligence as the applicable standard of care rather than medical malpractice, because the complaint took issue with the general safety and operation procedures surrounding the blood donation—facts within the common knowledge and experience of the jury—and did not raise questions requiring medical judgment.

On the contrary, *Baumann v. American National Red Cross*[52] involved a donor whose right median nerve was injured during phlebotomy. The plaintiff sued the American National Red Cross under an ordinary negligence theory, alleging failure to warn of the potential for injury to donors during phlebotomy and negligence in the phlebotomy procedure. The court held that the claim should have been brought under the state's medical malpractice statute, reasoning that the standard of care governing these types of claims clearly involves medical learning or principles and is not within the knowledge of most laypeople.

Informed Consent

The doctrine of informed consent has its origins in the legal theory of battery or nonconsensual touching.[53] Although this legal theory is sometimes referenced in case law involving the failure to obtain informed consent, more recent cases base the legal theory on negligence.[54] Whichever theory serves as the basis for the analysis, it is clear that the ethical principle of autonomy, or the individual's right to make choices about personal matters, is well ingrained in the legal system. Multiple cases in virtually every jurisdiction reinforce the legal obligation to obtain informed consent for most medical treatments or interventions, including blood transfusion.

With the exception of federal regulations applicable to patients participating in research protocols, the law of informed consent is governed by state law, which varies from jurisdiction to jurisdiction. Some states, notably California, New Jersey, and Pennsylvania, have enacted statutes that delineate specific steps that must be taken in the informed-consent process. In other states, informed-consent requirements have been developed through case law.

Failure to obtain informed consent also has become an issue in clinical trials. In a relatively recent case, *Wright v. Fred Hutchinson Cancer Research Center*,[55] patients and their families brought a class action against the hospital and four physicians after 80 of 82 patients receiving care under a certain protocol, designed to reduce the risk of GVHD, died. The plaintiffs claimed that the center failed to inform them adequately about the risks inherent in the T-cell–depletion protocol. Although the case never went to trial, apparently because of the inability to certify the class, one of the evidentiary rulings precluded summary judgment in favor of the cancer center, creating the inference that the center could have been found liable for failure to inform.

As informed consent for blood transfusion has become the standard of practice, the elements of effective informed consent have become more standardized. The process includes (1) disclosure of the risks and benefits of transfusion or related therapies, (2) presentation of the potential alternatives, (3) an opportunity to ask questions of learned professionals,[56] and (4) documentation of the consent. Although these elements are straightforward, identifying which risks must be disclosed has been the subject of significant case law and has resulted in the development of two different standards. The first and older standard requires the disclosure of risks that are considered to be material to the reasonable physician.[57] This standard, however, has been replaced in a majority of jurisdictions by a newer standard, which requires the disclosure of risks that would be considered to be material to a reasonable patient.[58]

The adoption of the "reasonable patient standard" has introduced additional issues for transfusion-medicine professionals. Specifically, (1) the relevant risks must be disclosed, (2) the disclosure must be in language understandable to the patient, and (3) a new informed-consent discussion is required if a substantial change in circumstances, whether medical or legal occurs.[56]

Who Has the Duty to Obtain Informed Consent?

Courts have not been consistent in deciding who specifically has the obligation to provide the information and to obtain informed consent. Generally, the obligation to obtain informed consent has been considered to be that of the treating physician, who is the professional most likely to have developed a relationship with the patient. In the transfusion setting, however, this question is more complex, and some courts have reasoned that a physician who refers a patient for surgery is not responsible for obtaining informed consent for transfusion; rather, it is the surgeon who performs the procedure who has the duty to obtain informed consent.[59] This line of cases does not automatically implicate all surgeons assisting in the surgery. Some cases have held the primary surgeon responsible, while refusing to hold assisting physicians responsible for the failure to obtain informed consent.[60] In some circumstances, however, physicians may delegate the duty to obtain informed consent to other health care providers.[61]

For the most part, hospitals have not been held to owe a duty to patients to obtain informed consent,[62] because the obligation to do so is generally that of the physician who ordered the transfusion. However, as the requirement to obtain informed consent becomes incorporated into the requirements of standard-setting organizations like the Joint Commission on the Accreditation of Healthcare Organizations (JCAHO)[63] hospitals increasingly will be held accountable for ensuring that informed consent is obtained.

Courts in several jurisdictions have relied on additional theories of liability, including the "corporate negligence theory,"[64] under which a hospital may be liable for failing properly to oversee the treatment of patients or require physicians with hospital privileges to obtain informed consent. Another theory is "respondeat superior," under which an employer is responsible for its employees and, particularly, has a duty to exercise reasonable care in selecting, retaining, and supervising medical staff.[65] In addition, an institution that voluntarily assumes this duty, but fails effectively to obtain the consent, can be held liable for injury relating to those failures, even in the absence of an original duty to obtain consent.

Separate from any specific duty to obtain informed consent, hospitals do have a duty to educate their physicians about risks, including the risks of transfusion. Hospitals are independently responsible for providing information sufficient to allow a treating physician to carry out his or her duty to obtain informed consent. In the transfusion setting, this means that hospitals must have information available to physicians on transfusion risks, as well as available alternatives to allogeneic transfusions.[66]

Alternatives

One of the elements of informed consent is the obligation to advise the patient of alternatives to the recommended therapy. This particular element raises some interesting questions about the obligation to provide information about alternatives to conventional transfusion therapy. Courts have had numerous opportunities to consider the liability of physicians for failing to recommend alternative procedures, such as autologous and directed donations, as well as other alternatives to allogeneic transfusion. This complex issue is based primarily on two questions: the standard of practice in the community (including the availability of the alternate therapy), and the hospital or blood bank's adherence to its own policies and procedures.

In one case, a California court held that a blood center could not be held liable for failing to disclose the option of a directed-donation program because the plaintiff had failed to show that these programs were standard practice in the community.[66] Interestingly, the blood center in this case did have a directed-donation program, but not for patients with the plaintiff's specific illness, which required multiple transfusions.

The outcome of these cases is often directly affected by the expert testimony presented. In *Spann v. Irwin Memorial Blood Centers*,[66] the plaintiffs failed to offer testimony regarding the standard of practice in the community. If expert testimony supporting the general availability of directed donations or other alternative therapies had been presented, it is possible that the testimony could have been sufficient to defeat a motion for summary judgment. This would have created a question of fact for the jury, provided that the failure to follow the standard practice was causally connected to the injury. It is, however, noteworthy that hospitals and blood-collection facilities have successfully defended against allegations that the failure to provide directed donations constitutes negligence by introducing evidence that directed donations are not necessarily safer, and possibly even less safe, than regular donations.[67]

In other cases, the interplay between the testimony of experts and the availability of the optional therapy determines the outcome of the case. In *Doe v. Johnston*,[68] the plaintiff offered testimony on the superiority of autologous transfusion, but conflicting evidence over the "reasonable availability" of the procedure in 1985 created a question of fact sufficient to uphold the trial court's denial of a request for a directed verdict in favor of the plaintiff.

As the type and availability of alternative therapies to blood transfusion continue to grow, the obligation to inform potential recipients about the availability of these therapies will increase. In addition to preoperative autologous donation, many hospitals now offer intraoperative blood salvage, postoperative blood salvage, and acute normovolemic hemodilution. Not every alternative is either appropriate for, or available to, every patient. To the extent that an option is available and appropriate for a particular procedure, and the patient is not informed of the option, any complication from an allogeneic unit can create potential liability for a physician or hospital.

Less clear is whether a hospital would be held liable for failing to make these alternative therapies available for patients. Case law from the HIV litigation, discussed earlier, suggests that a hospital would not be required to offer alternative therapies that are so new that they have not yet become accepted as the norm. To the extent that a hospital offering bloodless surgery is located in or near other hospitals, its physicians could rely on the fact that the patient has the option to choose to have a procedure performed at a different location. It is possible, however, that an expert witness testifying that the availability of these alternatives is now the standard of care could create a question of fact for the jury.

In still other cases involving an alleged failure to inform a plaintiff of alternative procedures, the determining issue is not the availability of the alternative, but a hospital or blood center's adherence to its existing internal policies. In *Doe v. American National Red Cross*,[69] a hospital that failed to inform a plaintiff about the option of directed donations was denied summary judgment, at least in part, because a policy allowing such donations existed within the hospital. Again, the outcome of many of these cases is fact-specific and depended not only on the availability of an alternative therapy, but also on the question whether the available therapy would be appropriate for the specific patient.

Medically Necessary Transfusions

Beginning in the 1980s, many plaintiffs brought cases against physicians and hospitals based on the theory that the transfusion that caused injury to the patient was not medically necessary. The lack of reference standards or universally accepted comprehensive transfusion guidelines, as well as regional variations in transfusion practice, contributed to the unpredictable outcome of these cases. In addition, expert testimony is critical to defining the appropriate standard of care in these cases. One of the most interesting and troubling cases for transfusing physicians is presented in Box 17–7.

Once a case challenging the medical necessity of a particular transfusion becomes a battle of the experts, the outcome is difficult to predict, but juries have found hospitals and physicians liable for injuries on the basis of expert testimony about the necessity of the transfusion.[71] Case dicta, as well as experience, underscore the importance of hospital policies and hospital transfusion guidelines, as well as the review of transfusion practice in the hospital transfusion committee.

Some courts, applying a broad definition of foreseeability, have allowed cases to proceed against physicians whose prior negligence required the transfusion that transmitted HIV.[72] In other cases, applying a narrower interpretation of foreseeability, courts have granted summary-judgment motions in favor of defendant physicians who provided negligent treatment that required transfusion because the outcome of the transfusion was not foreseeable.

BOX 17–7 *Illustrative Case*

Oiler v. Willke[70] demonstrates what can happen when expert testimony and a broad interpretation of a reasonably foreseeable injury coincide in the same case. *Oiler* involved a platelet transfusion that allegedly resulted in the transmission of human immunodeficiency virus (HIV). The plaintiff presented expert testimony that the platelet transfusion was unnecessary. Although the transfusion was administered in 1980, at a time when the transmissibility of HIV through blood transfusion was not yet established, the court ruled that the plaintiff had established a genuine issue of fact as to whether the transmission of HIV was foreseeable because the plaintiff had presented evidence that many viruses, including hepatitis, were known to be transmissible through blood transfusion.

Blood Administration

Now that the risk of transfusion-transmitted diseases has dramatically decreased because of donor screening and increasingly sensitive testing, more attention is being placed on injuries resulting from improper administration of blood and blood components. Currently, one of the leading causes of death relating to transfusion is mistransfusion, or administering the wrong unit to the wrong patient. Although not many cases have been reported, plaintiffs are most likely to be successful if they allege medical negligence in the transfusion of the unit. In *Walker v. Humana Medical Corporation*,[73] a phlebotomist failed to draw blood from the proper patient. The resulting transfusion caused a reaction due to the incompatible blood, and the court found sufficient evidence of wantonness, or knowledgeable malfeasance, to present the facts to a jury.

Theories of breach of contract or of implied warranty generally will not apply in these cases because usually it cannot be demonstrated that the unit of blood itself is defective. Although logic suggests that every case of mistransfusion results in a legal action, few legal cases or rulings involve these types of injuries, presumably because most of these cases are settled by hospitals out of court. Given the existence of devices that can prevent mistransfusion, constructing a successful legal defense to these cases is difficult.

PRIVACY AND SECURITY CONCERNS UNDER HIPAA

Invasion of Privacy

Invasion of privacy is the unwarranted appropriation or exploitation of one's personality, publicizing one's private affairs with which the public has no legitimate concern, or wrongful intrusion into one's private activities, in such a manner as to cause mental suffering, shame, or humiliation to a person of ordinary sensibilities.

Right to Privacy

Although not explicitly stated in the Constitution, "a right to be left alone" began to emerge in the late 1800s. This right has evolved into a liberty of personal autonomy protected by the 14th amendment of the United States Constitution. Along with the constitutional right of privacy, states have adopted statutory rights of privacy that limit access to personal information, and the Federal Trade Commission (FTC) protects the public's financial privacy through legislation such as the Right to Financial Privacy Act of 1978[74] and the more recent Financial Services Modernization Act of 1999.[75]

Most recently, federal and state privacy laws protect health-related information.

HIPAA

With the passage of the Health Insurance Portability and Accountability Act of 1996 (HIPAA),[76] as amended, which became effective for most "covered entities" on April 14, 2003, practices relating to the use and disclosure of medical information have been subject to increasing attention. The federal privacy regulations that implement portions of HIPAA ("Privacy Rules") were designed to combat fraud and abuse in health care, standardize the electronic exchange of administrative and financial data, and protect the privacy and security of individual health information.

Covered Entities

"Covered Entities" generally include health plans, health care clearinghouses, and health care providers.[77] A health care provider is a covered entity under HIPAA if it (1) meets the definition of "health care provider;" and (2) transmits health information in electronic form in connection with covered transactions. Independent blood suppliers who do not perform patient-related health care activities are specifically exempt from the provision of the act, as they engage in "activities related to the procurement or banking of blood, sperm, organs, or any other tissue for administration to patients."[78]

However, an entity's status as a "covered entity" requires a careful, fact-specific analysis of all of the activities provided by the facility in question. The Department of Health and Human Services (HHS) has stated, "the procurement or banking of organs, blood (including autologous blood) … or any other tissue or human product is not considered to be health care under this rule and the organizations that perform such activities would not be considered health care providers when conducting these functions."[79]

Under this definition, if a facility is involved in activities other than the procurement and banking of blood, such as laboratory testing used to diagnose or otherwise treat a patient, as opposed to simply performing blood screening, it may be providing patient-related services that bring it under the definition of "health care provider" under HIPAA. It is not clear whether a facility that performs cross-matching and other compatibility testing would be considered a health care provider. To be considered a covered entity, the health care provider must also meet the second criterion: it must be transmitting protected health information in electronic form in connection with one of the "standard transactions" listed in the rules.

Covered entities must comply with numerous and extensive requirements under the Privacy Rules, including administrative, physical, and technical safeguards under the HIPAA Security Rule,[80] which are designed to safeguard electronically protected health information. Generally, covered entities may use protected health information only as it relates to treatment, payment, or health care operations.[81] Covered entities must make reasonable efforts to limit the use or disclosure of, and requests for, patient health information (PHI) to the minimal amount necessary to accomplish the intended purpose. Covered entities are required to develop written policies and procedures that are summarized in a "Notice of Privacy Practices" that is publicly available.[82] Noncompliance with the Privacy Rules may result in civil and criminal penalties.[83]

Business Associates

Even facilities that are not covered entities under HIPAA may have to comply with certain requirements if they are "business associates." Covered Entities are required to enter into business associate agreements with persons and organizations that perform functions or activities on their behalf and receive PHI in connection with these services for other than treatment purposes. Common examples of business associates are accountants, consultants, administrators, and financial services. HIPAA specifically includes accreditation as an activity, giving rise to a business associate relationship.

Business associate agreements principally are designed to ensure that business associates and those acting on their behalf use the PHI only for the purposes that they are engaged to perform or as otherwise required by law; safeguard the information from disclosure and misuse; promptly report any disclosure to the Covered Entity; and assist the Covered Entity in complying with HIPAA requirements.

Criminal Penalties

In June 2005, the U.S. Department of Justice (DOJ) clarified who can be held criminally liable under HIPAA. Covered entities and those individuals that "knowingly" obtain or disclose individually identifiable health information in violation of the applicable regulations may face criminal liability. The DOJ interpreted the "knowingly" element of the HIPAA statute for criminal liability as requiring only knowledge of the actions that constitute an offense. Specific knowledge of an action being in violation of the HIPAA statute is not required.[84]

In 2004, the U.S. Attorney in Seattle announced that a hospital phlebotomist was being indicted for violating the HIPAA privacy law.[85] The phlebotomist had allegedly accessed the medical records of a patient with a terminal cancer condition, obtained credit cards in the patient's name, and run up more than $9,000 in charges. In a statement to the court, the patient said he "lost a year of life both mentally and physically dealing with the stress" that resulted from the phlebotomist's actions. The guilty individual signed a plea agreement and was sentenced to 16 months in jail. At the time, the DOJ trumpeted the first HIPAA criminal prosecution. The DOJ site announced: "This case should serve as a reminder that misuse of patient information may result in criminal prosecution."[85] Under its new legal opinion, however, the phlebotomist could not be prosecuted further under HIPAA because, arguably, he did not knowingly violate HIPAA. Whereas HIPAA protects the health information of individuals, it does not create a private cause of action for those aggrieved. State law, however, may provide other avenues of liability. Generally, HIPAA does not preempt state privacy laws or professional licensure requirements, so that determining compliance requires examining the relevant state's confidentiality laws.[86]

EXTRAPOLATION OF THE TRANSFUSION LEGAL EXPERIENCE

The legal precedents established in transfusion cases have application to other areas. Notably, the collection, processing, manipulation, and administration of cellular therapy products raise legal issues similar to those presented in transfusion cases. Although the actual requirements for cellular therapy donor screening and unit testing may ultimately differ from those applicable to blood donors and blood components, the case law concerning the appropriate negligence standard and the legal requirements for defining the standard of care against which actions are to be measured will influence the outcome of cellular therapy litigation.

An additional legal risk in the collection, processing and administration of cellular therapy products, not generally present in transfusion medicine, is the relative efficacy of processing protocols for cellular therapy products. Unlike blood components, which are basically licensed generic biologics, most cellular therapy products are developed under highly individualized collection, processing, manipulation, freezing, and/or thawing protocols. Although some of these protocols and methods are protected intellectual property, others are in the public domain and thus are available for use. One of the areas of legal concern will be the extent to which these different processes are associated with varying engraftment survival rates. As in the transfusion field, the testimony of experts will be key to the outcome of litigation in this area.

In the cellular therapies arena, the proliferation of clinical trials will also draw increased attention to the informed-consent process. The failure to have in place or to follow a well-thought-out process will most certainly lead to legal problems. In addition, given the vulnerability of expectant parents, issues related to informed consent for cord blood donation, particularly in cord blood banks that collect and store these units for use by the family, will pose legal concerns for institutions that provide this service.

Finally, facilities that store cord units for future use by the family may find that issues surrounding the obligation to store and, in some cases, dispose of these collected units may raise contract, as well as negligence, issues. Although the intricacies of contract law are beyond the scope of this chapter, facilities that store cord blood units should have all storage contracts carefully reviewed by legal counsel. Even the best contracts cannot completely protect a facility against legal liability in the event that a facility negligently loses or renders unusable a cord blood unit. In this event, as in the case of blood donor injuries, the actions or inactions of the facility are likely to be judged against an ordinary negligence standard.

DEFENDING AGAINST LEGAL RISKS

In addition to preventive measures for avoiding litigation, litigation strategies can help expedite resolution of issues and, if all else fails, affirmative defenses can be used effectively to defend against litigation.

Preventive Measures

One theory to be considered is that patients who have suffered from medical errors are motivated not so much by the prospect of economic compensation, as by the desire to ensure that the error is not repeated. A pilot mediation conducted under the sponsorship of the Massachusetts Board of Registration in Medicine confirms this theory and strongly suggests that private dispute resolution through mediation improves the outcome for all concerned. As Ed Dauer, one of mediation's key proponents suggests, "For its part, mediation, when properly employed, can be private, integrative, safe, nonjudgmental, and flexible in scope, process, and outcome. It can be a safe harbor with therapeutic potential, and can offer its participants the opportunity to address the source as well as the consequence of the immediate problem. Mediation may, in short, offer a process whose traditional attributes are consistent with, rather than antithetical to, the requisites of quality improvement."[87]

Some lawyers have embraced variations of these concepts in the form of "good-faith conferences" and "apology meetings." The good-faith conference is geared toward furnishing the plaintiff with the opportunity to vent his or her anger at the defendant. The conference may be a condition to settlement, or it may follow settlement. No apology is promised or expected, but apologies often develop during well-managed meetings. The apology meeting is similar, except that an apology from the defendant is expected, along with a therapeutic discussion.

Both types of meetings must be carefully planned and skillfully executed. It is imperative that all parties have a certain level of trust in one another and that all are committed to conducting the meeting in a civil and nonthreatening manner.

Litigation Strategies

It is not uncommon for plaintiffs in transfusion-related litigation to file suit against as many defendants as ethically possible to maximize the chances of finding a culpable "deep pocket." Typically, the treating physician and other medical professionals involved in the administration of transfusions, along with the hospital, the blood bank, and even AABB, will be named as defendants. Although the first reaction among co-defendants is to point fingers and assign blame, a more productive approach often is to work together on a common defense. Not only can this cooperative approach result in stronger defenses, but it can significantly reduce legal bills, as well.

Affirmative Defenses

Even if a plaintiff is able to prove all four elements of negligence, a defendant can raise defenses that minimize or defeat the plaintiff's claims. One such defense is that the plaintiff failed to bring the lawsuit within the legal time limits set by the jurisdiction where the case is being brought. This defense is referred to as the statute-of-limitations defense.

Another affirmative defense available in many jurisdictions is that the actions of the plaintiff contributed to the cause of the injury. This theory is called contributory negligence or comparative negligence on the part of the plaintiff. Contributory or comparative negligence is a legally contributing cause, in addition to the negligence of the defendant, in bringing about the plaintiff's harm.

A related affirmative defense is that an unforeseeable intervening event caused the injury, rather than the defendant's negligence.

LESSONS LEARNED

By applying the difficult lessons learned from the HIV-related transfusion litigation to cases appearing on the horizon, it is possible to avoid litigation, or at least minimize its impact. One key lesson is the importance to medical facilities of promptly implementing government recommendations and standards adopted by private organizations. Another lesson is to consider all available scientific evidence continually and to keep abreast of best practices, especially those relating to new techniques, technologies, and medical challenges, to anticipate the adoption of a practice as the standard of care.

Equally important, particularly in situations in which lack of consensus exists regarding how to manage a particular risk, is the demonstration that a facility is knowledgeable about the risks and has considered the available options.

Finally, efforts such as consensus conferences and workshops that attempt to establish a consensus or practice within the professional community are extremely important. Even such simple efforts as the development and adoption of a uniform donor-history questionnaire can ensure the recognition of clear standards of care.

Minimizing the risk of legal liability in the transfusion setting is not difficult, but in today's litigious society, eliminating that risk entirely is not possible. The most important preventive measures have been and remain using best practices, engaging in effective risk communication with patients, and taking swift corrective action when problems inevitably occur. Keeping current with standards of practice and effectively educating staff about those standards is essential to fending off legal claims. By taking these proactive steps, it will be possible to demonstrate, to the extent possible, that the physician or facility conformed to the currently accepted standard of care in the transfusion and cellular therapy communities. This will allow the professional to spend much less time defending past activities and devote considerably more valuable time to serving donors and patients.

REFERENCES

1. Speiser SM, Krause CF, Gans AW: The American Law of Torts. Rochester, N.Y.: Lawyers Cooperative Publishing Co, 1.4, 1983.
2. Restatement (Second) of Torts § 402A American Law Institute, 1964.
3. *Nestor v. Hospital Pavia*, et al: 2005 WL 348313 (D.P.R. 2005).
4. *Stanley v. McCarver*, 92 P.3d 849 (Ariz. 2004).
5. *Betesh v. United States*, 400 F.Supp. 238 (D.D.C. 1974).
6. *Dyer v. Trachtman*, 679 N.W.2d 311 (Mich. 2004).
7. *Reed v. Bojarski*, 764 A.2d 433 (N.J. 2001).
8. *Smith v. American Red Cross*, 886 F.Supp. 1494 (E.D. Mo. 1995).
9. *Snyder v. American Ass'n of Blood Banks*, 676 A.2d 1036 (N.J. 1996).
10. *Weigand v. University Hosp. of New York University Med. Ctr.*, 659 N.Y.S.2d 395 (N.Y. 1997).
11. *N.N.V. v. American Ass'n of Blood Banks*, 75 Cal.App.4th 1358, 1373 (Cal.App.4th Dist. 1999).
12. Keeton WP, Dobbs DB: Prosser and Keeton on Torts, 5th ed. West Grove, St. Paul, Minn.:1984.
13. *Osborn v. Irwin Memorial Blood Bank*, 5 Cal.App.4th 234 (Cal. App. 1st Dist. 1992), review denied (July 9, 1992).
14. *Boland v. Montefiore*, 800 N.Y.S.2d 343 (N.Y. Super. 2005).
15. Simmons KC: Recovery for emotional distress based on fear of contracting HIV or AIDS. ALR 5th 59:535, 1998.
16. *Lobowitz v. Albert Einstein Medical Center*, 623 A.2d 3 (Pa. Super. 1993).
17. *Doe v. Arts*, 823 A.2d 855 (N.J. Super. 2003).
18. *Goelz v. J.K. & Susie L. Wadley Research Institute & Blood Bank*, 350 S.W.2d 573 (Tex. Civ. App. 1961).
19. *Pneumocystis carinii* pneumonia among persons with hemophilia A. MMWR 1982;31:365.
20. Health and Human Services: New Release, March 4, 1985.
21. *Kirkendall v. Harbor Ins. Co.*, 698 F.Supp. 768 (W.D. Ark. 1988), aff'd, 887 F.2d 857 (8th Cir. 1989).
22. *Doe v. American Nat. Red Cross*, 866 F.Supp. 242 (D. Md. 1994).
23. *Zaccone v. American Red Cross*, 872 F.Supp. 457 (N.D. Ohio 1994).
24. Silliman C, Ambruso R, Boshkov L: Transfusion-related acute lung injury. Blood 2005;105:2266–2273.
25. *United Blood Services v. Quintana*, 827 P.2d 509, 520–21 (Colo. 1992).
26. *Ray v. American Nat. Red Cross*, 696 A.2d 399 (D.C. App. 1997).
27. Kleinman S, Caulfield T, Chan P, et al: Toward an understanding of transfusion-related acute lung injury: Statement of a consensus panel. Transfusion 2004;44:1774–1789.
28. National Blood Service, Hospitals & Science Website: Update on TRALI: reducing the risk. Blood Matters Winter 2003/4:14.
29. *Quijano v. United States*, 325 F.3d 564 (5th Cir. 2003).
30. McClear JA: Family wins tainted-blood suit. *The Detroit News*, October 16, 1997.
31. AABB. Standards for blood banks and transfusion services 22d ed., 2003.
32. AABB Association Bulletin 05–02: Bacterial contamination of platelets: summary for clinicians on potential management issues related to transfusion recipients and blood donors. AABB Bacterial Contamination Task Force, February 23, 2005.
33. Silva M: Summary of results of AABB bacterial contamination task force survey. Advisory Committee on Blood Safety and Availability Committee, Department of Health and Human Services, http://www.hhs.gov/bloodsafety/transcripts/ACBSA_Transcript_Jan_25_2005.pdf, January 25, 2005.
34. West Nile virus activity in the United States, September 26–October 2, 2002 and investigations of West Nile virus infections in recipients of blood transfusion and organ transplantation. MMWR 2002;51: 39–884.
35. AABB: Information regarding West Nile virus, www.aabb.org/pressroom/in_the_news/wnwnv100302.htm, October 3, 2002.
36. AABB Association Bulletin 02–09: Further information relating to voluntary withdrawal of frozen product to mitigate the risk of transfusion of West Nile virus through blood transfusion: Statement of the American Association of Blood Banks, America's Blood Centers, and the American Red Cross, December 18, 2002.
37. AABB Association Bulletin 02–10: Update on testing of frozen products for West Nile virus: Statement of the American Association of Blood Banks, America's Blood Centers, and the American Red Cross, December 24, 2000.
38. AABB Association Bulletin 03–06: Update on FDA West Nile virus recommendations, May 13, 2003.
39. AABB Association Bulletin 04–04: Joint statement of the American Association of Blood Banks, America's Blood Centers, and American Red Cross on implementation of individual donation nucleic acid amplification testing for West Nile virus, June 4, 2004.
40. Nakhasi H: Development of West Nile virus testing and donor screening as a model for screening bioterrorist agents. www.fda.gov/oc/initiatives/criticalpath/wnv.html, July 15, 2004.
41. FDA Talk Paper: New precautionary measures to reduce the theoretical risk of new variant CJD from blood products, T99-38, http://www.fda.gov/bbs/topics/ANSWERS/ANS00970.html, August 17, 1999.
42. FDA Guidance for industry: revised preventive measures to reduce the possible risk of Creutzfeldt-Jakob Disease (CJD) or variant Creutzfeldt-Jakob Disease (vCJD) by blood and blood products. January 9, 2002.
43. Blajchman MA: Allogeneic blood transfusions, immunomodulation, and postoperative bacterial infection: do we have the answers yet? Transfusion 1997;37:121–125.
44. Vamvakas EC: Transfusion-association cancer recurrence and postoperative infection: meta-analysis of randomized, controlled clinical trials. Transfusion 1996;36:175–186.
45. McAlister FA, Clark HD, Wells PS, Laupacis A: Perioperative allogeneic blood transfusion does not cause adverse sequelae in patients with cancer: a meta-analysis of unconfounded studies. Br J Surg 1998;85:171–178.
46. van de Watering LMG, Herrnans J, Houbiers JGA, et al: Beneficial effects of leukocyte depletion of transfused blood on postoperative complications in patients undergoing cardiac surgery: a randomized clinical trial. Circulation 1998;97:562–568.
47. AABB Association Bulletin 99–7: Leukocyte reduction. August 12, 1999.
48. Hillyer C, Silberstein L, Ness P, Anderson K (eds.): Blood Banking and Transfusion Medicine: Basic Principles and Transfusion Practice. Philadelphia, Churchill Livingstone/Elsevier Science, 2003:255.

49. King KE, Ness PM. Prevention of transfusion-associated graft-versus-host disease in undiagnosed severe combined immunodeficiency syndrome [Abstract]. Blood 1996;88:528a.
50. Maung ZT, Wood AC, Jackson GH, et al. Transfusion-associated graft-versus-host disease in fludarabine-treated B-chronic lymphocytic leukaemia. Br J Haematol 1994;88:649–652.
51. *McDonnell v. American Nat. Red Cross*, 2005 WL 1335128 (Mich. App. June 7, 2005) (unpublished opinion).
52. *Baumann v. American Nat. Red Cross*, 262 F.Supp.2d 965, 968 (C.D. Ill. 2003).
53. *Paulsen v. Gundersen*, 260 N.W. 448 (Wis. 1935).
54. *Scaria v. St. Paul Fire & Marine Ins. Co.*, 227 N.W.2d 647 (Wis. 1975).
55. *Wright v. Fred Hutchinson Cancer Research Center*, 206 FRD 679 (W.D. Wash. 2002).
56. Stowell C: Informed Consent for Blood Transfusion. Bethesda, Md.: American Association of Blood Banks, 1997:4–5.
57. *Sawyer v. Methodist Hospital*, 522 F.2d 1102 (6th Cir. 1975).
58. *Canterbury v. Spence*, 464 F.2d 772 (D.C. Cir.), cert. denied, 409 U.S. 1064 (1972).
59. *Douglass v. Alton Ochsner Medical Foundation*, 696 So.2d 136, (La. Ct. App. 5th Cir. 1997).
60. *Jones v. Philadelphia College of Osteopathic Medicine*, 813 F.Supp. 1125 (E.D. Pa. 1993).
61. *Smogor v. Enke*, 874 F.2d 295 (5th Cir. 1989).
62. *Goss v. Oklahoma Blood Institute*, 856 P.2d 998 (Okla. App. 1990).
63. JCAHO: Comprehensive Accreditation Manual for Hospitals. Oakbrook Terrace, Ill.: Joint Commission on Accreditation of Healthcare Organizations, 2005.
64. *Whittington v. Episcopal Hosp.*, 768 A.2d 1144 (Pa. Super. 2001).
65. *Howell v. Spokane & Inland Empire Blood Bank*, 785 P.2d 815, 823 (Wash. 1990).
66. *Spann v. Irwin Memorial Blood Centers*, 40 Cal.Rptr.2d 360 (1st Dist. 1995).
67. *Hoemke v. New York Blood Center*, 912 F.2d 550 (2d Cir. 1990).
68. *Doe v. Johnston*, 476 N.W.2d 28 (Iowa 1991), reh'g denied (October 23, 1991).
69. *Doe v. American Nat. Red Cross*, 848 F.Supp.1228 (S.D.W.Va. 1994).
70. *Oiler v. Willke*, 642 N.E.2d 667 (Ohio App. 4th Dist. 1994).
71. *Jeanne v. Hawkes Hosp. of Mt. Carmel*, 598 N.E.2d 1174 (Ohio App.10th Dist. 1991), case dismissed, 579 N.E.2d 210 (1991).
72. *Doe v. United States*, 737 F.Supp. 155 (D.R.I. 1990).
73. *Walker v. Humana Medical Corp.*, 415 So.2d 1107 (Ala. Civ. App.), on remand, 423 So.2d 891 (June 9, 1982).
74. 12 U.S.C.A. §§ 3401, et seq. (November 10, 1978).
75. 15 U.S.C.A. §§ 6701, et seq. (November 12, 1999).
76. Public Law 104–191(HR 3103) (August 21, 1996).
77. 45 C.F.R. § 160.103 (2003).
78. 65 Fed. Reg. 82462, 82571–82572 (December 28, 2000).
79. 65 Fed. Reg. 82477 (December 28, 2000).
80. 45 C.F.R. §§ 164.308 et seq. (current through November 17, 2005).
81. 45 C.F.R. § 164.506 (August 14, 2002).
82. 45 C.F.R. § 164.530 (August 14, 2002).
83. 42 U.S.C. § 1320d–5 (December 27, 2001).
84. Memorandum Opinion for the General Counsel Department of Health and Human Services and the Senior Counsel to the Deputy Attorney General (June 1, 2005).
85. Scott M: HIPAA gavel drops: A message to healthcare. Radiology Today Nov. 22, 2004;24:38.
86. 65 Fed. Reg. 82566 (December 28, 2000).
87. Dauer EA, Marcus LJ: Adapting mediation to link resolution of medical malpractice disputes with health care quality improvement. Law & Contemp Probs 1997;60:185–218.

D. Specific Blood Components

Chapter 18

Packed Red Blood Cells and Related Products

Sally A. Campbell-Lee • Paul M. Ness

Landsteiner[1] discovered the ABO system in 1901, more than 100 years ago. Since that time, the development of a safe and effective anticoagulant-preservative solution[2] and the efforts in World War II that led to current methods of organized blood collection[3] have promoted transfusion medicine to an essential aspect of clinical medicine. The appropriate use of red blood cell concentrates (commonly referred to as packed red blood cells, pRBCs) depends on knowledge of the physiology of RBC transfusion and the therapeutic options of various component manipulations (Table 18–1). This chapter covers the manufacturing, storage, and indications for whole blood, pRBCs, and related products.

COLLECTION

In 2001, nearly 15 million units of whole blood were collected in the United States.[4] Whole blood, composed of RBCs, leukocytes, platelets, and plasma, is collected into a closed, sterile system. The system consists of a phlebotomy needle, integral donor tubing, and several attached polyvinyl resin bags.[5] Within the polyvinyl resin bags is 63 mL of, most commonly, citrate, phosphate, and dextrose (CPD) or citrate, phosphate, dextrose, and adenine (CPDA-1) anticoagulant-preservative, which provides a shelf-life of 35 days when the contents are stored at 4°C. Including the anticoagulant-preservative, the volume of a unit of whole blood is approximately 510 mL (450 mL of blood plus 63 mL of anticoagulant),[6] although many blood centers now collect 500 mL of donor blood. Within 24 hours of collection, the platelets (if refrigerated) and granulocytes are dysfunctional, and several coagulation factors are at suboptimal levels.[7] To optimize factor activity and platelet recovery, preparation of fresh frozen plasma (FFP) and platelet concentrates must occur within 8 hours.[8]

One of the problems with the standard method of collecting whole blood is that the amount of anticoagulant-preservative is predetermined, but the exact amount of whole blood collected is not. Because of variability in donor hematocrits, different RBC masses are collected per unit, resulting in variable RBC mass provided per unit transfused.

Table 18–1 pRBC Characteristics and General Indications

Product	Manipulation/Comment	Indications
Whole blood	None	Trauma, massive surgical bleeding
pRBCs, unmodified	Volume reduced	Symptomatic anemia Hemorrhagic shock (with volume expanders)
pRBCs, leukoreduced	White blood cell reduction	Prevent transfusion reactions Reduce alloimmunization Reduce infectious diseases Minimize immunomodulation
pRBCs, washed	Plasma removal	Recurrent severe allergic reactions IgA deficiency with anti-IgA
pRBCs, irradiated	Inactivation of lymphocytes	Prevention of TAGVHD
pRBCs, frozen deglycerolized	Frozen with subsequent deglycerolization Facilitates long-term storage	Storage of rare RBC phenotypes Autologous storage
pRBCs, CMV seronegative	Tested and found to be negative serologically Also applies to leukocytes, platelets, and residual plasma	CMV-negative transplantation Low-birth-weight infants CMV-negative pregnant women In utero transfusion

CMV, cytomegalovirus; IgA, immunoglobulin A; RBC, red blood cell; TAGVHD, transfusion-associated graft-versus-host disease.

A more efficient method of collecting RBCs for transfusion has been developed. RBCs may be collected by apheresis, with the unwanted components returned to the donor. Apheresis has become commonplace in the collection of platelet concentrates and granulocytes. Modified apheresis equipment has been used to collect RBCs and plasma.[9] The MCS+ machine (Haemonetics Corp., Braintree, MA) was developed for RBC collection and is now approved by the U.S. Food and Drug Administration (FDA) for 2-unit apheresis with automated return of 500 mL of saline to the donor or collection of 1 unit of RBCs and 200 to 550 mL of plasma.[10] Other manufacturers have also developed automated RBC collection systems.

For whole blood collections, a donor must have a hematocrit of at least 38% or a hemoglobin level of 12.5 g/dL and must wait 56 days between donations.[11] The FDA criteria for allogeneic 2-unit apheresis red blood cell donation require a minimum hematocrit of 40% or a hemoglobin of 13.3 g/dL, with a minimum of 112 days between donations. Height and weight requirements ensure adequate donor RBC mass. For men, a minimum height of 5 feet 1 inch and weight of 130 pounds, and for women, 5 feet 5 inches and 150 pounds are required. The total volumes removed from the donor in 2-unit RBC apheresis (380 to 500 mL RBCs) are comparable to the total volumes removed during whole blood donation (405 to 495 mL). The percentage of total blood volume (8.7% to 10.5%) removed is less than the 15% total blood volume allowed in whole blood donation. RBC apheresis donors do not appear to have more symptomatic anemia than whole blood donors, and the most common reactions are attributable to citrate toxicity.[11] Additional details on this procedure can be found in Chapter 12.

The quality of apheresis-collected RBCs is comparable to that of manually collected RBCs. In a study by Holme and colleagues,[10] both 1-unit and 2-unit RBC apheresis was performed by using the MCS+ with CPD or CP2D preservative. After resuspension in AS-3 additive and storage for 42 days at 48°C, the apheresis units had slightly less hemolysis, lower supernatant potassium levels, and better tolerance for osmotic shock than did manually collected units, with no difference in RBC adenosine triphosphate (ATP) or 24-hour percentage recovery after autologous transfusion. The addition of an in-line white blood cell reduction filter now permits collection of 2 units of prestorage leukoreduced RBC concentrates.[12] On evaluation of RBCs collected by using the MCS+ with in-line filtration, the study showed that residual white blood cell counts were less than 0.4×10^6, below the current standard of 5.0×10^6.

RED BLOOD CELL PRODUCTS

Whole Blood

Although whole blood is rarely used, certain clinical situations exist in which it might be preferable to pRBCs. Whole blood can correct combined deficits in oxygen-carrying capacity and blood volume. Whole blood is thus potentially indicated in trauma and massive surgical bleeding when the blood type of the patient has been determined. This approach minimizes the use of RBCs and plasma from different donors, thus decreasing the risk of transfusion-transmitted infectious disease. In addition, one study demonstrated that a unit of fresh whole blood has a hemostatic effect equivalent to that of 8 to 10 platelet units[13]; this effect appears to be diminished after storage of the blood at 4–8°C for a period as short as 5 hours,[14] which makes whole blood impractical as a source of platelets.

Although fresh whole blood can be useful for patients who require both oxygen-carrying capacity and volume, adequate inventories are difficult to maintain. Most cases requiring whole blood involve trauma, emergency cardiovascular surgery, or liver transplantation, which can be difficult to predict. In addition, the community need for platelets and plasma must be considered. Therefore, although some have argued that whole blood should be used more often, even for certain elective surgeries, most trauma centers continue to manage their cases with pRBCs.[15]

Instead of whole blood, pRBCs and one of several volume expanders can increase oxygen-carrying capacity and volume. Volume can be replaced with crystalloid, which is not only sterile but also economical, in the setting of mild to moderate blood loss. With more massive transfusion, colloid oncotic pressure may have to be enhanced; colloid solutions such as albumin are preferred to plasma as no risk of transfusion-transmitted infectious disease exists. A study of patients massively transfused (defined as 10 or more units of RBC concentrates in 24 hours) and given crystalloid demonstrated that significant thrombocytopenia developed after 20 units of pRBCs. Significant prolongation of the prothrombin and partial thromboplastin times occurred after transfusion of 12 pRBCs.[16] Whether these laboratory values are actually associated with abnormal clinical bleeding deserves investigation.

Plasma is rarely indicated during massive transfusion unless a well-documented coagulopathy is found, as in liver failure or disseminated intravascular coagulation.[17] In some cases of trauma or cardiac surgery, platelet concentrates may be indicated as well to treat microvascular bleeding secondary to dilutional thrombocytopenia or platelet dysfunction secondary to bypass. When a pool of 6 random units or a single-donor apheresis unit of platelets is given, at least 300 mL of plasma is also infused, eliminating the need for concomitant administration of FFP.

pRBCs

pRBCs are manufactured by removal of the majority of plasma from a unit of whole blood. pRBCs have a volume of approximately 250 to 300 mL and a hematocrit of 65% to 80%. pRBCs prepared without further modifications contain white blood cells, platelets, and residual plasma. Transfusion of pRBCs is indicated in the treatment of anemia with symptomatic deficits of oxygen-carrying capacity and hemorrhagic shock when administered with volume expanders. One unit of pRBCs should raise the hemoglobin of an average adult by 1 g/dL and the hematocrit by 3%. For pediatric patients, the usual dose given is 3 mL/kg to raise the hemoglobin by 1 g/dL and the hematocrit by 3%.

PRESERVATION AND STORAGE

The ability of transfused RBCs to deliver oxygen to tissues and survive in the patient's circulation is the best measure of how well the RBCs were preserved and stored. Survival of transfused RBCs is acceptable when at least 75% of the transfused RBCs are present in the circulation for 24 hours.[6]

The development of blood preservatives provided a means to store RBCs to facilitate blood banking with minimally toxic anticoagulants. A long history of clinical development has provided preservative solutions that optimize storage length and in vivo function. The main areas that have been addressed are glucose, anticoagulation, ATP, and 2,3-diphosphoglycerate (2,3-DPG).

Glucose

Glucose is the main source of fuel for energy-requiring processes to preserve membrane function. Initially, dextrose was added to citrate as an energy source, but caramelization occurred during heat sterilization because of the alkaline pH.[18] The citrate and dextrose were thus sterilized separately and mixed before the blood was collected. In 1943, Loutit and Mollison[18] added citric acid, creating acid citrate dextrose (ACD) solution. This formulation decreased the pH, allowed sterilization without caramelization, and facilitated storage for up to 21 days. It was also noted that because of the decreased pH, the blood and preservative solution had to be mixed thoroughly during collection to avoid clot formation.[19] The most commonly used storage solution in the United States, CPDA-1, supplies 10.1 mmol per unit of glucose, compared with 9.4 and 8.1 mmol per unit in ACD-A and CPD storage solutions, respectively (Table 18–2). Most patients tolerate the glucose transfused. However, for many years, hyperglycemia seen during massive transfusion in orthotopic liver transplantation has been commonly attributed to the glucose contained in transfused RBCs.[20] A recent study of pediatric and adult patients questions this finding: 60 pediatric and 16 adult patients receiving orthotopic liver transplants were included in the study. Blood glucose levels in transfused and nontransfused patients were compared, and no difference was found between the two groups.[21]

Anticoagulation

Citrate has been used since the early 1900s as a stable, minimally toxic anticoagulant that also has preservative properties.[22] Citrate in preservative solutions also influences intracellular pH and provides buffering.

Citrate is part of the Krebs cycle of respiration and therefore occurs endogenously. It is metabolized by muscle, liver, and renal cortex and stored in bone. In massive transfusion, citrate has been considered to be a cause of cardiac arrhythmia because of its ability to decrease plasma ionized calcium through chelation, although clear evidence of toxicity resulting from hypocalcemia has been difficult to obtain. Citrate is metabolized rapidly, preventing systemic anticoagulation. However, certain conditions may place patients at risk for toxicity. Hypothermia, liver disease, and hypoparathyroidism are conditions in which patients may already have depressed ionized calcium or may not be able to metabolize the citrate rapidly.[23] Newborns without adequate calcium stores and immature livers may also be at risk. Because supplementation with intravenous calcium may be associated with its own toxicities, routine calcium administration is not recommended in massive transfusion.

Adenosine Triphosphate

The ATP content of pRBCs decreases with storage, from 4.18 μmol/g hemoglobin at collection in CPDA-1 to 2.40 μmol/g hemoglobin at 35 days of storage.[24] Changes in RBC shape and increased cell fragility have been noted in stored RBCs.[25] It was not until 1962 that a direct correlation was made between erythrocyte shape and ATP content.[26] The decrease in ATP with storage is associated with a change in erythrocyte shape from biconcave disc to spherocyte, as well as a decrease in membrane lipid content and an increase in cell rigidity. Therefore, ATP must be maintained during storage for appropriate post-transfusion survival of RBCs. The addition of adenine counteracts the loss of adenine groups and allows enough ATP for RBC survival.

2,3-Diphosphoglycerate

The concentration of erythrocyte 2,3-DPG in pRBCs also decreases with storage. The decrease is dependent on pH. In whole blood collected in CPDA-1, the pH decreases from 7.16 to 6.73 over 35 days as a result of lactic acid formation, and the 2,3-DPG concentration decreases markedly from 13.2 to 0.7 μmol/g hemoglobin.[24]

In the RBC, the glucose intermediate metabolite 1,3-DPG is transformed to 2,3-DPG by a mutase. The 2,3-DPG is then dephosphorylated to 3-phosphoglycerate by a phosphatase. The phosphatase is inactive at pH levels above 7.2 but is more active at the lower pH in older pRBCs, contributing to the decreased 2,3-DPG levels.[27]

Table 18–2 pRBC Storage and Additive Solutions

Substance Content (mmol/unit)	ACD-A*	CPDA-1*	CPD*	CP2D*	Adsol (AS-1)†	Nutri-cell (AS-3)†
Citrate	5.3	6.6	6.6	6.6	—	0.2
Phosphate	—	1.0	1.3	1.3		
Glucose	9.4	10.1	8.1	16.3	11.1	5.5
Adenine	—	0.128	—	—	0.21	0.22
NaCl	—	—	—	—	15.4	7.0
Na_2HPO_4	—	—	—	—	—	1.9
Na_3 citrate	—	—	—	—	—	1.9
Mannitol	—	—	—	—	4.1	—
pH	6.9	7.1	7.1	7.1	—	—
Volume (mL) per unit blood	67.5	63	63	63	100	100

*pRBC storage solutions.
†pRBC additive solutions.
From Hogman CF. Preparation and preservation of red cells. Vox Sang 1998;74(suppl 2):177.

The function of erythrocyte 2,3-DPG is to bind to deoxyhemoglobin and facilitate oxygen transport. When 2,3-DPG binds to deoxyhemoglobin, the deoxyhemoglobin molecule is stabilized, and the equilibrium between deoxyhemoglobin and oxyhemoglobin shifts toward deoxyhemoglobin. This interaction shifts the oxygen-dissociation curve to the right, decreasing the oxygen affinity of hemoglobin and enhancing oxygen delivery to tissues.[28] Therefore, with decreased 2,3-DPG levels, the oxygen dissociation curve is shifted to the left, decreasing oxygen delivery to tissues.

Although it may be feared that transfused RBCs beyond a certain date of storage are of limited benefit to the patient, it has been shown that 2,3-DPG is rapidly regenerated in transfused RBCs, with nearly complete restoration after 1 day. In addition, in hypoxia, lactic acid is produced, decreasing the pH and thus shifting the oxygen-dissociation curve back to the right.[29] An increase in cardiac output also occurs with hypoxia, increasing oxygen delivery. Therefor, for most patients requiring transfusion, decreased 2,3-DPG is of little consequence. For the patient who is in shock and cannot increase cardiac output to compensate, the current preservative solutions may not be optimal because no added component is available to slow the decrease in 2,3-DPG levels.

Additive and Rejuvenation Solutions

In 1983 an RBC additive solution, Adsol (Baxter, Round Lake, Ill.), also referred to as AS-1, was approved for use. Adsol consists of adenine (to help maintain ATP during storage), dextrose, saline, and mannitol. It contains 60% more adenine and approximately 2.5 times as much glucose as CPDA-1.[30] The addition of mannitol prevents excessive hemolysis over the storage period.[31] The increased glucose allows an adequate supply of energy for the RBCs beyond 35 days, and blood stored with Adsol is outdated in 42 days (Tables 18–2 and 18–3).[8] This decreases the number of pRBCs lost because of outdating and is helpful in shipping and storing autologous blood.

One of the added benefits of this preservative solution is that the amount of plasma recovered from a unit of whole blood can be maximized. Whole blood is collected into a system of multiple closed bags containing CPD. The whole blood is then centrifuged for separation, and sufficient plasma is removed to raise the hematocrit to approximately 85%. Then 100 mL of Adsol preservative solution is added to the pRBCs, with a resultant hematocrit of 60% to 70%. Because the final hematocrit is about 62%, the Adsol-preserved pRBCs are less viscous. The lower viscosity results in potentially faster flow rates, which are beneficial in emergency situations.[32] A second commonly used additive solution, AS-3, contains sodium chloride, phosphate, adenine, and glucose and is used similarly to AS-1.

Other additive solutions have been investigated. A solution containing adenine, dextrose, mannitol, sodium citrate, ammonium chloride, and inorganic phosphate was studied.[33] Levels of ATP were higher in this test solution, compared with those in Adsol, over 84 days of storage. 2,3-DPG levels were higher in the test solution, but not significantly, and hemolysis was higher in the Adsol units. It was thought that the higher ATP concentration in the test solution was due to the ammonium or phosphate ions or both.[30] In vivo survival was demonstrated in a second study by using a modification of the previous test solution (less ammonium chloride). The 24-hour chromium-51 viability was superior to that of Adsol at 8 or 9 weeks of storage. Preparation for transfusion required removal of supernatant with one washing step.[34] This additive solution appears to be suitable for extending pRBC shelf life, but confirmatory studies are necessary.

Rejuvenation solutions can restore some intracellular ATP and 2,3-DPG lost during storage. The current FDA-licensed solution contains pyruvate, inosine, phosphate, and adenine. This solution may be added only to pRBCs prepared from whole blood collected in CPD or CPDA-1. It may be added at any point between 3 days after collection and 3 days after expiration. This solution is not intended for intravenous use, and pRBCs must be washed before administration or used when thawing frozen units.[8] Rejuvenation of units stored in AS-1 or AS-3 has also been studied.[35] In one experiment, rejuvenation of the AS-1 and AS-3 pRBCs resulted in above-normal levels of ATP after one treatment but suboptimal levels of 2,3-DPG. A second treatment raised the 2,3-DPG levels to normal. The authors suggested that this may be due to the increased adenine in the storage solutions; the conversion of 1,3-DPG to 3-phosphoglycerate is favored, decreasing 1,3-DPG availability to make 2,3-DPG.[35] Currently, only units stored in CPD or CPDA-1 may be used for rejuvenation.

Table 18–3 42-Day Poststorage pRBC Characteristics after Resuspension in AS-3

Characteristic	Prestorage	Poststorage
pH	6.8	6.4
ATP (μmol/g Hb)	4.1	2.9
DPG (μmol/g Hb)	9.0	0.3
Potassium (mEq/L)	2.4	63
Glucose (mg/dL)	608	402
Plasma Hb (mg/dL)	39	372
Hemolysis (%)	—	0.61

ATP, adenosine triphosphate; DPG, 2,3-diphosphoglycerate; Hb, hemoglobin; pRBC, packed red blood cell.

Modified from Holme S, Elfath MD, Whitley P: Evaluation of in vivo and in vitro quality of apheresis-collected RBC stored for 42 days. Vox Sang 1998;75:212–217.

Temperature

RBC concentrates must be stored between 1° C and 6° C.[8] Storage at this temperature slows RBC metabolism and facilitates extended storage in blood banks. Liquid blood storage in CPDA-1 allows a shelf-life of up to 35 days. Even at 4–8° C, significant chemical changes take place during the storage period that may have clinical consequences for some patients. These changes are collectively known as the *storage lesion.*

No clinically significant change occurs in the plasma levels of sodium and chloride. However, the plasma potassium increases nearly eightfold over 28 days.[36] At a temperature of 4–8° C, the sodium-potassium pump is essentially nonfunctional, and intracellular and extracellular levels gradually equilibrate. In addition, the hemolysis that occurs during the storage period results in increased potassium in the supernatant. However, because the total volume of plasma in pRBCs is low (approximately 70 mL), the total potassium burden is only about 5.5 mEq at product expiration. Therefore, the potassium load is rarely a clinical problem except in the setting of preexisting hyperkalemia and renal failure or for very sick neonates. In these situations, fresher units of RBCs or washed RBCs may be used.

Storage Containers

The use of vinyl plastic blood bags and tubing in transfusion medicine is advantageous in the collection, processing, storage, and dispensing of blood components. In the early 1970s, however, reports surfaced about the potential toxicity of blood stored in bags with di(2-ethylhexyl)phthalate (DEHP). DEHP, the chemical that allows the vinyl plastic to be pliable, is referred to as a plasticizer. DEHP is added in large quantities to the plastic, approximately 40% by weight. It is not bound to the plastic but is dissolved in it. As a result, DEHP can leak into blood stored in the container and be transfused along with the blood. In 1970, Jaeger and Rubin[37] reported that 5 to 7 mg of DEHP could be isolated per 100 mL of blood. In addition, two patients were found to have DEHP at levels ranging from 0.069 to 0.270 mg per gram dry weight of tissue. A more recent evaluation of the levels of DEHP in stored blood components found that as storage time increased, the amount of DEHP detected ranged from 6.8 to 36.5 μg/mL in RBC concentrates. Whole blood products had the highest DEHP levels, compared with RBC concentrates, irradiated RBC concentrates, FFP, and platelet products.[38] Concern over the potential toxic effects of DEHP in humans has fueled a great deal of research and much debate. DEHP, identified as a carcinogen in rats and mice,[39] is ubiquitous in the environment. It caused a form of shock lung leading to death when administered to rats in intravenous form,[40] caused testicular atrophy in rats given dietary doses,[41] and led to lung injury in dogs and baboons transfused with stored blood.[42]

Because of an association with hepatomegaly, DEHP has also been linked to potential hepatocarcinogenicity. Hepatomegaly has been shown to be caused by proliferation of cellular organelles called peroxisomes. Peroxisomes are involved in the β-oxidation of fatty acids, producing hydrogen peroxide, which has been suggested to be the causative agent in the carcinogenicity of DEHP.[43] With all of this information, however, no direct causal link has been established between DEHP and cancer in humans.

Because of the concerns about toxicity, alternative materials for blood-storage containers have been under investigation for some time. A study comparing another plastic, poly(ethylene-co-ethyl acrylate) (EEA), with polyvinyl chloride (PVC) containing DEHP[44] found that blood stored in EEA containers had higher plasma hemoglobin and greater susceptibility to osmotic lysis than did blood stored in PVC containers. When DEHP was added to EEA containers, blood stored in EEA containers without DEHP had greater RBC osmotic fragility than did blood in EEA with DEHP or PVC containers.

PVC plasticized with butyryl-*n*-trihexyl-citrate (BTHC) has been introduced in place of DEHP. Use of BTHC has not become widespread. Less BTHC than DEHP leaches into the bag contents, and excellent 24-hour posttransfusion RBC recovery occurs with minimal hemolysis.[45]

FROZEN RED BLOOD CELL CONCENTRATES

RBCs can be frozen for long-term storage, at least 10 years, and probably longer for certain indications.[8] After pRBCs are prepared from whole blood, they are treated with glycerol as a cryoprotective agent. Because glycerol binds water, the formation of ice spicules from the solvent water within the unit, which would damage the RBCs, is prevented.[46] Another theory concerning the efficacy of glycerol is that it prevents cellular hypotonicity or hypertonicity, which may enhance cell lysis. The blood of donors who have sickle cell trait is unsuitable for freezing because hemolysis occurs during routine deglycerolization.[47]

Of three methods of freezing RBCs,[48] the most common one in the United States is the high-glycerol (40% to 50%) method. A low-glycerol method exists, but it has several disadvantages: liquid nitrogen must be used for storage, and the metal containers in which the plastic blood bags are placed before freezing can cause explosions if the liquid nitrogen leaks.[49] With a third method, agglomeration, the cells are deglycerolized with a low-ionic-strength saline solution. The cells clump and sediment in the bag, after which the supernatant is removed, and the cells are washed.[50]

When the glycerol solution has been added, the cells are frozen and stored at −65° C or below in a suitable freezer or in liquid nitrogen with a gas-phase temperature below −120° C.[8] To be transfused, the cells must be thawed and deglycerolized. One of the initial drawbacks of the high-glycerol method was that the procedure of thawing and removing the glycerol had many practical limitations. A simpler method of processing these cells for transfusion was developed by Meryman and Hornblower.[50] Their method requires only two cycles of centrifugation, washing with saline, and resuspension with isotonic saline containing glucose.

The remaining product contains few white cells or platelets, and 99.9% of the plasma is removed by the extensive washing during processing.[51] More than 90% of the donor's RBCs are recovered.[52] The 24-hour posttransfusion survival has been shown to be 85% to 90%.[53]

Posttransfusion survival and oxygen-carrying capacity of RBCs are affected by the amount of time spent between donation, refrigeration, and freezing.[46] Frozen cells have been shown to maintain prefreezing ATP and 2,3-DPG levels. The standard is to freeze within 6 days of collection, before these factors become significantly depleted. When it is necessary to freeze older units, rejuvenation with a solution containing pyruvate, glucose, phosphate, and adenine can be used.[54]

The major advantage of frozen RBCs is that rare blood types, such as (Oh) Bombay, can be stored. Patients with rare phenotypes may make autologous donations that can be frozen for later use. Cells from autologous donors can also be frozen if more units are required than can be collected in the maximum 42-day liquid storage period or if surgery is postponed.

For patients who become alloimmunized to multiple clinically significant RBC antigens, frozen RBCs from donors with rare phenotypes are useful. Among these patients are multiply transfused patients with sickle cell anemia who have multiple alloantibodies. African-Americans frequently lack antigens found on most donor RBCs from whites. During blood drives targeting the African-American community for the benefit of such patients, it is helpful to phenotype these RBCs and freeze the more uncommon types.

Because 99.9% of plasma is removed in processing frozen RBCs, patients who may have adverse events related to plasma components may also benefit from the use of frozen RBCs. For example, immunoglobulin A (IgA)-deficient patients with anti-IgA antibodies may have anaphylactoid reactions when exposed to donor plasma. In the past, patients who had multiple febrile nonhemolytic transfusion reactions that persisted despite removal of the buffy coat and treatment with medications also benefited from the more complete removal of cytokine-laden plasma and the leukoreduction that thawed frozen RBCs offered. Newer leukocyte reduction techniques have largely replaced this indication. Because of the high cost and cumbersome nature of freeze-thaw procedures, other more routine uses of frozen RBCs are difficult to justify. If a simpler means of preparation of frozen blood were available that avoided the limitations of the open systems now used, more widespread use could be envisioned.

CYTOMEGALOVIRUS-SERONEGATIVE RED BLOOD CELL CONCENTRATES

Cytomegalovirus (CMV) is a double-stranded DNA herpesvirus (human herpesvirus 5) that can be transmitted by transfusion. Forty percent to 100% of adults are seropositive for CMV, depending on socioeconomic status and geographic region.[55] Persistent and latent infection can result, as well as reactivation and reinfection. The first report of transfusion-transmitted CMV described a syndrome seen in patients 3 to 8 weeks after cardiopulmonary bypass. The syndrome consisted of fever, lymphocytosis, and splenomegaly.[56] A congenital syndrome including petechiae, hepatosplenomegaly, jaundice, and microcephaly has also been identified. Postnatal infection in children can cause hepatitis. In immunocompromised adults, infection with CMV can result in interstitial pneumonitis, hepatitis, encephalitis, gastroenteritis, thrombocytopenia, or leukopenia; in certain patients receiving transplants, these conditions are associated with a high fatality rate. In immunocompetent adults, fever and hepatitis may result, but most patients have an asymptomatic mononucleosis.[55]

Transfusion-transmitted CMV is of concern in immunocompromised patients. CMV-seronegative blood is often requested for CMV-negative bone-marrow transplant candidates or recipients, in utero transfusions, low-birth-weight premature infants of CMV-negative mothers, CMV-negative pregnant women, and rare cases of human immunodeficiency virus–positive, CMV-negative patients. CMV-negative recipients of solid organ transplants from CMV-negative donors are among the patients who may benefit but in whom the risk of using blood products not tested for CMV is not well established.[52]

The sites of CMV latency are thought to include CD34-positive progenitor cells and CD13- and CD14-positive monocytes.[55] Thus transfusion-transmitted disease can be mitigated by removal of leukocytes in the pRBCs. A study published in 1995 compared bedside leukoreduction and CMV-seronegative blood products in bone-marrow transplant recipients and suggested that filtration is an effective alternative to CMV-seronegative blood for the prevention of transfusion-transmitted CMV. A follow-up of 142 bone-marrow transplant recipients found that in 62 CMV-seronegative recipients of bone marrow from CMV-seronegative donors, supported with the use of leukocyte-reduced blood products, no documented CMV infection occurred.[57] The American Association of Blood Banks (AABB) has suggested that both approaches, leukocyte reduction and the use of CMV-seronegative blood, are essentially equivalent in the prevention of CMV transmission.[58]

LEUKOCYTE-REDUCED RED BLOOD CELL CONCENTRATES

Leukocyte-reduced RBCs are defined by the AABB as having less than 5×10^6 leukocytes in the final component. Early techniques of leukocyte reduction involved centrifugation, washing with saline, and removal of the buffy coat. A second-generation technique known as the spin-cool-filter method was introduced in the 1980s.[59] This method requires use of 1-week-old RBCs, which are centrifuged and then cooled for 4 hours to enhance microaggregate formation before passage through a microaggregate filter. Currently, filtration can be performed at the bedside or in the laboratory with attachable filters that reduce leukocytes more than 99.9% with less than 10% depletion of RBCs.[60]

Leukocyte-reduced RBCs are indicated primarily in the setting of repeated febrile nonhemolytic transfusion reactions. It was previously thought that these reactions were mediated only by antibodies to foreign leukocyte antigens.[61] Now increasing evidence suggests that cytokines produced by the leukocytes during storage also cause these reactions.[62,63] Prestorage leukocyte reduction has also been shown to reduce substantially the incidence of febrile nonhemolytic transfusion reactions.[64]

A second indication for leukocyte-reduced RBCs is the prevention of sensitization to human leukocyte antigens (HLAs) in bone-marrow transplant recipients and other patients who require frequent platelet transfusion. The Trial to Reduce Alloimmunization to Platelets (TRAP) study[65] demonstrated a reduction in alloimmunization in acute myelogenous leukemia patients who received leukocyte-reduced blood components. Platelet refractoriness, although low in the control group (16%), was reduced among patients receiving leukocyte-reduced products (7%).

As a third indication, CMV transmission is mitigated as compared with the transfusion of unscreened blood products[66–68] and may be comparable (as mentioned earlier), or better than the use of seronegative products. At the time of this writing, it is unclear whether using both leukoreduced, seronegative units is superior to using either alone. Last, the use of nucleic acid testing, though only in use on a research basis, may provide additional safety (see Chapter 46).

Finally, leukocyte-reduced RBCs may have another indication. The transfusion of allogeneic blood is thought by many scientists to be immunosuppressive, an effect termed transfusion-related immune modulation (TRIM). Several studies appear to document this effect, but some controversy remains. A correlation between pretransplantation allogeneic RBC transfusions and improved renal allograft survival has been known for many years.[69,70] Initial reports appeared before the availability of cyclosporine and other improvements in immunosuppression that made this phenomenon less clinically relevant. However, a subsequent study including patients receiving modern immunosuppressive regimens demonstrated that recipients of three unmodified allogeneic RBC transfusions had 90% 1-year and 79% 5-year graft survivals, compared with 82% and 70% 1- and 5-year survivals, respectively, for patients who received no transfusion, which suggests continued importance.[71]

Perioperative allogeneic RBC transfusion may also have an adverse effect on tumor recurrence.[72–74] The data on this effect are more controversial; Blajchman[75] observed that approximately 50% of the nonrandomized studies indicate an adverse effect of transfusion on tumor recurrence. Patients with colorectal cancer who received perioperative transfusions were shown to have longer hospital stays than those who did not receive transfusion,[76] but the effect in this study was attributed to a higher incidence of postoperative infection. In surgical patients, perioperative transfusion may also predispose to bacterial infection. A dose-response relation appears to exist between transfusion and the probability of infection; transfusion is the best predictor of infection, over such factors as extent of trauma, degree of blood loss, and presence of wound contamination,[77] although confounding factors have not been eliminated in many studies.

The mechanism for these effects may be related to the transfusion of contaminating white blood cells. The donor white blood cells could cause a downregulation of cellular immunity, mediated by secretion of T-helper 2 cytokines and inhibitors (interleukin-4, interleukin-10, and transforming growth factor-β), with resultant inhibition of the T-helper 1 response.[78] The potential benefit of leukocyte reduction appears to be supported by reports that patients having colorectal surgery who received leukocyte-reduced RBC transfusions had fewer infections and shorter hospital stays than did those who received unmodified RBCs.[78] Animal studies also appear to support this theory. In rabbits inoculated with VX-2 tumor cells, those that received unmodified allogeneic RBC transfusions had significantly more pulmonary metastases than did those that received 99.8% leukocyte-reduced blood.[79]

An editorial concerning TRIM stated, "prestorage WBC reduction is an intervention that is virtually risk-free and that, except for its cost, has no down side … the decision to implement universal prestorage WBC reduction need not be delayed until further evidence of efficacy becomes available."[80] The suggestion that leukocyte-reduced RBCs decrease the unwanted immunosuppressive effects of transfusion may be further proof that conversion to a leukocyte-reduced blood supply enhances patients' safety.

In light of these indications for leukoreduced RBCs, many centers have moved to universal prestorage leukoreduction. Some hospitals, however, use a selective leukodepletion policy based on lack of direct convincing evidence that leukoreduction offers benefits to patients not in certain categories. Data in support of this practice is available from a prospective randomized trial, which showed no benefit to conversion to a universally leukodepleted inventory, except for specific indications, such as a reduction in febrile transfusion reactions.[81] The cited study did, however, show a trend toward increased safety with leukoreduced units and may have been underpowered. One of the pitfalls of selective leukodepletion is the difficulty of recognizing which patients require leukodepletion in complex clinical settings; in addition, this study did not address the potential adverse long-term consequences of CMV infection or alloimmunization in the recipients. Without a community standard for universal leukodepletion, patients in groups that do qualify for certain protocols may be overlooked and will not receive these components.[82] Based on these concerns, the authors feel that universal leukodepletion offers safety advantages for all patients and guarantees the receipt of leukoreduced blood in such cases in which the specific indication is not recognized or may not have yet occurred.

WASHED PRBCs

Washed RBCs are prepared with isotonic saline by either manual or automated methods. Automation is more efficient, resulting in loss of fewer RBCs with each wash cycle. Because washing takes place in an open system, the product must be used within 24 hours.

Washing RBCs removes plasma proteins, some leukocytes, and remaining platelets. This product is indicated for patients who have had recurrent severe allergic transfusion reactions that are not prevented by antihistamines. Recipient IgE antibodies to donor plasma proteins mediate these reactions. Washed RBCs are also indicated for IgA-deficient patients who have formed anti-IgA antibodies. In these patients, transfusion of blood products containing plasma with IgA can result in anaphylaxis.[83]

In patients with paroxysmal nocturnal hemoglobinuria (PNH), a rare disorder in which RBCs are unusually sensitive to complement lysis, transfusion of washed RBCs has been advocated to prevent hemolysis. However, a report by Brecher and Taswell[84] on 23 patients with PNH seen over a 38-year period appears to show that this is a needless practice.[84] A total of 431 RBC products (94 whole blood, 208 pRBCs, 80 leukocyte-reduced RBCs, 38 washed RBCs, 5 frozen RBCs, and 6 intraoperatively salvaged units) were transfused with only one episode of hemolysis after transfusion. This single event was associated with transfusion of group O whole blood to a group AB individual. Although the need for washed RBCs in PNH is questionable, this disorder is rare, and changing established transfusion protocols may not be justified.

IRRADIATED PRBCs

RBCs are commonly irradiated by using a cesium 137 source. A dose of at least 2500 cGy must be delivered to each unit, and quality-control standards have been published to ensure that this dose is achieved with blood bank irradiators.[85] After irradiation, storage time is decreased to a maximum of 28 days[8] because of shortened RBC survival and increased potassium leakage. Please see Chapter 28 for additional and detailed information.

The purpose of irradiation of cellular blood products in transfusion medicine is to inactivate immunocompetent lymphocytes. Irradiated RBCs are indicated for the prevention of transfusion-associated graft-versus-host disease in immunocompromised patients, a frequently fatal complication. Neonates, patients with hematologic malignancies, patients with aplastic anemia, bone-marrow transplant recipients, and patients with congenital immune deficiency are susceptible to transfusion-associated graft-versus-host disease.[86] Graft-versus-host disease is also a potential hazard of directed donation from first-degree relatives who share HLA haplotypes.[87] See Chapter 53 for additional information regarding this phenomenon.

REFERENCES

1. Landsteiner K. Ueber Agglutinationserscheinungen normalen menschlichen Blutes. Wein Klin Wochenschr 1901;14:1132–1134.
2. Loutit JF, Mollison PL. Advantages of a disodium-citrate-glucose mixture as a blood preservative. Br Med J 1943;2:744–745.
3. Schmidt PJ. Charles Drew, a legend in our time. Transfusion 1997;37:234–236.

4. National Blood Data Resource Center. Comprehensive Report on Blood Collection and Transfusion in the United States in 2001. Bethesda, Md., National Blood Data Resource Center, 2002.
5. Walter C, Murphy W. A closed gravity technique for the preservation of whole blood in ACD solution utilizing plastic equipment. Surg Gynecol Obstet 1952;94:687–692.
6. Brecher M (ed). Technical Manual, 15th ed. Bethesda, Md., American Association of Blood Banks, 1999.
7. Baldini M, Costea N, Dameschek W. The viability of stored human platelets. Blood 1960;16:1669–1692.
8. Standards for Blood Banks and Transfusion Services, 23rd ed. Bethesda, Md., American Association of Blood Banks, 2005.
9. Knutson F, Rider J, Franck V, et al. A new apheresis procedure for the preparation of high-quality red cells and plasma. Transfusion 1999;39:565–571.
10. Holme S, Elfath M, Whitley P. Evaluation of in vivo and in vitro quality of apheresis-collected RBC stored for 42 days. Vox Sang 1998;75:212–217.
11. Shi P, Ness P. Two-unit red cell apheresis and its potential advantages over traditional whole-blood donation. Transfusion 1999;39:218–225.
12. Bandarenko N, Rose M, Kowalsky R, et al. In vivo and in vitro characteristics of double units of RBCs collected by apheresis with a single in-line WBC-reduction filter. Transfusion 2001;41:1373–1377.
13. Lavee J, Martinowitz U, Mohr R, et al. The effect of transfusion of fresh whole blood versus platelet concentrates after cardiac operations. J Thorac Cardiovasc Surg 1989;97:204–212.
14. Golan M, Modan M, Lavee J, et al. Transfusion of fresh whole blood stored (4°C) for short period fails to improve platelet aggregation of extracellular matrix and clinical hemostasis after cardiopulmonary bypass. J Thorac Cardiovasc Surg 1990;99:354–360.
15. Schmidt P. Whole blood transfusion. Transfusion 1984;24:368–369.
16. Leslie SD, Toy P. Laboratory hemostatic abnormalities in massively transfused patients given red blood cells and crystalloid. Am J Clin Pathol 1991;96:770–773.
17. National Institute of Health Consensus Conference. Fresh frozen plasma: indications and rules. Transfus Med Rev 1987;1:201–204.
18. Boral L, Henry JB. Clinical Diagnosis and Management by Laboratory Methods, 19th ed. Philadelphia, WB Saunders, 1996, p 802.
19. Loutit JF, Mollison PL. Advantages of a disodium-citrate-glucose mixture as a blood preservative. Br Med J 1943;2:744–745.
20. Atchison SR, Rettke SR, Fromme GA, et al. Plasma glucose concentrations during liver transplantation. Mayo Clin Proc 1989;64:241–245.
21. Cheng KW, Chen CL, Cheng YF, et al. Dextrose in the banked blood products does not seem to affect the blood glucose levels in patients undergoing liver transplantation. World J Gastroenterol 2005;11:87–89.
22. Rous P, Turner JR. The preservation of living red blood cells in vitro. J Exp Med 1996;23:219–248.
23. Howland W, Bellville J, Zucker M, et al. Massive blood replacement: Failure to observe citrate intoxication. Surg Gynecol Obstet 1957;105:529–540.
24. Moore GL, Peck CC, Sohmer PR, Zuck TF. Some properties of blood stored in anticoagulant CPDA-1 solution. Transfusion 1981;21:135–137.
25. Rapoport S. Dimensional, osmotic and clinical changes of erythrocytes in stored blood I: Blood preserved in sodium citrate, neutral and acid citrate-glucose (ACD) mixtures. J Clin Invest 1947;26:591–615.
26. Nakao K, Wada T, Kamiyama T, et al. A direct relationship between adenosine triphosphate level and in vivo viability of erythrocytes. Nature 1962;194:877–878.
27. Hogman C. Preparation and preservation of red cells. Vox Sang 1998; 74(suppl 2):177–187.
28. Harken A. The surgical significance of the oxyhemoglobin dissociation curve. Surg Gynecol Obstet 1997;144:935–955.
29. Beutler E. What is the clinical importance of alterations of the hemoglobin oxygen affinity in preserved blood, especially as produced by variations of red cell 2,3-DPG content? Vox Sang 1078;34:1130.
30. Mollison PL, Engelfriet CP, Contreras M. Blood Transfusion in Clinical Medicine, 10th ed. Boston, Blackwell Scientific, 1997, p 249.
31. Hogman CF. Additive system approach in blood transfusion: birth of the SAG and Sagman systems. Vox Sang 1986;51:339–340.
32. Heaton A, Miripol J, Aster R, et al. Use of Adsol preservation solution for prolonged storage of low viscosity AS-1 red blood cells. Br J Haematol 1984;57:467–478.
33. Greenwalt TJ, McGuinness CG, Dumaswala UJ, Carter HW. Studies in red blood cell preservation, 3: A phosphate-ammonium-adenine additive solution. Vox Sang 1990;58:94–99.
34. Greenwalt TJ, Dumaswala UJ, Dhingra N, et al. Studies in red blood cell preservation, 7: In vivo and in vitro studies with a modified phosphate-ammonium additive solution. Vox Sang 1993;65:87–94.
35. Brecher ME, Zylstra-Halling VW, Pineda AA. Rejuvenation of erythrocytes preserved with AS-1 and AS-3. Am J Clin Pathol 1991;96:767–769.
36. Latham J, Bove J, Weirich F. Chemical and hematologic changes in stored CPDA-1 blood. Transfusion 1982;22:158–159.
37. Jaeger R, Rubin R. Contamination of blood stored in plastic packs. Lancet 1970;29:151.
38. Inoue K, Kawaguchi M, Yamanaka R, et al. Evaluation and analysis of exposure levels of di(2-ethylhexyl)phthalate from blood bags. Clin Chim Acta 2005;358:159–166.
39. Kluwe W, Haseman J, Douglas J, Huff J. The carcinogenicity of dietary di-(2-ethylhexyl)phthalate (DEHP) in Fischer 344 rats and B6C3F1 mice. J Toxicol Environ Health 1982;10:797–815.
40. Schulz CO, Rubin RJ, Hutchins GM. Acute lung toxicity and sudden death in rats following the intravenous administration of the plasticizer, di-(2-ethylhexyl)phthalate, solubilised with tween surfactants. Toxicol Appl Pharmacol 1975;33:514–525.
41. Gray T, Butterworth K. Testicular atrophy produced by phthalate esters. Arch Toxicol Suppl 1980;4:452–455.
42. Bennet SH, Creelhoed GW, Aaron RK, et al. Pulmonary injury resulting from perfusion with stored bank blood in the baboon and dog. J Surg Res 1972;13:295–306.
43. Rubin RJ, Ness PM. What price progress? An update on vinyl plastic blood bags. Transfusion 1989;29:358–361.
44. Horowitz B, Stryker M, Waldman A, et al. Stabilization of red blood cells by the plasticizer, diethylhexylphthalate. Vox Sang 1985;48:150–155.
45. Hogman CF, Eriksson L, Ericson A, Reppucci AJ. Storage of saline-adenine-glucose- mannitol-suspe red cells in a new plastic container: polyvinylchloride plasticized with butyryl-*n*-trihexyl-citrate. Transfusion 1991;31:26–29.
46. Huggins C. Preparation and usefulness of frozen blood. Annu Rev Med 1985;36:499–503.
47. Meryman HT, Hornblower M. Freezing and deglycerolizing sickle-trait red blood cells. Transfusion 1976;16:627–632.
48. Boral L, Henry JB. Clinical Diagnosis and Management by Laboratory Methods, 19th ed. Philadelphia, WB Saunders, 1996, p 803.
49. Akerblom O, Hogman CF. Frozen blood: A method for low-glycerol, liquid nitrogen freezing allowing different postthaw deglycerolization procedures. Transfusion 1974;14:16–26.
50. Meryman HT, Hornblower M. A simplified procedure for deglycerolizing red blood cells frozen in a high glycerol concentration. Transfusion 1977;17:438–442.
51. Contreras TJ, Valeri CR. A comparison of methods to wash liquid-stored red blood cells and red blood cells frozen with high or low concentration of glycerol. Transfusion 1976;16:539–565.
52. Sayers M. Transfusion-transmitted viral infections other than hepatitis and human immunodeficiency virus infection: cytomegalovirus, Epstein-Barr virus, human herpes virus 6 and human parvovirus B19. Arch Pathol Lab Med 1994;118:346–349.
53. Valeri CR. Factors influencing the 24 hour post-transfusion survival and oxygen transport function of previously frozen red cells preserved with 40% glycerol and frozen at −80°C. Transfusion 1974;14:1–15.
54. Valeri CR, Zaroulis CG. Rejuvenation and freezing of outdated stored human red cells. N Engl J Med 1972;287:1307–1313.
55. Pamphilon DH, Rider JR, Barbara JAJ, Williamson LM. Prevention of transfusion-transmitted cytomegalovirus infection. Transfus Med 1999;9:115–123.
56. Kreel I, Zarroff LI, Canter JW. A syndrome following total body perfusion. Surg Gynecol Obstet 1960;111:317–321.
57. Pamphilon DH, Foot ABM, Adeodu A, et al. Prophylaxis and prevention of CMV infection in bone marrow allograft recipients: leucodepleted platelets are equivalent to those from CMV seronegative donors. Bone Marrow Transplant 1999;23(suppl 1):S66.
58. American Association of Blood Banks. Leukocyte Reduction for the Prevention of Transfusion-transmitted Cytomegalovirus (AABB Association Bulletin 97–2, 10–12). Bethesda, Md., American Association of Blood Banks Press, 1997.
59. Meryman HT, Hornblower M. The preparation of red cells depleted of leukocytes: Review and evaluation. Transfusion 1986;26:101–106.
60. Dzik WH. Leukoreduced blood components: Laboratory and clinical aspects. In Rossi EC, Simon TL, Moss GS, et al. (eds): Principles of Transfusion Medicine. Baltimore, Williams & Wilkins, 1995, p 353.
61. Payne R. Leukocyte agglutinins in human sera. Arch Intern Med 1957; 99:587–606.
62. Davenport RD, Kunkel SL. Cytokine roles in hemolytic and non-hemolytic transfusion reactions. Transfus Med Rev 1994;7:157–168.
63. Heddle NM, Kelton JG. Febrile non-hemolytic transfusion reactions. In Popovsky MA (ed): Transfusion Reactions. Bethesda, Md., AABB Press, 1996, p 45.
64. King KE, Shirey RS, Thoman SK, et al. Universal leukoreduction decreases the incidence of febrile nonhemolytic transfusion reactions to RBCs. Transfusion 2004;44:25–29.

65. The Trial to Reduce Alloimmunization to Platelets Study Group. Leukocyte reduction and ultraviolet B irradiation of platelets to prevent alloimmunization and refractoriness to platelet transfusions. N Engl J Med 1997;337:1861–1869.
66. Bowden RA, Slichter SJ, Sayers M, et al. A comparison of filtered leukocyte-reduced and cytomegalovirus (CMV) seronegative blood products for the prevention of transfusion-associated CMV infection after marrow transplant. Blood 1995;86:3598–3603.
67. Narvios AB, de Lima M, Shah H, Lichtiger B. Transfusion of leukoreduced cellular blood components from cytomegalovirus-unscreened donors in allogeneic hematopoietic transplant recipients: analysis of 72 recipients. Bone Marrow Transplant 2005;36:499–501.
68. Laupacis A, Brown J, Costello B, et al. Prevention of prosttransfusion CMV in the era of universal WBC reduction: a consensus statement. Transfusion 2001;41:560–569.
69. Opelz G, Sengar DP, Mickey MR, et al. Effect of blood transfusions on subsequent kidney transplants. Transplant Proc 1973;5:253–259.
70. Blajchman MA, Singal DP. Renal transplantation: the role of red blood cell antigens, histocompatibility antigens and blood transfusions on renal allograft survival. Transfus Med Rev 1983;3:171–179.
71. Opelz G, Vanrentergehm Y, Kirste G, et al. Prospective evaluation of pretransplant blood transfusion in cadaver kidney recipients. Transplantation 1997;63:964–697.
72. Schriemer PA, Longnecker DE, Mintz PD. The possible immunosuppressive effects of perioperative blood transfusion in cancer patients. Anesthesiology 1988;68:422–428.
73. Van Aken WG. Does perioperative blood transfusion promote tumor growth? Transfus Med Rev 1989;3:243–252.
74. Heiss MM, Jauch KW, Delanoff C, et al. Blood transfusion modulated tumor recurrence: A randomized study of autologous versus homologous blood transfusion in colorectal cancer. J Clin Oncol 1994;12:1859–1867.
75. Blajchman MA. Immunomodulatory effects of allogeneic blood transfusions: Clinical manifestations and mechanisms. Vox Sang 1988;74 (suppl 2):315.
76. Vamvakas EC, Carven JH. Allogeneic blood transfusion, hospital charges, and length of hospitalization: a study of 487 consecutive patients undergoing colorectal cancer resection. Arch Pathol Lab Med 1998;122:145–151.
77. Blumberg N, Heal J. Transfusion immunomodulation. In Anderson KC, Ness PM (eds): Scientific Basis of Transfusion Medicine, 2nd ed. Philadelphia, WB Saunders, 2000, p 430.
78. Blumberg N, Heal JM. Blood transfusion immunomodulation: the silent epidemic. Arch Pathol Lab Med 1998;122:117–119.
79. Blajchman MA, Bardossy L, Carmen R, et al. Allogeneic blood transfusion-induced enhancement of tumor growth: two animal models showing amelioration by leukocyte reduction and passive transfer using spleen cells. Blood 1993;81:1880–1882.
80. Blajchman MA. Transfusion-associated immunomodulation and universal white cell reduction: are we putting the cart before the horse? Transfusion 1999;39:665–670.
81. Dzik WH, Anderson JK, O'Neill EM, et al. A prospective, randomized clinical trial of universal WBC reduction. Transfusion 2002;42:1114–1122.
82. Ness PM, Lipton KS. Selective transfusion protocols: errors and accidents waiting to happen. Transfusion 2001;41:713–715.
83. Vyas GN, Holmdahl L, Perkins HA, Fudenberg HH. Serologic specificity of human anti-IgA and its significance in transfusion. Blood 1969;34:573–581.
84. Brecher ME, Taswell HF. Paroxysmal nocturnal hemoglobinuria and the transfusion of washed red cells: a myth revisited. Transfusion 1989;29:681–685.
85. Moroff G, Leitman SF, Luban NLC. Principles of blood irradiation, dose validation, and quality control. Transfusion 1997;37:1084–1092.
86. Leitman SF, Holland PV. Irradiation of blood products: indications and guidelines. Transfusion 1985;25:293–303.
87. Thaler M, Shamiss A, Orgad S, et al. The role of blood from HLA-homozygous donors in fatal transfusion associated graft versus host disease after open heart surgery. N Engl J Med 1989;321:25–28.

Chapter 19

Fresh Frozen Plasma and Related Products

Robert L. Crookes • Christopher D. Hillyer

Component therapy has had a profound impact on the practice of transfusion medicine. The extraction of various constituents, including plasma, from whole blood has led to increased efficacy and economic utilization of the blood supply. When only the component that is needed is transfused, the patient is spared untoward effects of other blood components. Plasma, both in the circulation and for transfusion, contains a variety of organic and inorganic elements with therapeutic value as described subsequently. However, the isolation, purification, and preparation for injection or transfusion of some specific plasma constituents [e.g., factor VIII (FVIII), albumin, immunoglobulins] have limited the use of fresh frozen plasma (FFP) in clinical practice. The use of FFP (and related plasma components) is now reserved for conditions requiring therapy in which replacement of multiple plasma constituents is needed or for which the specific constituent is not commercially available in a purified injectable or transfusable form.

PHYSIOLOGIC ROLE OF PLASMA

Plasma is the aqueous component of blood in which cellular elements and macromolecules are transported throughout the body and other constituents are maintained in a dynamic equilibrium with the extravascular compartment. The composition of plasma is influenced by gender, age, diet, and other individual and environmental characteristics.[1,2] The major component of plasma is water, which constitutes approximately 85% to 90% of the plasma volume. The solute component constitutes 0.3 mol/L, of which about 30% is made up of proteins, with colloids, crystalloids, clotting factors, hormones, vitamins, and trace elements making up the rest. Normal human plasma has a density of 1.055 to 1.063 g/mL and a pH that varies between 7.33 and 7.43 with respective temperature changes between 37°C and 4°C.[3]

Although human plasma contains a multitude of substances including ionic and nonionic solutes, the practice of transfusion medicine has exploited plasma mainly for its protein content. It is estimated that human plasma contains more than 700 different proteins with various physiologic characteristics and functions. Although some 120 proteins have been isolated, only a few are available for clinical use. The most abundant plasma protein is albumin, with a concentration between 3500 and 5000 mg/dL. Albumin is responsible for maintaining colloid oncotic pressure and serves as a major transport protein for endogenous and exogenous substances. Plasma proteins with immunologic functions include the immunoglobulin (Ig) family, of which IgG (5 to 14 mg/dL) is the most abundant, and the complement components, of which C3 (1.2 mg/dL) predominates quantitatively. In addition, plasma proteins include those involved in maintaining normal rheologic properties of blood (e.g., coagulation and fibrinolytic proteins).[4–6]

PLASMA COLLECTION, QUALITY, AND PROCESSING

Plasma can be obtained through centrifugation of whole blood, single-donor plasmapheresis, or as a by-product of cytapheresis [e.g., platelet or red blood cell (RBC); *concurrent plasma*]. One unit of plasma is defined as the amount of plasma obtained from centrifugation of 1 unit of whole blood, and it usually contains 180 to 300 mL. When plasma is obtained through single-donor plasmapheresis, the amount may be 2 to 3 times greater than that obtained from whole blood processing (500 to 800 mL). Most plasma that will be used as FFP or FP24 (see later) is collected from whole blood (or equivalent) donors, and thus donor safety, screening and testing measures apply.

The rapidity with which plasma is collected and stored determines its quality and subsequent use.[7,8] Thus several plasma products are available at various centers. Single-donor plasmapheresis can produce *source plasma* (or single-donor plasma) when it is stored at or below −18°C at variable times from its collection. Plasma prepared from whole-blood or apheresis collections and stored frozen within 8 hours of its collection (at −18°C or colder) is called *fresh frozen plasma (FFP).* Plasma separated from whole-blood donations and frozen below −18°C within 24 hours of collection (FP24) shows good retention of relevant coagulation factor activity. However, compared with historic data on FFP frozen within 8 hours, fibrinogen, FV, FVIII, and FXI were shown to be reduced in FP24 by 12%, 15%, 23%, and 7%, respectively.[9] This may be significant in certain clinical circumstances, such as in the treatment of neonates with coagulopathies. In general, however, FFP and FP24 are used interchangeably in many facilities throughout the United States, especially at large tertiary care hospitals with busy level 1 trauma centers.[10] *Thawed plasma* is prepared in a closed system from FFP or FP24. Centrifugation or sedimentation of whole blood can also produce *recovered plasma,* which is obtained from a whole-blood donation: *liquid plasma,* when collected and stored refrigerated within 5 days of the expiration date of whole blood: *Cryo-poor plasma* (*cryosupernatant plasma; CSP*), which is the plasma product remaining after the cryoprecipitate fraction is extracted from FFP through cold precipitation.

Both source plasma and recovered plasma may be used in the manufacture of various plasma derivatives. Source plasma can also be administered as component therapy, whereas recovered plasma, because of the less-stringent conditions of collection, processing, and storage, does not meet the standards for coagulation factor concentrations and therefore is not used as component therapy. Liquid plasma is no longer used in the United States. *Donor retested plasma (FFP-DR)* is FFP, or FP24, which has been placed in "quarantine" and released for transfusion only after the donor has donated a subsequent blood donation, which has been tested ("retested") and found to be negative for markers of transfusion-transmissible infection. The quarantine period is at least 56 days. FFP-DR is considered a safer product, as subsequent testing of the blood donor is expected to detect and eliminate plasma donations that are in an infectious window period.[11]

Virally inactivated plasma is pooled plasma subjected to a solvent-detergent process and is termed *solvent-detergent plasma* (SD plasma). This method is highly efficient at inactivating viruses by using a combination of organic solvent, tri(*n*-butyl)phosphate (TNBP), and a nonionic detergent, Triton X-100. The SD method is virucidal against lipid-enveloped viruses, including human immunodeficiency virus (HIV) types 1 and 2, hepatitis viruses (HBV, HCV, HGV), human T-cell leukemia/lymphoma virus (HTLV) types I and II, vesicular stomatitis virus, Sindbis virus, and Sendai virus, but does not inactivate parvovirus or hepatitis A virus.

SD plasma is pooled from approximately 2500 donors, which results in a standard unit of 200 mL of SD plasma with a coagulation factor profile similar to that of FFP.[12–16] In part due to its cost, and in part due to the lack of availability of virally inactivated RBC and platelet units, SD plasma is not used in the United States.

SD plasma is, however, not simply a virally inactivated equivalent of FFP.[17] Levels of factor V, factor VIII, protein S, antiplasmin, and antitrypsin are lower in SD plasma, and this is of potential clinical significance.[17–20] The serpin-type serine proteinase inhibitors such as antiplasmin, antitrypsin, and antithrombin, have a flexible reactive-site loop that can convert from the active conformation to the inactive latent or polymerized conformations when exposed to heat or detergents or both. Comparisons of conformational stability and inhibitory activity have shown that, in SD plasma, virtually 100% of antiplasmin and approximately 50% of antitrypsin are in either the latent or polymerized conformation and lack inhibitory activity, whereas in FFP, only the active conformation is present.[17] Leukocyte depletion of FFP may also result in losses of coagulation factor activity and in increases in markers of coagulation activation, depending on the type of filter used. This is unlikely to be clinically significant unless subsequent processing of plasma (such as pathogen inactivation) results in further losses of coagulation factors.[21]

CLINICAL CONSIDERATIONS

In clinical practice, FFP has been used as an exogenous source of proteins, specifically albumin, immunoglobulins, coagulation factors, and certain protease inhibitors. With the development of the fractionation method of Cohn and colleagues[22] and the consequent capability to administer individual plasma components, the use of FFP has been reserved for situations in which it is necessary to replace either multiple plasma constituents (e.g., multiple factor deficiency) or a plasma constituent not yet isolated. The randomized controlled trial evidence base for the clinical use of FFP is, however, limited.[23] Indications and contraindications are listed in Table 19–1.

THE USE OF FFP IN THE MANAGEMENT OF COAGULOPATHIES

Patients with a known underlying coagulopathy, as ascertained by an increase in the prothrombin time (PT >16 seconds) or partial thromboplastin time (PTT >55 seconds) exceeding 1.5 to 1.8 times the control value, have an increased risk for clinically significant bleeding. In these patients, administration of FFP has decreased the risk of bleeding and reduced or stopped active bleeding. Although FFP contains all coagulation factors at normal plasma concentrations, it must be recognized that its administration in physiologically tolerable quantities results in only a 20% to 30% increase in the levels of coagulation factors.

Coagulopathy of Liver Dysfunction

The liver is essential in maintaining normal hemostasis. First, as the principal site of protein synthesis, it supplies the majority of proteins involved in the coagulation and fibrinolytic

Table 19–1 Fresh Frozen Plasma: Indications and Contraindications

Indications	Contraindications
Coagulopathies[23]	Volume expansion
Liver disease[24–45]	Immunoglobulin replacement
Acute hepatocellular injury	Nutritional support
Chronic hepatic dysfunction	Reconstitution of pRBCs
Hepatic surgery[29–44]	Wound healing
Congenital factor deficiency*[46–50]	
Warfarin-induced coagulopathy[50–58]	
Dilution-induced coagulopathy[59–70]	
Disseminated intravascular coagulopathy[52,71–76]	
Replacement of other factor(s)[23]	
Plasma infusion or exchange[76–104] (TTP, HUS, HELLP)	
C1-esterase inhibitor deficiency*[105–107]	
Fluid replacement in TPE[108] (Refsum disease, frequent TPE, coagulopathy)	

*When factor concentrates are not available.

HELLP, hemolysis, elevated liver enzymes, and low platelets; HUS, hemolytic-uremic syndrome; pRBCs, packed red blood cells; TPE, therapeutic plasma exchange; TTP, thrombotic thrombocytopenic purpura.

pathways and their regulators (except FVIII, von Willebrand factor [vWF], tissue plasminogen activator, and plasminogen activator inhibitor). Second, a process important in the normal function of certain coagulation proteins (e.g., prothrombin; FVII, FIX, and FX; proteins C and S), vitamin K–dependent γ-carboxylation of glutamic acid residues, takes place in the liver. Third, the hepatic reticulum endothelial system is also involved in the clearance of activated coagulation factors, activation complexes, and fibrin and fibrinogen degradation by-products. Therefore the coagulopathy associated with hepatocellular injury has a complex pathogenesis including ineffective protein synthesis, consumption of coagulation factors and inhibitors, and impaired clearance of activated coagulation complexes.[24–26] In addition, end-stage liver disease is associated with a variable degree of thrombocytopenia secondary to hypersplenism[27] and a multifactorial thrombocytopathy.[28]

Impairment of hemostasis may also be encountered in hepatic surgery, including partial hepatic resection,[29] orthotopic liver transplantation (OLT), and peritoneovenous or LeVeen shunt placement. The coagulation disorder most frequently observed in these situations is acute and chronic disseminated intravascular coagulopathy (DIC) with a predominant fibrinolytic component.[30,31] The coagulopathy associated with OLT is usually more severe because of the underlying coagulopathy predating the transplantation, the profound hyperfibrinolysis characterizing the posttransplantation anhepatic phase, and, in some instances, the coagulopathy induced by massive transfusion during surgery.[32–35] The number of units of blood products transfused during OLT operations has decreased significantly for reasons that include the use of aprotinin to block fibrinolysis and the selective use of the thromboelastogram to monitor coagulation intraoperatively.[36] In liver transplantation patients, whole blood, when compared with component therapy (RBCs and FFP), has been reported to provide equally effective replacement therapy for blood loss and is associated with fewer donor exposures.[37] Plasmapheresis using FFP, or FFP and albumin (50%), as replacement fluid may provide an effective treatment option for primary hepatic allograft nonfunction immediately after liver transplantation and may obviate the need for retransplantation.[38]

It is well recognized that patients manifesting coagulopathy associated with liver disease or hepatic surgery are at increased risk for bleeding, especially during invasive procedures (e.g., liver biopsy, paracentesis). Therefore, FFP, either alone or in conjunction with other products (e.g., platelets, prothrombin complex, or antithrombin III concentrate), has been used to control active bleeding and to decrease the risk of bleeding complications during invasive procedures.[39–43] The efficacy of FFP in these situations is assessed clinically because laboratory evidence such as normalization of PT or PTT or improvement of the thromboelastogram may be lacking with the administration of usual quantities of FFP.[39,43,44] Recombinant activated factor VII (rFVIIa) is an antihemophilic factor that has shown promise in treating coagulopathy in liver disease and, in conjunction with FFP, is effective in transiently correcting laboratory parameters of coagulopathy in patients with fulminant hepatic failure.[45] In these patients, it facilitates the performance of invasive procedures and is associated with less frequent anasarca compared with conventional therapy.

Congenital Coagulation Factor Deficiency

The introduction of specific coagulation factor concentrates has limited the use of FFP. Currently, FFP is indicated for patients with rare familial isolated factor deficiencies (e.g., FV and FXI deficiency) for which no factor concentrate is commercially available.[46–49] In combined FV-FVIII deficiency, FFP is the only source of FV, and either FFP infusions or therapeutic plasma exchange (TPE) with FFP has been used to treat bleeding episodes. Congenital combined vitamin K–dependent factor deficiency can be treated with prothrombin complex concentrates, FFP, or occasionally high doses of vitamin K.[50] Dosages and schedules of FFP administration for congenital factor deficiencies and possible alternatives are listed in Table 19–2.

Warfarin-induced Coagulopathy

Vitamin K is a cofactor in the γ-carboxylation of the terminal glutamic acid residues of certain coagulation (e.g., factors II, VII, IX, and X) and regulatory (e.g., protein C and S)

Table 19–2 Uses of FFP in Congenital Factor Deficiencies

Deficient Factor	Half-life (hr)	FFP Dose	Hemostatic Plasma Level	Alternative Therapy
Prothrombin (FII)	72	15–20 mL/kg, followed by 3–6 mL/kg q 12–24 hr	>30%	PE with FFP Prothrombin complex concentrates*
Factor V (FV)	36	15–20 mL/kg, followed by 3–6 mL/kg q 12–24 hr	>25%	FFP infusions or TPE with FFP
Factor VII (FVII)	3–6			Prothrombin complex concentrates*
Major bleed		15–20 mL/kg followed by 5–10 mL/kg q 6–12 hr	15%–25%	FVII concentrates†
Mild bleed		5–10 mL/kg q 8–12 hr	5%–10%	
Factor X (FX)	40	15–20 mL/kg, followed by 3–6 mL/kg q 24 hr	10%–15%	Prothrombin complex*
Factor XI (FXI)	80	15–20 mL/kg, followed by 3–6 mL/kg q 12 hr	30%–40%	Cryosupernatant
Factor XIII (FXIII)	9 days	3–6 mL/kg q 4–6 wk	5%	Cryoprecipitate (1 U/10–20 kg q 3–4 wk) FXII concentration†

*Prothrombin complex concentrates contain variable amounts of FII, FVII, FIX, and FX.
†Concentrates available only in Europe.
FFP, fresh frozen plasma; FII, factor II; TPE, therapeutic plasma exchange.

proteins. This posttranslational modification of the coagulation proteins is essential for their binding to phospholipid surfaces through calcium and the subsequent formation of activation complexes.[51] By interfering with the recovery of the active form of vitamin K, warfarin or 4-hydroxycoumarin blocks the γ-carboxylation of these coagulation proteins, rendering them inactive.

Over-anticoagulation from excessive effects of warfarin can be reversed by a range of measures.[52] From the most mild to the most severe circumstances, these are withdrawing warfarin, giving vitamin K orally or parenterally, transfusing FFP, or administering prothrombin complex concentrate (FII, FVII, FIX, and FX or separate infusions of FII, FIX, and FX concentrate plus FVII concentrate or FFP).[53] The dose of vitamin K used to reverse over-anticoagulation depends on the international normalized ratio (INR).[54] Prothrombin complex concentrate (PCC), or FFP, should be used in such situations involving trauma, emergency surgical procedures, or active bleeding.[55,56] FFP is recommended only if major bleeding occurs and PCC is not available.[56,57] Makris et al.[57] showed that FFP contains insufficient concentrations of vitamin K factors to reverse warfarin effects completely. Treatment with FFP (15 mL/kg) and intravenous vitamin K (5 mg) will partially reverse anticoagulation, although the levels of individual factors will typically remain less than 20%, and larger doses should be given if possible. FFP should never be used for the reversal of warfarin when no evidence of severe bleeding exists.[56] Vitamin K and FFP often fails to achieve the desired correction of coagulopathy in urgent neurosurgical settings such as spontaneous or traumatic intracranial hemorrhage. A single dose of rFVIIa (120 mg/kg) was shown to provide rapid reversal of anticoagulation and should be considered when urgent neurosurgical intervention is required.[58]

Dilutional Coagulopathy

The replacement of one blood volume in 24 hours with packed red blood cells (pRBCs) and crystalloid or colloid solutions is defined as massive transfusion.[59] Leslie and Toy[60] found that massively transfused patients manifest a profound hemostatic disorder, as demonstrated by prolonged PT and PTT to twice control values and thrombocytopenia less than $50 \times 10^6/\mu L$, which are only in part due to hemodilution.[61,62] Although the number of units transfused, the degree of PT or PTT prolongation, and bleeding tendency are poorly correlated,[63,64] Ciavarella and colleagues[61] reported that increases in PT or PTT greater than 1.5 to 1.8 times control values are associated with decreases in some coagulation factors (e.g., fibrinogen, FV, FVIII) to below minimal hemostatic levels. Therefore the preceding laboratory changes, when associated with clinically significant coagulopathy, should be treated with FFP. Resuscitation from hemorrhagic shock can be successfully managed by restoration of blood loss with crystalloid and blood, and with FFP added to maintain coagulation proteins. In a canine hemorrhagic shock model, FFP has been demonstrated to prevent the reduction of coagulation factor levels, and unexpected postoperative bleeding has been observed in humans after the abandonment of routine supplementation of FFP for hemorrhagic shock.[65] Leukocyte adhesion to endothelial cells may contribute to microcirculatory disturbances during severe shock syndromes. When incubated with FFP, neutrophil adhesion to endothelial cells is decreased in vitro,[66] and the administration of FFP may attenuate the inflammatory response of endothelial cells in clinical situations in which dilution of plasma is found. In general, FFP should be considered when more than 50% of the blood volume has been replaced, and it is mandatory when more than 120% to 150% of the blood volume has been replaced with pRBCs or colloid solutions, or both, within a 24-hour period. In addition, platelets should be maintained above $50 \times 10^6/\mu L$ with transfusion of platelet concentrates, and other blood products (e.g., cryoprecipitate, specific factor concentrates) may be considered for replacement of coagulation factors when the volume of FFP becomes excessive.[67–69] The use of FFP in the pump prime in infants undergoing cardiopulmonary bypass surgery has been shown significantly to limit dilutional hypofibrinogenemia, decrease the transfusion of cryoprecipitate after bypass, and decrease overall exposure to blood products.[70]

Disseminated Intravascular Coagulopathy

Acute DIC is clinically characterized by a combination of diffuse microvascular hemorrhage and thrombosis. Abnormal activation of the coagulation cascade and thrombin generation leads to the consumption of procoagulant factors and platelets. All coagulation factors become depleted, but particularly fibrinogen, FV, FVIII, and FXIII.[52] Hyperfibrinolysis secondary to widespread fibrin deposition further exaggerates the coagulation factor consumption. A wide variety of disorders may lead to DIC, including sepsis, liver disease, trauma, obstetric complications, leukemia, metastatic malignancy, hypotension, and hypoperfusion.[71]

Because of the heterogeneous group of disorders that can trigger DIC, the gamut of clinical manifestations, and the lack of controlled clinical studies, the management of DIC is somewhat controversial. Therapy should be individualized and directed concomitant with the underlying disorder and the predominant clinical manifestation (e.g., hemorrhagic versus thrombotic diathesis). Component therapy, with platelet concentrates, FFP, or cryoprecipitate, should be considered in patients with prolonged PT and PTT and active bleeding or undergoing an invasive procedure. FFP should be administered at a dose of 10 to 15 mL/kg and its effect assessed clinically and with frequent PT-PTT measurements (every 6 hours). In patients with end-stage liver disease and DIC, FFP infusions may not correct PT-PTT abnormalities, and clinical responses may vary. Antifibrinolytic agents (e.g., ε-aminocaproic acid or tranexamic acid) in combination with heparin may be useful in patients with active bleeding who do not respond to coagulation factor replacement with FFP or cryoprecipitate and heparin infusions.[71,72] In clinical situations in which the thrombotic diathesis predominates (e.g., purpura fulminans), a trial of intravenous heparin with antithrombin III (AT-III) replacement may be appropriate.[73] Initial studies have demonstrated some benefit for the use of activated protein C concentrates in patients with purpura fulminans[74] and in those with DIC associated with meningococcemia,[75] although further studies are needed to confirm these results.

THE USE OF FFP AS REPLACEMENT OF OTHER FACTORS

Thrombotic Thrombocytopenic Purpura

Thrombotic thrombocytopenic purpura (TTP) is a clinical entity characterized by microangiopathic hemolytic anemia, thrombocytopenia, fever, and varying degrees of renal and neurologic dysfunction. Plasma exchange can induce remissions in approximately 80% of patients with idiopathic TTP; however, when thrombotic microangiopathy is associated with cancer, certain drugs, infections, or tissue transplantation, it carries a much worse prognosis.[76] The pathogenesis of idiopathic TTP has been shown, in many cases, to be due to an acquired autoimmune deficiency of a plasma metalloprotease, ADAMTS13 (a disintegrin and metalloproteinase with thrombospondin type 1 motif).[77–79] ADAMTS13 is a von Willebrand factor-cleaving protease (vWF-cp) responsible for the continuous degradation of ultralarge von Willebrand factor (ULVWF) multimers released from endothelial cells. Normally, ADAMTS13 cleaves ULFWF multimers within growing platelet aggregates, under flowing conditions, and this limits platelet thrombus formation. Plasma levels of vWF regulate ADAMTS13,[80] and the rate of VWF proteolysis is greater for blood group O VWF than for non-O VWF.[80,81] If ADAMTS13 is absent, either congenitally or because of acquired autoantibodies, platelet-rich microvascular thrombosis proceeds unchecked, and TTP ensues.[76,82,83] Severe deficiency of ADAMTS13 activity has been shown to define a distinct population of thrombotic microangiopathy patients.[84]

Plasma exchange is effective therapy for idiopathic TTP, probably because it replenishes the deficient ADAMTS13 and removes some of the pathogenic autoantibodies and endothelium-stimulating cytokines. Advances in assay methods should facilitate routine laboratory testing of ADAMTS13 for patients with thrombotic microangiopathy.[76,85,86] Severe ADAMTS13 deficiency is specific for idiopathic TTP and identifies a subgroup of patients with a high likelihood of response to plasma exchange. High-titer ADAMTS13 inhibitors correlate strongly with a high risk of relapsing disease. Patients with normal ADAMTS13 activity have a much worse prognosis, although many factors probably contribute to this difference.[76]

Infusion of FFP replaces the deficient or defective[87] metalloprotease, and therapeutic plasma exchange (TPE) with FFP or cryosupernatant removes much of the IgG metalloprotease inhibitor and simultaneously provides functional metalloprotease. The intrinsic VWF-cleaving protease activity of plasma-derived products correlates with their clinical efficacy.[85,88] VWF-cp activity is normal in FFP, CSP, and in virally inactivated components treated with methylene blue/light or by the solvent detergent process.[89] Current standard therapy for TTP is TPE with FFP as replacement fluid.[90–92] All patients do not respond initially to TPE with FFP, and in these recurrent or refractory TTP cases, the use of cryosupernatant plasma (CSP) lacking ULVWF multimers has been effective.[91–97] In the initial treatment of TTP in adults, the efficacy of FFP, compared with cryoprecipitate poor plasma, appears to be the same.[98] Other prospective studies have not shown an apparent advantage to the use of CSP in TTP.[99] Methylene blue–photoinactivated plasma seems to be less effective than FFP,[100,101] and reduced protein S activity in SD plasma may predispose to venous thromboembolism, especially if infused in large volumes.[89] A few patients with TTP have responded to simple infusions of FFP,[92,94,95] particularly patients who are HIV positive with a dominant microangiopathy.[102]

The standard therapy for TTP is daily exchanges with FFP or cryosupernatant replacing 1.0 to 1.5 plasma volumes. Plasma exchanges should be commenced at presentation and ideally within 24 hours of presentation.[103] The premature omission of a single plasma exchange may be associated with exacerbation. The total number of TPEs is dependent on the clinical response, and the daily schedule is continued until the serum lactic acid dehydrogenase is normal and the platelet count is greater than $100 \times 10^6/\mu L$ and continues to rise without the aid of TPE. A twice-daily (every 12 hours) schedule of TPE may be used in cases in which the patient's status is deteriorating despite an adequate daily regimen. The average number of TPEs necessary to achieve remission is approximately 16 procedures,[104] and more than 90% of patients have achieved clinical remission within 3 weeks of initiation of TPE.

C1-Esterase Inhibitor Deficiency

Deficiency of C1-esterase inhibitor, an important regulator of the complement system, is inherited in an autosomal dominant manner. Clinical manifestations of hereditary angioedema include swelling of the subcutaneous tissue and mucosa of the aerodigestive tract, leading to acute respiratory distress.[105] Replacement therapy with FFP infusions has been used during acute episodes of respiratory distress and before surgical interventions. C1-esterase inhibitor concentrates are available in Europe and will eventually replace the use of FFP in this rare condition.[106,107]

Fluid Replacement in TPE

In general, the volume of replacement fluids used in TPE is equal to the plasma volume removed, and for most situations, colloid or crystalloid solutions, or both, are acceptable fluid replacement. In addition to clinical conditions in which plasma is specifically indicated (e.g., TTP, Refsum disease), a few situations exist in which the use of FFP with TPE is preferred. Plasma exchange with FFP is indicated in all patients with significant underlying coagulopathy, including DIC, liver disease, and circulating anticoagulant, as well as in patients with iatrogenic coagulopathy, as observed in patients undergoing multiple TPEs within a short time.[108]

Investigational Uses of FFP

Coagulation factor replacement through the use of FFP, either as simple infusions or with plasma exchange, has been explored in fulminant meningococcemia,[109,110] in acute renal failure in the context of multiorgan failure,[111] and in the syndrome of hemolysis, elevated liver enzymes, and low platelets (HELLP).[112] FFP has been used successfully in the treatment of resistant, life-threatening angioedema due to an angiotensin-converting enzyme (ACE) inhibitor.[113]

PRACTICAL CONSIDERATIONS IN THE USE OF FFP

Although FFP is readily available for use in clinical practice, it must be recognized that its administration is not without risk. Although FFP contains albumin, coagulation proteins, immunoglobulins, and nutrients, no justification exists for its use in situations in which alternative therapy is safer and more efficacious. Therefore crystalloid or fractionated albumin solution is preferred to FFP for volume expansion in hypovolemic shock. A systematic review of randomized controlled trials of albumin administration in critically ill patients[114] concluded, however, that there was no evidence to indicate that albumin administration reduces mortality in critically ill patients with hypovolemia, burns, or hypoalbuminemia. In conditions involving a specific coagulation factor deficiency, including hemophilia A, replacement therapy with specific coagulation factor concentrates or recombinant proteins (e.g., FVIII) is recommended. Prophylactic replacement therapy with immunoglobulin fraction and the use of approved parenteral solutions to enhance the nutritional status of debilitated patients are also currently recommended alternatives to FFP. The efficacy of FFP in other clinical situations should be determined through clinical trials.[23]

The volume and schedule of FFP administration depend on the clinical situation for which it is intended and the patient's volume tolerance. The most common indication for the use of FFP is as a coagulation factor replacement, and the desired hemostatic level as determined by the specific coagulation factor level, PT or PTT, or clinical assessment should guide the dose, frequency, and duration of administration. It should also be noted that FFP requires 20 to 30 minutes to thaw, and subsequently the labile coagulation factors (FV, FVIII) decrease gradually (adequate for 24 hours after thawing). FFP should be thawed in a controlled environment between 34° C and 40° C. Thawing at higher temperatures may result in markedly decreased coagulation factor activity.[115] Therapy should be coordinated with the blood bank, especially when multiple FFP infusions are anticipated (e.g, supportive therapy in massive transfusion, during OLT). FFP contains isohemagglutinins, and therefore an ABO-compatible product should be administered. AB plasma may be used in cases in which the recipient's blood group is not known at the time of administration. Compatibility testing is not routinely performed.

For the use of FFP in mild to moderate coagulopathies (e.g., liver disease, DIC), it is recommended that a usual dose of 10 to 15 mL/kg be infused as rapidly as tolerated by the patient. The calculated dose in milliliters is used to determine approximately the whole number of units of FFP, knowing that a unit of FFP is 180 to 300 mL and a unit of SD plasma is 200 mL. The frequency and duration of FFP therapy depend primarily on the clinical response. Observed increments in coagulation factor levels have been shown to correlate with the dose of FFP, and in critically ill patients, higher doses (30 mL/kg) should be considered.[116]

In massive transfusion or during OLT, communication with the blood bank is essential to reserve sufficient quantities of FFP and ensure timely administration. In general, when more than 10 units of pRBCs has been transfused and abnormal hemostasis is observed, infusion of 4 units of FFP is recommended. To maintain coagulation factors above a critical hemostatic level, 4 units of FFP should be infused for every 6 units of pRBCs transfused thereafter. If the desired hemostasis is not achieved with this regimen, additional products may be considered, including cryoprecipitate, rFVIIa, AT-III concentrate, or prothrombin concentrate.

ALTERNATIVES

Many factor concentrates, including FVIII, prothrombin complex concentrate, activated FIX complex, recombinant factor VIIa, and AT-III, have been made available for clinical use, and a few others are at the investigational stage (e.g., C1-esterase inhibitor). Thus the use of FFP is limited to situations in which no specific therapeutic alternative exists.

POTENTIAL ADVERSE REACTIONS

Although FFP is considered an infrequent cause of major adverse reactions, the complexity of plasma proteins, the heterogeneity of its immunoglobulin content, and factors related to its processing and storage have the potential to cause a wide range of reactions with various pathophysiologic mechanisms (Table 19–3). Allergic reactions of variable degree, ranging from mild urticarial reactions to anaphylaxis and cardiopulmonary arrest, may be observed with FFP infusions. These reactions may be related to the immunologic differences between donor and recipient or to the processing and storage of plasma.

Patients with IgA deficiency who have anti-IgA antibodies (usually IgE) are at high risk for acute and potentially fatal allergic reactions when exposed to FFP containing IgA. Patients known to be IgA deficient should receive IgA-deficient plasma, available through the national registry.[117] High titers of an alloantibody in the donor plasma may induce a variety of clinical syndromes, depending on the specificity of the antibodies. When plasma contains reaginic antibodies to foreign antigens, an allergic-type reaction may ensue. Conversion to a positive direct antiglobulin test or even hemolysis can occur when plasma contains antibodies directed against RBCs (e.g., ABO isoantibodies). If FFP of the same ABO group is not available, FFP of a different ABO group may be transfused, provided that it does not possess high-titer anti-A or anti-B activity. Group O FFP should not be used in infants or neonates who are not group O because the relatively large volumes can lead to passive immune hemolysis.[52]

Less often, febrile allergic reactions may be due to undesirable contaminants in the donor plasma. The risk of exposure

Table 19–3 Potential Adverse Reactions to FFP

Potential Adverse Reactions to FFP
Immunologically mediated:
Alloimmunization: Rh1(D), other RBC antigens
Allergic reactions: IgA deficiency
Transfusion-related acute lung injury (TRALI): leukoagglutinins
Reaginic antibodies to exogenous antigens
Alloantibodies to platelets
Immunomodulation/immunosuppression
Transfusion-associated graft-versus-host disease (TA-GVHD)
Related to plasma contaminants:
Donor specific: medications, infectious
Processing/storage specific: cytokines, anaphylatoxins, plasticizers, preservatives
Related to infectious contaminants:
Bacterial contaminants
Viral contaminants
Leukocyte-associated: CMV, HTLV I/II
Non–leukocyte-associated: HIV, HBV, HCV, HAV, EBV, HHV-8, prions
Related to physiochemical characteristics:
Volume overload
Hypothermia

CMV, cytomegalovirus; EBV, Epstein-Barr virus; HAV, hepatitis A virus; HBV, hepatitis B virus; HHV, human herpesvirus; HIV, human immunodeficiency virus; HTLV, human T-cell lymphotropic virus; RBC, red blood cell.

to donor-specific contaminants such as infectious agents and medications has been reduced considerably by careful donor screening. Febrile nonhemolytic reactions may also be related to the quality of plasma after processing, including activation of proteolytic enzymes (e.g., kinins), generation of cytokines (e.g., interleukins-1, -6, and -8, and tumor necrosis factor) and anaphylatoxins (e.g., C3a, C5a), and the presence of preservatives and plasticizers.[118–121]

Transfusion-related Acute Lung Injury

Transfusion-related acute lung injury (TRALI) is an uncommon complication of allogeneic blood transfusion characterized by acute respiratory distress, severe hypoxemia, hypotension, and fever. Radiographic investigations typically reveal bilateral pulmonary infiltrates. Clinical signs and symptoms usually manifest within 6 hours of transfusion.[122–124] Both immunologic and nonimmunologic mechanisms have been postulated in the pathogenesis of TRALI. It has been hypothesized that significant numbers of TRALI cases are the result of two insults. The first, related to the clinical condition of the patient (e.g., in a setting of surgery, trauma, or severe infection) causes neutrophils to be "primed" but not activated, and the second, to the infusion of biologic-response modifiers such as biologically active lipids, cytokines, or leukoagglutinating alloantibodies within the blood component transfused.[123–127] It is unlikely, however, that biologically active lipids are responsible for all cases of TRALI because they have not been shown to be present in FFP, even though the transfusion of FFP has been linked to many cases of TRALI.[123,128–130] Whereas pathogenic alloantibodies are typically of donor origin, in fewer than 10% of cases, the alloantibodies may be of recipient origin, directed against donor-specific leukocyte alloantigens.[131,132] The alloantibodies usually thought responsible for TRALI have been identified as antigranulocyte, antihuman leukocyte antigen (anti-HLA), or anti HLA-DR antibodies,[122,128–132] although some have also been reported to be caused by antilymphocyte, antimonocyte,[133–136] or anti-immunoglobulin alloantibodies.[131,137,138] Alloantibodies to HLA class I and class II antigens have been detected in approximately 22% of blood components tested.[139] These antibodies may also pose a risk to transplant patients requiring transfusions by promoting allograft dysfunction or loss. Because of the higher frequency of alloantibodies in multiparous women,[140] the Blood Service in the United Kingdom has elected only to use plasma from male blood donors for the preparation of FFP. Pooled, SD plasma has been shown have undetectable levels of HLA antibodies.[141,142]

Leukocyte-associated Adverse Reactions

FFP has long been considered an acellular blood product with an infinitesimally small risk of leukocyte-associated complications, including transmission of cell-associated infections, alloimmunization, immunosuppression, or transfusion-associated graft-versus-host disease (TA-GVHD) in immunocompromised individuals. Several reports have documented the presence of leukocytes in FFP,[143–146] which has led to questions regarding their clinical relevance as well as the need for further processing (e.g., leukoreduction, irradiation) of FFP to reduce the risks of leukocyte-associated complications. Leukocytes have also been implicated in cytokine generation, which is responsible for febrile nonhemolytic transfusion reactions and lung injury.

Willis and colleagues[145] demonstrated that the number of leukocytes in FFP spanned a 3-logarithm range, depending on the method of preparation, with 43% of units obtained by the hard-spin method and 45.7% of units produced by the second-spin method containing more than 5×10^6 leukocytes. These values are higher than the American Association of Blood Banks cutoff standard ($<5 \times 10^6$ per red blood cell unit)[147] and far above the European cutoff standard ($< 1 \times 10^6$ per red blood cell unit)[148] for residual donor leukocytes in the final leukoreduced product. It had been assumed that the freezing process renders FFP practically devoid of viable leukocytes.[149] Wieding[143] and Bernvil[144] and their associates demonstrated that viable lymphocytes may be present, raising concern about possible adverse immunomodulation (e.g, TA-GVHD) in certain individuals at risk and pointing out the potential benefit of using irradiated FFP. Other investigators, using propidium iodide (PI) and fluorescein-conjugated antibodies to determine viability, have shown that the majority of leucocytes in FFP are PI-positive (dead) cells.[146] Nevertheless, a small but consistent population of PI-negative (live) cells was detected, including viable $CD3^+$ T cells. Both dead and live cells expressed HLA class I antigens. Approximately 38% of these cells expressed HLA class II antigens. These investigators concluded that transfusion of FFP is potentially alloimmunogenic owing to its residual leukocyte content and that leukocyte-reduction filters appear to be effective in suppressing the alloimmunogenicity of FFP. Although the viability of leukocytes may be important in the pathophysiologic mechanism of some adverse reactions, their destruction may release cytokines that are implicated in the pathophysiologic mechanism of febrile nonhemolytic reactions. A relation between exposure to allogenic plasma and the risk of postoperative pneumonia or wound infection or both was not detected in a retrospective study of patients undergoing coronary artery bypass surgery.[150]

FFP produced by certain methods may therefore contain enough leukocytes to be categorized as a cellular blood product and to justify the use of a leukoreduction filter. The use of prestorage leukodepletion filters decreases the overall leukocyte burden (viable and nonviable) in the blood component and decreases the concentration of cytokines and anaphylatoxins. Leukodepleted FFP may be indicated for certain individuals at risk for these complications, including immunosuppressed individuals and patients requiring massive transfusions.[121]

Infectious Potential

Although leukocytes have been shown to be present in FFP, transmission of cell-associated viruses including cytomegalovirus (CMV) and human lymphocytotropic viruses (HTLV-I and -II) has been associated with cellular blood components and not FFP, although some authorities remained concerned that transmission is possible. In addition to the use of donor questionnaires and serologic surrogate markers, the introduction of SD plasma, which efficiently inactivates lipid-encapsulated viruses including HBV, HCV, HGV, HTLV, and HIV, has eliminated a great majority of transfusion-transmitted pathogens.[151] Nonetheless, nonenveloped viruses, including parvovirus B19 and hepatitis A virus, still pose concerns regarding the safety of SD plasma, especially in immunodeficient individuals, pregnant women, and patients with chronic hemolytic anemias. Although SD plasma is a pooled product and may contain parvovirus B19 and hepatitis A virus, it also contains neutralizing antibody to these viruses, which may modify the risk of infectivity or its clinical significance. Furthermore, SD plasma is screened for these viruses by polymerase chain reaction, and lots with high viral loads are eliminated.[152,153] Other methods to reduce or inactivate pathogens in FFP have been developed. These include the treatment of plasma with methylene blue and white light[152] and the treatment of blood products such as platelet concentrates and FFP with psoralen and ultraviolet light.[154] As described earlier, FFP may be quarantined until after the donor has given a subsequent blood donation, is retested, and found to be negative for markers of transfusion-transmissible infection. This may obviate window-period infections.[11]

Another potential for transmission of infectious agents stems from the possibility of newly emerging pathogens in the donor pool, the presence of prions, or contamination during processing with agents not susceptible to inactivation by the SD process.[12–16] In the United Kingdom, it is recommended that the FFP given to neonates and children should be obtained from an area free of bovine spongiform encephalopathy (BSE) and be subjected to pathogen-reduction procedures.[52] In patients for whom pathogen-reduced plasma is being considered, the risks of HAV and parvovirus B19 transmission and their clinical sequelae should be weighed against the likely benefits. Patients likely to receive multiple units of FFP, such as those with a congenital coagulopathy, should be vaccinated against hepatitis A and B.[52]

REFERENCES

1. Lettellier G, Desjarlais F. Study of seasonal variations for eighteen biochemical parameters over a four-year period. Clin Biochem 1982;15:206–211.
2. Siest G. Human chemistry. In Siest G (ed): Reference Values in Human Chemistry: Effects, Analytical and Individual Variation, Food Intake, Drugs and Toxics: Applications in Preventive Medicine. Basel, Karger, 1973, p 134.
3. Gregersen MI, Rawson RA. Blood volume. Physiol Rev 1959;39:307–342.
4. Doweiko JP, Nompleggi DJ. Role of albumin in human physiology and pathophysiology. JPEN 1991;15:207–211.
5. Sorensen RU, Polmar SH. Immunoglobulin replacement therapy. Ann Clin Res 1987;19:293–304.
6. Alper CA. Inherited deficiencies of complement components in man. Immunol Lett 1987;14:175–181.
7. Myllyla G. Factors determining quality of plasma. Vox Sang 1998; 74:507–511.
8. Hellstern P, Haubelt H. Manufacture and composition of fresh frozen plasma and virus-inactivated therapeutic plasma preparations: correlation between composition and therapeutic efficacy. Thromb Res 2002;107(suppl 1):S3–58.
9. Cardigan R, Lawrie AS, Mackie IJ, et al. The quality of fresh-frozen plasma produced from whole blood stored at 4°C overnight. Transfusion 2005;45:1342–1348.
10. AABB Docket No. 2004N-0539. Establishing a docket for the development of plasma standards public workshop. www.fda.gov/ohrms/dockets.
11. McCarthy LJ, Danielson CF, Rothenberger SS, et al. Completely converting a blood service region to the use of safer plasma. Transfusion 2000;40:1264–1267.
12. Horowitz B, Bonomo R, Prince AM, et al. Solvent/detergent-treated plasma: a virus-inactivated substitute for fresh frozen plasma. Blood 1992;79:826–831.
13. Prince AM, Horowitz B, Brotman B, et al. Inactivation of hepatitis B and Hutchinson strain non-A, non-B hepatitis viruses by exposing to Tween 80 and ether. Vox Sang 1984;46:36–43.
14. Prince AM, Horowitz B, Brotman B, et al. Sterilization of hepatitis and HTLV-III viruses by exposure to tri(*n*-butyl)phosphate and sodium cholate. Lancet 1986;1:706–710.
15. Horowitz B, Wiebe ME, Lippin A, et al. Inactivation of viruses in labile blood derivatives: disruption of lipid-enveloped viruses by tri(*n*-butyl)phosphate detergent combinations. Transfusion 1985;25:516–522.
16. Pehta JC. Clinical studies with solvent detergent-treated products. Transfus Med Rev 1996;10:303–311.
17. Mast AE, Stadanlick JE, Lockett JM, et al. Solvent/detergent-treated plasma has decreased antitrypsin activity and absent antiplasmin activity. Blood 1999;94:3922–3927.
18. Doyle S, O'Brien P, Murphy K, et al. Coagulation factor content of solvent/detergent plasma compared with fresh frozen plasma. Blood Coagul Fibrinol 2003;14:283–287.
19. Nifong TP, Light J, Wenk RE. Coagulant stability and sterility of thawed S/D-treated plasma. Transfusion 2002;42:1581–1584.
20. Flamholz R, Jeon HR, Baron JM, et al. Study of three patients with thrombotic thrombocytopenic purpura exchanged with solvent/detergent-treated plasma: is its decreased protein S activity clinically related to their development of deep venous thromboses? J Clin Apheresis 2000;15:169–172.
21. Cardigan R, Sutherland J, Garwood M, et al. The effect of leucocyte depletion on the quality of fresh-frozen plasma. Br J Haematol 2001;114:233–240.
22. Cohn EJ, Gurd FRN, Surgenor DM, et al. A system for the separation of the components of human blood: qualitative procedures for the separation of protein components of human plasma. J Am Chem Soc 1950;72:465.
23. Stanworth SJ, Brunskill SJ, Hyde CJ, et al. Is fresh frozen plasma clinically effective? A systematic review of randomized controlled trials. Br J Haematol 2004;126:139–152.
24. Deutsch E. Blood coagulation disorder in liver diseases. Prog Liver Dis 1965;2:69.
25. Lechner K, Nissner H, Thaler E. Coagulation abnormalities in liver disease. Semin Thromb Hemost 1977;4:40–56.
26. Roberts HR, Cederbaum AI. The liver and blood coagulation: physiology and pathology. Gastroenterology 1972;63:279–320.
27. Aster RH. Pooling of platelets in the spleen: role in the pathogenesis of "hypersplenic" thrombocytopenia. J Clin Invest 1966;45:645–657.
28. Laffi G, Cominelli F, Ruggiero M, et al. Altered platelet function in cirrhosis of the liver: impairment of inositol lipid and arachidonic acid metabolism in response to agonists. Hepatology 1988;8:1620–1626.
29. Martin RC 2nd, Jarnagin WR, Fong Y, et al. The use of fresh frozen plasma after major hepatic resection for colorectal metastasis: is there a standard for transfusion? J Am Coll Surg 2003;196:402–409.
30. Harmon DC, Demirjan Z, Ellman L, et al. Disseminated intravascular coagulation in the peritoneovenous shunt. Ann Intern Med 1979; 90:774–776.
31. Ro JS. Hemostatic problems in liver surgery. Scand J Gastroenterol 1973; 8:71–81.
32. Bohmig HJ. The coagulation disorder of orthotopic hepatic transplantation. Semin Thromb Hemost 1977;4:57–82.
33. Lewis JH, Bontempo FA, Awad SA, et al. Liver transplantation: intraoperative changes in coagulation factors in 100 first transplants. Hepatology 1989;9:710–714.
34. Porte RJ, Bontempo FA, Knot EA, et al. Systemic effects of tissue plasminogen activator-associated fibrinolysis and its relation to thrombin generation in orthotopic liver transplantation. Transplantation 1989;47:978–984.
35. Ritter DM, Owen CA Jr, Bowie EJ, et al. Evaluation of preoperative hematology-coagulation screening in liver transplantation. Mayo Clin Proc 1989;64:216–223.
36. Gordon PC, James MF, Spearman CW, et al. Decreasing blood product requirements after orthoptic liver transplantation. S Afr J Surg 2002;40:46–48.
37. Laine E, Steadman R, Calhoun L, et al. Comparison of RBCs and FFP with whole blood during liver transplant surgery. Transfusion 2003;43:322–327.
38. Mandal AK, King KE, Humphreys SL, et al. Plasmapheresis: an effective therapy for primary allograft nonfunction after liver transplantation. Transplantation 2000;15:216–220.
39. McVay PA, Toy PTCY. Lack of increased bleeding after paracentesis and thoracocentesis in patients with mild coagulation abnormalities. Transfusion 1991;21:164–171.
40. Shanberge JN, Quattrochiocchi-Longe T. Analysis of fresh frozen plasma administration with suggestions for ways to reduce usage. Transfus Med 1992;2:189–194.
41. Stahl RL, Duncan A, Hooks MA, et al. A hypercoagulable state follows orthoptic liver transplantation. Hepatology 1990;12:553–558.
42. McNicol PL, Liu G, Harley ID, et al. Blood loss and transfusion requirements in liver transplantation: experience with the first 75 cases using thromboelastography. Anaesth Intensive Care 1994;22:666–671.

43. Spector I, Corn M, Ticktin HE. Effect of plasma transfusion on the prothrombin time and clotting factors in liver disease. N Engl J Med 1966;275:1032–1037.
44. Clayton DG, Miro AM, Kramer DJ, et al. Quantification of thromboelastographic changes after blood component transfusion in patients with liver disease in the intensive care unit. Anesth Analg 1995; 81:272–278.
45. Shami VM, Caldwell SH, Hespenheide EE, et al. Recombinant activated factor VII for coagulopathy in fulminant hepatic failure compared with conventional therapy. Liver Transplant 2003;9:138–143.
46. Seeler RA. Para hemophilia: Factor V deficiency. Med Clin North Am 1972;56:119.
47. Sharland M, Palton MA, Talbot S, et al. Coagulation factor deficiencies and abnormal bleeding in Noonan's syndrome. Lancet 1992;339:19–21.
48. Muntean W. Fresh frozen plasma in the pediatric age group and in congenital coagulation factor deficiency. Thromb Res 2002;107 (suppl 1):S29–S32.
49. Horowitz MS, Pehta JC. SD Plasma in TTP and coagulation factor deficiencies for which no concentrates are available. Vox Sang 1998;74(suppl 1):231–235.
50. Soff GA, Levin J. Familial multiple coagulation factor deficiencies, I: Review of the literature: differentiation of single hereditary disorders associated with multiple factor deficiencies from coincidental concurrence of single factor deficiency states. Semin Thromb Hemost 1981;7:112–148.
51. Nakao A, Suzuki Y, Isshiki K, et al. Clinical evaluation of plasma abnormal prothrombin (des-gamma-carboxy prothrombin) in hepatobiliary malignancies and other diseases. Am J Gastroenterol 1991;86:62–66.
52. British Committee for Standards in Haematology, Blood Transfusion Task Force. Guidelines for the use of fresh frozen plasma, cryoprecipitate and cryosupernatant. Br J Haematol 2004;126:11–28.
53. Baker RI, Coughlin PB, Gallus AS, et al. Warfarin reversal: Consensus guidelines, on behalf of the Australian Society of Thrombosis and Haemostasis. Med J Aust 2004;181:492–497.
54. Shetty H, Backhouse G, Bentley D, et al. Effective reversal of warfarin induced excessive anticoagulation with low dose vitamin K1. Thromb Haemost 1992;67:13–15.
55. Development Task Force of the College of American Pathologists. Practice parameters for the use of fresh-frozen plasma, cryoprecipitate and platelets. JAMA 1994;271:777–781.
56. Guidelines on oral anticoagulation, 3rd ed. Br J Haematol 1998;101: 374–387.
57. Makris M, Greaves M, Phillips WS, et al. Emergency oral anticoagulant reversal: the relative efficacy of infusions of fresh frozen plasma and clotting factor concentrate on correction of the coagulopathy. Thromb Haemost 1997;77:477–480.
58. Veshchev I, Elran H, Salame K. Recombinant coagulation factor VIIa for rapid preoperative correction of warfarin-related coagulopathy in patients with acute subdural hematoma. Med Sci Monit 2002;8: CS98–100.
59. Sawyer PR, Harrison CR. Massive transfusion in adults: diagnosis, survival, and blood bank support, Vox Sang 1990;58:199–203.
60. Leslie SD, Toy PT. Laboratory hemostatic abnormalities in massively transfused patients given red blood cells and crystalloid. Am J Clin Pathol 1991;96:770–773.
61. Ciavarella D, Reed RL, Counts RM, et al. Clotting factor levels and the risk of diffuse microvascular bleeding in the massively transfused patient. Br J Haematol 1987;67:365–368.
62. Hewson JR, Neame PB, Kumar N, et al. Coagulopathy related to dilution and hypotension during massive transfusion. Crit Care Med 1985;13:387–391.
63. Collins JA. Problems associated with the massive transfusion of stored blood. Surgery 1974;75:274–295.
64. Murray DJ, Olson J, Strauss R, et al. Coagulation changes during packed red cell replacement of major blood loss. Anesthesiology 1988; 69:839–845.
65. Ledgerwood AM, Lucas CE. A review of studies on the effects of hemorrhagic shock and resuscitation on the coagulation profile. J Trauma 2003;54:S68–S74.
66. Nohe B, Kiefer RT, Ploppa A, et al. The effects of fresh frozen plasma on neutrophil-endothelial interactions. Anesth Analg 2003;97:216–221.
67. Lundsgaard-Hansen P. Treatment of acute blood loss. Vox Sang 1992; 63:241–246.
68. Hiippala ST, Myllyla GJ, Vahtera EM. Hemostatic factors and replacement of major blood loss with plasma-poor red cell concentrates. Anesth Analg 1995;81:360–365.
69. Strauss RG. Clinical perspective of platelet transfusions: defining the optimal dose. J Clin Apheresis 1995;10:124–127.
70. McCall MM, Blackwell MM, Smyre JT, et al. Fresh frozen plasma in the pediatric pump prime: a prospective, randomized trial. Ann Thorac Surg 2004;77:983–987.
71. Bick RL. Disseminated intravascular coagulation. Hematol Oncol Clin North Am 1992;6:1259–1285.
72. Rubin RN, Colman RW. Disseminated intravascular coagulation: approach to treatment. Drugs 1992;44:963–971.
73. Vinazzer H. Therapeutic uses of antithrombin III in shock and disseminated intravascular coagulation. Semin Thromb Hemost 1989;15:347–352.
74. Dreyfus M, Masterson M, David M, et al. Replacement therapy with monoclonal antibody purified protein C concentrate in newborns with severe congenital protein C deficiency. Semin Thromb Hemost 1995;21:371–381.
75. Rintala E, Seppala OP, Kotilainen P, et al. Protein C in the treatment of coagulopathy of meningococcal disease [Letter]. Lancet 1996;347:1767.
76. Sadler JE, Moake JL, Miyata T, et al. Recent advances in thrombotic thrombocytopenic purpura. Hematology (Am Soc Hematol Educ Program) 2004;407–423.
77. Fujikawa K, Suzuki H, McMullen B, et al. Purification of human von Willebrand factor-cleaving protease and its identification as a new member of the metalloproteinase family. Blood 2001;98:1662–1666.
78. Gerritsen HE, Robles R, Lammle B, et al. Partial amino acid sequence of purified von Willebrand factor-cleaving protease. Blood 2001;98:1654–1661.
79. Soejima K, Mimura N, Hirashima M, et al. A novel human metalloprotease synthesized in the liver and secreted into the blood: possibly, the von Willebrand factor-cleaving protease? J Biochem 2001;130:475. Erratum in J Biochem 2001;130:519.
80. Mannucci PM, Capoferri C, Canciani MT. Plasma levels of von Willebrand factor regulate ADAMTS-13, its major cleaving protease. Br J Haematol 2004;126:213–218.
81. Bowen DJ. An influence of ABO blood group on the rate of proteolysis of von Willebrand factor by ADAMTS13. J Thromb Haemost 2003;1:33–40.
82. Veradier A, Obert B, Houllier A, et al. Specific von Willebrand factor-cleaving protease in thrombotic microangiopathies: a study of 111 cases. Blood 2001;98:1765–1772.
83. Levy GG, Motto DG, Ginsburg D. ADAMTS13 turns 3. Blood 2005;106:11–17.
84. Raife T, Atkinson B, Montgomery R, et al. Severe deficiency of VWF-cleaving protease (ADAMTS13) activity defines a distinct population of thrombotic microangiopathy patients. Transfusion 2004;44:146–150.
85. Furlan M, Lammle B. Assays of von Willebrand factor-cleaving protease: a test for diagnosis of familial and acquired thrombotic thrombocytopenic purpura. Semin Thromb Hemost 2002;28:167–172.
86. Rick ME, Austin H, Leitzman SF, et al. Clinical usefulness of a functional assay for the von Willebrand factor cleaving protease (ADAMTS 13) and its inhibitor in a patient with thrombotic thrombocytopenic purpura. Am J Hematol 2004;75:96–100.
87. Pimanda JE, Maekawa A, Wind T, et al. Congenital thrombotic thrombocytopenic purpura in association with a mutation in the second CUB domain of ADAMTS13. Blood 2004;103:627–629.
88. Allford SL, Harrison P, Lawrie AS, et al. von Willebrand factor-cleaving protease activity in congenital thrombotic thrombocytopenic purpura. Br J Haematol 2000;111:1215–1222.
89. Yarranton H, Lawrie AS, Purdy G, et al. Comparison of von Willebrand factor antigen, von Willebrand factor-cleaving protease and protein S in blood components used for treatment of thrombotic thrombocytopenic purpura. Transfus Med 2004;14:39–44.
90. Ruggenenti P, Remuzzi G. The pathophysiology and management of thrombotic thrombocytopenic purpura. Eur J Haematol 1996; 56:191–207.
91. Kwaan HC, Soff GA. Management of thrombotic thrombocytopenic purpura and hemolytic uremic syndrome. Semin Hematol 1997;34: 159–166.
92. Rock GA, Shumak KH, Buskard NA, et al. Comparison of plasma exchange with plasma infusion in the treatment of thrombotic thrombocytopenic purpura. N Engl J Med 1991;325:393–397.
93. Rock GA, Shumak KH, Sutton DMC, et al. Cryosupernatant as replacement fluid for plasma exchange in thrombotic thrombocytopenic purpura. Br J Haematol 1996;94:383–386.
94. Moschcowitz E. An acute febrile pleiochromic anemia and hyaline thrombosis of the terminal arterioles and capillaries: an undescribed disease. Thromb Haemost 1978;40:4–8.
95. Ruggenenti P, Galbusera M, Cornejo RP, et al. Thrombotic thrombocytopenic purpura: evidence that infusion rather than removal of plasma induces remission of the disease. Am J Kidney Dis 1993;21:314–318.
96. Obrador GT, Ziegler ZR, Shadduck RK, et al. Effectiveness of cryosupernatant therapy in refractory and chronic relapsing thrombotic thrombocytopenic purpura. Am J Hematol 1993;42:217–220.

97. Onundarson PT, Rowe JM, Heal JM, et al. Response to plasma exchange and splenectomy in thrombotic thrombocytopenic purpura. Arch Intern Med 1992;152:791–796.
98. Zeigler ZR, Shadduck RK, Gryn JF, et al. Cryoprecipitate poor plasma does not improve early response in primary adult thrombotic thrombocytopenic purpura (TTP). J Clin Apheresis 2001;16:19–22.
99. Rock G, Anderson D, Clark W, et al. Does cryosupernatant plasma improve outcome in thrombotic thrombocytopenic purpura? No answer yet. Br J Haematol 2005;129:79–86.
100. Alvarez-Larran A, Del Rio J, Ramirez C, et al. Methylene blue-photoinactivated plasma vs. fresh-frozen plasma as replacement fluid for plasma exchange in thrombotic thrombocytopenic purpura. Vox Sang 2004;86:246–251.
101. Barz D, Budde U, Hellstern P. Therapeutic plasma exchange and plasma infusion in thrombotic microvascular syndromes. Thromb Res 2002;107(suppl 1):S23–S27.
102. Novitzky N, Thompson J, Abrahams L, et al. Thrombotic thrombocytopenic purpura in patients with retroviral infection is highly responsive to plasma infusion therapy. Br J Haematol 2005;128:373–379.
103. British Society of Haematology. Guidelines on the diagnosis and management of thrombotic microangiopathic haemolytic anaemias. Br J Haematol 2004;120:556–573.
104. Sarode R, Gottschall JL, Aster RH, et al. Thrombotic thrombocytopenic purpura: early and late responders. Am J Hematol 1997;54:102–107.
105. Agostoni A, Cicardi M. Hereditary and acquired C1-inhibitor: biological and clinical characteristics in 235 patients. Medicine (Baltimore) 1992;71:206–215.
106. Fritsch S, Waytes TA, Kunschak M. Recovery and half-life of C1-inhibitor in prevention and treatment of acute attacks in hereditary angioedema. Thromb Haemost 1993;69:873.
107. Laxenaire MC, Audibert G, Janot C. Use of purified C1-esterase inhibitor in patients with hereditary angioedema. Anesthesiology 1990;72:956–957.
108. Leitman SF, Kucera E, McLeod B, et al. Guidelines for Therapeutic Hemapheresis. Bethesda, Md., American Association of Blood Banks, 1992.
109. Churchwell KB, McManus ML, Kent P, et al: Intensive blood and plasma exchange for treatment of coagulopathy in meningococcemia. J Clin Apheresis 1995;10:171–177.
110. Busund R, Straume B, Revhaug A. Fatal course in severe meningococcemia: clinical predictors and effect of transfusion therapy. Crit Care Med 1993;21:1699–1705.
111. Stegmayr BG, Jakobson S, Rydvall A, et al. Plasma exchange in patients with acute renal failure in the course of multiorgan failure. Int J Artif Organs 1995;18:45–52.
112. Martin JN, Files JC, Blake PG, et al. Postpartum plasma exchange for atypical preeclampsia-eclampsia as HELLP (hemolysis, elevated liver enzymes, and low platelets) syndrome. Am J Obstet Gynecol 1995;172:1107–1125.
113. Warrier MR, Copilevitz CA, Dykewicz MS, et al. Fresh frozen plasma in the treatment of resistant angiotensin-converting enzyme inhibitor angioedema. Ann Allergy Asthma Immunol 2004;92:573–575.
114. Cochrane Injuries Group Albumin Reviewers. Human albumin administration in critically ill patients: systematic review of randomised controlled trials. BMJ 1998;317:235–240.
115. Isaacs MS, Scheuermaier KD, Levy BL, et al. In vitro effects of thawing fresh-frozen plasma at various temperatures. Clin Appl Thromb Hemost 2004;10:143–148.
116. Chowdhury P, Saayman AG, Paulus U, et al. Efficacy of standard dose and 30 ml/kg fresh frozen plasma in correcting laboratory parameters of haemostasis in critically ill patients. Br J Haematol 2004;125: 69–73.
117. Pineda A, Taswell HF. Transfusion reactions associated with anti-IgA antibodies: report of four cases and review of the literature. Transfusion 1985;15:10–15.
118. Sack G, Snyder EL. Cytokine generation in stored platelet concentrates. Transfusion 1994;34:20–25.
119. Sonntag J, Stiller B, Walka MM, et al. Anaphylatoxins in fresh-frozen plasma. Transfusion 1997;37:798–803.
120. Myhre BA. Toxicological quandary of the use of bis(2-diethylhexyl) phthalate (DEHP) as plasticizer for blood bags. Ann Clin Lab Sci 1988;18:131–140.
121. Nielsen HJ, Reimert C, Pedersen AN, et al. Leukocyte-derived bioactive substances in fresh frozen plasma. Br J Anaesth 1997;78:548–552.
122. Popovsky MA, Moore SB. Diagnostic and pathogenetic considerations in transfusion-related acute lung injury. Transfusion 1985;25:573–577.
123. Webert KE, Blajchman MA. Transfusion-related acute lung injury. Transfus Med Rev 2003;17:252–262.
124. Kleinman S, Caulfield T, Chan P, et al. Toward an understanding of transfusion-related acute lung injury: statement of a consensus panel. Transfusion 2004;44:1774–1789.
125. Silliman CC, Boshkov LK, Mehdizadehkashi Z, et al. Transfusion-related acute lung injury: epidemiology and a prospective analysis of etiologic factors. Blood 2003;101:454–461.
126. Van Buren NL, Stroncek DF, Clay ME, et al. Transfusion-related acute lung injury caused by an NB2 granulocyte-specific antibody in a patient with thrombotic thrombocytopenic purpura. Transfusion 1990;30:42–45.
127. Silliman CC, Paterson AJ, Dickey WO, et al. The association of biologically active lipids with the development of transfusion-related acute lung injury: a retrospective study. Transfusion 1997;37: 719–726.
128. Kopko PM, Popovsky MA, MacKenzie MR, et al. HLA class II antibodies in transfusion-related acute lung injury. Transfusion 2001; 41:1244–1248.
129. Eastlund T, McGrath PC, Britten A, et al. Fatal pulmonary transfusion reaction to plasma containing donor HLA antibody. Vox Sang 1989;57:63–66.
130. Hashim SW, Kay HR, Hammond GL, et al. Noncardiogenic pulmonary edema after cardiopulmonary bypass: an anaphylactic reaction to fresh frozen plasma. Am J Surg 1984;147:560–564.
131. Engelfriet CP, Reesink HW. Transfusion-related acute lung injury (TRALI). Vox Sang 2001;81:269–283.
132. Bux J, Becker F, Seeger W, et al. Transfusion-related acute lung injury due to HLA-A2 specific antibodies in recipient and NBI-specific antibodies in donor blood. Br J Haematol 1996;93:707–713.
133. Flesch BK, Neppert J. Transfusion-related acute lung injury caused by human leucocyte antigen class II antibody. Br J Haematol 2003;116: 673–676.
134. Kopko PM, Paglieroni TG, Popovsky MA, et al. TRALI: Correlation of antigen-antibody and monocyte activation in donor-recipient pairs. Transfusion 2001;43:177–184.
135. Dooren MC, Ouwehand WH, Verhoeven AJ, et al. Adult respiratory distress syndrome after experimental intravenous gamma-globulin concentrate and monocyte-reactive IgG antibodies. Lancet 1998;352:1601–1602.
136. Paglieroni TG, Kopko PM, Popovsky MA. Monocyte antibody associated with transfusion related acute lung injury (TRALI). Blood 2001;98:57(abstr, suppl 1).
137. Saigo K, Sugimoto T, Tone K, et al. Transfusion-related acute lung injury in a patient with acute myelogenous leukaemia having anti-IgA2m[1] antibody. J Intern Med Res 1999;27:96–100.
138. Rizk A, Gorson KC, Kenney L, et al. Transfusion-related acute lung injury after the infusion of IVIG. Transfusion 2001;41:264–268.
139. Bray RA, Harris SB, Josephson CD, et al. Unappreciated risk factors for transplant patients: HLA antibodies in blood components. Hum Immunol 2004;65:240–244.
140. Popovsky MA, Davenport RD (eds). Transfusion-related acute lung injury: Femme fatale? Transfusion 2001;41:312–315.
141. Sinnott P, Bodger S, Gupta A, et al. Presence of HLA antibodies in single-donor-derived fresh frozen plasma compared with pooled, solvent detergent-treated plasma (Octaplas). Eur J Immunogenet 2004; 31:271–274.
142. Sachs UJ, Kauschat D, Bein G. White blood cell-reactive antibodies are undetectable in solvent/detergent plasma. Transfusion 2005; 45:1628–1631.
143. Wieding JU, Vehmeyer K, Dittman J, et al. Contamination of fresh-frozen plasma with viable white cells and proliferative stem cells [Letter]. Transfusion 1994;34:185.
144. Bernvill SS, Abdulatiff M, al-Sedairy S, et al. Fresh frozen plasma contains viable progenitor cells: should we irradiate? [Letter] Vox Sang 1994;67:405.
145. Willis JI, Lown JA, Simpson MC, et al. White cells in fresh-frozen plasma: evaluation of a new white cell-reduction filter. Transfusion 1998;38:645–649.
146. Hiruma K, Okuyama Y. Effect of leucocyte reduction on the potential alloimmunogenicity of leucocytes in fresh-frozen plasma products. Vox Sang 2001;80:51–56.
147. Menitove JE (ed.). Standards for Blood Banks and Transfusion Services, 19th ed. Bethesda, Md., American Association of Blood Banks, 1999, p 69.
148. British Committee on Standards in Haematology. Guidelines on the clinical use of leukocyte-depleted blood components. Transfus Med 1998;8:59–71.
149. Isbister JP. Adverse reactions to plasma and plasma components. Anaesth Intensive Care 1993;21:31–38.

150. Vamvakas EC, Carven JH. Exposure to allogeneic plasma and risk of postoperative pneumonia and/or wound infection in coronary artery bypass graft surgery. Transfusion 2002;42:107–113.
151. Horowitz B, Lazo A, Grossberg H, et al. Virus inactivation by solvent/ detergent treatment and the manufacture of SD plasma. Vox Sang 1998;74(suppl 1):203–206.
152. McOmish F, Yap PL, Simonds P, et al. Detection of hepatitis A virus (HAV) in coagulation factor concentrates using the polymerase chain reaction. Thromb Haemost 1993;69:939.
153. McOmish F, Yap PL, Jorda A, et al. Detection of parvovirus B19 in donated blood: A model system for screening by polymerase chain reaction. J Clin Microbiol 1993;31:323–328.
154. Mohr H, Knuver-Hopf J, Gravemann U, et al. West Nile virus in plasma is highly sensitive to methylene blue-light treatment. Transfusion 2004;44:886–890.

Chapter 20

Cryoprecipitate and Related Products

Leon L. Su • Lennart E. Lögdberg

Cryoprecipitate (cryoprecipitated antihemophilic factor, Cryo) is the common term for the cold-insoluble plasma proteins that precipitate in fresh frozen plasma (FFP) when it is thawed to between 1°C and 6°C and then centrifuged, collected, and refrozen. It is one of the four main blood components available in virtually every blood bank in the developed world, but paradoxically, it is likely the component most underutilized even in well-recognized clinical circumstances.

The main constituents of cryoprecipitate are the high-molecular-weight proteins fibrinogen, factor VIII, von Willebrand factor (vWF), factor XIII, and fibronectin. Initially developed in the mid-1960s by Judith Pool and colleagues,[1,2] cryoprecipitate revolutionized the treatment of hemophilia and von Willebrand disease (vWD), previously dependent on whole blood or fresh plasma. Cryoprecipitate, because of its concentrated factor VIII and factor VIII-vWF complex, could be pooled, and thus its transfusion could provide sufficient factor to prevent or treat serious bleeding with minimized risk of volume overload. In the decades after the introduction of cryoprecipitate, purified and recombinant factor concentrates were developed and eventually supplanted cryoprecipitate as the primary treatment for hemophilia and vWD in most cases.

Today, cryoprecipitate use has been redefined. It is used primarily to treat acquired fibrinogen deficiencies associated with active bleeding and either surgery or trauma with dilution from massive transfusion and fluid resuscitation. It also is used in congenital deficiency syndromes associated with bleeding or as prophylaxis against anticipated bleeding. Finally, cryoprecipitate is used as a source of fibrinogen, factor XIII, and fibronectin in the commercial production of tissue sealants as well as the institutional production of allogeneic and autologous fibrin glues. Whereas it is no longer routinely used as the primary treatment for hemophilia, vWD, and uremic coagulopathy, cryoprecipitate continues to have a role as second-line therapy in instances in which primary treatment is ineffective or not available.

PRODUCTION, PROCESSING, STORAGE, AND QUALITY CONTROL

The source and quality of plasma used to make cryoprecipitate is controlled by guidelines set forth by the Food and Drug Administration (FDA) as published in the Code of Federal Regulations (CFR).[3] Governing the quality of source plasma ensures that production of cryoprecipitate contains adequate amounts of biologically active product while minimizing contamination from infectious and cellular components. Current guidelines from the CFR allow source plasma to be obtained from whole-blood collection or plasmapheresis, although the vast majority of cryoprecipitate used for transfusion in the United States comes from whole-blood donors. Plasma donors are required to meet similar and additional eligibility requirements as whole-blood allogeneic donors. A sample of blood collected at the time of donation is tested for ABO phenotype and communicable infectious diseases. Pathogen-reduction techniques such as nanofiltration, solvent-detergent treatment, and methylene blue-photoactivation also may be used to treat source plasma to reduce further the risk of infectious disease transmission.

Preparation of plasma begins with separation of blood cells by centrifugation to create a cell-free product. If the collection is in CPD, CP2D, or CPDA-1, separated plasma must be frozen at a temperature less than or equal to −18°C within 8 hours of collection. For blood collected in ACD, separated plasma should be frozen within 6 hours of collection. Once frozen, cryoprecipitate can be made from FFP within 12 months of collection. The process resumes when FFP is thawed at 1°C to 6°C to allow formation of the cryoprecipitate. A final separation step using centrifugation or a plasma expressor removes the residual precipitate from the thawed plasma, where it is then placed in individual, sterile bags and resuspended in 10 to 15 mL (up to 20 mL in "wet cryo") of plasma.[4–8] After the extraction process, cryoprecipitate must be refrozen within 1 hour.

In addition to the traditional method of cryoprecipitation production outlined earlier, efforts to improve efficiency and quality control in component processing led to the development of a new automated device capable of generating cryoprecipitate from plasma. The CryoSeal FS system (Thermogenesis Corp. Rancho Cordova, Calif.), currently not for sale in the United States and pending FDA approval, is a compact, computerized device designed to produce fibrin sealant in the autologous preoperative setting.[9] Alternatively, the CryoSeal system is an automated device with tightly controlled temperature cycling capable of producing cryoprecipitate within 1 hour.[10,11] The fibrinogen and factor VIII content in cryoprecipitate prepared by the CryoSeal system is comparable to that with traditional production methods.[10,11] Advantages of the CryoSeal system over manual preparation include standardization and faster production of cryoprecipitate.

Current American Association of Blood Banks (AABB) Standards require cryoprecipitate to be stored at −18°C, transported in a frozen state, and used within 12 months of the original date of collection.[12] As a final measure to assure quality of cryoprecipitate, the CFR dictates that quality of antihemophilic factor and fibrinogen should be tested monthly on at least four representative containers of cryoprecipitate.[3] With every quality-assurance testing, the AABB Standard states that unpooled components of cryoprecipitated antihemophilic factor should contain a minimum of 150 mg of fibrinogen and 80 IU of coagulation factor VIII.[13]

PREPARATION, DOSAGE, AND ADMINISTRATION

Preparation

Before its administration, cryoprecipitate is thawed in a water bath at 30°C to 37°C for approximately 10 to 15 minutes. Pooling of cryoprecipitate bags is often done after thawing and before administration, as most adult patients are treated with multiple units (see later) of cryoprecipitate at once. Alternatively, pooling of cryoprecipitate can be performed before it is frozen and appropriately labeled as "Cryoprecipitated antihemophilic factor, pooled." To maximize the activity of the coagulation proteins, once thawed, cryoprecipitate cannot be refrozen and should be kept at temperatures of 20°C to 24°C for no longer than 6 hours.[14] To ensure sterility of the product, cryoprecipitate must be transfused within 4 hours if it is pooled.[12]

Cryoprecipitate contains a negligible amount of red blood cells and only a small amount of the isohemagglutinins anti-A and/or anti-B. Therefore compatibility testing and Rh testing are not required before its use in adults. Nevertheless, it is common practice for most institutions to provide ABO-compatible cryoprecipitate when available. In neonatal recipients, cryoprecipitate should be ABO-compatible because of the smaller plasma volumes in infants. Approximately 20 to 30 minutes must be allowed for thawing and pooling of cryoprecipitate units before administration. Prepooled units can often be thawed and ready for administration in about 10 to 15 minutes.

Dosing: First-line Indications

The dose of cryoprecipitate is based on several factors including its intended use, the desired target level of the specific factor to be repleted, and the approximate size of the recipient. For hypofibrinogemia, cryoprecipitate has been demonstrated to be an excellent source of therapeutic fibrinogen.[15,16] As a general guideline, the dose of cryoprecipitate necessary to replete a fibrinogen deficit may be estimated by using an empiric dose of 1 U of cryoprecipitate per 5 to 10 kg body weight, or alternatively, it may be calculated by using the following formula:

$$\text{Desired fibrinogen increment (g/L)} = (0.25 \times \text{number of units of cryoprecipitate})/\text{Plasma volume (L)}$$

This formula assumes 250 mg of fibrinogen per unit of cryoprecipitate and can be modified to reflect the actual fibrinogen content of the unit, if known.

A dose of 1 unit of cryoprecipitate per 10 kg body weight can be expected to increase the fibrinogen concentration by approximately 50 mg/dL in the absence of heavy consumption or bleeding. The frequency and duration of administration is based on the underlying condition. In acquired hypofibrinogenemia (e.g., L-asparaginase therapy, disseminated intravascular coagulation), a daily prophylactic regimen may be suitable. In conditions associated with hypofibrinogenemia and active bleeding (e.g., massive transfusion with bleeding), and when the measured fibrinogen is less than 100 g/dL, an initial pool of 10 units is needed, and up to three pools may be given in rapid succession. In this circumstance, frequent monitoring and replacement are recommended.

In congenital hypofibrinogenemia, fibrinogen replacement with cryoprecipitate should be reserved for episodes of active bleeding. In the normal steady state, fibrinogen has a half-life of approximately 3 days.[17] Although active bleeding may alter fibrinogen kinetics, a dosing schedule of cryoprecipitate infusion every 3 days may be an appropriate starting point for patients with congenital hypofibrinogenemia.

Because factor XIII has a long half-life (9 days) and levels of less than 5% are hemostatic, the recommended replacement dose and the frequency of cryoprecipitate administration in congenital factor XIII deficiency are 1 U per 10 to 20 kg body weight every 2 to 3 weeks.

Dosing: Second-line Indications

Cryoprecipitate can be used as a second-line treatment for hemophilia A when factor concentrates are unavailable. Typical regimens begin with a loading dose to achieve the desired factor VIII level, followed by maintenance doses every 8 to 12 hours. Larger doses may be necessary in cases with factor VIII inhibitor and can be adequately assessed and adjusted by monitoring factor VIII levels after treatment. The following formulas can be used to calculate the number of units of cryoprecipitate needed to achieve a target factor VIII level[4]:

Take the desired increase in factor VIII (percentage) and divide by 100 to obtain the desired factor VIII increase in units per milliliter. Factor VIII increase (in units per milliliter) multiplied with plasma volume (in milliliters) equals units of factor VIII needed. Assuming that each cryoprecipitate bag has a minimum of 80 U of factor VIII, the number of factor VIII units needed per 80 U per bag equals the number of bags or units of cryoprecipitate needed.

The quantity, quality, and activity of vWF in cryoprecipitate are variable. Therefore for the treatment of vWD and uremic coagulopathy, the replacement dose of vWF is estimated. For vWD, the usual recommendation is daily infusions of 1 U of cryoprecipitate per 10 kg body weight. In addition to clinical monitoring, appropriate laboratory studies should be performed to help individualize dosing strength and frequency of administration. For uremic coagulopathy, a similar dose of 1 U of cryoprecipitate per 10 kg body weight can be given as a one-time dose, with subsequent doses dependent on clinical and laboratory follow-up.

Preparation of Fibrin Glue/Sealants

Cryoprecipitate also may be used as a source of fibrinogen that can be added to a thrombin to form a *fibrin glue* or *sealant*. Fibrin glues and sealants are used as surgical hemostatic and adhesive agents that reproduce the final stages of the coagulation cascade to form fibrin clots. Fibrin glues and sealants can be divided into three categories including "home-made" preparations, commercially prepared fibrin sealants, and autologous fibrin sealant systems. Home-made glues have varying formulations that exist in the literature, but generally contain the basic components of cryoprecipitate, thrombin, and calcium chloride ($CaCl_2$).[18,19] Depending on how much fibrin glue is needed, common starting mixtures use 50 to 90 mL of cryoprecipitate combined with an equal volume of sterile solution containing 25,000 to 50,000 U of thrombin and 0.5 to 1 g of $CaCl_2$. Although home-made glues are effective as hemostatic and adhesive agents, they are not FDA approved for such applications. Furthermore, traditional home-made formulations that contain bovine thrombin have been associated with adverse effects; these include anaphylaxis to bovine proteins and the development of factor V inhibitors, leading to coagulopathy and increased morbidity and mortality.[20–22]

Commercially prepared fibrin sealants contain the same basic components as most home-made formulations, with a few differences. In the commercial production of fibrin sealants, fibrinogen is extracted from pooled human cryoprecipitate and combined with a fibrinolysis inhibitor solution. Separately, thrombin is prepared from pooled human plasma and is activated just before use by the addition of $CaCl_2$. By using a water bath (37°C), the fibrinogen concentrate/fibrinolytic inhibitor component is mixed with the thrombin/$CaCl_2$ solution to form a fibrin clot at the surgical surface. Whereas several commercially prepared fibrin sealants are available on the global market, only two are currently FDA approved and available for use in the United States. The first FDA-approved fibrin sealant, Tisseel (Baxter Healthcare, Deerfield, Ill.), was introduced in the United States in 1998, followed by a second-generation fibrin sealant, Crosseal (American Red Cross), in 2003. An important distinction between the commercially prepared fibrin solutions and the home-made fibrin glues is the viral inactivation/removal step of commercial fibrin solutions. The thrombin and fibrinogen components of Tisseel are freeze dried and heat treated as a means of viral inactivation.[23] Crosseal is produced by using a different viral-inactivation procedure in which the fibrinogen and thrombin components undergo solvent detergent treatment as well as pasteurization of the fibrinogen and nanofiltration of the thrombin.[24]

The last category of fibrin sealants is the autologous fibrin sealant systems. These fibrin solutions are automated devices that use autologous whole blood or plasma to create the protein components of the fibrin solution. The clear advantage of these systems is the elimination of infectious risk for human blood-borne diseases. Two of the fibrin-based systems, VivoStat[25] (Vivolution A/S) and AutoSeal (Harvest Technologies), produce a proprietary fibrin sealant within approximately 20 minutes by extracting fibrinogen and other sealant components directly from autologous whole blood. Another autologous fibrin-sealant system is the previously mentioned CryoSeal FS system that creates the two main components of a fibrin sealant, cryoprecipitate, and thrombin, from autologous blood within 1 hour.[9] All three systems are available in the global market but are currently not approved for use in the United States.

CRYOPRECIPITATE CONSTITUENTS AND THEIR STABILITY

Cryoprecipitate is a plasma-derived product that contains a higher concentration of fibrinogen as compared with FFP. Whereas AABB Standards indicate that cryoprecipitate must contain a minimum of 150 mg of fibrinogen, most cryoprecipitate products using current methods of extraction will contain higher amounts of fibrinogen near the order of 250 to 350 mg of fibrinogen per bag, representing a recovery rate of approximately 30% of the original fibrinogen content.[9,10,16] Cryoprecipitate also contains 80 to 120 U of factor VIII, with a higher rate of recovery near 50% of the original factor VIII content.[10] Additional components include 30 to 60 mg of fibronectin, and a variable percentage of the original plasma concentration of vWF (approximately 40% to 70%), and factor XIII (approximately 30%). Remaining components include small amounts of immunoglobulin G (IgG), IgM, and albumin.[26] Different processing factors including preservative solutions (e.g., CPDA-1, ACD), temperature, time of storage, rate of centrifugation, rate of freezing, and viral inactivation procedures (e.g., methylene blue plus light, solvent detergent) have all been shown to have varying effects on the overall fibrinogen, vWF, and factor VIII content, and thus should be evaluated if quality testing reveals below standard component levels in the final cryoprecipitate product.[27–33]

Interestingly, whereas expiration times set forth by AABB and FDA serve to ensure the quality and safety of cryoprecipitate components, several studies show that fibrinogen levels remain stable and adequate up to 24 hours after thaw at room temperature and in units kept up to 8 years in frozen storage.[14,34–36] In contrast, factor VIII levels appear less stable than fibrinogen over time, and whereas some studies show that it remains adequate up to 24 hours after thaw and in units stored frozen for up to 8 years, conflicting data indicate that the quality of factor VIII can be consistently verified only within the standard guidelines.[14,34–36] Decisions to extend the expiration of cryoprecipitate based on medical necessity, therefore, should take into consideration the intended use of the product, the duration of expiration, and the possible increased risk of infectious contamination.

PRIMARY AND SECONDARY INDICATIONS FOR CRYOPRECIPITATE USE

Because cryoprecipitate contains the highest concentration of fibrinogen, factor XIII, and vWF, it is most often used in the treatment of hemorrhagic disorders resulting from quantitative or qualitative deficits of these factors. As factor concentrates and recombinant factors have become more readily available and affordable, the use of cryoprecipitate has declined. Table 20–1 lists primary and secondary uses of cryoprecipitate in addition to common misuses and underutilization of cryoprecipitate.

Quantitative and Qualitative Fibrinogen Deficiency

The common coagulation pathway culminates in the formation of the fibrin clot through the action of thrombin on fibrinogen. Thus congenital abnormalities in fibrinogen synthesis, either hypofibrinogenemia/afibrinogenemia or dysfibrinogenemia, may result in spontaneous or posttraumatic hemorrhage of variable degree. Various clinical entities including hepatocellular disease, disseminated intravascular coagulopathy, and L-asparaginase therapy may be associated with clinically significant hypofibrinogenemia or dysfibrinogenemia. In general, fibrinogen levels greater than 100 mg/dL are considered to be adequate for hemostasis whereas fibrinogen levels below 100 mg/dL frequently are associated with severe bleeding.[37] Although fibrinogen levels lower than 100 mg/dL result in the prolongation of the prothrombin and activated partial thromboplastin time, correction of the fibrinogen deficit is typically required only during episodes of active bleeding or before surgical procedures.[38–40]

Table 20–1 Primary and Secondary Clinical Indications, Common Misuses, and Underutilization of Cryoprecipitate

Primary

Acquired/congenital hypofibrinogenemia[16,38–39,43–44,47]
Massive transfusion with bleeding[48–51]
Component for tissue sealants or fibrin glues[23–24,72–92]
Factor XIII deficiency[60–65]
Reversal of thrombolytic therapy[93,97]

Secondary

Hemophilia A[4,94]
von Willebrand disease[34,52–59]
Uremic coagulopathy[66–71]

Common Misuses[97,98]

Fibrinogen replacement with normal fibrinogen levels and no evidence of increased dysfunction or consumption
Reversal of warfarin therapy
Treatment of impaired surgical hemostasis in the absence of hypofibrinogenemia
Treatment of hepatic coagulopathy with multiple factor deficiencies

Common Underutilization[48–51]

Massive transfusion with bleeding

In a review, Humphries[41] reported that the most common use of cryoprecipitate as fibrinogen replacement is in acquired fibrinogen deficiency. Dose and frequency of administration depend on the rate of consumption or destruction of fibrinogen, and this can be assessed by monitoring the fibrinogen level. In certain coagulopathies, repletion of other coagulation proteins in addition to fibrinogen may necessitate the use of FFP.[16,42–47]

Massive Transfusion

The coagulopathy associated with massive transfusion in bleeding is often multifactorial. However, the primary cause is usually coagulation factor deficiencies from dilution and increased factor consumption, as in disseminated intravascular coagulation or normal coagulation.[48] Situations of major blood loss with massive transfusion often lead to an initial decrease in fibrinogen levels below 100 mg/dL after loss of 1.5 blood volumes followed by a decrease to less than 25% activity of labile coagulation factors after loss of two blood volumes.[49,50] In some cases, rapid consumption and dilution of fibrinogen is associated with massive transfusion and bleeding, FFP dosing without additional cryoprecipitate may not be sufficient to maintain hemostatic fibrinogen levels. Although FFP does contain fibrinogen, the amount provided this way may be insufficient to maintain adequate levels during massive transfusion and bleeding, in turn leading to delayed correction and excessive volumes.[51] As a result, use of cryoprecipitate should always be considered in massive transfusion with bleeding and should be given early in the course along with FFP.

von Willebrand Disease

The complex adhesive glycoprotein vWF is synthesized by megakaryocytes and endothelial cells and circulates in plasma as multimers of various molecular weights (500 to 10,000 kDa). vWF has two important hemostatic functions: (1) it mediates platelet adhesion to the subendothelium through its interaction with platelet glycoprotein Ib, and (2) it stabilizes factor VIII by complexing with it in circulation.[52,53] Therefore, both quantitative and qualitative abnormalities in vWF can result in increased bleeding tendency. Desmopressin acetate [1-deamino (8-D-arginine) vasopressin] (DDAVP) enhances the release of vWF from the endothelial cells and augments platelet activity. DDAVP is considered effective therapy in most types of vWD. In approximately 10% to 20% of patients with vWD, however, DDAVP is either ineffective (types 1 and 3) or contraindicated (types 2B and 2N), or the development of tachyphylaxis prevents its prolonged use. In these circumstances, cryoprecipitate can provide adequate replacement of both vWF and factor VIII:C to shorten the bleeding time and to control clinical bleeding.[54–57] In the past 20 years, lyophilized and pasteurized plasma concentrates (e.g., intermediate-purity and high-purity plasma-derived factor VIII concentrates) rich in high-molecular-weight vWF and factor VIII, have been developed and have largely replaced cryoprecipitate in the treatment of vWD.[58,59]

Factor XIII Deficiency

Through the dual action of thrombin, fibrinogen is converted into fibrin, and factor XIII is activated; this process facilitates the cross-linking of polymerized fibrin and α_2-antiplasmin to fibrin clots. In the neonatal period, deficiency of this hemostatic function (factor XIII deficiency) manifests as protracted umbilical stump bleeding, whereas later in life, postsurgical bleeding and delayed or abnormal (keloid) wound healing may be observed. Factor XIII also has been linked to the development of implantation tissue during pregnancy, and its deficiency is believed to be the cause of repeated miscarriages.[60] In these cases of factor XIII deficiency, prophylactic replacement therapy with plasma-derived factor XIII concentrates such as Fibrogammin P[61,62] (available in certain countries but currently not licensed in the United States) or cryoprecipitate is feasible.[63–65]

Uremic Coagulopathy

Many patients with uremia have evidence of abnormal primary hemostasis, as documented by a prolonged bleeding time and decreased platelet aggregation, findings suggesting an abnormal interaction between platelets and vascular endothelium.[66,67] Because vWF promotes normal interaction between platelets and subendothelium, the use of cryoprecipitate in uremic bleeding has been reported in a few small studies and case reports.[68–70] Janson and associates[68] described a significant reduction in bleeding time with improvement in uremic bleeding diathesis in a group of six patients. The beneficial effect of cryoprecipitate on uremic bleeding is transient and is observed in only up to 50% of patients.[71]

Fibrin Glue or Sealant

Fibrin glues and sealants are commonly used today to enhance local surgical hemostasis and to provide effective tissue adherence. The elastic property, tensile strength, and tissue adhesiveness of plasma fibrin glue or sealant has made it an important adjunct in microsurgical technique. As previously mentioned, many variations of fibrin glues/sealants are available, including home-made formulations, commercially prepared products, and autologous sealant devices, yet only two commercially prepared fibrin sealants are approved for specific use in the United States. Tisseel has been approved for use as an adjunct in conventional surgical hemostasis, cardiopulmonary bypass surgery, colostomy closure, and splenic injury repair.[23] Crosseal has been approved for use in hepatic surgery.[24,72,73] Although the efficacy of the two sealants have not been fully addressed in the literature, the composition and related adverse effects have been compared (Table 20–2). Tisseel incorporates a bovine aprotinin as the antifibrinolytic agent as opposed to Crosseal, which uses Tranexamic acid (a human-derived product). The advantage of using a bovine-free fibrin sealant such as Crosseal is that it does not carry the increased risk of anaphylactic reaction to bovine proteins[74] or the theoretic risk of bovine spongiform encephalopathy (BSE) transmission seen with Tisseel. One disadvantage of Crosseal is that there is an absolute contraindication to its use in procedures in which contact exists with the cerebrospinal fluid (CSF) or dura mater. Crosseal used in neurosurgical procedures on rabbits at doses equivalent to clinical use in patients demonstrated severe neurologic symptoms and death in the rabbits.[24]

A wide variety of investigational uses for fibrin glue and sealants are documented in the literature.[75–78] Although the approved uses of commercial sealants are limited, experimental or off-label uses of various fibrin tissue adhesives or sealants are numerous and are still expanding. Fibrin sealants have been used to achieve hemostatic control in patients with preexisting coagulopathy.[79] In cosmetic surgery, tissue fibrin adhesives have been used in lieu of sutures to reduce scar formation and in aiding skin-graft fixation in burn patients.[80–83] In various microsurgical techniques, fibrin sealants have been used to attain a fluid or air barrier, to maintain tissue adhesiveness, and as an adjunct in bone and cartilage repair.[84–89] As an extemporaneous fibrin glue, infusion of cryoprecipitate with thrombin into the renal pelvis facilitated the removal of small renal stones.[90] Applications of fibrin glues and sealants have also been investigated in repairing punctured fetal membranes as a potential treatment for premature rupture of membranes.[91] Similar to the concept of fibrin glue and sealants is the promising use of cryoprecipitate and platelets to form an "amniopatch" in the treatment of iatrogenic previable premature rupture of membranes.[92]

Other Uses

As a minimal-volume fibrinogen source, cryoprecipitate has been used to decrease bleeding during orthotopic liver transplantation and is indicated for reversal of thrombolytic therapy associated with bleeding.[93] In developing countries where factor concentrates are unavailable, cryoprecipitate can serve a primary role in the treatment of hemophilia A, if available.[94] As a source of fibronectin, cryoprecipitate was once believed to have potential in treating critically ill patients with organ failure and sepsis; however, it was proven not to have any such clinical benefit in several controlled studies.[95] In contrast, in a small, controlled study, Steinbaum and Cucinell[96] demonstrated a beneficial effect of cryoprecipitate containing fibronectin on wound healing. Further controlled

Table 20–2 Comparison of FDA-Approved Commercially Prepared Fibrin Sealants: Tisseel and Crosseal[23,24,74]

Tisseel	Crosseal
Approved Indications	
As adjunct to hemostasis in cardiopulmonary bypass surgery As a hemostatic agent in fully heparinized patients undergoing cardiopulmonary bypass surgery As adjunct in the closure of colostomies In the control of bleeding associated with splenic injury	As adjunct to hemostasis in liver surgery
Antifibrinolytic Agent	
Bovine aprotinin	Tranexamic acid
Contraindications	
Patients with a known hypersensitivity to bovine proteins or reactions to human blood products Injection into circulation or tissues Massive and brisk arterial bleed	Patients with known anaphylactic or severe systemic reactions to human blood products Surgical procedures in which contact with cerebrospinal fluid or dura mater could occur Injection into circulation or tissues Massive and brisk arterial bleeding
Potential Adverse Reactions	
Severe allergic/anaphylactoid reactions Thromboembolic events (if injected into circulation or tissue) Transmission of infectious agents (e.g., viruses)	Severe allergic/anaphylactoid reactions Transmission of infectious agents (e.g., viruses)

studies have yet to prove or disprove the use of fibronectin on wound healing, and its use in this area remains unclear.

COMMON MISUSES AND UNDERUTILIZATION OF CRYOPRECIPITATE

Audits of the use of cryoprecipitate have been reported in the literature and demonstrate that still considerable misuse of cryoprecipitate occurs in the clinical setting. Recent studies show patterns of inappropriate use involving up to 24% to 62% of all cryoprecipitate orders.[97,98] Commonly encountered misuses include fibrinogen replacement in patients with normal fibrinogen levels or who do not have current laboratory results *and* no evidence of increased dysfunction or consumption, reversal of warfarin therapy, treatment of impaired surgical hemostasis in the absence of hypofibrinogemia, and the treatment of hepatic coagulopathy with multiple factor deficiencies.

In addition, underutilization of cryoprecipitate in the setting of massive transfusion with bleeding commonly occurs in the intraoperative setting. The inappropriately low use of cryoprecipitate, and in some cases FFP, in the massive transfusion setting may stem from a once-held notion that coagulation deficiency occurred late in massive transfusion and after the development of thrombocytopenia. This belief, although probably valid when whole blood was used predominantly in massive transfusion, no longer reflects current practice, because today's blood products are mostly packed red blood cells (pRBCs) with significantly less plasma volumes.[48,50] As a result, coagulation deficiencies appear very early on in massive transfusion, with fibrinogen being one of the first coagulation proteins to fall below hemostatic levels.[49,50] Recent observations in the clinical setting suggest that during massive transfusion with bleeding, fibrinogen levels below 100 mg/dL may still persist despite repletion with pRBCs, FFP, and platelets, resulting in a persistent coagulopathy. Recognition of the rapid consumption and dilution of fibrinogen in the setting of massive transfusion and bleeding underscores the importance of frequent monitoring of fibrinogen levels and vigilant use of cryoprecipitate with other blood products to maintain hemostasis.

The incidence and pattern of inappropriate and insufficient use of cryoprecipitate signify an alarming misunderstanding of the use of cryoprecipitate among some clinicians and suggest the need for further education with respect to acceptable applications of this blood component.

POTENTIAL ADVERSE REACTIONS

Cryoprecipitate administration may be associated with nonspecific side effects related to its protein, cytokine, and isohemagglutinin content. Adverse reactions include fever, chills, and allergic reactions of variable severity. In situations in which large volumes of ABO-incompatible cryoprecipitate are given, adult recipients may develop a positive direct antiglobulin test (DAT), and in rare circumstances, hemolytic anemia.[4,99] Untoward effects of tissue fibrin adhesives such as home-made fibrin glues have been related to the source of thrombin, especially of bovine origin. These include the development of allergic-type reactions, some as severe as anaphylaxis, and factor V antibodies, which may lead to abnormal prothrombin times and postsurgical bleeding.[20–22]

SUMMARY

Cryoprecipitate is given primarily to treat acquired and congenital hypofibrinogenemia and is used in the production of fibrin glues and commercial sealants. Less frequently, it may be used to treat factor XIII deficiency and to reverse thrombolytic therapy. Cryoprecipitate may also be used as secondary treatment for hemophilia, vWD, and uremic coagulopathy or as initial treatment in situations in which specific factor concentrates or DDAVP are unavailable. Underutilization of cryoprecipitate in clinically appropriate circumstances and inappropriate use continue to occur at a high rate, according to institutional audits. This pattern of use underscores the need for continued education of ordering physicians on the appropriate use of cryoprecipitate.

REFERENCES

1. Pool JG, Shannon AE. Production of high potency concentrates of antihemophilic globulin in a closed bag system assay in vitro and in vivo. N Engl J Med 1965;273:1443–1447.
2. Hershgold EJ, Pool JG, Pappenhagen AR. The potent antihemophilic globulin concentrate derived from a cold insoluble fraction of human plasma: characterization and further data on preparation and clinical trial. J Lab Clin Med 1966;67:13–32.
3. Code of Federal Regulations, 21 CFR 640 Subpart F. Washington, D.C., Government Printing Office, 2004.
4. American Association of Blood Banks, America's Blood Centers, American Red Cross. Circular of information for the use of human blood and blood components, 2002, 26–28. http://www.fda.gov/cber/gdlns/circbld.pdf.
5. Brecher ME (ed). Technical Manual, 15th ed. Bethesda, Md., American Association of Blood Banks, 2005.
6. Myllyla G. Factors determining quality of plasma. Vox Sang 1998;74:507.
7. Allersma DP, Imambaks RMR, Meerhof LJ. Effect of whole blood storage on factor VIII recovery in fresh frozen plasma and cryoprecipitate. Vox Sang 1996;71:150.
8. Hughes C, Thomas KB, Schiff P, et al. Effect of delayed blood processing on the yield of factor VIII in cryoprecipitate and factor VIII concentrate. Transfusion 1988;28:566.
9. Buchta C, Dettke M, Funovics PT, et al. Fibrin sealant produced by the CryoSeal® FS System: Product chemistry, material properties and possible preparation in the autologous preoperative setting. Vox Sang 2004;86:257–262.
10. Gosselin RC, Larkin E, Owings JT, et al. CryoSeal™ System, a new device for generating cryoprecipitate from plasma. Clin Chem 1997;43:1782–1783.
11. Rock G, Berger R, Lange J, et al. A novel, automated method of temperature cycling to produce cryoprecipitate. Transfusion 2001;41:232–235.
12. AABB. 5.1.8A Standards for Blood Banks and Transfusion Services, 23rd ed. Bethesda, Md., American Association of Blood Banks, 2005, pp 58–59.
13. AABB. 5.7.5.14 Standards for Blood Banks and Transfusion Services, 23rd ed. Bethesda, Md., American Association of Blood Banks, 2005, p 30.
14. Saxena S, Odono V, Francis RB Jr, et al. Storage of thawed cryoprecipitated AHF is better at room temperature than at 1°C to 6°C for factor VIII content. Arch Pathol Lab Med 1991;115:343–345.
15. Sherman LA. In vivo stability of cryoprecipitate fibrinogen. Transfusion 1977;17:19–61.
16. Ness PM, Perkins HA. Cryoprecipitate as a reliable source of fibrinogen replacement. JAMA 1979;241:1690.
17. Thompson HW, Touris S, Giambartolomei S, et al. Treatment of congenital afibrinogenemia with cryoprecipitate collected through a plasmapheresis program using dedicated donors. J Clin Apheresis 1998;13:143–145.
18. Basu S, Marini CP, Bauman FG, et al. Comparative study of biological glues: cryoprecipitate glue, two-component fibrin sealant, and "French" glue. Ann Thorac Surg 1995;60:1255–1262.
19. Cohn SM, Feinstein AJ, Nicholas JM, et al. Recipe for poor man's fibrin glue. J Trauma 1998;44:507.
20. Berguer R, Staerkel RL, Moore EE, et al. Warning: Fatal reaction to the use of fibrin glue in deep hepatic wounds: case reports. J Trauma 1991;126:432.

21. Streiff MB, Ness PM. Acquired FV inhibitors: a needless iatrogenic complication of bovine thrombin exposure. Transfusion 2002;42:18–25.
22. Ortel TL, Mercer MC, Thames EH, et al. Immunologic impact and clinical outcomes after surgical exposure to bovine thrombin. Ann Surg 2001;233:88–96.
23. Tisseel VH, Kit Insert. Two-component fibrin sealant, vapor-heated, kit, manufactured by Osterreichisches Institut für Haemoderivate GES, M.B.H., Subsidiary of Immuno AG. Distributed by Baxter Healthcare Corporation, Deerfield, Ill., 1998.
24. American Red Cross. Crosseal fibrin sealant (human) package insert. Washington, DC, American Red Cross, 2003.
25. Dodd RA, Cornwell R, Holm NE, et al. The Vivostat® application system: a comparison with conventional fibrin sealant application systems. Tech Health Care 2002;10:401–411.
26. Allain JP. Non-factor VIII related constituents in concentrates. Scand J Haematol 1984;33:173–180.
27. Hornsey VS, Young DA, Docherty A, et al. Cryoprecipitate prepared from plasma treated with methylene blue plus light: increasing the fibrinogen concentration. Transfus Med 2004;14:569.
28. Farrugia A, Grasso S, Douglas S, et al. Modulation of fibrinogen content in cryoprecipitate by temperature manipulation during plasma processing. Transfusion 1992;32:755–759.
29. Farrugia A, Prowse C. Studies on the procurement of blood coagulation factor VIII: effects of plasma freezing rate and storage conditions on cryoprecipitate quality. J Clin Pathol 1985;38:433–437.
30. DePalma L, Criss VR, Luban NL. The preparation of fibrinogen concentrate for use as fibrin glue by four different methods. Transfusion 1993;33:717–720.
31. Keeling DM, Luddington R, Allain JP, et al. Cryoprecipitate prepared from plasma virally inactivated by the solvent detergent method. Br J Haematol 1997;96:194–197.
32. Piedras J, Sanchez-Montero PE, Herrera FM, et al. Effect of plasma freezing temperature, anticoagulant and time of storage on factor VIII: C activity in cryoprecipitate. Arch Med Res 1993;24:13–26.
33. Seghatchian J, Krailadsiri P. What's happening? The quality of methylene blue treated FFP and cryo. Transfus Apheresis Sci 2001;25:327–331.
34. Pomper GJ, Rick ME, Epstein JS, et al. Management of severe vWD with cryoprecipitate collected by repeated apheresis of a single dedicated donor. Transfusion 2003;43:1515–1521.
35. Saxena S, Odono V, Francis RB Jr, et al. Can storage of thawed cryoprecipitate be extended to more than six hours? Am J Clin Pathol 1990;94:203–206.
36. Spivey MA, Jeter EK, Lazarchick J, et al. Postfiltration factor VIII and fibrinogen levels in cryoprecipitate stored at room temperature and at 1 to 6°C. Transfusion 1992;32:340–343.
37. Fresh-frozen Plasma, Cryoprecipitate, and Platelets Administration Practice Guidelines, Development Task Force of the College of American Pathologists. Practice parameter for the use of fresh-frozen plasma, cryoprecipitate, and platelets. JAMA 1994;271:777–781.
38. Galanakis DK. Fibrinogen anomalies and disease: a clinical update. Hematol Oncol Clin North Am 1992;6:1171.
39. Mammen EF. Fibrinogen abnormalities. Semin Thromb Hemost 1983;9:1.
40. Forbes CD, Madhok R. Genetic disorders of blood coagulation: clinical manifestation and management. In Ratnoff OD, Forbes CD (eds): Disorders of Hemostasis. Philadelphia, WB Saunders, 1991, p 141.
41. Humphries JE. Transfusion therapy in acquired coagulopathies. Transfus Med 1994;8:1181.
42. Nusbacher J. Blood transfusion support in liver transplantation. Transfusion 1991;5:207.
43. Colman RW, Robboy SJ, Minna JD. Disseminated intravascular coagulation: a reappraisal. Annu Rev Med 1979;30:359.
44. Francis JL, Armstrong DJ. Acquired dysfibrinogenemia in liver disease. J Clin Pathol 1982;35:667.
45. Gilabert J, Estelles A, Asnar J, et al. Abruptio placentae and disseminated intravascular coagulation. Acta Obstet Gynecol Scand 1985;64:35.
46. Sutton DM, Hauser R, Kulapongs P, et al. Intravascular coagulation in abruptio placentae. Am J Obstet Gynecol 1971;109:604.
47. Al-Mondhiry H, Ehmann WC. Congenital afibrinogenemia. Am J Hematol 1994;46:343–347.
48. Ho AM, Karmakar MK, Dion PW. Are we giving enough coagulation factors during major trauma resuscitation? Am J Surg 2005;190:479–484.
49. Ciavarella D, Reed RL, Counts RB, et al. Clotting factor levels and the risk of diffuse microvascular bleeding in the massively transfused patient. Br J Haematol 1987;67:365–368.
50. Hiippala ST, Myllyla GJ, Vahtera EM. Hemostatic factors and replacement of major blood loss with plasma-poor red cell concentrates. Anesth Analg 1995;81:360–365.
51. Stainsby D, MacLennan S, Hamilton PJ. Management of massive blood loss: a template guide. Br J Anaesth 2000;85:387–491.
52. Fischer BE, Kramer G, Mitterer A, et al. Effect of multimerization of human and recombinant von Willebrand factor on platelet aggregation, binding to collagen and binding of coagulation factor VIII. Thromb Res 1996;84:55.
53. Sadler JE, Matsushita T, Dong Z, et al. Molecular mechanism and classification of von Willebrand disease. Thromb Haemost 1995;74:161.
54. Rodeghiero F, Castaman G, diBona E, et al. Consistency of responses to repeated DDAVP infusions in patients with von Willebrand's disease and hemophilia A. Blood 1989;74:1997.
55. Lusher JM. Response to 1-deamino-8-arginine vasopressin in von Willebrand disease. Haemostasis 1994;24:276.
56. Castaman G, Rodeghiero F. Current management of von Willebrand's disease: practical therapeutics. Drugs 1995;602:14.
57. Mannucci PM. Biochemical characteristics of therapeutic plasma concentrates used in the treatment of von Willebrand disease. Haemostasis 1994;24:285.
58. Mannucci PM, Tenconi PM, Castaman G, et al. Comparison of four virus-inactivated plasma concentrates for treatment of severe von Willebrand disease: a cross-over randomized trial. Blood 1992;79:3130.
59. Rodeghiero F, Castaman G, Meyer D, et al. Replacement therapy with virus-inactivated plasma concentrates in von Willebrand disease. Vox Sang 1992;62:193.
60. Asahina T, Kobayashi T, Okada Y, et al. Maternal blood coagulation factor XIII is associated with the development of cytotrophoblastic shell. Placenta 2000;21:388–393.
61. Gootenberg JE. Factor concentrates for the treatment of factor XIII deficiency. Curr Opin Hematol 1998;5:372–375.
62. Dreyfus M, Arnuti BB, Borg P, et al. Safety and efficacy of Fibrogammin P®)for the treatment of patients with severe FXIII deficiency [Abstract]. J Thromb Haemost 2003;1(suppl 1):abstract P0299.
63. Stirling D, Ludlam CA. Therapeutic concentrates for the treatment of congenital deficiencies of factors VII, XI, XIII. Semin Thromb Hemost 1993;19:48.
64. Fear JD, Miloszewski KJA, Losowsky MS. The half life of factor XIII in the management of inherited deficiency. Thromb Haemost 1983;49:102.
65. Rodeghiero F, Castaman GC, Di Bona E, et al. Successful pregnancy in a woman with congenital factor XIII deficiency treated with substitutive therapy. Blut 1987;55:45.
66. Remuzzi G. Bleeding disorders in uremia: pathophysiology and treatment. Adv Nephrol 1989;18:171.
67. Andrassy K, Ritz E. Uremia as a cause of bleeding. Am J Nephrol 1985;5:313.
68. Janson PA, Jubelirer SJ, Weinstein MJ, et al. Treatment of the bleeding tendency in uremia with cryoprecipitate. N Engl J Med 1980;303:1318.
69. Maierhoter W, Adams MB, Kleinman JG, et al. Treatment of the bleeding tendency in uremia with cryoprecipitate [Letter]. N Engl J Med 1981;305:645.
70. Juhl A. DDAVP, cryoprecipitate, and highly "purified" factor VIII concentrate in uremia. Nephron 1986;43:305.
71. Triulzi DJ, Blumberg N. Variability in response to cryoprecipitate treatment for hemostatic defects in uremia. Yale J Biol Med 1990;63:1.
72. Noun R, Elias D, Balladur P, et al. Fibrin glue effectiveness and tolerance after elective liver resection: a randomized trial. Hepatogastroenterology 1996;43:221–224.
73. Kohno H, Nagasue N, Chang YC, et al. Comparison of topical hemostatic agents in elective hepatic resection: a clinical prospective randomized trial. World J Surg 1992;16:966–969.
74. Shirai T, Shimota H, Chida K, et al. Anaphylaxis to aprotinin in fibrin sealant. Intern Med 2005;44:1088–1089.
75. Sierra DH. Fibrin sealant adhesive systems: a review of their chemistry, material properties and clinical applications. J Biomater Appl 1993; 7:309.
76. Spotnitz WD. Fibrin sealant in the United States: clinical use at the University of Virginia. Thromb Haemost 1995;74:482.
77. Martinowtz U, Spotnitz WD. Fibrin tissue adhesives. Thromb Haemost 1997;78:661.
78. Radosevich M, Goubran HA, Burnouf T. Fibrin sealant: Scientific rationale, production methods, properties, and current clinical use. Vox Sang 1997;72:133.
79. Martinowitz U, Schulman S, Horoszowski H, et al. Role of fibrin sealants in surgical procedures on patients with hemostatic disorders. Clin Orthop 1996;328:65.
80. Saltz R, Dimick A, Harris C, et al. Application of autologous fibrin glue in burn wounds. J Burn Care Rehabil 1989;10:504.
81. Saltz R, Guzman G. Aesthetic reconstruction of burned hands. Plast Surg 1992;11:23.

82. Marchac D, Pugash E, Gault D. The use of sprayed fibrin glue for face lifts. Eur J Plast Surg 1987;10:139.
83. Vogel A, O'Grady K, Toriumi DM. Surgical tissue adhesives in facial plastic and reconstructive surgery. Facial Plast Surg 1993;9:76.
84. Shirai T, Amano J, Takabe K. Thoracoscopic diagnosis and treatment of chylothorax after pneumonectomy. Ann Thorac Surg 1991;52:306.
85. Shaffrey CI, Spotnitz WD, Shaffrey ME, et al. Neurosurgical applications of fibrin glue: augmentation of dural closure in 134 patients. Neurosurgery 1990;26:207.
86. Martinowitz U, Ozer Y, Varon D, et al. Fibrin sealing in nerve repair. Thromb Haemost 1993;69:1287.
87. Egkher E, Spangler H, Spangler HP. Indications and limits of fibrin adhesive applied to traumatological patients. In Schlag G, Redl H (eds): Fibrin Sealant in Operative Medicine: Traumatology and Orthopaedics. Berlin, Springer, 1986, pp 7, 144.
88. Lagoutte FM, Gauthier L, Comte PRM. A fibrin sealant for perforated and pre-perforated corneal ulcers. Br J Ophthalmol 1989;73:757.
89. Kang DR. Fibrin tissue adhesive use in costal cartilage laryngotracheal reconstruction. Paper presented at the Cambridge Symposium on Tissue Sealants: Current Practice, Future Uses, La Jolla, Calif., 1996.
90. Fischer CP, Sonda LP, Dionko AC. Further experience with cryoprecipitate coagulum in renal calculus surgery: a review of 60 cases. J Urol 1981;126:432.
91. Reddy UM, Shah SS, Nemiroff RL, et al. In vitro sealing of punctured fetal membranes: potential treatment for midtrimester premature rupture of membranes. Am J Obstet Gynecol 2001;185:1090–1093.
92. Quintero RA, Morales WJ, Allen M, et al. Treatment of iatrogenic previable premature rupture of membranes with intra-amniotic injection of platelets and cryoprecipitate (amniopatch): preliminary experience. Am J Obstet Gynecol 1999;181:744–749.
93. Sane DC, Califf RM, Topol EJ. Bleeding during thrombolytic therapy for acute myocardial infarction: mechanisms and management. Ann Intern Med 1989;111:1010–1022.
94. Srivastava A. Factor replacement therapy in haemophilia: are there models for developing countries? Haemophilia 2003;9:391.
95. Powell FS, Doran JE. Current status of fibronectin in transfusion medicine: focus on clinical studies. Vox Sang 1991;60:193–202.
96. Steinbaum SS, Cucinell S. Effects of cryoprecipitate on the healing of chronic wounds. Mil Med 1994;159:105.
97. Pantanowitz L, Kruskall M, Uhl L. Cryoprecipitate patterns of use. Am J Clin Pathol 2003;119:874–881.
98. Schofield WN, Rubin GL, Dean MG. Appropriateness of platelet, fresh frozen plasma and cryoprecipitate transfusion in New South Wales public hospitals. Med J Aust 2003;178:117–121.
99. Goodnight SH Jr. Cryoprecipitate and fibrinogen [Editorial]. JAMA 1979;241:1716–1717.

Chapter 21
Albumin

Elizabeth E. Culler • Lennart E. Lögdberg

INTRODUCTION

Over the past 70 years, significant progress has been made in the isolation and purification of human plasma proteins for use as therapeutic products. This chapter focuses on albumin, the first such protein to be made commercially available through large-scale purification. The majority of this chapter will focus on the product Albumin (Human), a sterile solution of purified human plasma albumin, now dominating the therapeutic albumin market.[1] Less commonly used is Plasma Protein Fraction (Human), which is a sterile solution of albumin and globulin derived from human plasma.[1]

The development of a method to purify albumin was begun in 1940. By the end of 1941, human serum albumin (HSA) was put into clinical use on the battlefield.[2] The administration of human serum albumin proved so effective in the treatment of shock that the demand by the military resulted in the production of over 500,000 units in the United States by the end of World War II in 1945.[3]

In the decades following the war, albumin continued to be used in the treatment of shock but was also used experimentally in the treatment of various other conditions, such as malnutrition or hypoalbuminemia. Owing to the use of albumin for an expanding number of conditions and because of its significant cost, guidelines for albumin usage were established by the Division of Blood Diseases and Resources, National Heart and Lung Institute, National Institutes of Health, in 1975.[4] Since that time, further studies have prompted even more conservative albumin usage guidelines, such as those established by the University HealthSystem Consortium (UHC) in 2000.[5] Auditing of albumin transfusion practices, based on current guidelines, indicates substantial inappropriate use of this product.[6,7]

This chapter provides an overview of albumin products and begins by discussing plasma donation, the plasma industry, infectious disease testing, manufacturing methods, and regulatory aspects of albumin product production. This is followed by a review of the current guidelines for the therapeutic use of Albumin (Human), which is hereafter referred to as albumin. Finally, the adverse effect profile for the product will be summarized, including the risk of infectious disease transmission.

ALBUMIN, THE PROTEIN

Albumin is the quantitatively dominant plasma protein. A 66-kDa, water-soluble protein, it is synthesized in the liver at a rate of about 15 g/day and has a half-life of around 25 days.[8] In a healthy person with normal nutrition, albumin synthesis and catabolism are regulated by the colloid osmotic pressure.[9] An average 70-kg man contains about 320 g of albumin,[8] of which 35% to 40% is localized to the intravascular space, where it contributes about 80% of the colloidal osmotic pressure of plasma. Accordingly, albumin is important for physiologic maintenance and regulation of plasma volume.

In addition, albumin has a high negative charge[10] and a thiol group on the surface of the molecule that enables albumin to function effectively as a ligand binder, a radical scavenger, and a versatile transport protein.[11] Thus, albumin also serves as a major carrier for hormones, medications, enzymes, fatty acids, cholesterol, and many other substances.[9]

PLASMA DONATION AND COLLECTION

Albumin is derived from plasma collected either by whole blood donation (Recovered Plasma) or by apheresis (Source Plasma).[1] The following subsections discuss plasma collection and its regulation, plasma pooling, donor suitability, and prefractionation infectious disease testing. Refer to Chapter 12 for further information on these subjects and on the preparation and storage of Recovered Plasma and Source Plasma.

Regulation of Plasma Collection

The World Health Organization (WHO) has established guidelines for the collection and production of human plasma for fractionation.[12] In addition, regional or national regulatory authorities such as the U.S. Food and Drug Administration (FDA) and the Council of Europe are responsible for the establishment and enforcement of regulations pertaining to the safety and quality of the products in their respective areas.[13] The FDA inspects facilities that it licenses for plasma fractionation every 2 years. There are 26 facilities worldwide that are licensed by the FDA to produce plasma fractions for use in the United States.[14] In addition, almost all of the approximately 450 source plasma collection facilities in the world belong to the Plasma Protein Therapeutics Association (PPTA). The PPTA offers an International Quality Plasma Program (IQPP) certification requiring that facilities meet voluntary standards established by the PPTA. Approximately 90% of source plasma collection facilities around the world have qualified for IQPP certification. Source plasma facilities currently account for approximately 12 million liters of plasma production annually.[13]

Plasma Pooling

A donation of plasma by apheresis contains approximately 450 to 880 mL of plasma, while a donation of Recovered Plasma contains only around 100 to 260 mL of plasma.[12] Thus, albumin derived from pools of Source Plasma requires contributions from fewer donors than albumin derived from pools of Recovered Plasma. Because about 1 liter of plasma must be processed to produce 20 to 25 grams of albumin,[15] plasma from tens of thousands of donors must be pooled to make the production process efficient.

Donor Suitability

Pooling of the large number of plasma donations required to manufacture albumin allows a single infected donor unit the potential to transmit disease to a large number of final product recipients. Therefore, steps are added throughout the manufacturing process to limit infectious disease transmission. The initial step is to select appropriate donors by reviewing the donor's medical history and by conducting a medical examination. Although the WHO guidelines encourage the use of plasma from voluntary, nonremunerated donors,[12] many plasma collection facilities provide $15 to $25 per donation. To decrease the risk of infectious disease transmission, donors of Source Plasma must present themselves twice within a 6-month period to be considered acceptable by voluntary PPTA standards.[13] An "applicant donor" is an individual who comes in to donate and who has not qualified as a donor in the previous 6 months. Until the applicant donor screens negative for viral markers and passes the medical history screen on two separate occasions within a 6-month period, the initial donation is quarantined. When the donor successfully passes all tests twice within the 6-month period, the donor is considered "qualified" and the donations are used in manufacturing pools. When more than 6 months pass between donations, individuals are reclassified as "applicant donors" and must become qualified again. After donation, Source Plasma must be held for at least 60 days prior to pooling to allow time for investigation of any postdonation information that might become available.[13]

Infectious Disease Testing

After donors at low risk for infectious disease transmission have been selected, the plasma donations are screened using approved tests for hepatitis B surface antigen (HBsAg), anti–human immunodeficiency virus (HIV), and anti–hepatitis C virus (HCV).[12] The PPTA voluntary standards also require that nucleic acid testing (NAT) be performed for HIV, hepatitis B virus (HBV), HCV, and parvovirus B19. Manufacturing pools of plasma must contain less than 10^5 IU of parvovirus B19 DNA per milliliter according to PPTA standards.[13] Testing for HTLV-1 and HTLV-2 is not required because these are cell-associated viruses.[12]

The risk of infectious disease transmission is further reduced by the cold ethanol processing method and by filtration steps that eliminate microbes with diameters larger than 0.2 μm.[12] This is discussed below in the section on Commercial Albumin Preparations, Quality Specifications, and Formulations and the section on Infectious Potential.

MANUFACTURE OF ALBUMIN PRODUCTS

Development of a Technique for Plasma Fractionation

The development of a process for the isolation and purification of plasma components was driven by the need to provide blood products for casualties of World War II. In 1940, a meeting was held in Washington, D.C., to discuss the large number of blood products requested by the U.S. armed forces. Because of the limited supply, Dr. Edwin J. Cohn at the Harvard Medical School was asked to determine whether animal plasma could be used for human treatment.[16] Cohn developed a plasma fractionation technique (cold ethanol fractionation; see below) that he used to separate and characterize plasma components.[17]

Albumin, responsible for 80% of the colloid osmotic pressure of plasma, was the most suitable component for volume replacement.[18] Because bovine albumin was found to cause serum sickness in human recipients, the focus instead became the development of a human albumin preparation. Thus, treatment with a 25% human albumin solution was found to restore blood volume in volunteers made hypovolemic by removal of a measured volume of blood by venesection.[16] Further studies were cut short when the total albumin supply was needed at Pearl Harbor to treat burn victims.[16] The military experience with the product's clinical efficacy, ease of transport, and stability at a wide temperature range prompted initiation of mass production of albumin.[2] The 25% albumin solution used by the military contained sodium at a concentration of 300 mEq/L to maintain product stability. After the introduction of new stabilizers, the sodium content of albumin was reduced and the new product became known as "salt-poor albumin," a term still occasionally used within the medical community.[15] Currently the FDA requires that all albumin preparations contain 130 to 160 mEq/L of sodium.[1]

Producing plasma products during World War II was challenging. Of more than 12.5 million blood donations delivered to plasma processing facilities during this period, more than 204,800, or 1.6%, were ultimately rejected.[19] The biggest losses were due to bacterial contamination (>125,700 or 0.99% of the donations) or to breakage of the glass bottles used for plasma storage (>18,700 or 0.14% of the donations).[19] An investigation revealed that the main causes of bacterial contamination were the use of multiple technicians in the preparation process, break-in technique, nonsterile processing conditions, and, in some cases, collection facilities exceeding their capacity at the expense of quality. After these issues had been addressed, the rate of bacterial contamination was reduced.

Commercial Albumin Preparations, Quality Specifications, and Formulations

Because the implementation of new technology in albumin manufacturing requires a substantial capital investment and because the cold ethanol fractionation technique (see below) has a proven safety record, U.S. suppliers continue to use methods based on Cohn fractionation for albumin concentration and purification. In Europe, by comparison, some manufacturers have either incorporated chromatography into their production methods or switched to processes based exclusively on chromatographic purification methods.[20] The addition of chromatography to plasma processing has significantly increased the yield (80% to 85% vs 60% to 70%) and purity (>98% vs 95%) of albumin products when compared to cold ethanol fractionation.[10] In addition, chromatography has allowed significant reductions in the concentration of unwanted elements such as endotoxin, aluminum, and trace proteins.[10] It is uncertain whether these alternative purification schemes will be incorporated into commercial albumin production in the United States.

Cold Ethanol Fractionation

Albumin purification using Cohn fractionation begins with frozen plasma, which is thawed at a low temperature, permitting the removal of cryoprecipitate. The product then undergoes cold ethanol plasma fractionation, which relies on the manipulation of pH, ionic strength, temperature, protein concentration, and ethanol concentration to precipitate plasma fractions. The ethanol content is increased and the pH and temperature are decreased in a stepwise fashion with separation of fractions by centrifugation and filtration. Fibrinogen is precipitated in fraction I, immunoglobulins in fraction II + III, α_1-proteinase inhibitor, antithrombin III, and factor IX complex in fraction IV-1, and plasma protein fraction in fraction IV-4. Albumin, which has the highest solubility of the major proteins in plasma, precipitates in the final fraction (fraction V). The ethanol is then removed by ultracentrifugation or freeze-drying.[21]

After the albumin has been purified and within 24 hours of being placed in the final container, the product is heated to 60 ± 0.5°C for 10 to 11 hours.[1] This inactivates a variety of viruses, including HBV and HIV. Albumin does not denature under these conditions owing to the presence of 17 stabilizing disulphide bonds in its structure[18] and to the addition of stabilizing compounds (sodium caprylate or a combination of sodium acetyltryptophanate and sodium caprylate). All final containers of albumin are incubated at 20–35°C for at least 14 days after heat treatment. After the incubation period, each final container is examined for turbidity before it is released.[1] The label on the final product must state the sodium (range in mEq/L) and the protein concentration (4%, 5%, 20%, or 25%).[1] Table 21–1 summarizes the FDA regulations pertaining to the production of Albumin (Human) and Plasma Protein Fraction (Human) and also lists FDA-required testing on the final albumin products.

Toward Commercialization of Recombinant Albumin

Over the past couple of decades, efforts have been directed toward producing recombinant human albumin.[22,23] A recent phase I trial compared the safety, tolerability, and

Table 21–1 FDA Requirements for Manufacturing of Therapeutic-Grade Albumin (Human) and Plasma Protein Fraction (Human)

Characteristic	Albumin (Human)	Plasma Protein Fraction (Human)
Required Production Characteristics		
Source material	Recovered Plasma or Source Plasma	
Pasteurization	Heated within 24 hours of the filling of the final containers at 60 ± 0.5°C for 10–11 hours	
Incubation	Incubated in final containers at 20–35°C for at least 14 days	
Processing	The processing method should not affect the integrity of the product and should consistently produce a safe product	Components with an electrophoretic mobility similar to that of α globulin should account for ≤5% of the total protein when tested after the pasteurization step The product should contain <5% protein with a sedimentation coefficient greater than 7.0S
Stabilizer	Either 0.08 ± 0.016 mmol sodium caprylate or 0.08 ± 0.016 mmol sodium acetyltryptophanate and 0.08 ± 0.016 mmol sodium caprylate per gram of protein	
Preservative	None	
Required Tests on Final Products		
Protein concentration	The protein concentration of the final solution may be 4.0 ± 0.25%, 5.0 ± 0.30%, 20.0 ± 1.2%, or 25.0 ± 1.5%	5.0 ± 0.30%
Protein composition	≥96% of the total protein in the final product must consist of albumin, as determined by a Center for Biologics Evaluation and Research (CBER)–approved method	The protein composition of the final product must consist of ≥83% albumin and ≤17% globulins; ≤1% of the total protein should be gammaglobulin, as determined by a CBER-approved method
pH	When the final product is diluted to a concentration of 1% protein with sodium chloride 0.15 mol/L, the pH must be 6.9 ± 0.5	7.0 ± 0.3
Sodium concentration	130 to 160 mEq/L	
Potassium concentration	≤2 mEq/L	
Heat stability	The final product is inspected visually after it is heated to 57°C for 50 hours It must be not be visually different from an unheated control sample taken from the same lot	

From Code of Federal Regulations. Title 21 CFR 640. Washington, D.C., U.S. Government Printing Office, 2005 (revised annually).

hemodynamic responses in volunteers receiving either recombinant human albumin or human serum albumin.[24] Thirty participants in the double-blind, randomized trial received intravenous doses of 10g on day 1, 20g on day 22, and 50g on day 43 of either recombinant human albumin or human serum albumin. There were no significant differences in safety or tolerability between the two products. The serum albumin, colloid osmotic pressure, and hematocrit pre- and postinfusion were measured and were not significantly different between the groups receiving either recombinant human albumin or human serum albumin. Since recombinant human albumin is virus- and prion-free, there is incentive for manufacturers to continue the clinical development of this product.

DOSING AND ADMINISTRATION

Choosing a Product

Albumin solutions with protein concentrations of 5%, 20%, and 25% are currently available on the U.S. market. Because PPF solutions contain a greater proportion of proteins other than albumin, they are not often used. Thus, the focus of this section is on albumin solutions.

The infusion of 5% albumin solutions, which are iso-oncotic with human plasma, increases the plasma volume by the volume of albumin solution infused,[8] while the infusion of the hyperoncotic 25% albumin solutions causes the plasma volume to expand by 3.5 times the volume of albumin solution infused.[25] For treating pediatric patients or volume- or sodium-sensitive patients, the more concentrated 20% or 25% albumin solutions are more commonly used, whereas the 5% albumin solutions are especially useful for hypovolemic patients.[26] Dehydrated patients usually require additional fluids along with the 20% or 25% albumin solutions.[1]

If necessary, a 5% albumin solution can be prepared by diluting a 20% or 25% albumin solution with either normal saline or 5% dextrose. Sterile water should not be used to dilute albumin because the resulting hypotonic solution can cause hemolysis when infused. This has occurred in at least 10 patients with one reported death.[27] When large volumes of diluted albumin are required, normal saline is the diluent of choice, since the infusion of large volumes of albumin diluted with dextrose 5% can cause hyponatremia leading to cerebral edema.[28]

When choosing a product, clinicians must also consider the aluminum concentration. As mentioned in the section on Potential Adverse Effects, albumin products contain small amounts of aluminum, which can accumulate in premature infants or in patients with chronic renal failure.[10] Talecris Biotherapeutics produces low-aluminum formulations of 5%, 20%, and 25% human albumin, each of which has an aluminum content of less than 200 μg/L.[29–31]

Dose

According to the American Hospital Formulary Service (AHFS) Drug Information guide, a typical initial adult dose of albumin is 25 g, which can be repeated in 15 to 30 minutes depending on the patient's response. Up to 250 g of albumin may be infused in a 48-hour period.[26] However, because studies have used different end points to assess clinical improvement after the administration of albumin, no standard dose of albumin can be recommended to fit all clinical situations. When evaluating the appropriate dose of albumin to administer, study investigators have relied on parameters such as serum albumin level, urine output, pulse, blood pressure, hematocrit, and degree of venous and pulmonary congestion.[26]

Rate

There are no guidelines addressing the optimal infusion rate for albumin solutions. The infusion rate should be based on the patient's condition and is limited only by the capacity of the administration set when an albumin infusion is needed emergently. Because high rates of albumin infusion can cause circulatory overload and pulmonary edema, 5% albumin solutions are commonly started at a rate of 1 to 2 mL/min and are not usually infused at a faster rate than 4 mL/min, and 25% albumin solutions are not infused at rates faster than 1 mL/min.[26]

Administration

Albumin should be inspected for turbidity prior to administration. Although albumin does not have to be infused through a filter, some manufacturers either recommend or include a filter in administration sets to be used during albumin administration. Hospital policy also may require the use of a filter.[15] Administration must begin within 4 hours of entry into the container.[1]

Because blood group isohemagglutinins are removed from albumin products during preparation, albumin is given without regard to ABO type. The Code of Federal Regulations (CFR) does not address the measurement of isohemagglutinin titers in albumin products; however, the European Pharmacopoeia states that plasma products intended for intravenous use should have an isohemagglutinin titer of less than 1:64.[12]

CLINICAL CONSIDERATIONS

Hypoalbuminemia may result from the decreased production, altered distribution, increased metabolism, or excessive loss of albumin. Some causes of decreased albumin production are liver dysfunction, malnutrition, and malabsorption. Approximately 40 cases of congenital analbuminemia (defined as HSA < 1 g/L) have been reported in the literature; however, this disorder is usually associated with only mild signs and symptoms.[32] Hypoalbuminemia also may result from a redistribution of albumin to the extravascular space as a result of increased vascular permeability, as seen in inflammatory states. Thyrotoxicosis and pancreatitis are two conditions associated with increased albumin catabolism. Increased albumin loss occurs in patients with protein-losing gastroenteropathy and nephrotic syndrome.

Indication Guidelines for Albumin Usage

Although decreased albumin levels are present in many conditions, albumin infusion is not usually required to treat hypoalbuminemia. Rather, albumin infusions are used therapeutically for plasma expansion. Historically, this led to broad indications and widespread use of the product. Later studies showed albumin to be ineffective in many of these uses, leading to a still-ongoing evolution toward more

Table 21–2 **UHC Guidelines on Albumin Usage**

Clinical Situation or Condition	Recommendation for Albumin Use
Therapeutic plasma exchange	Albumin can be used as a replacement fluid for plasma exchanges of > 20 mL/kg for a single procedure, or > 20 mL/kg/week for multiple exchanges Nonprotein colloids or crystalloids can be considered for smaller exchanges
Cirrhosis and large-volume paracentesis	Albumin or nonprotein colloids may be used in patients who do not respond to sodium restriction and diuretic therapy and who require paracentesis of > 5 L
Nephrotic syndrome	For patients with acute severe peripheral or pulmonary edema in whom diuretic therapy is ineffective, albumin (25%) may be used in the short term along with diuretics
Ovarian hyperstimulation syndrome	Prophylactic albumin infusion is estimated to prevent one case of severe OHSS for every 18 women at risk[73]
Hemorrhagic or nonhemorrhagic shock	Albumin can be used when nonprotein colloids are contraindicated in adult patients who have not responded within 2 hours to the administration of 4 L of crystalloids
Maintenance of volume following hepatic resection	Albumin can be used when crystalloids are ineffective or when crystalloid administration causes clinically significant edema
Maintenance of volume during and after liver and kidney transplantation	Albumin can be used during or after surgery to control ascites and severe pulmonary and peripheral edema Albumin is used when the serum albumin is < 2.5 g/dL, pulmonary capillary wedge pressure is < 12 mm Hg, and hematocrit is > 30% The administration of albumin during or after kidney transplantation has not conclusively shown benefit
Thermal injury	Albumin can be used when nonprotein colloids are contraindicated in adult patients who have received more than 4 L of crystalloids within 18–26 hours of injury when burns cover > 30% of the patient's body surface area
Maintenance of cerebral perfusion pressure (CPP) in patients with vasospasm associated with subarachnoid hemorrhage, cerebral ischemia, or head trauma	Crystalloids are first-line therapy for patients with increased hematocrit For patients with hematocrit < 30%, packed RBCs can be used for CPP maintenance Albumin (25%) can be used to maintain CPP patients when cerebral edema is a concern
Postoperative volume expansion after cardiac surgery	Albumin may be used when nonprotein colloids are contraindicated in patients who have not responded to crystalloids
Hyperbilirubinemia of the newborn	Albumin could be useful as an adjuvant in exchange transfusion

From Technology assessment: albumin, nonprotein colloid, and crystalloid solutions. Oak Brook, JH, University HealthSystem Consortium, 2000. Aboulghar M, Evers JH, Al-Inany H. Intravenous albumin for preventing severe ovarian hyperstimulation syndrome. Cochrane Database Syst Rev 2002:CD001302.

conservative indication guidelines such as the most recent UHC guidelines for the use of albumin (summarized and updated in Table 21–2), nonprotein colloid, and crystalloid solutions.[5] Reflecting the liberal guidelines of the past, a 2003 report that examined albumin prescribing patterns in 53 member institutions of the University HealthSystem Consortium found that albumin was inappropriately used in 57.8% of adult patients and 52.2% of pediatric patients. In the report, which collected data on 1649 adult and 23 pediatric patients receiving albumin, two of the most common inappropriate uses of albumin were for intradialytic blood pressure support (159 patients) and for serum albumin values of <2 g/dL (142 patients).[6] The consensus of the panelists involved in creating the 2000 UHC guidelines for albumin use was that the available evidence did not support the use of albumin in these situations. Table 21–3 provides a list of common misuses of therapeutic albumin infusions.

In the following sections, we discuss alternatives to the use of albumin for plasma expansion and then summarize some of the well-recognized clinical indications for albumin infusions, noting that such infusions are often a secondary treatment option.

Alternatives to Albumin for Plasma Expansion

The two major categories of products that may be used for plasma expansion are crystalloids (e.g., 0.9% sodium chloride, Ringer's lactate) and colloids, including protein (e.g., albumin) and nonprotein substances (e.g., dextrans, gelatins, and starches). Crystalloids have not demonstrated a definite clinical advantage over albumin, but are considerably cheaper and are therefore widely used as first-line treatment.[33] Although nonprotein colloids have been associated with side effects such as alterations in hemostatic laboratory results, pruritus, and, rarely, with severe head and back pain, they also are less expensive than albumin and are preferred by some.[34–39] In those clinical conditions in which plasma expansion through albumin or nonprotein colloids has demonstrated equivalent patient outcomes, the 2000 UHC guidelines recommend the use of the latter due to their lower cost. Neither crystalloids nor colloids can be substituted for red blood cells when oxygen-carrying capacity is needed or for platelets or plasma when coagulopathy exists.[5]

Table 21–3 Common Misuses of Albumin Infusions
Intradialytic blood pressure support
Hypoalbuminemia
Impending hepatorenal syndrome
Increasing drug efficacy
Acute or chronic pancreatitis
Acute normovolemic hemodilution in surgery
Volume expansion in neonates, unless expansion with 10 mL/kg of crystalloids was unsuccessful

From Technology assessment: albumin, nonprotein colloid, and crystalloid solutions. Oak Brook, Ill: University HealthSystem Consortium, 2000. Tanzi M, Gardner M, Megellas M, et al. Evaluation of the appropriate use of albumin in adult and pediatric patients. Am J Health Syst Pharm 2003;60:1330–1335. Tarin Remohi MJ, Sanchez Arcos A, Santos Ramos B, et al. Costs related to inappropriate use of albumin in Spain. Ann Pharmacother 2000;34:1198–1205.

Clinical Usage of Albumin Infusions

Therapeutic Plasma Exchange

Albumin is commonly used as the replacement fluid in therapeutic plasma exchange (TPE) unless a condition exists that specifically requires factors present in fresh frozen plasma (FFP).[40] Albumin solutions have a lower probability of viral transmission and a decreased risk of citrate-induced hypocalcemia than FFP.[41] According to the Circular of Information, FFP should not be used when other volume expanders can safely and adequately replace blood volume.[42]

Although albumin is a frequently used replacement fluid in TPE, cryopoor plasma or FFP are the preferred replacement fluids in thrombotic thrombocytopenic purpura (TTP) and related disorders.[43] In TTP, a metalloprotease (ADAMTS-13) that usually cleaves von Willebrand factor (vWF) into multimers is rendered ineffective by antibody inhibitors or by mutations in the ADAMTS-13 gene.[44–48] This results in the accumulation of ultralarge von Willebrand factor multimers, which interact with platelets, causing aggregation.[45,47] Plasma exchange treats the disease by removing the metalloprotease inhibitor and the ultralarge von Willebrand factor multimers and by replacing functional ADAMTS-13 metalloprotease through FFP or cryopoor plasma. Cryopoor plasma contains fewer ultralarge von Willebrand factor multimers than FFP does and is, therefore, preferred by some.[43]

The use of FFP as the TPE replacement fluid may also be considered in patients undergoing treatment with angiotensin-converting enzyme (ACE) inhibitors. In such patients, plasma exchange with albumin is associated with atypical reactions such as flushing, hypotension, dyspnea, and bradycardia.[49]

Paracentesis

Ascites associated with cirrhosis follows elevated portal pressure that results from increased intrahepatic vascular resistance, leading to increased nitric oxide levels and systemic arterial vasodilatation.[50] In patients with ascites, the vasoconstrictor systems become activated in response and the kidney retains sodium, causing ascites and edema.[50] Approximately 10% of patients with ascites are refractory to first-line treatment, which consists of a sodium-restricted diet and high-dose diuretics.[51] These patients' treatment options include serial therapeutic paracenteses, transjugular intrahepatic portosystemic stent shunt (TIPS), peritoneovenous shunts, and liver transplantation.[51]

For cirrhotic patients with refractory ascites who require serial therapeutic paracenteses, controversy exists concerning whether volume expansion is useful and, if so, which expander is most effective. A study by Gines and colleagues found that paracentesis in cirrhotic patients with tense ascites without albumin infusion resulted in significant increases in blood urea nitrogen, plasma renin activity, and plasma aldosterone concentration, whereas patients who received postparacentesis albumin did not experience those changes.[52] There were no significant differences in mortality between the groups. On the other hand, it has been shown that a single paracentesis of 4 to 6 L may be performed as a short-term option without albumin infusion in patients with tense, diuretic-resistant ascites.[51,53] Thus, given the safety of paracentesis of smaller volumes, the guidelines released by the American Association for the Study of Liver Diseases (AASLD) in 1998 suggest that postparacentesis albumin infusion is unnecessary for removed volumes of less than 4 to 5 L but that an albumin infusion can be considered for larger volume paracenteses.[51]

Alternatives to serial paracentesis with albumin infusion have been studied, and none has clearly demonstrated a better patient outcome. Albumin infusion more effectively prevents hemodynamic deterioration than the infusion of other plasma expanders such as dextran 70 and polygeline after large-volume paracentesis.[54] Results are conflicting when comparing treatment of cirrhotic patients with ascites refractory to diuretic treatment, with either TIPS or large-volume paracenteses followed by albumin, using survival without transplantation as outcome.[55–57] Because no other treatment has demonstrated a superior patient outcome, the 1998 AASLD guideline advising that albumin infusion be considered for large-volume paracentesis still seems applicable.[51]

Cirrhosis and Spontaneous Bacterial Peritonitis

Albumin infusion may be beneficial for patients with cirrhosis and spontaneous bacterial peritonitis, as demonstrated in a study in which such patients received either antibiotics or antibiotics plus albumin infusion.[58] The latter group had less renal impairment and a lower mortality rate. This clinical benefit may due to the thiol-related antioxidant effect of albumin.[59]

Nephrotic Syndrome

The nephrotic syndrome is caused by increased permeability of the glomerular capillary basement membranes, resulting in a urine protein excretion rate of greater than 3.5 g/24 hr.[60] Nephrotic syndrome is associated with hypoalbuminemia, edema, renal dysfunction, and hyperlipidemia. The standard treatment consists of corticosteroid and cytotoxic therapies to treat the underlying disease and diuretic therapy with a sodium-restricted diet to reduce peripheral edema and improve quality of life. A few patients may become refractory to these treatments. In such patients, investigators have attempted to increase diuresis by administering albumin in combination with furosemide with some success.[61] In one study in which patients with hypoalbuminemia received either furosemide alone, albumin alone, or a mixture of the two, the latter regimen led to modest increases in sodium and volume excretion.[62] In contrast, more recent studies in nephrotic patients with hypoalbuminemia found no benefit in combining albumin with furosemide.[63,64] In fact, several detrimental effects have been linked to combined furosemide-albumin treatment, including response delays, frequent relapse to primary immunosuppressive therapy,[65] hypertension, respiratory distress, and electrolyte abnormalities.[66]

Given the above limitations, combining 25% albumin with diuretic drugs is primarily indicated for patients with nephrotic syndrome refractory to standard diuretic therapy with a sodium-restricted diet. Accordingly, the University Hospital Consortium Guidelines for the Use of Albumin, No-Protein Colloid, and Crystalloid Solutions recommend the short-term use of albumin with diuretics only for such refractory patients with acute, severe peripheral, or pulmonary edema.[67]

Ovarian Hyperstimulation Syndrome

Ovarian hyperstimulation syndrome (OHSS) is a complication of ovulation induction that occurs after the additional administration of human menopausal gonadotrophin (hMG) but rarely after the use of clomiphene citrate alone.[68] The incidence of severe OHSS is estimated to occur in 0.5% to 5% of in vitro fertilization cycles.[69] OHSS is graded as mild, moderate, or severe; in the last case, it can be fatal.[70,71] The pathophysiology of the syndrome is not yet clearly defined, but it is thought that the ovaries secrete vasoactive substances when final follicular maturation occurs, causing increased capillary permeability.[72] This results in the movement of protein-rich fluid out of the intravascular space, and patients can have vomiting, diarrhea, large ovarian cysts, thromboembolism, ascites, hydrothorax, hemoconcentration, oliguria, and anasarca.

Although the panelists involved in making the 2000 UHC guidelines concluded that there was not enough information on the pathophysiology of OHSS to recommend the use of albumin to prevent it, a recent meta-analysis demonstrated that albumin administration was effective in the prevention of severe OHSS.[73] The meta-analysis of five randomized controlled trials compared the use of human albumin with placebo or no treatment on patient outcome. The albumin dose ranged from 10 to 50 g and was given at 2 hours before, 1 hour before, or just after oocyte retrieval. Albumin infusion was estimated to prevent one case of severe OHSS for every 18 women at risk.

As an alternative treatment to albumin infusion, some clinicians have attempted to prevent OHSS by withholding gonadotropins (so-called coasting). A retrospective study comparing intravenous albumin and coasting found that the latter was as effective as albumin in preventing OHSS in high-risk patients but that pregnancy rates were lower.[74] Although prophylactic albumin infusion has been shown to prevent severe OHSS, it is unknown whether therapeutic albumin infusion for women with an established diagnosis of severe OHSS is effective.

Resuscitation and Volume Expansion in Critically Ill Patients

In the past, albumin was given for volume expansion in critically ill patients because it was assumed to be more effective than crystalloids at increasing plasma volume while minimizing interstitial volume expansion. However, Fleck and colleagues demonstrated that the rate of albumin loss from the vasculature to the tissue spaces was markedly increased in critically ill patients, such as those with cachectic cancer or septic shock and those who had undergone cardiac surgery,[75] suggesting that albumin administration may not be beneficial in these patient populations. Albumin infusion may also have detrimental effects and can cause renal dysfunction, decreased sodium clearance, and increased free water clearance in patients with hypovolemic shock.[76] It has been suggested that albumin inhibits platelet aggregation and enhances antithrombin III activity.[77,78]

In the late 1990s, a meta-analysis of 30 randomized controlled trials compared the use of albumin versus crystalloids or no albumin and found that when albumin was used to treat patients with hypovolemia, burns, or hypoalbuminemia the risk of death was 6% higher than in patients not treated with albumin.[33] The results prompted the FDA to issue a letter to health care providers on August 19, 1998, urging discretion in the use of albumin in the critically ill population.[79] Subsequently, a review of 17 studies found no difference in the incidence of pulmonary edema, length of hospital stay, and mortality in adult patients receiving crystalloids compared to those receiving albumin.[80] A meta-analysis of 55 trials conducted by Wilkes and Navickis[81] also did not show a significant difference in the mortality rate when albumin was administered versus crystalloids, no albumin, or lower doses of albumin. The patient populations studied included high-risk neonates, burn patients, patients with ascites, patients with hypoalbuminemia, and trauma patients, among others. The more recent Saline versus Albumin Fluid Evaluation (SAFE) trial[82] supported the conclusion of the Choi review and the Wilkes and Navickis meta-analysis.[80,81] The SAFE-trial randomly assigned 6997 ICU patients to receive either 4% albumin or saline for fluid resuscitation and found no significant differences in outcome in the number of days of mechanical ventilation, number of days in the ICU, length of the hospital stay, or in mortality rate at 28 days. The study included subgroups of patients with trauma, severe sepsis, and acute respiratory distress syndrome (ARDS); however, the study had insufficient power to draw conclusions regarding albumin use in these populations.[82] These studies prompted the FDA's Blood Products Advisory Committee (BPAC) to release an information sheet on May 16, 2005, indicating that the SAFE study resolved previous safety concerns and urging further studies on the use of albumin in burn patients and in patients with traumatic brain injury and septic shock.[83] An updated meta-analysis from the Cochrane Injuries Group concludes that that there is no evidence that albumin reduces mortality to a greater extent than much less expensive and equally safe options such as crystalloids in the overall critically ill patient population.[84] Table 21–2 lists subsets of critically ill patients (e.g., burn patients, patients in hemorrhagic or nonhemorrhagic shock, patients in particular postoperative situations, etc.) who may benefit from albumin administration according to UHC guidelines. In these situations, albumin is typically used when other treatments are ineffective.

POTENTIAL ADVERSE REACTIONS

The incidence of adverse reactions to albumin infusions is approximately 1 in 6600 infusions, with only 1 in 30,000 infusions being life threatening.[39] Most adverse reactions to albumin are mild and are either allergic in nature or are related to albumin's function as a volume expander. Some of the mild reactions that can occur include nausea, vomiting, increased salivation, chills, and febrile reactions.[85] Owing to albumin's role in increasing colloidal osmotic pressure and intravascular volume, rapid infusion can result in circulatory overload, pulmonary edema, and decreases in hematocrit and hemoglobin. Albumin, with its high negative charge, binds calcium and can also cause complications related to hypocalcemia.[86] In addition, because albumin contains aluminum in trace amounts, large doses can cause aluminum to accumulate in patients with chronic renal failure and lead to hypercalcemia, vitamin D–refractory osteodystrophy, anemia, and severe progressive encephalopathy.[8]

PPF preparations can cause allergic reactions and reactions related to intravascular volume expansion as well. PPF differs from other albumin-containing solutions because it includes a larger percentage of proteins other than albumin. PPF has been associated with hypocoagulability, which could be due to the platelet factor-4 and β-thromboglobulin present in the preparations. Owing to a higher concentration of contaminating proteins such as PKA, PPF causes more hypotensive episodes than albumin does and has been associated with metabolic acidosis in patients with renal dysfunction.[21]

INFECTIOUS POTENTIAL

Because plasma derivatives are made from pooled plasma from thousands of donors, reduction of infectious disease transmission is an important issue in plasma processing. The process of cold ethanol fractionation significantly reduces the concentration of viruses in plasma fractions. The pasteurization process also limits the transmission of infectious agents by denaturing viral proteins and nucleic acids, inactivating the viruses.[87–90] When plasma is deliberately spiked with viruses, the manufacturing process for the production of 25% albumin results in a global viral reduction ($\log_{10}$) of ≥17.8 for HIV; ≥16.3 for bovine viral diarrhea virus (BVDV), which is a model virus for HCV; and ≥16.4 for pseudorabies virus (PRV), which is a model virus for HBV.[91] The process results in a global viral reduction ($\log_{10}$) of 14.9 for reovirus, which is a small, nonenveloped virus; 7.8 for hepatitis A virus (HAV); and 6.8 for porcine parvovirus (PPV), which is a model virus for parvovirus B19.[91] There has never been a report of HIV or hepatitis C transmission through albumin infusion. One hepatitis B outbreak was reported in relation to PPF infusion in 1976,[92] but it probably resulted from a lack of uniform heating of the bulk product during the pasteurization process. Since 1977, the FDA has required that the heating step take place after the product is placed in individual containers.[1] Since that time, there have been no other reports of hepatitis B transmission through albumin products. Since albumin is acellular, cell-associated viruses such as CMV and Epstein-Barr virus are eliminated from the final product.

Cold ethanol fractionation and pasteurization reduces but does not eliminate the risk of bacterial contamination of albumin products. An outbreak of *Pseudomonas* bacteremia occurred in seven patients who had received albumin from the same lot in 1973. When 190 albumin vials from the suspected lot were cultured, one vial grew *Pseudomonas cepacia*. A subsequent experiment showed that, in addition to *P. cepacia*, *Escherichia coli*, *Bacillus subtilis*, *Candida albicans*, and *Staphylococcus epidermidis* also are able to grow in 25% albumin. In the experiment, *P. cepacia* remained viable in sealed vials of albumin kept at room temperature for 17 months after inoculation.[93] Although albumin solutions can support the growth of many types of bacteria, bacterial contamination of albumin products is rarely reported in the literature.

CONCLUSION

The development of therapeutic albumin formulations was critical for soldiers in need of volume support during World War II. Over the decades following that war, albumin was used in a wide variety of settings despite the relative lack of published evidence supporting its use in those situations. This led to the establishment of guidelines in 1975 that recommended more conservative use of albumin.[4] Since that time, studies have compared albumin with alternative fluids for volume expansion. When crystalloid administration was compared with albumin use in several clinical situations, no significant difference was demonstrated in terms of patient outcome.[80–82] Thus, usage guidelines for albumin have become even more conservative. Since albumin is more expensive than crystalloids and is a plasma derivative with related risks, crystalloids currently serve as first-line therapy for plasma expansion in most cases. The exceptions are those clinical scenarios in which albumin has demonstrated a significant clinical benefit over crystalloids, including large-scale therapeutic plasma exchange. At present, albumin is a valuable second-line treatment in many patients with conditions refractory to other plasma expanders.

REFERENCES

1. Code of Federal Regulations. Title 21 CFR 640. Washington, D.C., U.S. Government Printing Office, 2005 (revised annually).
2. Kendrick DB. The Bovine and Human Albumin Programs. In Coates JB (ed). Blood Program in World War II. Washington, D.C., U.S. Government Printing Office, 1964.
3. Kendrick DB. Byproducts of Plasma Fractionation. In Coates JB (ed). Blood Program in World War II. Washington, D.C., U.S. Government Printing Office, 1964.
4. Sgouris JT, Rene A (eds). Proceedings of the Workshop on Albumin. Washington, D.C., U.S. Government Printing Office, 1975.
5. Technology assessment: albumin, nonprotein colloid, and crystalloid solutions. Oak Brook, Ill., University HealthSystem Consortium, 2000.
6. Tanzi M, Gardner M, Megellas M, et al. Evaluation of the appropriate use of albumin in adult and pediatric patients. Am J Health Syst Pharm 2003;60:1330–1335.
7. Tarin Remohi MJ, Sanchez Arcos A, Santos Ramos B, et al. Costs related to inappropriate use of albumin in Spain. Ann Pharmacother 2000;34:1198–1205.
8. Immuno, U.S., Inc. Package insert for Albumin (Human) 5%, 1998.
9. Rothschild MA, Oratz M, Schreiber SS. Serum albumin. Hepatology 1988;8:385–401.
10. Matejtschuk P, Dash CH, Gascoigne EW. Production of human albumin solution: a continually developing colloid. Br J Anaesth 2000;85: 887–895.
11. Tullis JL. Albumin. 1. Background and use. JAMA 1977;237:355–360.
12. WHO Recommendations for the Production, Control, and Regulation of Human Plasma for Fractionation. Geneva, Switzerland, World Health Organization, 2005.
13. Plasma Protein Therapeutics Association, Available at http://www.plasmainfo.org. Accessed Jan. 3, 2006.
14. Testimony on Plasma Fractionator Industry FDA Regulation of Blood Safety by Thomas D. Roslewicz. Available at www.hhs.gov/asl/testify/t970605b.html. Accessed Jan. 3, 2006.

15. Baxter Albumin Therapy. Available at www.albumintherapy.com. Accessed Jan. 3, 2006.
16. Janeway CA. Human serum albumin: Historical review. In Sgouris JT, Rene A (eds). Proceedings of the Workshop on Albumin. Washington, D.C., U.S. Government Printing Office, 1975.
17. Cohn EJ, Strong LE, Hughes WL, et al. Preparation and properties of serum and plasma proteins. IV. A system for the separation into fractions of the protein and lipoprotein components of biological tissues and fluids. J Am Chem Soc 1946;68:459–475.
18. Finlayson JS. Physical and biochemical properties of human albumin. In Sgouris JT, Rene A (eds). Proceedings of the Workshop on Albumin. Washington, D.C., U.S. Government Printing Office, 1975.
19. Kendrick DB. The plasma program. In Coates JB (ed). Blood Program in World War II. Washington, D.C., U.S. Government Printing Office, 1964.
20. Curling JM, Berglof J, Lindquist LO, Eriksson S. A chromatographic procedure for the purification of human plasma albumin. Vox Sang 1977;33:97–107.
21. Finlayson J. Albumin products. Semin Thromb Hemost 1980;6:85–120.
22. Quirk AV, Geisow MJ, Woodrow JR, et al. Production of recombinant human serum albumin from Saccharomyces cerevisiae. Biotechnol Appl Biochem 1989;11:273–287.
23. Kobayashi K, Nakamura N, Sumi A, et al. The development of recombinant human serum albumin. Ther Apher 1998;2:257–262.
24. Bosse D, Praus M, Kiessling P, et al. Phase I comparability of recombinant human albumin and human serum albumin. J Clin Pharmacol 2005;45:57–67.
25. Immuno, U.S., Inc. Package insert for Albumin (Human) 25%, 1998.
26. McEvoy GK (ed). AHFS Drug Information. Bethesda, Md., American Society of Health-System Pharmacists, Inc., 2005.
27. Hemolysis Associated with 25% Human Albumin Diluted with Sterile Water—United States, 1994–1998. MMWR 1999;48:157–159.
28. USP DI Drug Information for the Healthcare Professional, 25th ed. Available at http://online.statref.com/document.aspx?fxid=6&docid=2. Accessed Jan. 3, 2006.
29. Talecris Biotherapeutics, Inc. Package insert for Plasbumin-5 (Low Aluminum), Albumin (Human) 5%, USP, 2005.
30. Talecris Biotherapeutics, Inc. Plasbumin-20 (Low Aluminum), Albumin (Human) 20%, USP, 2005.
31. Talecris Biotherapeutics, Inc. Plasbumin-25 (Low Aluminum), Albumin (Human) 25%, USP, 2005.
32. Koot BG, Houwen R, Pot DJ, Nauta J. Congenital analbuminaemia: biochemical and clinical implications—a case report and literature review. Eur J Pediatr 2004;163:664–670.
33. Human albumin administration in critically ill patients: systematic review of randomised controlled trials. Cochrane Injuries Group Albumin Reviewers. BMJ 1998;317:235–240.
34. Strauss RG, Pennell BJ, Stump DC. A randomized, blinded trial comparing the hemostatic effects of pentastarch versus hetastarch. Transfusion 2002;42:27–36.
35. Owen HG, Brecher ME. Partial colloid starch replacement for therapeutic plasma exchange. J Clin Apher 1997;12:87–92.
36. Kimme P, Jannsen B, Ledin T, et al. High incidence of pruritus after large doses of hydroxyethyl starch (HES) infusions. Acta Anaesthesiol Scand 2001;45:686–689.
37. Roberts JS, Bratton SL. Colloid volume expanders: problems, pitfalls and possibilities. Drugs 1998;55:621–630.
38. Vercueil A, Grocott MP, Mythen MG. Physiology, pharmacology, and rationale for colloid administration for the maintenance of effective hemodynamic stability in critically ill patients. Transfus Med Rev 2005;19:93–109.
39. Nearman HS, Herman ML. Toxic effects of colloids in the intensive care unit. Crit Care Clin 1991;7:713–723.
40. Leblond PF, Rock G, Herbert CA. The use of plasma as a replacement fluid in plasma exchange. Canadian Apheresis Group. Transfusion 1998;38:834–838.
41. Watson DK, Penny AF, Marshall RW, Robinson EA. Citrate induced hypocalcaemia during cell separation. Br J Haematol 1980;44:503–507.
42. American Association of Blood Banks, America's Blood Centers, and American Red Cross Circular of Information for the Use of Human Blood and Blood Components, July 2002.
43. Obrador GT, Zeigler ZR, Shadduck RK, et al. Effectiveness of cryosupernatant therapy in refractory and chronic relapsing thrombotic thrombocytopenic purpura. Am J Hematol 1993;42:217–220.
44. Levy GG, Nichols WC, Lian EC, et al. Mutations in a member of the ADAMTS gene family cause thrombotic thrombocytopenic purpura. Nature 2001;413:488–494.
45. Tao Z, Peng Y, Nolasco L, et al. Role of the CUB-1 domain in docking ADAMTS-13 to unusually large Von Willebrand factor in flowing blood. Blood 2005;106:4139–4145.
46. Zheng X, Chung D, Takayama TK, et al. Structure of von Willebrand factor-cleaving protease (ADAMTS13), a metalloprotease involved in thrombotic thrombocytopenic purpura. J Biol Chem 2001;276:41059–41063.
47. Tsai HM, Lian EC. Antibodies to von Willebrand factor-cleaving protease in acute thrombotic thrombocytopenic purpura. N Engl J Med 1998;339:1585–1594.
48. Furlan M, Robles R, Galbusera M, et al. von Willebrand factor-cleaving protease in thrombotic thrombocytopenic purpura and the hemolytic-uremic syndrome. N Engl J Med 339:1578–84, 1998.
49. Owen HG, Brecher ME. Atypical reactions associated with use of angiotensin-converting enzyme inhibitors and apheresis. Transfusion 1994;34:891–894.
50. Martin PY, Gines P, Schrier RW. Nitric oxide as a mediator of hemodynamic abnormalities and sodium and water retention in cirrhosis. N Engl J Med 1998;339:533–541.
51. Runyon BA. Management of adult patients with ascites due to cirrhosis. Hepatology 2004;39:841–856.
52. Gines P, Tito L, Arroyo V, et al. Randomized comparative study of therapeutic paracentesis with and without intravenous albumin in cirrhosis. Gastroenterology 1988;94:1493–1502.
53. Peltekian KM, Wong F, Liu PP, et al. Cardiovascular, renal, and neurohumoral responses to single large-volume paracentesis in patients with cirrhosis and diuretic-resistant ascites. Am J Gastroenterol 1997; 92:394–399.
54. Gines A, Fernandez-Esparrach G, Monescillo A, et al. Randomized trial comparing albumin, dextran 70, and polygeline in cirrhotic patients with ascites treated by paracentesis. Gastroenterology 1996;111:1002–1010.
55. Salerno F, Merli M, Riggio O, et al. Randomized controlled study of TIPS versus paracentesis plus albumin in cirrhosis with severe ascites. Hepatology 2004;40:629–635.
56. Gines P, Uriz J, Calahorra B, et al. Transjugular intrahepatic portosystemic shunting versus paracentesis plus albumin for refractory ascites in cirrhosis. Gastroenterology 2002;123:1839–1847.
57. Rossle M, Ochs A, Gulberg V, et al. A comparison of paracentesis and transjugular intrahepatic portosystemic shunting in patients with ascites. N Engl J Med 2000;342:1701–1707.
58. Sort P, Navasa M, Arroyo V, et al. Effect of intravenous albumin on renal impairment and mortality in patients with cirrhosis and spontaneous bacterial peritonitis. N Engl J Med 1999;341:403–409.
59. Quinlan GJ, Margarson MP, Mumby S, et al. Administration of albumin to patients with sepsis syndrome: a possible beneficial role in plasma thiol repletion. Clin Sci (Lond) 1998;95:459–465.
60. Orth SR, Ritz E. The nephrotic syndrome. N Engl J Med 1998;338: 1202–1211.
61. Inoue M, Okajima K, Itoh K, et al. Mechanism of furosemide resistance in analbuminemic rats and hypoalbuminemic patients. Kidney Int 1987;32:198–203.
62. Fliser D, Zurbruggen I, Mutschler E, et al. Coadministration of albumin and furosemide in patients with the nephrotic syndrome. Kidney Int 1999;55:629–634.
63. Chalasani N, Gorski JC, Horlander JC Sr, et al. Effects of albumin/furosemide mixtures on responses to furosemide in hypoalbuminemic patients. J Am Soc Nephrol 2001;12:1010–1016.
64. Akcicek F, Yalniz T, Basci A, et al. Diuretic effect of frusemide in patients with nephrotic syndrome: is it potentiated by intravenous albumin? BMJ 1995;310:162–163.
65. Yoshimura A, Ideura T, Iwasaki S, et al. Aggravation of minimal change nephrotic syndrome by administration of human albumin. Clin Nephrol 1992;37:109–114.
66. Haws RM, Baum M. Efficacy of albumin and diuretic therapy in children with nephrotic syndrome. Pediatrics 1993;91:1142–1146.
67. Vermeulen LC Jr, Ratko TA, Erstad BL, et al. A paradigm for consensus: The University Hospital Consortium guidelines for the use of albumin, nonprotein colloid, and crystalloid solutions. Arch Intern Med 1995;155:373–379.
68. Ovarian hyperstimulation syndrome. Fertil Steril 2004;82:S81–S86.
69. Klemetti R, Sevon T, Gissler M, Hemminki E. Complications of IVF and ovulation induction. Hum Reprod 2005;20:3293–3300.
70. Rabau E, David A, Serr DM, et al. Human menopausal gonadotropins for anovulation and sterility: results of 7 years of treatment. Am J Obstet Gynecol 1967;98:92–98.
71. Schenker JG, Weinstein D. Ovarian hyperstimulation syndrome: a current survey. Fertil Steril 1978;30:255–268.
72. Budev MM, Arroliga AC, Falcone T. Ovarian hyperstimulation syndrome. Crit Care Med 2005;33:S301–S306.
73. Aboulghar M, Evers JH, Al-Inany H. Intravenous albumin for preventing severe ovarian hyperstimulation syndrome. Cochrane Database Syst Rev 2002:CD001302.

74. Chen CD, Chao KH, Yang JH, et al. Comparison of coasting and intravenous albumin in the prevention of ovarian hyperstimulation syndrome. Fertil Steril 2003;80:86–90.
75. Fleck A, Raines G, Hawker F, et al. Increased vascular permeability: a major cause of hypoalbuminaemia in disease and injury. Lancet 1985;1:781–784.
76. Moon MR, Lucas CE, Ledgerwood AM, et al. Free water clearance after supplemental albumin resuscitation for shock. Circ Shock 1989;28:1–8.
77. Joorgensen KA, Stoffersen E. Heparin like activity of albumin. Thromb Res 1979;16:569–574.
78. Jorgensen KA, Stoffersen E. On the inhibitory effect of albumin on platelet aggregation. Thromb Res 1980;17:13–18.
79. Letter to Healthcare Providers. Available at http://www.fda.gov/cber/ltr/albumin.htm. Accessed Jan. 3, 2006.
80. Choi PT, Yip G, Quinonez LG, Cook DJ. Crystalloids vs. colloids in fluid resuscitation: a systematic review. Crit Care Med 1999;27:200–210.
81. Wilkes MM, Navickis RJ. Patient survival after human albumin administration: a meta-analysis of randomized, controlled trials. Ann Intern Med 2001;135:149–164.
82. Finfer S, Bellomo R, Boyce N, et al. A comparison of albumin and saline for fluid resuscitation in the intensive care unit. N Engl J Med 2004;350:2247–2256.
83. Safety of Albumin Administration in Critically Ill Patients. Available at http://www.fda.gov/cber/infosheets/albsaf051605.htm. Accessed Jan. 3, 2006.
84. Alderson P, Bunn F, Lefebvre C, et al. Human albumin solution for resuscitation and volume expansion in critically ill patients. Cochrane Database Syst Rev 2004;CD001208.
85. Aventis Behring L.L.C. Package insert for Albuminar-25 Albumin (Human) U.S.P., 25%, 2001.
86. Gales BJ, Erstad BL. Adverse reactions to human serum albumin. Ann Pharmacother 1993;27:87–94.
87. Erstad BL. Viral infectivity of albumin and plasma protein fraction. Pharmacotherapy 1996;16:996–1001.
88. McClelland DB. Safety of human albumin as a constituent of biologic therapeutic products. Transfusion 1998;38:690–699.
89. Yei S, Yu MW, Tankersley DL. Partitioning of hepatitis C virus during Cohn-Oncley fractionation of plasma. Transfusion 1992;32:824–828.
90. Scheiblauer H, Nubling M, Willkommen H, Lower J. Prevalence of hepatitis C virus in plasma pools and the effectiveness of cold ethanol fractionation. Clin Ther 1996;18:59–70.
91. Cai K, Gierman TM, Hotta J, et al. Ensuring the biologic safety of plasma-derived therapeutic proteins: detection, inactivation, and removal of pathogens. BioDrugs 2005;19:79–96.
92. Pattison CP, Klein CA, Leger RT, et al. An outbreak of type B hepatitis associated with transfusion of plasma protein fraction. Am J Epidemiol 1976;103:399–407.
93. Steere AC. Adverse reactions to albumin caused by bacterial contamination. In Sgouris JT, Rene A (eds). Proceedings of the Workshop on Albumin. Washington, D.C., U.S. Government Printing Office, 1975.

Chapter 22

IVIG and Derivatives

Elizabeth E. Culler • Lennart E. Lögdberg

INTRODUCTION

The immunoglobulins (Igs)[1] constitute a major class of structurally similar globular plasma proteins. Owing to their antibody activity they are the principal effector molecules of specific humoral immunity, but they also function as broad regulators of immune system activity. The elucidation of the biochemical structure of Ig proteins and their corresponding genes unraveled the molecular basis of antibody activity and diversity in the 1960s and 1970s.[2]

The diversity of Ig genes is known to be inherited in the germline, then magnified by recombination during embryonal development and expressed in each individual as a polyclonal B-lymphocyte repertoire.[2] Each B-lymphocyte clone carries its own unique cell surface Ig molecule and therefore a single antibody specificity. During an immune response, the provoking agent (antigen) interacts with and activates the B-cell clones that have a cell surface Ig containing a matching antibody combining site. Following activation, these B-cell clones differentiate into plasma cells, each of which mass-produces and releases soluble Ig molecules with the same or improved (by somatic mutation and further antigen-driven selection) antibody specificities as the parental B-cell clone.

The progress with respect to our molecular understanding of Ig has been paralleled, in the last few decades, by improved methods to select, produce, purify, and manufacture therapeutic Ig products. These methods include development of the hybridoma technology, allowing production of homogenous Ig molecules with predefined, single-antigen specificities (monoclonal antibodies [MABs]).[3] At present, there is a wide array of such products on the market, including both polyclonal and monoclonal preparations. The polyclonal products represent either attempts to capture representative sets of polyclonal Ig (mainly, intravenous immunoglobulin[IVIG]), or polyclonal Ig selected for particularly high titers of antibodies against a given antigen (hyperimmune globulin or hyper-Ig). Therapeutic MABs have mostly reached the market in the last decade.[4] Each MAB product has been selected to react with a specific pharmacologic target, usually a cell surface receptor or a soluble bioactive mediator.

Today, polyclonal Ig products have a wide range of therapeutic uses most falling within three broad clinical categories. IVIG is the main product for two of these: *replacement therapy* for patients with congenital or acquired deficiencies of humoral immunity (e.g., hypo- or agammaglobulinemia) and *immunomodulation.* Hyper-Ig preparations, by comparison, are therapies of choice for *transferring specific passive immunity,* particularly used in four situations: (1) prophylaxis or treatment of infectious diseases; (2) neutralization of toxins, venoms, or drug overdoses; (3) prevention of alloimmunization; and (4) selective immunosuppression.

At present, the FDA has approved the use of IVIG for six indications with nine products on the market.[5–13] However, because of its wide-ranging immunomodulatory effects, IVIG increasingly is being used off-label to treat a diverse assortment of diseases.[14,15] At present, the off-label use of IVIG exceeds the product's use for FDA-approved indications.[15] Similarly, a large number of hyper-Ig products are approved for their respective niche markets.

The development of therapeutic MABs represents a revolution in immunotherapy with all but 2 of the 17 marketed MAB products achieving FDA-approval in the last decade. Indications for these products include the treatment of organ allograft rejection, autoimmune or allergic diseases, and some types of malignant tumors. With over 400 additional MABs in clinical trials, Paul Ehrlich's now century-old dream of creating "magic bullets" for selective treatment of diseases is being realized.[16]

This chapter reviews the characteristics and clinical uses of the various Ig preparations that are FDA-approved for therapeutic administration in the United States.

DEVELOPMENT OF IMMUNOGLOBULINS FOR THERAPEUTIC USE: A SHORT HISTORY

Igs were first detected as antibody activity more than a century ago when, in 1890, Emil von Behring and Shibasabo Kitasato discovered that exposure of animals to diphtheria toxin induced them to produce soluble factors in plasma/serum that could transfer protection against diphtheria to "nonimmune" humans.[17] The factor responsible for this *passive immunity* was called "antitoxin." A decade later, Paul Ehrlich recognized that humans can also actively mount their own similar "antibody" responses specific to toxins or bacteria, providing the body with *active immunity* to the relevant pathogen.[16] He further suggested that such "magic bullets" might be involved in warding off tumors. Before the development of antibiotics and other antimicrobial drugs, passive serotherapy for infectious diseases became the first clinical use of Ig.

During World War II, cold ethanol fractionation was used to mass produce the protein fraction responsible for antibody activity (later shown to be polyclonal Ig).[18] As IV agents, however, these preparations caused chills, fever, and shock, later shown to be due to the presence of high-molecular-weight aggregates in the product.[19] Intramuscular (IM) administration of Ig using lower doses became the predominant mode of delivery and resulted in fewer side effects. In fact, this was the route used by Bruton when he successfully treated a patient with congenital agammaglobulinemia,[20] thus demonstrating, for the first time, the efficacy of exogenous Ig to confer global passive immunity and prevent infection in patients broadly deficient in humoral immunity.

Despite the limited doses of Ig that could be administered IM, this injection route continued to be the primary method of Ig administration until 1981, when a new processing method limited aggregate formation in the Ig preparations. This enabled the safe IV administration of large Ig doses[19] and rapidly led to the approval of IVIG formulations that now dominate the market.

In addition to the expanded use of IVIG in the modern era, hyper-Ig formulations also have been developed for the treatment of specific infectious diseases.[21] Like IVIG, the hyperimmune Igs are polyclonal Igs purified via fractionation of large plasma pools. However, in the latter case the pools are derived either[1] from specifically immunized (vaccinated) donors or[2] by preselecting specific high-titer plasma donations before pooling.

The hybridoma technology to develop murine MABs was described in 1975[3] and quickly led to attempts to develop therapeutic products. However, the first generation of therapeutic MAB candidates largely failed in clinical trials because of their tendency to provoke human anti-mouse antibody (HAMA) responses in the patients.[4] After many years of efforts to overcome the technologic difficulties, researchers are now proficient in creating and developing "near human" or fully human MABs with antibody specificity directed against human target molecules. This has resulted in FDA approval for clinical use of many products of this kind in the last decade.

IMMUNOGLOBULINS: PHYSICOCHEMICAL AND BIOLOGICAL ASPECTS

Ig proteins, then, are the family of molecules that carry antibody activity.[2] These proteins are synthesized and secreted by plasma cells, originating from resting B lymphocytes activated by antigen during an initial immune response. The B lymphocytes are "clonally selected" for activation by the antigen because they synthesize and express a cell surface Ig molecule reacting with sufficient avidity with the same antigen. This cell surface Ig is, in essence, of the same specificity as the soluble Ig molecule that their clonally expanded activated offspring—the plasma cell—will mass-produce.

The basic structure of an Ig molecule consists of two identical heterodimers, each comprising a larger (heavy [H]) and a smaller (light [L]) polypeptide chain linked by interchain disulfide bonds. The two heterodimers are kept together by disulfide bridges between the two H chains. Each H and L chain, in turn, is composed of a variable (V) and a constant (C) region, organized in globular units called Ig domains [V_H,C_{H1}, C_{H2}, C_{H3}, (C_{H4}), V_L, and C_L], the two V regions (V_H and V_L) together forming an antigen-binding site. The contact residues of this binding site are largely encoded by the so-called hypervariable regions of the V genes, whereas the rest of these genes are thought of as "framework regions."

The basis for antibody diversity, that is, that the immune system is intrinsically capable of mounting tailor-made antibodies to the universe of foreign antigens, is a combination of[1] inherited germline diversity of both V_H- and V_L-gene-families,[2] so-called junctional diversity, which occurs when IgC- and IgV-region genes recombine during development of B lymphocytes from their progenitor cells,[3] combinatorial diversity due to cooperation of diverse V_H- and V_L-gene products in creating the antigen-binding site, and[4] somatic hypermutation of hypervariable region V-gene codons during B-lymphocyte activation, combined with reselection by antigen of those B-lymphocyte clones that possess higher affinity Ig receptors.

There are five linked, but distinct, H-chain C genes (α, δ, ε, γ, and μ) on human chromosome 14 that can recombine with members of the same, linked V_H-gene family if selected during lymphocyte development and plasma cell differentiation. Each H-chain constant region confers different physicochemical and biological properties to the resulting plasma Ig molecule, leading to five Ig classes (or *isotypes*): IgA, IgD, IgE, IgG, and IgM. IgG is the predominant isotype in plasma (75% of plasma Ig). IgG, of which 55% is found extravascularly, is second only to albumin among plasma proteins in quantity, with a concentration of about 10 g/L. The plasma half-life of IgG is about 3 weeks, and it is the only Ig class that crosses the placenta. The plasma IgG of a donor represents a mixture of IgG species from thousands of different plasma cell clones and their precursors actively produced during the last several months prior to donation.

Enzymatic cleavage of the double IgG heterodimer yields two Fab′ fragments (V_H,$C\gamma_{H1}$- V_L,C_L) or one $(Fab')_2$ fragment (depending on the enzyme used) and one Fc fragment ($C\gamma_{H2}$, $C\gamma_{H3}$-$C\gamma_{H2}$, $C\gamma_{H3}$). Each Fab′ fragment contains an *a*ntigen-*b*inding site (V_H,V_L), a complete L chain (V_L, C_L), and the first part of the H-chain constant region (C_{H1}). The *c*rystallizable Fc-fragment consists of a homodimer of the remaining parts of the H-chain constant regions, which make up the binding site for (1) cellular receptors (Fc receptors) on various cells, such as monocyte/macrophages and granulocytes, and (2) proteins of the complement cascade.

The other four Ig classes have physicochemical and biological properties that are distinct from those of IgG, including their own Fc receptors on a variety of immune system–related effector cells. Thus, they likely fulfill important and unique functions in host defense, such as during the initiation of primary immune responses (IgD and IgM are the predominant receptor molecules on naive B lymphocytes) or when mucosal immunity is needed and they serve as secretory molecules.

However, IgG molecules appear to function as the main humoral basis of long-lasting immunity. This critical role and their high prevalence have made them the predominant Ig molecules selected for therapeutic development thus far. The bulk of the clinical experience has been with polyclonal IgG, but the last few years have witnessed a rapidly expanding clinical database of patients treated with FDA-approved MABs.

POLYCLONAL IMMUNOGLOBULINS

The original therapeutic use of Ig was as a transfer vehicle of passive immunity against specific infectious disease agents through serotherapy.[16] The idea of using polyclonal Ig to transfer *global* passive immunity to individuals with broad humoral immunodeficiency was realized much later. Whereas the latter use is a direct replacement therapy that relies on the therapeutic product to transfer broad representative humoral immunocompetence, the former use can be seen as a version of agent-specific passive protection during a vulnerable period, before otherwise immunocompetent individuals have mounted their own responses. In both cases, though, polyclonal Igs are used. In addition, in both cases, the therapeutic products are manufactured from plasma pools.

In the first case, the goal is to transfer specific antibodies against selected antigens using an Ig preparation with high titers against these antigens. This kind of Ig preparation is represented by the various commercialized *hyper-Ig products*. In conferring global passive immunity, by comparison, the goal is to create an Ig preparation with a representative spectrum of antibody titers reflecting average humoral immunocompetence. This kind of Ig preparation is represented by the *IVIG products* currently on the market.

Commercial Production

IVIG

IUIS/WHO GUIDELINES FOR IVIG PRODUCTION

FDA regulations regarding polyclonal Ig production were established for IM formulations only and have not been updated to cover IVIG products.[22] Unique specifications for IVIG production are determined for each manufacturer through negotiations prior to approval of the Biologics License Application.[15] Although each manufacturer produces IVIG using a different combination of steps, most manufacturers follow the general guidelines established for IVIG production by the IUIS/WHO (International Union of Immunological Societies/World Health Organization) in 1982[23]:

1. The *source* material should be plasma obtained from a pool of at least 1000 donors.
2. For *safety* purposes, the final products should be virtually free of prekallikrein activator, kinins, plasmin, accumulative preservatives, or potentially harmful contaminants. The IgA concentration and the level of IgG aggregates should be as low as possible.
3. To meet *quality control* guidelines, the products should contain at least 90% intact IgG. The IgG should maintain opsonin activity, complement binding, and other biological activities. The IgG subclasses should be present in similar proportions to those in normal pooled plasma. The antibody levels against at least two species of bacteria (or toxins) and two viruses (by neutralization) should be determined. There must be at least 0.1 IU of hepatitis B antibody per milliliter and a hepatitis A radioimmunoassay titer of at least 1:1000.
4. The manufacturer should *specify the contents* of the final product including the diluent and any other additive used. Any chemical modifications of the Ig made by the manufacturer should be described.

PLASMA COLLECTION FOR IVIG PRODUCTION

The process of plasma collection is regulated by the FDA.[22] Many plasma collection facilities belong to the Plasma Protein Therapeutics Association (PPTA), which offers an International Quality Plasma Program (IQPP) certification requiring that facilities meet voluntary standards established by the PPTA.[24] In addition, WHO has published guidelines pertaining to plasma collection.[25] Chapter 19 provides more detailed information on determining donor suitability for plasma collection, prefractionation infectious disease testing, and regulation of the plasma industry.

IVIG is derived from plasma collected either by whole blood donation (Recovered Plasma) or by apheresis (Source Plasma).[22] Plasma so obtained is pooled to serve as the starting material for IVIG production. Source plasma accounts for approximately 80% and plasma recovered from whole blood accounts for about 20% of the plasma used for the manufacture of IVIG.[15]

SIZE OF PLASMA POOLS

Although the IUIS/WHO regulations for IVIG set the minimum number of donors from which plasma should be obtained for immunoglobulin production at 1000,[23] currently there is not a similarly set maximum number of donors that can be pooled. The pool size is proprietary information and is unique to each manufacturer, but it is thought that plasma from several hundreds of thousands of donors are typically pooled to create IVIG products, leading to enhanced concerns about infectious disease transmission. In 1997, the Subcommittee on Human Resources of the House Committee on Government Reform and Oversight requested recommendations from the National Institute of Allergy and Infectious Diseases regarding the minimum donor pool size needed for safety and efficacy of immunoglobulin products.[26] An expert panel determined that there was not enough scientific data to set a minimum number of donors to ensure an effective product. Because of the proven safety record of the currently produced formulations and because limiting the donor size could limit the supply of the product, the panel decided not to recommend capping the donor size below that which is currently used.[26]

PROCESSING METHODS

In addition to differences in the source of plasma, manufacturers also differ in (1) the steps used to fractionate, purify, and stabilize Ig, (2) the methods used to inactivate and/or remove viruses from the preparations, and (3) the formulation of the final product.[27] This variation causes differences in composition between the brands of IVIG products, some of which can be clinically significant. Table 22–1 lists some of these differences in processing methods and final composition among marketed IVIG products.

In general, Igs are isolated from the plasma using modifications of the cold ethanol fractionation method (see Chapter 12). The product is further purified and the viral load is reduced by means of filtration steps (e.g., nanofiltration, ultrafiltration, depth filtration), chromatography, and precipitation. Viruses may be inactivated physically by heat (e.g., pasteurization) and chemical/enzymatic methods (e.g., incubation at low pH with or without enzymatic treatment, or treatment with methylene blue, psoralens, riboflavin, caprylate, or solvent detergents).[27]

Many of these steps not only limit viral transmission but also serve to reduce the concentration of IgG aggregates. Examples of such approaches are ion exchange chromatography, treatment with pepsin at a pH of 4, and use of polyethylene glycol (PEG) to precipitate aggregates. Simply maintaining the product at pH 4 during storage limits aggregate formation because IgG exists almost exclusively in a monomeric form at this pH.[28] The fraction of IgG aggregates in the product may also be limited by the addition of stabilizers such as sucrose, glucose, glycine, maltose, sorbitol, and albumin.[28]

Table 22–1 **Available IVIG* Preparations, Methods of Production, and Composition**

Product	Manufacturer	How Supplied	Method of Production	Additive	Osmolarity or Osmolality	pH	IgA Content
Carimune NF IV	ZLB Behring	Lyophilized, 1, 3, 6, or 12 g	Cold ethanol fractionation and depth filtration, pH4/pepsin, nanofiltration	1.67 g sucrose/g of protein, <20 mg sodium/g of protein	192–1074 mOsm/kg (depending on concentration and diluent used)	6.4–6.8	Trace
Flebogamma 5%	Grifols	Liquid, 10 mL (0.5 g), 50 mL (2.5 g), 100 mL (5.0 g), 200 mL (10.0 g)	Cold ethanol fractionation, polyethylene glycol precipitation, ion exchange chromatography, pasteurization at 60°C for 10 hours	50 mg/mL of D-sorbitol, <3.2 mEq sodium/L, ≤6 mg PEG/mL	240–350 mOsm/L	5.0–6.0	<0.05 mg/mL
Gammagard S/D	Baxter Healthcare	Lyophilized, 2.5 g, 5 g, 10 g	Cold ethanol fractionation, ultrafiltration, ion-exchange chromatography, solvent/detergent treatment	20 mg/mL of glucose, 22.5 mg/mL glycine, 3 mg/mL albumin, 8.5 mg sodium/mL, 2 mg PEG/mL	5% 636 mOsm/L, 10% 1250 mOsm/L	6.4–7.2	≤2.2 μg/mL
Gammagard liquid 10%	Baxter Healthcare	Liquid, 10 mL (1.0 g), 25 mL (2.5 g), 50 mL (5.0 g), 100 mL (10.0 g), 200 mL (20.0 g)	Cold ethanol fractionation, chromatography, solvent/detergent treatment, nanofiltration, low pH incubation	0.25 mol/L of glycine	240–300 mOsmol/kg	4.6–5.1	37 μg/mL
Gammar-P IV	ZLB Behring	Lyophilized, 1 g, 2.5 g, 5 g, 10 g	Cold ethanol fractionation, pasteurization at 60°C for 10 hours	50 mg/mL of sucrose, 3% albumin, 5 mg sodium/mL	5% 309 mOsm/L, 10% 600 mOsm/L	6.4–7.2	<25 μg/mL
Gamunex 10%	Talecris Biotherapeutics	Liquid, 10 mL (1.0 g), 25 mL (2.5 g), 50 mL (5.0 g), 100 mL (10.0 g), 200 mL (20.0 g)	Cold ethanol fractionation, caprylate precipitation/cloth filtration, caprylate incubation, depth filtration, column chromatography, low pH incubation	0.16–0.24 mol/L of glycine, trace sodium	258 mOsm/kg	4.0–4.5	0.046 mg/mL
Iveegam EN	Baxter Healthcare	Lyophilized, 0.5 g, 1 g, 2.5 g, 5 g	Cold ethanol fractionation, 12% alcohol precipitation, ion exchange chromatography, incubation with immobilized hydrolases, and PEG precipitation	50 mg/mL of glucose, 3 mg sodium/mL, <0.5 g PEG/dL	≥240 mOsm/L	6.4–7.2	Trace
Octagam	Octapharma USA	Liquid, 20 mL (1 g), 50 mL (2.5 g), 100 mL (5 g), 200 mL (10 g)	Cold ethanol fractionation, ultrafiltration, chromatography, S/D treatment, pH 4 treatment	100 mg/mL of maltose, ≤30 mmol sodium/L	310–380 mOsmol/kg	5.1–6.0	≤1 mg/mL
Polygam S/D	Baxter Healthcare	Lyophilized, 1 g, 3 g, 6 g, 12 g	Cold ethanol fractionation, ultrafiltration, ion-exchange chromatography, solvent/detergent treatment	1.67 g sucrose/g of protein, <20 mg sodium/g of protein	192–1074 mOsm/kg (depending on concentration and diluent used)	6.4–6.8	Trace

*IVIG should never be frozen.
Data from refs. 5 through 13.

Hyper-Ig

Hyper-Ig preparations are manufactured much in the same manner as IVIG, with the exception of the donor selection step. The plasma used for the manufacture is drawn from donors who have high titers of the Ig specificity of interest. The donors may have obtained immunity naturally, through prophylactic immunization, or through targeted immunization for the purpose of becoming a donor of hyper-Ig.[28] Following collection and pooling, donor plasma is fractionated and purified, then undergoes viral reduction steps as described in the section on IVIG production. Hyper-Ig products should contain at least fivefold increased titer of the antibody-specificity of interest, compared to otherwise quantitatively comparable standard preparations of IVIG, according to guidelines established by IUIS/WHO in 1982.[23]

Hyper-Ig products are usually derived from human plasma. Exceptions include several hyper-Ig products for neutralization of venoms or toxins, where immune plasma donors generally are not prevalent in the population, and the risk for adverse consequences on active immunization of volunteer donors is too high. Instead, hyper-Ig products directed toward such targets are derived from plasma from animals immunized against these substances.

Clinical Considerations

The rational for the therapeutic use of polyclonal Ig products is based on the paramount importance of Ig in immunity. Thus, in patients with acquired or congenital Ig deficiency (e.g., hypo- or agammaglobulinemia), these products are aids to globally supplement or replace the missing antigen-specific humoral effector components of the deficient immune system. Such treatment protects these patients against their otherwise increased susceptibility to infections. In other groups of patients, disease is caused by dysregulation of the immune system, pathology often being mediated by the activity of autoantibodies. Polyclonal Ig products, by causing immunomodulation, can provide alleviation of the disease in such patients. The mechanisms of Ig-induced immunomodulation are incompletely understood (see below). IVIGs are currently the products most often used, both for global Ig replacement and for Ig-induced immunomodulation, although hyper-Ig products can also be used for these purposes.[29] However, hyper-Igs have been developed with antigen-specific purposes in mind and are the products of choice for transfer of specific passive immunity for a variety of conditions, as described below.

Mechanism of Action

IVIG

IVIG preparations typically are prepared from plasma pools representing many thousands of human donors. Given the capability of the individual human immune system to produce an estimated up to 10^8 different antibody specificities toward unique antigen epitopes,[30] IVIG products contain a diverse collection of antibody specificities indeed. Therefore, it is not surprising that the mechanisms by which IVIGs exert their effects are incompletely understood.

Some of the known or possible mechanisms are[15,31] (1) classical elimination of opsonized infectious organisms by antibody-dependent cell-mediated cytotoxicity (ADCC) or by complement activation followed by lysis, (2) neutralization of soluble infectious proteins by immunocomplex formation and elimination through the reticuloendothelial system (RES), (3) anti-idiotypic regulation of autoreactive B lymphocytes or antibodies (IVIG contains a broad array of anti-idiotype autoantibodies that can interact with these cellular or humoral autoreactive agents), and (4) "Fc-receptor blockade," which can block clearing of autoantibody-opsonized cells (e.g., platelets in idiopathic thrombocytopenic purpura).

The first two of these mechanisms are important in conferring protection by IVIG to patients with humoral immunodeficiency. The last two are mechanisms by which IVIG causes broad immunomodulation.

HYPER-IG

Hyper-Igs contain high concentrations of Ig against specified antigens. Selected opsonized cellular targets are lysed through complement activation or by ADCC,[15,31] whereas soluble target antigens are bound in immunocomplexes and then eliminated by the RES. Because hyper-Igs are polyclonal Igs, they exert immunomodulation through the same mechanisms listed above for IVIG.

IVIG Products

IVIG products typically are used as either direct replacement of immunoglobulins (for primary or secondary immunodeficiencies) or for their immunomodulatory activity.

IVIG is available in liquid or lyophilized forms. The liquid form is convenient; however, the lyophilized form can be reconstituted to different concentrations and osmolalities as needed for each clinical situation.[32] The lyophilized form can be reconstituted with sterile water, 5% dextrose, and 0.9% saline; however, not all brands can be reconstituted with all diluents. No other medications or fluids should be mixed with the IVIG.[32]

When choosing which IVIG product to use, differences in product composition, such as the concentration of additives, IgA content, osmolarity or osmolality, and pH, should be considered (Table 22–2). The different processing methods can also impact the Ig content and function of the product (e.g., the use of solvent detergent treatment reduces the amount of IgG in the product).[15] However, the antibody titers and biological functions of the immunoglobulin preparations are not typically tested, making it more difficult to compare IVIG products.[15]

Despite the potentially clinically significant differences in the products, many hospital pharmacies stock only one formulation of IVIG, which is then used universally in the treatment of patients in the hospital. Only one randomized, double-blind, multicenter study has compared two different products. The study found that an IVIG prepared using caprylate/chromatography (Gamunex) prevented more validated sinopulmonary infections in patients with primary immunodeficiencies than did a solvent detergent–treated IVIG (Gamimune N, 10% which is no longer produced).[33]

Alternative Ig formulations have been developed for IM, IV, subcutaneous (SC), and oral administration. Only IM and IV products have been approved by the FDA, but the IV product dominates the market mainly owing to

Table 22–2 **Variables to Consider When Choosing an IVIG Product**

Variable	Clinical Significance
Sucrose	The FDA issued a warning letter stating that the administration of IVIGs containing sucrose may increase the risk of development of acute renal failure.[89]
Sorbitol	Patients with hereditary fructose intolerance who receive sorbitol- or fructose-containing solutions may develop irreversible multiple organ failure.
Glucose	Use caution when using glucose-containing preparations in patients with diabetes or renal dysfunction and in the elderly.
Glycine	Glycine-containing IVIG products are associated with increased frequency of vasomotor events.
Maltose	Some blood glucose monitoring systems may interpret maltose as glucose and give falsely elevated results, which can result in an iatrogenic insulin overdose.
Sodium	The concentration of sodium in the product is dependent on the concentration to which the product is reconstituted and the diluent used for reconstitution. Caution should be used when products with high sodium concentrations are given to patients with heart failure or renal dysfunction, neonates, young children, the elderly, and those at risk for thromboembolism.
pH	Use caution when administering low pH products to patients with compromised acid-base compensatory methods such as neonates or patients with renal dysfunction. There are reports that low-pH preparations may be associated with thrombophlebitis.
Osmolality and osmolarity	The osmolality and osmolarity of the product should be taken into account when treating patients with heart disease or renal dysfunction and for young children, the elderly, and those at risk for thromboembolism.
Volume	Use caution when infusing IVIG to volume-sensitive patients. Some formulations can be diluted to various concentrations, but when a smaller volume is used, the trade-off is that the osmolarity of the solution increases. Some volume-sensitive populations include patients with renal dysfunction and heart disease, the elderly, neonates, and small children.

advantages in dosing.[34] SC administration is an off-label use but may be helpful when venous access is difficult and offers the convenience of home self-administration by the patient. When IVIG and SC Ig therapy were compared in a randomized trial, there were no significant differences in clinical efficacy or in the incidence of adverse reactions.[35] Oral Ig preparations have also been developed and have been administered experimentally with the intent of neutralizing pathogenic microorganisms in the gastrointestinal tract; however, current evidence does not support their routine use.[36,37]

THERAPEUTIC USES

Because of the differences in preparation procedures, the FDA requires that each company demonstrate the efficacy of its product in clinical trials for each indication.[15] IVIG is generally used to either replace antibodies (in primary or secondary immunodeficiency syndromes) or as an immunomodulatory agent in autoimmune disorders. Table 22–3 lists the FDA-approved indications for each product along with the manufacturer's recommended dose. The high-dose regimens are not recommended for volume-sensitive patients. Although each IVIG preparation has not been approved by the FDA for all of the six uses, many clinicians use the preparations interchangeably. Besides the FDA-approved uses, IVIG has a wide variety of off-label uses. It is estimated that more than half of the IVIG prescribed annually is for a non-FDA-approved indication.[38]

FDA-Approved Indications

Primary Immunodeficiency Syndromes. Primary immunodeficiency syndromes are genetically determined disorders that may affect humoral immunity, cellular immunity, phagocytosis, complement function, or a combination of immune activities.[39] Disorders affecting specific humoral immunity (e.g., common variable immunodeficiency, X-linked agammaglobulinemia, and severe combined immunodeficiency) can result in decreased levels of IgG through disorders in B-cell differentiation or in antibody production and can predispose patients to recurrent sinus infections, otitis media, and bronchiectasis. Encapsulated bacteria such as *Streptococcus pneumoniae*, *Neisseria meningitidis*, and *Haemophilus influenzae* are usually the causative agents.[39] Prophylactic administration of immunoglobulins has been the mainstay of therapy to reduce the number and duration of infections.[39] The typical maintenance dose for adults is 400 to 600 mg/kg IVIG at monthly intervals.[5–13]

A study comparing high-dose (600 mg/kg every 4 weeks for adults or 800 mg/kg every 4 weeks for children) and low-dose (300 mg/kg every 4 weeks for adults or 400 mg/kg every 4 weeks for children) IVIG therapy found that high-dose therapy reduced the number and duration of infections.[40] No target serum IgG trough level has been established; however, a trough level of greater than 500 mg/dL was more protective against infection than a trough level of less than 500 mg/dL in one study.[41] Patients with active infections may require more frequent IVIG administration until the infection is cleared, followed by maintenance replacement therapy.[39,40,42] The use of IVIG and antibiotics in patients with primary immunodeficiency syndromes has significantly reduced the incidence and duration of infections in these patients, markedly improving their quality of life.

Secondary Immunodeficiencies. Secondary immunodeficiency syndromes are acquired disorders of the immune system, which may be caused by a hematologic malignancy, by an infection, or by immunosuppressive therapy. IVIG is approved by the FDA in the treatment of secondary immunodeficiencies caused by chronic lymphocytic leukemia (CLL), HIV infection, and immunosuppressive therapy related to bone marrow transplantation.

Table 22–3 **Recommended Doses for FDA-approved Indications for IVIG[5–13]**

Product	Primary Immunodeficiency	ITP	Secondary Immunodeficiency Due to CLL	Pediatric HIV Infection	Prevention of GVHD and Infection in Adult BMT	Kawasaki Syndrome
Carimune	200 mg/kg once a month; dose may be increased to 300 mg/kg, or frequency of dosing may be increased	400 mg/kg for 2–5 consecutive days. If platelet count does not respond, a single infusion of 400 mg/kg may be given. If response is still inadequate, a single infusion of 800–1000 mg/kg may be given.	×	×	×	×
Flebogamma	300–600 mg/kg body weight every 3–4 weeks	×	×	×	×	×
Gammagard S/D	300–600 mg/kg body weight every 3-4 weeks	A single dose of 1000 mg/kg. The need for additional doses can be determined by clinical response and platelet count. Up to three separate doses may be given on alternate days if required.	400 mg/kg every 3–4 weeks	×	×	Either a single 1000 mg/kg dose or a dose of 400 mg/kg for 4 consecutive days beginning within 7 days of the onset of fever. Also administer aspirin therapy (80–100 mg/kg/day in four divided doses)
Gammagard liquid 10%	300–600 mg/kg every 3–4 weeks	×	×	×	×	×

Gammar-P IV	Children and adolescents: starting doses of 200 mg/kg every 3 to 4 weeks Adults: 200 mg/kg to 400 mg/kg given every 3–4 weeks	×	×	×	×	×
Gamunex	300 and 600 mg/kg every 3–4 weeks	Either two doses of 1000 mg/kg given on consecutive days, or five doses of 400 mg/kg given daily for 5 days	×	×	×	×
Iveegam EN	200 mg/kg per month; the dose may be increased up to fourfold, or intervals between infusions can be shortened	×	×	×	×	Either 400 mg/kg daily for 4 consecutive days or a single dose of 2000 mg/kg given over a 10-hour period within 10 days of disease onset. Also, a dose of 100 mg/kg of aspirin should be administered daily through the 14th day of illness, then 3–5 mg/kg each day for 5 weeks
Octagam	300–600 mg/kg every 3–4 weeks	×	×	×	×	×

×, not an FDA-approved indication.

Hypogammaglobulinemia Associated with CLL. The use of prophylactic IVIG in patients with hypogammaglobulinemia associated with CLL has been shown to prevent recurrent bacterial infections.[43] Several studies have demonstrated that low-dose IVIG (250 mg/kg every 4 weeks in two studies[44,45] or 10 g every 3 weeks in another study[46]) is as effective as high-dose IVIG (400 mg/kg every 3 weeks) therapy in preventing infection. Although IVIG is approved by the FDA to treat hypogammaglobulinemia associated with CLL, there has been debate regarding the cost effectiveness of this measure.[47]

HIV Infection. Patients with advanced HIV infection demonstrate defects in cellular and humoral immunity, making them susceptible to life-threatening infections. In the early to mid-1990s, studies demonstrated that prophylactic IVIG administration in children with advanced HIV infection was associated with a decrease in the number of severe bacterial infections.[48] Spector and colleagues randomly assigned 255 children who were being treated with zidovudine to receive either 400 mg/kg IVIG or a placebo monthly and examined the 2-year rate of bacterial infections. The group concluded that, for children with advanced HIV disease treated with zidovudine, IVIG decreased the incidence of serious bacterial infection only in children who were not also receiving prophylactic trimethoprim-sulfamethoxazole.[49]

Studies conducted in the mid-1990s examining the use of prophylactic IVIG in adults with advanced HIV infection yielded conflicting results in terms of protection against infection and reduction of hospital stays.[50,51] However, no studies of IVIG effectiveness have been conducted in children or adults receiving more recent therapies such as HAART and prophylactic trimethoprim-sulfamethoxazole, so the benefits of adding IVIG to current treatment protocols are unknown.[48]

Allogeneic Bone Marrow Transplantation. Patients who have undergone bone marrow transplantation and immunosuppression are at risk for infectious complications. Several studies[52,53] have shown that allogeneic bone marrow transplant recipients who received IVIG experienced a reduction in graft-versus-host disease (GVHD) and transplantation-related mortality in the first 90 days after transplant. Monthly treatment from 90 days to 1 year post-transplantation resulted in no significant differences versus placebo in survival, incidence of obliterative bronchiolitis, severity of airflow obstruction, and incidence of or mortality due to chronic GVHD. In addition, treated patients experienced delayed humoral recovery.[54]

Because of the high cost of IVIG therapy, more recent studies have focused on finding the minimal IVIG dose necessary to reduce GVHD and transplantation-associated mortality. A 1999 study by Abdel-Mageed and coworkers found that patients receiving 250 mg/kg weekly from day −8 to day +111 did not differ significantly from patients receiving a 500 mg/kg course of IVIG in terms of event-free survival and frequency of infection. However, patients receiving the higher dose of IVIG had less acute GVHD.[55] In a multicenter, randomized, double-blind trial by Winston and colleagues, patients received either 100 mg/kg, 250 mg/kg, or 500 mg/kg doses of IVIG weekly for 90 days and then monthly until 1 year after transplantation. All three groups were similar in the incidence of chronic GVHD, type and frequency of infection, relapse of hematologic malignancy, and survival. As demonstrated in previous studies, there was less acute GVHD in patients treated with higher dose IVIG.[56] Because of the high cost of treatment and because IVIG has been associated with a delay in recovery of recipient humoral responses, the clinical benefit of IVIG use in bone marrow transplant recipients is questionable and may even delay engraftment.[54]

Immune Dysregulation

Idiopathic Thrombocytopenic Purpura. Idiopathic thrombocytopenic purpura (ITP) is caused by the removal of autoantibody-coated platelets by the RES. Practice guidelines from the American Society of Hematology do not recommend treating patients with ITP whose platelet counts are >50,000/μL.[57] When the platelet count is significantly decreased and treatment is indicated, glucocorticoids are the first-line therapy. When steroids are contraindicated or are ineffective, RhIG may be used in Rh-positive individuals who have a spleen (see Hyper-Ig section). IVIG is reserved for patients with platelet counts <50,000/μL who have severe, life-threatening bleeding or are refractory to initial therapy. Because the response to IVIG is rapid but temporary, the use of IVIG is typically reserved for situations in which the platelet count needs to be raised quickly, such as prior to surgery or during an acute hemorrhage.[57–59] In children with ITP, treatment is usually not required if the platelet count is >30,000/μL or if the patient is asymptomatic or has minor purpura.[59] IVIG may be used as initial therapy in children with platelet counts <10,000/μL and minor purpura, for children with platelet counts <20,000/μL and mucous membrane bleeding, and to treat severe, life-threatening bleeding.[57]

Kawasaki Disease. Kawasaki disease, also known as mucocutaneous lymph node syndrome, is an acute, self-limited childhood disorder manifested by fever, bilateral conjunctivitis, erythema or drying or fissuring of the lips and oral mucosa, edema or erythema of the peripheral extremities, rash, and cervical lymphadenopathy.[60] The etiology of Kawasaki disease is unknown, but the presentation and course of the disease, its occurrence in young children (median age of 2 years in the United States), the pattern of spread within a community, and the winter-spring seasonality of outbreaks suggest an infectious etiology. However, no microbial agent has been identified. An alternative hypothesis is that Kawasaki disease is an immunologic response to an infectious agent.[60]

For unknown reasons, Kawasaki disease is associated with systemic vasculitis. One of the most concerning complications of the disease is the development of coronary artery aneurysms in 15% to 25% of untreated children.[60] The vasculitis begins with endothelial cell swelling and subendothelial edema. Around 7 to 9 days after onset of the disease, the vessels are invaded by neutrophils and then by mononuclear cells, CD8+ T cells, and IgA plasma cells, resulting in destruction of the internal elastic lamina. This is ultimately followed by scar tissue formation.[60]

To prevent coronary artery complications, the American Heart Association Committee on Rheumatic Fever, Endocarditis, and Kawasaki Disease recommends the administration of daily doses of 80 to 100 mg/kg of aspirin along with IVIG.[60] Some clinicians reduce the dose to 3 to 5 mg/kg/day after the child has been afebrile for 48 to 72 hours, whereas others wait until day 14 of illness and 48 to 72 hours after the fever has subsided. If there is no evidence of coronary changes by 6 to 8 weeks after the onset of illness, the low-dose aspirin may be stopped, but if coronary abnormalities develop, aspirin might be continued indefinitely. A single infusion of 2 g/kg of IVIG is given with aspirin within 7 days of illness if possible.

Children treated before day 5 of illness are no more likely to develop cardiac abnormalities than are those treated on days 5 or 7 of illness. Children presenting after day 10 of illness who demonstrate persistent fever without other explanation or aneurysms and ongoing systemic inflammation are also treated with IVIG.[60] The mechanism by which IVIG prevents coronary artery complications is unknown, but some hypotheses include the neutralization of microbial agents and/or the modulation of immune activities including cytokine production, the downregulation of antibody production by B cells, and the modulation of T-cell activity.[60]

Off-Label IVIG Use

Hypogammaglobulinemia Associated with Multiple Myeloma. There is evidence that prophylactic IVIG use in patients with plateau-phase multiple myeloma is effective in preventing infection.[48] In a double-blind, multicenter trial, [82] patients with plateau-phase multiple myeloma were randomized to receive either 400 mg/kg of IVIG or a placebo monthly for 1 year. The patients receiving IVIG experienced significantly reduced incidence of recurrent infections.[61] A second study examined 25 patients with multiple myeloma and polyclonal immunoglobulins below the lower limit of normal or a recent history of recurrent infections. In the 2-year cross-over study, patients either received 300 mg/kg IVIG or no therapy. The data suggested that IVIG could be beneficial in preventing serious infections.[62]

Neonatal Prophylaxis and Treatment of Sepsis. Because maternal IgG crosses the placenta in the last 4 to 6 weeks of pregnancy, preterm infants have lower levels of maternal IgG and are more susceptible to infection compared with term infants. Although initial studies demonstrated clinical benefit in preterm infants treated with prophylactic IVIG, a subsequent randomized, controlled trial of 2400 preterm infants showed no evidence that IVIG prevented infections shortterm or long term or improved mortality.[63] A 2004 meta-analysis conducted by Ohlsson and Lacy also demonstrated no clinical benefit in terms of morbidity or mortality,[64] so the routine use of prophylactic IVIG in preterm neonates is not recommended.

Although the use of IVIG as adjuvant to antibiotics in the treatment of neonatal sepsis was associated with reduced mortality and a more rapid recovery in one study,[65] a meta-analysis conducted by Ohlsson and Lacy that examined administration of IVIG for suspected or subsequently proved infection in neonates did not find a statistically significant decrease in mortality for neonates treated with IVIG.[66]

Sepsis and Septic Shock in Adults. A meta-analysis of 27 clinical trials compared the use of IVIG versus placebo or no treatment on outcome in patients with bacterial sepsis or septic shock. Outcome measurements were mortality, bacteriologic failure rates, and duration of stay in hospital. Mortality was significantly reduced in patients who received IVIG; however, the number of patients studied was small.[67] Although the use of IVIG for sepsis or septic shock seems beneficial, further studies should be conducted before its routine use can be recommended.

Severe Anemia Due to Parvovirus. Parvovirus usually has only mild effects in immunocompetent individuals, but in the immunocompromised it may cause severe anemia and reticulocytopenia. Immunocompromised patients infected with parvovirus who receive IVIG experience an increase in hematocrit to greater than 40% and a resolution of symptoms.[68] The use of IVIG should be considered in this clinical situation.

Organ Transplantation. A retrospective study showed that the incidence of cytomegalovirus (CMV) infection in renal transplant patients treated with ganciclovir while in the hospital followed by 3 months of acyclovir was not significantly different from that of patients who received acyclovir followed by IVIG.[69] The subset of patients treated with gancyclovir who were CMV seronegative and who received a transplant from a CMV-seropositive donor had a lower incidence of CMV infection compared with the group receiving IVIG, so IVIG may be helpful in this situation.[69] Given the equivocal results of comparisons of antiviral agents with IVIG and given its expense and adverse effect profile, the use of IVIG in this situation is controversial.48 Early studies suggested that IVIG prophylaxis was beneficial in heart and lung transplantation; however, IgG-CMV-enriched preparations have not demonstrated benefit in heart and kidney transplant recipients.[70,71] Studies with a limited number of patients have suggested that IVIG could help reverse allograft rejection, but routine use of IVIG in this situation is not recommended.[72,73] IVIG has not shown consistent benefit when given to prevent infection in patients who have undergone solid organ transplant.

Post-transfusion Purpura. Post-transfusion purpura occurs when a person with an antiplatelet antibody is transfused with platelets expressing the corresponding antigen.[74] A sudden drop in platelet count occurs 5 to 14 days after transfusion. Post-transfusion purpura most commonly occur in women whose platelets do not express the HPA-1a (PlA1) platelet antigen and who have developed anti-HPA-1a antibodies through exposure due to pregnancy. The disease is usually self-limited, but life-threatening bleeding can occur and can be treated with high-dose IVIG (400 mg/kg/day) therapy, which produces a rapid increase in platelet count.[74]

Neonatal Alloimmune Thrombocytopenia (NAIT). NAIT occurs when maternal antibodies cross the placenta and destroy fetal platelets. The antibodies are usually directed toward an antigen inherited from the father (usually the Pl_{A1} antigen), which is not present on maternal platelets.[75,76] Several small studies have demonstrated an increase in fetal platelet counts when IVIG was administered. None of the patients experienced intracerebral hemorrhage (ICH).[75,76]

Multiple Sclerosis. A recent review of the seven studies in which IVIG was used to treat patients with relapsing-remitting sclerosis found that IVIG reduced the mean number of annual exacerbations and reduced disability.[77] Similarly, a Cochrane review of two randomized trials also concluded that the administration of IVIG resulted in a reduction in relapse rate and increased time to first relapse during treatment with IVIGs.[78] However, the Cochrane review points out that the number of available studies is limited and encourages future investigators to consistently use MRI findings and evidence of disease progression as end points.[78]

Chronic Inflammatory Demyelinating Polyradiculoneuropathy. Chronic inflammatory demyelinating polyradiculoneuropathy (CIDP) is a neurologic disorder caused by demyelination of the peripheral nerves that results in weakness and impaired sensation in the extremities. Although initially several double-blind studies[79,80] showed that IVIG stabilized symptoms and induced remissions compared with placebo in patients with CIDP, a meta-analysis involving 170 patients receiving IVIG versus placebo, plasma exchange, or corticosteroids that examined patient outcome in terms of disability score, the Medical Research Council sum score, electrophysiologic data, or walking distance demonstrated no statistically significant difference in outcome when patients were treated with IVIG versus plasma exchange and oral prednisolone. The decision to use IVIG versus steroids or plasma exchange as the first-line therapy can be made on an individual basis keeping in mind the pros and cons of each treatment.[81]

Guillain-Barré Syndrome. While some initial studies[82] reported clinical benefit in patients receiving IVIG for the treatment of Guillain-Barré syndrome, a Cochrane meta-analysis comparing a seven-grade disability scale in Guillain-Barré patients receiving IVIG versus plasma exchange 4 weeks after randomization found no statistically significant difference in the two treatments. The Cochrane review urges that more trials be conducted to determine the optimal dose of IVIG required for treatment. When deciding between the use of IVIG and plasma exchange, cost and availability have to be considered.[83]

Myasthenia Gravis. A meta-analysis of four studies compared short-term patient benefit when IVIG was administered compared with no treatment, placebo, or plasma exchange. None of the trials showed a significant difference between the treatments.[84] Currently, evidence does not support the routine use of IVIG for this indication.[84]

Multifocal Motor Neuropathy. A meta-analysis of four studies compared disability, strength, or conduction block in patients with multifocal motor neuropathy when IVIG was used versus placebo.[85] The analysis, which included 34 patients, showed that IVIG was associated with an increase in strength. Disability was improved but not significantly so. Because of the limited number of patients studied, there is currently not enough evidence to recommend the routine use of IVIG for this indication.[85]

IVIG INFUSION

For patients not previously exposed to IVIG, the initial rate of infusion is typically set at a rate such as 0.01 mL/kg/min for the first 30 minutes (using the lowest available concentration, usually 5%) and is gradually increased, with a rate in the range of 0.03 to 0.06 mL/kg/min tolerated by most adults.[5–13] Package inserts typically recommend a maximum infusion rate in the range of 0.06 to 0.10 mL/kg/min. Slow infusion rates are used for patients who have never been treated with IVIG, patients who are being treated with a different brand of IVIG than received previously, and patients who have not been exposed to IVIG in more than 8 weeks.[32] Patients at increased risk of developing renal insufficiency or thrombosis are also treated with slow infusion rates. Vital signs are monitored every 15 minutes for the first hour and every 30 to 60 minutes thereafter until the infusion is complete. The common adverse reactions occurring during infusion include headache, nausea, vomiting, chills, fever, and malaise and seem to be related to the rate and dose of infusion.[32]

About 90% to 98% of the protein content of IVIG is IgG.[5–13] The serum IgG level peaks immediately after infusion and drops to 40% to 50% of this level approximately 1 week later.[10] The mean half-life of the product is approximately 3 to 4 weeks, but the half-life varies according to the patient population being treated.[15] Because of the presence of small amounts of IgA, IgA-deficient patients could experience an anaphylactic reaction upon exposure to IVIG.[5–13] Epinephrine should be available during infusion in case an anaphylactic reaction occurs.

SPECIAL CONSIDERATIONS

Isohemagglutinins. The cold ethanol fractionation manufacturing process leaves only trace amounts of blood group isohemagglutinins in immunoglobulin preparations. Thus, the process abrogates the need for ABO and Rh testing before administration of the product. Because of the presence of low titers of IgG anti-A and anti-B antibodies in Ig preparations, their administration may cause a positive direct antiglobulin test[86] and may lead to low-grade hemolysis after high-dose IVIG therapy.[87,88]

False-Positive Serologic Testing. Caution should be used when interpreting serologic results from recipients of IVIG because the Ig infused via the IVIG product can cause false positives.[15] The presence of a suspected infection in a patient receiving IVIG may be confirmed using methods other than serologic testing such as PCR or by repeating serologic testing several weeks after the initial test and watching for an increase in titer.[15]

Risks for Acute Renal Failure. In 1999, the FDA distributed a letter alerting health care providers to reports associating IVIG use with renal dysfunction and acute renal failure.[89] Baseline blood urea nitrogen (BUN) and serum creatinine measurements should be drawn prior to the initiation of IVIG therapy and monitored periodically after the infusion. If patients develop signs of renal dysfunction, discontinuation of IVIG should be considered. Since sucrose-containing preparations have been most commonly implicated, these preparations should either not be used in those at risk or should be infused at a maximum rate of 3 mg sucrose/kg/min to well-hydrated patients.[89]

Hyper-Ig

The passive administration of Igs has been used to treat infectious diseases since the late 1800s.[16] With the advent of antibiotics, Igs were used less frequently; however, they continue to play a role in the prevention and treatment of infectious diseases. Hyper-Igs are concentrations of high titers of specific antibodies produced from the plasma of actively immunized individuals or from immunized animals (e.g., bovine, equine).

Although the majority of hyper-Ig formulations are used to treat infectious diseases, preparations are also available to prevent Rh alloimmunization, to modulate immune function, and to neutralize toxins and venoms.[21] The following sections discuss the clinical use of hyper-Ig.

HYPER-IG FOR THE TREATMENT OF INFECTIOUS DISEASES

Hepatitis A. Human plasma–derived hepatitis A Ig is obtained from donors who have obtained immunity naturally, prophylactically, or through targeted volunteer programs.[25] The Ig is administered to travelers who plan to travel to an endemic area for hepatitis A, to individuals after exposure, and to infants born to mothers infected with hepatitis A. However, the most effective method of prevention is vaccination prior to travel. A dose of 0.02 mL/kg of hepatitis A Ig is 85% to 90% effective in preventing clinical hepatitis when given prior to or within 2 weeks of exposure to the virus.[21]

Hepatitis B. A 0.06 mL/kg dose of hepatitis B Ig (HBIG) is administered to individuals who have been exposed to the virus by needle stick, sexual activity, or mucous membrane exposure. This Ig is prepared from donors with high anti-HBsAg who have obtained immunity naturally, prophylactically, or through targeted volunteer programs[25] and is 80% to 90% effective in preventing infection if given prior to or within 24 hours of exposure. It is also recommended that a 0.5-mL dose of HBIG be administered to infants born to hepatitis B–positive mothers. Studies have also shown benefit when HBIG and antiviral agents are administered for at least 6 months to prevent the recurrence of hepatitis B in liver transplant recipients.[21]

Respiratory Syncytial Virus (RSV). RSV-IGIV is a hyper-Ig produced from human donors with high titers of RSV-neutralizing antibody as determined by a proprietary assay. Alternatively, palivizumab, an MAB directed against the RSV surface F glycoprotein, may be used as prophylaxis against RSV.[21] Although not useful in treating RSV infection, both RSV-IGIB and palivizumab reduce RSV hospitalizations. Palivizumab is the preferred product because it is less expensive and is given intramuscularly instead of intravenously.[21] The American Academy of Pediatrics recommends that RSV prophylaxis be considered during RSV season for high-risk groups including children younger than 2 years old with chronic lung disease who have required treatment in the last 6 months, infants born at less than 32 weeks of gestation, and possibly children with congenital or acquired immunodeficiency.[21,90]

Cytomegalovirus. CMV Ig (CMVIG) is produced from individuals who are naturally immune to CMV with a high antibody titer.[25] CMV infection is of particular concern in patients who have undergone bone marrow transplantation or solid organ transplantation. Although a 1994 meta-analysis showed a decreased incidence of CMV lung infections as well as other symptoms related to CMV when patients were given anti-CMV Ig preparations,[91] subsequent studies of prophylactic IVIG or hyper-Ig CMV-IG to prevent CMV infection after bone marrow transplantation have yielded conflicting results. Studies of the co-administration of CMVIG and antiviral therapy to patients after solid organ transplantation for prophylaxis against CMV infection also have failed to show a clear benefit. Although used by some centers for high-risk patients, CMVIG preparations are not recommended as post-transplant prophylaxis at this time.[48,92,93] Some investigators have reported that the intraperitoneal administration of CMVIG to CMV-infected fetuses may be associated with clinical benefit.[21]

Varicella-Zoster Virus (VZV). VZV Ig is obtained from naturally immunized donors with high titer anti-VZV antibody titers.[25] A dose of 125 U/10 kg (minimum dose of 125 U and maximum dose of 625 U) is used to prevent or modify disease in immunocompromised adults or in adolescents or children who have not been vaccinated. VZVIG is most effective when given within 96 hours of exposure, but it also demonstrates effectiveness when given up to 10 days postexposure. VZVIG is also administered to infants whose mothers develop varicella between 5 days before and 2 days after delivery, infants born at less than 28 weeks of gestation or weighing less than 1000 g at birth if exposed, or infants born at greater than 28 weeks of gestation if exposed and the mother is seronegative.[21,94,95]

Rabies. Rabies Ig (RIG) is a hyper-Ig derived from human donors who have been immunized either prophylactically or through a targeted immunization program.[25] A 20 IU/kg dose of RIG is administered along with rabies vaccine to patients beginning up to 7 days after exposure. In addition, sterile saline is used to make a two- to threefold RIG dilution that is used to infiltrate the wound.[21,96–98]

Measles. A 0.25 mg/kg dose of human plasma–derived Ig for healthy individuals and a 0.5 mg/kg dose for immunocompromised patients is used to prevent or modify measles in infants younger than 1 year, nonimmunized pregnant women, and immunocompromised patients within 6 days of exposure.[21]

Vaccinia. Human vaccinia Ig is obtained from donors who have been immunized with booster immunizations of the smallpox vaccine.[25] Vaccinia Ig intravenous (Human) or VIGIV is used to treat serious complications of smallpox vaccination such as eczema vaccinatum, severe generalized vaccinia, and ocular vaccinia. Although smallpox vaccination is no longer routine, laboratory employees and health care workers who could potentially be exposed to smallpox or a related virus are immunized. Prior to the eradication of smallpox, VIGIV was used to prevent smallpox infection in exposed persons. A 0.6 mL/kg dose divided over 24 to 36 hours is administered IM and may be repeated in 2 to 3 days.[21,99]

PREVENTION OF ALLOIMMUNIZATION WITH RHIG

Licensed for use since 1968, RhIG is a hyper-Ig preparation of anti-D IgG used[1] to prevent alloimmunization resulting from exposure to Rh-positive red blood cells or[2] to treat ITP. The product is derived from human plasma obtained from donors who have natural immunity or who have volunteered to undergo immunization.[25]

RhIG is used to prevent Rh alloimmunization of Rh-negative individuals exposed to the Rh antigen through transfusion or pregnancy.[100] In these situations, the anti-D binds to the Rh-positive red cells, causing their destruction by the RES. This elimination of the highly antigenic Rh-positive red blood cells decreases the probability that the recipient of the red cells will become alloimmunized.

Alloimmunization can be prevented for Rh-negative patients who have received Rh-positive cellular blood products by administering 300 μg of RhIG when the patient has received up to 15 mL of Rh-positive red blood cells.[101–105] When the patient has been exposed to less than 2.5 mL of Rh-positive red blood cells, a dose of 50 μg can be administered.[106] The dose should be administered within 72 hours of exposure to the Rh-positive red blood cells. The 300-μg RhIG dose also is recommended for use in Rh-negative females experiencing abortion or threatened abortion, ectopic pregnancy, abdominal trauma, or obstetric manipulation (e.g., amniocentesis, chorionic villus sampling, percutaneous umbilical blood sampling).[106] Rh-negative pregnant patients also should receive a 300-μg dose as prophylaxis at 26 to 28 weeks' gestation as well as postpartum if the newborn is Rh-positive.[101–105]

MODULATION OF THE IMMUNE SYSTEM

RhIG. RhIG is used to treat ITP in Rh-positive patients with intact spleens. In such cases, the RES works to destroy Ig-coated cells and becomes less able to eliminate platelets.[29] For the treatment of ITP, the initial dose of RhIG is based on the patient's hemoglobin: 50 µg/kg of RhIG in cases where the hemoglobin is greater than or equal to 10 g/dL, and 25 to 40 µg/kg when the hemoglobin is in the range of 8 to 10 g/dL. Because the administration of anti-D (RhIG) results in a decrease in hemoglobin, it should be used with caution in patients with hemoglobin less than 8 g/dL. Patients who do not respond to the initial dose may receive a second dose of RhIG adjusted for their hemoglobin.[105]

Antithymocyte Ig. Antithymocyte Ig is a preparation of Ig derived from rabbits (Thymoglobulin) or horses (ATGAM) immunized with human thymocytes, resulting in the development of antibodies reacting with human T lymphocytes.[107,108] For the treatment of acute renal graft rejection, a 1.5-mg/kg dose of Thymoglobulin can be given daily for 7 to 14 days or a 10- to 15-mg/kg dose of ATGAM may be given daily for 14 days.[107,108] ATGAM may be used also to delay allograft rejection by giving a 15-mg/kg daily dose for 14 days, beginning just before or after transplantation, followed by a dose given every other day for 14 days. ATGAM can also be used to treat aplastic anemia with a 10- to 20-mg/kg dose given daily for 8 to 14 days.[108]

NEUTRALIZATION OF TOXINS WITH HYPER-IG

Diphtheria. Available through the CDC, diphtheria antitoxin (DAT) produced from horses immunized with diphtheria toxoid administered with antibiotics has proved effective in treating diphtheria.[109] The antitoxin is mixed in 250 to 500 mL of normal saline and administered IV over 2 to 4 hours. Dosages are as follows: 20,000 to 40,000 units for pharyngeal or laryngeal disease of 48 hours duration; 40,000 to 60,000 units for nasopharyngeal disease; 80,000 to 100,000 units for systemic disease of 3 or more days duration or for any patient with diffuse swelling of the neck; and 20,000 to 40,000 for skin lesions when treatment is indicated. Children are treated with the same doses as adults.[109]

Tetanus. Human hyper-Ig preparations of tetanus Ig (TIG) are derived from human donors who have been immunized either prophylactically or who have volunteered to undergo immunization for this purpose.[25] The final product contains no less than 250 tetanus antitoxin units per container using the U.S. Standard Antitoxin as the reference material.[110] A 250 IU intramuscular dose of TIG is administered to patients lacking immunity who sustain a contaminated wound, deep puncture wound, or wound associated with devitalized tissue. A 3000–6000 IU intramuscular dose of TIG is used for active disease. The patient should also be actively immunized at the time TIG is administered.[21,110]

Botulism. Human- and equine-derived botulism antitoxin formulations are available for the treatment of wound botulism or food-borne illness and are available as prophylaxis for individuals who have been exposed through tainted food.[111,112] The human plasma–derived product is obtained from donors immunized with pentavalent botulinum toxoid. The final product contains a titer of 15 IU/mL against type A toxin and 4 IU/mL against type B toxin. A 1-mL/kg intravenous infusion of botulism Ig is recommended for the treatment of infant botulism.[112]

TREATMENT OF DRUG OVERDOSE WITH HYPER-IG

Digitoxin or Digoxin. Ovine-derived digoxin immune Fab can be used to treat the life-threatening effects of digoxin or digitoxin overdose.[113] The administration of digoxin immune Fab is indicated for adult patients who have ingested digitalis doses of greater than 10 mg or pediatric patients who have ingested greater than 4 mg, patients with steady-state serum concentrations greater than 10 ng/mL, and patients with potassium concentrations greater than 5 mEq/L following overdose. Each vial contains 38 mg of digoxin-specific Fab fragments, which can neutralize 0.5 mg of digoxin or digitoxin. When an acute overdose of an unknown amount of digoxin or digitoxin occurs, 20 vials of digoxin immune Fab fragments should be administered to adults or children. In volume-sensitive patients, this may be reduced to 10 vials followed by close monitoring and additional doses if needed. For patients experiencing toxicity due to chronic therapy, a six-vial dose for adults and a one-vial dose for infants and small children is recommended.[113]

TREATMENT OF ENVENOMATION WITH HYPER-LG

Black Widow Spider (*Latrodectus mactans*). Patients with symptoms due to black widow spider bites are treated with black widow spider antivenin, which is obtained from horses immunized with the venom.[114] Adults and children are generally treated with one vial that contains not less than 6000 antivenin units. The dose may be given IM (usually in the anterolateral thigh) or may be diluted in 10–50 mL of saline and given IV over 15 minutes. Although one dose usually causes a resolution of symptoms in 1 to 3 hours, a second dose may be required.[114]

Pit Viper (crotalid). Patients who have been envenomed by pit vipers can be treated with polyvalent antivenin obtained from horses immunized with pit viper venom.[115] Reconstitution of each vial yields a 10-mL solution of antivenin. For minimal exposure to venom, 2 to 4 vials are administered, moderate exposure requires treatment with 5 to 9 vials, and 10 to 15 vials are used to treat severe exposure. The dose is typically given IV but may be given IM. When given IV, the dose is usually diluted 1:1 or 1:10 using sodium chloride. The first 5 to 10 mL are given slowly over 3 to 5 minutes and then increased as tolerated by the patient. The dose is most effective when given within 4 hours of the pit viper bite.[115]

Coral Snake (*Micrurus fulvius*). Antivenin directed against coral snake venom is produced by immunizing horses with venom from the eastern coral snake (*Micrurus fulvius fulvius*).[116] The resulting antivenin also neutralizes Texas coral snake (*Micrurus fulvius tenere*) venom but does not neutralize venom from the Arizona or Sonoran coral snake (*Micruroides euryxanthus*). Each vial is reconstituted to a 10-mL solution. Initial therapy should consist of the administration of 3 to 5 vials of *Micrurus fulvius* antivenin with the initial 1 to 2 mL given over 3 to 5 minutes. The administration rate is increased as tolerated by the patient. Additional doses may be given if needed.[116]

Adverse Reactions

IVIG

Because most adverse reactions associated with Ig infusion are reported as case reports, the true incidence of adverse events associated with Ig administration is unknown. Most reactions are mild, with the most common adverse reactions being headache, fever, malaise, myalgia, nausea, vomiting, chills, blood pressure changes, flushing, rash, diaphoresis, pruritus, bronchospasm, chest pain, back pain, and dizziness.[5–13] These symptoms typically occur as a result of either allergy or the rate of infusion. The most severe reactions that can occur in response to Ig infusion are anaphylaxis, aseptic meningitis, acute renal failure, and thromboembolism.[15,87]

1. Anaphylaxis can occur owing to the exposure of IgA-deficient patients to the small amount of IgA in the IVIG product. Epinephrine should always be available during IVIG infusion. Some manufacturers keep products with low IgA concentrations on their shelves particularly for the treatment of IgA-deficient patients.[5–13]
2. Another rare and severe reaction is aseptic meningitis, which is characterized by severe headache, nuchal rigidity, drowsiness, fever, photophobia, painful eye movements, and nausea and vomiting. Beginning 6 to 48 hours after infusion, patients with a history of migraine who have received high-dose Ig treatment appear to be most susceptible. The CSF demonstrates pleocytosis and elevated protein. The symptoms are reversible and typically resolve in hours to days.[15,87,88]
3. As mentioned previously, over 100 cases of acute renal failure (including at least 17 deaths) have been associated with the infusion of IVIG, particularly those formulations containing sucrose.[15,87] These patients should be infused slowly and monitored carefully for signs of renal dysfunction.
4. IVIG infusion has been associated with thromboembolic events such as deep venous thrombosis, myocardial infarction, cerebrovascular accidents, and pulmonary embolism and could be related to the increase in viscosity experienced after IVIG administration. Patients receiving large Ig doses at rapid rates, as well as elderly, overweight, or immobilized patients, and patients with cardiovascular disease are thought to be at highest risk for development of this complication.[15,87,88]

In addition to these adverse reactions that can occur with any of the IVIG products, specific adverse effects can occur in relation to individual products. The variables associated with the adverse effects as well as the at-risk populations are listed in Table 22–2.

Hyper-Ig. Because hyper-Igs contain many of the same elements as IVIG, they are associated with the same adverse effects (see above section). Unlike IVIG, because many hyper-Igs may be given IM, soreness at the site of injection may occur. Individual hyper-Ig products also have adverse effects specific to them.

RhIG. Because RhIG results in the destruction of Rh-positive red cells, administration of this hyper-Ig can result in anemia and renal insufficiency.[105] Intravascular hemolysis occurring after RhIG administration resulted in four deaths between May 1996 and April 1999.[105] The package inserts recommend adjusting the dose according to the patient's hemoglobin level.

Antithymocyte Globulin. Because antithymocyte globulin works by clearing human T lymphocytes from circulation, chronic use or overdosage of the drug can result in excessive immuno suppression that can put the patient at risk for infection or lymphoma.[107,108] In addition, the antibodies may crossreact with platelets and neutrophils, causing clearance of these cells. This can be reversed by reducing the dose of the hyper-Ig.

Digoxin Immune Fab. Because this hyper-Ig is used to treat digoxin or digitalis overdose, the abrupt withdrawal of the drug's effects may result in a rapid ventricular response if the patient is being treated for atrial fibrillation or congestive heart failure.[113] The reversal of the effects of digoxin or digitalis by digoxin immune Fab also results in hypokalemia.[113]

Animal-Derived Hyper-Ig. Animal-derived hyper-Igs carry the risk of serum sickness. Sensitivity testing should be conducted prior to their use.

Infectious Disease Transmission

IVIG

The effort to limit viral transmission begins by testing plasma donors for antibodies to HIV-1 and -2, HBsAg, and HCV, as well as performing NAT testing for HCV and HIV. As discussed in the section on commercial production of IVIG, the manufacturers pool the collected plasma and produce IVIG using the cold ethanol fractionation method, which significantly reduces the concentration of viruses (approximately 5 log).[15] The transmission of cell-associated viruses such as CMV, Epstein-Barr virus, and human T-cell leukemia/lymphoma virus type 1 is limited by this process, which results in an acellular product. Each manufacturer then adds additional steps (see Commercial Production) to further limit viral transmission. The transmission of HBV and HIV by IVIG has not been reported. However, by the mid-1990s, HCV had been transmitted by IVIG to over 450 people,[117,118] leading the FDA to require that each manufacturer test its viral reduction and inactivation steps by adding model viruses and testing the viral clearance at the end of each step in processing. Since that time, no additional cases of IVIG-transmitted hepatitis C have been reported.[15] According to package inserts of various IVIG products, the manufacturing process results in an overall viral log reduction of 9.6 to greater than 26 for HIV-1, 6.2 to greater than 16.8 for bovine viral diarrhea virus (a model virus for HCV), and 8.5 to greater than 25 for pseudorabies virus (a model virus for lipid enveloped DNA viruses such as the herpes and hepatitis B viruses). One virus that is difficult to eliminate and has been transmitted via IVIG is parvovirus, which is partially heat resistant and is resistant to solvent/detergent treatment. Although antibodies to parvovirus are valuable as a component of IVIG, their presence also indicates an increased risk for viral transmission, presenting a dilemma for manufacturers. At present, screening for antibodies to parvovirus is not required.[15] One other disease caused by an infectious agent that has caused concern in recent years is Creutzfeldt-Jakob disease. Models developed for prion disease indicate that there is probably a low chance of infectivity by blood transfusion. In addition, the concentration of the infectious agent is reduced by several logs during the manufacturing process.[119,120]

HYPER-IG

Because hyper-Igs are produced using the same methods that are used to produce IVIG, the infectious disease risk is similar (see above).

THERAPEUTIC MAB

The ability to mass produce homogeneous Ig with a single predefined specificity was realized by the adaptation of hybridoma technology for the creation, selection, and expansion of monoclonal cell lines derived from single B lymphocytes.[3]

Table 22–4 Monoclonal Antibodies Approved by FDA for Therapeutic Uses in the United States

Category	Subcategory	Composition	Target-Specificity	Generic Name/Trade Name	Main Clinical Application Area	FDA Approval
Murine	Unmodified	IgG2a	CD3	Muromonab-CD3/ Orthoclone OKT3	Immunosuppression (treatment of allograft rejection)	1986
Murine	Conjugate radiolabeled (yttrium 90)	IgG1/κ	CD20	Ibritumomab tiuxetan/ Zevalin	Oncology (treatment of relapsed or refractory low-grade B-cell non-Hodgkin's lymphoma)	2002
Murine	Conjugate radiolabeled (iodine 131)	IgG2a/λ	CD20	Tositumomab-I131/Bexxar	Oncology (treatment of relapsed or refractory low-grade B-cell non-Hodgkin's lymphoma)	2003
Near-Human	Chimeric Fab fragment	IgG1	GPIIb/IIIa	Abciximab/ReoPro	Anti-hemostasis (adjunct to percutaneous coronary intervention, for prevention of cardiac ischemic complications)	1994
Near-Human	Chimeric	IgG1/κ	CD20	Rituximab/Rituxan	Oncology (treatment of relapsed or refractory low-grade B-cell non-Hodgkin's lymphoma)	1997
Near-Human	Chimeric	IgG1/κ	CD25	Basiliximab/Simulect	Immunosuppression (prophylaxis of renal allograft rejection)	1998
Near-Human	Chimeric	IgG1/κ	TNFα	Infliximab/Remicade	Anti-inflammation (treatment of rheumatoid arthritis, Crohn's disease, ankylosing spondylitis, and psoriatic arthritis)	1998
Near-Human	Chimeric	IgG1/κ	Epidermal growth factor receptor (EGFR)	Cetuximab/Erbitux	Oncology (treatment of EGFR-expressing, metastatic colorectal carcinoma in patients who are refractory or intolerant to irinotecan-based chemotherapy)	2004
Near-Human	Humanized	IgG1/κ	CD25	Daclizumab/Zenapax	Immunosuppression (prophylaxis of renal allograft-rejection)	1997
Near-Human	Humanized	IgG1/κ	Respiratory syncytial virus	Palivizumab/Synagis	Anti-infection (prevention of serious lower respiratory tract infection in pediatric patients at high risk for RSV disease)	1998
Near-Human	Humanized	IgG1/κ	HER2	Trastuzumab/Herceptin	Oncology (treatment of metastatic breast cancer that overexpresses the HER2 protein)	1998

Near-Human	Humanized Conjugate immunotoxin (calicheamicin)	IgG4/κ	CD33	Gemtuzumab ozogamicin/ Mylotarg	Oncology (treatment of CD33-positive acute myeloid leukemia in first relapse in patients who are 60 years or older and not candidates for other cytotoxic chemotherapy)	2000
Near-Human	Humanized	IgG1/κ	CD52	Alemtuzumab/Campath-1H	Oncology (treatment of B-cell chronic lymphocytic leukemia (B-CLL) in patients who have been treated with alkylating agents and in whom fludarabine therapy has failed)	2001
Near-Human	Humanized	IgG1/κ	IgE	Omalizumab/Xolair	Allergy (treatment of moderate to severe persistent asthma of adults and adolescents with positive skin test or in vitro reactivity to a perennial aeroallergen and whose symptoms are inadequately controlled with inhaled corticosteroids)	2003
Near-Human	Humanized	IgG1/κ	CD11a	Efalizumab/Raptiva	Anti-inflammation (treatment of adult patients with chronic moderate to severe plaque psoriasis who are candidates for systemic therapy or phototherapy)	2003
Near-Human	Humanized	IgG1	Vascular endothelial growth factor	Bevacizumab/Avastin	Oncology (treatment of metastatic carcinoma of the colon or rectum when used in combination with intravenous 5-fluorouracil-based chemotherapy)	2004
Human	Phage-display	IgG1/κ	TNF-α	Adalimumab/Humira	Anti-inflammation (treatment of rheumatoid arthritis in adult patients with moderately to severely active disease and inadequate response to one or more DMARDs)	2002

Data from refs. 122–124, 130–142, 146.

The products, called monoclonal antibodies (MABs), were predicted to revolutionize drug therapy and the pharmaceutical industry by allowing new ways for selective therapeutic targeting. Using the relatively well-understood IgG molecule as a biocompatible homing device, it was argued, any cellular target accessible via the bloodstream could be reached and selectively targeted for destruction or interference.

The first step is to develop an MAB directed against a molecule that is selectively expressed on the surface of the cell in question (i.e., a molecular flag), regardless of whether the cell is foreign (such as an invading microorganism) or intrinsic (such as a tumor cell) to the body. Once attached to the target, destruction can be achieved by lethal substances attached to the MAB during its pharmaceutical production/formulation, such as radioisotopes or toxins, or by the destructive capabilities of the Ig nature of the MAB, such as complement-fixation or activation of phagocytes via Fc-receptor-dependent opsonization. Similarly, the MAB can inhibit extracellular molecular pathways through neutralization and elimination of soluble molecular targets. In short, the MAB was envisioned as fulfilling Paul Ehrlich's dream of a "magic bullet."

Thus, together with cytokines, MABs were important inspirations for the development of the biotechnology-based drug industry. The *first-generation* therapeutic products were murine MABs. Many went to clinical trials in the early to mid-1980s. It turned out that murine MABs, by and large, had a critical flaw with respect to repeated clinical use: they are detected as foreign by the human immune system.[121] The development of HAMAs dramatically reduced the in vivo half-life of the MAB development compounds in many patients, thereby reducing their effectiveness. Only one of the early lead candidates made it to market: anti-CD3 (OKT3/muromonab), used for the treatment of acute allograft rejection.[122] More recently, two murine anti-CD20 MABs have been approved as radionuclide-labeled conjugates and are used for treatment of refractory or relapsed, low-grade, non-Hodgkin's B-cell lymphoma.[123,124]

One solution to this problem has been to make more "human-like" MABs in order to reduce their immunogenicity. Technologies were refined to achieve this, and *second-generation* candidate therapeutic MABs emerged, including (1) chimeric MABs (human C regions, murine V regions),[125] (2) nonhuman primate MABs,[126,127] (3) humanized MABs (human C regions, humanized V regions (framework region amino acid residues are exchanged for consensus human, whereas murine hypervariable region amino acid residues are maintained),[128] and (4) a combination of 2 and 3, so-called primatized MABs (human C regions, nonhuman primate-based V regions).[129] Thirteen[130–142] of the 17 therapeutic MABs on the U.S. market belong to the second generation, five of which are chimeric[133–136,140] and eight humanized,[130–132,137–139,141,142] and all but one[135] were FDA-approved in the last decade. Table 22–4 presents an overview of these new Ig-products.

Third-generation therapeutic MABs, predominantly still in development, are fully human MAB proteins. Such MABs have been derived in several ways. The earliest intentionally created, completely human MABs were generated from immunized human B lymphocytes obtained from immunized hosts or through in vitro immunization. These B lymphocytes were immortalized either by EBV-transformation or fusion to a nonproducing heterohybridoma,[143] or both. Some antiviral human MABs (e.g., anti-CMV, anti-HBV) of this kind progressed relatively far in clinical trials[144] but ultimately were not brought to market. In addition, this approach to making completely human MABs faced serious challenges when the intention was to address human pharmaceutical targets.

Instead, two other approaches to human MAB-development emerged. One is based on displaying human Ig V-region repertoires on the surface of filamentous phage.[145] Such V-region libraries can be interrogated by antigens allowing affinity selection of interesting V-region candidate genes. In vitro affinity-maturation schemes have been invented, and full Ig-producing cassettes have been developed for resulting expression of selected V regions. A first fully human MAB, directed against the cytokine TNFα, was developed by this technique and has reached the market as an anti-inflammatory.[146]

Another angle to develop fully human MABs to human pharmaceutical targets is the generation of transgenic mice expressing human Ig genes. Such murine models were described by investigators at two California biotech companies in 1994.[147–149] There are now about 30 MABs in clinical testing based on human Ig V-region sequences derived from these transgenic mice.[148]

Overall, the MABs that currently have penetrated the market predominantly focus on targets in immunology/inflammation and oncology. The many MAB candidates in development have a similar profile. Although a detailed clinical profile of each of these MABs is beyond the scope of this chapter, it is predicted that this product line will continue to grow and increasingly intersect with transfusion medicine.[150]

CONCLUSION

A natural defense protein with a good safety profile, Ig derived from pooled human plasma is broadly used to confer passive immunity and to achieve immunomodulation. There are currently six FDA-approved indications for IVIG administration. Because of the expense of the product, the risks involved in IVIG administration, and the lack of studies supporting the growing number of off-label uses of IVIG, the decision to administer IVIG should be made carefully. A recent successful development in the field of Ig therapy is improved technology to produce and develop MABs for a variety of clinical markets. This offers the unprecedented possibility to intentionally and specifically clinically target bioactive mediators and receptors. Owing to the purity, specificity, and limited potential of infectious disease transmission of MABs, they now enjoy a consistently high success rate compared with other pharmaceutical development compounds. MAB products will likely both increase in existing markets and diversify into other applications. Given both the expense and versatility of MAB therapy, transfusion medicine physicians are likely to take an increasing role in consulting about their uses.

REFERENCES

1. Black CA. A brief history of the discovery of the immunoglobulins and the origin of the modern immunoglobulin nomenclature. Immunol Cell Biol 1997;75:65–68.
2. Kolar G, Capra J. Immunoglobulins: Structure and Function. In Paul WE (ed). Fundamental Immunology. Philadelphia, Lippincott Williams & Wilkins, 2003.
3. Kohler G, Milstein C. Continuous cultures of fused cells secreting antibody of predefined specificity. Nature 1975;256:495–497.
4. Reichert JM, Rosensweig CJ, Faden LB, Dewitz MC. Monoclonal antibody successes in the clinic. Nat Biotechnol 2005;23:1073–1078.
5. Carimune NF IV package insert. ZLB Bioplasma AG. Glendale, Calif., 2003.

6. Flebogamma 5% package insert. Instituto Grifols, S.A. Los Angeles, Calif., 2004.
7. Gammagard S/D package insert. Baxter Healthcare Corporation. Westlake Village, Calif., 2002.
8. Gamunex Immune Globulin I.V. 10% package insert. Bayer Corporation. Elkhart, Ind., 2003.
9. Gammar-P I.V. package insert. Aventis Behring. Kankakee, Ill., 2001.
10. Iveegam EN package insert. Baxter Healthcare Corporation. Glendale, Calif., 2000.
11. Gammagard Liquid package insert. Baxter Healthcare Corporation. Westlake Village, Calif., 2005.
12. Octagam package insert. Octapharma. Centreville, Va., 2005.
13. Polygam package insert. Baxter Healthcare. Deerfield, Ill., 1993.
14. Ratko TA, Burnett DA, Foulke GE, et al. Recommendations for off-label use of intravenously administered immunoglobulin preparations. University Hospital Consortium Expert Panel for Off-Label Use of Polyvalent Intravenously Administered Immunoglobulin Preparations. JAMA 1995;273:1865–1870.
15. Knezevic-Maramica I, Kruskall MS. Intravenous immune globulins: an update for clinicians. Transfusion 2003;43:1460–1480.
16. Waldmann TA. Immunotherapy: past, present and future. Nat Med 2003;9:269–277.
17. von Behring E, Kitasato S. Ueber das zustandekommen der diptherie-immunitat under der tetanus-immunitat bei thieren. Deutsche Med Wochenschrift Deutsche Med Wochenschrift 1890;16:1113–1114.
18. Cohn EJ, Strong LE, Hughes WL, et al. Preparation and properties of serum and plasma proteins. IV. A system for the separation into fractions of the protein and lipoprotein components of biological tissues and fluids. J Am Chem Soc 1946;68:459–475.
19. Barandun S, Isliker HL. Development of immunoglobulin preparations for intravenous use. Vox Sang 1986;51:157–160.
20. Bruton O. Agammaglobulinemia. Pediatrics 1952;52:722–728.
21. Keller MA, Stiehm ER. Passive immunity in prevention and treatment of infectious diseases. Clin Microbiol Rev 2000;13:602–614.
22. Code of Federal Regulations. Title 21 CFR 640. Washington, D.C., U.S. Government Printing Office, 2005 (revised annually).
23. Seligmann M, Cunningham-Rundles C, Hanson A, et al. IUIS/WHO notice: appropriate uses of human immunoglobulin in clinical practice. Clin Exp Immunol 1983;52:417–422.
24. Plasma Protein Therapeutics Association. Available at http://www.plasmainfo.org. Accessed 1/3/06.
25. WHO Recommendations for the Production, Control, and Regulation of Human Plasma for Fractionation. Geneva, Switzerland, World Health Organization, 2005.
26. Report of the Expert Panel on Donor Pool Size of Immunoglobulin Products. Available at http://www.niaid.nih. gov/dait/ivig1.html. Accessed 1/17/06.
27. Gelfand EW. Critical decisions in selecting an intravenous immunoglobulin product. J Infus Nurs 2005;28:366–374.
28. Teeling JL, Bleeker WK, Hack CE. History, biological mechanisms of action and clinical indications of intravenous immunoglobulin (IVIG) preparations. Rev Med Microbiol 2002;13:91–100.
29. Sandler SG, Tutuncuoglu SO. Immune thrombocytopenic purpura—current management practices. Expert Opin Pharmacother 2004;5:2515–2527.
30. Parslow TG. Immunoglobulins and immunoglobulin genes. In Parslow TG, Stites DP, Terr AI, Imboden JB (eds). Medical Immunology, 10th ed. New York, Lange Medical Books/McGraw-Hill Medical Publishing Division, 2001.
31. Kazatchkine MD, Kaveri SV. Immunomodulation of autoimmune and inflammatory diseases with intravenous immune globulin. N Engl J Med 2001;345:747–755.
32. Murphy E, Martin S, Patterson JV. Developing practice guidelines for the administration of intravenous immunoglobulin. J Infus Nurs 2005;28:265–272.
33. Roifman CM, Schroeder H, Berger M, et al. Comparison of the efficacy of IGIV-C, 10% (caprylate/chromatography) and IGIV-SD, 10% as replacement therapy in primary immune deficiency: a randomized double-blind trial. Int Immunopharmacol 2003;3:1325–1333.
34. Weiler CR. Immunoglobulin therapy: history, indications, and routes of administration. Int J Dermatol 2004;43:163–166.
35. Chapel HM, Spickett GP, Ericson D, et al. The comparison of the efficacy and safety of intravenous versus subcutaneous immunoglobulin replacement therapy. J Clin Immunol 2000;20:94–100.
36. Mohan P, Haque K. Oral immunoglobulin for the treatment of rotavirus infection in low birth weight infants. Cochrane Database Syst Rev 2003:CD003742.
37. Foster J, Cole M. Oral immunoglobulin for preventing necrotizing enterocolitis in preterm and low birth-weight neonates. Cochrane Database Syst Rev 2004:CD001816.
38. Nydegger UE, Mohacsi PJ, Escher R, Morell A. Clinical use of intravenous immunoglobulins. Vox Sang 2000;78:191–195.
39. Durandy A, Wahn V, Petteway S, Gelfand EW. Immunoglobulin replacement therapy in primary antibody deficiency diseases—maximizing success. Int Arch Allergy Immunol 2005;136:217–229.
40. Eijkhout HW, van Der Meer JW, Kallenberg CG, et al. The effect of two different dosages of intravenous immunoglobulin on the incidence of recurrent infections in patients with primary hypogammaglobulinemia: a randomized, double-blind, multicenter crossover trial. Ann Intern Med 2001;135:165–174.
41. Gelfand EW, Reid B, Roifman CM. Intravenous immune serum globulin replacement in hypogammaglobulinemia: a comparison of high-versus low-dose therapy. Monogr Allergy 1988;23:177–186.
42. Quartier P, Debre M, De Blic J, et al. Early and prolonged intravenous immunoglobulin replacement therapy in childhood agammaglobulinemia: a retrospective survey of 31 patients. J Pediatr 1999; 134:589–596.
43. Cooperative Group for the Study of Immunoglobulin in Chronic Lymphocytic Leukemia. Intravenous immunoglobulin for the prevention of infection in chronic lymphocytic leukemia: a randomized, controlled clinical trial. N Engl J Med 1988;319:902–907.
44. Gamm H, Huber C, Chapel H, et al. Intravenous immune globulin in chronic lymphocytic leukaemia. Clin Exp Immunol 1994;97:17–20.
45. Chapel H, Dicato M, Gamm H, et al. Immunoglobulin replacement in patients with chronic lymphocytic leukaemia: a comparison of two dose regimes. Br J Haematol 1994;88:209–212.
46. Jurlander J, Geisler CH, Hansen MM. Treatment of hypogammaglobulinaemia in chronic lymphocytic leukaemia by low-dose intravenous gammaglobulin. Eur J Haematol 1994;53:114–118.
47. Molica S, Musto P, Chiurazzi F, et al. Prophylaxis against infections with low-dose intravenous immunoglobulins (IVIG) in chronic lymphocytic leukemia: results of a crossover study. Haematologica 1996;81:121–126.
48. Mouthon L, Lortholary O. Intravenous immunoglobulins in infectious diseases: where do we stand? Clin Microbiol Infect 2003;9:333–338.
49. Spector SA, Gelber RD, McGrath N, et al. A controlled trial of intravenous immune globulin for the prevention of serious bacterial infections in children receiving zidovudine for advanced human immunodeficiency virus infection. Pediatric AIDS Clinical Trials Group. N Engl J Med 1994;331:1181–1187.
50. Kiehl MG, Stoll R, Broder M, et al. A controlled trial of intravenous immune globulin for the prevention of serious infections in adults with advanced human immunodeficiency virus infection. Arch Intern Med 1996;156:2545–2550.
51. Jablonowski H, Sander O, Willers R, et al. The use of intravenous immunoglobulins in symptomatic HIV infection: results of a randomized study. Clin Invest 1994;72:220–224.
52. Sullivan KM, Kopecky KJ, Jocom J, et al. Immunomodulatory and antimicrobial efficacy of intravenous immunoglobulin in bone marrow transplantation. N Engl J Med 1990;323:705–712.
53. Wolff SN, Fay JW, Herzig RH, et al. High-dose weekly intravenous immunoglobulin to prevent infections in patients undergoing autologous bone marrow transplantation or severe myelosuppressive therapy: a study of the American Bone Marrow Transplant Group. Ann Intern Med 1993;118:937–942.
54. Sullivan KM, Storek J, Kopecky KJ, et al. A controlled trial of long-term administration of intravenous immunoglobulin to prevent late infection and chronic graft-vs.-host disease after marrow transplantation: clinical outcome and effect on subsequent immune recovery. Biol Blood Marrow Transplant 1996;2:44–53.
55. Abdel-Mageed A, Graham-Pole J, Del Rosario ML, et al. Comparison of two doses of intravenous immunoglobulin after allogeneic bone marrow transplants. Bone Marrow Transplant 1999;23:929–932.
56. Winston DJ, Antin JH, Wolff SN, et al. A multicenter, randomized, double-blind comparison of different doses of intravenous immunoglobulin for prevention of graft-versus-host disease and infection after allogeneic bone marrow transplantation. Bone Marrow Transplant 2001;28:187–196.
57. George JN, Woolf SH, Raskob GE, et al. Idiopathic thrombocytopenic purpura: a practice guideline developed by explicit methods for the American Society of Hematology. Blood 1996;88:3–40.
58. Stasi R, Provan D. Management of immune thrombocytopenic purpura in adults. Mayo Clin Proc 2004;79:504–522.
59. Buchanan GR, Journeycake JM, Adix L. Severe chronic idiopathic thrombocytopenic purpura during childhood: definition, management, and prognosis. Semin Thromb Hemost 2003;29:595–603.

60. Newburger JW, Takahashi M, Gerber MA, et al. Diagnosis, treatment, and long-term management of Kawasaki disease: a statement for health professionals from the Committee on Rheumatic Fever, Endocarditis, and Kawasaki Disease, Council on Cardiovascular Disease in the Young, American Heart Association. Pediatrics 2004;114:1708–1733.
61. Chapel HM, Lee M, Hargreaves R, et al. Randomised trial of intravenous immunoglobulin as prophylaxis against infection in plateau-phase multiple myeloma. The UK Group for Immunoglobulin Replacement Therapy in Multiple Myeloma. Lancet 1994;343:1059–1063.
62. Musto P, Brugiatelli M, Carotenuto M. Prophylaxis against infections with intravenous immunoglobulins in multiple myeloma. Br J Haematol 1995;89:945–946.
63. Fanaroff AA, Korones SB, Wright LL, et al. A controlled trial of intravenous immune globulin to reduce nosocomial infections in very-low-birth-weight infants. National Institute of Child Health and Human Development Neonatal Research Network. N Engl J Med 1994;330:1107–1113.
64. Ohlsson A, Lacy JB. Intravenous immunoglobulin for preventing infection in preterm and/or low-birth-weight infants. Cochrane Database Syst Rev 2004:CD000361.
65. Haque KN, Remo C, Bahakim H. Comparison of two types of intravenous immunoglobulins in the treatment of neonatal sepsis. Clin Exp Immunol 1995;101:328–333.
66. Ohlsson A, Lacy JB. Intravenous immunoglobulin for suspected or subsequently proven infection in neonates. Cochrane Database Syst Rev 2004:CD001239.
67. Alejandria MM, Lansang MA, Dans LF, Mantaring JB. Intravenous immunoglobulin for treating sepsis and septic shock. Cochrane Database Syst Rev 2002:CD001090.
68. Mouthon L, Guillevin L, Tellier Z. Intravenous immunoglobulins in autoimmune- or parvovirus B19-mediated pure red-cell aplasia. Autoimmun Rev 2005;4:264–269.
69. Walton T, Sankari B, Wyner L. Comparison of ganciclovir- and immune globulin-containing regimens in preventing cytomegalovirus infection in patients with renal transplants. Am J Health Syst Pharm 1999;56:1831–1834.
70. Boland GJ, Ververs C, Hene RJ, et al. Early detection of primary cytomegalovirus infection after heart and kidney transplantation and the influence of hyperimmune globulin prophylaxis. Transpl Int 1993;6:34–38.
71. Sia IG, Patel R. New strategies for prevention and therapy of cytomegalovirus infection and disease in solid-organ transplant recipients. Clin Microbiol Rev 2000;13:83–121.
72. Montgomery RA, Zachary AA, Racusen LC, et al. Plasmapheresis and intravenous immune globulin provides effective rescue therapy for refractory humoral rejection and allows kidneys to be successfully transplanted into cross-match-positive recipients. Transplantation 2000;70:887–895.
73. Jordan SC, Quartel AW, Czer LS, et al. Posttransplant therapy using high-dose human immunoglobulin (intravenous gammaglobulin) to control acute humoral rejection in renal and cardiac allograft recipients and potential mechanism of action. Transplantation 1998; 66:800–805.
74. Ziman A, Klapper E, Pepkowitz S, et al. A second case of post-transfusion purpura caused by HPA-5a antibodies: successful treatment with intravenous immunoglobulin. Vox Sang 2002;83:165–166.
75. Jolly MC, Letsky EA, Fisk NM. The management of fetal alloimmune thrombocytopenia. Prenat Diagn 2002;22:96–98.
76. Silver RM, Porter TF, Branch DW, et al. Neonatal alloimmune thrombocytopenia: antenatal management. Am J Obstet Gynecol 2000;182:1233–1238.
77. Fergusson D, Hutton B, Sharma M, et al. Use of intravenous immunoglobulin for treatment of neurologic conditions: a systematic review. Transfusion 2005;45:1640–1657.
78. Gray OM, McDonnell GV, Forbes RB. Intravenous immunoglobulins for multiple sclerosis. Cochrane Database Syst Rev 2004:CD002936.
79. Hahn AF, Bolton CF, Zochodne D, Feasby TE. Intravenous immunoglobulin treatment in chronic inflammatory demyelinating polyneuropathy: a double-blind, placebo-controlled, cross-over study. Brain 1996;119:1067–1077.
80. Thompson N, Choudhary P, Hughes RA, Quinlivan RM. A novel trial design to study the effect of intravenous immunoglobulin in chronic inflammatory demyelinating polyradiculoneuropathy. J Neurol 1996;243:280–285.
81. Van Schaik IN, Winer JB, De Haan R, Vermeulen M. Intravenous immunoglobulin for chronic inflammatory demyelinating polyradiculoneuropathy. Cochrane Database Syst Rev 2002:CD001797.
82. Jackson MC, Godwin-Austen RB, Whiteley AM. High-dose intravenous immunoglobulin in the treatment of Guillain-Barre syndrome: a preliminary open study. J Neurol 1993;240:51–53.
83. Hughes RA, Raphael JC, Swan AV, Doorn PA. Intravenous immunoglobulin for Guillain-Barre syndrome. Cochrane Database Syst Rev 2004:CD002063.
84. Gajdos P, Chevret S, Toyka K. Intravenous immunoglobulin for myasthenia gravis. Cochrane Database Syst Rev 2003:CD002277.
85. van Schaik IN, van den Berg LH, de Haan R, Vermeulen M. Intravenous immunoglobulin for multifocal motor neuropathy. Cochrane Database Syst Rev 2005:CD004429.
86. Lichtiger B, Rogge K. Spurious serologic test results in patients receiving infusions of intravenous immune gammaglobulin. Arch Pathol Lab Med 1991;115:467–469.
87. Nydegger UE, Sturzenegger M. Adverse effects of intravenous immunoglobulin therapy. Drug Saf 1999;21:171–185.
88. Pierce LR, Jain N. Risks associated with the use of intravenous immunoglobulin. Transfus Med Rev 2003;17:241–251.
89. Letter to Healthcare Providers. Available at http://www.fda.gov/ cber/ ltr/igivrenal.htm. Accessed Jan. 19, 2006.
90. Meissner HC, Long SS. Revised indications for the use of palivizumab and respiratory syncytial virus immune globulin intravenous for the prevention of respiratory syncytial virus infections. Pediatrics 2003;112:1447–1452.
91. Messori A, Rampazzo R, Scroccaro G, Martini N. Efficacy of hyperimmune anti-cytomegalovirus immunoglobulins for the prevention of cytomegalovirus infection in recipients of allogeneic bone marrow transplantation: a meta-analysis. Bone Marrow Transplant 1994;13:163–167.
92. Ruutu T, Ljungman P, Brinch L, et al. No prevention of cytomegalovirus infection by anti-cytomegalovirus hyperimmune globulin in seronegative bone marrow transplant recipients. The Nordic BMT Group. Bone Marrow Transplant 1997;19:233–236.
93. Zikos P, Van Lint MT, Lamparelli T, et al. A randomized trial of high dose polyvalent intravenous immunoglobulin (HDIgG) vs. cytomegalovirus (CMV) hyperimmune IgG in allogeneic hemopoietic stem cell transplants (HSCT). Haematologica 1998;83:132–137.
94. Varicella Zoster Immune Globulin (Human) package insert. Cangene Corporation. Winnipeg, Canada, 2001.
95. Centers for Disease Control. Recommendations of the Immunization Practices Advisory Committee (ACIP) Varicella-Zoster Immune Globulin for the Prevention of Chickenpox. MMWR Morb Mortal Wkly Rep 1984;33:84–90, 95–100.
96. Centers for Disease Control. Human Rabies Prevention—United States, 1999 Recommendations of the Advisory Committee on Immunization Practices. MMWR Morb Mortal Wkly Rep 1999;48:1–21.
97. BayRab package insert. Bayer Healthcare. Elkhart, Ind., 1999.
98. Imogam Rabies–HT package insert. Aventis Pasteur. Swiftwater, Pa., 1999.
99. Vaccinia immune globulin intravenous (human) package insert. Massachusetts Public Health Biologic Laboratories. Jamaica Plain, Mass., 2005.
100. Bowman J. Thirty-five years of Rh prophylaxis. Transfusion 2003;43:1661–1666.
101. BayRho-D Full Dose package insert. Bayer Healthcare. Elkhart, Ind., 2000.
102. BayRho-D Mini-Dose package insert. Bayer Healthcare. Elkhart, Ind., 2000.
103. MICRhoGAM Ultra-Filtered package insert. Ortho-Clinical Diagnostics, Inc. Raritan, N.J., 2001.
104. Rhophylac I.V. package insert. ZLB Behring. Glendale, Calif., 2004.
105. WinRho SDF package insert. Cangene Corporation. Winnipeg, Canada, 2003.
106. Hartwell EA. Use of Rh immune globulin: ASCP practice parameter. American Society of Clinical Pathologists. Am J Clin Pathol 1998;110:281–292.
107. Thymoglobulin package insert. Genzyme Corporation. Cambridge, Mass., 2005.
108. Atgam lymphocyte immune globulin, anti-thymocyte globulin [equine] sterile solution package insert. Pharmacia & Upjohn Company. Kalamazoo, Mich., 2003.
109. Use of Diphtheria Antitoxin (DAT) for Suspected Diphtheria Cases. Available at http://www.cdc.gov/nip/vaccine/dat/protocol_032504.pdf. Accessed Jan. 17, 2006.
110. BayTet package insert. Bayer Healthcare. Elkhart, Ind., 2004.
111. Products Distributed by The Centers for Disease Control and Prevention. Available at http://www.cdc.gov/ncidod/srp/drugs/formulary.html. Accessed Jan. 17, 2006.

112. BabyBIG, Botulism Immune Globulin Intravenous (Human) (BIG-IV) package insert. Massachusetts Public Health Biologic Laboratories. Boston, Mass., 2003.
113. Digibind for Injection package insert. GlaxoSmithKline. Research Triangle Park, N.C., 2001.
114. Black widow spider antivenin package insert. Merck. Whitehouse Station, N.J., 2005.
115. Antivenin (Crotalidae) Polyvalent package insert. Wyeth-Ayerst. Marietta, Pa., 2001.
116. Antivenin (Micrurus fulvius) package insert. Wyeth-Ayerst. Marietta, Pa., 2001.
117. Meeks EL, Beach MJ. Outbreak of hepatitis C associated with intravenous immunoglobulin administration: United States, October 1993–June 1994. MMWR Morb Mortal Wkly Rep 1994;43: 505–509.
118. Rossi G, Tucci A, Cariani E, et al. Outbreak of hepatitis C virus infection in patients with hematologic disorders treated with intravenous immunoglobulins: different prognosis according to the immune status. Blood 1997;90:1309–1314.
119. Cai K, Gierman TM, Hotta J, et al. Ensuring the biologic safety of plasma-derived therapeutic proteins: detection, inactivation, and removal of pathogens. BioDrugs 2005;19:79–96.
120. Korneyeva M, Hotta J, Lebing W, et al. Enveloped virus inactivation by caprylate: a robust alternative to solvent-detergent treatment in plasma derived intermediates. Biologicals 2002;30:153–162.
121. Pendley C, Schantz A, Wagner C. Immunogenicity of therapeutic monoclonal antibodies. Curr Opin Mol Ther 2003;5:172–179.
122. Orthoclone OKT3 package insert. Ortho Biotech products, L.P. Raritan, N.J., 2003.
123. Zevlin package insert. Biogen Idec Inc. Cambridge, Mass., 2005.
124. Bexxar package insert. GlaxoSmithKline. Research Triangle Park, N.C., 2005.
125. Morrison SL, Johnson MJ, Herzenberg LA, Oi VT. Chimeric human antibody molecules: mouse antigen-binding domains with human constant region domains. Proc Natl Acad Sci U S A 1984;81:6851–6855.
126. Logdberg L, Kaplan E, Drelich M, et al. Primate antibodies to components of the human immune system. J Med Primatol 1994;23:285–297.
127. Ehrlich PH, Moustafa ZA, Harfeldt KE, et al. Potential of primate monoclonal antibodies to substitute for human antibodies: nucleotide sequence of chimpanzee Fab fragments. Hum Antibodies Hybridomas 1990;1:23–26.
128. Jones PT, Dear PH, Foote J, et al. Replacing the complementarity-determining regions in a human antibody with those from a mouse. Nature 1986;321:522–525.
129. Newman R, Alberts J, Anderson D, et al. "Primatization" of recombinant antibodies for immunotherapy of human diseases: a macaque/human chimeric antibody against human CD4. Biotechnology (N Y) 1992;10:1455–1460.
130. Zenapax for Injection package insert. Roche Laboratories. Basel, Switzerland, 2003.
131. Xolair package insert. Genentech, Inc. South San Francisco, Calif., 2003.
132. Synagis package insert. MedImmune. Gaithersburg, Md., 2004.
133. Simulect package insert. Novartis. East Hanover, N.J., 2003.
134. Rituxan package insert. Genentech, Inc. South San Francisco, Calif., 2004.
135. ReoPro package insert. Centocor B.V. Leiden, The Netherlands, 2003.
136. Remicade package insert. Centocor, Inc. Malvern, Pa., 2005.
137. Raptiva package insert. Genentech, Inc. South San Francisco, Calif., 2003.
138. Herceptin package insert. Genentech, Inc. South San Francisco, Calif., 2003.
139. Mylotarg package insert. Wyeth Laboratories. Philadelphia, Pa., 2005.
140. Erbitux package insert. ImClone Systems Incorporated. Branchburg, N.J., 2004.
141. Campath package insert. ILEX Pharmaceuticals, L.P. San Antonio, Tex., 2002.
142. Avastin package insert. Genentech, Inc. South San Francisco, Calif., 2004.
143. Ostberg L, Pursch E. Human X (mouse X human) hybridomas stably producing human antibodies. Hybridoma 1983;2:361–367.
144. Ostberg L. Human monoclonal antibodies in transplantation. Transplant Proc 1992;24:26–30.
145. McCafferty J, Griffiths AD, Winter G, Chiswell DJ. Phage antibodies: filamentous phage displaying antibody variable domains. Nature 1990;348:552–554.
146. Humira package insert. Abbott Laboratories. North Chicago, Ill., 2003.
147. Lonberg N, Taylor LD, Harding FA, et al. Antigen-specific human antibodies from mice comprising four distinct genetic modifications. Nature 1994;368:856–859.
148. Lonberg N. Human antibodies from transgenic animals. Nat Biotechnol 2005;23:1117–1125.
149. Green LL, Hardy MC, Maynard-Currie CE, et al. Antigen-specific human monoclonal antibodies from mice engineered with human Ig heavy and light chain YACs. Nat Genet 1994;7:13–21.
150. Ouwehand WH, Watkins NA, Garner SF, Smethurst PA. Monoclonal antibody therapies in transfusion medicine. Vox Sang 2004;87: 151–154.

Chapter 23
Platelets and Related Products

John M. Fisk • Patricia T. Pisciotto • Edward L. Snyder • Peter L. Perrotta

INTRODUCTION

Platelet transfusion therapy has dramatically improved since the 1950s when whole blood and freshly prepared, platelet-rich plasma were the only available sources of viable platelets. In parallel, technical advances also made over the past several decades have greatly facilitated the collection and storage of platelet concentrates. These include centrifugation procedures optimized to allow the separation of high numbers of functionally active platelets from whole blood donation, and the introduction of automated cell separators now widely used to collect even larger numbers of platelets from a single donor. Initially, the shelf life of platelets was very limited (<1 day) until improved storage containers and optimization of storage conditions allowed for longer (5- to 7-day) storage. This improvement was based on the development of gas-permeable containers that overcame the adverse effects of prolonged storage on platelet structure and function—the "platelet storage defect."

While platelets can be stored for up to 7 days and still have acceptable function and post-transfusion recovery, platelets stored at room temperature were kept only up to 5 days because of the increased risk of bacterial proliferation. However, recent advances in blood collection techniques and automated bacterial culture methodologies coupled with mandatory bacterial testing of all platelets have once again offered the possibility of extended room temperature platelet storage. In addition, many workers continue to investigate alternative techniques to store platelets (e.g., platelet-storage solutions, refrigerated storage) and explore possible platelet substitutes. The latter may be either derived from donor platelets or entirely synthetic.

Platelet transfusions are indicated for the prophylaxis or treatment of bleeding in patients who have low numbers of circulating platelets or functionally inactive platelets.[1] Indeed, thrombocytopenic bleeding was a major cause of death in patients with acute leukemia until stored platelet products became widely available.[2] Today, stored platelets are most commonly transfused to prevent bleeding in severely thrombocytopenic patients. These prophylactic platelet transfusions, largely provided to patients who receive intensive therapies for hematologic malignancies and solid tumors, are primarily responsible for the dramatic increase in the number of platelet transfusions over the past 20 years.[3] Despite the widespread use of platelets in clinical practice, there remains considerable variability in platelet transfusion practices.[4] Part of the difficulty in developing evidence-based guidelines for platelet transfusion therapy is that the relationship between a patient's platelet count and clinically significant bleeding remains only partially understood. Furthermore, the properties of transfused platelets that best correlate with hemostatic effectiveness are not fully defined. These characteristics, which are presumably related to the efficacy of platelet transfusions, are most likely affected by the techniques used to prepare and store platelet concentrates. Thus, despite efforts to standardize platelet transfusion therapy, practices are largely determined locally.

PHYSIOLOGIC ROLE OF PLATELETS

Platelets play a critical role in normal hemostatic processes by preserving vascular integrity and maintaining hemostasis. They accumulate at sites of vascular injury and form hemostatic "plugs." Platelets also participate in clot retraction and wound healing. The effectiveness of platelet transfusion therapy is at least partially explained by the role of endogenous platelets in normal hemostasis. The innate properties of platelets are related to their unique structure, composition, and ability to respond to a variety of stimuli. Their importance in both bleeding and thrombotic conditions has been elucidated over the past several decades. Therefore, one of the goals of transfusion practice is to prepare platelets that maintain these properties during their preparation and storage. Alternatively, novel substances that have many of the hemostatic properties of intact human platelets are being developed as potential alternatives to standard platelet concentrates.

Platelets circulate in the blood as small anucleate, membrane-encapsulated cell fragments. It was recognized in the early 1900s that platelets are derived from bone marrow megakaryocytes.[5] However, the overall process of platelet production, or *thrombopoiesis*, remained poorly understood.[6] Platelets appear on Wright-stained blood smears as small, oval to round bluish-gray bodies containing small purple-red granules. They normally range in size from 1.0 to 2.5 μm, or less than one half the diameter of a normal red cell. The platelet surface is covered by a thin glycocalyx that contains various membrane glycoproteins, mucopolysaccharides, glycolipids, and adsorbed plasma proteins. Sialic acid residues attached to lipids and proteins impart a net negative charge to the platelet surface that may play a role in minimizing the interaction between other platelets and negatively charged endothelial cells. The folded platelet external plasma membrane forms a surface connected canalicular or collecting system that allows plasma components to enter the platelet and internal granule contents to be released. It also greatly increases the surface area of the platelet. Sodium and calcium ATPase pumps within the plasma membrane are thought to control the platelet's ionic environment.

Platelet Structure

Platelets have a discoid shape when in a resting state. The discoid shape is likely maintained by a network of actin filaments near the plasma membrane and a circumferential band of microtubules composed of tubulin polymers and microtubule-associated proteins.[7] On activation, platelet actin can polymerize into microfilamentous bundles that contribute to platelet shape change. The intracellular signaling events that contribute to platelet adhesion and aggregation are becoming better understood.[8] Platelets contain both organelles found in other cells (lysosomes, peroxisomes) and platelet-specific organelles (dense bodies, α-granules). Electron-dense granules (dense bodies) contain storage pool adenosine diphosphate (ADP), adenosine triphosphate (ATP), serotonin, and a major portion of the platelet's calcium. α-Granules contain a variety of proteins including adhesive proteins (von Willebrand factor [vWF], fibrinogen, fibronectin, thrombospondin, P-selectin), anticoagulants (platelet factor 4, β-thromboglobulins), coagulation factors (factors V, XI, XIII, protein S), and growth factors for angiogenesis and repair (platelet-derived growth factor, transforming growth factor β, thrombospondin).[9] Each platelet contains from 2 to 7 small mitochondria that participate in oxidative metabolic processes and are able to undergo changes that are associated with cell injury and death.[10] α-Granules are the most numerous granules seen in platelets by electron microscopy.

Platelet Proteins and the Platelet Membrane

Platelets contain a large array of proteins; some are taken up into α-granules from plasma, whereas others are platelet specific. The most concentrated platelet-specific proteins include platelet factor 4 (PF4) and members of the β-thromboglobulin family. Both proteins can bind heparin. PF4, in particular, binds heparin with high affinity and can neutralize heparin's anticoagulant activity.[11] Other described activities of PF4 include chemotaxis for neutrophils and monocytes,[12] inhibition of megakaryocyte maturation,[13] potentiation of platelet aggregation in vitro,[14] and widespread immunomodulatory effects.[15]

The platelet plasma membrane serves two important roles in hemostasis: (1) it provides a means for cell-to-cell or cell-to-matrix interactions, and (2) it furnishes a surface that enhances the fluid phase of coagulation. Like other mammalian cells, the lipid bilayer consists of phospholipids (PLs) asymmetrically arranged between the outer and inner leaflets.[16] In a resting state, the outer leaflet is composed primarily of neutral phospholipids (PL, phosphatidylcholine, and sphingomyelin), while the inner leaflet is composed of negatively charged PL (phosphatidylserine [PS] and phosphatidylethanolamine [PE]). An ATP-dependent aminophospholipid translocase has been identified in platelet plasma membranes that rapidly transports PS and PE from the outer to the inner leaflet. Other mechanisms also help maintain the normal plasma membrane PL asymmetry.[17] Upon activation and increased intracellular Ca^{2+} levels, a "flip-flop" in the normal membrane PL distribution occurs that results in an increase in PS and PE exposure on the outer leaflet. This membrane alteration contributes to the procoagulant activity of platelets. Specifically, activated platelets participate in thrombin generation by providing a favorable external surface charge for the prothrombinase complex (X-Va), thereby localizing fibrin generation in close proximity to the platelet plug.[18]

The most important adhesive glycoproteins found in α-granules include fibrinogen and vWF. Presumably, these substances are released after platelets accumulate at sites of vascular injury. Since megakaryocytes do not produce fibrinogen, platelets accumulate fibrinogen from plasma through processes involving the $\alpha_{IIb}\beta_3$ integrin.[19] vWF is synthesized in megakaryocytes and endothelial cells and is stored in platelet α-granules. Platelet stores of vWF are high enough so that transfusion of platelets alone to patients with severe type 3 von Willebrand disease partially corrects their bleeding times.[20] The platelet membrane also contains a number of membrane glycoproteins (GPs), many of which function as adhesive proteins. These include the glycoprotein Ib-IX-V complex (GPIb-IX-V), which acts as a platelet receptor for vWF in platelet adhesion and facilitates the ability of thrombin, at low concentrations, to activate platelets.[21] The $\alpha_{IIb}\beta_3$ complex, also termed GpIIb/IIIa, spans the platelet membrane and is a functional receptor for fibrinogen, vWF, fibronectin, and vitronectin.[22] The glycoprotein Ia-IIa complex (GpIa-IIa, $\alpha_2\beta_1$) is the receptor for collagen,[23] and, finally, glycoprotein Ic-IIa (GPIc-IIa, $\alpha_5\beta_1$) is a receptor for fibronectin. The latter three glycoproteins are considered integrins, which are a large family of related heterodimers grouped based on their β-subunit structure. P-selectin (known as CD62P, GMP-140, and PADGEM) is an integral membrane protein found in α-granules that becomes expressed on the surface of activated platelets after granule release.[24] Also found in Weibel-Palade bodies of endothelial cells, P-selectin is an adhesive protein that mediates the attachment of neutrophils and monocytes to activated platelets.

Adhesion and Aggregation

Platelets normally circulate in a "resting" state without adhering to vessel walls for approximately 9 to 10 days before they are removed, primarily in the spleen. Transfused platelets do not usually circulate for this long. Platelets rapidly respond to appropriate stimuli, such as collagen exposed on denuded endothelium, by first adhering to the subendothelial matrix. They initially undergo physical changes that include assuming a more spherical shape. Platelet membranes then form multiple extended pseudopods, an event that dramatically increases their surface area. Interaction between agonists in the microenvironment and specific receptors on the platelet surface results in the transmission of signals from the outside of the cell to the interior, generating secondary messengers that induce protein phosphorylation and the opening of ion channels.[25] The ability of platelets to aggregate on surfaces coated with type 1 collagen has been utilized in in vitro tests designed to measure the functional capacity of transfused platelets.[26] This testing is currently available using automated methodologies.[27]

Adhesion, the binding of platelets to a nonplatelet surface, is the initial event in the formation of the platelet plug. Shear forces within the vessel influence the deposition of platelets on exposed endothelium.[28] At high shear stress, as encountered within the microcirculation, the primary adhesive event is mediated by the interaction of the subendothelium-bound vWF with the platelet GPIb receptor. vWF bound to the subendothelial matrix is believed to undergo a conformational change that exposes the binding site for the GPIb-IX-V complex.[29] The binding site for GPIb appears to reside in the A1 domain of vWF. This bond is transient, and the interaction induces a transmembrane flux of calcium ions, which results in a conformational change and activation of $\alpha_{IIb}\beta_3$. Activated $\alpha_{IIb}\beta_3$ binds irreversibly to vWF to allow firm adhesion of platelets to the vessel wall. The activated $\alpha_{IIb}\beta_3$ integrin recognizes and binds to the RGD (Arg-Gly-Asp) peptide sequences of circulating vWF and fibrinogen, resulting in platelet aggregation.[30] At low shear stresses normally found in larger vessels, the role of vWF in platelet adhesion is less significant.

A critical level of ATP is required for each aspect of platelet function, including shape change, aggregation, and the release reaction. ATP is generated, in part, when glucose is metabolized via the glycolytic and oxidative pathways. As platelets are stimulated, an increase in glycolysis and Krebs cycle metabolism serves to replenish depleted ATP. Platelet adhesion does not appear to be an energy-dependent function as very little ATP is consumed during primary adhesion.[31] ATP consumption mainly occurs during the early phases of platelet aggregation (e.g., shape change).[32] Adenine nucleotides present in platelets are found in two pools: ADP in the metabolic pool, which is constantly turning over, and storage pool ADP, which is found in the dense bodies and released during platelet activation. Plasma glucose metabolism generates approximately 15% of the ATP required during normal aerobic storage, largely via glycolytic catabolism to lactate.[33] Oxidative phosphorylation, perhaps utilizing plasma free fatty acids via β-oxidation, contributes the remaining 85%. Clearly, adequate O_2 and CO_2 exchange is important in maintaining aerobic capabilities of stored platelets. If deprived of oxygen, platelets increase lactate production via anaerobic glycolysis in an attempt to compensate for the loss of energy normally derived from oxidative phosphorylation. Thus, the ability to transport gases—mainly O_2—across the platelet storage bag is critical to normal platelet metabolism and to platelet survival during storage.

PREPARATION AND STORAGE OF PLATELETS

Techniques of Platelet Concentrate Preparation

Platelets are prepared from individual whole blood (WB) donations or are collected from a single donor by automated blood cell separators using apheresis technology.[34] Hereafter, the term *WB-derived platelets* (WB-Plts) is used for platelet concentrates made from either platelet-rich plasma or buffy coats (see below) and the term *apheresis-derived platelets* (AD-Plts) for those collected using automated methods from a single donor.

Whole blood is drawn through wide-bore, siliconized needles to minimize platelet and clotting factor activation and is immediately mixed with anticoagulant. Mechanical devices mix blood with anticoagulant as it is withdrawn and monitor collection volume.[35] Then platelet concentrates are prepared from whole blood using either the buffy coat (BC) or the platelet-rich plasma (PRP) methods (Fig. 23–1). The BC method is favored in Europe, whereas the PRP technique is preferred in the United States. In the PRP method, whole blood is first spun at a low speed (2200 × *g*) for 3 to 4 minutes within 8 hours of collection. The resulting PRP is then spun at a higher speed (4000 × *g*) for 5 minutes to pellet the platelets. All but about 60 mL of PRP is removed and the pellet is left undisturbed for about 1 hour.[36] The pellet is then resuspended by gentle kneading of the bag or by placing the unit on a platelet agitator.[37] Generally, the platelets smoothly resuspend within several hours after which they are stored under continuous gentle agitation. Research has shown that using a hard spin first to spin the platelets into a buffy coat on a cushion of red cells and then using a slow spin to isolate the platelets from the separated buffy coat yields a platelet product with less evidence of in vitro activation.[38] It is unclear whether differences in the properties of PRP and BC platelets affect in vivo survival and efficacy. Earlier studies suggested that 1-hour and 24-hour platelet increments were similar following transfusion of either product.[39] A more recent study comparing post-transfusion recovery and survival of radiolabeled WB-Plts prepared by the BC and PRP methods suggested equivalent in vitro and in vivo activity.[40]

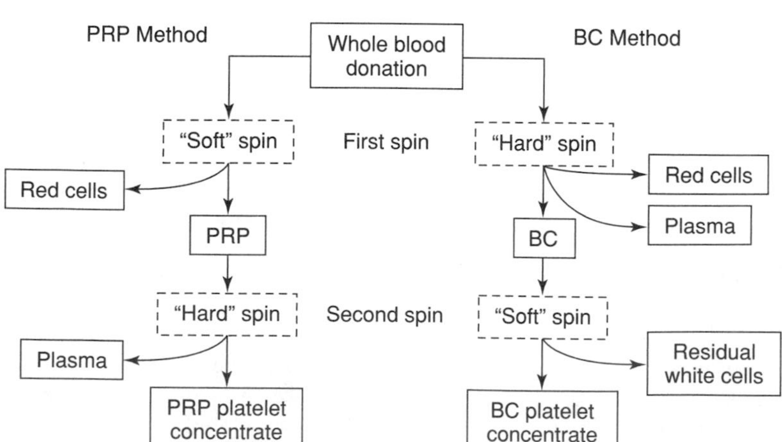

Figure 23–1 Methods for preparation of platelet-rich plasma (PRP)– and buffy coat (BC)–derived platelet concentrates.

Similar studies have compared AD-Plts with BC WB-Plts in terms of their in vitro hemostatic characteristics. Data from these studies support the contention that AD-Plts possess better in vitro hemostatic parameters including preservation of ADP and collagen-induced platelet aggregation and shorter closure times of the PFA 100 test system.[41,42] In vivo studies to ascertain therapeutic differences in these preparations remain to be performed.

Anticoagulant/Preservative Solutions

Citrate-based Storage Solutions

Platelets are prepared from whole blood drawn into one of several anticoagulant-preservative solutions, the most common being citrate-phosphate-dextrose solutions (CPD, CP2D) and CPD with adenine (CPDA-1). Citrate anticoagulates blood according to its ability to chelate calcium and thus inhibit the coagulation cascade. Phosphate serves as a buffer and dextrose as a source of energy. Adenine, which improves red cell survival by increasing cellular ATP levels, serves no purpose in platelet storage. EDTA cannot be used because it causes platelet structural changes associated with reduced in vivo viability and is toxic to humans. Heparin is not an acceptable alternative because it activates platelets, causing platelet clumping. It also causes systemic anticoagulation through its effect on antithrombin. The amount of citrate in the CPD or CPDA-1 preservative does not generally produce systemic anticoagulation or hypocalcemia in blood recipients because it is quickly metabolized to bicarbonate in the liver. AD-Plts are prepared in ACD-A (citric acid, trisodium citrate, dextrose) preservative using automated cell collectors. Citric acid is used to provide a lower pH. In some apheresis systems, platelets are collected as platelet-rich plasma and do not require resuspension, whereas other systems yield a concentrated platelet pellet that must be resuspended. AD-Plts are stored similarly to WB-Plts.

Alternative Storage Solutions

Although platelets stored in citrated plasma are satisfactory for clinical use, several investigators have evaluated other solutions that could extend the shelf life of platelet concentrates or improve their capacity to circulate in vivo after infusion.[43] The majority of these studies have evaluated storage media alternatives in PRP WB-Plts although synthetic storage medium has also been examined for stored BC WB-Plts.[38,44] The scientific basis for this came out of work performed in the 1990s demonstrating that the rate of in vitro platelet aging at 22°C was slowed to less than half of that associated with in vivo aging at 37°C, as determined by isotope labeling.[45] The reduced rate of aging closely paralleled the concomitant reduction in platelet metabolic rate. Thus, in theory, the normal 9- to 10-day platelet life span could be extended to 18 to 20 days or more under optimal storage conditions. Proposed interventional targets to achieve "optimal storage conditions" have included methods to (1) reduce platelet activation during collection, component preparation, and storage; (2) reduce platelet metabolism,[46] thereby decreasing the rates of in-storage glucose consumption and lactate production; and (3) ensure that glucose is not exhausted in the storage medium prior to component outdate.[47]

Most alternatives studied or currently under development are composed of buffered salt solutions containing various additives such as acetate and gluconate.[47–49] Acetate, like glucose and fatty acids, acts as a substrate for platelet metabolism and provides the highly desirable side effect of bicarbonate production during its consumption, which helps buffer pH. Glucose-free crystalloid solutions do not appear to maintain concentrate pH and are associated with reduced in vivo recovery after 5 days of storage.[50] Other investigators have suggested placing various additives in the platelet storage bag that inhibit platelet and coagulation factor activation such as prostaglandin E_1, theophylline, aprotinin, and hirudin.[51–53] Although platelet shelf life can possibly be extended with these additives, the potential for harmful side effects, especially in infants and pregnant women, has slowed their commercial development. Moreover, these solutions could not be deployed to extend the shelf life of stored platelets without the availability of suitably robust methods to detect and limit bacterial contamination.

Storage Temperature

Current Storage Standards

Liquid platelet concentrates were originally stored at 4° C until the late 1960s when it was discovered that products stored at room temperature had longer in vivo survival and greater hemostatic efficacy than those stored at the colder temperature.[54–56] In fact, the shelf life of liquid platelets stored at 22° C was extended from 5 to 7 days in 1984 by the U.S. Food and Drug Administration (FDA) owing to a combination of improved plastic storage containers and increased storage temperature. Within 2 years, however, a marked increased in the incidence of platelet transfusion–related bacterial sepsis prompted the FDA to reduce the maximum storage period back to its current 5-day limit.

The optimal liquid platelet storage temperature appears to be 20° C to 24° C with continuous gentle agitation. While colder storage temperatures demonstrably slow bacterial growth, platelets stored in the cold become activated and lose their normal discoid shape.[57] Development of spherical morphology on exposure to cold has long been recognized as evidence of irreversible physical damage.[58] Changes in platelet morphology have been observed even following short-term (24 hours) exposure to temperatures below 20° C, as may occur during platelet transport. The mechanism for these changes may be related to the release of calcium ions from platelet dense bodies or to influx of calcium across the platelet membrane, resulting in actin filament assembly and, subsequently, platelet activation.[59,60] Chilled platelets have recently been shown to undergo rapid clearing from the circulation by hepatic macrophages. This clearance is mediated by the $\alpha_M\beta_2$ integrin (a complement receptor type 3/Mac-1) that binds to clustered GP1b receptors on the surface of chilled platelets, resulting in rapid platelet phagocytosis.[61] Binding occurs through a lectin-mediated interaction with exposed β-*N*-acetylglucosamine (β-GlcNAc) residues on the GP1b complex. Enzymatic galactosylation of exposed β-GlcNAc residues, however, has been shown to inhibit $\alpha_M\beta_2$ binding, resulting in normalization of chilled platelet intravascular circulation time.[62]

Investigative Strategies for Extended Cold Storage

If changes in the platelet cytoskeleton can be prevented, long-term storage of liquid platelets could become feasible. Platelets treated with cytochalasin B, an inhibitor of new actin filament assembly, do not develop pseudopods or undergo spreading when cooled to 4°C.[63] Human platelets stored for 21 days at 4°C with EGTA-AM, a cytoplasmic Ca^{2+} chelator, and cytochalasin B remain responsive to ADP and thrombin in the presence of exogenous calcium. Other strategies have been developed to allow for preservation of platelet morphology and function during cold storage. These include trehalose, a disaccharide used during freeze-drying, and the antifreeze glycoproteins (AFGPs). The latter proteins are isolated from fish that have adapted to survive in the cold temperatures found in the polar regions. AFGPs reduce platelet activation that occurs when human platelets are stored in the cold.[57] Despite these observations, the future role of cold-stored platelets in clinical transfusion practice remains unclear.

Cryopreserved Platelets

Similarly, the use of cryopreserved platelets remains limited in clinical practice. Platelets frozen in a cryoprotectant solution of 5% to 6% dimethyl sulfoxide (DMSO) can be stored for a period of years at −80°C. Post-thaw ex vivo recovery has been reported to be 75%, with an in vivo 1-hour recovery in normal volunteers of 33% and 8-day survival.[64] The clinical utility of frozen platelets, however, is diminished by the lack of trained personnel and facilities at most hospitals for their preparation, storage, and reconstitution.[65] Thus, widespread adoption of the use of cryopreserved platelets currently appears unlikely. Some investigators, however, support their use in specialized circumstances, such as for autologous or allogeneic donation for subsequent transfusions to manage treatment-related thrombocytopenia in patients with malignancies.[66]

Platelet Storage Containers

Development of Gas-Permeable Plastic Storage Bags

The critical importance of oxygen-permeable containers was recognized shortly after the development of plastic bags for the storage of platelet concentrates. It was appreciated that if oxygen supply to the platelet was inadequate, then metabolism would shift from primarily aerobic to the anaerobic glycolytic pathway. This pathway produces high concentrations of lactic acid, which reacts with the bicarbonate buffer in the plasma. When bicarbonate is exhausted, at levels of 20 to 25 mmol/L of lactic acid, there is a rapid reduction in pH with a resultant loss of platelet viability. Adequate entrance of oxygen into the storage bag, conversely, allows platelets to maintain energy metabolism through mitochondrial oxidative phosphorylation.

Plastic bags originally developed to store platelet concentrates were composed of polyvinyl chloride (PVC) containing a di-2-ethylhexyl phthalate (DEHP) plasticizer and did not permit storage of platelets beyond 3 days. The walls of such plastic bags failed to allow sufficient CO_2 and oxygen exchange for platelets to sustain aerobic metabolism. After 3 days of storage, anaerobic metabolism would produce enough lactic acid that the pH of concentrates routinely fell below 6.0. These changes markedly reduced in vivo platelet recovery and survival.[33,67,68]

Storing platelets in gas-permeable storage bags that permitted the influx of oxygen and the efflux of carbon dioxide was found to ameliorate these untoward effects. It was later discovered that platelet concentrate pH can be adequately maintained for 5 days by storing 50 to 65 mL of PCS in more gas-permeable blood bags made of either PVC with a trimellitate, non-DEHP plasticizer such as TOTM (Fenwal PL1240 or Cutter CLX),[69] or blow-molded polyolefin (Fenwal PL732).[70] Other second-generation platelet storage bags were composed of thin-film PVC with a 2-DEHP plasticizer (XT-612; Terumo), and PVC with a citrate-based non-DEHP plasticizer (butyryl-tri-hexyl citrate [BTHC]; Fenwal PL2209). The latter compound, PL-2209, allows storage of 5–7 × 10^{11} platelets/bag in 400 mL of plasma for 5 days at 20°C to 24°C with acceptable in vitro and in vivo storage characteristics.[71]

Plasticizers and Potential Toxicity

Despite their use since the 1950s, there remain concerns regarding the potential toxicity of storage bags composed of PVC plastic with a DEHP plasticizer, which readily leaches into the blood product.[72–74] These concerns, which include the possible carcinogenicity of DEHP and its monoethylhexyl phthalate (MEHP) metabolite, have led to the development of various alternative plasticizers used in blood storage containers.[75,76] Studies have suggested that transfusing platelets stored in BTHC containing bags, for example, is safe.[77] BTHC leaches into plasma at a level 60% to 70% lower than does DEHP. Moreover, BTHC differs from the phthalate plasticizer in that BTHC is metabolized to physiologic compounds like citric acid, butyric acid, and hexanol. Extensive toxicology testing has shown that BTHC has a very low level of toxicity and that the plasticizer and its degradation products are rapidly eliminated from the body by pulmonary, fecal, and urinary routes. Although gas permeability of the material is slightly less than that of PL-732 plastic, there is sufficient transmission of oxygen into, and carbon dioxide out of, the container to ensure aerobic oxidative metabolism and maintenance of an acceptable pH.

Platelet Storage Agitation

In the late 1970s, it was found that platelets stored with gentle agitation maintained better morphology and in vitro functionality than platelets stored undisturbed.[78] Thus, platelets are now stored with continuous gentle agitation. Rotators are available in a face-over-face (circular) angle of rotation or in a flatbed configuration.[37] However, not all agitators are appropriate to store platelets collected in certain plastic containers. For example, platelets stored in PL732 blow-molded, polyolefin bags using 6-rpm elliptical rotators showed decreased post-transfusion recovery and survival.[70] These findings were thought to be related to platelet–plastic storage bag interactions at various shear stresses created with agitation. Platelet storage using any available storage bag–rotator combination is associated with increasing levels of CD62P over time and progressive release of β-thromboglobulin from α-granules. Agitation is also associated with discharge of cytosolic lactate dehydrogenase (LDH), suggesting that some degree of platelet lysis occurs during agitation.[79]

Apheresis-Derived Platelets

Development of Apheresis Collection Technologies

The development of automated instruments for platelet collection was, in part, motivated by the need to collect large numbers of platelets from a single donor.[80] It was clear during the earliest periods of platelet transfusion therapy that some patients did not demonstrate expected increases in platelet counts following transfusion. However, these patients often had better responses when transfused with platelets collected from HLA-identical siblings.[81] Later, platelets collected from unrelated donors that were HLA-identical to the recipient were also found of use in unrelated platelet-refractory patients.[82]

Advances in apheresis technology have resulted in improved collection efficiencies for various apheresis machines.[83,84] These instruments are highly automated and can also be used to collect granulocytes, red blood cells, and plasma.[85] Apheresis machines routinely collect 5 to 7×10^{11} platelets from a single donor. In fact, many centers are collecting two or three individual units from a single donor collection, each unit containing more than the 3×10^{11} platelets which many standards require for a single-donor apheresis unit.[86] The platelets are collected in larger storage containers that allow adequate transport of oxygen and maintenance of pH. Inability to provide adequate transport of oxygen into the storage bag and, to a lesser degree, adequate transport of carbon dioxide out, limits the number of platelets that can be stored. Currently available citrate-based plasticizer bags can store up to 7×10^{11} platelets in a bag. Like WB-Plts, apheresis products must also be stored at 20° C to 24° C with continuous gentle agitation. Generally, apheresis platelets are collected in ACD-A solutions rather than the standard whole blood anticoagulants CPD, CP2D, or CPDA-1. AD-Plts show in vitro characteristics comparable to, or better than, those of random-donor platelets prepared from whole blood donation.

Apheresis In-Process Leukoreduction

Refinements in apheresis technology now permit in-process leukoreduction capable of achieving a 3 to 4 log-order reduction in the number of residual leukocytes in an AD-Plt unit. This allows collection of highly enriched platelet products with white blood cell contamination levels low enough to allow the unit to be designated as "leukoreduced." This form of "process leukoreduction" appears to provide several direct benefits that include[1] minimizing the levels of various cytokines such as TNFα, which have been implicated in febrile transfusion reactions[87]; (2) reducing the risk of transfusion-related CMV transmission due to virally infected passenger leukocytes[88]; and (3) reducing the risk of platelet refractoriness and HLA alloimmunization.[89] An additional and oft-cited additional benefit is that of "limiting donor exposure." Most transfusion specialists do not believe that it is necessary to administer these products through leukoreduction filters to further reduce the number of white cells.

Autologous Platelet Donation

Several groups have explored the feasibility of autologous platelet donation. Platelets stored in the liquid phase at room temperature currently have a shelf life of only 5 days, making autologous donation impractical. However, platelets collected by apheresis and frozen preserved in DMSO can be stored at −80°C for long periods of time.[90] They are then thawed, washed, and resuspended in autologous plasma or other solutions before transfusion. Platelets prepared by this technique, however, do undergo a number of structural and metabolic changes that decrease their recovery and survival, as compared with liquid-stored platelet concentrates.[91] Furthermore, most patients cannot donate sufficient platelet units to support their needs, for instance, during a course of induction chemotherapy. It is possible, however, to store significant numbers of frozen autologous platelets for patients who are refractory to platelet transfusion, provided the blood bank is technically capable of preparing and storing these specialized products.[92]

Transfusion Practices: Use of Whole Blood–Derived versus Apheresis Platelets

The transfusion practice at a given hospital or medical institution with respect to the use of AD-Plts platelets versus WB-Plts is often dependent on local issues, such as economics, budgetary constraints, and the ability of the local blood supplier to provide these products. Blood collection centers vary in their ability to provide AD-Plts owing to the size and makeup of their donor population, as well as the extent of local facilities and expertise to support apheresis collection. Although an estimated 70% of all platelet transfusions in the United States are leukoreduced apheresis platelet units, blood collection agencies are still unable to meet 100% of the demand with AD-Plts, and the use of WB-Plts remains commonplace in many regions of the country. It is also worthy of note that while platelet collection by apheresis is well tolerated by most donors, hemodynamic instability and adverse reactions related to citrate toxicity (hypocalcemia) can occur.[93] Additionally, recent toxicologic studies investigating intravenous exposure to DEHP in a volunteer apheresis platelet donor demonstrated that exposure to the plasticizer and its metabolites could exceed the U.S. Environmental Protection Agency's Reference Dose (RfD) of 20 μg/kg/day for DEHP on the day of donation.[94] The authors recommended adoption of measures to protect donors from DEHP exposure, particularly potentially at-risk populations such as women in their reproductive years.

Volume-Reduced Platelets

Clinical Indications for Volume Reduction

Platelets prepared from whole blood collections are stored in donor plasma, which serves as a buffering agent. WB-Plts are typically suspended in 40 to 60 mL of plasma to maintain product pH greater than 6.0 for the duration of storage.[95] Volume-reducing platelets for neonates is not usually necessary, because adequate platelet increments are achieved by transfusing small volumes of platelets; 10 mL/kg is a standard dose for neonates.[96] There are specific clinical situations, however, in which volume-reduced platelets are considered. For example, transfusing plasma-incompatible platelets, a reasonably common adult transfusion practice, is of more potential harm to infants with smaller red cell volumes. The most dangerous scenario is when a group A infant is transfused with AD-Plts from a group O donor who carries high-titer anti-A.[96] For this reason, blood services that provide mainly AD-Plts may titer group O products before they are transfused to group A recipients. If ABO-compatible platelets are not available, plasma can be removed from the platelets by centrifugation and replaced with saline or albumin. Plasma removal is also considered when an antibody present in donor plasma is directed against an antigen present on a neonatal blood cell. This situation arises when an HPA-1a negative mother is the only source of antigen-negative platelets for her newborn with neonatal alloimmune thrombocytopenia due to anti-HPA-1a. Volume-reduced platelets may also be warranted when circulatory overload is a major concern, as part of an overall restriction of intravenous fluids.

Platelet Effects of Volume Reduction

Recentrifugation of platelets stored for up to 5 days at 1500 × *g* for 7 minutes, 2000 × *g* for 10 minutes, or 5000 × *g* for 6 minutes, followed by resuspension in 10 mL of plasma after a 1-hour rest period, results in a loss of 5% to 20% of the platelets.[97] At the latter two centrifuge speeds, in vivo survival of the platelets that tolerate centrifugation/resuspension appeared normal in healthy volunteers. Platelet loss is less than 15% after a shorter 20-minute rest period, when platelets are spun at lower speeds but for longer times (e.g., 580 × *g* for 20 minutes).[98] Platelets stored for 1 or 5 days either on a flatbed or an end-over-end tumbler agitator and then volume-reduced showed no adverse effects on in vitro function as assessed by morphology, response to hypotonic stress, aggregation, platelet factor 3 activity, pH, and discharge of lactate dehydrogenase (LDH). Acceptable platelet increments can also be obtained in critically ill thrombocytopenic neonates transfused with volume-reduced AD- or WB-Plts. The use of the softer spin technique to produce volume-reduced PCs has the advantage of more rapid availability of products. Recent studies have confirmed the adequacy of recentrifuged, volume-reduced platelets, although data from one study demonstrated a higher level of spontaneous activation (43.2%, control 33.8%) and impaired ADP-induced but not collagen-induced aggregability of treated AD-Plts versus control platelets.[99]

Use of Syringe Storage for Neonatal Transfusion

Neonates usually require small-volume transfusions; therefore, blood components are often dispensed or transfused with a syringe. For platelets to maintain an acceptable pH, it is imperative that the storage container allow sufficient gas exchange. Platelet concentrates stored for up to 5 days and then maintained in gas-impermeable polypropylene syringes for 6 hours showed increases in consumption of glucose and production of lactic acid.[100] The resultant decline in pH was associated with a switch from aerobic to anaerobic metabolism. Similar results were observed when platelets were stored in syringes for 6 hours at 37° C. The pH in all these situations, however, never fell below 6.5, which is within the accepted range for platelets stored in gas-permeable blood bags. Volume-reduced platelets produced by the soft-spin technique described above and stored in syringes for 6 hours at room temperature or 37° C were also evaluated.[101] Higher temperature storage produced the greatest and most rapid decline in pH. Other in vitro parameters of platelet function, such as morphology score, response to hypotonic stress, and LDH discharge were not adversely affected under the conditions studied. Therefore, it appears that PCs, either standard or volume-reduced, that are dispensed to neonatal nurseries in syringes for transfusion within 4 to 6 hours maintain acceptable in vitro platelet function.

STANDARDS AND QUALITY CONTROL OF PLATELET CONCENTRATE MANUFACTURE

Standards for Platelet Concentrates

In many respects, the standards for platelet products have evolved in parallel with advances in processing and storage conditions that allow longer storage of viable platelets. Quality assurance (QA) programs have been developed to monitor the composition and viability of platelets.[102] These procedures are designed to minimize the variability in end products—variability that can preclude determining the efficacy of platelet products. Standards for monitoring the quality of platelet products vary across countries and are specific for the preparation technique. Most standards require that platelet product testing include platelet numbers, pH, white cell numbers for leukoreduced products, and product volume (Table 23–1).[103] In the United States, WB-Plts must contain a minimum of 5.5×10^{10} platelets per bag; AD-Plts must contain at least 3.0×10^{11} platelets per bag. Platelet counts are commonly determined using automated hematology analyzers whose precision and accuracy is acceptable for this purpose. Flow cytometric methods have also been developed that allow for precise platelet enumeration.

Table 23–1 **Standards for Platelet Products**

	United States*		Europe†	
	Whole-Blood Derived	Apheresis Derived	Whole-Blood Derived	Apheresis Derived
Platelets ($\times 10^{10}$)	≥5.5	≥30	Varies#	Varies#
Volume (mL)	Not specified	Not specified	Not specified‖	Not specified‖
White cells ($\times 10^{6}$) to label leukoreduced	<0.83‡	<5.0‡	<1.0§	<1.0§
pH	>6.2	>6.2	6.4–7.4	6.4–7.4

*Data from American Association of Blood Banks. Technical manual, 14th ed. Bethesda, Md.: American Association of Blood Banks, 2002.
†Data from Guide to the Preparation, Use and Quality Assurance of Blood Components, 10th ed. Strasbourg, Council of Europe Publishing, 2004.
‡In 95% of units tested.
§Standard met if 90% of units tested fall within indicated values.
‖Volume must maintain product within specified pH for duration of storage.
#Platelet number within limits that comply with validated preparation and preservation conditions.

These utilize fluorescent dyes and monoclonal antibodies conjugated to fluorochromes.[104] These techniques, which require a flow cytometer or other instrument capable of detecting fluorescence, are not routinely used in platelet quality monitoring.

The volume of suspending plasma is not specified; however, the amount must be sufficient to maintain a pH greater than 6.0 for the duration of storage. Prior to pretransfusion release of a platelet concentrate, some investigators advocate inspecting the unit for the presence of the "swirling phenomenon" in which normal discoid platelets exposed to light and rotated display a characteristic appearance.[105] Presence of swirling, which suggests grossly normal platelet morphology, may correlate with acceptable pH values and adequate in vivo viability.[106,107] There is no requirement, however, to check for swirling prior to issue of platelet components. Finally, temperature control charts should document that platelets are stored at 20°C to 24°C in an uninterrupted manner.

Standards for Leukocyte Reduced Platelets

Allowable Levels of White Cell Contamination

Platelets may be designated as "PLATELETS LEUKOCYTES REDUCED" although the criterion for this designation differs between the United States and Europe. Current standards in the E.U. mandate that leukoreduced platelet units contain $<1 \times 10^6$ white cells per unit, whereas U.S. FDA standards allow $<5 \times 10^6$ white cells per unit, provided that a minimum of 85% of the original product be retained if leukoreduction filters are employed.

Methods for Determination of Residual White Cell Counts

Most blood collection centers continue to use manual methods to determine residual white blood cell counts for quality control (QC) purposes. Automated hematology analyzers that are commonly used in clinical laboratories utilize techniques based on the principles of impedance or light-scattering properties of cells suspended in a liquid medium. These techniques, however, lack the requisite precision and accuracy at very low residual white blood cell numbers that are commonly encountered in leukoreduced blood products—generally on the order of 5 cells/μL—and thus cannot be used for QC purposes. At present, residual white blood cell numbers are most commonly performed by manual chamber techniques. Larger volume (50 μL) Nageotte type hemacytometers using Turk's or Plaxan's staining solutions are typically employed.[108,109] The variability of chamber counts, however, is considerable,[110] which has prompted development of alternative techniques. These include methods based on flow cytometry, microvolume fluorimetry, and quantitative polymerase chain reaction.[111–114] Most flow cytometric methods developed to count residual leukocytes use dyes that stain nuclear components (propidium iodide) or leukocyte-specific antibodies (CD45) conjugated to a fluorochrome.

Quality Control Sampling Requirements

Current methods of leukoreduction (LR), when properly performed, consistently provide products that fulfill standards for white blood cell removal.[115] However, a proportion of products must be sampled within a QC program to document adequate LR.[116] Only a small number of the platelet products produced are actually sampled because it is not currently feasible to test all products. Typically, from 4 to 10 products per month, or 1% of all products collected, are tested for WC numbers. Concerns have been expressed that such sampling numbers and sampling frequencies are inadequate.[117] Ideally, the QC program should include a formal technique for statistical monitoring that is performed on a continuous basis. These steps could maximize the likelihood of detecting process failures. However, most facilities continue to test platelet products at weekly or monthly intervals.

Standards for Detection of Bacterial Contamination of Platelets

Current AABB Standards to Limit and Detect Bacterial Contamination

In the United States, inspecting and accrediting agencies such as the American Association of Blood Banks (AABB) have recently instituted standards that must be followed to limit and detect bacterial contamination of all platelet units. The 22nd edition of the AABB *Standards for Blood Banks and Transfusion Services* mandates that "blood bank or transfusion service shall have methods to limit and detect bacterial contamination of all platelet components" and that "the venipuncture site shall be prepared so as to minimize the risk of bacterial contamination. Green soap shall not be used."[118] Although originally scheduled for implementation by November 1, 2003, logistical concerns led to a revised implementation date of March 1, 2004, for the new standard. Additional AABB Association Bulletins were subsequently published to provide guidance and clarification regarding specifics of implementation. In addition, the College of American Pathologists (CAP) now includes testing for bacterial detection of platelets as part of its Transfusion Medicine Checklist as a Phase I requirement for laboratory accreditation.[119]

The requirements for additional measures to detect and limit bacterial contamination were prompted by growing concerns over transfusion-related bacterial sepsis and fatalities, particularly associated with platelet transfusions. In order to ensure appropriate in vivo function and survival, platelets are stored at 20°C to 24°C with gentle agitation in oxygen-permeable bags as previously described. These storage conditions render platelets particularly susceptible to bacterial contamination. Of the estimated 9 million platelet units transfused in the United States annually,[120] approximately 1:1000 to 1:3000 are bacterially contaminated—a figure that has remained remarkably consistent over numerous studies.[121–124]

Transfusion-Related Deaths Due to Bacterial Contamination

FDA statistics on transfusion-related fatalities underscore the seriousness of microbial contamination of blood products: 46 (17%) of the 277 reported transfusion-related deaths during the period 1990 to 1998 were due to bacterial sepsis.[125] Rates of serious, potentially life-threatening sepsis due to bacterially contaminated platelets have been estimated at 1:50,000 to 1:100,000 transfused units; rates of immediate fatality are estimated at 1:500,000.[120,126] Data on adverse outcomes of transfusion, however, remain limited, and these estimates may be low; prospective studies from the Johns Hopkins University Hospital[127] and University Hospital of Cleveland[128] reported the risk of fatality due to bacterially contaminated AD-Plts at 1:17,000 and 1:48,000, respectively.

Historically, rates of platelet transfusion-related sepsis have been closely tied to duration of product storage. Nearly all the platelet-transfusion related fatalities reported to the FDA in the late 1990s were with units that were 4 or 5 days old.[125] Recognition of this phenomenon gained widespread attention in the mid-1980s, as improvements in platelet storage containers led to an extension of the maximal platelet storage time from 3 to 5 days in 1982, and from 5 to 7 days the following year. Concurrent with longer platelet storage was a marked increase in the number of FDA-reported deaths due to bacterially contaminated platelets: four cases were reported in 1983 alone, compared with only a single case reported in the period from 1976 to 1979.[129] In response, the FDA reduced the allowable platelet storage duration back to 5 days in 1986, resulting in a decline in the rate of reported cases of bacterial sepsis due to contaminated products.

Through this period and into the mid-1990s, interest in the issue of bacterial contamination was largely eclipsed by greater concerns for viral transfusion-transmitted disease (TTD) risks, particularly human immunodeficiency virus (HIV) transmission. Improvements in donor screening and viral detection methods, particularly with the advent of nucleic acid amplification technology (NAT) based methods, led to a dramatic reduction in the risk of viral TTDs.[130] With reductions in the risk of HIV, hepatitis B (HBV), and hepatitis C (HCV) infection, attention once again turned to the issue of bacterial contamination, which had seen no significant reduction in rates in over a decade. Three FDA-sponsored workshops on bacterial contamination of platelets were convened to review the scope of the problem and discuss possible interventions.[125,131,132] Supporting the need for measures to curb rates of bacterial contamination were data from numerous national transfusion surveillance programs, including the BaCon Study (U.S.),[133] Serious Hazards of Transfusion (SHOT) study (U.K.),[134] and the French Haemovigilance System.[135]

Spectrum and Sources of Bacterial Contaminants

Gram-Positive versus Gram-Negative Bacterial Contamination

A broad spectrum of contaminants have been isolated in cases of platelet transfusion-associated sepsis including *Staphylococcus* spp., *Streptococcus* spp., *Bacillus* spp., *Escherichia coli*, *Salmonella* spp., *Serratia* spp., *Enterobacter* spp., and other organisms.[133,134] In a review of transfusion-transmitted bacterial infections, Wagner found that over half (56%) of all reported isolates in cases of bacterial contamination of platelets were gram-positive organisms, the majority of which were aerobes. He also noted differential representation of bacterial species in cases of clinical sepsis versus sepsis-related deaths. *Staphylococcus epidermidis* was more commonly encountered in cases of clinical sepsis than in septic fatalities, whereas *Klebsiella* spp. were only rarely encountered in cases of clinical sepsis but represented 17.3% of cases of septic fatalities. Overall, approximately 60% of sepsis-related deaths were due to gram-negative organisms. Based heavily on data from work done by Brecher and others,[136] a list of organisms required for bacterial contamination detection system clearance by the FDA was drafted. The list includes representatives of the most commonly isolated gram-positive and -negative organisms, aerobes and anaerobes, and the fungus *Candida albicans*.

Sources of Bacterial Contamination

Investigators in the aforementioned studies frequently noted that sources of bacterial contamination often could not be definitively identified, although considerable evidence pointed to three primary sources[137]:

1. Donor skin flora
2. Donor bacteremia (asymptomatic) at the time of collection
3. Contamination during product manufacture

Bacterial contamination by donor skin flora may occur as a result of several mechanisms including inadequate donor arm-skin disinfection,[138] scarring at the phlebotomy site with resultant harboring of bacteria,[139] and contamination of collections by phlebotomy needle-associated skin cores or flaps.[140] Asymptomatic donor bacteremia at the time of blood donation is a well-recognized phenomenon and has occurred in the setting of chronic enterocolitis infection, chronic gut infection, chronic osteomyelitis, and following medical or dental procedures.[141,142] Contaminated apheresis solutions, water baths, etc., have also been implicated as portals of bacterial contamination.[125]

Methods to Limit Bacterial Contamination of Platelets

Donor Phlebotomy Site Disinfection and Initial Collection Diversion

AABB standards mandate methods to both *limit* and *detect* bacterial contamination of platelet components. Although considerable recent effort has been devoted to developing more sensitive methods of bacterial detection, improvements in prevention of bacterial contamination have also been reported. Improved donor phlebotomy site disinfection and methods to divert an initial aliquot of blood have both been associated with decreased rates of skin flora contamination of blood products. McDonald and colleagues reported a 57% rate of reduction in bacterial contamination rates using a two-stage procedure with 70% isopropyl alcohol followed by 2% tincture of iodine, as compared with a one-stage process using 70% isopropyl alcohol and 0.5% chlorhexidine wipe system.[143] He also reported a 47% reduction in contamination rate using a collection bag system that allowed diversion of the first 20 mL of collection into a sampling pouch. When combined, improved donor arm preparation with diversion resulted in an overall 77% reduction in contamination. The results of these interventions are consistent with decreased bacterial contamination rates reported by other investigators.[138,144,145]

Methods to Detect Bacterial Contamination of Platelets

Numerous methods for detection of bacterial contamination of platelets are both in current clinical practice and in ongoing development. These vary widely with respect to analytical sensitivity, procedural complexity, turn-around time, cost, and time-to-detection characteristics. Comprehensive reviews of current and investigational technologies have recently been published.[126,137]

Culture-Based and Nonculture "Surrogate" Detection Methods

Current methodologies can be broadly divided into culture-based and nonculture ("surrogate") methods. In bacteriology, culture remains the "gold standard" for sterility testing,[146] and automated bacterial culture systems have been extensively investigated. Surrogate methods such as visual inspection for swirling, Gram staining, pH, and glucose analysis, while less sensitive, are generally faster and less costly. At present, culture-based methods tend to be utilized by blood collection facilities near the time of collection, whereas surrogate methods are more commonly employed in prerelease testing by hospital-based transfusion services.

Surrogate Bacterial Detection Methods: Visual Swirl, Reagent Strip pH and Glucose Semiquantification, and Direct Visualization of Organisms

Surrogate methods for detection of bacterial contamination are based on changes in platelet unit pH, glucose concentration, and platelet morphology due to activation that occurs in response to increasing levels of microbial contamination. In general, these methods lack analytical sensitivity and can only reliably detect heavily contaminated units. Presently, the AABB recommends use of surrogate methods only for prerelease testing owing to their poor analytical performance characteristics.[147,148]

Visual inspection for "swirling" can easily be performed by trained personnel. Loss of swirl occurs when pH drops sufficiently to inhibit platelet metabolism: the normally discoid platelets then become spherical. This shape change is associated with loss of visual "swirl." Although use of this method is simple, rapid, and noninvasive, it is highly subjective, difficult to validate, and has a detection sensitivity of $\geq 10^7$ colony-forming units (CFU)/mL.[148]

Multireagent strips ("urine dipsticks") for pH and glucose have shown similar levels of sensitivity ($>10^7$ CFU/mL), although some authors have reported greater sensitivities.[149] Validation studies for pH and glucose concentration are collection bag/preservative solution specific and have been reported for the Baxter PL732 CPD bag and the Medsep CLX CP2D bags. A pH of <7.0 and glucose of <250 mg/dL in the Baxter PL732 bags or ≤ 500 mg/dL for the Medsep CLX bags was predictive of bacterial contamination.[147]

Direct visualization of microorganisms using staining methods may also be employed. These generally utilize Gram's stain, Wright's stain, or acridine orange and have reported sensitivities of approximately 10^5 CFU/mL[106] for Wright's and Gram's stains and 10^4 CFU/mL for acridine orange.[126,147] Successful use of staining methods to interdict contaminated platelet units has been previously reported.[121]

Culture-Based Bacterial Detection Methods

Although culture remains the gold standard for bacterial detection and identification, its sensitivity in detecting bacterial contamination of blood products is affected by numerous factors including the growth characteristics of the contaminating organism, timing of specimen procurement, specimen volume, and degree of initial bacterial contamination. Numerous studies of culture-based detection systems have been performed. These have demonstrated that the timing of specimen collection is critically important to test sensitivity: cultures obtained on the day of collection invariably fail to demonstrate bacterially contaminated units that could develop clinically significant overgrowth during storage.[150] Because of the small sample volume normally obtained, reliable detection requires time for the organisms to proliferate to levels at which sampling would include adequate numbers of the organism. Currently, most detection system manufacturers recommend at least a 24-hour incubation period prior to sampling.

Current FDA-Approved Culture-Based Detection Systems

Of the various automated or semiautomated culture systems in use in clinical bacteriology laboratories, only two are presently FDA approved for QC testing for bacterial detection of platelet products in the United States: BacT/ALERT (bioMérieux, Durham, N.C.) and the Pall Enhanced Bacterial Detection System (eBDS) (Pall Corp., East Hills, N.Y.). The BacT/ALERT system uses broth bottles with colorimetric sensors that detect changes in CO_2 levels that occur with bacterial proliferation. Several investigators have validated its sensitivity and specificity in the detection of a wide variety of organisms.[151–154] The system reliably detects contamination levels of 10 CFU/mL or less in 12 to 26 hours, although slower growing organisms such as *Propionibacterium acnes* may take longer to detect.

The Pall eBDS system provides testing in an essentially closed system in which the inoculation receptacle is provided as a satellite bag connected to the main platelet component bag. A 5- to 6-mL sample is expressed from the storage bag into the inoculation bag and allowed to incubate. Following incubation, oxygen tension in the head space of the bag is measured: a drop in O_2 tension indicates bacterial contamination. Independent validation studies of the eBDS system have reported analytical sensitivities for 10 common bacterial contaminants of 96.5% at 24 hours and 100% at 30 hours.[155]

Laboratory Detection of Bacterial Contamination versus Clinical Outcomes

Despite promising early validation studies, clinical studies of culture-based as well as surrogate method bacterial detection strategies have revealed occasional discordance between laboratory findings and clinical outcomes. In 2005, te Boekhorst and coworkers reported their 2-year experience with universal bacterial screening of all pooled platelet concentrates using the BacT/ALERT system.[156] Of the 28,104 products tested, 203 generated a positive signal (0.72%) of which 184/203 were confirmed true positive (0.65%). Of these bacterially contaminated units, 113/184 had been transfused prior to positive screening, and none were associated with clinically detectable transfusion reaction. Conversely, two patients developed severe, life-threatening sepsis with *Bacillus cereus* that was cultured from both the patient and the platelet bag at the time of the reaction. In both cases, 7-day screening cultures were negative. Similar reports of negative screening results associated with severe or fatal septic transfusion reactions from contaminated platelet units have been reported.[120] This has led some investigators to call for stricter requirements for bacterial testing of platelet units.[157]

Extended Platelet Storage

With the institution of the new standards to both *limit* and *detect* bacterial contamination of platelet products, consideration is once again being given to increasing the maximum storage time of platelets to 7 days. Some have argued that the additional cost burden of mandatory culturing could be mitigated in part by the more favorable inventory situation that extended platelet storage would provide.[158] At present, only Gambro BCT AD-Plt technology has been cleared by the FDA for 7-day platelet storage.[159] This system requires use of an approved release test for bacterial contamination screening, as described in the manufacturer's instructions for use (IFU). Owing to the low incidence of bacterial contamination of platelet units, FDA approval has been coupled with mandatory postmarket surveillance study to estimate the performance of the bioMérieux BacT/ALERT Microbial System when used as a release test with Gambro AD-Plts.

CHANGES IN PLATELETS WITH STORAGE

Platelet-Storage Defect

The platelet-storage defect (PSD), or platelet-storage lesion (PSL), encompasses all untoward effects on platelet morphology, structure, and function with storage. These changes begin at the time of blood collection and component preparation and continuously progress during storage. The mechanisms responsible for the PSD are not fully understood but are clearly multifactorial. Development of the PSL is in general related to collection technique, storage conditions, and postcollection manipulation.[160] For example, centrifugation can affect platelet function by exposing platelets to shear stress conditions. Shear stresses not only produce a discharge of cytosolic LDH but also stimulate the platelet release reaction.[79] Release of β-thromboglobulin into the suspending plasma and appearance of P-selectin (CD62P, GMP-140) on the platelet membrane surface following platelet preparation are both evidence of platelet granule release.[161,162]

During storage, the metabolic activity of platelets and residual leukocytes continues to consume nutrients and produce harmful metabolic products. Activated clotting factors, cellular debris, and proteolytic enzymes found in the suspending plasma can adversely affect platelets. Many structural changes to the platelet cytoskeleton and surface membrane antigens that occur during storage also appear related to poorer in vivo post-transfusion recovery and survival.[163] A vast array of in vitro tests have been used to follow changes in platelets with processing and storage (Table 23–2). In general, only platelet numbers, concentrate volumes, pH at 5 days, and leukocyte content are routinely measured in transfusion practice. The remaining assays, primarily relegated to research settings, correlate to varying degrees with in vivo platelet survival. Techniques used to study in vivo platelet survival—mainly, radiolabeling or biotinylation of platelets prior to transfusion—are not commonly performed and have their own limitations.[164,165] Many of these supplemental assays cannot be applied to large-scale platelet production. Unfortunately, there is no single in vitro assay that can accurately predict in vivo recovery and survival of transfused platelets.

Table 23–2 **Analytic Methods for Characterizing Platelets and Quantifying the Platelet Storage Defect**

Type of Analysis	Method
Routine studies	Platelet number Concentrate volume pH Visual inspection, swirl Leukocyte content
Morphology and shape changes	Qualitative swirling Morphology score Mean platelet volume Osmotic recovery Extent of shape change
Metabolic activity	pH, pO_2, pCO_2, HCO_3 changes Lactate production Glucose consumption Intracellular calcium ATP/ADP ratio
Platelet aggregation	Spontaneous aggregation Response to dual agonists
Platelet activation	CD62 P-selectin expression Annexin V binding
Platelet lysis	Supernatant LDH content Lysate vWF:Ag levels
Miscellaneous	Cytokine levels Activated complement Bacterial growth
In vivo assays	Corrected count increment Radiolabeled survival Biotin-labeled survival

Platelet Activation during Preparation and Storage

A variety of markers have been employed to examine the platelet activation that occurs during the storage of platelet concentrates. These include proteins associated with the α-granule, such as β-thromboglobulin, platelet factor 4, and P-selectin; dense granule proteins such as serotonin; cytosolic enzymes such as LDH; and membrane ligands including GPIb and GPIIb/IIIa.[166,167] There is little evidence that the degree of platelet activation associated with routine platelet preparation and storage adversely affects the ability of transfused platelets to circulate, correct the bleeding time, produce acceptable corrected count increments, and arrest bleeding. In fact, activated platelets have been shown to continue to circulate and function in a nonhuman primate model of platelet transfusion.[168] However, it is likely that platelet activation attributed to the preparation and storage of platelets is partially responsible for their deterioration, as assessed by certain in vivo tests of platelet function.[169]

Platelet Activation and Expression of P-Selectin

P-selectin (CD62P, previously known as GMP-140 or PADGEM) is an important adhesive protein involved in platelet/leukocyte/endothelial interactions. Its functions are related to leukocyte attachment, rolling, and extravasation and the regulation of leukocyte cytokine synthesis.[170] This α-granule membrane protein is sequestered on the internal membrane of the α-granule in resting platelets. Platelet activation through most mechanisms results in fusion of the α-granule with the platelet membrane. P-selectin then becomes expressed on the outer surface of the platelet membrane.[171] Thus, the number of platelets that have undergone α-granule release can be estimated by measuring the total surface content of P-selectin.

Several investigators have used monoclonal antibodies directed against P-selectin to study platelet activation during PCS preparation and storage.[172] Platelet preparation by the PRP technique can result in P-selectin expression by approximately 20% of platelets. Platelet activation is in general lower, approximately 8%, when platelets are isolated from the buffy coat without pelleting.[173] Interestingly, approximately 50% of all platelets are activated after 5 days of storage, whether prepared by the PRP or buffy coat methods. These observations suggest that while platelet pelleting used in the PRP method causes significant α-granule release, an obligatory degree of platelet activation occurs during storage regardless of the preparative technique. In another study, it was found that the higher the platelet count in the platelet concentrate, the greater the percentage of activated platelets at any given time.[174] After 5 days of storage, platelet activation averaged 15% in less concentrated, stored platelets (1×10^9/mL) and 30% in more concentrated units (1.4×10^9/mL); these percentages increased to 60% and 70%, respectively, by 10 days of storage.

P-Selectin and Platelet Recovery/ Survival Studies

It has been suggested that activated, P-selectin-positive platelets might be preferentially removed from the circulation after transfusion. Activated platelets first bind to leukocytes and are then eliminated, presumably through the mononuclear phagocyte (reticuloendothelial) system. This hypothesis was tested by isolating platelets from normal donors, storing them for 2 to 4 days under standard blood bank conditions, and then reinfusing the platelets. Pretransfusion platelet P-selectin expression was determined, and in vivo survival was estimated by ^{111}In labeling.[161] Platelet recoveries at 1 hour demonstrated a modest inverse correlation with the percentage of activated platelets expressing P-selectin ($r^2 = 0.30$; $P < 0.05$). As in other studies of platelet survival, other factors (pH, temperature, agitation) in addition to activation may have influenced platelet recovery. The recovery of activated platelets after transfusion was also studied in thrombocytopenic cancer patients. By quantifying the percentage of activated platelets in patients before and after transfusion and in the platelet concentrate, the observed recovery of activated platelets was compared with the predicted recovery, which was based on the increment in platelet count after transfusion. The observed recovery of activated platelets was always lower than predicted, averaging 38% of the predicted values and implying that activated platelets may be preferentially cleared after transfusion. These data suggest that increased platelet activation as measured by P-selectin expression may be related to poorer in vivo survival.

Proteolysis of Platelet Cytoskeletal Proteins during Storage

The platelet cytoskeleton plays a major role in maintaining platelet shape. It also assures the integrity of the external platelet membrane, which carries several important receptors.[175,176] Platelet cytoskeletal proteins undergo a degree of degradation during storage. However, the contribution of this "proteolysis" to the progression of the platelet storage defect is largely unknown. Certainly, deterioration of cytoskeletal proteins could negatively impact platelet structure and function. Moreover, protein degradation may play a role in platelet microvesicle formation during platelet storage.[172,177] There are a large number of platelet cytoskeleton proteins including actin, actin-binding protein (ABP), talin, vinculin, gelsolin, tubulin, and myosin heavy chain. Of these, actin is present in greatest abundance, constituting 15% to 20% of total platelet protein.

Actin Breakdown during Platelet Storage

When platelet products are stored under blood bank conditions, actin is cleaved into at least two fragments of approximately 28 kDa.[178] Amino acid sequencing has identified that these proteins are formed when actin is cleaved at the N terminus of residues Thr-106 and Ala-114. Actin fragments are generated when platelets are stimulated by the calcium ionophore A23187, in a reaction that can be inhibited by nonspecific protease inhibitors.[179–181] This finding suggests that actin is proteolyzed by the calcium-dependent neutral protease calpain. Degradation of other platelet cytoskeletal proteins during storage like ABP, talin, and vinculin may also be related to calpain activation. Specifically, ABP degradation products have been seen on immunoblots of 1-day-old platelets, providing further evidence that platelet activation begins during actual platelet preparation. After 6 days of platelet storage under blood bank conditions, ABP undergoes additional degradation as reflected by further generation of lower molecular weight breakdown products.

Calpain Activation and Platelet Microvesicle Formation

Platelets are exposed to shear stresses during their separation from blood as well as during agitated storage. These, and other physical stresses, appear capable of stimulating calpain generation. Calpain activation during storage may also promote platelet microvesicle (PMV) formation. Microvesicles are fragments of platelet membrane that are continuously formed during platelet concentrate storage.[177] Presumably, activated calpain promotes PMV formation by degrading actin and other cytoskeletal proteins, leading to a weakening of the actin-cytoplasmic membrane interface with resultant formation of microvesicles.[182] Despite these observations, the overall contribution of such proteases in the deterioration of platelets with storage remains unclear.

Non-Caspase-Dependent Platelet Apoptosis

Recent data suggest that apoptosis, possibly mediated through non-caspase-dependent mechanisms, may also play a role in platelet cytoskeletal changes during storage.[183–186] Apoptosis—programmed cell death—was first described by Kerr and associates in 1972[187] and was long held to be solely a property of nucleate cells. Only relatively recently was it appreciated that anucleate platelets likewise possessed extranuclear apoptotic machinery.[188] Many of the changes commonly found in apoptosis have been identified in platelets including apoptotic morphology, loss of mitochondrial function, activation of the effector caspase 3, microparticle formation, and elaboration of phosphatidylcholine (PC) on the platelet surface. Research findings on platelet apoptosis were recently summarized in a review by Leytin and Freedman.[186]

Modulation of Glycoprotein Ib and IIb/IIIa Expression during Storage

Changes in the expression of platelet-specific glycoproteins, such as GPIb and GPIIb/IIIa, occur during platelet storage. Over time the extracellular portion of GPIb can be cleaved by thrombin or plasmin, resulting in increased levels of the glycosylated portion of GPIb, glycocalicin, in the cell-free supernatant.[189] Despite an increase in plasma glycocalicin, however, platelet surface GPIb content remains relatively constant, although a distinct subpopulation of GPIb-negative platelets does appear over time.[189] Investigators have postulated that surface GPIb may be replenished through relocation of GPIb to the surface from an intracellular pool or a sequestered surface population.

Storage Conditions and Expression of Platelet Surface Receptors

Storage conditions may play a significant role in platelet surface receptor changes. Platelet products stored on an elliptical rotator will loose nearly 50% of their surface GPIb, whereas membrane GPIb on platelets stored on a circular tumbler rotator do not significantly decrease.[172] Therefore, comparisons made between studies of stored platelet concentrates must take into account storage and preparation protocols. Postprocessing manipulation of platelet concentrates may also decrease surface GPIb. For example, PCs exposed to high-dose (10,000 mJ/cm^3) ultraviolet B (UV-B) irradiation have significantly reduced surface GPIb expression as compared to untreated PCs.[190] By contrast, UV-B at these doses does not appear to affect GPIIb/IIIa surface density. Filtering platelets through various leukocyte removal filters also does not appear to appreciably alter the surface expression of GPIb or GPIIb/IIIa.[191]

Seven days of storage on elliptical and tumbler rotators causes platelet surface GPIIb/IIIa to increase slightly as measured by ^{125}I-labeled monoclonal antibodies.[172] Studies using flow cytometry and monoclonal antibodies directed against GPIIb/IIIa have similarly demonstrated increasing GPIIb/IIIa expression during platelet storage.[173] After 5 days of storage, mean surface expression of GPIIb/IIIa increased by 50% to 70% from baseline; expression increased by 300% or more when storage was extended to 10 days. A separate study found that preparation of platelets, especially the pelleting step, was largely responsible for the initial increase in surface GpIIb/IIIa.[174] Increased surface GPIIb/IIIa paralleled increases in β-TG release and surface expression of P-selectin, both of which reflect α-granule release. Because α-granules contain a pool of GPIIb/IIIa, it seems likely that the increase in platelet surface expression of GpIIb/IIIa is due to relocation of this protein from α-granule stores to the platelet membrane. Alternatively, loss of surface GPIIb/IIIa may occur during platelet storage as a result of protease degradation or formation of microparticles from the platelet membrane.[177]

Thus, potential losses of both GPIb and GPIIb/IIIa during platelet storage can be at least partially compensated for by release of intracellular pools or by sequestration from other sources. For example, fresh plasma can restore platelet GPIb surface expression and is a possible explanation for the preservation of platelet function after transfusion.[192] Alternatively, GPIb could be relocated from platelet storage pools or sequestered at vascular surfaces. Interestingly, the levels of GPIb after storage, although low, are not as low as those seen on platelets collected from individuals with Bernard-Soulier syndrome—a hereditary absence of GPIb receptors associated with a bleeding tendency. Thus, a critical level of these surface receptors may be required for platelet adhesion to the corresponding ligand.

POSTCOLLECTION PROCESSING

Leukoreduction

Platelets, like red blood cells (RBCs), should be transfused through standard blood administration filters—either a 170-μm "clot filter" or a 20-μm "microaggregate filter." Both filters trap larger debris such as clots, while the smaller pore microaggregate filter additionally traps finer particulate matter such as small aggregates of dead cells and fibrin strands. Neither removes white blood cells (WBCs). Filtration of platelets through microaggregate filters results in loss of less than 5% of the platelets, a loss attributed to the filter's void volume.[193]

Leukoreduction—the differential removal of WBCs from cellular blood components—is generally agreed to be beneficial because of the range of adverse patient effects that may arise from contaminating donor leukocytes in blood products. The most commonly accepted complications associated with high levels of contaminating WBCs include febrile nonhemolytic transfusion reactions (FNHTRs),[194] alloimmunization,[195,196] and CMV transmission.[197]

Development of Leukoreduction Filters

In the 1990s, highly efficient filters were developed that were capable of removing 3 to 4 $\log_{10}$ or more of all WBCs found in a unit of RBCs or platelets.[198,199] These filters are generally manufactured from a polyester fiber matrix to which various polymer chemicals are linked. The size of the polymer affects the degree to which WBCs are exposed to its surface and, thus, the efficiency of leukocyte removal. Filters that are designed to leukoreduce RBC units cannot be used to filter platelets because these filters nonspecifically adsorb both WBCs and platelets.[200] Therefore, filters have been specifically designed for leukodepleting platelet concentrates.[201]

Leukoreduction Strategies

Many countries have instituted, or plan to institute, universal leukoreduction of all cellular blood components, including platelets.[202–204] This strategy imposes an additional cost burden, and the added expense must be thoughtfully weighed against the additional benefits to patient care and outcomes.[205] Leukocyte reduction using filtration can be performed at the time of transfusion using a bedside leukoreduction filter (e.g., Baxter SEPACELL Platelet Leukoreduction Filter). It may also be performed as part of component manufacture—so-called prestorage leukoreduction—using inline filters contained in blood collection sets (e.g., Pall Leukotrap RC PL Whole Blood Collection, Filtration, and Storage Systems).

Leukoreduction and Prevention of Transfusion-Transmitted CMV Infection

The use of leukoreduced (LR) blood components, particularly prestorage LR products, as "CMV safe" versus serologically tested "CMV seronegative" products has drawn considerable attention in those communities that treat at-risk patient populations—particularly those with hematologic malignancies,[206] solid organ[207] and stem cell[208] transplant recipients, AIDS patients,[209] and neonates.[210] CMV infection in these immunocompromised hosts has been associated with considerable morbidity and mortality. Studies conducted in the 1980s demonstrated that transfusion of blood products from CMV-seronegative donors significantly reduced the rate of transfusion-transmitted CMV (TT-CMV) infection.[211] For a period of time, many transfusion centers maintained dual inventories of CMV-seronegative and CMV-untested products. Later studies revealed that TT-CMV was mediated by passenger leukocytes harboring the virus.[212] With the advent of third-generation leukoreduction filters capable of removing 3-$\log_{10}$ WBCs, it was hypothesized that such reductions could lead to reduced rates of TT-CMV. This was confirmed by the landmark study by Bowden and colleagues[88] showing that the rates of CMV infection were nearly identical when seronegative stem cell transplant (SCT) patients were transfused with LR products versus seronegative products (2.4% vs 1.4%, $P = 0.50$). Much debate has ensued, and while data have demonstrated the effectiveness of leukoreduction in decreasing CMV antigenemia from donor blood and reducing TT-CMV rates,[213–215] some investigators continue to challenge the effectiveness of this strategy.[216,217]

Leukoreduction and Prevention of Febrile Nonhemolytic Transfusion Reactions

At the cellular level, lysosomal enzymes present in neutrophils are known to digest various platelet proteins. For example, elastase digests GPIb. During storage, the platelet NADPH oxidase system is activated, resulting in release of platelet-activating factor (PAF).[218] Cytokines released from lymphocytes are known to produce a variety of adverse effects in vivo. Platelet-poor supernatant plasma from stored platelet concentrates is more likely to produce febrile reactions than are platelets contained in the cellular fraction of the stored units of concentrates.[219] Other groups have shown that lymphocytes present in units of stored platelets produce cytokines such as interleukin-8 (IL-8), which may be partially responsible for febrile transfusion reactions.[220,221] Thus, removal of leukocytes before or early in storage (prestorage leukoreduction) may reduce this risk by removing the lymphocytes before they can synthesize or release various enzymes and cytokines.

Leukoreduction and Prevention of HLA Alloimmunization

Antigen-presenting cells (APCs) present in platelet concentrates appear to promote HLA alloimmunization that is responsible for one form of platelet refractoriness.[222] The adverse effects of neutrophilic enzyme discharge and lymphocyte cytokine release during platelet storage could be ameliorated by prestorage leukodepletion. Using a rabbit infusion model, it has been shown that supernatant plasma obtained from blood stored prior to filtration induces a significantly higher degree of alloimmunization than does plasma filtered before whole blood storage.[223] These results suggest that prefiltration may further decrease the incidence of HLA alloimmunization by preventing generation of soluble biological response modifiers, as well as by preventing the formation of platelet or RBC microparticles during storage. It is generally believed that viable donor APCs are needed to present donor HLA antigen to the recipient's T cells. Whether this mechanism would function with the infusion of plasma without donor APCs is not clear. In such cases, the recipient's APCs can also present transfused donor antigens. If so, removal of leukocytes before they shed HLA antigens into the stored plasma may be beneficial. Blood bags with RBC and platelet leukoreduction filters integrally attached so as to provide a closed system for prestorage leukocyte depletion at the time of collection are available and are being used more extensively.

Gamma Irradiation

Prevention of Transfusion-Associated Graft-versus-Host Disease

Cellular blood components are exposed to γ irradiation to prevent transfusion-associated graft-versus-host disease (TA-GVHD) in susceptible patients[224]—a nearly uniformly fatal complication of transfusion.[225] Until recently, the dose of irradiation used varied from 1500 to 5000 cGy (1 rad = 1 cGy), with most transfusion centers using doses between 1500 and 3500 cGy.[226] The FDA recommends that a dose of 2500 cGy be delivered to the mid-plane of a free-standing irradiation canister with a minimum dose of 1500 cGy delivered to any other point in the canister.[227] Platelets stored for 1 to 5 days and subsequently irradiated with 5000 cGy have been shown to maintain normal platelet function in vitro, morphology, platelet factor 3 activity, response to hypotonic stress and synergistic aggregation, β-thromboglobulin release, and thromboxane B_2 formation.[228] Irradiation with 5000 cGy causes a decrease in the initial recovery of fresh and stored platelets transfused into normal volunteers, although the platelets appear to survive normally.[229] In this study, the circulating platelets failed to neutralize the effects of aspirin on the recipient's bleeding time, however, the hemostatic effectiveness of these platelets in thrombocytopenic patients did not appear compromised. Subsequent studies have not confirmed any damaging effect of irradiation at these doses on platelets. Exposure of platelet concentrates to 3000 cGy followed by storage for 5 days has no significant effect on either in vivo platelet recovery or platelet survival.[230] Similarly, no detrimental effects on in vitro function were demonstrated in platelet units irradiated with 2000 cGy and stored for up to 5 days.[231] Evaluation of paired apheresis platelets stored for 5 days after receiving 2500 cGy on days 1 or 3 similarly showed no deleterious effects on in vivo recovery or survival or on in vitro properties of platelets.[232] In contrast to the negative effects of irradiating RBCs, which limits their shelf life, the 5-day storage period of irradiated platelets does not need to be shortened.[224] These observations are of practical importance because many transfusion services are not equipped to irradiate blood components just prior to transfusion. Therefore, they must maintain an inventory of irradiated platelets obtained from the collecting facility.

Ultraviolet Irradiation

Prevention of HLA Alloimmunization

Donor leukocytes contained in platelet products are considered to play a significant role in primary alloimmunization of recipients to class I major histocompatibility complex (MHC) antigens, which in turn may result in refractoriness-to-platelet transfusions.[233] It was originally shown over 30 years ago that lymphocytes exposed to sufficient doses of UV irradiation are unable to stimulate allogeneic cells in mixed lymphocyte culture (MLC) or to respond to mitogenic stimuli.[234] UV-C, which has the shortest wavelength (200 to 280 nm) and the greatest biological activity, has been found to induce the formation of pseudopods at the platelet surface and to cause a degree of platelet aggregation.[235] Medium wavelength UV-B light (280 to 320 nm) has been shown to inactivate leukocytes in PCs. The UV-B doses needed to irreversibly damage WBCs depends on the UV source, the type of plastic container used, and the cross-sectional depth of the platelet concentrate volume.[236] PCs irradiated with 3000 J/m^2 UV-B and then stored for 5 days experienced no adverse effects on pH, hypotonic stress, or aggregation responses.[237] In addition, transfusing healthy volunteers with autologous platelets irradiated at this dose and stored for 5 days reveals equivalent platelet recovery, half-life, and survival as compared to control nonirradiated platelets.[238] However, irradiating pooled PCs with high-dose UV-B (100,000 J/m^2) results in a significant decrease in morphology score and osmotic recovery after 96 hours of storage. Expression of GPIb also declines by 60% at 96 hours after irradiation at the higher dose, with no alterations in surface GPIIb-IIIa expression.[190] Therefore, long-term storage of platelets after higher-dose UV-B irradiation is not recommended.

Results of one small study suggested that in vivo recovery and survival of autologous PCs irradiated with high-dose UV-B (15,000 J/m^2) are modestly reduced as compared to control platelets (7 vs 7.75 days, $n=4$).[239] Differences of this magnitude would not be clinically relevant. In the Trial to Prevent Alloimmunization to Platelets (TRAP), UV-B irradiation at 1480 mJ/cm^2 was shown to be equivalent to leukofiltration for decreasing the incidence of refractoriness to platelet transfusions in patients with acute myelogenous leukemia.[240] Long-wavelength UV-A (320 to 400 nm) light by itself is insufficient to inactivate leukocytes. However, UV-A at low doses activates 8-methoxypsoralen (8-MOP), transforming it into a potent DNA cross-linking agent capable of abolishing MLC activity.[241] Pretreating PCs with 8-MOP and UV-A irradiation can reduce the allogenicity of class I MHC antigen in mice without affecting platelet aggregation responses.[242]

Photochemical Treatment and Pathogen Reduction

The risk of viral TTD has steadily decreased with advances in donor screening and testing.[243] Despite these improvements, however, there remains a small residual risk of viral, bacterial, or protozoal transmission. Many potentially serious infectious agents are not directly screened for, and emerging pathogens such as West Nile virus demonstrate the ongoing potential for new risks to the blood supply.[244–246] Stringent donor screening and TTD testing offer significant, but incomplete, protection and are associated with both time and cost burdens that have prompted many experts in the field to champion for adoption of pathogen reduction (PR) strategies.[247] PR technology is already in active use in Europe,[248] although efficacy and patient safety concerns have slowed adoption in the United States.[249]

Spectrum of Pathogen Reduction Technologies

PR technologies encompass a heterogenous group of methods that differ with respect to their chemical and biological characteristics, the spectrum of pathogens against which they have activity, their efficacy of inactivation, and the blood components to which the method may be applied. The highly effective techniques developed to inactivate viruses in plasma, such as solvent and detergent treatment and heat sterilization,[250,251] are too harsh and cannot be applied to cellular blood components. Thus, alternative methods to inactivate infectious pathogens in cellular blood components such as platelets and RBCs are undergoing clinical development.[252]

Psoralen-Based Pathogen Reduction

Currently, one of the most actively investigated systems for PR of platelets utilizes the novel psoralen amotosalen HCl (previously known as S-59), which is photoactivated by long-wavelength (UV-A) ultraviolet light. Psoralens, a family of naturally occurring, small planar molecules, readily pass through cell membranes and viral capsids and reversibly intercalate into helical regions of DNA and RNA. On exposure to UV-A light, covalent crosslinks to the pyrimidines thymidine and cytosine form, resulting in blockage of DNA replication and RNA transcription of nucleic acids.[253] This results in the effective inactivation of viruses,[254,255] bacteria,[256] protozoa,[257] and leukocytes.[258] Photochemical treatment with amotosalen has been shown to be capable of inactivating high concentrations of cell-free HIV, proviral HIV, duck hepatitis B virus (a surrogate for HBV), bovine viral diarrhea virus (a surrogate for HCV), CMV, gram-positive bacteria, and gram-negative bacteria.[259,260] This technique can also inactivate *Trypanosoma cruzi, Plasmodium malariae, Borrelia burgdorferi*, and rickettsiae in PCs.[261]

Optimal PR using amotosalen requires resuspension of the platelets in a plasma-reduced medium, since plasma has been shown to interfere with the inactivation of viruses.[262] Additionally, after UV-A exposure, residual amotosalen remains in the product; although amotosalen is not mutagenic in the absence of UV-A,[263] the use of an S-59 reduction device or similar method is routinely practiced to remove unspent psoralen. Specific photochemical treatment (PCT) methods for platelets using amotosalen are well described.[256] The resulting products contain very low levels of residual amotosalen and free photoproducts. Following PR, the platelet products can be stored under routine conditions.

The safety profile of PR methods using amotosalen appears quite good. Extensive preclinical toxicologic studies have been performed using amotosalen-treated platelets and have shown no evidence of toxicologically significant CNS, renal, cardiac, or reproductive toxicity.[264,265] In addition, clinical trials of the INTERCEPT (S-59 psoralen system) system conducted in Europe[266] and the United States[267,268] have shown therapeutic equivalence between conventional and amotosalen-treated platelet products, as well as similar adverse reaction profiles. Data also suggest that amotosalen treatment may prevent transfusion-associated GVHD.[269–271]

Riboflavin-Based Pathogen Reduction

A second candidate PR system for use with platelets involves the use of riboflavin (vitamin B_2), an essential nutrient whose photoactivation properties have been extensively studied.[272] Riboflavin, like amotosalen, readily intercalates between DNA and RNA bases. On exposure to UV light in the 280- to 360-nm range, several photolytic processes occur including oxidation of guanosine through direct electron transfer, production of singlet oxygen, and generation of hydroxyl radicals. These collectively result in single-strand breaks and the formation of covalent adducts that inhibit replication.[273] Effective PR using riboflavin/UV-A methodologies have been reported against a broad spectrum of pathogens including porcine parvovirus, cell-associated and cell-free HIV-1, intracellular HIV-1, gram-positive and -negative bacteria, and West Nile virus.[274,275] Preclinical toxicologic studies have shown no significant toxicity.[276]

Clinical studies with the Mirasol PRT (riboflavin/UV) system have shown some differences between PCT-treated platelet units and control units. In a study of leukoreduced apheresis platelets by Aubuchon and colleagues,[277] riboflavin/UV-treated platelet units demonstrated in vitro evidence of increased glycolysis and decreased pH during 5-day storage as compared to control platelet units, although glucose was not completely exhausted during this time and pH (7.02 ± 0.10, control 7.38 ± 0.07) was maintained at a level that did not interfere with platelet metabolism. Differences were likewise noted with in vivo parameters: treated platelets showed diminished recovery (50.0% ± 18.9, control 66.5% ± 13.4) and survival (104 ± 26 hours, control 142 ± 26 hours) compared with controls. These data were similar to those from previously published studies.[274,278]

Other Pathogen Reduction Agents

Other agents capable of photoinactivating viruses such as merocyanine 540 (MC 540), a heterocyclic polymethine dye, have adverse effects on platelet structure and function. In both the presence and absence of visible light, MC 540 has deleterious in vitro effects on platelets that include inhibition of platelet aggregation, a more precipitous decline in pH, and poorer morphology scores during platelet storage.[279,280] Thus, photoinactivation techniques must be rigorously evaluated to ensure that they do not harm platelet membranes or result in loss of normal platelet function.

BIOLOGICAL RESPONSE MODIFIERS

Febrile Reactions and Biological Response Modifiers

Pathogenesis of Febrile Nonhemolytic Transfusion Reactions

Many adverse effects of platelet transfusion therapy are related to the elaboration of various biologically active molecules by the constituents of platelet products or the blood recipient. These substances, often termed *biological response modifiers* (BRMs), are clearly involved in the pathophysiology of common nonhemolytic febrile transfusion reactions,[281,282] which occur in 4% to 30% of platelet transfusions. They also play a role in more severe immunohemolytic and septic transfusion reactions. The pathogenesis of febrile reactions was originally attributed to the presence of antibodies in the transfusion recipient that react with donor leukocytes.[283] Following binding of these antibodies to donor leukocytes, fever ensues through a cytokine-mediated inflammatory response that results in release of interleukin 1 (IL-1). Fever is then produced through IL-1 stimulated synthesis of prostaglandin E_2 (PGE_2) in the thermoregulatory center of the hypothalamus.[284]

Subsequent data, however, demonstrated that cytokines present in the plasma portion of PCs act as the primary agent for the development of febrile reactions.[285] Following platelet preparation, whether by the platelet-rich plasma, buffy coat, or apheresis methods, there is continued elaboration of cytokines by viable donor leukocytes.[286] PCs contain not only WBCs but a vast array of soluble proteins that have biological activity. It is not entirely understood what stimulates WBCs to produce cytokines during platelet storage. Platelets themselves could contribute to these reactions through the release of platelet-specific cytokines following activation or damage to platelets with component preparation and storage.[287] The major classes of BRMs include complement fragments, interleukins, chemokines, arachidonic acid metabolites, kininogens, and histamines (Table 23–3). There is also a wide array of other biologically active and inorganic compounds that are similarly capable of interacting with humoral and cellular receptors.

Biological Response Modifiers in Platelet Products

Direct and indirect evidence suggest a key role for BRMs in febrile, nonhemolytic transfusion reactions to platelet infusions. FNHTRs are seen in patients who are receiving their first blood transfusion and have not been pregnant.[288] Presumably, these patients would not have developed a secondary immune response from a prior exposure to foreign blood constituents. The incidence of platelet transfusion reactions may be related to the duration of platelet storage: reaction rates can be nearly double in 3- to 5-day-old platelets as compared to 1- to 2-day-old products.[219] These findings have been attributed to reactive substances contained in the plasma portion of stored platelet concentrates. Specifically, supernatant levels of IL-1β and IL-6 strongly correlate with the frequency of febrile reactions. Similar relationships between storage duration and febrile reaction rates have been found following transfusion of nonfiltered pooled platelet concentrates.[289] The incidence of allergic reactions does not appear related to storage time.

Specific chemical mediators thought to play a role in FNHTRs include cytokines, complement fragments, antibodies, and cell adhesion molecules.[290] Donor leukocytes can continue to produce cytokines after they are infused into a recipient, the so-called passenger leukocyte effect. Cytokines are synthesized and elaborated by donor leukocytes during storage, after which these preformed cytokines are infused during transfusion.[291] The latter mechanism, in vitro cytokine production during platelet storage, has received increasing support as the mechanism responsible for the majority of FNHTR.[292] Accordingly, many investigators have focused their research on modulating the effects of BRMs in platelet therapy. Most efforts are directed at limiting the formation of

Table 23–3 Biological Response Modifiers (BRMs) Found in Platelet Concentrates

Class	Examples
Complement fragments	C3a, C5a
Cytokines	
Interleukins	TNF-α, IL-6, IL-10, IFN-γ, IL-10, IL-4, TGF-β
Chemokines	IL-8, MCP-1, RANTES, β-TG, NAP-2, MIP-1β
Monokines	IL-1, IL-8, TNF-α, IL-6, IL-12
Anti-inflammatory cytokines	IL-1 receptor antagonist
Kininogens	Bradykinin
Histamine	
Other BRMs	Prostaglandins, nitric oxide, leukotrienes (LTB4), platelet activating factor

BRMs during platelet collection and processing, decreasing the formation of BRMs during platelet storage, and removing BRMs prior to or during platelet transfusion. Many of these techniques involve collecting platelets with little WBC contamination (process leukoreduction) or removing leukocytes from PCs shortly after their preparation (prestorage leukoreduction).

Leukoreduction and Biological Response Modifiers

Our understanding of the effects of BRMs in platelet therapy is largely derived from studies of leukoreduced blood components. Third-generation leukoreduction filters eliminate approximately 99.9% ($<5 \times 10^6$ leukocytes remaining per unit) of the WBCs found in a unit of whole blood. Generally recognized benefits of leukoreduction include reducing the incidence of febrile reactions, preventing transmission of cytomegalovirus, and decreasing alloimmunization to HLA antigens. Leukoreducing blood products, however, does not prevent allergic reactions.[293] Prestorage leukoreduction of RBCs has been shown to further reduce the likelihood of FNHTRs as compared to the use of bedside leukoreduction filters.[294] This study also suggested that FNHTRs are more common following infusions of single-donor apheresis platelets than of RBC transfusions—a finding that may be related to the storage of platelets at room temperature.

Several groups have shown that prestorage leukoreduction of blood components slows the accumulation of cytokines in platelet products and RBCs during storage. It is now clear that prestorage leukoreduction decreases the incidence and severity of FNHTRs by minimizing the production of cytokines by residual leukocytes. In particular, levels of IL-8 in PCs prepared by the platelet-rich plasma method and leukoreduced shortly after collection are much lower than in nonleukoreduced PCs after 5 days' storage.[220] Reductions of RANTES and C3a are also seen when PCs are filtered through third-generation filters that reliably reduce WBC numbers by 4 $\log_{10}$ per unit filtered.[295] The filter used in the latter study (PXL-8; Pall Corp.) did not remove the proinflammatory cytokines IL-1β and IL-6.

Direct Removal of Biological Response Modifiers by Leukoreduction Filters

The ability of certain platelet leukoreduction filters to remove the anaphylatoxins C3a and C5a, as well as the chemokines IL-8 and RANTES chemokines, has been studied. Levels of C3a, C5a, IL-8, and RANTES were reduced by filtration through the two bedside leukoreduction filters examined (PXL-8 and PXL-A; Pall Corp., East Hills, N.Y.), but not through a prestorage platelet filter (Sepacell PLS-5A; Asahi, Toyko, Japan).[296] IL-1β was not removed by any of these filters. These experiments, which used WBC-free plasma, demonstrate that binding of WBCs to filters is not necessary for the trapping or degradation of most BRMs. Earlier in vitro studies showed that C5a can be removed from plasma by peripheral blood leukocytes that contain high-affinity binding sites for C5a.[297] The binding of C5a to leukocyte receptors likely represents a physiologic mechanism that protects cells from this potent anaphylatoxin. Similarly performed studies have shown little accumulation of IL-1β, IL-6, IL-8, or TNF-α in leukoreduced platelet concentrates.[221] Data from additional studies have shown that the frequency of reactions is significantly higher in patients receiving poststorage WBC-reduced platelets (25.8%) than plasma-depleted platelets (17.0%).[298] In this study, IL-6 levels of platelet products appeared to be associated with the risk of reaction; however, IL-6 levels were not measured in patients during or after transfusion, and other cytokines that have been implicated in febrile reactions were not examined.

Hypotensive Reactions to Platelet Transfusions: Role of Bradykinin

Severe hypotensive reactions have been reported following platelet transfusion therapy.[299] The most serious reactions appear to occur in patients receiving angiotensin-converting enzyme (ACE) inhibitors who are transfused with platelets through a bedside leukoreduction filter.[300] The reactions were more common when filters bearing a net negative surface charge were used. While the pathogenesis of this syndrome remains unclear, it appears in some cases to be due to activation of factor XII and the prekallikrein-kinin cascade by negatively charged surfaces, resulting in bradykinin production.[301] Bradykinin (BK) produces adverse in vivo effects such as hypotension, abdominal pain, and facial flushing, without fever or chills. In most cases, it is possible to distinguish these reactions from febrile reactions and transfusion-related acute lung injury. However, these reactions must be promptly recognized.

ACE is identical to kininase II, an enzyme that degrades bradykinin. Accordingly, blocking kininase II prolongs the half-life of bradykinin such that clinical symptoms can develop in susceptible patients.[302] BK levels have been directly measured in donors undergoing plasmapheresis procedures[301] and in patients transfused with platelets through leukoreduction filters.[303] In the latter study, platelet-recipient BK levels transiently increased during the first 5 minutes when platelets were administered through a negatively charged filter (PL-50H; Pall Corp., Glen Cove, N.Y.). BK levels were particularly high in two patients with diminished ACE-inhibitor activity. Since bradykinin has a half-life of 15 to 30 seconds, prestorage leukoreduction, as opposed to bedside leukoreduction, should eliminate reactions due to BK generation from contact with the filter biomaterials. Such patients could benefit from receiving blood that has been either prestorage or in-laboratory leukoreduced, as opposed to being infused through a bedside leukoreduction filter.

In addition, a metabolic abnormality that affects des-Arg^9-BK degradation has been identified in several patients with severe hypotensive transfusion reactions.[304,305] Des-Arg^9-BK is an active metabolite of BK that is primarily inactivated by ACE and aminopeptidase P. With ACE inhibition, the half-life of des-Arg^9-BK, not BK, has been shown to be significantly higher in patients with pronounced hypotensive transfusion reactions when compared to control transfusion recipients. These findings suggest that failure to metabolize active vasodilatory peptides could contribute to transfusion reactions. However, they do not imply that bedside leukoreduction of blood components is absolutely contraindicated in patients on ACE inhibitors.

PLATELET TRANSFUSION THERAPY

Early in the 20th century, freshly drawn whole blood was the only source of viable platelets.[306] Although whole blood was neither a convenient nor an optimal source of platelets, such transfusions reportedly reduced bleeding times and halted hemorrhage in thrombocytopenic patients. Platelet products became widely available only after the development of plastic collection and storage containers in the late 1960s and early 1970s, which allowed the separation of platelets from whole blood.[307] These products contained large numbers of viable platelets in a relatively small volume. Oncology patients utilize the majority of platelet products produced, and the increasing number of platelets used over the past two decades was in patients being supported during chemotherapy. Significant numbers of platelet products are also provided to trauma, surgical, and solid-organ transplant patients.

Indications for Platelet Transfusion

Platelet transfusion therapy is indicated for the prophylaxis or treatment of bleeding in patients with rapidly decreasing or critically decreased circulating platelet counts or in patients with functionally abnormal platelets.[1] In practice, most platelets are transfused to nonbleeding thrombocytopenic patients as a prophylactic measure.[308] Thrombocytopenia can result from myriad causes including marrow suppression (e.g., due to drugs, irradiation, infiltration, intrinsic marrow disease such as myelofibrosis), massive transfusion (dilutional thrombocytopenia), or immune destruction (e.g., immune thrombocytopenic purpura, thrombotic thrombocytopenic purpura, neonatal alloimmune thrombocytopenia). Patients with congenital or acquired platelet disorders, such as Bernard-Soulier syndrome or platelet storage pool deficiency, may also benefit from platelet transfusion. These individuals will frequently have normal platelet counts but diminished platelet function that is inadequate for normal hemostasis. Platelet transfusions are also considered in disseminated intravascular coagulation (DIC), during or following cardiopulmonary bypass, and to support patients undergoing extracorporeal membrane oxygenation (ECMO).

Despite vast clinical experience, few trials have been conducted to investigate the effectiveness of platelet transfusion therapy in controlling and preventing thrombocytopenic bleeding.[309,310] Thus, practices followed for platelet therapy often vary between and within medical facilities. This has resulted in a number of clinical controversies that have not been entirely resolved (Table 23–4). For example, it is unclear at what platelet count a nonbleeding patient should receive prophylactic platelet transfusions. Additionally, the optimal dose of platelets for an individual patient has not been clearly defined. Some practitioners advocate larger doses of platelets than those routinely provided (e.g., 10 WB-Plts instead of 4 to 6 WB-Plts). A variety of separation techniques have been developed to prepare platelets, each of which has certain advantages and disadvantages. Platelets isolated by each of the commonly used methods, however, have been successfully used in the clinical arena. Finally, a number of strategies have been employed to manage platelet refractory patients. These patients are often difficult to manage, and they can consume large quantities of platelets.

Table 23–4 Clinical Controversies in Platelet Transfusion Therapy

Topic	Controversy
Prophylactic platelet transfusions	Higher versus lower platelet transfusion triggers
Platelet dosing	Larger versus smaller platelet doses
Platelet preparation and product selection	ABO-matched versus unmatched platelet concentrates
	Fresh versus stored platelet concentrates
	Single donor platelets by apheresis versus pooled donor platelet concentrates
	Decreased exposure to infectious agents in single donor units
Platelet refractory patients	Crossmatched versus HLA-selected platelets

Prophylactic Platelet Transfusion

It is now generally accepted that the decision to transfuse platelets, or any blood product, should almost never be based solely on transfusion thresholds (or "transfusion triggers"). Patient factors should always be considered when deciding when an individual patient should be transfused. These factors may include the patient's primary disease, the presence of fever or sepsis, concurrent medications, and overall coagulation status.[311] Until recently, physicians typically transfused platelets to maintain a patient's platelet count above 20,000/μL. This level was believed necessary to prevent spontaneous bleeding.[312] However, serious spontaneous bleeding is unusual unless platelet counts fall below 5000/μL in the absence of other irregularities (e.g., aspirin use, decreased clotting factors) of the hemostatic system.[313] In fact, the earliest studies of the effectiveness of prophylactic platelet transfusions were limited by the widespread use of aspirin as an antipyretic agent, before the antiplatelet effects of this drug were recognized.

Determination of Optimal Platelet Transfusion "Trigger"

Other difficulties have hindered efforts to determine an optimal prophylactic platelet transfusion "trigger." First, serious thrombocytopenic hemorrhage is unusual, even at extremely low platelet counts. This fact was recognized early in the history of platelet transfusion therapy. Results of an early small clinical trial suggested that RBC usage and major bleeding were no different in patients who received prophylactic platelet transfusions at the 20,000/μL threshold as compared to those transfused only when bleeding from sites other than the skin or mucous membranes occurred.[314] Second, it is difficult to quantify minor clinical bleeding. Investigators have estimated stool RBC loss by ^{51}Cr RBC labeling as an indicator of spontaneous bleeding. One study using such a technique found that patients with aplastic anemia did not have significantly elevated stool blood loss until platelet levels dropped below 5000/μL.[315] Finally, platelet counts, as determined by automated counters or manual methods, are less reliable in severely thrombocytopenic patients.

During the past decade, a number of studies have been performed that were designed to more clearly define platelet transfusion thresholds. In one of the earlier studies, Gmur and colleagues prospectively followed 102 consecutive patients with acute leukemia.[316] Patients with platelet levels <6000/μL received prophylactic platelet transfusions, whereas those with levels >20,000/μL were transfused only when major bleeding developed or before invasive procedures. Intermediate thresholds included 6000 to 11,000/μL for patients with minor bleeding or fever and 11,000 to 20,000/μL for those with coagulation disorders and prior to minor procedures. Overall, 31 episodes of major bleeding occurred on 1.9% of total study days when platelet counts were <10,000/μL and on 0.07% of study days when counts were 10,000 to 20,000/μL. The investigators suggested that prophylactic levels of 5000/μL were safe in the absence of fever or bleeding. However, it was noted that several serious bleeds occurred in patients in the 6000 to 10,000/μL groups who did not receive prophylactic transfusions.

Bleeding Risk and Platelet Transfusion Needs in Thrombocytopenic Patients

Numerous prospective trials have compared the bleeding risks and platelet transfusion needs of thrombocytopenic patients. Most of these have grouped patients using 10,000/μL and 20,000/μL thresholds. In a nonrandomized trial, Gil-Fernandez and coworkers found no difference in bleeding using the 10,000/μL or 20,000/μL threshold in 190 bone marrow transplant recipients.[317] Heckman and associates randomized 78 patients with acute leukemia to the 10,000/μL or 20,000/μL threshold and could demonstrate no difference in bleeding between these two levels.[318] Similarly, Wandt and associates were unable to demonstrate a difference in bleeding risk when they prospectively compared transfusion thresholds in 105 patients with acute myeloid leukemia (AML).[319] Finally, in a large, randomized, multi-institution study of 255 patients with newly diagnosed AML, Rebulla and colleagues found no difference in major bleeding or in RBC transfusions when patients were transfused at the 10,000/μL or 20,000/μL threshold.[320] Although most of these studies were limited to patients with acute leukemia, similar studies performed in other patient groups, such as those with severe aplastic anemia[321] or following allogeneic marrow transplantation,[322] have shown that platelet thresholds can be safely lowered.

These studies suggest that there are no clear differences in serious hemorrhage or hemorrhagic death when the platelet transfusion trigger is set below 20,000/μL. When lower prophylactic platelet transfusion thresholds are used, recipients are exposed to less donor blood and the potential complications of such a transfusion. Despite the results of these studies, there remains no clear consensus on the clinical indications for prophylactic platelet transfusion. Accordingly, there is wide variation in the thresholds selected for prophylactic platelet transfusions.[323] For most patients, the lower 10,000/μL threshold is likely as safe as higher levels. Patients with other risk factors for bleeding such as fever and sepsis are probably best transfused at higher thresholds, although specific triggers for these groups of patients have not been defined. In addition, profound anemia can alter hemostatic capabilities and, accordingly, should be avoided in severely thrombocytopenic patients.[324] Platelet counts above 20,000/μL are indicated prior to invasive procedures. Typically, platelet counts are increased to >50,000/μL before lumbar puncture, indwelling catheter insertion, thoracentesis, liver biopsy, or transbronchial biopsy.[325] However, some data suggest that adults with acute leukemia may tolerate lumbar puncture (LP) without serious complication when platelet counts are ≥20,000/μL,[326] and children with acute lymphoblastic leukemia may tolerate LP without serious complication with platelet counts <10,000/μL.[327] Platelet transfusions are usually not necessary before bone marrow aspiration/biopsy if adequate surface pressure can be applied to the site after the procedure.

Platelet Dosing

Doses of platelets, as determined by the number of platelets in single or pooled PCs, have not been standardized. In practice, a single dose of transfused platelets generally contains approximately 3×10^{11} platelets, corresponding to 1 AD-Plt product or 5 to 6 pooled WB-Plt units. The optimal adult dose of platelets has not been clearly established, and doses are often determined based on factors unrelated to efficacy, such as cost and availability.[328–330] For example, an adult's body weight is not usually considered when determining the number of platelets to administer. In general, the higher a patient's post-transfusion platelet increment, the longer the interval will be before the next platelet transfusion is required. Endogenously produced platelets normally survive approximately 9 to 10 days in the absence of diseases that decrease platelet survival. Transfused platelets do not circulate this long in thrombocytopenic patients, as they are more rapidly consumed, for instance, to maintain vascular integrity. At platelet counts below 100,000/μL, a direct relationship exists between lower platelet counts and shorter platelet life span in the circulation.[331] For this reason, patients undergoing chemotherapy for various malignancies often require platelet transfusions at least every 3 days.[331] During periods of severe bone marrow hypoplasia, daily platelet transfusions are often required.

Large/Infrequent versus Small/Frequent Platelet Dosing Strategies

Several transfusion specialists advocate transfusing doses of platelets larger than the standard 6 WB-Plt pool, albeit at longer intervals between transfusions (e.g., 10–12 WB-Plt units every 2–3 days). The rationale for this practice is largely based on decreasing the number of individual transfusion episodes. This is more convenient in outpatient settings. As expected, it is possible to obtain higher post-transfusion platelet increments by transfusing higher platelet numbers.[332,333] However, it is unclear whether this practice is more effective than standard platelet doses in reducing the risk of spontaneous bleeding. Alternatively, smaller doses of platelets transfused at shorter intervals (e.g., 3–4 WB-Plt per transfusion) may reduce the total number of platelets required during a patient's thrombocytopenic period.[334] This strategy could decrease the overall number of platelets needed for a large patient population and decrease the number of exposures for an individual patient. Thus, smaller platelet doses may be more economical, but this practice has been criticized for possibly increasing the number of individual transfusions, which increases overall costs.[335] Therefore, an "optimal" dose of platelets has not been clearly defined, and transfusion practices will likely remain largely based on local preferences, which will often be heavily influenced by costs and supply.

Platelet Preparation and Product Selection

Platelet Surface Antigens and Immune Considerations

Platelets express a wide variety of surface antigens including the ABH, Lewis, P, and Ii blood group antigens; MHC class I HLA-A, -B, and -C antigens; and platelet-specific, human platelet antigens (HPAs).[336,337] Those that are most relevant to allogeneic platelet survival are the ABH, class I HLA, and HPA antigens. Interestingly, the presence of recipient antibodies directed against these antigens does not imply that all platelets carrying these antigens will be rapidly destroyed. Platelet survival is clearly decreased when recipients with higher-titer anti-A or anti-B IgG antibodies in their plasma are transfused with platelets carrying one of these antigens. This incompatibility can be avoided by using ABO-identical platelets and should be considered as a first step in patients who are not responding appropriately to platelet transfusions.[338] Unfortunately, ABO-identical platelets are often not available during blood shortages. Transfusing ABO-incompatible, apheresis-derived platelets does not usually produce measurable hemolysis in adults, although significant hemolysis has been reported, especially in patients with small plasma volumes.[339,340]

Efficacy and Availability of Platelet Preparations

There appears to be little difference in the efficacy of platelet transfusions whether the concentrates are prepared from platelet-rich plasma or from buffy coats or are collected by apheresis.[341] The decision to use any of these products—or a mixture of such products—is often based largely on cost and availability. Advocates of BC WB-Plts, the technique widely practiced in Europe, note that cytokine production is lower in such concentrates.[342] BC WB-Plts have also been reported as less activated immediately after preparation. However, this difference is not appreciable after storage for 48 hours, and transfusing such products does not imply improved 5-day post-transfusion platelet recovery.[40,174] Thus, although various in vitro measurements of platelet concentrates compared by any technique may differ, these differences are not usually associated with decreased platelet survival in vivo. Human transfusion studies are difficult to perform and compare for several reasons, one being that thrombocytopenic patients often have extremely variable responses to platelet transfusion.[343]

Use of Apheresis Platelet Products

Many blood centers provide only platelets collected from apheresis donors on the basis of several theoretical benefits. AD-Plt transfusions decrease donor exposure, which theoretically could reduce the risk of transfusion-associated infection. Donor testing, however, has improved to the point that the most important human viruses are reliably detected in potentially infectious blood donors. NAT for viruses has dramatically reduced the risk of viral transmission, primarily by shortening the "window period" from the time of initial infection to the earliest point of detection.[243] This fact makes "limiting donor exposure" more difficult to justify. Use of AD-Plt products has also not been shown to reduce rates of alloimmunization,[89] although the benefits of leukoreduction have clearly been established.[344] Platelets prepared by apheresis are usually more expensive than those prepared from single whole-blood donations because of equipment and personnel costs for such a collection. Finally, there are risks to the apheresis platelet donors themselves inherent to this collection technique.[345]

Management of Platelet-Refractory Patients

It has long been recognized that a subset of patients who receive long-term platelet therapy develop progressively poorer responses to transfusion, marked by the rapid destruction of transfused platelets.[346] Platelet refractoriness arises from any condition that results in premature removal of platelets from the circulation. These conditions are often classified as immune-mediated and nonimmune-mediated based on the presumed mechanism of platelet destruction (Table 23–5).[343,347] Overall, nonimmune platelet destruction caused by splenomegaly (platelet sequestration), antibiotic treatment (e.g., amphotericin B), and infection are more common than immune-mediated causes.[348,349] From a practical standpoint, the effects of amphotericin B on platelet survival can be mitigated by transfusing platelets at least 2 hours after completing amphotericin infusion.[350] Antibody-related platelet destruction is most often related to the development of HLA-specific antibodies in response to foreign donor HLA antigens.[81,351] Presumably, these antibodies coat donor platelets that carry antigens these immunoglobulins are capable of recognizing.[352] The antibody-coated platelets are then removed by the reticuloendothelial system or through mechanisms involving platelet activation and deposition on endothelial surfaces.[353] Less commonly, patients develop platelet-specific antibodies.[354,355]

Table 23–5 Conditions Associated with Rapid Destruction of Transfused Platelets

Immune-Mediated	Non-Immune-Mediated
HLA class I alloantibodies	Splenomegaly
Platelet-specific alloantibody formation	Drugs (amphotericin B, other antibiotics)
Platelet-specific autoantibodies	Sepsis and fever
Circulating immunocomplexes	Disseminated intravascular coagulation
	Graft-versus-host disease

Strategies used to manage platelet refractory patients vary across institutions and are often based on the availability of specialized testing and platelet products.[356] Initial evaluation should include determination of several recent 1-hour, post-transfusion corrected count increments (CCIs)[357] to assess response to transfusion and review of the patient's chart to rule out nonimmune etiologies of refractoriness. In confirmed refractory but uncomplicated nonbleeding patients, it may be possible to simply withhold platelet transfusion and defer unnecessary invasive procedures. In patients in whom platelet transfusion is unavoidable—such as those with active bleeding or prior to an invasive procedure—several strategies have been advocated.

Large-Volume, ABO-Compatible, and Fresh Platelet Transfusion

A first maneuver can simply be to increase the number of platelets transfused (e.g., 6–12 random donor platelets per pool or 2 single-donor platelets by apheresis). Additionally, ABO-compatible platelets can be used, particularly in group O patients with known high titers of anti-ABO antibodies.[358] In practice, ABO-compatible platelets may not be readily available, although their potential benefit has long been established.[359] Likewise, "fresh platelets" less than 48 hours postcollection have been advocated based on storage time versus post-transfusion recovery studies.[360] Data supporting this strategy are less well established, and the requirement for mandatory TTD and bacterial testing has all but staunched the availability of fresh platelet products. If these relatively simple methods have been exhausted without benefit, more specialized platelet products may be required, including HLA-selected, HLA antigen-negative, and crossmatch-compatible platelet products.

HLA-Selected ("HLA-Matched") Platelets

In patients for whom HLA-selected platelets are being considered, identification of anti-HLA antibodies in the patient should, ideally, be documented owing to the difficulties frequently encountered in obtaining such products. Provision of HLA-selected platelets requires that the patient be HLA typed; it also necessitates communication with the blood supplier to identify potential donors. The HLA system is extremely polymorphic and thus, a pool of 1000 to 3000 or more HLA-typed donors is needed to maximize the likelihood of an ideal platelet "match."[361] Platelet products are usually collected by apheresis and selected on the basis of degree of match for HLA-A and HLA-B types of donor and recipient, which is expressed as a match grade of A–D and R (random).[362] The best CCIs occur with grade A (4-antigen match), B1U (3-antigen match, 1 antigen unknown), and B2U (2-antigen match, 2 antigens unknown), although mismatches for some antigens that are poorly expressed on platelets, such as B44 or B45, have not been associated with poor response. HLA-C antigens are only weakly expressed by platelets, and mismatch of this antigen does not appear to significantly influence platelet survival.[363] The use of HLA-selected platelets in patients who are not alloimmunized for the purpose of preventing HLA alloimmunization does not appear warranted.[364,365]

HLA Antigen-Negative Platelets

Alternatively, if anti-HLA antibodies are present, their specificities can be determined and matched donors selected whose platelets lack the corresponding antigen. This method has been termed the *antibody specificity prediction* (ASP) method.[366] Comparison of platelets selected by the ASP method versus HLA-selected, crossmatched, and random (control) platelets demonstrated therapeutic equivalence for the ASP-matched, HLA-selected, and crossmatched products and superiority to randomly selected platelets. An additional benefit of the ASP method is the relative greater ease with which donors can be identified from a pool of potential donors.

Crossmatched Platelets

An alternative to HLA-selected or HLA antigen-negative platelets is crossmatch-compatible platelets. Platelet crossmatching may be performed using a solid phase system that involves incubating a sample of patient serum or plasma with donor platelets that have been anchored to the solid medium; reactivity is determined using indicator RBCs.[367] Flow cytometric methods have also been described.[368,369] Similarly to traditional RBC crossmatching, compatibility is based on the presence or absence of reactivity. In theory, crossmatching is more "sensitive" than HLA matching owing to the detection of *any* reactive antiplatelet antibodies, including anti-HLA, anti-HPA, antiplatelet glycoprotein (e.g., GPIIb), and anti-ABO. An incompatible platelet crossmatch predicts a poor response (platelet increment) in over 90% of transfusions. Conversely, a compatible crossmatch does not guarantee good survival—a compatible crossmatch is predictive of a successful transfusion only 50% to 60% of the time.[370,371] For this reason, large collection facilities may combine multiple approaches: platelet units are selected for crossmatch based on the class I HLA types of the recipient and potential donor. This approach is also of potential use in the unusual patient who has developed both HLA and platelet-specific antibodies. Other approaches that have been proposed to transfuse heavily alloimmunized patients include techniques to reduce class I HLA antigen expression on platelets.[372,373] These methods, which are largely based on eluting HLA antigens, are not available for routine clinical practice.

PLATELET SUBSTITUTES

Several products have been explored as alternatives to liquid platelet concentrates stored at 22°C. These "platelet substitutes" are, in general, either derived from platelets themselves or synthetic in nature. Platelet substitutes are designed to mimic the normal hemostatic properties of intact human platelets. Other advantageous properties of platelet substitutes include (1) an ability to retain efficacy when sterilized to prevent bacterial or viral infection; (2) a long, biologically active shelf life; (3) few specialized storage requirements; and (4) ease of preparation and administration. Substitutes should be hemostatically effective in vivo without causing dangerous thromboses and, in addition, be nonimmunogenic. Novel products derived from human platelets include platelet-derived microparticles, lyophilized platelets, and cryopreserved (frozen) platelets. Synthetic platelet substitutes include RBCs carrying surface-bound fibrinogen or surface-bound arginine-glycine-aspartic acid (RGD) peptides, fibrinogen-coated microspheres, and liposome-based agents.[65,374]

Platelet-Derived Microparticles

Platelet microparticles (PMPs) are platelet membrane microvesicles that form spontaneously during platelet storage. They have also been identified in fresh frozen plasma and cryoprecipitate. PMPs are strongly procoagulant and retain many of the biological properties of intact platelets. Specifically, they can both adhere to vascular endothelium and enhance platelet adhesion.[375] PMPs range in size from 0.1 to 1.0 μm in diameter and are identified based on their expression of surface receptors for platelet/endothelial interactions including glycoprotein IIb/IIIa, Ib/IX, and P-selectin.[170] Early studies in the late 1950s using infusions of platelets disrupted by sonication were discouraging.[376] This product had no apparent hemostatic effect in thrombocytopenic dogs and produced significant tachycardia and hypotension in recipients. More recently, human "infusible platelet membranes" (Cyplex; Cypress Bioscience, San Diego, Calif.) have been developed and tested in animal models.[377] This material is prepared from outdated platelets which are lysed by freeze-thawing, virally heat inactivated for 20 hours at 60°C, and finally sonicated. The fragments are then formulated with a preservative solution, lyophilized, and stored at 4°C; the product is reported stable for 3 years. The resulting spherical vesicles measure <1 μm in diameter and express detectable GPIb but not GPIIb/IIIa. This preparation has a phospholipid content similar to that of natural platelets, retains so-called platelet factor 3 (PF3) activity, and may have reduced class I HLA expression.[378] Studies have demonstrated shortening of the bleeding time in thrombocytopenic rabbits.[377] There is preliminary evidence that platelet membrane fragments prepared in this fashion are tolerated by human recipients and possess hemostatic effectiveness.[379] Human phase I and II clinical trials have shown no appreciable toxicity. This product, however, has not been licensed by the FDA because of the difficulties in demonstrating efficacy. Measurement of postinfusion platelet count increments is not possible because they consist of platelet fragments that are not routinely measured. In addition, it is difficult to quantify the effects of any platelet substitute in thrombocytopenic patients who typically have other conditions associated with a bleeding tendency.

Lyophilized Platelets

The process of lyophilization—rapidly freezing a substance at an extremely low temperature and then dehydrating in a high vacuum—has been investigated as a means of long-term platelet storage. In fact, studies of rehydrated lyophilized platelets were originally performed in the 1950s. Unfortunately, these studies failed to demonstrate hemostatic efficacy in animal models of thrombocytopenia.[380] A more recently developed lyophilization procedure appears to allow better preservation of platelet structure.[381] This technique involves fixing washed platelets in 1.8% paraformaldehyde, followed by freezing in 5% albumin, and lyophilization at −20°C to −40°C. The resulting "fixed and lyophilized" platelets retain important hemostatic properties after rehydration in studies of thrombocytopenic rats and canine models of von Willebrand disease. Their ultrastructure by electron microscopy is similar to that of fresh platelets, and they also express the glycoprotein surface receptors GPIb and GPIIb-IIIa, albeit at decreased concentration. Reconstituted, lyophilized platelets appear capable of supporting thrombin generation and facilitating fibrin deposition of exposed vascular endothelium in a vascular perfusion model.[382]

More recent data from human and baboon subjects suggests possible poorer in vivo and in vitro performance characteristics. In a study by Valeri and colleagues using paraformaldehyde-treated lyophilized reconstituted platelets,[383] human lyophilized platelets failed to aggregate to the dual agonists arachidonic acid and adenosine diphosphate (4% aggregation vs 84% fresh control); weakly aggregated with ristocetin (27% aggregation vs 93% fresh control); and failed to produced thromboxane A_2, increase surface expression of P-selectin, increase surface expression of GP IIb/IIIa, or decrease expression of GP Ib with agonist stimulation. However, the lyophilized platelets did demonstrate greater accumulation of factor V (FV) on their surface after recalcification as compared with fresh controls. Thus, modifications to the platelet membrane during processing appeared to interfere with both platelet aggregation and thromboxane production.

Additional data from this group looking at in vivo characteristics show similar differences between fresh control platelets and reconstituted lyophilized platelets.[384] Survival studies in a baboon model using either biotin-X-N-hydroxysuccinimide or ^{111}In oxine–labeled platelets showed marked differences in in vivo survival; whereas fresh platelets showed greater than 50% survival at 48 hours postinfusion and remained detectable at 6 days, reconstituted lyophilized platelets were rapidly cleared from the circulation and undetectable beyond 15 minutes. Similarly to the prior study, the lyophilized platelets demonstrated greater procoagulant activity immediately following infusion than fresh controls. Levels of surface-bound FV were five times greater at 1 minute postinfusion in lyophilized platelets than in fresh controls.

At present, the clinical use of lyophilized platelets remains unclear owing to concerns regarding the toxicity, in vivo survival (short in vivo life span), thrombogenicity, and reticuloendothelial blockade of such preparations. Clinical trials utilizing reconstituted lyophilized platelets have not, as yet, been performed.

Cryopreserved Platelets

Cryopreservation has been used to store RBCs units since the 1960s. However, similar techniques evaluated for preserving platelets at low temperatures have been less successful. Platelets that are frozen or stored for prolonged periods at 4°C demonstrate abnormalities in aggregation, hypotonic stress response, clot retraction, and most importantly in vivo survival. These changes are related to irreversible cytoskeletal and membrane alterations.[385] Adverse effects of freezing platelets could be minimized by using high concentrations of a cryoprotectant; however, cryoprotectants themselves can harm platelets. These effects can result from direct chemical damage and osmotic changes that develop as the cryoprotectant crosses the cell membrane.

Cryopreservative Agents

A number of compounds have been evaluated as potential platelet cryoprotective agents including glucose, dimethyl sulfoxide (DMSO, Me_2SO), propylene glycol, polyvinylpyrrolidone, hydroxyethyl starch, polyethylene glycol, ethylene glycol, and others.[386] Propane-1,2-diol (propylene glycol), which is an effective agent for other hematopoietic elements, has a higher permeability rate than glycerol and is an ineffective platelet cryoprotectant.[387] Glycerol, used extensively for RBC cryopreservation, has little direct toxic chemical effects on platelets at the concentrations needed for effective protection. However, this compound enters the cell relatively slowly, resulting in severe osmotic damage. Use of a 5% glycerol–4% glucose solution may minimize freeze-thaw platelet loss and in initial studies, preserved platelet function.[388] Despite these precautions, adverse effects of freezing on in vitro platelet function have been demonstrated. This damage consists of platelet morphologic and ultrastructural changes, decreased ATP levels, an inability to undergo the release reaction or aggregation, decreased recovery from hypotonic stress, and decreased in vivo recovery.[389,390] Modifications of the original procedure, including optimization of the platelet count prior to freezing and use of a nonplasma diluent, did improve in vitro function.[391] Attempts to adapt platelet cryopreservation using glucose-glycerol solutions for clinical use have, as yet, been unsuccessful.[392]

DMSO-Based Cryopreservation

DMSO, used widely as a cryopreservative for human progenitor (stem) cells, rapidly penetrates the platelet membrane and has less of an osmotic effect than glucose-glycerol. In addition, both in vitro and in vivo studies suggest that DMSO is a more effective cryoprotective agent than glycerol.[393] Long-term studies have shown that DMSO-preserved platelets remain functional when stored for 3 years at −80°C.[394] However, cryopreservation with 5% to 6% DMSO does result in a clear loss of platelet structure and function in terms of platelet morphology, aggregation responses, and platelet recovery following transfusion.[395] The average post-transfusion recovery of cryopreserved platelets is approximately 50% to 70% that of fresh platelets; those platelets that do survive the freeze-thaw cycle appear to circulate normally.[379] The nearly 50% of platelets that are damaged during cryopreservation become unresponsive to various platelet agonists. In addition, there is a decrease in the content of secretory granules and an almost complete absence of the metabolic activity typically seen after platelet activation. It has been postulated that these findings reflect a defect in the stimulus-response coupling mechanisms that follow plasma membrane damage. Although these effects generally appear equally distributed among subpopulations of platelets, larger platelets may be most capable of retaining normal aggregatory responses.[396] Platelets stored frozen in liquid nitrogen with DMSO as a cryoprotectant have lower adhesive capacity in vitro as compared with fresh platelets from the same platelet unit.[397]

Platelet concentrates cryopreserved using DMSO are in use clinically as an alternative to conventional liquid stored platelets. However, this use is limited because the technique is relatively time consuming, laborious, and quite costly.[386] In addition, they must be washed before transfusion to remove DMSO, which can produce clinical side effects such as nausea, vomiting, and local vasospasm. Frozen platelets have generally been reserved for banking of autologous platelets from patients with acute leukemia who have become heavily alloimmunized and, hence, refractory to allogeneic platelet products. The efficacy of cryopreserved and liquid-preserved platelets has also been compared in cardiopulmonary bypass surgery.[398] Cryopreserved platelets appeared effective in minimizing blood loss and the need to transfuse blood products. However, these authors suggest that procoagulant activity, rather than common in vitro measures of platelet quality (aggregation, hypotonic stress, etc.), more accurately reflects the ability of cryopreserved platelets to maintain hemostasis. This argument has been further buttressed by data showing that thawed cryopreserved platelets, while possessing diminished capacity for aggregation to common agonists, generate significantly higher levels of thromboxane A2, a potent vasoconstrictor and platelet aggregator, when compared with conventionally stored platelet controls.[399]

DMSO Cryopreservation with Platelet-Stabilizing Agents

Solutions containing platelet-stabilizing agents (e.g., ThromboSol [Life Cell, The Woodlands, Tx.] containing amiloride, adenosine, and nitroprusside) have been developed that allow reducing the DMSO concentration while preserving recovery and survival on transfusion.[400,401] These solutions allow using only 2% DMSO while better maintaining platelet viability and both in vitro and in vivo function. Other investigators have reported the use of epinephrine[402] and varying combinations of Composol PS (Fresenius Kabi AG, Bad Homburg, Germany) and plasma[403] with DMSO that likewise demonstrate acceptable post-thaw in vitro and in vivo characteristics. Platelet cryopreservation using a combination of trehalose, a simple disaccharide sugar, supplemented with phosphate demonstrates preservation of the platelet plasma membrane, metabolic activity, and aggregation response to thrombin following cryopreservation.[404]

Synthetic Platelet Alternatives

Arg-Gly-Asp (RGD)–Based Platelet Substitutes

Several approaches to the creation of "platelet substitutes"—hemostatically active synthetic products that do not rely on the use of platelets or platelet fragments, yet possess properties similar to intact platelets—have been attempted. One such approach makes use of peptides containing Arg-Gly-Asp (RGD) sequences that mimic those normally found on fibrinogen. RGD motifs present on fibrinogen act as the primary binding sites for the platelet integrin on the surface glycoprotein GPIIb-IIIa and are responsible for the cross-linking of activated platelets that results in formation of the primary platelet plug at the site of vascular injury. Because binding occurs only to activated GPIIb-IIIa molecules, reactivity is limited to activated platelets normally present only at sites of vascular disruption. Peptides containing RGD sequences have been successfully covalently bound to RBCs.[405] The clinical application of this method, however, appears doubtful at present; although RBCs coated with RGD-bearing peptides are able to cause platelet agglutination in vitro, in vivo studies have failed to demonstrate adequate hemostatic efficacy.[406]

Fibrinogen-Coated Albumin Microcapsules

A second approach makes use of fibrinogen adsorbed onto carrier albumin microcapsules. At least two commercial formulations are in development—Synthocytes (Quadrant Healthcare, Nottingham, U.K.) and Haemaplax (Haemostatix, Leicester, U.K.). These products, also referred to more generically as fibrinogen-coated albumin microcapsules (FAMs), readily stimulate platelet activation and aggregation in vitro[407] and shorten bleeding time (BT) and reduce bleeding in thrombocytopenic rabbit models.[408] The results of human phase IIa trials using Synthocytes have not yet been reported.[409]

Liposome-Based Strategies

A third strategy has been to use liposome-based agents bearing either covalently bound fibrinogen or platelet glycoproteins such as recombinant GPIbα,[410] or infusion of procoagulant liposomes with activated factor Xa.[379] In vitro tests have shown that GPIbα-liposomes can mediate vWF accumulation on subendothelial tissues and enhance platelet function. Intravenous infusions of procoagulant liposomes in conjunction with activated factor Xa have been studied in hemophiliac dogs; however, this strategy had unacceptable toxic effects. Other platelet substitutes being studied include inert polyacrylonitrile beads coated with fibrinogen.[378]

Although many of these products face long research and development times, problems with current platelet preparations and antigenicity of certain formulations of thrombopoietic cytokines are encouraging many companies to further pursue development of these products.

THROMBOPOIETIC GROWTH FACTORS

Clinical Success of Recombinant Hematopoietic Growth Factors

Hematopoietic growth factors have enjoyed tremendous clinical successes as witnessed by the widespread use of recombinant erythropoietin to treat anemias due to chemotherapy,[411] myelodysplasia,[412] or chronic kidney diseases[413] and the use of granulocyte-colony stimulating factor[414] (G-CSF) in the treatment of patients with hematologic disorders[415] and infectious diseases.[416,417] Their use in clinical medicine has been to help limit exposure of patients to allogenic blood components and the short- and long-term adverse effects—such as platelet alloimmunization and iron overload[418]—that can occur with chronic exposure. The isolation, characterization, and subsequent synthesis of erythropoietin by recombinant technology, for example, has reduced the need for chronic RBC transfusions in certain patient populations. A similar agonist that would stimulate endogenous production of platelets in thrombocytopenic hosts has yet to be developed, although the current limitations and risks inherent in platelet transfusion therapy continue to drive development of such an agent.[419]

Potential Benefits of Recombinant Thrombopoietic Growth Factors

Thrombopoietic growth factors have the potential to stimulate platelet apheresis donors, to increase stem cell harvest yields, and to expand progenitor cells ex vivo.[420] There are rapid developments in the use of growth factors including FLT-3 ligand, c-Mpl ligand (thrombopoietin), and various combinations of growth factors. Interleukin-11 (IL-11), a 199-amino-acid protein coded for on chromosome 19q, directly stimulates the proliferation of hematopoietic stem cells and megakaryocyte progenitors and induces increased megakaryocyte maturation. A commercial form of IL-11 was approved by the FDA in 1997 for preventing severe thrombocytopenia in patients receiving myelosuppressive chemotherapy. However, IL-11 effects on platelet production are modest, and it is not recommended for patients with myeloid leukemias.[421]

Growth Factors and Megakaryocytopoiesis

Megakaryocytopoiesis—the production of platelets by bone marrow megakaryocytes—is under the control of a large host of cytokines and growth factors including IL-1, IL-3, IL-6, IL-11, erythropoietin, granulocyte-macrophage colony stimulating factor (GM-CSF), fibroblast growth factor (FGF), stem cell factor (SCF), leukemia inhibitory factor (LIF), and thrombopoietin.[422,423] Of these, thrombopoietin (TPO), a relatively lineage-specific trophic factor, is the most potent.[424] Although TPO messenger RNA (mRNA) has been detected in numerous organs, particularly the liver and kidney,[425,426] data from liver transplantation studies, in which pretransplant undetectable TPO levels were restored to normal following successful transplantation, suggest that essentially all TPO is synthesized in the liver.[427] In normal individuals, TPO production appears relatively constant[428]; variations in plasma concentration are due to binding, internalization, and subsequent degradation of TPO by c-Mpl[429] (the thrombopoietin receptor) expressing cells, such as hematopoietic stem cells, megakaryocytes, and platelets. Clinically, this results in an inverse relationship between circulating platelet counts and plasma TPO concentration. The thrombocytopenia associated with chemotherapy, for example, results in a net loss of MPL-expressing cells, resulting in elevated TPO levels due to diminished consumption.[430] This normal inverse relationship, however, is disrupted in a variety of pathologic states such as reactive thrombocytosis[431] and essential thrombocytosis[432] and in myeloproliferative disorders that result in down-regulation of the MPL receptor,[433] all of which lead to elevated TPO levels in the face of thrombocytosis.

Thrombopoietin

TPO is synthesized as a 353-amino-acid precursor protein that undergoes subsequent removal of a 21-amino-acid sequence and posttranslational glycosylation to generate the mature 95-kDa molecule. Two functional domains have been identified: a receptor-binding domain that shares significant sequence homology to erythropoietin and a carbohydrate-rich carboxyl terminus that helps maintain protein stability.[434] The TPO receptor, c-Mpl, was discovered during study of the viral oncogene v-Mpl in the myeloproliferative (Mpl) leukemia virus.[435] Once the receptor was identified, the ligand (TPO) was rapidly isolated and cloned by several independent laboratories.[436–439] Binding of TPO to target cells results in receptor dimerization and activation of intracellular signaling pathways that include the Janus kinase (JAK)–signal transducers and activators of transcription (STAT) and Ras cascades.[440] The physiologic effects of TPO include increasing the size, ploidy, and number of marrow megakaryocytes and the elaboration of megakaryocyte-specific surface markers[441]; it does not appear involved in the release of platelets from mature megakaryocytes.[442] TPO also exerts trophic effects on erythroid and myeloid precursors in synergy with other growth factors, such as erythropoietin and stem cell factor.[439]

Recombinant Thrombopoietin

Development of rhTPO and PEG-rHuMGDF

Since TPO was first identified and cloned, two recombinant forms have been developed that have undergone extensive clinical testing: rhTPO and PEG-rHuMGDF.[443] The former, rhTPO (Pharmacia, Peapack, N.J.; formerly developed by Genentech, South San Francisco, Calif.), shares exact amino acid sequence homology with endogenous TPO; it is produced in mammalian cells and glycosylated. PEG-rHuMGDF (Amgen, Thousand Oaks, Calif.) is produced in *E. coli* and consists of the first 163 amino acids of endogenous TPO—the receptor-binding domain—that is conjugated to a 20-kDa polyethylene glycol moiety that confers prolonged circulatory half-life. Both formulations possess all of the biological properties of native TPO. Using a baboon model, research has shown that PEG-MGDF does not increase platelet secretory granule membrane protein P-selectin expression nor increase the binding of annexin V to platelet membranes.[444] In addition, direct exposure of platelets to various concentrations of PEG-rHuMGDF does not appear to hasten or retard development of the platelet storage defect as defined by a battery of in vitro tests of platelet structure and function.[445]

Clinical Studies of rhTPO and PEG-rHuMGDF

Both rhTPO and PEG-rHuMGDF are potent stimulators of platelet production in humans. Their clinical use in the treatment of oncology patients has recently been reviewed by Kuter and Begley.[443] It was observed that both forms of recombinant TPO have a half-life in excess of 40 hours, and increases in circulating platelet counts are generally not seen until at least 5 days after administration, with a peak effect normally present 10 to 12 days after administration. The time lag to effect is likely due to the fact that TPO exerts most of its effects on precursor cells and has little physiologic effect on mature megakaryocytes. In all clinical trials, TPO appeared well tolerated with minimal side effects reported from phase I dose-escalation studies.

Use of Recombinant TPO following Nonmyeloablative versus Myeloablative Chemotherapy

A significant difference in the degree of beneficial effects from the use of post-treatment recombinant TPO has been noted between nonmyeloablative and myeloablative chemotherapy regimens. Studies addressing the ability of PEG-rHuMGDF to hasten hematologic recovery following nonmyeloablative chemotherapy for lung cancer, sarcomas, and gynecologic malignancies have generally shown modest benefits, including a reduction in the chemotherapy-related platelet count nadir, duration of thrombocytopenia, and number of platelet transfusions required.[446–448] Data from pediatric oncology trials in patients with recurrent or refractory solid tumors also suggest a promising role for recombinant TPO in reducing the severity of chemotherapy-associated thrombocytopenia.[449]

Myeloablative protocols in patients with leukemia or those undergoing hematopoietic progenitor cell (HPC) transplantation, however, have been disappointing. In aggregate, treatment with recombinant TPO in the setting of myeloablative chemotherapy in all studies failed to reduce the time to platelet recovery as marked by a platelet count of 20×10^9/L or greater or reduce the number of platelet transfusions needed prior to marrow reconstitution,[450–452] although a moderate increase in peak platelet counts and a reduction in the time to full platelet recovery were seen with both rhTPO and PEG-rHuMGDF. The reason for this is unclear, although a possible explanation is that the elevated levels of endogenous TPO commonly encountered with myeloablation may already have saturated available c-Mpl receptors.[443]

Adverse Effects of Neutralizing Antithrombopoietin Antibodies

In addition, the development of neutralizing antibodies against endogenous thrombopoietin has plagued clinical testing of thrombopoietic growth factors, in particular, PEG-rHuMGDF. These antibodies have caused severe thrombocytopenia in healthy volunteers and in oncology patients undergoing intensive chemotherapy.[453] This adverse effect has not been reported with rhTPO. One explanation offered for this observation is that PEG-rHuMGDF, which is truncated, nonglycosylated, and pegylated, is more immunogenic than the full-length glycosylated rhTPO form.[443] Additionally, rhTPO is generally administered intravenously while PEG-rHuMGDF is given as a subcutaneous injection. Because TPO is a potent mobilizer of dendritic cells, it has been postulated that the subcutaneous route of administration may also increase immunogenicity.

Treatment of HIV-Related Thrombocytopenia with Recombinant TPO

While the utility of recombinant TPO in hematologic malignancies appears unclear, its use in the setting of HIV-related thrombocytopenia appears more promising. PEG-rHuMGDF is effective in increasing platelet counts in chimpanzees with HIV-related thrombocytopenia.[444] In addition, case reports and small studies with HIV-infected patients likewise suggest improved thrombocytopenia following treatment with PEG-rHuMGDF.[443] These platelets, produced in response to PEG-rHuMGDF administration, demonstrate the expected responses to platelet agonists and ATP release in vivo, and their function is abrogated by aspirin.[454]

Mobilization for Platelet Apheresis Collection with Recombinant TPO

Likewise, recombinant TPO has shown potential benefits in mobilization of platelets for apheresis collection.[455] Studies with normal plateletpheresis donors have shown that PEG-rHuMGDF given as a single 2-μg/kg dose produced a doubling of the platelet count 9 to 14 days after administration. A single 3-μg/kg dose reliably produced a platelet count of 600×10^9/L. Single intravenous doses of PEG-rHuMGDF produced higher platelet elevations on day 5 after administration, whereas daily administration for 5 days produced a more prolonged thrombocytosis. Platelets collected by apheresis following PEG-rHuMGDF also were shown to have normal in vitro aggregation characteristics and produced expected increases in corrected count increments in thrombocytopenic recipients.

Use of Recombinant TPO in Autologous Marrow Transplantation

Finally, thrombopoietic growth factors have also been used in combination with other growth factors, such as FLT-3 ligand, to produce megakaryocytic progenitors ex vivo that can then be administered to autologous donors.[456–458] Other cytokines are under development that are designed to mimic the effects of TPO. A peptide agonist has been described that is a 14-amino-acid peptide with a high affinity for the thrombopoietin receptor.[459] This molecule was shown to be equipotent to the 332-amino-acid natural cytokines in cell-based assays. These small molecules that can activate receptors, replacing the need for large peptide ligands, may open the way for production of new types of hematopoietic stem cell growth factors.[460]

CONCLUSIONS

For the foreseeable future, clinicians will continue to rely on AD- and WB-Plts for the prophylaxis or treatment of bleeding in thrombocytopenic patients. Recently enacted AABB standards now stipulate mandatory bacterial detection for all platelet products, a move designed to address the relatively high incidence of bacterial contamination of platelets and the lower, but more serious, risk of septic transfusion reaction and sepsis-related deaths. With this additional testing has come renewed interest in extending the maximum shelf life of platelets from the current 5-day limit to 7 days, to help ease the economic and inventory burdens blood collection centers and transfusion facilities now face. It has also led many workers in the field to petition for accelerated development, validation, and adoption of pathogen reduction technologies, particularly in light of the ongoing emergence of new, potentially serious transfusion-transmitted diseases, such as West Nile virus.

Despite many advances in understanding of the basic biology of platelets, their translation into clinical practice has remained slow. Many basic questions remain unanswered, such as whether in vitro platelet tests can reliably predict in vivo function, how to determine a given patient's risk of bleeding, or what constitutes best platelet transfusion practice. The present pace of development of platelet substitutes likewise remains slow, despite some encouraging animal model data. This is also true for improvements in platelet storage methodologies. The use of recombinant thrombopoietin, despite its disappointing performance with myeloablative therapies, has shown demonstrable benefit in a variety of clinical scenarios. Clearly, a number of basic and clinical questions remain whose answers have the potential of dramatically affecting patient care and the ability to offer therapies now limited by intractable thrombocytopenia.

REFERENCES

1. AABB. Circular of Information for the Use of Human Blood and Blood Components. Bethesda, Md., AABB, 2002.
2. Hersh EM, Bodey GP, Boyd AN, Freireich EJ. Causes of death in acute leukaemia: a ten year study of 414 patients from 1954–1963. JAMA 1965;193:99–103.
3. Wallace EL, Churchill WH, Surgenor DM, Cho GS, McGurk S. Collection and transfusion of blood and blood components in the United States, 1994. Transfusion 1998;38:625–636.
4. Schiffer CA, Anderson KC, Bennett CL, et al. Platelet transfusion for patients with cancer: clinical practice guidelines of the American Society of Clinical Oncology. J Clin Oncol 2001;19:1519–1538.
5. Wright JH. The histogenesis of blood platelets. J Morphol 1910; 21:263.
6. Bruno E, Hoffman R. Human megakaryocyte progenitor cells. Semin Hematol 1998;35:183–191.
7. Fox JE. The platelet cytoskeleton. Thromb Haemost 1993;70:884–893.
8. Abrams CS. Intracellular signaling in platelets. Curr Opin Hematol 2005; 12:401–405.
9. Holt JC, Niewiarowski S. Biochemistry of alpha granule proteins. Semin Hematol 1985;22:151–163.
10. Perrotta PL, Perrotta CL, Snyder EL. Apoptotic activity in stored human platelets. Transfusion 2003;43:526–535.
11. Rucinski B, Niewiarowski S, Strzyzewski M, Holt JC, Mayo KH. Human platelet factor 4 and its C-terminal peptides: heparin binding and clearance from the circulation [erratum in Thromb Haemost 1991;66:269]. Thromb Haemost 1990;63:493–498.
12. Deuel TF, Senior RM, Chang D, Griffin GL, Heinrikson RL, Kaiser ET. Platelet factor 4 is chemotactic for neutrophils and monocytes. Proc Natl Acad Sci USA 1981;78:4584–4587.
13. Gewirtz AM, Calabretta B, Rucinski B, Niewiarowski S, Xu WY. Inhibition of human megakaryocytopoiesis in vitro by platelet factor 4 (PF4) and a synthetic COOH-terminal PF4 peptide. J Clin Invest 1989;83:1477–1486.
14. Capitanio AM, Niewiarowski S, Rucinski B, et al. Interaction of platelet factor 4 with human platelets. Biochim Biophys Acta 1985;839: 161–173.
15. Zucker MB, Katz IR, Thorbecke GJ, Milot DC, Holt J. Immunoregulatory activity of peptides related to platelet factor 4. Proc Natl Acad Sci USA 1989;86:7571–7574.
16. Bevers EM, Comfurius P, Dekkers DW, Harmsma M, Zwaal RF. Transmembrane phospholipid distribution in blood cells: control mechanisms and pathophysiological significance. Biol Chem 1998;379:973–986.
17. Comfurius P, Senden JM, Tilly RH, Schroit AJ, Bevers EM, Zwaal RF. Loss of membrane phospholipid asymmetry in platelets and red cells may be associated with calcium-induced shedding of plasma membrane and inhibition of aminophospholipid translocase. Biochim Biophys Acta 1990;1026:153–160.
18. Rosing J, van Rijn JL, Bevers EM, van Dieijen G, Comfurius P, Zwaal RF. The role of activated human platelets in prothrombin and factor X activation. Blood 1985;65:319–332.
19. Harrison P, Wilbourn B, Cramer E, et al. The influence of therapeutic blocking of Gp IIb/IIIa on platelet alpha-granular fibrinogen. Br J Haematol 1992;82:721–728.
20. Castillo R, Escolar G, Monteagudo J, Aznar-Salatti J, Reverter JC, Ordinas A. Hemostasis in patients with severe von Willebrand disease improves after normal platelet transfusion and normalizes with further correction of the plasma defect. Transfusion 1997;37:785–790.
21. Kieffer N, Phillips DR. Platelet membrane glycoproteins: functions in cellular interactions. Annu Rev Cell Biol 1990;6:329–357.
22. Nachman RL, Leung LL. Complex formation of platelet membrane glycoproteins IIb and IIIa with fibrinogen. J Clin Invest 1982;69: 263–269.
23. Nieuwenhuis HK, Akkerman JW, Houdijk WP, Sixma JJ. Human blood platelets showing no response to collagen fail to express surface glycoprotein Ia. Nature 1985;318:470–472.
24. Berman CL, Yeo EL, Wencel-Drake JD, Furie BC, Ginsberg MH, Furie B. A platelet alpha granule membrane protein that is associated with the plasma membrane after activation: characterization and subcellular localization of platelet activation-dependent granule-external membrane protein. J Clin Invest 1986;78:130–137.
25. Clemetson KJ. Platelet activation: signal transduction via membrane receptors. Thromb Haemost 1995;74:111–116.
26. Eriksson L, Kristensen J, Olsson K, Bring J, Hogman CF. Evaluation of platelet function using the in vitro bleeding time and corrected count increment of transfused platelets: comparison between platelet concentrates derived from pooled buffy coats and apheresis. Vox Sang 1996;70:69–75.
27. Jilma B. Platelet function analyzer (PFA-100): a tool to quantify congenital or acquired platelet dysfunction. J Lab Clin Med 2001;138:152–163.
28. Weiss HJ. Flow-related platelet deposition on subendothelium. Thromb Haemost 1995;74:117–122.
29. Perutelli P, Biglino P, Mori PG. von Willebrand factor: biological function and molecular defects [see comments]. Pediatr Hematol Oncol 1997;14:499–512.
30. Ruggeri ZM. Mechanisms initiating platelet thrombus formation [erratum in Thromb Haemost 1997;78:1304] [see comments]. Thromb Haemost 1997;78:611–616.
31. Lyman B, Rosenberg L, Karpatkin S. Biochemical and biophysical aspects of human platelet adhesion to collagen fibers. J Clin Invest 1971;50:1854–1863.
32. Holmsen H, Setkowsky CA, Day HJ. Effects of antimycin and 2-deoxyglucose on adenine nucleotides in human platelets: role of metabolic adenosine triphosphate in primary aggregation, secondary aggregation and shape change of platetets. Biochem J 1974;144:385–396.
33. Kilkson H, Holme S, Murphy S. Platelet metabolism during storage of platelet concentrates at 22°C. Blood 1984;64:406–414.
34. Moroff G, Holme S. Concepts about current conditions for the preparation and storage of platelets. Transfus Med Rev 1991;5:48–59.
35. Murphy S, Heaton WA, Rebulla P. Platelet production in the Old World—and the New. Transfusion 1996;36:751–754.
36. Mourad N. A simple method for obtaining platelet concentrates free of aggregates. Transfusion 1968;8:48.
37. Snyder EL, Pope C, Ferri PM, Smith EO, Walter SD, Ezekowitz MD. The effect of mode of agitation and type of plastic bag on storage characteristics and in vivo kinetics of platelet concentrates. Transfusion 1986;26:125–130.
38. Fijnheer R, Veldman HA, van den Eertwegh AJ, et al. In vitro evaluation of buffy-coat-derived platelet concentrates stored in a synthetic medium. Vox Sang 1991;60:16–22.
39. Bishop D, Tandy N, Anderson N, Bessos H, Seghatchian MJ. A clinical and laboratory study of platelet concentrates produced by pooled buffy coat and single donor apheresis technologies. Transfus Sci 1995; 16:187–188.
40. Keegan T, Heaton A, Holme S, Owens M, Nelson E, Carmen R. Paired comparison of platelet concentrates prepared from platelet-rich plasma and buffy coats using a new technique with 111In and 51Cr. Transfusion 1992;32:113–120.
41. Bock M, Rahrig S, Kunz D, Lutze G, Heim MU. Platelet concentrates derived from buffy coat and apheresis: biochemical and functional differences. Transfus Med 2002;12:317–324.
42. Vasconcelos E, Figueiredo AC, Seghatchian J. Quality of platelet concentrates derived by platelet rich plasma, buffy coat and apheresis. Transfus Apheresis Sci 2003;29:13–16.
43. Murphy S. The efficacy of synthetic media in the storage of human platelets for transfusion. Transfus Med Rev 1999;13:153–163.
44. Bertolini F, Rebulla P, Riccardi D, Cortellaro M, Ranzi ML, Sirchia G. Evaluation of platelet concentrates prepared from buffy coats and stored in a glucose-free crystalloid medium. Transfusion 1989;29: 605–609.
45. Holme S, Heaton A. In vitro platelet ageing at 22 degrees C is reduced compared to in vivo ageing at 37°C. Br J Haematol 1995;91: 212–218.
46. Badlou BA, Ijseldijk MJ, Smid WM, Akkerman JW. Prolonged platelet preservation by transient metabolic suppression. Transfusion 2005; 45:214–222.
47. Gulliksson H. Defining the optimal storage conditions for the long-term storage of platelets. Transfus Med Rev 2003;17:209–215.
48. Rock G, White J, Labow R. Storage of platelets in balanced salt solutions: a simple platelet storage medium. Transfusion 1991;31:21–25.
49. Gulliksson H, Eriksson L, Hogman CF, Payrat JM. Buffy-coat-derived platelet concentrates prepared from half-strength citrate CPD and CPD whole-blood units: comparison between three additive solutions: in vitro studies. Vox Sang 1995;68:152–159.
50. Murphy S, Kagen L, Holme S, et al. Platelet storage in synthetic media lacking glucose and bicarbonate. Transfusion 1991;31:16–20.
51. Bode AP, Holme S, Heaton WA, Swanson MS. Extended storage of platelets in an artificial medium with the platelet activation inhibitors prostaglandin E1 and theophylline. Vox Sang 1991;60:105–112.
52. Bode AP, Norris HT. The use of inhibitors of platelet activation or protease activity in platelet concentrates stored for transfusion. Blood Cells 1992;18:361–380; discussion 381–362.
53. Mrowiec ZR, Oleksowicz L, Zuckerman D, et al. Buffy coat platelets stored in apyrase, aprotinin, and ascorbic acid in a suspended bag: combined strategies for reducing platelet activation during storage. Transfusion 1996;36:5–10.

54. Murphy S, Gardner FH. Effect of storage temperature on maintenance of platelet viability—deleterious effect of refrigerated storage. N Engl J Med 1969;280:1094–1098.
55. Slichter SJ, Harker LA. Preparation and storage of platelet concentrates. II. Storage variables influencing platelet viability and function. Br J Haematol 1976;34:403–419.
56. Filip DJ, Aster RH. Relative hemostatic effectiveness of human platelets stored at 4 degrees and 22 degrees C. J Lab Clin Med 1978;91:618–624.
57. Vostal JG, Mondoro TH. Liquid cold storage of platelets: a revitalized possible alternative for limiting bacterial contamination of platelet products. Transfus Med Rev 1997;11:286–295.
58. White JG, Krivit W. An ultrastructural basis for the shape changes induced in platelets by chilling. Blood 1967;30:625–635.
59. Hartwig JH. Mechanisms of actin rearrangements mediating platelet activation. J Cell Biol 1992;118:1421–1442.
60. Hoffmeister KM, Falet H, Toker A, Barkalow KL, Stossel TP, Hartwig JH. Mechanisms of cold-induced platelet actin assembly. J Biol Chem 2001;27:27.
61. Hoffmeister KM, Felbinger TW, Falet H, et al. The clearance mechanism of chilled blood platelets. Cell 2003;112:87–97.
62. Hoffmeister KM, Josefsson EC, Isaac NA, Clausen H, Hartwig JH, Stossel TP. Glycosylation restores survival of chilled blood platelets. Science 2003;301:1531–1534.
63. Winokur R, Hartwig JH. Mechanism of shape change in chilled human platelets. Blood 1995;85:1796–1804.
64. Melaragno AJ, Carciero R, Feingold H, Talarico L, Weintraub L, Valeri CR. Cryopreservation of human platelets using 6% dimethyl sulfoxide and storage at −80° C: effects of 2 years of frozen storage at −80°C and transportation in dry ice. Vox Sang 1985;49:245–258.
65. Blajchman MA. Novel platelet products, substitutes and alternatives. Transfus Clin Biol 2001;8:267–271.
66. Vadhan-Raj S, Currie LM, Bueso-Ramos C, Livesey SA, Connor J. Enhanced retention of in vitro functional activity of platelets from recombinant human thrombopoietin-treated patients following long-term cryopreservation with a platelet-preserving solution (ThromboSol) and 2% DMSO. Br J Haematol 1999;104:403–411.
67. Murphy S, Gardner FH. Platelet storage at 22° C: role of gas transport across plastic containers in maintenance of viability. Blood 1975;46:209–218.
68. Moroff G, Friedman A, Robkin-Kline L. Factors influencing changes in pH during storage of platelet concentrates at 20–24° C. Vox Sang 1982;42:33–45.
69. Snyder EL, Ezekowitz M, Aster R, et al. Extended storage of platelets in a new plastic container. II. In vivo response to infusion of platelets stored for 5 days. Transfusion 1985;25:209–214.
70. Murphy S, Kahn RA, Holme S, et al. Improved storage of platelets for transfusion in a new container. Blood 1982;60:194–200.
71. Snyder EL, Aster RH, Heaton A, et al. Five-day storage of platelets in a non-diethylhexyl phthalate-plasticized container. Transfusion 1992; 32:736–741.
72. Jaeger RJ, Rubin RJ. Migration of a phthalate ester plasticizer from polyvinyl chloride blood bags into stored human blood and its localization in human tissues. N Engl J Med 1972;287:1114–1118.
73. Jaeger RJ, Rubin RJ. Di-2-ethylhexyl phthalate, a plasticizer contaminant of platelet concentrates. Transfusion 1973;13:107–111.
74. Sasakawa S, Mitomi Y. Di-2-ethylhexylphthalate (DEHP) content of blood or blood components stored in plastic bags. Vox Sang 1978;34:81–86.
75. Rock G, Secours VE, Franklin CA, Chu I, Villeneuve DC. The accumulation of mono-2-ethylhexylphthalate (MEHP) during storage of whole blood and plasma. Transfusion 1978;18:553–558.
76. Peck CC, Odom DG, Friedman HI, et al. Di-2-ethylhexyl phthalate (DEHP) and mono-2-ethylexyl phthalate (MEHP) accumulation in whole blood and red cell concentrates. Transfusion 1979;19:137–146.
77. Gulliksson H, Shanwell A, Wikman A, Reppucci AJ, Sallander S, Uden AM. Storage of platelets in a new plastic container: polyvinyl chloride plasticized with butyryl-n-trihexyl citrate. Vox Sang 1991;61:165–170.
78. Holme S, Vaidja K, Murphy S. Platelet storage at 22° C: effect of type of agitation on morphology, viability, and function in vitro. Blood 1978;52:425–435.
79. Snyder EL, Hezzey A, Katz AJ, Bock J. Occurrence of the release reaction during preparation and storage of platelet concentrates. Vox Sang 1981;41:172–177.
80. Graw RG, Jr., Herzig GP, Eisel RJ, Perry S. Leukocyte and platelet collection from normal donors with the continuous flow blood cell separator. Transfusion 1971;11:94–101.
81. Yankee RA, Grumet FC, Rogentine GN. Platelet transfusion: the selection of compatible platelet donors for refractory patients by lymphocyte HL-A typing. N Engl J Med 1969;281:1208–1212.
82. Thorsby E, Helgesen A, Gjemdal T. Repeated platelet transfusions from HL-A compatible unrelated and sibling donors. Tissue Antigens 1972;2:397–404.
83. Burgstaler EA, Pineda AA, Wollan P. Plateletapheresis: comparison of processing times, platelet yields, and white blood cell content with several commonly used systems. J Clin Apheresis 1997;12:170–178.
84. Yockey C, Murphy S, Eggers L, et al. Evaluation of the Amicus Separator in the collection of apheresis platelets. Transfusion 1998;38:848–854.
85. Elfath MD, Whitley P, Jacobson MS, et al. Evaluation of an automated system for the collection of packed RBCs, platelets, and plasma. Transfusion 2000;40:1214–1222.
86. Standards for Blood Banks and Transfusion Services, 23rd ed. Bethesda, Md., AABB Press, 2005.
87. Chalandon Y, Mermillod B, Beris P, et al. Benefit of prestorage leukocyte depletion of single-donor platelet concentrates. Vox Sang 1999;76:27–37.
88. Bowden RA, Slichter SJ, Sayers M, et al. A comparison of filtered leukocyte-reduced and cytomegalovirus (CMV) seronegative blood products for the prevention of transfusion-associated CMV infection after marrow transplant. Blood 1995;86:3598–3603.
89. The Trial to Reduce Alloimmunization to Platelets Study Group. Leukocyte reduction and ultraviolet B irradiation of platelets to prevent alloimmunization and refractoriness to platelet transfusions. N Engl J Med 1997;337:1861–1869.
90. Bock M, Schleuning M, Heim MU, Mempel W. Cryopreservation of human platelets with dimethyl sulfoxide: changes in biochemistry and cell function. Transfusion 1995;35:921–924.
91. Funke I, Wiesneth M, Koerner K, et al. Autologous platelet transfusion in alloimmunized patients with acute leukemia. Ann Hematol 1995;71:169–173.
92. Torretta L, Perotti C, Pedrazzoli P, et al. Autologous platelet collection and storage to support thrombocytopenia in patients undergoing high-dose chemotherapy and circulating progenitor cell transplantation for high-risk breast cancer. Vox Sang 1998;75:224–229.
93. McLeod BC, Price TH, Owen H, et al. Frequency of immediate adverse effects associated with apheresis donation. Transfusion 1998;38:938–943.
94. Koch HM, Bolt HM, Preuss R, Eckstein R, Weisbach V, Angerer J. Intravenous exposure to di(2-ethylhexyl)phthalate (DEHP): metabolites of DEHP in urine after a voluntary platelet donation. Arch Toxicol 2005:1–5.
95. Holme S, Heaton WA, Moroff G. Evaluation of platelet concentrates stored for 5 days with reduced plasma volume. Transfusion 1994; 34:39–43.
96. Blanchette VS, Kuhne T, Hume H, Hellmann J. Platelet transfusion therapy in newborn infants. Transfus Med Rev 1995;9:215–230.
97. Simon TL, Sierra ER. Concentration of platelet units into small volumes. Transfusion 1984;24:173–175.
98. Moroff G, Friedman A, Robkin-Kline L, Gautier G, Luban NL. Reduction of the volume of stored platelet concentrates for use in neonatal patients. Transfusion 1984;24:144–146.
99. Schoenfeld H, Muhm M, Doepfmer UR, Kox WJ, Spies C, Radtke H. The functional integrity of platelets in volume-reduced platelet concentrates. Anesth Analg 2005;100:78–81.
100. Pisciotto PT, Snyder EL, Napychank PA, Hopfer SM. In vitro characteristics of volume-reduced platelet concentrate stored in syringes. Transfusion 1991;31:404–408.
101. Pisciotto PT, Snyder EL, Snyder JA, et al. In vitro characteristics of white cell-reduced single-unit platelet concentrates stored in syringes. Transfusion 1994;34:407–411.
102. Sweeney J. Quality assurance and standards for red cells and platelets. Vox Sang 1998;74:201–205.
103. Menitove J (ed). Standards for blood banks and transfusion services (19th ed.). Bethesda, Md., American Association of Blood Banks, 1999.
104. Dickerhoff R, Von Ruecker A. Enumeration of platelets by multiparameter flow cytometry using platelet-specific antibodies and fluorescent reference particles. Clin Lab Haematol 1995;17:163–172.
105. Bertolini F, Murphy S. A multicenter inspection of the swirling phenomenon in platelet concentrates prepared in routine practice. Biomedical Excellence for Safer Transfusion (BEST) Working Party of the International Society of Blood Transfusion. Transfusion 1996;36:128–132.
106. Bertolini F, Murphy S. A multicenter evaluation of reproducibility of swirling in platelet concentrates. Biomedical Excellence for Safer Transfusion (BEST) Working Party of the International Society of Blood Transfusion. Transfusion 1994;34:796–801.
107. Bertolini F, Agazzi A, Peccatori F, Martinelli G, Sandri MT. The absence of swirling in platelet concentrates is highly predictive of poor post-transfusion platelet count increments and increased risk of a transfusion reaction. Transfusion 2000;40:121–122.

108. Lutz P, Dzik WH. Large-volume hemocytometer chamber for accurate counting of white cells (WBCs) in WBC-reduced platelets: validation and application for quality control of WBC-reduced platelets prepared by apheresis and filtration. Transfusion 1993;33:409–412.
109. Moroff G, Eich J, Dabay M. Validation of use of the Nageotte hemocytometer to count low levels of white cells in white cell-reduced platelet components. Transfusion 1994;34:35–38.
110. Finch SJ, Chen JB, Chen CH, et al. Process control procedures to augment quality control of leukocyte-reduced red cell blood products. Stat Med 1999;18:1279–1289.
111. Dzik WH, Ragosta A, Cusack WF. Flow-cytometric method for counting very low numbers of leukocytes in platelet products. Vox Sang 1990;59:153–159.
112. Adams MR, Johnson DK, Busch MP, Schembri CT, Hartz TP, Heaton WA. Automatic volumetric capillary cytometry for counting white cells in white cell-reduced plateletpheresis components. Transfusion 1997;37:29–37.
113. Dzik S, Moroff G, Dumont L. A multicenter study evaluating three methods for counting residual WBCs in WBC-reduced blood components: Nageotte hemocytometry, flow cytometry, and microfluorometry. Transfusion 2000;40:513–520.
114. Dijkstra-Tiekstra MJ, van der Meer PF, Pietersz RN, de Wildt-Eggen J. Multicenter evaluation of two flow cytometric methods for counting low levels of white blood cells. Transfusion 2004;44: 1319–1324.
115. Sirchia G, Rebulla P, Sabbioneda L, Garcea F, Greppi N. Optimal conditions for white cell reduction in red cells by filtration at the patient's bedside. Transfusion 1996;36:322–327.
116. Seghatchian J, Krailadsiri P. Current methods for the preparation of platelet concentrates: laboratory and clinical aspects. Transfus Sci 1997;18:27–32.
117. Dumont LJ, Dzik WH, Rebulla P, Brandwein H. Practical guidelines for process validation and process control of white cell-reduced blood components: report of the Biomedical Excellence for Safer Transfusion (BEST) Working Party of the International Society of Blood Transfusion (ISBT). Transfusion 1996;36:11–20.
118. Standards for Blood Banks and Transfusion Services, 23rd ed. Bethesda, Md., AABB Press, 2005.
119. Transfusion Medicine Checklist. In Sarewitz SJ (ed). Laboratory Accreditation Program Inspection Checklists. College of American Pathologists, 2003.
120. Fatal Bacterial Infections Associated with Platelet Transfusions—United States, 2004. MMWR Morb Mortal Wkly Rep 2005;54:168–170.
121. Yomtovian R, Lazarus HM, Goodnough LT, Hirschler NV, Morrissey AM, Jacobs MR. A prospective microbiologic surveillance program to detect and prevent the transfusion of bacterially contaminated platelets. Transfusion 1993;33:902–909.
122. Lee CK, Ho PL, Lee KY, et al. Estimation of bacterial risk in extending the shelf life of PLT concentrates from 5 to 7 days. Transfusion 2003;43:1047–1052.
123. Macauley A, Chandrasekar A, Geddis G, Morris KG, McClelland WM. Operational feasibility of routine bacterial monitoring of platelets. Transfus Med 2003;13:189–195.
124. Larsen CP, Ezligini F, Hermansen NO, Kjeldsen-Kragh J. Six years' experience of using the BacT/ALERT system to screen all platelet concentrates, and additional testing of outdated platelet concentrates to estimate the frequency of false-negative results. Vox Sang 2005;88:93–97.
125. Lee JH. Workshop on bacterial contamination of platelets. Bethesda, Md., Center for Biologics Evaluation and Research (CBER), Food and Drug Administration, 1999.
126. Blajchman MA, Goldman M, Baeza F. Improving the bacteriological safety of platelet transfusions. Transfus Med Rev 2004;18:11–24.
127. Ness P, Braine H, King K, et al. Single-donor platelets reduce the risk of septic platelet transfusion reactions. Transfusion 2001;41:857–861.
128. Engelfriet CP, Reesink HW, Blajchman MA, et al. Bacterial contamination of blood components. Vox Sang 2000;78:59–67.
129. Morrow JF, Braine HG, Kickler TS, Ness PM, Dick JD, Fuller AK. Septic reactions to platelet transfusions: a persistent problem. JAMA 1991;266:555–558.
130. Uhl L. Infectious risks of blood transfusion. Curr Hematol Rep 2002;1:156–162.
131. Klein HG, Dodd RY, Ness PM, Fratantoni JA, Nemo GJ. Current status of microbial contamination of blood components: summary of a conference. Transfusion 1997;37:95–101.
132. Center for Biologics Evaluation and Research. Safety and Efficacy of Methods for Reducing Pathogens in Cellular Blood Products Used in Transfusion. Bethesda, Md., Center for Biologics Evaluation and Research (CBER), Food and Drug Administration, 2002.
133. Kuehnert MJ, Roth VR, Haley NR, et al. Transfusion-transmitted bacterial infection in the United States, 1998 through 2000. Transfusion 2001;41:1493–1499.
134. Williamson L, Cohen H, Love E, Jones H, Todd A, Soldan K. The Serious Hazards of Transfusion (SHOT) initiative: the UK approach to haemovigilance. Vox Sang 2000;78(Suppl 2):291–295.
135. Rebibo D, Hauser L, Slimani A, Herve P, Andreu G. The French Haemovigilance System: organization and results for 2003. Transfus Apheresis Sci 2004;31:145–153.
136. Brecher ME, Means N, Jere CS, Heath D, Rothenberg S, Stutzman LC. Evaluation of an automated culture system for detecting bacterial contamination of platelets: an analysis with 15 contaminating organisms. Transfusion 2001;41:477–482.
137. Wagner SJ. Transfusion-transmitted bacterial infection: risks, sources and interventions. Vox Sang 2004;86:157–163.
138. Lee CK, Ho PL, Chan NK, Mak A, Hong J, Lin CK. Impact of donor arm skin disinfection on the bacterial contamination rate of platelet concentrates. Vox Sang 2002;83:204–208.
139. Anderson KC, Lew MA, Gorgone BC, Martel J, Leamy CB, Sullivan B. Transfusion-related sepsis after prolonged platelet storage. Am J Med 1986;81:405–411.
140. Kojima K, Togashi T, Hasegawa K. Subcutaneous fatty tissue can stray into a blood bag. Vox Sang 1998;74(Suppl 1):Abstract 1205.
141. Grossman BJ, Kollins P, Lau PM, et al. Screening blood donors for gastrointestinal illness: a strategy to eliminate carriers of Yersinia enterocolitica. Transfusion 1991;31:500–501.
142. Goldman M, Blajchman MA. Blood product-associated bacterial sepsis. Transfus Med Rev 1991;5:73–83.
143. McDonald CP, Roy A, Mahajan P, Smith R, Charlett A, Barbara JA. Relative values of the interventions of diversion and improved donor-arm disinfection to reduce the bacterial risk from blood transfusion. Vox Sang 2004;86:178–182.
144. Wagner SJ, Robinette D, Friedman LI, Miripol J. Diversion of initial blood flow to prevent whole-blood contamination by skin surface bacteria: an in vitro model. Transfusion 2000;40:335–338.
145. de Korte D, Marcelis JH, Verhoeven AJ, Soeterboek AM. Diversion of first blood volume results in a reduction of bacterial contamination for whole-blood collections. Vox Sang 2002;83:13–16.
146. AuBuchon JP, Cooper LK, Leach MF, Zuaro DE, Schwartzman JD. Experience with universal bacterial culturing to detect contamination of apheresis platelet units in a hospital transfusion service. Transfusion 2002;42:855–861.
147. Dodd RY, Lipton KS. Guidance on Implementation of New Bacterial Reduction and Detection Standard. AABB Association Bulletin No. 03-10. Bethesda, Md., AABB, 2003, p. 8.
148. Dodd RY, Lipton KS. Further Guidance on Methods to Detect Bacterial Contamination of Platelet Components. AABB Association Bulletin No. 03–12. Bethesda, Md., AABB, 2003, p. 41.
149. Werch JB, Mhawech P, Stager CE, Banez EI, Lichtiger B. Detecting bacteria in platelet concentrates by use of reagent strips. Transfusion 2002;42:1027–1031.
150. Brecher ME, Hay SN. Bacterial contamination of blood components. Clin Microbiol Rev 2005;18:195–204.
151. Brecher ME, Hay SN, Rothenberg SJ. Evaluation of a new generation of plastic culture bottles with an automated microbial detection system for nine common contaminating organisms found in PLT components. Transfusion 2004;44:359–363.
152. Brecher ME, Heath DG, Hay SN, Rothenberg SJ, Stutzman LC. Evaluation of a new generation of culture bottle using an automated bacterial culture system for detecting nine common contaminating organisms found in platelet components. Transfusion 2002;42:774–779.
153. McDonald CP, Rogers A, Cox M, et al. Evaluation of the 3D BacT/ALERT automated culture system for the detection of microbial contamination of platelet concentrates. Transfus Med 2002; 12:303–309.
154. McDonald CP, Roy A, Lowe P, Robbins S, Hartley S, Barbara JA. Evaluation of the BacT/Alert automated blood culture system for detecting bacteria and measuring their growth kinetics in leucodepleted and non-leucodepleted platelet concentrates. Vox Sang 2001;81:154–160.
155. Ortolano GA, Freundlich LF, Holme S, et al. Detection of bacteria in WBC-reduced PLT concentrates using percent oxygen as a marker for bacteria growth. Transfusion 2003;43:1276–1285.
156. te Boekhorst PA, Beckers EA, Vos MC, Vermeij H, van Rhenen DJ. Clinical significance of bacteriologic screening in platelet concentrates. Transfusion 2005;45:514–519.
157. Yomtovian R, Brecher ME. pH and glucose testing of single-donor apheresis platelets should be discontinued in favor of a more sensitive detection method. Transfusion 2005;45:646–648.

158. Dumont LJ, AuBuchon JP, Whitley P, et al. Seven-day storage of single-donor platelets: recovery and survival in an autologous transfusion study. Transfusion 2002;42:847–854.
159. Substantially Equivalent 510(k) Device Information: COBE Spectra Apheresis System & Trima Automated Blood Component Collection System. In: Center for Biologics Evaluation and Research. U.S. Food and Drug Administration, Department of Health and Human Services, Rockville, Md., 2005.
160. Seghatchian J, Krailadsiri P. The platelet storage lesion [see comments]. Transfus Med Rev 1997;11:130–144.
161. Rinder HM, Murphy M, Mitchell JG, Stocks J, Ault KA, Hillman RS. Progressive platelet activation with storage: evidence for shortened survival of activated platelets after transfusion. Transfusion 1991;31:409–414.
162. Triulzi DJ, Kickler TS, Braine HG. Detection and significance of alpha granule membrane protein 140 expression on platelets collected by apheresis [see comments]. Transfusion 1992;32:529–533.
163. Chernoff A, Snyder EL. The cellular and molecular basis of the platelet storage lesion: a symposium summary. Transfusion 1992;32: 386–390.
164. Snyder EL, Moroff G, Simon T, Heaton A. Recommended methods for conducting radiolabeled platelet survival studies. Transfusion 1986; 26:37–42.
165. Heilmann E, Friese P, Anderson S, et al. Biotinylated platelets: a new approach to the measurement of platelet life span. Br J Haematol 1993;85:729–735.
166. Rinder HM, Bonan JL, Rinder CS, Ault KA, Smith BR. Dynamics of leukocyte-platelet adhesion in whole blood. Blood 1991;78:1730–1737.
167. Murphy S, Rebulla P, Bertolini F, et al. In vitro assessment of the quality of stored platelet concentrates. The BEST (Biomedical Excellence for Safer Transfusion) Task Force of the International Society of Blood Transfusion. Transfus Med Rev 1994;8:29–36.
168. Michelson AD, Barnard MR, Hechtman HB, et al. In vivo tracking of platelets: circulating degranulated platelets rapidly lose surface P-selectin but continue to circulate and function. Proc Natl Acad Sci U S A 1996;93:11877–11882.
169. Metcalfe P, Williamson LM, Reutelingsperger CP, Swann I, Ouwehand WH, Goodall AH. Activation during preparation of therapeutic platelets affects deterioration during storage: a comparative flow cytometric study of different production methods. Br J Haematol 1997;98:86–95.
170. Dumont LJ, VandenBroeke T, Ault KA. Platelet surface P-selectin measurements in platelet preparations: an international collaborative study. Biomedical Excellence for Safer Transfusion (BEST) Working Party of the International Society of Blood Transfusion (ISBT). Transfus Med Rev 1999;13:31–42.
171. McEver RP. GMP-140: a receptor for neutrophils and monocytes on activated platelets and endothelium. J Cell Biochem 1991;45:156–161.
172. George JN, Pickett EB, Heinz R. Platelet membrane glycoprotein changes during the preparation and storage of platelet concentrates. Transfusion 1988;28:123–126.
173. Fijnheer R, Modderman PW, Veldman H, et al. Detection of platelet activation with monoclonal antibodies and flow cytometry: changes during platelet storage. Transfusion 1990;30:20–25.
174. Fijnheer R, Pietersz RN, de Korte D, et al. Platelet activation during preparation of platelet concentrates: a comparison of the platelet-rich plasma and the buffy coat methods. Transfusion 1990;30:634–638.
175. Fox JE, Reynolds CC, Morrow JS, Phillips DR. Spectrin is associated with membrane-bound actin filaments in platelets and is hydrolyzed by the Ca^{2+}-dependent protease during platelet activation. Blood 1987; 69:537–545.
176. Pollard TD, Cooper JA. Actin and actin-binding proteins: a critical evaluation of mechanisms and functions. Annu Rev Biochem 1986; 55:987–1035.
177. Bode AP, Orton SM, Frye MJ, Udis BJ. Vesiculation of platelets during in vitro aging. Blood 1991;77:887–895.
178. Snyder EL, Horne WC, Napychank P, Heinemann FS, Dunn B. Calcium-dependent proteolysis of actin during storage of platelet concentrates. Blood 1989;73:1380–1385.
179. Robey FA, Freitag CM, Jamieson GA. Disappearance of actin binding protein from human blood platelets during storage. FEBS Lett 1979;102:257–260.
180. Tsujinaka T, Sakon M, Kambayashi J, Kosaki G. Cleavage of cytoskeletal proteins by two forms of Ca^{2+} activated neutral proteases in human platelets. Thromb Res 1982;28:149–156.
181. Fox JE, Goll DE, Reynolds CC, Phillips DR. Identification of two proteins (actin-binding protein and P235) that are hydrolyzed by endogenous Ca^{2+}-dependent protease during platelet aggregation. J Biol Chem 1985;260:1060–1066.
182. Wiedmer T, Shattil SJ, Cunningham M, Sims PJ. Role of calcium and calpain in complement-induced vesiculation of the platelet plasma membrane and in the exposure of the platelet factor Va receptor. Biochemistry 1990;29:623–632.
183. Brown SB, Clarke MC, Magowan L, Sanderson H, Savill J. Constitutive death of platelets leading to scavenger receptor-mediated phagocytosis. A caspase-independent cell clearance program. J Biol Chem 2000;275:5987–5996.
184. Seghatchian J, Krailadsiri P. Platelet storage lesion and apoptosis: are they related? Transfus Apheresis Sci 2001;24:103–105.
185. Seghatchian J, de Sousa G. Blood cell apoptosis/necrosis: some clinical and laboratory aspects. Ann N Y Acad Sci 2003;1010:540–547.
186. Leytin V, Freedman J. Platelet apoptosis in stored platelet concentrates and other models. Transfus Apheresis Sci 2003;28:285–295.
187. Kerr JF, Wyllie AH, Currie AR. Apoptosis: a basic biological phenomenon with wide-ranging implications in tissue kinetics. Br J Cancer 1972;26:239–257.
188. Vanags DM, Orrenius S, Aguilar-Santelises M. Alterations in Bcl-2/Bax protein levels in platelets form part of an ionomycin-induced process that resembles apoptosis. Br J Haematol 1997;99:824–831.
189. Michelson AD, Adelman B, Barnard MR, Carroll E, Handin RI. Platelet storage results in a redistribution of glycoprotein Ib molecules: evidence for a large intraplatelet pool of glycoprotein Ib. J Clin Invest 1988;81:1734–1740.
190. Snyder EL, Beardsley DS, Smith BR, et al. Storage of platelet concentrates after high-dose ultraviolet B irradiation. Transfusion 1991; 31:491–496.
191. Bertolini F, Rebulla P, Porretti L, Sirchia G. Comparison of platelet activation and membrane glycoprotein Ib and IIb-IIIa expression after filtration through three different leukocyte removal filters. Vox Sang 1990;59:201–204.
192. Michelson AD, Barnard MR. Plasmin-induced redistribution of platelet glycoprotein Ib. Blood 1990;76:2005–2010.
193. Snyder EL, Mosher DF, Hezzey A, Golenwsky G. Effect of blood transfusion on in vivo levels of plasma fibronectin. J Lab Clin Med 1981;98:336–341.
194. Yazer MH, Podlosky L, Clarke G, Nahirniak SM. The effect of prestorage WBC reduction on the rates of febrile nonhemolytic transfusion reactions to platelet concentrates and RBC. Transfusion 2004;44:10–15.
195. Kao KJ. Effects of leukocyte depletion and UVB irradiation on alloantigenicity of major histocompatibility complex antigens in platelet concentrates: a comparative study. Blood 1992;80:2931–2937.
196. Meryman HT. Transfusion-induced alloimmunization and immunosuppression and the effects of leukocyte depletion. Transfus Med Rev 1989;3:180–193.
197. Bowden RA, Slichter SJ, Sayers MH, Mori M, Cays MJ, Meyers JD. Use of leukocyte-depleted platelets and cytomegalovirus-seronegative red blood cells for prevention of primary cytomegalovirus infection after marrow transplant. Blood 1991;78:246–250.
198. Kickler TS, Bell W, Drew H, Pall D. Depletion of white cells from platelet concentrates with a new adsorption filter. Transfusion 1989;29:411–414.
199. Sirchia G, Wenz B, Rebulla P, Parravicini A, Carnelli V, Bertolini F. Removal of white cells from red cells by transfusion through a new filter. Transfusion 1990;30:30–33.
200. Kao KJ, Mickel M, Braine HG, et al. White cell reduction in platelet concentrates and packed red cells by filtration: a multicenter clinical trial. The Trap Study Group. Transfusion 1995;35:13–19.
201. Snyder EL, DePalma L, Napychank P. Use of polyester filters for the preparation of leukocyte-poor platelet concentrates. Vox Sang 1988; 54:21–23.
202. Beckman N, Sher G, Masse M, et al. Review of the quality monitoring methods used by countries using or implementing universal leukoreduction. Transfus Med Rev 2004;18:25–35.
203. Blackall DP. The Canadian Universal Leukoreduction Program. Curr Hematol Rep 2003;2:493–494.
204. Hebert PC, Fergusson DA. Evaluation of a universal leukoreduction program in Canada. Vox Sang 2002;83(Suppl 1):207–209.
205. Fisk JM, Snyder EL. Universal pre-storage leukoreduction—a defensible use of hospital resources: the Yale-New Haven Hospital experience. Dev Biol (Basel) 2005;120:39–44.
206. Manna A, Cordani S, Canessa P, Pronzato P. CMV infection and pneumonia in hematological malignancies. J Infect Chemother 2003; 9:265–267.
207. Rowshani AT, Bemelman FJ, van Leeuwen EM, van Lier RA, ten Berge IJ. Clinical and immunologic aspects of cytomegalovirus infection in solid organ transplant recipients. Transplantation 2005;79:381–386.
208. Moss P, Rickinson A. Cellular immunotherapy for viral infection after HSC transplantation. Nat Rev Immunol 2005;5:9–20.

209. Lim JB, Kwon OH, Kim HS, et al. Adoptive immunotherapy for cytomegalovirus (CMV) disease in immunocompromised patients. Yonsei Med J 2004;45(Suppl):18–22.
210. Enright AM, Prober CG. Herpesviridae infections in newborns: varicella zoster virus, herpes simplex virus, and cytomegalovirus. Pediatr Clin North Am 2004;51:889–908, viii.
211. Bowden RA, Sayers M, Flournoy N, et al. Cytomegalovirus immune globulin and seronegative blood products to prevent primary cytomegalovirus infection after marrow transplantation. N Engl J Med 1986;314:1006–1010.
212. Stoddart CA, Cardin RD, Boname JM, Manning WC, Abenes GB, Mocarski ES. Peripheral blood mononuclear phagocytes mediate dissemination of murine cytomegalovirus. J Virol 1994;68:6243–6253.
213. Lipson SM, Shepp DH, Match ME, Axelrod FB, Whitbread JA. Cytomegalovirus infectivity in whole blood following leukocyte reduction by filtration. Am J Clin Pathol 2001;116:52–55.
214. Dumont LJ, Luka J, VandenBroeke T, Whitley P, Ambruso DR, Elfath MD. The effect of leukocyte-reduction method on the amount of human cytomegalovirus in blood products: a comparison of apheresis and filtration methods. Blood 2001;97:3640–3647.
215. Narvios AB, de Lima M, Shah H, Lichtiger B. Transfusion of leukoreduced cellular blood components from cytomegalovirus-unscreened donors in allogeneic hematopoietic transplant recipients: analysis of 72 recipients. Bone Marrow Transplant 2005;36:499–501.
216. Nichols WG, Price TH, Gooley T, Corey L, Boeckh M. Transfusion-transmitted cytomegalovirus infection after receipt of leukoreduced blood products. Blood 2003;101:4195–4200.
217. Vamvakas EC. Is White Blood Cell Reduction Equivalent to Antibody Screening in Preventing Transmission of Cytomegalovirus by Transfusion? A Review of the Literature and Meta-Analysis. Transfus Med Rev 2005;19:181–199.
218. Silliman CC, Dickey WO, Paterson AJ, et al. Analysis of the priming activity of lipids generated during routine storage of platelet concentrates. Transfusion 1996;36:133–139.
219. Heddle NM, Klama L, Singer J, et al. The role of the plasma from platelet concentrates in transfusion reactions [see comments]. N Engl J Med 1994;331:625–628.
220. Stack G, Snyder EL. Cytokine generation in stored platelet concentrates. Transfusion 1994;34:20–25.
221. Aye MT, Palmer DS, Giulivi A, Hashemi S. Effect of filtration of platelet concentrates on the accumulation of cytokines and platelet release factors during storage [see comments]. Transfusion 1995;35:117–124.
222. Claas FH, Smeenk RJ, Schmidt R, van Steenbrugge GJ, Eernisse JG. Alloimmunization against the MHC antigens after platelet transfusions is due to contaminating leukocytes in the platelet suspension. Exp Hematol 1981;9:84–89.
223. Blajchman MA, Bardossy L, Carmen RA, Goldman M, Heddle NM, Singal DP. An animal model of allogeneic donor platelet refractoriness: the effect of the time of leukodepletion. Blood 1992;79:1371–1375.
224. Moroff G, Luban NL. The irradiation of blood and blood components to prevent graft-versus-host disease: technical issues and guidelines. Transfus Med Rev 1997;11:15–26.
225. Schroeder ML. Transfusion-associated graft-versus-host disease. Br J Haematol 2002;117:275–287.
226. Anderson KC, Goodnough LT, Sayers M, et al. Variation in blood component irradiation practice: implications for prevention of transfusion-associated graft-versus-host disease. Blood 1991;77:2096–2102.
227. Guidance for Industry—Gamma irradiation of blood and blood components: a pilot program for licensing. CBER Office of Communication, Training, and Manufacturers Assistance, U.S. Department of Health and Human Services, Food and Drug Administration, Rockville, Md., 2000.
228. Moroff G, George VM, Siegl AM, Luban NL. The influence of irradiation on stored platelets. Transfusion 1986;26:453–456.
229. Button LN, DeWolf WC, Newburger PE, Jacobson MS, Kevy SV. The effects of irradiation on blood components. Transfusion 1981;21:419–426.
230. Read EJ, Kodis C, Carter CS, Leitman SF. Viability of platelets following storage in the irradiated state: a pair-controlled study. Transfusion 1988;28:446–450.
231. Rock G, Adams GA, Labow RS. The effects of irradiation on platelet function. Transfusion 1988;28:451–455.
232. Sweeney JD, Holme S, Moroff G. Storage of apheresis platelets after gamma radiation. Transfusion 1994;34:779–783.
233. Pamphilon DH. The rationale and use of platelet concentrates irradiated with ultraviolet-B light. Transfus Med Rev 1999;13:323–333.
234. Lindahl-Kiessling K, Safwenberg J. Inability of UV-irradiated lymphocytes to stimulate allogeneic cells in mixed lymphocyte culture. Int Arch Allergy Appl Immunol 1971;41:670–678.
235. Doery JC, Dickson RC, Hirsh J. Induction of aggregation of human blood platelets by ultraviolet light: action spectrum and structural changes. Blood 1973;42:551–555.
236. Kahn RA, Duffy BF, Rodey GG. Ultraviolet irradiation of platelet concentrate abrogates lymphocyte activation without affecting platelet function in vitro. Transfusion 1985;25:547–550.
237. Pamphilon DH, Corbin SA, Saunders J, Tandy NP. Applications of ultraviolet light in the preparation of platelet concentrates. Transfusion 1989;29:379–383.
238. Pamphilon DH, Potter M, Cutts M, et al. Platelet concentrates irradiated with ultraviolet light retain satisfactory in vitro storage characteristics and in vivo survival. Br J Haematol 1990;75:240–244.
239. Andreu G, Boccaccio C, Lecrubier C, et al. Ultraviolet irradiation of platelet concentrates: feasibility in transfusion practice. Transfusion 1990;30:401–406.
240. The Trial to Reduce Alloimmunization to Platelets Study Group Leukocyte reduction and ultraviolet B irradiation of platelets to prevent alloimmunization and refractoriness to platelet transfusions. [see comments]. N Engl J Med 1997;337:1861–1869.
241. Kraemer KH, Levis WR, Cason JC, Tarone RE. Inhibition of mixed leukocyte culture reaction by 8-methoxypsoralen and long-wavelength ultraviolet radiation. J Invest Dermatol 1981;77:235–239.
242. Grana NH, Kao KJ. Use of 8-methoxypsoralen and ultraviolet-A pretreated platelet concentrates to prevent alloimmunization against class I major histocompatibility antigens. Blood 1991;77:2530–2537.
243. Allain JP, Bianco C, Blajchman MA, et al. Protecting the blood supply from emerging pathogens: the role of pathogen inactivation. Transfus Med Rev 2005;19:110–126.
244. Kleinman S, Glynn SA, Busch M, et al. The 2003 West Nile virus United States epidemic: The America's Blood Centers experience. Transfusion 2005;45:469–479.
245. Macedo de Oliveira A, Beecham BD, Montgomery SP, et al. West Nile virus blood transfusion-related infection despite nucleic acid testing. Transfusion 2004;44:1695–1699.
246. Nash D, Mostashari F, Fine A, et al. The outbreak of West Nile virus infection in the New York City area in 1999. N Engl J Med 2001;344:1807–1814.
247. Klein HG. Pathogen inactivation technology: Cleansing the blood supply. J Intern Med 2005;257:224–237.
248. van Rhenen D, Gulliksson H, Cazenave JP, et al. Transfusion of pooled buffy coat platelet components prepared with photochemical pathogen inactivation treatment: the euroSPRITE trial. Blood 2003;101: 2426–2433.
249. Epstein JS, Vostal JG. FDA approach to evaluation of pathogen reduction technology. Transfusion 2003;43:1347–1350.
250. Rubinstein AI, Rubinstein DB, Coughlin J. Combined solvent-detergent and 100°C (boiling) sterilizing dry-heat treatment of factor VIII concentrates to assure sterility. Vox Sang 1991;60:60.
251. Powell JS, Bush M, Harrison J, et al. Safety and efficacy of solvent/detergent-treated antihaemophilic factor with an added 80°C terminal dry heat treatment in patients with haemophilia A. Haemophilia 2000;6:140–149.
252. Corash L. Pathogen reduction technology: methods, status of clinical trials, and future prospects. Curr Hematol Rep 2003;2:495–502.
253. Hanson CV. Photochemical inactivation of viruses with psoralens: an overview. Blood Cells 1992;18:7–25.
254. Jauvin V, Alfonso RD, Guillemain B, Dupuis K, Fleury HJ. In vitro photochemical inactivation of cell-associated human T-cell leukemia virus Type I and II in human platelet concentrates and plasma by use of amotosalen. Transfusion 2005;45:1151–1159.
255. Lin L, Hanson CV, Alter HJ, et al. Inactivation of viruses in platelet concentrates by photochemical treatment with amotosalen and long-wavelength ultraviolet light. Transfusion 2005;45:580–590.
256. Lin L, Dikeman R, Molini B, et al. Photochemical treatment of platelet concentrates with amotosalen and long-wavelength ultraviolet light inactivates a broad spectrum of pathogenic bacteria. Transfusion 2004;44:1496–1504.
257. Van Voorhis WC, Barrett LK, Eastman RT, Alfonso R, Dupuis K. *Trypanosoma cruzi* inactivation in human platelet concentrates and plasma by a psoralen (amotosalen HCl) and long-wavelength UV. Antimicrob Agents Chemother 2003;47:475–479.
258. Hossain MS, Roback JD, Lezhava L, Hillyer CD, Waller EK. Amotosalen-treated donor T cells have polyclonal antigen-specific long-term function without graft-versus-host disease after allogeneic bone marrow transplantation. Biol Blood Marrow Transplant 2005;11:169–180.
259. Lin L, Londe H, Janda JM, Hanson CV, Corash L. Photochemical inactivation of pathogenic bacteria in human platelet concentrates. Blood 1994;83:2698–2706.

260. Lin L, Cook DN, Wiesehahn GP, et al. Photochemical inactivation of viruses and bacteria in platelet concentrates by use of a novel psoralen and long-wavelength ultraviolet light. Transfusion 1997;37:423–435.
261. Corash L. Inactivation of viruses, bacteria, protozoa, and leukocytes in platelet concentrates. Vox Sang 1998;74:173–176.
262. Moroff G, Wagner S, Benade L, Dodd RY. Factors influencing virus inactivation and retention of platelet properties following treatment with aminomethyltrimethylpsoralen and ultraviolet A light. Blood Cells 1992;18:43–54; discussion 54–46.
263. Wollowitz S. Fundamentals of the psoralen-based Helinx technology for inactivation of infectious pathogens and leukocytes in platelets and plasma. Semin Hematol 2001;38:4–11.
264. Ciaravino V. Preclinical safety of a nucleic acid-targeted Helinx compound: a clinical perspective. Semin Hematol 2001;38:12–19.
265. Ciaravi V, McCullough T, Dayan AD. Pharmacokinetic and toxicology assessment of INTERCEPT (S-59 and UVA treated) platelets. Hum Exp Toxicol 2001;20:533–550.
266. van Rhenen DJ, Vermeij J, Mayaudon V, Hind C, Lin L, Corash L. Functional characteristics of S-59 photochemically treated platelet concentrates derived from buffy coats. Vox Sang 2000;79:206–214.
267. McCullough J, Vesole DH, Benjamin RJ, et al. Therapeutic efficacy and safety of platelets treated with a photochemical process for pathogen inactivation: the SPRINT Trial. Blood 2004;104:1534–1541.
268. Snyder E, Raife T, Lin L, et al. Recovery and life span of 111indium-radiolabeled platelets treated with pathogen inactivation with amotosalen HCl (S-59) and ultraviolet A light. Transfusion 2004; 44:1732–1740.
269. Grass JA, Hei DJ, Metchette K, et al. Inactivation of leukocytes in platelet concentrates by photochemical treatment with psoralen plus UVA. Blood 1998;91:2180–2188.
270. Grass JA, Wafa T, Reames A, et al. Prevention of transfusion-associated graft-versus-host disease by photochemical treatment. Blood 1999;93: 3140–3147.
271. Bhattacharyya S, Chawla A, Smith K, et al. Multilineage engraftment with minimal graft-versus-host disease following in utero transplantation of S-59 psoralen/ultraviolet a light-treated, sensitized T cells and adult T cell-depleted bone marrow in fetal mice. J Immunol 2002;169:6133–6140.
272. Kumar V, Lockerbie O, Keil SD, et al. Riboflavin and UV-light based pathogen reduction: extent and consequence of DNA damage at the molecular level. Photochem Photobiol 2004;80:15–21.
273. Dardare N, Platz MS. Binding affinities of commonly employed sensitizers of viral inactivation. Photochem Photobiol 2002;75:561–564.
274. Ruane PH, Edrich R, Gampp D, Keil SD, Leonard RL, Goodrich RP. Photochemical inactivation of selected viruses and bacteria in platelet concentrates using riboflavin and light. Transfusion 2004;44:877–885.
275. Corbin F III. Pathogen inactivation of blood components: current status and introduction of an approach using riboflavin as a photosensitizer. Int J Hematol 2002;76(Suppl 2):253–257.
276. Hardwick CC, Herivel TR, Hernandez SC, Ruane PH, Goodrich RP. Separation, identification and quantification of riboflavin and its photoproducts in blood products using high-performance liquid chromatography with fluorescence detection: a method to support pathogen reduction technology. Photochem Photobiol 2004;80:609–615.
277. Aubuchon JP, Herschel L, Roger J, et al. Efficacy of apheresis platelets treated with riboflavin and ultraviolet light for pathogen reduction. Transfusion 2005;45:1335–1341.
278. Li J, de Korte D, Woolum MD, et al. Pathogen reduction of buffy coat platelet concentrates using riboflavin and light: comparisons with pathogen-reduction technology-treated apheresis platelet products. Vox Sang 2004;87:82–90.
279. Prodouz KN, Lytle CD, Keville EA, Budacz AP, Vargo S, Fratantoni JC. Inhibition by albumin of merocyanine 540-mediated photosensitization of platelets and viruses. Transfusion 1991;31:415–422.
280. Dodd RY, Moroff G, Wagner S, et al. Inactivation of viruses in platelet suspensions that retain their in vitro characteristics: comparison of psoralen-ultraviolet A and merocyanine 540-visible light methods. Transfusion 1991;31:483–490.
281. Heddle NM. Febrile nonhemolytic transfusion reactions to platelets. Curr Opin Hematol 1995;2:478–483.
282. Lin JS, Tzeng CH, Hao TC, et al. Cytokine release in febrile nonhaemolytic red cell transfusion reactions. Vox Sang 2002;82:156–160.
283. Payne R. The association of febrile transfusion reactions with leukoagglutanins. Vox Sang 1957;2:233.
284. Conti B, Tabarean I, Andrei C, Bartfai T. Cytokines and fever. Front Biosci 2004;9:1433–1449.
285. Muylle L. The role of cytokines in blood transfusion reactions. Blood Rev 1995;9:77–83.
286. Hartwig D, Hartel C, Hennig H, Muller-Steinhardt M, Schlenke P, Kluter H. Evidence for de novo synthesis of cytokines and chemokines in platelet concentrates. Vox Sang 2002;82:182–190.
287. Edvardsen L, Taaning E, Dreier B, Christensen LD, Mynster T, Nielsen HJ. Extracellular accumulation of bioactive substances during preparation and storage of various platelet concentrates. Am J Hematol 2001;67:157–162.
288. Chambers LA, Kruskall MS, Pacini DG, Donovan LM. Febrile reactions after platelet transfusion: the effect of single versus multiple donors [see comments]. Transfusion 1990;30:219–221.
289. Sarkodee-Adoo CB, Kendall JM, Sridhara R, Lee EJ, Schiffer CA. The relationship between the duration of platelet storage and the development of transfusion reactions. Transfusion 1998;38:229–235.
290. Snyder EL. The role of cytokines and adhesive molecules in febrile nonhemolytic transfusion reactions. Immunol Invest 1995;24:333–339.
291. Ferrara JL. The febrile platelet transfusion reaction: a cytokine shower [editorial; comment]. Transfusion 1995;35:89–90.
292. Heddle NM, Klama LN, Griffith L, Roberts R, Shukla G, Kelton JG. A prospective study to identify the risk factors associated with acute reactions to platelet and red cell transfusions. Transfusion 1993;33:794–797.
293. Paglino JC, Pomper GJ, Fisch GS, Champion MH, Snyder EL. Reduction of febrile but not allergic reactions to RBCs and platelets after conversion to universal prestorage leukoreduction. Transfusion 2004;44:16–24.
294. Federowicz I, Barrett BB, Andersen JW, Urashima M, Popovsky MA, Anderson KC. Characterization of reactions after transfusion of cellular blood components that are white cell reduced before storage. Transfusion 1996;36:21–28.
295. Snyder EL, Mechanic S, Baril L, Davenport R. Removal of soluble biologic response modifiers (complement and chemokines) by a bedside white cell-reduction filter. Transfusion 1996;36:707–713.
296. Geiger TL, Perrotta PL, Davenport R, Baril L, Snyder EL. Removal of anaphylatoxins C3a and C5a and chemokines interleukin 8 and RANTES by polyester white cell-reduction and plasma filters. Transfusion 1997;37:1156–1162.
297. Oppermann M, Gotze O. Plasma clearance of the human C5a anaphylatoxin by binding to leucocyte C5a receptors. Immunology 1994;82:516–521.
298. Heddle NM, Klama L, Meyer R, et al. A randomized controlled trial comparing plasma removal with white cell reduction to prevent reactions to platelets. Transfusion 1999;39:231–238.
299. Hume HA, Popovsky MA, Benson K, et al. Hypotensive reactions: a previously uncharacterized complication of platelet transfusion? [See comments.] Transfusion 1996;36:904–909.
300. Hild M, Soderstrom T, Egberg N, Lundahl J. Kinetics of bradykinin levels during and after leucocyte filtration of platelet concentrates. Vox Sang 1998;75:18–25.
301. Perseghin P, Capra M, Baldini V, Sciorelli G. Bradykinin production during donor plasmapheresis procedures. Vox Sang 2001;81:24–28.
302. Mair B, Leparc GF. Hypotensive reactions associated with platelet transfusions and angiotensin-converting enzyme inhibitors. Vox Sang 1998;74:27–30.
303. Shiba M, Tadokoro K, Sawanobori M, Nakajima K, Suzuki K, Juji T. Activation of the contact system by filtration of platelet concentrates with a negatively charged white cell-removal filter and measurement of venous blood bradykinin level in patients who received filtered platelets [see comments]. Transfusion 1997;37:457–462.
304. Cyr M, Hume HA, Champagne M, et al. Anomaly of the des-Arg9-bradykinin metabolism associated with severe hypotensive reactions during blood transfusions: a preliminary study. Transfusion 1999;39: 1084–1088.
305. Arnold DM, Molinaro G, Warkentin TE, et al. Hypotensive transfusion reactions can occur with blood products that are leukoreduced before storage. Transfusion 2004;44:1361–1366.
306. Duke WW. The relation of blood platelets to hemorrhagic disease: description of a method for determining the bleeding time and coagulation time and report of 3 cases of hemorrhagic disease relieved by transfusion. JAMA 1910;55:1185–1192.
307. Tobin JR Jr, Friedman IA. Platelet transfusion with use of blood in plastic bags from routine storage. JAMA 1960;172:50–52.
308. Pisciotto PT, Benson K, Hume H, et al. Prophylactic versus therapeutic platelet transfusion practices in hematology and/or oncology patients. Transfusion 1995;35:498–502.
309. Hunt BJ. Indications for therapeutic platelet transfusions. Blood Rev 1998;12:227–233.
310. Stanworth SJ, Hyde C, Heddle N, Rebulla P, Brunskill S, Murphy MF. Prophylactic platelet transfusion for haemorrhage after chemotherapy and stem cell transplantation. Cochrane Database Syst Rev 2004: CD004269.

311. Ancliff PJ, Machin SJ. Trigger factors for prophylactic platelet transfusion. Blood Rev 1998;12:234–238.
312. Gaydos LA, Freireich EJ, Mantel N. The quantitative relation between platelet count and hemorrhage in patients with acute leukemia. N Engl J Med 1962;13:283–290.
313. Beutler E. Platelet transfusions: the 20,000/μL trigger. Blood 1993; 81:1411–1413.
314. Solomon J, Bofenkamp T, Fahey JL, Chillar RK, Beutel E. Platelet prophylaxis in acute non-lymphoblastic leukaemia. Lancet 1978;1:267.
315. Slichter SJ, Harker LA. Thrombocytopenia: mechanisms and management of defects in platelet production. Clin Haematol 1978;7:523–539.
316. Gmur J, Burger J, Schanz U, Fehr J, Schaffner A. Safety of stringent prophylactic platelet transfusion policy for patients with acute leukaemia. Lancet 1991;338:1223–1226.
317. Gil-Fernandez JJ, Alegre A, Fernandez-Villalta MJ, et al. Clinical results of a stringent policy on prophylactic platelet transfusion: non-randomized comparative analysis in 190 bone marrow transplant patients from a single institution. Bone Marrow Transplant 1996;18:931–935.
318. Heckman KD, Weiner GJ, Davis CS, Strauss RG, Jones MP, Burns CP. Randomized study of prophylactic platelet transfusion threshold during induction therapy for adult acute leukemia: 10,000/μL versus 20,000/μL. J Clin Oncol 1997;15:1143–1149.
319. Wandt H, Frank M, Ehninger G, et al. Safety and cost effectiveness of a 10×10^9/L trigger for prophylactic platelet transfusions compared with the traditional 20×10^9/L trigger: a prospective comparative trial in 105 patients with acute myeloid leukemia. Blood 1998;91:3601–3606.
320. Rebulla P, Finazzi G, Marangoni F, et al. The threshold for prophylactic platelet transfusions in adults with acute myeloid leukemia. Gruppo Italiano Malattie Ematologiche Maligne dell'Adulto. N Engl J Med 1997;337:1870–1875.
321. Sagmeister M, Oec L, Gmur J. A restrictive platelet transfusion policy allowing long-term support of outpatients with severe aplastic anemia. Blood 1999;93:3124–3126.
322. Diedrich B, Remberger M, Shanwell A, Svahn BM, Ringden O. A prospective randomized trial of a prophylactic platelet transfusion trigger of 10×10^9 per L versus 30×10^9 per L in allogeneic hematopoietic progenitor cell transplant recipients. Transfusion 2005;45:1064–1072.
323. Murphy MF, Murphy W, Wheatley K, Goldstone AH. Survey of the use of platelet transfusions in centres participating in MRC leukaemia trials. Br J Haematol 1998;102:875–876.
324. Ho CH. The hemostatic effect of packed red cell transfusion in patients with anemia. Transfusion 1998;38:1011–1014.
325. Murphy MF, Brozovic B, Murphy W, Ouwehand W, Waters AH. Guidelines for platelet transfusions. British Committee for Standards in Haematology, Working Party of the Blood Transfusion Task Force. Transfus Med 1992;2:311–318.
326. Vavricka SR, Walter RB, Irani S, Halter J, Schanz U. Safety of lumbar puncture for adults with acute leukemia and restrictive prophylactic platelet transfusion. Ann Hematol 2003;82:570–573.
327. Howard SC, Gajjar A, Ribeiro RC, et al. Safety of lumbar puncture for children with acute lymphoblastic leukemia and thrombocytopenia. JAMA 2000;284:2222–2224.
328. Rinder HM, Arbini AA, Snyder EL. Optimal dosing and triggers for prophylactic use of platelet transfusions. Curr Opin Hematol 1999;6:437–441.
329. Tinmouth AT, Freedman J. Prophylactic platelet transfusions: which dose is the best dose? A review of the literature. Transfus Med Rev 2003;17:181–193.
330. Schlossberg HR, Herman JH. Platelet dosing. Transfus Apheresis Sci 2003;28:221–226.
331. Hanson SR, Slichter SJ. Platelet kinetics in patients with bone marrow hypoplasia: evidence for a fixed platelet requirement. Blood 1985;66:1105–1109.
332. Klumpp TR, Herman JH, Innis S, et al. Factors associated with response to platelet transfusion following hematopoietic stem cell transplantation. Bone Marrow Transplant 1996;17:1035–1041.
333. Norol F, Bierling P, Roudot-Thoraval F, et al. Platelet transfusion: a dose-response study. Blood 1998;92:1448–1453.
334. Hersh JK, Hom EG, Brecher ME. Mathematical modeling of platelet survival with implications for optimal transfusion practice in the chronically platelet transfusion-dependent patient [see comments]. Transfusion 1998;38:637–644.
335. Ackerman SJ, Klumpp TR, Guzman GI, et al. Economic consequences of alterations in platelet transfusion dose: analysis of a prospective, randomized, double-blind trial. Transfusion 2000;40:1457–1462.
336. Kelton JG, Smith JW, Horsewood P, et al. ABH antigens on human platelets: expression on the glycosyl phosphatidylinositol-anchored protein CD109. J Lab Clin Med 1998;132:142–148.
337. Rozman P. Platelet antigens: the role of human platelet alloantigens (HPA) in blood transfusion and transplantation. Transpl Immunol 2002;10:165–181.
338. Lee EJ, Schiffer CA. ABO compatibility can influence the results of platelet transfusion: results of a randomized trial. Transfusion 1989;29:384–389.
339. McManigal S, Sims KL. Intravascular hemolysis secondary to ABO incompatible platelet products: an underrecognized transfusion reaction. Am J Clin Pathol 1999;111:202–206.
340. Larsson LG, Welsh VJ, Ladd DJ. Acute intravascular hemolysis secondary to out-of-group platelet transfusion. Transfusion 2000;40:902–906.
341. Rebulla P. In vitro and in vivo properties of various types of platelets. Vox Sang 1998;74 (Suppl 2):217–222.
342. Flegel WA, Wiesneth M, Stampe D, Koerner K. Low cytokine contamination in buffy coat-derived platelet concentrates without filtration. Transfusion 1995;35:917–920.
343. Ishida A, Handa M, Wakui M, Okamoto S, Kamakura M, Ikeda Y. Clinical factors influencing posttransfusion platelet increment in patients undergoing hematopoietic progenitor cell transplantation—a prospective analysis. Transfusion 1998;38:839–847.
344. Seftel MD, Growe GH, Petraszko T, et al. Universal prestorage leukoreduction in Canada decreases platelet alloimmunization and refractoriness. Blood 2004;103:333–339.
345. Despotis GJ, Goodnough LT, Dynis M, Baorto D, Spitznagel E. Adverse events in platelet apheresis donors: a multivariate analysis in a hospital-based program. Vox Sang 1999;77:24–32.
346. Howard JE, Perkins HA. The natural history of alloimmunization to platelets. Transfusion 1978;18:496–503.
347. Bishop JF, McGrath K, Wolf MM, et al. Clinical factors influencing the efficacy of pooled platelet transfusions. Blood 1988;71:383–387.
348. Doughty HA, Murphy MF, Metcalfe P, Rohatiner AZ, Lister TA, Waters AH. Relative importance of immune and non-immune causes of platelet refractoriness. Vox Sang 1994;66:200–205.
349. Bock M, Muggenthaler KH, Schmidt U, Heim MU. Influence of antibiotics on posttransfusion platelet increment. Transfusion 1996;36:952–954.
350. Hussein MA, Fletcher R, Long TJ, Zuccaro K, Bolwell BJ, Hoeltge A. Transfusing platelets 2 h after the completion of amphotericin-B decreases its detrimental effect on transfused platelet recovery and survival. Transfus Med 1998;8:43–47.
351. Novotny VM, van Doorn R, Witvliet MD, Claas FH, Brand A. Occurrence of allogeneic HLA and non-HLA antibodies after transfusion of prestorage filtered platelets and red blood cells: a prospective study. Blood 1995;85:1736–1741.
352. Green D, Tiro A, Basiliere J, Mittal KK. Cytotoxic antibody complicating platelet support in acute leukemia: response to chemotherapy. JAMA 1976;236:1044–1046.
353. Brandt JT, Julius CJ, Osborne JM, Anderson CL. The mechanism of platelet aggregation induced by HLA-related antibodies. Thromb Haemost 1996;76:774–779.
354. Kurz M, Greinix H, Hocker P, et al. Specificities of anti-platelet antibodies in multitransfused patients with haemato-oncological disorders. Br J Haematol 1996;95:564–569.
355. Legler TJ, Fischer I, Dittmann J, et al. Frequency and causes of refractoriness in multiply transfused patients. Ann Hematol 1997;74:185–189.
356. McFarland JG. Alloimmunization and platelet transfusion. Semin Hematol 1996;33:315–328.
357. Wood L, Jogessar V, Ward P, Jacobs P. Estimation and predictive use of the corrected count increment—a proposed clinical guideline. Transfus Apher Sci 2005;32:117–124.
358. Slichter SJ. Algorithm for managing the platelet refractory patient. J Clin Apheresis 1997;12:4–9.
359. Aster RH. Effect of anticoagulant and ABO incompatibility on recovery of transfused human platelets. Blood 1965;26:732–743.
360. Peter-Salonen K, Bucher U, Nydegger UE. Comparison of posttransfusion recoveries achieved with either fresh or stored platelet concentrates. Blut 1987;54:207–212.
361. Bolgiano DC, Larson EB, Slichter SJ. A model to determine required pool size for HLA-typed community donor apheresis programs. Transfusion 1989;29:306–310.
362. AABB Technical Manual, 14th ed. Bethesda, Md., AABB Press, 2002.
363. Mueller-Eckhardt G, Hauck M, Kayser W, Mueller-Eckhardt C. HLA-C antigens on platelets. Tissue Antigens 1980;16:91–94.
364. Messerschmidt GL, Makuch R, Appelbaum F, et al. A prospective randomized trial of HLA-matched versus mismatched single-donor platelet transfusions in cancer patients. Cancer 1988;62:795–801.
365. Schonewille H, Haak HL, van Zijl AM. Alloimmunization after blood transfusion in patients with hematologic and oncologic diseases. Transfusion 1999;39:763–771.

366. Petz LD, Garratty G, Calhoun L, et al. Selecting donors of platelets for refractory patients on the basis of HLA antibody specificity. Transfusion 2000;40:1446–1456.
367. O'Connell BA. Case report: solid-phase platelet crossmatching to support the alloimmunized patient. Immunohematology 1995;11:150–152.
368. Skogen B, Christiansen D, Husebekk A. Flow cytometric analysis in platelet crossmatching using a platelet suspension immunofluorescence test. Transfusion 1995;35:832–836.
369. Kohler M, Dittmann J, Legler TJ, et al. Flow cytometric detection of platelet-reactive antibodies and application in platelet crossmatching. Transfusion 1996;36:250–255.
370. von dem Borne AE, Ouwehand WH, Kuijpers RW. Theoretic and practical aspects of platelet crossmatching. Transfus Med Rev 1990;4: 265–278.
371. Friedberg RC, Donnelly SF, Mintz PD. Independent roles for platelet crossmatching and HLA in the selection of platelets for alloimmunized patients. Transfusion 1994;34:215–220.
372. Bertolini F, Porretti L, Corsini C, Rebulla P, Sirchia G. Platelet quality and reduction of HLA expression in acid-treated platelet concentrates. Br J Haematol 1993;83:525–527.
373. Novotny VM, Doxiadis, II, Brand A. The reduction of HLA class I expression on platelets: a potential approach in the management of HLA-alloimmunized refractory patients. Transfus Med Rev 1999;13:95–105.
374. Blajchman MA. Substitutes and alternatives to platelet transfusions in thrombocytopenic patients. J Thromb Haemost 2003;1:1637–1641.
375. Owens MR, Holme S, Cardinali S. Platelet microvesicles adhere to subendothelium and promote adhesion of platelets. Thromb Res 1992;66:247–258.
376. Hjort PF, Perman V, Cronkite EP. Fresh, disintegrated platelets in radiation thrombocytopenia: correction of prothrombin consumption without correction of bleeding. Proc Soc Exp Biol Med 1959;102:31–35.
377. Chao FC, Kim BK, Houranieh AM, et al. Infusible platelet membrane microvesicles: a potential transfusion substitute for platelets. Transfusion 1996;36:536–542.
378. Lee DH, Blajchman MA. Novel platelet products and substitutes. Transfus Med Rev 1998;12:175–187.
379. Alving BM, Reid TJ, Fratantoni JC, Finlayson JS. Frozen platelets and platelet substitutes in transfusion medicine. Transfusion 1997;37: 866–876.
380. Fliedner TM, Sorensen DK, Bond VP. Comparative effectiveness of fresh and lyophilized platelets in controlling irradiation hemorrhage in the rat. Proc Soc Exp Biol Med 1958;99:731–733.
381. Read MS, Reddick RL, Bode AP, et al. Preservation of hemostatic and structural properties of rehydrated lyophilized platelets: potential for long-term storage of dried platelets for transfusion. Proc Natl Acad Sci USA 1995;92:397–401.
382. Bode AP, Read MS, Reddick RL. Activation and adherence of lyophilized human platelets on canine vessel strips in the Baumgartner perfusion chamber. J Lab Clin Med 1999;133:200–211.
383. Valeri CR, Macgregor H, Barnard MR, Summaria L, Michelson AD, Ragno G. In vitro testing of fresh and lyophilized reconstituted human and baboon platelets. Transfusion 2004;44:1505–1512.
384. Valeri CR, Macgregor H, Giorgio A, Ragno G. Circulation and distribution of 111-In-oxine-labeled autologous baboon platelet aggregates and buffy coat. Transfus Apheresis Sci 2005;32:139–146.
385. Reid TJ, LaRussa VF, Esteban G, et al. Cooling and freezing damage platelet membrane integrity. Cryobiology 1999;38:209–224.
386. Gao DY, Neff K, Xiao HY, et al. Development of optimal techniques for cryopreservation of human platelets. I. Platelet activation during cold storage (at 22 and 8 degrees C) and cryopreservation. Cryobiology 1999;38:225–235.
387. Arnaud FG, Pegg DE. Cryopreservation of human platelets with propane-1,2-diol. Cryobiology 1990;27:130–136.
388. Dayian G, Pert JH. A simplified method for freezing human blood platelets in glycerol-glucose using a statically controlled cooling rate device. Transfusion 1979;19:255–260.
389. Kotelba-Witkowska B, Schiffer CA. Cryopreservation of platelet concentrates using glycerol-glucose. Transfusion 1982;22:121–124.
390. Redmond Jd, Bolin RB, Cheney BA. Glycerol-glucose cryopreservation of platelets: in vivo and in vitro observations. Transfusion 1983;23:213–214.
391. Dayian G, Harris HL, Vlahides GD, Pert JH. Improved procedure for platelet freezing. Vox Sang 1986;51:292–298.
392. Arnaud FG, Pegg DE. Cryopreservation of human platelets with 1.4 m glycerol at −75° C in PVC blood packs. Thromb Res 1990;57:919–924.
393. Taylor MA. Cryopreservation of platelets: an in-vitro comparison of four methods. J Clin Pathol 1981;34:71–75.
394. Daly PA, Schiffer CA, Aisner J, Wiernik PH. Successful transfusion of platelets cryopreserved for more than 3 years. Blood 1979;54:1023–1027.
395. van Prooijen HC, van Heugten JG, Mommersteeg ME, Akkerman JW. Acquired secretion defect in platelets after cryopreservation in dimethyl sulfoxide. Transfusion 1986;26:358–363.
396. van Prooijen HC, van Heugten JG, Riemens MI, Akkerman JW. Differences in the susceptibility of platelets to freezing damage in relation to size. Transfusion 1989;29:539–543.
397. Owens M, Cimino C, Donnelly J. Cryopreserved platelets have decreased adhesive capacity. Transfusion 1991;31:160–163.
398. Khuri SF, Healey N, MacGregor H, et al. Comparison of the effects of transfusions of cryopreserved and liquid-preserved platelets on hemostasis and blood loss after cardiopulmonary bypass. J Thorac Cardiovasc Surg 1999;117:172–183; discussion 183–174.
399. Valeri CR, Macgregor H, Ragno G. Correlation between in vitro aggregation and thromboxane A2 production in fresh, liquid-preserved, and cryopreserved human platelets: effect of agonists, pH, and plasma and saline resuspension. Transfusion 2005;45:596–603.
400. Currie LM, Livesey SA, Harper JR, Connor J. Cryopreservation of single-donor platelets with a reduced dimethyl sulfoxide concentration by the addition of second-messenger effectors: enhanced retention of in vitro functional activity. Transfusion 1998;38:160–167.
401. Currie LM, Lichtiger B, Livesey SA, Tansey W, Yang DJ, Connor J. Enhanced circulatory parameters of human platelets cryopreserved with second-messenger effectors: an in vivo study of 16 volunteer platelet donors. Br J Haematol 1999;105:826–831.
402. Xiao H, Harvey K, Labarrere CA, Kovacs R. Platelet cryopreservation using a combination of epinephrine and dimethyl sulfoxide as cryoprotectants. Cryobiology 2000;41:97–105.
403. Dijkstra-Tiekstra MJ, de Korte D, Pietersz RN, Reesink HW, van der Meer PF, Verhoeven AJ. Comparison of various dimethylsulphoxide-containing solutions for cryopreservation of leucoreduced platelet concentrates. Vox Sang 2003;85:276–282.
404. Nie Y, de Pablo JJ, Palecek SP. Platelet cryopreservation using a trehalose and phosphate formulation. Biotechnol Bioeng 2005;92:79–90.
405. Coller BS, Springer KT, Beer JH, et al. Thromboerythrocytes: in vitro studies of a potential autologous, semi-artificial alternative to platelet transfusions. J Clin Invest 1992;89:546–555.
406. Lee DH, Blajchman MA. Novel treatment modalities: new platelet preparations and substitutes. Br J Haematol 2001;114:496–505.
407. Davies AR, Judge HM, May JA, Glenn JR, Heptinstall S. Interactions of platelets with Synthocytes, a novel platelet substitute. Platelets 2002;13:197–205.
408. Levi M, Friederich PW, Middleton S, et al. Fibrinogen-coated albumin microcapsules reduce bleeding in severely thrombocytopenic rabbits. Nat Med 1999;5:107–111.
409. Update of Platelet Substitutes. ANH Bulletin. Sugar Land, Tex., Hematicus, 2004.
410. Kitaguchi T, Murata M, Iijima K, Kamide K, Imagawa T, Ikeda Y. Characterization of liposomes carrying von Willebrand factor-binding domain of platelet glycoprotein Ibalpha: a potential substitute for platelet transfusion. Biochem Biophys Res Commun 1999;261: 784–789.
411. Desai J, Demetri GD. Recombinant human erythropoietin in cancer-related anemia: an evidence-based review. Best Pract Res Clin Haematol 2005;18:389–406.
412. Lichtin A. The ASH/ASCO clinical guidelines on the use of erythropoietin. Best Pract Res Clin Haematol 2005;18:433–438.
413. Choukroun G, Martinez F. Benefits of erythropoietin in renal transplantation. Transplantation. 2005;79:S49–50.
414. Basu S, Dunn A, Ward A. G-CSF: function and modes of action (Review). Int J Mol Med 2002;10:3–10.
415. von Aulock S, Diterich I, Hareng L, Hartung T. G-CSF: boosting endogenous production—a new strategy? Curr Opin Investig Drugs 2004;5:1148–1152.
416. Cheng AC, Stephens DP, Currie BJ. Granulocyte-colony stimulating factor (G-CSF) as an adjunct to antibiotics in the treatment of pneumonia in adults. Cochrane Database Syst Rev 2004:CD004400.
417. Carr R, Modi N, Dore C. G-CSF and GM-CSF for treating or preventing neonatal infections. Cochrane Database Syst Rev 2003:CD003066.
418. Vichinsky E. Consensus document for transfusion-related iron overload. Semin Hematol 2001;38:2–4.
419. Webb IJ, Anderson KC. Risks, costs, and alternatives to platelet transfusions. Leuk Lymphoma 1999;34:71–84.
420. Kuter DJ. Thrombopoietins and thrombopoiesis: a clinical perspective. Vox Sang 1998;74:75–85.
421. Tepler I, Elias L, Smith JW, 2nd, et al. A randomized placebo-controlled trial of recombinant human interleukin-11 in cancer patients with severe thrombocytopenia due to chemotherapy. Blood 1996;87: 3607–3614.

422. Caen JP, Han ZC, Bellucci S, Alemany M. Regulation of megakaryocytopoiesis. Haemostasis 1999;29:27–40.
423. Avraham H, Price DJ. Regulation of megakaryocytopoiesis and platelet production by tyrosine kinases and tyrosine phosphatases. Methods 1999;17:250–264.
424. Kaushansky K, Drachman JG. The molecular and cellular biology of thrombopoietin: the primary regulator of platelet production. Oncogene 2002;21:3359–3367.
425. Kaushansky K. Thrombopoietin. N Engl J Med 1998;339:746–754.
426. Sungaran R, Markovic B, Chong BH. Localization and regulation of thrombopoietin mRNa expression in human kidney, liver, bone marrow, and spleen using in situ hybridization. Blood 1997;89:101–107.
427. Peck-Radosavljevic M, Wichlas M, Zacherl J, et al. Thrombopoietin induces rapid resolution of thrombocytopenia after orthotopic liver transplantation through increased platelet production. Blood 2000;95:795–801.
428. Folman CC, de Jong SM, de Haas M, von dem Borne AE. Analysis of the kinetics of TPO uptake during platelet transfusion. Transfusion 2001;41:517–521.
429. Vigon I, Mornon JP, Cocault L, et al. Molecular cloning and characterization of MPL, the human homolog of the v-mpl oncogene: identification of a member of the hematopoietic growth factor receptor superfamily. Proc Natl Acad Sci USA 1992;89:5640–5644.
430. Engel C, Loeffler M, Franke H, Schmitz S. Endogenous thrombopoietin serum levels during multicycle chemotherapy. Br J Haematol 1999;105:832–838.
431. Folman CC, Ooms M, Kuenen BB, et al. The role of thrombopoietin in post-operative thrombocytosis. Br J Haematol 2001;114:126–133.
432. Werynska B, Ramlau R, Podolak-Dawidziak M, et al. Serum thrombopoietin levels in patients with reactive thrombocytosis due to lung cancer and in patients with essential thrombocythemia. Neoplasma 2003;50:447–451.
433. Kaushansky K. Etiology of the myeloproliferative disorders: the role of thrombopoietin. Semin Hematol 2003;40:6–9.
434. Foster DC, Sprecher CA, Grant FJ, et al. Human thrombopoietin: gene structure, cDNA sequence, expression, and chromosomal localization. Proc Natl Acad Sci USA 1994;91:13023–13027.
435. Wendling F, Tambourin P. The oncogene V-MPL, a putative truncated cytokine receptor which immortalizes hematopoietic progenitors. Nouv Rev Fr Hematol 1991;33:145–146.
436. Bartley TD, Bogenberger J, Hunt P, et al. Identification and cloning of a megakaryocyte growth and development factor that is a ligand for the cytokine receptor Mpl. Cell 1994;77:1117–1124.
437. Lok S, Kaushansky K, Holly RD, et al. Cloning and expression of murine thrombopoietin cDNA and stimulation of platelet production in vivo. Nature 1994;369:565–568.
438. de Sauvage FJ, Hass PE, Spencer SD, et al. Stimulation of megakaryocytopoiesis and thrombopoiesis by the c-Mpl ligand. Nature 1994;369:533–538.
439. Kuter DJ, Beeler DL, Rosenberg RD. The purification of megapoietin: a physiological regulator of megakaryocyte growth and platelet production. Proc Natl Acad Sci USA 1994;91:11104–11108.
440. Fishley B, Alexander WS. Thrombopoietin signalling in physiology and disease. Growth Factors 2004;22:151–155.
441. Kaushansky K, Lok S, Holly RD, et al. Promotion of megakaryocyte progenitor expansion and differentiation by the c-Mpl ligand thrombopoietin. Nature 1994;369:568–571.
442. Choi ES, Hokom MM, Chen JL, et al. The role of megakaryocyte growth and development factor in terminal stages of thrombopoiesis. Br J Haematol 1996;95:227–233.
443. Kuter DJ, Begley CG. Recombinant human thrombopoietin: basic biology and evaluation of clinical studies. Blood 2002;100:3457–3469.
444. Harker LA, Marzec UM, Novembre F, et al. Treatment of thrombocytopenia in chimpanzees infected with human immunodeficiency virus by pegylated recombinant human megakaryocyte growth and development factor. Blood 1998;91:4427–4433.
445. Snyder E, Perrotta P, Rinder H, Baril L, Nichol J, Gilligan D. Effect of recombinant human megakaryocyte growth and development factor coupled with polyethylene glycol on the platelet storage lesion. Transfusion 1999;39:258–264.
446. Basser RL, Rasko JE, Clarke K, et al. Randomized, blinded, placebo-controlled phase I trial of pegylated recombinant human megakaryocyte growth and development factor with filgrastim after dose-intensive chemotherapy in patients with advanced cancer. Blood 1997;89:3118–3128.
447. Vadhan-Raj S, Murray LJ, Bueso-Ramos C, et al. Stimulation of megakaryocyte and platelet production by a single dose of recombinant human thrombopoietin in patients with cancer. Ann Intern Med 1997;126:673–681.
448. Vadhan-Raj S, Verschraegen CF, Bueso-Ramos C, et al. Recombinant human thrombopoietin attenuates carboplatin-induced severe thrombocytopenia and the need for platelet transfusions in patients with gynecologic cancer. Ann Intern Med 2000;132:364–368.
449. Angiolillo AL, Davenport V, Bonilla MA, et al. A phase I clinical, pharmacologic, and biologic study of thrombopoietin and granulocyte colony-stimulating factor in children receiving ifosfamide, carboplatin, and etoposide chemotherapy for recurrent or refractory solid tumors: a Children's Oncology Group experience. Clin Cancer Res 2005;11:2644–2650.
450. Archimbaud E, Ottmann OG, Yin JA, et al. A randomized, double-blind, placebo-controlled study with pegylated recombinant human megakaryocyte growth and development factor (PEG-rHuMGDF) as an adjunct to chemotherapy for adults with de novo acute myeloid leukemia. Blood 1999;94:3694–3701.
451. Schiffer CA, Miller K, Larson RA, et al. A double-blind, placebo-controlled trial of pegylated recombinant human megakaryocyte growth and development factor as an adjunct to induction and consolidation therapy for patients with acute myeloid leukemia. Blood 2000;95:2530–2535.
452. Nash RA, Kurzrock R, DiPersio J, et al. A phase I trial of recombinant human thrombopoietin in patients with delayed platelet recovery after hematopoietic stem cell transplantation. Biol Blood Marrow Transplant 2000;6:25–34.
453. Kuter DJ. Future directions with platelet growth factors. Semin Hematol 2000;37:41–49.
454. O'Malley CJ, Rasko JE, Basser RL, et al. Administration of pegylated recombinant human megakaryocyte growth and development factor to humans stimulates the production of functional platelets that show no evidence of in vivo activation. Blood 1996;88:3288–3298.
455. Kuter DJ, Goodnough LT, Romo J, et al. Thrombopoietin therapy increases platelet yields in healthy platelet donors. Blood 2001;98: 1339–1345.
456. Bertolini F, Battaglia M, Pedrazzoli P, et al. Megakaryocytic progenitors can be generated ex vivo and safely administered to autologous peripheral blood progenitor cell transplant recipients. Blood 1997;89: 2679–2688.
457. Yagi M, Ritchie KA, Sitnicka E, Storey C, Roth GJ, Bartelmez S. Sustained ex vivo expansion of hematopoietic stem cells mediated by thrombopoietin. Proc Natl Acad Sci USA 1999;96:8126–8131.
458. Piacibello W, Sanavio F, Garetto L, et al. Extensive amplification and self-renewal of human primitive hematopoietic stem cells from cord blood. Blood 1997;89:2644–2653.
459. Cwirla SE, Balasubramanian P, Duffin DJ, et al. Peptide agonist of the thrombopoietin receptor as potent as the natural cytokine. Science 1997;276:1696–1699.
460. Li C, Cheng DS, Zhou YR, Chen TM, Huang PT. [Synthesis and function analysis of a new thrombopoietin (TPO) mimic peptide]. Zhongguo Shi Yan Xue Ye Xue Za Zhi 2003;11:128–131.

Chapter 24
Granulocytes

Thomas H. Price

INTRODUCTION

Infection associated with severe neutropenia continues to be a major limiting factor in the application of aggressive chemotherapeutic regimens and hematopoietic stem cell transplantation.[1–3] In the Trial to Reduce Alloimmunization to Platelets, 7% of patients undergoing induction therapy for acute myelocytic leukemia died of infection.[4] The spectrum of these therapy-related infections has shifted since the 1980s. Improved antibiotic regimens have reduced the incidence of refractory bacterial infection, and fungal infections have emerged as the principal infectious cause of mortality and morbidity.[5–7] Prophylactic use of fluconazole has reduced the incidence of disseminated *Candida* infection, and the leading cause of mortality has become infection with invasive molds such as *Aspergillus, Fusarium,* and *Zygomyces.*[5,8–10] The incidence of invasive *Aspergillus* infection in patients undergoing allogeneic bone marrow transplantation is approximately 15%, with a mortality rate of 30% to 80%.[5,7,11] *Fusarium* infection in these patients is associated with a 70% mortality rate.[9]

If these infections occur during periods of neutropenia, the provision of normally functioning neutrophils is a logical approach to the problem. The first reports of modern neutrophil transfusion therapy occurred in the mid-1960s, with large numbers of neutrophils obtained from donors with chronic myelocytic leukemia. The development of apheresis equipment shortly thereafter allowed the collection of transfusion doses of neutrophils from hematologically normal donors, and favorable clinical reports ushered in an era of enthusiasm for this therapeutic approach. A series of controlled trials followed that, on aggregate, indicated efficacy in terms of a survival advantage for patients given transfusions.

In spite of these results, granulocyte transfusion therapy all but disappeared from clinical use from about 1985 to 1995. This change in attitude occurred for several reasons. Improvement in antibiotic and general supportive care rendered refractory bacterial infection a less common clinical problem. Reports also surfaced of adverse effects of granulocyte transfusion, particularly adverse pulmonary reactions. Finally, and probably most important, the clinical results in most patients were, at best, marginal.

This unimpressive clinical efficacy had two probable causes. First, the dose of neutrophils supplied to patients with the best standard collection techniques, even in the mid-1990s ($20–30 \times 10^9$), was probably inadequate. Normal neutrophil production in an average-sized adult is approximately 60×10^9 cells per day in the uninfected state.[12] Although reliable quantitative information is lacking, the normal bone marrow is probably capable of increasing production severalfold in the presence of severe infection. Thus, the number of neutrophils routinely provided to patients undergoing neutrophil transfusion therapy was likely only about one tenth of the normal need. The second problem is that neutrophils rapidly undergo apoptosis after collection, a phenomenon that may be responsible for both the failure of the transfused cells to circulate and the short shelf life of these components.

Since the mid-1990s interest in granulocyte support therapy has been rekindled with the availability of granulocyte colony-stimulating factor (G-CSF), a cytokine that may be administered to granulocyte donors to increase the number of cells that can be collected.[3,13] G-CSF also inhibits neutrophil apoptosis, and this feature raises the possibility that in vitro and in vivo survival of these cells may be enhanced.

In this chapter, the features of traditional granulocyte transfusion are discussed first, including issues such as collection, storage, indications, evidence of efficacy, and adverse effects. This is followed by a discussion of the more recent experience using G-CSF to stimulate donors to obtain greatly increased numbers of cells for transfusion.

TRADITIONAL GRANULOCYTE TRANSFUSION THERAPY

Procurement of Granulocytes

Donor Selection

Granulocyte donors are selected from pools of community apheresis donors, or, perhaps more commonly, they are family members or friends of the patient. The ABO blood group is not important for granulocyte compatibility,[14] but donors should be ABO compatible with the patient because of the relatively large number of red blood cells contained in a typical granulocyte concentrate. Donors should be generally healthy and must meet the AABB and the United States Food and Drug Administration (FDA) standards for blood donation. There should be no contraindication to their receiving the institution's stimulation regimen (e.g., corticosteroids) for increasing the donor's blood neutrophil count. Infectious disease screening and testing must be the same as for any blood product, but modifications are often made in the timing of this testing to accommodate the need to transfuse the granulocytes as soon as possible after collection. In some centers, blood for infectious disease testing is drawn up to 24 hours before leukapheresis so that release of the cells will not be delayed.

CYTOMEGALOVIRUS (CMV) STATUS

If the patient is CMV seronegative, the donor should also be CMV seronegative, since most granulocyte recipients are in a patient population that requires CMV-safe components. The incidence of CMV transmission appears to be higher with granulocyte concentrates than with other cellular blood products because the latent virus resides in the leukocytes,[15,16] and the risk of transmission can be nearly eliminated by selecting seronegative donors. Needless to say, leukocyte reduction (leukoreduction), a technique available to render other blood components relatively CMV-safe, is not appropriate for granulocyte concentrates.

LEUKOCYTE COMPATIBILITY

If the patient is not alloimmunized, it is probably not necessary to select granulocyte donors on the basis of HLA or granulocyte typing or to perform leukocyte compatibility testing.[17] However, convincing evidence indicates that alloimmunized recipients who are transfused with incompatible leukocytes are more likely to experience adverse pulmonary reactions or febrile transfusion reactions.[18–22] In addition, the infused granulocytes will be rapidly cleared from the circulation and will be ineffective.[17,18,21,22–26] The difficulty is in knowing which patients are alloimmunized. Leukocyte antibodies detected in the laboratory do not necessarily correlate well with clinical evidence of alloimmunization, such as the ability of the transfused cells to circulate or to accumulate at sites of inflammation. In addition, reliable detection of clinically significant antibodies requires that a panel of sophisticated tests be performed,[19,24] tests that are not available in most institutions. In the absence of such results, a common approach is to attempt to gauge the likelihood of alloimmunization on the basis of information such as the patient's history of febrile transfusion reactions, response to random donor platelet transfusions, and results of a lymphocytotoxic antibody screen. If these results are normal, it is not likely that the patient is alloimmunized. Significant abnormalities in these parameters do not necessarily mean that the patient will have difficulty with granulocyte transfusions, but they do suggest that the physician proceed gingerly and also consider further clinical or laboratory evaluation.

Collection Procedure

Granulocytes are collected from donors by a leukapheresis procedure. Historically, two methods have been used: filtration and centrifugation. In the former, the donor's blood was passed over nylon wool filters to which the neutrophils adhered; the cells were subsequently eluted from the columns. Although large numbers of granulocytes could be collected by this technique, subsequent studies showed that the cells were functionally impaired.[27–29] In addition, the process itself activated complement and was associated with transfusion reactions in recipients and with occasional and sometimes serious adverse effects in donors.[30,31] This technique is no longer in use. For centrifugal leukapheresis, the cells are separated from other components by centrifugation. Numerous acceptable cell separators are on the market for this purpose. Usually, 7 to 10 L of the donor's blood are processed in a procedure that takes approximately 3 hours.

RED CELL SEDIMENTATION

It is necessary to add a red blood cell (RBC) sedimenting agent to the donor's blood to effect adequate separation of the granulocytes from the RBCs. Hydroxyethyl starch has traditionally been used for this purpose, and in modern cell separating machines this allows for 30% to 50% efficiency in granulocyte collection. Two preparations of hydroxyethyl starch are available for this purpose. Hetastarch, a high-molecular-weight compound, was the substance used originally, but it was shown to persist in the circulation for months. This persistence led to a concern for its safety, although long-term effects were not actually observed. The lower molecular weight version, pentastarch, was shown to have a much more rapid elimination time and appeared to function equivalently for the purposes of granulocyte collection.[32] Many collection centers switched to pentastarch as a result of these findings. More recent controlled studies showed, however, that collection efficiency is much greater when the high-molecular-weight preparation of hydroxyethyl starch is used.[33] Whichever agent is used, it must be infused continuously for as long as the collection proceeds in order to maintain the effect.

DONOR STIMULATION

In an effort to increase the number of granulocytes collected, donors are routinely stimulated with corticosteroids to mobilize cells from the marrow storage pool and to increase the circulating granulocyte count, thereby increasing the number of granulocytes that can be collected. Numerous stimulation regimens have been proposed, the most successful using up to 60 mg prednisone or 8 mg dexamethasone, which raises the donor's neutrophil count two- to threefold from baseline values.[34,35] Short-term administration of such doses of corticosteroids are well tolerated by most donors; persons with medical contraindications to such medications, such as active peptic ulcer disease or diabetes, should not be donors. Even higher donor granulocyte counts can be obtained by stimulation with G-CSF, a strategy discussed later in this chapter.

Cell Concentrate

Granulocyte concentrates are not licensed by the FDA and therefore have no defined regulatory specifications. AABB standards require that at least 75% of concentrates contain at least 10×10^9 granulocytes,[36] a value intended to serve as a benchmark for adequate collection technique but not to imply that 10×10^9 granulocytes is an adequate clinical dose. With the techniques discussed earlier, including adequate corticosteroid stimulation of the donor, mean yields of 20–30×10^9 granulocytes are typically achieved. Depending on the particular cell separator used, the granulocytes are suspended in 200 to 400 mL plasma and contain 10 to 30 mL red blood cells and 1–6×10^{11} platelets.

The functional capabilities of granulocytes obtained by these techniques have been the subject of many reports. In vitro and in vivo studies have shown repeatedly that cells collected by centrifugal apheresis are normal or nearly normal functionally, and the characteristics are not compromised by the use of hydroxyethyl starch or by stimulation of normal donors with corticosteroids.[27,37,38]

Storage of Neutrophils

After collection, granulocytes rapidly undergo apoptosis,[3,39,40] and this process greatly limits the ability to store the cells before transfusion. Although the hardier cell functions persist after a few days of liquid storage, the more sensitive ones, such as the ability to migrate, deteriorate more quickly.[41,42] In vivo studies have shown that blood recovery and survival are adversely affected by as little as 24 hours of storage, and the ability of the transfused cells to localize to areas of inflammation is decreased as much as 75% after 8 to 24 hours of storage.[27,43] As a result of these observations, granulocytes should be administered as soon as possible after collection. In the event that this is not possible, the cells should be stored without agitation for no more than 24 hours.[36,44] The preponderance of evidence to date indicates that the cells should be maintained at room temperature for any period of storage.[41,45]

Transfusion of Granulocytes

Once the decision is made to initiate granulocyte support, the physician should strive to provide daily granulocyte transfusions until the patient's infection clears or until the patient's neutrophil count has returned to at least 500/μL. Data are insufficient to determine whether higher neutrophil counts would be more appropriate as stopping points for certain clinical conditions. Outside these parameters, it is generally not appropriate to stop and start transfusion support on the basis of the patient's daily clinical status.

Granulocyte concentrates usually contain 10 to 30 mL red blood cells, enough to cause a hemolytic transfusion reaction if the donor and patient are incompatible. Therefore, AABB standards require that an RBC crossmatch be performed before transfusion.[36]

Granulocyte preparations contain viable lymphocytes, and graft-versus-host disease has been reported after granulocyte transfusion.[46] Although this complication can easily be prevented by gamma-irradiation of the component, the decision to irradiate granulocyte concentrates routinely has been debated in the past. Those who opposed routine irradiation noted that graft-versus-host disease is an extremely rare complication, expressed concern that irradiation may compromise the integrity of the cells, and argued that, as with any other blood product, the decision to irradiate the cells should be based on clinical evaluation of the patient.[47] However, in regard to the last concern, most studies suggest that standard irradiation does not impair neutrophil function.[48–51] Since most patients receiving granulocyte transfusions are to some degree immunosuppressed and since transfusion-related graft-versus-host disease is almost uniformly fatal, it is recommended that granulocyte concentrates always be irradiated before transfusion.

Granulocytes should be administered through a standard blood administration set filter (170 μm) and infused over 1 to 2 hours. As mentioned above, the use of a leukoreduction filter is contraindicated. Administration of antipyretics or corticocosteroids is appropriate for patients who experience symptoms such as chills and fever; routine prophylaxis with these agents is not recommended except for patients who have previously experienced such symptoms.

CLINICAL EFFICACY OF NEUTROPHIL TRANSFUSION THERAPY

Neutropenia

Early Studies

The first reports of treating infected neutropenic patients with granulocyte transfusions occurred in the 1960s. In these studies, granulocytes were harvested from donors with chronic myelocytic leukemia by a manual leukapheresis technique whereby leukocyte-rich plasma was prepared from individual units of donor blood by sedimenting the red blood cells. Schwarzenberg and associates[52] treated 33 patients with various malignant diseases and reported that approximately half showed a favorable response. In several of the patients, the postinfusion rise in the patient's neutrophil count persisted, and the Philadelphia chromosome could be demonstrated in the patient's marrow cells, findings suggesting that a temporary graft had occurred. Morse and associates[53] used a similar technique and transfused 40 patients with leukopenia, most of whom had acute leukemia. Following 81 transfusions given to patients who were febrile before the transfusion, more than half of the patients were afebrile by 36 hours after the transfusion. Lowenthal and colleagues[54] collected granulocytes from normal donors and those with chronic myelocytic leukemia by continuous-flow centrifugation and treated 41 febrile patients with acute leukemia or aplastic anemia. Two thirds of the patients responded by defervescence. Response was more likely in those patients with proven or probable bacterial or fungal infection than in those with fever of unknown origin.

With the development of the automated cell separator, it became possible to collect large numbers of granulocytes from normal donors, and the use of donors with chronic myelocytic leukemia fell into disuse. A flurry of reports of granulocyte transfusion therapy in patients with neutropenia then followed. The aggregate experience was reviewed by Strauss[55] and is summarized in Table 24–1. In this review, patients were categorized by the infection for which the transfusions were begun and were counted only once. All patients with documented fungal infection were categorized as such, whether or not they fit into other categories. After these patients were excluded, all patients with sepsis were listed only in the sepsis section. The number of patients indicated in Table 24–1 represents the number of patients who could actually be evaluated for treatment efficacy, sometimes a much smaller number than actually treated. Therapy was considered successful if so indicated by the authors of the study. Although these results indicate the general experience with granulocyte transfusion therapy, care must be taken to not overinterpret the data. The number of patients often was small, and the studies represented were heterogeneous, with different inclusion criteria, granulocyte preparations, and criteria for success.

Controlled Trials

Included in the foregoing aggregate experience were seven controlled trials, reported between 1972 and 1982, designed

Table 24–1 Treatment of Neutropenic Patients with Granulocyte Transfusions

Infection	*N*	Success (%)
Bacterial sepsis	206	62
Sepsis, organism unspecified	39	46
Pneumonia, organism unspecified	11	64
Invasive fungal infection	77	36
Localized infection	47	83
Nonspecific fever	85	75

Adapted from Strauss RG. Granulocyte (neutrophil) transfusion. In McLeod BC, Price TH, Weinstein R (eds). Apheresis: Principles & Practice, 2nd ed. Bethesda, Md., AABB Press, 2003, pp 237–252.

to assess the efficacy of therapeutic granulocyte transfusion in adults.[56–62] In each of these studies, neutropenic patients with clinical evidence of infection who were treated with granulocyte transfusions were compared with a group of similar patients who received only conventional antibiotic therapy. All but two of the studies were randomized trials; in those that were not,[56,58] patients were assigned to the control group if no suitable granulocyte donor could be identified. When patient survival was compared, three of the studies showed a clear beneficial effect of transfusion. Higby and associates[57] treated patients with clinically evident infection with four daily transfusions and found that 15 of 17 treated patients and 5 of 19 control patients survived until day 20. Vogler and Winton[59] studied 30 patients with documented infection who had failed to respond to at least 72 hours of appropriate antibiotic therapy; survival to 22 days was 59% in the transfused group and 31% in the control group. Herzig and associates[61] treated 27 patients with documented gram-negative septicemia; 75% (12 of 16) of the treated group survived compared with 36% (5 of 14) of the control group. When these results were further analyzed, the survival advantage was entirely in the subset of patients who did not recover bone marrow function.

Two of the controlled trials showed no statistically significant overall beneficial effect of transfusion, but subset analysis suggested efficacy in certain groups. In the study of Graw and colleagues[56] of patients with documented gram-negative septicemia, overall survival was not improved in the treatment group, but survival was improved for those who received at least four transfusions. In the other study with partial benefit, that of Alavi and colleagues,[60] no advantage of granulocyte transfusion was apparent for the overall patient population; however, in the subgroup with persistent bone marrow failure, 75% of the transfused patients survived compared with 20% of the controls.

In two of the controlled studies, no benefit to transfusion was identified. Fortuny and associates[58] treated 58 febrile episodes in 39 patients with acute nonlymphocytic leukemia. Survival of the episode was 78% in the transfused group versus 80% in the control group. Winston and colleagues[62] studied 95 neutropenic patients with documented infections; 63% (30 of 48) of the transfused patients and 72% (34 of 47) of the controls survived the infection.

In trying to understand the somewhat disparate results of these controlled trials, it is useful to keep in mind that the number of patients involved in many of the studies was relatively small, and the study designs and evaluation parameters were different. Whether efficacy was demonstrated may have been primarily influenced by the survival of the control group. In those trials in which the control group did well, it would be difficult to demonstrate that additional benefit was provided by transfusion therapy, even if the therapy itself was generally useful. As discussed later, subsequent analysis of these studies also suggested that the positive studies generally were those in which larger numbers of functional neutrophils were provided, as well as those in which some attempt was made to take leukocyte compatibility into account.[63,64] Moreover, by modern standards, only one of the controlled studies[59] provided adequate numbers of functional neutrophils as a transfusion dose. In four of the studies, cells were collected by filtration leukapheresis, a technique now known to produce damaged cells.

Despite the foregoing caveats, the aggregate message from the controlled therapeutic trials is that, in the proper clinical circumstances, granulocyte transfusion therapy is likely beneficial, a conclusion that is bolstered by meta-analysis.[64] The current standard indications for granulocyte transfusion therapy were derived from these controlled trials—namely, that patients are severely neutropenic, that they have a documented infection, and that the infection has not responded to appropriate antimicrobial therapy. These clinical criteria, although developed over 20 years ago, still seem eminently reasonable.

Fungal Infection

No systematic studies have been conducted to evaluate the role of granulocyte transfusion therapy in the treatment of documented fungal infection. Experimental studies in dogs suggested that transfused neutrophils may be effective. Ruthe and associates[65] used a dog *Candida* sepsis model to show that the extent of infection could be reduced by granulocyte transfusions. Chow and coworkers[66] developed a *Candida* meningitis model in dogs and showed that transfused neutrophils were capable of migrating into the cerebrospinal space and increasing survival.

Reports of granulocyte transfusions in patients with fungal infection have mostly consisted of case reports.[67,68] Bhatia and associates[69] conducted a retrospective study of granulocyte transfusion therapy in 87 patients who were undergoing bone marrow transplantation and who had various systemic fungal infections. No beneficial effect of transfusion was seen. It is difficult to draw conclusive answers from this study for several reasons: it was a retrospective study in which patient entry was controlled only by the patient's physician; the control group and the treatment group were not comparable; the dose of granulocytes delivered was largely unknown and was probably inadequate because the granulocyte donors were not stimulated with corticosteroids; and the collection parameters were not optimal. Clinical trials are obviously needed to address the issue of efficacy in fungal infection. In the meantime, it is probably reasonable to provide granulocytes to patients with a serious systemic fungal infection that is refractory to conventional therapy.

Prophylactic Transfusion

If granulocytes are effective in treating an established infection, it would seem logical that they could even be more effective in preventing infection in neutropenic patients. Numerous controlled trials of prophylactic granulocyte support were reported from 1977 to 1984 and were summarized by Strauss.[70] As with the trials of therapeutic transfusion, positive effects were limited to those in which larger doses of granulocytes were provided. The effects were modest, however, and some studies reported a high rate of adverse effects.[20,71] Cost-effectiveness analysis contemporary to these studies showed that provision of prophylactic support was also very expensive.[72]

Neonatal Sepsis

Bacterial sepsis occurs in 1 to 10 per 1000 neonates and is associated with an average mortality of approximately 20%.[70] A contributing factor to this high mortality is relative dysfunction of neonatal neutrophils, cells that have been shown to exhibit quantitative abnormalities in chemotaxis, adhesion, and oxidative metabolism.[70] As a result, neonates with sepsis whose blood neutrophil counts are less than 3000/μL and who have diminished marrow neutrophil stores have a high mortality in spite of antibiotic treatment.[73] The efficacy of granulocyte transfusion therapy in the setting of neonatal sepsis was evaluated in six controlled trials[74–79] and reviewed by Strauss.[70] In four of the six studies, a survival benefit was identified in patients who received granulocyte transfusions, although subsequent meta-analysis concluded that the studies were so heterogeneous that no definite conclusion could be reached about efficacy.[64]

In the study of Laurenti and associates,[74] which was controlled but not randomized, 20 neonates with sepsis received 2 to 15 granulocyte transfusions, and these patients were compared with 18 similar patients who did not receive transfusions. Survival was 90% in the transfused group and 28% in the control group. The granulocytes were collected by filtration leukapheresis and, for half of the transfused patients, were stored for up to 2 days before transfusion; these features would suggest that the cells were probably nonfunctional. Christensen and colleagues[75] randomized 16 neonates with bacterial infection and depleted marrow neutrophil storage pools. All the transfused patients (7 of 7) and 11% (1 of 9) of the controls survived. Cairo and associates[76] randomized 23 newborns with clinical sepsis; those who received transfusions were transfused every 12 hours for a total of 5 transfusions. Survival of the transfused group (13 of 13) was significantly higher than that of the control group (6 of 10). When analysis was limited to those patients with positive blood cultures, there was still a survival advantage to those who received transfusions (100% vs 57%), but the difference was no longer statistically significant.

In a subsequent randomized study, Cairo and associates compared granulocyte transfusion therapy with intravenous immune globulin treatment in the same clinical population.[77] Again, all the neonates who received transfusions (21 of 21) survived, whereas only 64% (9 of 14) of those treated with immune globulin survived. In the remaining two studies,[78,79] no survival advantage was seen with transfusion, but in both studies the granulocytes were prepared from units of whole blood, rather than by leukapheresis, and this makes the viability of the cells suspect.

In summary, the role of granulocyte transfusion therapy in neonatal sepsis is not clear. As a practical approach, it is probably reasonable to recommend that in institutions experiencing high mortality in this clinical situation, granulocyte support be considered in neonates with sepsis who have blood neutrophil counts less than 3000/μL with evidence that the marrow storage pool is depleted.

Granulocyte Function Disorders

Patients with severe neutrophil dysfunction, who may have normal or even elevated blood neutrophil counts, may also benefit from granulocyte transfusion therapy. Some investigators have reported, usually as single case studies, apparent clinical success in treatment of antibiotic-resistant bacterial or fungal infection in patients with disorders such as chronic granulomatous disease and leukocyte adhesion deficiency.[80–84] Although few patients have these disorders and controlled trials have not been performed, efficacy of such therapy can be very convincing with an individual patient who has recurring infections. At the Puget Sound Blood Center in Seattle, the author treated a patient with leukocyte adhesion deficiency (originally described by Bowen and associates[84]) over the course of 15 to 20 years. He was repeatedly unable to clear bacterial infections until he received a course of granulocyte transfusion therapy. The indications for transfusion in patients with neutrophil function disorders are not firmly established. The physician should probably be conservative, however, because these patients ordinarily have immune systems that are otherwise functional, and alloimmunization can be a significant problem.[19]

Adverse Effects

Fever and chills are fairly commonly seen after the administration of granulocytes. Precise figures are not available, but the incidence depends on the likelihood of alloimmunization.[19] As an approximation, nonimmunized patients can expect to experience mild to moderate fever or chills with about 10% of transfusions. Routine premedication is not necessary, but for those patients experiencing reactions, premedication with acetaminophen or corticosteroids often prevents recurrences. Moderate to severe pulmonary reactions can occur in these patients, but true transfusion reactions are often difficult to distinguish from other conditions such as fluid overload or underlying pulmonary disease.[85] Wright and associates[86] reported a high incidence of severe pulmonary reactions in patients receiving both granulocyte transfusions and amphotericin B, a finding that several investigators have failed to confirm.[22,85,87,88] Nevertheless, it remains common practice to space the administration of amphotericin from that of granulocytes by several hours.

In addition to affecting the ability to provide effective granulocyte support, alloimmunization may be a complication of such support. The incidence likely depends on the integrity of the patient's immune system as well as the tests used to detect antibody. Stroncek and colleagues[19] reported that approximately 75% of patients with chronic granulomatous disease who receive repeated courses of granulocyte support will develop clinically significant antibodies. Other studies have detected leukocyte antibodies after granulocyte transfusion in 40% to 80% of patients with acute leukemia or various marrow failure states.[89,90] In the study of Price and colleagues[91] baseline incidence of alloimmunization, as measured by the presence of HLA antibodies, was approximately 10% in patients undergoing hematopoietic stem cell transplantation. After a course of granulocyte transfusions, another 25% developed HLA antibodies, but the presence of these antibodies appeared to have no effect on the posttransfusion neutrophil increments observed or on the incidence of transfusion reactions. Adkins and associates, on the other hand, reported that patients with preexisting lymphocytotoxic antibodies eventually experienced reduced neutrophil increments after a series of prophylactic neutrophil transfusions.[92]

As previously discussed, graft-versus-host disease, a highly fatal but unusual complication of granulocyte transfusion therapy, can be prevented by gamma-irradiation (2500 cGy) of the concentrate.

GRANULOCYTE TRANSFUSION THERAPY USING DONORS STIMULATED WITH G-CSF

Granulocyte Dose

An important reason for the unimpressive efficacy of traditional granulocyte transfusion therapy is the inadequacy of the cell dose usually provided. Evidence of the importance of dose comes from several quarters. First, in the early, uncontrolled trials of granulocyte transfusion therapy, in which large doses of cells could be obtained from donors with marked leukocytosis, clinical responses were reported to be associated with the dose delivered. Morse and associates[53] observed that the increase in the patient's neutrophil count was directly related to the dose of cells provided and was detectable only if the dose exceeded $10^{10}/m^2$. The clinical response, as defined by defervescence, was also proportional to the dose, the fraction of patients responding ranging from 30% to 100% with mean doses of $2.6 \times 10^{10}/m^2$ and $15.6 \times 10^{10}/m^2$, respectively. Lowenthal and colleagues[54] reported that patients with clinical responses received, on average, four times as many cells as patients without responses. Second, retrospective analysis of the controlled trials of therapeutic granulocyte transfusion therapy suggested that higher doses of cells were provided in the studies that showed efficacy.[63,64] Third, the experience with the provision of granulocytes to neonates, in whom the relative dose is much higher because of the size of these patients, suggests that efficacy is determined by dose. Finally, studies in animals indicated the importance of dose. Appelbaum and associates[93] examined the clinical effect of granulocyte support in dogs with *Pseudomonas* sepsis and showed that dogs receiving 10^8 cells/kg did not survive the infection, whereas 100% (5 of 5) survived when they were given 2×10^8 cells/kg. Epstein and Chow[94] provided granulocytes to dogs with *Candida albicans* meningitis and showed a direct relationship between the dose of cells administered, the blood granulocyte increments, and the number of granulocytes migrating to the cerebrospinal fluid.

Actions of G-CSF

With the availability of recombinant G-CSF, the possibility of greatly increasing the number of granulocytes for collection and thus for transfusion raised the hope that the efficacy of granulocyte transfusion therapy could be improved.[3,13] When administered to normal subjects, G-CSF causes a rapid dose-dependent increase in the neutrophil count, beginning within 2 hours and peaking at approximately 12 hours.[95] This phenomenon is the result of the rapid release of neutrophils from the marrow storage pool into the blood. When given daily, G-CSF also stimulates the proliferation of granulocyte precursors and accelerates the transit time of the developing cells through the maturation pool into the blood.[96] G-CSF also affects neutrophil function. It increases phagocytosis as well as bactericidal and fungicidal activity.[39,97,98] It primes neutrophils and enhances their metabolic responses to second agonists.[39] It affects the expression of cell surface proteins such as CD64, CD35, CD14, and CD11/18,[38,98,99] proteins that are important in cell adhesion processes. G-CSF also inhibits neutrophil apoptosis,[39,101] a finding that may explain, in part, the prolonged blood survival of neutrophils from subjects given the drug.[96]

Stimulation of Donors with G-CSF

The use of G-CSF to stimulate normal granulocyte donors has been reported by numerous investigators (Table 24–2). In most of these studies, G-CSF was administered repeatedly to donors who were family members or friends of the patient who received the transfusions, although in the study of Price and associates,[91] the donors were community apheresis donors who were recruited to donate for patients whom they did not know. The dose of G-CSF in these studies ranged from 5 to 10 μg/kg, and it resulted in granulocyte concentrates containing an average of 40 to 60×10^9 cells. Leitman and associates[102] and Price and colleagues[91] achieved substantially higher average yields (80×10^9 cells) by administering both G-CSF and dexamethasone (8 mg) to normal subjects. Liles and coworkers[103] determined that the addition of corticosteroids resulted in higher donor blood neutrophil counts, irrespective of the dose of G-CSF, and the maximum neutrophil counts occurred approximately 12 hours after stimulation. Administration of G-CSF, with or without corticosteroids, is well tolerated by donors.[104,105] Most donors experience mild to moderate bone aching, headache, or insomnia. In one study, 98% of donors were willing to undergo future G-CSF stimulation.[91]

Because G-CSF has been shown to inhibit neutrophil apoptosis,[39,101] this cytokine may be useful in lengthening the acceptable storage time for neutrophils and thereby improving the logistics of granulocyte therapy programs. Whether this will turn out to be true awaits further studies.

Hematologic Effect in Recipients

In marked contrast to the situation in traditional granulocyte transfusion therapy, the postinfusion neutrophil increments seen in patients receiving these large doses of cells are quite substantial. Hester and associates[106] reported a mean post-transfusion neutrophil increment of $0.6 \times 10^3/\mu L$ after infusion of 40×10^9 granulocytes, and the value remained higher than the baseline value for 24 hours. In the study of Adkins and colleagues,[107] patients received a mean granulocyte dose

Table 24–2 Granulocyte Colony-Stimulating Factor (G-CSF)–Stimulated Granulocyte Collections

	N	G-CSF	Donor PMN ($10^3/\mu L$)	PMN Yield (10^9)
Caspar et al[124]	22	300 μg	20	44
Hester et al[106]	124	5 μg/kg/day	24–36	41
Bensinger et al[125]	58	5 μg/kg/day	15–40	42
Jendiroba et al[126]	221	5 μg/kg/day	—	42
	179	5 μg/kg/day or every other day	—	46
Adkins et al[107]	29	5 μg/kg/day	20–30	51
Grigg et al[116]	55	10 μg/kg/day	—	59
Leitman et al[102]	7	5 μg/kg Dexa 8 mg	28	78
Price et al[91]	175	600 μg Dexa 8 mg	31	82

Dexa, dexamethasone; PMN, polymorphonuclear leukocytes.

of 51 × 10^9 and exhibited a mean post-transfusion neutrophil increment of 1 × 10^3/μL, a value that was maintained for 1 to 1.5 days. With even higher cell doses (mean 82 × 10^9), as reported Price and coworkers,[91] post-transfusion neutrophil increments were 2.6 × 10^3/μL, with an average next morning count of 2.6 × 10^3/μL. It thus appears that donors stimulated with G-CSF and corticosteroids are able to provide enough granulocytes to sustain a normal or near-normal blood neutrophil count in the most severely neutropenic patients. Strong evidence indicates that these granulocytes are also capable of migrating to extravascular sites. Dale and associates[108] showed that neutrophils collected from G-CSF–stimulated normal donors were able to accumulate in skin chambers. Adkins and colleagues[109] reported that ^{111}In-labeled granulocytes obtained from G-CSF–stimulated donors were able to localize to areas of infection in neutropenic recipients. Price and coworkers[91] measured buccal neutrophil accumulation in neutropenic granulocyte recipients and demonstrated the ability of the transfused cells to migrate to the extravascular compartment.

Recipient Adverse Effects

Transfusion of granulocytes obtained from G-CSF–stimulated donors has generally been well tolerated by recipients. In the study of Adkins and associates,[107] 29 HLA-matched transfusions were administered to 10 patients. After one of the transfusions, the patient experienced dyspnea, cough, and the sensation of a large tongue, all of which disappeared after treatment with antihistamines. No febrile or other respiratory reactions were seen. Hester and associates[106] reported adverse pulmonary reactions in approximately 5% of transfusions, reactions characterized by varying degrees of dyspnea, hypoxia, and changes on the chest radiograph. In the study of Price and associates,[91] chills and fever were seen in only about 10% of patients. These reactions were mild to moderate and were preventable in subsequent transfusions by treatment with antipyretics or corticosteroids. No changes were seen in blood oxygen saturation measured before and after the transfusions. Although this experience is encouraging, the likelihood of alloimmunization is low in the groups of patients studied to date. Similar results may not occur with transfusion of multitransfused patients with intact immune systems, such as those with neutrophil function disorders.

Clinical Efficacy

The evidence that providing large numbers of granulocytes from G-CSF–stimulated donors is clinically efficacious is limited to case reports[110–114] and small uncontrolled series.[91,106,115,116] Hester and associates[106] transfused 15 patients with fungal infection and reported that 60% responded. Eighty-three percent of patients (15 of 18) with established bacterial or fungal infection recovered in the series reported by Taylor and colleagues.[115] Results were more discouraging in the study of Grigg and associates,[116] in which 3 of 3 patients with bacterial infection survived, but 5 of 5 with fungal infection died. Kerr and colleagues prophylactically transfused G-CSF/dexamethasone–stimulated granulocytes in nine allogeneic stem cell transplant patients considered to be at high risk for the development of invasive fungal infection.[117] Six of the patients had previous invasive *Aspergillus* infection, and two had prolonged neutropenia. Results were compared to that of 18 control patients. Patients receiving prophylactic granulocytes were significantly less likely to develop fever (25% vs 100%) and the mean number of days with fever was less (2.5 vs 7.1). Of the six patients in whom it possible to judge response radiographically, four improved and two worsened. In a prospective uncontrolled study, Lee and associates[118] treated 32 patients with neutropenia-related infection with a mean of 3.8 G-CSF–stimulated granulocyte transfusions. Clinical responses were reported in 80%, 67%, and 50% of fungal, gram-negative bacterial, and gram-positive bacterial infections, respectively. The fate of infused Tc99m-labeled granulocytes was measured in two responders and two nonresponders; the cells localized to the area of infection in both responders but failed to so localize in the nonresponders, suggesting that efficacy depends on the cells' ability to home to the site of infection.

Peters and coworkers[119] administered granulocyte transfusions to 30 children with documented infection. Fifty-eight percent of the granulocyte concentrates were from G-CSF–stimulated donors. Since the patients were children, the average dose of granulocytes per kilogram was relatively high. In this uncontrolled series, recovery from bacterial and fungal infection was 82% and 54%, respectively. Rutella and colleagues[120] treated 20 patients with a variety of bacterial and fungal infections with G-CSF–stimulated granulocytes. Overall, 50% of patients responded, response rates being equivalent for those with bacterial or fungal infection. However, no patient with a localized invasive fungal infection responded. Price and associates[91] treated 19 bone marrow transplant recipients with a variety of bacterial and fungal infections. Infection resolved in 8 of 11 patients with invasive bacterial infections or candidemia; none of the eight patients with invasive mold infection, however, survived 30 days to document clearance of infection. More recently, Nichols and associates reported on a phase II multicenter feasibility trial in which 39 patients with neutropenia and documented infection were treated with daily granulocyte transfusions from G-CSF–stimulated donors.[121] A microbial response was observed in 38%, 60%, and 40% of patients with invasive mold infection, tissue bacterial infection, and bacteremia/fungemia, respectively.

In a retrospective case-controlled study, Hubel and colleagues examined the effect of G-CSF–stimulated granulocyte transfusion therapy on the course of infection and on overall survival in 74 patients undergoing bone marrow transplantation.[122] These results were compared to those of a matched cohort of 74 patients who received antimicrobial therapy alone. The fraction of patients with progressive infection was actually greater in the transfused group (57% vs 39%), although the difference was not statistically significant for patients with fungal infection. No differences were seen in the overall survival rate. These negative results must be interpreted with caution. This study was not a prospective randomized study, the "controls" were partly historical, and the patients selected to receive granulocyte transfusions were likely to have had more severe illness. Regardless, these data do not provide clear evidence that granulocyte transfusions are clinically effective.

In another case-controled study, Safdar and associates[123] analyzed 491 patients with candidemia. Twenty-nine of these patients received granulocyte transfusions; 429 did not. Short-term survival was comparable (48% in the transfused group, 45% in the control group) in spite of the fact that a number of risk factors for higher mortality were more common in the patients receiving granulocytes (e.g., longer duration of neutropenia, higher incidence of breakthrough invasive fungal infection). The authors interpreted these findings to be supportive of the notion that the transfusions were effective.

Of note, many of these trials were conducted prior to the availability of antifungal agents that are more effective and less toxic than conventional amphotericin B, including the third-generation triazole voriconazole. It is possible that the administration of more effective therapy would allow the incremental benefit of granulocyte therapy to be more clearly demonstrated, but this hypothesis remains to be proved.

CONCLUSION

Many studies have shown that G-CSF (with or without corticosteroid) stimulation of normal donors causes marked neutrophilia and permits the collection of large numbers of functional granulocytes for transfusion. G-CSF is well tolerated by the donors, although mild side effects are fairly common, and more serious adverse events can occur. The transfusion of these large numbers of granulocytes usually results in a substantial increase in the patient's blood neutrophil count. Transfusion reactions can occur and are usually mild, although serious pulmonary reactions occur in approximately 5% of patients, an incidence that may depend on the frequency of alloimmunization. These reactions do not seem to be more common or severe than those seen with the administration of granulocytes obtained without donor G-CSF stimulation. The remaining critical question is whether the transfusion of large doses of granulocytes is clinically effective in eradication of infection or in prolonging patient survival. Evidence for efficacy to date is only anecdotal or based on small, uncontrolled series. Some of these series have suggested efficacy, impressing some clinicians that the therapy is useful; others have shown no effect. The current situation is one of clinical equipoise. It is not clear whether this rather expensive therapy would be advantageous, disadvantageous, or neutral, given that clinical efficacy is uncertain and there are known possible adverse effects for both donor and patient. Clarification will only be possible by means of a large-scale, randomized, controlled clinical efficacy trial. Such a trial is in its final planning stages within the National Heart, Lung, and Blood Institute's Transfusion Medicine/Hemostasis Network and may be under way by the time of publication of this text.

REFERENCES

1. Pizzo PA. Management of fever in patients with cancer and treatment-induced neutropenia. N Engl J Med 1993;328:1323–1332.
2. Hughes WT, Armstrong D, Bodey GP, et al. 1997 Guidelines for the use of antimicrobial agents in neutropenic patients with unexplained fever. Clin Infect Dis 1997;25:551–573.
3. Dale DC, Liles WC, Price TH. Renewed interest in granulocyte transfusion therapy. Br J Haematol 1997;98:497–501.
4. Trial to Reduce Alloimmunization to Platelets Study Group. Leukocyte reduction and ultraviolet B irradiation of platelets to prevent alloimmunization and refractoriness to platelet transfusions. N Engl J Med 1997;337:1861–1869.
5. Grow WB, Moreb JS, Roque D, et al. Late onset of invasive aspergillus infection in bone marrow transplant patients at a university hospital. Bone Marrow Transplant 2002;29:15–19.
6. Marr KA, Carter RA, Crippa F, et al. Epidemiology and outcome of mould infections in hematopoietic stem cell transplant patients. Clin Infect Dis 2002;34:909–917.
7. Marr KA, Boeckh M, Carter RA, et al. Combination antifungal therapy for invasive aspergillosis. Clin Infect Dis 2004;39:797–802.
8. Wingard JR. Fungal infections after bone marrow transplant. Biol Blood Marrow Transplant 1999;5:55–68.
9. Boutati EI, Anaissie EJ. *Fusarium*, a significant emerging pathogen in patients with hematologic malignancy: ten years' experience at a cancer center and implications for management. Blood 1997;90:999–1008.
10. Imhof A, Balajee A, Fredricks DN, et al. Breakthrough fungal infections in stem cell transplant recipients receiving voriconazole. Clin Infect Dis 2004;39:743–746.
11. Herbrecht R, Denning DW, Patterson TF, et al. Voriconazole versus amphotericin B for primary therapy of invasive aspergillosis. N Engl J Med 2002;347:408–415.
12. Dancey JT, Deubelbeiss KA, Harker LA, et al. Neutrophil kinetics in man. J Clin Invest 1976;58:705–715.
13. Strauss RG. Neutrophil (granulocyte) transfusions in the new millennium. Transfusion 1998;38:710–712.
14. McCullough J, Clay M, Loken M, et al. Effect of ABO incompatibility on the fate in vivo of 111-indium granulocytes. Transfusion 198828:358–361.
15. Winston DJ, Ho WG, Howell CL, et al. Cytomegalovirus infections associated with leukocyte transfusions. Ann Intern Med 1980;93: 671–675.
16. Hersman J, Meyers JD, Thomas ED, et al. The effect of granulocyte transfusions on the incidence of cytomegalovirus infection after allogeneic marrow transplantation. Ann Intern Med 1982;96:149–152.
17. Dutcher JP, Schiffer CA, Johnston GS, et al. Alloimmunization prevents the migration of transfused indium-111-labeled granulocytes to sites of infection. Blood 1983;62:354–360.
18. Dutcher JP, Riggs JR, Fox JJ, et al. Effect of histocompatibility factors on pulmonary retention of indium-111-labeled granulocytes. Am J Hematol 1990;33:238–243.
19. Stroncek DF, Leonard K, Eiber G, et al. Alloimmunization after granulocyte transfusions. Transfusion 1996;36:1009–1015.
20. Schiffer CA, Aisner J, Daly PA, et al. Alloimmunization following prophylactic granulocyte transfusion. Blood 1979;54:766–774.
21. Goldstein IM, Eyre HJ, Terasaki PI, et al. Leukocyte transfusions: role of leukocyte alloantibodies in determining transfusion response. Transfusion 1971;11:19–24.
22. Dutcher JP, Kendall J, Norris D, et al. Granulocyte transfusion therapy and amphotericin B: adverse reactions? Am J Hematol 1989;31: 102–108.
23. Westrick MA, Debelak-Fehir KM, Epstein RB. The effect of prior whole blood transfusion on subsequent granulocyte support in leukopenic dogs. Transfusion 1977;17:611–614.
24. McCullough J, Clay M, Hurd D, et al. Effect of leukocyte antibodies and HLA matching on the intravascular recovery, survival, and tissue localization of 111-indium granulocytes. Blood 1986;67:522–528.
25. McCullough J, Weiblen BJ, Clay ME, et al. Effect of leukocyte antibodies on the fate of in vivo of indium-111-labeled granulocytes. Blood 1981;58:164–170.
26. Appelbaum FR, Trapani RJ, Graw JR: Consequences of prior alloimmunization during granulocyte transfusion. Transfusion 1977;17: 460–464.
27. Price TH, Dale DC. Blood kinetics and in vivo chemotaxis of transfused neutrophils: effect of collection method, donor corticosteroid treatment, and short-term storage. Blood 1979;54:977–986.
28. Wright DG, Kauffmann JC, Chusid MJ, et al. Functional abnormalities of human neutrophils collected by continuous flow filtration leukapheresis. Blood 1975;45:901–911.
29. McCullough J, Weiblen BJ, Deinard AR, et al. In vitro function and post-transfusion survival of granulocytes collected by continuous-flow centrifugation and by filtration leukapheresis. Blood 1976;48: 315–326.
30. Nusbacher J, Rosenfeld SI, MacPherson JL, et al. Nylon fiber leukapheresis: associated complement component changes and granulocytopenia. Blood 1978;51:359–365.
31. Wiltbank TB, Nusbacher J, Higby DJ, et al. Abdominal pain in donors during filtration leukapheresis. Transfusion 1977;17:159–162.
32. Strauss RG, Hester JP, Vogler WR, et al. A multicenter trial to document the efficacy and safety of a rapidly excreted analog of hydroxyethyl starch for leukapheresis with a note on steroid stimulation of granulocyte donors. Transfusion 1986;26:258–264.
33. Lee J-H, Leitman SF, Klein HG. A controlled comparison of the efficacy of hetastarch and pentastarch in granulocyte collections by centrifugal leukapheresis. Blood 1995;86:4662–4666.
34. Hinckley ME, Huestis DW. Premedication for optimal granulocyte collection. Plasma Ther 1981;2:149–152.
35. Winton EF, Vogler WR. Development of a practical oral dexamethasone premedication schedule leading to improved granulocyte yields with the continuous-flow centrifugal blood cell separator. Blood 1978; 52:249–253.
36. Standards Committee of the American Association of Blood Banks. In Klein HG (ed). Standards for Blood Banks and Transfusion Services, 23rd ed. Bethesda, Md., American Association of Blood Banks, 2004.

37. Glasser L, Huestis DW, Jones JF. Functional capabilities of steroid-recruited neutrophils harvested for clinical transfusion. N Engl J Med 1977;297:1033–1036.
38. Price TH. Neutrophil transfusion: in vivo function of neutrophils collected using cell separators. Transfusion 1983;23:504–507.
39. Dale DC, Liles WC, Summer WR, et al. Granulocyte colony-stimulating factor: role and relationships in infectious diseases. J Infect Dis 1995;172:1061–1075.
40. Colotta F, Re F, Mantovani A. Granulocyte transfusions from granulocyte colony-stimulating factor-treated donors: also a question of cell survival? Blood 1993;82:2258.
41. Lane TA, Windle B. Granulocyte concentrate function during preservation: effect of temperature. Blood 1979;54:216–225.
42. McCullough J, Carter SJ, Quie PG. Effects of anticoagulants and storage on granulocyte function in bank blood. Blood 1974;43:207–217.
43. McCullough J, Weiblen BJ, Fine D. Effects of storage of granulocytes on their fate in vivo. Transfusion 1983;23:20–24.
44. Glasser L, Lane TA, McCullough J, et al. Panel VII: Neutrophil concentrates-functional considerations, storage, and quality control. J Clin Apheresis 1983;1:179–184.
45. McCullough J, Weiblen BJ, Peterson PK, et al. Effects of temperature on granulocyte preservation. Blood 1978;52:301–310.
46. Anderson KC, Weinstein HJ. Transfusion-associated graft-versus-host disease. N Engl J Med 1990;323:315–321.
47. McCullough J. Granulocyte transfusion. In Petz LD, Swisher SN, Kleinman S, et al (eds). Clinical Practice of Transfusion Medicine, 3rd ed. New York, Churchill Livingstone, 1996, pp 413–432.
48. Valerius NH, Johansen KS, Nielsen OS, et al. Effect of in vitro x-irradiation on lymphocyte and granulocyte function. Scand J Haematol 1981;27:9–18.
49. Eastlund DT, Charbonneau TT. Superoxide generation and cytotactic response of irradiated neutrophils. Transfusion 1988;28:368–370.
50. Wolber RA, Duque RE, Robinson JP, et al. Oxidative product formation in irradiated neutrophils: a flow cytometric analysis. Transfusion 1987;27:167–170.
51. Button LN, DeWolf WC, Newburger PE, et al. The effects of irradiation on blood components. Transfusion 1981;21:419–426.
52. Schwarzenberg L, Mathé G, de Grouchy J, et al. White blood cell transfusions. Isr J Med Sci 1965;1:925–956.
53. Morse EE, Freireich EJ, Carbone PP, et al. The transfusion of leukocytes from donors with chronic myelocytic leukemia to patients with leukopenia. Transfusion 1966;6:183–192.
54. Lowenthal RM, Grossman L, Goldman JM, et al. Granulocyte transfusions in treatment of infections in patients with acute leukaemia and aplastic anaemia. Lancet 1975;1:353–358.
55. Strauss RG. Granulocyte transfusion. In McLeod BC, Price TH, Drew MJ (eds). Apheresis: Principles and Practice. Bethesda, Md., AABB Press, 1997, pp 195–209.
56. Graw RG, Herzig GH, Perry S, et al. Normal granulocyte transfusion therapy: treatment of septicemia due to gram-negative bacteria. N Engl J Med 1972;287:367–371.
57. Higby DJ, Yates JW, Henderson ES, et al. Filtration leukapheresis for granulocyte transfusion therapy: clinical and laboratory studies. N Engl J Med 1975;292:761–766.
58. Fortuny IE, Bloomfield CD, Hadlock DC, et al. Granulocyte transfusion: a controlled study in patients with acute nonlymphocytic leukemia. Transfusion 1975;15:548–557.
59. Vogler WR, Winton EF. A controlled study of the efficacy of granulocyte transfusions in patients with neutropenia. Am J Med 1977;63:548–555.
60. Alavi JB, Root RK, Djerassi I, et al. A randomized clinical trial of granulocyte transfusions for infection in acute leukemia. N Engl J Med 1977;296:706–711.
61. Herzig RH, Herzig GP, Graw RG, et al. Successful granulocyte transfusion therapy for gram-negative septicemia: a prospectively randomized controlled study. N Engl J Med 1977;296:701–705.
62. Winston DJ, Ho WG, Gale RP. Therapeutic granulocyte transfusions for documented infections: a controlled trial in ninety-five infectious granulocytopenic episodes. Ann Intern Med 1982;97:509–515.
63. Strauss RG. Therapeutic granulocyte transfusions in 1993. Blood 1993;81:1675–1678.
64. Vamvakas EC, Pineda AA. Meta-analysis of clinical studies of the efficacy of granulocyte transfusions in the treatment of bacterial sepsis. J Clin Apheresis 1996;11:1–9.
65. Ruthe RC, Andersen BR, Cunningham BL, et al. Efficacy of granulocyte transfusions in the control of systemic candidiasis in the leukopenic host. Blood 1978;52:493–497.
66. Chow HS, Sarpel SC, Epstein RB. Pathophysiology of *Candida albicans* meningitis in normal, neutropenic, and granulocyte transfused dogs. Blood 1980;55:546–551.
67. Spielberger RT, Falleroni MJ, Coene AJ, et al. Concomitant amphotericin B therapy, granulocyte transfusions, and GM-CSF administration for disseminated infection with *Fusarium* in a granulocytopenic patient. Clin Infect Dis 1993;16:528–530.
68. Swerdlow B, Deresinski S. Development of *Aspergillus* sinusitis in a patient receiving amphotericin B treatment with granulocyte transfusions. Am J Med 1984;76:162–166.
69. Bhatia S, McCullough J, Perry EH, et al. Granulocyte transfusions: efficacy in treating fungal infections in neutropenic patients following bone marrow transplantation. Transfusion 1994;34:226–232.
70. Strauss RG. Granulocyte transfusions. In Rossi EC, Simon TL, Moss GS, et al (eds). Principles of Transfusion Medicine, 2nd ed. Baltimore, Md., Williams & Wilkins, 1996, pp 321–328.
71. Strauss RG, Connett JE, Gale RP, et al. A controlled trial of prophylactic granulocyte transfusions during initial induction chemotherapy for acute myelogenous leukemia. N Engl J Med 1981;305:597–603.
72. Rosenshein MS, Farewell VT, Price TH, et al. The cost effectiveness of therapeutic and prophylactic leukocyte transfusion. N Engl J Med 1980;302:1058–1062.
73. Christensen RD, Anstall HB, Rothstein G. Deficiencies in the neutrophil system of newborn infants, and the use of leukocyte transfusions in the treatment of neonatal sepsis. J Clin Apheresis 1982;1:33–41.
74. Laurenti F, Ferro R, Isacchi G, et al. Polymorphonuclear leukocyte transfusion for the treatment of sepsis in the newborn infant. J Pediatr 1981;98:118–123.
75. Christensen RD, Rothstein G, Anstall HB, et al. Granulocyte transfusions in neonates with bacterial infections, neutropenia, and depletion of mature marrow neutrophils. Pediatrics 1982;70:1–6.
76. Cairo MS, Rucker R, Bennetts GA, et al. Improved survival of newborns receiving leukocyte transfusions for sepsis. Pediatrics 1984;74:887–892.
77. Cairo MS, Worcester C, Rucker RW, et al. Randomized trial of granulocyte transfusions versus intravenous immune globulin therapy for neonatal neutropenia and sepsis. J Pediatr 1992;120:281–285.
78. Baley JE, Stork EK, Warkentin PI, et al. Buffy coat transfusions in neutropenic neonates with presumed sepsis: a prospective, randomized trial. Pediatrics 80:712–720, 1987.
79. Wheeler JG, Chauvenet AR, Johnson CA, et al. Buffy coat transfusions in neonates with sepsis and neutrophil storage pool depletion [abstract]. Pediatrics 1987;79:422–425.
80. Pflieger H, Arnold R, Bhaduri S, et al. Beneficial effect of granulocyte transfusions in patients with defects in granulocyte function and severe infections. Scand J Haematol 1979;22:33–41.
81. Buescher ES, Gallin JI. Leukocyte transfusions in chronic granulomatous disease: persistence of transfused leukocytes in sputum. N Engl J Med 1982;307:800–803.
82. Yomtovian R, Abramson J, Quie P, et al. Granulocyte transfusion therapy in chronic granulomatous disease: report of a patient and review of the literature. Transfusion 1981;21:739–743.
83. Dougherty SH, Peterson PK, Simmons RL. Granulocyte transfusion as adjunctive therapy for qualitative granulocytopenia: multiple liver abscesses in a patient with chronic granulomatous disease. Arch Surg 1983;118:873–874.
84. Bowen TJ, Ochs HD, Altman LC, et al. Severe recurrent bacterial infections associated with defective adherence and chemotaxis in two patients with neutrophils deficient in a cell-associated glycoprotein. J Pediatr 1982;101:932–940.
85. Dana BW, Durie BG, White RF, et al. Concomitant administration of granulocyte transfusions and amphotericin B in neutropenic patients: absence of significant pulmonary toxicity. Blood 1981;57:90–94.
86. Wright DG, Robichaud KJ, Pizzo PA, et al. Lethal pulmonary reactions associated with the combined use of amphotericin B and leukocyte transfusions. N Engl J Med 1981;304:1185–1189.
87. Bow EJ, Schroeder ML, Louie TJ. Pulmonary complications in patients receiving granulocyte transfusions and amphotericin B. Can Med Assoc J 1984;130:593–597.
88. Karp DD, Ervin TJ, Tuttle S, et al. Pulmonary complications during granulocyte transfusions: incidence and clinical features. Vox Sang 1982;42:57–61.
89 Pegels JG, Bruynes ECE, Engelriet CP, et al. Serological studies in patients on platelet- and granulocyte-substitution therapy. Br J Haematol 1982;52:59–68.
90. Arnold R, Goldmann SF, Pflieger H. Lymphocytotoxic antibodies in patients receiving granulocyte transfusion. Vox Sang 1980;38:250–258.
91. Price TH, Bowden RA, Boeckh M, et al. Phase I/II trial of neutrophil transfusions from donors stimulated with G-CSF and dexamethasone for treatment of patients with infections in hematopoietic stem cell transplantation. Blood 2000;95:3302–3309.
92. Adkins DR, Goodnough LT, Shenoy S, et al. Effect of leukocyte incompatibility on neutrophil increment after transfusion of granulocyte

colony-stimulating factor-mobilized prophylactic granulocyte transfusions and on clinical outcomes after stem cell transplantation. Blood 2000;95:3605–3612.

93. Appelbaum FR, Bowles CA, Makuch RW, et al. Granulocyte transfusion therapy of experimental *Pseudomonas* septicemia: study of cell dose and collection technique. Blood 1978;52:323–331.
94. Epstein RB, Chow HS. An analysis of quantitative relationships of granulocyte transfusion therapy in canines. Transfusion 1981;21:360–362.
95. Chatta GS, Price TH, Allen RC, et al. Effects of in vivo recombinant methionyl human granulocyte colony-stimulating factor on the neutrophil response and peripheral blood colony-forming cells in healthy young and elderly adult volunteers. Blood 1994;84:2923–2929.
96. Price TH, Chatta GS, Dale DC. Effect of recombinant granulocyte colony-stimulating factor on neutrophil kinetics in normal young and elderly humans. Blood 1996;88:335–340.
97. Liles WC, Huang JE, van Burik JH, et al. Granulocyte colony-stimulating factor administered in vivo augments neutrophil-mediated activity against opportunistic fungal pathogens. J Infect Dis 1997;175:1012–1015.
98. Gaviria JM, van Burik J-A, Dale DC, et al. Comparison of interferon-gamma, granulocyte colony-stimulating factor, and granulocyte-macrophage colony-stimulating factor for priming leukocyte-mediated hyphal damage of opportunistic fungal pathogens. J Infect Dis 1999;179: 1038–1041.
99. Liles WC, Rodger ER, Dale DC. Differential regulation of human neutrophil surface expression of CD14, CD11b, CD18, and L-selection following the administration of G-CSF in vivo and in vitro [abstract]. Clin Res 1994;42:304A.
100. Stroncek DF, Jaszcz W, Herr GP, et al. Expression of neutrophil antigens after 10 days of granulocyte-colony-stimulating factor. Transfusion 1998;38:663–668.
101. Liles WC. Regulation of apoptosis in neutrophils: fast track to death? J Immunol 1995;155:3289–3291.
102. Leitman SF, Yu M, Lekstrom J. Pair-controlled study of granulocyte colony stimulating factor (G-CSF) plus dexamethasone (DEXA) for granulocytapheresis donors [abstract]. Transfusion 1995;35:53S.
103. Liles WC, Huang JE, Llewellyn C, et al. A comparative trial of granulocyte-colony-stimulating factor and dexamethasone, separately and in combination, for the mobilization of neutrophils in the peripheral blood of normal volunteers. Transfusion 1997;37:182–187.
104. Stroncek DF, Clay ME, Petzoldt ML, et al. Treatment of normal individuals with granulocyte-colony-stimulating factor: donor experiences and the effects on peripheral blood CD34+ cell counts and on the collection of peripheral blood stem cells. Transfusion 1996;36:601–610.
105. Anderlini P, Przepiorka D, Seong D, et al. Clinical toxicity and laboratory effects of granulocyte-colony-stimulating factor (filgrastim) mobilization and blood stem cell apheresis from normal donors, and analysis of charges for the procedures. Transfusion 1996;36:590–595.
106. Hester JP, Dignani MC, Anaissie EJ, et al. Collection and transfusion of granulocyte concentrates from donors primed with granulocyte stimulating factor and response of myelosuppressed patients with established infection. J Clin Apheresis 1995;10:188–193.
107. Adkins D, Spitzer G, Johnston M, et al. Transfusions of granulocyte-colony-stimulating factor-mobilized granulocyte components to allogeneic transplant recipients: analysis of kinetics and factors determining posttransfusion neutrophil and platelet counts. Transfusion 1997;37:737–748.
108. Dale DC, Liles WC, Llewellyn C, et al. Neutrophil transfusions: kinetics and functions of neutrophils mobilized with granulocyte colony-stimulating factor (G-CSF) and dexamethasone. Transfusion 1998; 38:713–721.
109. Adkins D, Goodgold H, Hendershott L, et al. Indium-labeled white blood cells apheresed from donors receiving G-CSF localize to sites of inflammation when infused into allogeneic bone marrow transplant recipients. Bone Marrow Transplant 1997;19:809–812.
110. Leitman SF, Oblitas JM, Emmons R, et al. Clinical efficacy of daily G-CSF-recruited granulocyte transfusions in patients with severe neutropenia and life-threatening infections [abstract]. Blood 1996; 88(Suppl 1):331A.
111. Clarke K, Szer J, Shelton M, et al. Multiple granulocyte transfusions facilitating successful unrelated bone marrow transplantation in a patient with very severe aplastic anemia complicated by suspected fungal infection. Bone Marrow Transplant 1995;16:723–726.
112. Di Mario A, Sica S, Salutari P, et al. Granulocyte colony-stimulating factor-primed leukocyte transfusions in Candida tropicalis fungemia in neutropenic patients. Haematologica 1997;82:362–363.
113. von Planta M, Ozsahin H, Schroten H, et al. Greater omentum flaps and granulocyte transfusions as combined therapy of liver abscess in chronic granulomatous disease. Eur J Pediatr Surg 1997;7:234–236.
114. Catalano L, Fontana R, Scarpato N, et al. Combined treatment with amphotericin-B and granulocyte transfusion from G-CSF-stimulated donors in an aplastic patient with invasive aspergillosis undergoing bone marrow transplantation. Haematologica 1997;82:71–72.
115. Taylor K, Moore D, Kelly C, et al. Safety and logistical use of filgrastim (FG) mobilized granulocytes (FMG) in early management of severe neutropenic sepsis (SNS) in acute leukemia (AL)/autograft [abstract]. 1996;Blood 88(Suppl 1):349A.
116. Grigg A, Vecchi L, Bardy P, et al. G-CSF-stimulated donor granulocyte collections for prophylaxis and therapy of neutropenic sepsis. Aust N Z J Med 1996;26:813–818.
117. Kerr JP, Liakopolou E, Brown J, et al. The use of stimulated granulocyte transfusions to prevent recurrence of past severe infections after allogeneic stem cell transplantation. Br J Haematol 2003;123:114–118.
118. Lee JJ, Song HC, Chung IJ, et al. Clinical efficacy and prediction of response to granulocyte transfusion therapy for patients with neutropenia-related infections. Haematologica 2004;89:632–633.
119. Peters C, Minkov M, Matthes-Martin S, et al. Leucocyte transfusions from rhG-CSF or prednisolone stimulated donors for treatment of severe infections in immunocompromised neutropenic patients. Br J Haemotol 1999;106:689–696.
120. Rutella S, Pierelli L, Piccirillo N, et al. Efficacy of granulocyte transfusions for neutropenia-related infections: retrospective analysis of predictive factors. Cytotherapy 2003;5:19–30.
121. Nichols WG, Strauss RG, Ambruso D, et al. G-CSF-stimulated granulocyte transfusions from unrelated community donors for severe infections during neutropenia: a phase II multicenter trial of feasibility and efficacy. Blood 2003;102:978a.
122. Hubel K, Carter RA, Liles WC, et al. Granulocyte transfusion therapy for infections in candidates and recipients of HPC transplantation: a comparative analysis of feasibility and outcome for community donors versus related donors. Transfusion 2002;42:1414–1421.
123. Safdar A, Hanna HA, Boktour M, et al. Impact of high-dose granulocyte transfusions in patients with cancer with candidemia. Cancer 2004;101:2859–2865.
124. Caspar CB, Seger RA, Burger J, et al. Effective stimulation of donors for granulocyte transfusions with recombinant methionyl granulocyte colony-stimulating factor. Blood 1993;81:2866–2871.
125. Bensinger WI, Price TH, Dale DC, et al. The effects of daily recombinant human granulocyte colony-stimulating factor administration on normal granulocyte donors undergoing leukapheresis. Blood 1993;81:1883–1888.
126. Jendiroba DB, Lichtiger B, Anaissie E, et al. Evaluation and comparison of three mobilization methods for the collection of granulocytes. Transfusion 1998;38:722–728.

Chapter 25
Coagulation Factor Preparations

James C. Zimring • Alexander Duncan

This chapter introduces the different types of coagulation factor concentrates that are available, the advantages and disadvantages of utilizing different products, and the indications for their use. Detailed information on dosing and administration of a given product should be obtained from the published guidelines for that product.

REPLACEMENT THERAPY FOR COAGULATION FACTOR DEFICIENCIES

Since the initial descriptions of hemophilia and von Willebrand disease, it has been appreciated that the coagulation system is made up of discrete factors, the absence of which can result in life-threatening bleeding. Early attempts to replace such factors consisted of transfusing plasma. However, the low concentrations of coagulation factors in normal plasma are a limiting factor to this approach, since there is a maximal rate of plasma infusion and total volume that a patient can tolerate. Treatment of specific factor deficiencies was improved with the introduction of relatively crude fractions of plasma that effectively concentrated the desired factors (i.e., cryoprecipitate). However, such products contain only certain factors (predominantly vWF, VIII, XIII, and fibrinogen). In addition, multiple pooled units of cryoprecipitate carry the risk of transmitting infectious disease from donors.[1] Further advances in factor purification provided concentrates of factors VIII and IX for the treatment of hemophilia A and hemophilia B, respectively. Modern concentrates are now subjected to pathogen inactivation techniques, which minimizes but does not eliminate the risk of infection.[2,3] More recently, recombinant DNA technology has allowed the expression of human coagulation factors in vitro, which essentially eliminates the risk of transmitting human pathogens that could co-purify from donor plasma. However, since some products are stabilized with human albumin, it has been suggested that a risk of transmission of selected pathogens, such as parvovirus B19 and prions remains a possibility.[2] The current move to albumin free stabilizers may address this issue.[4–6]

PURIFIED VERSUS RECOMBINANT COAGULATION FACTORS

Prior to the advent of recombinant DNA technology, the only available source of human coagulation factors was purification from plasma donors. The advantage to this approach is that the factors are derived from their natural biological source, which results in a biochemically authentic factor. However, there are a number of distinct disadvantages to purifying coagulation factor concentrates from human donors. There is always the concern of transmitting infectious agents from the donor into the recipient. Indeed, before HIV was identified as the causative agent of AIDS, a large number of hemophilia patients were infected from HIV-tainted purified factor VIII. Current purified human factor VIII is obtained only from donors who screen negative for the known transmissible pathogens. However, this will not protect factor VIII recipients from unidentified emerging pathogens that may enter the blood supply in the future. For this reason, there are ongoing efforts to perfect sterilization techniques that would potentially inactivate all pathogens. Since coagulation factors are proteins, these techniques focus on methodologies that do not damage proteins, such as cross-linking of nucleic acids (DNA or RNA) or disrupting membranes of lipid-enveloped pathogens. However, such techniques will not inactivate prions, since, like coagulation factors, prions are also proteins. Thus, transmission of spongiform encephalopathies remains a concern.[7,8]

The advent of recombinant DNA technology has allowed the cloning of cDNAs and the ectopic expression of human proteins in cell culture. This process allows for the expression and purification of large quantities of the protein products of human genetic sequences and essentially eliminates the risk of pathogen transmission from human donors. A residual risk of infection from pathogens of animal origin remains, since animal serum typically is required to culture the cell lines producing the factors. In addition, albumin of human or animal origin has been required to stabilize recombinant factors. These additives provide a potential residual source for introducing infectious material. However, recent advances have circumvented these technical limitations. For example, in 2003 the U.S. Food and Drug Administration (FDA) approved a recombinant factor VIII product expressed in Chinese hamster ovary cells, which has never come into contact with products from human or animals. Although it is still theoretically possible that undetected pathogens harbored in the cell lines themselves may infect human recipients, recombinant factors expressed in serum-free systems without albumin additives are as close to being pathogen free as is possible in culture-based systems.

Despite the above attributes, there are several disadvantages to utilizing recombinant factors. These products are typically expressed from nonhuman cell lines, such as Chinese hamster ovary cells. Thus, in patients who have hypersensitivity to mice or hamsters, allergic side effects can theoretically be observed. Although it is rare to observe allergic reactions to recombinant products,[9] anaphylaxis after administration of recombinant factor VIII has been reported, but it is unclear whether the reaction was due to hypersensitivity to contaminants in the factor VIII preparation.[10] Thus, allergic reactions remain a possibility, and known hypersensitivity to animals from which the expressing cell lines are derived is considered a contraindication to utilizing factors expressed in such cell lines.

An additional issue is that human gene products expressed in cell lines may have different post-translational modifications (glycosylation, phosphorylation, etc.) from the naturally occurring material. This can introduce neo-epitopes that may constitute a foreign entity to the host immune system. Thus, it is possible that recipients of recombinant factors may develop antibody inhibitors against foreign "non-natural" epitopes on the recombinant factor. Although the above concerns may cause problems in the case of certain recombinant factors, current preparations of recombinant factor VIII do not show increased frequency of inhibitor induction in previously untreated patients.[11] However, it has been reported that the change from one factor VIII preparation to another may increase risk of anti–factor VIII antibodies, perhaps as a result of neoantigen exposure.[12]

HUMAN VERSUS ANIMAL COAGULATION FACTORS

The sequences of coagulation factors are sufficiently conserved in nonhuman mammals that purified coagulation factors from nonhuman sources can be used in some settings to treat factor deficiency states. There is a slightly decreased risk of viral transmission of pathogens, since most viruses are species specific. However, some cases of viral transmission may occur,[13] and numerous porcine pathogens may potentially contaminate tissues or products of porcine origin.[14] In addition, there is a theoretical concern that introduction of undetected animal viruses into humans may result in novel recombination with human viruses, which could lead to the generation of new human infectious entities. The greatest utility for coagulation factors of nonhuman origin has been limited cross-reactivity with antibody inhibitors against human coagulation factors. In particular, porcine factor VIII has been used to circumvent antibody inhibitors against human factor VIII (see below).

FACTORS USED TO TREAT BLEEDING DIATHESES

Treatment of Congenital Hemophilia A

Replacement therapy with factor VIII has long been the treatment for patients with hemophilia A. A wide variety of human factor VIII replacement products are available including both recombinant factor VIII and factor VIII products purified from human plasma. In addition, modified factor VIII and porcine factor VIII can be used in the context of anti–factor VIII antibody inhibitors (see below). Currently, recombinant products are the treatment of choice because they confer the lowest risk of infectious disease transmission and may reduce the risk of inhibitor development.

Recombinant Factor VIII Products

Recombinant factor VIII was first approved by the FDA for human use in 1992. Although these early products were produced from cell lines, they required that the cells be cultured in media containing animal serum and that the products be stabilized with albumin of animal origin. Advances in cell culture technology have resulted in FDA approval of recombinant factor VIII expressed in a culture system to which no animal serum or products are added.

Recombinant factors provide the lowest risk of transmission of infectious agents, especially factors expressed in culture systems that do not require the addition of serum. As mentioned above, hypersensitivity to mice or hamsters can be a contraindication, because it may lead to allergic reactions to co-purifying proteins or monoclonal antibodies. Although isolated incidents of allergic reactions after recombinant factor VIII administration have been reported,[10] sensitivity to mouse or hamster contaminants has not been observed.[15] Overall, recombinant factor VIII products are well tolerated and highly efficacious in the treatment of factor VIII deficiency.

It is worth noting that unlike partially purified human factor VIII (e.g., Humate-P), in which case von Willebrand factor (vWF) co-purifies with factor VIII, recombinant factor VIII contains no vWF. Accordingly, while partially purified factor VIII can be used to treat von Willebrand disease (vWD) in addition to factor VIII deficiency, recombinant factor VIII is not a viable treatment for vWD.

Purified Factor VIII Products

Prior to the advent of recombinant factor VIII, patients with hemophilia A were treated with purified factor VIII isolated from plasma of human donors. Initially, procedures for producing partially purified plasma fractions highly enriched for factor VIII were utilized. To minimize the risk of infectious disease transmission, such products are subjected to treatments that typically inactivate pathogens, such as pasteurization or chemical inactivation with solvent and detergents. In addition to factor VIII, these enriched products also have high amounts of vWF that co-purifies with factor VIII. Thus, these products are also useful in treating certain forms of vWD (see below).

Further progress in purifying factor VIII was made with implementation of affinity purification using monoclonal antibodies to human factor VIII. Isolation of factor VIII by this procedure results in a highly purified product. Only a small quantity of vWF co-purifies with factor VIII by this approach. Accordingly, this product is not useful for the treatment of vWD. Purification and pathogen inactivation limit the chance of transmitting pathogens from the donor. In addition, small amounts of monoclonal antibody may be present in the final factor VIII preparation, which can result in allergic reactions in patients who have hypersensitivity to mice or hamsters.

Although rare, the type 2N vWD (Normandy) consists of a mutation in vWF that no longer stabilizes factor VIII.[16] In this case, the half-life of factor VIII decreases to the point that only very low levels of circulating factor VIII persist. Thus, it is possible for a patient with type 2N vWD to be misdiagnosed as having hemophilia A, since factor VIII levels are very low and vWF antigen is normal. In such a case, partially purified factor VIII (e.g., Humate-P) will correct the defect due to the co-purification of vWF. However, highly purified or recombinant factor VIII will have no efficacy in this setting, since vWF is largely removed during the purification process.

Cryoprecipitate

Cryoprecipitate contains a concentrate of factors VIII, vWF, XIII, and fibrinogen. In the United States, current use of cryoprecipitate is almost exclusively limited to the replacement of fibrinogen in hypofibrinogenemic patients. However, prior to the advent of purified factor VIII, cryoprecipitate was the mainstay of treatment for hemophilia A. In settings in which recombinant and purified factor VIII are not available, cryoprecipitate still is used to treat hemophilia A. Likewise, cryoprecipitate also has vWF and can be used to treat vWD, if vWF-containing factor VIII products are not available. However, unlike the partially purified factor VIII preparations, cryoprecipitate is not routinely subjected to pathogen inactivation treatments. Depending on the donor populations and screening procedures, the lifetime risk of contracting HIV infection from treatment of hemophilia with monthly infusions of cryoprecipitate has been estimated from 2% to 40%.[1] Accordingly, use of cryoprecipitate for treatment of hemophilia A and vWD should be limited to circumstances in which no other factor VIII product is available.

Treatment of Anti–Factor VIII Antibody Inhibitors

Antibodies against factor VIII can result in rapid clearance or functional inactivation of factor VIII.[17] Anti–factor VIII antibodies are most commonly seen in hemophilia A patients who mount a humoral immune response against replacement factor VIII. Since the factor VIII gene is either absent or altered in hemophilia A patients, wild-type factor VIII is not recognized as self. Thus, generation of antibodies to factor VIII represents an appropriate immune response to a foreign protein. However, spontaneous anti–factor VIII antibodies can also arise in patients without congenital hemophilia.[18] In these cases, the anti–factor VIII antibodies are autoantibodies against the patient's own factor VIII. This state has been referred to as acquired hemophilia.

In either of the above scenarios, the patient can have profoundly decreased factor VIII levels that are refractory to treatment with factor VIII replacement, since the antibodies neutralize the transfused factor that is given. The level of anti–factor VIII antibodies can be determined by running a Bethesda assay. Inhibitors that have low Bethesda assay levels (<5 units) can usually be overcome by administration of very large doses of factor VIII. However, in the case of inhibitors with a high level Bethesda assay, overcoming the inhibitor with factor VIII is not possible. In such cases, several products can be given, as detailed below.

Porcine Factor VIII

The utility of porcine factor VIII is its limited cross-reactivity with antibodies against human factor VIII. Thus, in a hemophilia A patient who has formed anti–human factor VIII antibodies, or in a patient with an autoantibody against factor VIII, porcine factor VIII may circumvent such an inhibitor.[19,20] Levels and potency of anti–factor VIII antibody inhibitors can be determined by a Bethesda assay. Values of Bethesda assays specific for human versus porcine factor VIII activities can be juxtaposed to determine whether a given patient's anti–factor VIII antibody cross-reacts with porcine factor VIII. Some patients who are initially responsive to porcine factor VIII rapidly develop antibodies against porcine factor VIII and may become refractory to subsequent treatment. At present, porcine factor VIII no longer is available in North America.

Mutant Factor VIII

A second strategy to circumvent anti–factor VIII antibodies is the expression of novel recombinant forms of human factor VIII in which the immunodominant epitopes have been modified or deleted. A number of different modifications have been made and are in the process of being developed for human use. Like porcine factor VIII, these products should have good efficacy in patients with anti–factor VIII antibodies. However, whether patients treated with altered factor VIII will subsequently develop antibodies to neo-epitopes introduced by the modification remains to be determined.

Recombinant Factor VIIa

Recombinant factor VIIa (rFVIIa), commercially called NovoSeven, functions in theory by promoting hemostasis through the tissue factor pathway. Since factor VIII is not involved in the tissue factor pathway of coagulation, anti–factor VIII inhibitors do not interfere with extrinsic pathway coagulation. This clever approach has shown efficacy in treating anti–factor VIII inhibitors. Since rFVIIa requires tissue factor to promote clot formation, it works selectively at sites of injury or bleeding. Accordingly, the risk of eliciting a thrombosis or consumptive coagulopathy is decreased. The exact mechanism by which rFVIIa functions is likely more complicated than simple tissue factor pathway activation, as interactions with the platelet surface appear to play a role in the clinical efficacy of rFVIIa.

rFVIIa has clear efficacy for the treatment of anti–factor VIII inhibitors and factor VII deficiency, which are the current FDA-approved indications for this drug. However, rFVIIa is being used with increasing frequency for off-label treatment of a wide variety of clinical bleeding situations including trauma, surgery, hepatic coagulopathy, Glanzmann thrombasthenia, Bernard-Soulier syndrome, and reversal of over-anticoagulation with warfarin sodium (Coumadin) and fondaparinux.[21,22] In addition, rFVIIa is used prophylactically to lower INR prior to mildly invasive procedures such as a liver biopsy in a patient with hepatic coagulopathy. The potential efficacy in these settings suggests that factor VIIa has mechanisms of action in addition to extrinsic pathway activation. Reports of small groups of patients and isolated cases have suggested efficacy of rFVIIa in each of the above settings, and it has been suggested that rFVIIa can essentially be used as a universal hemostatic agent.[23] However, there have also been reports of limited efficacy and several instances of increased morbidity or mortality from rVIIa usage.[24–27] In general, the utility and danger of using rFVIIa in these off-label settings has yet to be tested by clinical trials with sufficient size and proper randomization to allow evidence-based decisions.[28] Careful attention should be paid to ongoing studies that assess the benefit and risk of rFVIIa usage for the above indications.

Prothrombin Complex Concentrates (PCCs)

Prothrombin complex concentrates (also known as factor IX complex concentrates) consist of plasma fractions that are significantly enriched for the vitamin K–dependent clotting factors. A number of different methodologies for preparation of PCCs have been described, leading to a variety of products that have been available since the 1960s. Because PCCs contain large amounts of factor IX, they have been used in the treatment of hemophilia B. In addition, since PCCs contain all the vitamin K dependent–factors, they can achieve rapid reversal of overmedication with warfarin sodium without requiring the large volume and slow administration time of multiple FFP units. PCCs also have efficacy in overcoming factor VIII inhibitors, likely by a mechanism similar to that of rFVIIa, in which the extrinsic pathway promotes clotting in a FVIII–independent manner.

Although PCCs have good efficacy for promoting hemostasis in the context of an anti–factor VIII inhibitor, adverse events have been observed with a greater frequency than for other treatments such as rFVIIa.[29] Such events include thrombosis, thrombophlebitis, pulmonary embolism, and disseminated intravascular coagulation (DIC) and can lead to significant morbidity and mortality.[29] It has been argued that since the methodology for manufacturing PCCs has improved, adverse events are less frequent. Nonetheless, the safety profile of PCCs remains inferior to that of other treatments such as rFVIIa.

Treatment of Congenital Hemophilia B

Congenital hemophilia B is a deficiency of factor IX, for which the only existing therapy is replacement of factor IX with factor IX concentrates. Like factor VIII concentrates for the treatment of hemophilia A (see above), factor IX concentrates are available both as human plasma–derived product and as a recombinant human product expressed in tissue culture.[30] PCCs also contain considerable amounts of factor IX and were the mainstay of treatment for hemophilia B in the past. However, while PCCs can achieve hemostasis in a patient with factor IX deficiency, they are no longer the product of choice given the high rate of adverse thrombotic events described above.

The same issues of safety, efficacy, and cost apply to factor IX concentrates. Both plasma-derived and recombinant factor IX show excellent efficacy in the treatment of hemophilia B.[30] However, since the plasma-derived product comes from multiple donors, there is a risk of disease transmission. Purified factor IX is obtained from screened donors, and the product is subjected to treatments to inactivate known human pathogens. Nevertheless, the risk of infection, although low, is not zero. Moreover, emerging pathogens, which are not currently screened and against which the inactivation procedures may be ineffective, are a persistent concern. Thus, when possible, the recombinant factor is the product of choice.

Treatment of Factor XI Deficiency (Hemophilia C)

Deficiency of factor XI is a rare genetic disorder found predominantly in individuals of Ashkenazi Jewish or French Basques descent.[31,32] The bleeding diathesis that accompanies factor XI deficiency is typically milder than that seen in hemophilia A or B. However, bleeding can become a problem during invasive procedures, surgeries, dental procedures, childbirth, and injuries. Interestingly, the extent and frequency of bleeding does not correlate with the levels of factor XI.[31] Thus, a bleeding history is typically more predictive of the need for prophylaxis than a measurement of plasma factor XI levels alone. Treatment of factor XI deficiency can be achieved by infusing large volumes of fresh frozen plasma (FFP), often in combination with inhibitors of fibrinolysis.[33] Owing to the dilute nature of fresh frozen plasma (FFP), volume overload may be limiting. Although not currently available in the United States, there is a plasma-derived factor XI product.[34] However, use of plasma-derived factor XI concentrates has been associated with thrombosis in up to 10% of patients treated,[34] especially in the elderly, and DIC has also been observed. Thus, there is considerable risk to the use of factor XI concentrates. It has been suggested that treatment with inhibitors of fibrinolysis are therefore contraindicated in conjunction with factor XI concentrates. Recently, rFVIIa has shown potential efficacy in the treatment of both congenital factor XI deficiency and acquired deficiency due to anti-XI autoantibodies.[31,34–37]

Treatment of von Willebrand Disease (vWD)

von Willebrand factor (vWF) is a multifunctional protein that is intimately involved in platelet-initiated clotting at the site of vascular injury.[38,39] Through separate protein domains, vWF binds to subendothelial collagen that is exposed after vessel injury and to glycoprotein Ib on platelets. vWF is synthesized as a multimer, resulting in a high-avidity molecule with multiple binding sites. Thus, when multimeric vWF binds to collagen, it provides a high-avidity docking site for circulating platelets. In this way, vWF is the lynchpin of platelet-initiated clotting.

Defects in vWF result in disorders of platelet-based hemostasis, collectively referred to as vWD. A variety of mutations have resulted in the description of at least six distinct subtypes of vWD.[40] A detailed description of vWD subtypes is outside the scope of this chapter. However, specifics of each subtype will be referred to as they relate to factor-based replacement treatments.

Types 1 and 3 vWD are quantitative defects due to decreased levels of vWF. Type 1 has moderately decreased levels of vWF, whereas levels of vWF are extremely low or absent in type 3 vWD. Mature vWF is stored in the Weibel-Palade bodies of endothelial cells. The administration of DDAVP (desmopressin) results in a sudden release of vWF from the Weibel-Palade bodies. Thus, in the case of type 1 vWD, DDAVP may cause sufficient increases in endogenous vWF release such that no replacement therapy is needed. Since essentially no vWF is synthesized in type 3 vWD, DDAVP has no efficacy in this setting. Thus, administration of replacement vWF is indicated in type 3 vWD patients and in type 1 patients who do not have an adequate response to DDAVP or who require prolonged therapy. Type 2 vWD is a qualitative defect in which vWF levels are typically normal or only slightly decreased, but the function of vWF is defective.[41] Thus, DDAVP may have only limited efficacy in type 2 vWD, since higher levels of a malfunctioning molecule are being induced. In the case of type 2B vWD, DDAVP has been considered to be contraindicated because the defective vWF in this case has an increased binding affinity for platelets. Thus, increasing the levels of the pathologic vWF may induce thrombosis. There also can be a decrease in platelets in type 2B vWD patients after DDAVP administration. However, this relative contraindication has been challenged in some clinical settings, suggesting that DDAVP may have efficacy in type 2B vWD.[42,43]

In addition to the different subtypes of vWD, there is a platelet-type vWD (also called *pseudo-vWD*), which is similar to type 2B vWD because the disease is caused by an increased affinity between platelets and vWF. However, in the case of pseudo-vWD, it is a mutation in the glycoprotein Ib on the platelet membrane that causes the gain in affinity.[44] In this setting, appropriate treatment is the transfusion of normal platelets. The administration of vWF would have no efficacy, since it is not the vWF that is defective.

Current highly purified factor VIII preparations contain only low amounts of residual vWF, while less stringently purified factor VIII products maintain a large amount of functional vWF. In particular, Humate-P (Aventis Behring) is a purified VIII/vWF complex that is FDA approved for the treatment of vWD. Humate-P has excellent efficacy in all subtypes of vWD.[45–50] Humate-P is not used to treat pseudo (platelet-type) vWD, since this is a defect in glycoprotein Ib and not in vWF. As for all purified products, there is a residual risk of infectious disease. However, like most plasma-derived products, Humate-P undergoes pathogen inactivation. Currently, no recombinant form of vWF is available. Rare occurrences of thrombosis in vWD patients receiving Humate-P have been reported but are infrequent. Elevated levels of factor VIII in vWD patients may be a risk factor for thrombosis during Humate-P therapy.

Prior to the advent of Humate-P, cryoprecipitate was the replacement factor of choice for vWD, since the factor VIII/vWF complex is significantly enriched in cryoprecipitate. Thus, if Humate-P is unavailable, cryoprecipitate is a viable source of vWF for the treatment of vWD. However, because cryoprecipitate has less vWF and is not subjected to pathogen inactivation procedures, Humate-P should always be the treatment of choice.

Factor XIII

Factor XIII enzymatically crosslinks fibrin after clot formation. This cross-linking contributes significantly to the structural integrity of clots. Accordingly, deficiencies in factor XIII do not interfere with clot formation, but resulting clots are unusually fragile and therefore less effective in maintaining hemostasis.[51] The typical symptom is unusually delayed hemorrhaging after primary hemostasis is achieved.[51] Excessive bleeding from the cut umbilical cord of a newborn is associated with factor XIII deficiency.[52] In addition, there is an increased risk of intracranial hematoma formation.[51]

A recombinant form of factor XIII is currently in human clinical trials and not yet available in the United States. However, factor XIII purified from human plasma is available. As mentioned above, the risk of infection from donors is minimized by pathogen inactivation techniques, but it is not zero. In the absence of purified factor XIII, cryoprecipitate can be used because factor XIII is found in cryoprecipitate. However, since cryoprecipitate is not pathogen inactivated, purified factor XIII is the treatment of choice.

Fibrinogen

As described above, cryoprecipitate can be used as a source of concentrated factor VIII, vWF, and factor XIII when the corresponding purified factor preparations are unavailable. However, the purified factors are the preferred treatment, and cryoprecipitate is seldom substituted. In contrast, cryoprecipitate is the preferred method for replacing fibrinogen, since purified or recombinant factors are not available. Hypofibrinogenemia can be observed as a result of a congenital defect, hepatic disease, or a consumptive process. Cryoprecipitate is also useful in the treatment of bleeding secondary to inactivation of platelets by metabolic waste products that accumulate during renal failure (uremic platelet syndrome).[53] The risk of disease transmission is decreased by donor screening. However, since cryoprecipitate does not routinely undergo pathogen inactivation, chronic use of cryoprecipitate is not recommended when a purified factor product is available (e.g., Humate-P for vWD).

Factors Used to Treat Thrombophilia and Sepsis

Antithrombin

Antithrombin (AT), also called *antithrombin III*, is a naturally occurring protease inhibitor that serves to maintain balance in the coagulation system predominantly by inactivating a number of coagulation factors, including IIa and Xa. In addition, enhancement of AT activity is the mechanism by which heparin achieves its anticoagulant effect. Antithrombin levels can be decreased by a congenital defect or a consumptive process. In either case, AT purified from human plasma is commercially available. In addition to its role as an anticoagulant, AT has anti-inflammatory properties.[54] There is interest in the use of AT to treat the inflammatory component of conditions such as sepsis.[55] As for other purified plasma products, the risk of infectious disease transmission is minimized by pathogen inactivation techniques.

Activated Protein C

Protein C is a natural anticoagulant that, together with its cofactor protein S, inactivates coagulation factors Va and VIIIa. There is a recombinant form of activated protein C (APC) that is available for use in humans (Xigris). However, APC is not used to treat the thrombophilia of protein C deficiency, which is typically managed by pharmacologic anticoagulation or protein C replacement (see below). Rather, APC is FDA approved for use in the treatment of adults with severe sepsis only when such patients have a high risk of death as defined by the APACHE II criteria.[56] Although prospective clinical trials have demonstrated that use of APC increases survival in this population,[57] it is not clear whether this is due to anticoagulant activity, since APC also has anti-inflammatory and anti-apoptotic properties. However, while the mechanism of efficacy in treating sepsis may or may not involve APCs anticoagulant properties, such properties appear to be involved in APC toxicity, since bleeding is the most serious side effect of APC use. Accordingly, APC is contraindicated in patients with increased risk of bleeding in anatomically fragile sites such as the central nervous system. Such conditions were exclusion criteria from the phase III trial of APC for treating sepsis.[57]

Protein C Concentrates

Plasma-derived protein C concentrates have been produced in Europe for the treatment of congenital protein C deficiency.[57–59] The heterozygous form of the deficiency is one of the classic causes of congenital thrombophilia but rarely needs protein C replacement, since most patients are adults and the deficiency is controlled by oral anticoagulant therapy. The homozygous form of the disease causes severe thrombotic events, often at birth, and protein C concentrate can be lifesaving in this setting.[57–59] Although not yet FDA approved, the product may be acquired for compassionate use in the United States.

Recombinant Thrombomodulin

Thrombomodulin is an endothelial cell surface protein that binds thrombin and activates protein C, which subsequently downregulates thrombin generation by inactivating factors V and VIII.[60] It is being developed for the treatment of septic DIC in a way that parallels the use of the recombinant activated protein C mentioned previously.[61]

REFERENCES

1. Evatt B, Austin H, Leon G, Ruiz-Saez A, de Bosch N. Hemophilia treatment: Predicting the long-term risk of HIV exposure by cryoprecipitate. Haemophilia 2000;6(Suppl 1):128–132.
2. Schlesinger KW, Ragni MV. Safety of the new generation recombinant factor concentrates. Expert Opin Drug Saf 2002;1:213–223.
3. Kasper CK. Concentrate safety and efficacy. Haemophilia 2002;8:161.
4. Tarantino MD, Collins PW, Hay CR, et al, and RAHF-PFM Clinical Study Group. Clinical evaluation of an advanced category antihaemophilic factor prepared using a plasma/albumin-free method: pharmacokinetics, efficacy, and safety in previously treated patients with haemophilia A. Haemophilia 2004;10:428–437.
5. Osterberg T, Fatouros A, Mikaelsson M. Development of freeze-dried albumin-free formulation of recombinant factor VIII SQ. Pharm Res 1997;14:892.
6. Ewenstein BM, Collins P, Tarantino MD, et al. Hemophilia therapy innovation: development of an advanced category recombinant factor VIII by a plasma/albumin-free method. Proceedings of a Special Symposium at the XIXth Congress of the International Society on Thrombosis and Haemostasis, July 12–18, 2003, Birmingham, U.K. Semin Hematol 2004;41:1.
7. Ironside JW, Head MW. Variant Creutzfeldt-Jakob disease: risk of transmission by blood and blood products. Haemophilia 2004;4:64.
8. Cervenakova L, Brown P, Hammond DJ, Lee CA, Saenko EL. Factor VIII and transmissible spongiform encephalopathy: the case for safety. Haemophilia 2002;8:63.
9. Brackmann HH, Aygoren E, Scharrer I, Schwaab R, Hammerstein U, Oldenburg J. Two years' experience with two recombinant factor VIII concentrates. Blood Coagul Fibrinolysis 1993;4:421–424.
10. Shopnick RI, Kazemi M, Brettler DB, et al. Anaphylaxis after treatment with recombinant factor VIII. Transfusion 1996;36:358.
11. Lusher J, Abildgaard C, Arkin S, et al. Human recombinant DNA-derived antihemophilic factor in the treatment of previously untreated patients with hemophilia A: final report on a hallmark clinical investigation. J Thromb Haemost 2004;2:574–583.
12. Prowse CV, MacGregor IR. Neoantigens and antibodies to factor VIII. Blood Rev 1998;12:99.
13. Soucie JM, Erdman DD, Evatt BL, et al. Investigation of porcine parvovirus among persons with hemophilia receiving Hyate:C porcine factor VIII concentrate. Transfusion 2000;40:708.
14. Paul PS, Halbur P, Janke B, et al. Exogenous porcine viruses. Curr Top Microbiol Immunol 2003;278:125.
15. Lusher JM. First and second generation recombinant factor VIII concentrates in previously untreated patients: recovery, safety, efficacy, and inhibitor development. Semin Thromb Hemost 2002;28:273–276.
16. Nishino M, Yoshioka A. The revised classification of von Willebrand disease including the previously masqueraded female hemophilia A (type 2N) [erratum in Int J Hematol 1997;66:31]. Int J Hematol 1997;66:21.
17. Jacquemin MG, Saint-Remy JM. Factor VIII alloantibodies in hemophilia. Curr Opin Hematol 2004;11:146.
18. Zakarija A, Green D. Acquired hemophilia: diagnosis and management. Curr Hematol Rep 2002;1:27.
19. Lee CA. The evidence behind inhibitor treatment with porcine factor VIII. Pathophysiol Haemost Thromb 2002;1:5.
20. Garvey MB. Porcine factor VIII in the treatment of high-titre inhibitor patients. Haemophilia 2002;1:5.
21. Ghorashian S, Hunt BJ. "Off-license" use of recombinant activated factor VII. Blood Rev 2004;18:245.
22. Midathada MV, Mehta P, Waner M, Fink LM. Recombinant factor VIIa in the treatment of bleeding. Am J Clin Pathol 2004;121:124.
23. Hedner U. NovoSeven as a universal haemostatic agent. Blood Coagul Fibrinolysis 2000;11(Suppl 1):S107–S111.
24. Basso IN, Keeling D. Myocardial infarction following recombinant activated factor VII in a patient with type 2A von Willebrand disease. Blood Coagul Fibrinolysis 2004;15:503.
25. Hayashi T, Tanaka I, Shima M, et al. Unresponsiveness to factor VIII inhibitor bypassing agents during haemostatic treatment for life-threatening massive bleeding in a patient with haemophilia A and a high responding inhibitor. Haemophilia 2004;10:397.
26. Roberts HR, Monroe DM III, Hoffman M. Safety profile of recombinant factor VIIa. Semin Hematol 2004;41:101.
27. Clark AD, Gordon WC, Walker ID, Tait RC. 'Last-ditch' use of recombinant factor VIIa in patients with massive haemorrhage is ineffective. Vox Sang 2004;86:120.
28. Zimring JC. Appropriate use of recombinant factor VIIa: an expanding and unanswered question [see comment]. Transfusion 2004;44:1544.
29. Kohler M. Thrombogenicity of prothrombin complex concentrates. Thromb Res 1999;95:15.
30. Di Paola J. Product selection issues in the management of hemophilia B. Blood Coagul Fibrinolysis 2004;15(Suppl 2):S17–S18.
31. O'Connell NM. Factor XI deficiency—from molecular genetics to clinical management. Blood Coagul Fibrinolysis 2003;14(Suppl 1):S59–S64.
32. Kitchens CS. Factor XI: a review of its biochemistry and deficiency. Semin Thromb Hemost 1991;17:55–72.
33. Bolton-Maggs PH. Factor XI deficiency and its management. Haemophilia 2000;1:100.
34. Salomon O, Seligsohn U. New observations on factor XI deficiency. Haemophilia 2004;4:184.
35. Bern MM, Sahud M, Zhukov O, Qu K, Mitchell W Jr. Treatment of factor XI inhibitor using recombinant activated factor VIIa. Haemophilia 2005;11:20.
36. Lawler P, White B, Pye S, et al. Successful use of recombinant factor VIIa in a patient with inhibitor secondary to severe factor XI deficiency. Haemophilia 2002;8:145.
37. Billon S, Le Niger C, Escoffre-Barbe M, Vicariot M, Abgrall JF. The use of recombinant factor VIIa (NovoSeven) in a patient with a factor XI deficiency and a circulating anticoagulant. Blood Coagul Fibrinolysis 2001;12:551.
38. Meyer D, Girma JP. von Willebrand factor: structure and function. Thromb Haemost 1993;70:99.
39. Ruggeri ZM. Structure of von Willebrand factor and its function in platelet adhesion and thrombus formation. Best Pract Res Clin Haematol 2001;14:257–279.
40. Ruggeri ZM. Structure and function of von Willebrand factor: relationship to von Willebrand's disease. Mayo Clin Proc 1991;66:847.
41. Fressinaud E, Mazurier C, Meyer D. Molecular genetics of type 2 von Willebrand disease. Int J Hematol 2002;75:9.
42. Casonato A, Steffan A, Pontara E, et al. Post-DDAVP thrombocytopenia in type 2B von Willebrand disease is not associated with platelet consumption: failure to demonstrate glycocalicin increase or platelet activation. Thromb Haemost 1999;81:224.
43. McKeown LP, Connaghan G, Wilson O, Hansmann K, Merryman P, Gralnick H. 1-Desamino-8- arginine-vasopressin corrects the hemostatic defects in type 2B von Willebrand's disease. Am J Hematol 1996;51:158.
44. Tait AS, Cranmer SL, Jackson SP, Dawes IW, Chong BH. Phenotype changes resulting in high-affinity binding of von Willebrand factor to recombinant glycoprotein Ib-IX: analysis of the platelet-type von Willebrand disease mutations. Blood 2001;98:1812.
45. Czapek EE, Gadarowski JJ Jr, Ontiveros JD, Pedraza JL. Humate-P for treatment of von Willebrand disease. Blood 1988;72:1100.
46. Thompson AR, Gill JC, Ewenstein BM, Mueller-Velten G, Schwartz BA, Humate PSG. Successful treatment for patients with von Willebrand disease undergoing urgent surgery using factor VIII/VWF concentrate (Humate-P). Haemophilia 2004;10:42.
47. Gill JC, Ewenstein BM, Thompson AR, Mueller-Velten G, Schwartz BA, Humate PSG. Successful treatment of urgent bleeding in von Willebrand disease with factor VIII/VWF concentrate (Humate-P): use of the ristocetin cofactor assay (VWF:RCo) to measure potency and to guide therapy. Haemophilia 2003;9:688.
48. Lillicrap D, Poon MC, Walker I, Xie F, Schwartz BA; Association of Hemophilia Clinic Directors of Canada. Efficacy and safety of the factor VIII/von Willebrand factor concentrate, haemate-P/humate-P: ristocetin cofactor unit dosing in patients with von Willebrand disease. Thromb Haemost 2002;87:224–230.
49. Dobrkovska A, Krzensk U, Chediak JR. Pharmacokinetics, efficacy and safety of Humate-P in von Willebrand disease. Haemophilia 1998;3:33.
50. Berntorp E, Nilsson IM. Use of a high-purity factor VIII concentrate (Hemate P) in von Willebrand's disease. Vox Sang 1989;56:212.
51. Board PG, Losowsky MS, Miloszewski KJ. Factor XIII: inherited and acquired deficiency. Blood Rev 1993;7:229.
52. Anwar R, Minford A, Gallivan L, Trinh CH, Markham AF. Delayed umbilical bleeding—a presenting feature for factor XIII deficiency: clinical features, genetics, and management. Pediatrics 2002;109:E32.

53. Couch P, Stumpf JL. Management of uremic bleeding [see comment]. Clin Pharm 1990;9:673.
54. Wiedermann ChJ, Romisch J. The anti-inflammatory actions of antithrombin—a review. Acta Medica Austriaca 2002;29:89–92.
55. Opal SM. Therapeutic rationale for antithrombin III in sepsis. Crit Care Med 2000;28(9 Suppl):S34–S37.
56. Parrillo JE. Severe sepsis and therapy with activated protein C [see comment]. N Engl J Med 2005;353:1398.
57. Bernard GR, Vincent JL, Laterre PF, et al. Recombinant human protein C Worldwide Ev aluation in Severe Sepsis (PROWESS) study group. Efficacy and safety of recombinant human activated protein C for severe sepsis [see comment]. N Engl J Med 2001;344:699–709.
58. Salonvaara M, Kuismanen K, Mononen T, Riikonen P. Diagnosis and treatment of a newborn with homozygous protein C deficiency. Acta Paediatrica 2004;93:137.
59. Sanz-Rodriguez C, Gil-Fernandez JJ, Zapater P, et al. Long-term management of homozygous protein C deficiency: replacement therapy with subcutaneous purified protein C concentrate. Thromb Haemost 1999;81:887.
60. Van de Wouwer M, Collen D, Conway EM. Thrombomodulin-protein C-EPCR system: integrated to regulate coagulation and inflammation. Arterioscler Thromb Vasc Biol 2004;24:1374–1383.
61. Maruyama I. Recombinant thrombomodulin and activated protein C in the treatment of disseminated intravascular coagulation. Thromb Haemost 1999;82:718.

Chapter 26

Leukocyte-Reduced Products

Walter H. Dzik • Zbigniew M. Szczepiorkowski

Recipient exposure to allogeneic donor leukocytes can result in several complications of blood transfusion. To reduce the likelihood of these complications, leukoreduction of red blood cells (RBCs) and platelets is widely practiced. This chapter addresses the basis for the adverse effects of recipient exposure to donor leukocytes and presents the evidence supporting the scientific foundation for leukoreduction of cellular blood products. In particular, we address the biophysical mechanisms involved in the preparation of leukoreduced RBCs and platelets and the biologic mechanisms accounting for febrile nonhemolytic reactions, primary human leukocyte antigen (HLA) alloimmunization, transmission and reactivation of cytomegalovirus (CMV), transfusion-associated immunosuppression, and the adverse effects from transfusion of leukoreduced blood. The reader is referred to other sources for a discussion of additional aspects of leukoreduction, including device evaluations, quality control and cell-counting methods, cost effectiveness, and operational issues.[1–3]

TECHNOLOGIES FOR THE PREPARATION OF LEUKOREDUCED BLOOD

Achieving a 10,000-fold reduction in the leukocyte content of blood requires specialized technologies of leukofiltration or apheresis collection. Numerous factors affect the performance of leukofiltration, including the temperature of filtration, the speed of blood flow through the filter, the number of leukocytes presented to the filter, the protein content of the suspending medium, the platelet content of blood, the use of a rinse step after filtration, the storage age of the blood, and the presence of hemoglobin S in the RBCs to be filtered. Standards in the United States require that leukoreduced components be prepared by a method known to reduce donor leukocytes to residual levels of $<5 \times 10^6$ white blood cells (WBCs) per unit for RBCs and apheresis platelets and $<8.3 \times 10^5$ WBCs/unit for whole blood–derived platelets. Methods to produce leukoreduced apheresis platelets should produce products with $>3 \times 10^{11}$ platelets.

Leukofilter Device Design

Removal of leukocytes from whole blood, packed RBCs, or platelets depends on a combination of barrier filtration and cell adsorption to the filter material. Certain principles of design are common to leukofiltration devices.[4] A large surface area of filter medium is required to allow sufficient opportunity for contact of blood leukocytes with the medium. This requirement for surface area can be met through the use of filter media composed of fibers with a very small diameter (microfibers) or open-cell media that are geometrically like a sponge.

Two different approaches to manufacturing such nonwoven media have been commercially viable. The first is a dry formation process in which a polymer (typically a polyester or polyolefin) is melted and extruded through very fine nozzles into a turbulent gas stream at high velocity to produce a microfiber. The synthetic microfiber is simultaneously stretched and cooled to form thin strands of fibers in a process akin to the making of cotton candy. The microfibers are then collected, matted, and heat compressed to a controlled density. Some variation of this basic technique is used in products from Pall Corporation, Asahi Medical Company, Fresenius AG, and MacoPharma, among others.

A second approach is to prepare superfine glass fiber membranes.[5] Foam-like structures with open-cell geometry contain interconnecting voids that allow a circuitous flow passage. The manufacture of such media derives from principles used in the manufacture of sponges. For example, filters from Terumo Corporation are made with the use of a porous polyurethane medium that exhibits an open-cell architecture.

Because they offer an effective pore size that is extremely small, filter media must be designed to have a hydrophilic surface. Otherwise, the material will fail to "wet" as blood encounters the medium owing to the inherent surface tension of blood. The synthetic materials used in leukoreduction filters—polyester and polyolefin microfibers, porous polyurethane, and glass microfibers—are all naturally hydrophobic. Manufacturers modify the surface chemistry of these materials to increase their ability to "wet." Although prefiltration rinsing with a more hydrophilic liquid (e.g., saline rinse) can wet the filter medium, prerinsing introduces an inconvenience that manufacturers of filters generally wish to avoid.

The volume of blood left inside the filter after filtration is referred to as the "hold-up volume." Filters that have a hard external housing often include a venting step at the end of filtration, which allows sterile air to enter the filter and displace blood that would otherwise have been held up in the device. One manufacturer (MacoPharma, Tourcoing, France) packages the filter medium in a flexible plastic housing that collapses under atmospheric pressure as blood drains out of the filter. U.S. Food and Drug Administration (FDA) guidelines require that the filtration process result in loss of no more than 15% of the original amount of therapeutic blood elements.[6]

The filtration medium is packaged in an external housing, and it is essential that the medium completely fill the housing, allowing no opportunity for the path of blood to flow around the filter (bypass) and thereby circumvent the leukodepletion medium. To appreciate the stringency required, consider that the leukocyte content of an entire unit of leukoreduced RBC is equal to the leukocyte content of only one drop (100 μL) of nonleukoreduced blood.

Mechanisms of Leukoreduction

Barrier Filtration

Simple barrier filtration, in which the effective pore size of the filter medium is smaller than the size of the leukocyte, is a major mechanism used by leukoreduction filters. Modern leukoreduction filters have an effective pore size on the order of 4 μm. This space is sufficient for passage of platelets and deformable erythrocytes but is able to retain leukocytes. Because effective leukoreduction by barrier-based filtration is tightly linked to the deformability of blood cells, factors affecting cell deformability have an impact on filter performance. Increased leukocyte deformability at higher temperatures probably accounts for the poorer performance of leukofiltration when it is applied to room temperature RBCs compared with refrigerated RBCs (see Biophysical Reasons for Reduced Performance of Leukofiltration, below).

Cell Adhesion

Contact-mediated adhesion between leukocytes and the filter medium also contributes to the performance of leukofiltration devices. For contact to occur, there must be a sufficient dwell time of the blood with the medium. For the cells not to detach from the medium, shear forces of the flowing blood must not be too strong. High flow rates can result in insufficient contact and excess detachment of leukocytes from the medium. Because cell adhesion to filter media involves a complex surface chemistry that is not fully understood, filter media development has been largely determined by experimentation. The nature of the fluid in which cells are suspended, including the plasma protein content and the platelet content, affects the adhesion of leukocytes to synthetic media. Steneker[7] demonstrated that during leukofiltration of fresh RBCs the presence of viable platelets improves the performance of leukofiltration. This has been attributed to sticking of platelets to protein-coated fibers in the filter medium, with subsequent binding of leukocytes to these activated platelets. Ledent and Berlin[8] demonstrated that replacement of plasma with crystalloid can decrease the performance of leukofiltration, presumably by decreasing the concentration of adhesive plasma proteins that participate in leukocyte adhesion to the medium.

Leukofiltration of platelet concentrates presents the added complexity that platelets are naturally adhesive under shear conditions in a plasma environment, as a result of von Willebrand factor–mediated platelet adhesion. Therefore, manufacturers of leukoreduction filters designed for platelets have further modified the surface chemistry of the filter media to decrease binding of platelets to the filter. For example, Nishimura and colleagues[9] documented that by adjusting the molar ratio of positively charged diethyl-amino ethyl methacrylate to negatively charged hydroxyethyl methacrylate, the net surface charge on the filter medium could be adjusted to optimize leukocyte adhesion but minimize platelet adhesion to the medium.

Biophysical Reasons for Reduced Performance of Leukofiltration

The reduced efficiency of leukofiltration applied to warmed RBCs compared with cold RBCs has repeatedly been demonstrated. For example, Beaujean and coworkers[10] split RBCs (storage age, 2 to 10 days) into two equal aliquots, which were then filtered at either 4°C or 37°C. The mean postfiltration leukocyte content was 10-fold higher for units filtered at 37°C. Ledent and Berlin[8] found leukocyte content to be 100-fold higher among units filtered at 37°C compared with 4°C. Sirchia and colleagues[11] studied filtration under conditions designed to mimic bedside use. They found that cold RBCs warmed to room temperature within 90 minutes after removal of the units from the refrigerator. They also documented that as the blood warmed, filtration performance declined, and units failed to meet minimum standards for leukoreduced blood ($<5 \times 10^6$ WBCs/unit). The failure was striking with units containing as much as 100-fold more leukocytes than the upper threshold level for leukoreduction. The performance failure associated with bedside leukoreduction is very important to the interpretation of major clinical trials of leukoreduction technology. For example, both the CMV prevention trial of Bowden and associates[12] and the HLA alloimmunization trial of Williamson and coworkers[13] used bedside filtration with filters subsequently determined to have reduced performance under warm conditions. The performance of newer versions of leukoreduction filters may be less sensitive to temperature. Van der Meer and colleagues demonstrated enhanced performance at 4°C, but the difference between the results at 4°C and at 22°C was less than that seen in earlier studies.[14]

Several other factors may reduce the effectiveness of leukofiltration. Excess shear force and resulting cell detachment from the filter medium may be an important consideration when bedside leukofiltration is combined with mechanical blood delivery systems that may "pull" blood through the filter at excessive rates. Postfiltration rinsing of filters may also occur during bedside transfusion and has been documented to result in leukocyte detachment. Filtration of excessive volumes of blood or of blood containing excessive numbers of leukocytes can overwhelm the capacity of the filter medium, leading to ineffective leukoreduction.

Leukofiltration of RBCs has been shown to be less effective if the donor blood carries hemoglobin AS (sickle trait).[15,16] Poor leukofiltration is believed to result from reduced red cell deformability among hemoglobin AS erythrocytes under conditions of reduced oxygen tension and pH, such as occur within the filter. Stroncek and colleagues showed that increasing the oxygen tension of hemoglobin AS blood prevented the poor filtration performance.[16] Decreased deformability of red cells containing hemoglobin S at low oxygen tensions is presumed either to directly "clog" the filter or to reduce the effective area of filter medium available for retention of leukocytes. Because sickle trait is relatively common in some donor populations, the frequency of failure of leukoreduction by filtration may be higher than expected.

Leukoreduced Components Prepared by Apheresis

Modern apheresis devices are able to collect concentrates of platelets or RBCs that are leukoreduced during collection; this is referred to as process leukoreduction. Several devices are licensed for collection of one or more components (for review see ref. 17).

The Amicus apheresis system (Baxter Healthcare, Round Lake, Ill.) is a widely used apheresis system for the preparation of leukoreduced platelets. The device incorporates three design features to achieve leukoreduction: active interface control, autoelutriation, and fluid flow dynamics. An optical interface detector is positioned within the separation chamber to monitor changes in the platelet interface. The system recirculates some of the donor plasma into the interface in order to separate platelets from leukocytes by elutriation. Just as a wind blows lightweight leaves but not heavy objects across a street, plasma pumped through the interface dislodges the platelets but not the leukocytes into the collection path. The collection path for platelet collection is in the opposite direction to the flow path for the return of RBCs and plasma to the donor, promoting further separation between donor platelets and donor leukocytes.

The Trima Accel automated system separates platelets from donor whole blood using a single-stage channel design. Whole blood enters the channel and separates under centrifugation into component layers. Platelets are drawn out through a specially designed conical-shaped chamber (LRS chamber) while plasma and RBCs are returned to the donor. The LRS chamber, originally developed for the COBE Spectra System, combines centrifugal separation technology with saturated fluidized particle-bed dynamics to achieve a natural separation of WBCs from platelets. White cells are separated from the platelets according to the fluid dynamics of the separation chamber, the sedimentation velocity of the platelet and white cell components, and the plasma flow rate through the chamber. These dynamics result in a flow geometry that traps donor leukocytes in the lower levels of the LRS chamber while allowing platelets in the upper levels of the chamber to exit toward the platelet collection/storage bag. Under some donor collection conditions, leukocytes can spill out of the chamber into the collection product. The Trima System uses a computerized on-line process that monitors for conditions known to increase the risk of WBC contamination in the platelet product.

Quality Control of Leukoreduction

Because any leukoreduction process may fail, standards for quality control testing exist. No common standard exists for all nations, however. For example, in the United States the American Association of Blood Banks standards require that 95% of the units sampled meet threshold requirements for residual leukocyte content.[18] In Europe, the threshold level of residual leukocytes is $<1 \times 10^6$/unit.[19] Validation of new leukoreduction methods or devices and ongoing quality control evaluation requires counting methods specifically designed for the extremely low concentration of white cells found in leukoreduced blood components. A variety of techniques are available based on microscopy, flow cytometry, and the polymerase chain reaction.[20] No standards address the relative proportion of residual leukocyte subpopulations in leukoreduced blood. Although different leukocyte subpopulations are relevant for different biologic effects attributed to donor leukocytes, there is no convincing clinical outcomes evidence that any particular leukoreduction technique is superior to any other for removal of specific leukocyte subpopulations.[21,22] Currently, all methods of leukoreduction that meet the threshold standard for total number of residual donor leukocytes are considered equivalent.

In addition to the reduced performance of leukofiltration resulting from filtration at higher temperature or in the presence of hemoglobin S blood, quality control studies of leukoreduction have documented occasional process problems with both leukofiltration and apheresis technologies. For example, Kao and colleagues[23] reported quality control data from the Trial to Reduce Alloimmunization to Platelets (TRAP). Using a propidium iodide stain and microscopic chamber counting, they found that 7% of apheresis platelets and 5% of pooled platelets contained more than 5×10^6 residual donor leukocytes. For RBCs, 0.3% to 2.7% of units failed to meet leukoreduction standards depending on the particular leukofilter used. In addition, they reported substantial losses of platelets and RBCs as a result of the process of leukofiltration. Although quality control monitoring of apheresis platelets documents reliable performance of collection systems,[17] as with leukofiltration, the apheresis process can fail. Sudden changes in the rate of blood entering the machine or pauses in blood flow during collection will disturb the centrifugal separation of blood in the chambers and may interrupt the controlled flow paths upon which the cells travel during separation. These interruptions can lead to "spillover" of leukocytes into the platelet collection stream. Manufacturers have attempted to engineer alarms into the software that will alert operators to conditions that might result in the failure to collect a leukoreduced product. The leukocyte content of these collections can then be tested to determine whether the product is leukoreduced. Although refinements in filter design and apheresis technology have improved leukoreduction, there remains value in continuous quality monitoring of blood component preparation and modification.

CLINICAL INDICATIONS FOR LEUKOREDUCED BLOOD COMPONENTS

Three prominent clinical indications for leukoreduced cellular blood components are (1) to reduce the frequency of febrile nonhemolytic transfusion reactions among patients with a prior history of such reactions, (2) to decrease the incidence of HLA sensitization and platelet refractoriness among patients with hematologic malignancy, and (3) to reduce the risk of transfusion-transmitted CMV infection among susceptible recipients[24] (Box 26–1). Leukocyte-reduction technology has also been applied to other clinical situations in the absence of strong evidence but with an expectation of benefit.

Universal Leukoreduction

Use of leukocyte reduction for all cellular components is controversial[25] (Box 26–2). Several countries adopted policies

BOX 26–1 ***Indications for Leukoreduced Blood Components***

- Reduce rate of recurrent febrile nonhemolytic transfusion reactions (FNHTRs)
- Reduce rate of HLA alloimmunization among hematology-oncology patients
- Reduce rate of cytomegalovirus transmission to susceptible recipients

BOX 26–2 *Pros and Cons of Universal Leukoreduction*

Pro:

- Patients with selected indications to receive leukoreduced blood will be more likely to receive leukoreduced units
- Inventory management is streamlined

Con:

- Large clinical studies fail to demonstrate clear or consistent benefit of leukoreduction on proposed transfusion-associated immunosuppression
- Adds >$500 million each year to health care costs
- May adversely affect adequacy of blood supply in setting of recalls of leukoreduction devices; may interfere with supply of blood donors of African ancestry (sickle trait blood)
- Removes physician choice from product selection

in favor of universal leukoreduction for different reasons. The decision was linked to a program of hemovigilance in France, to concern over the potential for spread of transmissible spongiform encephalopathies by donor leukocytes in the United Kingdom, and to a general reorganization of blood services in Canada. In the United States, the Blood Product Advisory Committee of the FDA voted in 1998 in favor of universal leukoreduction in the absence of any consideration of cost to the health care system and sponsored a conference in 1999 that was geared toward implementation of universal leukoreduction. However, such implementation was never mandated, and studies estimated that universal leukoreduction would cost more than $500 million per year in the United States with uncertain benefit. Nevertheless, despite the absence of any regulatory mandate, some major blood suppliers in the United States elected to sell only leukoreduced products, and thus the proportion of leukoreduced blood components has gradually increased to more than 50% in the United States.

The potential benefit of universal leukoreduction among surgical patients was investigated in a retrospective multicenter study conducted in Canada.[26] The study was not a prospective randomized trial, but rather compared outcomes in two cohorts of patients—one cohort transfused prior to the implementation of universal leukoreduction ($N = 6982$) and the other cohort transfused after universal leukoreduction ($N = 7804$). The study did not examine outcomes among all transfusion recipients (universal impact) but rather focused on three groups of more critically ill patients: those with trauma, those undergoing cardiac surgery, and those undergoing major orthopedic surgery. Because these patient groups receive large numbers of transfusions, they were expected to be most likely to demonstrate any beneficial effect of leukoreduction. Prior to adjustment for potential confounders the authors found a slightly lower risk of overall mortality (unadjusted odds ratio = 0.87, 95% CI, 0.76–0.99, $P = 0.04$) among cohort 2 (leukoreduced group). However, when the results were adjusted for the effects of cardiac medications, the adjusted odds ratio failed to show a statistically significant benefit for leukoreduction. Moreover, within each of the three major patient categories studied (trauma, cardiac surgery, orthopedic surgery), the adjusted odds of death were not statistically different in the cohort of patients receiving leukoreduced components compared with the cohort receiving control RBCs. Finally, it was noted that unadjusted mortality rates also declined among *nontransfused* patients during the two periods of observation. Major secondary outcomes included infections, length of stay in intensive care, or total hospital length of stay—none of which were statistically different in the two cohorts of patients. In particular, the authors noted that the lack of effect on infectious complications argued against a transfusion-related immunosuppression effect. No difference was seen in the two groups for the proportion of patients requiring ventilation support, hemodynamic support, or renal dialysis. In addition, there was no observed beneficial effect of leukoreduction among the subgroups of patients receiving larger doses of blood (>5 units per patient) compared with those receiving fewer transfusions.

One large prospective randomized clinical trial specifically examined the potential benefit of conversion from selective leukoreduction to universal leukoreduction.[27] This single center study randomized 2780 patients to receive either prestorage leukoreduced RBCs and prestorage leukoreduced apheresis platelets (for patients needing platelets) versus nonleukoreduced RBCs (buffy coat not removed) and nonleukoreduced pooled whole blood–derived platelets. All patients (adult, pediatric, medical, and surgical) not meeting standard criteria for leukoreduced blood (see Box 26–1) were eligible. Because individual patient consent was not required, the study had the advantage that all eligible candidates were automatically enrolled (no exclusions). The primary outcome measures were in-hospital mortality, length-of-stay in hospital following transfusion, and total hospital costs. The study found no difference among primary outcomes for patients assigned to leukoreduced versus nonleukoreduced blood components. This large trial was powered to have an 85% chance to detect a 15% difference in the primary outcome with a 95% confidence. Several secondary outcomes were examined all of which also showed no benefit to leukoreduction. These included antibiotic use to treat infection following transfusion (all patients) or to treat postoperative infection (surgical subset), length of stay in intensive care, postoperative length of stay, or readmission rates to hospital. There was a statistically nonsignificant trend toward fewer febrile nonhemolytic reactions in the group assigned to receive leukoreduced blood. Subset analysis restricted to heavily transfused patients failed to show any advantage for leukoreduced blood. The study provided randomized, controlled trial evidence for a lack of measurable benefit resulting from conversion to universal leukoreduction.

Prevention of Febrile Nonhemolytic Transfusion Reactions by Leukoreduction

One of the first indications for the use of leukocyte filters was prevention of febrile nonhemolytic transfusion reactions (FNHTRs). Original studies suggested that the frequency of FNHTRs to packed RBCs is reduced when the residual leukocyte content is less than 5×10^8 WBCs/unit.[28–32] Although FNHTRs are one of the most common transfusion reactions experienced by recipients of blood components, they are also relatively easy to manage. Many, but not all, FNHTRs can be prevented by leukoreduction of blood components.

Fever is a hallmark and part of the clinical definition of FNHTR. In addition to fever, patients may experience chills, rigors, cold, a sense of discomfort, headache, and nausea. Because the pathophysiology of fever involves a rigor/chill response before the temperature rises, the initial signs of an FNHTR may be only rigors without temperature elevation. Therefore, the presence of early-onset fever should not be required to diagnose an FNHTR.[33,34] FNHTRs tend to develop toward the end of a transfusion, and in 10% to 20% of cases reactions are noted after the transfusion has been discontinued. Such clinical observations underline the fact that reactions are dose related and require time to develop.

Pathophysiology of Fever

Fever is one of the oldest signs and symptoms recognized in medicine. Fever results from cytokine generation by activated monocytes, macrophages, and Kupffer cells. The involved cytokines, including interleukin-1β (IL-1β), IL-6, interferon-β (IFN-β), and tumor necrosis factor-α (TNF-α), are polypeptides that act on the organum vasculosum of lamina terminalis (OVLT).[35] The OVLT interacts with the preoptic area of the hypothalamus. In the case of TNFα, the induction of cyclooxygenase-2 in brain blood vessels leads to increased production of prostaglandins (mainly prostaglandin E_2)[36] and subsequently to fever.[37] Engel and associates[38] reported the peripheral blood levels of cytokines measured in patients with fever and neutropenia. The median peak concentration for IL-6 was 400 pg/mL (range, 100 to 41,000 pg/mL); for IL-8, it was 1025 pg/mL (range, 600 to 26,000 pg/mL); for TNFα, less than 10 pg/mL; and for IL-1β, 17 pg/mL (range, <10 to 36 pg/mL).

Incidence and Mechanisms of FNHTR

The reported incidence of FNHTR depends on the transfused component. Transfusions of nonleukoreduced RBCs are associated with 0.5% to 6.0% risk, whereas transfusions of platelet concentrates carry a risk as high as 20% to 30%.[39–41] This significant difference between RBCs and platelet concentrates can be attributed to different mechanisms involved in development of febrile reactions.

FNHTR CAUSED BY DESTRUCTION OF TRANSFUSED DONOR LEUKOCYTES

First proposed in the 1960s, the original hypothesized mechanism suggests that donor leukocytes react with recipient antileukocyte antibodies, causing the donor cells to release endogenous pyrogens (cytokines) (Fig. 26–1). This mechanism is consistent with the prevention of FNHTRs by leukoreduction of donor blood, and it is supported by studies of de Rie and colleagues,[42] Decary and colleagues,[43] Perkins and colleagues,[44] Brubaker,[45] and others[46] that documented the high prevalence of antilymphocyte or antigranulocyte antibodies in the sera of patients who experienced FNHTRs. However, the mechanism fails to account for the fact that FNHTRs are more common among recipients of platelets compared with packed RBCs, and it failed to explain the observation that FNHTRs may occur among men with no history of prior transfusions. In addition, the mechanism can be challenged because leukocytes are not known to store IL-1 and TNF[47] suitable for "immediate release" upon destruction by recipient antibody. Finally, the original mechanism fails to explain why patients with anti-HLA antibodies have febrile reactions when transfused with leukocyte-reduced platelet concentrates.

FNHTRS CAUSED BY PASSIVE TRANSFER OF CYTOKINES

In a series of simple and well-designed experiments, Heddle and associates[48] focused attention on the plasma constituent of stored platelet concentrates, rather than the platelets themselves, as the source of febrile reactions after transfu-

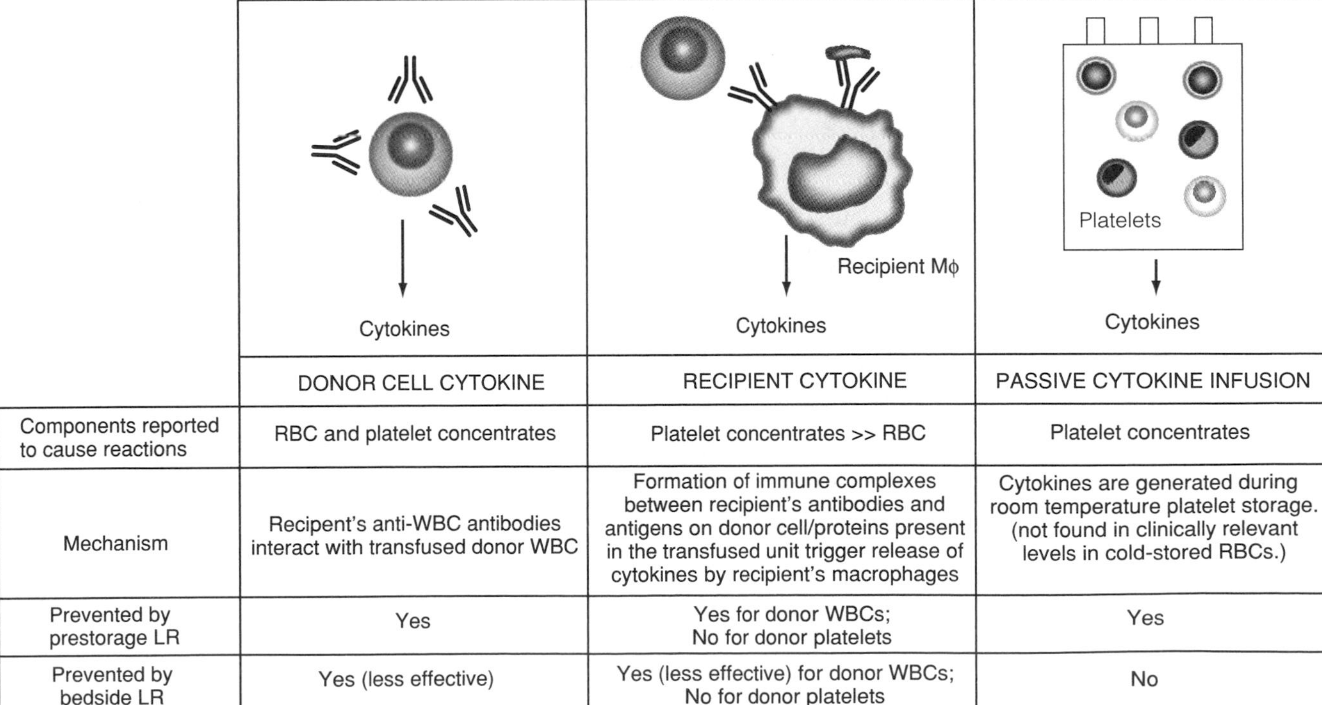

	DONOR CELL CYTOKINE	RECIPIENT CYTOKINE	PASSIVE CYTOKINE INFUSION
Components reported to cause reactions	RBC and platelet concentrates	Platelet concentrates >> RBC	Platelet concentrates
Mechanism	Recipent's anti-WBC antibodies interact with transfused donor WBC	Formation of immune complexes between recipient's antibodies and antigens on donor cell/proteins present in the transfused unit trigger release of cytokines by recipient's macrophages	Cytokines are generated during room temperature platelet storage. (not found in clinically relevant levels in cold-stored RBCs.)
Prevented by prestorage LR	Yes	Yes for donor WBCs; No for donor platelets	Yes
Prevented by bedside LR	Yes (less effective)	Yes (less effective) for donor WBCs; No for donor platelets	No

Figure 26–1 Mechanisms underlying febrile nonhemolytic transfusion reactions. (Adapted from Klein HG, Dzik WH, Slichter SJ, Hillyer CD, Silberstein LE. Leukocyte-reduced Blood Components: Current Status. Educational Program, American Society of Hematology, 1998, pp 154–177.)

sion of platelet concentrates. The authors selected 4- and 5-day-old platelet concentrates. Using centrifugation, the platelet-poor plasma was separated from the platelet pellet, which was resuspended in fresh plasma. Patients were then transfused with both components in random sequence, with a 2-hour washout period between transfusions. Signs and symptoms suggestive of FNHTR were assessed. Transfusions of the platelet-poor plasma obtained from stored platelet concentrates were associated with a significantly higher rate of FNHTR, compared with the resuspended platelet pellets. The authors concluded that soluble substances that had accumulated in the plasma during platelet storage were primarily responsible for febrile reactions in the older platelet concentrates. Increased levels of two cytokines, IL-1β and IL-6, were present in stored platelets and correlated with the frequency of observed reactions.

Mechanism of cytokine accumulation in platelet concentrates. Cytokines include a large family of molecules involved in innate immunity and cell signaling. After release by mononuclear phagocytes, T lymphocytes, and several other cell types, cytokines bind to specific receptors on target cells. Cytokine receptor chains cluster, and their intracellular portions are phosphorylated by Janus kinases (Jaks). The phosphorylation step is required for the Src homology–2 (SH-2) portion of the Jak to bind to the receptor. SH-2 facilitates binding of a signal transducer and activator of transcription (STAT) protein. After phosphorylation, these STAT proteins form homodimers, which migrate to the nucleus and bind to nuclear factors such as nuclear factor-κB (NF-κB) or activation protein–1 (AP-1) transcription factors. The transcription factors then activate genes involved in innate immunity.[49]

A number of reports showed increased accumulation of cytokines, especially IL-1β, IL-6, IL-8, TNF-α, and RANTES (regulated on activation, normal T expressed and secreted), with prolonged storage of platelet concentrates.[50–52] Increased cytokine levels were observed especially on the fourth and fifth day of storage. Stack and Snyder[51] assayed 2-, 3-, 4-, and 5-day-old platelet concentrates for IL-1β, IL-6, IL-8, and TNFα. Although IL-8 was the cytokine most frequently detected, IL-8 is not regarded as a fever-producing cytokine. Increased IL-1β was observed in the units with elevated IL-8. In general, the highest levels of IL-8 were found in the units with the longest storage times and highest leukocyte counts. Only 8% and 10% of tested units showed detectable levels of IL-6 and TNFα, respectively. Leukoreduction before storage prevented the accumulation of IL-8 and IL-1β to day 5 of storage. This study underscored the importance of storage time and initial number of leukocytes before storage in the generation of cytokines.

Palmer and coworkers[53,54] combined results of their two studies and showed that cytokine accumulation during storage of platelet concentrate correlated with the number of leukocytes present before storage. Units with a leukocyte concentration greater than 100/μL resulted in detectable levels of IL-8 and IL-1β. Although prestorage leukoreduction prevented cytokine accumulation, leukoreduction had no beneficial effect on markers of platelet activation such as P-selectin, transforming growth factor-β1 (TGF-β1), platelet-derived growth factor AB (PDGF-AB), von Willebrand factor, and serotonin. These results were confirmed in a study by Fujihara and colleagues,[55] who showed that accumulation of platelet-derived RANTES and TGF-β1 was independent of leukocyte concentration but correlated with platelet concentration.

Monocyte activation. Monocytes are a major constituent of the leukocyte population in platelet concentrates. They are also capable of secreting cytokines, namely IL-1β, IL-6, and TNFα. Several authors have investigated monocyte activation in platelet concentrates as a potential explanation for cytokine accumulation. Muller-Steinhardt and associates[56] studied the influence of storage time, temperature, and type of anticoagulant on the capability of mononuclear cells to secrete cytokines. Mononuclear cells were harvested on days 1, 3, and 5 from platelet concentrates stored under routine conditions, and the response to mitogenic stimulants, such as lipopolysaccharide (LPS), phytohemagglutinin, and staphylococcal enterotoxin B, was evaluated by measuring secretion of IL-1β, IL-2, IL-6, and IFNα. The ability of monocytes to secrete cytokines did not change significantly during the first 3 days of storage and decreased to 25% to 50% of original levels by day 5 of storage. Mitogenic response of mononuclear cells was significantly higher at 37°C than at 22°C. These findings showed that under normal storage conditions mononuclear cells in platelet concentrates preserve the ability to synthesize and secrete cytokines for at least 5 days. Heddle and coworkers[57] demonstrated that cytokine accumulation during storage is temperature dependent. Platelet concentrates were split into two identical portions, one of which was stored for 5 days at 22°C and the other at 4°C. Cytokines failed to accumulate in the aliquots stored at 4°C.

Grey and associates[58] reported in vivo activation of monocytes in platelet concentrates. They analyzed platelet concentrates for leukocyte and monocyte total count, CD14 and CD16 monocyte-associated antigen expression, and IL-1β and IL-6 concentrations on days 1, 2, 3, 4, and 5. The analyzed monocytes expressed increased levels of CD14 (LPS receptor) and CD16 (FcRIII), which are both markers of activation, starting on the first day of storage. On day 3, more than 50% of platelet concentrates had an increased IL-6 concentration. The elevation of IL-6 and IL-1β correlated with the number of monocytes in the unit on day 1. However, increased IL-6 levels occurred earlier during storage. Several hypotheses have sought to explain the delay between monocyte activation and detectable elevation of interleukins. TNFα and IL-1 are known to induce IL-1 synthesis and together with PDGF can stimulate IL-6 synthesis.[59] Both IL-1α and IL-1β were found in the cytoplasm of resting and thrombin-activated platelets.[60] It is possible that the cumulative effect of PDGF and IL-1 derived from platelets reaches a threshold concentration necessary to trigger monocytes to generate additional cytokines such as IL-8 and IL-6. This hypothesis is supported by the findings by Aye and colleagues[53] indicating that, despite uniform release of PDGF from platelets during preparation and storage, only components with high leukocyte content had a detectable level of cytokines.

Mononuclear cells in stored platelet concentrates may be activated by other mechanisms. Activation of monocytes by the plastic used in storage bags was studied by El-Kattan and coworkers.[61] Whole blood–derived platelets were stored in plastic bags made of polyolefin (POF), and apheresis platelets were stored in the bags made of polyvinyl chloride (PVC). Mononuclear cells showed preferential adherence to POF compared with PVC. This adherence was associated with increased mean cytokine levels (IL-1β, TNF, IL-6) that were 11- to 48-fold higher in POF bags compared with PVC bags.

FNHTRS CAUSED BY CYTOKINE PRODUCTION BY RECIPIENT MACROPHAGES

A third mechanism for FNHTRs depends on cytokine release by the recipients' own macrophages (see Fig. 26–1). It has been proposed that recipient antibody bound to donor-cell antigen may form an immunocomplex that serves to activate recipient macrophages to release inflammatory cytokines.[62] This mechanism does not depend on release of preformed stored cytokines contained within donor leukocytes but acknowledges that immunocomplexes are a known stimulus for macrophage activation. Indirect support for this hypothesis comes from a number of observations, including the development of fever among alloimmunized recipients of prestorage leukoreduced platelets; fever after transfusion of platelets to patients with immune thrombocytopenia or drug-induced thrombocytopenia; fever among recipients of incompatible RBC transfusions; and the fever reactions to the cellular portion of platelet concentrates seen in the study by Heddle and associates[48] cited earlier.

CYTOKINE CONCENTRATIONS IN VIVO AND IN VITRO

Sacher[63] attempted to establish the causality between cytokines and FNHTR. IL-6 levels were measured in vivo before and after transfusion in a group of 42 patients. Acute transfusion reactions occurred in 26 patients. The mean post-transfusion IL-6 level was 3.7-fold higher than in pretransfusion specimens. Patients without acute reactions had insignificant increases in IL-6 levels. Unfortunately, the concentration of IL-6 in the transfused components was not measured, leaving uncertainty as to the origin of the cytokine elevation (i.e., a blood component or the recipient).

In the absence of conclusive clinical trials, one may question which cytokines found in platelet concentrates may cause FNHTRs. The amount of TNF-α known to cause fever and chills is approximately 5 to 10 μg/m,[2] or 8500 to 17,000 ng of TNF-α for a 70-kg person.[64,65] In order to achieve such an amount after transfusion of a blood component, the amount of TNF-α present should be approximately 28,000 to 56,000 ng/L in a 300-mL unit, or 170,000 to 340,000 ng/L in a 50-mL unit. However, the measured levels of TNF-α in platelet concentrates were far below this level, with the highest reported concentration being 1890 ng/L and the median concentration in the range of 42 to 571 ng/L.[51–53] The data suggest that passive transfer of TNF-α cannot be solely responsible for symptoms observed in patients with FNHTR. The situation is slightly different for the other endogenous pyrogen, IL-1. This cytokine can cause clinical symptoms at concentrations as low as 10 to 100 ng/kg, corresponding to 700 to 7000 ng in a 70-kg recipient.[66–68] The maximum measured levels of accumulated IL-1 in platelet concentrates vary from 143 to 26,000 ng/L, with medians ranging from 14 to 5250 ng/L.[51–53] These median values correspond to 0.7 to 260 ng in a 50-mL unit or 4.2 to 1560 ng in a 300-mL unit. Passive transfer of such quantities of IL-1 might be able to cause fever in a 70-kg person.

Cytokine accumulation during storage of RBCs is not likely to contribute to FNHTRs. The measured levels of cytokines are substantially lower than found in the platelet concentrates.[69] Stack and coworkers[70] analyzed levels of IL-1β, IL-6, and IL-8 in leukoreduced and nonleukoreduced RBCs. Over 42 days of storage, IL-1β accumulated in the nonleukoreduced units from the baseline of 0 ng/L to 5 to 13 ng/L. Thus, a 42-day-old RBC with 125 mL of supernatant would passively transfer 0.6 to 1.6 ng of IL-1. These values are substantially below the 700 to 7000 ng required to achieve fever levels (see above).

SUMMARY OF THE MECHANISMS OF FNHTRS

FNHTRs to RBCs are best explained by release of recipient cytokines (immunocomplex mechanism). In particular, cytokines do not accumulate during refrigerated storage of red cells to levels considered sufficient to induce a clinical febrile response.[69,70] In contrast, FNHTRs to platelets that have not undergone prestorage leukocyte reduction can be attributed to either accumulation of cytokines during storage or to release of recipient cytokines (immunocomplex mechanism). When prestorage leukoreduced platelets are implicated in FNHTRs, the most likely mechanism is the immunocomplex in which donor platelets are the target of recipient antibodies. Such reactions may be a clinical tip-off to the presence of HLA antibodies and refractoriness.

Clinical Evaluation of FNHTRs

Studies[30,31] in chronically transfused patients with thalassemia have documented that leukoreduction is a highly effective means to prevent FNHTRs to RBCs. Current methods of leukoreduction—whether done before storage, just before blood issue, or at the bedside—are capable of reducing the residual donor leukocyte concentration to levels well below those that result in FNHTRs. Moreover, owing to refrigerated blood storage (and in contrast to platelet concentrates), RBCs do not accumulate clinically important levels of cytokines during storage. Indeed, fever reactions to properly leukoreduced RBCs are sufficiently rare that patients who receive leukoreduced RBCs and experience fever should be evaluated for the presence of hemolytic reactions due to RBC blood group incompatibility and for the presence of bacterial contamination of the transfused product. In contrast to RBCs and as described earlier, FNHTRs to platelet concentrates are much more common and are not completely eliminated by leukoreduction. Patients experiencing FNHTRs to platelet concentrates should be evaluated for platelet increments, for evidence of alloimmunization, for drug-induced platelet refractoriness, for bacterial contamination of platelets, and for passive transfer of antibodies to ABO antigens from donor to recipient.

Prevention of HLA Alloimmunization

Alloimmunization to HLA donor antigens is a well-recognized complication of blood transfusion. Clinical consequences of HLA alloimmunization include FNHTRs, renal allograft rejection, and platelet refractoriness. There are many nonimmune causes of platelet refractoriness, including fever, use of amphotericin B, drug-related antiplatelet antibodies, hypersplenism, consumptive coagulopathy, and idiopathic thrombocytopenic purpura. Because these conditions contribute to platelet refractoriness, no studies have documented that prevention of alloimmunization by leukoreduction prevents *bleeding complications* due to platelet refractoriness. Nevertheless, prevention of HLA alloimmunization is generally regarded as an important benefit of leukoreduction.

After the demonstration in rodents by Claas and colleagues that leukocytes and not platelets are responsible for primary alloimmunization,[71] leukoreduction of blood components was the subject of numerous clinical trials assessing alloimmunization to donor HLA antigens. The reported rate of anti-HLA alloimmunization due to unmodified components in randomized controlled trials varied from 20% to 50% in the control arm, with median incidence of 42%.[72] Meta-analysis of eight controlled, randomized trials demonstrated a 70% reduction in the incidence of HLA alloimmunization in the group of patients who received leukoreduced blood components.[13,72–79] The same report identified a corresponding reduction in platelet refractoriness. The currently recommended level of leukoreduction to prevent allosensitization is less than 5×10^6 WBCs/unit (3 to 17 WBCs/μL).[80,81]

Immune recognition of foreign donor cells requires at least three fundamental elements: binding of the antigen to the antigen receptor, binding of costimulatory molecules mediating cell–cell contact, and local elaboration of cytokines and appropriate cytokine receptors. In whole blood, the majority (70%) of class I HLA antigen is found on the surface of platelets, which express 50,000 to 100,000 copies at their surface.[82,83] The rest of the HLA molecules are distributed among RBCs (3%), granulocytes (2%), lymphocytes (2%), and plasma (23%). Platelet concentrates contain approximately 3.4 mg of HLA molecules, of which 3.2 mg (94%) are associated with platelets, 0.2 mg is in plasma, and 17 μg are present on leukocytes.[82] Therefore, most of the HLA antigens in nonleukoreduced platelet concentrates are found on the platelets themselves. For this reason, it may seem counterintuitive that leukoreduction decreases the risk of alloimmunization.

The recipient of platelet concentrates is exposed to different forms of HLA antigens: soluble class I/II antigens in the plasma, class I/II antigens on cell fragments shed from leukocytes and platelets during processing and storage, class I antigens present on intact platelets, and class I/II antigens expressed on leukocytes. The route by which the antigen presentation occurs influences the likelihood of alloimmunization. Indeed, an important feature of transfusion-induced alloimmunization is the availability of two different sets of antigen-presenting cells (APCs): those of donor origin and those of recipient origin. Stimulation of recipient T or B cells by donor APCs has been called "direct" alloimmunization. In contrast, stimulation by recipient APCs, presenting peptides of donor origin, has been called "indirect" alloimmunization. The data derived from clinical trials of leukoreduction and from basic research suggest that the direct alloimmunization pathway plays a more important role in transfusion-induced alloimmunization.[82]

Direct Alloimmunization Pathway

Direct alloimmunization refers to the process by which recipient immune cells respond directly to donor HLA antigens without the processing of donor antigens by recipient APCs. The mixed lymphocyte reaction is an in vitro example of direct T-cell recognition. Direct sensitization to donor class I antigens results when the recipient is exposed to donor cells bearing class II structures. The route by which donor peptides derived from class I antigens are directly presented has not been precisely delineated. Class II–positive donor cells might carry within the peptide-binding groove oligopeptides representing the cell's own HLA class I antigen. It is known, for example, that a proportion of the endogenous peptides eluted from major histocompatibility class (MHC) molecules are from degraded self-MHC molecules.[84,85] In addition, donor CD4+ T cells were shown in a rodent transfusion model to serve as direct APCs to recipient CD8+ cells.[86]

Kao and del Rosario provided additional direct experimental evidence for the importance of HLA class II cells in transfusion-induced alloimmunization to class I MHC antigens.[87] Using a rodent transfusion system, they compared alloantigen response to transfusion of unmodified donor mononuclear cells versus transfusion of mononuclear cells that were first depleted of cells bearing class II MHC antigens. Alloantibodies against class I MHC antigens were generated in 100% of mice infused with unmodified mononuclear cells, whereas only 25% of mice transfused with the modified components became alloimmunized. This study confirmed the validity of direct immunization mediated by donor APCs and also showed variability in response among different strains.

Clinical studies of transfusion-induced HLA alloimmunization suggest that donor class I peptides presented by class II cells are more immunogenic than intact class I molecules found on donor platelets. The failure of platelets to directly provoke immunization presumably reflects the absence of critical costimulatory molecules on platelets. For example, Gouttefangeas and coworkers showed that HLA class I molecules from platelets cannot directly induce allogeneic CD8+ cytotoxic T-cell response in vitro.[88] Moreover, pure platelet suspensions are unable to stimulate cells in a mixed lymphocyte reaction. Because leukoreduction depletes blood of cells bearing the combination of HLA antigens and costimulatory molecules, and because neither RBCs nor platelets display the combination of class I antigen, costimulatory molecule, and relevant cytokine, leukoreduction of RBCs or platelets prevents direct HLA alloimmunization.

Indirect Allorecognition Pathway

Indirect allorecognition refers to the process by which recipient APCs first engulf donor cells and then process donor antigen for redisplay to the recipient immune system. Donor cells, cell fragments, and soluble donor antigens undergo endocytosis by phagocytosis, macropinocytosis, or a clathrin-mediated process.[89] The proteins are degraded to small peptides within a specialized lysosomal compartment termed the *MHC class II compartment* of the recipient APCs. The peptides are then loaded onto class II molecules as follows. The MHC invariant chain (Ii), a chaperone molecule that guides α and β chains of class II molecules from the endoplasmic reticulum, is digested proteolytically. A fragment of Ii, the class II–associated Ii peptide (CLIP), remains associated with αβ dimers and occupies the peptide-binding groove. In addition, HLA-DM stabilizes the αβ complex and facilitates binding of the peptides to the peptide-binding groove. The allogeneic peptides are then loaded into the MHC class II groove, replacing CLIP or HLA-DM.[90] Empty class II molecules—those that contain neither peptide, invariant chain, nor HLA-DM—are unstable and are degraded in the low pH compartment of the lysosomes. Because HLA-DM is found at a fivefold lower concentration than HLA class II in the late endosomal compartments, excess self-HLA class II molecules are presumably degraded and their peptide fragments recycled.

Since transfusion typically results in alloimmunization to class I HLA antigens, trafficking of class I molecules in donor APCs is of special interest to transfusion science. Although no evidence currently documents that class I peptides are concentrated in the MHC class II compartment, current technical limitations make it hard to determine the proportion of peptides bound to class II that originated from class II compared with class I molecules.[91] However, Turley and colleagues reported that class I HLA molecules can accompany class II HLA molecules from the endoplasmic reticulum, where the class I molecules may be potentially degraded and their peptides loaded onto class II structures ultimately expressed on the surface of the cell.[92]

Expression of costimulatory molecules by APCs is presumably required for transfusion alloimmunization. Both CD80 and CD86 can bind to CD28 found on T-helper (Th) lymphocytes, thereby promoting T-cell activation. Activated helper T cells in turn increase their expression of CD40 ligand (CD40L) and the IL-2 receptor. CD40L interacts with CD40 present on B cells to induce activation of B cells and expression of B7-2, and later B7-1, on the surface. Resting B cells do not express CD80/CD86 on their membrane, but on activation, either by cytokines or by activated T lymphocytes, B cells are able to fully interact with T cells and follicular dendritic cells in germinal centers. In addition, a profile of cytokines secreted by T cells is needed for B-cell activation and antibody synthesis. A Th1 response is associated with increased secretion of IL-2 and IFN-γ whereas a Th2 response is characterized by secretion of IL-4, -5, -10, and -13. The cytokines generated by T cells allow for B-cell proliferation, maturation, and antibody production.

Investigators have attempted to dissect the pathway of antigen processing by recipient APCs in response to transfusion. Bang and colleagues[93] developed a system in which allogeneic platelets were incubated with the recipient's APCs in the presence of various compounds that potentially affect intracellular peptide processing, such as IFN-γ, aminoguanidine, L-arginine, colchicine, ammonium chloride, chloroquine, brefeldin A, and a cytosolic proteasome inhibitor (MG115). The pulsed APCs (enriched spleen macrophages) were then injected into recipients, and antidonor IgG production was evaluated. Forty-five percent of recipients developed alloantibodies after two infusions, and all recipients were alloimmunized by the sixth transfusion. Two patterns of response were observed. The first was consistent with the classic endosome-dependent processing of exogenous antigen and resulted in production of IgG1 antibodies. The second pattern was insensitive to both chloroquine and pH, suggesting a nonendosomal pathway, and led to an IgG2a alloimmune response.

Clinical Studies of Leukoreduced Components to Prevent Alloimmunization

There have been eight prospective, randomized, clinical trials of filter-leukoreduced blood components to prevent platelet alloimmunization. The populations studied were patients with chronic thrombocytopenia and, in most of the investigations, acute myelogenous leukemia. As reviewed by Heddle[94] and by Vamvakas,[72] these trials varied greatly in experimental design. For example, they differed in such fundamental issues as exclusion criteria, definition of alloimmunization and platelet refractoriness, methods of leukoreduction, consistency of leukoreduction, and numbers and types of patients enrolled. The majority of studies showed that fewer patients in the study arm receiving leukoreduced components developed lymphocytotoxic antibodies (Table 26–1). However, this difference between groups was less pronounced when the researchers looked at clinically significant platelet refractoriness. Not surprisingly, these studies documented that alloimmunization to platelet-specific antigens was not affected by leukoreduction.

The largest and the most authoritative prospective randomized trial was the TRAP study, which enrolled 268 patients with acute myelogenous leukemia.[79] The results demonstrated conclusively that leukoreduction of blood components reduces the rate of alloimmunization among patients with leukemia. The study also demonstrated that leukoreduced, pooled, whole blood–derived platelets are as effective as apheresis platelets for the prevention of alloimmunization. Although the rate of HLA alloimmunization was higher among patients with a history of prior pregnancy, compared with never-pregnant patients, the alloimmunization rate among previously pregnant patients was lower in the leukoreduced arms than in the control arm. The finding that patients who were previously pregnant might benefit from leukoreduction differed from the results of other studies that showed lack of efficacy of leukoreduction for such patients.[78] Despite the size of the TRAP trial, the measured

Table 26–1 Prospective Randomized Controlled Trials in Hematology-Oncology Patients Using Leukocyte Reduction (LR) to Prevent Primary Alloimmunization

			Patients with Lymphocytotoxic Antibodies (%)		Patients with Platelet Antibodies (%)		Patients with Platelet Refractoriness (%)	
Author	**Year**	**No. of Patients**	**Control**	**LR**	**Control**	**LR**	**Control**	**LR**
Elghouzzi et al[193]	1981	160	28	15	NT	NT	NA	NA
Schiffer et al[74]	1983	56	42	20	NT	NT	19	16
Murphy et al[195]	1986	50	48	16	10	11	23	5
Sniecinski et al[73]	1988	40	50	15	35	15	50	15
Andreu et al[75]	1988	69	31	12	NT	NT	47	21
Oksanen et al[77]	1991	31	26	13	33	31	26	13
van Marwijk Kooy et al[76]	1991	53	42	7	NT	NT	46	11
Lane and Myllyla[194]	1994	46	35	11	NT	NT	NA	NA
Williamson et al[13]	1994	123	38	22	NT	NT	30	26
TRAP trial[79]	1997	268	45	18	11	6	16	7

Adapted from Klein HG, Dzik WH, Slichter S, et al. Leukocyte-reduced Blood Components: Current Status. Educational Program, American Society of Hematology, 1998, pp 154–177.

rate of platelet refractoriness was low: 16% in the control arm and 7% in the study arm ($P = 0.03$). Platelet refractoriness was strictly defined as corrected count increments of less than 5000/μL on two sequential transfusions. The study defined the primary outcome as concurrent development of both antibodies and platelet refractoriness. Platelet refractoriness (defined as described) that was present within 2 weeks after the development of antibodies constituted alloimmune platelet refractoriness. By these criteria, 13% of patients in the control arm and 3% of those in the treatment arm had alloimmune platelet refractoriness ($P = 0.004$).

A recent study on the value of prestorage leukoreduction on alloimmunization comes from Canada.[95] In this one center study a retrospective analysis was performed on 617 patients with hematologic malignancies who were treated with chemotherapy and/or stem cell transplantation. The authors note that the level of alloimmunization strongly correlates with history of previous transfusion of nonleukoreduced components, pregnancy, and transfusion of more than 13 doses of platelets. This study carries a number of caveats including its retrospective design; multi–year span, which may have affected treatment outcomes; and population of patients who routinely receive leukoreduced components in the United States. It is then difficult to interpret the observed decrease of alloimmunization. Though the number of patients with pre-existing antibodies was small, there was no evidence that universal leukoreduction affected their level of alloimmunization.

The collective results from existing clinical trials support the use of leukoreduced components to prevent primary alloimmunization in patients with acute myelogenous leukemia who are receiving induction chemotherapy. However, there have been few studies of leukoreduction and alloimmunization in other patient groups. Because treatment of leukemia is itself immunosuppressive, the impact of leukoreduction may be different in other patient groups, and the efficacy of leukoreduction for prevention of HLA alloimmunization among nonleukemic patients has not been formally demonstrated.

The prevention of alloimmunization in immunocompetent patients has not been studied extensively. We can get a glimpse of the potentially complicated issues from two recently published reports. The group from Leiden studied the influence of buffy coat depletion with additional pre- or poststorage leukoreduction on formation of new anti-WBC and/or anti-RBC alloantibodies in patients undergoing cardiac surgery.[96] Approximately 75% of patients in this study had no detectable antibodies against WBC or RBC prior to transfusion. After a single transfusion episode with multiple units of either buffy coat–depleted RBCs, prestorage leukoreduced RBCs, or poststorage leukoreduced RBCs, approximately 10% of patients in each group developed anti-WBC antibodies. In addition, the patients who were alloimmunized prior to transfusion increased their panel reactivity in almost 30% of cases, again without significant difference between study arms. This study raises a question of a failure of leukoreduction to protect nonimmunosuppressed patients from developing both anti-WBC and anti-RBC antibodies. An interesting observation was published by Ohto and colleagues.[97] The group performed a multicenter randomized trial of bedside leukoreduced (average content of 0.3×10^6 WBC/unit) versus buffy coat–depleted (average content 1234×10^6 WBC/unit) RBCs administered to nonimmunocompromised patients undergoing cardiac surgery. The authors noted lack of statistically significant difference between the groups with the rate of alloimmunization of 17% and 5%, respectively. This somewhat counterintuitive result may reflect the competence of the immune system in the study groups. These two reports raise an important question of generalizability of leukoreduction as a means to prevent alloimmunization in both immunosuppressed and immunocompetent individuals. Additional studies are clearly needed to answer this important question.

Cytomegalovirus: Transmission and Reactivation

CMV is a member of the herpes family of DNA viruses and is a significant pathogen for immunocompromised individuals. Approximately 2 decades of clinical and basic research provide evidence that CMV can be transmitted by donor leukocytes and that transmission can be reduced by leukoreduction. Clinical trials documenting the effectiveness of leukoreduction as a means to reduce the risk of transmission of CMV have been reviewed elsewhere.[98,99] Testing of donors for evidence of antibodies to CMV is another widely practiced method for reducing the risk of CMV transmission by blood components. Please see Chapter 46 for a detailed discussion.

Clinical Trials of Transfusion-Transmitted CMV and Leukoreduction

From among the many studies on transfusion-transmitted CMV, two clinical trials stand out. Both were large studies and involved bone marrow transplant patients.

Bowden and associates performed a prospective, randomized trial of leukoreduction versus CMV serologic screening for prevention of transfusion-transmitted CMV.[12] Patients undergoing bone marrow transplantation (BMT) who were CMV seronegative were randomly assigned to receive either CMV-seronegative nonleukoreduced blood components ($N = 252$) versus CMV-untested leukoreduced blood products ($N = 250$). The primary outcome was CMV infections occurring after day 21 from transplant. This outcome was selected because infectious outcomes before day 21 of transplant were considered to be the result of exposure *prior* to the study period. The primary analysis found no difference in the rate of CMV infection (CMV− = 0 1.3% vs LR = 2.4%, $P = 1.00$) or CMV disease (CMV− = 0% vs LR = 2.4%, $P = 1.00$). The study was designed to have 80% power to detect a 5% difference between the two study arms with 95% confidence. In a secondary analysis that included all events during days 0 to 100, there was still no statistical difference in the rate of CMV infection, but the rate of CMV disease was lower in the CMV-seronegative arm (CMV− = 0% vs LR = 2.4%, $P = 0.03$). The authors concluded that leukofiltration was an effective alternative to the use of seronegative blood components for prevention of transfusion-transmitted CMV. The study sparked lively controversy on the difference between the primary and the secondary analysis of the data.[100] It was also noted that patients could receive up to 6 units of "nonstudy" blood and remain in their original assigned arm although these violations appeared to account for only one infection in each arm.

The interpretation of the Bowden paper involves two important details. Firstly, RBCs in the leukoreduced arm were leukofiltered at the bedside. It was not known at the time of the study that bedside leukoreduction of RBCs has a very high failure rate.[11] Thus, patients assigned to the leukoreduction arm of the study received products that had far inferior leukoreduction compared with today's technology. On the other hand, the sensitivity of assays for CMV serologic screening has remained stable since the Bowden trial. Thus, if the trial were repeated today, it would be reasonable to expect an even lower rate of CMV transmission in the leukoreduction arm. The Bowden study also provides some insight into the issue of HLA refractoriness and fatal hemorrhagic outcomes. While higher rates of HLA alloimmunization and platelet refractoriness would be expected to have occurred in the patients randomized to receive *nonleukoreduced* blood, there was no observed impact of study arm assignment to overall survival. Thus, any degree of benefit from leukoreduction regarding prevention of fatal bleeding due to platelet refractoriness was so small as to be undetectable in a trial of 500 BMT patients. Although the Bowden study remains the best clinical trial to date on the topic of CMV transfusion-transmitted CMV, its findings need to be interpreted in light of the technology used to prepare leukoreduced blood.

A second major study among BMT patients was the report by Nichols and colleagues, who took an entirely different approach and reached opposite conclusions.[101] They compared CMV infection in two cohorts of patients. One cohort was treated from 1994 to 1996 and received mostly CMV-seronegative blood components. When these were not available for individual patients, the patients received leukofiltered blood from CMV-positive donors. The second cohort was patients treated from 1996 to 2000 who received similar blood components except that platelet support was provided with apheresis platelets collected on machines designed to produce leukoreduced platelets (process leukoreduced apheresis platelets). The study design was, therefore, a comparison of "before versus after" introduction of apheresis leukoreduced platelets. The principal finding of this study was that the incidence of transfusion-transmitted CMV was 1.7% in the first cohort versus 4.0% in the second cohort ($P = 0.05$). Because the two cohorts were sequential in time, the results are subject to other confounding factors that differed during the two periods. Furthermore, the incidence of CMV in the "before" cohort (1.7%) may have been unusually low that year by chance. This is suggested by the authors' observation that the usual background incidence of transfusion-transmitted CMV in their population is 2% for patients transfused exclusively with CMV-seronegative donor blood. The authors did find that patient exposure to leukofiltered blood from CMV-seropositive donors was marginally higher during period two. For example, the mean number of leukofiltered RBCs from CMV-seropositive donors was 0.08 units in period one and 0.15 in period two ($P = \text{NS}$).

Analysis of the data provided complex results. Using univariate analysis for the cohort 2 patients, the odds of CMV infection by transfusion rose weakly in association with receiving CMV *seronegative RBCs* (OR = 1.00–1.02, $P = 0.05$). A positive odds ratio was also found for cohort 2 patients who were transfused with process leukoreduced apheresis platelets from CMV seropositive donors, but the association was also rather weak (OR = 1.00–1.06, $P = 0.05$). However, in multivariate analysis of the same cohort 2 data, the above-mentioned associations with higher odds of CMV infection were no longer significant, but a third factor was associated with higher odds of CMV infection—namely, transfusion with leukofiltered RBCs from a CMV-positive donor. This latter finding is unexpected because the principal change in blood support between cohort 1 and cohort 2 did not involve RBCs but rather was a change from leukofiltered platelets to process leukoreduced apheresis platelets. One possible explanation is that the use of leukofiltered RBCs from CMV-seropositive donors may simply have been a marker (correlate) for sicker patients whose increased transfusion demands resulted in the blood bank selecting CMV-seropositive donors. Indeed, patients acquiring CMV from transfusion had a statistically higher overall blood requirement than those not acquiring CMV infection.

It is difficult to make firm policy decisions based on the Nichols study. Although the authors' conclusions were that serologic screening might be superior to leukofiltration, other interpretations of the findings are possible: leukofiltration of platelets might be superior to process leukoreduction by apheresis, the use of CMV-seropositive leukofiltered RBCs might have been a correlate for sicker patients, patients from cohort 1 may have had by chance an unusually low background incidence of CMV, or the results may have been confounded by other influences.

Comparative trials of leukoreduction versus CMV serotesting have not shown a clear benefit of one method over the other. Although a meta-analysis concluded that serologic testing was superior,[102] that analysis was dominated by results of the Bowden trial and the Nichols trial. As noted above, the Bowden study used bedside leukofiltration prior to the discovery that bedside leukofiltration has a high failure rate and the Nichols trial was a "before-versus-after" study design with several methodological weaknesses.

CMV Is Present in Blood Donors as a Latent Infection in Mononuclear Cells

Almost all studies of the epidemiology of CMV infection identify that the virus is common in healthy individuals and that the prevalence of serologic markers for prior infection increases with age. Although carriers of CMV may intermittently shed virus in their saliva, they do not have continuous viremia. Rather, CMV is present in latent form—the viral genome is present, but gene expression is limited and infectious virus is not produced. Blood cells, endothelial cells, tissue macrophages, stromal cells, and neural cells are all sites of CMV latency.

Leukoreduction reduces the likelihood of transfusion-transmitted CMV because the virus is tropic for leukocytes and is not found in erythrocytes, platelets, or plasma of healthy blood donors. CMV DNA is difficult to recover from leukocyte DNA of healthy carriers. Whereas CMV is found in polymorphonuclear leukocytes of patients with *active* infection, viral DNA is found in mononuclear cells of healthy donors.[103,104] Polymerase chain reaction (PCR) has been used to demonstrate that blood monocytes and macrophages (rather than T and B cells) are the principal sites of latent CMV infection. In particular, it appears that CMV is tropic for peripheral blood cells expressing either CD13 antigen[105] or CD14 antigen.[106]

Using reverse transcriptase PCR, Taylor-Wiedeman and colleagues[107] demonstrated that monocytes from latently infected, healthy, seropositive individuals failed to transcribe CMV genes. However, when the cells were cultured in vitro after exposure either to granulocyte-monocyte colony-stimulating factor plus hydrocortisone or to phorbol 12-myristate 13-acetate plus hydrocortisone, they differentiated into macrophages and expressed messenger RNA for the CMV early-intermediate gene. However, late CMV gene transcripts were not produced, and the cells failed to shed complete virus, suggesting an arrest in productive viral transcription at the early gene phase.

Few Mononuclear Cells in Healthy Donors Harbor CMV

Among healthy blood donors, the proportion of mononuclear cells infected with CMV bears directly on the likelihood that 3- to 4-log leukoreduction will prevent CMV transmission by transfusion. Earlier studies reported that CMV immediate-early gene transcripts were present in 0.03% to 2% of peripheral blood mononuclear cells from healthy seropositive individuals.[108] Subsequently, Slobedman and Mocarski[109] analyzed the proportion of infected cells by PCR and in situ hybridization and by quantitative competitive PCR. Using normal donors undergoing granulocyte colony-stimulating factor mobilization of hematopoietic progenitors, they found that 0.004% to 0.01% of mononuclear cells contained viral genomes at a copy number of 2 to 13 genomes per infected cell. Among healthy blood donors who are not undergoing growth factor–mediated mobilization, the proportion of infected cells presumably would be lower. These findings generate a plausible explanation for the ability of leukoreduction to reduce the transmission of CMV. If a unit of blood contains approximately 10^7 monocytes and if 1 in 10,000 to 1 in 100,000 monocytes are infected, then the unit contains 10^3 to 10^2 latently infected cells. Therefore, a 3- to 4-log leukoreduction may be expected to render the unit noninfectious. However, in vitro experiments in which units were spiked with CMV-infected fibroblasts failed to show complete clearance of CMV transcripts when the leukofiltered blood was tested by PCR.[110] On the other hand, it is unlikely that clinical infections in humans result from exposure to a single latently infected cell, even though the threshold level required to acquire infection is not known. For example, quantitative studies of the level of viremia in patients after liver transplantation have documented that levels greater than 10^4 genomes per milliliter are required for infections to become symptomatic.[111]

Seronegative Healthy Subjects May Test Positive for CMV DNA

Although serologic testing has proved of great practical value for reducing transfusion-related CMV, some investigators have reported that a minority of serologically negative samples may be positive for CMV DNA when tested by PCR. CMV-seronegative, PCR-positive blood donors could account for the finding that patients supported with CMV-seronegative units experience a 1% to 4% rate of CMV transmission, as measured by CMV seroconversion, viremia, or viruria.[112] However, the actual incidence of CMV DNA-positive seronegative donors remains uncertain. In the largest study to date, Roback and colleagues[113] used two previously validated PCR assays and found that none of 514 CMV seronegative donor samples were DNA positive. This result is in sharp contrast to Bevan and associates[114] who studied 312 CMV-seronegative samples and found that 25% were positive for CMV DNA. There is no clear explanation for these different results although numerous methodological details sharply affect the performance of the tests. For example, Rahbar and co-workers[115] reported that CMV-seronegative blood donors lacked antibodies to the laboratory strain AD 169—a strain commonly used as the antigen target in serologic assays, but that 36% of these CMV "seronegative" individuals had antibodies to clinical isolates of CMV prepared from infected patients. On the other hand, Krajden and colleagues[116] found that the method of DNA extraction affected the performance of CMV DNA tests. Among 101 samples obtained from CMV-seropositive blood donors, the frequency of a positive PCR result was 0%, 1%, or 8% depending on which of three different kits were used to isolate DNA for testing.

Infection with Multiple CMV Strains Has Not Been Shown to Result from Transfusion

Molecular typing methods have demonstrated that some patients are infected with more than one strain of CMV. Using restriction enzyme analysis, Chou[117] compared the patterns of isolates among 36 pairs of recipients of CMV-seropositive renal allografts. Although material from the kidney donors was not analyzed, they found paired recipients who shared the same kidney donor also demonstrated a common CMV strain that was not present in the recipients before the transplant. Follow-up studies confirmed that solid organ transplants were capable of infecting recipients with a second strain of CMV.[118] Multiple-strain infection was also reported by Chandler and colleagues,[119] who found molecular evidence for multiple-strain infection among four of eight women attending a clinic for sexually transmitted diseases. Spector and associates[120] reported multiple-strain infection in two persons with serologic evidence of infection with the human immunodeficiency virus (HIV) who were diagnosed with acquired immunodeficiency syndrome. However, the interpretation of studies of second-strain infection has been confounded by the fact that strain mutations develop under the selective pressure of antiviral therapy.[121] These mutations lead to a different pattern of restriction digest, which can be misinterpreted as a second independent strain.

Recognition of second-strain infection via organ transplantation or multiple sexual contacts raises the possibility of transfusion-transmitted second-strain infection and the question of whether CMV-seropositive transfusion recipients should receive CMV–reduced risk blood components. The risk of second-strain infection by transfusion remains only theoretical to date, because no such cases have been reported. Using restriction endonuclease analysis, Winston and coworkers[122] observed no second-strain infections in a study of 18 allogeneic bone marrow transplant recipients who developed CMV during the course of their treatment.

Reactivation of Latent CMV by Transfusion of Allogeneic Donor Leukocytes

Decades ago, the hypothesis was put forward that allogeneic transfusion would result in an in vivo mixed lymphocyte reaction and that this immunologic stimulus might result in reactivation of latent CMV infection.[123] The hypothesis that allogeneic donor leukocytes would result in viral reactivation in the recipient following transfusion was definitively tested in the Viral Activation Transfusion Study (VATS).[124] The study was a multicenter, randomized, double-blind trial comparing the effects of allogeneic blood with and without leukoreduction on the outcomes of 531 patients already infected with HIV-1 and CMV. A total of 3864 units of RBCs were transfused. The primary study outcome measures were mortality and plasma levels of HIV (RNA assay) measured 7 days after transfusion. The results showed no survival advantage with the use of leukoreduced blood, with 151 deaths in the leukoreduced group and 138 deaths in the control group. Median survival was 13 months (leukoreduced) versus 20.5 months (control), $P = NS$. When adjusted for baseline prognostic factors (CD4 count and plasma HIV RNA level) survival was statistically worse in the leukoreduced group (relative hazard for death 1.35 compared with nonleukoreduced, 95% CI, 1.06–1.72). The use of leukoreduced blood did not delay the time to onset of new opportunistic infections and had no effect on the frequency of transfusion reactions. No changes were seen in plasma HIV RNA levels after transfusion. In addition, there was no advantage to leukoreduction for a variety of secondary outcome measures including CMV DNA levels, CD4 cell counts, cell activation assays, or plasma cytokine levels. This study provided substantial evidence against the hypothesis that donor leukocytes cause clinical viral reactivation. Because HIV-infected individuals are at high risk for immune breakdown, the failure to observe increased infections in the control group relative to the leukoreduced group also cast doubt on the role for leukoreduction as a means to abrogate any proposed immunosuppressive effect of transfusion. In summary, the available clinical evidence fails to support a role for leukoreduction in the prevention of viral reactivation.

Donor Leukocytes and Immunosuppression

Allogeneic blood transfusion has been suggested to induce a mild state of immunosuppression. The original suggestion for this effect arose from the observation in 1973 by Opelz and associates[125] that allogeneic transfusions given before renal transplantation resulted in improved allograft survival. Although the allograft effect was confirmed by numerous subsequent reports, including studies conducted in the era of modern antirejection therapy,[126] the exact mechanism has never been conclusively explained. In 1981 Gantt[127] questioned whether transfusions might also down-regulate host antitumor immunity, thereby resulting in either an increased rate of tumor relapse or a shorter interval from primary tumor resection to time of relapse. Subsequently, the hypothesis of transfusion-related immunosuppression was extended to include concern that transfusion might increase the frequency of postoperative bacterial infections. A detailed account of the possible immunosuppressive effects of transfusion was published by Vamvakas and Blajchman.[2]

Common Themes in Experimental Studies of Transplant Tolerance and Transfusion

Four themes regularly appear in experimental studies of transfusion and immune tolerance to organ transplantation: recipient immune conditioning, the histocompatibility relationship between donor and recipient, the presentation of antigen, and the persistence of donor antigen. First, experimental induction of transplant tolerance appears to require proper *"conditioning" of the recipient.* Conditioning regimens usually consist of mild immunosuppression with anti–T cell globulins, chemotherapy, or corticosteroids. Presumably these agents weaken the immune response in such a way as to prevent the transfused cells or proteins from provoking alloimmunization and to allow the transfused cells or proteins to persist within the recipient long enough to induce tolerance.

Second, antigen-specific tolerance induction appears to depend on the proper *relationship between the MHC antigens of the donor and those of the recipient.* Transfusions from donors who are highly mismatched at MHC loci appear more likely to provoke alloimmunization than immunosuppression. Immune tolerance may depend on partial histocompatibility matching of donor and recipient. However, the details of the MHC relationship required for the induction of tolerance are poorly defined and appear to vary among species and with the experimental conditions. In human studies, HLA class II antigen matching appears to be particularly relevant. For example, van Twuyver and associates[128] studied 23 untransfused, first-time renal allograft recipients, each of whom was deliberately transfused before transplantation with donor fresh blood containing approximately 7×10^8 leukocytes. After transfusion, cytotoxic T-cell precursors directed against donor antigen targets were measured. Ten patients demonstrated a significant decline in the level of antidonor T-cell response at 1 month after transfusion. Nine of them were found to share one HLA haplotype (HLA-B and HLA-DR match) with their donor. In contrast, those patients transfused with mismatched blood maintained strong anti–T cell responsiveness after transfusion.

Third, the *dose and molecular presentation of transfused antigens* may affect whether the recipient response is directed toward alloimmunization or tolerance. Evidence for the induction of tolerance by infusion of large intravenous doses of antigen (high-zone tolerance) has existed for years in experimental immunology. The molecular presentation of donor antigen may also play a critical role in the immune response of the transfusion recipient, and there is evidence supporting a role for both cell-associated antigen and soluble antigen as agents for the induction of experimental tolerance. Experimental work from several laboratories has demonstrated that soluble HLA antigens can downregulate in vitro immune responses by several different mechanisms.[129] For example, peptides from the nonpolymorphic 3 region of the class I HLA molecule were able to inhibit the differentiation of cytotoxic T cells in response to an alloantigen stimulus,[130] and soluble HLA peptides can inhibit NK cells.[130] Soluble HLA antigen or other factors released from leukocytes form the basis for the hypothesis that prestorage leukoreduction would reduce an immunosuppressive effect of transfusion. However, Dzik and colleagues[131] found no evidence that the measured soluble HLA antigens differ in units of RBCs stored with or without prestorage leukoreduction. In contrast, Ghio and associates[132] measured increased concentrations of soluble class I HLA antigens and soluble Fas ligand in units of RBCs and platelets during storage. They found that concentrations of soluble antigens and Fas ligand were proportionate to the number of residual donor leukocytes in the blood components.

Finally, the *persistence of donor antigen* in the recipient is a common finding in experimental models for the induction of transplant tolerance.[133] Studies have focused on "microchimerism"—the persistence of low levels of donor cells in the graft recipient. There appears to be little doubt that microchimerism accompanies tolerance. However, it is uncertain whether the persistence of donor cells contributes to the induction of tolerance or is merely a consequence of tolerance. Microchimerism after clinical solid organ transplantation is unquestionably present and has been verified by numerous assays. Microchimerism with fetal cells may also exist in women after normal pregnancy and delivery.[134] Whether microchimerism develops after blood transfusion is controversial. Lee and colleagues[135] reported evidence for extended microchimerism after blood transfusion. Using a PCR assay directed against donor-type HLA genes, they detected donor signal in one recipient for up to 1.5 years after transfusion. Of note, the transfusions occurred in the setting of trauma and included infusions of fresh blood. In follow-up studies, Lee and colleagues reported that recipients of leukoreduced blood also demonstrated microchimerism.[136]

Immunologic Mechanisms Suggested for Transfusion-related Immunosuppression

At various times, one or more of the following four immunologic mechanisms has been suggested as mechanisms for a proposed immunosuppressive effect of blood transfusion: clonal deletion, anergy, active suppression, and indirect effect via viral transmission.

CLONAL DELETION

Central thymic tolerance to self-antigens develops when T cells are deleted during thymic education. Thymic tolerance to foreign antigens can be induced by the inoculation of MHC peptide into the recipient thymus. These peptides are presumably taken up by recipient APCs and displayed as if they were self-antigens. For example, Chowdhury and colleagues[137] were able to induce prolonged cardiac allograft acceptance in a rat model by intrathymic injection of synthetic class I allopeptides. Whether central tolerance is relevant for blood transfusion is unknown. It is conceivable that donor HLA peptide present in blood becomes localized in the recipient thymus gland. Because the thymus involutes with age, the role of central thymic tolerance may be more relevant for pediatric transfusions than for those given to adults.

T-cell clones may also undergo deletion outside the environment of the thymus gland. Activation-induced apoptosis occurs when T cells respond to antigen via their T-cell receptor but are not sustained by costimulatory molecules or by proper cytokine support. Normally, for any given environmental antigen, only approximately 1 in 10^5 to 1 in 10^6 T cells have a matching T-cell receptor and are able to respond to the antigen. However, in the setting of an allogeneic HLA stimulus, such as occurs with organ transplantation or blood transfusion, approximately 1% to 10% of T cells are able to respond. This remarkable finding is the basis of the strong blastogenic response of the routine mixed lymphocyte culture. It is possible that this large activation signal leads to considerable activation-induced apoptosis of recipient cells and subsequent peripheral clonal deletion.

DEVELOPMENT OF CELLULAR ANERGY

Multiple lines of experimental evidence demonstrate that immune activation of T cells depends on the cell's receiving not only a primary signal (the antigen signal) but also a secondary signal known as a costimulatory signal. Certain costimulatory molecules send an activation signal, whereas others send an anergy signal. One hypothesis concerning the immunomodulatory effect of blood transfusion suggests that during refrigerated blood storage donor leukocytes undergo alterations that result in anergy signals to recipient T cells. There is little direct experimental evidence to support this contention, although Minchef and coworkers,[138] using a rodent transfusion model, reported that refrigerated storage resulted in both necrosis and apoptosis of donor cells. Other experimental evidence has also suggested that apoptotic cells are directly immunosuppressive.[139]

INDUCTION OF SUPPRESSOR CELLS

One important hypothesis for the immunosuppressive effect of blood transfusion suggests that transfusion may drive the recipient toward T-cell suppression. In a series of experiments in mice, Chen and associates[140] showed evidence for tolerance induced by a suppressor T cell found in the spleen. BALB/c mice (H-2d) were donors of cardiac allografts to MHC-disparate CBA/Ca (H-2k) recipients. In the absence of any conditioning, the recipients promptly rejected the cardiac allografts. Transplant tolerance was induced by pretransplantation blood transfusion from the donor after conditioning with nonlytic antilymphocyte globulin. Under these conditions, the animals retained the cardiac allografts for more than 100 days. Splenic lymphocytes taken from these tolerant animals were then transferred to naive CBA/Ca animals, which were then tolerant of BALB/c heart allografts in the absence of any immunosuppression. In fact, tolerance could be transferred successfully through nine passages of splenic lymphocytes into new animals. The suppressor cell was localized to the CD4+ subset of T cells. Studies, such as this one, that demonstrate adoptive transfer of tolerance argue strongly in favor of a suppressor cell mechanism. Similar findings were reported by Yang and colleagues,[141] who suggested than the CD45RC+ subset of CD4+ T cells accounted for the immunosuppression.

More direct experimental evidence that allogeneic blood transfusion can induce suppressor T cells in recipients comes from the studies of Blajchman and colleagues,[142,143] who examined the potential of transfusions to promote tumor growth in animals. In one series of experiments, animals were first transfused with either unmodified allogeneic blood, leukoreduced allogeneic blood, or syngeneic blood (as a control). After the transfusions, the animals were challenged with an injection of tumor cells. After a waiting period, the animals were sacrificed and the number of pulmonary metastases were counted. The investigators found that transfusion with unmodified blood promoted increased numbers of pulmonary metastases, compared with leukoreduced or syngeneic blood. Moreover, spleen cells transferred to naive animals from animals that had received unmodified allogeneic blood transfusions promoted greater numbers of pulmonary metastases than did spleen cells transferred from animals that had not been transfused or had received transfusion of leukoreduced blood. These findings argue for the induction of suppressor spleen cells in the animals who had received unmodified donor blood.

Further evidence for splenic suppressor cells induced by blood transfusion was presented by Kao.[144] He was able to induce humoral immune nonresponsiveness in CBA mice (H-2k) using transfusions of ultraviolet B–irradiated leukocytes from BALB/c (H-2d) donor mice. Ultraviolet B irradiation is known to interfere with the expression of costimulatory molecules (see earlier discussion). When spleen cells from the tolerant animals were transferred to naive CBA recipients, the recipients also became tolerant to BALB/c donor antigens. Presumably, the transferred cells suppressed the ability of CBA recipients to form a humoral immune response.

In humans, direct evidence for the induction of Th2-type suppressor cells by blood transfusion is lacking. However, Kirkley and associates[145] reported in vitro cytokine release in 43 patients transfused with either allogeneic or autologous blood at the time of hip surgery. Mean levels of IL-10 and IL-4 released in vitro were slightly higher among recipients of allogeneic blood, suggesting polarization by allogeneic transfusion toward a Th2 phenotype. However, other studies of transfused patients have not found statistically significant differences in cytokine profiles as a result of transfusion.[146,147]

Clinical Studies of Immunosuppression and Leukocyte Depletion

Whether blood transfusion results in a clinically measurable increase in tumor recurrence or postoperative bacterial infection has never been adequately resolved. The issue is difficult to address experimentally in human subjects. A large number of observational studies have documented that patients who receive transfusions are more likely than their untransfused counterparts to develop tumor recurrence or bacterial infection. This observation, however, represents a correlation and does not imply that the transfusions resulted in these adverse effects. Rather, blood transfusion may simply be a marker that correlates with severity of disease. Moreover, the finding that transfusion correlates with tumor recurrence or bacterial infection does not imply that leukoreduction would have a beneficial effect on the frequency of these complications. The effect of leukoreduction has been addressed by randomized, prospective, blinded clinical trials in which patients are assigned to receive either leukoreduced or nonleukoreduced blood components. In addition, trials that examine outcomes in cohorts of patients transfused before versus after implementation of leukoreduction have been reported. Summarized below and in Table 26–2 are large clinical studies published after the year 2000.

Transfusion and Cancer Recurrence

It was proposed in the 1990s that transfusion would increase the rate of cancer recurrence. This hypothesis was supported by preclinical animal experiments that involved deliberate inoculation of tumor cells[142,143] and by retrospective reports in humans showing an association between transfusion at the time of cancer surgery and the subsequent development of recurrent cancer. However, well-designed clinical trials have not supported the hypothesis that leukoreduction would affect tumor biology. For example, van de Watering and colleagues provided results on long-term cancer recurrence among 697 patients with colorectal cancer who were randomized to receive either leukoreduced or nonleukoreduced (buffy coat–depleted) blood components.[148] They found that the 5-year survival rates (65% leukoreduced; 64% control) and 5-year cancer recurrence rates (28% leukoreduced; 28% control) were nearly identical in the two groups. The study provided randomized controlled trial evidence that leukocyte reduction at the time of cancer surgery did not affect the rate of cancer recurrence.

Transfusion and Postoperative Infection

NONCARDIAC SURGERY

The hypothesis that recipient exposure to donor leukocytes induced some form of immunosuppression was also extensively investigated as a potential cause for post-transfusion infection in surgical patients. Initially, retrospective studies found an association between higher rates of postoperative infection among transfused patients compared with untransfused patients. However, as with cancer recurrence, such studies may have only identified that transfusion was a marker of more serious illness.

Because earlier studies suggested that patients undergoing colorectal surgery were more likely to benefit from leukoreduction technology, Titlestad and colleagues performed a prospective randomized trial in 279 such patients who were randomized prior to transfusion to receive either leukoreduced or nonleukoreduced RBCs.[149] Because only a minority of patients required transfusion, the number of transfused patients receiving leukoreduced RBCs ($N = 48$) or nonleukoreduced RBCs ($N = 64$) was modest. The authors found that the rate of postoperative infection was not different in the two groups. In addition, there was no effect of leukoreduction on mortality or hospital length of stay.

Baron and colleagues[150] recorded infection rates following abdominal aortic surgery in a cohort of patients ($N = 192$) transfused before implementation of leukoreduction and compared them with infection rates of a subsequent cohort of patients ($N = 195$) transfused after implementation of leukoreduction. The two cohorts showed no difference in rates of postoperative infection (leukoreduced 27% [95% confidence of 21–33%] versus control 31% [95% confidence of 25–38%]); no difference in the proportion with severe infection or pneumonia; no differences in either total hospital length of stay or intensive care stay, and no difference in overall mortality.

Van Hilten and colleagues[151] reported a large prospective randomized clinical study that examined infection rates among patients undergoing aortic aneurysm or gastrointestinal cancer surgery. Among 1200 patients randomized prior to transfusion, 545 were transfused. Among those transfused, the two groups were balanced between those randomized to receive leukofiltered products ($N = 237$) or nonfiltered products ($N = 257$). Among transfused patients, there was no statistical difference between leukoreduced versus nonleukoreduced groups for postoperative infection. There was also no effect of leukoreduction on the incidence of multiorgan failure or death. Median length of stay in intensive care was lower in the patients assigned to receive leukoreduced blood, but mean overall hospital length of stay was not different between the two groups.

In the largest prospective randomized trial, Dzik and coworkers[27] randomly assigned all transfused patients who did not meet standard criteria for leukoreduced blood to receive either leukofiltered components ($N = 1355$ patients) or nonleukoreduced components ($N = 1425$ patients). Patients included both surgical and medical patients with no exclusions. Any infection sufficiently severe to cause treating physicians to begin antibiotic therapy was recorded. The results showed no difference between the two groups for the proportion of patients who were treated with antibiotics after transfusion (leukoreduced = 66%; control 68%, $P = 0.42$) and showed no difference for the duration of antibiotic therapy. There was also no difference when antibiotic use was analyzed for the postoperative period among surgical patients. Subgroup analysis also found no effect of leukoreduction on the proportion of patients receiving antibiotics (or the duration of antibiotic therapy) among specific patient groups, including colorectal surgery ($N = 110$), noncardiac surgery ($N = 1087$), and nonsurgical patients ($N = 1077$). There was also no effect of leukoreduction on mortality rates or various measures of hospital length of stay.

Table 26–2 Clinical Trials of Leukoreduction (LR) Published after the Year 2000 That Investigate Clinical Evidence for Immunosuppression and Infection

Author	Year	Design	Patient Population	Non-LR (N)*	LR (N)*	Infection	Mortality	Length of Stay (LOS)
Tilestad et al[149]	2001	RCT	Colorectal	64	48	No effect	No effect	No effect
Baron et al[150]	2002	Before vs after	Aortic surgery	192	195	No effect	No effect	No effect
Dzik et al[27,139]	2002	RCT	All patients	1425	1355	No effect	No effect	No effect
Hebert et al[26]	2003	Before vs after	Trauma, cardiac, orthopedic	6982	7804	No effect	No effect (adjusted OR)§	No effect
van Hilten et al[151]	2004	RCT	Aortic; GI surgery	257	237	No effect	No effect	LR = ↓ ICU LOS; No effect on hospital LOS
Bracey et al[155]	2002	RCT	Cardiac	159	136	No effect	No effect	No effect
Wallis et al[153]	2002	RCT	Cardiac	163	174	Inconsistent effect†	No effect	No effect
Dzik et al[27,139]	2002	RCT	Cardiac	260	246	No effect	No effect	No effect
Volkova et al[156]	2002	Before vs after	Cardiac	416; 317	484	Inconsistent effect‡	No effect	No effect
Hebert et al[26]	2003	Before vs after	Cardiac	4476	5050	No effect	No effect	Not stated
Fung et al[157]	2004	Before vs after	Cardiac	501	645	No effect	No effect	LR = ↓ hospital LOS
Llewelyn et al[159]	2004	Before vs after	Cardiac and orthopedic	997	1098	LR = ↑ rate in cardiac	LR ↑ Cardiac; LR ↓ Ortho	No effect
Bilgin et al[154]	2004	RCT	Heart valve	216	216	LR = ↓ rate	No effect	No effect

*Number of patients shows *transfused* patients. Several studies randomized more patients not all of whom were transfused.
†LR group had lower in-hospital rate of nonserious infections, but LR group had higher rate of infections postdischarge.
‡Infection rates declined ($p < 0.05$) when switched from LR to non-LR.
§Unadjusted odds ratio for mortality significantly lower for LR group, but significance not found when odds ratio adjusted for effect of cardiac medications.

CARDIAC SURGERY

Interest in a possible beneficial effect of leukocyte reduction more specific for cardiac surgery patients originated from the early report of van de Watering and colleagues.[152] They randomly assigned more than 900 patients undergoing cardiac surgery to three groups. Among those transfused, patients received either prestorage leukofiltered RBCs ($N = 283$), poststorage leukofiltered RBCs ($N = 280$), or buffy coat–depleted but not extensively leukoreduced RBCs ($N = 303$). The primary outcome of the study was infection complications, and the authors found no effect of leukoreduction on the frequency of infection outcomes ($P = 0.15$). An unexpected finding was a lower 60-day mortality (3.5%) in either of the leukofiltered arms compared with the nonleukoreduced blood arm (7.9%); $P = 0.025$. Although van de Watering found no evidence that transfusion increased the rate of postoperative infection, the authors noted that the difference in mortality was only apparent among patients receiving more than 3 units of RBCs and appeared to be due to different rates of wound dehiscence or multiorgan failure.

Three prospective randomized trials published since 2000 examined infection rates and mortality among cardiac surgery patients. Wallis and associates[153] reported results among 510 transfused patients assigned to receive control RBCs ($N = 163$); buffy coat–depleted RBCs ($N = 173$), or leukofiltered RBCs ($N = 174$). Although patients were randomized prior to transfusion, significantly fewer patients assigned to receive control RBCs were transfused. Among transfused patients, they found that use of control RBCs was associated with more events coded as infection ($P = 0.02$). However, when events coded as urinary tract infection were excluded, there was no significant difference among the three groups; $P = 0.25$. Following discharge from hospital, a significantly higher rate of infection requiring antibiotic treatment was found among patients assigned to receive leukoreduced blood (47%) compared with control RBCs (34%); $P = 0.01$. The authors concluded that no evidence was found that leukocyte reduction reduced postsurgical infection rates.

Bilgin and colleagues[154] conducted a second clinical trial in cardiac surgery focusing on patients undergoing valve-replacement surgery (with or without bypass grafting). Patients were randomly assigned to receive either buffy coat–depleted RBCs ($N = 216$) or leukofiltered RBCs ($N = 216$). Multiple outcomes were compared with no statistical correction for multiple comparisons. Among transfused patients, infection rates were higher in patients assigned to buffy coat–depleted blood (mean odds ratio = 1.64; 95% CI, 1.08–2.49). However, in-hospital mortality, frequency of multiorgan failure, length of stay in intensive care, overall length of stay in hospital, or 90-day mortality were all not significantly different between the two groups.

Bracey and co-workers conducted a prospective randomized trial in cardiac surgery patients at the Texas Heart Institute.[155] Patients were randomized prior to transfusion. Transfused patients assigned to receive control blood components ($N = 159$) or leukoreduced RBCs ($N = 136$) were balanced for preoperative risk factors, surgical procedures, and dose of transfusion. The authors found no difference in the two groups for in-hospital infections or infections during the first 3 months after discharge. There was also no difference in the two groups for mortality, intensive care length of stay, or overall hospital length of stay.

The prospective trial of Dzik and colleagues[27] included all patients undergoing cardiac surgery during the study period. Patients ($N = 246$) received transfusion with leukoreduced blood compared with patients ($N = 260$) who received nonleukoreduced components. Infection rates, measured by the clinical decision to administer antibiotic therapy, were not different in the two groups.

In addition to the above randomized trials, four studies in cardiac surgery patients examined outcomes among a cohort of patients transfused before implementation of leukoreduction compared with outcomes in a subsequent cohort of patients transfused after implementation of leukoreduction.

Volkova and associates[156] reported a study based on three sequential cohorts of patients: those receiving nonleukoreduced blood ($N = 416$), then a cohort receiving transfusion following implementation of leukocyte-reduced blood ($N = 484$), and finally a cohort transfused following return to the use of nonleukocyte-reduced blood ($N = 317$). They noted that mean hospital length of stay decreased progressively with each subsequent time interval (15.9 days, 14.1 days, and 12.1 days). Thus, the implementation of leukoreduction in 1992 was associated with a reduced length of stay, but the discontinuation of leukoreduction and a return to nonleukoreduced blood was also associated with a further decreased length of stay. This finding suggests that hospital length of stay was simply decreasing independently of blood policy and demonstrates that "before-versus-after" study designs can produce misleading conclusions. Observed rates of infection were not reduced with implementation of leukocyte reduction but declined in the third cohort after the switch from leukoreduced to nonleukoreduced blood.

In the study by Fung and colleagues[157] 501 patients received unfiltered blood products.[158] The following year, 645 patients received leukofiltered products. No significant changes were seen in the rate of mediastinitis, operative mortality, or stay in intensive care. There was a statistically significant decrease in postoperative hospital length of stay. This study also did not identify an immunosuppressive effect of donor leukocytes as measured by infection rates.

Llewelyn and colleagues[159] reported outcomes among cardiac surgery and orthopedic surgery patients in 11 hospitals before implementation of leukoreduction ($N = 997$) and compared these to outcomes following implementation ($N = 1098$). The proportion of all transfused patients with suspected or proved infection was unchanged before and after implementation of leukoreduction (odds ratio 0.83; 95% CI, 0.77–1.02). Among cardiac patients, use of leukoreduced blood was statistically associated with a *higher* rate of proved infections ($P = 0.004$). Overall postoperative length of stay was also not affected by leukoreduction. Subgroup analysis showed no effect related to dose of blood transfused. Mortality rates among cardiac surgery patients were increased following implementation of leukocyte reduction ($P = 0.031$) but were decreased among orthopedic patients. The authors concluded that leukoreduction did not improve outcomes.

The large Canadian study that examined outcomes before versus after implementation of leukoreduction included cardiac patients.[26] Patients in cohort 1 ($N = 4475$) were transfused with nonleukoreduced blood, and those in cohort 2 ($N = 5050$) received leukoreduced blood. There was no effect of leukoreduction on the adjusted odds of death and no observed effect of leukoreduction on infectious complications.

Taken together, the findings of clinical studies in surgery patients since 2000 fail to demonstrate that leukocyte reduction has any significant or consistent effect on the incidence of postoperative infection. Whether allogeneic transfusion by itself (with or without donor leukocytes) causes an immunosuppression not seen in untransfused individuals is not resolved by these studies. However, the finding that leukoreduction fails to change infection outcomes argues against a role for donor leukocytes in any proposed immunosuppressive effect on bacterial defenses. The studies provide conflicting results regarding overall hospital length of stay among cardiac patients assigned to receive leukoreduced blood components, and the extent to which any findings can be attributed to leukoreduction (especially in before-versus-after study designs) is difficult to determine. The early observation by van de Watering of decreased mortality in a subgroup of cardiac valve patients receiving leukoreduced blood compared with nonleukoreduced blood was not substantiated in any subsequent study. In summary, the clinical trials data since the year 2000 suggest that transfusion-related immunosuppression, if it does exist, may be mediated by factors other than donor leukocytes.

ADVERSE REACTION TO FILTRATION AND LEUKOCYTE REDUCED COMPONENTS

Administration of leukocyte-reduced components is generally safe with a few adverse effects. Now, when the process of leukoreduction occurs mostly during, or shortly after, component collection, the profile of adverse reactions has changed. When bedside leukoreduction was commonplace, the main observed adverse reaction was hypotensive episodes due to bradykinin production upon activation of the contact phase. With the increased use of prestorage leukoreduced components, this type of reaction is less likely to occur; however, the manufacturing process may now play a more important role as a cause of observed reactions. This section discusses three types of reported adverse reactions: (1) hemolysis due to leukoreduction, (2) hypotensive reactions due to contact system activation, and (3) hypotensive reactions to prestorage leukoreduced components.

Hemolysis Due to Prestorage Filtration

There has been a concern that prestorage leukoreduction may lead to an increased level of hemolysis in stored RBC components. First reports posted on transfusion medicine discussion group[160] in 2001 described increased hemolysis in segments of leukoreduced units versus nonleukoreduced units. The ensuing discussion did not identify a cause for hemolysis but raised awareness of this potential manufacturing problem. However, no adverse clinical sequelae were reported related to hemolysis. After this initial report the FDA continued to receive reports of hemolysis in RBC and WBC components following leukocyte reduction using a high-efficiency filter. Because of this information, Pall Medical decided to perform a voluntary market recall of their Leukotrap SC RC.[161] Additional units were recalled in February 2005. The hemolysis has been reported both immediately following filtration as well as 24 to 48 hours after leukocyte removal. The cause of this phenomenon is unclear at this time. Gyongyossy-Issa and associates[162] analyzed the influence of ambient temperature at which filters are used on the degree of hemolysis. The results supported a notion that when the leukoreduction is performed at 4° C in a strictly controlled environment, hemolysis can be avoided. Janatpour and co-workers[158] studied three different methods for determination of hemolysis in segments and the unit. They split the units into two aliquots, one of which was leukoreduced, and measured plasma hemoglobin using (1) a HemoCue Plasma/Low Hb Photometer system, (2) a tetramethyl-benzidine (TMB) chemical method, and (3) a free Hb visual comparator. They concluded that visual criteria overestimate the degree of hemolysis. Other methods could be more objective, raising the question whether a visual inspection of hemolysis can be used as the part of the quality control of the unit prior to distribution.

Although there were no reported clinical side effects of the increased hemolysis postfiltration, this scenario underscores the need for postmarketing surveillance of WBC filters and the quality of components. It remains to be seen if increased hemolysis translates into clinically detectable side effects. However, even without such adverse events, transfusion services should remain vigilant in detecting potential problems with any blood components. This proactive approach should be able to identify manufacturing problems early on and eliminate them in a timely manner.

Hypotensive Reactions to Bedside Leukoreduction

There have been several case reports of severe hypotension, occasionally accompanied by skin flushing and loss of consciousness, developing in patients who received bedside filtered blood components.[163–170] Although the reported incidence of these reactions is relatively low and is decreasing as fewer products are transfused using bedside filtration, some reactions have been severe and illustrate an interesting phenomenon. Four clinical features intersect to result in these reactions: transfusion of plasma-containing blood components; use of a bedside leukoreduction filter; use of a filter whose medium carries a net negative charge; and, most importantly, the concurrent administration of angiotensin-converting enzyme (ACE) inhibitors to the recipient. The sudden elaboration of bradykinin was a prime suspect as the cause of these reactions because bradykinin had previously been implicated in anaphylactic reactions observed among patients receiving ACE inhibitors and undergoing low-density lipoprotein apheresis or hemodialysis.[171–173]

Implication of Kinins and Activation of the Contact Pathway in the Pathogenesis of Hypotensive Reactions

Two related vasodilator peptides—the nonapeptide bradykinin and the decapeptide lysyl-bradykinin (kallidin)—exert strong hypotensive effects in humans. Both peptides are metabolized by kininase I, a carboxypeptidase that removes one amino acid (arginine) from the carboxyterminal end. Kininase II, also known as ACE, removes two amino acids (phenylalanine and arginine) from the carboxyterminal end, rendering the peptides inactive. Bradykinin and lysyl-bradykinin are formed from two precursor proteins: high-molecular-weight kininogen, or HMWK (approximately 110,000 D), and low-molecular-weight kininogen, or LMWK (approximately 68,000 D) (Fig. 26–2). The physiologic function of both

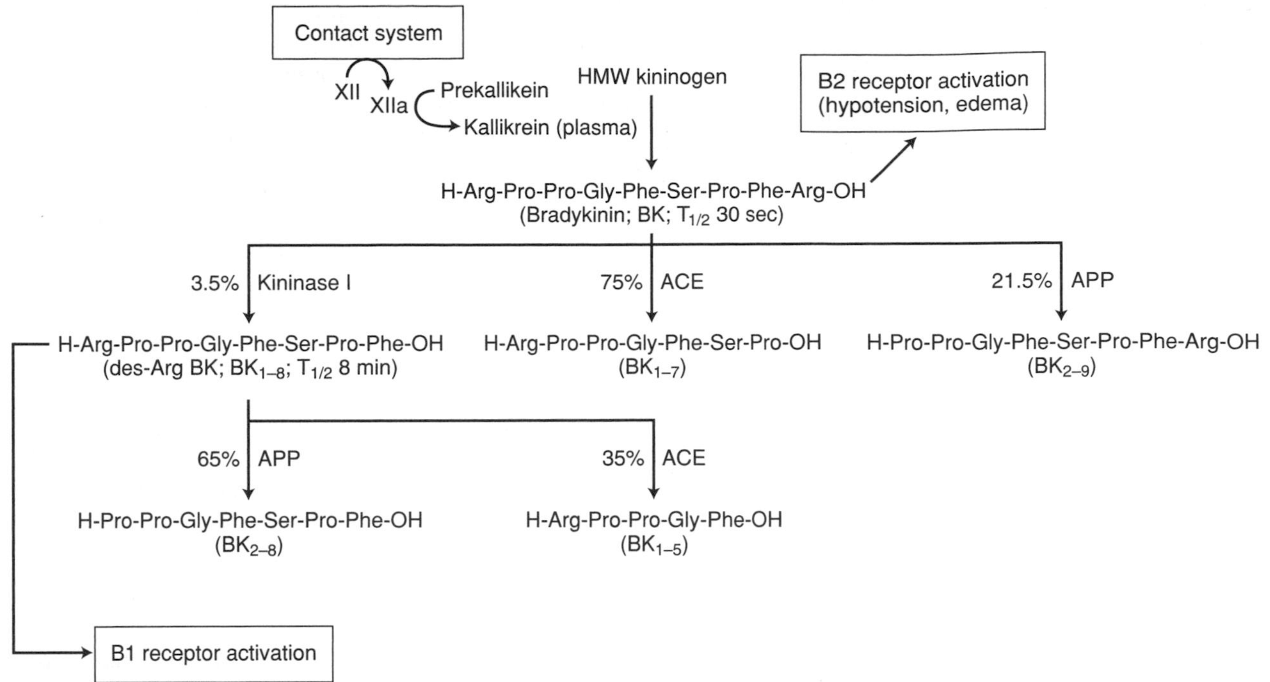

Figure 26–2 Simplified diagram representing synthesis and catabolism of bradykinin. The contact system upon activation through contact with a negatively charged surface (e.g., glass, kaolin, dextran sulfate, blood filter, dialysis membrane) leads to activation of the intrinsic coagulation cascade and to bradykinin (BK) generation. The active components of this pathway include kallikrein, bradykinin (acts through B2 receptor), and des-Arg9 bradykinin (acts through B1 receptor), all labeled in boldface. The other metabolites of bradykinin are inactive. The inhibition of the major pathway of catabolism by ACE inhibitors results in prolongation of the half-life ($T_{1/2}$) of active components and clinical signs and symptoms. ACE, angiotensin-converting enzyme; APP,. aminopeptidase; HMW, high molecular weight; LMW, low molecular weight.

kinins is exerted through their action on two receptors, B1 and B2. These receptors were cloned and identified as serpentine receptors coupled to G proteins. Because bradykinin and lysyl-bradykinin are primarily tissue hormones, their concentration in the circulation is usually low. Reported physiologic levels vary from less than 3 to 55 pg/mL.[174,175] Both peptides are responsible for contraction of visceral smooth muscles, but they relax vascular smooth muscles through the action of nitric oxide. In addition to the effect on smooth muscle cells, the kinins cause increased capillary permeability, accumulation of leukocytes, and pain after injection under the skin. Bradykinin acting on the B2 receptor triggers nitric oxide formation, which activates guanylate cyclase in smooth muscle cells, leading to increased concentrations of cyclic guanosine monophosphate (cGMP) and smooth muscle relaxation.[176] Previous studies have shown that bradykinin also activates phospholipase A_2, phospholipase C, protein kinases, and prostaglandins, thereby resulting in the accumulation of cGMP and cyclic adenosine monophosphate in cells.[177] Although bradykinin can activate tissue mast cells, leading to release of histamine,[178] histamine release does not account for the full vasodilatory effects of bradykinin. Dachman and colleagues[179] demonstrated a residual vasodilatory effect even in the presence of a histamine$_1$ receptor antagonist (brompheniramine) and a histamine$_2$ receptor antagonist (cimetidine).

In healthy individuals, approximately 95% of injected bradykinin is metabolized during the first passage through the lungs. Pulmonary kininases rapidly degrade bradykinin, thereby preventing its effect on the arterial circulation. Indeed, these pulmonary kininases may normally provide transfusion recipients with protection against bradykinin-induced vasodilation. However, pulmonary breakdown of bradykinin is significantly diminished among patients with genetically low activity of pulmonary kininases and patients receiving ACE inhibitor medications. In addition, patients undergoing cardiopulmonary bypass are at increased risk for bradykinin-mediated hypotensive reactions, because during the bypass venous blood flow is diverted around the pulmonary circulation. The largest series of severe hypotensive reactions accompanying bedside leukoreduction filtration was reported among patients undergoing cardiopulmonary bypass.[165]

The vasodilatory effect of bradykinin was studied in several experimental settings. Forearm blood flow increased after doses of 10 and 100 ng/min.[180,181] Icatibant, a B2-kinin receptor antagonist, was used to demonstrate dose-dependent vasodilation in response to bradykinin. With increased dosage of icatibant, blood flow diminished significantly. N(G)-monomethyl-L-arginine, a specific inhibitor of nitric oxide synthase, was used to demonstrate that bradykinin-induced vasodilation is mediated in part by nitric oxide.[180]

Bonner and colleagues[182] reported on the hemodynamic effects of bradykinin on the systemic and pulmonary circulation in normotensive and hypertensive subjects. Bradykinin was injected intravenously and intra-arterially at doses ranging from 42.4 to 6413 ng/kg. Bradykinin lowered blood pressure by decreasing systemic vascular resistance. ACE inhibitors potentiated this effect by approximately 20- to 50-fold. Systolic blood pressure declined by more than 20 mm Hg when the arterial bradykinin concentration reached at least 100 pg/mL. The study demonstrated that the physiologic effect of bradykinin is very rapid, with a hypotensive effect demonstrable within seconds after administration.

Activation of Contact System During Passage of Blood through Leukoreduction Filters

Because bradykinin elaboration would occur if the contact system were activated, investigators have examined whether leukofiltration could induce contact activation of blood. Studies have measured either an increase in bradykinin or its stable metabolite 1,5-bradykinin or a decrease in the substrates HMWK or LMWK. Although direct measurement of bradykinin is more appealing, bradykinin is technically difficult to assay owing to ex vivo activation of the contact system. Shiba and coworkers[183] measured bradykinin during leukofiltration of platelet concentrates, using a negatively charged filter and a positively charged filter. After filtration through the negatively charged filter, decreased levels of prekallikrein and increased levels of bradykinin were observed. The bradykinin level was inversely related to the activity of ACE in the platelet concentrates. The same group studied the effects of storage time, plasma dilution, and filtration on contact-system activation in packed RBCs preserved in mannitol-adenine phosphate solution.[184] The authors noted an increase in the bradykinin level, up to 500 pg/mL on the 10th day of storage. The level decreased to 200 pg/mL during the subsequent 5 days and remained at this low level until the end of the storage time. A significantly decreased level of ACE activity was noted in the packed RBCs stored in solutions containing mannitol. Filtration using two different negatively charged filters generated bradykinin levels up to 6000 pg/mL. The authors concluded that mannitol may act as an ACE inhibitor, slowing down catabolism of bradykinin and leading to its accumulation in stored RBCs. Hild and colleagues[185] studied generation of bradykinin during leukofiltration of platelets using three different filters—negatively charged, positively charged, and neutral. Only the negatively charged filter contributed significantly to bradykinin production. The levels of bradykinin detected in the eluate varied from less than 200 pg/mL to as much as 10,000 pg/mL in samples collected after the processing of 50 and 100 mL of platelet concentrates. The final concentration in units ranged from 200 to 2500 pg/mL. Interestingly, bradykinin present after filtration was rapidly metabolized; after 60 minutes of storage, the bradykinin level was below the limit of detection. However, when an ACE inhibitor was added to the storage bag, bradykinin levels remained elevated for as long as 90 minutes.[185] Significant differences in bradykinin production were observed among the donors, so that some components generated measurable levels of bradykinin but others did not. The highest bradykinin levels (>20,000 pg/mL) were observed after leukofiltration of apheresis platelets. Scott and associates[186] investigated bradykinin generation by negatively charged filters by measuring substrates of the contact system during leukoreduction of apheresis platelets. The number of WBCs before leukoreduction varied from 0.5 to 1000 cells/μL. Two different leukocyte filters were used. Measurements of the cleavage products of HMWK and LMWK were used as markers of contact-phase activation and the potential for bradykinin production. Although no significant changes were detected in kininogen cleavage products, the assay could not exclude conversion of small amounts (<5%) of kininogen to kinin. The authors concluded that clinically significant activation of the contact system did not occur as a result of leukofiltration. However, they did observe a temporary decrease in kininogen levels with one of the studied filters. The interpretation of this study is difficult because, on a molar basis, kininogen is a very abundant molecule. Therefore, conversion of a minor fraction of kininogen could result in very significant levels of bradykinin.

Why is it that not all patients react uniformly when given bedside transfusions while receiving ACE inhibitors? Cyr and colleagues[187] studied the influence of ACE inhibitor medication on the in vitro generation of bradykinin and its active metabolite des-Arg9-bradykinin. The in vitro half-life of bradykinin and of des-Arg9-bradykinin was measured in the presence of an ACE inhibitor in serum from four patients who had experienced hypotensive reactions during blood transfusions of leukoreduced products. Although the half-life of bradykinin did not differ between the patients and controls, the degradation of des-Arg9-bradykinin was significantly slower in the patient samples (1549 vs 661 seconds). The authors proposed the hypothesis that an anomalous metabolism of des-Arg9-bradykinin might contribute to selection of patients who experience clinical reactions to bedside leukodepletion.

On the basis of the published studies, bradykinin produced during bedside filtration of platelets seems to be responsible for reactions during bedside leukofiltration in patients taking ACE inhibitor medications. Reactions to RBC components may be less likely, because cold storage of RBCs inhibits contact activation enzymes and because RBCs contain less plasma and kininogens. Concern regarding hypotensive reactions among patients receiving blood components filtered at the bedside prompted the FDA to issue a letter to physicians in May 1999. The FDA recommended use of blood products leukoreduced at the time of collection or during laboratory storage whenever available.

Hypotensive Reactions to Prestorage Leukoreduced Components

Arnold and colleagues[188] report two patients who developed hypotensive reactions after receiving prestorage leukoreduced components. Both patients were taking ACE inhibitors. This observation puts in question the assumption (as discussed above) that only bedside filters can activate the contact system to a sufficient degree to cause bradykinin generation with subsequent development of hypotension. A hypothesis was put forward that the ACE inhibitors present during the collection of the autologous (or allogeneic) unit were responsible for bradykinin accumulation during leukodepletion. This hypothesis would require significant contact phase activation with significant accumulation of bradykinin. Additional studies are needed to answer this question.

Similar reactions have been observed and reported in the patients undergoing therapeutic plasmapheresis, even if the replacement fluid consisted only of 5% albumin, though it was more common to observe such reaction with fresh frozen plasma. Owen and Brecher[189] performed a retrospective study to identify all patients who developed "atypical reactions" while undergoing therapeutic plasma exchange over the course of 12 years. The authors concluded that the use of ACE inhibitors was associated with symptomatic hypotension during the procedure and recommended that ACE inhibitors be discontinued at least 24 hours prior to apheresis procedure. Thus, it seems plausible that the patients undergoing therapeutic plasmapheresis with albumin as a replacement fluid are at increased risk for hypotension if concomitantly on ACE inhibitors.[189–192]

REFERENCES

1. Dzik S, Aubuchon J, Jeffries L, et al. Leukocyte reduction of blood components: public policy and new technology. Transfus Med Rev 2000;14:34–52.
2. Vamvakas EC, Blajchman MA (eds). Immunomodulatory Effects of Blood Transfusion. Bethesda, Md., American Association of Blood Banks Press, 1999.
3. Miller JP, Aubuchon JP. Leukocyte-reduced and cytomegalovirus-reduced risk blood components. In Mintz PD (ed). Practice Guidelines for Transfusion Therapy. Bethesda, Md., American Association of Blood Banks Press, 1998, pp 163–189.
4. Dzik S. Leukodepletion blood filters: filter design and mechanisms of leukocyte removal. Transfus Med Rev 1993;7:65–77.
5. Zou Y, Sun Q, Li A, et al. Efficiency of leukocyte removal by filters made of superfine glass fiber membranes. Vox Sang 1999;76:22–26.
6. US Food and Drug Administration, Center for Biologics Evaluation and Research. Available at http://www.fda.gov/cber/gdlns/preleuk.htm. Accessed March 28, 2006.
7. Steneker I. Leukocyte Depletion from Fresh Red Cell Concentrates by Fiber Filtration: Filtration Mechanisms. Amsterdam, VU University Press, 1992.
8. Ledent E, Berlin G. Factors influencing white cell removal from red cell concentrates by filtration. Transfusion 1996;36:714–718.
9. Nishimura T, Kuroda T, Mizoguchi Y, et al. Advanced methods for leukocyte removal by blood filtration. In Brozovic B (ed). The Role of Leukocyte Depletion in Blood Transfusion Practice: Proceedings of the International Workshop. Oxford, Blackwell Scientific, 1989, pp 35–40.
10. Beaujean F, Segier JM, le Forestier C, Duedari N. Leukocyte depletion of red cell concentrates by filtration: influence of blood product temperature. Vox Sang 1992;62:242–243.
11. Sirchia G, Rebulla P, Sabbioneda L, Garcea F, Greppi N. Optimal conditions for white cell reduction in red cells by filtration at the patient's bedside. Transfusion 1996;36:322–327.
12. Bowden RA, Slichter SJ, Sayers M, et al. A compar ison of filtered leukocyte-reduced and cytomegalovirus (CMV) seronegative blood products for the prevention of transfusion-associated CMV infection after marrow transplant. Blood 1995;86:3598–3603.
13. Williamson LM, Wimperis JZ, Williamson P, et al. Bedside filtration of blood products in the prevention of HLA alloimmunization: a prospective randomized study. Alloimmunisation Study Group. Blood 1994;83:3028–3035.
14. van der Meer PF, Pietersz RN, Nelis JT, Hinloopen B, Dekker WJ, Reesink HW. Six filters for the removal of white cells from red cell concentrates, evaluated at 4°C and/or at room temperature. Transfusion 1999;39:265–270.
15. Schuetz AN, Hillyer KL, Roback JD, Hillyer CD. Leukoreduction filtration of blood with sickle cell trait. Transfus Med Rev 2004;18:168–176.
16. Stroncek DF, Byrne KM, Noguchi CT, Schechter AN, Leitman SF. Increasing hemoglobin oxygen saturation levels in sickle trait donor whole blood prevents hemoglobin S polymerization and allows effective white blood cell reduction by filtration. Transfusion 2004;44:1293–1299.
17. Burgstaler EA. Blood component collection by apheresis. J Clin Apheresis 2006, in press.
18. Silva MA (ed). Standards for Blood Banks and Transfusion Services, 23rd ed. Bethesda, Md., American Association of Blood Banks, 2005.
19. Beckman N, Sher G, Masse M, et al. Review of the quality monitoring methods used by countries using or implementing universal leukoreduction. Transfus Med Rev 2004;18:25–35.
20. van der Meer PF, Gratama JW, van Delden CJ, et al. Comparison of five platforms for enumeration of residual leucocytes in leucoreduced blood components. Br J Haematol 2001;115:953–962.
21. Triulzi DJ, Meyer EM, Donnenberg AD. WBC subset analysis of WBC-reduced platelet components. Transfusion 2000;40:771–780.
22. Roback JD, Bray RA, Hillyer CD. Longitudinal monitoring of WBC subsets in packed RBC units after filtration: implications for transfusion transmission of infections. Transfusion 2000;40:500–506.
23. Kao KJ, Mickel M, Braine HG, et al. White cell reduction in platelet concentrates and packed red cells by filtration: a multicenter clinical trial. The Trap Study Group. Transfusion 1995;35:13–19.
24. Ratko TA, Cummings JP, Oberman HA, et al. Evidence-based recommendations for the use of WBC-reduced cellular blood components. Transfusion 2001;41:1310–1319.
25. Vamvakas EC, Blajchman MA. Universal WBC reduction: the case for and against. Transfusion 2001;41:691–712.
26. Hebert PC, Fergusson D, Blajchman MA, et al. Clinical outcomes following institution of the Canadian universal leukoreduction program for red blood cell transfusions. JAMA 2003;289:1941–1949.
27. Dzik WH, Anderson JK, O'Neill EM, Assmann SF, Kalish LA, Stowell CP. A prospective, randomized clinical trial of universal WBC reduction. Transfusion 2002;42:1114–1122.
28. Mintz PD. Febrile reactions to platelet transfusions. Am J Clin Pathol 1991;95:609–612.
29. Dzieczkowski JS, Barrett BB, Nester D, et al. Characterization of reactions after exclusive transfusion of white cell-reduced cellular blood components. Transfusion 1995;35:10–25.
30. Sirchia G, Rebulla P, Parravicini A, Carnelli V, Gianotti GA, Bertolini F. Leukocyte depletion of red cell units at the bedside by transfusion through a new filter. Transfusion 1987;27:402–405.
31. Sirchia G, Wenz B, Rebulla P, Parravicini A, Carnelli V, Bertolini F. Removal of white cells from red cells by transfusion through a new filter. Transfusion 1990;30:30–33.
32. Wenz B. Microaggregate blood filtration and the febrile transfusion reaction: a comparative study. Transfusion 1983;23:95–98.
33. Heddle NM, Kelton JG. Febrile nonhemolytic transfusion reactions. In Popovsky MA (ed). Transfusion Reactions. Bethesda, Md., American Association of Blood Banks Press, 1996, pp 45–80.
34. Brecher ME (ed). Technical Manual,15th ed. Bethesda, Md., American Association of Blood Bank Press, 2005.
35. Luheshi GN. Cytokines and fever. Mechanisms and sites of action. Ann NY Acad Sci 1998;856:83–89.
36. Cao C, Matsumura K, Yamagata K, Watanabe Y. Cyclooxygenase-2 is induced in brain blood vessels during fever evoked by peripheral or central administration of tumor necrosis factor. Brain Res Mol Brain Res 1998;56:45–56.
37. Ganong WF. Central regulation of visceral function. In Ganong WF. Review of Medical Physiology, 19th ed. Stamford, Conn., Appleton and Lange, 1999, p 242.
38. Engel A, Kern WV, Murdter G, Kern P. Kinetics and correlation with body temperature of circulating interleukin-6, interleukin-8, tumor necrosis factor alpha and interleukin-1 beta in patients with fever and neutropenia. Infection 1994;22:160–164.
39. Menitove JE, McElligott MC, Aster RH. Febrile transfusion reaction: what blood component should be given next? Vox Sang 1982;42: 318–321.
40. Chambers LA, Kruskall MS, Pacini DG, Donovan LM. Febrile reactions after platelet transfusion: the effect of single versus multiple donors. Transfusion 1990;30:219–221.
41. Heddle NM, Klama LN, Griffith L, Roberts R, Shukla G, Kelton JG. A prospective study to identify the risk factors associated with acute reactions to platelet and red cell transfusions. Transfusion 1993;33: 794–797.
42. de Rie MA, van der Plas-van Dalen CM, Engelfriet CP, von dem Borne AE. The serology of febrile transfusion reactions. Vox Sang 1985;49:126–134.
43. Decary F, Ferner P, Giavedoni L, et al. An investigation of nonhemolytic transfusion reactions. Vox Sang 1984;46:277–285.
44. Perkins HA, Payne R, Ferguson J, Wood M. Nonhemolytic febrile transfusion reactions. Quantitative effects of blood components with emphasis on isoantigenic incompatibility of leukocytes. Vox Sang 1966;11:578–600.
45. Brubaker DB. Clinical significance of white cell antibodies in febrile nonhemolytic transfusion reactions. Transfusion 1990;30:733–737.
46. Thulstrup H. The influence of leukocyte and thrombocyte incompatibility on nonhaemolytic transfusion reactions. I. A retrospective study. Vox Sang 1971;21:233–250.
47. Arend WP, Joslin FG, Massoni RJ. Effects of immune complexes on production by human monocytes of interleukin 1 or an interleukin 1 inhibitor. J Immunol 1985;134:3868–3875.
48. Heddle NM, Klama L, Singer J, et al. The role of the plasma from platelet concentrates in transfusion reactions. N Engl J Med 1994;331:625–628.
49. Abbas AK, Lichtman AN, Pober JS. Cytokines in Cellular and Molecular Immunology, 3rd ed. Philadelphia, WB Saunders, 1997.
50. Muylle L, Joos M, Wouters E, De Bock R, Peetermans ME. Increased tumor necrosis factor alpha (TNF alpha), interleukin 1, and interleukin 6 (IL-6) levels in the plasma of stored platelet concentrates: relationship between TNF alpha and IL-6 levels and febrile transfusion reactions. Transfusion 1993;33:195–199.
51. Stack G, Snyder EL. Cytokine generation in stored platelet concentrates. Transfusion 1994;34:10–25.
52. Muylle L. Ex vivo production in blood components: relevant and irrelevant. Paper presented at the 21st International Symposium on Blood Transfusion, Gronigen, 1996.
53. Aye MT, Palmer DS, Giulivi A, Hashemi S. Effect of filtration of platelet concentrates on the accumulation of cytokines and platelet release factors during storage. Transfusion 1995;35:117–124.

54. Palmer DS, Aye MT, Dumont L, et al. Prevention of cytokine accumulation in platelets obtained with the COBE spectra apheresis system. Vox Sang 1998;75:115–123.
55. Fujihara M, Ikebuchi K, Wakamoto S, Sekiguchi S. Effects of filtration and gamma radiation on the accumulation of RANTES and transforming growth factor-beta 1 in apheresis platelet concentrates during storage. Transfusion 1999;39:498–505.
56. Muller-Steinhardt M, Kirchner H, Kluter H. Impact of storage at 22°C and citrate anticoagulation on the cytokine secretion of mononuclear leukocytes. Vox Sang 1998;75:12–17.
57. Heddle NM, Tan M, Klama L, Schroeder J. Factors affecting cytokine production in platelet concentrates [abstract]. Transfusion 1994;34(Suppl):67S.
58. Grey D, Erber WN, Saunders KM, Lown JA. Monocyte activation in platelet concentrates. Vox Sang 1998;75:110–114.
59. Molloy RG, Mannick JA, Rodrick ML. Cytokines, sepsis, and immunomodulation. Br J Surg 1993;80:289–297.
60. Hawrylowicz CM, Howells GL, Feldmann M. Platelet-derived interleukin 1 induces human endothelial adhesion molecule expression and cytokine production. J Exp Med 1991;174:785–790.
61. El-Kattan I, Anderson J, Yun JK, et al. Mononuclear cell (MC) adhesion to platelet storage bag plastic polymers correlates with cytokine levels [abstract]. Transfusion 1995;35(Suppl):44S.
62. Dzik WH. Is the febrile response to transfusion due to donor or recipient cytokine? [letter] Transfusion 1992;32:594.
63. Sacher RA, Boyle L, Freter CE. High circulating interleukin 6 levels associated with acute transfusion reaction: cause or effect? Transfusion 1993;33:962–963.
64. Schiller JH, Storer BE, Witt PL, et al. Biological and clinical effects of intravenous tumor necrosis factor-alpha administered three times weekly. Cancer Res 1991;51:1651–1658.
65. Agosti JM, Coombs RW, Collier AC, et al. A randomized, double-blind, phase I/II trial of tumor necrosis factor and interferon-gamma for treatment of AIDS-related complex (Protocol 025 from the AIDS Clinical Trials Group). AIDS Res Hum Retroviruses 1992;8:581–587.
66. Tewari A, Buhles WC Jr, Starnes HF Jr. Preliminary report: effects of interleukin-1 on platelet counts. Lancet 1990;336:712–714.
67. Crown J, Jakubowski A, Kemeny N, et al. A phase I trial of recombinant human interleukin-1 beta alone and in combination with myelosuppressive doses of 5-fluorouracil in patients with gastrointestinal cancer. Blood 1991;78:1420–1427.
68. Dinarello CA. Interleukin-1 and interleukin-1 antagonism. Blood 1991;77:1627–1652.
69. Jacobi KE, Wanke C, Jacobi A, Weisbach V, Hemmerling TM. Determination of eicosanoid and cytokine production in salvaged blood, stored red blood cell concentrates, and whole blood. J Clin Anesth 2000;12:94–99.
70. Stack G, Baril L, Napychank P, Snyder EL. Cytokine generation in stored, white cell-reduced, and bacterially contaminated units of red cells. Transfusion 1995;35:199–203.
71. Claas FH, Smeenk RJ, Schmidt R, van Steenbrugge GJ, Eernisse JG. Alloimmunization against the MHC antigens after platelet transfusions is due to contaminating leukocytes in the platelet suspension. Exp Hematol 1981;9:84–89.
72. Vamvakas EC. Meta-analysis of randomized controlled trials of the efficacy of white cell reduction in preventing HLA-alloimmunization and refractoriness to random-donor platelet transfusions. Transfus Med Rev 1998;12:258–270.
73. Sniecinski I, O'Donnell MR, Nowicki B, Hill LR. Prevention of refractoriness and HLA-alloimmunization using filtered blood products. Blood 1988;71:1402–1407.
74. Schiffer CA, Dutcher JP, Aisner J, Hogge D, Wiernik PH, Reilly JP. A randomized trial of leukocyte-depleted platelet transfusion to modify alloimmunization in patients with leukemia. Blood 1983;62:815–820.
75. Andreu G, Dewailly J, Leberre C, et al. Prevention of HLA immunization with leukocyte-poor packed red cells and platelet concentrates obtained by filtration. Blood 1988;72:964–969.
76. van Marwijk Kooy M, van Prooijen HC, Moes M, Bosma-Stants I, Akkerman JW. Use of leukocyte-depleted platelet concentrates for the prevention of refractoriness and primary HLA alloimmunization: a prospective, randomized trial. Blood 1991;77:201–205.
77. Oksanen K, Kekomaki R, Ruutu T, Koskimies S, Myllyla G. Prevention of alloimmunization in patients with acute leukemia by use of white cell-reduced blood components—a randomized trial. Transfusion 1991;31:588–594.
78. Sintnicolaas K, van Marwijk Kooij M, van Prooijen HC, et al. Leukocyte depletion of random single-donor platelet transfusions does not prevent secondary human leukocyte antigen-alloimmunization and refractoriness: a randomized prospective study. Blood 1995;85:824–828.
79. The Trial to Reduce Alloimmunization to Platelets Study Group. Leukocyte reduction and ultraviolet B irradiation of platelets to prevent alloimmunization and refractoriness to platelet transfusions. N Engl J Med 1997;337:1861–1869.
80. Fisher M, Chapman JR, Ting A, Morris PJ. Alloimmunisation to HLA antigens following transfusion with leucocyte-poor and purified platelet suspensions. Vox Sang 1985;49:331–335.
81. Petranyi GG, Padanyi A, Horuzsko A, Rethy M, Gyodi E, Perner F. Mixed lymphocyte culture: evidence that pretransplant transfusion with platelets induces FcR and blocking antibody production similar to that induced by leukocyte transfusion. Transplantation 1988;45:823–824.
82. Kao KJ, Luz de Rosario M. Platelet alloimmunization. In Anderson KC, Ness P (eds). Scientific Basis of Transfusion Medicine: Implications for Clinical Practice. Philadelphia, WB Saunders, 2000, pp 409–419.
83. Kao KJ, Cook DJ, Scornik JC. Quantitative analysis of platelet surface HLA by W6/32 anti-HLA monoclonal antibody. Blood 1986;68:627–632.
84. Rudensky A, Preston-Hurlburt P, Hong SC, Barlow A, Janeway CA Jr. Sequence analysis of peptides bound to MHC class II molecules. Nature 1991;353:622–627.
85. Chicz RM, Urban RG, Gorga JC, Vignali DA, Lane WS, Strominger JL. Specificity and promiscuity among naturally processed peptides bound to HLA-DR alleles. J Exp Med 1993;178:27–47.
86. Fast LD. Recipient elimination of allogeneic lymphoid cells: donor $CD4^+$ cells are effective alloantigen-presenting cells. Blood 2000;96:1144–1149.
87. Kao KJ, del Rosario ML. Role of class-II major histocompatibility complex (MHC)-antigen-positive donor leukocytes in transfusion-induced alloimmunization to donor class-I MHC antigens. Blood 1998;92:690–694.
88. Gouttefangeas C, Diehl M, Keilholz W, Hornlein RF, Stevanovic S, Rammensee HG. Thrombocyte HLA molecules retain nonrenewable endogenous peptides of megakaryocyte lineage and do not stimulate direct allocytotoxicity in vitro. Blood 2000;95:3168–3175.
89. Mellman I, Turley SJ, Steinman RM. Antigen processing for amateurs and professionals. Trends Cell Biol 1998;8:231–237.
90. Vogt AB, Kropshofer H. HLA-DM—an endosomal and lysosomal chaperone for the immune system. Trends Biochem Sci 1999;24:150–154.
91. Gould DS, Auchincloss H Jr. Direct and indirect recognition: the role of MHC antigens in graft rejection. Immunol Today 1999;20:77–82.
92. Turley SJ, Inaba K, Garrett WS, et al. Transport of peptide-MHC class II complexes in developing dendritic cells. Science 2000;288:522–527.
93. Bang KW, Speck ER, Blanchette VS, Freedman J, Semple JW. Unique processing pathways within recipient antigen-presenting cells determine IgG immunity against donor platelet MHC antigens. Blood 2000;95:1735–1742.
94. Heddle NM. The efficacy of leukodepletion to improve platelet transfusion response: a critical appraisal of clinical studies. Transfus Med Rev 1994;8:15–28.
95. Seftel MD, Growe GH, Petraszko T, et al. Universal prestorage leukoreduction in Canada decreases platelet alloimmunization and refractoriness. Blood 2004;103:333–339.
96. van de Watering L, Hermans J, Witvliet M, Versteegh M, Brand A. HLA and RBC immunization after filtered and buffy coat-depleted blood transfusion in cardiac surgery: a randomized controlled trial. Transfusion 2003;43:765–771.
97. Ohto H, Nomizu T, Kuroda F, Hoshi T, Rokkaku Y. HLA alloimmunization of surgical patients by transfusion with bedside leukoreduced blood components. Fukushima J Med Sci 2003;49:45–54.
98. Hillyer CD, Emmens RK, Zago-Novaretti M, Berkman EM. Methods for the reduction of transfusion-transmitted cytomegalovirus infection: filtration versus the use of seronegative donor units. Transfusion 1994;34:929–934.
99. Smith DM, Shoos-Lipton K. Leukocyte Reduction for the Prevention of Transfusion-Transmitted Cytomegalovirus. Bethesda, Md., American Association of Blood Banks Press, 1997.
100. Landaw EM, Kanter M, Petz LD. Safety of filtered leukocyte-reduced blood products for prevention of transfusion-associated cytomegalovirus infection [letter]. Blood 1996;87:4910.
101. Nichols WG, Price TH, Gooley T, Corey L, Boeckh M. Transfusion-transmitted cytomegalovirus infection after receipt of leukoreduced blood products. Blood 2003;101:4195–4200.
102. Vamvakas EC. Is white blood cell reduction equivalent to antibody screening in preventing transmission of cytomegalovirus by transfusion? A review of the literature and meta-analysis. Transfus Med Rev 2005;19:181–199.
103. Taylor-Wiedeman J, Hayhurst GP, Sissons JG, Sinclair JH. Polymorphonuclear cells are not sites of persistence of human cytomegalovirus in healthy individuals. J Gen Virol 1993;74(pt 2):265–268.

104. Taylor-Wiedeman J, Sissons JG, Borysiewicz LK, Sinclair JH. Monocytes are a major site of persistence of human cytomegalovirus in peripheral blood mononuclear cells. J Gen Virol 1991;72(pt 9):2059–2064.
105. Larsson S, Soderberg-Naucler C, Moller E. Productive cytomegalovirus (CMV) infection exclusively in CD13-positive peripheral blood mononuclear cells from CMV-infected individuals: implications for prevention of CMV transmission. Transplantation 1998;65:411–415.
106. Bolovan-Fritts CA, Mocarski ES, Wiedeman JA. Peripheral blood CD14+ cells from healthy subjects carry a circular conformation of latent cytomegalovirus genome. Blood 1999;93:394–398.
107. Taylor-Wiedeman J, Sissons P, Sinclair J. Induction of endogenous human cytomegalovirus gene expression after differentiation of monocytes from healthy carriers. J Virol 1994;68:1597–1604.
108. Stanier P, Taylor DL, Kitchen AD, Wales N, Tryhorn Y, Tyms AS. Persistence of cytomegalovirus in mononuclear cells in peripheral blood from blood donors. BMJ 1989;299:897–898.
109. Slobedman B, Mocarski ES. Quantitative analysis of latent human cytomegalovirus. J Virol 1999;73:4806–4812.
110. Visconti MR, Pennington J, Garner SF, Allain JP, Williamson LM. Assessment of removal of human cytomegalovirus from blood components by leukocyte depletion filters using real-time quantitative PCR. Blood 2004;103:1137–1139.
111. Cope AV, Sabin C, Burroughs A, Rolles K, Griffiths PD, Emery VC. Interrelationships among quantity of human cytomegalovirus (HCMV) DNA in blood, donor-recipient serostatus, and administration of methylprednisolone as risk factors for HCMV disease following liver transplantation. J Infect Dis 1997;176:1484–1490.
112. Miller WJ, McCullough J, Balfour HH Jr, et al. Prevention of cytomegalovirus infection following bone marrow transplantation: a randomized trial of blood product screening. Bone Marrow Transplant 1991;7:227–234.
113. Roback JD, Drew WL, Laycock ME, Todd D, Hillyer CD, Busch MP. CMV DNA is rarely detected in healthy blood donors using validated PCR assays. Transfusion 2003;43:314–321.
114. Bevan IS, Daw RA, Day PJ, Ala FA, Walker MR. Polymerase chain reaction for detection of human cytomegalovirus infection in a blood donor population. Br J Haematol 1991;78:94–99.
115. Rahbar AR, Sundqvist VA, Wirgart BZ, Grillner L, Soderberg-Naucler C. Recognition of cytomegalovirus clinical isolate antigens by sera from cytomegalovirus-negative blood donors. Transfusion 2004;44: 1059–1066.
116. Krajden M, Shankaran P, Bourke C, Lau W. Detection of cytomegalovirus in blood donors by PCR using the digene SHARP signal system assay: effects of sample preparation and detection methodology. J Clin Microbiol 1996;34:29–33.
117. Chou SW. Acquisition of donor strains of cytomegalovirus by renal-transplant recipients. N Engl J Med 1986;314:1418–1423.
118. Chou SW. Reactivation and recombination of multiple cytomegalovirus strains from individual organ donors. J Infect Dis 1989;160:11–15.
119. Chandler SH, Handsfield HH, McDougall JK. Isolation of multiple strains of cytomegalovirus from women attending a clinic for sexually transmitted disease. J Infect Dis 1987;155:655–660.
120. Spector SA, Hirata KK, Newman TR. Identification of multiple cytomegalovirus strains in homosexual men with acquired immunodeficiency syndrome. J Infect Dis 1984;150:953–956.
121. Baldanti F, Simoncini L, Sarasini A, et al. Ganciclovir resistance as a result of oral ganciclovir in a heart transplant recipient with multiple human cytomegalovirus strains in blood. Transplantation 1998;66:324–329.
122. Winston DJ, Huang ES, Miller MJ, et al. Molecular epidemiology of cytomegalovirus infections associated with bone marrow transplantation. Ann Intern Med 1985;102:16–20.
123. Lang DJ. Cytomegalovirus infections in organ transplantation and post transfusion: an hypothesis. Arch Gesamte Virusforsch 1972;37: 365–377.
124. Collier AC, Kalish LA, Busch MP, et al. Leukocyte-reduced red blood cell transfusions in patients with anemia and human immunodeficiency virus infection: the Viral Activation Transfusion Study, a randomized controlled trial. JAMA 2001;285:1592–1601.
125. Opelz G, Sengar DP, Mickey MR, Terasaki PI. Effect of blood transfusions on subsequent kidney transplants. Transplant Proc 1973;5: 253–259.
126. Opelz G, Vanrenterghem Y, Kirste G, et al. Prospective evaluation of pretransplant blood transfusions in cadaver kidney recipients. Transplantation 1997;63:964–967.
127. Gantt CL. Red blood cells for cancer patients [letter]. Lancet 1981;2:363.
128. van Twuyver E, Mooijaart RJ, ten Berge IJ, et al. Pretransplantation blood transfusion revisited. N Engl J Med 1991;325:1210–1213.
129. Murphy B, Krensky AM. HLA-derived peptides as novel immunomodulatory therapeutics. J Am Soc Nephrol 1999;10:1346–1355.
130. Clayberger C, Lyu SC, DeKruyff R, Parham P, Krensky AM. Peptides corresponding to the CD8 and CD4 binding domains of HLA molecules block T lymphocyte immune responses in vitro. J Immunol 1994;153:946–951.
131. Dzik S, Szuflad P, Eaves S. HLA antigens on leukocyte fragments and plasma proteins: prestorage leukoreduction by filtration. Vox Sang 1994;66:104–111.
132. Ghio M, Contini P, Mazzei C, et al. Soluble HLA class I, HLA class II, and Fas ligand in blood components: a possible key to explain the immunomodulatory effects of allogeneic blood transfusions. Blood 1999;93:1770–1777.
133. Starzl TE, Zinkernagel RM. Antigen localization and migration in immunity and tolerance. N Engl J Med 1998;339:1905–1913.
134. Bianchi DW, Zickwolf GK, Weil GJ, Sylvester S, DeMaria MA. Male fetal progenitor cells persist in maternal blood for as long as 27 years postpartum. Proc Natl Acad Sci USA 1996;93:705–708.
135. Lee TH, Paglieroni T, Ohto H, Holland PV, Busch MP. Survival of donor leukocyte subpopulations in immunocompetent transfusion recipients: frequent long-term microchimerism in severe trauma patients. Blood 1999;93:3127–3139.
136. Lee TH, Paglieroni T, Utter GH, et al. High-level long-term white blood cell microchimerism after transfusion of leukoreduced blood components to patients resuscitated after severe traumatic injury. Transfusion 2005;45:1280–1290.
137. Chowdhury NC, Murphy B, Sayegh MH, et al. Acquired systemic tolerance to rat cardiac allografts induced by intrathymic inoculation of synthetic polymorphic MHC class I allopeptides. Transplantation 1996;62:1878–1882.
138. Mincheff MS, Getsov SI, Meryman HT. Mechanisms of alloimmunization and immunosuppression by blood transfusions in an inbred rodent model. Transplantation 1995;60:815–821.
139. Dzik S, Mincheff M, Puppo F. Apoptosis, transforming growth factor-beta, and the immunosuppressive effect of transfusion. Transfusion 2002;42:1221–1223.
140. Chen ZK, Cobbold SP, Waldmann H, Metcalfe S. Amplification of natural regulatory immune mechanisms for transplantation tolerance. Transplantation 1996;62:1200–1206.
141. Yang CP, McDonagh M, Bell EB. CD45RC+ CD4 T cell subsets are maintained in an unresponsive state by the persistence of transfusion-derived alloantigen. Transplantation 1995;60:192–199.
142. Blajchman MA, Bardossy L, Carmen R, Sastry A, Singal DP. Allogeneic blood transfusion-induced enhancement of tumor growth: two animal models showing amelioration by leukodepletion and passive transfer using spleen cells. Blood 1993;81:1880–1882.
143. Bordin JO, Bardossy L, Blajchman MA. Growth enhancement of established tumors by allogeneic blood transfusion in experimental animals and its amelioration by leukodepletion: the importance of the timing of the leukodepletion. Blood 1994;84:344–348.
144. Kao KJ. Induction of humoral immune tolerance to major histocompatibility complex antigens by transfusions of UVB-irradiated leukocytes. Blood 1996;88:4375–4382.
145. Kirkley SA, Cowles J, Pellegrini VD Jr, Harris CM, Boyd AD, Blumberg N. Cytokine secretion after allogeneic or autologous blood transfusion [letter]. Lancet 1995;345:527.
146. Quintiliani L, Iudicone P, Di Girolamo M, et al. Immunoresponsiveness of cancer patients: effect of blood transfusion and immune reactivity of tumor infiltrating lymphocytes. Cancer Detect Prev 1995;19:518–526.
147. Tietze M, Kluter H, Troch M, Kirchner H. Immune responsiveness in orthopedic surgery patients after transfusion of autologous or allogeneic blood. Transfusion 1995;35:378–383.
148. van de Watering LM, Brand A, Houbiers JG, Klein Kranenbarg WM, Hermans J, van de Velde C. Perioperative blood transfusions, with or without allogeneic leucocytes, relate to survival, not to cancer recurrence. Br J Surg 2001;88:267–272.
149. Titlestad IL, Ebbesen LS, Ainsworth AP, Lillevang ST, Qvist N, Georgsen J. Leukocyte-depletion of blood compon ents does not significantly reduce the risk of infectious complications. Results of a double-blinded, randomized study. Int J Colorectal Dis 2001;16:147–153.
150. Baron JF, Gourdin M, Bertrand M, et al. The effect of universal leukodepletion of packed red blood cells on postoperative infections in high-risk patients undergoing abdominal aortic surgery. Anesth Analg 2002;94:529–537.
151. van Hilten JA, van de Watering LM, van Bockel JH, et al. Effects of transfusion with red cells filtered to remove leucocytes: randomised controlled trial in patients undergoing major surgery. BMJ 2004;328:1281–1291.

152. van de Watering LM, Hermans J, Houbiers JG, et al. Beneficial effects of leukocyte depletion of transfused blood on postoperative complications in patients undergoing cardiac surgery: a randomized clinical trial. Circulation 1998;97:562–568.
153. Wallis JP, Chapman CE, Orr KE, Clark SC, Forty JR. Effect of WBC reduction of transfused RBCs on postoperative infection rates in cardiac surgery. Transfusion 2002;42:1127–1134.
154. Bilgin YM, van de Watering LM, Eijsman L, et al. Double-blind, randomized controlled trial on the effect of leukocyte-depleted erythrocyte transfusions in cardiac valve surgery. Circulation 2004;109:2755–2760.
155. Bracey AW, Radovancevic R, Nussmeier NA, et al. Leukocyte-reduced blood in open heart surgery patients: effects on outcome [abstract]. Transfusion 2002;42(Suppl):5S.
156. Volkova N, Klapper E, Pepkowitz SH, Denton T, Gillaspie G, Goldfinger D. A case-control study of the impact of WBC reduction on the cost of hospital care for patients undergoing coronary artery bypass graft surgery. Transfusion 2002;42:1123–1126.
157. Fung MK, Rao N, Rice J, Ridenour M, Mook W, Triulzi DJ. Leukoreduction in the setting of open heart surgery: a prospective cohort-controlled study. Transfusion 2004;44:30–35.
158. Janatpour KA, Paglieroni TG, Crocker VL, DuBois DJ, Holland PV. Visual assessment of hemolysis in red blood cell units and segments can be deceptive. Transfusion 2004;44:984–989.
159. Llewelyn CA, Taylor RS, Todd AA, Stevens W, Murphy MF, Williamson LM. The effect of universal leukoreduction on postoperative infections and length of hospital stay in elective orthopedic and cardiac surgery. Transfusion 2004;44:489–500.
160. California Blood Bank Society. Available at http://www.cbbsweb.org/enf/enetcomm2001.html. Accessed March 28, 2006.
161. US Food and Drug Administration, Center for Biologics Evaluation and Research. Available at http://www.fda.gov/cber/recalls/leukpal022305.htm. Accessed March 28, 2006.
162. Gyongyossy-Issa MI, Weiss SL, Sowemimo-Coker SO, Garcez RB, Devine DV. Prestorage leukoreduction and low-temperature filtration reduce hemolysis of stored red cell concentrates. Transfusion 2005;45:90–96.
163. Sano H, Koga Y, Hamasaki K, Furuyama H, Itami N. Anaphylaxis associated with white-cell reduction filter [letter]. Lancet 1996;347:1053.
164. Fried MR, Eastlund T, Christie B, Mullin GT, Key NS. Hypotensive reactions to white cell-reduced plasma in a patient undergoing angiotensin-converting enzyme inhibitor therapy. Transfusion 1996;36:900–903.
165. Mair B, Leparc GF. Hypotensive reactions associated with platelet transfusions and angiotensin-converting enzyme inhibitors. Vox Sang 1998;74:27–30.
166. Yenicesu I, Tezcan I, Tuncer AM. Hypotensive reactions during platelet transfusions. Transfusion 1998;38:410; author reply 413–415.
167. Sweeney JD, Dupuis M, Mega AP. Hypotensive reactions to red cells filtered at the bedside, but not to those filtered before storage, in patients taking ACE inhibitors. Transfusion 1998;38:410–411; author reply 413–415.
168. Abe H, Ikebuchi K, Shimbo M, Sekiguchi S. Hypotensive reactions with a white cell-reduction filter: activation of kallikrein-kinin cascade in a patient. Transfusion 1998;38:411–412; author reply 413–415.
169. Belloni M, Alghisi A, Bettini C, Soli M, Zampieri L. Hypotensive reactions associated with white cell-reduced apheresis platelet concentrates in patients not receiving ACE Inhibitors. Transfusion 1998;38:412–415.
170. Myers T, Uhl L, Kruskall MS. Association between angiotensin-converting enzyme (ACE) inhibitors and hypotensive transfusion reactions [abstract]. Transfusion 1996;36(Suppl):60S.
171. Verresen L, Waer M, Vanrenterghem Y, Michielsen P. Angiotensin-converting-enzyme inhibitors and anaphylactoid reactions to high-flux membrane dialysis. Lancet 1990;336:1360–1362.
172. Olbricht CJ, Schaumann D, Fischer D. Anaphylactoid reactions, LDL apheresis with dextran sulphate, and ACE inhibitors. Lancet 1992;340:908–909.
173. Davidson DC, Peart I, Turner S, Sangster M. Prevention with icatibant of anaphylactoid reactions to ACE inhibitor during LDL apheresis [letter]. Lancet 1994;343:1575.
174. Nielsen F, Damkjaer Nielsen M, Rasmussen S, Kappelgaard AM, Giese J. Bradykinin in blood and plasma: facts and fallacies. Acta Med Scand Suppl 1983;677:54–59.
175. Scicli AG, Mindroiu T, Scicli G, Carretero OA. Blood kinins, their concentration in normal subjects and in patients with congenital deficiency in plasma prekallikrein and kininogen. J Lab Clin Med 1982;100:81–93.
176. Berridge MJ. Inositol trisphosphate and diacylglycerol: two interacting second messengers. Annu Rev Biochem 1987;56:159–193.
177. Sung CP, Arleth AJ, Shikano K, Berkowitz BA. Characterization and function of bradykinin receptors in vascular endothelial cells. J Pharmacol Exp Ther 1988;247:8–13.
178. Mousli M, Bueb JL, Bronner C, Rouot B, Landry Y. G protein activation: a receptor-independent mode of action for cationic amphiphilic neuropeptides and venom peptides. Trends Pharmacol Sci 1990;11:358–362.
179. Dachman WD, Ford GA, Blaschke TF, Hoffman BB. Mechanism of bradykinin-induced venodilation in humans. J Cardiovasc Pharmacol 1993;21:241–248.
180. O'Kane KP, Webb DJ, Collier JG, Vallance PJ. Local L-NG-monomethyl-arginine attenuates the vasodilator action of bradykinin in the human forearm. Br J Clin Pharmacol 1994;38:311–315.
181. Cockcroft JR, Chowienczyk PJ, Brett SE, Bender N, Ritter JM. Inhibition of bradykinin-induced vasodilation in human forearm vasculature by icatibant, a potent B2-receptor antagonist. Br J Clin Pharmacol 1994;38:317–321.
182. Bonner G, Preis S, Schunk U, Toussaint C, Kaufmann W. Hemodynamic effects of bradykinin on systemic and pulmonary circulation in healthy and hypertensive humans. J Cardiovasc Pharmacol 1990;15(Suppl 6):S46–S56.
183. Shiba M, Tadokoro K, Sawanobori M, Nakajima K, Suzuki K, Juji T. Activation of the contact system by filtration of platelet concentrates with a negatively charged white cell-removal filter and measurement of venous blood bradykinin level in patients who received filtered platelets. Transfusion 1997;37:457–462.
184. Shiba M, Tadokoro K, Nakajima K, Juji T. Bradykinin generation in RC-MAP during storage at 4°C and leukocyte removal filtration. Thromb Res 1997;87:511–520.
185. Hild M, Soderstrom T, Egberg N, Lundahl J. Kinetics of bradykinin levels during and after leucocyte filtration of platelet concentrates. Vox Sang 1998;75:18–25.
186. Scott CF, Brandwein H, Whitbread J, Colman RW. Lack of clinically significant contact system activation during platelet concentrate filtration by leukocyte removal filters. Blood 1998;92:616–622.
187. Cyr M, Hume HA, Champagne M, et al. Anomaly of the des-Arg9-bradykinin metabolism associated with severe hypotensive reactions during blood transfusions: a preliminary study. Transfusion 1999;39:1084–1088.
188. Arnold DM, Molinaro G, Warkentin TE, et al. Hypotensive transfusion reactions can occur with blood products that are leukoreduced before storage. Transfusion 2004;44:1361–1366.
189. Owen HG, Brecher ME. Atypical reactions associated with use of angiotensin-converting enzyme inhibitors and apheresis. Transfusion 1994;34:891–894.
190. Reutter JC, Sanders KF, Brecher ME, Jones HG, Bandarenko N. Incidence of allergic reactions with fresh frozen plasma or cryo-supernatant plasma in the treatment of thrombotic thrombocytopenic purpura. J Clin Apher 2001;16:134–138.
191. Perseghin P, Capra M, Baldini V, Sciorelli G. Bradykinin production during donor plasmapheresis procedures. Vox Sang 2001;81:24–28.
192. Molinaro G, Adam A, Lepage Y, Hammerschmidt D, Koenigbauer U, Eastlund T. Hypotensive reaction during staphylococcal protein A column therapy in a patient with anomalous degradation of bradykinin and Des-Arg9-bradykinin after contact activation. Transfusion 2002;42:1458–1465.
193. Elghouzzi MH, Vedrenne JB, Jullien AM, Delcey D, Nadal M, Habibi B. Etude technique immunologique et clinique des performances de filtration du sang a la l'aide de l'appareill Erypur. Rev Fr Transfus Immunohematol 1981;24:579–595.
194. Lane TA, Myllyla G. Leukocyte-depleted blood products. In Leikola J, Lundgaard-Hansen P (eds). Current Studies in Hematology and Blood Transfusion. Basel, Karger, 1994;60:1–145.
195. Murphy MF, Metcalfe P, Thomas H, et al. Use of leucocyte-poor blood components and HLA-matched platelet donors to prevent HLA alloimmunization. Br J Haematal 1986;62:529–534.

Chapter 27

Virus-Safe Products: Pathogen Reduction and Inactivation

Laurence Corash

INTRODUCTION

Transfusion of blood components continues to be implicated in transmission of viral, bacterial, and protozoan diseases,[1] and the landscape of these infections and technologies to inactivate contaminating pathogens has continued to evolve. This review focuses on technologies that have reached the clinical trial phase. In the past 5 years, threats to blood safety from the emergence of new pathogens, migration of donor populations from regions with unusual endemic infectious agents, and increased recognition of problems in averting transfusion of labile components contaminated with recognized pathogens continue to emphasize the need for robust pathogen inactivation technologies. Since the previous edition of this text, new technologies for the prevention of transfusion-transmitted infections have been introduced into clinical practice, providing an opportunity to assess the practical efficacy of these technologies.

The residual risk for human immunodeficiency virus (HIV) and hepatitis C virus (HCV) transmission by transfusion varies by geographic region.[2] Continued improvements in donor screening with the introduction of nucleic acid testing (NAT) have decreased the risks for HIV and HCV to very low levels, ranging from 1:400,000 to 1:5,540,000 per donation.[3,4] However, greater risks remain for hepatitis B virus (HBV), ranging from 1:102,000 to 1:220,000,[3,5] and in some regions NAT has failed to detect significant numbers of donations with low levels of virus.[6] Although the risks per donation for HIV and HCV have diminished substantially with NAT, it is important to recall that many patients receive multiple transfusions for support of intensive therapies, and the residual risk of transfusion-transmitted infection increases with the number of donor exposures.

While it is commonly recognized that HIV, HCV, HBV, cytomegalovirus (CMV), and human T-lymphotropic viruses (HTLV) can be transmitted through cellular components, other pathogens are also emerging as potentially significant transfusion-associated infectious agents.[7] For example, transmission of protozoan infections due to trypanosomes,[8–10] *Leishmania*,[11] and *Babesia* have been documented.[12] Although protozoan agents have typically been thought of as unimportant transfusion-associated infections, recent experience with *Babesia* indicates seroprevalence rates among blood donors as high as 4%.[13]

Over the past 5 years, experience with conventional methods to prevent transfusion-associated transmission of infectious pathogens has demonstrated the continuing need for technologies to further improve the safety of blood transfusion.[14] The West Nile virus epidemic illustrates the limitations of testing as a reactive strategy to prevent transfusion transmission of an emerging pathogen.[15] Despite the rapid deployment of a sensitive test to detect infected blood donors, not all cases can be prevented owing to low copy numbers of virus in some infectious donors.[16,17] In addition, other viruses with early-phase low viral burdens may escape detection by sensitive methods.[18] For cell-associated viruses such as CMV and HTLV, leukoreduction technologies may be inadequate to ensure compete removal of infected cells as demonstrated by both in vitro[19,20] and in vivo studies.[21]

With the introduction of widespread culturing of platelet components to detect bacteria, the data indicate a prevalence greater than previously expected.[22] Within the last 5 years four studies have reported experience with culturing approximately 200,000 platelet components. The rates of contamination have ranged from 0.3% to 0.7% (3–7 per 1000 units) depending on volume cultured and use of both aerobic and anaerobic cultures.[23–26] More importantly, these studies demonstrated that the majority of the contaminated components were not interdicted before transfusion. Reported cases of serious transfusion-transmitted sepsis are infrequent and are generally due to highly contaminated units.[27] However, the true prevalence of platelet transfusion-transmitted infections encompassing all clinical consequences remains unknown.[22] Only one prospective study of 3584 platelet transfusions in 161 bone marrow transplant patients has been conducted and demonstrated a risk of symptomatic bacteremia in 1 per 16 patients, 1 per 350 transfusions, and 1 per 2100 platelet units.[28] These frequencies are significant considering that over 8 million units of platelet concentrates are transfused annually in the United States alone.[29] Despite the implementation in 2004 of requirements for bacterial detection of platelet components in the United States, at least three deaths due to transfusion of contaminated platelet components have been reported to the CDC.[30]

The logistics and costs of continued expansion of testing processes—for example, NAT and bacterial cultures—to further improve blood safety have been questioned.[23,31,32] The impact of bacterial detection methods has delayed release of platelet units and shortened the effective shelf life, leading to increased rates of expiration.[33] Furthermore, testing remains a reactive strategy to ensure blood component safety, since new pathogens may enter the donor population before adequate tests can be implemented. A complementary approach to improving the safety of blood component transfusion is

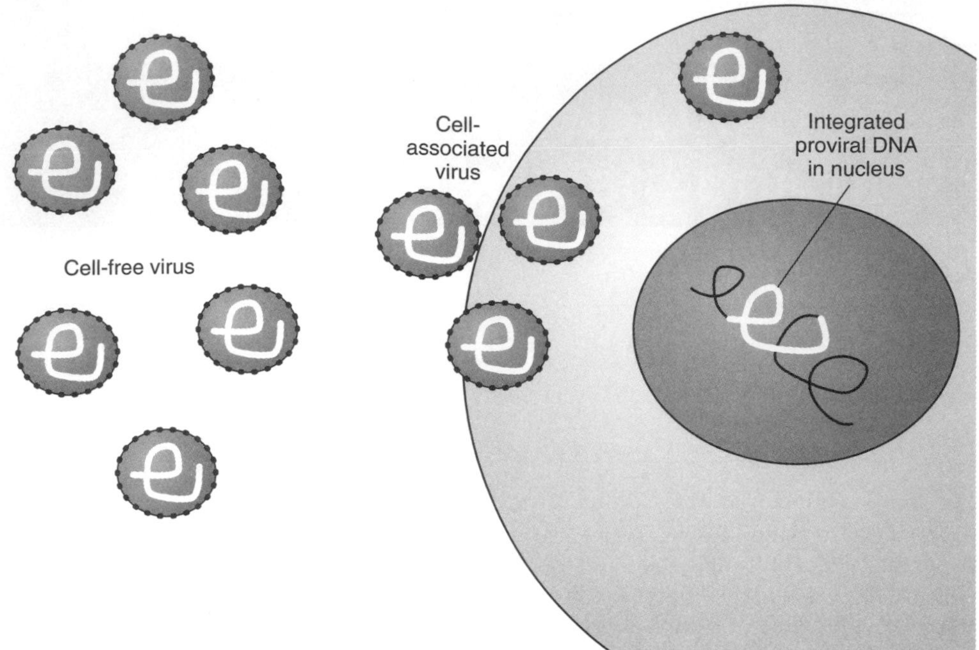

Figure 27–1 Infectious pathogens (e.g., viruses) may be present in the plasma as cell-free virus, associated with cell membranes, in the cell cytoplasm, or in the nucleus. Moreover, some viruses (e.g., retroviruses) may integrate nucleic acid sequences into host genomic DNA. A robust pathogen inactivation technology should be effective in each of these compartments.

inactivation of infectious pathogens in blood components. Treatment of plasma fractions with the solvent detergent process has demonstrated the benefits of this approach.[34] A robust inactivation technology that is compatible with current blood component processing procedures offers the potential for significantly improving transfusion safety. To be highly effective, a successful technology must inactivate pathogens in extracellular, intracellular, and nuclear compartments (Fig. 27–1). In the last case, inactivation also must be effective against pathogen nucleic acid sequences integrated into donor leukocytes.

Furthermore, a technology capable of inactivating residual leukocytes may confer additional benefits owing to inhibition of critical leukocyte functions, including cytokine synthesis, lymphocyte proliferation, and antigen presentation. Donor leukocytes may be associated with a variety of adverse immune events ranging in severity from febrile transfusion reactions to alloimmunization and graft-versus-host disease.[35,36] Recently, studies have shown that massively transfused patients may develop stable microchimerism, the significance of which is unclear.[37] Although a number of measures have been implemented to reduce the likelihood of these adverse immune reactions, a robust nucleic acid targeted pathogen inactivation process offers the potential to inactivate leukocytes as well as infectious pathogens.

SYSTEMS FOR INACTIVATION OF PATHOGENS IN PLATELET CONCENTRATES

Considerable effort has been devoted to developing methods for pathogen inactivation in platelet concentrates (Tables 27–1 and 27–2). The potential processes are divided into two basic groups: nucleic acid targeted and photodynamic methods. Both methods utilize photochemical reactions in an ex vivo treatment process combining a photo reactive compound and ultraviolet (UV) light. Nucleic acid targeting using psoralen compounds has been extensively investigated and is discussed in detail below, since a method using the novel psoralen amotosalen has undergone clinical trials and been commercialized. The photodynamic methods generally result in lower levels of pathogen inactivation and are associated with more platelet injury.[38] These technologies will not be reviewed further (see Table 27–2), with the exception of the riboflavin method, which has advanced to clinical trials.

The psoralen-based methods generally rely on nucleic acid–specific adduct formation,[39] in contrast to photodynamic processes that tend to utilize the production of active oxygen species in addition to nucleic acid reactions as the primary mechanism for pathogen inactivation.[40] Psoralens are low-molecular-weight, planar furocoumarins (Fig. 27–2). In the absence of UV light, psoralens reversibly intercalate into helical regions of DNA and RNA, under equilibrium kinetics. Upon illumination with UVA (320 to 400 nm), psoralens react with pyrimidine bases to form covalent mono-adducts and cross-links with nucleic acids (Fig. 27–3). Bacteria,[41] protozoa,[42,43] viruses,[44] and nucleated cells[45] with genomes that have been modified by psoralens are unable to replicate.

Early investigations with psoralen-mediated pathogen inactivation were conducted with 8-methxyopsoralen (8-MOP)[46] based on the history of prior human use to treat psoriasis and cutaneous T-cell lymphoma. These initial studies by Lin and co-workers established the principle of psoralen-mediated pathogen inactivation, but 8-MOP photochemical treatment was not a sufficiently rapid process for treatment of platelet concentrates in clinical use.[46,47]

Table 27–1 Psoralen Methods Used to Inactivate Pathogens and Leukocytes in Platelet Concentrates

Photoreactive Agent	Target	Reference
8-MOP	fd, R17, FeLV, *Escherichia coli, Staphylococcus aureus*	46
8-MOP	MCMV, FeRTV	132
8-MOP	HIV	133
8-MOP	DHBV	134
8-MOP	12 pathogenic bacteria	135
AMT	VSV	136
AMT	HIV	137, 138
AMT	VSV, Sindbis	139
PSR-Br	Bacteriophage	140, 141
Amotosalen	Pathogenic bacteria	67
Amotosalen	Leukocytes	45
Amotosalen	HIV, DHBV, BVDV	67
	CMV, bacteria	41, 44

8-MOP, 8-methoxypsoralen; AMT, aminomethyltrimethyl psoralen; PSR-Br, brominated psoralens; fd, bacteriophage; R17, bacteriophage; FeLV, feline leukemia virus; MCMV, murine cytomegalovirus; FeRTV, feline rhinotracheitis virus; HIV, human immunodeficiency virus; HSV, herpes simplex virus; DHBV, duck hepatitis B virus; VSV, vesicular stomatitis virus; Sindbis, Sindbis virus; BVDV, bovine viral diarrhea virus; CMV, cytomegalovirus.

Two laboratories investigated the use of aminomethyltrimethylpsoralen (AMT), a synthetic psoralen with enhanced nucleic acid–binding efficiency (see Table 27–2). Although AMT has increased nucleic acid–binding affinity compared with 8-MOP, it exhibits mutagenicity in the absence of light and thus has an unfavorable toxicology profile. Several classes of new psoralens have been synthesized that offer potential advantages over AMT and 8-MOP. The halogenated psoralens do not appear to be sufficiently effective for viral inactivation and in preliminary studies demonstrated adverse effects on platelet viability.[48,49]

Table 27–2 Photodynamic Methods Used to Inactivate Pathogens in Platelet Concentrates

Photoreactive Agent	Target	Reference
UVB	Poliovirus	142
Merocyanine 540	VSV	143
Merocyanine 540	HSV, MS2, F6	136
Methylene blue	Unspecified	144
Phthalocyanines	VSV	145
Riboflavin	HIV, WNV, PPV	55

UVB, ultraviolet B light (280–320 nm; VSV, vesicular stomatitis virus; HSV, herpes simplex virus; MS2, bacteriophage; F6, bacteriophage; HIV, human immunodeficiency virus; WNV, West Nile virus; PPV, postpolio virus.

AMT   Amotosalen

Figure 27–2 Structures of aminomethyltrimethylpsoralen (AMT) and amotosalen.

A new amino psoralen, amotosalen, was synthesized and shown to be highly effective for inactivation of pathogenic viruses, bacteria, and leukocytes in platelet concentrates with preservation of in vitro platelet function properties (Table 27–3). Lin and co-workers reported that human platelet concentrates (300 mL) contaminated with high titers of HCV($10^{4.5}$) and HBV($10^{5.5}$) and treated with amotosalen did not transmit hepatitis after transfusion into naive chimpanzees. Jordan and colleagues have shown that amotosalen treatment effectively prevents transfusion-transmitted CMV infection in a sensitive murine model.[50] Other studies demonstrated that amotosalen inactivates high levels of T cells, inhibits leukocyte cytokine synthesis during platelet storage, and inhibits nucleic acid amplification.[45,51] More importantly, treatment of T cells with the amotosalen process prevented transfusion-associated graft-versus-host disease (TA-GVHD) in both immunocompetent and immunocompromised murine bone marrow transplant models.[52] Amotosalen treatment of platelet concentrates

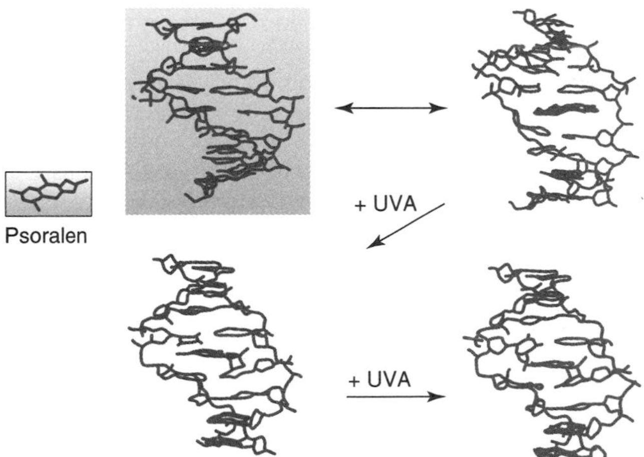

Figure 27–3 The mechanism of amotosalen binding to nucleic acid. In the dark, psoralens intercalate into helical regions of nucleic acid, either DNA or RNA. This phase is a reversible equilibrium process without covalent addition to nucleic acid. During illumination with long wavelength ultraviolet light (UVA), mono-adducts and di-adducts between amotosalen and pyrimidine form. Both types of adducts inhibit the function of polymerases and block nucleic acid replication.

Table 27–3 **Summary of Amotosalen Pathogen Inactivation in Platelet Concentrates**

Pathogen	Strain	Inactivation Achieved
HIV-1	IIIB, cell-free	$>10^{6.2}$ pfu/mL
	IIIB, cell-associated	$>10^{6.1}$ pfu/mL
	Integrated provirus*	No p24 expression using 0.1 μM Amotosalen + 1 J/cm²
	Clinical isolate Z84, cell-free†	$>10^{3.4}$ TCID50/mL
HIV-2	Clinical isolate CBL20, cell-free†	$>10^{2.5}$ TCID50/mL
HBV	MS-2‡	$>10^{5.5}$ CID50/mL
	DHBV as a model	$>10^{6.2}$ ID50/mL
HCV	Hutchinson‡	$>10^{4.5}$ CID50/mL
	BVDV as a model	$>10^{6.0}$ pfu/mL
HCMV	AD169, cell-associated	$>10^{5.9}$ pfu/mL
	AD169, cell-associated*	Below limit of detection using 1.5 μM S59 + 1.4 J/cm²
	MCMV as a model, Smith strain, cell-associated*	$>10^{3.3}$–$10^{5.1}$ ID_{50}/mL
Bacteria	*Staphylococcus epidermidis*	$>10^{6.6}$ cfu per unit
	Listeria monocytogenes	$>10^{6.3}$ cfu per unit
	Corynebacterium minutissimum	$>10^{6.3}$ cfu/mL
	Streptococcus pyogenes	$>10^{6.8}$ cfu per unit
	Staphylococcus aureus	$10^{6.6}$ cfu per unit
	Escherichia coli	$>10^{6.4}$ cfu per unit
	Yersinia enterocolitica	$>10^{5.9}$ cfu/mL
	Serratia marcescens	$>10^{6.7}$ cfu per unit
	Salmonella choleraesuis	$>10^{6.2}$ cfu/mL
	Enterobacter cloacae	$10^{5.9}$ cfu/mL
	Klebsiella pneumoniae	$>10^{5.6}$ cfu per unit
	Pseudomonas aeruginosa	$10^{4.5}$ cfu/mL
	Bacillus cereus	$>10^{3.6}$, $\leq 10^{3.9}$ cfu per unit

HIV, human immunodeficiency virus; HBV, hepatitis B virus; HCV, hepatitis C virus; HCMV, human cytomegalovirus, DHBV, duck hepatitis B virus; BVDV, bovine viral diarrhea virus, MCMV, murine cytomegalovirus; pfu, plaque-forming units; ID_{50} infectious dose which is measured from an endpoint dilution that causes infection in 50% of inoculated animals; cfu, colony-forming units; $TCID_{50}$, tissue culture infectious dose, which is measured from an endpoint dilution that causes infection in 50% of inoculated samples; CID_{50}, chimpanzee infectious dose, which is measured from an endpoint dilution that causes infection in 50% of inoculated chimpanzees.

* Three studies are indicated: the HIV-1 provirus inactivation was performed in cell culture medium and the other two studies were performed with platelet sample size less than 300 mL.

†Highest titers possible.

‡The infectivity of the MS-2 strain of HBV and the Hutchinson strain of HCV was measured in susceptible chimpanzees.

effectively blocks PCR mediated amplification of mitochondrial DNA sequences without impairment of ATP levels.[53,54]

A photochemical treatment process using riboflavin (Fig. 27–4) and a combination of UVB and UVA light (5 J/cm²: 265–370 nm) has been developed for platelet components suspended in donor plasma without the use of a platelet additive solution.[55] Photodynamic reactions involving the generation of active oxygen species are a critical aspect of riboflavin pathogen inactivation mechanism.[40] Earlier studies had used this process with additive solutions, but the system evaluated in clinical trials requires suspension of platelets in 100% donor plasma.[56] This process has demonstrated activity against enveloped viruses, a nonenveloped model virus, and two species of bacteria.[55] Earlier studies showed capacity for the inactivation of protozoa.[57] In vitro aspects of platelet function and hemostatic function assessed in an ex vivo system have shown conservation of function after riboflavin treatment.[58] The process appears to produce comparable effects on in vitro platelet properties for apheresis and pooled buffy coat platelet components.[59] Recently, preliminary data were reported describing the inactivation of lymphocytes using a murine immunodeficiency model.[60]

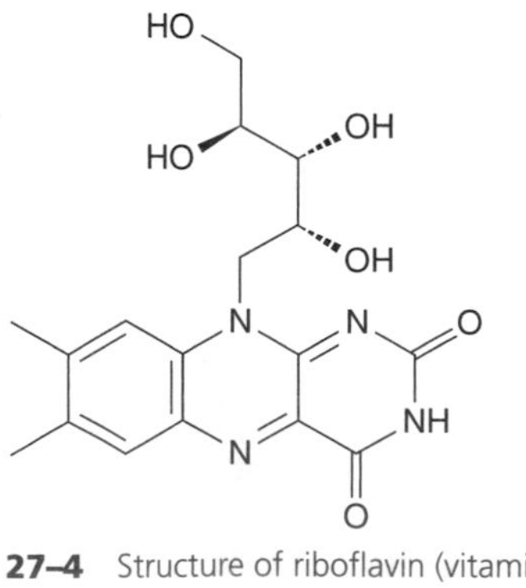

HO, HO, OH, OH, N, N, O, NH, N, O

Figure 27–4 Structure of riboflavin (vitamin B_2).

Clinical Experience with Platelets Prepared with Amotosalen Photochemical Treatment

Amotosalen, formerly known as S-59, treatment of platelet components has been extensively evaluated in clinical trials[61–64] and has been introduced into practice in Europe.[65] The prototype system is a closed system with a series of plastic containers that are carried through a sequence of processing steps (Fig. 27–5). A pooled buffy-coat or single-donor platelet concentrate, suspended in approximately 35% plasma and 65% platelet additive solution, is connected to a container of amotosalen. The platelet concentrate is passed through the amotosalen container into a PL 2410 Plastic

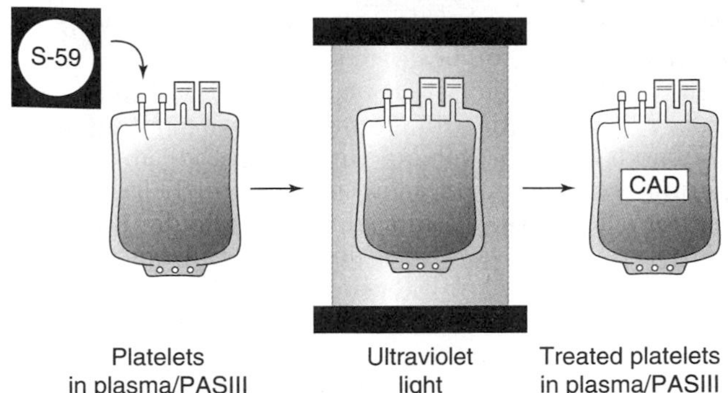

Figure 27–5 The amotosalen process for treatment of platelet concentrates. In a series of connected containers, amotosalen is added to the platelet concentrate suspended in approximately 300 mL of 35% plasma and 65% of a platelet additive solution (PAS III, Intersol). The platelet concentrate is illuminated with a 3 J/cm^2 treatment for approximately 3 minutes. After illumination, the platelet concentrate is transferred to another plastic container containing the compound absorption device (CAD). Platelets are incubated with shaking in the CAD for at least 4 hours to lower the levels of residual amotosalen and free photoproducts, followed by transfer to a final plastic container for 5 to 7 days of storage at 20–24°C. The final transfused dose of residual amotosalen ranges from 25 to 50 μg per 300 mL of platelet concentrate.

container (Baxter Healthcare Corp., Round Lake, Ill.). The platelet concentrate containing amotosalen (150 μmol/L) is illuminated with long wavelength UVA light for 3 minutes (3 J/cm^2 treatment) with reciprocal shaking at 20 °C to 24 °C in a microprocessor controlled light source. After illumination, the platelets are transferred to a compound absorption device (CAD) to passively reduce the residual amotosalen to low levels (<0.5 μmol/L). The CAD consists of resin beads integrated into PL 2410 Plastic. After CAD exposure for a minimum of 4 hours, the platelets are transferred to a final PL 2410 Plastic container for storage for 5 to 7 days under conventional platelet storage conditions with reciprocal shaking at 20°C to 24 °C.

Phase 1 and 2 studies with amotosalen-treated, 5-day-old platelets transfused in healthy subjects have shown adequate viability.[63] The average post-transfusion recovery of 5-day-old treated platelets was 42.5% with an average life span of 4.8 days. Interestingly, the rate of radiolabel elution from treated platelets was greater than that of control platelets (3.3% vs 2.1%). In these studies, treated platelets were well tolerated during and after transfusion of full therapeutic doses (300 mL, 3.0×10^{11} platelets) in healthy subjects. This study also provided information regarding the peak plasma amotosalen concentrations after transfusion and the kinetics of amotosalen clearance, including the area under the curve (AUC) and terminal half-life. The median peak amotosalen plasma level was less than 1 ng/mL and rapidly fell to concentrations below the limits of quantitative measurement.

A clinical trial was conducted to evaluate the hemostatic therapeutic efficacy of amotosalen-treated platelet concentrates and to expand the safety experience in a spectrum of patients requiring platelet transfusion support.[66] In this randomized, double-blinded crossover trial, patients received double-dose transfusions (>6.0×10^{11} platelets) of amotosalen-treated platelets and standard platelets in random order. Based on the daily platelet count, platelet transfusions were ordered by physicians blinded to the type of platelet product. Platelet counts and cutaneous template bleeding times were performed prior to each platelet transfusion, and 1 and 24 hours following each study platelet transfusion. In addition, secondary end points included clinical hemostasis before and after transfusion, the frequency of transfusion reactions, corrected count increments, and adverse events. Prior to platelet transfusion, the average platelet count was less than 13×10^9/L and the median bleeding time was greater than 30 minutes. After transfusion of amotosalen-treated platelets, the average platelet count increased to 53.2 $\times 10^9$/L and the median bleeding time decreased to 15 minutes. Control platelet transfusions demonstrated an average posttransfusion platelet count of 63.3×10^9/L with a median bleeding time of 12 minutes. The improvements in bleeding times persisted for up to 24 hours after platelet transfusion. The amotosalen-treated platelets were well tolerated.

A randomized, controlled, double-blinded clinical trial was initiated using pooled whole-blood buffy coat platelets stored up to 5 days after preparation with amotosalen treatment or by conventional methods using either plasma or a mixture of plasma and an approved additive solution (T-Sol; Baxter, La Chatre, France) as the suspension medium.[62] This study enrolled 103 patients at four European centers. The experimental platelet concentrates were pooled, treated with amotosalen, and then stored for up to 5 days before transfusion. Patients were randomized to receive all platelet transfusions of the assigned type for up to 8 weeks of transfusion support with an additional 4-week period of surveillance for adverse events. The primary endpoint of this trial was the corrected count increment (CCI) 1 hour following platelet transfusion. Secondary end points included the CCI 24 hours after transfusion, clinical hemostasis, the frequency of platelet transfusion, the frequency of acute transfusion reactions, the frequency of refractoriness to platelet transfusion, the frequency of platelet associated bacteremia, and overall safety.

The average dose of experimental platelets was significantly lower than that of conventional platelets (3.9×10^{11} vs 4.3 $\times 10^{11}$, $P < 0.001$). This study demonstrated that for up to the first eight transfusions the mean 1-hour CCI was not different between treatment groups (13,400 ± 5400 vs 14,900 ± 6,200, $P = 0.11$). When analyzed by linear regression using 1-hour count increments and transfused dose for all transfusions, equal doses of treated and conventional platelets did not differ significantly with respect to 1-hour post-transfusion count increments (mean difference = 1.5 $\times 10^9$/L: 95% CI: −3.1 to 6.1×10^9/L, $P = 0.53$).

For up to the first eight transfusions, the 24-hour CCI results were statistically lower for treated platelets (7400 ± 5500 vs 10,600 ± 7100, $P = 0.02$). However, when analyzed by linear regression using 24-hour count increments for all transfusions, equal doses of treated and conventional platelets were not different (mean difference = 2.6×10^9/L: 95% CI: −1.3 to 6.5×10^9/L, $P = 0.19$). The mean interval between transfusions was not different between treatment groups (3.0 ± 1.2 vs 3.4 ± 1.2 days, $P = 0.13$). The treatment groups were not different with respect to hemostasis, alloimmunization, or safety.

A second clinical trial was conducted to compare the therapeutic efficacy and safety of amotosalen-treated apheresis platelets with conventional platelets.[61] This study utilized a noninferiority design to evaluate specifically the hemostatic efficacy of platelets treated with a photochemical (PCT) pathogen inactivation process in comparison to conventional platelets. It was a controlled, double-blinded trial in which 645 patients were transfused at 12 clinical centers. Single-donor platelets were collected on the Amicus cell separator system and prepared with either photochemical treatment[41,44,67] or conventional methods. Patients were randomized to receive all platelet transfusion support of the assigned treatment type for up to 4 weeks. Patients who required additional platelet transfusion support after the initial 4-week period were invited to enroll into a second transfusion cycle for up to 4 weeks. The primary end point of this trial was the frequency of grade 2 bleeding (WHO scoring system[68]) in the two treatment groups. Grade 2 bleeding was selected as the primary end point, since it is primarily a reflection of platelet function in transfusion-dependent thrombocytopenic patients.[69–72] Secondary end points included grade 3 and 4 bleeding, time to the first grade 2 bleeding event, days of grade 2 bleeding, 1- and 24-hour platelet count increments, the interval between platelet transfusions, the frequency of acute transfusions reactions, the frequency of platelet associated bacterial sepsis, the rate of refractoriness to platelet transfusion, the number of platelet transfusions and red cell transfusions, and safety.

Analysis of data from this study showed that the incidence of grade 2 bleeding and higher grade bleeding (grade 3 and 4) was equivalent for patients supported with treated platelets and conventional platelets.[61] The median time to the first grade 2 bleeding event was 8 days and not different between the treatment groups.[61] The mean 1-hour and 24-hour CCI values were significantly lower for patients in the experimental group. Using longitudinal linear regression analysis, when equal doses of PCT and control platelets were transfused, the 1-hour post-transfusion count was estimated to be 10.4×10^9/L lower and the average time to the next transfusion was 0.4 days shorter for treated platelets. The average 1-hour increment, 24-hour count increment, and interval to the next transfusion for amotosalen-treated platelets were similar to those observed for conventional platelets in the TRAP trial.[73]

The mean number of platelet transfusions required per patient was greater for the PCT group compared with the control group; however, owing to processing and sampling losses the proportion of platelet doses below 3.0×10^{11} was significantly greater for the PCT group (20% vs 12%, $P < 0.01$).[61] Subsequently, a poststudy analysis to examine in greater detail the effect of platelet dose consistency on the number of platelet transfusions and bleeding was performed.[74] This analysis showed that when patients were transfused with all doses containing $>3.0 \times 10^{11}$ platelets of either PCT or conventional platelets, the number of platelet transfusions required for support was not different between the PCT and control groups. Similarly, when patients transfused with one or more doses of either PCT or control platelets were compared, the number of platelet transfusions required for support remained similar between the groups. Despite the differences in numbers of transfusions required, the count increments and transfusion intervals for PCT platelets were, respectively, lower and shorter for PCT platelets consistent with qualitative differences observed in phase 1 studies of platelet viability.[63]

Because the initial clinical trials were conducted with a prototype processing set that resulted in poor control of platelet doses, a study with an optimized integrated processing set configuration was carried out.[75] This was a smaller randomized controlled trial than the prior studies in which the trend for lower count increments and shorter transfusion intervals with PCT platelets persisted; however, more transfusions of PCT platelet components were not required for support of patients compared with conventional platelets.[75] With the introduction of PCT platelets into routine clinical use in Europe as of 2003, experience has been extended to examine the impact of the PCT process on platelet utilization and donor resources in a broader patient population and under routine operating conditions.[65] Preliminary reports of these studies with apheresis platelets have shown a minimal or only modest impact on platelet utilization.

Another important aspect of the use of platelet products prepared with pathogen inactivation methods has been to evaluate the safety profile of these products including the potential for induction of antibody responses to potential neoantigens. Reports of clinical trials conducted with platelets treated with amotosalen and UVA light have indicated that the safety profile of the treated platelets is similar to that of conventional platelets.[61,62,76] The cumulative experience in these trials has involved 412 patients transfused with 3736 doses of PCT platelets.[77] While differences in some specific adverse events have been observed,[76] no consistent differences or trends in system organ class adverse events were detected. Patients enrolled in the phase 3 clinical trials were primarily recruited from populations with hematologic and oncologic disorders associated with high morbidity and mortality rates and treated with intensive therapies with recognized substantial adverse event rates. In all these studies, the mortality rate for patients transfused with amotosalen-treated platelets has been comparable to that of conventional platelet components.[61,62,75,76] After the introduction of amotosalen-treated platelets into routine clinical practice in Europe, a hemovigilance reporting system was initiated to examine the incidence of acute reactions in the 24-hour post-transfusion period for 5000 transfusions of amotosalen-treated platelets. Preliminary analysis of 2512 transfusions has confirmed a low rate of acute transfusion reactions and tolerability of the treated platelets.[78]

Clinical Experience with Platelets Treated with Riboflavin and UV Light

A phase 1 clinical trial in healthy subjects has been conducted to assess the viability of autologous platelets treated with riboflavin (50 µmol/L) and ultraviolet light (5.0 J/cm^2, 265–370 nm) and stored in autologous plasma for 5 days.[79] The pH and metabolic parameters of the treated platelets were well maintained during storage. The average post-transfusion recovery (%) of the treated platelets was statistically lower than that of untreated autologous platelets (50.0 ± 18.9 vs 66.5 ± 13.4, $P < 0.05$) and the average survival (hours) was statistically reduced (104 ± 26 vs 142 ± 26, $P < 0.05$). While the viability of riboflavin-treated platelets was different from that of untreated platelets, in vitro studies of hemostasis suggested that functionality was adequately retained.[58] Further studies in thrombocytopenic patients are required to demonstrate that therapeutic efficacy has been retained and that the treated platelets are well tolerated after repeated transfusions.

POTENTIAL SYSTEMS FOR INACTIVATION OF PATHOGENS IN RED CELL CONCENTRATES

A number of laboratories have investigated the application of pathogen inactivation to red cell concentrates (Table 27–4). Red cells present a difficult environment for pathogen inactivation owing to the light absorbance by hemoglobin and the viscosity of packed red cells. To date, most research efforts have explored the use of photodynamic methods, although photodynamic-associated damage may increase during prolonged red cell storage. Additional significant defects of the photodynamic systems include incomplete inactivation of pathogens, damage to red cells resulting in hemolysis and potassium leakage, increased binding of immunoglobulins, long treatment times, and the necessity to work at a reduced hematocrit or in thin-layer configurations to facilitate light activation. Recent work suggests that cellular damage due to active oxygen species can be ameliorated by the inclusion of scavengers or quenchers of active oxygen species,[80,81] but this modification further complicates the treatment process. More recently, several groups have developed nucleic acid–targeted processes that do not require light activation. The latter approach offers the potential to minimize nonspecific damage by active oxygen species to red cells and plasma proteins.

The initial red cell studies were conducted with porphyrin-based compounds and dyes such as merocyanine 540, methylene blue, and phthalocyanine (see Table 27–4). Each method had limited viral inactivation capacity and induced various levels of red cell injury. Subsequently, Wagner and colleagues described the use of a new phenothiazine compound, 1,9-dimethylmethylene blue (DMMB), which exhibited an improved inactivation spectrum compared with methylene blue and demonstrated less hemolysis and less immunoglobulin binding during storage after treatment.[82] The photodynamic damage due to 1,9-DMMB was diminished by the use of dipyridamole.[83] More recently, another photodynamic process which uses a thiopyrylium dye and dipyridamole to control oxidative membrane damage has been described.[84] None of these methods have reached the clinical trial stage.

Two groups have explored using nucleic acid targeted compounds that do not require photo-activation for nucleic acid inactivation. INACTINE (PEN 110), a nucleic acid–targeted compound, was reported to inactivate viruses, bacteria, and leukocytes in red cell suspensions.[85–87] The INACTINEs are stable monoalkylators that are immediately active upon addition to blood or red cell concentrates (Fig. 27–6). Red cells treated with PEN 110 were stored for 28 days, radiolabeled, and then transfused into chimpanzees. PEN 110 demonstrated no effect on the viability of chimpanzee red cells.[88]

PEN 110 was studied in a phase 1 trial of 12 healthy subjects to examine the effect of treatment on post-transfusion red cell recovery and life span. This trial was designed as a crossover study and utilized autologous red cells stored for 28 days before transfusion. In vitro studies were conducted with treated and control red cells stored for 42 days. In this study the PEN 110–treated red cells were exposed to sodium thiosulfate as a quenching reagent and washed before transfusion. Post-transfusion dual radiolabel recovery (%) was comparable to that of untreated cells (85.0 ± 5.0 vs 85.9 ± 2.7%), as was the half-life (days) (31.9 ± 8.2 vs 32.9 ± 3.3).[89] Over 42 days of storage, PEN 110–treated red cells demonstrated reduced metabolic activity, but cell-free hemoglobin levels and extracellular potassium levels remained within acceptable limits.

A phase 2 study was performed to evaluate the viability of PEN 110–treated red cells after 35 or 42 days of storage.[90] Healthy subjects (12 per treatment and storage cohort) were randomized to receive either treated or untreated autologous red cells stored for the assigned storage period. In this study, thiosulfate quenching was not used and the treated red cells were washed extensively prior to storage to remove residual PEN 110. These studies demonstrated comparable post-transfusion recoveries (%) after 42 days of storage as measured by a single radiolabel method (82.9 ± 5.7 vs 86.3 ± 8.7), but half-life of the PEN 110–treated red cells was reduced by approximately 30%. In vitro studies demonstrated a trend for decreased 2,3-DPG and ATP levels of treated cells compared with control cells. Subsequently, PEN 110–treated red cells were used in a phase 3 clinical trial for patients requiring transfusion support of acute and chronic anemia. These studies were halted when patients developed antibodies to the treated red cells. However, these studies have not been further described, and development of this technology was suspended.

Table 27–4 Methods Used to Inactivate Pathogens in Red Cell Concentrates

Reactive Agent	Target	Reference
Dihematoporphyrin	HIV, HSV, CMV, SIV, *Trypsnosoma cruzi*	146
Benzoporphyrin A	VSV, FeLV	147
Merocyanine 540	Friend LV	148
Merocyanine 540	HSV-1	149
Merocyanine 540	*Plasmodium falciparum*	150
Methylene blue	VSV	151
Methylene blue	VSV, Φ6, Sindbis, M13	152
Phthalocyanines	VSV	153
Phthalocyanines	VSV, Sindbis	145
PSR-Br	Φ6	154
Hypericin	HIV	155
1,9-DMMB	VSV, PRV, BVDV, Φ6, R17, EMC	82
Thiopyrylium	VSV, PRV, BVDV, HIV, DHBV	84
INACTINE	Porcine parvovirus, BVDV, HIV-1, VSV	156
S-303	HIV, DHBV, BVDV, bacteria	91

HIV, human immunodeficiency virus; HSV, herpes simplex virus; CMV, cytomegalovirus; SIV, simian immunodeficiency virus; VSV, vesicular stomatitis virus; FeLV, feline leukemia virus; Friend LV, Friend erythroleukemia virus; Φ6, bacteriophage; Sindbis, Sindbis virus; PSR-Br, brominated psoralen; PRV, pseudorabies virus; BVDV, bovine viral diarrhea virus; EMC, encephalo-myocarditis virus; R17, bacteriophage; DMMB, dimethylmethylene blue.

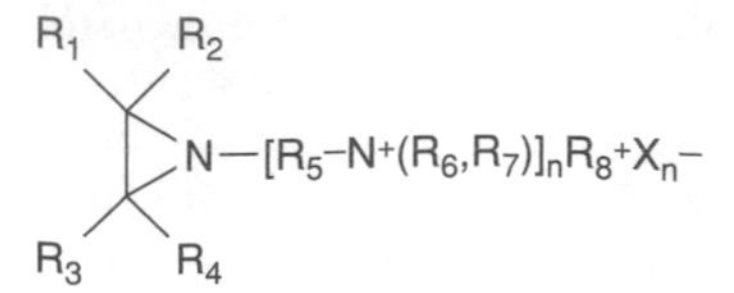

$$R_1R_2\text{-}C,\ R_3R_4\text{-}C\ (\text{aziridine})\ N-[R_5-N^+(R_6,R_7)]_nR_8{}^+X_n{}^-$$

Figure 27–6 Structure of INACTINE compounds. PEN 110 is a member of the class.

Cook and colleagues developed a class of compounds known as anchor linker effectors (ALE) and frangible anchor linker effectors (FRALE) for inactivation of pathogens in red cell concentrates.[91] The FRALE compounds are composed of three moieties (Fig. 27–7): a nucleic acid–targeted intercalator group, an effector group for covalent addition to nucleic acid, and a central frangible bond facilitating compound degradation. The FRALES are stable at low pH and are activated by a pH shift upon addition to packed red cells suspended in residual plasma and a red cell additive solution at neutral pH. The FRALE compounds rapidly degrade to a negatively charged, inactive species after reaction, thus preventing further binding to DNA and RNA (Fig. 27–8). The lead compound, S-303 (100 µg/mL), upon addition to packed red cells (60% hematocrit), inactivated high titers of cell-free and cell-associated HIV, DHBV, VSV, HSV, BVDV, and both gram-negative and gram-positive bacteria.[92] Using a murine transfusion model, S-303–treated red cells exhibited post-transfusion recovery and life span comparable to those of untreated red cells.[91] In a second series of studies, dog red cells treated with S-303 exhibited post-transfusion recovery and life span comparable to those of untreated red cells.[92] Dogs transfused multiple times with allogeneic S-303–treated red cells failed to develop antibodies to S-303–treated autologous red cells, but some dogs did develop alloantibodies to untreated donor cells indicating an intact alloimmune response not directed against S-303–treated red cells. Other dogs transfused with S-303–treated red cells (10 mL/kg) 12 times over a 1-month period had no clinical or histopathologic evidence of toxicity. In addition, replacement of 80% of the blood volume of dogs with S-303–treated red cells using treatment concentrations up to 500 µg/mL resulted in no toxicity. S-303–treated red cells and S-300, the breakdown product of S-303, were not carcinogenic in a repeated transfusion study of transgenic heterozygous p53 knockout mice.[93]

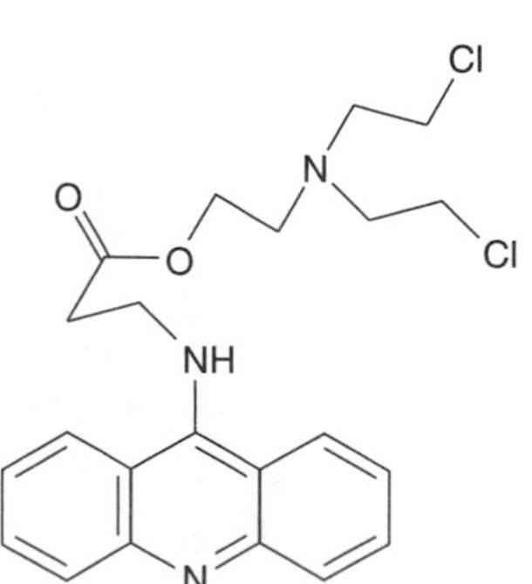

Figure 27–7 Structure of the frangible anchor linker effector (FRALE) compound S-303. The molecule consist of three parts: an anchor for nucleic acid intercalation, an effector region for covalent addition to nucleic acid, and a labile, "frangible" linker to facilitate S-303 degradation.

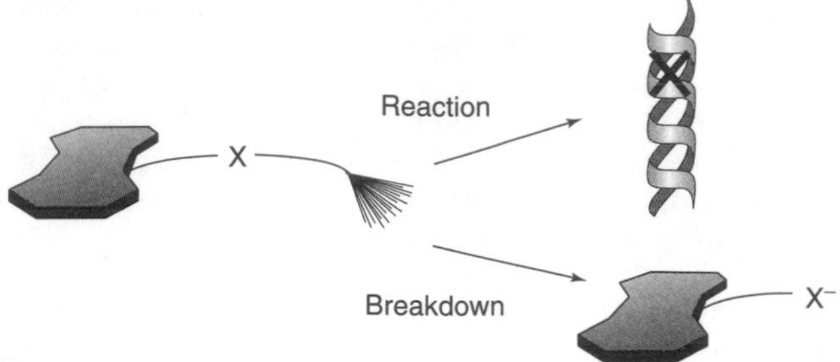

Figure 27–8 Mechanism of action for FRALE compounds. After addition to red blood cells, S-303 rapidly attaches to nucleic acid and then degrades to S-300, a negatively charged compound that does not bind to nucleic acid.

A prototype S-303 system was designed to inactivate infectious pathogens in plastic containers (Fig. 27–9). Using a closed system with a series of connected containers, S-303 (200 µmol/L) and glutathione (2 mmol/L) were incubated with red blood cell concentrates (200–250 mL). The red cells were incubated at room temperature for 8 hours, during which time pathogen inactivation was completed and S-303 degraded to the inert compound S-300. After incubation, the treated red cells were transferred to a plastic storage container with an integral CAD for storage for 35 to 42 days at 4°C. Evaluation of in vitro red cell properties after 42 days of storage demonstrated no differences in the following parameters: red cell ATP levels, extracellular potassium, hemolysis, and glucose consumption.[91] S-303–treated red cells advanced through preclinical safety studies and entered the clinical phase in 1998.

Three clinical trials with S-303–treated red cells have been completed in healthy subjects. The first was a controlled, two-arm, randomized trial in which the post-transfusion viability of S-303–treated, autologous red cells stored for 35 days after treatment was compared to that of untreated red cells stored for 35 days.[94] The study was designed to detect small differences in post-transfusion recovery. Twenty-one subjects were enrolled into the S-303 treatment group and 22 into the control group. The average post-transfusion recovery of

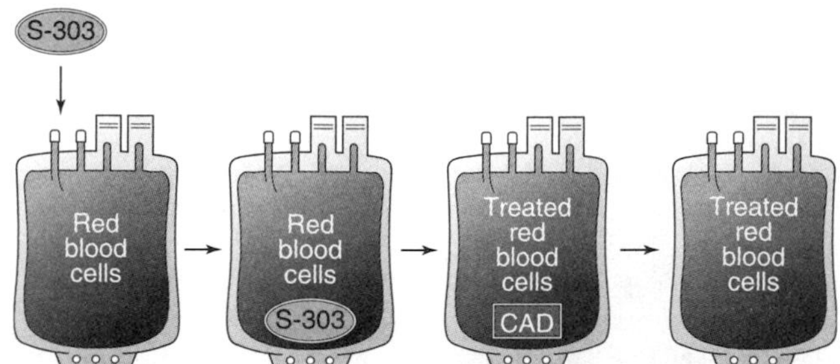

Figure 27–9 The prototype FRALE S-303 process for treatment of red blood cell concentrates. The treatment is conducted in a closed system. S-303 is maintained at low pH and is activated by addition to red cell concentrates at neutral pH. The inactivation process is conducted in full-sized units ranging in hematocrit from 60% to 80%. After addition of S-303 to the red cells, the plastic container is incubated at room temperature for 6 to 8 hours to complete pathogen inactivation. Following pathogen inactivation, the red cells are transferred to a plastic container with a compound absorption device (CAD) to reduce the levels of S-300. The red cells remain in contact with the CAD for up to 35 days of storage at 4° C.

35-day-old S-303 red cells was statistically lower than that of control red cells (78.7 ± 5.7% vs 83.9 ± 6.1%, $P = 0.002$), but recovery for both types exceeded 75%, the generally accepted threshold for viability of stored red cells. No adverse events were observed following transfusion of S-303 red cells.

A second phase 1 study was conducted in which the viability and potential immune response of healthy subjects to multiple exposures to autologous S-303–treated red cells were evaluated.[95] Subjects from the first study, of either treatment group, were invited to participate. The second study was initiated approximately 6 months after completion of the first study; thus, there was an interval of 6 to 9 months before the next transfusion exposure. In the second study, each subject donated a unit of blood that was processed into packed red cells. All the units were treated with S-303 and stored for 35 days. At four times, approximately 7 days apart, during the 35-day storage period, subjects were transfused with an aliquot of autologous S-303–treated red cells. The final aliquot on day 35 was radiolabeled with 51-Cr to measure post-transfusion viability. The red cell recovery 24 hours after transfusion of S-303–treated red cells was compared with each subject's red cell recovery in the first study. Sixteen subjects received control red cells in the first study and S-303 red cells in the second study. The average red cell recovery in the first study with control cells was 82.6 ± 6.4%, which was not statistically different from the average recovery of 84.3 ± 6.4% after transfusion of S-303 cells in the second study ($P = 0.30$). Twelve subjects received S-303 red cells in the first study, with an average recovery of 77.5 ± 6.6%, and after transfusion in the second study, these subjects demonstrated an average recovery of 79.2 ± 6.6%. After exposure to either four or five aliquots of S-303–treated red cells, no subjects developed antibodies directed against S-303 red cells.[95]

A third phase 1 study was conducted in 29 healthy subjects using a randomized crossover design to measure both post-transfusion recovery and life span of autologous S-303–treated red cells compared with control red cells processed with conventional methods.[96] Both types of red cells were stored for 35 days. The study was designed to detect small differences in red cell viability. A small difference in 24-hour post-transfusion recovery of S-303–treated red cells was detected compared with conventional red cells (81.7 ± 6.3% vs 84.5 ± 6.2%, $P = 0.048$). However, mean half-life was identical (37.4 ± 8.9 vs 37.4 ± 6.7 days, $P = 1.0$).

On the basis of the three phase 1 red cell clinical trials, phase 3 clinical trials were initiated to evaluate the therapeutic efficacy and safety of S-303–treated red cells in patients for the two major indications for red cell transfusion: acute and chronic anemia. For the indication of acute anemia, a randomized, two-arm controlled study to evaluate the response to transfusion in 200 patients undergoing cardiovascular surgical procedures was initiated.[97] The primary end point of this study was the composite incidence of renal failure, myocardial infarction, and death as a reflection of tissue oxygenation efficacy during correction of acute anemia. For the therapeutic indication of chronic anemia, a randomized, two-period crossover study enrolling patients with thalassemia and sickle cell anemia requiring chronic transfusion support was initiated. The primary end point of this study was the consumption of hemoglobin (g/kg body weight per day) over approximately 6 months.[98] Both studies were under way when two patients in the chronic trial developed positive crossmatch reactivity to S-303–treated red cells.[99] The sponsor elected to suspend both studies until the mechanism of the immunologic response could be elucidated.

Evaluation of sera from two patients with consistently reactive crossmatches to S-303–treated red cells confirmed that the reactivity was directed against the acridine (anchor moiety) portion of S-303.[99] The antibody was low titer and did not promote red cell phagocytosis in a monocyte-macrophage ingestion assay.[100] No patients in the acute anemia trial developed crossmatch reactivity with S-303–treated red cells. Prior to detection of positive crossmatch reactivity in the two chronic study patients, 148 patients completed the acute anemia study. Analysis of results from the study demonstrated that the primary end point was met, as well as all secondary end points.[97] The treated red cells were well tolerated and the safety profile was comparable to that of conventional red cells. In the chronic trial, no patients completed the study, but an interim analysis of data suggested that S-303–treated red cells were similar to conventional red cells for transfusion support of chronic anemia.[98] Further investigation of the S-303 process resulted in development of a modified process using an increased concentration of glutathione. Additional clinical trials are required to demonstrate that this modified process avoids cross-reactivity and alloimmunization in chronically transfused patients.

SYSTEMS FOR INACTIVATION OF PATHOGENS IN PREPARATION OF FRESH FROZEN PLASMA

The solvent detergent (SD) process for inactivation of enveloped viruses in plasma used for transfusion was introduced into clinical practice.[101] The SD process is generally highly effective against enveloped viruses, although very recently new evidence has been reported to suggest that some enveloped viruses, such as vaccinia, may be resistant to SD treatment.[102] Moreover, since SD treatment is not effective against nonenveloped viruses, concern has been expressed over the potential for transmission of these pathogens as a result of pooling with failure to inactivate resistant viruses.[103] Despite these issues, solvent detergent fresh frozen plasma (SD-FFP) has demonstrated therapeutic efficacy for replacement of congenital[104] and acquired coagulation factor deficiencies.[105,106] Furthermore, since SD-FFP does not contain high-molecular-weight multimers of von Willebrand factor (vWF), it has been advocated for use during therapeutic plasma exchange (TPE) therapy of thrombotic thrombocytopenic purpura (TTP).[104] Transfusion of SD-FFP has been well tolerated with a low incidence of transfusion reactions and adverse events.[107]

With increasing experience, other studies with SD-FFP documented mild to marked decreased levels of antithrombotic proteins: protein S and plasmin inhibitor.[108] Mast and co-workers confirmed that SD-FFP has markedly reduced levels of the antithrombotic proteins antiplasmin and antitrypsin and that these reduced levels are due to conformational changes induced by detergent treatment.[109] The clinical significance of these observations was unclear when initially reported, but subsequent reports indicated that there was an increased incidence of thrombotic events after large volume exposure during liver transplantation[110] and TPE for TTP.[111,112]

The SD process utilizes pooled plasma from 100 to 2500 donors and is not amenable to a single-unit viral inactivation process. In Europe, a single-unit treatment process using the phenothiazine dye methylene blue (MB) and long wavelength visible light has been used in clinical practice for preparation of fresh frozen plasma (MB-FFP).[113] MB exhibits limited binding affinity for nucleic acid; rather, the predominant mechanism of action is photodynamic via production of active oxygen species. More importantly, methylene blue is not effective against intracellular viruses owing to conversion to the inactive leuko–methylene blue species. Certain coagulation proteins, primarily factor VIII and fibrinogen, are sensitive to MB treatment and undergo a decrease in functional activity during treatment ranging from 30% to 40% of the levels in untreated plasma.[113] More recent studies with a commercial system using both fresh and frozen plasma with leukocyte reduction and a device to reduce the residual levels of MB demonstrated decreases in factor VIII activity ranging from 24% to 29%.[114] MB-FFP did provide adequate levels of fibrinogen, factor VIII, factor XIII, and vWF in cryoprecipitate, and the corresponding cryosupernatant fraction was depleted of the high-molecular-weight vWF multimers.[115]

MB-FFP has been well tolerated when transfused into healthy subjects.[116] Reports of randomized, controlled clinical trials for MB-FFP for the major therapeutic indications of FFP use are limited, despite transfusion of more than 1 million units in Europe.[117] A single study compared the usage of SD and MB-FFP in cardiac surgery patients and reported improved levels of protein S and α_2-antiplasmin with MB-FFP.[118] Several reports have indicated that MB-FFP use for TPE to treat TTP resulted in reduced efficacy.[119,120] A more generalized experience with MB-FFP was reported based on a retrospective analysis of three 1-year periods before and after adoption of MB-FFP.[121] This study indicated that use of MB-FFP resulted in increased use of FFP and cryoprecipitate owing to reduced hemostatic efficacy of the treated plasma. These observations have yet to be confirmed by additional studies.

A photochemical method using amotosalen and UVA light has been developed to inactivate viruses in single units of plasma prepared as FFP. Using a prototype configuration, with 3 J/cm² of UVA delivered in approximately 3 minutes, the average log reduction of virus was cell associated–HIV 6.4 ± 0.2, cell-free HIV >5.9 (95% CI), DHBV 5.4 ± 0.4, and BVDV 6.7 ± 0.4 after only 0.5 J/cm.[2] Because the amotosalen process is nucleic acid–targeted, it has demonstrated some inactivation efficacy of several nonenveloped viruses (e.g., rotavirus, calicivirus, and blue tongue virus). After PCT, FFP units were treated for 1 hour with a CAD to reduce residual amotosalen concentration followed by freezing (−20 °C). Coagulation activity of thawed amotosalen FFP units was compared with matched-control FFP units without PCT or CAD. Retained factor activities (% of control ± SD) were clottable fibrinogen, 87 ± 3%; factor V, 98 ± 2%; factor VII, 86 ± 2%; factor VIII, 73 ± 4%; factor IX, 95 ± 4%; factor X, 98 ± 4%; and factor XI, 91 ± 5%.[122] This system has been modified to treat up to 650 mL of plasma in a single process using a flow instead of a batch CAD to shorten processing time.[123] This system is compatible with either apheresis plasma collections[124] or pools of 2 or 3 units of whole blood–derived plasma.

Plasma prepared with the prototype system has been evaluated in a series of clinical trials. A single blinded, crossover, stepwise ascending dose clinical trial (100–1000 mL) was conducted in 15 healthy subjects. No adverse events were attributed to transfusion of amotosalen FFP at any dose and no clinically significant changes in post-transfusion coagulation, chemistry, or hematology profiles.[125,126] Peak post-transfusion levels (9 ± 1 ng/mL) of amotosalen were determined immediately after transfusion of 1000 mL of treated plasma and 18 to 24 hours later (0.52 ± 0.1 ng/mL).

In a second study, using a randomized crossover design, Hambleton and colleagues compared the pharmacokinetics of factor VII and the post-transfusion recoveries of factors II, VII, IX, and X in 27 healthy subjects after transfusion of conventional and treated FFP. Subjects received a 4-day regimen (7.5 mg/day) of warfarin prior to each study transfusion to suppress endogenous factor VII levels.[127] At the start of the study, subjects donated 2 L of FFP by apheresis collection. One liter of plasma was treated with amotosalen and frozen at −18 °C; the other liter was prepared as standard FFP and stored at −18 °C. Each subject received both types of FFP in random order. Prior to each transfusion, subjects were given 4 days of warfarin therapy followed by transfusion of 1 L of amotosalen FFP or untreated FFP. Warfarin therapy resulted in reduction of factor VII levels to approximately 30% of normal. No statistical differences (Wilcoxon signed-rank test) of clearance, recovery, half-life, or mean residence time (MRT) for factor VII were observed between amotosalen and control FFP.[127] No differences in recoveries of other factors (II, IX, and X) were observed. Transfusion of amotosalen FFP provided acceptable coagulation factor preservation without adverse effects. The anticoagulant challenge crossover trial demonstrated that transfusion of amotosalen FFP yielded therapeutic coagulation factor increments similar to those of standard FFP.

A phase 2 randomized, controlled, pilot study of amotosalen FFP was completed in 13 patients with acquired coagulopathy to evaluate the response of prolonged prothrombin (PT) and partial thromboplastin times (PTT) to transfusion with amotosalen FFP. Patients with a diagnosis of acquired coagulopathy undergoing minor invasive procedures were randomized to transfusion with either amotosalen FFP or conventional FFP.[128] The average PT and PTT were prolonged before FFP transfusion and responded similarly to transfusion with either amotosalen or conventional FFP. The response lasted 8 to 12 hours, and amotosalen FFP demonstrated acceptable control of bleeding in patients undergoing invasive procedures, such as liver biopsy. Peak post-transfusion plasma levels of amotosalen were 3.10 ± 1.65 ng/mL.

A phase 3 clinical trial program for amotosalen FFP was conducted to assess therapeutic efficacy and safety for the major indications for FFP transfusion: congenital coagulopathy, acquired coagulopathy, and therapeutic plasma exchange. The first study evaluated the post-transfusion recovery and clearance of specific coagulation factors in 34 patients with congenital coagulopathies requiring FFP transfusion.[129] This open-label, single arm study enrolled patients with deficiencies of factors I, II, V, VII, X, XI, and protein C. Enrolled patients received at least one transfusion of amotosalen FFP (suggested dose of 15 mL/kg) to measure the recovery and clearance of the specified deficient clotting factor. Patients were eligible to receive additional amotosalen FFP transfusions as required to manage active bleeding or for prophylaxis during surgical procedures. This study demonstrated that the post-transfusion clearance of factors V, VII, X, XI, and protein C was comparable to reported values.[129] The clearance of factors I, II, and XIII were shorter than the reported values but provided acceptable post- transfusion recoveries for support of patients.[129] Pretransfusion prolonged prothrombin times (PT) and PTT corrected after transfusion of amotosalen FFP.[129] Seventy-seven transfusions were administered for management of active bleeding or for prophylaxis against bleeding during surgical procedures. In each case, acceptable hemostasis was achieved after transfusion.[129] Some patients received repeated transfusions of amotosalen FFP over 2 years. Peak plasma levels of amotosalen immediately after transfusion were 8.42 ± 2.72 ng/mL, similar to those observed in healthy subjects. The treated plasma was well tolerated, and the adverse event profile was similar to that reported for conventional plasma.

A controlled, double-blinded, randomized study of 121 patients with acquired coagulopathy, largely due to chronic liver disease, was conducted to evaluate therapeutic efficacy and safety for this indication.[130] Prior to elective surgical procedures, including liver transplantation, patients were randomized to receive either conventional FFP or amotosalen FFP for up to 7 days of support. The primary end point of this study was the response of PT and PTT to FFP transfusion. This study demonstrated correction of the PT and PTT responses on a dose- and patient weight–adjusted basis, hemostasis, and use of blood products comparable to that of patients supported with conventional FFP. The mean incremental recovery for factor VII was not different between the treatment groups (0.69 ± 1.80 vs 0.48 ± 0.76 IU/dL/IU/kg). After large doses of amotosalen FFP, peak post-transfusion plasma levels of amotosalen (5.4 ± 3.5 ng/mL) were lower than those of nonbleeding healthy subjects. Transfusion of amotosalen FFP was well tolerated in this patient group.

A double-blinded randomized study of patients with TTP was subsequently carried out.[131] In this study, 35 patients were assigned to receive up to 30 days of TPE with either conventional FFP or amotosalen FFP. The primary end point was the proportion of patients in remission in each treatment group after 30 days of TPE. Patients who failed to reach remission after 30 days of TPE were eligible to continue TPE for an additional 30 days. The rates of remission were not different between the treatment groups (82 vs 89%, $P = 0.66$). In addition, time to remission, relapse rates, and time to relapse were not different for patients treated with amotosalen FFP. Despite the exposure to large volumes of amotosalen FFP, peak plasma levels were within the same range as the other patient groups (5.4 ± 3.6 ng/mL). As in the other studies, amotosalen FFP was well tolerated and the safety profile was similar to that for patients supported with conventional FFP.

CONCLUSIONS

New threats to the safety and availability of labile blood components continue to evolve. To meet these challenges, new tests and increased donor restrictions have been implemented, but transfusion-transmitted infections persist. Robust pathogen inactivation systems for treatment of each blood component have been developed and are in various stages of clinical trials in the United States and Europe. However, progress has been slow, and problems have been encountered during development. Despite these hurdles, systems for treatment of platelets and plasma are in clinical use, and as experience is gained these technologies may result in a paradigm shift for prevention of transfusion-transmitted infections. The availability of pathogen inactivation systems for all blood components, ultimately, may permit modification of current testing strategies to take advantage of a stratified, integrated approach to transfusion safety by using pathogen inactivation and a modified testing strategy to achieve higher levels of blood component transfusion safety. As new pathogens of clinical importance are identified in the donor population, both pathogen inactivation and testing strategies will require further modification to meet new challenges.

REFERENCES

1. Dodd RY. Will blood products be free of infectious agents? In Nance SJ (ed). Transfusion Medicine in the 1990s. Arlington, Va., American Association of Blood Banks, 1990, pp 223–251.
2. Laperche S. Blood safety and nucleic acid testing in Europe. Euro Surveill 2005;10:3–4.
3. Alvarez do Barrio M, Gonzalez Diez R, Sanchez Hernandez JM, Oyonarte Gomez S. Residual risk of transfusion-transmitted viral infections in Spain, 1997–2002, and impact of nucleic acid testing. Euro Surveill 2005;10:20–22.
4. Offergeld R, Faensen D, Ritter D, Hamouda O. Human immunodeficiency virus, hepatitis C and hepatitis B infections among blood donors in Germany, 2000–2002: risk of virus transmission and the impact of nucleic acid testing. Euro Surveill 2005;10:8–11.
5. Busch MP, Kleinman SH, Nemo GJ. Current and emerging infectious risks of blood transfusions. JAMA 2003;289:959–962.
6. Satake M. Lookback study for transfusion-related HBV infection in Japan. Transfusion 2005;45(Suppl 3):9A–10A.
7. McQuiston JH, Childs JE, Chamberland ME, Tabor E. Transmission of tick-borne agents of disease by blood transfusion: a review of known and potential risks in the United States. Transfusion 2000;40:274–284.
8. Schmunis GA. *Trypanosoma cruzi,* the etiologic agent of Chagas disease: status in the blood supply in endemic and nonendemic countries. Transfusion 1991;31:547–557.
9. Grant IH, Gold JM, Wittner M, et al. Transfusion-associated acute Chagas disease acquired in the United States. Ann Intern Med 1989;111:849–851.
10. Nickerson P, Orr P, Schroeder ML, Sekla L, Johnston JB. Transfusion-associated *Trypanosoma cruzi* infection in a nonendemic area. Ann Intern Med 1989;111:851–853.
11. Riera C, Muncunill J, Fisa R, et al. Asymptomatic infection by *Leishmania infantum* in blood donors from the Balearic Islands, Spain. Transfusion 2005;45(Suppl 3):18A.
12. Leiby DA, Gill JE. Transfusion-transmitted tick-borne infections: a cornucopia of threats. Transfus Med Rev 2004;18:293–306.
13. Linden JV, Wong SJ, Chu FK, Schmidt GB, Bianco C. Transfusion-associated transmission of babesiosis in New York State. Transfusion 2000;40:285–289.
14. Petersen LR, Epstein JS. Problem solved? West Nile virus and transfusion safety. N Engl J Med 2005;353:516–517.
15. Iwamoto M, Jernigan DB, Guasch A, et al. Transmission of West Nile virus from an organ donor to four transplant recipients. N Engl J Med 2003;101:2196–2203.
16. Busch MP, Cagliotti S, Robertson EF, et al. Screening the blood supply for West Nile virus RNA by nucleic acid amplification testing. N Engl J Med 2005;353:460–467.
17. Stramer SL, Fang CT, Foster GA, Wagner AG, Brodsky JP, Dodd RY. West Nile virus among blood donors in the United States, 2003 and 2004. N Engl J Med 2005;353:451–459.
18. Fiebig EW, Hildebrant CM, Smith RI, Conra s EA, Vos MC, Vermeij H, van Rhenen DJ. Clinical significance of bacteriologic screening in platelet concentrates. Transfusion 2005;45:514–519.
19. Visconti Mr, Pennington J, Garner SF, Allain JP, Williamson LM. Assessment of removal of human cytomegalovirus from blood components by leucocyte depletion filters using real-time quantitative PCR. Blood 2004;103:1137–1139.
20. Pennington J, Taylor GP, Sutherland J, et al. Persistence of HTLV-I in blood components after leukocyte depletion. Blood 2002;100:677–681.
21. Nichols WG, Price TH, Gooley T, Corey L, Boeckh M. Transfusion-transmitted cytomegalovirus infection after receipt of leukoreduced blood products. Blood 2003;101:4195–4200.
22. Blajchman MA. Bacterial contamination of cellular components: risks, sources, and control. Vox Sang 2004;87(Suppl 1):S98–S103.
23. Te Boekhorst PA, Beckers EA, Vos MC, Vermeij H, van Rhenen DJ. Clinical significance of bacteriologic screening in platelet concentrates. Transfusion 2005;45:514–519.

24. Munksgaard L, Albjerg L, Lillevang ST, Gahrn-Hansen B, Georgsen J. Detection of bacterial contamination of platelet components: six years' experience with the BactT/ALERT system. Transfusion 2004;44:1166–1173.
25. Claeys H, Logghe F, Vandekerchove B, et al. Four-year experience with routine bacterial screening of platelet concentrates.Transfus Med 2003;1(Suppl 1):S326.
26. Larsen CP, Ezligini F, Hermansen NO, Kjeldsen-Kragh J. Six years' experience of using the BactT/ALERT system to screen all platelet concentrates, and additional testing of outdated platelet concentrates to estimate the frequency of false-negative results. Vox Sang 2005;88:93–97.
27. Sapatnekar S, Wood EM, Miller JP, et al. Methicillin-resistant *Staphylococcus aureus* sepsis associated with the transfusion of contaminated platelets: a case report. Transfusion 2001;41:1426–1430.
28. Chiu EK, Yuen KY, Lie AK, et al. A prospective study of symptomatic bacteremia following platelet transfusion and of its management. Transfusion 1994;34:950–954.
29. Sullivan MT, McCullough J, Schreiber GB, Wallace EL. Blood collection and transfusion in the United States in 1997. Transfusion 2002;42:1253–1260.
30. Srinivasan A. Septic transfusion reactions despite implementation of methods to reduce bacterial contamination. Paper presented at the Advisory Committee on Blood Safety and Availability, Bethesda, Md., 2005.
31. Laperche S, Pillonel J. Residual risk of transfusion-transmitted HIV, HCV, and HBV infections in France and impact of NAT. Vox Sang 2004;87(Suppl 3):S23.
32. Blajchman MA, Beckers EA, Dickmeiss E, Lin L, Moore G, Muylle L. Bacterial detection of platelets: current problems and possible resolutions. Transfus Med Rev 2005;19:259–272.
33. Benjamin RJ. Bacterial detection in platelet components and the rationale for pathogen inactivation: a blood center perspective. J Clin Apher 2005;20:117–122.
34. Horowitz B, Wiebe ME, Lippin A, Stryker MH. Inactivation of viruses in labile blood derivatives. I. Disruption of lipid-enveloped viruses by tri(n-butyl)phosphate detergent combinations. Transfusion 1985;25:516–522.
35. Heddle NM, Kalma L, Singer J, et al. The role of plasma from platelet concentrates in transfusion reactions. N Engl J Med 1994;331:625–628.
36. Ohto H, Anderson KC. Survey of transfusion-associated graft-versus-host disease in immunocompetent recipients. Transfus Med Rev 1996;10:31–43.
37. Lee TH, Parlieroni T, Utter GH, et al. High-level long-term white blood cell microchimerism after transfusion of leukoreduced blood components to patients resuscitated after severe traumatic injury. Transfusion 2005;45:1280–1290.
38. Ben-Hur E, Moor ACE, Margolis-Nunno H, et al. The photodecontamination of cellular blood components: mechanisms and use of photosensitization in transfusion medicine. Transfus Med Rev 1996;10:15–22.
39. Wollowitz S. Targeting DNA and RNA in pathogens: mode of action of amotoslaen HCl. Transfus Med Hemother 2004;31(Suppl 1):11–16.
40. Kumar V, Lockerbie O, Keil SD, et al. Riboflavin and UV-light based pathogen reduction: extent and consequence of DNA damage at the molecular level. Photochem Photobiol 2004;80:15–21.
41. Lin L, Dikeman R, Molini B, et al. Photochemical treatment of platelet concentrates with amotosalen and UVA inactivates a broad spectrum of pathogenic bacteria. Transfusion 2004;44:1496–1504.
42. Van Voorhis WC, Barrett LK, Eastman RT, Alfonso R, Depuis K. *Trypanosoma cruzi* inactivation in human platelet concentrates and plasma by a psoralen (amotosalen HCl) and long-wavelength UV. Antimicrob Agents Chemother 2003;47:475–479.
43. Eastman RT, Barrett LK, Dupuis K, Buckner FS, Van Voorhis WC. Leishmania inactivation in human pheresis platelets by a psoralen (amotosalen HCl) and long-wavelength ultraviolet irradiation. Transfusion 2005;45:1459–1463.
44. Lin L, Hanson CV, Alter HJ, et al. Inactivation of viruses in platelet concentrates by photochemical treatment with amotosalen and long-wavelength ultraviolet light. Transfusion 2005;45:580–590.
45. Grass JA, Hei DJ, Metchette K, et al. Inactivation of leukocytes in platelet concentrates by psoralen plus UVA. Blood 1998;91:2180–2188.
46. Lin L, Wiesehahn GP, Morel PA, Corash L. Use of 8-methoxypsoralen and long wavelength ultraviolet radiation for decontamination of platelet concentrates. Blood 1989;74:517–525.
47. Alter HJ, Morel PA, Dorman BP, et al. Photochemical decontamination of blood components containing hepatitis B and non-A, non-B virus. Lancet 1988;2:1446–1450.
48. Goodrich RP, Yerram NR, Tay GB, et al. Selective inactivation of viruses in the presence of human platelets: UV sensitization with psoralen derivatives. Proc Natl Acad Sci USA 1994;91:5552–5556.
49. Goodrich RP, Yerram NR, Crandall SL, Sowemimo-Coker SO. In vivo survival of platelets subjected to virus inactivation protocols using psoralen and coumarin photosensitizers. Blood 1995;86(Suppl 1):354A.
50. Jordan CT, Saakadze N, Newman JL, et al. Photochemical treatment of platelet concentrates with amotosalen hydrochloride and ultraviolet A light inactivates free and latent cytomegalovirus in a murine transfusion model. Transfusion 2004;44:1159–1165.
51. Hei DJ, Grass J, Lin L, Corash L, Cimino G. Elimination of cytokine production in stored platelet concentrate aliquots by photochemical treatment with psoralen plus ultraviolet A light. Transfusion 1999; 39:239–248.
52. Grass JA, Wafa T, Reames A, et al. Prevention of transfusion-associated graft-versus-host disease by photochemical treatment. Blood 1999;93: 3140–3147.
53. Bruchmiller I, Janetzko K, Bugert P, et al. Polymerase chain reaction inhibition assay documenting the amotosalen-based photochemical pathogen inactivation process of platelet concentrates. Transfusion 2005;45:1464–1472.
54. Van Rhenen DJ, Vermeij J, Mayaudon V, Hind C, Lin L, Corash L. Functional characteristics of S-59 photochemically treated platelet concentrates derived from buffy coats. Vox Sang 2000;79:206–214.
55. Ruane PH, Edrich R, Gampp D, Keil SD, Leonard L, Goodrich RP. Photochemical inactivation of selected viruses and bacteria in platelet concentrates using riboflavin and light. Transfusion 2004;44:877–885.
56. Goodrich RP. The use of riboflavin for the inactivation of pathogens in blood products. Vox Sang 2000;78(Suppl 2):211–215.
57. Lippert L, Watson R, Doane S, Reddy H, Goodrich R. Inactivation of *Plasmodium falciparum* by riboflavin and light. Vox Sang 2002;83 (Suppl 2):163.
58. Perez-Pujol S, Tonda R, Lozano M, et al. Effects of a new pathogen-reduction technology (Mirasol PRT) on functional aspects of platelet concentrates. Transfusion 2005;45:911–919.
59. Li J, de Korte D, Woolum MD, et al. Pathogen reduction of buffy coat platelet concentrates using riboflavin and light: comparisons with pathogen-reduction technology-treated apheresis platelet products. Vox Sang 2004;87:82–90.
60. Fast LD, DiLeone GR, Li J, Goodrich RP. Mirasol PRT treatment of human white blood cells prevents the development of xenogeneic graft versus host disease. Transfusion 2005;45(3 Suppl):28A–29A.
61. McCullough J, Vesole DH, Benjamin RJ, et al. Therapeutic efficacy and safety of platelets treated with a photochemical process for pathogen inactivation: the SPRINT trial. Blood 2004;104:1534–1541.
62. Van Rhenen D, Gulliksson H, Cazenave JP, et al. Transfusion of pooled buffy coat platelet components prepared with photochemical pathogen inactivation treatment: the euroSPRITE trial. Blood 2003; 101:2426–2433.
63. Snyder E, Raife T, Lin L, et al. Recovery and lifespan of 111 indium-radiolabeled platelets treated with pathogen inactivation with amotosalen HCl (S-59) and ultraviolet A light. Transfusion 2004;44:1732–1740.
64. Snyder E, McCullough J, Slichter SJ, et al. Clinical safety of platelets photochemically treated with amotosalen HCl and ultraviolet A light for pathogen inactivation: the SPRINT trial. Transfusion 2005;45:1864–1875.
65. Osselaer JC, Doyen C, Sonet A, et al. Routine use of platelet components prepared with photochemical treatment (INTERCEPT platelets): impact on clinical outcomes and costs. Blood 2004;104:3629.
66. Slichter SJ, Raife TJ, Davis K, et al. Platelets photochemically treated with amotosalen HCl and ultraviolet A light correct prolonged bleeding times in thrombocytopenic patients. Transfusion 2005;45: 1864–1875.
67. Lin L, Cook DN, Wiesehahn GP, et al. Photochemical inactivation of viruses and bacteria in platelet concentrates by use of a novel psoralen and long-wavelength ultraviolet light. Transfusion 1997;37:423–435.
68. Miller AB, Hoogstraten B, Staquet M, Winkler A. Reporting results of cancer treatment. Cancer 1981;47:207–214.
69. Rebulla P, Finazzi G, Marangoni F, et al. The threshold for prophylactic platelet transfusions in adults with acute myelogenous leukemia. N Engl J Med 1997;337:1870–1875.
70. Heddle NM, Cook RJ, Webert KE, Sigouin C, Rebulla P. Methodological issues in the use of bleeding as an outcome in transfusion medicine studies. Transfusion 2003;43:742–752.
71. Corash L. How much do we know about the platelet transfusion threshold? Transfusion 2003;43:691–693.
72. Heddle NM, Cook RJ, Rebulla P, Slichter SJ, Sigouin C, Murphy MF. Bleeding in patients with acute leukemia. Vox Sang 2002;83(Suppl 2):8.
73. Slichter SJ, Davis K, Enright H, et al. Factors affecting posttransfusion platelet increments, platelet refractoriness, and platelet transfusion intervals in thrombocytopenic patients. Blood 2005;105:4106–4114.

74. Murphy S, Snyder E, Cable R, et al. Platelet dose consistency and its effect on the number of platelet transfusions for support of thrombocytopenia: an analysis of the SPRINT trial of platelets photochemically treated with amotosalen HCl and ultraviolet A light. Transfusion 2006;46:24–33.
75. Janetzko K, Cazenave JP, Kluter H, et al. Therapeutic efficacy and safety of photochemically treated apheresis platelets processed with an optimized integrated set. Transfusion 2005;45:1443–1452.
76. Snyder E, McCullough J, Slichter SJ, et al. Clinical safety of platelets photochemically treated with amotosalen HCl and ultraviolet A light for pathogen inactivation: the SPRINT trial. Transfusion 2005;45:1864–1875.
77. Lin L, Conlan MG, Tessman J, Cimino G, Porter S. Amotosalen interactions with platelet and plasma components: absence of neoantigen formation after photochemical treatment. Transfusion 2005;45:1610–1620.
78. Osselaer JC, Bueno JL, Messe N, Jacquet M, Castro E, Flament J. Prospective active hemovigilance plan for INTERCEPT platelets in Europe: a status report. Vox Sang 2005;89:137.
79. AuBuchon JP, Herschel L, Roger J, et al. Efficacy of apheresis platelets treated with riboflavin and ultraviolet light for pathogen reduction. Transfusion 2005;45:1335–1341.
80. Rywkin S, Ben-Hur E, Reid ME, Oyen R, Ralph H, Horowitz B. Selective protection against IgG binding to red cells treated with phthalocyanines and red light for virus inactivation. Transfusion 1995;35:414–420.
81. Ben-Hur E, Rywkin S, Rosenthal I, Geacintov NE, Horowitz B. Virus inactivation in red cell concentrates by photosensitization with phthalocyanines: protection of red cells but not of vesicular stomatitis virus with a water-soluble analogue of vitamin E. Transfusion 1995; 35:401–406.
82. Wagner SJ, Skirpchenko A, Robinette D, Mallory DA, Cincotta L. Preservation of red cell properties after virucidal phototreatment with dimethylmethylene blue. Transfusion 1998;38:729–737.
83. Besselink GA, van Engelenburg FA, Korsten HG, et al. The band III ligand dipyridamole protects human RBCs during photodynamic treatment while extracellular virus inactivation is not affected. Transfusion 2002;42:728–733.
84. Wagner SJ, Skripchenko A, Cincotta L, Thompson-Montgomery D, Awatefe H. Use of a flexible thiopyrylium photosensitizer and competitive inhibitor for pathogen reduction of viruses and bacteria with retention of red cell storage properties. Transfusion 2005; 45:752–760.
85. Fast LD, DiLeone G, Edson CM, Purmal A. PEN 110 treatment functionally inactivates the PBMNCs present in RBC units: comparison to the effects of exposure to gamma irradiation. Transfusion 2002;42:1318–1325.
86. Jayarama V, Lazo A, Marcello J, et al. Inactine PEN 110 inactivates cell-free and cell-associated CMV in red cell concentrates. Transfusion 2003;43(Suppl 9):8A.
87. Ohagen A, Gibaja V, Aytay S, Horrigan J, Lunderville D, Lazo A. Inactivation of HIV in blood. Transfusion 2002;42:1308–1317.
88. Edson CM, Purmal A, Brown F, Valeri CR, Budowsky E, Chapman JR. Viral inactivation of red blood cell concentrates by Inactine: mechanism of action and lack of effect on red cell physiology. Transfusion 1999;39(Suppl 1):108S.
89. AuBuchon JP, Pickard CA, Herschel LH, et al. Production of pathogen-inactivated red cell concentrates using PEN 110 chemistry: a phase I clinical study. Transfusion 2002;42:146–152.
90. Snyder E, Mintz P, Burks S, et al. Pathogen inactivated red blood cells using Inactine technology demonstrate 24-hour posttransfusion recovery equal to untreated red cells after 42 days of storage. Blood 2001;98(Suppl 1):109A.
91. Cook D, Stassinopoulos A, Merritt J, et al. Inactivation of pathogens in packed red blood cell (PRBC) concentrates using S-303. Blood 1997;90(Suppl 1):409A.
92. Cook D, Stassinopoulos A, Wollowitz S, et al. In vivo analysis of packed red blood cells treated with S-303 to inactivate pathogens. Blood 1998;92(Suppl 1):503A.
93. Ciaravino V, McCullough T, Woods N, Sullivan T. Absence of carcinogenicity in a 26-week intravenous study with S-303-treated mouse red blood cells in C57BL/6TAC-TRP53TML heterozygote mice. Blood Bank Transfus Med 2003;1(Suppl 1):S365.
94. Greenwalt TJ, Hambleton J, Wages D, et al. Viability of red blood cells treated with a novel pathogen inactivation system. Transfusion 1999;39(Suppl 1):109S.
95. Hambleton J, Greenwalt T, Viele M, et al. Posttransfusion recovery after multiple exposures to red blood cell concentrates (RBCS) treated with a novel pathogen inactivation (PI) process. Blood 1999;94(Suppl 1):376A.
96. Wages D, Hambleton J, Viele M, et al. RBCs treated with Helinx pathogen inactivation have recovery and half-life comparable to conventional RBCS in a randomized crossover trial. Hematol J 2002;3 (Suppl 1):171.
97. Benjamin RJ, McCullough J, Mintz PD, et al. Therapeutic efficacy and safety of red blood cells treated with a chemical process (S-303) for pathogen inactivation: a phase III clinical trial in cardiac surgery patients. Transfusion 2005;45:1739–1749.
98. Conlan MG, Vichinsky E, Snyder E, et al. S-303 pathogen inactivated red blood cells in patients with hemoglobinopathies participating in chronic RBC programs: preliminary safety and efficacy results. Vox Sang 2005;89(Suppl 1):121.
99. Conlan MG, Lin J, Stassinopoulos A. Investigation of immunoreactivity observed after transfusion of S-303 RBCs in 2 phase III clinical trials in support of acute or chronic anemia. Transfusion 2005;45 (Suppl 3):29A.
100. Arndt PA, Garratty G. A retrospective analysis of the value of monocyte monolayer assay results for predicting the clinical significance of blood group alloantibodies. Transfusion 2004;44:1273–1281.
101. Horowitz B, Bonomo R, Prince AM, Chin SN, Brotman B, Shulman RW. Solvent/detergent treated plasma: a virus-inactivated substitute for fresh frozen plasma. Blood 1992;79:826–831.
102. Roberts P. Resistance of vaccinia virus to inactivation by solvent/detergent treatment of blood products. Biologicals 2000;28:29–32.
103. Luban NL. Human parvovirus: implications for transfusion medicine. Transfusion 1994;34:821–827.
104. Horowitz MS, Pehta JC. SD plasma in TTP and coagulation factor deficiencies for which no concentrates are available. Vox Sang 1998;74(Suppl 1):231–235.
105. Haubelt H, Blome M, Kiessling AH, et al. Effects of solvent/detergent-treated plasma and fresh frozen plasma on haemostasis and fibrinolysis in complex coagulopathy following open-heart surgery. Vox Sang 2002;82:9–14.
106. Williamson LM, Llewelyn CA, Fisher NC, et al. A randomized trial of solvent/detergent-treated and standard fresh-frozen plasma in the coagulopathy of liver disease and liver transplantation. Transfusion 1999;39:1227–1234.
107. Baudoux E, Margraff U, Coenen A, et al. Hemovigilance: clinical tolerance of solvent-detergent treated plasma. Vox Sang 1998;74(Suppl 1):237–239.
108. Beeck H, Hellstern O. In vitro characterization of solvent/detergent-treated human plasma and quarantine fresh frozen plasma. Vox Sang 1998;74(Suppl 1):219–223.
109. Mast AE, Stadanlick JE, Lockett JM, Dietzen DJ. Solvent/detergent-treated plasma has decreased antitrypsin activity and absent antiplasmin activity. Blood 1999;94:3922–3927.
110. Beach KJ. Reported Serious Adverse Events in Liver Transplant Patients. V.I. Technologies Inc. Available at http://www.fda.gov/medwatch/safety/2000/plassd.pdf. Accessed March 28, 2006.
111. Yarranton H, Cohen H, Pavord SR, Benjamin S, Hagger D, Machin SJ. Venous thromboembolism associated with management of acute thrombotic thrombocytopenic purpura. Br J Haematol 2003;121:778–785.
112. Flamholz R, Jeon HR, Baron JM, Baron BW. Study of three patients with thrombotic thrombocytopenic purpura exchanged with solvent/detergent-treated plasma: is its decreased protein S activity clinically related to their development of deep venous thrombosis? J Clin Apher 2000;15:169–172.
113. Mohr H, Lambrecht B, Knueyer-Hopf J. Virus inactivated single-donor fresh plasma preparations. Infusionsther Transfusionsmed 1992;19:79–83.
114. Garwood M, Cardigan RA, Drummond O, et al. The effect of methylene blue photoinactivation and methylene blue removal on the quality of fresh-frozen plasma. Transfusion 2003;43:1238–1247.
115. Aznar JA, Bonanad S, Montoro JM, et al. Influence of methylene blue photoinactivation treatment on coagulation factors from fresh frozen plasma, cryoprecipitates, and cryosupernatants. Vox Sang 2000; 79:156–160.
116. Simonsen AC, Sorensen H. Clinical tolerance of methylene blue virus-inactivated plasma. A randomized crossover trial in 12 healthy volunteers. Vox Sang 1999;77:210–217.
117. Williamson LM, Cardigan R, Prowse CV. Methylene blue-treated fresh-frozen plasma: what is the contribution to blood safety? Transfusion 2003;43:1322–1329.
118. Wieding JU, Rathberger J, Zenjer D. Prospective, randomized trial and controlled study on solvent detergent versus methylene blue virus inactivated plasma. Transfusion 1999;39:23S.
119. Alvarez-Larran A, Del Rio J, Ramirez C, et al. Methylene blue-photoinactivated plasma vs fresh frozen plasma as replacement fluid for plasma exchange in thrombotic thrombocytopenic purpura. Vox Sang 2004;86:246–251.

120. de la Rubria J, Arriaga F, Linares D, et al. Role of methylene blue-treated or fresh-frozen plasma in the response to plasma exchange in patients with thrombotic thrombocytopenic purpura. Br J Haematol 2001;114:721–723.
121. Atance R, Pereira A, Ramirez B. Transfusing methylene blue-photoinactivated plasma instead of FFP is associated with an increased demand for plasma and cryoprecipitate. Transfusion 2001;41:1548–1552.
122. Alfonso R, Lin C, Dupuis K, et al. Inactivation of viruses with preservation of coagulation function in fresh frozen plasma. Blood 1996;88(Suppl 1):526A.
123. Singh Y, Sawyer L, Pinkoski L, et al. Photochemical treatment of plasma with amotosalen and UVA light inactivates pathogens while retaining coagulation function. Transfusion 2006;46:1168–1177.
124. Hervig T, Cazenave JP, Schlenke P, et al. INTERCEPT plasma: process validation studies in three European blood centers. Hematologica 2005;90:246.
125. Wages D, Smith D, Walsh J, et al. Transfusion of therapeutic doses of virally inactivated fresh frozen plasma in healthy subjects. Blood 1997;90(Suppl 1):409A.
126. Wages D, Radu-Radurescu L, Adams M, et al. Quantitative analysis of coagulation factors in response to transfusion of S-59 photochemically treated fresh frozen plasma (S-59 FFP) and standard FFP. Blood 1998;92(Suppl 1):503A.
127. Hambleton J, Wages D, Radu-Radulescu L, et al. Pharmacokinetic study of FFP photochemically treated with amotosalen (S-59) and UV light compared to FFP in healthy volunteers anticoagulated with warfarin. Transfusion 2002;42:1302–1307.
128. Wages D, Bass N, Keefe E, et al. Treatment of acquired coagulopathy by transfusion of fresh frozen plasma (FFP) prepared using a novel, single unit photochemical. Blood 1999;94(Suppl 1):247A.
129. de Alarcon P, Benjamin R, Dugdale M, et al. Fresh frozen plasma prepared with amotosalen HCl (S-59) photochemical pathogen inactivation (PCT-FFP): transfusion of patients with congenital factor deficiencies. Transfusion 2005;45:1362–1372.
130. Mintz PD, Bass NM, Petz LD, et al. Photochemically treated fresh frozen plasma for transfusion of patients with acquired coagulopathy of liver disease. Blood 2006;107:3753–3760.
131. Mintz PD, Neff A, MacKenzie M, et al. Therapeutic plasma exchange (TPE) for thrombotic thrombocytopenic purpura (TTP) using plasma prepared with photochemical treatment (INTERCEPT plasma). Blood 2004;104:239A.
132. Londe H, Damonte P, Corash L, Lin L. Inactivation of human cytomegalovirus with psoralen and UVA in human platelet concentrates. Blood 1995;86(Suppl 1):544A.
133. Lin L, Londe H, Hanson CV, et al. Photochemical inactivation of cell-associated human immunodeficiency virus in platelet concentrates. Blood 1993;82:292–297.
134. Eble BE, Corash L. Photochemical inactivation of duck hepatitis B virus in human platelet concentrates: a model of surrogate human hepatitis B virus infectivity. Transfusion 1996;36:406–418.
135. Lin L, Londe H, Janda JM, et al. Photochemical inactivation of pathogenic bacteria in human platelet concentrates. Blood 1994;83:2698–2706.
136. Dodd RY, Moroff G, Wagner S, et al. Inactivation of viruses in platelet suspensions that retain their in vitro characteristics: comparison of psoralen-ultraviolet A and merocyanine 540-visible light methods. Transfusion 1991;31:483–490.
137. Margolis-Nunno H, Williams B, Rywkin S, Geacintov N, Horowitz B. Virus sterilization in platelet concentrates with psoralen and ultraviolet A light in the presence of quenchers. Transfusion 1992;32:541–547.
138. Benade LE, Shumaker J, Xu Y, Chen X, Dodd RY. Inactivation of free and cell-associated human immunodeficiency virus in platelet suspensions by aminomethyltrimethylpsoralen and ultraviolet light. Transfusion 1994;34:680–684.
139. Margolis-Nunno M, Williams B, Rywkin S, Horowitz B. Photochemical virus sterilization in platelet concentrates with psoralen derivatives. Thromb Haemost 1991;65:1162.
140. Yerram N, Forster P, Goodrich T, et al. Comparison of virucidal properties of brominated psoralen with 8-methoxy psoralen (8-MOP) and aminomethyl trimethyl psoralen (AMT) in platelet concentrates. Blood 1993;82(Suppl 1):402A.
141. Rai S, Kasturi C, Grayzar J, et al. Dramatic improvements in viral inactivation with brominated psoralens, napthalenes, and anthracenes. Photochem Photobiol 1993;58:59–65.
142. Prodouz KN, Fratantoni JC, Boone EJ, Bonner RF. Use of laser-UV for inactivation of virus in blood products. Blood 1987;70:589–592.
143. Prodouz KN, Lytle CD, Keville EA, Budacz AP, Vargo S, Fratantoni JC. Inhibition by albumin of merocyanine 540-mediated photosensitization of platelets and viruses. Transfusion 1991;31:415–422.
144. Klein-Struckmeier A, Mohr H. Virus inactivation by methylene blue light in thrombocyte concentrates. Vox Sang 1994;67(Suppl 2):36.
145. Horowitz B, Rywkin S, Margolis-Nunno H, et al. Inactivation of viruses in red cell and platelet concentrates with aluminum phthalocyanine (AlPc) sulfonates. Blood Cells 1992;18:141–150.
146. Matthews JL, Sogandres-Bernal F, Judy M, et al. Inactivation of viruses with photoactive compounds. Blood Cells 1992;18:75–89.
147. North J, Neyndorff H, King D, Levy JG. Viral inactivation in blood and red cell concentrates with benzoporphyrin derivative. Blood Cells 1992;18:129–140.
148. Sieber F, Krueger GJ, O'Brien JM, Schober SL, Sensenbrenner LL, Sharkis SJ. Inactivation of friend erythroleukemia virus and friend virus-transformed cells by merocyanine 540-mediated photosensitization. Blood 1989;73:345–350.
149. O'Brien JM, Gaffney DK, Wang TP, Sieber F. Merocyanine 540-sensitized photoinactivation of enveloped viruses in blood products: site and mechanism of phototoxicity. Blood 1992;80:277–285.
150. Smith OM, Dolan SA, Dvorak JA, Wellems TE, Sieber F. Merocyanine 540-sensitized photoinactivation of human erythrocytes parasitized by Plasmodium falciparum. Blood 1992;80:21–24.
151. Wagner SJ, Storry JR, Mallory DA, Stromberg RR, Benade LE, Friedman LI. Red cell alterations associated with virucidal methylene blue phototreatment. Transfusion 1993;33:30–36.
152. Wagner SJ, Robinette D, Storry J, Chen XY, Shumaker J, Benade L. Differential sensitivities of viruses in red cell suspensions to methylene blue photosensitization. Transfusion 1994;34:521–526.
153. Horowitz B, Williams B, Rywkin S, et al. Inactivation of viruses in blood with aluminum phthalocyanine derivatives. Transfusion 1991;31:102–108.
154. Yerram N, Platz MS, Forster P, Goodrich T, Goodrich R. Selective viral inactivation in RBC, platelets, and plasma using a novel psoralen derivative plus ultraviolet A (UVA) light. Transfusion 1993;33(Suppl 9):50S.
155. Lavie G, Mazur Y, Lavie D, et al. Hypericin as an inactivator of infectious viruses in blood components. Transfusion 1995;35:392–400.
156. Zhang QX, Edson C, Budowsky E, Purmal A. Inactine: a method for viral inactivation in red blood cell concentrates. Transfusion 1998;38(Suppl 10):75S.

Chapter 28

Irradiated Products

Naomi L. C. Luban • Edward C. C. Wong

INTRODUCTION

Transfusion-associated graft-versus-host disease (TA-GVHD), an often fatal alloimmune complication mediated by donor T cells in the blood component, was first reported in the 1960s in individuals with hematologic malignancies and in infants with congenital immunodeficiencies who developed "runting disease" after blood transfusion.[1]

Since these early reports, the spectrum of individuals at risk has expanded, the pathogenesis has been partially elucidated, and preventive strategies have been established.[2–4] Despite these advances, many unanswered questions remain. For example, there are no adequate estimates of prevalence. In Japan, an estimated annual incidence of one TA-GVHD case per 212 transfusions has been calculated based on homozygosity for one-way human leukocyte antigen (HLA) haplotype sharing, the use of familial donors, and the use of fresh rather than stored red blood cells (RBCs).[5] In the United Kingdom and Canada, in contrast, risk estimates are much lower as determined by adverse transfusion outcome reporting. The *S*erious *H*azards *o*f *T*ransfusion (SHOT) study in the United Kingdom has identified only 13 cases from 1996 to present, although all were fatal.[6] In Canada, mathematical modeling by Kleinman and colleagues estimated the magnitude of risk to be between 1:12,893 and 1:21,157, but based on cases reported and other factors a true risk of less than 1 per million units transfused is cited.[7] No incidence figures are available for the United States, and it is likely that under-recognition and under-reporting are common. Additionally, while the pathogenesis of TA-GVHD partially resembles that of GVHD in the setting of hematopoietic stem cell transplantation, further, more detailed investigations of TA-GVHD have been hindered by the lack of well-established animal models. Instead, investigators typically utilize the classic parent-to-F1 hybrid mouse model of GVHD, which may or may not provide the correct tool for TA-GVHD investigations.[8]

Given the almost uniform lethality of TA-GVHD, extensive clinical investigations have fortunately led to the development of pretransfusion irradiation methods that uniformly prevent TA-GVHD. The technical and regulatory aspects of these methodologies are addressed in detail in this chapter. Since irradiation devices are not available in all transfusion settings, attention has recently focused on alternative approaches to prevention. Data are accumulating to suggest that filtration and nucleic acid–targeted pathogen reduction technologies may remove or inactivate donor leukocytes, respectively, to the extent that TA-GVHD is also prevented, although further study and validation are required.

PATHOGENESIS OF TA-GVHD

Three prerequisites for the development of GVHD in the transplant setting have been proposed: (1) differences in histocompatibility between recipient and donor, (2) presence of immunocompetent cells in the graft, and (3) inability of the host to reject the immunocompetent cells. A similar set of circumstances underlie TA-GVHD. First, in almost all cases, leukocytes in homologous blood components are mismatched with the transfusion recipient at HLA and minor histocompatibility loci. Second, transfused donor leukocytes are immunologically functional, except in circumstances in which they have been specifically inactivated (e.g., following gamma-irradiation). And third, the commonality between many of the patients at risk for TA-GVHD is their inability to reject transfused leukocytes, either due to immune immaturity (low-birth-weight neonates) or iatrogenic immunosuppression (transplant recipients). The development of TA-GVHD in additional clinical settings illustrates the importance of these factors. For example, most immunocompetent recipients destroy transfused donor T cells through lymphocytolysis and therefore do not develop TA-GVHD. However, transfusion from an HLA homozygous donor to an HLA heterozygous, but immunocompetent, recipient who shares one HLA haplotype may result in failure of recognition of the donor cells as foreign.[9,10] This so-called "one-way HLA match" is often responsible for the development of TA-GVHD in immunocompetent recipients, such as might occur in familial (directed) blood transfusions, in populations with limited HLA diversity, and when HLA-matched platelet transfusions are administered. In these cases, the non-self HLA or minor histocompatibility antigens of the host, or both, stimulate clonal expansion of donor T cells and the induction of an inflammatory response that is ultimately responsible for clinical manifestations of TA-GVHD.

Studies of the pathogenesis of TA-GVHD, both in vitro experiments as well as animal investigations, have begun to define roles for donor leukocyte subsets in the process. Among leukocytes, donor T cells play the most prominent role in disease pathogenesis. CD4+ T cells (sometimes known as T-helper cells) can be functionally divided into Th1 and Th2 subsets. Th1 CD4 T cells secrete interleukin-2 (IL-2), while Th2 CD4 T cells produce IL-4, IL-5, IL-6, IL-10, IL-13, and lesser amounts of tumor necrosis factor–α (TNFα). Th1 and Th2 both produce IL-3 and granulocyte-macrophage colony-stimulating factor. The type 1 cell is proinflammatory and induces cell-mediated immunity, whereas the type 2 cell is considered anti-inflammatory. Differentiation toward Th1 or Th2 is a complicated process that involves early exposure to IL-4 or IL-12, the type of antigen-presenting cells, costimulating molecules, and the presence of macrophages and their unique cytokines.

On the basis of their work in mice, Ferrera and colleagues proposed a three-step process for the development of acute GVHD in the transplant setting, including the involvement of T-cell subsets. In this model (Fig. 28–1), host tissue damaged through irradiation or chemotherapy secretes TNFα and IL-1, which enhance recognition of host histocompatibility antigens by donor T cells. Donor T-cell activation results in proliferation of Th1 T cells and secretion of IL-2 and TNFα, which in turn further activate T cells and induce cytotoxic T- lymphocyte (CTL) and natural killer (NK) responses.

Additional studies have shown that donor and residual host phagocytes are stimulated to produce IL-1, TNFα, and the free radical nitric oxide (NO), which has further deleterious effects on host tissues. In addition, NO up-regulates alloreactivity and mediates the cytotoxic function of macrophages.[11] A secondary triggering signal initiates a subsequent stage in the disease process wherein lipopolysaccharide (LPS) stimulates gut-associated macrophages and lymphocytes, stimulates keratocytes and dermal fibroblasts, and further promotes the inflammatory response and end-organ damage that are classic hallmarks of the disorder.

Whether the development of TA-GVHD is dependent on similar mechanisms remains an open question. To begin to address this question, the importance of CD4 and CD8 T cells in the pathogenesis of TA-GVHD has been studied by Fast and coworkers[12] in a mouse model and by Nishimura and associates[13] in a patient with TA-GVHD. Their findings are further supported by clinical correlation in patients with human immunodeficiency virus (HIV) infection and acquired immunodeficiency syndrome (AIDS).[14] In the mouse, depletion of CD4+ cells increases the number of donor cells needed to induce TA-GVHD, whereas depletion of CD8+ or NK cells, or both, decreases the number of donor cells needed to induce the disorder. In HIV and AIDS, there has been only one report of TA-GVHD[15] despite widespread use of supportive transfusion and profound immunosuppression. This observation is consistent with the concept that

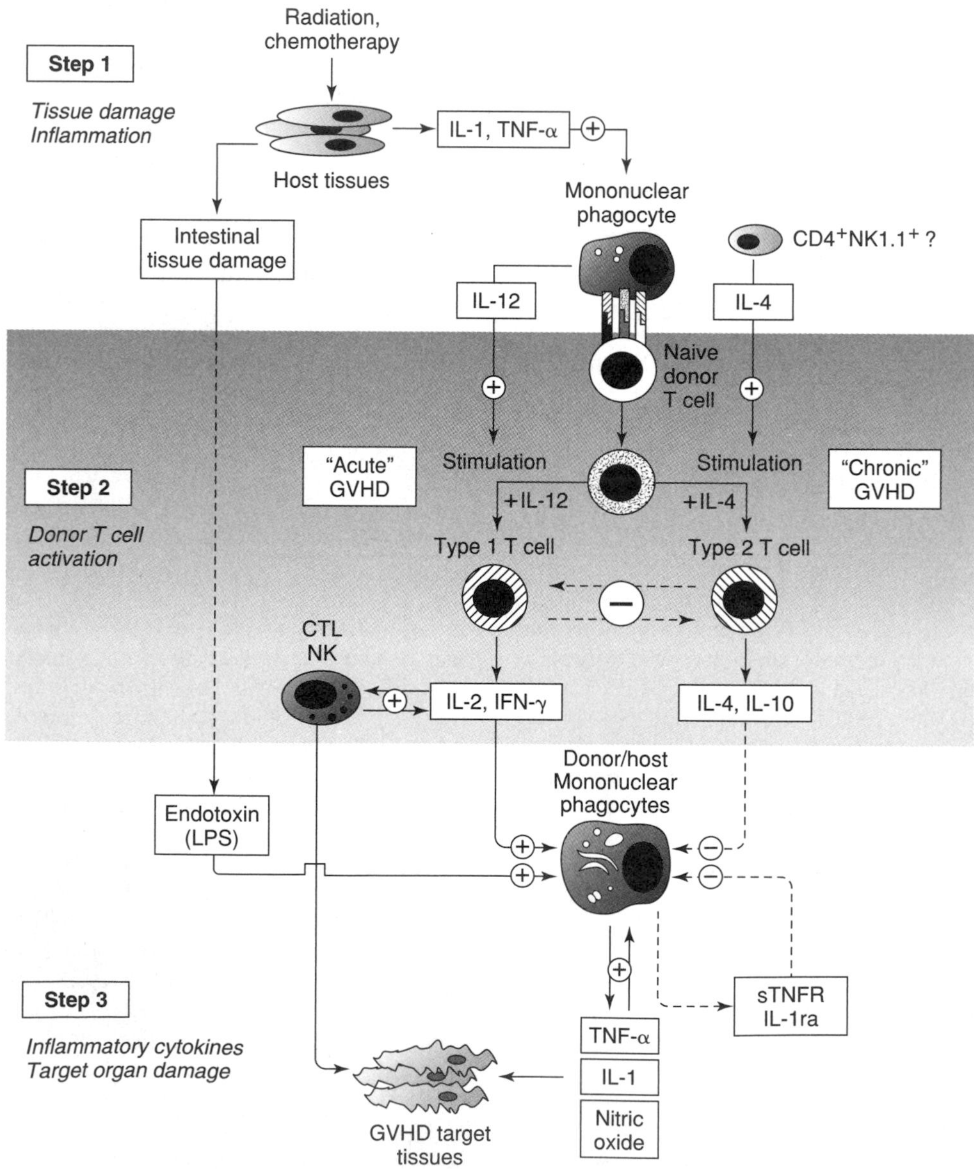

Figure 28–1 Proposed interactions between T-cell cytokines and mononuclear phagocyte–derived cytokines during graft-versus-host disease (GVHD). IFN, interferon; IL-1, interleukin-1; LPS, lipopolysaccharide; sTNFR, soluble tumor necrosis factor receptor; TNFα, tumor necrosis factor–α.

early depletion of CD4 may well protect against establishment of TA-GVHD. Additionally, expansion and activation of NK and CD8+ lymphocytes against HIV-infected CD4 T cells may limit the development of the GVHD process.

Since donor leukocytes must persist to cause TA-GVHD, other investigators have evaluated clearance of leukocytes after transfusion.[16] In 1996, Busch and colleagues[17] demonstrated a thousand-fold expansion of donor lymphocytes in the circulation of otherwise healthy recipients 3 to 5 days after transfusion for elective orthopedic procedures. Within 2 weeks, the allogeneic cells were cleared. In contrast, in a study of adult trauma victims who received large numbers (4 to 18 units) of fresh-packed RBCs, 8 of 10 had long-term persistence of donor leukocytes with confirmed microchimerism (MC). Two of the eight had persistence of MC when studied as long as 1.5 years after transfusion.[18] These studies have been further expanded in additional patients transfused for acute trauma who received nonleukoreduced[17] or leukoreduced[19] products. That MC in some cases persisted for years[18] recently has been confirmed and attributed to a single donor source from which leukocytes expanded over time.[18,20] These studies suggest that transfusion during a period of diminished lymphocyte responsiveness may result in a microchimeric state with persistence of functional donor leukocytes, possibly with long-term consequences.

Wang-Rodriquez and associates[21] studied post-transfusion immune modulation in 14 premature infants and identified two of six female infants, transfused with nonleukodepleted RBCs, who experienced transient MC detected by Y chromosome PCR amplification. In both, these cells were cleared by 2 weeks after transfusion. An additional three infants who received leukodepleted RBCs also had transient MC.

Vietor and coworkers[22] studied 9 surviving recipients of intrauterine transfusion whose donors were still available for testing. Using fluorescence in situ hybridization, PCR of Y chromosome–specific sequences, and assays for the frequencies of CTL and T-helper lymphocyte precursors, they detected true MC in 6 of 7 young adults studied 20 years after transfusion. Reed and colleagues[23] have developed sequence-specific amplification of DRB1, which permitted identification of minor chimeric populations at the 0.01% level. The establishment of stable MC and identification of its biological consequences are critical for pediatric patients who are expected to live to adulthood and may well be stable transfusion-induced chimeras, an intriguing and at the same time potentially worrisome occurrence. The persistence of MC may predispose to autoimmune disease,[24–26] chronic GVHD, and recurrent abortion[27] and may serve as an allogeneic stimulus of latent viral reactivation in the recipient.

In a mouse system, allogeneic male donor WBCs derived from C57BL/6 mice persisted in female BALB/c recipient mice and their survival was unaffected by irradiation. Although the experimental model could not differentiate nonproliferative from proliferative WBC, these data set the stage for additional studies on MC and post-transfusion WBC kinetics. Fast and colleagues studied the effects of different forms of irradiation on murine splenocytes to better understand inhibition of both in vitro and in vivo proliferative responses. Among their findings was that the genotype of the donor-recipient pair regulates recipient alloantibody formation, a conclusion suggested by studies of prolonged MC in humans.[19] They also showed that the accelerated elimination of donor cells from recipient lymphoid compartments might be due to altered expression of cell surface molecules like CD31, CD47, and CD200, a phenomenon yet to be confirmed in human studies.

CLINICAL MANIFESTATIONS OF TA-GVHD

Fever, anorexia, nausea, vomiting, and diarrhea typically develop 7 to 10 days post-transfusion. Skin manifestations of TA-GVHD are variably severe and begin as an erythematous maculopapular eruption that may proceed to erythroderma with bullae and frank desquamation. Gastrointestinal bleeding is commonly seen, usually as bloody diarrhea. Hepatic dysfunction with transaminitis and hyperbilirubinemia, including a progressively increasing direct fraction, is also seen. In contrast to acute GVHD in the setting of allogeneic transplantation, TA-GVHD leads to severe pancytopenia because donor T cells attack marrow hematopoietic cells. This often results in the death of the patient. The diagnosis typically is made at postmortem examination and is based on pathognomonic histopathologic findings of donor lymphocyte infiltration and expansion in skin, lymph nodes, liver, and the gastrointestinal tract.[28]

DIAGNOSIS OF TA-GVHD

Clinical suspicion may warrant a skin biopsy, which often reveals vacuolization of the epidermal basal cell layer, dermal-epithelial layer separation, and formation of bullae. Other findings include mononuclear cell migration into the epidermis, hyperkeratosis, and dyskeratosis. Liver biopsies may reveal eosinophilic infiltration and degeneration of small bile ducts, peripheral inflammation, and lymphocyte infiltration. The bone marrow findings are classically those of "empty marrow," with pancytopenia, fibrosis, and some lymphocytic infiltration.

Definitive confirmation of TA-GVHD is more complicated. Several methods have been utilized to identify lymphocytes of foreign origin in the patient's circulation or in affected tissues. Serologic HLA typing, DNA-based HLA class II typing, karyotype analysis, restriction fragment length polymorphism analysis using probes from both HLA and non-HLA regions, and genetic fingerprinting have all been used.[29–33] Fibroblast and buccal mucosal cells of the recipient are often needed, as the lymphocytolysis accompanying the disorder prohibits standardized serologic HLA typing using recipient lymphocytes. Alternatively, parental or familial specimens may be necessary to deduce a recipient's HLA type.[34] Donor lymphocytes in attached remaining segments from suspected blood products often require PCR amplification and sequence-specific oligonucleotide probe methodologies to provide confirmation of donor cell origin.[35]

GROUPS AT RISK FOR TA-GVHD

Patients in whom TA-GVHD may develop have been described in a number of reviews,[2–4,10,11,36,37] and this remains an area of active discussion. For example, on the basis of two reports of TA-GVHD in older infants with severe combined immunodeficiency,[18,35] it has been recommended that infants well past the neonatal age group be considered at risk.[38,39] Because of the lack of adequate animal models and laboratory tests to identify individual TA-GVHD risk, many reports stratify the need for irradiation using such terms as *clearly indicated* or *probably indicated*.[3,36,37] In reality, the spectrum of individuals at risk is likely to grow as intensive immunomodulatory therapies expand beyond oncologic disease and transplantation (Table 28–1).

THERAPY FOR TA-GVHD

The rapid progression of clinical manifestations of the disorder and similarity of clinical presentation to that of viral, drug-related, or disease-related enteropathy and hepatocellular damage contribute to the high mortality rates. Anecdotal success has been reported with immunosuppressive treatment including cytoxan, antithymocyte globulin, and high-dose corticosteroids. Recently, the serum protease inhibitor nafamostat mesylate has been used with some success.[40,41] The effectiveness of hematopoietic stem cell transplantation is mixed.[35,42]

PREVENTION OF TA-GVHD

Irradiation

Among methodologies (e.g., irradiation, photoinactivation, pegylation, and ultraviolet [UV] light) that can be used to prevent TA-GVHD, only irradiation of whole blood and cellular components is currently accepted by the U.S. Food and Drug Administration (FDA). Exposure of cellular components to ionizing radiation results in the inactivation of T cells by damage to nuclear DNA either directly or through generation of ions and free radicals that have damaging biological actions. Irradiation prevents post-transfusion donor T-cell proliferation in response to host antigen-presenting cells, which, in turn, abrogates GVHD.[43–46] Two types of ionizing radiation—gamma rays and x-rays—are equivalent in inactivating T cells in blood components at a given absorbed dose. Gamma rays originate from the radioactive decay process within the atomic nucleus of cesium 137 (^{137}Cs) or cobalt 60 (^{60}Co). Freestanding blood bank gamma-irradiators, which are the predominant instruments for blood component irradiation, use either of these two isotopes as the irradiation source.

In contrast, x-rays are generated from the interaction of a beam of electrons with a metallic surface. Linear accelerators typically used to generate x-rays for clinical radiation therapy (teletherapy) may serve as an irradiation source for blood and blood components. The FDA has also approved the use of a freestanding x-ray machine (Rad-Source RS3000, Coral Springs, Fla.) for irradiation of blood components.

Instrumentation for Irradiation

The basic operating principles and configurations of a freestanding irradiator with either a ^{137}Cs source or a linear accelerator are shown schematically in Figure 28–2. With a freestanding ^{137}Cs irradiator, blood components are contained within a metal canister that is positioned on a rotating turntable. Continuous rotation allows the gamma rays, originating from one to four closely positioned pencil sources, to penetrate all portions of the blood component. The number of sources and their placement depend on the instrument and model. The speed of rotation of the turntable is also specific to each model. A lead shield encloses the radiation chamber, protecting the operator from radiation exposure. Freestanding irradiators employing ^{60}Co as the source of gamma rays are comparable except that the canister containing the blood component does not rotate during the irradiation process; rather, tubes of ^{60}Co are placed in a circular array around the entire canister within the lead chamber. When freestanding irradiators are used, the gamma rays are attenuated as they pass through air and blood but at different rates.[45] The magnitude of attenuation is greater with ^{137}Cs than with ^{60}Co sources.

Linear accelerators generate a beam of x-rays over a field of given dimensions. Routinely, the field is projected on a tabletop structure. The blood component is placed (flat) between two sheets of biocompatible plastic several centimeters thick. The plastic on the top of the blood component (i.e., nearer to the radiation source) generates electronic equilibrium of the secondary electrons at the point where they pass through the component container. The plastic sheet on the bottom of the blood component provides radiation backscattering that helps ensure homogeneous delivery of the x-rays. The blood component is usually left stationary during delivery of the entire x-ray dose. Alternatively, it may be inverted when half of the dose has been delivered, although additional data on this practice are needed. Guidance is available on the FDA website (http://www.fda.gov/cder/guidelines.htm).[47] In June 1999, the FDA licensed the first x-ray irradiator based on principles utilized in standard x-ray machines. This irradiator does not require federal or nuclear regulatory licensing or reporting, a shielded room for operation, or special floor reinforcement.

Table 28–1 Clinical Indications for Irradiated Products

In Fetus/Infant
Intrauterine transfusion
Prematurity
Congenital immunodeficiency
Exchange transfusion for erythroblastosis
In Child/Adult
Congenital immunodeficiency
Hematologic malignancy or solid tumor (neuroblastoma, sarcoma, Hodgkin's disease where ablative chemotherapy and/or radiotherapy is administered)
Peripheral blood stem cell or marrow transplant
Recipient of familial blood donation
Human leukocyte antigen–matched products
Lupus or any other condition requiring fludarabine
Potential Indications
Recipient and donor pair from a genetically homogeneous population
Other patients with hematologic malignancy or solid tumor receiving immunosuppressive agents
Infant/child with congenital heart disease with 22 qll deletions, other than DiGeorge syndrome
Recipient and donor pair from genetically less homogeneous populations
Those receiving "less intensive" immunosuppressive regimens
No/Limited Indications
Patients infected with HIV
Term infants
Obstetric, surgical, and general medicine patients

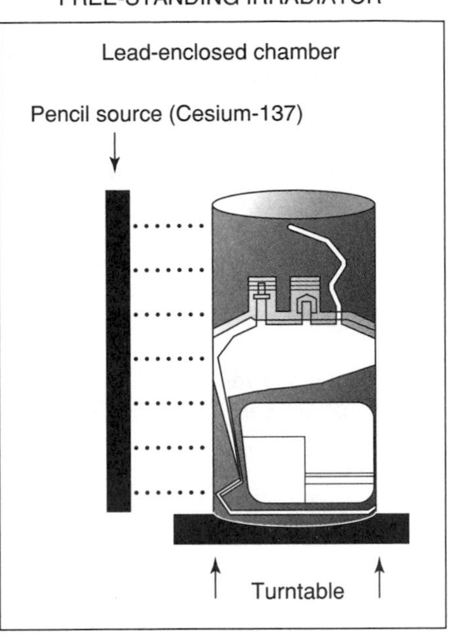

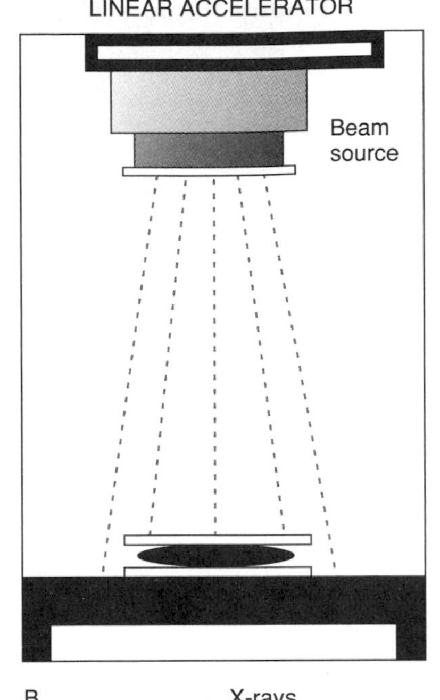

Figure 28–2 Diagrammatic views of two common types of instrumentation used for blood irradiation. **A**, Configuration of a freestanding irradiator using a cesium 137 source. **B**, Configuration of a linear accelerator.

Components to Be Irradiated

The content of viable T lymphocytes is the single most important factor in determining whether a blood component can induce TA-GVHD. On the basis of animal models and estimates from the clinical bone marrow transplant literature, 5×10^4 to 1×10^5 T cells per kilogram produces GVHD in ablated hosts[46]; a greater number is probably needed in a nonablated recipient. The content of T lymphocytes in each blood component differs depending on the donor's initial lymphocyte count, the method of collection, and any post-collection manipulation and processing. There are probably sufficient lymphocytes in almost all blood products to induce TA-GVHD in a susceptible recipient (Table 28–2). As storage time increases, fewer viable lymphocytes can be isolated from RBC and platelet concentrates. However, a detailed analysis of lymphocyte subsets in different blood products has not been produced, making assessment of the TA-GVHD risk for a specific class of product and a subcategory of patients difficult. Further, there could be a cumulative or synergistic effect of viable T cells present in the multiple transfusions received by a given patient whose own immunologic status fluctuates with time from treatment and infectious disease state.

For patients at risk for GVHD, all components that might contain viable T cells should be irradiated. These include units of whole blood and cellular components (RBCs, platelets, granulocytes), whether prepared from whole blood or by apheresis (Table 28–3). All types of RBCs should be irradiated, whether they are suspended in citrated plasma or in an additive solution. Data support retention of the quality of irradiated RBCs after subsequent freezing and thawing.[48,49] If frozen/thawed RBC units are intended for GVHD-susceptible individuals and have not been previously irradiated, they should be irradiated because it is known that such components contain viable T cells.[50] Filtered RBC products should also be irradiated. Extensive leukoreduction

Table 28–2 White Blood Cell (WBC) Content of Different Blood Components

Component	Volume (approximate)* (mL)	Average WBC Content
Whole blood	500	$1–2 \times 10^9$
Red blood cells	250	$10^8–10^9$
Washed red blood cells	180	$<5 \times 10^8$
Frozen deglycerolized red blood cells	250	$10^6–10^7$
Red blood cells, pheresis	300	$10^8–10^9$
Platelet concentrate (whole blood–derived)	50–75	4×10^7
Platelets, pheresis	200–500	$10^6–10^8$*
Fresh frozen plasma	220	$0.6 \times 10^6 – 1.5 \times 10^7$
Granulocytes, pheresis	220	$>1 \times 10^{10}$

*Less with new modified chambers.

Data from Brechner ME (ed). Technical Manual. Bethesda, Md., American Association of Blood Banks, 2005; Dzik WH. Leukoreduced blood components: Laboratory and clinical aspects. In Slonim TL, Dzik WH, Snyder EL, Stowell CP, Strauss RG (eds). Rossi's Principles of Transfusion Medicine, 3rd ed. Philadelphia, Lippincott, 2002, pp 270–287.

Table 28–3 Blood Components Requiring Irradiation for Patients at Risk of Graft-versus-Host Disease

Products *Known* to Contain Viable T Cells
Whole blood
Packed red blood cells (pRBCs)
Frozen/deglycerolized RBCs
Leukoreduced pRBCs
Platelet concentrates, pooled
Platelets, pheresis
Granulocytes
Nonfrozen plasma (fresh plasma)
Products That *May* Contain Viable T Cells
Fresh frozen plasma
Frozen plasma (e.g., FP24)
Products *Unlikely* to Contain Viable T Cells
Cryoprecipitate
SD-plasma
"Pathogen-reduced" products (in development)

through filtration may decrease the potential for GVHD and serve as an alternative to irradiation in the future when filtration technology is improved and questions about the minimum level of viable T cells that can lead to GVHD are resolved. However, there have been reports of TA-GVHD in patients who received leukoreduced but not irradiated RBCs, although the extent of leukoreduction was not uniformly quantified in such reports.[51–54]

Irradiated RBCs undergo enhanced efflux of potassium during storage at 1°C to 6°C,[55,56] which is not affected by prestorage leukoreduction.[57] Washing of RBC units before transfusion to reduce the supernatant potassium load is not typically warranted in most cases, because post-transfusion dilution prevents increases in plasma potassium.[58] On the other hand, when irradiated RBCs are used for neonatal exchange transfusion or the equivalent of a whole blood exchange is anticipated, RBC washing should be considered to prevent the possible adverse cardiotoxicity caused by hyperkalemia associated with irradiation and storage.[59] In this regard, recent studies have provided guidance on storage of irradiated and washed packed RBCs: storage at 4° C for 3 hours postirradiation and washing will produce units with less than 5 mEq of potassium per liter.[60]

Platelet components that have low levels of leukocytes because of apheresis collection or leukofiltration, or both, should also be irradiated if intended for transfusion to susceptible patients because, as with RBC transfusions, the minimum number of T cells that induces TA-GVHD has not yet been delineated.

In contrast, there is controversy about irradiation of fresh frozen plasma. It is generally accepted that the freezing and thawing processes destroy the T cells that are present in such plasma. However, two brief articles have suggested that immunocompetent progenitor cells may be present in frozen/thawed plasma, and the authors recommended that frozen/thawed plasma be irradiated.[61,62] Further studies are needed to validate these findings and to assess whether the number of immunocompetent cells present in thawed fresh frozen plasma is sufficient to induce TA-GVHD. In the rare instances in which nonfrozen plasma (termed *fresh plasma*) is transfused, it should certainly be irradiated because of the presence of a sizable number (approximately 1×10^7) of viable lymphocytes.

Blood components containing lymphocytes that are homozygous for an HLA haplotype that is shared with the recipient, whether that recipient is immunocompromised or immunocompetent, pose a specific risk for TA-GVHD. This circumstance occurs when first- and second-degree relatives serve as directed donors[10,11,37,39] and when HLA-matched platelet components donated by related or unrelated individuals are transfused.[63,64] Irradiation of blood components must be performed in these situations.

One group has evaluated lymphocyte cell surface activation markers over time to determine whether older red blood cells (4 days or more) had alterations that could account for the reduced frequency of TA-GVHD as compared with "fresh" blood transfusion. They demonstrated reduced expression of CD3, CD4, CD28, CD2, and CD45 and less responsiveness in a mixed lymphocyte culture (MLC) by day 4 of storage.[65] Additional studies are warranted, however, to confirm these findings using techniques more sensitive than MLC. In addition, the number and specific subtype of T cells present in a product that induce TA-GVHD may depend on the patient's immunocompetence at the time of transfusion. It is likely that the greater the degree of immunosuppression, the fewer viable T cells are required to produce GVHD in susceptible patients. It has also been suggested that CTLs or IL-2–secreting precursors of helper T cells may be more predictive of GVHD than the number of proliferating T cells alone.

Storage of Red Blood Cells and Platelets after Irradiation

RED BLOOD CELLS

Irradiation of RBCs is not a benign process. The viability in vivo of irradiated RBCs, evaluated as the 24-hour recovery, is reduced during storage compared with that of nonirradiated RBCs.[66–70] This reduced viability has raised questions concerning the maximum storage time for RBCs after irradiation. Davey and colleagues[66] found that the 24-hour recovery for RBCs preserved in a solution containing adenine, sodium chloride, dextrose, and mannitol (Adsol) and treated with 3000 cGy on day 0 was 68.5% ± 8.1% (mean ± standard deviation [SD]) after 42 days of storage compared with 78.4% ± 7.1% for control, nontreated RBCs. Subsequent studies employed total storage periods of 21 to 35 days after irradiation on day 0 or day 1. After storage for 35 days, the mean (± SD) 24-hour recovery for irradiated (3000 cGy) and control Adsol-preserved RBCs was 78.0% ± 6.8% and 81.8% ± 4.4%, respectively. In studies with a 28-day storage period, the values for irradiated (2500 cGy) and control Adsol-preserved RBCs were 78.6% ± 5.9% and 84.2% ± 5.1%, respectively.[68] In a study which compared x-ray to gamma-irradiation with CPDA1 red cells, slight increases in extracellular potassium were noted in gamma-irradiated cells with no differences in lymphocyte inhibition as measured by MLC; RBC survival and viability studies were not included in this report.[69]

Moroff and colleagues[70] evaluated the effect of irradiation on Adsol-preserved RBCs stored from day 1 to 28 (irradiated day 1, protocol 1), day 14 to 28 (irradiated day 14, protocol 2), day 14 to 42 (irradiated day 14, protocol 3), and day 26 to 28 (irradiated day 26, protocol 4). In comparison with previous work, these investigations were unique because RBCs were studied after being irradiated for various times in storage and then examined after further storage. For protocol 1, the mean ± SD recovery was 84.2% ± 5.1% for control RBCs and 78.6% ± 5.9% for irradiated RBCs (n=16; P 0.01). With protocol 3, the recoveries were 76.3% ± 7.0% for control RBCs and 69.5% ± 8.6% for irradiated RBCs (n=16; P<0.01). Protocols 2 and 4 demonstrated comparable 24-hour recoveries for control and irradiated RBCs. Long-term RBC survival was comparable for control and irradiated RBCs in all protocols, confirming previous data showing that long-term survival of RBCs is minimally influenced by irradiation. On the basis of multiple linear regression analysis, only the length of storage after irradiation had a significant effect on the 24-hour recovery. No effect was related to day of irradiation or total storage time.

Most RBC properties such as adenosine triphosphate (ATP) levels and the amount of hemolysis were altered to only a small extent compared with control values with extended storage after irradiation, but potassium leakage from the RBCs during storage was substantially enhanced by irradiation.[70] Despite elevated potassium levels, the irradiation-induced changes in RBC viability and potassium leakage were not complementary. On the basis of analysis of these studies, FDA guidelines call for a 28-day maximum storage period for RBCs after irradiation, irrespective of the day of storage on which the treatment was performed, with the provision that the total storage time not exceed that for nonirradiated RBCs.[47]

The etiology of the RBC irradiation lesion has never been completely elucidated. Lipid peroxidation and RBC membrane protein array appear unaffected[71] whereas purine nucleotides decrease over time.[72] While the actual structural changes that make RBCs sensitive to irradiation-induced oxidative damage and result in potassium leakage are not yet clarified, addition of antioxidants such as dipyridamole, Trolox, and mannitol to RBCs prior to irradiation is under consideration in Japan.[73]

PLATELETS

In contrast to RBCs, platelets appear to be relatively unaffected by irradiation. The storage period at 20°C to 24°C for irradiated platelet components does not need to be modified. Neither in vitro nor in vivo platelet properties are influenced to any extent by irradiation. Many studies have confirmed that platelet properties are retained immediately after conventional levels of irradiation and at the conclusion of a 5-day storage period, whether irradiation is performed before storage or in the middle of storage.[74–81] One report, however, has indicated some differences in selected in vitro parameters between irradiated and control platelets after storage.[80]

Selection of Radiation Dose

In the past, there were no standards pertaining to the radiation dose that should be used. A survey in 1989 indicated that a range of radiation dose levels between 1500 and 5000 cGy (1 rad = 1 cGy) were being used, with the majority of facilities employing 1500 cGy.[82] These reported radiation doses were typically estimates and retrospective calculations because most facilities were not performing any type of dosimetry measurements. Furthermore, these values may be different from current values determined through careful dose mapping because there was previously no standardized way of calculating or reporting radiation dose. The selection of 1500 cGy as the target radiation dose was based on studies in the 1970s showing that 500 cGy abrogated the MLC response of isolated lymphocytes.[83–85]

Later studies from our laboratory with a more sensitive limiting dilution assay (LDA) indicated that 2500 cGy (measured at the internal midplane of a component) is the most appropriate dose.[86,87] In these experiments, RBC and platelet components were irradiated in their original plastic containers (blood bags) with increasing radiation doses. The author's laboratory selected LDA as a tool to study the effect of gamma-irradiation for several reasons. LDA measures the clonogenic potential of both CD4+ and CD8+ T cells in a functional assay. It provides a quantification at low T-cell numbers and has been used to determine residual, functional T cells in bone marrow purged of T cells, thus providing a clinical correlate of prevention of GVHD.[88] Assays of T-cell proliferation using MLC, mitogens, or detection of T cells by flow cytometry can detect up to a 2 logarithm (log) reduction in viable cells. PCR techniques are capable of detecting up to a 6-log reduction but cannot distinguish between viable and nonviable cells and hence are not informative if T cells are inactivated but remain in the sample. While the LDA assay may fail to detect an as yet undescribed human T-cell subset that contributes to GVHD, it is nonetheless an appropriate assay for selection of radiation doses for platelet pheresis and RBC components to abrogate TA-GVHD.

In the authors' studies, after each radiation dose, samples were removed and the clonogenic proliferation of T cells was measured by LDA. With RBC units, 500 cGy had a minimal influence, whereas 1500 cGy inactivated T-lymphocyte proliferation by approximately 4-log; however, some growth was still observed in each experiment. Increasing the dose to 2000 cGy resulted in no T-lymphocyte proliferation in all but one experiment. No proliferation was observed after 2500 cGy in any experiment.[86] In a subsequent study using platelet pheresis components with sufficient T cells to perform the LDA, the effects of 1500 and 2500 cGy were again evaluated.[87] With 1500 cGy, substantial inactivation was measured; however, some growth was still observed in all experiments. As noted with the RBC experiments, 2500 cGy resulted in complete abrogation of clonogenic T-lymphocyte proliferation. Other laboratories used more traditional assay methods to assess T-lymphocyte inactivation and suggested a radiation dose of between 2800 to 3000 cGy. Based on their review, the FDA has recommended that the irradiation process deliver 2500 cGy to the internal midplane of a free-standing irradiation instrument canister, with a minimum of 1500 cGy at any other point within the canister.[47]

Quality Assurance Measures

The instrument being used for irradiation must be documented to be operating appropriately and it must be confirmed that blood components have been irradiated. To ensure that the irradiation process is being conducted correctly, specific procedures are recommended for freestanding irradiators and linear accelerators, as summarized in Table 28-4 and discussed in detail in a published review.[89]

Dose mapping measures the delivery of irradiation within a simulated blood component or over an area in which a blood component is placed. This applies to a radiation field when a linear accelerator is used or to the canister of a freestanding irradiator. Dose mapping is the primary means of ensuring that the irradiation process is being conducted correctly. It documents that the intended dose of irradiation is being delivered at a specific location (such as the central midplane of a canister), and it describes the variation of the delivered radiation dose

Table 28–4 **Quality Assurance Guidelines for Irradiating Blood Components**

Dose
2500 cGy to the central midplane of a canister (freestanding irradiator) or to the center of an irradiation field (linear accelerator) with a minimum of 1500 cGy
Dose Mapping (Freestanding Irradiators)
Routinely, once a year (^{137}Cs) or twice a year (^{60}Co) and after major repairs, using a fully filled canister (water/plastic) with a dosimetry system to map the distribution of the absorbed dose
Dose Mapping (Linear Accelerators)
Yearly dose mapping with an ionization chamber and a water phantom recommended; more frequent evaluation of instrument conditions to ensure consistency of x-rays
Correction for Radioisotopic Decay
With ^{137}Cs as the source, annually With ^{60}Co as the source, quarterly
Turntable Rotation (Freestanding ^{137}Cs Irradiators)
Daily verification
Storage Time for Red Blood Cells after Irradiation
For up to 28 days; total storage time cannot exceed maximum storage time for unirradiated red blood cells
Storage Time for Platelets after Irradiation
No change related to irradiation procedure

Adapted from Moroff G, Luban NLC. The irradiation of blood and blood components to prevent graft-versus-host disease: Technical issues and guidelines. Transfus Med Rev 1997;11:15–26.

within a simulated component or over a given area. This allows conclusions to be drawn about the maximum and minimum doses being delivered. Dose mapping should be performed with sensitive dosimetry techniques. Several commercially available systems have been developed (see Dosimetry Systems in Use, below).

Other quality assurance measures include routine confirmation that the turntable is operating correctly (for ^{137}Cs irradiators), measurements to ensure that the timing device is accurate, and periodic lengthening of the radiation time to correct for source decay. With linear accelerators, it is necessary to measure the characteristics of the x-ray beam to ensure consistency of delivery. Confirming that a blood component has, in actuality, been irradiated is also an important part of a quality assurance program. Several firms have developed indicator labels for this purpose.

Dose Mapping with Freestanding Irradiators

For freestanding irradiators, a dose-mapping procedure measures the dose delivered throughout the circular canister in which the blood component is placed. To establish a two-dimensional map, a dosimetry system is placed in a canister that is completely filled with a blood/tissue-compatible phantom composed of water or an appropriate plastic such as polystyrene.[90,91] The dosimetry material is placed within the phantom in a predetermined way. This approach provides data showing the minimum levels of irradiation that would be absorbed by a blood component placed in the canister and recognizes that maximum attenuation occurs when the canister is completely filled with a blood-compatible material. The absorbed dose at the central midplane of a canister (i.e., at the center point) may be decreased by 25% (from 3100 to 2500 cGy) in a ^{137}Cs irradiator (JL Shepherd and Associates, San Francisco, Calif.) when the loading of the canister is changed from 0% (air) to 100% (with blood components).[92] An irradiation-sensitive film dosimetry system (International Specialty Products) was used in this study.

Other studies have shown that the variability in the dose delivered to the interior of simulated blood phantoms depended on the model of the ^{137}Cs freestanding irradiator.[93,94] An immobilized grid of thermoluminescent dosimeters in a plastic sheet was placed within the simulated blood units to measure dose delivery. A spacer in the bottom of the canister increased the minimum level of irradiation within the simulated blood units, as expected from the results of full-canister dose mapping involving a phantom.[94] The variability with ^{137}Cs irradiation is influenced by a number of factors, including the blood-compatible environment. Cumulatively, these studies underscored the need for consistency in loading the canister.

When an irradiator is purchased, the distributor provides a central dose level that is determined in a blood-compatible environment. In the 1970s and 1980s, manufacturers provided a central dose that was determined in air, resulting in the use of timer settings that provided a dose level somewhat less than was expected. Since the issuance of the FDA guidelines in July 1993 and the use of dose mapping, it has been necessary to readjust irradiation times with some instruments because the attenuation effect had not been considered previously.

The dose map can also be used to assess whether the turntable of a ^{137}Cs irradiator is rotating in an appropriate manner. The occurrence of comparable readings at the two edges of the two-dimensional map, as depicted in the theoretical dose map, indicates that the canister is rotating evenly in front of the ^{137}Cs source. If the turntable were not rotating, the dose levels at the edge of the map closest to the source would be much higher than those on the opposite edge (i.e., the side farthest from the source).

Dosimetry Systems in Use

The radiation dose delivered can be measured by a variety of dosimetry systems. Several commercial systems have been introduced to the market; each system consists of a phantom that fills the canister and a sensitive dosimeter. These dosimeters are referred to as routine dosimeters. They are calibrated against standard systems, usually at national reference laboratories such as the National Institute of Standards and Technology in the United States. The routine dosimeter measurement systems were initially developed for use with ^{137}Cs irradiators because this is the predominant irradiation source for blood. Subsequently, they were also developed for use with ^{60}Co irradiators.

Thermoluminescent dosimeters (TLD chips) are one type of routine dosimeter. TLD chips are small plastic chips with millimeter dimensions having a crystal lattice that absorbs ionizing radiation. Specialized equipment is used to release and measure the energy absorbed by the TLD chip at the time of the test irradiation. In one commercially available system, chips are placed at nine different locations within a polystyrene phantom that fits into the canister for the IBL 437C irradiator (CIS US, Inc., Bedford, Mass.). The timer setting routinely used with the instrument is also used in the test procedure.

Two alternative systems use radiochromic film. On exposure to irradiation, the film darkens, resulting in an increase in optical density. The optical density, determined at various locations on the film, is linearly proportional to the absorbed radiation dose. Standard films that are irradiated at a given dose level with a source calibrated at a national reference laboratory provide the means to assess the absolute level of absorbed irradiation. This type of dosimeter is basically an x-ray film comparable with that used in clinical practice. With this device, the map that is developed identifies the absorbed radiation dose measured at a large number of locations.

In one such system, a film contained in a thin watertight casement is placed into the canister (International Specialty Products, Wayne, N.J.). This approach is being used with a variety of irradiators. The canister is filled completely with water before the irradiation procedure. This system provides a direct readout of the dose that is delivered throughout the canister. The timer setting used routinely is employed for the test procedure. In a second system, a film having different irradiation-sensitive characteristics is embedded between two halves of a circular-fitting polystyrene plastic phantom (Nordion International, Kanata, Ontario, Canada). Irradiation of specialized films is performed with a number of timer settings, each longer than that used routinely. The map produced is normalized for a central midplane dose of 2500 cGy. The time to produce the 2500 cGy is predetermined with a different dosimeter system, the Fricke system, in which absorbed radiation causes a change in the state of an iron salt that can be assessed spectrophotometrically.

Another approach to irradiation dose mapping employs a solid-state electronic dosimeter that is technically referred to as a metal oxide semiconductor field effect transistor (MOSFET). A board contains a number of small transistors in an arrangement that provides data for a dose map. The board is placed between two halves of a circular polystyrene phantom that fits into the canister. This dosimeter absorbs and stores the radiation dose imparted to it electronically. Irradiation causes the formation of holes in the metal oxide layer that become trapped within the transistor. The magnitude of the holes is evaluated by measuring the voltage across the transistor with a voltmeter. The voltages measured are converted to absorbed dose.

With each dosimetry system, measurements are used to express the absorbed radiation dose in grays (or centigrays).

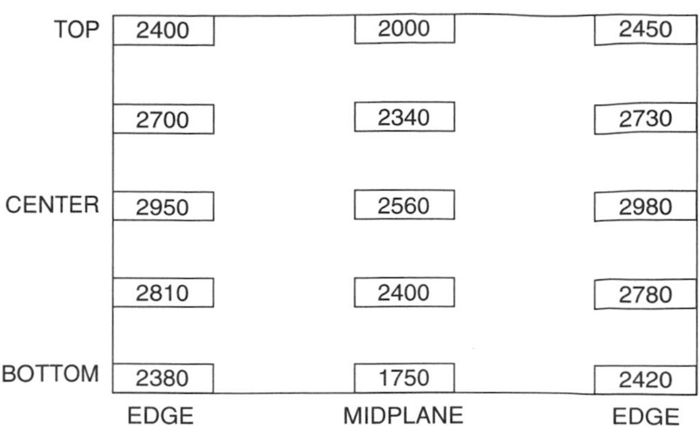

Figure 28–3 Two-dimensional dose map showing the irradiation dose distribution through a fully filled canister of a freestanding cesium 137 irradiator.

All dosimetry measurements are associated with a degree of uncertainty or possible error. The magnitude of the uncertainty depends on the kind of dosimeter used. For most dosimeters, the level is ±5% of the measured value. For a central absorbed dose level of 2560 cGy (see theoretical dose map in Fig. 28–3), the value could be as high as 2788 cGy or as low as 2432 cGy. Correspondingly, a measured value of 2400 cGy could be as high as 2520 cGy or as low as 2380 cGy. Because the measured value could in actuality meet the 2500 cGy standard, it is appropriate to accept a value of 2400 cGy as meeting the current standard. The same approach should be used when evaluating the minimum value on a dose map. Albeit arbitrary and cautious, the actual minimum on an irradiation dose map should not be below 1500 cGy.

Other Measures with Freestanding Irradiators

CORRECTION FOR ISOTOPIC DECAY

It is important to lengthen the time of irradiation periodically to correct for decay of the isotopic source that emits the gamma-irradiation. Previously, this was the only major quality assurance measure that was performed routinely. With the 30-year half-life of ^{137}Cs, annual lengthening of the timer setting is appropriate. On the other hand, since the half-life of ^{60}Co is only 5 years, the time of irradiation should be increased on a quarterly basis. The additional seconds of irradiation that are needed can be calculated using formulas that can be found in a physics textbook. Alternatively, distributors of irradiators provide a chart that specifies the appropriate setting as a function of calendar time.

TURNTABLE ROTATION

For ^{137}Cs irradiators, it is essential that the turntable operate at a constant speed in a circular pattern to ensure that all parts of a blood component are exposed equally to the source. Daily verification of turntable rotation is an appropriate quality assurance measure. With some freestanding irradiator models, rotation of the turntable can be observed before the door of the compartment in which the canister is positioned is closed. In other models, it can be observed only indirectly by ensuring that an indicator light is operating appropriately. With some older models, there have been occasional reports that the turntable failed to rotate because of mechanical problems. Such problems should not be encountered with the newer models because of changes in the turntable mechanisms.

ASSESSING RADIOACTIVITY LEAKAGE

Irradiators are constructed so that the isotopic sources are contained in a chamber heavily lined with a protective lead shield to prevent leakage of radioactivity. Accordingly, gamma-irradiators are considered to be safe instruments. Although there have been no reports of source leakage of radioactivity, periodic measurements are warranted. Attaching a film badge to the outside of the irradiator, using a Geiger counter periodically, and performing a wipe test of the inside of the chamber where the canister is positioned at least semiannually are typical measures.

Dose Mapping with Linear Accelerators

Linear accelerators that are used to provide radiation therapy are carefully monitored to ensure appropriateness of dose to an irradiation field. When blood components are treated with x-rays, the instrument settings are different from those used to treat oncology patients. Hence, additional periodic quality control measures, primarily to assess the dose delivered to blood components, are needed to ensure that linear accelerators are being operated appropriately when used for blood irradiation.

Currently, there are no commercially available systems for assessing the dose delivered throughout the area of an irradiation field in which blood components are placed for treatment with x-rays. An ideal dosimeter for this purpose would be made of a tissue-compatible plastic phantom containing appropriate dosimeter material that could be placed at the correct distance from the source. An alternative approach might involve use of a blood bag filled with water (simulating a blood unit) containing TLD chips, as described earlier. In comparative studies using such simulated blood units, it was determined that radiation delivery was more uniform with linear accelerators than with ^{137}Cs freestanding irradiators.[93] This uniformity reflects the relative homogeneity of x-ray beams. One group of investigators has developed a phantom with TLD chips that can serve as both a dose monitor and a temperature monitor, a critical issue when multiple units are held out of refrigeration during irradiation.[95]

In the absence of an available system modified for irradiation of blood bags, the dose delivered throughout an irradiation field should be mapped with the dosimetric measuring system known as an ionization chamber. The ionization chamber is used to calibrate linear accelerators for use with patients. In addition, on a yearly basis, dose mapping should be performed using a tissue-compatible phantom. In view of the widely divergent conditions that are employed during the operation of linear accelerators, other parameters pertaining to the x-ray beam should be evaluated on at least a quarterly basis to provide assurance that the instrument is being used appropriately for the irradiation of blood components.

When setting a linear accelerator for blood component irradiation, the following should be measured: (1) the distance between the x-ray source and the position where the blood components are to be placed, (2) consistency of the strength of the x-ray beam, and (3) intensity of the x-ray beam. The distance between the source and position on the table where blood components will be placed (referred to as the target) can be evaluated easily with a calibrated measuring device. This is a simple task that can be performed routinely. The consistency of beam output can be evaluated by measuring the beam current. Beam intensity can be evaluated by measuring the ionization current in a monitoring ionization chamber array, which can be expressed in terms of the number of photons delivered per square centimeter. These parameters should be assessed routinely as part of quality control programs used by radiation physicists. A code of blood practice was published in 1994 by the Radiation Therapy Committee of the American Association of Physicists in Medicine for the quality control of radiotherapy accelerators.[96,97]

Unusual Geometries

Dose delivery can be influenced by several physical and geometrical factors. The greatest influence on delivery is the geometry of the sample being irradiated. The authors' laboratory used gel dosimetry to measure three-dimensional radiation dose distributions in blood containers with irregular geometries, such as syringes, platelet bags, and small-volume red cell bags.[98] This approach, while technically complex, permits "imaging" of the actual dose delivered.

Confirmation That Irradiation Occurred

It is important to have positive confirmation that the irradiation process has taken place. For example, irradiation would not occur if an operator failed to initiate the electronically controlled irradiation process or there was an instrumentation malfunction. A radiation-sensitive indicator label has been developed specifically for this purpose (International Specialty Products, Wayne, N.J.). The label containing a radiation-sensitive filmstrip is placed on the external surface of the blood component. Irradiation causes distinct visually observable changes in the label that can be readily assessed by the operator, which represents a permanent visual record that the irradiation process has taken place. The reliability of this type of indicator has been documented in a multisite study.[99]

Two versions of the indicator label have been manufactured. They differ in the range of irradiation needed to cause a change in the radiation-sensitive film. The ratings for these indicators are 1500 and 2500 cGy. The ratings serve as an approximate guideline for the amount of absorbed radiation needed to change the window completely from reddish to opaque. Because the indicator labels are designed and used to confirm that the irradiation process has occurred, the authors' laboratory utilizes the 1500 cGy label as the most appropriate tool to perform this quality control measure. This is based on the routinely observed pattern of dose distribution to a blood component in a canister of a freestanding irradiator. Despite a targeted central dose of 2500 cGy, there are spots at which the dose is less. If the theoretical dose map presented in Figure 28–3 is used as an example, there is a spot that receives only 1800 cGy. If the label rated 2500 cGy was located on the external surface of a component, there might be minimal changes in the appearance of the radiation-sensitive film window. This would result in a judgment that the blood component was not irradiated when in actuality it was treated satisfactorily.

New Methods

Photochemical treatment (PCT) using psoralens and long-wavelength UV irradiation (UVA) have been developed to reduce the risks of bacterial and viral contaminants of platelet transfusions (see Chapter 27 for further discussion of pathogen inactivation technologies). Psoralens bind reversibly to nucleic acids by intercalation and, after UVA illumination, form covalent monoadducts and crosslinks with RNA and DNA. The process modifies bacterial and viral genomes sufficiently to prevent replication. Among a broad group of compounds, the psoralen S-59 has been shown to be particularly effective in inactivating bacteria and viruses without adversely affecting platelet function in vitro and in vivo.[100] Clinical trials confirm adequate in vivo survival, lack of adverse effects, and equivalence to standard platelet units.[101]

The use of S-59 and PCT has been studied for possible inactivation of leukocytes in platelet concentrates.[102,103] PCT inactivation of T cells was evaluated with four assay systems. These included T-cell quantitation, inhibition of cytokine synthesis, modification of leukocyte genomic DNA by quantification of psoralen-DNA adducts, and inhibition of replication of T cells using PCR amplification of genomic DNA sequences. This work built on previous studies in which IL-8, a marker of cytokine generation in platelet concentrates, was significantly reduced in pools treated with PCT compared with those treated with irradiation.[102,103]

A more detailed study by Grass and coworkers[103] compared PCT with irradiation at 2500 cGy; cytokine synthesis was not inhibited, and induction of DNA strand breaking was inhibited less than with S-59 and PCT. LDA was used to confirm inactivation of T cells in the platelet concentrates. The efficacy of S-59 and PCT was further supported by a study of transfusion-induced GVHD in a murine F1 hybrid model.[104,105] No GVHD was noted in mice receiving splenocytes treated with either 2500 cGy or S-59 at 150 μmol/L and UVA at 2.1 J/cm. Another set of experiments was performed to study the use of PCT to prevent GVHD in an immunocompromised mouse model.[106] Taken together, these studies suggest that PCT may well be an alternative to irradiation and may provide a mechanism to prevent an increase in cytokine concentration in platelet concentrates. The limitation of PCT methodology is the need for UVA penetration, which is not currently possible with RBC products.

REFERENCES

1. von Fliedner V, Higby DJ, Kim U. Graft-versus-host reaction following blood product transfusion. Am J Med 1972;72:951–961.
2. Anderson KC, Weinstein HJ. Transfusion-associated graft-versus-host disease. N Engl J Med 1990;323:315–321.
3. Webb IJ, Anderson KC. Transfusion-associated graft-versus-host disease. In Anderson KC, Ness PM (eds). Scientific Basis of Transfusion Medicine. Philadelphia, WB Saunders, 2000, pp 420–425.
4. Linden JV, Pisciotto PT. Transfusion-associated graft-versus-host disease and blood irradiation. Transfus Med Rev 1992;6:116–123.
5. Yasuura K, Okamoto H, Matsuura A. Transfusion-associated graft-versus-host disease with transfusion practice in cardiac surgery. J Cardiovasc Surg (Torino) 2000;41:377–380.
6. Serious Hazards of Transfusion. Available at *http://www.shotuk.org.* Accessed March 29, 2006.
7. Kleinman S, Chan P, Robillard P. Risks associated with transfusion of cellular blood components in Canada. Transfus Med Rev 2003;17:120–162.
8. Ferrera JM, Krenger W. Graft-versus-host disease: the influence of type 1 and type 2 T cell cytokines. Transfus Med Rev 1998;12:1–17.
9. McMilan KD, Johnson RL. HLA-homozygosity and the risk of related-donor transfusion-associated graft-versus-host disease. Transfus Med Rev 1993;7:37–41.
10. Petz LD, Calhoun L, Yam P, et al. Transfusion-associated graft-versus-host disease in immunocompetent patients: report of a fatal case associated with transfusion of blood from a second-degree relative, and a survey of predisposing factors. Transfusion 1993;33:742–750.
11. Worrall NK, Lazenby WD, Misko TP, et al. Modulation of in vivo alloreactivity by inhibition of inducible nitric oxide synthetase. J Exp Med 1995;181:63–70.
12. Fast LD, DiLeone G, Edson CM, et al. PEN110 treatment functionally inactivates the PBMNCs present in RBC units: comparison to the effects of exposure to gamma irradiation. Transfusion 2002;42: 1318–1325.
13. Nishimura M, Uchida S, Mitsunaga S, et al. Characterization of T-cell clones derived from peripheral blood lymphocytes of a patient with transfusion-associated graft-versus-host disease: FAS-mediated killing by CD4+ and CD8+ cytotoxic T-cell clones and tumor necrosis factor beta production by CD4+ T-cell clones. Blood 1997;89:1440–1445.
14. Ammann AJ. Hypothesis: absence of graft-versus-host disease in AIDS is a consequence of HIV-1 infection of CD4+ T cells. J Acquir Immune Defic Syndr 1993;6:1224–1227.
15. Klein C, Fraitag S, Foulon E, et al. Moderate and transient transfusion-associated cutaneous graft versus host disease in a child infected by human immunodeficiency virus. Am J Med 1996;101:445–446.
16. Lee TH, Reed W, Mangawang-Montalvo L, et al. Donor WBCs can persist and transiently mediate immunologic function in a murine transfusion model: effects of irradiation, storage, and histocompatibility. Transfusion 2001;41:637–642.
17. Lee TH, Donegan E, Slichter S, Busch MP. Transient increase in circulating donor leukocytes after allogeneic transfusions in immunocompetent recipients compatible with donor cell proliferation. Blood 1996;85:1207–1214.
18. Lee TH, Paglieroni T, Ohto H, et al. Survival of donor leukocyte subpopulations in immunocompetent transfusion recipients: frequent long term microchimerism in severe trauma patients. Blood 1999;93:3127–3139.
19. Lee TH, Paglieroni T, Utter GH, et al. High-level long-term white blood cell microchimerism after transfusion of leukoreduced blood components to patients resuscitated after severe traumatic injury. Transfusion 2005;45:1280–1290.
20. Utter GH, Owings JT, Lee TH, et al. Microchimerism in transfused trauma patients is associated with diminished donor-specific lymphocyte response. J Trauma 2005;58:925–931; discussion 931–932.
21. Wang-Rodriguez J, Fry E, Fiebig E, et al. Immune response to blood transfusion in very-low-birthweight infants. Transfusion 2000;40: 25–34.
22. Vietor HE, Hallensleben E, van Bree SP, et al. Survival of donor cells 25 years after intrauterine transfusion. Blood 2000;95:2709–2714.
23. Reed WF, Lee TH, Trachlenberg E, et al. Detection of microchimerism by PCR as a function of amplification strategy. Transfusion 2001;41:39–44.
24. Nelson J, Furst D, Maloney S, et al. Microchimerism and HLA compatible relationships of pregnancy in scleroderma. Lancet 1998;351: 559–562.
25. Arlett CM, Smith JB, Jimenez SA. Identification of fetal DNA and cells in skin lesions from women with systemic sclerosis. N Engl J Med 1998;333:1186–1191.
26. Evans PC, Lambert N, Maloney S, et al. Long-term fetal microchimerism in peripheral blood mononuclear cell subsets in healthy women and women with scleroderma. Blood 1999;93:2033–2037.
27. Daya S, Gunby J, Clark DA. Intravenous immunoglobulin therapy for recurrent spontaneous abortion: a meta-analysis. Am J Reprod Immunol 1998;39:69–76.
28. Brubaker DB. Immunopathogenic mechanisms of posttransfusion graft versus host disease. Proc Soc Exp Biol Med 1993;202:122–147.
29. Blundell EL, Pamphilon DH, Anderson NA, et al. Transfusion-associated graft-versus-host disease, monoclonal gammopathy and PCR. Br J Haematol 1992;82:622–623.
30. Capon SM, DePond WD, Tyan DB, et al. Transfusion associated graft-versus-host disease in an immunocompetent patient. Ann Intern Med 1991;114:1025–1026.
31. Drobyski W, Thibodeau S, Truitt RL, et al. Third-party-mediated graft rejection and graft-versus-host disease after T-cell-depleted bone marrow transplantation, as demonstrated by hypervariable DNA probes and HLA-DR polymorphism. Blood 1989;74:2285–2294.
32. Kunstmann E, Bocker T, Roewer L, et al. Diagnosis of transfusion-associated graft-versus-host disease by genetic fingerprinting and polymerase chain reaction. Transfusion 1992;32:766–770.
33. Depalma L, Bahrami KR, Kapur S, et al. Amplified fragment length polymorphism analysis in the evaluation of posttransfusion graft versus host disease. J Thorac Cardiovasc Surg 1994;108:182–184.
34. Wang L, Juji T, Tokunaga K, et al. Polymorphic microsatellite markers for the diagnosis of graft-versus-host disease. N Engl J Med 1994;330:398–401.
35. Friedman DF, Kwittken P, Cizman B, et al. DNA-based HLA typing of nonhematopoietic tissue used to select the marrow transplant donor for successful treatment of transfusion-associated graft-versus-host disease. Clin Diagn Lab Immunol 1994;1:590–596.
36. Higgins MJ, Blackall DP. Transfusion-associated graft-versus-host disease: a serious residual risk of blood transfusion. Curr Hematol Reports 2005;4:470–476.

37. Kanter MH. Transfusion-associated graft-versus-host disease: do transfusions from second-degree relatives pose a greater risk than those from first-degree relatives? Transfusion 1992;32:323–327.
38. Luban NL, DePalma L. Transfusion-associated graft-versus-host disease in the neonate—expanding the spectrum of disease [editorial]. Transfusion 1996;36:101–103.
39. Ohto H, Anderson KC. Post-transfusion graft-versus-host disease in Japanese newborns. Transfusion 1996;36:117–123.
40. Van Royen-Kerkhof A, Wulffraat NM, Kamphuis SS, et al. Nonlethal transfusion associated graft-versus-host disease in a severe combined immunodeficient patient. Bone Marrow Transplant 2003;32: 1027–1030.
41. Juji T, Nishimura M, Tadokoro K. Treatment of posttransfusion graft-versus-host disease. Vox Sang 2000;78(Suppl 2):277–279.
42. Hutchinson K, Kopko PM, Muto KN, et al. Early diagnosis and successful treatment of a patient with transfusion-associated GVHD in autologous peripheral blood progenitor cell transplantation. Transfusion 2002;42:1567–1572.
43. Shlomchik WD, Couzens MS, Tang CB, et al. Prevention of graft versus host disease by inactivation of host antigen-presenting cells. Science 1999;285:412–415.
44. Gorlin JB, Mintz PD. Transfusion-associated graft-vs-host-disease. In Mintz PD (ed). Transfusion Therapy: Clinical Principles and Practice, Bethesda, Md., American Association of Blood Banks, 2005, pp 579–591.
45. Fearon TC, Luban NL. Practical dosimetric aspects of blood and blood product irradiation. Transfusion 1986;26:457–459.
46. Korngold R. Biology of graft-versus-host disease. Am J Pediatr Hematol Oncol 1993;15:18–37.
47. U.S. Food and Drug Administration, Center for Biologics Evaluation and Research. Available at http://www.fda.gov/cber/guidelines.htm. Accessed March 29, 2006.
48. Suda BA, Leitman SF, Davey RJ. Characteristics of red cells irradiated and subsequently frozen for long term storage. Transfusion 1993; 33:389–392.
49. Miraglia CC, Anderson G, Mintz PD. Effect of freezing on the in vivo recovery of irradiated red cells. Transfusion 1994;34:775–778.
50. Crowley JP, Skrabut EM, Valeri CR. Immunocompetent lymphocytes in previously frozen washed red cells. Vox Sang 1974;26:513–517.
51. Akahoshi M, Takanashi M, Masuda M, et al. A case of transfusion-associated graft-versus-host disease not prevented by white cell-reduction filters. Transfusion 1992;32:169–172.
52. Heim MU, Munker R, Sauer H, et al. Graft versus host Krankheit: GVH mit letalem Ausgang nach der Gabe von gefilterten Erythrozytenkonzentraten [Graft versus host disease with fatal outcome after administration of filtered erythrocyte concentrates]. Beitr Infusionsther 1992;30:178–181.
53. Hayashi H, Nishiuchi T, Tamura H, et al. Transfusion associated graft-versus-host disease caused by leukocyte filtered stored blood. Anesthesiology 1993;79:1419–1421.
54. Anderson KC. Leukodepleted cellular blood components for prevention of transfusion-associated graft-versus-host disease. Transfus Sci 1995;16:265–268.
55. Ramirez AM, Woodfield DG, Scott R, et al. High potassium levels in stored irradiated blood. Transfusion 1987;27:444–445.
56. Rivet C, Baxter A, Rock G. Potassium levels in irradiated blood [letter]. Transfusion 1989;29:185.
57. Swann ID, Williamson LM. Potassium loss from leukodepleted red cells following gamma-irradiation. Vox Sang 1996;70:117–118.
58. Strauss RG. Routine washing of irradiated red cells before transfusion seems unwarranted. Transfusion 1990;30:675–677.
59. Luban NL, Strauss RG, Hume HA. Commentary on the safety of red cells preserved in extended-storage media for neonatal transfusion. Transfusion 1991;31:229–235.
60. Weiskopf RB, Schnapp S, Rouine-Rapp K, et al. Extracellular potassium concentrations in red blood cell suspensions after irradiation and washing. Transfusion 2005;45:1295–1301.
61. Wielding JU, Vehmeyer K, Dittman J, et al. Contamination of fresh-frozen plasma with viable white cells and proliferable stem cells [letter]. Transfusion 1994;34:185–186.
62. Bernvill SS, Abdulatiff M, Al-Sedairy S, et al. Fresh frozen plasma contains viable progenitor cells—should we irradiate [letter]? Vox Sang 1994;67:405.
63. Benson K, Marks AR, Marshall MJ, et al. Fatal graft-versus-host disease associated with transfusions of HLA-matched, HLA-homozygous platelets from unrelated donors. Transfusion 1994;34:432–437.
64. Grishaber JE, Birney SM, Strauss RG. Potential for host transfusion-associated graft-versus-host disease due to apheresis platelets matched for HLA class I antigens. Transfusion 1993;33:910–914.
65. Chang H, Voralia M, Bali M, et al. Irreversible loss of donor blood leucocyte activation may explain a paucity of transfusion-associated graft-versus-host disease from stored blood. Br J Haematol 2000;111:146–156.
66. Davey RJ, McCoy NC, Yu M, et al. The effect of pre-storage irradiation on post-transfusion red cell survival. Transfusion 1992;32:525–528.
67. Mintz PD, Anderson G. Effect of gamma irradiation on the in vivo recovery of stored red blood cells. Ann Clin Lab Sci 1993;23:216–220.
68. Moroff G, Holme S, Heaton A, et al. Effect of gamma irradiation on viability of AS-1 red cells [abstract]. Transfusion 1992;32(Suppl):70S.
69. Janatpour K, Denning L, Nelson K, et al. Comparison of x-ray vs. gamma irradiation of CPDA-1 red cells. Vox Sang 2005;89:215–219.
70. Moroff G, Holme S, AuBuchon JP, et al. Viability and in vitro properties of AS-1 red cells after gamma irradiation. Transfusion 1999;39:128–134.
71. Cicha I, Suzuki Y, Tateishi N, et al. Gamma-ray-irradiated red blood cells stored in mannitol-adenine-phosphate medium: rheological evaluation and susceptibility to oxidative stress. Vox Sang 2000;79:75–82.
72. Leitner GC, Neuhauser M, Weigel G, et al. Altered intracellular purine nucleotides in gamma-irradiated red blood cell concentrates. Vox Sang 2001;81:113–118.
73. Hirayama J, Abe H, Azuma H, et al. Leakage of potassium from red blood cells following gamma ray irradiation in the presence of dipyridamole, trolox, human plasma, or mannitol. Biol Pharm Bull 2005;28:1318–1320.
74. Moroff G, George VM, Siegl AM, et al. The influence of irradiation on stored platelets. Transfusion 1986;26:453–456.
75. Espersen GT, Ernst E, Christiansen OB, et al. Irradiated blood platelet concentrates stored for five days: evaluation by in vitro tests. Vox Sang 1988;55:218–221.
76. Duguid JK, Carr R, Jenkins JA, et al. Clinical evaluation of the effects of storage time and irradiation on transfused platelets. Vox Sang 1991;60:151–154.
77. Read EJ, Kodis C, Carter CS, et al. Viability of platelets following storage in the irradiated state. A paired-controlled study. Transfusion 1988;28:446–450.
78. Rock G, Adams GA, Labow RS. The effects of irradiation on platelet function. Transfusion 1988;28:451–455.
79. Sweeney JD, Holme S, Moroff G. Storage of apheresis platelets after gamma irradiation. Transfusion 1994;34:779–783.
80. Seghatchian MJ, Stivala JF. Effect of 25 Gy gamma irradiation on storage stability of three types of platelet concentrates: a comparative analysis with paired controls and random preparation. Transfus Sci 1995;16:121–129.
81. Bessos H, Atkinson A, Murphy WG, et al. A comparison of in vitro storage markers between gamma-irradiated and non-irradiated apheresis platelet concentrates. Transfus Sci 1995;16:131–134.
82. Anderson KC, Goodnough LT, Sayers M, et al. Variation in blood component irradiation practice: implications for prevention of transfusion-associated graft-versus-host disease. Blood 1991;77:2096–2102.
83. Sprent J, Anderson RE, Miller JF. Radiosensitivity of T and B lymphocytes. II. Effect of irradiation on response of T cells to alloantigens. Eur J Immunol 1974;4:204–210.
84. Valerius NH, Johansen KS, Nielsen OS, et al. Effect of in vitro x-irradiation on lymphocyte and granulocyte function. Scand J Hematol 1981; 27:9–18.
85. Rosen NR, Weidner JG, Bold HD, et al. Prevention of transfusion-associated graft-versus-host disease: selection of an adequate dose of gamma irradiation. Transfusion 1993;33:125–127.
86. Pelszynski MM, Moroff G, Luban NL, et al. Effect of gamma-irradiation of red blood cell units on T-cell inactivation as assessed by limiting dilution analysis: implications for preventing transfusion-associated graft-versus-host disease. Blood 1994;83:1683–1689.
87. Luban NL, Drothler D, Moroff G, et al. Irradiation of platelet components: inhibition of lymphocyte proliferation assessed by limiting dilution analysis. Transfusion 2000;40:348–352.
88. Quinones RR, Gutierrez RH, Dinndorf PA, et al. Extended cycle elutriation to adjust T-cell content in HLA-disparate bone marrow transplantation. Blood 1993;82:307–317.
89. Moroff G, Luban NL. The irradiation of blood and blood components to prevent graft-versus-host disease: technical issues and guidelines. Transfus Med Rev 1997;11:15–26.
90. Masterson ME, Febo R. Pre-transfusion blood irradiation: clinical rationale and dosimetric considerations. Med Phys 1992;19:649–657.
91. Leitman SF. Dose, dosimetry and quality improvements of irradiated blood components [editorial]. Transfusion 1993;33:447–449.
92. Perkins JT, Papoulias SA. The effect of loading conditions on dose distribution within a blood irradiator [abstract]. Transfusion 1994; 34:75S.

93. Moroff G, Luban NLC, Wolf L, et al. Dosimetry measurements after gamma irradiation with cesium-137 and linear acceleration sources [abstract]. Transfusion 1993;33:52S.
94. Luban NL, Fearon T, Leitman SF, et al. Absorption of gamma irradiation in simulated blood components using cesium irradiators [abstract]. Transfusion 1995;35:63S.
95. Goes EG, Covas DT, Haddad R, et al. Quality control system for blood irradiation using a teletherapy unit. Vox Sang 2004;86:105–110.
96. Kutcher GJ, Coia L, Gillin M, et al. Comprehensive QA for radiation oncology: report of AAPM Radiation Therapy Committee Task Group 40. Med Phys 1994;21:581–618.
97. Nath R, Biggs PJ, Bova FJ, et al. AAPM code of practice for radiotherapy accelerators: report of AAPM Radiation Therapy Task Group 45. Med Phys 1994;21:1093–1121.
98. Fearon T, Criss VR, Luban NLC. Blood irradiator dosimetry with BANG polymer gels. Transfusion 2005;45:1658–1662.
99. Leitman SF, Silberstein L, Fairman RM, et al. Use of a radiation-sensitive film label in the quality control of irradiated blood components [abstract]. Transfusion 1992;32:4S.
100. Lin L, Cook DN, Wiesehahn GP, et al. Photochemical inactivation of viruses and bacteria in human platelet concentrates using a novel psoralen and long wavelength UV light. Transfusion 1997;37:423–435.
101. Corash L, Lin L. Novel processes for inactivation of leukocytes to prevent transfusion-associated graft-versus-host disease. Bone Marrow Transplant 2004;33:1–7.
102. Hei DJ, Grass J, Lin L, et al. Elimination of cytokine production in stored platelet concentrate aliquots by photochemical treatment with psoralen plus ultraviolet A light. Transfusion 1999;39:239–248.
103. Grass JA, Hei DJ, Metchette K, et al. Inactivation of leukocytes in platelet concentrates by psoralen plus UVA. Blood 1998;91:2180–2188.
104. Grass JA, Wafa T, Reames A, et al. Prevention of transfusion-associated graft-versus-host disease by photochemical treatment. Blood 1999;93: 3140–3147.
105. Fast LD. The effect of exposing murine splenocytes to UVB light, psoralen plus UVA light, or gamma-irradiation on in vitro and in vivo immune responses. Transfusion 2003;43:576–583.
106. Grass J, Delmonte J, Wages D, et al. Prevention of transfusion-associated graft vs. host disease (TA-GVHD) in immunocompromised mice by photochemical treatment (PCT) of donor T cells. Blood 1997;90(Suppl 1):207A.
107. Brechner ME (ed). Technical Manual. Bethesda, Md., American Association of Blood Banks, 2005.
108. Dzik WH. Leukoreduced blood components: laboratory and clinical aspects. In Slonim TL, Dzik WH, Snyder EL, Stowell CP, Strauss RG (eds). Rossi's Principles of Transfusion Medicine, 3rd ed. Philadelphia, Lippincott, 2002, pp 270–287.

Chapter 29

Washed and Volume-Reduced Blood Components

S. Gerald Sandler • Viviana V. Johnson • Jayashree Ramasethu

INTRODUCTION

Standard red blood cell (RBC) or platelet components may be washed or volume-reduced to make them more suitable for patients who have special transfusion requirements. In the United States, blood components for transfusion are standardized to comply with applicable federal statutes and regulations of the Food and Drug Administration (FDA).[1] Typically, community blood centers collect blood from donors and supply hospital transfusion services with standard FDA-licensed blood components. Some hospital transfusion services modify RBC or platelet components by washing with 0.9% sodium chloride ("normal saline") or by centrifugation to reduce the volume of plasma or anticoagulant-preservative solution. While the rationale for transfusing these modified blood components in selected recipients may be medically sound, the methods for their preparation are often not standardized and their therapeutic efficacy is not well established.

Washed or volume-reduced blood components may be considered to be the latest step in the process of improving the match between the blood products that are collected from donors and the products that are needed by individual patients. In 1937, two decades after the introduction of blood transfusions of stored whole blood,[2] concentrated RBCs were introduced as an alternative to whole blood for anemic patients who were at risk for hypervolemia.[2,3] Early experience transfusing concentrated RBC components established lower rates of adverse transfusion reactions compared with conventional whole blood.[4] The subsequent development of sterile plastic collection bags and refrigerated centrifuges facilitated the separation of whole blood collections into RBC, plasma, and platelet components. This advance made it possible to match standardized blood components to *categories* of patients, but these generic blood components did not always meet the requirements of *individual* patients. The introduction of washed or volume-reduced blood components allowed physicians to further customize blood transfusions for the requirements of specific patients.

The following chapter summarizes current indications and methods for preparing washed or volume-reduced RBC and platelet components. The methods for preparing the modified blood components may vary in technical detail, depending on the specific RBC or platelet component selected for washing or volume reduction. In this chapter, the generic term RBC component applies to all RBC-containing components that are categorized as Red Blood Cells in the FDA-approved Circular of Information.[1] The term platelet component applies to either Platelets (random donor platelet concentrates) or Platelets Pheresis (apheresis platelets), as described in the Circular of Information.[1]

WASHED RED BLOOD CELLS

Transfusion services may wash standard RBC components using automated cell washing systems to prepare Washed Red Blood Cells for selected patients. This procedure decreases their risk of adverse effects from constituents of plasma (i.e., plasma proteins, antibodies, electrolytes), from constituents of anticoagulant-preservative-storage solutions (i.e., citrate, adenine, dextrose, mannitol), and from glycerol, which is occasionally used to freeze RBC units (Table 29–1). Washing RBC components removes approximately 90% of leukocytes, 20% to 90% of platelets, and nearly all plasma proteins, including unwanted donor antibodies.[5] In many situations, RBC components are washed to decrease the potassium concentration or remove potentially allergenic plasma proteins. During intraoperative salvage of shed blood, recovered RBCs are washed to remove clots, leukocytes, platelets, cellular debris, and heparin. Previously, RBC components were routinely washed before transfusion in patients with paroxysmal nocturnal hemoglobinuria (PNH), but recent studies demonstrate that this precaution is unnecessary (see below).

Indications for Washed Red Blood Cells

Large-Volume or Rapid Transfusion to Newborns and Other Small Children

Small-volume transfusions (<25 mL/kg) of CPDA-1"packed" RBC components or RBC components in extended-storage media (AS-1 [ADSOL]; Baxter Healthcare Corporation, Deerfield, Ill.; AS-3 [Nutricel]; Medsep Corporation, Covina, Calif.; AS-5 [Optisol]; Terumo Corporation, Somerset, N.J.) may be safely transfused to small children, including newborns and preterm infants.[6] However, large-volume transfusions (>25 mL/kg) of conventionally stored RBC components, particularly if transfused rapidly, may cause acute hyperkalemia, cardiac arrest, and death.[7] During refrigerated storage of RBC components, potassium leaks from the intracellular fluid of RBCs, increasing potassium concentration in the plasma (or in the anticoagulant-preservative solution) to levels that are potentially dangerous for rapid transfusions in susceptible recipients.

Table 29–1 Clinical Indications and Rationale for Washed RBC Components

Clinical Indication	Rationale
Large-volume or rapid transfusion	Particularly in newborns and small children, decreases risk of hyperkalemia and cardiac arrhythmias
Following gamma irradiation and storage	Decreases potassium in plasma or additive solution
Allergic or anaphylactic reaction	Removes allergenic plasma proteins, whether or not they are specifically identified
Intraoperative salvaged autologous blood	Removes clots, cellular debris, and heparin and suspends shed RBCs in saline solution
T-activation	During ongoing hemolysis, reduces further hemolysis by eliminating IgM anti-T present in normal donors' plasma
Paroxysmal nocturnal hemoglobinuria	No longer recommended

The potassium concentration in plasma of CPDA-1 RBC components increases from 4.2 mmol/L to nearly 80 mmol/L during the 35-day storage period.[6] For a 1-kg newborn, a conventional transfusion (15 mL/kg) of 42-day stored AS-1 RBCs (hematocrit of 80%) may have a potassium *concentration* as high as 50 mEq/L, but the *total potassium content* is only 0.15 mEq. While that relatively high concentration of potassium is tolerable and safe if the component is transfused slowly (over 2 to 4 hours), the same component could present a potentially fatal acute potassium load if transfused rapidly in a small child or susceptible adult. Rapid transfusions of stored RBC components in such patients may increase potassium acutely and, therefore, require washed or freshly collected RBC components. Typical situations include exchange transfusions, extracorporeal membrane oxygenation (ECMO), cardiopulmonary bypass, or solid organ transplantation.[8–10] Washed RBC components should also be considered for large-volume (>25 mL/kg) or rapid transfusions in newborns and other small children with renal failure, hyperkalemia, or severe acidosis.

Some physicians are also concerned that the doses of certain additives in extended-storage solutions (AS-1, AS-3, AS-5) may exceed known limits for safety for large-volume transfusions in small children.[11] These concerns derive from the theoretical possibility that constituents in the storage media could contribute to hyperosmolality, hyperglycemia, hypernatremia, or hyperphosphatemia. For that reason, some transfusion services routinely wash or volume-reduce RBC components stored in additive solutions for large-volume or rapid transfusions in newborns or other small children.

Transfusion of RBC Components following Gamma Irradiation

To prevent transfusion-associated graft-versus-host disease (TA-GVHD) in immunocompromised or other patients who are at risk, transfusion services (or blood centers) routinely gamma-irradiate blood components with a dose of 2000 to 3000 cGy. Although gamma-irradiation is highly effective for preventing TA-GVHD, irradiation has adverse effects on RBC survival, plasma hemoglobin concentration, and RBC ATP.[12–15] Plasma potassium concentration nearly doubles during the 48 hours after RBC components are irradiated with 3000 cGy.[12] Gamma-irradiation increases passive permeability of RBC membrane lipid bilayers, resulting in a progressive, reciprocal increase in intracellular sodium and decrease in intracellular potassium.[13] AABB *Standards* requires RBC components to outdate no longer than 28 days from the date of irradiation.[16] While washing irradiated RBC components reduces potassium concentration in the supernatant, it does not arrest the process. From the time irradiated RBC components are stored following washing, potassium concentration increases in a time-dependent fashion, which is more rapid than for nonirradiated RBC components. The potassium concentration in irradiated and washed RBC components may reach a critical concentration of 5 mEq/L after only 3 hours of storage at 4°C, compared with 6 hours for nonirradiated washed RBC components.[17]

Allergic or Anaphylactic Reactions

Mild, first-time allergic transfusion reactions (hives, flushing, pruritus) often seem to be *product*-related, rather than *patient*-related. These reactions typically respond to antihistamines and do not recur when additional plasma-containing blood components are transfused. In contrast, some chronically transfused persons develop more serious and generalized allergic reactions (bronchospasm, rash, nausea, vomiting, or diarrhea) that are not prevented by, or respond to, treatment with antihistamines. Transfusing washed RBC components usually prevents allergic reactions in such patients.

If acute allergic reactions progress to life-threatening anaphylaxis, bronchospasm, and hypotension, a diagnosis of an immunoglobulin A (IGA) anaphylactic reaction should be considered.[18] Conventionally, that diagnosis is made by demonstrating IGA deficiency (by a highly sensitive passive hemagglutination inhibition assay) and the presence of anti-IgA (by passive hemagglutination assay).[19] However, we advise caution when interpreting results of IgA hemagglutination assays because they may yield nonspecific results.[20] The same hemagglutination assay that is used to diagnose *patients* with IgA anaphylactic reactions detected IgA deficiency and the presence of anti-IgA in 1:1200 asymptomatic healthy *blood donors*.[19] Clearly, this number of healthy persons at risk for an IgA anaphylactic reaction greatly exceeds the incidence of IgA anaphylactic transfusion reactions in clinical practice. Nonetheless, if the diagnosis of IgA deficiency is made, RBCs and platelets can be washed with high volumes of saline (4–6 L) to effectively remove plasma antibodies. Washed RBC and platelet components have been transfused successfully in persons with IgA deficiency and anti-IgA who had a history of anaphylactic transfusion reactions when blood components from IgA-deficient donors were not available.[21,22] Other severe generalized reactions to plasma-containing blood components that may be abrogated by washing components prior to transfusion include transfusion-related acute lung injury (TRALI), leukocyte-mediated cytokine reactions, and anaphylaxis in persons with ahaptoglobinemia and antihaptoglobin.[23]

Intraoperative Salvage of Shed RBCs

Intraoperative salvage of shed RBCs has been used for more than four decades to reduce the number of allogeneic blood transfusions in trauma and surgery associated with large-volume blood loss.[24–26] Typically, shed blood is aspirated from the sterile surgical field, anticoagulated using a heparin-saline solution, and washed with 0.9% sodium chloride in an automated cell salvage machine. The effluent containing clots, leukocytes, platelets, cellular debris, and heparin is discarded. Saline-washed concentrated autologous RBCs are returned to the patient. When suitable wash volumes are used, activated coagulation factors, cytokines, and heparin are substantially reduced.[27–32]

An alternative method of salvaging shed autologous RBCs involves collecting heparinized sanguineous drainage from the chest, large joints, or other sites that is returned directly (unwashed) from collection canisters.[33–36] Postoperative infusion of unwashed filtered blood has been reported to be effective and without clinically relevant complications in orthopedic patients.[33,34] However, this method is controversial, because such drainage may contain procoagulant material, variable amounts of anticoagulant, and unsterile debris.[35] Even *saline-washed* salvaged RBCs collected under optimal conditions may contain residual biologically active materials capable of causing increased vascular permeability, acute respiratory distress syndrome, or disseminated intravascular coagulation.[36,37] These complications, which have been described as the "salvaged blood syndrome," can be averted by standardizing aspiration methods, controlling saline wash volumes, and monitoring for an abnormal accumulation of debris on the inner wall of the rotating bowl.[36]

T-Activation of RBCs

Immune-mediated hemolysis has been reported following transfusion of plasma-containing blood components to patients whose RBC T-crypt antigens have been exposed by bacterial infection.[38–40] T-activation occurs when bacterial neuraminidase removes *N*-acetyl neuraminic acid and exposes RBC T-crypt antigens. Exposed T-crypt antigens bind with IgM anti-T, a normal constituent of adult plasma, resulting in RBC agglutination (polyagglutination) and hemolysis. T-activation has been reported to occur in a wide range of bacterial infections, including necrotizing enterocolitis, septicemia, hemolytic uremic syndrome, and *Streptococcus pneumoniae* infection. T-activation should be suspected in children who have the onset of intravascular hemolysis following transfusion of plasma-containing blood components.

T-activation has been diagnosed less frequently in recent years because many hospital transfusion services now use non-plasma-containing monoclonal typing reagents instead of traditional plasma-derived blood typing reagents (anti-A, -B, and -A,B). Previously, some cases of clinically unrecognized polyagglutination due to T-activation were detected during routine compatibility testing using plasma-derived ABO typing reagents. Discrepancies in forward and reverse ABO typing results caused by polyagglutination or in vitro hemolysis suggested T-activation. T-activation is confirmed by specific agglutination tests using *Arachis hypogaea* and *Glycine soja* lectins. To prevent further hemolysis in patients who have active hemolysis and polyhemagglutination, RBC (or platelet) components should be washed using 0.9% sodium chloride before transfusion. Exchange transfusion with plasma-reduced components may be necessary for infants with T-activation and ongoing hemolysis.[39]

In patients with T-activation, some physicians recommend completely avoiding transfusions of fresh frozen plasma, platelets, or other plasma-containing blood products. Others question the clinical importance of T-activation and recommend that if plasma-containing components are indicated, they should not be withheld.[41] Recommendations, which are based on case reports, are conflicting and there are neither evidenced-based guidelines nor results of a randomized, controlled clinical trial to direct practice. The authors concur with the preponderance of clinical evidence, which favors not withholding plasma-containing blood components when they are indicated. The authors do not recommend that transfusion services, which routinely use murine or other monoclonal blood typing reagents, consider adding human plasma–derived typing reagents as a screening procedure to detect T-activation.

Paroxysmal Nocturnal Hemoglobinuria

PNH is an uncommon stem cell disorder manifested by complement-mediated hemolytic anemia, thrombophilia, and marrow failure.[42–44] The mainstay of managing the typical Coombs-negative, treatment-resistant, intravascular hemolytic anemia is RBC transfusions.[45] Promising results have been reported for managing hemolysis using eculizumab, a humanized monoclonal antibody to complement C5.[46] However, the role for this new treatment has yet to be defined.

In 1948, Dacie reported that blood transfusions exacerbated complement-mediated intravascular hemolysis in patients with PNH, increasing hemoglobinuria and hemoglobinemia.[47] As a consequence, some hematologists request washed RBC components for routine transfusions in patients with PNH. Admittedly, post-transfusion hemolysis is rare in patients with PNH when washed RBC components are transfused,[47] although it has been reported.[48,49] However, it should be noted that most PNH patients do not experience hemolysis after RBC transfusions, even when whole blood is transfused.[50] A retrospective review of 23 PNH patients who were transfused with a total of 556 units of whole blood, packed RBCs, leukocyte-poor RBCs, washed RBCs, frozen RBCs, and intraoperatively salvaged RBCs, identified only one case of post-transfusion hemolysis.[51] This case occurred after transfusion of group O whole blood to a group AB-positive recipient. This specific serologic incompatibility is similar to that in the 1948 case reported by Dacie, which is the origin of the practice of washing RBC components before transfusion to patients with PNH.[47] Based on this large-scale study, a supporting opinion from the PNH Interest Group,[52] as well as the authors' own uneventful personal experiences transfusing patients with PNH with unwashed AS-1 RBCs, we believe that transfusing washed RBC components to PNH patients is unwarranted.

Methods for Preparing Washed Red Blood Cells

RBC components may be washed manually using a refrigerated centrifuge or, more commonly, an automated cell washer. Washing an RBC component using 1 to 2 L of 0.9% sodium chloride removes approximately 99% of plasma proteins, electrolytes, and antibodies but may result in loss of up to 20% of the RBCs depending on the protocol.[53] Rarely, recipients who have acute reactions to even small quantities of residual plasma require RBC components that have been washed using 4 to 6 L of saline. If the objective of washing is to remove leukocytes, platelets, and plasma, the cell washer may be programmed to remove the buffy coat, which will increase loss of RBCs. If RBC components are already leukocyte-reduced prior to washing, there is no requirement to remove the buffy coat and RBC loss will be minimized. Most transfusion services use cell washers with an "open" system, which limits the duration of refrigerated storage (1°C–6°C) to 24 hours.

Alternatives to Washed Red Blood Cells

For certain clinical situations, there may be alternatives to washed RBC components for reducing the potassium concentration or removing plasma proteins. For rapid transfusions in small infants, reconstituted whole blood (i.e., RBCs resuspended in fresh-frozen plasma shortly before transfusion), should dilute supernatant potassium to a safe concentration. According to the AABB Pediatric Hemotherapy Committee, "reconstituted whole blood...or whole blood (<5 days old) may be given [to infants and children <18 years] without the need for further justification in the setting of massive transfusions."[54]

Additionally, selecting an RBC component stored in AS-1, AS-3, or AS-5 preservative-storage solutions, rather than as packed CPDA-1–anticoagulated RBCs in plasma, should reduce the *concentration* of plasma proteins to a level tolerable for most patients with mild, recurrent allergic reactions.

VOLUME-REDUCED RED BLOOD CELL COMPONENTS

Hospital transfusion services may prepare volume-reduced RBC components for newborns or other small children who require transfusions but whose capacity to receive additional intravenous fluids is limited. Volume-reduction methods are intended primarily for AS-1 and AS-3 RBC components (hematocrit 60%) because "packed" CPDA-1 RBC components (hematocrit 75% to 80%) are already concentrated.

Indications for Volume-Reduced RBC Components

Volume-reduced RBC components are indicated when the intended recipient has a need for RBC transfusion (e.g., symptomatic anemia), but the patient's circulatory system cannot tolerate the additional volume. In adults, this situation may be the consequence of renal or cardiac insufficiency. In newborns, it may result from competition between intravenous nutrition protocols, medications, and blood components for the relatively small volume that the infant's circulation can tolerate. Transfusion of volume-reduced RBC components in volume-sensitive infants and small children is controversial. Not all physicians agree that recentrifugation of conventional RBC components with additive solutions (hematocrit 60%) to prepare volume-reduced RBCs (hematocrit 85% to 87%) is a clinically meaningful procedure. Alternatives to volume-reduction of RBC components include transfusing less volume or selecting ("packed") CPDA-1 RBC components, which have a higher hematocrit.

Methods for Preparing Volume-Reduced Red Blood Cells

AS-3 Red Blood Cells

Conventional Red Blood Cells are prepared by removing supernatant plasma from Whole Blood following a "heavy spin" (5000 × *g*, 5 minutes).[55] Removing 225–250 mL of plasma results in an RBC component with a hematocrit of 70% to 80%. The hematocrit of the final component may be decreased by removing proportionally less plasma.[55] Strauss and colleagues developed a method to prepare multiple aliquots of RBCs for neonatal transfusions with hematocrit >90% using RBC components stored at 4°C for as long as 42 days.[56] For this method, donor blood is collected in a primary bag containing CP2D anticoagulant (Leukotrap RC System, Miles Inc., Elkhart, Ind.), which is centrifuged at 5000 × *g* for 5 minutes. Platelet-rich plasma is transferred to a second bag, which is disconnected. Extended storage media (100 mL) (Nutricel, AS-3, Miles) is added to the storage bag, and after mixing, the RBCs are transferred via the leukocyte-reduction filter to another storage bag. A cluster of small-volume bags is attached to the storage bag using a sterile connecting device. When a transfusion is ordered, the storage bag is centrifuged in an inverted position to pack the AS-3 RBC component to a hematocrit of approximately 90%. Strauss modified the original method to centrifuge at 4000 × *g* for 4 minutes, not faster as in the original description.[57] The volume of RBCs requested flows from the bottom of the storage bag through the outlet tubing into one of the small-volume bags. The aliquot is disconnected, and the residual contents of the storage bag are mixed thoroughly and returned to storage until the next aliquot is required. During storage, AS-3 RBCs are mixed and resuspended weekly. In the original study, measurements of extracellular potassium, hemoglobin, and lactic dehydrogenase from repeatedly mixed and centrifuged units that were stored in inverted position were comparable to those of uncentrifuged, conventionally stored AS-3 RBCs.[56]

AS-1 Red Blood Cells

The method described above for AS-3 RBC components has been modified to prepare AS-1 RBC components with hematocrits of approximately 85% to 87% after storage at 4°C for as long as 42 days.[58] For this method, AS-1 RBC components (Adsol, Baxter Healthcare Corp., Deerfield, Ill.) are processed and stored by conventional methods with hematocrits of approximately 60%. When a transfusion is requested, the AS-1 RBC component is centrifuged in an inverted position at 4000 × *g* for 4 minutes. Aliquots are removed, as above. During storage, the primary AS-1 RBC component is remixed and stored until another transfusion is ordered and aliquots are removed. We concur with the authors of this method, who caution that "... this technique may not be desired by all centers, and if it is adopted, quality control studies should be performed to ensure the quality and sterility of the RBC aliquots."[58]

Inverted Gravity Sedimentation

Storing RBC components in the refrigerator "upside down" (inverted gravity sedimentation) will concentrate AS-1 RBC components to a hematocrit of approximately 68% by 72 hours.[59] This simple manipulation provides a method for volume-reducing AS-1 RBC components in transfusion services that may not have access to an appropriate refrigerated centrifuge.

WASHED PLATELET COMPONENTS

Washed platelet components contain less plasma, but the procedure also decreases the total platelet content and may decrease platelet function. Therefore, washing platelet components is not recommended, except for relatively limited clinical indications[60] (Table 29–2).

Indications for Washed Platelet Components

Recurrent Allergic or Anaphylactic Transfusion Reactions

Patients who require washed RBC components because of recurrent allergic or anaphylactic transfusion reactions may also require washed platelet components (see above).

Neonatal Alloimmune Thrombocytopenia

Neonatal alloimmune thrombocytopenia (NAIT) is a potentially fatal disease of the fetus or newborn that may occur when there is serologic incompatibility for human platelet antigens (HPAs) between mother and fetus. More than 16 different HPAs have been implicated in NAIT.[61] Approximately 90% of cases of NAIT in Caucasians of European ancestry present in an HPA-1a–positive newborn or fetus of an HPA-1a–negative mother who has developed anti-HPA-1a.[62] Approximately 6% to 19% of cases of NAIT in Caucasians are due to anti-HPA-5b and 0% to 2% are due to anti-HPA-1b.[63,64] Mothers of Asian ancestry whose newborns have NAIT most often have antibodies specific for HPA-4 antigens.[65]

One approach to managing an at-risk pregnancy consists of using periumbilical blood sampling (PUBS) to monitor fetal platelet counts after 20 weeks of gestation and infusing the mother with intravenous immune globulin (IVIG) (1 g/kg) weekly to decrease the risk of fetal thrombocytopenia.[66] In this protocol, adding dexamethasone (1.5 mg) to weekly infusions of IVIG did not improve the response rate. In an alternative approach, the fetus's platelet count is measured at 20 weeks of gestation and the mother receives weekly infusions of IVIG (1 mg/kg) if the fetus is thrombocytopenic.[67] A second PUBS is performed at 26 weeks, and if the fetus remains thrombocytopenic, prednisone (60 mg daily) is added to weekly IVIG infusions. PUBS is repeated before delivery and, if thrombocytopenic, the fetus is transfused with platelets.[67]

Since maternal platelets are serologically compatible with the offending antibody in NAIT, the mother is a potential source of platelets for transfusion in the newborn.[68] However, maternal platelets are collected in the mother's plasma, which contains the offending antibody. Therefore, it is necessary to wash the maternal platelet component and resuspend the maternal platelets in compatible plasma, 0.9% sodium chloride, or a platelet storage solution. Platelet components may be washed by manual or automated methods using 0.9% sodium chloride, with or without adding ACD-A.[69] Such washing may result in loss of as many as 33% of the original platelets.[70] Since washing presently requires an "open" system, and since platelets must be stored at 20°C to 24°C, washed platelet components must be transfused within 4 hours.

A limited number of blood centers are able to supply HPA-matched platelet components collected from HPA-typed and qualified donors.[70] Usually, the donor panels are limited to HPA-1a–negative platelet donors, since this is the most frequently required HPA phenotype. In some blood centers, these platelet donors are scheduled for platelet apheresis collections at frequent intervals, so that their platelet components qualify for "emergency release" protocols (provided that recent test results are acceptable). In the authors' experience, serologically compatible platelet components collected from such call-in donors may be collected and emergency-released faster than collecting, testing, and processing platelet components from the postpartum mother. Donors of less common HPA phenotypes are more difficult to identify and recruit. When maternal platelets or HPA-matched platelets from allogeneic donors are transfused, conventional doses of platelets (10 mL/kg) should be adequate for most clinical situations. Nevertheless, monitoring post-transfusion platelet counts is essential, given the serious consequences of inadequate dosing in thrombocytopenic newborns.

Out-of-Group Platelet Components

In many hospitals, platelet components from group O donors are transfused to group A, B, or AB recipients if ABO group-specific platelet components are not available. Usually, the small volume of donor plasma, representing a "minor-type" ABO incompatibility, does not cause overt hemolysis. Recipients of out-of-group platelet transfusions may develop a weakly positive direct antiglobulin test result, but that is typically the only evidence of incompatibility. Occasionally,

Table 29–2 Clinical Indications and Rationale for Washed Platelet Components

Clinical Indication	Rationale
Allergic or anaphylactic reactions	Removes allergenic plasma proteins, whether or not they have been specifically identified
Febrile nonhemolytic transfusion reactions	May be effective in some adults but unproved in children
Neonatal alloimmune thrombocytopenia	Removes maternal alloantibodies from platelet components collected from the mother, whether or not serologic specificity has been identified
Out-of-group platelets	Eliminates risk of hemolysis due to anti-A or -B when compatible platelet components are not available for susceptible progenitor cell transplantation or newborn recipients
T-activation	During ongoing hemolysis, reduces further hemolysis by eliminating IgM anti-T present in normal donors' plasma
Paroxysmal nocturnal hemoglobinuria	No longer recommended

acute intravascular hemolysis may occur (e.g., when ABO-incompatible apheresis platelet components from donors who have high-titer anti-A/A,B have been transfused to A_1 recipients).[71,72] As clinical practice shifts from transfusing pools of random donor platelet concentrates (where a high-titer unit is diluted) to transfusing more single-donor (apheresis) platelet components,[71] more cases of hemolysis may be identified. Some transfusion services perform anti-A/anti-A,B titers on group O single-donor platelet components prior to an "out-of-group" transfusion.[73] However, there is lack of agreement as to what titer is clinically relevant and whether IgM or IgG antibody is more significant.[73] Although washing of out-of-group platelet components removes incompatible plasma, the process may decrease platelet function,[74] requires considerable skill and experience,[59] and is not practiced routinely.

In some hospitals, the practice of washing (or volume-reducing) platelet components to prevent anti-A/A,B or anti-B hemolysis is limited to transfusions in progenitor cell transplant (PCT) recipients and newborns. In PCT recipients, transfusion support between myeloablation and engraftment may require washed or volume-reduced platelet components to avoid anti-A/A,B– or anti-B–associated hemolysis. Plasma in platelet concentrates may represent a significant percentage of a newborn's blood volume, placing newborns at higher risk than adults for ABO-related hemolysis. Some hospitals routinely wash or volume-reduce out-of-group platelet components for newborns.

Methods for Washing Platelet Components

Methods have been developed for manual and automated washing using blood cell processors.[75–77] Washed platelet components have a threefold increase in spontaneous activation, as well as impaired ADP-induced aggregation, compared with unwashed platelet components.[74] Washing platelets requires skill and experience to minimize platelet loss, activation, and clumping.[78] Automated cell processors are more likely to deliver a consistent result and are recommended. Kalman and Brown developed a protocol using the IBM 2991 Blood Cell Processor, which removed a mean of 99.6% of plasma proteins following a 1500-mL wash using 0.9% sodium chloride. That cell processor is currently marketed as the COBE 2991 Blood Cell Processor (COBE Laboratories, Lakewood, Colo.).

Washed platelet components should be used immediately after washing owing to lack of substrates to support platelet metabolism during storage. In vitro studies of new additive solutions for washing platelets suggest that a postwash storage duration of up to 48 hours may be feasible.[79]

VOLUME-REDUCED PLATELET COMPONENTS

Indications for Volume-Reduced Platelet Components

There are two indications for transfusing volume-reduced platelets: to prevent circulatory overload and to lessen the volume of any potentially adverse constituents in the plasma of platelet components. Volume-reduction can be achieved either during collection and processing of collections (primary volume reduction) or subsequently by recentrifugation of stored platelet components (secondary volume reduction).[79] Additional concentration of standard platelet components is controversial.

Hypervolemia

A typical argument to support the availability of such "super- or hyper-concentrated" platelet components for newborns is that a standard 50-mL unit of random donor platelet components represents more than half the blood volume of a 1-kg infant and may precipitate circulatory overload.[80] In vitro studies of recentrifuged, volume-reduced platelet components demonstrated satisfactory viability, and in vivo studies have demonstrated satisfactory survival of 51r-labeled concentrated platelets and post-transfusion platelet count increments.[81,82] Arguments against routinely reducing the volume of standard platelet components focus on the reliability of transfusing 5 to 10 mL/kg of standard platelet concentrates or apheresis platelets to increase the platelet count to $>100 \times 10^9$ L.[83] A secondary concern is that while satisfactory concentration of platelets may be achieved by experienced research technologists in a limited study, technologists working in routine transfusion service operations may not be able to achieve that level of quality control. A transfusion service undertaking recentrifugation of platelets must take special precautions to control for platelet loss, clumping, and dysfunction caused by additional handling.[78]

The AABB Pediatric Hemotherapy Committee published the results of a national survey of neonatal transfusion practices, noting that "because of the potential for harm, institutions transfusing volume-reduced platelets should monitor both the quality of the final product (i.e., the number of platelets, degree of clumping, and function) and in vivo effects such as post-transfusion increment in platelet count and adverse reactions, including altered vital signs and pulmonary distress."[84] The Committee made the observation that 61% of respondents reported a final desired volume of 10 to 15 mL, and an additional 30% desired 18 to 25 mL, both volumes being within the range likely to achieve the targeted platelet count increase using an unmodified platelet concentrate.

Recurrent Febrile Nonhemolytic Transfusion Reactions

In adults, the incidence of febrile nonhemolytic transfusion reactions (FNHTRs) is decreased when plasma-reduced platelet components are transfused.[85,86] This effect, similar to that of prestorage leukoreduction, is attributed to decreased leukocyte-derived proinflammatory cytokines, which accumulate in plasma of stored platelet components.[86,87] In children, a randomized, prospective, crossover study compared the frequency of acute reactions to post storage plasma-removed platelet components and to standard platelets.[88] Study platelet components were prepared by removing plasma from stored components and replacing it with an equal volume of ABO-compatible fresh frozen plasma (FFP). While there was a trend toward lower frequency of FNHTRs with post storage plasma removal, the results were not statistically significant.[88] The investigators could not explain why FNHTRs occurred less frequently in children than in adults. On the basis of these findings, the authors do not recommend removing plasma (with or without replacement using FFP) as a method to reduce the incidence of FNHTRs in children.

We believe that routine recentrifugation of platelet components is neither necessary nor prudent. As stated by the

Table 29–3 **Methods for Preparation of Secondary Volume-Reduced Platelet Components**

Method	Starting Platelet Component	*N*	Volume of Final Platelet Component (mL)	Platelet Count of Final Platelet Component (×10⁹/mL)	In Vitro Platelet Function Studied after Volume Reduction	In Vivo Platelet Efficacy Studied after Volume Reduction
Moroff et al, 1984[80]	Random donor	12	15–20	Not reported	Yes	No
Pisciotto et al, 1991[95]	Random donor	6	20–25	2.32	Yes	Yes
Ali et al, 1994[96]	Random donor	20	30–35	Not reported	No	Yes
Holme et al, 1994[81]	Random donor	20	30–34; 35–50	1.95; 1.39	Yes	Yes
Rock et al, 1998[97]	Random donor	12	10	2.38	Yes	No
Zilber et al, 2003[98]	Random donor	21	10, 20	Not reported	Yes	No
Schoenfeld et al, 2005[99]	Single donor (apheresis)	20	90	1.90	Yes	No

Modified from Schoenfeld H, Spies C, Jakob C. Volume-reduced platelet concentrates. Current Hematol Rep 2006;5:82–88.

AABB Committee on Pediatric Hemotherapy, " . . . volume reduction of platelet concentrates . . . should be reserved for special infants for whom marked reduction of all intravenous fluids is truly needed."[84]

Methods to Volume-Reduce Platelet Components

Primary Volume Reduction

Primary volume reduction of platelet concentrates occurs at the time of collection and processing of platelet components. Several studies have shown that platelet collections may be concentrated beyond current standards using new, high-efficiency apheresis collection devices with or without specialized platelet storage solutions.[89–93] Schoenfeld has evaluated and compared these experimental platelet components.[99] Since most hospital transfusion services do not have facilities to collect or adequately monitor the efficacy of such components, this discussion focuses on selective secondary volume reduction of standard platelet components.

Secondary Volume Reduction

Secondary volume reduction occurs after storage by recentrifugation to remove plasma and resuspend platelets in a decreased volume for immediate transfusion.[94] There is no standard method for preparing volume-reduced platelet concentrates. The functional characteristics of secondary volume-reduced platelet components prepared by different methods have been studied (Table 29–3).[80–81,95–99] If secondary volume reduction of platelet components is necessary, the authors recommend the method of Moroff and colleagues.[80] This method uses standard platelet concentrates that may be stored for as long as 5 days before recentrifugation, a standard blood bank refrigerated centrifuge, and manual resuspension of the centrifuged platelets.

Methods for collecting platelets by apheresis and storing them in platelet additive solutions in a reduced volume of plasma have also been developed. Proponents report that decreased plasma reduces allergic and febrile transfusion reactions, facilitates ABO-incompatible platelet transfusions, and is the preferred approach for some pathogen-inactivation methods.[100–103]

REFERENCES

1. Circular of Information for the Use of Human Blood and Blood Components. Available at http://www.aabb.org/Documents/About_Blood/Circulars_of_Information/coi0702.pdf. Accessed March 29, 2006.
2. Robertson LB. Transfusion of whole blood: a suggestion for its more frequent employment in war surgery. Br Med J 1917;2:38–40.
3. Castellanos A. La transfusion de globules. Arch Med Infant 1937;6:319.
4. MacQuaide DH, Mollison PL. Treatment of anaemia with concentrated red cell suspensions. Br Med J 1940;2:555.
5. Friedberg RC, Chester A. Stem cell transplantation. In Mintz PD (ed). Transfusion Therapy: Clinical Principles and Practice. Bethesda, Md., American Association of Blood Banks, 2005, p 290.
6. Strauss RG. Data-driven blood-banking practices for neonatal RBC transfusions. Transfusion 2000;40:1528–1540.
7. Hall TL, Barnes A, Miller JR, et al. Neonatal mortality following transfusion of red cells with high plasma potassium levels. Transfusion 1993;33:606–609.
8. Luban NL. Massive transfusion in the neonate. Transfus Med Rev 1995;9:200–214.
9. Scanlon JW, Krakaur R. Hyperkalemia following exchange transfusion. J Pediatr 1980;96:108–110.
10. Estrin JA, Belani KG, Karnavas AG, et al. A new approach to massive blood transfusion during pediatric liver resection. Surgery 1986;99:664–670.
11. Luban NL, Strauss RF, Hume HA. Commentary on the safety of red cells preserved in extended storage media for neonatal transfusions. Transfusion 1991;31:229–235.
12. Ramirez AM, Woodfield DG, Scott R, et al. High potassium levels in stored irradiated blood [letter]. Transfusion 1987;27:444–445.
13. Brugnara C, Churchill WH. Effect of irradiation on red cell cation content and transport. Transfusion 1992;32:246–252.
14. Davey RJ, McCoy NC, Yu M, et al. The effect of prestorage irradiation on posttransfusion red cell survival. Transfusion 1992;32:525–528.
15. Moore GL, Ledford ME. Effects of 4000 rad irradiation on the in vitro storage properties of packed red cells. Transfusion 1985;25:583–585.
16. Silva MA (ed). Standards for Blood Banks and Transfusion Services, 23rd ed. Bethesda, Md., American Association of Blood Banks, 2005.
17. Weiskopf RB, Schnapp S, Rouine-Rap K, et al. Extracellular potassium concentrations in red blood cell suspensions after irradiation and washing. Transfusion 2005;45:1295–1301.
18. Sandler SG, Malloy D, Malamut D, et al. IgA anaphylactic transfusion reactions. Transfus Med Rev 1995;9:1–8.
19. Sandler SG, Eckrich R, Malamut D, et al. Hemagglutination assays for diagnosis and prevention of IgA anaphylactic transfusion reactions. Blood 1994;84:2031–2035.
20. Sandler SG. How I manage patients suspected of having had an IgA anaphylactic transfusion reaction. Transfusion 2006;46:10–13.
21. Rogers RL, Javed TA, Ross RE, et al. Transfusion management of an IgA deficient patient with anti-IgA and incidental correction of IgA deficiency after allogeneic bone marrow transplantation. Am J Hematol 1998;57:326–330.

22. Meena-Leist CE, Fleming DR, Heye M, et al. The transfusion needs of an autologous bone marrow transplant patient with IgA deficiency. Transfusion 1999;39:457–459.
23. Sandler SG, Yu H, Rassai N. Risks of blood transfusion and their prevention. Clin Adv Hematol Oncol 2003;1:120–124.
24. Sandler SG, Silvergleid AJ (eds). Autologous Transfusion. Arlington, Va., American Association of Blood Banks, 1983, pp 1–9.
25. Kruger LM, Colbert JM. Intraoperative autologous transfusion in children undergoing spinal surgery. J Pediatr Orthop 1985;5:330–332.
26. Estrin JA, Belani KG, Karnavas AG, et al. A new approach to massive blood transfusion during pediatric liver resection. Surgery 1986;99:664–670.
27. Burman JF, Westlake AS, Davidson SJ, et al. Study of five cell salvage machines in coronary artery surgery. Transfus Med 2002;12:173–179.
28. McShane AJ, Power C, Jackson JF, et al. Autotransfusion: quality of blood prepared with a red cell processing device. Br J Anaesth 1987;59:1035–1039.
29. Yawn DH, Bull B. Intraoperative salvage: quality of products. In Maffei LM, Thurer RL (eds). Autologous Blood Transfusion: Current Issues. Arlington, Va., American Association of Blood Banks, 1988, pp 43–55.
30. Boldt J, Klind D, von Bormann B, et al. Blood conservation in cardiac operations: cell separation versus hemofiltration. J Thorac Cardiovasc Surg 1989;97:832–840.
31. Williams GD, Ramamoorthy C, Totzek FR, et al. Comparison of the effects of red cell separation and ultrafiltration on heparin concentration during pediatric cardiac surgery. J Cardiothorac Vasc Anesth 1997;11:840–844.
32. Reents W, Babin-Ebell J, Misoph MR, et al. Influence of different autotransfusion devices on the quality of salvaged blood. Ann Thorac Surg 1999;68:8–62.
33. Munoz M, Garcia-Vallejo JJ, Ruiz MD, et al. Transfusion of postoperative shed blood: laboratory characteristics and clinical utility. Eur Spine J 2004;13(Suppl 1):S107–S113.
34. Strumper EW, Weber S, Gielen-Wijffels R, et al. Clinical efficacy of postoperative autologous transfusion of filtered shed blood in hip and knee arthroplasty. Transfusion 2004;44:1567–1571.
35. De Haan J, Boonstra PW, Monnik SH, et al. Retransfusion of suctioned blood during cardiopulmonary bypass impairs hemostasis. Ann Thorac Surg 1995;59:901–907.
36. Bull BS, Bull MH. The salvaged blood syndrome. Blood Cells 1990;16:5–23.
37. Ramirez G, Romero A, Garcia-Vallejo JJ, et al. Detection and removal of fat particles from postoperative salvaged blood in orthopedic surgery. Transfusion 2002;42:66–75.
38. Van Loghem JJ, van der Hart M, Land ME: Polyagglutinability of red cells as a cause of severe haemolytic transfusion reaction. Vox Sang 1955;5:125.
39. Williams RA, Brown EF, Hurst D, et al. Transfusion of infants with activation of erythrocyte T antigen. J Pediatr 1989;115:949–953.
40. Ramasethu J, Luban NL. T activation. Br J Haematol 2001;112: 259–263.
41. Eder AF, Manno CS. Does red-cell T activation matter? Br J Haematol 2001;114:25–30.
42. Paeker C, Omine M, Richards S, et al. Diagnosis and management of paroxysmal nocturnal hemoglobinuria. Blood 2005;106:3699–3709.
43. Hillmen P, Lewis SM, Bessler M, et al. Natural history of paroxysmal nocturnal hemoglobinuria. N Engl J Med 1995;333:1253–1258.
44. Smith LJ. Paroxysmal nocturnal hemoglobinuria. Clin Lab Sci 2004;17:172–177.
45. Rosse WF, Nishimura J. Clinical manifestations of paroxysmal nocturnal hemoglobinuria: present state and future problems. Int J Hematol 2003;77:113–120.
46. Hill A, Hillmen P, Richards SJ, et al. Sustained response and long-term safety of eculizumab in paroxysmal nocturnal hemoglobinuria. Blood 2005;106:2559–2565.
47. Dacie JV. Transfusion of saline-washed red cells in nocturnal haemoglobinuria (Marchiafava-Micheli disease). Clin Sci 1947;7:65.
48. Baranett EC, Dunlop JB, Pullar TH. Chronic haemolytic anemia with paroxysmal haemoglobinuria (Marchiafava syndrome): report of a case improved by splenectomy. NZ Med J 1951;50:39.
49. Hirsch J, Ungar B, Robinson JS. Paroxysmal nocturnal haemoglobinuria: an acquired dyshaemopoiesis. Aust Ann Med 1964;13:24.
50. Manchester RC. Chronic hemolytic anemia with paroxysmal hemoglobinuria. Ann Intern Med 1945;23:935.
51. Brecher ME, Taswell HF. Paroxysmal nocturnal hemoglobinuria and the transfusion of washed red cells: a myth revisited. Transfusion 1989;29:681.
52. Parker C, Omine M, Richards S, et al. Diagnosis and management of paroxysmal nocturnal hemoglobinuria. Blood 2005;106:3699–3708.
53. Brecher ME (ed). Technical Manual, 15th ed. Bethesda, Md., American Association of Blood Banks, 2005, p 193.
54. Blanchette VS, Hume HA, Levy GJ, et al. Guidelines for auditing pediatric blood transfusion practices. Am J Dis Child 1991;145:787–796.
55. Brecher ME (ed). Technical Manual, 15th ed. Bethesda, Md., American Association of Blood Banks, 2005, p 804.
56. Strauss RG, Villhauer PJ, Cordle DG. A method to collect, store, and issue multiple aliquots of packed red blood cells for neonatal transfusions. Vox Sang 1995;68:77–81.
57. Personal communication. RG Strauss to SG Sandler. May 15, 2003.
58. Strauss RG, Burmeister F, Johnson K, et al. AS-1 red cells for neonatal transfusions: a randomized trial assessing donor exposure and safety. Transfusion 1996;36:873–878.
59. Sherwood WC, Clapper C, Wilson S. The concentration of AS-1 RBCs after gravity sedimentation for neonatal transfusion. Transfusion 2000;40:618–619.
60. Sandler SG, Ramasethu J. Washed and volume-reduced components. In Hillyer C, Strauss RG, Luban NL (eds). Handbook of Pediatric Transfusion Medicine. San Diego, Elsevier Academic Press, 2004, pp 113–120.
61. Skupski DW, Bussel JB. Alloimmune thrombocytopenia. Clin Obstet Gynecol 1999;42:335–348.
62. Uhrynowska M, Maslanka K, Zupanska B. Neonatal thrombocytopenia: incidence, serological and clinical observations. Am J Perinatol 1997;14:415–418.
63. McFarland JG. Platelet and neutrophil alloantigen genotyping in clinical practice. Transfus Clin Biol 1998;5:13–21.
64. Kroll H, Keifel V, Santoso S. Clinical aspects and typing of platelet alloantigens. Vox Sang 1998;74(Suppl 2):345–354.
65. Stroncek D. Neonatal alloimmune neutropenia and alloimmune thrombocytopenia. In Herman JH, Manno CS (eds). Pediatric Transfusion Therapy. Bethesda, Md., American Association of Blood Banks, 2002, pp 109–127.
66. Bussel JB, Berkowitz RL, Lynch L, et al. Antenatal management of alloimmune thrombocytopenia with intravenous gamma-globulin: a randomized trial of the addition of low-dose steroid to intravenous gamma-globulin. Am J Obstet Gynecol 1996;174:1414–1423.
67. Johnson JA, Ryan G, al-Musa A, et al. Prenatal diagnosis and management of neonatal alloimmune thrombocytopenia. Semin Perinatol 1997;1:45–52.
68. Adner MM, Fisch GR, Starobin SG, et al. Use of "compatible" platelet transfusions in treatment of congenital isoimmune thrombocytopenic purpura. N Engl J Med 1969;280:244–246.
69. Pineda AA, Zylstra VW, Clare DE, et al. Viability and functional integrity of washed platelets. Transfusion 1989;29:524–527.
70. Ranasinghe E, Walton JD, Hurd C, et al. Provision of platelet support for fetuses and neonates affected by severe fetomaternal alloimmune thrombocytopenia. Br J Haematol 2001;117:482–483.
71. Larsson L, Welsh VJ, Ladd DJ. Acute intravascular hemolysis secondary to out-of-group platelet transfusion. Transfusion 2000;40:902–906.
72. Pierce RN, Reich LM, Mayer K. Hemolysis following platelet transfusions from ABO incompatible donors. Transfusion 1985;25:60–62.
73. Josephson CD, Mullis NC, Van Demark C, et al. Significant numbers of apheresis-derived group O platelet units have "high-titer" anti-A/A,B: implications for transfusion policy. Transfusion 2004;44:805–808.
74. Schoenfeld H, Muhm M, Doepfmer U, et al. Platelet activity in washed platelet concentrates. Anesth Analg 2004;99:17–20.
75. Mustard JF, Perry DW, Ardlie N, Packham MA. Preparation of washed platelets from humans. Br J Haematol 1972;22:193–204.
76. Silvergleid AJ, Hafleigh E, Harbin M, et al. Clinical value of washed-platelet concentrates in patients with non-hemolytic transfusion reactions. Transfusion 1977;17:33–37.
77. Kalman ND, Brown DJ. Platelet washing with a blood cell processor. Transfusion 1982;22:125–127.
78. Smogorzewska A, Dzik W. Volume-reduced apheresis platelets. Transfusion 2005;45:651.
79. Schoenfeld H, Spies C, Jakob C. Volume-reduced platelet concentrates. Curr Hematol Rep 2006;5:82–88.
80. Moroff G, Friedman A, Robkin-Kline L, et al. Reduction of the volume of stored platelet concentrates for use in neonatal patients. Transfusion 1984;24:144–146.
81. Holme S, Heaton WA, Moroff G, et al. Evaluation of platelet concentrates stored for 5 days with reduced plasma volume. Transfusion 1994;34:39–43.
82. Simon TL, Sierra ER. Concentration of platelet units into small volumes. Transfusion 1984;24:173–175.

83. Strauss RG. Neonatal transfusion. In Anderson KC, Ness PM (eds). Scientific Basis of Transfusion Medicine: Implications for Clinical Practice, 2nd ed. Philadelphia, WB Saunders, 2000, pp 321–336.
84. Strauss RG, Levy GJ, Sotelo-Avila C, et al. National survey of neonatal transfusion practices. II. Blood component therapy. Pediatrics 1993;91:530–536.
85. Heddle NM, Klama L, Meyer R, et al. A randomized controlled trial comparing plasma removal with white cell reduction to prevent reactions to platelets. Transfusion 1999;39:231–238.
86. Heddle NM, Klama L, Singer J, et al. The role of the plasma from platelet concentrates in transfusion reactions. N Engl J Med 1994;331: 625–628.
87. Muylle L, Wouters E, Peetermans ME. Febrile reactions to platelet transfusion: the effect of increased interleukin 6 levels in concentrates prepared by the platelet-rich plasma method. Transfusion 1996;36:886–890.
88. Couban S, Carruthers J, Andreou P, et al. Platelet transfusions in children: results of a randomized, prospective, crossover trial of plasma removal and a prospective audit of WBC reduction. Transfusion 2002;42:753–758.
89. Vetlesen A, Mirlashari MR, Torsheim IA, Kjeldsen-Kragh J. Platelet activation and residual activation potential storage of hyperconcentrated platelet products in two different additive solutions. Transfusion 2005;45:1349–1355.
90. Allen DL, Samol J, Benjamin S, et al. Survey of the use and clinical effectiveness of HPA-1a/5b-negative platelet concentrates in proven or suspected platelet alloimmunization. Transfus Med 2004;14:409–417.
91. Dumont LJ, Krailadsiiri P, Seghatchian J, et al. Preparation and storage characteristics of white cell-reduced platelet concentrates collected by an apheresis system for transfusions in utero. Transfusion 2000;40:91–100.
92. Dumont LJ, Beddard R, Whitley P, et al. Autologous transfusion recovery of WBC-reduced high-concentration platelet concentrates. Transfusion 2002;42:1333–1339.
93. Rinder HM, Snyder EL, Tracey JB, et al. Reversibility of severe metabolic stress in stored platelets after in vitro plasma rescue or in vivo transfusion: restoration of secretory function and maintenance of platelet survival. Transfusion 2003;43:1230–1237.
94. Simon TL, Sierra ER. Concentration of platelet units into small volumes. Transfusion 1984;24:173–175.
95. Pisciotto PT, Snyder EL, Napychank PA, et al. In vitro characteristics of volume-reduced platelet concentrate stored in syringes. Transfusion 1991;31:404–408.
96. Ali AM, Warkentin TE, Bardossy L, et al. Platelet concentrates stored for 5 days in a reduced volume of plasma maintain hemostatic function and viability. Transfusion 1994;34:44–47.
97. Rock G, Haddad SA, Poon AO, et al. Reduction of plasma volume after storage of platelets in CP2D. Transfusion 1998;38:242–246.
98. Zilber M, Friedman Z, Shapiro H, et al. The effect of plasma depletion of platelet concentrates on platelet aggregation and phosphatidylserine expression. Clin Appl Thromb Hemost 2003;9:39–44.
99. Shoenfeld H, Muhm M, Doepfmer UR, et al. The functional integrity of platelets in volume-reduced platelet concentrates. Anesth Analg 2005;100:78–81.
100. Ringwald J, Walz S, Zimmermann R, et al. Hyperconcentrated platelets stored in additive solution: aspects on productivity and in vitro quality. Vox Sang 2005;89:11–18.
101. Isola H, Kientz D, Aleil B, et al. In vitro evaluation of Haemaonetics MCS+ apheresis platelet concentrates treated with photochemical pathogen inactivation following plasma volume reduction using the INTERCEPT Preparation Set. Vox Sang 2006;90:128–130.
102. Janetzko K, Lin L, Eichler H, et al. Implementation of the INTERCEPT Blood System for Platelets into routine blood bank manufacturing procedures: evaluation of apheresis platelets. Vox Sang 2004;86: 239–245.
103. Gulliksson H. Defining the optimal storage conditions for the long-term storage of platelets. Transfus Med Rev 2003;17:209–215.

Chapter 30

Blood Management: Conservation, Salvage, and Alternatives to Allogeneic Transfusion

Beth Shaz

INTRODUCTION

Blood management is the term given to the practice of minimizing allogeneic blood use while maximizing patient outcome. The four main tenets of blood management are (1) to focus on guideline-driven proper use of banked blood and minimizing its inappropriate use, (2) to utilize pharmaceutical preparations that prevent, minimize, or control blood loss, usually in the operative setting, (3) to employ blood conservation methods, and (4) to have a multidisciplinary approach. Blood conservation includes preoperative (preoperative autologous donation), intraoperative (hemodilution and blood salvage), and postoperative (blood salvage) techniques. A multidisciplinary approach makes use of the entire team of health care providers in the uniform goal of minimizing transfusion in the treatment of patients. This approach incorporates addressing preoperative anemia, using meticulous anesthetic and surgical techniques intraoperatively, and avoiding overphlebotomy postoperatively. This chapter focuses on these four topics.

GUIDELINE-DRIVEN BLOOD PRODUCT USE

Although the blood supply in developed countries has become increasingly safe, mortality and morbidity continue to be associated with transfusions. The risks of transfusion are detailed in subsequent chapters. The risk of transfusion must be weighed against the benefit. A retrospective review of patients who declined blood transfusion showed an increase in morbidity and mortality in proportion to decreasing hemoglobin at a hemoglobin level below 8 g/dL.[1] Therefore, for each patient, depending on co-morbidities, a transfusion threshold should exist. Creating restrictive transfusion criteria reduces the likelihood of transfusion with an average savings of a single unit per transfused patient.[2] Prior to creation of the guidelines, perform an audit to understand the established transfusion practice. Transfusion guidelines should be created by a multidisciplinary team based on evidence in the literature (an example is shown in Fig. 30–1). Prior to implementation of the guidelines, education is required to ensure the guidelines are understood and followed. After implementing the guidelines, perform a repeat audit to guarantee they are being followed. This practice can also identify areas that need continued improvement.[3,4]

PHARMACEUTICAL PREPARATIONS THAT DECREASE BLOOD LOSS

Desmopressin

Desmopressin (DDAVP; 1-deamino-8-D-arginine-vasopressin) is a vasopressin analog that increases the circulating levels of factor VIII and von Willebrand factor in patients with hemophilia A and von Willebrand disease, respectively.[5] Side effects of DDAVP include hypotension, hyponatremia, headache, and decreased urine output.[6] The Cochrane collaboration reviewed 25 clinical trials of DDAVP use in adult elective surgery without underlying bleeding disorders and concluded that DDAVP does not reduce blood loss, risk of allogeneic transfusion, volume of red blood cells (RBCs) transfused, or mortality. The majority of the studies were performed in cardiac surgery patients.[7]

Antifibrinolytics

Aprotinin

Aprotinin, a proteinase inhibitor obtained from bovine lung, inhibits multiple mediators of inflammatory responses, fibrinolysis, and thrombin generation.[6] Aprotinin inhibits kallikrein at higher doses and plasmin at lower doses (Fig. 30–2). Anaphylactic reactions are possible, especially when patients are reexposed to aprotinin; therefore, a test dose is required.[6] In the Cochrane database of systematic reviews, aprotinin reduces the need for allogeneic blood transfusion, bleeding, and the need for reexploration in cardiac bypass surgery patients.[8] Considerations in the use of aprotinin include the following: use of half versus full dose, use in surgeries other than bypass, use of aprotinin versus lysine analogs, and cost.

Aprotinin has been administered in several dose sizes: the kallikrein-inhibiting full dose ("full Hammersmith"), the plasmin-inhibiting half-dose, and a pump-prime-only dose.[8] All three doses decrease blood transfusion, both in the number of products received and the percentage of patients transfused. This also held true when patients were stratified for risk of bleeding. There is a concern of an increased risk of myocardial infarction with the pump-prime-only dose.[9] A study of the cost effectiveness of the high and low doses in coronary artery bypass patients found that in primary CABG patients aprotinin was cost neutral, whereas in repeat CABG patients both doses resulted in cost savings over placebo ($4483 for the low dose and $6044 for the high dose; 2005 USD).[10]

South Glasgow University Hospitals NHS Trust
Southern General Hospital

GUIDELINES FOR BLOOD TRANSFUSION

This guideline promotes best practice regarding blood use within the Southern General Hospital. Recent audit revealed widespread differences in practice and confusion as to when and how to prescribe blood.

INDICATIONS FOR TRANSFUSION

1. Acute Blood Loss

An acute blood loss of greater than 20% of blood volume (about 1000 mls blood) will often need a transfusion. Do not delay ordering blood in situations where blood loss is acute and rapid. If blood loss is very rapid, the hospital Major Haemorrhage Protocol should be activated by dialing 3333.

2. For Surgical Patients

Consider transfusion if:

- Pre-operative haemoglobin is less than 80 g/l and the surgery is associated with the probability of major blood loss.
- Post-operative haemoglobin falls below 70 g/l.
- Pre-operative anaemia MUST be investigated, as medical management may be more appropriate than transfusion.

3. Anaemia in Active Myocardial Infarction (Hb below 100g/l)

These patients are among the few who may benefit feom a Hb above 80. Transfusion to an Hb of 100 g/l is acceptable but to overshoot to 110 may be excessive. Evaluate effect of each unit as it is given.

4. Anaemia in Other Patients (Hb below 100 g/l but above 70 g/l)

Consider transfusion in normovolaemic patients ONLY if they have symptomatic anaemia. Symptoms and signs of anaemia include:

- Shortness of breath for no other reason
- Angina
- Syncope/postural hypotension
- ST depression on ECG
- Tachycardia for no other reason

Transfusion above 100 g/l is very rarely indicated and WILL be questioned by haematology staff.

- Think before transfusion. Blood is expensive and potentially dangerous if used inappropriately.
- Reassess after each unit given. Do you need to give more?
- Stop if symptoms/signs shown above resolve.
- Stop if you have reached an adequate Hb i.e. above 80 g/l in symptomless patients (100 g/l in acute MI).

Transfusion or Not?

Acute blood loss over 20% volume
Consider transfusion immediately Consider dialing 3333 for Major Haemorrhage
Patient anaemic? (Hb below 100 g/l)
Surgical
Medical
Pre-op investigate
Post-op Hb below 80
No acute MI Hb 70–100
Acute MI
Transfuse to Hb of 100 g/l
Symptoms or signs*
Yes
No
Do not transfuse unless Hb below 70
Hb below 70
Transfuse, but evaluate after each unit
No symptoms or signs*
Do not transfuse
Symptoms or signs* or Hb below 70
Transfuse, but evaluate after each unit

Figure 30–1 Example of guidelines for red cell transfusion. (From Garrioch M, Sandbach J, Pirie E, Morrison A, Todd A, Green R. Reducing red cell transfusion by audit, education and a new guideline in a large teaching hospital. Transfus Med 2004;14:27.)

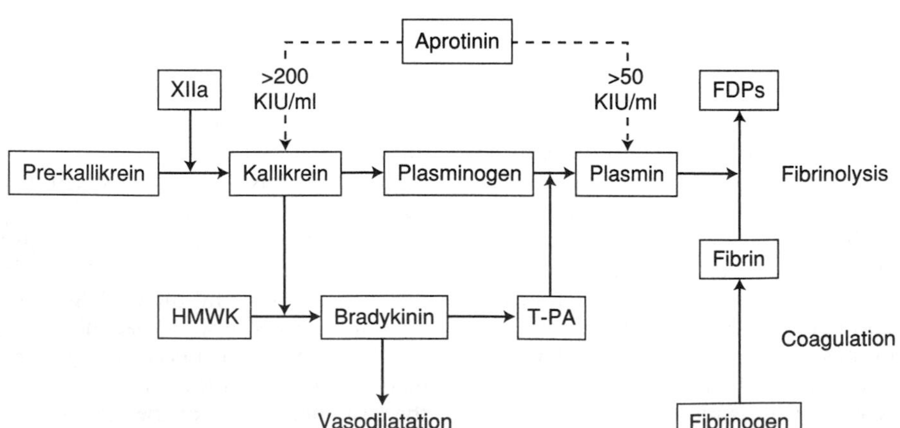

Figure 30–2 Aprotinin inhibition. (From Porte RJ, Hendriks HG, Slooff MJ. Blood conservation in liver transplantation: The role of aprotinin. J Cardiothorac Vasc Anesth 2004;18(4 Suppl):31S–37S.)

Aprotinin has been used in other surgeries including orthopedic surgery, liver transplantation, liver resection, and vascular surgery.[8] In liver transplantation, studies have demonstrated a decrease in transfusion with no difference in mortality.[11,12] In major orthopedic surgery, there are conflicting data about the usefulness of aprotinin, and the studies consist of small numbers of patients with varying procedures.[13–15] Small trials have shown decreased transfusion rates with aprotinin versus placebo in orthognathic surgery[16] and major thoracic surgery.[17,18] In summary, aprotinin has not been extensively studied in noncardiac surgery but may be beneficial if substantial blood loss is predicted.

e-Aminocaproic Acid (EACA) and Tranexamic Acid (TXA)

TXA and EACA are synthetic lysine analogs that inhibit fibrinolysis. These drugs block the lysine-binding site on the plasminogen molecule, which inhibits the formation of plasmin and therefore inhibits fibrinolysis. In the Cochrane database of systematic reviews, TXA, but not EACA, statistically significantly reduces the rate of allogeneic transfusion.[8]

There are only a handful of trials with small numbers of patients using EACA to decrease the rate of transfusion, and a few more trials using TXA. A small study demonstrated a small but statically significant decrease in transfusion rate in scoliosis repair in EACA versus placebo.[19] A similar study with TXA showed decreased blood loss, with no difference in transfusion.[20] The use of TXA versus placebo reduced the total number of packed red cell units transfused in patients receiving coronary artery bypass grafting on and off pump.[21] No difference in transfusion rates in total knee replacement was seen with the use of TXA or aprotinin.[22,23] Multiple small trials with either TXA or EACA for a variety of surgeries have demonstrated conflicting data on their ability to decrease allogeneic red cell transfusion, but in general more benefit has been seen in procedures associated with greater blood loss.

Comparison of Antifibrinolytics

Antifibrinolytics decrease the need for allogeneic transfusion. Aprotinin is the most expensive but the most frequently studied of the antifibrinolytics. The Ischemia Research and Education Foundation recently published an observational study involving 4374 patients undergoing cardiac revascularization. They compared aprotinin, aminocaproic acid, and tranexamic acid with no agent and discovered that aprotinin was associated with serious end-organ damage involving the heart, brain, and kidney. There was a dose-response relationship for aprotinin with increased death, renal dysfunction, and cardiovascular events at a higher dose. All three antifibrinolytics reduced blood loss equally, but aminocaproic acid and tranexamic acid were not associated with serious end-organ damage.[24] In a recent study in cardiac surgery patients of aprotinin versus tranexamic acid versus control, aprotinin significantly decreased the likelihood of allogeneic transfusion.[25] A similar study in coronary artery bypass patients receiving aspirin showed no significant difference between aprotinin, TXA, and EACA on blood loss or transfusion.[26] In the Cochrane review, no clinical significant difference between TXA and aprotinin on transfusion could be found, but there is significant heterogeneity in the trials.[8] In orthotopic liver transplantation, use of TXA versus aprotinin showed no difference in transfusion or mortality.[27]

Most of the data on antifibrinolytics is in cardiac surgery patients. There is a debate about its use in primary surgeries, where blood loss should not be substantial and the drug may therefore be of limited benefit. The second most common use in the literature is in orthopedic surgery, where it can be beneficial in surgeries with substantial blood loss. Few trials in orthotopic liver transplantation have shown a decrease in transfusion, but there are multiple case reports of thrombotic complications with its use.[28]

Recombinant Factor VIIa (rFVIIa)

Factor VIIa binds to tissue factor to activate factors IX and X, thereby activating factor V, which converts prothrombin to thrombin. Thrombin activates platelets and factors VII, V, and XI. This creates a thrombin burst, which converts fibrinogen to fibrin for clot formation (Fig. 30–3).[29] Recombinant activated factor VII (rFVIIa) is licensed for use to control bleeding in hemophilia with inhibitors, but there are case series demonstrating its success in controlling severe or refractory bleeding in nonhemophilic patients as well. One randomized controlled study in patients undergoing retropubic prostatectomy demonstrated a reduction in blood loss, number of units transfused, and likelihood of transfusion.[30] rFVIIa did not reduce blood loss or transfusion in trauma patients undergoing pelvic reconstruction.[31] A third trial of rFVIIa versus placebo in patients receiving liver resection demonstrated no change in transfusion or blood loss.[32] In a recent trial of its use in intracranial hemorrhage, there was an increased rate of thrombosis, especially as the dose was escalated.[33] rFVIIa may decrease blood loss and decrease transfusion needs in cases of large blood loss but carries a risk of thrombosis and a high cost.

Fibrin Sealant

Fibrin sealant is the combination of thrombin and fibrinogen mixed with calcium to form fibrin, which is used as a topical hemostatic agent. Products may contain antifibrinolytics (aprotinin) to reduce fibrinolysis or factor XIII to increase strength of the clot (Fig. 30–4).[34] A variety of commercially and individually produced fibrin sealants are available. Bovine thrombin products are commonly used but have a risk for allergic reactions and antibody formation. Antibodies to bovine thrombin cross-react with human factor V, leading to factor V deficiency and risk for hemorrhage.[35] In contrast, human thrombin, though virally inactivated, has a small risk for transfusion-transmitted disease. Currently, two fibrin sealant products consisting of human fibrinogen, human thrombin, calcium chloride, and aprotinin (bovine) are commercially available in the United States. Alternatively, automated devices exist to produce fibrin sealant from autologous plasma.[36] Another option is autologous fibrin glue prepared from the cryoprecipitated portion of autologous plasma; after thawing, this material is mixed with bovine thrombin immediately before application to the surgical field. A disadvantage of fibrin sealant is the time it takes to prepare, especially autologous products, and also the time for the clot to form.[34] Fibrin sealants have been studied in a number of surgeries, including prostatectomy, lung resection, liver resection, carotid endarterectomy, cardiac surgery, and orthopedic surgery.[34] In the Cochrane database of systematic reviews, fibrin sealants reduced allogeneic transfusion and decreased intraoperative and postoperative blood loss, but most trials were small and unblinded, resulting in less reliable data.[37]

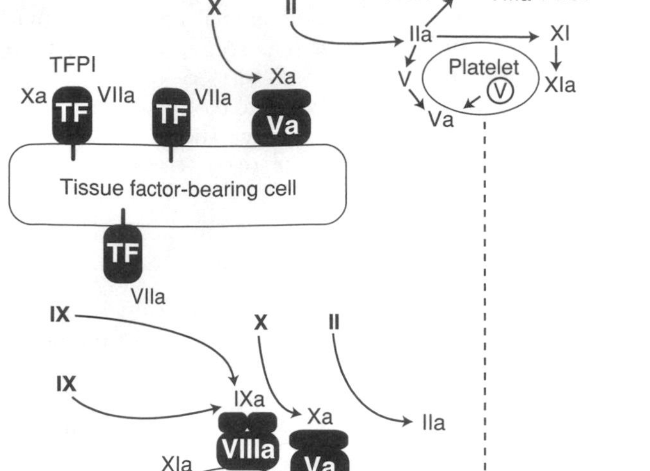

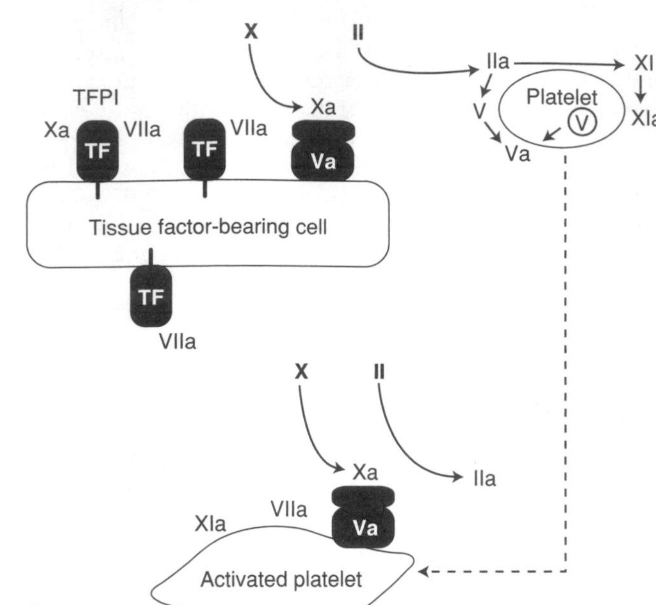

Figure 30–3 Role of FVIIa in coagulation. **A,** Coagulation is initiated when coagulation proteins and platelets come into contact with the extravasculature. Factor VII binds to tissue factor, is activated, and activates both factor IX and factor X. The factor Xa forms a complex with factor Va on the tissue factor–bearing cell and activates a small amount of thrombin. This thrombin acts to amplify the initial coagulation signal by activating platelets, causing release of factor V, activating factor V, cleaving factor VIII and releasing it from vWF, and activating factor XI. In the propagation phase, factor IXa, formed by factor VIIa/tissue factor or generated on the platelet surface by factor XIa, forms a complex with factor VIIIa to activate factor X on the platelet surface, where, in complex with factor Va and in the presence of prothrombin, it is protected from inhibition. Formation of the factor Xa/Va complex results in a burst of thrombin generation. **B,** In hemophilia, the initiation and amplification phases proceed normally. The propagation phase is absent or significantly decreased because factor Xa cannot be generated on the platelet surface. High-dose factor VIIa acts to partially restore platelet surface factor Xa generation so that factor Xa/Va complex formation proceeds and the propagation phase is improved relative to the hemophilic state. (From Roberts HR, Monroe DM, White GC. The use of recombinant factor VIIa in the treatment of bleeding disorders. Blood 2004;104:3858–3864.)

BLOOD CONSERVATION

Autologous Blood

Autologous blood can be collected from a patient in advance of anticipated blood loss (preoperative donation) or at the start of the procedure (acute normovolemic hemodilution); in addition, shed blood can be salvaged for reinfusion both during surgery and in the postoperative period (Table 30–1). As early as the late 19th century, the concept of using a patient's own blood as a source of transfusable RBCs was born of necessity because allogeneic transfusions were fraught with immunologic risks. Early authors proposed the recovery of blood shed during childbirth, ectopic pregnancy, and splenectomy.[38,39] With the discovery of the ABO blood group system, the development of approaches for storage of blood and preparation of components, and the need during two world wars for a large and immediately available blood supply, interest in autologous blood waned. The appearance in the early 1980s of the human immunodeficiency virus (HIV) as a transfusion-transmissible complication of allogeneic transfusion fostered a recurrence of interest in autologous blood techniques. As the risk of transfusion decreased and understanding of the risks and costs of autologous donation increased, there has been a decline in the utilization of preoperative blood donation.[40] Blood collection statistics bear out this trend: donations of blood for autologous use increased from 28,000 units in 1982 to a peak of 1,117,000 units in 1992 and have currently decreased to 651,000 units in 1999 (Fig. 30–5).[41–44]

Preoperative Erythropoietin

Erythropoietin is a 165-amino-acid glycoprotein hormone, which is synthesized in fetal liver and adult kidney as a response to hypoxia to stimulate erythropoiesis. Erythropoietin receptors have been identified on both hematopoietic and other (brain, heart, liver, and retina, vascular endothelium, gastrointestinal tract, and reproductive tract) tissues. Therefore, erythropoietin likely mediates additional activities, such as having a protective antiapoptotic effect.[45] Erythropoietin corrects anemia caused by renal failure, cancer, cancer therapy, and HIV.[46] Erythropoietin is contraindicated in patients with uncontrolled hypertension. Adverse events associated with its use include thrombotic events, hypertension, seizures, and rare cases of pure red cell aplasia.[6] Erythropoietin can be used preoperatively, with or without preoperative blood donation, or with acute normovolemic hemodilution in elective surgery.[46] Two to four weeks is necessary for adequate erythropoietin-stimulated erythropoiesis to occur.[46] Depending on the estimated blood loss, patient's blood volume, and amount of time prior to surgery, erythropoietin may be useful.

Because erythropoietin increases the preoperative hemoglobin, it can be used in mildly anemic patients preoperatively to decrease the risk of transfusion in elective surgeries with moderate blood loss.[47] Erythropoietin given perioperatively decreases the number of intraoperative and postoperative transfusions and results in improved 1-year survival rate.[48] One study demonstrated that patients receiving daily erythropoietin (300 IU/kg or 100 IU/kg subcutaneously beginning 10 days prior to orthopedic surgery for a total of

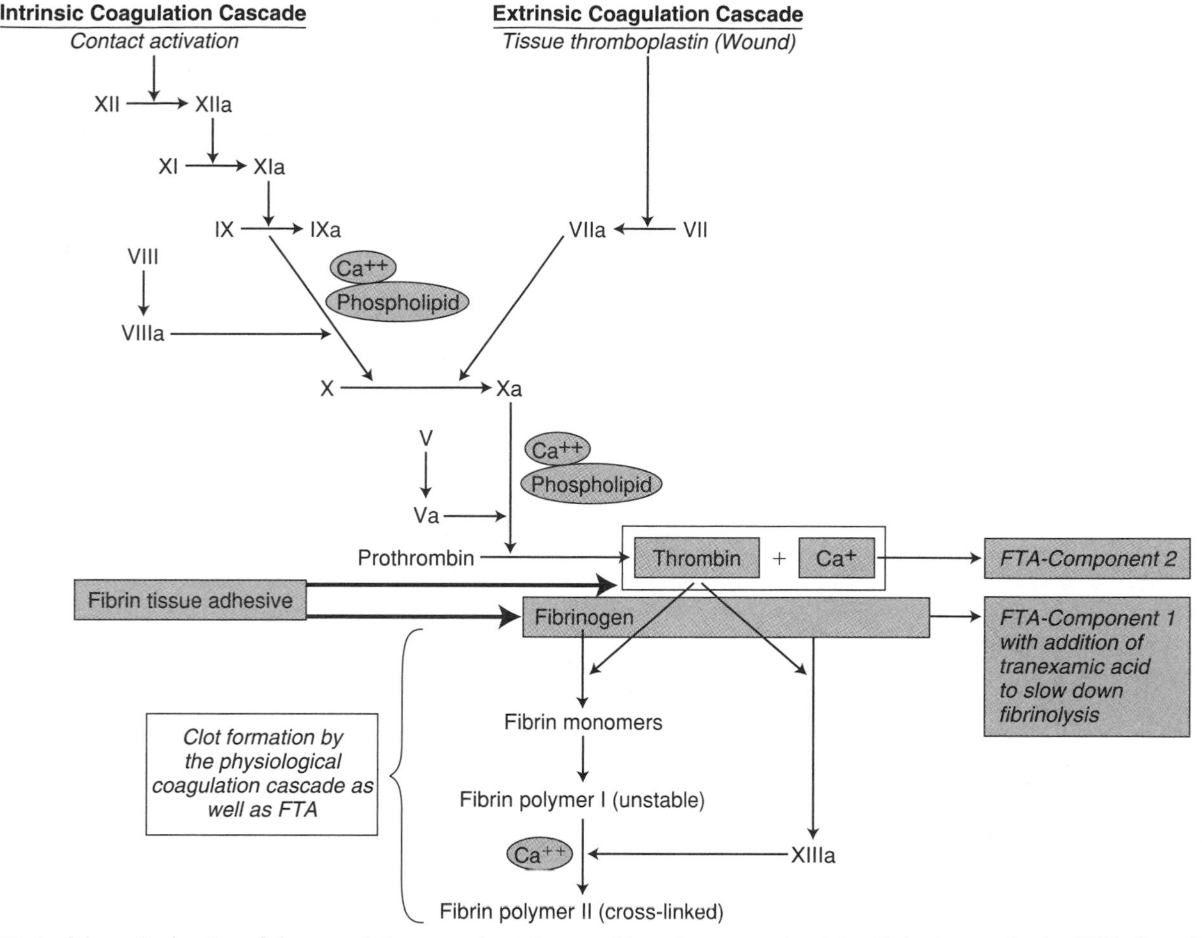

Figure 30–4 Schematic drawing of the coagulation cascade and composition of components of the fibrin tissue adhesive (FTA). (From Levy O, Martinowitz U, Oran A, Tauber C, Horoszowski H. The use of fibrin tissue adhesive to reduce blood loss and the need for blood transfusion after total knee arthroplasty. A prospective, randomized, multicenter study. J Bone Joint Surg Am 1999;81:1580–1588.)

15 doses) versus placebo perioperatively had significantly decreased transfusion rates. This improvement was significant even in patients with a preoperative hemoglobin level above 13 g/dL.[49] An earlier study with erythropoietin given daily perioperatively to patients undergoing elective hip replacement showed a decreased transfusion rate with erythropoietin compared with placebo, but the patients who benefited most had a hemoglobin below 13.5 g/dL at baseline.[50] Preoperative erythropoietin has also been shown to decrease allogeneic transfusion in anemic patients receiving elective open heart surgery or gastrointestinal cancer resection.[51] In anemic patients who are not eligible to donate autologous blood preoperatively, erythropoietin decreases the likelihood of allogeneic blood transfusion.

Iron supplementation maximizes the benefit of erythropoietin used either orally or intravenously.[52] Other major

Table 30–1 Indications for Autologous Blood Techniques

Surgical Procedure	Preoperative Donation	Perioperative Salvage	Acute Normovolemic Hemodilution
Vascular surgery (intra-abdominal procedures)	Yes	Yes	Yes
Open heart surgery	Yes	Yes	Yes
Total hip surgery	Yes	No*	No*
Total knee surgery	Yes	Yes†	No*
Scoliosis surgery	Yes	Yes	Yes
Radical prostatectomy	Yes	Yes‡	Yes
Liver resection/transplantation	Yes	Yes	Yes
Placenta previa	Yes	No§	No*

*Need not conclusively established.
†Intraoperative salvage is unnecessary when a tourniquet is used; postoperative salvage may be of value in cementless procedures.
‡Hypothetical risk of cancer spread after transfusion of intraoperatively salvaged blood.
§The safety of blood containing amniotic fluid has not been conclusively established.

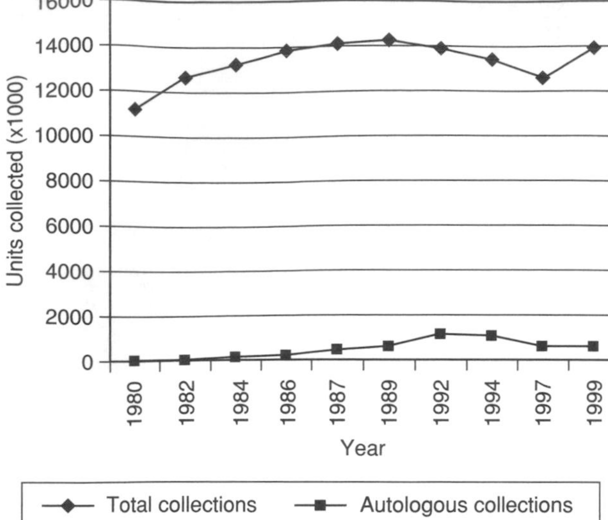

Figure 30–5 Units of total whole blood or red cell collections compared with units of autologous whole blood or red cell collections over time.

causes of hyporesponsiveness to erythropoietin include folic acid, vitamin B_{12}, vitamin C deficiency, infection, inflammatory states, and chronic blood loss.[53]

Erythropoietin has also been used in combination with preoperative autologous blood donation to increase the number of units donated or with other blood conservation strategies, as discussed in the sections on Indications for Autologous Whole Blood Collection in Combination with Erythropoietin and Acute Normovolemic Hemodilation in Combination with Erythropoietin.

Preoperative Iron Supplementation

Correcting iron deficiency anemia prior to surgery should decrease the likelihood of the need for allogeneic transfusion.[54] Iron therapy is not beneficial in non–iron-deficient patients without concomitant erythropoietin.[52] A preliminary study shows a decrease in allogeneic blood transfusion with an accompanied reduction in morbidity-mortality rate and length of hospital stay with the use of intravenous iron preoperatively in patients undergoing displaced subcapital hip fracture repair.[55]

Advantages and Disadvantages of Autologous Blood Transfusion

Advantages

In the past, autologous donations have been viewed as a strategy for obtaining blood to augment short allogeneic supplies. More relevant in current times is the use of autologous blood to eliminate the risk of transfusion-transmitted microorganisms, in particular HIV and hepatitis viruses. The institution of increasingly sensitive tests for such infections, including nucleic acid testing, has softened the impact of this argument; however, the risk of future incursions into the blood supply by new infectious agents remains a threat. Immunologic complications, such as antibody-mediated hemolysis and leukocyte-associated febrile reactions, are eliminated with the use of autologous blood. Supported by human and animal data, some authors also believe that allogeneic transfusions induce immunosuppression in the recipient and that autologous blood may not.[56] Only prospective observational studies have been performed to answer the question of allogeneic versus autologous blood transfusion and the risk of postoperative infection.[57–59] Other advantages include the stimulation of erythropoiesis in the repeatedly bled autologous donor, which could speed recovery from postoperative anemia.[60] Intraoperatively salvaged RBCs are typically transfused back to the patient within a few hours after collection, thereby precluding the acquired membrane defects and enzyme deficiencies (2,3-diphosphoglycerate and adenosine triphosphate) that develop during refrigeration (the "storage lesion").[61]

Disadvantages

Autologous techniques are not without drawbacks. Although an ideal preoperative donation schedule should allow sufficient time for compensatory erythropoiesis to occur, some individuals develop donation-induced anemia at the time of admission for surgery. Concerns regarding complications of donation in patients with underlying cardiac disease have been raised[62] although it can be difficult in such settings to distinguish between an untoward effect of blood letting and the natural history of the baseline condition. Clerical errors, including release of the wrong unit of blood, still occur.[63] Finally, although it is rare, autologous blood may itself pose infectious risks. *Yersinia enterocolitica*, a common cause of community-acquired diarrhea, persists in the bloodstream for many weeks after infection and can grow at refrigerator temperatures; an individual who donates blood during this time period can be made severely ill by later transfusion of the component.[64]

Costs of Autologous Blood Techniques

As the allogeneic blood supply has become safer, more attention has been focused on the costs associated with autologous transfusion techniques. Costs come from unused autologous collections (e.g., when a patient has donated enough blood to match the mean number of components used by others undergoing the procedure but requires less). This problem is magnified by overcollection and unnecessary utilization (e.g., in plastic surgery) and by the extra work involved in deviation from routine, large-scale allogeneic collection practices.[65] In one hypothetical cost-utility analysis of patients undergoing primary elective hip replacement, the cost effectiveness of autologous transfusion per quality-adjusted life-year (QALY) was estimated at an extremely high 3.4 million. However, if allogeneic transfusions were assumed to increase the risk of postoperative bacterial infection, a possibility suggested by some workers,[66–68] the cost of using autologous blood fell to less than $50,000 per QALY, and the procedure became dominant (cheaper to use than allogeneic blood) as the infection risk rose.[69] Some authors have suggested that autologous blood could be kept cost effective by streamlining collection and processing, including forgoing infectious disease testing of autologous donors.[70,71] Reducing costs through the intentional use of autologous blood by a recipient other than the donor ("crossover") is not recommended. Only 30% of collections are typically eligible for allogeneic use, and the costs, complexity, and risk of error of the transition all serve to negate the value.[72]

Preoperative Autologous Donation

Indications for Autologous Whole Blood Collection

The decision to use preoperative autologous blood donations should be predicated on the type of surgery, the amount of time available for donation and hematopoietic reconstitution, the patient's hematocrit, and the predicted vigor of the erythropoietic response to donation. Patients planning to undergo elective orthopedic surgery are ideal candidates for autologous transfusion, because they require moderate amounts of blood during and immediately after surgery, and they typically have sufficient time prior to surgery to make multiple donations.[73–75] Open heart surgery and vascular surgery are other procedures in which autologous blood collections have led to reduction or elimination of allogeneic blood use.[6] The use of preoperative autologous blood donation has also been reported for a variety of other surgical procedures, including radical prostatectomies, hysterectomies, and other gynecologic procedures, gastrointestinal surgery, and neurosurgery.[76,77] Donors of bone marrow for transplantation undergo multiple iliac crest aspirations and may develop a moderate anemia; advance donation of autologous blood forestalls the need for allogeneic transfusions.[78] As surgical techniques change, the need for blood transfusions may be affected, and in such instances the role of autologous blood should be reexamined. Radical prostatectomy is a case in point: ten years ago many hospitals encouraged patients undergoing the procedure to donate autologous blood,[79,80] but today in some hands fewer than 2% of patients require blood, and autologous blood donations may be superfluous.[81,82] Blood transfusion is also rarely necessary in plastic surgical procedures, and the collection of autologous blood in such cases is often frivolous.[83]

Autologous blood can be collected from a pregnant woman for use during childbirth. The expanded maternal blood volume contributes a substantial safety cushion, and the donation process appears safe for both mother and fetus.[84] However, the use of blood transfusions in uncomplicated pregnancies is low (1%) even in patients undergoing cesarean section (3.3%).[85–87] A role for autologous collections may exist for patients with placenta previa, in which the likelihood of transfusion may exceed 25%, and the condition is often identified with sufficient time for advance blood donations.[88] In addition, autologous blood has been collected from patients with unusual antibodies discovered during the pregnancy.[89]

Long-term frozen storage of autologous RBCs in the absence of an anticipated transfusion episode is both ineffective and expensive. An exception is the storage of blood by individuals with high-frequency or complex alloantibodies, for whom stockpiling of rare autologous units may be beneficial. Even here, however, the likelihood that such blood would be helpful is slim. To be of value, sufficient autologous blood would have to be available to meet the needs of an unexpected emergency; furthermore, delays in sending the blood expeditiously to the hospital where it is needed and in preparing units (thawed and washed free of the glycerol cryoprotectant) would make its use unwieldy.

Indications for Autologous Whole Blood Collection in Combination with Erythropoietin

Preoperative erythropoietin and preoperative autologous donation have the equivalent likelihood of allogeneic red cell transfusion.[90–92] The superiority of adding erythropoietin to preoperative autologous donation was demonstrated in a three-arm study of preoperative erythropoietin alone, erythropoietin plus preoperative autologous donation, versus preoperative autologous donation alone in patients undergoing total joint arthroplasty with an initial hemoglobin of ≤14.0 g/dL. Allogeneic transfusion rates were lowest in patients who had received erythropoietin and predonated autologous blood (11% vs 28% or 33%).[93]

When large blood loss is expected and multiple units of autologous blood are needed, erythropoietin increases the number of preoperative autologous blood units that can be donated.[47] In one study, orthopedic patients with a baseline hematocrit of ≤39% were requested to donate six weekly autologous units. Erythropoietin (six weekly doses) versus placebo significantly increased the number of units donated (4.5 vs 3.0), resulting in fewer patients who received erythropoietin being transfused allogeneic blood (26% vs 38%).[94] An earlier small study in women undergoing total hip replacement with hematocrit <40% showed donation of more units with erythropoietin versus placebo (4.1 vs 2.8 units) resulted in less transfused allogeneic blood (0.4 vs 1.2 units). This study had an aggressive donation schedule, with one donation every 3 to 4 days for 3 weeks, and a high transfusion rate of 4 units on average.[95] A similar study in spine surgery showed benefit in erythropoietin with autologous donation, evidenced by a decrease in allogeneic blood and hospital stay.[96] A single small study in patients with iron deficiency anemia (hematocrit ≤ 33%) and gastrointestinal cancer showed an increase in autologous unit donation and a trend toward decrease of allogeneic blood transfusion with the use of intravenous iron and erythropoietin preoperatively versus intravenous iron alone.[97] A small study in patients undergoing coronary artery bypass surgery demonstrated that erythropoietin increased the number of autologous units collected and decreased the rate of allogeneic blood transfusion.[98]

Other studies have demonstrated an increase in autologous units donated preoperatively with the use of erythropoietin but no significant decrease in allogeneic blood transfusion. In patients undergoing hysterectomy, erythropoietin increased the number patients able to donate 3 units in 2 weeks but did not decrease the transfusion of allogeneic blood.[99] Patients undergoing resection of rectal cancer were able to donate more red cells (4 units in 2 weeks) if treated with erythropoietin, but there was no difference in autologous or allogeneic transfusions.[100] Multiple studies show no use for erythropoietin in combination with preoperative autologous donation in nonanemic patients undergoing surgery, even with large blood needs.[101–103]

Clearly determining which patients are most likely to benefit from erythropoietin with or without preoperative autologous donation depends on the estimated blood loss for a surgical procedure, the patient's ability to donate autologous blood, the amount of time available prior to surgery, the baseline hematocrit, and the patient's blood volume. A single institution's experience with a tailored program of no preoperative autologous donation in patients with hematocrits greater than 39%, autologous blood donation (2 weekly donations) in patients with hematocrits between 37% and 39%, and erythropoietin if the hematocrit was less than 37% (3 weekly doses preoperatively) showed a decrease in transfusion (88% vs 57%), especially in patients with hematocrits greater than 39%, (majority of the patients).[104] This study proved the concept of tailoring preoperative treatment based on a patient's baseline hematocrit.

Indications for Other Autologous Components

Although autologous plasma is easily prepared from whole blood, little need exists for plasma in most elective surgery.[105] Autologous platelet-rich plasma can be prepared at the start of open heart surgery, using apheresis equipment before bypass, to be returned to the patient after heparin reversal.[106] Because thrombocytopenia or an acquired platelet defect can occur after blood passes through the membrane oxygenator,[107] the theoretical advantages of transfusing platelet-rich plasma should include improvement in hemostasis and reduced transfusion requirements. Although initial studies of this approach provided supportive data,[106,108–110] later prospective, blinded protocols were not able to demonstrate a reduction in blood use in either primary heart surgery or reoperations.[111,112] In addition, the harvesting of platelet-rich plasma has been followed by intraoperative heparin resistance, possibly owing to release of platelet factor 4 and other procoagulants from platelets damaged during the collection.[113] The Cochrane Database of systematic reviews identified 19 trials of platelet-rich plasmapheresis in mostly cardiac surgery patients for which allogeneic transfusion data were available. They concluded that platelet-rich plasmapheresis reduces allogeneic transfusion, but there was heterogeneity in the studies and the majority was unblinded; therefore, the procedure is not justified at this time.[114]

Collecting Autologous Blood

Autologous blood donations are well tolerated by a variety of ostensibly high-risk donors, including the elderly,[76,115] children,[116] pregnant women,[117,118] and patients with atherosclerotic coronary artery disease.[119] One group reported an increased frequency of serious reactions among autologous donors at blood collection facilities, although this may reflect an intentionally conservative approach to patients (compared with the "normal" volunteers to which donor centers are accustomed).[120] A weekly phlebotomy schedule fosters some degree of RBC regeneration before surgery (in one study, a mean of 522 mL of RBCs donated over 3 weeks resulted in a mean RBC production of 351 mL).[121] However, the most important medical problem associated with autologous donation is anemia developing during the collection interval. When this occurs, it is typically as a result of marginal iron stores and insufficient erythropoietic response (with little or no increase in serum erythropoietin levels), probably because the hematocrit of most donors is not allowed to fall below 30%.[122] This situation may be improved by the administration of recombinant human erythropoietin.[123] Many variables affect the response of blood donors to this drug, including route of administration, adequacy of iron stores, and method of iron supplementation (oral vs parenteral).[124,125] Especially in the United States, the expense of recombinant human erythropoietin has limited its use to situations in which autologous blood donation might otherwise be difficult or impossible (e.g., in a patient who is already anemic).[94,95] An alternative approach employs RBC apheresis—collection of two units of RBCs (without plasma)—because each collection enhances the rate of compensatory erythropoiesis.[126] Other advantages of RBC apheresis include increased time between donation and surgery, which allows more time for compensation for the red cell loss, and savings in time and cost.[127]

Provided that the donor has satisfactory iron stores and that bone marrow erythropoiesis can occur in a timely fashion, blood may be comfortably collected from an autologous donor on a weekly schedule. Oral ferrous sulfate is commonly prescribed (325 mg three times daily) although the amount absorbed may not be sufficient to counter the iron lost with the donations.[128,129] In non–iron-deficient patients undergoing preoperative autologous blood donation, oral or intravenous iron versus no iron did not increase the number of units donated or decrease the need for allogeneic transfusion.[130] The shelf life of refrigerated whole blood is limited to 42 days with current formulations of anticoagulant-preservative solutions, and a schedule for multiple donations is usually fits into this 6-week window. Alternatively, some or all of the units can be frozen at −65°C, with glycerol as a cryopreservative, for up to 10 years. Although frozen units allow collections to occur over a longer period, the flexibility of utility at the time of surgery is affected: thawing and deglycerolizing takes a few hours, and the thawed units have an outdate of 24 hours.

Intraoperative Autologous Transfusion: Blood Salvage

Several techniques have been developed for the salvage and reinfusion of blood lost during an operative procedure. Interest in intraoperative salvage has been spurred by the introduction of pumps, separation chambers for washing RBCs, and increasing automation of the collection process.[131,132] The simplest approach—direct reinfusion without washing—involves collection of blood under low vacuum pressure in a plastic bag seated within a hard outer canister. An anticoagulant, usually citrate, is added. As soon as the bag is full, or within 4 hours after the start of the collection (to prevent bacterial growth), the contents of the bag are reinfused through a standard blood filter to the patient (Fig. 30–6). RBCs shed into a surgical field, already poten-

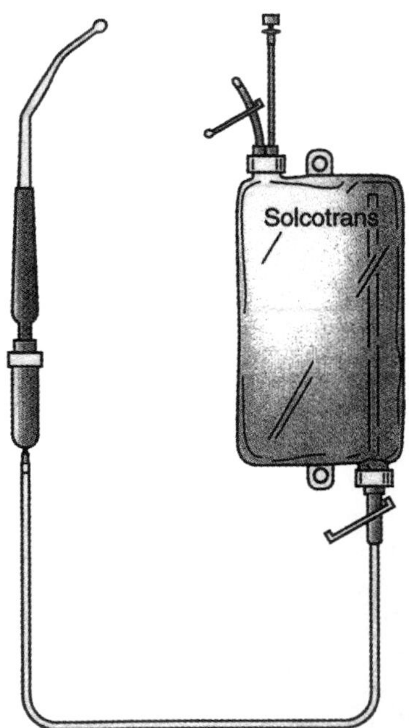

Figure 30–6 Equipment for direct reinfusion of perioperatively salvaged blood without washing. A 600-mL plastic bag is seated within the rigid plastic outer shell. A suction aspirator wand and filter are connected to the bottom port; vacuum suction is connected to the top left port. The top right port is connected to a blood filter for transfusion to the autologous recipient. (From Solco Basle, Rockland, Mass., and Williams & Wilkins, with permission.)

tially damaged by their travail, are accompanied by activated coagulation factors and platelets, cellular debris and soluble factors released from injured tissue cells, pharmaceuticals applied to the field, and irrigant solutions. Despite this scenario, salvaged blood has been reinfused directly into patients with few untoward consequences.

Alternatively, the contents of the bag can be washed with saline. Devices that include a reservoir for collecting the salvaged blood and a centrifuge for washing are available (Fig. 30–7) to collect and process large volumes (e.g., 225 mL of RBCs with a final hematocrit of 50% in less than 3 minutes).[133] With these techniques, intraoperative blood salvage has become practical in situations in which blood loss may be extremely rapid, such as trauma or liver transplantation. Approximately half of the blood lost during a surgical procedure can be recovered; the rest is irretrievably absorbed by drapes and sponges or damaged during collection.[134]

Complications of intraoperative salvage are surprisingly infrequent. The hematocrit of salvaged unprocessed blood is typically low because of a combination of dilution from irrigation fluids and some degree of mechanical hemolysis.[135] Free hemoglobin levels may exceed 1000 mg/dL, and in the recipient this can result in hemoglobinemia and hemoglobinuria (Table 30–2). Nevertheless, renal sequelae are uncommon.[136] The survival of chromium 51–labeled salvaged cells is normal in most patients, presumably because damaged cells are cleared during processing.[137,138]

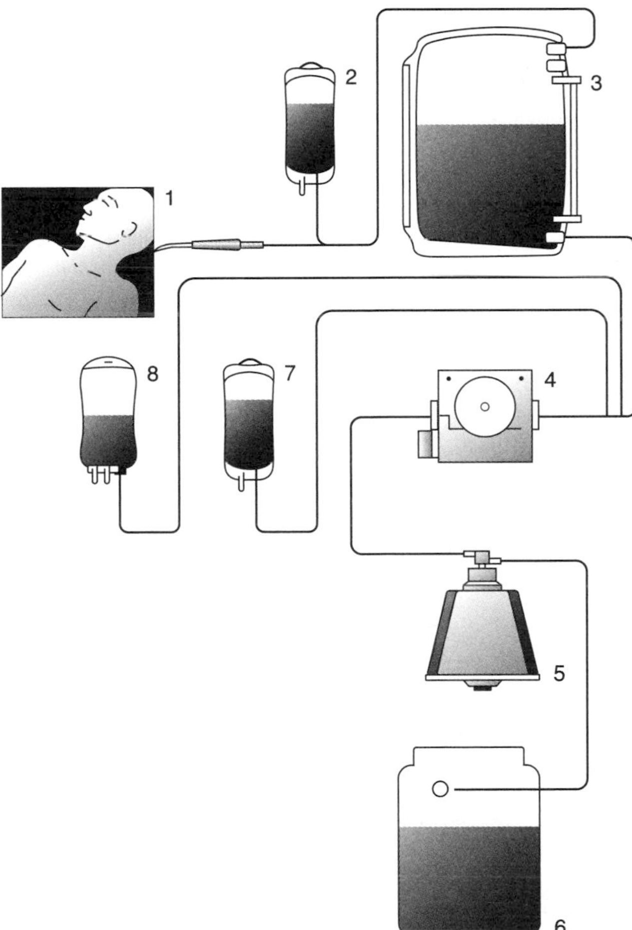

Figure 30–7 Schematic of an instrument used for collection and washing of perioperatively salvaged blood. Shed blood is suctioned from the operative field (1), an anticoagulant is added (2), and the blood moves past a mesh filter into a reservoir (3). A pump (4) forces the blood into a spinning plastic centrifuge bowl (5). With separation, plasma flows into a waste bag (6); saline (7) is continuously pumped into the bowl to wash the packed red blood cells. At the completion of washing, the red blood cells are moved into a reinfusion bag (8) for return to the patient. (From Haemonetics, Braintree, Mass., and Williams & Wilkins, with permission.)

Coagulation abnormalities are often observed in recipients of large volumes of salvaged blood and include hypofibrinogenemia, elevated fibrin degradation products, thrombocytopenia, and prolonged prothrombin and partial thromboplastin times.[139,140] In general, this clinical picture is related to a combination of the characteristics of the salvaged blood and hemodilution in the recipient. After exposure to serosal surfaces in the operative field, blood becomes depleted of coagulation factors and platelets; in the case of unwashed autologous blood, fibrin degradation products accumulate.[141] Although the clinical picture can resemble that of disseminated intravascular coagulation, which in theory might be initiated by phospholipids and other materials released from damaged blood cells, no evidence exists to support a cause-and-effect relationship.

Other substances in salvaged blood include fat, fibrin, and microaggregates. Infusion of unprocessed blood has not been shown to be harmful in either animals or humans, possibly because of the removal of most particulate matter by standard blood filters.[142,143] Pharmaceutical contaminants, such as heparin, topical antibiotics, hemostatic agents, and biologic substances such as tissue enzymes and hormones, can be removed, but usually not completely, by washing.[144,145] Bacterial contamination during the collection and processing of autologous blood is inevitable owing to environmental organisms such as coagulase-positive and -negative staphylococci, propionibacteria, and *Corynebacterium* species. Administration of antibiotics to the patient reduces the microorganisms but does not eliminate them,[146] and complete removal of bacteria after collection also is not possible, even when the washing solution includes antibiotics.[147] There is no apparent clinical significance to such low levels of contamination. Larger bacterial counts are of more concern. Collection of blood from a contaminated site, such as that associated with spilled intestinal contents, is probably contraindicated, although some authors have argued that, if no other blood is available, such transfusions may be lifesaving and worth the risk.[148,149] Tumor cells have also been found in salvaged blood during cancer surgery; their malignant potential is unknown, and many consider cancer another contraindication.[150,151]

Finally, although it is uncommon, the collection process can be associated with fatal air embolism; such events were originally reported in association with a device that allowed reservoir contents to be pumped directly into a venous catheter, without an air detection system.[152] Although instruments with this design are no longer marketed, rare fatalities are still reported. A 1997 report cautioned that external pressure devices magnify the risk of air embolism and should never be used with perioperatively salvaged blood except if absolutely necessary and under close supervision.[153]

The collection and transfusion of intraoperatively salvaged blood has been associated with substantial reductions in allogeneic transfusions (>50%), particularly in spine surgery,[154,155] hip replacement,[156] and vascular procedures such as aortic reconstruction.[157] During cardiac surgery, the largest volume of blood that can be processed for return to the patient comes from the membrane oxygenator. Although this blood technically is not shed, in that it is removed from the

Table 30–2 **Characteristics of Perioperatively Salvaged Blood Compared with Banked Blood and Normal Patient Values***

Component	Hematocrit	Free Hemoglobin (mg/dL)	Platelet Count (per mm³)	Coagulation Factors	Fibrin Degradation Products
Salvaged blood, unwashed	Low (25%)	Very high (≥200)	Low (100,000)	Low (35%–75%)	High (300 mg/dL)
Salvaged blood, washed	High (60%)	Low (<50)	Very low (<10,000)	Absent	Absent
Allogeneic blood (packed red blood cells)	High (60%)	Variable with age of component	Low and dysfunctional (100,000)	Low (35%–75%)	Increased
Normal patient	Normal (40%)	<5	300,000	100%	<10 mg/dL

*Typical results of laboratory tests are given. The transfusion of large volumes of salvaged blood could result in similar alterations in the recipient.

From Noon GP. Intraoperative autotransfusion. Surgery 1978;84:719–721, and Silva R, Moore EE, Bar-Or D, et al. The risk:benefit ratio of autotransfusion: Comparison to banked blood in a canine model. J Trauma 1984;24:557–564. Used with permission.

extracorporeal circuit at the end of surgery, the processing is helpful in concentrating RBCs and removing cardioplegia solution.[158,159] In liver transplantation, volumes as large as 25 units have been salvaged,[160–162] and salvage during trauma is also feasible.[147,163,164] The collection of autologous blood during cesarean section carries theoretical risks associated with transfusing amniotic fluid; however, an analysis of 139 women who received processed salvaged blood identified no increased incidence of obstetric complications.[165] Blood has also been recovered from the hemoperitoneum in association with ectopic pregnancy,[166] during radical prostatectomy,[167] and during splenectomy.[168] Intraoperatively salvaged blood has been a useful adjunct in the treatment of some Jehovah's Witnesses, whose literal acceptance of the Bible includes abstention from routine allogeneic blood transfusions. In this situation, an uninterrupted circuit between the salvaged blood processor and the patient facilitates acceptance.[169]

Postoperative Autologous Transfusion: Blood Salvage

Both canister systems and RBC processors can be used to collect postoperative blood drainage, such as that from the mediastinum after heart surgery,[170] from the peritoneal cavity after hepatic injury,[171] or from the knee or hip site after orthopedic procedures.[172] Blood salvaged from a serosal cavity has little residual fibrinogen and few platelets, and clotting is usually not a problem; therefore, the addition of anticoagulants to the collection is usually not necessary.[173] Despite the substantial levels of free hemoglobin in the salvaged blood, RBCs survive normally, as documented by studies involving radiolabeled markers.[174]

In addition to free hemoglobin, the salvaged blood may be contaminated with tissue exudate, bone, bone marrow, and other biologic and surgical materials; nevertheless, most patients tolerate the infusions well. Bioactive substances measured in the unwashed drainage include histamine, interleukin-6 and other cytokines, prostaglandins, and activated complement components; however, these levels have not been associated with transfusion reactions, and levels in patients after infusion are not significantly altered.[175–177] Similarly, methyl methacrylate (used as a cement in orthopedic surgery) and its breakdown product, methanol, can be measured in blood salvaged postoperatively from the surgical site; however, these materials have not been detected in recipients after transfusion.[178] Occasional complications do occur, however, including respiratory distress,[179] hypotension with anaphylaxis,[180] and fever.[181] The last more likely to occur when the product is collected over a long time interval (6 to 12 hours). The pathophysiology of these events remains unclear.

After open heart surgery, mediastinal blood may contain very high levels of cardiac muscle enzymes, especially creatine phosphokinase, as well as lactate dehydrogenase from hemolyzed RBCs.[141,182] The reinfusion of shed mediastinal blood can result in increased levels of these enzymes and can confound the diagnosis of myocardial infarction in the postoperative period.[183,184] The volume of RBCs actually salvaged is often small and the effect on reducing transfusions debatable. Infusion of shed mediastinal blood after cardiac operations appears to have the potential to reduce the volume of allogeneic blood required (by 1.4 units in one study).[185] In other situations, the benefit is less clear. Although the volume of postoperative drainage is often substantial in orthopedic procedures,[186,187] much of the collection is plasma and other serosanguineous fluids rather than RBCs. One study reported a mean total collection of only 55 ± 29 mL of RBCs in drains after hip surgery.[188] Orthoplasty procedures performed without cement are associated with larger perioperative blood losses, and postoperative salvage may be more effectively used in such cases.[189]

Acute Normovolemic Hemodilution

The collection of autologous blood at the start of surgery, for return to the patient at the end of the procedure, had its origins in open-heart surgery. The original goal was prevention of postoperative coagulopathies through ex vivo maintenance of a supply of platelets undamaged by exposure to the membrane oxygenator.[190,191] However, additional advantages to the intentionally created anemia were also identified. Hemodilution can contribute to a reduction in RBC loss. In simplest terms, a patient with a hematocrit of 45% and a 2 L blood loss during surgery loses roughly 900 mL of RBCs, whereas a similar patient with a hematocrit of 20% loses only 400 mL of RBCs. More elaborate mathematical modeling studies have been published that take into account the dynamic nature of the patient's RBC mass as it is affected by blood loss, fluid replacement, and blood transfusions (Fig. 30–8).[192,193] Hemodilution is probably less expensive to

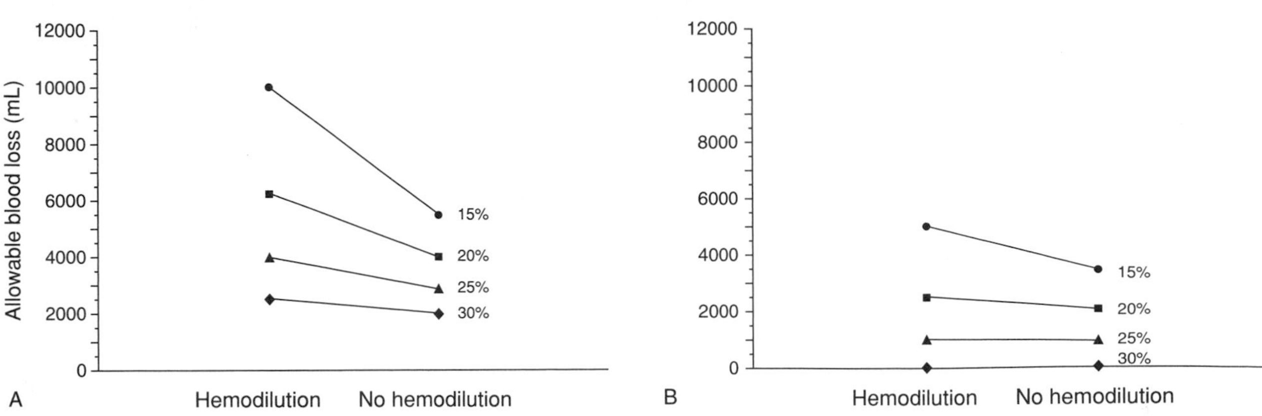

Figure 30–8 The volume of surgical blood loss (*y*-axis) that could occur before transfusion of allogeneic blood is needed in a patient of either 45% (**A**) or 30% (**B**) blood loss with a starting hematocrit and a blood volume of 5 L who either has or has not undergone isovolemic hemodilution. Each curve represents a different target hematocrit (the hemodilution end point, which is then maintained during surgery with autologous blood). (From Weiskopf RB. Mathematical analysis of isovolemic hemodilution indicates that it can decrease the need for allogeneic blood transfusion. Transfusion 1995;35:37–41. Used with permission.)

accomplish than preoperative autologous blood donation, and it may be the only option available when surgery is performed in other than elective settings.[194]

The technique involves removal of blood into standard collection bags with citrate anticoagulation (unless the patient is already heparinized) and replacement of lost volume with either crystalloids or colloids. Close monitoring of the patient's cardiovascular status is necessary during the hemodilution process. Units are stored in the operating room during surgery and reinfused as needed, in reverse order of collection, reserving the bags with the highest concentration of RBCs for the end of the procedure, after blood loss has been controlled.

In orthopedic and cardiovascular surgery, reductions in allogeneic blood use have been reported after extreme hemodilution (reduction of the patient's RBC mass by as much as 50%).[193,195] More modest hemodilution (e.g., removal of 2 units of blood at the beginning of surgery) may also be beneficial, according to some workers,[196,197] but this is not accepted by others.[192,198,199] The severity of the anemia could affect oxygen transport, although the concomitant drop in blood viscosity, and compensatory cardiac output increases, could restore oxygen delivery. However, one group has provided evidence that hemodilution may jeopardize patients at risk for myocardial infarction.[200] Further clinical studies appear necessary to resolve the continued controversy over the value of hemodilution in contemporary transfusion practice.[201,202]

Acute Normovolemic Hemodilution in Combination with Erythropoietin

Erythropoietin can be used preoperatively in conjunction with acute normovolemic hemodilution. A three-armed study looked at preoperative autologous donation (3 units) versus erythropoietin plus acute normovolemic hemodilution versus acute normovolemic hemodilution alone in patients undergoing prostatectomy. The investigation showed similar allogeneic transfusion rates with the lowest cost in the acute normovolemic hemodilution alone arm.[203] Mathematical modeling predicts preoperative erythropoietin will be most beneficial when used in conjunction with acute normovolemic hemodilution, especially in patients with small blood volumes and mild anemia.[204] This is confirmed in a study of elective open-heart surgery patients receiving erythropoietin or placebo preoperatively with intraoperative isovolemic hemodilution. In the erythropoietin group, more patients were able to have intraoperative isovolemic hemodilution, fewer patients received allogeneic blood transfusion, and the total mean transfusion per patient was lower. Further analysis showed blood loss, age, baseline hematocrit, as well as preoperative treatment with erythropoietin, to be independent predictors of the need for allogeneic blood transfusion.[205]

MULTIDISCIPLINARY APPROACH TO BLOOD MANAGEMENT

To decrease allogeneic transfusion, communication between all health care providers must occur. The likelihood of blood transfusion is decreased if the care of the patient is optimized before, during, and after surgery.

Preoperative Factors

The strongest predictor of a patient needing blood during an elective surgery is the baseline hematocrit, with other significant contributing factors being the patient's blood volume and red cell loss during the procedure.[181,206,207] Optimization of the patient's hemoglobin prior to surgery will decrease the chance of transfusion. Iron or erythropoietin may be indicated, depending on the cause of the patient's anemia. Preoperative anemia additionally increases perioperative infection and mortality, which may be a result of increase risk of allogeneic blood transfusion.[208]

The correction of impaired hemostasis should decrease blood loss and, therefore, decrease the need for transfusion. Impaired hemostasis can be corrected by discontinuing anticoagulants and antiplatelet agents in a timely manner or treating the cause of the impaired hemostasis. In a retrospective study, the frequency of blood transfusion was higher in patients without preoperative correction of primary hemostasis than in patients with correction.[209] In another retrospective study in cardiac surgery patients, preoperative use of antithrombotics (enoxaparin, clopidogrel, or GP IIb/IIIa inhibitors) increased transfusion, but uniquely preoperative enoxaparin increased postoperative bleeding and the need for reexploration.[210]

Intraoperative Factors

Intraoperative factors to reduce allogeneic transfusion include preventing hypothermia, optimizing surgical technique, and controlling hemostasis. Surgical techniques that reduce bleeding include laparoscopic, robotic, or endovascular approaches.[211] Surgical instruments that maximize coagulation include the ultrasonic scalpel and argon beam coagulator.

Controlled Hypotension

Controlled hypotension has been shown in some small studies to decrease blood loss and transfusion in orthopedic surgery.[212,213] Combining controlled hypotension with other banked blood saving techniques, such as hemodilution, may increase the likelihood of avoiding transfusion.[214] Other studies have not shown a benefit with controlled hypotension alone.[215] The concern with controlled hypotension is that it may produce end-organ ischemia, especially in patients with atherosclerosis. The decrease in blood loss as a result of controlled hypotension may not outweigh its risk of ischemia.[211]

Normothermia

Central body temperature decreases after induction of general anesthesia, which may increase blood loss and transfusion requirements. In a small study of patients undergoing major abdominal surgery, active warming with forced air showed reduced blood loss and blood product use.[216] Two studies show conflicting results in mild hypothermia affecting blood loss in total hip arthroplasty.[217,218] Studies demonstrate conflicting results regarding blood loss and transfusion requirements with normothermia versus hypothermia cardiopulmonary bypass.[219,220] In summary, no definitive answer is available about maintaining normothermia to decrease blood loss.

Postoperative Factors

Phlebotomy

Patients in the intensive care unit have a mean blood draw of approximately 40 mL a day with a total volume of 760 mL. Patients with arterial lines have a total blood loss of approximately 900 mL. These large losses from phlebotomy contribute to increased transfusion requirements.[221]

REFERENCES

1. Carson JL, Noveck H, Berlin JA, Gould SA. Mortality and morbidity in patients with very low postoperative Hb levels who decline blood transfusion. Transfusion 2002;42:812–818.
2. Hill SR, Carless PA, Henry DA, et al. Transfusion thresholds and other strategies for guiding allogeneic red blood cell transfusion. Cochrane Database Syst Rev 2002;CD002042.
3. Mallett SV, Peachey TD, Sanehi O, Hazlehurst G, Mehta A. Reducing red blood cell transfusion in elective surgical patients: the role of audit and practice guidelines. Anaesthesia 2000;55:1013–1019.
4. Garrioch M, Sandbach J, Pirie E, Morrison A, Todd A, Green R. Reducing red cell transfusion by audit, education, and a new guideline in a large teaching hospital. Transfus Med 2004;14:25–31.
5. Oliver WC Jr, Santrach PJ, Danielson GK, Nuttall GA, Schroeder DR, Ereth MH. Desmopressin does not reduce bleeding and transfusion requirements in congenital heart operations. Ann Thorac Surg 2000;70:1923–1930.
6. Physicians' Desk Reference, 59th ed. Montvale, NJ, Thomson PDR, 2005.
7. Carless PA, Henry DA, Moxey AJ, et al. Desmopressin for minimising perioperative allogeneic blood transfusion. Cochrane Database Syst Rev 2004;CD001884.
8. Henry DA, Moxey AJ, Carless PA, et al. Anti-fibrinolytic use for minimising perioperative allogeneic blood transfusion. Cochrane Database Syst Rev 2001;CD001886.
9. Lemmer JH Jr, Dilling EW, Morton JR, et al. Aprotinin for primary coronary artery bypass grafting: a multicenter trial of three dose regimens. Ann Thorac Surg 1996;62:1659–1667.
10. Smith PK, Datta SK, Muhlbaier LH, Samsa G, Nadel A, Lipscomb J. Cost analysis of aprotinin for coronary artery bypass patients: analysis of the randomized trials. Ann Thorac Surg 2004;77:635–642.
11. Findlay JY, Rettke SR, Ereth MH, Plevak DJ, Krom RA, Kufner RP. Aprotinin reduces red blood cell transfusion in orthotopic liver transplantation: a prospective, randomized, double-blind study. Liver Transpl 2001;7:802–807.
12. Porte RJ, Molenaar IQ, Begliomini B, et al. Aprotinin and transfusion requirements in orthotopic liver transplantation: a multicentre randomised double-blind study. EMSALT Study Group. Lancet 2000;355:1303–1309.
13. Amar D, Grant FM, Zhang H, Boland PJ, Leung DH, Healey JA. Antifibrinolytic therapy and perioperative blood loss in cancer patients undergoing major orthopedic surgery. Anesthesiology 2003;98: 337–342.
14. Samama CM, Langeron O, Rosencher N, et al. Aprotinin versus placebo in major orthopedic surgery: a randomized, double-blinded, dose-ranging study. Anesth Analg 2002;95:287–293.
15. Jeserschek R, Clar H, Aigner C, Rehak P, Primus B, Windhager R. Reduction of blood loss using high-dose aprotinin in major orthopaedic surgery: a prospective, double-blind, randomised and placebo-controlled study. J Bone Joint Surg Br 2003;85:174–177.
16. Stewart A, Newman L, Sneddon K, Harris M. Aprotinin reduces blood loss and the need for transfusion in orthognathic surgery. Br J Oral Maxillofac Surg 2001;39:365–370.
17. Bedirhan MA, Turna A, Yagan N, Tasci O. Aprotinin reduces postoperative bleeding and the need for blood products in thoracic surgery: results of a randomized double-blind study. Eur J Cardiothorac Surg 2001;20:1122–1127.
18. Kyriss T, Wurst H, Friedel G, Jaki R, Toomes H. Reduced blood loss by aprotinin in thoracic surgical operations associated with high risk of bleeding: a placebo-controlled, randomized phase IV study. Eur J Cardiothorac Surg 2001;20:38–41.
19. Florentino-Pineda I, Thompson GH, Poe-Kochert C, Huang RP, Haber LL, Blakemore LC. The effect of amicar on perioperative blood loss in idiopathic scoliosis: the results of a prospective, randomized double-blind study. Spine 2004;29:233–238.
20. Sethna NF, Zurakowski D, Brustowicz RM, Bacsik J, Sullivan LJ, Shapiro F. Tranexamic acid reduces intraoperative blood loss in pediatric patients undergoing scoliosis surgery. Anesthesiology 2005;102:727–732.
21. Casati V, Della VP, Benussi S, et al. Effects of tranexamic acid on postoperative bleeding and related hematochemical variables in coronary surgery: comparison between on-pump and off-pump techniques. J Thorac Cardiovasc Surg 2004;128:83–91.
22. Veien M, Sorensen JV, Madsen F, Juelsgaard P. Tranexamic acid given intraoperatively reduces blood loss after total knee replacement: a randomized, controlled study. Acta Anaesthesiol Scand 2002;46:1206–1211.
23. Engel JM, Hohaus T, Ruwoldt R, Menges T, Jurgensen I, Hempelmann G. Regional hemostatic status and blood requirements after total knee arthroplasty with and without tranexamic acid or aprotinin. Anesth Analg 2001;92:775–780.
24. Mangano DT, Tudor IC, Dietzel C; the Multicenter Study of Perioperative Ischemia Research Group and the Ischemia Research and Education Foundation. The risk associated with aprotinin in cardiac surgery. N Engl J Med 2006;354:353–365.
25. Diprose P, Herbertson MJ, O'Shaughnessy D, Deakin CD, Gill RS. Reducing allogeneic transfusion in cardiac surgery: a randomized double-blind placebo-controlled trial of antifibrinolytic therapies used in addition to intra-operative cell salvage. Br J Anaesth 2005;94:271–278.
26. Landymore RW, Murphy JT, Lummis H, Carter C. The use of low-dose aprotinin, epsilon-aminocaproic acid, or tranexamic acid for prevention of mediastinal bleeding in patients receiving aspirin before coronary artery bypass operations. Eur J Cardiothorac Surg 1997;11:798–800.

27. Dalmau A, Sabate A, Koo M, et al. The prophylactic use of tranexamic acid and aprotinin in orthotopic liver transplantation: a comparative study. Liver Transpl 2004;10:279–284.
28. Xia VW, Steadman RH. Antifibrinolytics in orthotopic liver transplantation: current status and controversies. Liver Transpl 2005;11:10–18.
29. Spahn DR, Tucci MA, Makris M. Is recombinant FVIIa the magic bullet in the treatment of major bleeding? Br J Anaesth 2005;94:553–555.
30. Friederich PW, Henny CP, Messelink EJ, et al. Effect of recombinant activated factor VII on perioperative blood loss in patients undergoing retropubic prostatectomy: a double-blind placebo-controlled randomised trial. Lancet 2003;361:201–205.
31. Raobaikady R, Redman J, Ball JA, Maloney G, Grounds RM. Use of activated recombinant coagulation factor VII in patients undergoing reconstruction surgery for traumatic fracture of pelvis or pelvis and acetabulum: a double-blind, randomized, placebo-controlled trial. Br J Anaesth 2005;94:586–591.
32. Lodge JP, Jonas S, Oussoultzoglou E, et al. Recombinant coagulation factor VIIa in major liver resection: a randomized, placebo-controlled, double-blind clinical trial. Anesthesiology 2005;102:269–275.
33. Wernet D, Mayer G. Isoagglutinins following ABO-incompatible bone marrow transplantation. Vox Sang 1992;62:176–179.
34. Milne AA. Clinical impact of fibrin sealants. Vox Sang 2004;87(Suppl 2):29–30.
35. Neschis DG, Heyman MR, Cheanvechai V, Benjamin ME, Flinn WR. Coagulopathy as a result of factor V inhibitor after exposure to bovine topical thrombin. J Vasc Surg 2002;35:400–402.
36. Buchta C, Dettke M, Funovics PT, et al. Fibrin sealant produced by the CryoSeal FS System: product chemistry, material properties, and possible preparation in the autologous preoperative setting. Vox Sang 2004;86:257–262.
37. Carless PA, Henry DA, Anthony DM. Fibrin sealant use for minimising perioperative allogeneic blood transfusion. Cochrane Database Syst Rev 2003;CD004171.
38. Highmore W. Practical remarks on an overlooked source of blood supply for transfusion in postpartum hemorrhage, suggested by a recent fatal case. Lancet 1874;1:89.
39. Theis HJ. Zur Behandlung der Estrauteringraviditar. Zentralbl Gynaekol 1914;38:1191–1193.
40. Brecher ME, Goodnough LT. The rise and fall of preoperative autologous blood donation. Transfusion 2001;41:1459–1462.
41. Surgenor DM, Wallace EL, Hao SL, Chapman RH. Collection and transfusion of blood in the United States, 1982–1988. N Engl J Med 1990;322:1646–1651.
42. Wallace EL, Churchill WH, Surgenor DM, et al. Collection and transfusion of blood and blood components in the United States, 1992. Transfusion 1995;35:802–812.
43. Sullivan MT, Wallace EL. Blood collection and transfusion in the United States in 1999. Transfusion 2005;45:141–148.
44. Sullivan MT, McCullough J, Schreiber GB, Wallace EL. Blood collection and transfusion in the United States in 1997. Transfusion 2002;42:1253–1260.
45. Lewis LD. Preclinical and clinical studies: a preview of potential future applications of erythropoietic agents. Semin Hematol 2004;41(4 Suppl 7):17–25.
46. Goodnough LT, Monk TG, Andriole GL. Erythropoietin therapy. N Engl J Med 1997;336:933–938.
47. Monk TG. Preoperative recombinant human erythropoietin in anemic surgical patients. Crit Care 2004;8(Suppl 2):S45–S48.
48. Kosmadakis N, Messaris E, Maris A, et al. Perioperative erythropoietin administration in patients with gastrointestinal tract cancer: prospective randomized double-blind study. Ann Surg 2003;237: 417–421.
49. Faris PM, Ritter MA, Abels RI. The effects of recombinant human erythropoietin on perioperative transfusion requirements in patients having a major orthopaedic operation. The American Erythropoietin Study Group. J Bone Joint Surg Am 1996;78:62–72.
50. Canadian Orthopedic Perioperative Erythropoietin Study Group. Effectiveness of perioperative recombinant human erythropoietin in elective hip replacement. Lancet 1993;341:1227–1232.
51. Podesta A, Carmagnini E, Parodi E, et al. Elective coronary and valve surgery without blood transfusion in patients treated with recombinant human erythropoietin (epoetin-alpha). Minerva Cardioangiol 2000;48:341–347.
52. Olijhoek G, Megens JG, Musto P, et al. Role of oral versus IV iron supplementation in the erythropoietic response to rHuEPO: a randomized, placebo-controlled trial. Transfusion 2001;41:957–963.
53. Drueke T. Hyporesponsiveness to recombinant human erythropoietin. Nephrol Dial Transplant 2001;16(Suppl 7):25–28.
54. Okuyama M, Ikeda K, Shibata T, Tsukahara Y, Kitada M, Shimano T. Preoperative iron supplementation and intraoperative transfusion during colorectal cancer surgery. Surg Today 2005;35:36–40.
55. Cuenca J, Garcia-Erce JA, Martinez AA, et al. Role of parenteral iron in the management of anaemia in the elderly patient undergoing displaced subcapital hip fracture repair: preliminary data. Arch Orthop Trauma Surg 2005;125:342–347.
56. Blajchman MA. Transfusion-associated immunomodulation and universal white cell reduction: are we putting the cart before the horse? Transfusion 1999;39:665–670.
57. Innerhofer P, Walleczek C, Luz G, et al. Transfusion of buffy coat-depleted blood components and risk of postoperative infection in orthopedic patients. Transfusion 1999;39:625–632.
58. Innerhofer P, Klingler A, Klimmer C, Fries D, Nussbaumer W. Risk for postoperative infection after transfusion of white blood cell-filtered allogeneic or autologous blood components in orthopedic patients undergoing primary arthroplasty. Transfusion 2005;45:103–110.
59. Westphal RG. Transfusion of buffy coat-depleted blood components and risk of postoperative infection in orthopedic patients. Transfusion 2000;40:381–383.
60. Owings DV, Kruskall MS, Thurer RL, Donovan LM. Autologous blood donations prior to elective cardiac surgery: safety and effect on subsequent blood use. JAMA 1989;262:1963–1968.
61. Wolfe LC, Byrne AM, Lux SE. Molecular defects in the membrane skeleton of blood bank-stored red cells: abnormal spectrin-protein 4.1-actin complex formation. J Clin Invest 1986;78:1681–1686.
62. Spiess BD, Sassetti RJ, McCarthy RJ, Narbone RF, Tuman KJ, Ivankovich AD. Autologous blood donation: hemodynamics in a high-risk patient population. Transfusion 1992;32:17–22.
63. Linden JV. Autologous blood errors and incidents [abstract]. Transfusion 1994;34:28S.
64. Haditsch M, Binder L, Garbriel C, Muller-Uri P, Wartschinger R, Mittermayer H. Yersinia enterocolitica septicemia in autologous blood transfusion. Transfusion 1994;34:907–909.
65. Etchason J, Petz L, Keeler E, et al. The cost-effectiveness of preoperative autologous blood donations. N Engl J Med 1995;332:719–724.
66. Heiss MM, Mempel W, Jauch KW, et al. Beneficial effect of autologous blood transfusion on infectious complications after colorectal cancer surgery. Lancet 1993;342:1328–1333.
67. Busch OR, Hop WC, van Papendrecht MA, Marquet RL, Jeekel J. Blood transfusion and prognosis in colorectal cancer. N Engl J Med 1993;328:1372–1376.
68. Jensen LS, Kissmeyer-Nielsen P, Wolff B, Qvist N. Randomised comparison of leucocyte-depleted versus buffy-coat-poor blood transfusion and complications after colorectal surgery. Lancet 1996;348:841–845.
69. Sonnenberg FA, Gregory P, Yomtovian R, et al. The cost-effectiveness of autologous transfusion revisited: implications of an increased risk of bacterial infection with allogeneic transfusion. Transfusion 1999;39:808–817.
70. Kruskall MS, Yomtovian R, Dzik WH, Friedman KD, Umlas J. On improving the cost-effectiveness of autologous blood transfusion practices. Transfusion 1994;34:259–264.
71. Kruskall MS. Cost effectiveness of autologous blood donation. N Engl J Med 1995;333:461–462.
72. Blum LN, Allen JR, Genel M, Howe JP. Crosover use of donated blood for autologous transfusion: report of the Council on Scientific Affairs, American Medical Association. Transfusion 1998;38:891–895.
73. Haugen RK, Hill GE. A large-scale autologous blood program in a community hospital: a contribution to the community's blood supply. JAMA 1987;257:1211–1214.
74. Woolson ST, Marsh JS, Tanner JB. Transfusion of previously deposited autologous blood for patients undergoing hip-replacement surgery. J Bone Joint Surg Am 1987;69:325–328.
75. Woolson ST, Pottorff G. Use of preoperatively deposited autologous blood for total knee replacement. Orthopedics 1993;16:137–141.
76. Kruskall MS, Glazer EE, Leonard SS, et al. Utilization and effectiveness of a hospital autologous preoperative blood donor program. Transfusion 1986;26:335–340.
77. Toy PT, Strauss RG, Stehling LC, et al. Predeposited autologous blood for elective surgery. N Engl J Med 1987;316:517–520.
78. Thompson HW, McCullough J. Use of blood components containing red cells by donors of allogeneic bone marrow. Transfusion 1986;26:98–100.
79. Peters CA, Walsh PC. Blood transfusion and anesthetic practices in radical retropubic prostatectomy. J Urol 1985;134:81–83.
80. Toy PT, Menozzi D, Strauss RG, Stehling LC, Kruskall M, Ahn DK. Efficacy of preoperative donation of blood for autologous use in radical prostatectomy. Transfusion 1993;33:721–724.

81. Koch MO, Smith JA Jr. Blood loss during radical retropubic prostatectomy: is preoperative autologous blood donation indicated? J Urol 1996;156:1077–1080.
82. Goh M, Kleer CG, Kielczewski P, Wojno KJ, Kyungmann K, Oesterling JE. Autologous blood donation prior to anatomical radical retropubic prostatectomy: is it necessary? Urology 1996;49:569–574.
83. Kruskall MS. Autologous blood transfusions and plastic surgery [editorial]. Plast Reconstr Surg 1989;84:662–664.
84. Kruskall MS. Controversies in transfusion medicine: the safety and utility of autologous donations by pregnant patients. Transfusion 1990;30:168–171.
85. Larsen R, Titlestad K, Lillevang ST, Thomsen SG, Kidholm K, Georgsen J. Cesarean section: is pretransfusion testing for red cell alloantibodies necessary? Acta Obstet Gynecol Scand 2005;84:448–455.
86. Combs CA, Murphy EL, Laros RK. Cost-benefit analysis of autologous blood donation in obstetrics. Obstet Gynecol 1992;80:621–625.
87. Andres RL, Piacquadio KM, Resnik R. A reappraisal of the need for autologous blood donation in the obstetric patient. Am J Obstet Gynecol 1990;163:1551–1553.
88. Klapholz H. Blood transfusion in contemporary obstetric practice. Obstet Gynecol 1990;75:940–943.
89. Katz AR, Ali V, Ross PJ, Gammon E. Management of a rare blood type: O "Bombay" in pregnancy. Obstet Gynecol 1981;57:16S–17S.
90. Hardwick ME, Morris BM, Colwell CW Jr. Two-dose epoetin alfa reduces blood transfusions compared with autologous donation. Clin Orthop Relat Res 2004;23:240–244.
91. Stowell CP, Chandler H, Jove M, Guilfoyle M, Wacholtz MC. An open-label, randomized study to compare the safety and efficacy of perioperative epoetin alfa with preoperative autologous blood donation in total joint arthroplasty. Orthopedics 1999;22(Suppl 1):S105–S112.
92. Chun TY, Martin S, Lepor H. Preoperative recombinant human erythropoietin injection versus preoperative autologous blood donation in patients undergoing radical retropubic prostatectomy. Urology 1997;50:727–732.
93. Bezwada HP, Nazarian DG, Henry DH, Booth RE Jr. Preoperative use of recombinant human erythropoietin before total joint arthroplasty. J Bone Joint Surg Am 2003;85:1795–1800.
94. Price TH, Goodnough LT, Vogler WR, et al. Improving the efficacy of preoperative autologous blood donation in patients with low hematocrit: a randomized, double-blind, controlled trial of recombinant human erythropoietin. Am J Med 1996;101:22S–27S.
95. Mercuriali F, Zanella A, Barosi G, et al. Use of erythropoietin to increase the volume of autologous blood donated by orthopedic patients. Transfusion 1993;33:55–60.
96. Shapiro GS, Boachie-Adjei O, Dhawlikar SH, Maier LS. The use of epoetin alfa in complex spine deformity surgery. Spine 2002;27:2067–2071.
97. Braga M, Gianotti L, Vignali A, et al. Evaluation of recombinant human erythropoietin to facilitate autologous blood donation before surgery in anaemic patients with cancer of the gastrointestinal tract. Br J Surg 1995;82:1637–1640.
98. Kulier AH, Gombotz H, Fuchs G, Vuckovic U, Metzler H. Subcutaneous recombinant human erythropoietin and autologous blood donation before coronary artery bypass surgery. Anesth Analg 1993;76:102–106.
99. Hyllner M, Avall A, Swolin B, Bengtson JP, Bengtsson A. Autologous blood transfusion in radical hysterectomy with and without erythropoietin therapy. Obstet Gynecol 2002;99:757–762.
100. Rau B, Schlag PM, Willeke F, Herfarth C, Stephan P, Franke W. Increased autologous blood donation in rectal cancer by recombinant human erythropoietin (rhEPO). Eur J Cancer 1998;34:992–998.
101. Avall A, Hyllner M, Bengtson JP, Carlsson L, Bengtsson A. Recombinant human erythropoietin in preoperative autologous blood donation did not influence the haemoglobin recovery after surgery. Acta Anaesthesiol Scand 2003;47:687–692.
102. De Pree C, Mermillod B, Hoffmeyer P, Beris P. Recombinant human erythropoietin as adjuvant treatment for autologous blood donation in elective surgery with large blood needs (≥ 5 units): a randomized study. Transfusion 1997;37:708–714.
103. Cazenave JP, Irrmann C, Waller C, et al. Epoetin alfa facilitates presurgical autologous blood donation in non-anaemic patients scheduled for orthopaedic or cardiovascular surgery. Eur J Anaesthesiol 1997;14:432–442.
104. Couvret C, Laffon M, Baud A, Payen V, Burdin P, Fusciardi J. A restrictive use of both autologous donation and recombinant human erythropoietin is an efficient policy for primary total hip or knee arthroplasty. Anesth Analg 2004;99:262–271.
105. Consensus conference. Fresh-frozen plasma: indications and risks. JAMA 1985;253:551–553.
106. Giordano GF, Rivers SL, Chung GK, et al. Autologous platelet-rich plasma in cardiac surgery: effect on intraoperative and postoperative transfusion requirements. Ann Thorac Surg 1988;46:416–419.
107. Harker LA, Malpass TW, Branson HE, Hessel EA, Slichter SJ. Mechanism of abnormal bleeding in patients undergoing cardiopulmonary bypass: acquired transient platelet dysfunction associated with selective alpha-granule release. Blood 1980;56:824–834.
108. Boldt J, von Bormann B, Kling D, Jacobi M, Moosdorf R, Hempelmann G. Preoperative plasmapheresis in patients undergoing cardiac surgery procedures. Anesthesiology 1990;72:282–288.
109. Davies GG, Wells DG, Mabee TM, Sadler R, Melling NJ. Platelet-leukocyte plasmapheresis attenuates the deleterious effects of cardiopulmonary bypass. Ann Thorac Surg 1992;53:274–277.
110. DelRossi AJ, Cernaianu AC, Vertrees RA, et al. Platelet-rich plasma reduces postoperative blood loss after cardiopulmonary bypass. J Thorac Cardiovasc Surg 1990;100:281–286.
111. Tobe CE, Vocelka C, Sepulvada R, et al. Infusion of autologous platelet rich plasma does not reduce blood loss and product use after coronary artery bypass. J Thorac Cardiovasc Surg 1993;105:1007–1014.
112. Ereth MH, Oliver WC, Beynen FMK, et al. Autologous platelet-rich plasma does not reduce transfusion of homologous blood products in patients undergoing repeat valvular surgery. Anesthesiology 1993;79:540–547.
113. Wickey GS, Keifer JC, Larach DR, Diaz MR, Williams DR. Heparin resistance after intraoperative platelet-rich plasma harvesting. J Thorac Cardiovasc Surg 1992;103:1172–1176.
114. Carless PA, Rubens FD, Anthony DM, O'Connell D, Henry DA. Platelet-rich plasmapheresis for minimising perioperative allogeneic blood transfusion. Cochrane Database Syst Rev 2003;CD004172.
115. Greenwalt TJ. Autologous and aged blood donors. JAMA 1987;257:1220–1221.
116. Silvergleid AJ. Safety and effectiveness of predeposit autologous transfusions in preteen and adolescent children. JAMA 1987;257:3403–3404.
117. Kruskall MS, Leonard S, Klapholz H. Autologous blood donation during pregnancy: analysis of safety and blood utilization. Obstet Gynecol 1987;70:938–941.
118. McVay PA, Hoag RW, Hoag MS, Toy PT. Safety and use of autologous blood donation during the third trimester of pregnancy. Am J Obstet Gynecol 1989;160:1479–1486.
119. Goldfinger D, Capon S, Czer L, et al. Safety and efficacy of preoperative donation of blood for autologous use by patients with end-stage heart or lung disease who are awaiting organ transplantation. Transfusion 1993;33:336–340.
120. Popovsky MA, Whitaker B, Arnold NL. Severe outcomes of allogeneic and autologous blood donation: frequency and characterization. Transfusion 1995;35:734–737.
121. Kasper SM, Gerlich W, Buzello W. Preoperative red cell production in patients undergoing weekly autologous blood donation. Transfusion 1997;37:1058–1062.
122. Kickler TS, Spivak JL. Effect of repeated whole blood donations on serum immunoreactive erythropoietin levels in autologous donors. JAMA 1988;260:65–67.
123. Goodnough LT, Price TH, Rudnick S, Soegiarso RW. Preoperative red cell production in patients undergoing aggressive autologous blood phlebotomy with and without erythropoietin therapy. Transfusion 1992;32:441–445.
124. Brugnara C, Chambers LA, Malynn E, Goldberg MA, Kruskall MS. Red blood cell regeneration induced by subcutaneous recombinant erythropoietin: iron-deficient erythropoiesis in iron-replete subjects. Blood 1993;81:956–964.
125. Rutherford CJ, Schneider TJ, Dempsey H, Kirn DH, Brugnara C, Goldberg MA. Efficacy of different dosing regimens for recombinant human erythropoietin in a simulated perisurgical setting: the importance of iron availability in optimizing response. Am J Med 1994;96:139–145.
126. Smith KJ, James DS, Hunt WC, McDonough W, Quintana R. A randomized, double-blind comparison of donor tolerance of 400 mL, 200 mL, and sham red cell donation. Transfusion 1996;36:674–680.
127. Hocker P. Red cell apheresis in autologous preoperative blood donation. Transfus Apher Sci 2001;24:75–78.
128. Monsen ER, Critchlow CW, Finch CA, Donohue DM. Iron balance in super donors. Transfusion 1983;23:221–225.
129. Lieden G, Hoglund S, Ehn L. Iron supplement to blood donors. II: Effect of continuous iron supply. Acta Med Scand 1975;197:37–41.
130. Weisbach V, Skoda P, Rippel R, et al. Oral or intravenous iron as an adjuvant to autologous blood donation in elective surgery: a randomized, controlled study. Transfusion 1999;39:465–472.

131. Wilson JD, Utz DC, Taswell HF. Autotransfusion during transurethral resection of the prostate: technique and preliminary clinical evaluation. Mayo Clin Proc 1969;44:374–386.
132. Long GW, Glover JL, Bendick PJ, et al. Cell washing versus immediate reinfusion of intraoperatively shed blood during abdominal aortic aneurysm repair. Am J Surg 1993;166:97–102.
133. Williamson KR, Taswell HF. Intraoperative blood salvage: a review. Transfusion 1991;31:662–675.
134. O'Hara PJ, Hertzer NR, Santilli PH, Beven EG. Intraoperative autotransfusion during abdominal aortic reconstruction. Am J Surg 1983;145:215–220.
135. Aaron RK, Beazley RM, Riggle GC. Hematologic integrity after intraoperative allotransfusion: comparison with bank blood. Arch Surg 1974;108:831–837.
136. Brener BJ, Raines JK, Darling RC. Intraoperative autotransfusion in abdominal aortic resections. Arch Surg 1973;107:78–84.
137. Ansell J, Parrilla N, King M, et al. Survival of autotransfused red blood cells recovered from the surgical field during cardiovascular operations. J Thorac Cardiovasc Surg 1982;84:387–391.
138. Buth J, Raines JK, Kolodny GM, Darling RC. Effect of intraoperative autotransfusion on red cell mass and red cell survival. Surg Forum 1975;26:276–278.
139. Stillman RM, Wrezlewicz WW, Stanczewski BS, Chapa L, Fox MJ, Sawyer PN. The haematological hazards of autotransfusion. Br J Surg 1976;63:651–654.
140. Moore EE, Dunn EL, Breslich DJ, Galloway WB. Platelet abnormalities associated with massive autotransfusion. J Trauma 1980;20:1052–1056.
141. Griffith LD, Billman GF, Daily PO, Lane TA. Apparent coagulopathy caused by infusion of shed mediastinal blood and its prevention by washing of the infusate. Ann Thorac Surg 1989;47:400–406.
142. Dorang LA, Klebanoff G, Kemmerer WT. Autotransfusion in long-segment spinal fusion: an experimental model to demonstrate the efficacy of salvaging blood contaminated with bone fragments and marrow. Am J Surg 1972;123:686–688.
143. Bennett SH, Geelhoed GW, Terrill RE, Hoye RC. Pulmonary effects of autotransfused blood: a comparison of fresh autologous and stored blood with blood retrieved from the pleural cavity in an in situ lung perfusion mode. Am J Surg 1973;125:696–702.
144. Umlas J, O'Neill TP. Heparin removal in an autotransfusor device. Transfusion 1981;21:70–73.
145. Paravicini D, Thys J, Hein H. Use of neomycin-bacitracin irrigating solution with intraoperative autotransfusions during orthopedic operations. Arzneimittelforschung 1983;33:997–999.
146. Wollinsky KH, Oethinger M, Buchele M, Kluger P, Puhl W, Mehrkens HH. Autotransfusion bacterial contamination during hip arthroplasty and efficacy of cefuroxime prophylaxis: a randomized controlled study of 40 patients. Acta Orthop Scand 1997;68:225–230.
147. Rumisek JD, Weddle RL. Autotransfusion in penetrating abdominal trauma. In Hauer JM, Thurer RL, Dawson RB (eds). Autotransfusion. New York, Elsevier, 1981, pp 105–113.
148. Timberlake GA, McSwain NE. Autotransfusion of blood contaminated by enteric contents: a potentially life-saving measure in the massively hemorrhaging trauma patient? J Trauma 1988;28:855–857.
149. Ozmen V, McSwain NE Jr, Nichols RL, Smith J, Flint LM. Autotransfusion of potentially culture-positive blood (CPB) in abdominal trauma: preliminary data from a prospective study. J Trauma 1992;32:36–39.
150. Yaw PB, Sentany M, Link WJ, Wahle WM, Glover JL. Tumor cells carried through autotransfusion: contraindication to intraoperative blood recovery? JAMA 1975;231:490–491.
151. Lane TA. The effect of storage on the metastatic potential of tumor cells collected in autologous blood: an animal model. Transfusion 1989;29:418–420.
152. Duncan SE, Klebanoff G, Rogers W. A clinical experience with intra operative autotransfusion. Ann Surg 1974;180:296–304.
153. Linden JV, Kaplan HS, Murphy MT. Fatal air embolism due to perioperative blood recovery. Anesth Analg 1997;84:422–426.
154. Lennon RL, Hosking MP, Gray JR, Klassen RA, Popovsky MA, Warner MA. The effects of intraoperative blood salvage and induced hypotension on transfusion requirements during spinal surgical procedures. Mayo Clin Proc 1987;62:1090–1094.
155. Kruger LM, Colbert JM. Intraoperative autologous transfusion in children undergoing spinal surgery. J Pediatr Orthop 1985;5:330–332.
156. Bovill DF, Moulton CW, Jackson WST, Hensen JK, Barcellos RW. The efficacy of intraoperative autologous transfusion in major orthopedic surgery: a regression analysis. Orthopedics 1986;9:1403–1407.
157. Hallett JW Jr, Popovsky M, Ilstrup D. Minimizing blood transfusions during abdominal aortic surgery: recent advances in rapid autotransfusion. J Vasc Surg 1987;5:601–606.
158. Keeling MM, Gray LA, Brink MA, Hillerich VK, Bland KI. Intraoperative autotransfusion: experience in 725 consecutive cases. Ann Surg 1983;197:536–541.
159. McCarthy PM, Popovsky MA, Schaff HV, et al. Effect of blood conservation efforts in cardiac operations at the Mayo Clinic. Mayo Clin Proc 1988;63:225–229.
160. Dzik WH, Jenkins R. Use of intraoperative blood salvage during orthotopic liver transplantation. Arch Surg 1985;120:946–948.
161. Van Voorst SJ, Peters TG, Williams JW, Vera SR, Britt LG. Autotransfusion in hepatic transplantation. Am Surg 1985;51:623–626.
162. Williamson KR, Taswell HF, Rettke SR, Krom RAF. Intraoperative autologous transfusion: its role in orthotopic liver transplantation. Mayo Clin Proc 1989;64:340–345.
163. Reul GJ Jr, Solis RT, Greenberg SD, Mattox KL, Whisennand HH. Experience with autotransfusion in the surgical management of trauma. Surgery 1974;76:546–555.
164. Smith RS, Meister RK, Tsoi EK, Bohman HR. Laparoscopically guided blood salvage and autotransfusion in splenic trauma: a case report. J Trauma 1993;34:313–314.
165. Rebarber A, Lonser R, Jackson S, Copel JA, Sipes S. The safety of intraoperative autologous blood collection and autotransfusion during cesarean section. Am J Obstet Gynecol 1998;179:715–720.
166. Merrill BS, Mitts DL, Rogers W, Weinberg PC. Autotransfusion: intraoperative use in ruptured ectopic pregnancy. J Reprod Med 1980;24:14–16.
167. Klimberg I, Sirois R, Wajsman Z, Baker J. Intraoperative autotransfusion in urologic oncology. Arch Surg 1986;121:1326–1329.
168. Witte CL, Esser MJ, Rappaport WD. Updating the management of salvageable splenic injury. Ann Surg 1992;215:261–265.
169. Spence RK, Alexander JB, DelRossi AJ, et al. Transfusion guidelines for cardiovascular surgery: lessons learned from operations in Jehovah's Witnesses. J Vasc Surg 1992;16:825–831.
170. Johnson RG, Rosenkrantz KR, Preston RA, Hopkins C, Daggett WM. The efficacy of postoperative autotransfusion in patients undergoing cardiac operations. Ann Thorac Surg 1983;36:173–179.
171. Semkiw LB, Schurman DJ, Goodman SB, Woolson ST. Postoperative blood salvage using the Cell Saver after total joint arthroplasty. J Bone Joint Surg Am 1989;71:823–827.
172. Reiner DS, Tortolani AJ. Postoperative peritoneal blood salvage with autotransfusion after hepatic trauma. Surg Gynecol Obstet 1991;173:501–504.
173. Glover JL, Broadie TA. Intraoperative autotransfusion. World J Surg 1987;11:60–64.
174. Schmidt H, Lund JO, Nielsen SL. Autotransfused shed mediastinal blood has normal erythrocyte survival. Ann Thorac Surg 1996;62:105–108.
175. Jensen CM, Pilegaard R, Hviid K, Nielsen JD, Nielsen HJ. Quality of reinfused drainage blood after total knee arthroplasty. J Arthroplasty 1999;14:312–318.
176. Schmidt H, Bendtzen K, Mortensen PE. The inflammatory cytokine response after autotransfusion of shed mediastinal blood. Acta Anaesthesiol Scand 1998;42:558–564.
177. Mottl-Link S, Russlies M, Klinger M, Seyfarth M, Ascherl R, Gradinger R. Erythrocytes and proinflammatory mediators in wound drainage. Vox Sang 1998;75:205–211.
178. Hand GC, Henderson M, Mace P, Sherif N, Newman JH, Goldie DJ. Methyl methacrylate levels in unwashed salvage blood following unilaterial total knee arthroplasty. J Arthroplasty 1998;13:576–579.
179. Woda R, Tetzlaff JE. Upper airway oedema following autologous blood transfusion from a wound drainage system. Can J Anaesth 1992;390:290–292.
180. Dich-Nielsen JO, Rajan RM, Jensen JJ. An anaphylactoid reaction following infusion of salvaged unwashed drain blood. Can J Anaesth 1998;45:189.
181. Faris PM, Ritter MA, Keating EM, Valeri CR. Unwashed filtered shed blood collected after knee and hip arthroplasties: a source of autologous red blood cells. J Bone Joint Surg Am 1991;73:1169–1178.
182. Klebanoff G. Early clinical experience with a disposable unit for the intraoperative salvage and reinfusion of blood loss (intraoperative autotransfusion). Am J Surg 1970;120:718–722.
183. Schmidt H, Mortensen PE, Folsgaard SL, Jensen EA. Cardiac enzymes and autotransfusion of shed mediastinal blood after mycoardial revascularization. Ann Thorac Surg 1997;63:1288–1292.
184. Nguyen DM, Gilfix BM, Dennis F, et al. Impact of transfusion of mediastinal shed blood on serum levels of cardiac enzymes. Ann Thorac Surg 1996;62:109–114.
185. Kilgore ML, Pacifico AD. Shed mediastinal blood transfusion after cardiac operations: a cost-effectiveness analysis. Ann Thorac Surg 1998;65:1248–1254.

186. Gannon DM, Lombardi AV, Mallory TH, Vaughn BK, Finney CR, Niemcryk S. An evaluation of the efficacy of postoperative blood salvage after total joint arthroplasty. J Arthroplasty 1991;1:109–114.
187. Majkowski RS, Currie IC, Newman JH. Postoperative collection and reinfusion of autologous blood in total knee arthroplasty. Ann R Coll Surg Engl 1991;73:381–384.
188. Umlas J, Foster RR, Dalal SA, O'Leary SM, Garcia L, Kruskall MS. Red cell loss following orthopedic surgery: the case against postoperative blood salvage. Transfusion 1994;34:402–406.
189. Martin JW, Whiteside LA, Milliano MT, Reedy ME. Postoperative blood retrieval and transfusion in cementless total knee arthroplasty. J Arthroplasty 1992;7:205–210.
190. Cooley DA, Beall AC Jr, Grondin P. Open-heart operations with disposable oxygenators, 5 per cent dextrose prime, and normothermia. Surgery 1962;52:713–719.
191. Petry AF, Jost T, Sievers H. Reduction of homologous blood requirements by blood-pooling at the onset of cardiopulmonary bypass. J Thorac Cardiovasc Surg 1994;107:1210–1214.
192. Brecher ME, Rosenfeld M. Mathematical and computer modeling of acute normovolemic hemodilution. Transfusion 1994;34:176–179.
193. Weiskopf RB. Mathematical analysis of isovolemic hemodilution indicates that it can decrease the need for allogeneic blood transfusion. Transfusion 1995;35:37–41.
194. Monk TG, Goodnough LT, Brecher ME, et al. Acute normovolemic hemodilution can replace preoperative autologous blood donation as a standard of care for autologous blood procurement in radical prostatectomy. Anesth Analg 1997;85:953–958.
195. Milam JD, Austin SF, Nihill MR, Keats AS, Cooley DA. Use of sufficient hemodilution to prevent coagulopathies following surgical correction of cyanotic heart disease. J Thorac Cardiovasc Surg 1985;89:623–629.
196. Ness PM, Bourke DL, Walsh PC. A randomized trial of perioperative hemodilution versus transfusion of preoperatively deposited autologous blood in elective surgery. Transfusion 1992;32:226–230.
197. Johnson LB, Plotkin JS, Kuo PC. Reduced transfusion requirements during major hepatic resection with use of intraoperative isovolemic hemodilution. Am J Surg 1998;176:608–611.
198. Pliam MB, McGoon DC, Tarhan S. Failure of transfusion of autologous whole blood to reduce banked-blood requirements in open-heart surgical patients. J Thorac Cardiovasc Surg 1975;70:338–343.
199. Sherman MM, Dobnik DB, Dennis RC, Berger RL. Autologous blood transfusion during cardiopulmonary bypass. Chest 1976;70:592–595.
200. Weisel RD, Charlesworth DC, Mickleborough LL, et al. Limitations of blood conservation. J Thorac Cardiovasc Surg 1984;88:26–38.
201. Goodnough LT, Monk TG, Brecher ME. Acute normovolemic hemodilution should replace the preoperative donation of autologous blood as a method of autologous-blood procurement. Transfusion 1998;38:473–476.
202. Rottman G, Ness PM. Acute normovolemic hemodilution is a legitimate alternative to allogeneic blood transfusion. Transfusion 1998;38:477–480.
203. Monk TG, Goodnough LT, Brecher ME, Colberg JW, Andriole GL, Catalona WJ. A prospective randomized comparison of three blood conservation strategies for radical prostatectomy. Anesthesiology 1999; 91:24–33.
204. Brecher ME, Goodnough LT, Monk T. Where does preoperative erythropoietin therapy count? A mathematical perspective. Transfusion 1999;39:392–395.
205. Sowade O, Warnke H, Scigalla P, et al. Avoidance of allogeneic blood transfusions by treatment with epoetin beta (recombinant human erythropoietin) in patients undergoing open-heart surgery. Blood 1997;89:411–418.
206. de Andrade JR, Jove M, Landon G, Frei D, Guifoyle M, Young DC. Baseline hemoglobin as a predictor of risk of transfusion and response to epoetin alfa in orthopedic surgery patients. Am J Orthop 1996;25:533–542.
207. Faris PM, Spence RK, Larholt KM, Sampson AR, Frei D. The predictive power of baseline hemoglobin for transfusion risk in surgery patients. Orthopedics 1999;22(Suppl 1):S135–S140.
208. Dunne JR, Malone D, Tracy JK, Gannon C, Napolitano LM. Perioperative anemia: an independent risk factor for infection, mortality, and resource utilization in surgery. J Surg Res 2002;102:237–244.
209. Koscielny J, von Tempelhoff GF, Ziemer S, et al. A practical concept for preoperative management of patients with impaired primary hemostasis. Clin Appl Thromb Hemost 2004;10:155–166.
210. McDonald SB, Renna M, Spitznagel EL, et al. Preoperative use of enoxaparin increases the risk of postoperative bleeding and re-exploration in cardiac surgery patients. J Cardiothorac Vasc Anesth 2005;19:4–10.
211. Shander A. Surgery without blood. Crit Care Med 2003;31(Suppl 12): S708–S714.
212. Thompson GE, Miller RD, Stevens WC, Murray WR. Hypotensive anesthesia for total hip arthroplasty: a study of blood loss and organ function (brain, heart, liver, and kidney). Anesthesiology 1978; 48:91–96.
213. Niemi TT, Pitkanen M, Syrjala M, Rosenberg PH. Comparison of hypotensive epidural anaesthesia and spinal anaesthesia on blood loss and coagulation during and after total hip arthroplasty. Acta Anaesthesiol Scand 2000;44:457–464.
214. Shapira Y, Gurman G, Artru AA, et al. Combined hemodilution and hypotension monitored with jugular bulb oxygen saturation, EEG, and ECG decreases transfusion volume and length of ICU stay for major orthopedic surgery. J Clin Anesth 1997;9:643–649.
215. Karakaya D, Ustun E, Tur A, et al. Acute normovolemic hemodilution and nitroglycerin-induced hypotension: comparative effects on tissue oxygenation and allogeneic blood transfusion requirement in total hip arthroplasty. J Clin Anesth 1999;11:368–374.
216. Bock M, Muller J, Bach A, Bohrer H, Martin E, Motsch J. Effects of preinduction and intraoperative warming during major laparotomy. Br J Anaesth 1998;80:159–163.
217. Johansson T, Lisander B, Ivarsson I. Mild hypothermia does not increase blood loss during total hip arthroplasty. Acta Anaesthesiol Scand 1999;43:1005–1010.
218. Schmied H, Kurz A, Sessler DI, Kozek S, Reiter A. Mild hypothermia increases blood loss and transfusion requirements during total hip arthroplasty. Lancet 1996;347:289–292.
219. Stensrud PE, Nuttall GA, de Castro MA, et al. A prospective, randomized study of cardiopulmonary bypass temperature and blood transfusion. Ann Thorac Surg 1999;67:711–715.
220. Birdi I, Regragui IA, Izzat MB, Bryan AJ, Angelini GD. Effects of cardiopulmonary perfusion temperature: a randomized, controlled trial. Ann Thorac Surg 1995;60:747.
221. Smoller BR, Kruskall MS. Phlebotomy for diagnostic laboratory tests in adults: pattern of use and effect on transfusion requirements. N Engl J Med 1986;314:1233–1235.

Chapter 31

Blood Substitutes: Basic Principles and Practical Aspects

Robert M. Winslow

INTRODUCTION

Replacement of blood after acute loss has two main goals: restitution of blood volume and delivery of oxygen to tissues. In contrast, administration of red blood cells in chronic anemia or hypoxia is aimed only at restitution of oxygen delivery to tissues. Non-oxygen-carrying solutions such as saline, Ringer's lactate, albumin, dextran, and the starches are widely used to replace lost blood volume in surgery and trauma, and they can be used satisfactorily to expand blood volume. The term *red blood cell substitutes* (or just *blood substitutes*) usually refers to oxygen-carrying solutions that can both expand the blood volume and oxygenate tissues. These solutions contain a delivery system for oxygen—commonly modified hemoglobin or perfluorocarbon emulsions—and they are intended to carry out the primary function of red blood cells: transport of oxygen to tissues. To be both clinically and economically useful, such solutions should be free of antigens (i.e., not necessary to crossmatch), sterile, and have a long shelf life.

Development of a blood substitute has been an elusive goal: for centuries, an alternative to allogeneic blood for transfusion has been sought by scientists, the military, and industry. Early attempts included the use of milk, wine, gum, and red blood cell hemolysates.[1] In the modern era (since about 1965), three general types of products have been under development: modified hemoglobin solutions, perfluorocarbon emulsions, and lipid vesicle–encapsulated hemoglobin. None is as yet approved for clinical use.

The current forces driving the development of red blood cell substitutes are the perceived danger of transfusion of allogeneic blood (Table 31–1) as well as the diminishing numbers of donors of allogeneic blood. In fact, blood is safer now than it ever has been.[2] However, the aggregate risks listed in Table 31–1 are frightening to many patients, their families, and their doctors, and the demand for a safe and efficacious alternative is increasing. Beyond the risks listed in Table 31–1, in regions of the world where the frequency of human immunodeficiency virus infection is high, development of these solutions would be particularly important. Furthermore, the risks listed in Table 31–1 are for the United States; in other parts of the world, additional risks include contamination of blood with parasites, prions, other retroviruses, tick-borne illnesses, and malaria. Bacterial infections represent a growing risk as the length of time blood can be stored is increased, because the risk of contamination is proportionate to storage time.

Because of the risks of allogeneic blood transfusion, and because of the large markets that could be generated for red blood cell substitutes, considerable efforts have been expended by industry and academia to develop safe products. It is likely that red blood cell substitutes will find their way into clinical practice within the next decade. What is still not clear is what their clinical indications will be.

PRINCIPLES

It is not possible to reproduce the human red blood cell. Therefore, in designing a solution that can be used as an alternative, consideration must be given to the properties of the red cell that are critical and that can be simulated by a synthetic product. Some of these are enumerated below.

Oxygen Transport

Clearly, a red cell substitute must transport oxygen, but must a substitute transport oxygen in the same way as red blood cells do? Oxygen affinity and cooperativity of cell-free or encapsulated hemoglobin may be very different from that of red blood cells. Perfluorocarbons carry oxygen physically dissolved, rather than chemically bound, and therefore the dissociation curve is linear. Whether these factors are important, physiologically or clinically, is still not understood well, and assumptions are deeply rooted. Only extensive clinical experience will allow definite conclusions to be drawn.

Plasma Retention

The normal red blood cell half-life is about 30 days. However, the plasma half-life of cell-free hemoglobin may be only 12 to 24 hours, and that of encapsulated or surface-modified hemoglobin and perfluorocarbon emulsions may be 24 to 48 hours. Are these times clinically useful? If the effect of a red blood cell substitute is so short that a transfusion with allogeneic blood is only delayed rather than eliminated, then the usefulness of the product may be diminished.

Efficacy

It will be necessary to demonstrate efficacy for any red blood cell substitute to be used clinically. At present, it is taken as a matter of faith that a solution carrying oxygen will be more useful than one with no oxygen carrier, if it is without side

Table 31–1 Estimated Risk of Transfusion Transmission of Viral Agents

Virus	Risk Per Unit Transfused
HIV-1 and -2	1:2,000,000–3,000,000
Hepatitis B	1:100,000–200,000
Hepatitis C	1:1,000,000–2,000,000
HTLV-I and -II	1:641,000 (cellular components)
Parvovirus B19	1:20,000 (most recipients immune)
West Nile virus	Range 1:10,000 to 1:150 depending on region of epidemic
Bacterial contamination	1:5,000,000

Data from Klein HG. Transfusion medicine. In Blood Substitutes. Winslow R (ed). London, Elsevier, 2006, pp 17–33.

effects. However, conclusive demonstrations will be necessary because no red blood cell substitute currently being developed is without side effects. For example, if a particular substitute increases systemic pressure and vascular resistance (as many hemoglobin-based solutions do), this property could counteract any increase in oxygen transported. At present, the U.S. Food and Drug Administration (FDA) has accepted reduced use of allogeneic blood as a valid end point for clinical testing and licensure, but whether this is sufficient for widespread clinical use by physicians will not be known until products are actually on the market.[3]

Toxicity

No drug is without toxicity or side effects, and blood substitutes are no exception. Unmodified hemoglobin has vasoconstrictor properties that could limit its use in shock and trauma and in patients with ischemic disease. Lipid vesicles and perfluorocarbon emulsions stimulate macrophages to elaborate cytokines that can produce diverse effects, including fever, flulike symptoms, and thrombocytopenia.

Commercial Viability

A red blood cell substitute should be competitive with allogeneic red blood cells in effect, toxicity, and cost. The cost of providing human red blood cells for transfusion is complex and difficult to determine with accuracy, but it is probably in the range of $250 to $500 per unit. The technology required for the production of red blood cell substitutes is complex and possibly expensive, but the final cost of a product whose safety and efficacy are equivalent to those of banked blood will need to be in the same range.

PRODUCTS

Hemoglobin-Based Products

The red blood cell substitute products that have gained the most attention are based on hemoglobin, a complex molecule consisting of four polypeptide chains, each one made up of about 140 amino acids. Normally, hemoglobin is packaged in the red blood cell; when free in solution, it is fragile: the oxygen-binding iron atom tends to oxidize, it is unstable and toxic, and is excreted by the kidneys as the subunits dissociate. Over the years, the strategy for making a hemoglobin-based red blood cell substitute has been based on crosslinking hemoglobin to correct these problems.[4]

Hemoglobin has the desirable property of high capacity to bind oxygen and to release it cooperatively. However, free in solution, hemoglobin has several unique properties:

1. Its oxygen affinity is high because outside the red blood cell the allosteric effectors, 2,3-diphosphoglycerate and adenosine triphosphate, for example, are not present.
2. Its effectiveness as an oxygen carrier is limited because it dissociates into half-molecules (dimers). Haptoglobin is rapidly saturated, and excess dimers are quickly removed from the circulation by the kidney after filtration in the glomerulus.
3. Once it is filtered, a high concentration of protein in the renal tubules can cause tubular obstruction, oxidative damage, and consequent renal failure.
4. Cell-free hemoglobin binds nitric oxide, an endothelium-derived relaxing factor that may contribute to vasoconstriction.
5. Iron, when released from hemoglobin, can promote the formation of toxic oxygen radicals and bacterial growth.

Thus, to be an effective oxygen carrier in the cell-free state, hemoglobin must be chemically modified. Whether all these features must be resolved completely for a product to be useful is uncertain. Reactions currently used in the production of hemoglobin-based red cell substitutes employ chemical modification at one or more sites on the surface of the protein.[5] The dimensions and reactivity of the crosslinking reagents determine differences in the reactions. Because the function of hemoglobin in binding and releasing oxygen is intricately connected to a structural transition, it is not surprising that the oxygen half-saturation pressure and yield are variable. Even small differences among structures of the reagents can yield products with quite different properties. In addition, the conditions of the reaction are important, not only in regard to the state of ligation (i.e., oxygen saturation) but also the presence of agents or molecules that lack or compete for certain reactive sites.

A further complication of these reactions is that many nonhemoglobin proteins, copurified with hemoglobin, contain reactive groups and may also be modified to produce new, potentially toxic contaminants. It is understandable that it has been difficult to produce "pure" modified hemoglobin for toxicity studies when most processes start with relatively crude "stroma-free" hemoglobin.[6] One classification of the various types of modified hemoglobins is given in Table 31–2.

An illustrative example of a crosslinked hemoglobin is a product studied intensively by the U.S. Army and numerous academic laboratories.[7] Crosslinking of hemoglobin isolated from outdated human blood was carried out with bis(3,5-dibromosalicyl)fumarate (DBBF),[8] and it was called αα-Hb by the Army and DCLHb (proposed trade name HemAssist) by Baxter Healthcare, which produced it in commercial quantities. The reaction results in a 4-carbon covalent link between adjacent α-chains at position 99 (Lys $\alpha_1$99–Lys $\alpha_2$99) (Fig. 31–1). This covalently crosslinked hemoglobin cannot break down into subunits in the circulation and therefore cannot be excreted as filtered globin chains. Since αα-Hb was developed by the Army, its properties, toxicity,

Table 31–2 Classes of Hemoglobin-Based Red Cell Substitutes

Class	Examples (see also Table 31-3)	Molecular Radius* (nm)	Intravascular Persistence (h)	Oncotic Pressure	Viscosity	Vasoactivity
Crosslinked tetramers	Diaspirin crosslinked hemoglobin (DCLHb) αα-Hb rHb1.1 (Optro)	2.7	~12	Low	Low	Marked
Polymerized tetramers	HemoPure Hemolink PolyHem e	4.9	~12–24	Low	Low	Moderate
Surface-modified tetramers	Pyridoxalated hemoglobin polyoxyethylene Polyethylene glycol–hemoglobin MP4	~10	~24–48	Moderate-high	Moderate-high	Mild

*Data from Vandegriff K, McCarthy M, Rohlfs R. Winslow R. Colloid osmotic properties of modified hemoglobins: chemically cross-linked versus polyethylene glycol surface–conjugated. Biophys Chem 1997;69:23–30.

and physiologic effects have been reported in the open, peer-reviewed literature.[9] It is therefore a useful model to understand the complexities of the research and development that has taken place over the past 2 decades.

Production of αα-Hb is complex.[10] Stroma-free hemoglobin is separated from red blood cell membranes by osmotic lysis. It is then deoxygenated to achieve the proper molecular conformation for crosslinking, and the 2,3-diphosphoglycerate pocket is blocked reversibly with an allosteric effector. After crosslinking with DBBF, it is heated to pasteurize it and also to remove unreacted hemoglobin, then passed through a series of cross-flow filters. Finally, it is sterilized by filtration through a 0.2-μm filter.

The product has an oxygen equilibrium curve with an oxygen half-saturation pressure under physiologic conditions (i.e., P50) of 28 mm Hg. The degree of cooperativity (the slope of the dissociation curve) is similar to that of blood (Hill coefficient 2.62 for blood, 2.31 for crosslinked hemoglobin), and the Bohr[11] and carbon dioxide[12] effects are essentially intact.

Based on its oxygen equilibrium curve, this product should have in vivo oxygen transport properties similar to those of whole blood; its oxygen equilibrium curve is closer to that of red blood cells than that of other types of red blood cell substitutes (Fig. 31–2). The intravascular persistence is markedly extended in the rat: uncrosslinked hemoglobin has a half-life of about 1.2 hours, and crosslinked hemoglobin has a half-life of about 4.3 hours. In the rabbit, the persistence is longer, approximately 16 hours for crosslinked hemoglobin, for the monkey about 14 hours, and for the pig about 7 hours.[13] No doubt exists that cell-free hemoglobin transports oxygen. Many studies in the literature have demonstrated the ability of hemoglobin solutions to resuscitate animals in lethal hemorrhagic shock.[4]

DCLHb was studied extensively in clinical trials. However, the product was found to be severely vasoactive; it raised blood pressure and increased systemic and pulmonary vascular resistance.[14,15] Phase III clinical trials were disappointing; trials in trauma[16] and in stroke[17] both showed reduced survival in patients who received the product.

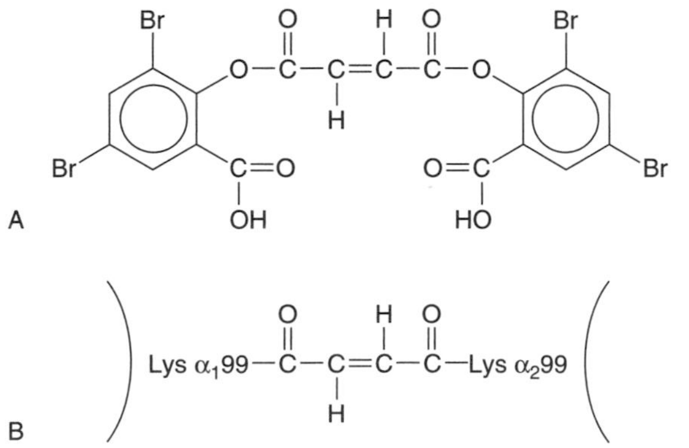

Figure 31–1 Structure of the crosslinker, bis(2,3-dibromosalicyl) fumarate (DBBF; **A**) and crosslinked hemoglobin (**B**). The brominated acetyl groups of the DBBF are leaving groups in the reaction, which results in a 4-carbon bridge between the two α-chain polypeptide subunits of hemoglobin.

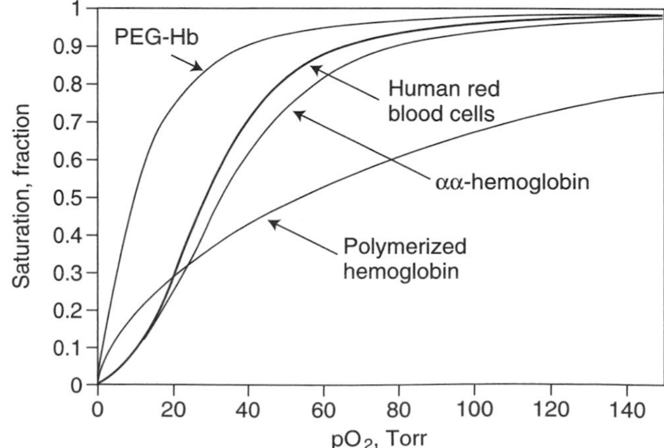

Figure 31–2 Oxygen equilibrium curves for some representative red cell substitutes. Note the large difference between the curves for PEG-Hb, *O*-raffinose polymerized hemoglobin, and red blood cells.

Closely related to αα-hemoglobin is a recombinant product (rHb1.1, Optro) produced in *Escherichia coli*.[18] Starting material for hemoglobin modification can also be produced in transgenic animals.[19] Hemoglobin additionally can be polymerized by means of various polyfunctional reagents to yield molecules with markedly increased molecular weights. One example is human hemoglobin, reacted first with pyridoxal 5′-phosphate and then polymerized with glutaraldehyde.[20] This product has a reduced colloidal osmotic (oncotic) pressure and longer intravascular persistence compared with smaller molecules, but the polymerization reaction is notoriously difficult to control.[21,22]

Large molecules, such as hemoglobin coupled to polyethylene glycol,[23,24] starch,[25] or dextran[26] may have prolonged plasma retention times, may have reduced interactions with the reticuloendothelial systems and may extravasate less readily than smaller molecules. The same result can be achieved by directly linking hemoglobin molecules to create large polymers[27] or by use of naturally occurring large polymers such as found in the earthworm.[28] In addition to reduced extravasation, these large molecules have reduced diffusivity in the plasma, which in turn reduces vasoconstriction by limiting oxygen supply to arterial walls.

Liposome-Encapsulated Hemoglobin

Because hemoglobin is normally packaged inside a membrane, it seems intuitively correct that encapsulated hemoglobin would be the ultimate solution to the red blood cell substitute problem. In 1957, Thomas Chang reported the use of microencapsulated hemoglobin as artificial red blood cells.[29] Since that time, dramatic results have been reported in the complete exchange transfusion of laboratory animals,[30,31] but progress toward development of an artificial red blood cell for human use has been slow because of difficulties with reticuloendothelial and other macrophage stimulation.[32] Other problems include maintaining sterility, limiting hemoglobin oxidation, and the economics of large-scale production.

In the years that have followed Chang's initial descriptions of encapsulated hemoglobin, much work with lipid vesicles (liposomes) has been done. Liposomes have served as models for understanding natural cell membranes. They also have been used investigationally as vehicles for gene transfer, as targeted carriers, for pharmacologic agents, and even as lubricants for degenerated joint surfaces. The most extensively studied liposomes used to encapsulate hemoglobin are composed of phospholipid in combination with cholesterol and other lipids that confer flexibility and stability, such as ganglioside GM_1 or cholesterol.[33] When injected into animals, such liposomes are rapidly coated with immunoglobulin G, albumin, and other opsonins.[34] Newer formulations include the use of surface components such as polyethylene glycol or dextran, which can stabilize the liposomes in the circulation.[35] Hemoglobin vesicles (HbV) are being developed in Japan and may enter clinical trials soon.[36]

The limitations to the development of liposome-encapsulated hemoglobin as a red blood cell substitute are difficulties in stabilizing the final product and the massive scale that would be required to produce a commercial product. The size of most liposome particles is approximately 0.2 to 1.0 μm, too large to be filter-sterilized. In addition, neither the liposome nor its hemoglobin contents can withstand pasteurization temperature without some type of stabilizer. Other potential approaches to the solution of these problems could include polymerizable phospholipids[37] and other polymers.[38]

Perfluorocarbon-Based Products

Fluosol-DA (Fluosol, Green Cross Corp., Osaka, Japan) was approved for marketing by the FDA for use in coronary angioplasty in 1990, but manufacture was discontinued in 1995 and the product was withdrawn for multiple reasons: efficacy was marginal, the product was technically difficult to use, and new developments in coronary angioplasty (the indication for which it was approved) made its use obsolete. Newer perfluorocarbon emulsions were developed by industry that carried more oxygen than did previous products[39]; however, regardless of oxygen capacity, a fundamental difference exists between perfluorocarbon- and hemoglobin-based red blood cell substitutes: oxygen is transported by perfluorocarbons as dissolved gas, whereas hemoglobin carries oxygen chemically bound to the protein itself. Because of the nature of the binding of oxygen by hemoglobin, oxygen is not released until hemoglobin reaches regions of the circulation where pO_2 is low (i.e., ischemic tissue). In contrast, the release of oxygen from perfluorocarbon emulsions is linear with pO_2, which means that the bulk of the dissolved oxygen will be lost from the circulation before the product reaches ischemic or hypoxic tissue. One product, Oxygent (Alliance Pharmaceutical Corp.) is an emulsion of perflubron and egg yolk phospholipid that contains about five times more fluorocarbon than Fluosol-DA does and therefore five times more dissolved oxygen. Oxygent underwent extensive phase 2 clinical testing but in critical phase 3 trials of hemodilution and perioperative autologous blood collection, there was a higher incidence of stroke in treated patients compared with controls.[40] Development of Oxygent was subsequently scaled back, and it is questionable whether trials will continue.

SAFETY

Demonstration of safety of red blood cell substitutes is a critical issue, because the risks of transfusion of allogeneic blood are well known (see Table 31–1). To be used, a substitute should be at least as safe as red blood cells, unless a decisive therapeutic advantage can be demonstrated.

In a review of almost a century of clinical trials with red blood cell substitutes, reported side effects involved renal dysfunction and systemic symptoms (fever, chills, nausea, headache, flushing, vomiting, allergic reactions, tachycardia, bradycardia, hypertension, rigors, low back pain, chest pain, abdominal pain, decreased platelets, and increased partial thromboplastin time).[4] Many of these effects could be explained by the depletion of nitric oxide, in the case of hemoglobin-based products, or by stimulation of macrophages, in the case of liposomes or perfluorocarbon emulsions. Many are smooth muscle effects, and some involve macrophages and platelets. Preclinical animal studies with hemoglobin-based solutions clearly have not been completely successful in predicting human reactions to the products.[41]

Cell-free hemoglobin is widely distributed in the tissues after administration. Studies of the distribution of cross-linked hemoglobin in the intact animal show that significant amounts of hemoglobin are retained in the kidney, spleen, liver, adrenal gland, lung, heart, brain, and muscle well after any hemoglobin is detected in plasma.[42–44] Thus, cell-free hemoglobin is distributed in almost every tissue of the body, and there could be unpredictable or unknown toxic effects. Extensive histologic studies were carried out in animals after exchange transfusion and summarized.[4]

The effect of cell-free hemoglobin of most concern is its known ability to cause vasoconstriction and hypertension. This vasoconstriction can be mediated in part by the reaction of hemoglobin with nitric oxide, an endothelium-derived relaxing factor.[45] Nitric oxide is synthesized from arginine in endothelial (and other) cells by an enzyme, nitric oxide synthase, which produces nitric oxide and citrulline. It binds to a heme group in guanylate cyclase that activates cyclic guanosine monophosphate. Nitric oxide diffuses rapidly out of endothelial cells into the vessel lumen, the interstitial space, and smooth muscle cells, where it binds to a heme group in guanylate cyclase, activating cyclic guanosine monophosphate and moving calcium from the unbound to bound state. The result is smooth muscle relaxation. Nitric oxide also stimulates platelets and polymorphonuclear leukocytes and macrophages. Hemoglobin binds nitric oxide very tightly, more tightly in fact than it binds oxygen, whether hemoglobin is in the red blood cell or free in solution.[46] The reaction is virtually irreversible. Whether this interaction of hemoglobin with nitric oxide will limit clinical usefulness of hemoglobin-based red blood cell substitutes remains to be determined.

Nitric oxide binding by cell-free hemoglobin is not the sole explanation for its vasoconstrictor activity, however.[47] In addition to its effect as a scavenger of nitric oxide, cell-free hemoglobin may induce vasoconstriction by disrupting normal autoregulation of vascular tone. In other words, it may make oxygen so readily available to regulatory arterioles that reflexive vasoconstriction could occur that paradoxically limits blood flow.[48,49] This concept is suggested by direct observation in the microcirculation[50] and has led to new design strategies for cell-free red blood cell substitutes.[51] Perfluorocarbon emulsions have the most extensive history of use in humans. Fluosol-DA was approved by the FDA for use in coronary angioplasty and therefore was given to many human patients. Similar formulations have been used on the battlefield in China and Afghanistan, although data are generally not available. Perfluorocarbon emulsions have also been tested in humans as imaging agents. The principal toxicity of perfluorocarbon emulsions appears to be in their stimulation of macrophages.[52,53] This can result in pulmonary hypertension and elaboration of thromboxane in swine and could lead to nonspecific symptoms such as fever, chills, and flulike symptoms in humans.

Biocompatibility studies with liposome-encapsulated hemoglobin have been generally favorable,[31] but such products tend to be removed from the circulation by the phagocytic cells of the reticuloendothelial system.[54] This situation leads to significant enlargement of the liver and spleen. Current research is aimed at prolongation of the intravascular persistence to minimize this problem.[55]

EFFICACY

It seems intuitively obvious that a plasma expander that carries oxygen would be superior to one that does not, and experimental proof of this concept should be relatively straightforward. However, the problem of efficacy can be appreciated by considering the difficulties in showing efficacy for red blood cell transfusions. The problem is a lack of clear end points: no single measure of oxygen transport is accurate and easily obtainable. It may be possible to show improved clinical outcome after transfusion of red blood cells to patients with extremely low hematocrits, but the bulk of allogeneic blood is given intraoperatively in response to blood loss and hemodynamic instability, not severe anemia.

Most demonstrations of efficacy in animals have been either by exchange transfusions with test material or by resuscitation from shock. Resuscitation from shock is exceedingly complex, however, and the most urgent requirement is for volume replacement.[56] Clinical trials involving trauma patients are particularly difficult to design because of the problems of controls and informed consent. Future clinical trials will most likely be aimed at, for example, reduced use of allogeneic blood, rather than at specific oxygen transport parameters, which may be controversial, at best. For example, one trial with Fluosol-DA during surgical procedures showed that its use did not reduce the need for allogeneic blood transfusions in the postoperative period.[57]

CLINICAL TRIALS

Early trials with various cell-free hemoglobin solutions were reviewed and showed an array of side effects involving every organ of the body.[4] However, most of these are mild or reversible, and only one death in more than 211 patients was reported in the early literature; this patient was terminally ill and would likely have died even without the administration of hemoglobin.[58]

Certain red blood cell substitute products are in various stages of advanced clinical trials (Table 31–3). The greatest concern for hemoglobin-based products is that the known vasoactivity of the solutions could lead to hypertension or underperfusion of ischemic tissue. A major concern with

Table 31–3 Red Cell Substitutes in Clinical Trials

Product (Manufacturer)	Composition	Indication	Clinical Testing Stage
Hemopure (BioPure)	Glutaraldehyde–polymerized bovine hemoglobin	Local perfusion	II
PolyHeme (Northfield)	Glutaraldehyde–polymerized human hemoglobin	Trauma	III
Hemospan (Sangart)	PEG–human hemoglobin	Elective surgery	III
Synthetic blood	Perfluorocarbon emulsion	Sickle cell anemia	II

perfluorocarbon emulsions appears to be thrombocytopenia.[59] No liposome-based product has yet been approved for use in human trials.

At this time, trauma trials are underway with Northfield's PolyHeme,[60] but advanced trials of several hemoglobin products, including HemAssist (Baxter),[16,17] HemoPure (Biopure), and Hemolink (Hemosol) have been abandoned. One new product, Sangart's Hemospan, based on PEG-modified human hemoglobin,[61] has successfully completed phase 2 testing.

IMPLICATIONS AND FUTURE APPLICATIONS

Potential Clinical Applications

The need for red blood cell substitutes to replace all use of allogeneic blood is both unnecessary and naive. The red blood cell substitute candidates now being developed will probably be used initially in surgical procedures to provide a margin of safety and perhaps to reduce or eliminate transfusions of 1 to 2 units of allogeneic blood.

Many clinical applications in addition to hemodilution for the products now being developed will be targeted by industry (Table 31–4). Applications for perfluorocarbon emulsions other than as red blood cell substitutes could surpass their use in trauma, surgery, and shock. For example, emulsions have been shown to increase the radiosensitivity of solid tumors,[62] to be excellent nuclear magnetic resonance and ultrasound imaging agents,[63] to be capable of removing gaseous microemboli during cardiopulmonary bypass,[64] and to measure tissue pO_2.[65]

Availability in the Future

It seems unlikely that cell-free hemoglobin as a red blood cell substitute with vasoactive effects will be accepted broadly by clinicians. Indeed, vasoconstriction is a hallmark of the shock state, but hemoglobin solutions with reduced vasoactivity could be successful. Perfluorocarbon emulsions may be used as imaging enhancers, liquid-breathing agents, or adjuncts to radiotherapy of solid tumors. The low cost and simplicity of production of perfluorocarbon emulsions are favorable qualities for commercialization.

Liposome-encapsulated hemoglobin may be the ultimate solution to the red blood cell substitute problem, but to be successful, an inexpensive and simple process has to be developed, and any problems of reticuloendothelial blockade and engorgement of organs such as liver and spleen must be thoroughly studied and understood.

The present commercial climate is such that few, if any, of these products are being used in scientific studies that can be evaluated in the peer-reviewed literature until they are approved for use by the FDA. This situation has retarded development in the past and is likely to do so in the future.[41]

Table 31–4 Potential Clinical Applications for Red Cell Substitutes

Hemodilution, elective surgery
Trauma
Chronic anemia
Ischemic disease (angioplasty, stroke)
Red cell incompatibility (rare blood types)
Extracorporeal circulation (bypass)
Cell culture media
High-blood-use surgery
Cardioplegia
Tumor oxygenation
Organ transplantation
Bone marrow transplantation support
Sickle cell anemia
Oxygen delivery and circulation research

REFERENCES

1. Winslow R. Historical background. In Winslow R (ed). Blood Substitutes. London, Elsevier, 2006, pp 5–16.
2. AuBuchon JP. Meeting transfusion safety expectations. Ann Intern Med 2005;143:537–538.
3. Silverman T, Aebersold P, Landow L, Lindsey K. Regulatory perspectives on clinical trials for oxygen therapeutics in trauma and transfusion practice. In Winslow R (ed). Blood Substitutes. London, Elsevier, 2006, pp 34–41.
4. Winslow R. Hemoglobin-based Red Cell Substitutes. Baltimore, Md., Johns Hopkins University Press, 1992.
5. Winslow R. Hemoglobin modification. In Winslow R (ed). Blood Substitutes. London, Elsevier, 2006, pp 341–353.
6. Christensen S, Medina F, Winslow R, Snell S, Zegna A, Marini M. Preparation of human hemoglobin Ao for possible use as a blood substitute. J Biochem Biophys Methods 1988;17:143–154.
7. Winslow R. αα-Crosslinked hemoglobin. In Winslow R (ed). Blood Substitutes. London, Elsevier, 2006, pp 386–398.
8. Walder J, Chatterjee R, Arnone A. Electrostatic effects within the central cavity of the hemoglobin tetramer. Fed Proc 1982;41:651.
9. Winslow RM. αα-Crosslinked hemoglobin: was failure predicted by preclinical testing? Vox Sang 2000;79:1–20.
10. Winslow R, Chapman K. Pilot-scale preparation of hemoglobin solutions. Methods Enzymol 1994;231:3–16.
11. Vandegriff K, Medina F, Marini M, Winslow R. Equilibrium oxygen binding to human hemoglobin cross-linked between the alpha chains by bis(3,5-dibromosalicyl) fumarate. J Biol Chem 1989;264: 17824–17833.
12. Vandegriff K, Benazzi L, Ripamonti M, et al. Carbon dioxide binding to human hemoglobin cross-linked between the alpha chains. J Biol Chem 1991;266:2697–2700.
13. Hess J, Fadare S, Tolentino L, Bangal N, Winslow R. The intravascular persistence of cross-linked human hemoglobin. In Brewer G (ed). The Red Cell: Seventh Ann Arbor Conference. New York, Alan R. Liss, 1989, pp 351–360.
14. Hess J, Macdonald V, Brinkley W. Systemic and pulmonary hypertension after resuscitation with cell-free hemoglobin. J Appl Physiol 1993;74:1769–1778.
15. Winslow RM, Gonzales A, Gonzales M, et al. Vascular resistance and the efficacy of red cell substitutes in a rat hemorrhage model. J Appl Physiol 1998;85:993–1003.
16. Sloan EP, Koenigsberg M, Gens D, et al. Diaspirin cross-linked hemoglobin (DCLHb) in the treatment of severe traumatic hemorrhagic shock: a randomized controlled efficacy trial. JAMA 1999;282:1857–1864.
17. Saxena R, Wijnhoud AD, Carton H, et al. Controlled safety study of a hemoglobin-based oxygen carrier, DCLHb, in acute ischemic stroke. Stroke 1999;30:993–996.
18. Hoffman S, Looker D, Roehrich J, et al. Expression of fully functional tetrameric human hemoglobin in *Escherichia coli.* Proc Natl Acad Sci USA 1990;87:8521–8525.
19. Sharma A, Martin MJ, Okabe JF, et al. An isologous porcine promoter permits high level expression of human hemoglobin in transgenic swine. Biotechnology (NY) 1994;12:55–59.
20. Gould S, Sehgal L, Sehgal H, Moss G. Artificial blood: current status of hemoglobin solutions. Crit Care Clin 1992;8:293–309.
21. Marini M, Moore G, Fishman R, et al. Reexamination of the polymerization of pyridoxylated hemoglobin with glutaraldehyde. Biopolymers 1990;29:871–882.
22. Marini M, Moore G, Fishman R, et al. A critical examination of the reaction of pyridoxal 5-phosphate with human hemoglobin Ao. Biopolymers 1989;28:2071–2083.
23. Nho K, Glower D, Bredehoeft S, Shankar H, Shorr R, Abuchowski A. PEG-bovine hemoglobin: safety in a canine dehydrated hypovolemic-hemorrhagic shock model. Artif Cells Blood Substit Immobil Biotechnol 1992;20:511–524.

24. Malchesky P, Takahashi T, Iwasaki K, Harasaki H, Nose Y. Conjugated human hemoglobin as a physiological oxygen carrier—pyridoxylated hemoglobin polyoxyethylene conjugate (PHP). Int J Artif Organs 1990;13:442–450.
25. Chavez-Negrete A, Oropeza MV, Rojas MM, Villanueva T, Campos MG. Starch-hemoglobin induces contraction on isolated rat aortic rings. Artif Cells Blood Substit Immobil Biotechnol 2004;32:549–561.
26. Wong J. Rightshifted dextran-hemoglobin as blood substitute. Artif Cells Blood Substit Immobil Biotechnol 1988;16:237–245.
27. Matheson B, Razynska A, Kwansa H, Bucci E. Appearance of dissociable and cross-linked hemoglobins in the renal hilar lymph. J Lab Clin Med 2000;135:459–464.
28. Barnikol WK, Potzschke H. Haemoglobin hyperpolymers, a new type of artificial oxygen carrier—the concept and current state of development [in German]. Anasthesiol Intensivmed Notfallmed Schmerzther 2005;40:46–58.
29. Chang T. Red blood cell substitutes: microencapsulated hemoglobin and cross-linked hemoglobin including pyridoxylated polyhemoglobin conjugated hemoglobin. Artif Cells Blood Substit Immobil Biotechnol 1988;16:11–29.
30. Djordjevich L, Mayoral J, Ivankovich A. Synthetic erythrocytes: cardiorespiratory changes during exchange transfusions. Anesthesiology 1985;63:A109.
31. Hunt C, Burnette R, MacGregor R, Strubbe A, Lau D, Taylor N. Synthesis and evaluation of a prototypal artificial red cell. Science 1985;230:1165–1168.
32. Rudolph A. Encapsulated hemoglobin: current issues and future goals. Artif Cells Blood Substit Immobil Biotechnol 1994;22:347–360.
33. Farmer M, Gaber B. Liposome-encapsulated hemoglobin as an artificial oxygen-carrying system. Methods Enzymol 1987;149:184–200.
34. MacGregor R, Hunt C. Artificial red cells: a link between the membrane skeleton and RES detectability? Artif Cells Blood Substit Immobil Biotechnol 1990;18:329–343.
35. Allen T, Hansen C, Martin F, Redemann C, Yau-Young A. Liposomes containing synthetic lipid derivatives of poly(ethylene glycol) show prolonged circulation half-times in vivo. Biochim Biophys Acta 1991;1066:29–36.
36. Sakai H, Sou K, Takeoka S, Kobayashi K, Tsuchida E. Hemoglobin vesicles as a molecular assembly: characteristics of preparation process and performances as artificial oxygen carriers. In Winslow R (ed). Blood Substitutes. London, Elsevier, 2006, pp 514–522.
37. Nakachi O, Tokuyama S, Satoh T, Tsuchida E. Characteristics of polylipid/Hb vesicles (ARC) (in vitro and in vivo test). Artif Cells Blood Substit Immobil Biotechnol 1992;20:635–640.
38. Yu WP, Chang TM. Submicron polymer membrane hemoglobin nanocapsules as potential blood substitutes: preparation and characterization. Artif Cells Blood Substit Immobil Biotechnol 1996;24:169–183.
39. Long C, Long D, Riess J, Follana R, Burgan A, Mattrey R. Preparation and application of highly concentrated perfluorooctylbromide fluorocarbon emulsions. Artif Cells Blood Substit Immobil Biotechnol 1988;16:441–442.
40. Keipert P. Oxygent, a perfluorochemical-based oxygen therapeutic for surgical patients. In Winslow R (ed). Blood Substitutes. London, Elsevier, 2006, pp 312–323.
41. Naval Research Advisory Committee. Delivery of Artificial Blood to the Military. Washington, D.C., U.S. Navy, 1992.
42. Keipert P, Verosky M, Triner L. Plasma retention and metabolic fate of hemoglobin modified with an interdimeric covalent cross link. Trans Am Soc Artif Intern Organs 1989;35:153–159.
43. Keipert PE, Gomez CL, Gonzales A, Macdonald VW, Hess JR, Winslow RM. Diaspirin cross-linked hemoglobin: tissue distribution and long-term excretion after exchange transfusion. J Lab Clin Med 1994;123:701–711.
44. Hsia J, Song D, Er S, et al. Pharmacokinetic studies in the rat on a o-raffinose polymerized human hemoglobin. Artif Cells Blood Substit Immobil Biotechnol 1992;20:587–595.
45. Palmer R, Ferrige A, Moncada S. Nitric oxide release accounts for the biological activity of endothelium-derived relaxing factor. Nature 1987;327:524–526.
46. Gibson QH, Roughton FJ. The kinetics and equilibria of the reactions of nitric oxide with sheep hemoglobin. J Appl Physiol 1956;136:123–134.
47. Rohlfs RJ, Bruner E, Chiu A, et al. Arterial blood pressure responses to cell-free hemoglobin solutions and the reaction with nitric oxide. J Biol Chem 1998;273:12128–12134.
48. Vandegriff K, Winslow R. A theoretical analysis of oxygen transport: a new strategy for the design of hemoglobin-based red cell substitutes. In Winslow R, Vandegriff K, Intaglietta M (eds). Blood Substitutes: Physiological Basis of Efficacy. New York, Birkhäuser, 1995, pp 143–154.
49. Winslow RM, Vandegriff KD. Hemoglobin oxygen affinity and the design of red cell substitutes. In Winslow RM, Vandegriff KD, Intaglietta M (eds). Advances in Blood Substitutes: Industrial Opportunities and Medical Challenges. Boston, Birkhäuser, 1997, pp 167–188.
50. Intaglietta M, Johnson P, Winslow R. Microvascular and tissue oxygen distribution. Cardiovasc Res 1996;32:632–643.
51. Winslow R. Current status of blood substitute research: towards a new paradigm. J Intern Med 2003;253:508–517.
52. Ingram D, Forman M, Murray J. Phagocytic activation of human neutrophils by the detergent component of fluosol. Am J Pathol 1992;140:1081–1087.
53. Bucala R, Kawakami M, Cerami A. Cytotoxicity of a perfluorocarbon blood substitute to macrophages in vitro. Science 1983;220:965–967.
54. Beach M, Morley J, Spiryda L, Weinstock S. Effects of liposome encapsulated hemoglobin on the reticuloendothelial system. Artif Cells Blood Substit Immobil Biotechnol 1992;20:771–776.
55. Flaim S. Perflubron-based emulsion: efficacy as temporary oxygen carrier. In Winslow RM, Vandegriff KD, Intaglietta M (eds). Advances in Blood Substitutes: Industrial Opportunities and Medical Challenges. Boston, Birkhäuser, 1997, pp 91–132.
56. Pope A, French G, Longnecker DE. Fluid Resuscitation: State of the Science for Treating Combat Casualties and Civilian Injuries. Washington, D.C., National Academy Press, 1999.
57. Gould S, Rosen A, Sehgal L, Sehgal H, Langdale L, Krause L. Fluosol-DA as a red-cell substitute in acute anemia. N Engl J Med 1986;314:1653–1656.
58. Amberson W, Jennings J, Rhode C. Clinical experience with hemoglobin-saline solutions. J Appl Physiol 1949;1:469–489.
59. Kaufman R. Clinical development of perfluorocarbon-based red cell substitutes. In Winslow R, Vandegriff K, Intaglietta M (eds). Blood Substitutes: Physiological Basis of Efficacy. New York, Birkhäuser, 1995, pp 53–75.
60. Gould S, Moore E, Hoyt D, et al. The first randomized trial of human polymerized hemoglobin as a blood substitute in acute trauma and emergent surgery. J Am Coll Surg 1998;187:113–120.
61. Vandegriff KD, Malavalli A, Wooldridge J, Lohman J, Winslow RM. MP4, a new nonvasoactive PEG-Hb conjugate. Transfusion 2003;43:509–516.
62. Teicher B, Herman T, Menon K. Enhancement of fractionated radiation therapy by an experimental concentrated perflubron emulsion (Oxygent) in the Lewis lung carcinoma. Artif Cells Blood Substit Immobil Biotechnol 1992;20:899–902.
63. Mattrey R. Perfluorooctylbromide: a new contrast agent for CT, sonography, and MR imaging. Am J Radiol 1988;152:247–252.
64. Blauth C, Smith P, Newman S, et al. Retinal microembolism and neuropsychological deficit following clinical cardiopulmonary bypass: comparison of a membrane and bubble oxygenator. A preliminary communication. Eur J Cardiothorac Surg 1989;3:135–138; discussion 139.
65. Mason R, Shukla H, Antich P. Oxygent: a novel probe of tissue oxygen tension. Artif Cells Blood Substit Immobil Biotechnol 1992;20:929–932.

Section III

Transfusion Medicine

A. Transfusion in Specific Clinical Settings

Chapter 32

Red Cell Transfusion in Perioperative and Critically Ill Patients

Paul C. Hébert • Alan Tinmouth • Jeffrey L. Carson

RED CELL UTILIZATION IN PERIOPERATIVE AND CRITICAL CARE

Despite concerns regarding transfusion-transmitted viruses, allogeneic red blood cell (RBC) transfusions clearly save lives in the perioperative and critical care setting. Indeed, hemoglobin binds and transports more than 98% of all oxygen delivered to peripheral tissues. Therefore, RBC transfusions are a lifesaving measure that maintain oxygen transport during severe anemia. Severe anemia has been shown to increase mortality rates from 1.3%, when hemoglobin concentrations exceed 120 g/L, to more than 33%, when hemoglobin concentrations are less than 60 g/L[1] in perioperative patients refusing allogeneic RBC transfusions. A limited number of studies describe the overall patient population requiring allogeneic RBC transfusions.[1–3] In a 1992 survey conducted in 61 Toronto area hospitals, 65% of RBCs transfused were administered to patients undergoing operative procedures categorized as digestive and abdominal, cardiovascular, and musculoskeletal.[2] Brien and colleagues[3] documented that 56% of all allogeneic RBCs were administered to surgical patients while a study by Ghali[1] documented that 69% of RBCs were transfused into surgical patients. In general, cardiovascular surgical procedures, orthopedic procedures (e.g., total hip and knee replacement), and selected gynecologic (e.g., radical hysterectomy) and urologic procedures (e.g., radical prostatectomy) were noted to have a high proportion of patients requiring allogeneic RBC transfusions.[2] In patients undergoing elective aortic aneurysm repair and coronary revascularization, up to 50% to 80% received RBCs.[2] In a recent study examining transfusion practice in critically ill patients, the authors documented that an average of 25% of all patients receive RBC transfusions, with a range of 20.4% to 53.4%.[4] Thus, albeit difficult to quantify, perioperative and critical care still consume a large proportion of the blood supply.

Allogeneic RBC transfusions are complex biological products prepared from donated blood and may be considered unique in many respects compared with other health interventions. Decisions concerning the use of RBC transfusion in the treatment of anemia and hemorrhage require a clear understanding of both risks and benefits of both the condition and treatment of patients. Although we have developed a much clearer appreciation for the infectious and immunomodulatory risks of RBC transfusion over the past two decades, the risks of anemia in many clinical settings and the benefits of RBC transfusion are still inadequately characterized. It is commonly assumed that the most significant risk associated with anemia is the harm resulting from the decreases in oxygen-carrying capacity and plasma volume. The development of adverse health consequences from anemia will, in part, depend on the capacity of the individual patient to compensate for these changes. The benefit of transfusion is derived from the capacity of donor RBCs to correct these deficits and possibly provide additional benefits such as increasing oxygen delivery to supranormal ranges. Such a framework highlights the concept that RBC transfusions have a number of tradeoffs between risks and benefits. With the exception of patients who refuse blood for religious reasons, it is impossible to separately analyze these competing risks and benefits for patients outside a randomized clinical trial.

ADAPTATION TO ANEMIA AND TRANSFUSIONS

In anemia, O_2-carrying capacity is decreased but tissue oxygenation is typically preserved, even at hemoglobin levels well below 100 g/L. Following the development of anemia, adaptive changes occur, including a shift in the oxyhemoglobin dissociation curve, hemodynamic alterations, and microcirculatory alterations. The shift to the right of the oxyhemoglobin dissociation curve in anemia is primarily the result of increased synthesis of 2,3-diphosphoglyerate (DPG) in red cells.[5–18] This rightward shift enables more O_2 to be released to the tissues at a given pO_2, offsetting the effect of reduced O_2-carrying capacity of the blood. In vitro studies have also demonstrated rightward shifts in the oxyhemoglobin dissociation curve with decreases in temperature and pH.[19] Although clinically important shifts have been documented in a number of studies, measurements of hemoglobin O_2 saturation are generally performed on arterial specimens processed at standardized temperatures and pH. Therefore, current measurement techniques will not reflect O_2-binding affinity in the patient's microcirculatory environment, which is potentially affected by temperature, pH, and some disease processes.[19,20]

Several hemodynamic alterations also occur following the development of anemia. The most important determinant of cardiovascular response is the patient's volume status or, more specifically, left ventricular preload. The combined effects of hypovolemia and anemia often occur as a result of blood loss. Tissue hypoxia or anoxia may occur as a result of either decreased blood flow (stagnant hypoxia) or decreased O_2-carrying capacity (anemic hypoxia).[21–24] The body primarily attempts to preserve O_2 delivery to vital organs through increased myocardial contractility and heart rate as well as increased arterial and venous vascular tone mediated through increased sympathetic activity. In addition, central and regional reflexes redistribute organ blood flow. The adrenergic system plays an important role in altering blood flow to and within specific organs. The renin-angiotensin-aldosterone hormone system is stimulated to retain both water and sodium. Losses ranging from 5% to 15% in blood volume result in variable increases in resting heart rate and diastolic blood pressure measures. Orthostatic hypotension is often a sensitive indicator of relatively small losses in blood volume that are not sufficient to cause a marked blood pressure fall. Larger losses result in progressive increases in heart rate and decreases in arterial blood pressure accompanied by evidence of end-organ hypoperfusion. The increased sympathetic tone diverts an ever decreasing global blood flow or cardiac output away from the splanchnic, skeletal, and skin circulation toward the coronary and cerebral circulation. Once vital organ systems such as the kidneys, central nervous system, and heart are affected, the patient is considered in hypovolemic shock. Although the American College of Surgeons' Committee on Trauma[25] categorizes the cardiovascular and systemic response to acute blood loss according to degrees of blood loss, many of these responses are modified by patient characteristics such as age, comorbid illnesses, pre-existing volume status and hemoglobin values, use of medications having cardiac (i.e., β-blockers) or peripheral vascular effects (i.e., antihypertensives), and rapidity of blood loss.

The compensatory changes in cardiac output have been the most thoroughly studied cardiovascular consequence of normovolemic anemia. When intravascular volume is stable or increased following the development of anemia (as opposed to hypovolemic anemia and shock), increases in cardiac output have been consistently reported. Indeed, an inverse relationship between hemoglobin levels (or hematocrit) and cardiac output has been clearly established in well-controlled laboratory studies.[26–32] Similar clinical observations were made in the perioperative setting[33–40] and in chronic anemia.[26,41–43] Recently, the rise in cardiac output with progressive decreases in hemoglobin concentrations was clearly established in healthy awake volunteers (Fig. 32–1).[43a] These adaptive responses observed in clinical studies may be affected by major comorbid illnesses such as cardiac disease and age, lack of appropriate control patients, and significant weaknesses in study design. Researchers have also attempted to determine the level of anemia at which cardiac output begins to rise. Reported thresholds for this phenomenon identified in primary clinical and laboratory studies range from 70 to 120 g/L.[26,28,44–47]

Two major mechanisms are thought to primarily modulate the physiologic processes underlying the increased cardiac output during normovolemic anemia: (1) reduced blood viscosity and (2) increased sympathetic stimulation of the cardiovascular effectors.[24,29,48–50] Blood viscosity exerts major effects on both preload and afterload, two of the major determinants of cardiac output[48,51,52] while sympathetic stimulation primarily increases the two other determinants: heart rate and contractility. As opposed to hypovolemic anemia, the effects of blood viscosity appear to predominate in this setting.[51–53]

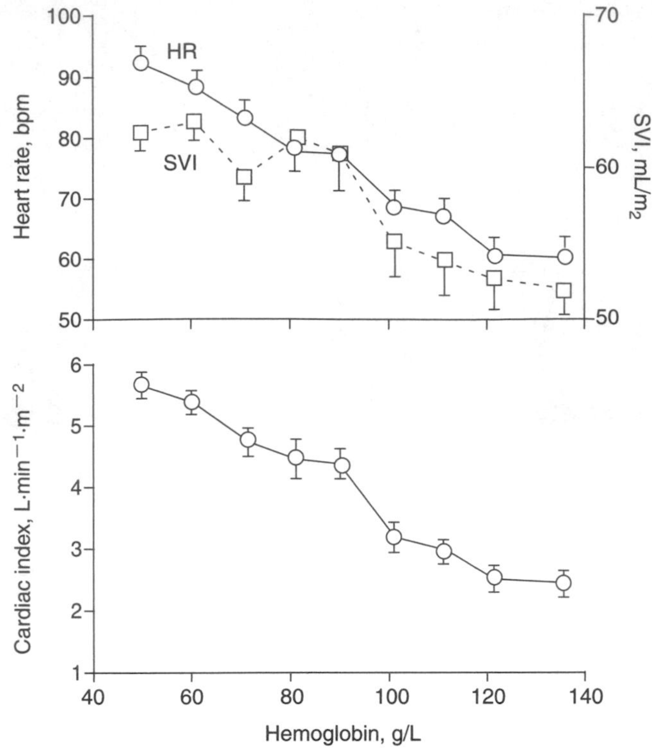

Figure 32–1 Acute isovolemic reduction of hemoglobin concentration to 50 g/L increased heart rate (HR). (From Weiskopf RB, Viele MK, Feiner J, et al. Human cardiovascular and metabolic response to acute, severe, isovolemic anemia. JAMA 1998;279:217–221.)

There are complex interactions between blood flow, blood viscosity, and cardiac output. In vessels, blood flow alters blood viscosity, and in turn blood viscosity modulates cardiac output. Under experimental conditions in rigid hollow cylinders, blood flow is directly related to the diameter and the pressure difference between the ends of the cylinder and inversely related to its length and the blood viscosity (Poiseuille-Hagen law).[24,48,49] Blood is not a Newtonian fluid (i.e., its viscosity will change according to blood flow velocity). Thus, viscosity is highest in postcapillary venules, where flow is lowest, and viscosity is lowest in the aorta, where flow is highest. In postcapillary venules, there is a disproportionate decrease in blood viscosity as anemia worsens, and as a consequence, venous return is significantly increased. If cardiac function is normal, the increase in venous return or left ventricular preload will be the most important determinant of the increase in cardiac output during normovolemic anemia. Interestingly, if viscosity is maintained during anemia using colloidal solutions of known high viscosity other than red cells, these cardiovascular effects are attenuated.[51] Decreased left ventricular afterload, another cardiac consequence of decreased blood viscosity, may also be an important mechanism for the increase in cardiac output as anemia worsens.[51]

Investigators[29,44,51,52,54–56] have observed alterations not only in viscosity during anemia but also in sympathetic stimulation. Reviews and guidelines indicate that anemia also results in an increase in heart rate.[28,48,57] This physiologic response is thought to be predominantly mediated through aortic chemoreceptors[29,50] and release of catecholamines.[27,29,54,58,59] However, primary laboratory studies,[59,60] studies of perioperative normovolemic hemodilution,[33–35] and studies of chronic anemia[41,42] have not consistently demonstrated significant increases in heart rate following moderate degrees of anemia. In a detailed review by Spahn and colleagues,[48] there appeared to be some differences in species responses as well as between awake and anesthetized patients. In three poorly controlled studies in children, there are conflicting results as to whether the increase in cardiac output is mostly a consequence of increased heart rate[42,61] or stroke volume.[62] In summary, the increase in cardiac output is more dependent on stroke volume and to a lesser extent on heart rate in most clinical settings. If indeed increased heart rate does occur from normovolemic anemia, one of its major consequences will be to adversely affect coronary blood flow by decreasing diastole, the time when the left ventricular myocardium is perfused.[63,64]

The sympathetic stimulation may also result in increased cardiac output through enhanced myocardial contractility[65,66] and increased venomotor tone.[29,67] The effects of anemia on left ventricular contractility in isolation have not been clearly determined given the complex changes in preload, afterload, and heart rate. Only one before and after hemodilution study used load-independent measures to document increased left ventricular contractility.[66] Chapler and Cain[29] have summarized several well-controlled studies indicating that venomotor tone is increased and that it results from stimulation of the aortic chemoreceptors. If sympathetic stimulation is significant in the specific clinical setting, then contractility will be enhanced from stimulation of the β-adrenergic receptors.[48,54,56,65]

Under experimental laboratory conditions, several investigators[58,68–72] have observed significant increases in coronary blood flow directly related to the degree of normovolemic anemia. In addition, these same studies do not appear to demonstrate significant shifts in the distribution of coronary flow between endocardium and epicardium in a normal coronary circulation during moderate degrees of anemia. Furthermore, significant alterations in flow distribution between major organs following acute hemodilution have been documented.[28,29,53,60,68,72–76] Disproportionate increases in coronary and cerebral blood flow were noted during observation of simultaneous decreases in blood flow to the splanchnic circulation.

The inverse relationship between cardiac output and hemoglobin levels has led investigators to determine the hemoglobin level that maximizes O_2 transport. Richardson and Guyton,[77] evaluating the effects of hematocrit on cardiac performance in a canine model, established optimal O_2 transport to occur between hematocrit values of 40% and 60%. Others determined maximum O_2 delivery to be in the lower end of the range, at a hematocrit value of 40% to 45% (132 to 150 g/L).[68,72,78] However, one of the most widely quoted studies addressing this topic from Messmer and colleagues[45] found that optimal O_2 transport occurred at hematocrit values of 30% (hemoglobin = 100 g/L). Unfortunately, global indices of optimal O_2 delivery will mask any differences in blood flow between specific organs.[53,58,79,80] In addition, attempting to identify a single optimal hemoglobin that maximizes O_2 delivery neglects consideration of the large number of factors interfering with adaptive mechanisms in patients other than healthy young adults with anemia.

Will the transfusion of allogeneic red cells reverse any adaptive response to acute or chronic normovolemic anemia? Given that O_2-carrying capacity is not impaired in the red cell storage process and that blood viscosity is restored following a transfusion, the cardiovascular consequences should be reversed if there has been no irreversible ischemic damage. However, the storage process alters red cell properties, which in turn may impair flow and O_2 release from hemoglobin[5,14] in the microcirculation.

NATURAL HISTORY OF UNCORRECTED ANEMIA IN PATIENTS

Numerous laboratory experiments indicate that extreme hemodilution is well tolerated in healthy animals. Animals subjected to acute hemodilution tolerate decreasing hemoglobin concentration down to 50 to 30 g/L, with ischemic electrocardiographic changes and depressed ventricular function occurring, respectively, at these levels of hemoglobin concentration.[81] However, acute hemodilution is less well tolerated in experimental animal models of coronary stenosis, with ischemic electrocardiographic changes and depressed cardiac function occurring at hemoglobin concentrations between 70 and 100 g/L. Human data regarding the limits of anemia tolerance are inadequate and often conflicting. For example, Leung and colleagues[82] found electrocardiographic changes that may have been indicative of myocardial ischemia in 3 of 55 conscious resting volunteers subjected to acute isovolemic hemodilution to hemoglobin concentration of 50 g/L.

Although the above experimental data provide insight to the human physiologic response to acute anemia, they are of limited applicability in the perioperative setting, where many of the factors that influence oxygen consumption including muscle activity, body temperature, heart rate, sympathetic activity, and metabolic state are altered. Instead, it is more appropriate to determine the risk of withholding RBC transfusions in the perioperative setting. From a systematic review completed for the Canadian Guidelines on red cells, Hébert et al[83] identified numerous reports of severe anemia being well tolerated in surgical patients.[84–96] Additional reports or case series[94,97–99] describe successful outcomes in patients with chronic anemia as a result of renal failure. Finally, descriptive studies in patients refusing red cell transfusion[85–87,93] and from regions experiencing limited blood supplies[88,100] have demonstrated that patients can survive surgical interventions with hemoglobin levels as low as 45 g/L.

In some of these studies, there appears to be an association between preoperative hemoglobin concentrations, intraoperative estimated blood loss, and postoperative mortality.[86,87] Indeed, there were no reported deaths in more than 100 major elective surgical patients when preoperative hemoglobins were greater than 80 g/L and the estimated blood loss was less than 500 mL. In a single center series of 542 Jehovah's Witness patients undergoing a cardiac surgical procedure, the overall mortality was 10.7% and only 2.2% of the deaths observed were considered to be a direct consequence of anemia. More recently, Viele and Weiskopf[96] identified 134 Jehovah's Witness patients who had a hemoglobin concentration less than 80 g/L or hematocrit below 24% who were treated for various medical and surgical conditions without the use of blood or blood components. There were 50 reported deaths, 23 of which were attributed primarily or exclusively to anemia, defined as deaths with hemoglobin concentration below 50 g/L. For those patients dying of anemia, 60% were more than 50 years old. However, in 27 survivors with hemoglobin concentration below 50 g/L, 65% were less than 50 years of age. While publication bias must be kept in mind when examining these data, young healthy patients may survive without transfusion at hemoglobin concentrations in the range of 50 g/L. From these data, it is clear that extreme anemia is tolerated in the perioperative setting but also appears to increase the risk of death. However, these observations should not be interpreted as support for a restrictive or conservative transfusion strategy, especially since most of the literature related to tolerance of anemia has not explored patient characteristics that predispose patients to adverse outcomes from moderate to severe anemia.

ANEMIA IN HIGH-RISK GROUPS

A number of risk factors for adverse outcomes associated with anemia have been identified in clinical practice guidelines[57,101,102] and reviews.[28,30,49] Anemia is believed to be less well tolerated in older patients, the severely ill, and patients with clinical conditions such as coronary, cerebrovascular, or respiratory disease. However, the clinical evidence confirming that these factors are independently associated with an increased risk of adverse outcome is lacking. One small case control study following high-risk vascular surgery suggests an increase in postoperative cardiac events with increasing severity of anemia.[90] In perioperative[103] and critically ill patients[104] two large cohort studies have documented that increasing degrees of anemia were associated with a disproportionate increase in mortality rate in the subgroup of patients with cardiac disease. In 1958 Jehovah's Witness patients,[103] the adjusted odds of death increased from 2.3 (95% CI of 1.4 to 4.0) to 12.3 (95% CI of 2.5 to 62.1) as preoperative hemoglobin concentrations declined from the range of 100 to 109 g/L to 60 to 69 g/L in patients with cardiac disease (Fig. 32–2). There was not a significant increase

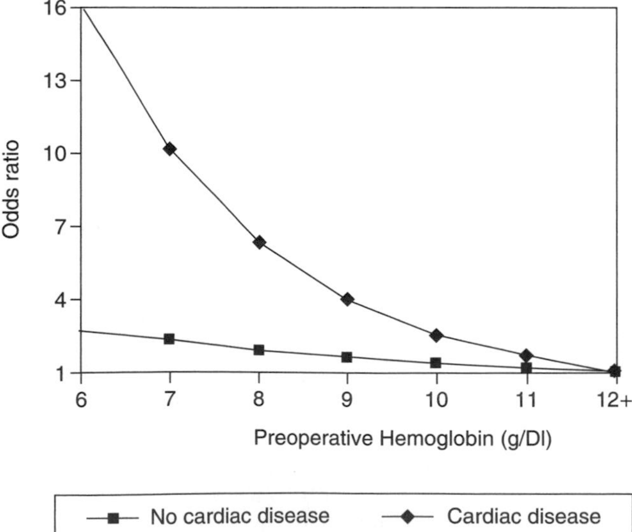

Figure 32–2 Adjusted odds ratio for mortality by cardiovascular disease and preoperative hemoglobin. (Adapted from Carson JL, Duff A, Poses RM, et al. Effect of anemia and cardiovascular disease on surgical mortality and morbidity. Lancet 1996;348:1055–1060.)

in mortality in noncardiac patients with comparable levels of anemia. In a separate study of critically ill patients,[104] patients with cardiac disease and hemoglobin concentrations less than 95 g/L also had a trend toward increased mortality (55% vs 42%, $P = 0.09$) compared with anemic patients with other diagnoses. Although both cohort studies were retrospective and may not have controlled for a number of important confounders, the evidence suggests that anemia increases the risk of death in patients with significant cardiac disease. Severity of illness also appears to be a risk factor in the critically ill.[86,104] Two retrospective studies document that the degree of blood loss contributes to perioperative mortality.[86,104] However, no studies have examined the independent contribution of age, cerebrovascular disease, and respiratory disease to an increased mortality risk in anemic patients. This relationship may well be complex given that age and cerebrovascular disease are risk factors associated with coronary artery disease. Smoking and related respiratory diseases may have similar associations to cardiac disease. Therefore, the association between anemia and increased rates of adverse outcomes in these patients can best be described as speculative at this time.

THE BENEFITS (AND POTENTIAL RISKS) OF TRANSFUSION

Four large observational studies specifically designed to compare clinical outcomes at varying hemoglobin concentrations in transfused and nontransfused patients were conducted in various clinical settings. In the first, Hébert et al[104] used a combined retrospective and prospective cohort design to examine 4470 critically ill patients admitted to six Canadian tertiary level intensive care units (ICUs) during 1993. In patients with cardiac diagnoses (ischemic heart disease, arrhythmia, cardiac arrest, and cardiac and vascular surgical procedures) there was a trend toward increased mortality when hemoglobin concentrations were less than 95 g/L. Furthermore, analysis of a subgroup of 202 patients with anemia, an Acute Physiology and Chronic Health Evaluation II (APACHE II) score greater than 20, and a cardiac diagnosis revealed that transfusion of 1 to 3 units or 4 to 6 units of RBCs was associated with a significantly lower mortality rate when compared with patients who did not receive transfusion (55% no transfusions vs 35% 1 to 3 units or 32% 4 to 6 units, respectively, $P = 0.01$). Although the design of the analysis attempted to control for the confounding influence of disease severity, it is quite possible that the complex interrelationship between disease severity, the number of transfusions, and the degree of anemia may have resulted in a spurious association between a cardiovascular diagnosis and the reported mortality risk with anemia.

Wu and associates[105] retrospectively studied Medicare records of 78,974 patients older than age 65 who were hospitalized with a primary diagnosis of acute myocardial infarction. The authors then categorized patients according to their hematocrit on admission. Although anemia, defined in the study as a hematocrit less than 39%, was present in nearly half the patients, only 3680 patients received an RBC transfusion. Lower admission hematocrit values were associated with increased 30-day mortality, with mortality rate approaching 50% among patients with a hematocrit of 27% or lower who did not receive an RBC transfusion. Unfortunately, this study did not have any data on nadir hemoglobins and their relationship to mortality. Interestingly, whereas RBC transfusion was associated with a reduction in 30-day mortality for patients who received at least one RBC transfusion if their admitting hematocrit was less than 33%, RBC transfusion was associated with increased 30-day mortality for patients whose admitting hematocrit values were 36.1% or higher. In the analysis, these associations were present even when adjustments were made for clinical patient factors including APACHE II scores, location of myocardial infarction and presence of congestive heart failure, and treatment factors including use of reperfusion therapies, aspirin, and β-adrenergic blockade.

In the only study exclusively focusing on the perioperative period, Carson and colleagues[106] attempted to determine the effect of perioperative transfusion on 30- and 90-day postoperative mortality with a retrospective cohort study involving 8787 patients with hip fractures undergoing repair between 1983 and 1993 in 20 different U.S. hospitals. This was a large, high-risk, elderly (median age, 80.3 years) population with extensive coexisting disease and with an overall 30-day mortality rate of 4.6%. A total of 3699 patients (42%) received a perioperative transfusion within 7 days of the surgical repair. After controlling for hemoglobin concentrations, cardiovascular disease, and other risk factors for death, the results suggested that patients who had hemoglobin concentrations as low as 80 g/L and did not receive transfusion were no more likely to die than those with similar hemoglobin concentration levels who received a transfusion. With hemoglobin concentrations < 80 g/L, nearly all patients received a transfusion, which did not allow investigators to draw conclusions about the effect of transfusion at these lower hemoglobin concentration levels. However, as the authors point out, despite the large sample size, inadequate power may still explain the inability to detect a reduction in mortality related to transfusion; they estimated that the study would need to be 10 times larger to detect a 10% difference in 30-day mortality with 80% power.

More recently, Vincent and colleagues[107] completed a prospective observational cross-sectional study involving 3534 patients admitted to 146 Western European ICUs during a 2-week period in November 1999. Thirty-seven percent of these patients received RBC transfusions during their ICU admission with the overall transfusion rate increasing to 41.6% over a 28-day period. For those patients who were transfused, the mean pretransfusion hemoglobin concentration was 84 ± 13 g/L. In an effort to control for confounding created by illness severity and the need for transfusion, these investigators employed a strategy of matching transfused and nontransfused patients based on their propensity to receive a transfusion, thereby defining two well-balanced groups (516 patients in each group) to determine the influence of RBC transfusions on mortality. Using this approach, the associated risk of death was increased instead of decreased by 33% for patients who received a transfusion compared with similar patients who did not receive blood. However, as pointed out in the accompanying editorial,[108] the results may have differed if the propensity scores were derived separately for categories of pretransfusion hemoglobin concentrations (e.g., <80, 80–100, and >100 g/L) instead of hemoglobin concentrations at ICU admission. For example, if one were to consider groups of patients with pretransfusion hemoglobin concentrations less than 60 g/L, it is unlikely that the observed 33% increase in mortality would hold true, or blood transfusion would never be recommended.

Unfortunately, as evidenced by a recent systematic review, there is a paucity of clinical trials comparing restrictive and liberal transfusion policies to examine efficacy of RBC transfusion. Carson and coworkers[109] were able to identify only 10 randomized clinical trials of adequate methodological quality in which different RBC transfusion triggers were evaluated. Included were a total of 1780 surgery, trauma, and ICU patients enrolled in trials conducted over the past 40 years. The transfusion triggers evaluated in these trials varied between 70 and 100 g/L. Data on mortality or hospital length of stay were available in only six trials (Fig. 32–3). Conservative transfusion triggers were not associated with an increase in mortality; on average, mortality was one fifth lower (RR 0.80; 95% CI 0.63, 1.02) with conservative compared with liberal transfusion triggers. Likewise, cardiac morbidity and length of hospital stay did not appear to be adversely affected by the lower use of red cell transfusions. There were insufficient data on potentially relevant clinical outcomes such as stroke, thromboembolism, multiorgan failure, delirium, and infection or delayed wound healing to perform any pooled analysis. Carson and colleagues[109] stated that the data were insufficient to address the full range of risks and benefits associated with different transfusion thresholds, particularly in patients with coexisting disease. They also noted that their meta-analysis was dominated by a single trial: the

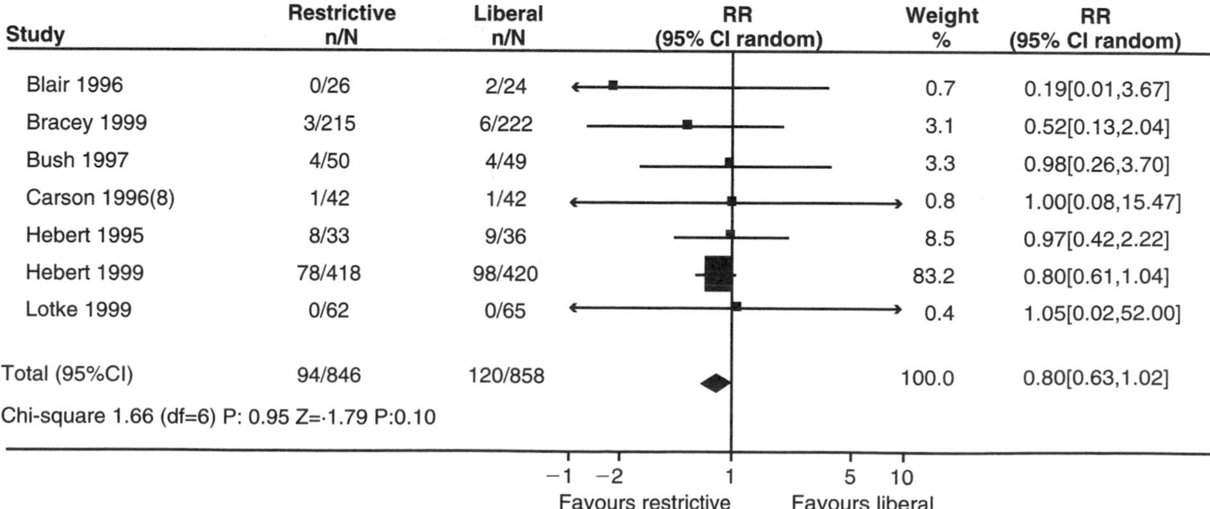

Study
Restrictive n/N
Liberal n/N
RR (95% CI random)
Weight %
RR (95% CI random)
Blair 1996 0/26 2/24 0.7 0.19[0.01,3.67]
Bracey 1999 3/215 6/222 3.1 0.52[0.13,2.04]
Bush 1997 4/50 4/49 3.3 0.98[0.26,3.70]
Carson 1996(8) 1/42 1/42 0.8 1.00[0.08,15.47]
Hebert 1995 8/33 9/36 8.5 0.97[0.42,2.22]
Hebert 1999 78/418 98/420 83.2 0.80[0.61,1.04]
Lotke 1999 0/62 0/65 0.4 1.05[0.02,52.00]
Total (95%CI) 94/846 120/858 100.0 0.80[0.63,1.02]
Chi-square 1.66 (df=6) P: 0.95 Z=-1.79 P:0.10
−1 −2 1 5 10
Favours restrictive
Favours liberal

Figure 32–3 Effect of restrictive transfusion triggers on 30-day, all-cause mortality. (Adapted from Carson JL, Hill S, Carless P, et al. Transfusion triggers: a systematic review of the literature. Transfus Med Rev 2002;16:87–199.)

Transfusion Requirements in Critical Care (TRICC) trial,[110] which enrolled 838 patients and was the only individual trial identified that was adequately powered to evaluate the impact of different transfusion strategies on mortality and morbidity.

The TRICC study[110] documented an overall nonsignificant trend toward decreased 30-day mortality (18.7% vs 23.3%, $P=0.11$) and significant decreases in mortality among patients who were less acutely ill (8.7% vs 16.1%, $P=0.03$) in the group treated using a hemoglobin transfusion trigger of 70 g/L compared with a more liberally transfused group that received 54% more red cell transfusions. The investigators also noted that the 30-day mortality rates were significantly lower with the restrictive transfusion strategy among patients who were less acutely ill (APACHE II scores less than 20) and among patients who were less than 55 years of age (Fig. 32–4).

A number of additional questions arose from the TRICC trial. The investigators were particularly interested in the risks and benefits of anemia and transfusion in patients with cardiovascular disease and in patients attempting to wean from mechanical ventilation. In the first of these subgroup analyses,[111] 357 patients (43%) were identified with cardiovascular disease. Of these, 160 had been in the restrictive RBC transfusion group and 197 in the liberal transfusion strategy group. The two groups were fairly equally balanced with regard to baseline characteristics and concurrent therapies with a few exceptions: there was less frequent diuretic use in the restrictive group (43% vs 58%, $P<0.01$) and the use of epidural anesthetics was greater in the restrictive group (8% vs 2%, $P<0.01$). Overall, in this subgroup analysis, there was no significant difference in mortality rate between the two treatment groups. However, there was a nonsignificant ($P=0.3$) decrease in overall survival rate in the restrictive group for patients with confirmed ischemic heart disease, severe peripheral vascular disease, or severe comorbid cardiac disease.

The subgroup analysis of patients receiving mechanical ventilation was limited to 713 (85% of the 838 patients in the TRICC trial who required invasive mechanical ventilatory support).[112] Of these, 357 had been in the restrictive RBC transfusion group and 356 in the liberal group. The mean duration of mechanical ventilation was 8.3 ± 8.1 days in the restrictive group and 8.8 ± 8.7 days in the liberal group ($P = 0.48$). Ventilator-free days were 17.5 ± 10.9 and 16.1 ± 11.4 in the restrictive and liberal RBC transfusion groups, respectively ($P = 0.09$). Eighty-two percent of the patients in the restrictive transfusion group were considered successfully weaned and extubated for at least 24 hours, compared with 78% for the liberal group ($P = 0.19$). Among the 219 patients who required mechanical ventila-

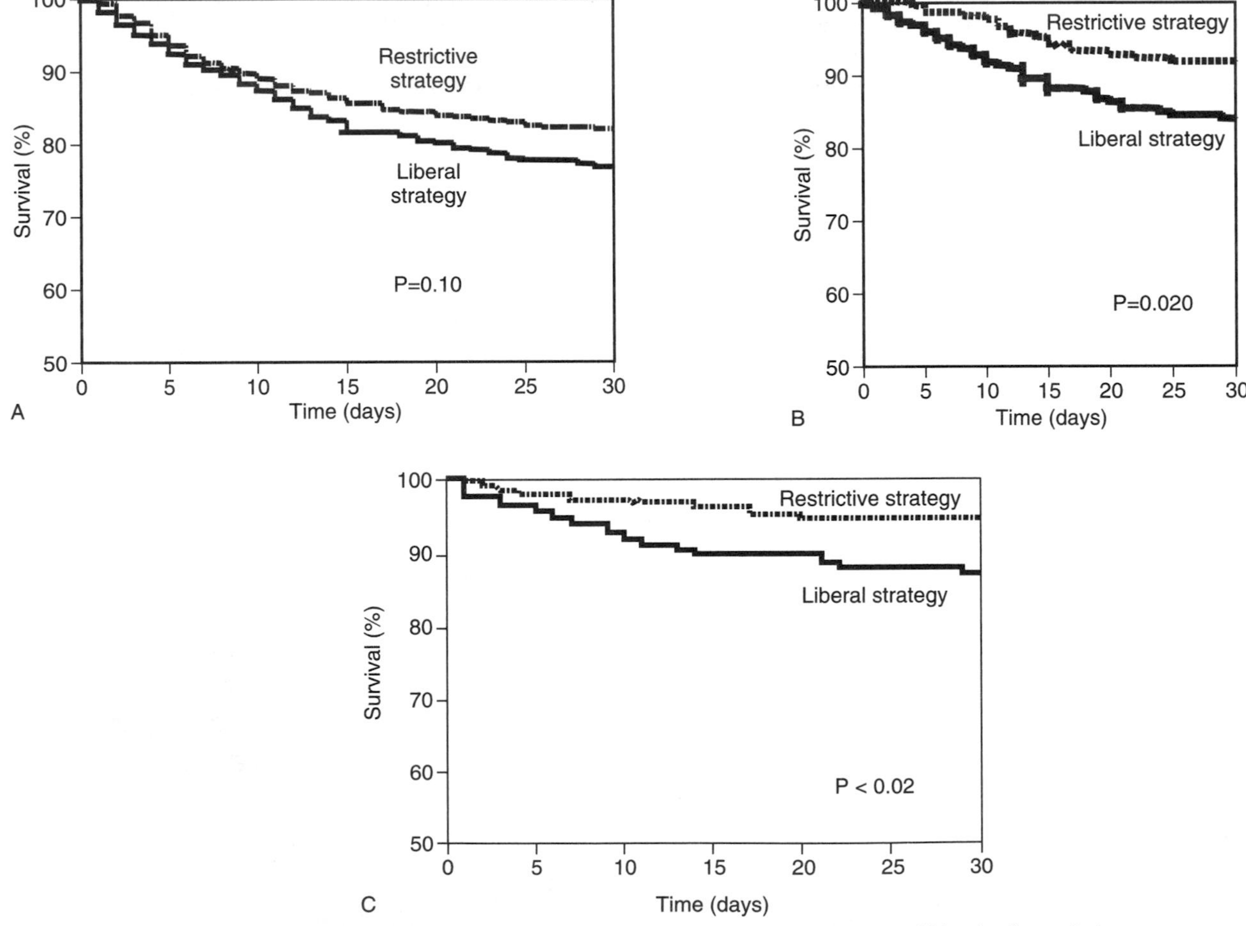

Figure 32–4 ICU survival over 30 days in study patients in the restrictive and liberal allogeneic red blood cell transfusion strategy groups. Graph **A** illustrates Kaplan-Meier survival curves for all patients in both study groups. There is a trend toward lower mortality in patients in the restrictive group (*dotted line*) compared with the liberal group (*solid line*) ($P=0.10$). In the subgroup with an APACHE II score less than 20 (graph **B**), fewer patients died in the restrictive group than in the liberal group ($P=0.02$). There were also significant differences in survival between groups in the subgroup with ages less than 55 years ($P=0.02$), as depicted in graph **C**. (Adapted from Hébert PC, Wells G, Blajchman M, et al. A multicenter, randomized, controlled clinical trial of transfusion requirements in critical care. N Engl J Med 1999;340:409–417.)

tion for more than 7 days, there were no differences in the time to successful weaning (Fig. 32–5). The independent effects of RBC transfusions and hemoglobin concentration were also examined. Each additional transfusion was associated with an increased duration of mechanical ventilation (RR = 1.10; 95% CI 1.14 to 1.06, $P < 0.01$) adjusting for the effect of age, APACHE II score, and comorbid illnesses. Hemoglobin concentrations did not influence the duration of mechanical ventilation (RR = 0.99; 95% CI 1.01 to 0.98, $P = 0.45$). Complications including pulmonary edema and ARDS were increased in patients in the liberal strategy group.

Even though a large RCT has been completed, a number of questions remain. One of the most important is why the liberal RBC transfusion strategy failed to improve 30-day mortality and rates of organ failure in critically ill patients. It is conceivable that the greater number of allogeneic RBC units in the liberal group significantly depressed host immune responses[112,113] or resulted in altered microcirculatory flow as a consequence of prolonged RBC storage times.

Following the publication of the TRICC trial, a study published by Rivers and colleagues[114] documented that early use of goal-directed care based on a mixed central venous saturation decreased mortality from 46.5% in the control group to 30.5% in the goal-directed therapy group ($P = 0.009$). As one of the many interventions in patients with early septic shock, hematocrit concentrations were increased beyond 30% if the central venous saturations fell below 70%. As a consequence of goal-directed therapy, 64% of patients compared with 18.5% of the control group received RBC transfusions ($P < 0.0001$). There are significant differences in patient populations between the study conducted by Rivers and colleagues and the TRICC trial. The early goal-directed therapy study does highlight the need to perform additional studies in subpopulations of critically ill patients.

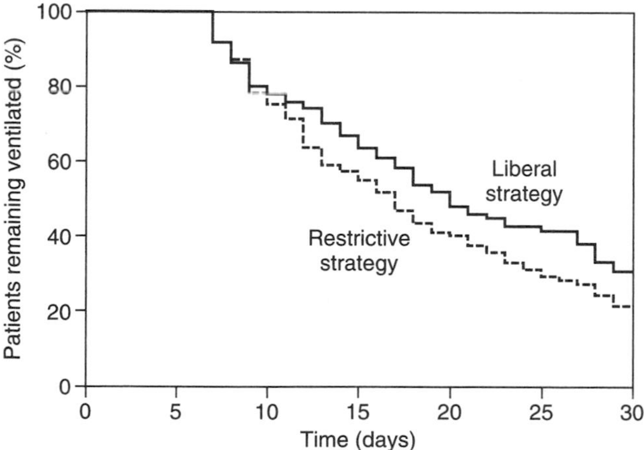

Figure 32–5 Time remaining on mechanical ventilation in the 283 patients requiring mechanical ventilation for >1 week. The time to successful weaning from mechanical ventilation is illustrated using Kaplan-Meier survival curves in patients who required mechanical ventilation for >1 week. Weaning success is defined as remaining off mechanical ventilation, once extubated, during the 30 days of observation. The hatched line refers to the restrictive group and the solid line to the liberal group. Survival curves were not statistically different when compared using a log rank test (P=0.08). (Adapted from Hébert PC, McDonald BJ, Tinmouth A. Overview of transfusion practices in perioperative and critical care. Can J Anesth 2003;50:565–575.)

ALTERNATIVES TO TRANSFUSION

Numerous strategies have been explored and recommended to decrease or to eliminate the need for blood transfusions during major surgery and critical illness. Some are relatively benign, but others carry risks that must be weighed against the benefit of red cell administration. Alternatives include decreasing the use of medications that result in perioperative bleeding such as nonsteroidal anti-inflammatory drugs and acetylsalicylic acid (ASA); avoidance of unnecessary phlebotomies and the use of blood conservation strategies such as pediatric test tubes and arterial line reinfusion set-ups; medications to decrease blood loss, such as antifibrinolytic agents; and medications to increase hemoglobin production. In addition to a restrictive transfusion strategy, the two most useful approaches to decrease red cell transfusions in critically ill patients appear to be blood conservation techniques such as decreased phlebotomies and erythropoietin therapy. Other therapeutic strategies are better suited to patients undergoing high-risk surgical procedures.

Decreased red cell production is one of the causes of anemia in the critically ill. Indeed, critical illness is characterized by a blunted erythropoietin production and response.[115] This blunted response appears to result from inhibition of the erythropoietin gene by inflammatory mediators.[116,117] It has also been shown that these same inflammatory cytokines directly inhibit red cell production by the bone marrow and may produce distinct abnormalities of iron metabolism.[118,119] In patients with multiple organ failure, recombinant human erythropoietin therapy (600 units/kg) has been shown to stimulate erythropoiesis.[120] Similarly, in a small, randomized, placebo-controlled trial (160 patients), therapy with recombinant human erythropoietin resulted in an almost 50% reduction in RBC transfusions versus placebo.[121] Erythropoietin was given at a dose of 300 units/kg daily for 5 days followed by every other day therapy until ICU discharge. Despite receiving fewer RBC transfusions, patients in the recombinant human erythropoietin group had a significantly greater increase in hematocrit.

Recently, the efficacy of recombinant human erythropoietin in the critically ill was evaluated in a large, randomized, controlled trial of 1302 critically ill patients.[122] Recombinant human erythropoietin was given weekly at a dose of 40,000 units. All patients received three weekly doses, and patients who remained in the ICU on study day 21 received a fourth dose. Treatment with recombinant human erythropoietin resulted in a 10% reduction in the number of patients receiving any RBC transfusions. The authors reported a 60.4% rate of transfusions following randomization in the placebo group compared with 50.5% in the recombinant human erythropoietin group (odds ratio of 0.67 with 95% CI of 0.54 to 0.83, $P<0.0004$) and a 20% reduction in the total number of RBC units transfused in patients receiving recombinant human erythropoietin ($P< 0.001$). All clinical outcomes including mortality rates, rates of organ failure, and length of stay in ICU and the hospital were comparable between groups (all P values >0.05). Taken together, these studies[121–123] demonstrate that recombinant human erythropoietin therapy in critically ill patients results in a decrease in red cell transfusion and an increase in hemoglobin level. These observations are consistent with the hypothesis that the anemia in the critically ill is similar to the anemia of chronic disease and is characterized, at least in part, by a relative erythropoietin deficiency.[124] However, erythropoietin therapy has yet to be shown to improve clinical outcomes.

CONCLUSION

Despite the frequent use of red cell transfusions, only one large randomized trial has examined red cell administration perioperatively and in the critical care setting. However, the TRICC trial does not provide sufficient evidence to determine optimal transfusion practice in postoperative care, in critically ill children, or in patients with myocardial infarction or acute coronary syndromes. In addition, most transfusion practice guidelines published prior to the completion of the TRICC trial[110] are now dated and need to have expert opinion informed by solid evidence in diverse clinical settings. During the next several years, randomized trials should provide additional evidence in support of bedside decision making. For example, three transfusion studies will be evaluating transfusion triggers including one in premature infants, another in critically ill children, and a third following high-risk patients who require operative repair of a hip fracture. At this time, high-quality clinical evidence is not yet available for many decisions related to red cell transfusions and alternatives such as human recombinant erythropoietin. The authors anticipate that risks and benefits of red cells and alternatives will be better elucidated in the coming years.

REFERENCES

1. Ghali WA, Palepu A, Paterson WG. Evaluation of red blood cell transfusion practices with the use of preset criteria. Can Med Assoc J 1994;150:1449–1454.
2. Chiavetta JA, Herst R, Freedman J, Axcell TJ, Wall AJ, Van Rooy SC. A survey of red cell use in 45 hospitals in central Ontario, Canada. Transfusion 1996;36:699–706.
3. Brien WF, Butler RJ, Inwood MJ. An audit of blood component therapy in a Canadian general teaching hospital. Can Med Assoc J 1989;140: 812–815.
4. Hutton B, Fergusson D, Tinmouth A, McIntyre L, Kmetic A, Hébert PC. Transfusion rates vary significantly amongst Canadian medical centres. Can J Anaesth 2005;52:581–590.
5. Sugerman HJ, Davidson DT, Vibul S, Delivoria-Papadopoulos M, Miller LD, Oski FA. The basis of defective oxygen delivery from stored blood. Surg Gynecol Obstet 1970;137:733–741.
6. Parris WC, Kambam JR, Blanks S, Dean R. The effect of intentional hemodilution on P_{50}. J Cardiovasc Surg 1988;19:560–562.
7. Oski FA, Marshall BE, Cohen PJ, Sugerman HJ, Miller LD. Exercise with anemia: the role of the left-shifted or right-shifted oxygen-hemoglobin equilibrium curve. Ann Intern Med 1971;74:44–46.
8. Oski FA, Gottlieb AJ, Delavoria-Papadopoulos M, Miller WW. Red-cell 2,3-diphosphoglycerate levels in subjects with chronic hypoxemia. N Engl J Med 1969;280:1165–1166.
9. Brecher ME, Zylstra-Halling VW, Pineda AA. Rejuvenation of erythrocytes preserved with AS-1 and AS-3. Am J Clin Pathol 1991;96: 767–769.
10. Chanutin A, Curnish RR. Effect of organic and inorganic phosphates on the oxygen equilibrium of human erythrocytes. Arch Biochem Biophys 1967;121:96–102.
11. Myburgh JA, Webb RK, Worthley LI. The P50 is reduced in critically ill patients. Intensive Care Med 1991;17:355–358.
12. Iapichino G, Radrizzani D, Solca M, et al. Restoration of blood 2,3-diphosphoglycerate levels in multi-transfused patients: effect of organic and inorganic phosphate. Int Surg 1984;69:113–116.
13. Rodman T, Close HP, Purcell MK. The oxyhemoglobin dissociation curve in anemia. Ann Intern Med 1960;52:295–309.
14. Kennedy AC, Valtis DJ. The oxygen dissociation curve in anemia of various types. J Clin Invest 1954;33:1372–1381.
15. Kahn RC, Zaroulis C, Goetz W, Howland WS. Hemodynamic oxygen transport and 2,3-diphosphoglycerate changes after transfusion of patients in acute respiratory failure. Intensive Care Med 1986;12:22–25.
16. Studzinski T, Czarnecki A, Gluszak A. Effect of acute posthaemorrhagic anaemia on the level of 2,3-diphosphoglycerate (2,3-DPG) in the erythrocytes of sheep. Acta Physiol Pol 1980;31:365–373.
17. Benesch R, Benesch RE. The effect of organic phosphates from human erythrocytes on the allosteric properties of hemoglobin. Biochem Biophys Res Commun 1967;26:162–167.
18. Benesch R, Benesch RE, Yu CI. Reciprocal binding of oxygen and diphosphoglycerate by human hemoglobin. Proc Natl Acad Sci USA 1968;59:526–532.
19. Wyman J. Hemoglobin function. In Bunn HF, Forget BG (eds). Hemoglobin: Molecular, Genetic and Clinical Aspects. Philadelphia, WB Saunders, 1986, pp 37–60.
20. Bohr C, Hasselbalch KA, Krogh A. Über einen in biologischer Beziehung wichtigen Einfluss, den die Kohlensäurespannung des Blutes auf dessen Sauerstoffbinding übt. Scand Arch Physiol 1904;16:402–412.
21. Snyder JV. Oxygen transport: the model and reality. In Snyder JV, Pinsky MR (eds). Oxygen Transport in the Critically Ill. Chicago, Year Book Medical Publishers, 1987, pp 3–15.
22. Schumacker PT, Samsel RW. Oxygen delivery and uptake by peripheral tissues: physiology and pathophysiology. Crit Care Clin 1989;5: 255–269.
23. Finch CA, Lenfant C. Oxygen transport in man. N Engl J Med 1972;286: 407–415.
24. Tuman KJ. Tissue oxygen delivery: the physiology of anemia. Anesthesiol Clin North Am 1990;8:451–469.
25. Alexander RH, Ali J, Aprahamian C, et al. Advanced Trauma Life Support: Program for Physicians, 5th ed. Chicago, American College of Surgeons, 1993.
26. Brannon ES, Merrill AJ, Warren VJ, Stead EA. The cardiac output in patients with chronic anemia as measured by the technique of right atrial catheterization. J Clin Invest 1945;24:332–336.
27. Bowens C Jr, Spahn DR, Frasco PE, Smith LR, McRae RL, Leone BJ. Hemodilution induces stable changes in global cardiovascular and regional myocardial function. Anesth Analg 1993;76:1027–1032.
28. Welch HG, Meehan KR, Goodnough LT. Prudent strategies for elective red blood cell transfusion. Ann Intern Med 1992;116:393–402.
29. Chapler CK, Cain SM. The physiologic reserve in oxygen carrying capacity: studies in experimental hemodilution. Can J Physiol Pharmacol 1985;64:7–12.
30. Cane RD. Hemoglobin: how much is enough? Crit Care Med 1990;18: 1046–1047.
31. Duke M, Abelmann WH. The hemodynamic response to chronic anemia. Circulation 1969;39:503–515.
32. Crystal GJ, Salem MR. Myocardial oxygen consumption and segmental shortening during selective coronary hemodilution in dogs. Anesth Analg 1988;67:500–508.
33. Laks H, Pilon RN, Klovekorn WP, Anderson WP, MacCallum JR, O'Connor NT. Acute hemodilution: its effect on hemodynamics and oxygen transport in anesthetized man. Ann Surg 1974;180: 103–109.
34. Shah DM, Prichard MN, Newell JC, Karmody AM, Scovill WA, Powers SR Jr. Increased cardiac output and oxygen transport after intraoperative isovolemic hemodilution: a study in patients with peripheral vascular disease. Arch Surg 1980;115:597–600.
35. Rosberg B, Wulff K. Hemodynamics following normovolemic hemodilution in elderly patients. Acta Anaesthesiol Scand 1981;25:402–406.
36. Rose D, Coutsoftides T. Intraoperative normovolemic hemodilution. J Surg Res 1981;31:375–381.
37. Boldt J, Kling D, Weidler B, et al. Acute preoperative hemodilution in cardiac surgery: volume replacement with a hypertonic saline-hydroxyethyl starch solution. J Cardiothorac Vasc Anesth 1991;5: 23–28.
38. Mouren S, Baron JF, Hag B, Arthaud M, Viars P. Normovolemic hemodilution and lumbar epidural anesthesia. Anesth Analg 1989;69: 174–179.
39. Herregods L, Foubert L, Moerman A, Francois K, Rolly G. Comparative study of limited intentional normovolaemic haemodilution in patients with left main coronary artery stenosis. Anaesthesia 1995;50:950–953.
40. Welch M, Knight DG, Carr MH, Smyth JV, Walker MG. The preservation of renal function by isovolemic hemodilution during aortic operations. J Vasc Surg 1993;18:858–866.
41. Duke M, Herbert VD, Abelmann WH. Hemodynamic effects of blood transfusion in chronic anemia. N Engl J Med 1964;271:975–980.
42. Cropp GJ. Cardiovascular function in children with severe anemia. Circulation 1969;39:775–784.
43. Roy SB, Bhatia ML, Mathur VS, Virmani S. Hemodynamic effects of chronic severe anemia. Circulation 1963;28:346–356.

43a. Weiskopf RB, Viele MK, Feiner J, et al. Human cardiovascular and metabolic response to acute, severe, isovolemic anemia. JAMA 1998;279:217–221.
44. Woodson RD, Auerbach S. Effect of increased oxygen affinity and anemia on cardiac output and its distribution. J Appl Physiol 1982;53:1299–1306.
45. Messmer K, Lewis DH, Sunder-Plassmann L, Klovekorn WP, Mendler N, Holper K. Acute normovolemic hemodilution. Eur Surg Res 1972;4:55–70.
46. Whitaker W. Some effects of severe chronic anaemia on the circulatory system. Quart J Med 1956;25:175–183.
47. Messmer K. Hemodilution: possibilities and safety aspects. Acta Anaesthesiol Scand 1988;32:49–53.
48. Spahn DR, Leone BJ, Reves JG, Pasch T. Cardiovascular and coronary physiology of acute isovolemic hemodilution: a review of nonoxygen-carrying and oxygen-carrying solutions. Anesth Analg 1994;78:1000–1021.
49. Crosby ET. Perioperative haemotherapy. I. Indications for blood component transfusion. Can J Anaesth 1992;39:695–707.
50. Hatcher JD, Chiu LK, Jennings DB. Anemia as a stimulus to aortic and carotid chemoreceptors in the cat. J Appl Physiol 1978;44:696–702.
51. Murray JF, Escobar E, Rapaport E. Effects of blood viscosity on hemodynamic responses in acute normovolemic anemia. Am J Physiol 1969;216:638–642.
52. Fowler NO, Holmes JC. Blood viscosity and cardiac output in acute experimental anemia. J Appl Physiol 1975;39:453–456.
53. Baer RW, Vlahakes GJ, Uhlig PN, Hoffman JIE. Maximum myocardial oxygen transport during anemia and polycythemia in dogs. Am J Physiol 1987;252:H1086–H1095.
54. Escobar E, Jones NL, Rapaport E, Murray JF. Ventricular performance in acute normovolemic anemia and effects of beta blockade. Am J Physiol 1966;211:877–884.
55. Kowalyshyn TJ, Prager D, Young J. Preoperative hemoglobin requirements. Anesth Analg 1972;51:75–79.
56. Glick G, Plauth WH Jr, Braunwald E. Role of the autonomic nervous system in the circulatory response to acutely induced anemia in unanesthetized dogs. J Clin Invest 1964;43:2112–2124.
57. American Society of Anesthesiologists Task Force on Blood Component Therapy. Practice guidelines for blood component therapy. Anesthesiology 1996;84:732–747.
58. Murray JF, Rapaport E. Coronary blood flow and myocardial metabolism in acute experimental anaemia. Cardiovasc Res 1972;6:360–367.
59. Hatcher JD, Jennings DB, Parker JO, Garvock WB. The role of a humoral mechanism in the cardiovascular adjustments over a prolonged period following the production of acute exchange anaemia. Can J Biochem Physiol 1963;41:1887–1899.
60. Race D, Dedichen H, Schenk WG Jr. Regional blood flow during dextran-induced normovolemic hemodilution in the dog. J Thorac Cardiovasc Surg 1967;53:578–586.
61. Martin E, Ott E. Extreme hemodilution in the Harrington procedure. Bibl Haematol 1981;47:322–337.
62. Fontana JL, Welborn L, Mongan PD, Sturm P, Martin G, Bunger R. Oxygen consumption and cardiovascular function in children during profound intraoperative normovolemic hemodilution. Anesth Analg 1995;80:219–225.
63. Neill WA, Phelps NC, Oxendine JM, Mahler DJ, Sim DN. Effect of heart rate on coronary blood flow distribution in dogs. Am J Cardiol 1973;32:306–312.
64. Neill WA, Oxendine J, Phelps N, Anderson RP. Subendocardial ischemia provoked by tachycardia in conscious dogs with coronary stenosis. Am J Cardiol 1975;35:30–36.
65. Rodriguez JA, Chamorro GA, Rapaport E. Effect of isovolemic anemia on ventricular performance at rest and during exercise. J Appl Physiol 1974;36:28–33.
66. Habler OP, Kleen MS, Podtschaske AH, et al. The effect of acute normovolemic hemodilution (ANH) on myocardial contractilty in anesthetized dogs. Anesth Analg 1996;83:451–458.
67. Chapler CK, Stainsby WN, Lillie MA. Peripheral vascular responses during acute anemia. Can J Physiol Pharmacol 1981;59:102–107.
68. Fan FC, Chen RY, Schuessler GB, Chien S. Effects of hematocrit variations on regional hemodynamics and oxygen transport in the dog. Am J Physiol 1980;238:H545–H552.
69. Brazier J, Cooper N, Maloney JV Jr, Buckberg G. The adequacy of myocardial oxygen delivery in acute normovolemic anemia. Surgery 1974;75:508–516.
70. Bassenge E, Schmid-Schonbein H, von Restorff W, Volger E. Effect of hemodilution on coronary hemodynamics in conscious dogs: a preliminary report. Int Symp Rottach-Egern. Basel, Karger, 1972, pp 174–183.
71. Crystal GJ, Rooney MW, Salem MR. Myocardial blood flow and oxygen consumption during isovolemic hemodilution alone and in combination with adenosine-induced controlled hypotension. Anesth Analg 1988;67:539–547.
72. Jan KM, Heldman J, Chien S. Coronary hemodynamics and oxygen utilization after hematocrit variations in hemorrhage. Am J Physiol 1980;239:H326–H332.
73. Noldge GF, Priebe HJ, Geiger K. Splanchnic hemodynamics and oxygen supply during acute normovolemic hemodilution alone and with isoflurane-induced hypotension in the anesthetized pig. Anesth Analg 1992;75:660–674.
74. Noldge GF, Priebe HJ, Bohle W, Buttler KJ, Geiger K. Effects of acute normovolemic hemodilution on splanchnic oxygenation and on hepatic histology and metabolism in anesthetized pigs. Anesthesiology 1991;74:908–918.
75. Levy PS, Quigley RL, Gould SA. Acute dilutional anemia and critical left anterior descending coronary artery stenosis impairs end organ oxygen delivery. J Trauma 1996;41:416–423.
76. Krieter H, Bruckner UB, Kefalianakis F, Messmer K. Does colloid-induced plasma hyperviscosity in haemodilution jeopardize perfusion and oxygenation of vital organs? Acta Anaesthesiol Scand 1995;39:236–244.
77. Richardson TQ, Guyton AC. Effects of polycythemia and anemia on cardiac output and other circulatory factors. Am J Physiol 1959;197:1167–1170.
78. Jan KM, Chien S. Effect of hematocrit variations on coronary hemodynamics and oxygen utilization. Am J Physiol 1977;233:H106–H113.
79. Kiel JW, Shepherd AP. Optimal hematocrit for canine gastric oxygenation. Am J Physiol 1989;256:H472–H477.
80. Kiel JW, Riedel GL, Shepherd AP. Effects of hemodilution on gastric and intestinal oxygenation. Am J Physiol 1989;256:H171–H178.
81. Wilkerson DK, Rosen AL, Sehgal LR, Gould SA, Sehgal HL, Moss GS. Limits of cardiac compensation in anemic baboons. Surgery 1988;103:665–670.
82. Leung JM, Weiskopf RB, Feiner J, et al. Electrocardiographic ST-segment changes during acute, severe isovolemic hemodilution in humans. Anesthesiology 2000;93:1004–1010.
83. Expert Working Group. Guidelines for red blood cell and plasma transfusion for adults and children. Report of the expert working group. Can Med Assoc J 1997;156(Suppl 11):S1–S24.
84. Bayer WL, Coenen WM, Jenkins DC, Zucker ML. The use of blood and blood components in 1,769 patients undergoing open-heart surgery. Ann Thorac Surg 1980;29:117–122.
85. Gollub S, Bailey CP. Management of major surgical blood loss without transfusion. JAMA 1966;198:149–152.
86. Carson JL, Spence RK, Poses RM, Bonavita G. Severity of anaemia and operative mortality and morbidity. Lancet 1988;1:727–729.
87. Spence RK, Carson JA, Poses R, et al. Elective surgery without transfusion: influence of preoperative hemoglobin level and blood loss on mortality. Am J Surg 1990;159:320–324.
88. Fullerton WT, Turner AG. Exchange transfusion in treatment of severe anaemia in pregnancy. Lancet 1962;282:75–78.
89. Kawaguchi A, Bergsland J, Subramanian S. Total bloodless open heart surgery in the pediatric age group. Circulation 1984;70:1–30.
90. Nelson AH, Fleisher LA, Rosenbaum SH. Relationship between postoperative anemia and cardiac morbidity in high-risk vascular patients in the intensive care unit. Crit Care Med 1993;21:860–866.
91. Lunn JN, Elwood PC. Anaemia and surgery. BMJ 1970;3:71–73.
92. Gopalrao T. Should anemia stop surgery? Int Surg 1971;55:250–255.
93. Ott DA, Cooley DA. Cardiovascular surgery in Jehovah's Witnesses: report of 542 operations without blood transfusion. JAMA 1977;238:1256–1258.
94. Graves CL, Allen RM. Anesthesia in the presence of severe anemia. Rocky Mountain Med J 1974;67:35–40.
95. Simmons CW Jr, Messmer BJ, Hallman GL, Cooley DA. Vascular surgery in Jehovah's Witnesses. JAMA 1970;213:1032–1034.
96. Viele MK, Weiskopf RB. What can we learn about the need for transfusion from patients who refuse blood? The experience with Jehovah's Witnesses. Transfusion 1994;34:396–401.
97. Slawson KB. Anaesthesia for the patient in renal failure. Br J Anaesth 1972;44:277–282.
98. Aldrete JA, Daniel W, O'Higghins JW, Homatas J, Starzl TE. Analysis of anesthetic-related morbidity in human recipients of renal holografts. Anesth Analg 1971;50:321–329.
99. Samuel JR, Powell D. Renal transplantation: anesthetic experience of 100 cases. Anaesthesia 1970;25:165–176.
100. Alexiu O, Mircea N, Balaban M, Furtunescu B. Gastrointestinal haemorrhage from peptic ulcer: an evaluation of bloodless transfusion and early surgery. Anaesthesia 1975;30:609–615.

101. Audet AM, Goodenough LT. Practice strategies for elective red blood cell transfusion. Ann Intern Med 1992;116:403–406.
102. Consensus Conference (National Institutes of Health). Perioperative red blood cell transfusion. JAMA 1988;260:2700–2703.
103. Carson JL, Duff A, Poses RM, et al. Effects of anaemia and cardiovascular disease on surgical mortality and morbidity. Lancet 1996;348:1055–1060.
104. Hébert PC, Wells G, Tweeddale M, et al. Does transfusion practice affect mortality in critically ill patients? Transfusion Requirements in Critical Care (TRICC) Investigators and the Canadian Critical Care Trials Group. Am J Respir Crit Care Med 1997;155:1618–1623.
105. Wu WC, Rathore SS, Wang Y, Radford MJ, Krumholz HM. Blood transfusion in elderly patients with acute myocardial infarction. N Engl J Med 2001;345:1230–1236.
106. Carson JL, Duff A, Berlin JA, et al. Perioperative blood transfusion and postoperative mortality. JAMA 1998;279:199–205.
107. Vincent JL, Baron JF, Reinhart K, et al. Anemia and blood transfusion in critically ill patients. JAMA 2002;288:1499–1507.
108. Hébert PC, Fergusson DA. Red blood cell transfusions in critically ill patients. JAMA 2002;288:1525–1526.
109. Carson JL, Hill S, Carless P, Hébert PC, Henry D. Transfusion triggers: a systematic review of the literature. Transfus Med Rev 2002;16:187–199.
110. Hébert PC, Wells G, Blajchman MA, et al. A multicenter, randomized, controlled clinical trial of transfusion requirements in critical care. N Engl J Med 1999;340:409–417 [erratum appears in N Engl J Med 1999;340:1056].
111. Hébert PC, Yetisir E, Martin C, et al. Is a low transfusion threshold safe in critically ill patients with cardiovascular diseases? Crit Care Med 2001;29:227–234.
112. Bordin JO, Heddle NM, Blajchman MA. Biologic effects of leukocytes present in transfused cellular blood products. Blood 1994;84:1703–1721.
113. van de Watering LM, Hermans J, Houbiers JG, et al. Beneficial effects of leukocyte depletion of transfused blood on postoperative complications in patients undergoing cardiac surgery: a randomized clinical trial. Circulation 1998;97:562–568.
114. Rivers E, Nguyen B, Havstad MA, et al. Early goal-directed therapy in the treatment of severe sepsis and septic shock. N Engl J Med 2001;345:1368–1377.
115. Rodriguez RM, Corwin HL, Gettinger A, Corwin MJ, Gubler D, Pearl RG. Nutritional deficiencies and blunted erythropoietin response as causes of the anemia of critical illness. J Crit Care 2001;16:36–41.
116. Frede S, Fandrey J, Pagel H, Hellwig T, Jelkmann W. Erythropoietin gene expression is suppressed after lipopolysaccharide or interleukin-1 beta injections in rats. Am J Physiol 1997;273(3 pt 2):R1067–R1071.
117. Jelkmann W. Proinflammatory cytokines lowering erythropoietin production. J Interferon Cytokine Res 1998;18:555–559.
118. Means RT Jr, Krantz SB. Progress in understanding the pathogenesis of the anemia of chronic disease. Blood 1992;80:1639–1647.
119. Krantz SB. Pathogenesis and treatment of the anemia of chronic disease. Am J Med Sci 1994;307:353–359.
120. Gabriel A, Kozek S, Chiari A, et al. High-dose recombinant human erythropoietin stimulates reticulocyte production in patients with multiple organ dysfunction syndrome. J Trauma 1998;44:361–367.
121. Corwin HL, Gettinger A, Rodriguez RM, et al. Efficacy of recombinant human erythropoietin in the critically ill patient: a randomized, double-blind, placebo-controlled trial. Crit Care Med 1999;27:2346–2350.
122. Corwin HL, Gettinger A, Pearl RG, et al. Efficacy of recombinant human erythropoietin in critically ill patients: a randomized controlled trial. JAMA 2002;288:2827–2835.
123. Silver MJ, Bazzan A, Corwin H, Gettinger A, Corwin MJ. A randomized double blind placebo controlled trial of recombinant human erythropoietin in long term acute care patients. Crit Care Med 2003;31(Suppl):A167.
124. Corwin HL, Krantz SB. Anemia of the critically ill: "acute" anemia of chronic disease. Crit Care Med 2000;28:3098–3099.

Chapter 33

Post-Transfusion Red Blood Cell and Platelet Survival and Kinetics: Basic Principles and Practical Aspects

Richard J. Davey • James P. AuBuchon

Investigating the fate of transfused blood cells can offer important information for the manufacturers of blood collection and storage systems, the transfusion specialists who collect and prepare the units, and patients with disorders involving reduced survival or abnormal trafficking of these cells. Tracking the recovery and survival of blood cells also allows for validation of systems' capabilities (and their improvement with innovations) as well as diagnostic procedures that can lead to therapeutic interventions for a variety of disorders.

The clinical and research applications of these techniques have led to their adoption by many medical centers. However, the technical complexity and regulatory requirements for handling radionuclides have limited their availability. Newer techniques that avoid the use of radioactive substances are under study and may eventually play a larger role in clinical applications as well as in trials of new blood collection, processing, and storage systems.

RADIONUCLIDES IN TRANSFUSION MEDICINE

Gray and Sterling[1] described the first clinically useful red cell radiolabel, chromium-51, in 1950. Fisher and colleagues[2] introduced technetium-99m as a cell label in 1967, and the importance of indium-111 was recognized after an evaluation of leukocyte radiolabels by McAfee and Thakur[3] in 1976. Other cell radiolabels have also been evaluated and used, with varying degrees of success. However, the vast majority of blood cell survival and imaging studies are performed with either chromium-51 (^{51}Cr), technetium-99m (^{99m}Tc), or indium-111 (^{111}In).

Each of the three commonly used radionuclides has advantages and disadvantages that affect its applicability in clinical and research settings. Investigators should have an understanding of fundamentals of nuclear medicine and radiation biophysics to use these materials appropriately. Desirable characteristics of a blood cell radiolabel include factors that relate to recipient safety as well as ease and reproducibility of use (Table 33–1).

The selection of an appropriate radionuclide requires familiarity with the radioactive half-life, elution characteristics, and gamma-photon energy (Table 33–2). The optimal range for detection of photoelectric events in a standard gamma-counting instrument (gamma counter) is 100 to 300 keV. The "yield" of gamma-photon emissions is the number of photons emitted per 100 radioactive decays. A high yield means that a lower radiation dose can be used to achieve adequate detection levels.

Chromium-51

^{51}Cr is a useful red cell label and also has utility as a platelet label. Advantages of this radionuclide include ease of red cell labeling, excellent red cell uptake, low toxicity, and low and stable elution rate. ^{51}Cr is produced in a reactor by neutron activation. It decays by electron capture, with a radioactive half-life of 27.7 days. The principal gamma-photon emission occurs by electron capture at 320 keV, slightly above the optimum detection range of standard gamma counters. The high energy and low yield (9.8%) of gamma-photon emissions from decay of this radionuclide necessitate a larger (typically 3-inch) NaI crystal for efficient detection in a gamma counter. Otherwise, a larger dose of this radionuclide may be necessary to achieve adequate counts.

The quite long radioactive half-life of ^{51}Cr makes it suitable for most red cell survival and recovery studies. However, this long half-life poses difficulties when multiple studies need to be performed in a short amount of time, since the overlapping survival curves make separation of the individual studies difficult. This problem can be addressed by correcting for residual radiation, by separating studies until the nuclide decays, or by using alternative radionuclides.[4]

Table 33–1 **Desirable Characteristics of Blood Cell Radiolabels**
Minimal radiation dose to the recipient
Nontoxic to the recipient
Nontoxic to the cell
Specific for the cell
No metabolism of the label by the cell
Radioactive half-life appropriate for the study
Radioactive emissions suitable for efficient detection or imaging
Minimal manipulation of the cell required
No elution of the label
No relabeling of other cells in vivo

Table 33–2 **Major Features of Radionuclides Used for Blood Cell Labeling**

	^{51}Cr	^{99m}Tc	^{111}In
Radioactivity half-life	27.7 days	6.0 hours	2.8 days
Major γ-photon emissions (yield)	320 keV (9.8%)	140 keV (90%)	173 and 247 keV (90%, 94%)
Elution rate (red cells)	1% per day	1% to 7% per hour	4% to 8% per day
Target organ*	Spleen	Total body	Spleen
Suitable for imaging?	No	Yes	Yes

*Target organ is dependent on cell type and clinical or experimental situation as well.

^{51}Cr is supplied as sodium radiochromate ($Na_2{}^{51}CrO_4$) for cell labeling purposes. Hexavalent chromate labels red cells by first binding rapidly and reversibly to the red cell membrane. After reduction to the trivalent state, the chromic ion binds more slowly and firmly to the β-globin chain of intracellular hemoglobin (and probably to other intracellular ligands as well). Labeling efficiency is about 90%. Younger red cells take up slightly more label than do older cells.

Chromium elutes from red cells in two phases. There is an early loss of 1% to 4% of the label within 24 hours, which may represent elution of a loosely bound fraction of the label.[5] Garby and Mollison[6] found that subsequent elution varies from 0.56% to 2.04% per day, similar to the 0.70% to 1.55% reported by Bentley and associates.[7] An estimated elution rate of 1% per day is satisfactory for most investigational and clinical purposes.[8] Trivalent chromium that elutes from the labeled cells is rapidly excreted in the urine and does not relabel other cells in vivo.

Moroff and colleagues[9] have described the technical steps for labeling red cells with ^{51}Cr for the evaluation of blood storage and preservation systems. The International Committee for Standardization in Hematology[10] has described a slightly different technique suitable for labeling red cells for the determination of transfusion compatibility.

Baldini and colleagues[11] first described the use of ^{51}Cr as a platelet radiolabel. The platelet-labeling efficiency of chromium-51 is low (9%) compared with its red cell labeling efficiency (90%). Therefore, it is important that platelet preparations be free of red cells before being labeled.[12] A procedure for labeling platelets with ^{51}Cr, which is more difficult than that for red cells, has been described by Snyder and colleagues.[13] Further useful refinements were developed by Heaton, Holme, and colleagues.[14,15] Unfortunately, the dose of ^{51}Cr required for imaging studies, which require a high yield of gamma-photon emissions, is typically unacceptably high for most other applications in transfusion medicine.

Technetium-99m

^{99m}Tc, which is widely employed as an imaging agent in nuclear medicine, is another useful red cell label. This metastable radionuclide is produced in a molybdenum generator as a product of molybdenum-99 decay. ^{99m}Tc decays, in turn, to ^{99}Tc, with a half-life of 6.02 hours. In doing so, ^{99m}Tc emits a gamma-photon at 140 keV, which falls within the optimal range of gamma counters. The high yield (90%) of this radionuclide is useful for external imaging. Because of the frequent use of this radionuclide in imaging procedures, many hospitals maintain a generator on site, and thus there is a readily available and inexpensive source of ^{99m}Tc for cell labeling applications.

^{99m}Tc, as pertechnetate, diffuses across the red cell membrane into the cell, where it binds to hemoglobin and other intracellular ligands with a labeling efficiency of about 90%. The short half-life of ^{99m}Tc precludes its use for long-term red cell survival studies. In fact, groups of samples must be counted rapidly, and, even with that, a correction must be made for radioactive decay that occurs during the counting procedure. However, because of its short half-life, ^{99m}Tc is useful as a red cell label when a series of survival studies must be performed for transfusion compatibility. This radionuclide is also useful for the accurate determination of red cell volume as part of red cell recovery studies (using ^{51}Cr) or in patients being investigated for possible pathologic expansion of their red cell mass (e.g., polycythemia).

This nuclide also has a high and variable rate of elution. The use of stannous compounds as intracellular reducing agents in the labeling process has permitted firmer binding of ^{99m}Tc, but elution rates of 4% per hour with considerable variation may be expected.[16,17] Heaton and colleagues[18] have described the technical steps necessary to minimize variability in labeling and elution with this nuclide. Its use as a platelet label has received little attention, however, primarily because its short half-life would prevent determination of postinfusion survival over the following 5 to 10 days, a parameter that is essential in the assessment of the effects of platelet collection and storage conditions.

Indium-111

^{111}In can be used as a label for red cells, platelets, and leukocytes. It is prepared in a cyclotron by proton bombardment of a cadmium target. It has two major gamma-photon emissions—173 keV (90.5% yield) and 247 keV (94% yield)—which are excellent for counting in a gamma counter and for external imaging. The radioactive half-life of the nuclide is 2.83 days, making it appropriate for leukocyte imaging studies that extend over several days.

^{111}In must be complexed with a lipophilic chelating agent if it is to traverse cell membranes and label intracellular proteins. Although several lipophilic chelates have been studied, 8-hydroxyquinoline (oxine) is the only agent currently licensed for this purpose in the United States. Technical procedures have been published for labeling red cells,[19] platelets,[13] and leukocytes[20] with ^{111}In.

Although ^{111}In is a nonselective label, it is preferentially taken up by platelets. Reduced uptake is observed by leukocytes, and still less by red cells.[21] Cell preparations therefore must be free of extraneous elements before being labeled. Like ^{99m}Tc, ^{111}In has a high and variable rate of elution from red cells. AuBuchon and Brightman[19] have shown that 8% to 10% of the label elutes within 24 to 48 hours, with a 4% per day loss after that time. This problem with elution renders ^{111}In unsuitable for red cell studies without a specific correction factor,[22] but ^{111}In is useful for determining red cell volume when precision is not critical.

BLOOD CELL LIFE SPAN AND SURVIVAL STUDIES

Red Cells

The red cell life span (110 to 120 days) was first approximated by differential absorption techniques[23] and subsequently confirmed by radioisotopic labeling studies using cohort (marrow) labels[24] and random (peripheral blood) labels.[6] When chromium-51 is used as the label, the time at which the recovered counts are 50% of the originally injected counts is the T_{50}Cr, normally 31 ± 6 days. Correction for elution will yield the true red cell life span. The T_{50}Cr is also useful for evaluating the extent of hemolysis in chronic hemolytic anemia. Modest reductions in the T_{50}Cr can indicate a substantial increase in the rate of red cell destruction.[25]

Red cell life span studies also have been conducted to assess the therapeutic benefit of transfused units that are enriched in young red cells ("neocytes"). The transfusion of such units has the theoretical benefit of reducing the iron burden in patients who undergo frequent transfusions by increasing the number of long-lived red cells in the circulation.[26] Chromium-51 life span studies have demonstrated that neocytes survive 30% to 60% longer in the circulation than do red cells derived from standard red cell units.[27,28] However, because neocyte units contain only about half the hemoglobin of standard units, their use results in only a modest reduction in transfusion requirements.[29,30] Additionally, since they are costly to prepare, neocyte transfusions have not achieved wide clinical acceptance.

In contrast to long-term life span studies, short-term red cell survival studies are useful in identifying patterns of immune red cell destruction. These studies are clinically important when standard pretransfusion serologic testing cannot clearly identify or characterize red cell alloantibodies or autoantibodies in a transfusion recipient. The various factors that contribute to immune red cell destruction have been discussed in detail elsewhere.[31–33] Of primary importance are the immunoglobulin class and subclass of the recipient red cell alloantibody[34] and the extent to which that antibody activates complement.[35,36]

Four characteristic survival patterns can be recognized in a 24-hour red cell survival study conducted to determine transfusion compatibility (Fig. 33–1). They are (1) normal survival, (2) extravascular destruction characterized by a "two-component" survival curve, (3) extravascular destruction characterized by a "single exponential" survival curve, and (4) intravascular destruction.

Normal Survival

The normal range for recovery of fresh, compatible red cells is ≥97% at 60 minutes and 95% to 100% at 24 hours.

Extravascular Destruction Characterized by a "Two-Component" Survival Curve

Most immunoglobulin M (IgM) red cell alloantibodies and some IgG alloantibodies (e.g., anti-Jk^{a}) can activate complement. IgM antibodies directly activate complement, with 20 to 40 IgM molecules per red cell being required to initiate red cell clearance. IgG antibodies can activate complement if two or more molecules are physically adjacent on the red cell membrane[37]; thus, many more IgG molecules are required for complement activation to occur. In most cases, the kinetics of complement activation result in generation of the membrane-bound C3b fragment but not the final C5b-C9 "membrane attack" complex. Plasma factor I, with plasma factor H as a cofactor, cleaves C3b to C3bi. Red cell–bound C3b and C3bi adhere to the complement receptors CR1 and CR3 on reticuloendothelial system (RES) macrophages in the liver and spleen. These red cells may thus be removed from the circulation by either antibody-dependent cell-mediated cytotoxicity or complete phagocytosis, or they may sustain membrane damage through partial phagocytosis. Alternatively, C3bi may be degraded before red cell damage occurs.[38,39]

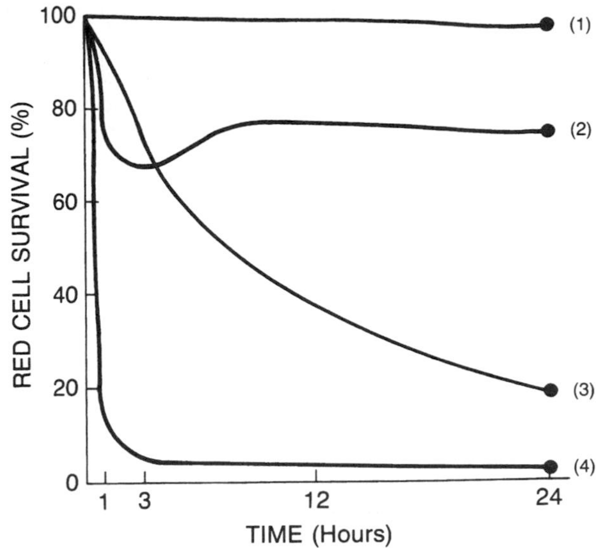

Figure 33–1 Red cell survival patterns representing different mechanisms of immune red cell destruction. (1), Normal survival; (2), two-component curve with partial complement activation to C3b→C3d,g; (3), single exponential curve characteristic of IgG non-complement-activating antibodies; (4), complete complement activation to C5b-C9 complex with intravascular hemolysis.

Plasma factors I and H further cleave C3bi to C3c, which detaches from the cell, and C3d,g, which remains attached to the cell membrane. Because C3d,g binds weakly to CR3 receptors, most red cells coated with C3d,g detach from RES macrophages and survive relatively normally.[40] The inactive C3d,g fragments may protect the red cell from further complement-mediated damage by occupying complement-binding sites. A "two-component" recovery curve, therefore, represents the early loss of C3b-coated red cells and more normal survival of those cells on whose membranes C3b has degraded to C3d,g. A "two-component" survival curve with more than 70% recovery at 24 hours indicates that the patient can safely receive larger quantities of similar red cells with little risk of rapid immune hemolysis.

Extravascular Destruction Characterized by a "Single Exponential" Survival Curve

Many IgG red cell alloantibodies (e.g., Rh antibodies) do not activate complement. Instead, there is progressive removal of sensitized red cells with a survival curve described by a single exponential. Factors such as the concentration and IgG subclass of the antibody determine the rate of removal of the cells. The efficiency of the four IgG subclasses in binding Fc receptors on RES macrophages is $IgG_3 > IgG_1 > IgG_2 > IgG_4$. IgG1 is present in higher titer than the other subclasses and is most often involved in IgG-mediated red cell destruction.[34] Red cell survival studies that demonstrate an IgG-mediated "single exponential" pattern of cell destruction indicate that the transfusion of similar cells may result in a delayed hemolytic transfusion reaction.

Intravascular Destruction

IgM antibodies that are efficient activators of complement, such as anti-A and anti-B, can drive the kinetics of the reaction to the formation of the terminal C5b-C9 "membrane attack" complex. Insertion of this complex into the red cell membrane results in loss of membrane integrity and osmotic lysis of the cell. Transfused cells that generate complement activation of this magnitude are usually hemolyzed within minutes.

Synergistic Effect of Complement and IgG

Complement and IgG appear to act synergistically in promoting red cell opsonization. Studies have demonstrated that the addition of complement to red cells sensitized with IgG alone will enhance phagocytosis.[41,42] A hybrid red cell survival curve may occur when both IgM and IgG antibodies are active. There is a rapid loss of a minor population of the cells from IgM-mediated complement activation, and a slower phase of cell destruction mediated primarily by the IgG antibody.

Platelets

Most studies of platelet life span and kinetics have been performed with chromium-51 and/or indium-111 using labeling procedures defined by the ICSH[43] and Heaton and Holme.[15] The low labeling efficiency, long half-life, and poor imaging characteristics of ^{51}Cr have led to preferential use of ^{111}In when a single platelet label is required.[44] However, serial studies in a subject using a single label may not be possible, since platelet kinetics vary over time. By using both chromium and indium labels for simultaneous infusion, a reduction in this variability is seen, and a more accurate estimation of the difference between platelets stored in a standard (or licensed) system and those in a test system can be achieved.[45] Using "dual-label" approaches in a protocol can allow simultaneous storage and labeling of test and control platelets (e.g., in different bag types). This technique has also been used to create novel approaches to the timing of collections, such as in a study where whole blood–derived platelets stored for 5 days were compared with those stored for 7 days. The test (7-day) platelets were derived from a unit collected on day 0 (with reinfusion of the red cells), and the control (5-day) platelets were derived from a collection 2 days later. Platelets from both study arms were labeled and infused simultaneously.[46]

Standard technical methods for preparation of radiolabeled platelets have been published by the ICSH and others.[13,15,47] The major drawback of ^{111}In-oxine is its high affinity for red cells, leukocytes, and plasma proteins, primarily transferrin. The washing and centrifugation steps necessary to prepare a "clean" platelet preparation cause a substantial loss of platelets (≈40%) and a "collection injury" that can distort test results if not performed carefully. Other compounds that form lipophilic complexes with ^{111}In, notably, acetylacetone,[48] tropolone,[49] and 2-mercaptopyridine-N-oxide (merc),[50] have been extensively studied as possible alternative agents to overcome this problem. Tropolone is widely used in Europe, but oxine remains the only licensed agent in the United States.

Heaton and colleagues contributed to the advancement of platelet labeling accuracy by developing a technique for determining the amount of radionuclide that elutes from platelets shortly after labeling and infusion.[15] With this "elution correction," the recovery curves for platelets labeled with ^{111}In are coincident with those labeled with ^{51}Cr. This procedure is the basis of the standard platelet radiolabeling protocol adopted by the Biomedical Excellence for Safer Transfusion (BEST) Collaborative.[51]

There are four methods for the calculation of platelet life span—linear, exponential, weighted mean, and γ-function (multiple hit)—each of which yields slightly different results. The γ-function analysis is the recommended method[13,43] and the most frequently used, but investigators often report their results using one or more additional statistical methods. An easy-to-use computer program that models platelet survival by a variety of techniques performs these calculations in a standardized, validated manner.[52,53] These calculations can also be performed on statistical analysis software to achieve the same results. The area under the survival curve has also been reported, but some believe this measure places an inordinate weight on the survival parameter.[54]

Because no radioactive tracer selectively labels newly formed platelets, cohort studies have not been practical to measure platelet production. Instead, the kinetics of normal platelet production has been measured indirectly by determining the turnover rate of circulating platelets (platelet count divided by platelet survival corrected for recovery). Estimates of daily platelet production in the steady state using this method have ranged from 35,000–66,000/μL of blood.[55] The life span of human platelets ranges between 8 and 12 days; Harker and Finch[56] found it to be 9.5 ± 0.6 days. Senescent platelets are removed from the circulation by RES macrophages in the liver and spleen and, to a lesser extent, by bone marrow and lungs.[57,58]

There is also evidence of a fixed platelet requirement necessary to maintain vascular integrity. Hanson and Slichter[59] have proposed that 82% of platelet turnover in normal persons is due to senescence, and 18% (≈7100 platelets/μL/day) is due to the fixed requirement. The fixed requirement becomes an increasingly large component of platelet removal as thrombocytopenia from bone marrow hypoplasia worsens. Thus, platelet life span correlates directly with the platelet count; an accelerated reduction in life span is noted as platelet counts decrease below 50,000/μL. The shortened platelet life span observed in thrombocytopenic patients, therefore, does not necessarily indicate an increased platelet destruction rate.

Patients with increased peripheral platelet destruction, such as those with idiopathic thrombocytopenic purpura,[60] have platelet life spans that are shorter than predicted by Hanson and Slichter's model.[59] Thus, platelet life span studies using ^{111}In are useful in discriminating between thrombocytopenia caused by decreased platelet production and that caused by increased platelet destruction (Fig. 33–2). Platelet life span studies are not generally useful in the alloimmunized patient, however. Post-transfusion platelet counts usually provide the clinician with the information necessary for the management of these patients.

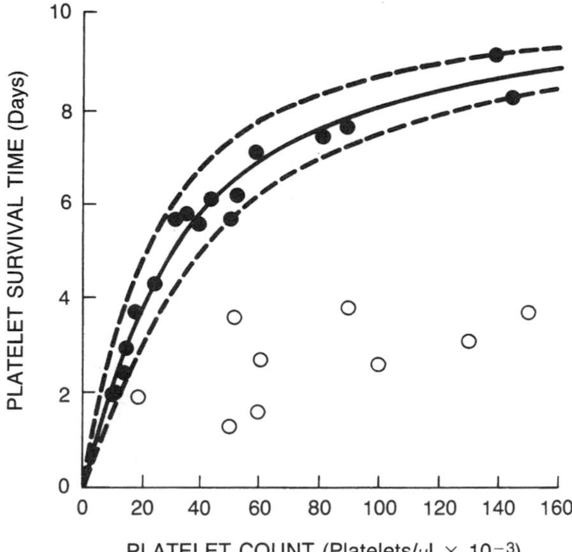

Figure 33–2 Relationship between the survival of ^{111}In-labeled autologous platelets and the circulating platelet count. *Solid circles* identify patients with impaired platelet production (hypoplasia; $n = 17$). *Open circles* identify patients with increased peripheral platelet destruction (ITP; $n = 9$). *Solid line* is best fit to data from the hypoplastic patient group. Platelet survival could be predicted by platelet count in the hypoplastic patient. The "fixed requirement" is increasingly apparent in this group at platelet counts below 50,000/μL. (Adapted from Tomer A, Harker LA. Megakaryocytopoiesis and platelet kinetics. In Rossi EC, Simon TL, Moss GS [eds]. Principles of Transfusion Medicine. Baltimore, Williams & Wilkins, 1991, p 175.)

Leukocytes

Although granulocytes, lymphocytes, and monocytes derive from a common pluripotent stem cell, they have widely variant functions and kinetics. Radionuclides have permitted the study of the normal kinetics of these various leukocyte classes.[61] ^{111}In-oxine is now the nuclide of choice for leukocyte radiolabeling. Because labeling with ^{111}In-oxine is nonselective, the leukocytes of interest must be separated from other cells and plasma before being labeled.[62]

Granulocytes

Studies done with granulocytes labeled with diisopropylfluorophosphate demonstrated that the circulating cells had a half-life of 3.8 to 6.7 hours. About half of the injected cells were recoverable in the circulation, with the remainder constituting a "marginating pool" of cells.[63,64] More recent studies done with ^{111}In-labeled granulocytes have shown a mean recovery of 30% of the labeled cells and a mean circulating half-life of 5.0 hours.[65] Imaging studies have shown that labeled and transfused granulocytes transiently sequester in the lungs. The extent and duration of the pulmonary sequestration appear to be more severe when the labeled cells are suspended in saline rather than plasma.[66] Alloimmunized patients demonstrate a more prolonged and intense pulmonary sequestration phase than do normal subjects.[67] In addition, HLA (human leukocyte antigen)– and granulocyte-specific antibodies appear to reduce the intravascular half-life of transfused granulocytes[68] and to impair their ability to migrate to a site of active infection.[69]

Lymphocytes

The extreme radiosensitivity of lymphocytes has hampered the conduct of kinetic and imaging studies. Autologous lymphocytes labeled with a low dose of ^{111}In (>20 μCi/10^8 cells) move rapidly from the circulation and sequester in the lung, liver, and spleen. A more gradual accumulation of radiolabel in the lymph nodes follows.[70] These findings are consistent with studies indicating that most lymphocytes are part of a large recirculating pool consisting of long-lived, nondividing cells.[71,72] Lymphocytes in this pool migrate from the circulation to the various lymphoid tissues, where they have opportunity to interact with foreign antigen. The migration patterns are not random but are modified by the lymphocyte class and immunologic history of the cell. T cells preferentially migrate to lymph nodes, whereas B cells tend to migrate to mucosal lymphoid tissue.[72] Lymphocytes collected from a specific type of lymphoid tissue (e.g., gut mucosa) move to that tissue because of "homing receptors" expressed on the cell after specific antigenic stimulation.[73]

Activated Mononuclear Cells

Kinetic studies of human monocytes have been limited because of the difficulty of obtaining a homogeneous collection of cells and because of technical problems with cell activation and clumping during preparation. However, monocytes prepared by leukapheresis, density gradient separation, and countercurrent elutriation have been activated with interferon-γ and infused intraperitoneally in patients with peritoneal spread of colorectal cancer.[74] In two patients, ^{111}In-labeled cells remained in the peritoneal cavity for up to 5 days after infusion, supporting the observation of clinical improvement in a larger group of patients treated with unlabeled activated monocytes.

A subpopulation of peripheral blood lymphocytes activated with the cytokine interleukin-2 has been found to exhibit antitumor activity. These lymphokine-activated killer cells presumably migrate to tumor sites, but cell trafficking and imaging studies have been inconclusive.[75] Lymphocytes directly harvested from tumor sites (tumor-infiltrating lymphocytes), however, have been shown to localize at tumor sites and persist in the circulation after activation.[76]

PROTOCOLS TO EVALUATE COMPONENT COLLECTION, PROCESSING, AND STORAGE SYSTEMS

The two critical advances that led to modern blood preservation techniques were the introduction of acid-citrate-dextrose in 1943[77] and the development of plastic blood containers in the early 1950s. Now, blood components are stored in various anticoagulant-preservative or additive solutions, in plastic containers with differing characteristics, and at nonphysiologic temperatures for extended periods. The advent of pathogen inactivation systems offers great potential for improving transfusion safety but at potential risk of injury to the cells during the process. For this reason, the safety and efficacy of new or modified storage conditions must be determined by both in vitro and in vivo evaluation of cell function and viability.

A variety of biochemical, hematologic, and functional parameters are often measured across the storage period in

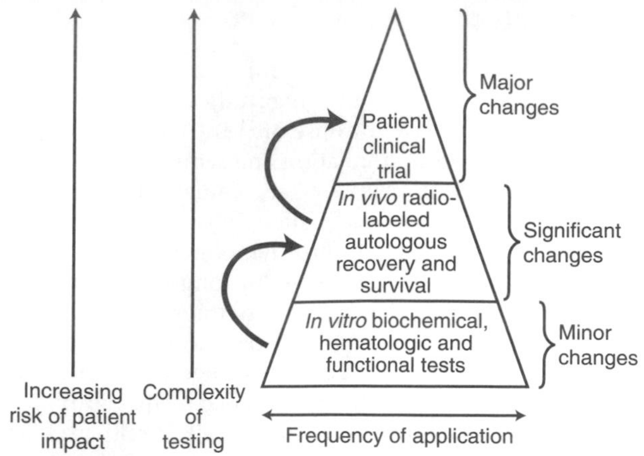

Figure 33–3 Scheme for progressive analysis of new blood component. A representation of the progressive analysis of a new blood component illustrating (1) the stepwise nature of investigation (beginning with in vitro testing and culminating with clinical trials) and (2) application of different degrees of scrutiny based on the extent to which the new component differed from previously investigated ones. Note that major changes would involve more extensive investigation using more complex testing techniques in response to an increase in the risk of (adverse) patient impact. More commonly encountered, simpler changes to a collection or storage system would more likely require only in vitro testing. Successful testing (indicative of safety and efficacy) at one level of the pyramid would be used to justify moving to the next "higher" level of testing, were that required. (Adapted from a presentation by Dr. Jaro Vostal.[79] Reprinted with permission from AuBuchon JP. Radioisotopic reflections. Transfusion 2005;45:28S–32S.)

an attempt to predict the in vivo outcome after transfusion. It is known, for example, that retention of at least half the original adenosine triphosphate (ATP) concentration in red cells is necessary for adequate recovery and that a $pH_{22°C} \geq 6.2$ for platelets is required in order to retain viability. Beyond these notable exceptions, however, few strong correlations between any in vitro parameters and life span in circulation after storage have been identified.[78] Therefore, documentation of the in vivo recovery (and, for platelets, survival) remains necessary whenever a substantial change in collection, processing, or storage is being proposed. The FDA has described the role of in vitro and in vivo testing as part of a "pyramid" of trials leading to approval of a new device or protocol[79] (Fig. 33–3). Radiolabeled kinetic studies thus remain a critical feature of this approach, which allows definitive documentation in a relevant (human) system and ensures that patients are likely to receive sufficient therapeutic benefit from the component under study.

Red Cells

The 24-hour post-transfusion recovery of red cells stored under experimental conditions is the standard measure of acceptability used in the United States. The FDA requires that a mean of 75% or more of the transfused red cells be recovered 24 hours after infusion. The lower bound of the 95% confidence interval is expected to be at least 70%. Although these criteria have never been encoded in federal regulations or statutes, they have become the accepted measures to obtain licensure. Long-term survival is not a parameter usually measured, since, at least before the advent of pathogen inactivation technologies, postinfusion longevity was assumed to be normal providing the red cell showed acceptable 24-hour survival.[80] Other measures, such as poststorage ATP and supernatant hemoglobin levels, contribute to the assessment of storage condition acceptability. Red cell recovery data have been important in studies evaluating the effect of gamma-irradiation,[81,82] blood bag plasticizing agents,[83] and prestorage leukocyte reduction[84] on stored red cells.

The technique for performing post-transfusion recovery studies to assess new storage conditions differs in important ways from red cell recovery studies to assess transfusion compatibility. As noted in Table 33–3, autologous red cells are chosen for storage studies, thereby avoiding the risks of transmissible disease and transfusion reactions inherent in allogeneic transfusions. The shape of the recovery curve is most important in transfusion compatibility studies. However, the recovery percentage at 24 hours is of prime importance for studies evaluating storage systems.

Because an accurate determination of 24-hour recovery is necessary, the method of establishing the zero-time point (100% recovery) is of critical importance. A direct measurement of the zero-time recovery value is not possible, however, because an infused blood sample is not completely mixed until approximately 3 minutes after transfusion in a normal person.[85] Senescent infused cells and cells damaged during storage are removed from the circulation by the spleen, with loss of these cells beginning immediately after infusion. By 3 minutes, a significant loss of the infused cells may have occurred that is not detected if the 3-minute sample is regarded as representing 100% survival. In this case, the radioactive counts in the 3-minute sample would be

Table 33–3 **Features of Red Cell Survival Studies to Evaluate Transfusion Compatibility and Red Cell Storage Systems**

Purpose of Evaluation	Features of Study
Transfusion compatibility	Allogeneic cells—chosen by specific phenotype Fresh cells (<5 days old)—avoid storage lesion Small volume infused (1 to 3 mL)—reduces risk of transfusion reaction Zero-time (100% recovery) point determined after mixing is complete (3–5 minutes) Interpretation—shape of 24-hour survival curve predictive of clinical significance of recipient antibody
Red cell storage	Autologous cells—avoid risks of allogeneic transfusion Larger volume infused (10–15 mL)—easy to manipulate and smaller radiation dose per cell Zero-time (100% recovery) point determined by independent red cell mass study (double-label method) or back-extrapolation (single-label method) Interpretation—precise determination of recovery at 24 hours (>75% mean recovery required)

falsely low and the 24-hour recovery value falsely elevated. Two methods for calculating the zero-time recovery value are useful in red cell storage evaluation studies: the single-label and the double-label techniques.

Single-Label Technique with Back-Extrapolation

The in vivo destruction of damaged stored red cells begins immediately and can be assumed to continue at a first-order rate. If so, the extrapolation of the logarithm of the post-transfusion counts to the *y*-intercept should yield an accurate determination of the zero-time counts, or the 100% recovery point. Beutler and West[86] compared the red cell mass calculated by the extrapolation method with the red cell mass determined independently using red cells labeled with ^{99m}Tc.[86] They found that extrapolation using fresh red cells yielded red cell mass values that were almost identical to those determined independently. When red cells had been stored for 35 to 49 days, however, there was a consistent overestimation of red cell mass (0.6% to 3.6%) by the extrapolation method, suggesting that the kinetics of the early removal of stored red cells is not described solely by a first-order rate equation (Fig. 33–4).

The removal of damaged and senescent red cells occurs within 15 to 20 minutes of transfusion. Moroff and colleagues[9] have shown that there is a break in the recovery curve at 15 minutes, with red cells persisting after that time having more normal survival. The recovery points used for extrapolation to the *y*-intercept, therefore, should be those obtained after 5 minutes, to ensure complete mixing, and before 15 minutes, to avoid the break in the recovery curve. Moroff and colleagues[9] and others[32,87] have described in detail the technique and interpretation of red cell recoveries using the single-label method.

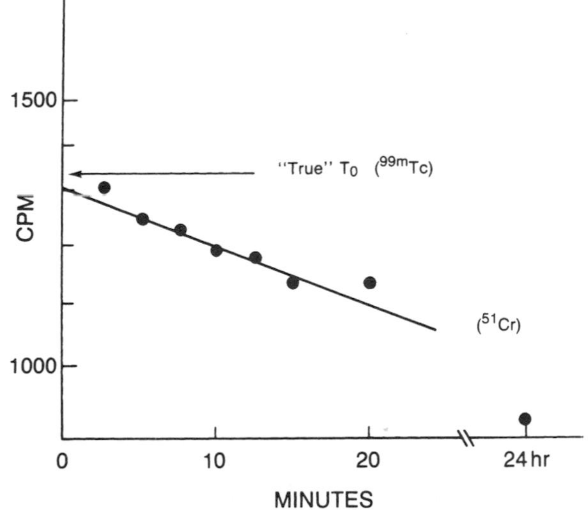

Figure 33–4 Two methods to calculate the counts per minute (CPM) at zero-time (T_0) for determination of red cell mass. With the single-label technique *(solid dots)*, the ^{51}Cr-labeled test cells are infused and samples are obtained at 5, 7.5, 10, 12.5, and 15 minutes after infusion. A regression line is plotted, and the y-intercept (T_0) is determined. In the double-label technique, an independent, or "true," measure of T_0 is determined *(arrow)* with fresh autologous red cells labeled with ^{99m}Tc. The single-label regression technique underestimates CPM at T_0 and, therefore, overestimates 24-hour red cell recovery, with the error increasing as red cell storage time increases. (Adapted from Beutler E, West C. Measurement of the viability of stored red cells by the single-isotope technique using ^{51}Cr. Transfusion 1984;24:100.)

Double-Label Technique with Direct Measurement of the Red Cell Mass

An accurate determination of the recipient's red cell mass provides the correct volume of dilution for the experimental red cell sample. Simultaneous infusion of fresh, autologous red cells labeled with ^{99m}Tc and stored experimental red cells labeled with ^{51}Cr permits this determination. The fresh, autologous red cells labeled with ^{99m}Tc are not removed by the spleen. Early samples, obtained after complete mixing, can be used to determine an accurate red cell mass. Subsequent samples counted for the ^{51}Cr-labeled experimental cells can be compared with zero-time ^{51}Cr determination calculated from the counts of ^{51}Cr injected and the volume of dilution or red cell mass. The major gamma-photon emissions of ^{51}Cr and ^{99m}Tc permit simultaneous counting of these radionuclides. Alternatively, the red cell mass can be determined and the ^{99m}Tc be allowed to decay before the samples are counted for ^{51}Cr.

The double-label method is accurate when properly performed. However, it is technically more difficult than the single-label method, especially in the preparation of the ^{99m}Tc-labeled cells. Heaton and colleagues, who have described the double-label technique in detail, have stressed the importance of keeping the ^{99m}Tc-labeled sample at 4° C to retard elution of the label before infusion.[18] Nevertheless, the most appropriate means of determining blood volume at the time of a radiolabeled red cell recovery infusion remains open for debate. Since the general adoption of the double-label approach 20 years ago, the ^{99m}Tc double-label approach has been found to differ slightly but consistently from the ^{51}Cr single-label approach even when good red cell recovery is noted.[88] Single-label recoveries appear to be about 1% to 2% *lower* than double-label calculation techniques. The single-label technique is simpler, cheaper, and exposes subjects to less radioactivity, but the double-label technique affords an independent opportunity to confirm the blood volume should an unexpected problem befall the interpretation of the ^{51}Cr recovery curve.

Platelets

The evaluation of platelet storage and preservation has been complex and challenging. Investigators generally conduct studies using normal volunteer subjects, with each subject serving as his or her own control. Data are usually reported as platelet recovery at 1 to 3 hours and as platelet survival or half-life over several days. Both ^{51}Cr and ^{111}In are suitable radiolabels for platelet storage studies,[89–91] and double labeling with ^{111}In and ^{51}Cr is well established.[15,92] Platelet recovery and survival studies have been critical to the development of plastics that permit 5-day platelet storage,[93,94] to the identification of the optimal temperature for platelet storage,[95,96] to the determination of proper agitation of the platelet concentrates,[97] and to the comparison of manual platelet preparation with automated plateletpheresis techniques.[98] These studies have traditionally compared a new approach for collection, processing, or storage with an established one.

Unlike red cell studies, however, there is no established criterion of acceptable performance. The test system has usually been accepted if (1) the statistical analysis failed to show a statistical difference in comparison to an established (i.e., previously licensed) method, or (2) a difference was documented but it was not regarded as being *clinically* significant.

There are obvious limitations to this approach. Trials involving radionuclide injections in normal subjects are usually small ($N < 25$) to limit exposure to radioactivity and costs and, as a result, have limited power to detect real differences that may be present. When differences are detected, the definition of what is a clinically relevant difference has remained subjective. Repetitive comparisons—as today's "test" system becomes tomorrow's "control system"—may lead inevitably to a "creeping inferiority"[54] of platelet components that could negatively affect patient care. Arbitrary standards for recovery and survival of platelets could be developed, but one would still need to validate a laboratory's techniques.

An alternative standard based on fresh platelets has been proposed by Murphy.[54] The control arm for trials would always be the infusion of fresh (autologous) platelets. Test platelets would be expected to demonstrate at least two thirds the recovery and half the survival of the standard-setting fresh platelets. The actual protocol design for this kind of trial has received much discussion.[99] Currently utilized apheresis platelets meet the criterion proposed by Murphy,[100] as do both apheresis[101] and whole blood–derived platelets[46] stored for 7 days. This approach needs to be tested through additional studies, but it has promise to permit clear regulatory decisions as well as to increase the assurance of platelet transfusion efficacy for patients.

Granulocytes

Granulocytes collected by a variety of techniques and labeled with ^{111}In migrate to sites of infection. They demonstrate a similar kinetic pattern in the lung, liver, and spleen.[102,103] McCullough and colleagues[104] demonstrated that post-transfusion granulocyte migration to skin window chambers was impaired when the cells were stored for 8 hours at 1° C to 6° C or for 24 hours at 22° C. Granulocytes stored for 8 hours at 22° C, however, migrated as well as unstored controls.

IMAGING AND OTHER DIAGNOSTIC APPLICATIONS

Blood cells labeled with appropriately chosen radionuclides migrate to sites of disease where they can be detected by collimated scintillation cameras. These devices consist of a sodium iodide crystal that interacts with collimated gamma-photons emitted from the source. Visible light is produced, which is recorded by photomultiplier tubes and converted into an image by means of a dedicated computer interfaced with the camera. The imaging of radiolabeled granulocytes is especially useful in clinical medicine, and the imaging of platelets and red cells can also be important in selected situations.

Red Cells

The diagnostic uses of imaged radiolabeled red cells include the localization and sizing of the spleen or accessory spleen, blood pool scanning, and the detection of gastrointestinal bleeding and vascular anomalies such as hemangiomas. Colloids such as rhenium sulfur labeled with ^{99m}Tc are often used to determine spleen size and location. Radiolabeled colloids also image the liver. On occasion, it is desirable to image the spleen alone, especially when an enlarged liver interferes with splenic images or when an accessory spleen is suspected. For these needs, red cells damaged by heat and labeled with ^{99m}Tc localize in the spleen without significant hepatic uptake.[105]

The blood pool can be imaged, and related red cell kinetics determined, with red cells labeled with ^{111}In. Quantitative sequential counting and imaging are possible, focusing on a selected target organ such as the spleen. This procedure can determine the rate of splenic sequestration when increased peripheral destruction of red cells is suspected (Fig. 33–5). However, this technique is infrequently utilized.

A common use of radionuclide labeling of autologous red cells is for the determination of red cell mass (or volume) in the diagnosis of polycythemic states. ^{99m}Tc provides the requisite information with a relatively small dose of radioactivity. Samples need only be acquired over the first 15 to 30 minutes after reinfusion.

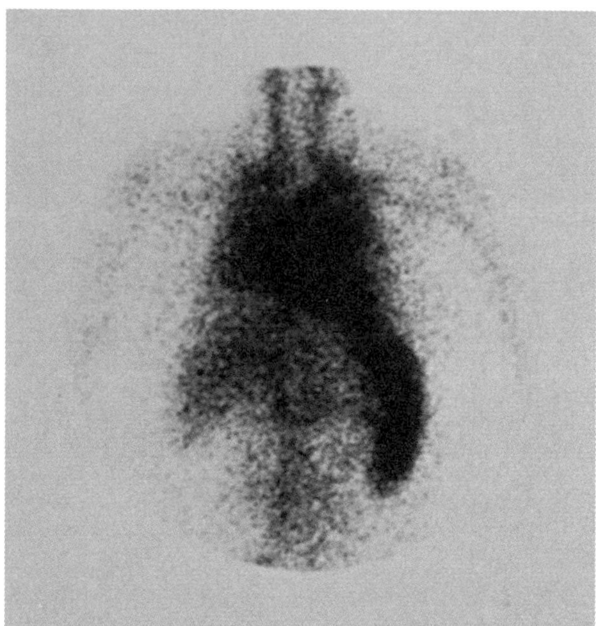

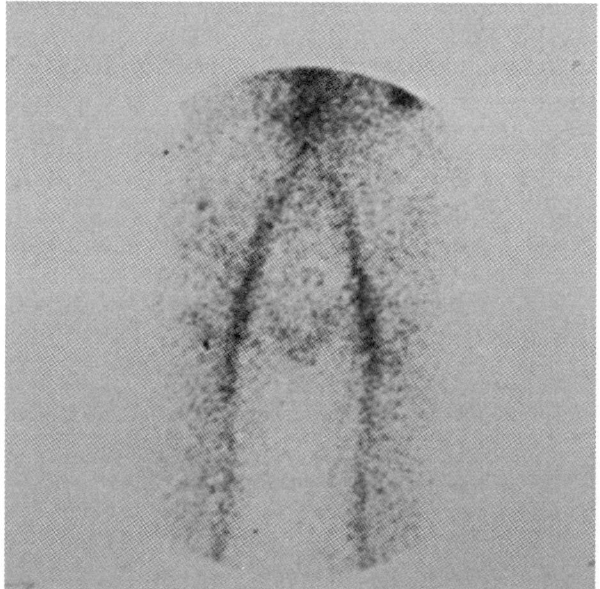

Figure 33–5 ^{111}In-labeled red cell blood pool scan. The heart, great vessels, liver, and enlarged spleen are clearly imaged. Differential counting over selected organs can identify sites of red cell sequestration.

Platelets

Platelets labeled with ^{111}In can be detected and imaged at the sites of their deposition, such as in intravascular thrombi. An actively forming clot incorporates platelets. Therefore, radiolabeled platelets are useful in identifying areas of *new* thrombus formation but do not label older thrombi. A venogram is often used to confirm a positive platelet scan. However, platelet scanning is reliable as a single diagnostic test and is especially useful in patients who are allergic to intravenous contrast material. Applications for the use of radiolabeled platelets include detection of venous, arterial, and intraventricular thrombi, pulmonary emboli, and aneurysms.[106,107] In addition, this technique can aid in the evaluation of the status of renal transplants[108] and arterial grafts.[109] If a suspicious area is identified on the early scans, the site is followed for several days to note whether the area persists or increases in activity as blood pool activity decreases. In a prospective study of gynecologic patients at high risk, 29% demonstrated increased platelet deposition in the major veins or lungs that were presumptive sites of thrombus formation.[110]

Granulocytes

^{111}In-labeled granulocytes are used to identify areas of infection and inflammation, such as suspected abscesses[111] or osteomyelitis,[112] or to evaluate a fever of unknown origin.[113] ^{111}In is usually preferred over gallium-67 citrate, an agent that is incorporated into phagocytic cells in vivo, because of the former's superior image quality and the absence of accumulation of the tracer in the gastrointestinal and urinary systems.[114] The technique for preparing granulocytes for imaging studies has been described by Loken and colleagues.[20] For most imaging studies in adults, 1 to 3×10^8 granulocytes are labeled with 400 to 500 μCi of indium-111. Autologous cells are used whenever possible, but allogeneic granulocytes must be used for patients with granulocytopenia or functional granulocyte defects.

FUTURE DIRECTIONS AND NEW APPLICATIONS

The necessity to identify and label formed hematopoietic blood elements, and to follow their in vivo kinetic and localization patterns, will continue as specialized cells designed for targeted clinical applications are developed. For example, mononuclear cells modified for adoptive immunotherapy of cancer is an exciting area in which knowledge of in vivo cell behavior after reinfusion is incomplete.[115–117]

Direct in vivo labeling of cells avoids damage to cells that may occur during in vitro labeling procedures. Coller[118] has described a monoclonal antiplatelet antibody that binds to platelet glycoprotein IIb-IIIa in vivo. This monoclonal antibody can be radiolabeled for localization of thrombi and other vascular lesions.

Improvements in the currently used radionuclides will enhance their clinical utility. Specifically, new chelates of ^{111}In and modifications in labeling procedure using ^{99m}Tc could reduce the high rates of elution that complicate their use. Stannous glucoheptonate, for example, results in a more stable ^{99m}Tc red cell label than can be achieved with the standard method using stannous citrate.

Nonradioactive isotopes avoid the delivery of an absorbed radiation dose to the recipient, and a variety have been developed. ^{50}Cr binds easily to red cells but is cumbersome to produce and detect. Heaton and colleagues[119,120] have demonstrated, however, that ^{52}Cr can be detected using advanced atomic absorption spectrophotometric techniques and is comparable to ^{51}Cr in red cell volume and post-transfusion survival studies. The scrupulous cleanliness and analytic technology required, however, put this technique beyond all but the most determined investigators. Red cells also can be labeled with biotin and then detected with a fluorescent or radioactive tag attached to streptavidin in ex vivo analysis. This technique has been used to determine blood volume and to track the survival of transfused red cells. The results correlate closely with ^{51}Cr-labeled red cells, but the subject is not exposed to radioactivity.[121,122] The ability to apply this technique to patients usually not suitable for studies with radionuclides, such as neonates, opens new avenues for investigation. For example, biotin-avidin studies have shown that hematocrit correlates well with blood volume in very-low-birth-weight infants and have provided useful measures of the effect of immediate umbilical cord clamping in preterm neonates.[123,124] However, the technique is not without drawbacks. For example, antibodies against biotinylated red cells, which have transiently appeared in some recipients, could potentially alter results in multiply tested individuals.[125]

Other groups have applied novel experimental techniques for the determination of blood volume and red cell survival. The dilution of fluorescein-labeled hydroxyethyl starch has been used to calculate blood volume accurately.[126] Additionally, the circulating proportion of antigenically distinct allogeneic red cells (usually antigen positive in a background of autologous negative cells) has been successfully tracked by flow cytometry.[127] However, the accuracy of this technique appears to be limited, particularly at very low proportions of the transfused cells.[128] These techniques remain experimental but worthy of further exploration as methods for performing in vivo labeling and kinetic studies without radiation exposure to the subject.

The necessity to perform and accurately interpret cell survival, kinetic, and imaging studies will increase as new cell storage and preservation systems are introduced and new clinical applications for standard and modified blood cells are developed. Close collaboration between specialists in transfusion medicine and other disciplines, especially nuclear medicine, will permit the opportunities in this exciting area to be fully explored.

REFERENCES

1. Gray SJ, Sterling K. The tagging of red cells and plasma proteins with radioactive chromium. J Clin Invest 1950;29:1604–1613.
2. Fisher J, Wolfe R, Leon A. Technetium-99m as a label for erythrocytes. J Nucl Med 1967;8:229–232.
3. McAfee JG, Thakur ML. Survey of radioactive agents for in vitro labeling of phagocytic leukocytes. I. Soluble agents. J Nucl Med 1976; 17:480–487.
4. Yoshida T, Bitensky MW, Pickard CA, Herschel LH, Roger J, AuBuchon JP. Nine-week storage of red blood cells in AS3 under oxygen-depleted conditions. Transfusion 1999;39:109S.
5. Mollison PL, Veall N. The use of the isotope 51 Cr as a label for red cells. Br J Haematol 1955;1:62–74.
6. Garby L, Mollison PL. Deduction of mean red cell life-span from 51 Cr survival curves. Br J Haematol 1971;20:527–536.
7. Bentley SA, Glass HI, Lewis SM, Szeur L. Elution correction in 51 Cr red cell survival studies. Br J Haematol 1974;26:179–184.

8. Mollison PL, Engelfriet CP, Contreras M. Blood Transfusion in Clinical Medicine, 8th ed. Oxford, Blackwell, 1987, p 104.
9. Moroff G, Sohmer PR, Button LN. Proposed standardization of methods for determining the 24-hour survival of stored red cells. Transfusion 1984;24:109–114.
10. International Committee for Standardization in Hematology. Recommended method for radioisotope red-cell survival studies. Br J Haematol 1980;45:659–666.
11. Baldini M, Costea N, Dameshek W. The viability of stored human platelets. Blood 1960;16:1669–1692.
12. Eyre HJ, Rosen PJ, Perry S. Relative labeling of leukocytes, erythrocytes and platelets in human blood by 51 Cr. Blood 1970;36:250–253.
13. Snyder EL, Moroff G, Simon T, Heaton A. Recommended methods for conducting radiolabeled platelet survival studies. Transfusion 1986; 26:37–42.
14. Heaton WA. Evaluation of posttransfusion recovery and survival of transfused red cells. Transfus Med Rev 1992;6:153–169.
15. Holme S, Heaton A, Roodt J. Concurrent label method with 111 In and 51 Cr allows accurate evaluation of platelet viability of stored platelet concentrates. Br J Haematol 1993;84:717–723.
16. Jones J, Mollison PL. A simple and efficient method of labeling red cells with (99m)Tc for determination of red cell volume. Br J Haematol 1978;38:141–148.
17. Holt JT, Spitalnik SL, McMican AE, et al. A technetium-99m red cell survival technique for in vivo compatibility testing. Transfusion 1983;23:148–151.
18. Heaton WA, Keegan T, Holme S, Momoda G. Evaluation of 99m technetium/51 chromium posttransfusion recovery of red cells stored in saline, adenine, glucose, and mannitol for 42 days. Vox Sang 1989;57:37–42.
19. AuBuchon JP, Brightman A. Use of indium-111 as a red cell label. Transfusion 1989;29:143–147.
20. Loken MK, Clay ME, Carpenter RT, et al. Clinical use of indium-111 labeled blood products. Clin Nucl Med 1985;10:902–911.
21. Mountford PJ, Allsopp MJ, Hall FM, et al. Leucocyte and contaminant cell-bound activities resulting from the labeling of leucocytes with indium-111 oxine. Eur J Nucl Med 1985;10:304–307.
22. AuBuchon JP. Radioisotopic reflections. Transfusion 2005;45:28S–32S.
23. Callender ST, Powell EO, Witts LJ. The life-span of the red cell in man. J Pathol Bacteriol 1945;57:129–139.
24. Berlin NI. Determination of red cell life span. JAMA 1964;188:375–378.
25. Mollison PL. Determination of red cell survival using 51 Cr. In Bell CA (ed). A Seminar on Immune-mediated Cell Destruction. Washington, D.C., American Association of Blood Banks, 1981, pp 45–69.
26. Propper RD, Button LN, Nathan DG. New approaches to the transfusion management of thalassemia. Blood 1980;55:55–60.
27. Corash L, Klein H, Deisseroth A, et al. Selective isolation of young erythrocytes for transfusion support of thalassemia major patients. Blood 1981;57:599–606.
28. Simon TL, Sohmer P, Nelson EJ. Extended survival of neocytes produced in a new system. Transfusion 1989;29:221–225.
29. Cohen AR, Schmidt JM, Martin MB, et al. Clinical trial of young red cell transfusions. J Pediatr 1984;104:865–868.
30. Marcus RE, Wonke B, Bantok HM, et al. A prospective trial of young red cells in 48 patients with transfusion-dependent thalassemia. Br J Haematol 1985;60:153–159.
31. Engelfriet CP, von dem Borne AE, Beckers D, et al. Immune destruction of red cells. In Bell CA (ed). A Seminar on Immune-mediated Cell Destruction. Washington, D.C., American Association of Blood Banks, 1981, pp 93–130.
32. Davey RJ. Mechanisms of premature red cell destruction. In Judd WJ, Barnes A (eds). Clinical and Serological Aspects of Transfusion Reactions. Arlington, Va., American Association of Blood Banks, 1982, pp 1–35.
33. Mollison PL. Survival curves of incompatible red cells. Transfusion 1986;26:43–50.
34. Garratty G. Factors affecting the pathogenicity of red cell allo- and autoantibodies. In Nance ST (ed). Immune Destruction of Red Blood Cells. Arlington, Va., American Association of Blood Banks, 1987, pp 114–122.
35. Garratty G. The significance of complement in immunohematology. CRC Crit Rev Clin Lab Sci 1984;20:25–56.
36. Freedman J. The significance of complement on the red cell membrane. Transfus Med Rev 1987;1:58–70.
37. Jaffe CJ, Atkinson JP, Frank MM. The role of complement in the clearance of cold agglutinin-sensitized erythrocytes in man. J Clin Invest 1976;58:942–949.
38. Lachmann PJ, Pangburn MK, Oldroyd RG. Breakdown of C3 after complement activation. J Exp Med 1982;156:205–276.
39. Lachmann PJ, Voak D, Oldroyd RG, et al. Use of monoclonal anti-C3 antibodies to characterize the fragments of C3 that are found on erythrocytes. Vox Sang 1983;45:367–372.
40. Atkinson JP, Frank MM. Studies on the in vivo effects of antibody: interaction of IgM antibody and complement in the immune clearance and destruction of erythrocytes in man. J Clin Invest 1974; 54:339–348.
41. Gaither TA, Vargas I, Inada S, Frank MM. The complement fragment C3d facilitates phagocytosis by monocytes. Immunology 1987; 62:405–411.
42. Ehlenberger AG, Nussenzweig V. The role of membrane receptors for C3b and C3d in phagocytosis. J Exp Med 1977;145:357–371.
43. International Committee for Standardization in Hematology. Recommended methods for radioisotope platelet survival studies. Blood 1977;50:1137–1144.
44. Thakur ML, Walch MJ, Malek HL, Gottschalk A. Indium-111-labeled human platelets: improved method, efficacy, and evaluation. J Nucl Med 1981;22:381–385.
45. Holme S. Storage and quality assessment of platelets. Vox Sang 1998;74(Suppl 2):207–216.
46. AuBuchon JP, Taylor H, Holme S, Nelson E. In vitro and in vivo evaluation of the leukoreduced platelets stored for 7 days in CLX containers. Transfusion 2005;45:1356–1361.
47. International Committee for Standardization in Hematology. Recommended method for indium-111 platelet survival studies. J Nucl Med 1988;29:564–566.
48. Mathias CJ, Heaton WA, Welch MJ, et al. Comparison of 111 In-oxine and 111 In-acetyl acetone for the labeling of cells: in vivo and in vitro biological testing. Int J Appl Radiat Isot 1981;32:651–656.
49. Dewanjee MK, Rao SA, Rosemark JA, et al. Indium-111 tropolone, a new tracer for platelet labeling. Radiology 1982;145:149–153.
50. Thakur ML, McKenney SL, Park CH. Simplified and efficient labeling of human platelets in plasma using indium-111-2- mercaptopyridine-N-oxide: preparation and evaluation. J Nucl Med 1985;26:510–517.
51. Biomedical Excellence for Safer Transfusion Collaborative. Platelet radiolabeling procedure. Transfusion 2005;45(Suppl), in press.
52. Lötter MG, Rabe W, Le R, et al. A computer program in compiled Basic for the IBM personal computer to calculate the mean platelet survival time with the multiple hit and weighted mean methods. Comput Biol Med 1988;18:305–315.
53. AuBuchon JP, Dumont L, Murphy S, et al. Comparison of computerized formulae for determination of platelet recovery and survival. Transfusion 2005;45:1237–1238.
54. Murphy S. Radiolabeling of PLTs to assess viability: a proposal for a standard. Transfusion 2004;44:131–133.
55. Paulus JM, Aster RH. Platelet kinetics: production distribution, lifespan, and fate of platelets. In Williams W, Beutler E, Erslev A, Lichtman M (eds). Hematology, 3rd ed. New York, McGraw-Hill, 1983, pp 1185–1196.
56. Harker LA, Finch CA. Thrombokinetics in man. J Clin Invest 1969; 48:963–974.
57. Heyns AD, Lotter MG, Badenhorst PN, et al. Kinetics, distribution and sites of destruction of indium-111-labelled human platelets. Br J Haematol 1980;44:269–280.
58. Klonizakis I, Peters AM, Fitzpatrick ML, et al. Radionuclide distribution following injection of In-111-labelled platelets. Br J Haematol 1980;46:595–602.
59. Hanson SR, Slichter SJ. Platelet kinetics in patients with bone marrow hypoplasia: evidence for a fixed platelet requirement. Blood 1985;66:1105–1109.
60. Tomer A, Harker LA. Megakaryocytopoiesis and platelet kinetics. In Rossi EC, Simon TL, Moss GS (eds). Principles of Transfusion Medicine. Baltimore, Md., Williams & Wilkins, 1991, p 175.
61. Read EJ. Leukocyte radiolabeling. In Davey RJ, Wallace ME (eds). Diagnostic and Investigational Uses of Radiolabeled Blood Elements. Arlington, Va., American Association of Blood Banks, 1987, pp 93–114.
62. McAfee JG, Subramanian G, Gagne G. Technique of leukocyte harvesting and labeling: problems and perspectives. Semin Nucl Med 1984; 12:83–106.
63. Athens JW, Haab OP, Raab SO, et al. Leukokinetic studies. IV. The total blood, circulating and marginal granulocyte pools and granulocyte turnover rate in normal subjects. J Clin Invest 1961;40:989–995.
64. Alexanian R, Donahue DM. Neutrophilic granulocyte kinetics in normal man. J Appl Physiol 1965;20:803–808.
65. Weiblen BJ, Forstrom L, McCullough J. Studies of the kinetics of indium-111-labeled granulocytes. J Lab Clin Med 1979;94:246–255.
66. Savermuttu SH, Peters AM, Danpure HJ, et al. Lung transit of 111 indium-labelled granulocytes: relationship to labelling techniques. Scand J Haematol 1983;30:151–160.

67. Dutcher JP, Fox JJ, Riggs C, et al. Pulmonary retention of indium-111-labeled granulocytes in alloimmunized patients. Blood 1982;58:177A.
68. McCullough J, Clay M, Hurd D, et al. Effect of leukocyte antibodies and HLA matching on the intravascular recovery, survival, and tissue localization of 111 In granulocytes. Blood 1986;67:522–528.
69. Dutcher JP, Schiffer CA, Johnston CS, et al. Alloimmunization prevents the migration of transfused indium-111-labeled granulocytes to sites of infection. Blood 1983;62:354–360.
70. Read EJ, Keenan AM, Carter CS, et al. In vivo traffic of indium-111-oxine labeled human lymphocytes collected by automated apheresis. J Nucl Med 1990;31:999–1006.
71. Ford WL, Gowans JL. The traffic of lymphocytes. Semin Hematol 1969;6:67–83.
72. Butcher EC. The regulation of lymphocyte traffic. Curr Top Microbiol Immunol 1986;128:85–122.
73. Gallatin M, St. John TP, Siegelman M, et al. Lymphocyte homing receptors. Cell 1986;44:673–680.
74. Stevenson HC, Keenan AM, Woodhouse C, et al. Fate of interferon-activated killer blood monocytes adoptively transferred into the peritoneal cavity of patients with peritoneal carcinomatosis. Cancer Res 1987;47:6100–103.
75. Mazumder A, Eberlein TJ, Grimm EA, et al. Phase I study of the adoptive immunotherapy of human cancer with lectin activated autologous mononuclear cells. Cancer 1984;53:896–905.
76. Fisher B, Packard BS, Read EJ, et al. Tumor localization of adoptively transferred indium-111 labeled tumor infiltrating lymphocytes in patients with metastatic melanoma. J Clin Oncol 1989;7:250–261.
77. Loutit JF, Mollison PL. Advantages of a disodium-citrate-glucose mixture as a blood preservative. 1943;2:744.
78. Murphy S, Rebulla P, Bertolini F, for the BEST (Biomedical Excellence for Safer Transfusion) Task Force of the ISBT. In vitro assessment of the quality of stored platelet concentrates. Transfus Med Rev 1994;8:29–36.
79. Vostal J, at December 13, 2003, Meeting of the Blood Products Advisory Committee. Available at http://www.fda.gov/ ohrms/dockets/ac/03/transcripts/4014T2.htm. Accessed March 29, 2006.
80. Snyder E, Mintz P, Burks S, et al. Pathogen inactivated red blood cells using INACTINE technology demonstrate 24-hour posttransfusion recovery equal to untreated red cells after 42 days of storage. Blood 2001;98:709A.
81. Davey RJ, McCoy NC, Yu M, et al. The effect of pre-storage irradiation on posttransfusion red cell survival. Transfusion 1992;32:525–528.
82. Moroff G, Holme S, AuBuchon JP, Heaton A, Sweeney J, Friedman LI. Viability and in vitro properties of gamma-irradiated AS-1 red blood cells. Transfusion 1999;39:128–134.
83. AuBuchon JP, Estep TN, Davey RJ. The effect of the plasticizer di-2-ethylhexylphthalate on the survival of stored red cells. Blood 1988; 71:448.
84. Brecher ME, Pineda AA, Torloni AS, et al. Prestorage leukocyte depletion: effect on leukocyte and platelet metabolites, erythrocyte lysis, metabolism, and in vivo survival. Semin Hematol 1991;28 (Suppl 5):3.
85. Mollison PL, Engelfriet CP, Contreras M. Blood Transfusion in Clinical Medicine, 8th ed. Oxford, Blackwell, 1987, pp 71–73.
86. Beutler E, West C. Measurement of the viability of stored red cells by the single-isotope technique using ^{51}Cr. Transfusion 1984;24:100–104.
87. Garratty G. Predicting the clinical significance of alloantibodies and determining the in vivo survival of transfused red cells. In Judd JW, Barnes A (eds). Clinical and Serological Aspects of Transfusion Reactions. Arlington, Va., American Association of Blood Banks, 1982, pp 91–120.
88. Pickard C, AuBuchon JP, Tosteson AN, Holme S. Influence of gender and collection order on radiolabeled red blood cell recovery. Transfusion 1995;35:6S.
89. Heaton WA. Indium-111 (111 In) and chromium-51 (51 Cr) labeling of platelets. Are they comparable? Transfusion 1986;26:16–19.
90. Snyder EL. Effect of storage conditions on radiolabeling of stored platelet concentrates. Transfusion 1986;26:6–8.
91. Moroff G, Simon TL. Use of radioisotopically labeled platelets to determine the survival characteristics of stored platelets. Transfusion 1986;26:1–6.
92. Keegan T, Heaton A, Holme S, et al. Paired comparison of platelet concentrates prepared from platelet-rich plasma and buffy coats using a new technique with 111 In and 51 Cr. Transfusion 1992;32:113–120.
93. Murphy S, Kahn RA, Holme S, et al. Improved storage of platelets for transfusion in a new container. Blood 1982;60:194–200.
94. Simon TL, Nelson EJ, Carmen R, Murphy S. Extension of platelet concentrate storage. Transfusion 1983;23:207–212.
95. Murphy S, Sayar SN, Gardner FH. Storage of platelet concentrates at 22°C. Blood 1970;35:549–557.
96. Filip DJ, Aster RH. Relative hemostatic effectiveness of human platelets stored at 4° and 22°C. J Lab Clin Med 1978;91:618–624.
97. Snyder EL, Pope C, Ferri PM, et al. The effect of mode of agitation and type of plastic bag on storage characteristics and in vivo kinetics of platelet concentrates. Transfusion 1986;26:125–130.
98. Buchholz DH, Porten JH, Menitove JE, et al. Description and use of the CS-3000 blood cell separator for single-donor platelet collection. Transfusion 1983;23:190–196.
99. FDA Workshop: Use of Radiolabeled Platelets for Assessment of In Vivo Viability of Platelet Products. Available at http://www.fda.gov/cber/minutes/radioplt050304.pdf. Accessed March 29, 2006.
100. AuBuchon JP, Herschel LH, Roger J, Murphy S. Preliminary validation of a new standard of efficacy for stored platelets. Transfusion 2004;44:36–41.
101. AuBuchon JP, Herschel L, Roger J. Further evaluation of a new standard of efficacy for stored platelet. Transfusion 2005;45:1143–1150.
102. Alavi JB, Alavi A, Staum MM. Evaluation of infection in neutropenic patients with indium-111-labeled donor granulocytes. Clin Nucl Med 1980;5:397–400.
103. Anstall HB, Coleman RE. Donor leukocyte imaging in granulocytopenic patients with suspected abscesses. J Nucl Med 1982;23:319–321.
104. McCullough J, Weiblen BJ, Fire D. Effect of storage on granulocytes and their fate in vivo. Transfusion 1983;23:20–24.
105. Sty JR, Conway JJ. The spleen: development and functional evaluation. Semin Nucl Med 1985;15:276–298.
106. Powers WJ, Siegel BA. Thrombus imaging with indium-111 platelets. Semin Thromb Hemost 1983;9:115–131.
107. Smith EO, Snyder EL. Radiolabeled platelets. In Davey RJ, Wallace ME (eds). Diagnostic and Investigational Uses of Radiolabeled Blood Elements. Arlington, Va., American Association of Blood Banks, 1987, pp 79–84.
108. Sinzinger HF, Leithner CW. The use of indium-111-labeled platelets in the management of renal transplant patients. In Thakur ML, Ezekowitz MD, Hardeman MR (eds). Radiolabeled Cellular Blood Elements. New York, Plenum Press, 1985, pp 201–228.
109. Hanson SR, Kotz HF, Pieters H, Heyns AD. Analysis of indium-111 platelet kinetics and imaging in patients with aortic grafts and abdominal aortic aneurysms. Arteriosclerosis 1990;10:1037–1044.
110. Clark-Pearson DL, Coleman RE, Siegel R, et al. Indium-111 platelet imaging for the detection of deep venous thrombosis and pulmonary embolism in patients without symptoms after surgery. Surgery 1985;98:98–104.
111. Segal AW, Arnot RN, Thakur ML, Lavender JP. Indium-111-labeled leukocytes for localization of abscesses. Lancet 1976;2:1056–1058.
112. King AD, Peters AM, Stuttle AW, Lavender JP. Imaging of bone infection with labelled white blood cells: role of contemporaneous bone marrow imaging. Eur J Nucl Med 1990;17:148–151.
113. Davies SG, Garvie NW. The role of indium-labelled leukocyte imaging in pyrexia of unknown origin. Br J Radiol 1990;63:850–854.
114. Froelich JW, Swanson D. Imaging of inflammatory processes with labeled cells. Semin Nucl Med 1984;14:128–140.
115. Dummer R, Becker JC, Eilles C, Schafer E, Borner W, Burg GT. Cells migrate to tumour sites after extracorporeal interleukin 2 stimulation and reinfusion in a patient with metastatic melanoma. Br J Dermatol 1993;128:399–403.
116. Quillien V, Moisan A, Lesimple T, Leberre C, Toujas L. Biodistribution of 111 indium-labeled macrophages infused intravenously in patients with renal carcinoma. Cancer Immunol Immunother 2001;50:477–482.
117. Lesimple T, Moisan A, Carsin A, et al. Injection by various routes of melanoma antigen-associated macrophages: biodistribution and clinical effects. Cancer Immunol Immunother 2003;52:438–444.
118. Coller B. Theoretical considerations in designing monoclonal antibodies for imaging thrombi with platelet directed antibodies. Presented at Colloquium on Coronary Thrombosis, the Future of Imaging Techniques. Oklahoma City, Oklahoma Cardiovascular Institute, 1984.
119. Heaton WA, Hanbury CM, Keegan TE, et al. Studies with nonradioisotopic sodium chromate. I. Development of a technique for measuring red cell volume. Transfusion 1989;29:696–702.
120. Heaton WA, Keegan T, Hanbury CM, et al. Studies with nonradioisotopic sodium chromate. II. Single-and double-label 52 Cr/51 Cr posttransfusion recovery estimations. Transfusion 1989;29:703–707.
121. Mock DM, Lankford GL, Widness JA, Burmeister LF, Kahn D, Strauss RG. Measurement of red cell survival using biotin-labeled red cells measured against 51 Cr-labeled red cells. Transfusion 1999;39:156–162.
122. Mock DM, Lankford GL, Widness JA, Burmeister LF, Kahn D, Strauss RG. RBCs labeled at two biotin densities permit simultaneous and

repeated measurements of circulating RBC volume. Transfusion 2004;44:431–437.
123. Mock DM, Bell EF, Lankford GL, Widness JA. Hematocrit correlates well with circulating red blood cell volume in very low birth weight infants. Pediatr Res 2001;50:525–531.
124. Strauss RG, Mock DM, Johnson K, et al. Circulating RBC volume, measured with biotinylated RBCs, is superior to the Hct to document the hematologic effects of delayed versus immediate umbilical cord clamping in preterm neonates. Transfusion 2003;43:1168–1172.
125. Cordle DG, Strauss RG, Lankford G, Mock DM. Antibodies provoked by the transfusion of biotin-labeled red cells. Transfusion 1999;39:1065–1069.
126. Massey EJ, de Souza P, Findlay G, et al. Clinically practical blood volume assessment with fluorescein-labeled HES. Transfusion 2004;44: 151–157.
127. Nance SJ, Garratty G. Application of flow cytometry to immunohematology. J Immunol Methods 1987;101:127–131.
128. Kumpel BM, Austin EB, Lee D, Jackson DJ, Judson PA, Chapman GE. Comparison of flow cytometric assays with isotopic assays of 51 chromium-labeled cells for estimation of red cell clearance or survival in vivo. Transfusion 2000;40:228–239.

Chapter 34

Transfusion of the Patient with Congenital Coagulation Defects

Suzanne Shusterman • Catherine S. Manno

INTRODUCTION

Tremendous progress has been made over the past few decades in the diagnosis and management of congenital bleeding disorders. Accurate diagnosis by genetic testing is widely available for most cases of severe hemophilia. Recombinant factor VIII (FVIII) and factor IX (FIX) concentrates have been licensed and are now commonly used in the management of bleeding episodes or, in prophylaxis regimens, for the prevention of bleeding episodes. This chapter reviews the clinical and laboratory features of hemophilia A and B, von Willebrand disease (vWD), and other less common congenital bleeding disorders. Treatment options for bleeding episodes and for prevention of bleeding are presented. Although certain clinical challenges, such as the management of patients with high-titer inhibitors, still exist, the outlook for children born today with hemophilia and other congenital bleeding disorders is brighter than ever before.

HEMOPHILIA A AND HEMOPHILIA B

Hemophilia A and hemophilia B are serious congenital clotting disorders caused by deficiencies in FVIII and FIX, respectively. Both diseases have an X-linked recessive pattern of inheritance. The incidence of hemophilia A (classic hemophilia) is 1 in 5000 male births, and the incidence of hemophilia B (Christmas disease) is approximately 1 in 30,000 to 50,000 male births.[1]

Hemophilia is a clinically heterogeneous disorder with severity and symptoms dependent on an individual's factor activity level. FVIII and FIX activity levels are measured in international units (IU/mL), with 1 IU/mL corresponding to 100% of the factor found in 1 mL of normal plasma. Normal FVIII and FIX activity levels range from 0.5 to 1.5 IU/mL (50% to 150%), with measurements lower than this range defining three levels of clinical severity of hemophilia. Patients with mild hemophilia have factor activity levels of approximately 0.05 to 0.30 IU/mL (5% to 30%) and tend to have bleeding difficulties only after severe trauma or surgical procedures. Moderate hemophilia is defined by factor activity levels between 0.01 and 0.05 IU/mL (1% to 5%) and is characterized by bleeding with moderate trauma and rarely spontaneous bleeding. Persons with factor activity levels of less than 0.01 IU/mL (<1%) are designated as having severe hemophilia and can bleed spontaneously into joints and soft tissues.[1] Affected boys and men tend to have the same factor levels and similar clinical manifestations of disease as other family members.[3]

Although most patients with hemophilia A have a positive family history, 20% to 30% of affected persons have no previous family history of disease.[2] A common presentation in the absence of a positive family history is excessive bleeding after circumcision. Hemophilia should also be suspected in any male patient with a history of spontaneous bleeding into joints or muscles, or excessive bleeding with surgery and trauma. Children may have excessive bruising. The diagnosis of hemophilia is made by direct assay of FVIII or FIX activity in plasma, which can even be performed on umbilical cord blood. The cloning of the genes for FVIII and IX on the X chromosome has made carrier and prenatal diagnosis of hemophilia possible in most families. Nearly half of patients with severe hemophilia A have an inversion in the FVIII gene at intron 22,[4,5] and five percent of patients have an inversion in intron 1.[6] If these mutations are not present, carriers can be identified for both hemophilia A and B by direct sequence analysis or linkage analysis, provided that affected and unaffected family members are available. Direct gene mutation and linkage analysis can also be performed in the prenatal period by chorionic villus sampling at 10 to 12 weeks' gestation or amniocentesis after 15 weeks' gestation.[4] If genetic analysis is not possible, fetal blood sampling, when available, can be used to assay plasma FVIII levels.[7] There is no single dominant mutation responsible for hemophilia B, so direct sequence analysis is often performed to identify carriers or make a prenatal diagnosis. FIX plasma assays are less reliable in making the definitive diagnosis before or at birth because of normally low levels of vitamin K–dependent factors in the prenatal and postnatal periods.[8]

Therapeutic Options for Factor Replacement in Hemophilia

Historical Perspective

Before the availability of specialized products to replace specific clotting factor deficiencies, patients with hemophilia were treated with whole blood or fresh frozen plasma. Many patients died of hemorrhage or were incapacitated with progressive joint disease because transfusions were either unavailable or contained inadequate amounts of factor. In the 1960s, fractionation of large pools of plasma allowed crude separation of FVIII and FIX from other plasma proteins. Cryoprecipitate, that portion of a unit of fresh frozen plasma that precipitates during thawing at 4°C to 6°C, contains FVIII, von Willebrand factor (vWF), FXIII, and fibrinogen and was the first concentrate available for more specific factor replacement for hemophilia A.[9,10] Prothrombin complex concentrates (PCCs), containing FII, FVII, FIX, and FX, were developed for treatment of hemophilia B in 1967.[11]

In the 1970s, efforts were focused on improving solubility, yield (units of clotting factor recovered from plasma), and purity of clotting factor preparations. Lyophilized specific FVIII and FIX concentrates became commercially available, and their ease of storage and reconstitution made home infusion for early signs of hemorrhage possible, thus markedly improving the quality of life of patients with hemophilia.[2,10,12] These concentrates, however, were prepared from pooled plasma obtained from 2000 to 200,000 mostly paid donors,[9] and by 1980, the transmission of hepatitis from these concentrates was recognized.[2] In 1982, the first case of acquired immunodeficiency syndrome in a patient with hemophilia was reported; by 1988, the prevalence of seropositivity for human immunodeficiency virus (HIV) was 77% in patients with severe hemophilia A and 42% in patients with hemophilia B.[3,13–15] As a result of the tragic transmission of HIV and hepatitis to so many patients with hemophilia, by the mid-1980s, the major goal of factor concentrate development was further improvement of product purity and elimination of viral transmission.[16]

Purification Methods

The purity of factor concentrates is classified according to specific activity, the ratio of clotting protein to nonclotting protein contained in a factor concentrate.[17] Improved separation techniques have resulted in the availability of increasingly pure products. Cryoprecipitate is a low-purity concentrate.[1] The first specific factor concentrates made in the 1970s were intermediate-purity products with specific activity levels between 1 and 10 IU/mg total protein.[10] High-purity concentrates with a specific activity ranging from 50 to 150 IU/mg total protein were later produced using ion exchange, affinity, or gel filtration chromatography to improve removal of contaminating proteins.[16] The use of monoclonal antibodies to FVIII or FIX in combination with immunoaffinity chromatography produces very high-purity products (specific activity from 200 to 2000 IU/mg total protein).[16] In addition to enhancing the separation of clotting from nonclotting proteins, purification processes partially separated the clotting proteins from contaminating transfusion-transmitted viruses.[12,16]

Virus Inactivation Methods

Purification techniques alone are not sufficient to eliminate the risk of viral contamination from plasma-derived factor concentrates. Since the mid-1980s, all concentrates made in the United States have undergone some form of viral inactivation, either physical or chemical.[3] HIV is exquisitely heat labile, and effective eradication can be accomplished with heat or a combination of heat and pressure.[3,18] Hepatitis viruses are more resistant to heat inactivation than HIV, although the degree of eradication improves with increased temperature, moisture, and length of heating.[16] One problem with heat treatment of factor concentrates is a reduction in factor yield. HIV and hepatitis B and C viruses are lipid-coated viruses and are readily inactivated with a combination of solvent and detergent treatments. Plasma-derived FVIII concentrates treated with solvent and detergent were first licensed in 1985, and the combination of the solvent tri-*n*-butyl phosphate and the detergent polysorbate-80 is now widely used.[16] No transmission of lipid-coated viruses has been seen in clinical trials using solvent-detergent treated products,[19] and product yield is high in these preparations.[18] Hepatitis A and parvovirus B19, however, are not lipid-coated; as such, they elude inactivation with solvent-detergent combinations and therefore remain potential contaminants in plasma-derived concentrates.[3,12,20]

Factor VIII Concentrates

Many different specific FVIII concentrates are licensed in the United States (Table 34–1). All products have undergone viral attenuation.[3] Plasma-derived products of high and very high purity (the latter including immunoaffinity purified) and recombinant products (ultra-pure) are available today.[1] Certain plasma-derived FVIII products contain vWF and fibrinogen in addition to FVIII,[3] which allows them to also be used for treatment of vWD. In 1984, two biotechnology companies (Genentech, San Francisco, and Genetics Institute, Boston) cloned and expressed the FVIII gene, which made the production of recombinant FVIII (rFVIII) possible.[21,22] After this, first-generation rFVIII products were developed and licensed by the U.S. Food and Drug Administration (FDA) for use in patients with FVIII deficiency in the United States.[12,23] All first-generation products contained trace amounts of hamster proteins and mouse immunoglobulin G.[12] However, development of antibodies against rodent protein or transmission of animal viruses to recipients of these products has not been reported.[17] Their biochemical profiles are similar to those of plasma-derived FVIII.

After preclinical safety evaluations, clinical studies with rFVIII (Recombinate and Kogenate) were performed in previously untreated patients to assess efficacy, safety, and inhibitor formation.[24,25] Both rFVIII products were found to have clinical efficacy equal to intermediate- or high-purity plasma-derived products and were well tolerated. Both studies in previously untreated patients showed a higher incidence of inhibitor formation than previously described; however, prior estimates were collected retrospectively and included patients with mild hemophilia as well as extensively pretreated patients, all of which likely contributed to previous underestimation of the risk of inhibitor formation.[24,25] In addition, longitudinal follow-up of previously untreated patients in both rFVIII trials demonstrated that the inhibitors were transient in more than 50% of those in whom they developed.[26]

Although first-generation recombinant FVIII products are not derived from human plasma and are ultra-pure, they required the addition of a stabilizer such as human albumin to prevent the highly concentrated clotting proteins from adhering to the surface of the container.[27] These concentrates have specific activity greater than 3000 IU/mg protein before the addition of human albumin.[28] Safety concerns about the addition of albumin have been raised, although none of the first-generation recombinant products have been associated with hepatitis transmission, HIV transmission, or transmission of any other known infectious disease. Recent rFVIII product development has focused on decreasing or eliminating use of human albumin. Second-generation FVIII products use only a small amount of human albumin in the production process and instead include sugar as an alternative stabilizer.[3] These products include Kogenate SF (sucrose formulated) and Helixate FS[29] as well as ReFacto, which is a B-domain-deleted rFVIII product.[30,31] In 2003, Advate was licensed as

Table 34–1 Factor VIII Concentrates Available in the United States in 2005

Product	Manufacturer	Method of Viral Inactivation or Depletion	Stabilizer	Specific Activity of Final Product*
A. Recombinant Factor VIII Concentrates				
Recombinate	Baxter Hyland Immuno	IAC	Human albumin	1.65–19
Bioclate	Baxter Hyland Immuno†	IAC	Human albumin	1.65–19
Kogenate	Bayer	IAC	Human albumin	8–30
Helixate	Bayer†	IAC	Human albumin	8–30
Kogenate SF	Bayer	IAC	Sucrose	4000
Helixate SF	Bayer†	IAC	Sucrose	4000
ReFacto	Pharmacia Upjohn AB‡	IAC, SD1	Sucrose	11,200–15,5000
B. Very High-Purity (Immunoaffinity-Purified) Plasma-Derived Factor VIII Concentrates				
Hemophil-M	Baxter Hyland Immuno	IAC, SD1		2–15
Monarc-M	Baxter Hyland Immuno§	IAC, SD1		2–15
Monoclate-P	Aventis Behring	IAC, P		5–10
C. High- and Intermediate-Purity Plasma-Derived Factor VIII Concentrates‖				
Alphanate SD	Alpha Therapeutics	IAC, SD2		8–30
Humate-P	Aventis Behring	P		1–2
Koate-DVI	Bayer	SD2, DH		9–22
D. Porcine Factor VIII Products¶				
Hyate:C	Ipsen, Inc.	P		>50

IAC, immunoaffinity chromatography, SD1, solvent–detergent (TNBP and Triniton X-100); P, pasteurization (60°C 10 h); DH, dry heat (72°C, 72 h); SD2 (TNBP and polysorbate-80).
*IU factor VIII/mg total protein, including stabilizer.
†Distributed by Aventis Behring.
‡Distributed by Genetics Institute.
§Manufactured from American Red Cross–collected plasma, distributed by American Red Cross.
‖Contain von Willebrand factor.
¶For use in patients with inhibitors to factor VIII.

a rFVIII with structure homologous to the previous product Recombinate but made without addition of exogenous human or animal proteins. Efficacy and safety have been demonstrated in patients for the treatment of hemophilia A without increased immunogenicity.[32]

Factor IX Concentrates

Three types of factor concentrates are available for treatment of patients with FIX deficiency: PCCs, coagulation FIX concentrates, and recombinant FIX (rFIX) (Table 34–2).

Prothrombin complex concentrates, also known as FIX complex concentrates, contain FIX as well as prothrombin, FVII, and FX, some of which becomes activated during preparation.[17] PCCs are low-purity products with a specific activity less than 50 IU/mg total protein.[1] When PCCs are used at frequent intervals or for prolonged periods, they have been associated with paradoxic thrombotic complications, such as myocardial infarction, venous thromboembolism, and disseminated intravascular coagulation.[16,33] These problems are caused either by the presence of activated factors that serve to trigger coagulation or by accumulation of high levels of the factors.[16] High-purity FIX concentrates, also known as coagulation FIX concentrates, were first licensed in 1992.[16] They are purified by immunoaffinity or gel chromatography, contain only FIX, and have little or no thrombotic potential.[16,17] High-purity concentrates are preferred over PCCs, particularly when frequent replacement is required, such as in surgical patients or in clinical situations associated with an increased risk of thrombosis, as in patients with advanced liver disease.[12] FIX concentrates currently available in the United States include Alphanine SD and Mononine.[16,34,35]

The gene for FIX was cloned in 1982 and was successfully transfected into Chinese hamster ovary cells, a process leading to rFIX production in 1985 by Genetics Institute.[36–39] Initially, rFIX was tested in a canine model and in previously treated patients and was shown to have clinical efficacy comparable to that of plasma-derived products, with a low thrombogenic potential even at high doses.[37,40] Inhibitor formation was also low; only 1 of 44 previously treated patients developed a low-titer inhibitor that was detectable for 11 months.[41]

In October 1995, a trial of rFIX in previously untreated patients was initiated. Although the final results of this trial are not yet published, preliminary reports show good clinical efficacy with no adverse effects, including no viral transmission. The only difference detected between plasma-derived and rFIX in these initial studies was that recovery of rFIX is approximately 20% less than in the plasma-derived products. Poorer than anticipated recovery has been attributed to minor differences in post-translational modifications between rFIX and plasma-derived products.[40] One rFIX concentrate, BeneFix, is currently available in the United States. The specific activity of BeneFix is greater than 200 to 360 IU/mg protein, and the final preparation does not contain human albumin.[28]

Nonconcentrate Therapeutic Options for Hemophilia

Desmopressin

Desmopressin (DDAVP, 1-deamino-8-d-arginine vasopressin) is a synthetic analog of vasopressin that stimulates

Table 34–2 Factor IX Concentrates Available in the United States in 2005

Product	Manufacturer	Method of Viral Inactivation or Depletion	Stabilizer	Specific Activity of Final Product*
A. Recombinant Factor IX Concentrates				
BeneFIX	Genetics Institute	IAC, UF	Sucrose	>200
B. Coagulation Factor IX Concentrates (Human Plasma Derived)				
Alphanine SD	Alpha	DAC, SD, NF		230
Mononine	Aventis Behring	IAC, ST, UF		>160
C. Factor IX Complex Concentrates (Prothrombin Complex Concentrates), Human Plasma Derived				
Bebulin VH	Baxter Hyland Immuno	VH		2
Konyne 80	Bayer	DH		1.25
Profilnine SD	Alpha	SD		4.5
Proplex T	Baxter Hyland Immuno	DH		3.9
D. Activated Factor IX Complex Concentrates (Activated Prothrombin Complex Concentrates), Human Plasma Derived				
Autoplex-T	Baxter Hyland Immuno†	DH		5
FEIBA VH	Baxter Hyland Immuno	VH		0.8

*IU factor VIII/mg total protein, including stabilizer.
†Distributed by Nabi.
DAC, dual-affinity chromatography; DH; dry heat (72°C, 72 h); IAC, immunoaffinity chromatography; NF, nanofiltration; SD, solvent-detergent (TNBP and polysorbate-80); ST, sodium thiocyanate; UF, ultrafiltration; VH, vapor heat (10h, 60°C 1190 mbar pressure plus 1h, 80°C 1375 mbar).

endothelial cell release of FVIII, vWF, and plasminogen activator. It is often useful for patients with mild hemophilia, in whom it may provide a therapeutic elevation of factor levels. DDAVP, at a dose of 0.3 μg/kg, is diluted in 10 to 50 mL of saline, and is administered intravenously over 15 to 30 minutes.[42,42] Side effects include facial flushing, mild headaches, nausea, and lightheadedness.[3] DDAVP can rarely cause inappropriate water retention and subsequent hyponatremia that can be avoided with fluid restriction after treatment.[2,3] A concentrated nasal spray (Stimate) is also available that is given at a dose of 300 μg (one spray in each nostril) for patients weighing 50 kg or more and 150 μg (one spray in one nostril) for patients weighing less than 50 kg.[17,42]

Antifibrinolytic Therapy

Antifibrinolytic therapy inhibits clot lysis and stabilizes clot formation by saturating the fibrin-binding sites on plasminogen and preventing its attachment to a developing clot.[44] Antifibrinolytic therapy is particularly helpful in the treatment of oral hemorrhage because saliva contains a high concentration of fibrinolytic proteins, so clot formation is rendered more difficult. Two antifibrinolytic agents—aminocaproic acid (Amicar) and tranexamic acid (Cyklokapron)—are in clinical use. Amicar is recommended at a dose of 100 mg/kg every 6 hours either orally or intravenously and is available both as a syrup and as a tablet.[2] The recommended dose of Cyklokapron is 25 mg/kg orally (as a tablet only) or 10 mg/kg intravenously every 8 hours.[2] These drugs are contraindicated in patients who have received PCCs or activated PCCs within 12 hours because of the possibility for enhanced thrombosis.[3]

Therapeutic Contraindications

Patients with hemophilia and other congenital coagulopathies should avoid the use of drugs that interfere with platelet function. These drugs include, but are not limited to, aspirin and nonsteroidal anti-inflammatory agents.[17]

Clinical Management

General Principles

The goal of hemophilia care is to prevent morbidity caused by both acute blood loss and chronic, repeated bleeding episodes. Treatment or prevention of acute hemorrhage requires intravenous replacement of FVIII or FIX to hemostatic plasma levels. Factor concentrate infusions can be given to induce and to maintain hemostasis at the time of a bleeding episode, an approach known as *on-demand therapy*, or at prescribed intervals to prevent hemorrhage, an approach known as *prophylactic therapy*, the long-term benefits of which have been documented over the past two decades. Once only recommended for patients in northern Europe, prophylaxis regimens are now broadly prescribed in developed nations where factor concentrates are widely available.

Factor Dosing

The dose of concentrate required for factor replacement is calculated on the basis of the volume of distribution, the half-life of the specific concentrate, the patient's type and severity of hemophilia, and the severity of the particular bleeding episode.[2,3] Based on the severity of a specific bleeding episode, the minimum plasma factor level required to sustain hemostasis is determined. Potentially severe bleeding episodes that are life-threatening or limb-threatening require factor replacement to maintain a plasma factor level of 50% to 100% of normal. As discussed later, depending on the specific situation, these levels may need to be maintained for several days. Less severe bleeding episodes require factor replacement to reach a plasma factor level of 30% to 50% of normal. Under these circumstances, usually only a few doses of factor are required to control bleeding.[3]

The dose of concentrate required to reach these plasma factor goals is calculated using the volume of distribution ofthe specific factor concentrate. In general, 1 IU of plasma-derived FVIII concentrate per kilogram raises the plasma factor level by 1% in children, whereas 1 IU of plasma-derived factor concentrate per kilogram raises the plasma factor level by 2% in adults.[45] Using rFVIII, 1 IU of factor concentrate raises the plasma factor level by 2% in both children and adults.[46] For FIX products, 1 IU of plasma-derived FIX concentrate per kilogram raises the plasma factor level by 1%,[17] and 1 IU of rFIX concentrate per kilogram raises the patient's plasma level by approximately 0.6%.[40] The volume of distribution of rFIX is variable among patients, and therefore a recovery study should be done for each patient to determine the optimal dosing regimen.[2]

Subsequent dosing of factor concentrate is based on the half-life of the specific concentrate. Both factors have an initial short half-life secondary to diffusion that becomes longer with repeat dosing. The initial half-life of FVIII is 6 to 8 hours, and the subsequent half-life is 8 to 12 hours. The initial half-life of FIX is 4 to 6 hours, and the subsequent half-life is 18 to 24 hours.

Treatment of Acute Bleeding Episodes (On-Demand Therapy)

Early treatment of bleeding episodes is essential to limit the amount of blood loss and the subsequent tissue damage caused by chronic blood exposure. Replacement factor recommendations for a specific bleeding episode depend on its location and the potential for complications secondary to blood loss. Laboratory measurements of the partial thromboplastin time (PTT) and FVIII or FIX levels are important guides to successful therapy and should be ordered when managing a serious bleeding episode such as intracranial hemorrhage. Management of common bleeding problems in hemophilia is discussed later, and factor replacement guidelines for specific hemorrhages are listed in Table 34–3.

Intracranial Hemorrhage

Intracranial hemorrhage is a major cause of morbidity and mortality in patients with hemophilia. Patients with severe factor deficiency are at higher risk of central nervous system bleeding than are patients with higher baseline factor levels. Before prophylaxis was widely practiced, about half of all cases of intracranial hemorrhage were not preceded by head trauma. Given the consequence of delayed or absent treatment, all patients with moderate or severe hemophilia with any type of head injury or a significant headache should be treated immediately with a factor replacement of 100%. Patients with a history of significant trauma should then be evaluated with a computed tomography scan. If the scan shows no sign of hemorrhage, the patient should be admitted to an inpatient setting for observation and should receive one to two subsequent 50% corrections to protect against possible delayed or slow bleeding.[42] Patients with mild hemophilia generally need factor replacement only after severe trauma. Management of actual intracranial bleeding requires prolonged maintenance of 100% of normal factor levels and includes the same life support measures and indications for surgery used in children without coagulation disorders.

Joint Bleeding

Hemarthroses are the most common cause of progressive morbidity in hemophilia. Bleeding into a joint space may occur in the absence of known trauma in patients with severe disease. The joints most commonly involved are the knees, elbows, and ankles.[2] To limit long-term joint damage, initial replacement therapy should be instituted as early as possible to raise the plasma factor level to 50% to 70%. For minor or early joint bleeding, an additional factor replacement should be given to maintain a plasma factor level of 30% for approximately 24 hours. For late or significant joint hemorrhage or bleeding in a joint that has been the site of recurrent hemorrhages (target joint), a factor level of 30% should be maintained for 36 to 48 hours. In addition, for all hemarthroses, the joint should be immobilized with a splint for 48 to 72 hours. These recommendations apply to all hemarthroses, regardless of the severity of an individual patient's disease. Children who have had more than one spontaneous hemarthrosis in a single joint are good candidates for future prophylaxis because they are likely to develop progressive joint disease in the affected joint and elsewhere without it.

Muscle Bleeding

Most muscle hemorrhages are superficial and are easily controlled with a single dose of replacement therapy to 30%

Table 34–3 Factor Replacement Guidelines for Common Bleeding Problems in Hemophilia

Type of Bleeding	Target Factor Level (IU/dL)	Duration of Factor Replacement	Comments
Intracranial	0.8–1.0	10–14 days	Secondary prophylaxis to prevent recurrent bleeding
Head trauma, no intracranial hemorrhage	1.0 initially, then 0.5 –1.0 if significant trauma	24–36 hours	Computed tomography scan even if normal exam for significant trauma
Joints	0.5–0.7 initially, then 0.3–0.5	24–48 hours	Immobilize for 48–72 hours
Deep muscle	0.7–1.0 initially, then 0.3–0.5	5–7 days	Hospitalize, bed rest, monitor for blood loss
Superficial muscle	0.3	12–24 hours	Immobilize for 24–48 hours
Oral mucosa	0.3	12–24 hours	Antifibrinolytics or topical therapy may be sufficient
Persistent hematuria	0.3–0.5	Until hematuria clears	Bed rest, adequate hydration, no antifibrinolytics, consider renal ultrasound
Trauma or surgery	1.0 initially, then 0.5–0.7	7–14 days	Shorter duration for minor procedure; recovery study preoperatively

correction, if correction is necessary at all. However, substantial blood loss can occur with internal muscle bleeding into large cavities such as the thigh or the iliopsoas. These hemorrhages should be treated with an initial 70% correction, and plasma factor levels should be maintained at more than 30% for several days while healing occurs. These severe muscle hemorrhages are best treated with hospital admission and bed rest. The patient's hemoglobin level should be checked initially and later, as clinically indicated, because significant blood loss can occur with minimal swelling, particularly with thigh hemorrhages.

Mouth Bleeding

Oral bleeding is particularly common in young children with hemophilia and may occur with primary tooth eruption or in association with loose deciduous teeth. In addition, bleeding can occur after trauma, leading to a laceration of the tongue or frenulum. Antifibrinolytic therapy or local measures such as topical thrombin, pressure, or ice may be sufficient to control bleeding. However, if these measures are not adequate, factor concentrate replacement should be given to obtain a 30% correction. If bleeding persists or recurs, additional replacement doses may be required.

Hematuria

Painless, atraumatic hematuria can occur in patients with severe hemophilia. Bed rest and increased fluid intake is sufficient initial treatment. If symptoms persist for more than 24 hours, bed rest should be continued and the plasma factor level should be corrected to 30% until the bleeding clears. If the patient has a history of trauma, bleeding is persistent, or bleeding occurs in a patient with mild or moderate hemophilia, an ultrasound scan should be performed to look for an intracapsular or intrarenal hemorrhage so that appropriate factor replacement can be given.

Soft Tissue Bleeding

Soft tissue hemorrhages do not require factor replacement unless they lead to compression of critical organs. For example, a soft tissue hemorrhage in the neck could lead to airway compression. In this situation, 100% correction should be given immediately, and appropriate measures should be taken to ensure airway patency.

Prophylactic Therapy

The major long-term morbidity of hemophilia is joint disease caused by repeated exposure of the synovium to blood. Blood acts as an irritant in a joint and leads to synovial membrane proliferation, which, in turn, makes the joint more susceptible to repeated injury and bleeding. Recurrent bleeding then causes chronic synovitis, damage to the underlying cartilage, and finally erosion of the bone.[47] Before the availability of specific factor concentrates, people with severe hemophilia had an average of 30 to 35 joint hemorrhages per year, and 90% developed subsequent degenerative joint disease.[48,49] The introduction of specific factor concentrates, which allowed earlier and more complete treatment of hemarthrosis, markedly decreased the incidence of hemophilic arthropathy, but it did not eliminate it entirely, thus necessitating an alternative treatment strategy.

Dr. Nilsson and colleagues in Malmo, Sweden, first developed the concept of prophylaxis in 1958.[47] Based on the observation that people with moderate and mild hemophilia rarely developed joint disease, these investigators hypothesized that by giving regular factor infusions with the goal of maintaining a factor level of at least 1% in patients with severe hemophilia, they could in a sense convert severe disease to mild or moderate disease and could prevent frequent hemorrhage and subsequent arthropathy.[50,51] These investigators published several case series demonstrating the benefits of their theory, and their data have been confirmed by others around the world.[47,52,53] A longitudinal, uncontrolled outcome study from 21 centers in the United States, Europe, and Japan published in 1994 reported that patients with severe hemophilia who were treated with adequate prophylaxis experienced a reduced number of hemorrhages and a reduced rate of joint degeneration, whereas patients receiving on-demand treatment had signs of progressive joint deterioration.[54]

Two prophylactic treatment strategies have been developed that vary according to the timing of initiation of regular infusions relative to joint status. *Primary prophylaxis* is defined as the initiation of regular factor concentrate infusions before the development of recurrent joint bleeding and clinical or radiologic abnormalities.[55] *Secondary prophylaxis* indicates the initiation of regular factor concentrate infusions after the development of chronic clinical or radiologic abnormalities in a particular joint, considered a "target" joint.[56] Until recently, secondary prophylaxis was the treatment strategy most commonly used in the United States. It has been shown to be beneficial in preventing frequent rebleeding in a target joint and to improve results on orthopedic examination and quality of life.[52,57,58] However, eventual joint deterioration, as evidenced by radiologic evaluation, is not stopped in most cases by secondary prophylaxis.[54] In contrast, primary prophylaxis has been shown to prevent permanent, chronic joint damage. An update of the Swedish prophylaxis experience demonstrates that boys who began primary prophylaxis at a mean age of 1.2 years had no clinical or radiologic evidence of joint damage when they were evaluated 3 to 12 years after the initiation of therapy.[51,53]

In 1994, the National Hemophilia Foundation's Medical and Scientific Advisory Counsel recommended that primary prophylaxis be the treatment of choice for severe hemophilia.[2] However, this recommendation has met several obstacles. Smith and colleagues[59] compared 27 boys receiving prophylactic factor concentrate infusions with 70 boys receiving episodic infusions over a 2-year interval and showed that the median cost of prophylaxis is at least three times the cost of on-demand therapy. One way to decrease the cost of prophylaxis, as suggested by Carlsson and colleagues,[60] is to give prophylactic factor infusions more frequently; therefore, smaller doses are required to maintain a factor trough level higher than the baseline value. The cost of recombinant factor concentrate for prophylaxis on a three times weekly schedule for a 70-kg man is approximately $100,000 a year.

Another major obstacle to prophylaxis is venous access. Placement of central venous access devices is often necessary to provide consistent venous access in young children receiving prophylaxis; this is associated with an increased risk of infection compared with intermittent intravenous access.[61,62] The incidence of central line infections in a survey of 81 hemophilia treatment centers from 33 states was 28% in patients receiving prophylaxis.[63] A third concern preventing the widespread adoption of prophylaxis is that frequent early exposure to large quantities of factor may stimulate inhibitor formation. Conversely, early regular factor infusion may prevent inhibitor formation because it may mimic immune tolerance.[28,51]

When prophylaxis is implemented, factor should be administered at a dose to maintain a trough factor activity of more than 1%, and recombinant factor should be given to minimize the risk of infection.[47,60] In general, this requires doses of rFVIII every other day or three times a week and twice-weekly dosing of rFIX.

Surgical Procedures

The goal of hemophilia care for elective surgery is to maintain factor levels of 50% to 70% throughout the surgical procedure and the postoperative period.[42] A factor recovery study should be done preoperatively to ensure that the patient has the expected response to therapy and to predict the half-life of the concentrate accurately. Regular factor infusion should continue 2 to 7 days postoperatively and then can be tapered.[42]

Treatment of Newborns

The newborn with unsuspected hemophilia born to a woman with no family history may pass through the newborn period with no clinical evidence of disease.[64] The likelihood of excess bleeding at circumcision is 50%[65]; bleeding from circumcision often prompts a diagnostic workup and definitive diagnosis. Male children born to obligate carrier mothers or those infants diagnosed prenatally with hemophilia present a perplexing question of management. Some practitioners recommend prophylactic infusion of factor concentrate in either case, to prevent neonatal intracranial hemorrhage that could result from a vaginal delivery. Others recommend immediate measurement of neonatal factor levels and concomitant head ultrasounds to rule out intracranial hemorrhage.[66,67]

Treatment for Patients with Inhibitors

One of the greatest challenges in the management of hemophilia is the development of inhibitors, high-affinity neutralizing immunoglobulin G antibodies directed against FVIII or FIX.[2] Based on both prospective and retrospective studies, inhibitor development occurs in 21% to 33% of patients with severe hemophilia A[28] and in 1% to 4% of patients with hemophilia B.[26] Most inhibitors form in young children who have had less than 20 treatment days and occur more often in black patients than in white patients.[26] There is also an increased incidence of inhibitors in brothers of boys who have already developed an inhibitor, a finding suggesting a genetic predisposition.[68] Patients with severe hemophilia are more likely to develop inhibitors than those with milder forms of disease. This may be because the low levels of factor produced in patients with mild and moderate hemophilia induce immune tolerance, whereas in severely affected patients, the endogenous factor level is so low that infused factor is regarded as a foreign protein and more easily provokes an immune response.[69] Among patients with severe hemophilia, there is a higher rate of inhibitor development among persons with large gene mutations that lead to undetectable factor levels. The rate of inhibitor development is lower in patients with severe hemophilia with missense mutations and small deletions in whom circulating, but abnormal, factor is present.[70,71]

The development of an inhibitor should be suspected when the patient has decreased clinical response to factor replacement; it can also be found in an asymptomatic person during routine laboratory screening.[69] The presence of an inhibitor is confirmed using the Bethesda assay, which measures the titer of neutralizing antibody and is reported in Bethesda Units (BU). One BU is defined as the amount of inhibitor needed to inactivate 50% of the FVIII or FIX in a mixture of inhibitor-containing plasma and normal plasma.[72] Inhibitor patients are classified as high responders or low responders, depending on the extent of amnestic response on repeat exposure to the factor against which the inhibitor has formed.[28] Patients with high-responder inhibitors develop an increased antibody level within a few days of repeat exposure to FVIII or FIX, whereas low-responder inhibitors only minimally increase after repeat exposure to factor. High-responder inhibitors have antibody titers greater than 10 BU and are also called *high-titer inhibitors*, whereas low responders have titers lower than 10 BU and are referred to as *low-titer inhibitors*.[26] The inhibitor titer level is a useful guide for determining the optimal replacement therapy. Specific treatment recommendations for patients with hemophilia A with inhibitors are outlined in Table 34–4.

Patients with low-titer inhibitors can be treated for acute hemorrhage with higher doses of their specific replacement therapy.[2] Patients often require doses two to three times higher than the normal replacement dose to effect hemostasis. FVIII or FIX levels should be monitored before and after treatment, along with the aPPT and clinical measurements, to help assess the treatment's usefulness. Adjuvant measures, including restriction of limb motion and bed rest, should also be used to preserve fragile clots.

First-line treatment of hemorrhage in patients with high-titer inhibitors is aimed at bypassing the factor against which the inhibitor is directed, using either activated PCCs (aPCCs), which contain FII, FVII, FIX, and FX, or rFVIIa. aPPCs are effective in stopping bleeding in approximately half of the inhibitor patients treated.[73] PCCs and aPCCs should be infused at doses of 50 to 100 IU/kg every 12 to 24 hours, with the maximum dose not to exceed 200 IU/kg in 24 hours.[26] As described previously, aPPCs can be associated with thrombotic complications with repeat dosing. In addition, patients with hemophilia B occasionally develop an increased inhibitor titer or a severe allergic response when they are treated with these products containing FIX and therefore must be monitored closely.[74] Recombinant activated FVIIa (rFVIIa; (NovoSeven) also bypasses FVIII and FIX by activating the extrinsic pathway of the clotting cascade. rFVIIa is thought to initiate hemostasis only at the site of tissue injury and therefore should not be thrombogenic.[75] In addition, rFVIIa is not plasma derived and is not associated with an anamnestic response. A drawback to using rFVIIa is its short half-life, which requires dosing every 2 to 3 hours, a feature that makes treatment cumbersome and costly.[76] Laboratory coagulation parameters have not been shown to correlate directly with the establishment of hemostasis when one uses bypassing agents. Dosing is therefore empiric, based largely on clinical response.

None of the transfusion options for patients with high-titer inhibitors are as reliable as specific factor replacement, and therefore elimination of inhibitors with immune tolerance therapy is a major emphasis of management. Immune tolerance therapy involves regular exposure to high doses of FVIII or FIX for weeks to years with or without concurrent immunosuppressive therapy. Several available immune tolerance therapy regimens are available, with an overall success rate of 60% to 80%, but these regimens often require central venous access and can be time intensive and costly.[2] Data from the North American immune tolerance therapy registry shows a higher efficacy and shorter interval to inhibitor elimination

Table 34–4 Treatment of Hemorrhage in Patients with Hemophilia with Inhibitors

Type of Patient	Titer at Time of Hemorrhage	Minor Hemorrhage: Agent	Minor Hemorrhage: Dosage	Major Hemorrhage: Agent/Method	Major Hemorrhage: Dosage
High responder	<10BU	PCC	75 IU/kg q12h	Human FVIII	100–200 IU/kg, q12h*
		aPCC	75 IU/kg q12h	Porcine FVIII	50–200 IU/kg*†
				aPCC	75–100 IU/kg q12h
				rFVIIa	90–120 μg/kg q2h
	>10BU	PCC	75 IU/kg q12h	Porcine FVIII	50–200 IU/kg*†
		aPCC	75 IU/kg q12h	aPCC	75–100 IU/kg q12h
				rFVIIa	90–120 μg/kg q2h
				Plasmapheresis and high-dose human FVIII	100–200 IU/kg q12h
Low responder	<5 BU	Human FVIII	50–75 IU/kg q 8–12 h	Human FVIII	100–200 IU/kg*
	<10 BU	PCC	75 IU/kg q12h	Human FVIII	100–200 IU/kg q12h*
		aPCC	75 IU/kg q12h	Porcine FVIII	20–50 IU/kg*†
				aPCC	50–100 IU/kg q12h
				rFVIIa	60–120 μg/kg q2h

*Monitor FVIII levels.

†Use porcine FVIII only if porcine FVIII inhibitor level <20 BU.

aPCC, activated prothrombin complex concentrates; BU, Bethesda units; FVIII, factor VIII; PCC, prothrombin complex concentrates; rFVIII, recombinant factor VIII.

From Manno CS: Treatment options for bleeding episodes in patients undergoing immune tolerance therapy. Haemophilia 1999;5:33–41.

when immune tolerance therapy is initiated when the inhibitor titer is low.[77] Other data show improved outcomes when the interval between inhibitor detection and starting immune tolerance therapy is short.[77] It is therefore important to start immune tolerance therapy as soon as a patient's high-titer, high-response status is confirmed. Once immune tolerance has been achieved, management of bleeding episodes can be the same as before inhibitor development. An international immune tolerance study is currently assessing optimal dose and interval for patients with high-titer inhibitors.[78]

Comprehensive Hemophilia Care

Patients with hemophilia have lifelong disease punctuated by hospitalization and the need for expensive intravenous medication. The management of such complicated patients is best supervised by a multidisciplinary expert team that includes a hematologist, a hemophilia nurse specialist, a physical therapist, a social worker, an orthopedist, and a dentist. Regular clinic visits for evaluation by these health care providers give the patient with hemophilia a solid foundation for managing the long-term medical and psychosocial issues associated with chronic disease.

Gene Therapy

Hemophilia is an attractive disease for a gene therapy approach for several reasons.[79] First, small increases in circulating levels of FVIII or FIX through expression of a successfully transferred gene would likely result in significant reduction of bleeding episodes. Second, tight regulation of transgene expression is not necessary because normal levels of FVIII and FIX extend to 150%. Gene therapy trials using numerous different viral and nonviral approaches to transfer the recombinant gene to human cells, including liver and muscle cells, have been completed, demonstrating no major safety problems but no long-term efficacy either.[79,80] Whether a gene therapy approach will be safe or effective has yet to be determined.[81]

VON WILLEBRAND DISEASE

Von Willebrand disease is the most common congenital coagulation disorder, occurring in approximately 1% to 2% of the population.[82,83] It is actually a collection of disorders caused by either quantitative or qualitative abnormalities of vWF, a glycoprotein that is important in both primary and secondary hemostasis.[84] In contrast to hemophilia, mucosal bleeding, especially epistaxis and menorrhagia, and easy bruising are the most frequent clinical signs, although more significant bleeding can occur with trauma or surgery. Bleeding symptoms are often most severe in children and adolescents.[85] vWD occurs at the same rate in male and female patients and is generally inherited as an autosomal trait with variable penetrance.[86] In contrast to hemophilia, bleeding symptoms may vary among members of affected families.[85]

Structure and Function of von Willebrand Factor

The gene for vWF is located on chromosome 12 and is 178 kb in length with 52 exons.[87] There is also a pseudogene on chromosome 22 with 97% homology.[88] vWF is initially transcribed as a large, single-chain protein with 2813 amino acids (prepro VFW) that undergoes a series of modifications to become the mature multimeric vWF.[85] First, a small signal peptide is removed to form pro-vWF. Next, the remaining peptide undergoes glycosylation, sulfation, and dimer formation, leading to the formation of vWF multimers of various sizes ranging in molecular weight from 500 to 20,000 kD.[89] vWF is the largest soluble protein in humans. Its plasma concentration and functional activity are generally expressed either as a percentage of normal or as units per milliliter related to a normal plasma pool calibrated against an international plasma standard for vWF.[89]

Von Willebrand factor is synthesized in endothelial cells and megakaryocytes. In endothelial cells, vWF is stored in

Weibel-Palade bodies and is secreted into the plasma or subendothelial matrix, predominantly as high-molecular-weight multimers.[90] Platelet vWF, consisting of mostly low-molecular-weight multimers, is synthesized in the megakaryocyte and is stored in platelet α granules.[89] vWF multimers with the highest molecular weight are most effective in hemostasis because they have a large surface area with a high concentration of binding sites for various ligands and receptors.[89]

Von Willebrand factor is important in both primary and secondary hemostasis. It is a cofactor in platelet adhesion and a participant in platelet aggregation. In response to vascular injury, a conformational change occurs in plasma vWF that allows it to bind to platelet glycoprotein Ib.[85,90] Platelets then adhere to the site of endothelial damage and become activated after interactions with subendothelial components such as collagen. Platelet activation causes release of stored platelet components, including vWF from α granules, and expression of activated glycoprotein IIb/IIIa, the receptor that is involved in platelet aggregation.[90] Platelet vWF can bind to glycoprotein IIb/IIIa to facilitate aggregation, although fibrinogen is the main cofactor in this reaction.[85] vWF also plays an important role in the coagulation cascade, by acting as a carrier protein for FVIII so that it is protected from proteolytic cleavage in the plasma.[90] Deficiency of vWF causes FVIII to have a reduced half-life and leads to a deficiency in plasma FVIII. In addition, vWF plays a role in stimulating FVIII release into plasma. This is shown in vitro, where cells transfected with the FVIII gene express rFVIII more efficiently when vWF is present in the media or is cotransfected along with FVIII. In addition, in vivo, when plasma from FVIII-deficient patients is infused into patients with vWD, an increase in FVIII in the patients with vWD is seen.[85]

Classification

As is evident from the previous discussion, vWF plays several critical roles in platelet function and thrombus formation. For vWF to function normally, several requirements must be met, including the presence of high-molecular-weight multimer forms, the appropriate release of activated vWF, and the presence of binding sites for platelet glycoproteins, FVIII, and constituents of the subendothelial cell matrix. Abnormalities of any of these components can lead to vWD, with particular deficiencies leading to different clinical phenotypes. In addition, because the vWF locus is autosomal and the protein is polymeric, the phenotype of a particular patient with vWD is the result of interactions between two different alleles and protein products that lead to the further clinical heterogeneity of this disorder.[91] More than 20 subtypes of vWD have been identified so far.[92] The current classification system for vWD, approved by the Subcommittee on vWF at the 39th Annual Meeting of the Scientific and Standardization Committee of the International Society of Thrombosis and Haemostasis in 1993, attempts to simplify this clinical heterogeneity by classifying patients based on pathophysiology, clinical behavior, and genetic abnormalities.[91] This classification scheme is based on the principle that all vWD is the result of mutations of the vWF locus. In the scheme are three major categories of vWD: type 1 disease, a partial quantitative deficiency of vWF; type 2 disease, a qualitative deficiency of vWF; and type 3 disease, a complete quantitative deficiency of vWF. The clinical course and genetic implications can be predicted by type. Mixed phenotypes can exist, resulting from compound heterozygosity.[91]

Type 1

Type 1 disease is most common and accounts for 70% to 80% of patients diagnosed with vWD.[89,93] Patients with type 1 disease have a mild to moderate decrease in plasma levels of vWF with a normal vWF multimer pattern. Type 1 disease is usually inherited in an autosomal dominant pattern. Clinically, patients with type 1 disease usually have only mild symptoms and are often only identified during routine preoperative screening tests.[85,89]

Type 2 (2A, 2B, 2M, and 2N)

Type 2 vWD disease is diagnosed in 15% to 20% of affected patients and is characterized by a qualitative defect in vWF caused by missense mutations and small inframe deletions or insertions.[84,89] Typically, patients have more significant bleeding symptoms than are seen in type 1 disease. Family history is often positive with this diagnosis, with both autosomal dominant and recessive patterns of inheritance seen.[89] Type 2 disease can be further classified into four variants according to the particular vWF abnormality.

Type 2A vWD is the most frequent subtype and is characterized by decreased vWF platelet-dependent function and an absence of high- and intermediate-molecular-weight vWF multimers as demonstrated on agarose gel electrophoresis.[84,91] This multimer abnormality can result from either abnormal synthesis of vWF or increased breakdown of circulating vWF. Type 2A vWD is usually inherited as a dominant trait.[90,91]

Type 2B is a rarer form of vWD in which an abnormal vWF has excessive affinity for platelet glycoprotein Ib. This causes excessive platelet activation and removal from the circulation and leads to variable thrombocytopenia as well as decreased plasma concentrations of vWF.[84,86] Thrombocytopenia may be intermittent and is often exacerbated by stress such as infection.[86] Type 2B is inherited as a dominant trait and is associated with absence of high-molecular-weight multimers.[84,93]

Type 2M disease describes patients with decreased platelet-dependent function that is similar to type 2A disease, except high-molecular-weight multimers are not absent. Decreased platelet function is instead caused by structural or functional defects in binding regions of the vWF protein. Like type 2A and 2B disease, this type is usually inherited as a dominant trait.[84,93]

Type 2N disease (also known as vWD Normandy) refers to patients with vWF variants with decreased binding affinity for FVIII. This leads to decreased survival of FVIII in the circulation and a moderate to severe reduction of FVIII plasma levels with normal vWF levels. Affected persons therefore have a mild hemophilia phenotype. This type usually has an autosomal recessive inheritance.[84–86]

Type 3

Type 3 vWD is characterized by near-complete deficiency of vWF (less than 10%) as well as a secondary deficiency of FVIII, resulting in a severe bleeding disorder with abnormalities in both primary and secondary hemostasis.[93] This type of vWD is very rare, with a prevalence of 1 to 3 cases per 1 million, and is inherited as an autosomal recessive disorder.[94]

Diagnosis

Von Willebrand disease should be suspected in patients with a history of increased bruising, prolonged bleeding after minor trauma, or mucosal bleeding, particularly epistaxis and menorrhagia, and is supported by a family history of abnormal bleeding. Initial screening tests include prothrombin time (PT), PTT, platelet count, and bleeding time. The PT is usually normal, whereas the PTT may be prolonged by a decrease in FVIII.[93] The platelet count is also usually normal, although, as described earlier, thrombocytopenia can be present in patients with type 2B disease.[86] The bleeding time, which is usually prolonged secondary to abnormal platelet function, may be normal in patients with type 1 disease with normal platelet vWF content, but it is rarely used today in the diagnostic workup.[93] All these screening tests may be normal in persons with vWD, so further testing may be needed when suspicion of disease is significant.[95]

Specific tests used to evaluate patients for vWD include vWF antigen, FVIII assay, vWF activity (also known as *ristocetin cofactor activity*), and vWF multimer analysis. Because normal physiologic variation can occur in plasma levels of vWF, FVIII, and vWF activity, repeated plasma measurements over time may be necessary to establish a diagnosis of disease.[86,95] Results of these tests vary according to type of vWD.

Von Willebrand factor antigen is decreased in type 1 disease, decreased or normal in type 2 disease, and undetectable in type 3 disease.[93] vWF is an acute phase reactant, and factors such as pregnancy, exercise, infection, and cigarette smoking, as well as medications, including corticosteroids, birth control pills, and DDAVP, can increase plasma concentrations of vWF and need to be taken into consideration when one evaluates test results.[86] In addition, vWF antigen varies with ABO blood types and therefore should be interpreted in reference to values specific for the patient's blood type; persons with blood group O have the lowest mean vWF antigen level.[96] FVIII levels are normal or mildly decreased in patients with types 1 and 2 vWD.[93] In contrast, patients with type 2N and type 3 vWD can have an extremely low FVIII level.[86] The ristocetin cofactor activity assay measures the vWF function, specifically the interaction of vWF with platelet glycoprotein Ib. Patients with type 1 and type 3 vWD tend to have a decrease in vWF activity that is proportional to their decrease in vWF antigen, whereas those with type 2 disease have a more substantial decrease in vWF activity than vWF antigen.[86,93] Studies have shown that measurement of vWF activity is the most sensitive test for diagnosing type 1 vWD.[82,95] Finally, the vWF can be separated by agarose gel electrophoresis into high-, intermediate-, and low-molecular-weight multimers. All the multimers are present in type 1 disease and are absent in type 3 disease. In type 2 vWD, gel electrophoresis can vary with disease type, but generally shows a reduction in high- and intermediate-weight multimer.[86] Table 34–5 summarizes the laboratory findings according to vWD type.

Therapeutic Products

Superficial bleeding, particularly in type 1 vWD, can usually be managed by applying local pressure, ice, or a local topical hemostatic agent. Systemic therapy is generally reserved for bleeding at sites not controllable by local measures or as prophylaxis before and after surgical treatment. The two main approaches to systemic therapy of vWD are increasing the release of endogenous vWF and exogenous replacement of vWF. Selecting the appropriate therapy for an individual patient depends on the specific type of vWD and clinical treatment goal.[44]

Desmopressin

As previously discussed, DDAVP, a synthetic analog of vasopressin, causes immediate endothelial cell release of vWF, FVIII, and plasminogen activator.[43] It is effective in patients with vWD who have adequate stores of functional vWF. Therefore, it is useful in type 1 disease but ineffective in type 3 disease. DDAVP can be used in some patients with type 2A vWD, but it is not recommended in patients with type 2B disease because it can exacerbate thrombocytopenia.[90,97] Patients with type 2N disease generally have high FVIII levels in response to DDAVP, but the released FVIII has a shorter than normal half-life that limits its therapeutic utility in major bleeding episodes.[97] DDAVP is given at the same dose used in mild FVIII deficiency, either intravenously or as a concentrated nasal spray (Stimate). Infusion of 0.3 μg/kg body weight results in an average three- to fivefold increase in vWF and FVIII; nasal dosing is slightly less effective.[43,90] Before therapeutic use, patients should have a trial to measure individual response to DDAVP.[98] Response to DDAVP is generally consistent over time, and family members usually have similar responses.[99] DDAVP is used preferentially over plasma-derived products in patients who have an adequate response, because it does not carry risks of viral transmission. In addition, DDAVP is substantially less expensive than exogenous vWF replacement.[43]

Table 34–5 Laboratory Findings in von Willebrand Disease According to Subtype

Study	Type 1	Type 2A	Type 2B	Type 2M	Type 2N	Type 3
von Willebrand factor antigen	↓	↓	+/– ↓	↓	↓	Absent
Ristocetin cofactor activity	↓	↓↓↓	+/– ↓	↓↓↓	↓	Absent
Factor VIII	↓	Normal	Normal	Normal	↓↓	Absent
Ristocetin-induced platelet aggregation	+/–↓	↓↓	Normal	↓	Normal	Absent
Multimers	Normal distribution	Absent intermediate and high-molecular-weight multimers	Absent high-molecular-weight multimers	Normal	Normal	Absent

Adapted from Montgomery RR, Gill JC, Scott JP. Hemophilia and von Willebrand disease. In Nathan DH, Orkin SH (eds). Naton and OSKI's Hematology of Infancy and Childhood, vol 2, 5th ed. Philadelphia, WB Saunders, 1998, p 1646.

Desmopressin may not be useful when prolonged hemostasis is required. When it is administered more often than once every 24 to 48 hours, decreased effectiveness may be observed because of depletion of storage pools (tachyphylaxis).[99] Therefore, when DDAVP is used for several days, coagulation parameters should be followed closely (vWF, FVIII, and ristocetin cofactor) to monitor the need for alternative replacement therapy.

Exogenous von Willebrand Factor Replacement

Exogenous replacement of vWF is used in patients in whom DDAVP is not effective, including most patients with type 2B, type 2M, and type 3 vWD, as well as those with type 1 and 2A disease who do not show adequate response in a DDAVP trial. Fresh frozen plasma contains both FVIII and vWF; however, the large volumes required to achieve hemostasis limit its clinical use.[98] Cryoprecipitate, containing vWF, FVIII, and fibrinogen, was the treatment of choice for patients with vWD from the early 1960s until the early 1980s.[44,100] The development of products with higher purity that are more convenient to store, have decreased volumes of infusion, and have undergone viral inactivation subsumed the need for cryoprecipitate. However, if other alternatives are not available, transfusion of cryoprecipitate will produce hemostasis.[90] Each bag of cryoprecipitate contains 80 to 100 IU of vWF, and the usual starting dose is 1 bag/10 kg body weight every 12 to 24 hours.[90,98] Cryoprecipitate from a single donor who has been pretreated with DDAVP contains supraphysiologic amounts of vWF and is another treatment option.[85]

The early plasma-derived FVIII concentrates were not effective in treating vWD because the vWF multimers were partially proteolyzed; this resulted in a loss of functional high-molecular-weight multimers.[44] In addition, high-purity plasma-derived (monoclonal antibody-derived) FVIII as well as rFVIII cannot be used to treat vWD because they do not contain appreciable amounts of vWF.[90] Two plasma-derived, virus-inactivated FVIII concentrates available in the United States contain sufficient amounts of functional vWF: Humate-P and Alphanate.[90,100,101] The latter product is not yet licensed by the FDA for use in vWD. In general, dosing for vWD is in units of ristocetin cofactor. In addition, a recombinant vWF concentrate is currently under development.[94]

Adjunctive Treatment

As previously described for hemophilia treatment, antifibrinolytic therapy, which inhibits lysis of newly formed clots, is also useful in the treatment of vWD. Aminocaproic acid and tranexamic acid, the agents most commonly used, are given at the same doses used in hemophilia. Both agents may be useful alone in mild type 1 disease or as adjuncts in the treatment of oral hemorrhage, epistaxis, gastrointestinal bleeding, and menorrhagia. These agents may increase the risk of thrombosis and are contraindicated in patients with a known pre-existing prothrombotic state and in the treatment of genitourinary bleeding.[90,98]

Estrogen causes an increase in plasma vWF. This effect is variable and is not dose related; therefore, it is not widely clinically applicable. However, estrogen therapy, particularly in the form of oral contraceptives, is useful in reducing the severity of menorrhagia, a common problem in women with vWD.[98] As previously discussed, patients with vWD should avoid drugs that interfere with platelet function.

RARE INHERITED CONGENITAL CLOTTING DISORDERS REQUIRING TRANSFUSION THERAPY

Fibrinogen Deficiencies

Congenital afibrinogenemia is a rare disorder, with an estimated incidence of 1 to 2 per 1 million that is inherited as an autosomal recessive trait with the gene located on chromosome 4.[102,103] It is characterized by virtual absence of fibrinogen secondary to deficient liver cell synthesis. Symptoms range from minimal bleeding to life-threatening hemorrhage, and are commonly seen in the newborn period and include hematomas or intracranial hemorrhage from birth trauma, bleeding from the umbilicus, and excessive bleeding after circumcision. Similar to hemophilia, spontaneous hemorrhage and excessive post-traumatic and postsurgical bleeding are seen and can result in excessive ecchymoses, hemarthroses, gastrointestinal bleeding, and intracranial hemorrhage.[102,104] In addition, menstrual bleeding can be severe, and first-trimester spontaneous abortion is common.[102,105] Laboratory screening tests that use clot formation as an endpoint, including thrombin time, PT, and PTT, are markedly prolonged. Definitive diagnosis is made by measurement of plasma fibrinogen, which is undetectable by both functional and immunologic assays.

Dysfibrinogenemia is characterized by structural fibrinogen defects causing alterations in the conversion of fibrinogen to fibrin. Approximately 250 cases have been reported, and the disorder is inherited as an autosomal dominant trait.[106] Dysfibrinogenemias can be associated with either hemorrhage or thromboses, or they can be asymptomatic.[103,106] The bleeding symptoms most commonly seen are ecchymoses, epistaxis, menorrhagia, and mild to moderate postoperative or post-traumatic bleeding. Symptoms are generally mild, although they can be more severe in patients with homozygous gene mutations. Results of screening tests are variable; the PT and PTT can be normal or prolonged. The thrombin time is prolonged in dysfibrinogenemias associated with hemorrhage, whereas it can be shortened or prolonged in those conditions associated with thromboses. More definitive diagnosis is made by measurement of fibrinogen; levels are normal or increased by immunologic assay, but they are reduced by functional assays.[104,106,107]

For both quantitative and qualitative fibrinogen deficiencies, cryoprecipitate can be used as replacement therapy for significant episodic bleeding. Cryoprecipitate should be administered at a dose to raise the fibrinogen level to between 50 and 100 mg/dL.[102] A typical bag of cryoprecipitate contains 200 to 300 mg of fibrinogen in a volume of 10 to 20 mL.[3] Because the half-life of fibrinogen is 80 hours, dosing is required only every other day.[104] Prophylactic replacement of fibrinogen, practical because of the long half-life of fibrinogen, should be considered for patients with severe symptoms.[108]

Prothrombin Deficiency

Prothrombin deficiency is a very rare autosomal recessive disorder that results from either an absolute protein deficiency or production of an abnormal protein.[109] It is characterized by mild symptoms, including mucocutaneous bleeding and hemorrhage after surgery or trauma. The PT is moderately prolonged, the PTT is normal or mildly prolonged, and the thrombin time is normal. Definitive diagnosis is made by immunologic and functional prothrombin assays.[104,109]

Therapy is usually not required. Fresh frozen plasma or PCCs can be used to treat clinically significant bleeding. The half-life of prothrombin is 48 to 120 hours.[103] Plasma prothrombin levels greater than 20 to 30 U/dL are generally sufficient to stop bleeding.[109]

Factor V Deficiency

Factor V deficiency occurs in less than 1 per 1 million persons and is associated with a mild to moderate bleeding tendency.[104] It is inherited as an autosomal recessive disease. Symptoms, generally only seen in homozygotes, consist mainly of mucocutaneous bleeding, including menorrhagia, and ecchymoses. Both the prothrombin and PTT are prolonged, with a normal thrombin time. Definitive diagnosis is made by a specific FV assay, with deficiency defined as FV levels lower than 20 U/dL.[110]

Fresh frozen plasma should be used to treat severe bleeding episodes and trauma and as prophylaxis for major surgery. For treatment, the FV level should be initially raised to 25% to 30% of normal using a 20 mL/kg dose of plasma followed by infusions of 6 mL/kg every 12 hours.[109] FV is more labile in frozen plasma than other hemostatic factors, and therefore fresh frozen plasma that is less than 1 to 2 months old should be used.[109]

Several families with combined deficiency of FV and FVIII have been reported.[111] Symptoms are usually milder than in hemophilia A because of higher baseline levels of FVIII. Treatment should include fresh frozen plasma in addition to FVIII concentrates.

Factor VII Deficiency

Factor VII deficiency, resulting from either a protein deficiency or production of a nonfunctional protein, occurs in 1 in 1 million persons and is inherited in an autosomal recessive pattern with high penetrance and variable expressivity.[112] Laboratory evaluation of patients with FVII deficiency reveals a prolonged PT with a normal PTT and thrombin time, a pattern that distinguishes FVII deficiency from other inherited clotting disorders. The diagnosis is confirmed by measuring FVII activity using a tissue factor-dependent one-stage technique. The clinical expression of the disease is generally correlated with the degree of factor deficiency, although reports exist of patients with extremely low FVII levels who present without a history of bleeding.[113] Patients with FVII levels greater than 10% to 15% rarely have significant bleeding problems, whereas patients with levels lower than 1% can have severe bleeding symptoms.[112] The most serious complication of FVII deficiency is intracranial hemorrhage, which occurs most frequently during the first year of life, particularly in the first postnatal week.[114] Mucous membrane bleeding, including excessive bruising, epistaxis, gastrointestinal bleeding, and menorrhagia, is the most common manifestation of FVII deficiency. Hemarthroses, in a pattern similar to what is seen in hemophilia, also occur occasionally.[114]

Treatment is required for severe bleeding episodes and before surgical procedures. PCCs have previously been the mainstays of therapy for FVII deficiency. Replacement doses are calculated to raise the FVII level to more than 15%. FVII concentrations vary among commercially available PCCs and among different lots produced by a single manufacturer, so it is important to monitor the patient's PT and FVII level carefully.[112] As discussed previously, patients receiving PCCs need to be monitored for an increased risk of developing thromboses. Recombinant FVIIa has more recently been shown to be effective as a more specific treatment without an accompanying risk of thrombosis.[115] Studies have shown efficacy of rFVIIa as treatment for intracranial hemorrhage and as prophylaxis for surgical procedures, and these features make rFVIIa the likely treatment of choice for FVII deficiency in the future.[116,117]

Factor X Deficiency

Factor X deficiency results from either a protein deficiency or production of a functionally abnormal protein.[109] It is inherited as an autosomal recessive trait, although some heterozygotes can have bleeding with severe trauma or major surgery. Symptoms generally correlate with the severity of the deficiency and consist mainly of mucocutaneous and post-traumatic bleeding. Hemarthrosis and intracranial hemorrhage have been reported in severely affected patients. Laboratory evaluation reveals prolonged PT and PTT. Diagnosis is confirmed with FX immunologic and functional assays.

Factor X replacement should be given as needed for severe bleeding and trauma as well as before major surgical procedures. The half-life of transfused FX is between 24 and 48 hours. FX is found in both fresh frozen plasma and PCCs.[104] Fresh frozen plasma is given at an initial dose of 10 to 20 mL/kg, followed every 12 hours by a dose of 3 to 6 mL/kg to reach a target plasma FX level of 20 to 30 IU/dL.[109] PCCs contain a variable concentration of FX that can be measured in a specific preparation before elective use.[109] PCCs are more practical to use in situations such as major surgery, when sustained hemostasis is necessary and would require large volumes of plasma infusions. As previously mentioned, when using PCCs, the risk of thrombosis should be considered and monitored.

Factor XI Deficiency

Factor XI deficiency, sometimes called hemophilia C, is a relatively rare disorder distinguished by a variable bleeding tendency in affected individuals. It is inherited as an autosomal trait and is seen most commonly among persons of Ashkenazi Jewish descent, with an 8% frequency of heterozygosity.[118] Three different point mutations in the FXI gene account for nearly all cases of FXI deficiency among Ashkenazi Jews.[119] FXI deficiency is most often detected in association with a positive family history or secondary to a prolonged PTT found during a routine presurgical evaluation. The diagnosis is confirmed with a plasma FXI assay.

Factor XI levels correlate with the genotype. Severe deficiency (FXI levels lower than 15 to 20 IU/dL) is seen in homozygotes or compound heterozygotes, and partial deficiency (FXI levels from 20 to 60 IU/dL) is seen in heterozygotes. Bleeding tendency, however, does not correlate with genotype.[120] Excessive bleeding is most commonly seen in association with severe deficiency, but it can also be seen in patients with partial deficiency. A compilation of studies shows abnormal bleeding in 30% to 50% of patients with partial deficiency.[121] In general, bleeding symptoms are mild or absent, only occurring in association with trauma or surgery, particularly tonsillectomy. Epistaxis, soft tissue hemorrhage, bleeding after dental extractions, and menorrhagia can also be seen in affected persons.

Fresh frozen plasma is most commonly given as treatment for severe bleeding episodes or as prophylaxis for major surgery. The half-life of FXI in plasma is approximately 45 hours. As an alternative treatment, two specific FXI concentrates are available in Europe.[118] Both have been shown to be hemostatically effective and virally safe, but they have been associated with an increased occurrence of thrombotic events, particularly in older patients with pre-existing vascular disease and when these concentrates are given at very high doses.[122,123] These products may be useful in selected patients without pre-existing hypercoagulable states at doses less than 30 IU/kg.[118] Bleeding from minor procedures such as dental extraction can be controlled with local measures or antifibrinolytic agents (aminocaproic acid and tranexamic acid) at the same doses that are used for hemophilia and vWD.[118]

Contact Factor Deficiencies

Deficiencies of the contact factors—FXII, prekallikrein, and high-molecular-weight kininogen—are not associated with bleeding symptoms.[104] Because these factors are necessary for the initiation of the intrinsic pathway, the PTT is markedly prolonged, frequently beyond what is seen in hemophilia, whereas the PT is normal. Both FXII and prekallikrein deficiencies are inherited as autosomal recessive traits.[104] Patients are usually identified during routine preoperative screening, and definitive diagnosis is made with specific contact factor assays. Treatment is not necessary.

Factor XIII Deficiency

Factor XIII deficiency is an autosomal recessive disorder. FXIII is also known as *fibrin-stabilizing factor* and is responsible for crosslinking of the fibrin polymer. Deficiency of FXIII is associated with reduced clot stability, and therefore ecchymoses or hematomas are usually seen 24 to 36 hours after trauma. FXIII deficiency is associated with severe bleeding, particularly delayed intracranial hemorrhage with minimal trauma. Other symptoms of FXIII deficiency include delayed separation of the umbilical stump in the neonatal period (at more than 3.5 to 4 weeks), poor wound healing, and recurrent spontaneous abortions in women secondary to severe decidual bleeding. Screening tests are normal, including bleeding time, PT, PTT, and thrombin time. Clots from affected persons appear more friable than normal. When the condition is suspected clinically, diagnosis of homozygous patients is made using a urea clot solubility assay or by measuring plasma levels of FXIII subunit proteins.[124]

Fresh frozen plasma is usually used for hemostasis in FXIII deficiency.[109] It is given at a dose of 5 to 10 mL/kg. Because the half-life of FXIII is very long (3 to 6 days), one dose is generally sufficient. Cryoprecipitate also contains FXIII and can also be used to treat acute bleeding episodes.[109] Patients with severe bleeding symptoms can receive either product as prophylaxis every 2 to 4 weeks. In addition, two plasma-derived FXIII concentrates are currently produced (by Centeon in the United States and Bio Products Laboratory in the UK).[125] These are not yet available for general distribution in the United States.

CONCLUSION

Accurate and early diagnosis, comprehensive clinical care, and the availability of factor concentrates that are manufactured with limited risk of transmitting blood-borne viruses and minimal risk of thrombosis have all contributed to improved outcomes for patients with congenital bleeding disorders. Despite these advances, patients with severe hemophilia require tremendous dedication and support to successfully manage their disease. The promise of gene transfer, which could allow for amelioration or elimination of the phenotypic abnormalities seen in severe hemophilia, is still in the future.

REFERENCES

1. Soucie JM, Evatt B, Jackson D. Occurrence of hemophilia in the United States: The Hemophilia Surveillance System Project Investigators. Am J Hematol 1998;59:288–294.
2. DiMichele D. Hemophilia 1996. New approach to an old disease. Pediatr Clin North Am 1996;43:709–736.
3. Kasper CK. Hereditary plasma clotting factor disorders and their management. Haemophilia 2000;6:13–27.
4. Goodeve AC. Advances in carrier detection in haemophilia. Haemophilia 1998;4:358–364.
5. Lillicrap D. Molecular diagnosis of inherited bleeding disorders and thrombophilia. Semin Hematol 1999;36:340–351.
6. Bagnall RD, Waseem N, Green PM, Giannelli F. Recurrent inversion breaking intron 1 of the factor VIII gene is a frequent cause of severe hemophilia A. Blood 2002;99168–174.
7. Tedgard U. Carrier testing and prenatal diagnosis of haemophilia: utilisation and psychological consequences. Haemophilia 1998;4:365–369.
8. Andrew M, Brooker LA. Blood component therapy in neonatal hemostatic disorders. Transfus Med Rev 1995;9:231–250.
9. DiMichele D, Neufeld EJ. Hemophilia: a new approach to an old disease. Hematol Oncol Clin North Am 1998;12:1315–1344.
10. Hoyer LW. Hemophilia A. NEJM 1994;330:38–47.
11. Hoag MS, Johnson FF, Robinson JA, Aggeler PM. Treatment of hemophilia B with a new clotting-factor concentrate. NEJM 1969;280:581–586.
12. Mannucci PM. Modern treatment of hemophilia: from the shadows towards the light. Thromb Haemost 1993;70:17–23.
13. Centers for Disease Control and Prevention. Update on acquired immune deficiency syndrome (AIDS) among patients with hemophilia A. MMWR Morb Mortal Wkly Rep 1982;31:644–646, 652,.
14. Berntorp E. Impact of replacement therapy on the evolution of HIV infection in hemophiliacs. Thromb Haemost 1994;71:678–683.
15. Brettler DB. Comments on the development of inhibitor antibodies in patients using recombinant factor VIII concentrates. Semin Hematol 1991;28:45–46.
16. Kasper CK, Lusher JM. Recent evolution of clotting factor concentrates for hemophilia A and B: Transfusion Practices Committee. Transfusion 1993;33:422–434.
17. Lusher JM. Transfusion therapy in congenital coagulopathies. Hematol Oncol Clin North Am 1994;8:1167–1180.
18. Mannucci PM. Clinical evaluation of viral safety of coagulation factor VIII and IX concentrates. Vox Sang 1993;64:197–203.
19. Horowitz MS, Rooks C, Horowitz B, Hilgartner MW. Virus safety of solvent/detergent-treated antihaemophilic factor concentrate. Lancet 1988;2:186–189.
20. Ludlam CA. Viral safety of plasma-derived factor VIII and IX concentrates. Blood Coagul Fibrinolysis 1997;8(Suppl):S19–S23.
21. Toole JJ, Knopf JL, Wozney JM, et al. Molecular cloning of a cDNA encoding human antihaemophilic factor. Nature 1984;312:342–347.
22. Wood WI, Capon DJ, Simonsen CC, et al. Expression of active human factor VIII from recombinant DNA clones. Nature 1984;312:330–337.
23. Schwartz RS, Abildgaard CF, Aledort LM, et al. Human recombinant DNA-derived antihemophilic factor (factor VIII) in the treatment of hemophilia A: recombinant Factor VIII Study Group. NEJM 1990;323:1800–1805.
24. Lusher JM, Arkin S, Abildgaard CF, Schwartz RS. Recombinant factor VIII for the treatment of previously untreated patients with hemophilia A: safety, efficacy, and development of inhibitors. Kogenate Previously Untreated Patient Study Group. NEJM 1993;328: 453–459.

25. Bray GL, Gomperts ED, Courter S, et al. A multicenter study of recombinant factor VIII (Recombinate): safety, efficacy, and inhibitor risk in previously untreated patients with hemophilia A. The Recombinate Study Group. Blood 1994;83:2428–2435.
26. Manno CS. Treatment options for bleeding episodes in patients undergoing immune tolerance therapy. Haemophilia 1999;5:33–41.
27. Mannucci PM, Tuddenbam EG. The hemophilias: progress and problems. Semin Hematol 1999;36:104–117.
28. Hilgartner MW, Manno CS, Nuss R, Di Michele DM. Pediatric issues in hemophilia. In Proceedings of the American Society of Hematology. San Diego, American Society of Hematology, 1997, pp 46–60.
29. Abshire TC, Brackmann HH, Scharrer I, et al. Sucrose formulated recombinant human antihemophilic factor VIII is safe and efficacious for treatment of hemophilia A in home therapy: International Kogenate-FS Study Group. Thromb Haemost 2000;83:811–816.
30. Berntorp E. Second generation, B-domain deleted recombinant factor VIII. Thromb Haemost 1997;78:256–260.
31. Sandberg H, Almstedt A, Brandt J, et al. Structural and functional characteristics of the B-domain-deleted recombinant factor VIII protein, r-VIII SQ. Thromb Haemost 2001;85:93–100.
32. Tarantino MD, Collins PW, Hay CR, et al. Clinical evaluation of an advanced category antihaemophilic factor prepared using a plasma/albumin-free method: pharmacokinetics, efficacy, and safety in previously treated patients with haemophilia A. Haemophilia 2004;10: 428–437.
33. Kohler M, Hellstern P, Lechler E, et al. Thromboembolic complications associated with the use of prothrombin complex and factor IX concentrates. Thromb Haemost 1998;80:399–402.
34. Goldsmith JC, Kasper CK, Blatt PM, et al. Coagulation factor IX: Successful surgical experience with a purified factor IX concentrate. Am J Hematol 1992;40:210–215.
35. Shapiro AD, Ragni MV, Lusher JM, et al. Safety and efficacy of monoclonal antibody purified factor IX concentrate in previously untreated patients with hemophilia B. Thromb Haemost 1996;75:30–35.
36. Bond M, Jankowski M, Patel H, et al. Biochemical characterization of recombinant factor IX. Semin Hematol 1998;35:11–17.
37. Brinkhous KM, Sigman JL, Read MS, et al. Recombinant human factor IX: replacement therapy, prophylaxis, and pharmacokinetics in canine hemophilia B. Blood 1996;88:2603–2610.
38. Choo KH, Gould KG, Rees DJ, et al. Molecular cloning of the gene for human anti-haemophilic factor IX. Nature 1982;299:178–180.
39. Kurachi K, Davie EW. Isolation and characterization of a cDNA coding for human factor IX. Proc Natl Acad Sci USA 1982;79:6461–6464.
40. White G, Shapiro A, Ragni M, et al. Clinical evaluation of recombinant factor IX. Semin Hematol 1998;35:33–38.
41. White GC 2nd, Beebe A, Nielsen B. Recombinant factor IX. Thromb Haemost 1997;78:261–265.
42. Furie B, Limentani SA, Rosenfield CG. A practical guide to the evaluation and treatment of hemophilia. Blood 1994;84:3–9.
43. Mannucci PM. Desmopressin (DDAVP) in the treatment of bleeding disorders: the first 20 years. Blood 1997;90:2515–2521.
44. Logan LJ. Treatment of von Willebrand's disease. Hematol Oncol Clin North Am 1992;6:1079–1094.
45. Manno CS, Butler RB, Cohen AR. Low recovery in vivo of highly purified factor VIII in patients with hemophilia. J Pediatr 1992;121:814–818.
46. Kelly KM, Butler RB, Farace L, et al. Superior in vivo response of recombinant factor VIII concentrate in children with hemophilia A. J Pediatr 1997;130:537–540.
47. Lusher JM. Prophylaxis in children with hemophilia: is it the optimal treatment? Thromb Haemost 1997;78:726–729.
48. Ahlberg A. Haemophilia in Sweden. VII. Incidence, treatment and prophylaxis of arthropathy and other musculo-skeletal manifestations of haemophilia A and B. Acta Orthop Scand Suppl 1965;3:132.
49. Aronstam A, Kirk PJ, McHardy J, et al. Twice weekly prophylactic therapy in haemophilia A. J Clin Pathol 1977;30:65–67.
50. Gruppo RA. Prophylaxis for hemophilia: state of the art or state of confusion [editorial]? J Pediatr 1998;132:915–917.
51. Nilsson IM, Berntorp E, Lofqvist T, Pettersson H. Twenty-five years' experience of prophylactic treatment in severe haemophilia A and B. J Intern Med 1992;232:25–32.
52. Liesner RJ, Khair K, Hann IM. The impact of prophylactic treatment on children with severe haemophilia. Br J Haematol 1996;92:973–978.
53. Lofqvist T, Nilsson IM, Berntorp E, Pettersson H. Haemophilia prophylaxis in young patients: a long-term follow-up. J Intern Med 1997;241:395–400.
54. Aledort LM, Haschmeyer RH, Pettersson H. A longitudinal study of orthopaedic outcomes for severe factor-VIII-deficient haemophiliacs: The Orthopaedic Outcome Study Group. J Intern Med 1994;236: 391–399.
55. Ljung RC. Prophylactic infusion regimens in the management of hemophilia. Thromb Haemost 1999;82:525–530.
56. Manco-Johnson MJ, Nuss R, Geraghty S, et al. Results of secondary prophylaxis in children with severe hemophilia. Am J Hematol 1994;47:113–117.
57. Aledort L. Inhibitors in hemophilia patients: current status and management. Am J Hematol 1994;47:208–217.
58. Manco-Johnson MJ, Nuss R, Geraghty S, Funk S. A prophylactic program in the United States: experience and issues. Semin Hematol 1994;31:10–12.
59. Smith PS, Teutsch SM, Shaffer PA, et al. Episodic versus prophylactic infusions for hemophilia A: a cost-effectiveness analysis. J Pediatr 1996;129:424–431.
60. Carlsson M, Berntorp E, Bjorkman S, Lindvall K. Pharmacokinetic dosing in prophylactic treatment of hemophilia A. Eur J Haematol 1993;51:247–252.
61. Blanchette VS, Al-Musa A, Stain AM, et al. Central venous access devices in children with hemophilia: an update. Blood Coagul Fibrinolysis 1997;8(Suppl):S11–S14.
62. Bollard CM, Teague LR, Berry EW, Ockelford PA. The use of central venous catheters (Portacaths) in children with haemophilia. Haemophilia 2000;6:66–70.
63. Ragni MJ, Hord JD, Blatt J. Central venous catheter infection in haemophiliacs undergoing prophylaxis or immune tolerance with clotting factor concentrate. Haemophilia 1997;3:90–95.
64. Conway JH, Hilgartner MW. Initial presentations of pediatric hemophiliacs. Arch Pediatr Adolesc Med 1994;148:589–594.
65. Baehner RL, Strauss HS. Hemophilia in the first year of life. NEJM 1966;275:524–528.
66. Buchanan GR. Factor concentrate prophylaxis for neonates with hemophilia. J Pediatr Hematol Oncol 1999;21:254–256.
67. Kulkarni R, Lusher JM, Henry RC, Kallen DJ. Current practices regarding newborn intracranial haemorrhage and obstetrical care and mode of delivery of pregnant haemophilia carriers: a survey of obstetricians, neonatologists and haematologists in the United States, on behalf of the National Hemophilia Foundation's Medical and Scientific Advisory Council. Haemophilia 1999;5:410–415.
68. Hoyer LW. Why do so many haemophilia A patients develop an inhibitor? Br J Haematol 1995;90:498–501.
69. Hoyer LW. Factor VIII inhibitors. Curr Opin Hematol 1995;2:365–371.
70. Hay CR. Why do inhibitors arise in patients with haemophilia A? Br J Haematol 1999;105:584–590.
71. Tuddenham EG, McVey JH. The genetic basis of inhibitor development in haemophilia A. Haemophilia 1998;4:543–545.
72. Kasper CK, Aledort L, Aronson D, et al. Proceedings: A more uniform measurement of factor VIII inhibitors. Thromb Diath Haemorrh 1975;34:612.
73. Leissinger CA. Use of prothrombin complex concentrates and activated prothrombin complex concentrates as prophylactic therapy in haemophilia patients with inhibitors. Haemophilia 1999;5:25–32.
74. Green D. Complications associated with the treatment of haemophiliacs with inhibitors. Haemophilia 1999;5:11–17.
75. Santagostino E, Gringeri A, Mannucci PM. Home treatment with recombinant activated factor VII in patients with factor VIII inhibitors: the advantages of early intervention. Br J Haematol 1999;104:22–26.
76. Teitel JM. Recombinant factor VIIa versus aPCCs in haemophiliacs with inhibitors: treatment and cost considerations. Haemophilia 1999; 5:43–49.
77. DiMichele DM. Immune tolerance: a synopsis of the international experience. Haemophilia 1998;4:568–573.
78. Conversation with Dr. CRM Hay and Dr. DM DiMichele on December 21, 2005. Untitled abstract: "International Randomized Immune Tolerance (ITI) Study: Progress Report."
79. Kay MA, High K. Gene therapy for the hemophilias. Proc Natl Acad Sci USA 1999;96:9973–9975.
80. Herzog RW, High KA. Adeno-associated virus-mediated gene transfer of factor IX for treatment of hemophilia B by gene therapy. Thromb Haemost 1999;82:540–546.
81. Kay MA, Manno CS, Ragni MV, et al. Evidence for gene transfer and expression of factor IX in haemophilia B patients treated with an AAV vector. Nat Genet 2000;24:257–261.
82. Rodeghiero F, Castaman G, Dini E. Epidemiological investigation of the prevalence of von Willebrand's disease. Blood 1987;69:454–459.
83. Werner EJ, Broxson EH, Tucker EL, et al. Prevalence of von Willebrand disease in children: a multiethnic study. J Pediatr 1993;123:893–898.

84. Ginsburg D. Molecular genetics of von Willebrand disease. Thromb Haemost 1999;82:585–591.
85. Werner EJ. von Willebrand disease in children and adolescents. Pediatr Clin North Am 1996;43:683–707.
86. Batlle J, Torea J, Rendal E, Fernandez MF: The problem of diagnosing von Willebrand's disease. J Intern Med Suppl 1997;740:121–128.
87. Mancuso DJ, Tuley EA, Westfield LA, et al. Structure of the gene for human von Willebrand factor. J Biol Chem 1989;264:19514–19527.
88. Mancuso DJ, Tuley EA, Westfield LA, et al. Human von Willebrand factor gene and pseudogene: structural analysis and differentiation by polymerase chain reaction. Biochemistry 1991;30:253–269.
89. Schneppenheim R, Thomas KB, Sutor AH. Von Willebrand disease in childhood. Semin Thromb Hemost 1995;21:261–275.
90. Phillips MD, Santhouse A. von Willebrand disease: Recent advances in pathophysiology and treatment. Am J Med Sci 1998;316:77–86.
91. Sadler JE. A revised classification of von Willebrand disease: for the Subcommittee on von Willebrand Factor of the Scientific and Standardization Committee of the International Society on Thrombosis and Haemostasis. Thromb Haemost 1994;71:520–525.
92. Sadler JE, Matsushita T, Dong Z, et al. Molecular mechanism and classification of von Willebrand disease. Thromb Haemost 1995;74: 161–166.
93. Federici AB. Diagnosis of von Willebrand disease. Haemophilia 1998;4: 654–660.
94. Schwarz HP, Turecek PL, Pichler L, et al. Recombinant von Willebrand factor. Thromb Haemost 1997;78:571–576.
95. Werner EJ, Abshire TC, Giroux DS, et al. Relative value of diagnostic studies for von Willebrand disease. J Pediatr 1992;121:34–38.
96. Gill JC, Endres-Brooks J, Bauer PJ, et al. The effect of ABO blood group on the diagnosis of von Willebrand disease. Blood 1987;69:1691–1695.
97. Mannucci PM. Treatment of von Willebrand's disease. J Intern Med Suppl 1997;740:129–132.
98. Mannucci PM. Treatment of von Willebrand disease. Int J Clin Lab Res 1998;28:211–214.
99. Mannucci PM. Desmopressin: a nontransfusional form of treatment for congenital and acquired bleeding disorders. Blood 1988;72: 1449–1455.
100. Menache D, Aronson DL. New treatments of von Willebrand disease: plasma derived von Willebrand factor concentrates. Thromb Haemost 1997;78:566–570.
101. Lubetsky A, Schulman S, Varon D, et al. Safety and efficacy of continuous infusion of a combined factor VIII–von Willebrand factor (vWF) concentrate (Haemate-P) in patients with von Willebrand disease. Thromb Haemost 1999;81:229–233.
102. al-Mondhiry H, Ehmann WC. Congenital afibrinogenemia. Am J Hematol 1994;46:343–347.
103. Hilgartner M, Corrigan JJ. Coagulation disorders. In Miller DR, Baehner RL (eds). Blood Diseases of Infancy and Childhood, 7th ed. Philadelphia, Mosby, 1995, pp 924–986.
104. Blanchette VS, Dean J, Lillicrap D. Rare congenital hemorrhagic disorders. In Lilleyman JS, Hann IM, Blanchette VS (eds). Pediatric Hematology, 2nd ed. Philadelphia, Churchill Livingstone, 1999, pp 611–628.
105. Kobayashi T, Kanayama N, Tokunaga N, et al. Prenatal and peripartum management of congenital afibrinogenaemia. Br J Haematol 2000; 109:364–366.
106. Haverkate F, Samama M. Familial dysfibrinogenemia and thrombophilia: report on a study of the SSC Subcommittee on Fibrinogen. Thromb Haemost 1995;73:151–161.
107. Martinez J. Congenital dysfibrinogenemia. Curr Opin Hematol 1997; 4:357–365.
108. Rodriguez RC, Buchanan GR, Clanton MS. Prophylactic cryoprecipitate in congenital afibrinogenemia. Clin Pediatr 1988;27:543–545.
109. Bauer KA. Rare hereditary coagulation factor abnormalities. In Nathan DG, Orkin SH (eds). Nathan and Oski's Hematology of Infancy and Childhood, vol 2, 5th ed. Philadelphia, WB Saunders, 1998, pp 1660–1675.
110. Mammen EF. Factor V deficiency. Semin Thromb Hemost 1983;9: 17–18.
111. Seligsohn U, Ramot B. Combined factor-V and factor-VIII deficiency: report of four cases. Br J Haematol 1969;16:475–486.
112. Ingerslev J, Kristensen HL. Clinical picture and treatment strategies in factor VII deficiency. Haemophilia 1998;4:689–696.
113. Triplett DA, Brandt JT, Batard MA, et al. Hereditary factor VII deficiency: heterogeneity defined by combined functional and immunochemical analysis. Blood 1985;66:1284–1287.
114. Ragni MV, Lewis JH, Spero JA, Hasiba U. Factor VII deficiency. Am J Hematol 1981;10:79–88.
115. Bauer KA. Treatment of factor VII deficiency with recombinant factor VIIa. Haemostasis 1996;26:155–158.
116. Mariani G, Testa MG, Di Paolantonio T, et al. Use of recombinant, activated factor VII in the treatment of congenital factor VII deficiencies. Vox Sang 1999;77:131–136.
117. Wong WY, Huang WC, Miller R, et al. Clinical efficacy and recovery levels of recombinant FVIIa (NovoSeven) in the treatment of intracranial haemorrhage in severe neonatal FVII deficiency. Haemophilia 2000;6:50–54.
118. Bolton-Maggs PH. The management of factor XI deficiency. Haemophilia 1998;4:683–688.
119. Asakai R, Chung DW, Ratnoff OD, Davie EW. Factor XI (plasma thromboplastin antecedent) deficiency in Ashkenazi Jews is a bleeding disorder that can result from three types of point mutations. Proc Natl Acad Sci USA 1989;86:7667–7671.
120. Asakai R, Chung DW, Davie EW, Seligsohn U. Factor XI deficiency in Ashkenazi Jews in Israel. NEJM 1991;325:153–158.
121. Bolton-Maggs PH, Young Wan-Yin B, McCraw AH, et al. Inheritance and bleeding in factor XI deficiency. Br J Haematol 1988;69:521–528.
122. Bolton-Maggs PH, Colvin BT, Satchi BT, et al. Thrombogenic potential of factor XI concentrate. Lancet 1994;344:748–749.
123. Mannucci PM, Bauer KA, Santagostino E, et al. Activation of the coagulation cascade after infusion of a factor XI concentrate in congenitally deficient patients. Blood 1994;84:1314–1319.
124. Anwar R, Miloszewski KJ. Factor XIII deficiency. Br J Haematol 1999;107:468–484.
125. Gootenberg JE. Factor concentrates for the treatment of factor XIII deficiency. Curr Opin Hematol 1998;5:372–375.

Chapter 35

Transfusion of the Patient with Acquired Coagulation Defects

Barbara Alving*

Patients who develop bleeding disorders because of underlying systemic disease, autoantibody formation, or as a result of complications of anticoagulant use can be effectively treated with strategies that may include, in addition to blood products, one or more hemostatic agents as well as newer immunosuppressive agents. This chapter discusses the diagnosis and treatment of the following acquired coagulopathies: those related to underlying systemic disorders such as liver disease and renal failure; disseminated intravascular coagulation (DIC); formation of autoantibodies to coagulation factors VIII, V, II, or XIII; and coagulopathies associated with anticoagulants and the newer antiplatelet agents.

APPROACH TO THE PATIENT WITH A COAGULOPATHY

Patient Evaluation

The evaluation of the patient with an apparent or possible coagulopathy includes a review of the past and present illness as well as use of medications and a physical examination. Patients who have developed autoantibodies to a clotting factor such as factor VIII may have no complaints other than easy bruising or unexpected excessive bleeding with minor trauma. For these patients, laboratory data may be the first indication of the etiology of a bleeding disorder.

Screening tests are an integral part of the initial evaluation (Table 35–1). If the activated partial thromboplastin time (aPTT) and prothrombin time (PT) are prolonged, then performing mixing studies to assess for the presence of an inhibitor and measuring coagulation factor levels are appropriate. If DIC is suspected, the levels of D-dimer, a late plasmin digest of crosslinked fibrin, should also be measured. Increased levels indicate that thrombin has been generated in sufficient quantities to activate factor XIII, which induces crosslinking of fibrin, and that plasmin has also been generated to degrade the fibrin. This process is consistent with the generalized activation of the coagulation and fibrinolytic system that occurs in DIC.

The complete blood count, along with evaluation of the peripheral smear, may reinforce the possibility of sepsis (e.g., toxic granulations and Döhle bodies in the neutrophils) and also help to determine whether or not an apparent thrombocytopenia is real or due to platelet clumping in ethylenediaminetetraacetic acid (EDTA).

Hemostatic Support, Including Blood Products

In the surgical setting, a realistic goal is to provide sufficient hemostatic support to allow the patient to undergo surgery or other invasive procedures without undue risk. Thus, complete correction of coagulation laboratory abnormalities may not be possible or even desirable. For example, replacement of factor VII, which has a half-life of 2 to 6 hours, by infusion of plasma could lead to excessive volume expansion and pulmonary edema.

A critical factor for patients who require invasive procedures such as line placement is the skill of the operator. In one retrospective review of patients who had received arterial, pulmonary artery, or central venous lines, the authors found that hemostatic complications were rare and were related more to the experience of the operator than to the underlying hemostatic defect.[1] They concluded that only patients with severe hemostatic defects require correction of the abnormalities before line placement.

For major surgery in patients with coagulopathies, hemostasis is best managed if there is close communication among the consultants, the surgeons, the personnel of the coagulation laboratory, and the staff of the blood bank (or pharmacy) who are responsible for supplying the products.[2] Examples of two newer products that are being used to provide hemostasis in a wide variety of clinical settings are fibrin sealant and recombinant factor VIIa (rFVIIa).

Products, such as fibrin sealant, that provide localized hemostasis can be used as adjuvants for systemic therapy in patients with coagulopathies. In the United States, one commercial product is now available (Tisseel). It is indicated for patients who are undergoing reoperative coronary artery bypass surgery or who have bleeding from sites, such as the spleen, where bleeding cannot be controlled by sutures. The product is composed of human fibrinogen (75 to 115 mg/mL) and human thrombin (500 IU/mL), both of which are virally inactivated.[3] The thrombin is solubilized in calcium chloride (40 mM), which stimulates crosslinking of the clot by factor XIII in the product (or patient). The product also contains aprotinin, a bovine-derived

*This chapter was written by Dr. Alving in her private capacity. The views expressed in this article do not necessarily represent the views of the National Institutes of Health, Department of Health and Human Services, or the United States. All material in this chapter is in the public domain, with the exception of any borrowed figures or tables.

Table 35–1 **Laboratory Testing for Patients with an Acquired Coagulopathy**

Perform complete blood count, aPTT, PT, and thrombin time; measurement of fibrinogen concentration; and test for D-dimer as appropriate.
If thrombin time is prolonged, evaluate for heparin (perform reptilase time, add heparinase to sample). If heparin is present, check to be sure that the patient is not excessively anticoagulated or has developed a heparin-like inhibitor.
If aPTT is prolonged, perform "correction" studies. Mix equal volumes of patient and normal plasma and repeat the aPTT immediately and after 1 hour's incubation at 37° C. The values for the mixing study should be within 5 seconds of the control value of the normal plasma aPTT.
An aPTT that becomes more prolonged with incubation is suggestive of an inhibitor to a specific factor. An aPTT that is initially prolonged and remains prolonged to the same degree at 1 hour is suggestive of a lupus anticoagulant.
Measure factor levels to be sure that a true deficiency of a coagulation factor is recognized, even if the diagnosis is "lupus anticoagulant."
Consider the presence of an inhibitor to factor XIII if bleeding persists and the screening studies are normal. This requires a special test for the solubility of the clot in urea and monochloroacetic acid.

aPTT, activated partial thromboplastin time; PT, prothrombin time.

protein that directly inhibits plasmin, which is included to increase clot stability.

A much less expensive form of this product can be made by mixing cryoprecipitate in one syringe (fibrinogen concentration, 10 to 15 mg/mL) and bovine thrombin (1000 IU/mL) in the second syringe. However, this preparation contains a lower concentration of fibrinogen and has not undergone viral inactivation. Furthermore, the bovine thrombin may be contaminated with bovine factor V, which can stimulate production of antibodies in the recipient that crossreact with human factor V, inducing a potentially severe bleeding disorder several days after surgery.[4–6] Currently, the bovine thrombin preparation with the lowest degree of contamination with factor V is that produced for Jones Medical Industries, St. Louis.[7]

Efficacy data for the commercial fibrin sealant were derived in part from a study in which 333 patients from 11 centers in the United States who were undergoing reoperative cardiac surgery or emergency resternotomy were randomly assigned to receive fibrin sealant or conventional hemostatic agents; the end point for efficacy was the number of bleeding episodes controlled at 5 minutes.[8] The success rate for fibrin sealant was 92.6% compared with 12.4% for conventional topical agents ($p < 0.001$). Fibrin sealant also rapidly controlled bleeding episodes that did not initially respond to conventional hemostatic agents in 82% of patients.

In addition to use in cardiac surgery and trauma, fibrin sealants have been used as adhesives to seal dural leaks in neurosurgery, to promote union of middle ear bones in otolaryngology, and as a matrix to repair bone defects.[3] Although randomized, blinded studies have not been done, fibrin sealant has been applied to sites of dental extractions in individuals with hemophilia; this treatment, combined with the use of an antifibrinolytic agent, has reduced or eliminated the need for systemic factor VIII replacement.[9,10] This combined therapy would potentially be efficacious in patients with coagulation factor inhibitors as well as those with severe thrombocytopenia who require dental extraction. Outside the operating room, these sealants may also be applicable to providing local hemostasis in the critical care setting in patients with coagulopathies who have a localized site of bleeding. In a randomized, prospective evaluation of fibrin sealant in neonates undergoing extracorporeal membrane oxygenation, application of fibrin sealant at the cannulation sites reduced the risk for any bleeding and was associated with a shorter duration of hemorrhage with less blood loss.[11]

Fibrin sealants produced by several manufacturers (in both the United States and Europe) are undergoing or will be undergoing clinical trials in the United States. Differences may include methods of viral inactivation and presence or absence of a fibrinolytic inhibitor in the product. In addition, companies are developing other forms of sealants or adhesives composed of collagen and thrombin and devices that allow production of autologous fibrin sealant in the operating room.

Recombinant activated factor VII (rFVIIa, NovoSeven) is approved by the U.S. Food and Drug Administration (FDA) for use in individuals with hemophilia (factor VIII or IX deficiency) who have inhibitors and are actively bleeding or at high risk to bleed. During the past few years it has gained widespread use as a "universal hemostatic agent," although clinical trials to define the dose and efficacy in multiple situations have not yet been performed.

The "off-label" applications that are reported in the literature include treatment of bleeding episodes and/or prevention of bleeding related to surgery in patients with platelet disorders (qualitative and/or quantitative), liver disease (cirrhosis, transplantation), surgery and trauma, and reversal of warfarin therapy.[12–16] For patients with hemophilia who have inhibitors, the dose of rFVIIa is usually 90 µg/kg given every 2 hours (half life, approximately 3 hours). The best doses to be used for continuous infusion are still being determined. For patients with factor VII deficiency, the most effective doses are 20 to 25 µg/kg. An international registry is being used to record experience on the doses used in patients with platelet disorders and hepatic failure as well as orthotopic liver transplantation.

In trauma and surgery, antecodotal reports suggest that in patients with excessive uncontrolled bleeding, one or two infusions of rFVIIa at doses ranging from 20 to 120 µg/kg can have a significant hemostatic effect.[12–16] The incidence of thrombosis has been estimated to be 1% to 2%.[14]

COAGULOPATHIES IN SYSTEMIC DISORDERS

Liver Disease

Pathophysiology and Laboratory Evaluation

Patients with liver disease may have a complex coagulopathy consisting of impaired coagulation factor synthesis, increased fibrinolytic activity, and thrombocytopenia.[17] In patients with splenomegaly related to cirrhosis and portal hypertension, 90% of the circulating platelets can be sequestered in the spleen, with platelet counts decreasing to as low as 30,000 to 40,000/μL. The thrombocytopenia may be due in part to decreased platelet production because of reduced levels of circulating thrombopoietin, which is synthesized in the liver.[18] In one study of 44 patients with cirrhosis and thrombocytopenia, thrombopoietin levels were undetectable in 89%; however, after undergoing liver transplantation, 94% had detectable levels of thrombopoietin and all had resolution of the thrombocytopenia.[18] In patients undergoing portal decompression or splenectomy, thrombocytopenia often persists, indicating that a defect in thrombopoietin production is present in addition to splenic sequestration. A further reduction in platelet count is usually due to additional factors such as coexisting immune thrombocytopenia.[17] Patients may also have platelet dysfunction due to the effects of increased plasmin on platelet receptors. Increased levels of nitric oxide may also induce some degree of platelet dysfunction.[19]

The liver is the site of production for almost all coagulation factors, including the inhibitors protein C, protein S, and antithrombin. Von Willebrand factor (vWF) and tissue plasminogen activator (t-PA) are produced by endothelial cells. The factor VIII activity is usually increased in liver disease, which may reflect activation of the molecule or increased synthesis at sites other than the liver.[17] Factor VII, which has the shortest half-life of the coagulation factors (2 to 6 hours), is the first to be decreased in liver disease. To be functional, factors II, VII, IX, and X as well as protein S and protein C must undergo γ-carboxylation, which is mediated by vitamin K. However, liver disease causes impairment of γ-carboxylation that cannot be reversed with vitamin K1.[20]

Patients with liver disease, including those with hepatomas, may have an acquired dysfibrinogenemia caused by synthesis of a fibrinogen molecule that has impaired polymerization because of an increased sialic acid content.[21] The fibrinogen levels are usually normal; however, PT, aPTT, and thrombin time are prolonged. One case has been reported in which acquired dysfibrinogenemia was part of a paraneoplastic manifestation of renal cell carcinoma and resolved after the tumor was removed.[22] Acquired dysfibrinogenemia is not associated with a bleeding diathesis, and patients with this abnormality do not need any treatment before invasive procedures.

Although inhibitors of the coagulation system are decreased in patients with hepatic disease, a thrombotic state does not usually occur. Liver disease is associated with hyperfibrinolysis, as defined by increased activity of t-PA and elevation of D-dimer. In one study of cirrhotic patients, those with elevated t-PA and D-dimer had a significantly higher rate of gastrointestinal bleeding than those who did not have these laboratory findings.[23] Patients with ascites and hyperfibrinolysis were also at higher risk for bleeding than those without ascites. The authors postulated that hyperfibrinolysis results in part from activation of the coagulation system, resulting in release of t-PA in the presence of fibrin. Decreased clearance of t-PA as well as reduced levels of α_2-antiplasmin, which is synthesized in the liver and is the major inhibitor of plasmin, could result in continued plasmin generation and a bleeding diathesis.

The assessment of bleeding risk in a patient with liver disease includes measurement of the platelet count, PT, aPTT, fibrinogen level, and D-dimer. Although measurement of t-PA or the euglobulin clot lysis time is desirable, these tests are usually not available in a hospital setting. The PT is also reported as an International Normalized Ratio (INR), which was originally developed to standardize anticoagulation among patients taking warfarin. A study of 29 patients with liver impairment (INR, 1.5 to 3.5) was conducted with three different thromboplastin reagents (International Sensitivity Index, 0.86 to 2.53).[24] The mean INR for the patient plasmas as determined with the three different reagents ranged from 1.88 to 2.63, depending on the reagent. In contrast, the three reagents gave the same INR in plasmas from patients taking warfarin. Thus, INR values are not well standardized for patients with liver disease and can vary depending on the reagent. However, this is also true for the measurement of the PT with the different reagents. Patients with liver disease may have only a prolonged PT (normal aPTT and thrombin time), reflecting a decrease in factor VII, which is the first factor to be reduced in liver disorders because of its short half-life.

The bleeding time does not predict gastrointestinal bleeding in patients with cirrhosis.[25] Furthermore, mild to moderate coagulopathy is not associated with prolonged bleeding after liver biopsy, as assessed by measurement of the bleeding time at the biopsy site; even if the studies are normal, patients may still bleed at the biopsy site.[26] Although controlled studies in 21 patients with cirrhosis (platelet counts, 45,000 to 286,000/μL) have shown that desmopressin (DDAVP) at a dose of 0.3 μg/kg significantly shortens the prolonged bleeding time for up to 4 hours, its role in prophylaxis has not been well defined.[27] Nonetheless, DDAVP would be a reasonable choice for a hemostatic agent if there were concerns about platelet function.[27,28]

Product Support

Guidelines for prophylaxis in patients with liver disease who are undergoing invasive procedures are summarized in Table 35–2. These suggestions are empirical and are based on many factors. For example, in a retrospective study of patients undergoing percutaneous liver biopsy, McVay and Toy[29] found that mild elevations of PT or aPTT were not associated with bleeding. Risk factors for bleeding were malignancy (hepatoma) and multiple passes. These authors concluded that PT and aPTT prolonged to less than 1.5 times the midnormal range do not require treatment and that a platelet count above 50,000/μL is satisfactory.

For patients in whom standard percutaneous biopsy is contraindicated, such as those who have ascites, portal hypertension, and coagulopathy, laparoscopic liver biopsy can be performed successfully using direct pressure and topical Gelfoam and thrombin to achieve hemostasis.[30] In these patients there appears to be no correlation between the risk of bleeding and the prophylactic administration of fresh frozen plasma (FFP) or platelets. The advantage of laparoscopic liver biopsy is the ability to place direct pressure along with hemostatic agents.

There is usually little or no need to infuse FFP in an individual who has only a prolonged PT and a normal aPTT because factor VII levels of 10% or greater are sufficient for hemostasis. If PT and aPTT are prolonged and the patient has not responded to empirical treatment with vitamin K1 at a dose of 10 mg/day subcutaneously for 3 days,[17] measurement of levels of factors IX, X, and V (a non-vitamin K–dependent factor) provides a good assessment of liver function with respect to synthesis of coagulation factors. On occasion,

Table 35–2 **Management of Patients with Liver Disease**

Prophylaxis before Procedures	
Platelet count < 50,000/μL	Administer platelets to increase to 50,000–75,000/μL (six platelet concentrates or one apheresis platelet product)
Fibrinogen < 100 mg/dL	Administer cryoprecipitate to maintain fibrinogen > 100 mg/dL (7–10 units)
Coagulation Factor Deficiency	
Prolonged PT and aPTT	Administer vitamin K, 10 mg daily subcutaneously for 3 days, and then FFP if factor VII is <10% or other factors are >50%
Prolonged PT, normal aPTT	No treatment beyond vitamin K, if factor VII is >10%
Prolonged thrombin time (dysfibrinogenemia)	No treatment if fibrinogen > 100 mg/dL

aPTT, activated thromboplastin time; FFP, fresh frozen plasma; PT, prothrombin time.

abnormalities are simply due to dysfibrinogenemia, which can be detected by a prolonged thrombin time and reptilase time. If the latter is the case, no plasma treatment is needed.[22] Preoperative replacement for patients with severe factor VII deficiency consists of infusion of plasma at a dose of 5 to 10 mL/kg beginning preoperatively (in time to achieve a level of 10%) and continued during and after surgery for at least 1 to 2 days.

The Actively Bleeding Liver Disease Patient

Screening tests for a patient with liver disease who is actively bleeding consist of measurement of the platelet count, PT (INR)/aPTT, fibrinogen level, and D-dimer.[19] Even in the presence of laboratory abnormalities, the most frequently established causes for bleeding are site-specific tears in esophageal varices or gastrointestinal ulcers. Thus, sites for bleeding should be sought as well as establishment of an improved coagulation profile.

For patients who have hemostatic defects and are bleeding or are to undergo a major procedure, therapy does not have to be aimed at complete correction of laboratory values; however, the hematocrit should be maintained at greater than 30%, the platelet count greater than 50,000/μL, and the fibrinogen level greater than 100 mg/dL.

The best source of fibrinogen is cryoprecipitate, which contains approximately 250 mg in each bag. The volume of distribution for the fibrinogen is 30% greater than the intravascular volume. Thus, to increase the fibrinogen level by 50 mg/dL in a 70-kg individual, seven bags of cryoprecipitate would be required.

In patients undergoing rapid blood loss, rFVIIa can be combined with FFP. Factor VIIa has not been used extensively in patients with liver disease, and appropriate doses are being explored.[13–15] In one series of 10 consecutive patients with alcoholic cirrhosis and esophageal bleeding, infusion of rFVIIa (80 μg/kg) corrected the prolonged PT for 2 to 4 hours and controlled the bleeding; the clinical response lasted for at least 24 hours in half of the patients.[31] Prothrombin complex concentrates (PCCs) are not recommended, because they may be associated with thrombosis.[17] If a patient is oozing diffusely from sites of minor trauma and fibrinolysis is suspected, antifibrinolytic therapy can be tried after an initial evaluation for DIC and urinary tract bleeding. The antifibrinolytic agent aminocaproic acid can be given intravenously at doses of 4 to 5 grams over 1 hour followed by 1 g/hr for 8 hours. The oral dose is 4 g every 4 hours.[19] If tranexamic acid is given orally, the dose is 25 mg/kg every 6 to 8 hours. The intravenous dose is 10 mg/kg as a bolus and then 10 mg/kg administered over 6 to 8 hours.[19]

Uremia

One of the most common sources of bleeding in uremia is the gastrointestinal tract. Studies have shown, however, that the causes of gastrointestinal bleeding in patients with uremia are not different from the causes in those who are not uremic,[32] and the frequency of rebleeding is similar for both groups. The frequency of angiodysplasia may be twice as high in patients with renal failure compared to those without and may account for 19% to 32% of episodes of gastrointestinal bleeding in patients who have chronic renal insufficiency.[32] Patients who have occult gastrointestinal blood loss may develop iron deficiency and have a reduced response to erythropoietin. Thus, adequate attention should be given to iron replacement in an anemic patient who appears to be erythropoietin-resistant. Drugs such as low-dose aspirin may have a potentiating effect on the degree of bleeding.[19,33]

Patients who are uremic usually have a normal PT and aPTT and platelet count. However, they may have prolonged bleeding times; the degree of prolongation appears to correlate with clinical bleeding.[34] The platelet dysfunction has multiple causes, including exposure to increased levels of nitric oxide, which inhibit function.[33,35,36] In addition, platelets may have a storage pool defect, reduced production of prostaglandin, and decreased adhesion because of a decrease in expression of the receptor glycoprotein IIb/IIIa (GPIIb/IIIa), which is a binding site for vWF as well as fibrinogen.[37] The vessel wall in patients with uremia may produce an increased amount of prostaglandin I_2, which impairs platelet adhesion.[38] Plasma factors, not well characterized, may also inhibit platelet adhesion and aggregation in vivo.[39]

Multiple strategies can be used to reduce the excessive bleeding associated with uremia (Table 35–3). Platelet function can be maximized rheologically by maintaining the hematocrit at 30%.[40] The prolonged bleeding time can also be corrected by administration of DDAVP at a dose of 0.3 μg/kg intravenously or subcutaneously. The effect begins 1 hour after administration and persists for approximately 4 hours.[40,41] In uremic patients, the terminal half-life of DDAVP can range from 8 to 16 hours (mean, 9.7 hours).[42] Thus, clearance is decreased to 25% of that in individuals with normal renal function and the half-life prolonged 2 to 3 times. DDAVP should not be used more frequently than once in 24 hours; repeated doses are not efficacious and can result in hyponatremia and seizures. DDAVP works through release of presynthesized vWF from endothelial cells.

A double-blind, randomized trial of intravenous conjugated estrogens administered at a dose of 0.6 mg/kg/day for 5 days to six patients with uremia and prolonged bleeding

Table 35–3 **Hemostatic Options for Patients with Uremia**

Goal	Treatment	Comments
Maintain hematocrit 27%–32%	Erythropoietin	Monitor for hypertension; maintain adequate iron stores; check iron stores if patient resistant to erythropoietin.
Acutely enhance platelet function	DDAVP, 0.3 μg/kg IV	Administer no more frequently than once in 24 hours. Monitor for hyponatremia to avoid seizures.
Chronic enhancement of platelet function	Conjugated estrogens, 0.6 mg/kg/day IV for 4–5 days; or transdermal 17β-estradiol, 50–100 μg/24 hours applied as patch every 3–5 days for 2 months	Monitor for adverse effects: fluid retention, hot flashes.

DDAVP, desmopressin.

times found that the bleeding time was partially corrected by 6 to 48 hours after the first dose, with a peak effect at 5 to 7 days and a duration as long as 14 days.[43] Transdermal estrogen was efficacious in reducing or stopping bleeding in a series of six patients with renal failure, prolonged bleeding times, and excessive bleeding from telangiectasia of the gastrointestinal tract.[44] The estrogen was administered as 17β-estradiol (Estraderm) in a skin patch that delivered 50 or 100 μg/day. In these patients, the mean bleeding time decreased from 14 to 7 minutes. The effects were noted at 24 hours and persisted at 17 days (total duration of administration was 2 months). No adverse effects were noted.[44] Vigano and colleagues postulate that the prolonged effect of estrogens is due to their ability to enter endothelial cells, which are known to have estrogen receptors, and alter their function so that improved hemostasis occurs.[45] Other studies have shown that administration of estrogen inhibits endothelial nitric oxide production.[36]

In renal dialysis patients, graft thrombosis is a frequent event; secondary prevention includes administration of aspirin, warfarin, or heparin depending on the clinical situation; low-molecular-weight (LMW) heparin is not used because of its prolonged half-life in patients with renal failure.[46]

Disseminated Intravascular Coagulation

Disseminated intravascular coagulation is associated with clinical conditions, such as sepsis, acute brain injury, or abruptio placentae, that induce expression of tissue factor and overwhelming activation of the coagulation system, with a resulting fibrinolytic response. The clinical manifestations of DIC are variable and depend on whether microvascular thrombosis with fibrin formation is the prominent feature or the major component is the fibrinolytic response to fibrin formation.[47] The clinical manifestations determine which hemostatic therapy, if any, is needed. In general, the most critical factor in the resolution of DIC is the ability to control the condition responsible for the initiation of the process.

The laboratory evaluation of DIC includes measurement of the platelet count, PT, aPTT, and D-dimer. An abnormality in any one of these tests is not specific for DIC. Rather, the test results are combined with the clinical setting to make a diagnosis. Serial coagulation tests are especially useful in establishing a diagnosis. If a patient is actively bleeding, blood products such as platelets, FFP, and cryoprecipitate may need to be administered. There is no evidence that administration of blood components increases the severity of the DIC.[47]

Sepsis

Thrombocytopenia may be a prominent aspect of sepsis and can be due to DIC or to hemophagocytosis.[48,49] Patients with hemophagocytosis also have elevated levels of ferritin and lactate dehydrogenase in addition to thrombocytopenia. The process resolves with treatment of the underlying condition.

Disseminated intravascular coagulation in sepsis is due in part to interleukin-6-induced expression of tissue factor, which generates procoagulant activity. The fibrinolytic response to fibrin formation is reduced because interleukin-6 also increases the expression of plasminogen activator inhibitor-1, the major inhibitor of t-PA. Thus, the major manifestation in sepsis may be microvascular fibrin deposition. The efficacy of heparin in this setting has not been demonstrated. Although administration of antithrombin III concentrates initially suggested promise in the treatment of sepsis, a phase III international trial of antithrombin III showed no effect on 28-day all-cause mortality in adult patients with severe sepsis and septic shock who received the concentrate within 6 hours of symptoms.[50]

Activated protein C (drotrecogin alfa [activated]) is approved for patients with severe sepsis; however, it does not appear to be beneficial in patients with severe sepsis who are at low risk for death.[51,52] In this population, it is associated with an increase in the rate of serious bleeding compared to placebo (2.4% vs 1.2%, $p = 0.02$).[51]

Acute Leukemia and DIC

Although DIC can be associated with any type of leukemia, it is most frequently associated with acute promyelocytic leukemia because the promyelocytes are rich in releasable tissue factor. The plasmin which is generated in DIC is initially inhibited by α_2-antiplasmin, its major inactivator.[47] However, with time, the α_2-antiplasmin is depleted, allowing plasmin activity to remain unchecked. This results in ongoing fibrinolysis and excessive bleeding.

The laboratory diagnosis of α_2-antiplasmin deficiency can be confirmed by a specific assay for α_2-antiplasmin that consists of measuring the rate at which plasmin added to patient plasma undergoes inhibition. Treatment is usually empirical and consists of administration of an antifibrinolytic agent such as oral aminocaproic acid or tranexamic acid.[53,54] Although the antifibrinolytic agents can be used alone, heparin is generally administered as an adjunctive agent at a dose of 300 to 500 U/hr to prevent continued generation of thrombin. A critical aspect of management of patients with acute promyelocytic leukemia is to maintain a platelet count of 50,000/μL or greater.

A combination of heparin and antifibrinolytic agents is also useful in patients with DIC related to solid tumors, such as prostatic carcinoma. Efficacy of treatment can be monitored clinically and by the increase in fibrinogen levels followed by an increase in platelets in 24 to 48 hours.

Obstetrical Conditions

Disseminated intravascular coagulation can occur with abruptio placentae, amniotic fluid embolism, retained placenta, preeclampsia, acute fatty liver, and in utero fetal death.[55] These processes are all associated with the release of tissue factor from the dead fetus or necrotic placenta. DIC is clinically noted by excessive or spontaneous bleeding combined with decreases in fibrinogen levels and platelet counts and increases in D-dimer.

The best treatment is to accomplish delivery as soon as possible. Blood products are given as needed until this can be achieved. The contraction of the myometrium and removal of the source of tissue factor are the two most important factors in controlling the DIC.[55] With proper treatment, the coagulopathy reverses in hours and no further treatment is required. The only obstetrical condition associated with DIC for which heparin has been efficacious is the rare condition in which fetal death has occurred in one of two or more fetuses carried by the mother. Full-dose intravenous heparin has been administered to allow the maturation and delivery of the other viable fetuses.[56,57]

AUTOANTIBODIES AGAINST COAGULATION FACTORS

Acquired antibodies to specific blood coagulation factors have been reported in association with a variety of conditions, including infections, malignancy, pregnancy, and autoimmune disorders.[58,59] The antibodies, which are usually of the immunoglobulin G (IgG) isotype, may not be detected until the patient undergoes a hemostatic challenge such as surgery, or they may develop in the postoperative period, causing increased morbidity and even mortality. Inhibitors should be suspected in patients who have sustained trauma or who have undergone a surgical procedure and yet continue to bleed excessively for no apparent reason. The first manifestation of an inhibitor may not be apparent for 4 to 5 days after surgery. A review of serial coagulation studies may show an increasingly prolonged aPTT or both PT and aPTT with no apparent explanation (i.e., not corrected by empirical use of vitamin K1 or FFP or, in the case of individuals with known hemophilia, decreased recovery immediately after infusion and shortened half-life of infused factor VIII). Evaluation of coagulation screening studies and measurement of appropriate factor levels can establish the diagnosis so that appropriate blood product replacement can be provided and immunosuppressive therapy initiated.

The antibodies most commonly associated with excessive bleeding are those that develop against factor VIII in a patient with or without hemophilia A. Postoperative patients may also develop an antibody against factor V, which may be due to exposure to bovine thrombin preparations that contain factor V. Patients may also develop lupus anticoagulants; in the critical care setting, these are usually IgM antibodies that are directed against phospholipid-binding proteins such as prothrombin. They are not associated with excessive bleeding unless the patient also has a true deficiency of prothrombin in association with the lupus anticoagulants. The essential goals for the successful treatment of patients with inhibitors are to establish the initial diagnosis and then plan for appropriate factor replacement as well as for immunosuppression to eliminate the inhibitor.

For patients who are not known to have hemophilia but who have a progressive prolongation of aPTT and continued or excessive bleeding with surgery, further evaluation should include a mixing study to test for the presence of an inhibitor and measurement of coagulation factors XII, XI, IX, and VIII. These tests can be followed by a Bethesda assay, which will provide an estimate of the inhibitor titer. The results are less accurate for those patients who have autoantibodies to factor VIII than for those who have alloantibodies (congenital hemophilia). One Bethesda unit (BU) is the reciprocal of the dilution of patient's plasma that destroys 50% of the factor VIII in normal plasma after incubation for 2 hours at 37° C. For example, a titer of 40 BU indicates that at a 1:40 dilution the patient's plasma can inhibit 50% of the factor VIII in normal plasma.

Factor VIII Deficiency

For patients who have hemophilia and known alloantibodies, exposure to factor VIII during the surgical procedure increases the antibody titer, resulting in a poor response to factor VIII by the fourth or fifth postoperative day. In these patients, serial aPTT and factor VIII measurements can be performed so that appropriate changes in therapy can be made if necessary. Depending on the clinical setting and the inhibitor titer, treatment choices include human factor VIII, rFVIIa, or activated PCCs.

Autoantibodies to factor VIII generally occur in individuals after age 50 and are first suspected when the patient presents with a complaint of new-onset bruising or bleeding into the soft tissues or from the gastrointestinal tract.[58] Associated conditions include rheumatoid arthritis, the postpartum period, allergies, asthma, autoimmune disorders, and malignancy; however, in approximately 50% of patients, no other medical disorders are identified.[58,59] In 1981, Green and Lechner[58] reported that major bleeding occurred in as many as 87% of patients with an acquired factor VIII antibody and resulted in death in 22%. With the advent of improved recognition and treatment of inhibitors, in terms of both treatment of bleeding episodes and use of immunosuppression, these data should now be improved.

Although antibodies to factor VIII can disappear spontaneously, the general approach is to begin immunosuppressive therapy to increase the factor VIII level to normal levels. Several therapies have been used with different degrees of success. Green and coworkers[60] reported a response rate of 30% to oral prednisone alone at a dose of 1 mg/kg of body weight administered daily for 3 to 6 weeks. The responders tended to have lower Bethesda titers than nonresponders (median, 3 BU vs 50 BU), although responses did occur in three patients with titers of 33, 52, and 240 BU. They also concluded that cyclophosphamide at an oral dose of 2 mg/kg daily is an efficacious therapy for patients who cannot tolerate prednisone.[60] In a follow-up publication, Green[61] reported an 80% response rate in 10 patients treated only with prednisone; their initial titers ranged from less than 1 BU to 27 BU. Patients who did not respond to steroids or had adverse effects all responded to single-agent cyclophosphamide.

In a report of nine consecutive patients (ages 50 to 79) with inhibitor titers ranging from 2.5 to 1040 BU, Shaffer and Phillips[62] described complete remission in 2 to 10 weeks with combined treatment with oral cyclophosphamide (100 to 200 mg/day) and prednisone (50 to 80 mg/day) with slow tapering of these doses when the inhibitor titer was no longer detectable. Cyclosporine has also been used successfully in a limited number of patients at a dose that provides therapeutic serum levels (150 to 350 ng/mL).[63]

The most promising treatment to eliminate factor VIII autoantibodies appears to be rituximab, a monoclonal antibody against CD20, which removes CD20+ B lymphocytes from the circulation. The dose generally used is 375 mg/m^2 IV every week for 4 weeks with or without prednisone.[64] This treatment may reduce the duration of exposure to cytotoxic treatment for these patients. Based on their experience in a limited case series, Aggarwal and colleagues have suggested a treatment algorithm for older patients with autoimmune hemophilia.[64] They recommend prednisone alone for those with a Bethesda titer of <5BU, and addition of rituximab to prednisone for those with low to intermediate titers (<30 BU). For those with higher titers, a combination of prednisone, cyclophosphamide, and rituximab may be required. Patients with very high titers may need to be treated with regimens that are used for chronic lymphocytic leukemia.[64]

A general approach to the use of coagulation factor components in patients with acquired factor VIII inhibitors is summarized in Table 35–4. For patients with an inhibitor titer that is less than 5 BU, factor VIII concentrates can still be used to neutralize the antibody and achieve a hemostatic level of factor VIII.[65] For those with a higher titer, other options exist, such as activated PCCs (Feiba and Autoplex T) and rFVIIa. In the United States, rFVIIa has largely replaced the use of PCCs.

In a retrospective French study of use of Feiba in 60 patients with inhibitors (most of whom had congenital hemophilia), efficacy was rated as excellent in 81% of bleeding episodes, which included surgical procedures, and poor in 17%.[66] The treatment was well tolerated in 98% of episodes; the doses infused were 65 to 100 U/kg at 6- to 12-hour intervals (total, 65 to 510 U/kg/day).

In patients with high-titer inhibitors, rFVIIa has been efficacious at a dose of 90 µg/kg administered intravenously every 2 hours during surgery and for 48 hours postoperatively, followed by every 2 to 6 hours for the next 3 days.[67] Factor VIIa has also been tested for home use in the treatment of mild to moderately severe bleeding episodes in the joints, muscles, or mucocutaneous tissues in patients with hemophilia A or B with inhibitors.[68] In this study, patients received rFVIIa (90 µg/kg) intravenously at 3-hour intervals within 8 hours of the onset of the episode. If the dose was considered effective after one to three applications, one additional injection was provided. rFVIIa was considered effective in 92% of bleeding episodes after a mean of 2.2 injections. The time from onset of bleeding to the first injection in the successfully treated episodes was 1.1±2.0 hours (standard deviation).

Several papers have described the use of sequential or alternative doses of activated PCCs and rFVIIa in patients with hemophilia and inhibitors who were actively bleeding.[69,70] Activated PCCs have been given in doses ranging from 35 to 80 U/kg alternating every 6 hours with rFVIIa (80 to 225 µg/kg).[69] If sequential therapy is to be undertaken, the patients should undergo serial laboratory monitoring for DIC. Additional studies need to be done to confirm the safety and efficacy of this treatment.

Factor V Deficiency

Antibodies to factor V are rare and are first manifested clinically as unexpected bleeding or bruising in a patient with a prolonged PT and aPTT. Multiple reports have described postoperative patients who have experienced significant bleeding related to factor V antibodies.[4–7] The coagulopathy develops as a result of exposure of the patient to bovine thrombin during surgery. Bovine thrombin, which is a commonly used hemostatic agent, contains multiple impurities, including bovine factor V. Patients develop antibodies to the bovine factor V, which then crossreact with their endogenous factor V, causing a marked inhibition of factor V activity.[5] Patients may also develop antibodies to the bovine thrombin. However, these antibodies do not crossreact with human thrombin and are of no clinical significance.

Patients who have antibodies to factor V have a prolonged PT and aPTT that are not corrected when the tests are repeated with a 1:1 mix of normal and patient's plasma. The prolongation of the PT and aPTT becomes even greater when the tests are repeated after incubation of patient's and normal plasma for 1 or 2 hours at 37°C. Measurement of

Table 35–4 Treatment of Bleeding Episodes in Patients with Inhibitors to Factor VIII

If Bethesda titer is <5 BU, use recombinant factor VIII concentrates; monitor factor VIII activity. Because Bethesda titers are not highly accurate in nonhemophiliac patients with an inhibitor, recombinant factor VIII may also be effective if the titer is >5 BU. The factor VIII activity is the best guide for treatment. An initial high dose may be required to neutralize the inhibitor in vivo, and then lesser doses may provide satisfactory activity. If possible, factor VIII should be the first choice for treatment.

Recombinant factor VIIa can be used at a dose of 90 µg/kg every 2 hours for the duration of bleeding and for several days thereafter. Choice of recombinant factor VIIa over activated prothrombin complex concentrates may be based on experience of the physician, cost, and availability. The two treatments have not been directly compared. Disadvantage of the activated prothrombin complex concentrates is potential for inducing thrombosis.

Activated prothrombin complex concentrates (Feiba 75–100 U/kg every 8–12 hours or Autoplex 50–75 U/kg every 8–12 hours) can be used for soft tissue bleeds and other bleeding episodes. Efficacy is judged by patient's response. For soft tissue bleeds, patients can be treated every 8 hours for 48 hours followed by every 12 hours for the next 48 hours.

coagulation factors shows a decrease in factor V. An antibody to bovine thrombin is detected by a prolongation of the thrombin time if bovine thrombin is used in the test system. The test remains abnormal when repeated with a 1:1 mix of normal and patient's plasma. The thrombin time is normal, however, if human thrombin is used in the test system.

The majority of patients in whom an antibody to factor V develops do not have clinical symptoms and the PT and aPTT become normal within 3 to 6 weeks after exposure to thrombin. For patients who are actively bleeding, FFP is the first choice for replacement of factor V. Infusion of platelets is a second option because they contain approximately 20% of the body stores of factor V, although they may not provide hemostasis in all situations.[71] Treatment with rFVIIa may also be an option for these patients.

Corticosteroids, cyclophosphamide, and vincristine have been used alone or in combination for suppression of antibodies. Corticosteroids have mostly been used alone as first-line therapy with success. Methylprednisolone at an initial dose of 1 to 1.5 mg/kg is usually given for 2 to 3 weeks and then tapered slowly over the next several weeks.[7] Cyclophosphamide and vincristine have been added to prednisone to suppress the antibody production successfully in cases with acquired factor VIII inhibitors; similar success has been achieved in some cases with factor V inhibitors. The use of rituximab has not been described in this clinical setting.

Factor II Deficiency

Autoantibodies to prothrombin usually occur in association with lupus anticoagulants, which are antibodies to phospholipid-binding proteins such as prothrombin or β_2-glycoprotein I.[72] Lupus anticoagulants are associated with the antiphospholipid syndrome, systemic lupus erythematosus (SLE), and infections as well as use of medications, such as procainamide (Pronestyl). In some patients with lupus anticoagulants, a true deficiency of prothrombin has also been recognized; this appears to be due to IgG antibodies that selectively bind prothrombin without neutralizing its activity. The antibodies do not interfere with the proteolytic cleavage of prothrombin or with the activity of thrombin. They appear to induce true prothrombin deficiency by binding to prothrombin in vivo and causing increased clearance.[73–75]

The majority of patients with lupus anticoagulants and SLE or other autoimmune connective tissue disorders may have IgG autoantibodies to prothrombin, although only 30% of patients with antibodies have a detectable prothrombin deficiency.[72] Antiprothrombin antibodies are more likely to occur in patients with an aPTT that is significantly prolonged (at least 50 seconds; normal range, 22 to 30 seconds).[74] Bleeding symptoms are correlated with the level of functional prothrombin and occur in patients with a prothrombin activity of 10% or lower.[74] In some cases, the first manifestation of lupus is the development of a lupus anticoagulant with true prothrombin deficiency. A significant decrease in the prothrombin activity related to antibody formation can occur at any time in a patient who has a lupus anticoagulants and underlying SLE or primary antiphospholipid syndrome. For patients with a lupus anticoagulants who are receiving warfarin, the first manifestation of an antibody to prothrombin that induces a significant decrease in the prothrombin activity may be a gradually increasing INR with no other apparent etiology.

Lupus anticoagulants and clinically significant hypoprothrombinemia have been associated with viral illnesses in children.[76] In these cases, the antibody disappeared spontaneously. The antibody production can usually be suppressed by administration of corticosteroids with or without adjunctive agents such as azathioprine; with this treatment, the PT can become normal as soon as 7 days after initiation of treatment.[73,75] For example, a 3-year-old girl with a viral illness and severe hypoprothrombinemia that resulted in epistaxis and gastrointestinal hemorrhage was treated successfully with intravenous methylprednisolone daily for 3 days followed by oral prednisone.[77] For a patient who is actively bleeding and has a severe prothrombin deficiency, treatment options are FFP or PCCs. Although not reported, rFVIIa could also be used.

Factor XIII Deficiency

Factor XIII deficiency may be due to the formation of autoantibodies that occur spontaneously or in association with drugs such as penicillin, isoniazid, or diphenylhydantoin or with autoimmune disorders.[78,79] The inhibitor is not detected on routine screening tests and can be confirmed only by finding rapid lysis of a clot that has been prepared from recalcified plasma and placed in 1% monochloroacetic acid or urea. Treatment consists of immunosuppressive agents and administration of cryoprecipitate if the patient is actively bleeding.

Laboratory monitoring of therapy can be done serially and qualitatively by assessing the time required for solubilization of a clot derived from patient plasma in urea or monochloroacetic acid.[80,81] Successful immunosuppression with rituximab has been reported in one patient with an apparent ciprofloxacin-induced antibody.[82]

COAGULOPATHIES RELATED TO ANTICOAGULANT ADMINISTRATION

Warfarin

The frequency of bleeding in patients who are receiving warfarin ranges from 8 to 16 per hundred patient-years, with major bleeding occurring in 1.3 to 2.7 patients per hundred years.[83] Patients at increased risk for bleeding are the elderly; those who have comorbid conditions such as cardiac, cerebrovascular, renal or hepatic disease; and those who have just recently been started on warfarin therapy or who have increased or fluctuating INRs.[84] One of the most important factors that predicts the risk for major bleed is a history of bleeding, especially if the site is in the gastrointestinal tract.[85]

Maintenance daily doses of warfarin can range from 4 mg up to 90 mg or higher in rare circumstances. Overall, more than 40% of the variability in warfarin dose requirements may be explained by genetic factors, use of concomitant specific medications such as amiodarone, age, and body surface area.[86] Two examples of the influence of genetic variation affecting dose requirements are related to the polymorphisms in the gene that codes for the cytochrome P450 complex *(CYP)*, which is responsible for metabolizing the potent "S" form of warfarin. Individuals who have polymorphisms in the *CYP2C9* gene, which produces the protein that metabolizes "S" warfarin, may have reduced catabolism of the "S" form and therefore have greatly reduced dose requirements.[86] Another genetic determinant of warfarin requirement is due to polymorphisms in the vitamin K epoxide reductase complex subunit 1 *(VKORC1)* gene, which affects the activity of vitamin K epoxide reductase complex. This complex, which is the target of warfarin, is responsible for regenerating reduced vitamin K so that it can serve as a cofactor for γ-carboxylation of coagulation factors. Polymorphisms in the gene can confer marked resistance or increased sensitivity to warfarin.[87]

The main strategies for treating warfarin overdose, depending on the degree of overanticoagulation and the clinical site of bleeding, include administration of vitamin K1, rFVIIa, PCCs, or FFP if the other products are not available (Table 35–5).[85] PCCs, which contain factors II, VII, and X in addition to factor IX and are virally inactivated, were originally developed for treatment of individuals with hemophilia B. Although PCCs are no longer used for this purpose, they are effective for use in the emergency correction of coagulation factor deficiencies in individuals who have major bleeding and are anticoagulated with warfarin.[88]

Approximately 50% to 90% of intracranial hemorrhages in patients receiving warfarin anticoagulation occur at a time when the INR is within the target range.[84] The mortality associated with intracranial bleeding is 16% to 68% and is influenced by the rapidity with which normalization of the coagulation factor deficiencies occurs.

The preferred replacement therapy in intracranial hemorrhage is rFVIIa or PCCs (25 to 50 U/kg). When PCCs were compared with infusion of 800 mL of FFP in a small study of patients with intracranial hemorrhage who were also anticoagulated with warfarin, the coagulation factor levels were raised into the normal range with the PCCs but not with FFP.[84] The INR can be corrected four to five times more quickly with the PCCs than with FFP. The elimination half-lives of the coagulation factors are as follows: factor II (58 hours), factor VII (5 hours), factor IX (19 hours), and factor X (35 hours); thus, repeated infusion may be necessary if the factor deficiency has not been reversed in 24 hours by the administration of vitamin K. Factor VII is in low concentration in some PCCs relative to the other coagulation factors, and it has a short half-life. The importance of replacing the factor VII level to values greater than 10% is unknown. FFP can be used to achieve minimal levels of 10% if this is deemed necessary. For some patients, especially those with mechanical heart valves, resuming anticoagulant therapy is critical; one report of 15 patients showed that this could be done safely.[89]

In a prospective case series, Deveras and Kessler administered rFVIIa to 13 patients (some of whom were actively bleeding) who needed rapid reversal of excessive warfarin anticoagulation.[90] rFVIIa was effective in doses ranging from 15 to 20 μg/kg. The cost of the product was approximately $1.40/μg at the time of this study. The product initially was administered at a dose as high as 90 μg/kg; however, lower doses were found to be effective. None of the patients sustained any adverse side effects from rVIIa. The INR value does not reflect the efficacy of the treatment; rather, patients who receive rFVIIa need to be clinically evaluated.

For patients who have ingested rat poison containing a superwarfarin such as brodifacoum, prolonged treatment with daily oral vitamin K is needed because the half-life of the superwarfarin is 16 to 36 days.[91] Oral vitamin K has a bioavailability of 10% to 60% and is therefore given at a dose three to five times greater than the parenteral dose. Initially, oral vitamin K may have to be taken every 6 to 8 hours and then tapered to a daily dose.

Heparin Preparations (Unfractionated Heparin, LMW Heparin, and Pentasaccharide)

According to one study, risk factors for bleeding are the same for patients receiving unfractionated heparin or LMW heparin and include the performance status of the patient as determined by World Health Organization criteria, history of a bleeding tendency, cardiopulmonary resuscitation, recent trauma or surgery, body surface area, and total dose of anticoagulant administered in 24 hours.[92] The bleeding risk may also be increased in older patients (>70 years).[93,94]

For unfractionated heparin, reversal of anticoagulant activity can be achieved by slow infusion (over 10 minutes) of protamine sulfate, which neutralizes 100 units of heparin for every milligram of protamine administered. Assuming that heparin has a half-life of 60 minutes, the protamine dose can be calculated in a patient receiving a constant IV infusion by adding the heparin dose infused during each of the past 3 hours.[95] The risk for anaphylaxis with protamine sulfate is approximately 1% and may be higher in diabetics who have taken NPH insulin or in patients who have allergies to fish or have undergone a vasectomy. Patients at risk for anaphylaxis should be pretreated with corticosteroids and with antihistamines.[96] For LMW heparin, protamine neutralizes only about 60% of the anti-factor Xa activity. If LMW heparin is administered within 2 hours of the bleeding episode, then protamine can be given based on a calculated dose of 1 mg for every 100 anti-factor Xa units given. This can be repeated at half the dose if bleeding continues.

Table 35–5 Guidelines for Reversal of Warfarin Anticoagulation*

Major bleeding	Stop warfarin Infuse rFVIIa or PCC (50 U/kg) or FFP (15 mL/kg) if rFVIIa or PCCs are not available Give vitamin K1 10 mg by slow IV infusion
INR > 9 (with no or minor bleeding)	Stop warfarin Restart when INR therapeutic Give vitamin K1 5–10 mg orally

FFP, fresh frozen plasma; PCC, prothrombin complex concentrates.

Adapted from Ansell J, Hirsh J. Poller L, et al. The pharmacology and management of the vitamin K antagonists. The Seventh ACCP Conference on Antithrombotic and Thrombolytic Therapy. Chest 2004;126:204S–233S (www.chestjournal.org).

The role of rFVIIa in reducing bleeding in this setting has not yet been clearly defined.[96] However, one preliminary report describes the use of rFVIIa in three patients with hypercoagulability who were anticoagulated with enoxaparin and were bleeding from the site of a kidney biopsy, femoral pseudoaneurysm, and arthroplasty, respectively.[16] The patients each received rFVIIa as a single infusion in doses that ranged from 20 to 30 μg/kg. All patients had required multiple infusions of FFP and packed red blood cells before administration of rFVIIa.

LMW heparin, when administered subcutaneously, has a plasma half-life of 3 to 6 hours. Since the approval of enoxaparin (Lovenox) in 1993 for prophylaxis after total hip or knee replacement at a dose of 30 mg subcutaneously every 12 hours, the FDA has received reports of more than 30 patients who experienced spinal or epidural hematomas in conjunction with LMW heparin prophylaxis and spinal or epidural anesthesia. The mean age of the patients was 74 years, and 75% were women. The procedures were predominantly orthopedic (hip or knee replacement), and more than 80% of the patients were receiving LMW heparin twice daily. Published guidelines have emphasized that in patients receiving LMW heparin preoperatively, needle placement for epidural or spinal anesthesia should occur no sooner than 12 hours after the last dose.[97–99] Subsequent dosing should be delayed for at least 2 hours after needle placement. Epidural catheters should be removed 12 to 24 hours after the last LMW heparin dose, with subsequent dosing delayed by at least 2 hours.[97,98] In addition, enoxaparin should be used whenever possible as a once-daily dose,[99] and other antiplatelet or anticoagulant agents should not be administered at the same time.

Fondaparinux (Arixtra) is a synthetic heparin pentasaccharide that inhibits factor Xa through its action on antithrombin; it does not inhibit thrombin, however.[100] In the United States, fondaparinux has been approved for the prevention of postoperative deep venous thrombosis. It has a half-life of 18 hours, allowing it to be administered subcutaneously once daily. Because it is excreted renally, it is contraindicated in patients with renal insufficiency. Recent studies, both in vitro and in vivo, have provided evidence that fondaparinux can be used in patients with heparin-induced thrombocytopenia (HIT), since it does not interact with platelet factor 4. Abstracts and case series have reported a normalization of platelet counts and no complications of bleeding or thrombosis in patients with HIT who received fondaparinux (generally at a dose of 2.5 mg daily).[101,102] There is no well-tested antidote for fondaparinux; however, one study in 16 normal volunteers who received fondaparinux (10 mg subcutaneously) followed 2 hours later by rFVIIa (90 μg/kg) reported normalization of thrombin generation for 2 to 6 hours after rFVIIa administration.[103]

Thrombin Inhibitors (Lepirudin, Bivalirudin, and Argatroban)

Lepirudin (Refludan), which is a recombinant protein, is approved for use in patients with HIT and associated thrombosis to prevent further complications. In one study, patients with HIT received lepirudin at a dose of 0.4 mg/kg as a bolus followed by continuous infusion of 0.15 mg/kg/hr; if they had received thrombolytic therapy, the dose was decreased to 0.2 mg/kg (bolus) followed by 0.1 mg/kg/hr continuous infusion. For prophylaxis, they received a dose of 0.1 mg/kg/hr as a continuous infusion.[104] The treated patients were compared with historical controls; the combined end point of mortality, limb amputation, and new thromboembolic events was reduced by 50% ($p = 0.014$) at day 7 and at day 35 in the group receiving lepirudin. Bleeding events and transfusions were not increased in the treated group compared with the historical controls. Current dosing recommendations are 0.4 mg/kg as a bolus with 0.15 mg/kg/hr (up to weight of 110 kg). The dose can be monitored with the aPTT, and recommendations are to maintain the aPTT at 1.5 to 2.5 times the median value for the normal range.

In normal volunteers, lepirudin, which is excreted and perhaps metabolized by the kidneys, has a half-life of approximately 2 hours. Pharmacokinetic studies in patients with renal failure who were undergoing dialysis showed that after a single dose of lepirudin (0.08 to 0.2 mg/kg) followed by five additional dialyses without further dosing, the half-life was increased to 52 hours.[105] The distribution volume was also lower in hemodialysis patients than in normal volunteers. Lepirudin has been used successfully to maintain anticoagulation during dialysis when given once before dialysis at a dose of 0.08 mg/kg.[106] However, subsequent dosing would require adjustment because of the prolonged half-life. The manufacturer recommends that dosing be reduced by 50% for both bolus and infusion for patients with a creatinine value of 1.5 to 2.0 mg/dL. Reductions would be even greater for those with more severe renal impairment.

The use of lepirudin in five patients who required bypass surgery has also been reported.[107] In these patients the dose was monitored by a coagulation-based assay, and infusions were given to maintain the plasma levels above 2 μg/mL. In patients receiving lepirudin for deep venous thrombosis, the plasma level at steady state was approximately 0.6 μg/mL.[108] In one patient who experienced severe lepuridin-induced bleeding after bypass surgery, the infusion of rFVIIa at a dose of 60 μg/kg had a major hemostatic impact compared to previous infusions of packed red cells, platelets, and FFP.[109]

With time, patients can develop antilepirudin antibodies that cause a further prolongation of the aPTT. In this situation, the dose needs to be reduced.[110]

The thrombin inhibitor bivalirudin (Angiomax) is a peptide modeled after hirudin; bilvalirudin has a half-life of 25 minutes and undergoes minor renal metabolism (20%). It is approved in the United States for percutaneous coronary angioplasty but can also be used in patients with HIT and is undergoing testing in these patients in cardiac surgery.[110]

Argatroban, a thrombin-specific inhibitor that has been used in more than 300 patients with HIT, is an arginine-based synthetic molecule. Argatroban has a half-life of 40 minutes in normal individuals. Unlike lepirudin, argatroban does not require dose adjustment in patients with renal disease.[111] Argatroban, which is cleared by the liver, requires dose reduction in patients with significant hepatic dysfunction. It is administered in weight-based doses, adjusted to maintain the aPTT 1.5 to 3 times the baseline value. Argatroban has been used successfully in patients with HIT who required repeated dialysis[112] and in a patient with HIT and thrombosis who required coronary stent implantation.[113]

The thrombin-specific inhibitors, unlike unfractionated heparin, prolong the PT as well as the aPTT. In patients who are undergoing conversion to warfarin while receiving argatroban or hirudin, these agents can be discontinued several hours before a PT is determined to ensure an accurate indication of the INR.

Clinical experience with these agents in critically ill patients who are receiving multiple other drugs as well as anesthetic agents is limited and is not well described in the literature. Thus, dosing in critically ill patients should be established with caution. In a retrospective chart review of 65 patients admitted to a medical or surgical intensive care unit who received argatroban for more than 24 hours, the authors concluded that doses of argatroban that are only 50% of those recommended should be used in patients with acute renal failure, sepsis, or one organ system failure even if the alanine transaminase, bilirubin, and INR are normal.[114] They suggest that the metabolism of argatroban may be delayed in these patients due to passive hepatic congestion or due to the effects of other drugs.

BLEEDING INDUCED BY ANTIPLATELET AGENTS

Agents That Inhibit the Platelet GPIIb/IIIa Receptor (Abciximab, Tirofiban, and Eptifibatide)

The most potent antiplatelet agents in clinical practice today are those that block the interaction between fibrinogen and platelet glycoprotein IIb/IIIa (GPIIb/IIIa), thus mimicking the bleeding diathesis seen in patients with Glanzmann thrombasthenia. Abciximab (ReoPro) is a Fab fragment of chimeric human–murine monoclonal antibody c7E3, which is used in patients undergoing percutaneous transluminal angioplasty (PTCA) and those with unstable angina with PTCA planned in 24 hours.[115] Treatment of patients undergoing angioplasty or stent procedures with abciximab significantly reduced the combined end point of death, repeated myocardial infarction, and need for urgent revascularization during 30 days compared with those undergoing stent procedures in the absence of abciximab.[115] Two newer GPIIb/IIIa inhibitors have also been licensed. One is tirofiban (Aggrastat), a tyrosine derivative that is indicated for patients with unstable angina or non–Q wave myocardial infarction (with or without PTCA).[116,117] The other is eptifibatide (Integrelin), a cyclic heptapeptide that is indicated for patients with unstable angina or non–Q wave myocardial infarction (with or without PTCA) and for patients undergoing PTCA.[118]

The risk for bleeding with these agents is in part due to their pharmacokinetics. Abciximab, which has a high affinity for GPIIb/IIIa, has a biologic half-life of 8 hours; in comparison, 1 hour after completion of the infusion of eptifibatide, the bleeding time becomes normal.[119] The antiplatelet effect of tirofiban is also short-lived after completion of infusion, although in patients with renal failure the biologic effect is more prolonged. Platelet function is inhibited when more than 80% of the GPIIb/IIIa receptors are blocked. For patients who are bleeding, the drugs should be discontinued immediately and 8 to 10 units of platelet concentrates (or one apheresis platelet unit) administered. The drug redistributes to the receptors of the infused platelets, thus lowering the occupancy of the receptors of the entire platelet pool and resulting in normalization of platelet function.

In patients who have received abciximab within 12 hours of requiring an emergent bypass procedure, platelet infusions should be administered prophylactically to prevent excessive bleeding.[120] This recommendation is based on the observation that patients who underwent bypass surgery within 12 hours of abciximab experienced threefold greater blood loss than those who underwent surgery more than 12 hours after receiving the drug (1300 vs 400 mL, respectively).[121] These patients required platelet infusions, red blood cells, and FFP. The recommendation for preoperative platelet infusions probably does not apply for tirofiban or eptifibatide because of their shorter duration of action.

The GPIIb/IIIa inhibitors can cause an acute thrombocytopenia that occurs as soon as several hours after the initiation of drug infusion.[122] For patients receiving abciximab, the incidence may be as high as 1% with the first exposure to the drug and 4% on repeat exposure.[123] The incidence of thrombocytopenia with administration of tirofiban and eptifibatide has not been well defined. The platelet counts for patients who are to receive the GPIIb/IIIa inhibitors should be measured before the infusion and within 2 to 6 hours after infusion.[122,124] If the platelet count is reduced, the peripheral blood smear should be checked to rule out pseudothrombocytopenia due to platelet agglutination occuring in the presence of EDTA. True thrombocytopenia is due to preformed antibodies that are directed against the GPIIb/IIa receptor in the presence of the GPIIb/IIIa inhibitors. The treatment for a bleeding episode is infusion of platelets, regardless of the platelet count. The drug will be redistributed among the receptors of the infused platelets and circulating platelets, thereby allowing normalization of platelet function if receptor occupancy on the platelets is less than 80%.

Agents That Inhibit the Platelet ADP Receptor (Clopidogrel and Ticlopidine)

The thienopyridines ticlopidine and clopidogrel inhibit platelet function by blocking the adenosine diphosphate (ADP) receptor.[125] Although ticlopidine has been widely employed to prevent stent closure after angioplasty and as secondary prevention against stroke in patients with cerebrovascular disease, its relatively poor safety profile has resulted in diminished use. Adverse events in patients receiving ticlopidine have included neutropenia, agranulocytosis, aplastic anemia, and thrombotic thrombocytopenic purpura.[126] In contrast, clopidogrel appears to have an excellent safety profile.

In a large, randomized, blinded trial in patients with atherosclerotic vascular disease, clopidogrel reduced the combined risk of ischemic stroke, myocardial infarction, and vascular death by 8.7% compared with aspirin ($p < 0.05$).[127] Patients treated with clopidogrel had fewer gastrointestinal ulcers and fewer gastrointestinal bleeding episodes than those treated with aspirin. Clopidogrel is indicated for the reduction of atherosclerotic events (myocardial infarction, stroke, and vascular death) in patients with atherosclerosis documented by recent stroke, myocardial infarction, or peripheral vascular disease.

Both clopidogrel and ticlopidine require metabolism by the hepatic cytochrome P450-1A enzyme system to acquire activity.[125] When clopidogrel was given at a dose of 300 to 400 mg orally, it caused maximal inhibition of platelet function within 2 hours.[128] With a daily dose of 75 mg, the same degree of inhibition was achieved at 3 to 7 days. Recovery of platelet function occurs over 3 to 5 days after discontinuation of either drug. Specific treatment for bleeding related to these agents is not well described. Administration of desmopressin, however, may shorten the bleeding time and provide temporary hemostasis.[129] Otherwise, supportive care and infusion of platelets may be needed in patients who are taking clopidogrel or ticlopidine and have a major bleeding episode.

SUMMARY

Acquired coagulation disorders range from subtle to catastrophic. Most can be quickly diagnosed by the history and appropriate laboratory testing, which is usually available in a tertiary hospital. Measurement of specific coagulation factors is much more useful than random infusion of FFP. A major problem is having the appropriate blood components available for the patient. If a hospital does not routinely stock coagulation factor concentrates, the patient should be transferred to a hospital where the specialty care can be provided; in addition, the hospital should know how to arrange for a core of specialty products that may be required on an emergent basis. The appropriate use of the newer products, such as rFVIIa, is still under investigation; cost and availability are two concerns for many hospitals. Because multiple options are available for the treatment of patients with acquired bleeding disorders, communication and collaboration among the services involved in the diagnosis and management of these patients will maximize the potential for good outcomes.

REFERENCES

1. DeLoughery TG, Liebler JM, Simonds V, Goodnight SH. Invasive line placement in critically ill patients: do hemostatic defects matter? Transfusion 1996;36:827–831.
2. Alving B, Alcorn K. How to improve transfusion medicine: a treating physician's perspective. Arch Pathol Lab Med 1999;123:492–495.
3. Jackson MR, Alving BM. Fibrin sealant in preclinical and clinical studies. Curr Opin Hematol 1999;6:415–419.
4. Rapaport SI, Zivelin A, Minow RA, et al. Clinical significance of antibodies to bovine and human thrombin and factor V after surgical use of bovine thrombin. Am J Clin Pathol 1992;97:84–91.
5. Zehnder JL, Leung LK. Development of antibodies to thrombin and factor V with recurrent bleeding in a patient exposed to topical bovine thrombin. Blood 1990;76:2011–2016.
6. Ortel TL, Mercer MC, Thames EH, et al. Immunologic impact and clinical outcomes after surgical exposure to bovine thrombin. Ann Surg 2001;233:88–96.
7. Christie RJ, Carrington L, Alving BA. Postoperative bleeding induced by topical bovine thrombin: report of two cases. Surgery 1997;121: 708–710.
8. Rousou J, Levitsky S, Gonzalez-Lavin L, et al. Randomized clinical trial of fibrin sealant in patients undergoing resternotomy or reoperation after cardiac operations: A multicenter study. J Thorac Cardiovasc Surg 1989;97:194–203.
9. Martinowitz U, Schulman S. Fibrin sealant in surgery of patients with hemorrhagic diathesis. Thromb Haemost 1995;74:486–492.
10. Rakocz M, Mazar A, Varon D, et al. Dental extractions in patients with bleeding disorders. The use of fibrin glue. Oral Surg Oral Med Oral Pathol 1993;75:280–282.
11. Atkinson JB, Gomperts ED, Kang R, et al. Prospective, randomized evaluation of the efficacy of fibrin sealant as a topical hemostatic agent at the cannulation site in neonates undergoing extracorporeal membrane oxygenation. Am J Surg 1997;173:479–484.
12. Aggarwal A, Malkovska V, Catlett JP, Alcorn K. Recombinant activated factor VII (rFVIIa) as salvage treatment for intractable hemorrhage. Thromb J 2004;2:9.
13. Franchini M, Zaffanello M, Veneri D. Recombinant factor VIIa. An update on its clinical use. Thromb Haemost 2005;93:1027–1035.
14. Levi M, Peters M, Buller H. Efficacy and safety of recombinant factor VIIa for treatment of severe bleeding: a systematic review. Crit Care Med 2005;33:883–890.
15. Roberts HR, Monroe DM, White GC. The use of recombinant factor VIIa in the treatment of bleeding disorders. Blood 2004;104:3858–3864.
16. Firozvi K, Acs P, Baidas S, et al. Efficacious and safe use of recombinant activated factor VII (rFVIIa) in patients with enoxaparin (ENOX)-induced bleeding and preexisting hypercoagulable states. Blood 2004;104:300a (abstract).
17. Martinez J, Barsigian C. Coagulopathy of liver failure and vitamin K deficiency. In Loscalzo J, Schafer AL (eds). Thrombosis and Hemorrhage, 2nd ed. Philadelphia, Williams & Wilkins, 1998, pp 987–1004.
18. Martin TG III, Somberg KA, Meng YG, et al. Thrombopoietin levels in patients with cirrhosis before and after orthotopic liver transplantation. Ann Intern Med 1997;127:285–288.
19. DeLoughery T. Management of bleeding with uremia and liver disease. Curr Opin Hematol 1999;6:329–333.
20. Blanchard RA, Furie BC, Jorgensen M. Acquired vitamin K-dependent carboxylation deficiency in liver disease. NEJM 1981;305:242–248.
21. Gralnick HR, Givelber H, Abrams E. Dysfibrinogenemia associated with hepatoma: increased carbohydrate content of the fibrinogen molecule. NEJM 1978;299:221–226.
22. Dawson NA, Barr CF, Alving BM. Acquired dysfibrinogenemia. Paraneoplastic syndrome in renal cell carcinoma. Am J Med 1985;78: 682–686.
23. Violi F, Basili S, Ferro D, et al. Association between high values of D-dimer and tissue-plasminogen activator activity and first gastrointestinal bleeding in cirrhotic patients. Thromb Haemost 1996;76:177–183.
24. Kovacs MJ, Wong A, MacKinnon K, et al. Assessment of the validity of the INR system for patients with liver impairment. Thromb Haemost 1994;71:727–730.
25. Basili S, Ferro D, Leo R: Bleeding time does not predict gastrointestinal bleeding in patients with cirrhosis. J Hepatol 1996;24:574–580.
26. Dillon JF, Simpson KJ, Hayes PC. Liver biopsy bleeding time: an unpredictable event. J Gastroenterol Hepatol 1994;9:269–271.
27. Mannucci PM, Vicento V, Vianello L, et al. Controlled trial of desmopressin in liver cirrhosis and other conditions associated with a prolonged bleeding time. Blood 1986;67:1148–1153.
28. Burroughs AK, Matthews K, Qadiri M, et al. Desmopressin and bleeding time in patients with cirrhosis. BMJ 1985;291:1377–1381.
29. McVay PA, Toy PTCY. Lack of increased bleeding after liver biopsy in patients with mild hemostatic abnormalities. Am J Clin Pathol 1990;94:747–753.
30. Inabet WB, Dcziel DJ. Laparoscopic liver biopsy in patients with coagulopathy, portal hypertension, and ascites. Am Surg 1995;61:603–606.
31. Eiglersen E, Melsen T, Ingerslev J, et al. Recombinant activated factor VII (rFVIIa) acutely normalizes prothrombin time in patients with cirrhosis during bleeding from oesophageal varices. Scand J Gastroenterol 2001;36:1081–1085.
32. Tomori K, Nakamoto H, Kotaki S, et al. Gastric angiodysplasia in patients undergoing maintenance dialysis. Adv Periton Dialys 2003;19:136–142.
33. Boccardo P, Remuzzi G, Galbusera M. Platelet dysfunction in renal failure. Semin Thromb Hemostas 2004;30:579–589.
34. Steiner RW, Coggins SC, Carvalho ACA. Bleeding time in uremia: a useful test to assess clinical bleeding. Am J Hematol 1979;7:107–117.
35. Noris M, Benigni A, Boccardo P, et al. Enhanced nitric oxide synthesis in uremia: implications for platelet dysfunction and dialysis hypotension. Kidney Int 1993;44:445–450.
36. Noris M, Remuzzi G: Uremic bleeding: closing the circle after thirty years of controversies. Blood 1999;94:2569–2574.
37. Sreedhara R, Itagaki I, Hakim RM. Uremic patients have decreased shear-induced platelet aggregation mediated by decreased availability of glycoprotein IIb-IIIa receptors. Am J Kidney Dis 1996;27:355–364.
38. Zachee P, Vermylen J, Boogaerts MA. Hematologic aspects of end-stage renal failure. Ann Hematol 1994;69:33–40.
39. Rabelink TJ, Zwaginga JJ, Koomans HA, Sixma JJ. Thrombosis and hemostasis in renal disease. Kidney Int 1994;46:287–296.
40. Bolan CD, Alving BM. Pharmacologic agents in the management of bleeding disorders. Transfusion 1990;30:541–551.
41. Mannucci PM. Desmopressin (DDAVP) in the treatment of bleeding disorders: the first 20 years. Blood 1997;90:2515–2521.
42. Ruzicka H, Bjorkman S, Lethagen S, Sterner G. Pharmacokinetics and antidiuretic effect of high-dose desmopressin in patients with chronic renal failure. Pharmacol Toxicol 2003;92:137–142.
43. Livio M. Mannucci PM, Vigano G, et al. Conjugated estrogens for the management of bleeding associated with renal failure. NEJM 1986;315:731–735.
44. Sloand JA, Schiff MS. Beneficial effect of low-dose transdermal estrogen on bleeding time and clinical bleeding in uremia. Am J Kidney Dis 1995;26:22–26.
45. Vigano G, Gaspari F, Locatelli M, et al. Dose-effect and pharmacokinetics of estrogens given to correct bleeding time in uremia. Kidney Int 1988;34:853–858.

46. Lo D, Rabbat C, Clase C. Thromboembolism and anticoagulant management in hemodialysis patients: a practical guide to clinical management. Thromb Res 2005 (in press).
47. Levi M. Current understanding of disseminated intravascular coagulation. Br J Haematol 2004;124:567–576.
48. Francois B, Trimoreau F, Vignon P, et al. Thrombocytopenia in the sepsis syndrome: role of hemophagocytosis and macrophage colony-stimulating factor. Am J Med 1997;103:114–120.
49. Baker GR, Levin J. Transient thrombocytopenia produced by administration of macrophage colony-stimulating factor: investigations of the mechanism. Blood 1998;91:89–99.
50. Warren BL, Eid A, Singer P, et al. High-dose antithrombin III in severe sepsis. A randomized controlled trial. JAMA 2001;286:1869–1878.
51. Abraham E, Laterre P-F, Garg R, et al. Drotrecogin alfa (activated) for adult with severe sepsis and a low risk of death. NEJM 2005;353: 1332–1341.
52. Parrillo JE. Severe sepsis and therapy with activated protein C. NEJM 2005;353:1398–1400.
53. Schwartz BS, Williams EC, Conlan MG, Mosher DF. ε-Aminocaproic acid in the treatment of patients with acute promyelocytic leukemia and acquired α2-plasmin inhibitor deficiency. Ann Intern Med 1986;105:873–877.
54. Avvisati G, ten Cate JW, Buller HR, Mandelli F. Tranexamic acid for control of haemorrhage in acute promyelocytic leukemia. Lancet 1989;2:122–124.
55. Bern MM. Acquired and congenital coagulation defects encountered during pregnancy and in the fetus. In Bern MM, Frigoletto FD Jr (eds). Hematologic Disorders in Maternal-Fetal Medicine. New York, Wiley-Liss, 1990, pp 395–447.
56. Romero R, Duffy TP, Berkowitz RL, et al. Prolongation of a preterm pregnancy complicated by death of a single twin in utero and disseminated intravascular coagulation. Effects of treatment with heparin. NEJM 1984;310:772–774.
57. Skelly H, Marivate M, Norman R, et al. Consumptive coagulopathy following fetal death in a triplet pregnancy. AJOG 1982;142:595–596.
58. Green D, Lechner K. A survey of 215 non-hemophilic patients with inhibitors to factor VIII. Thromb Haemost 1981;45:200–203.
59. Michiels JJ, Hamulyak K, Nieuwenhuis HK, et al. Acquired haemophilia A in women postpartum: management of bleeding episodes and natural history of the factor VIII inhibitor. Eur J Haematol 1997;59:105–109.
60. Green D, Rademaker AW, Briet E. A prospective, randomized trial of prednisone and cyclophosphamide in the treatment of patients with factor VIII autoantibodies. Thromb Haemost 1993;70:753–757.
61. Green D. Oral immunosuppressive therapy for acquired hemophilia [letter]. Ann Intern Med 1998;128:325.
62. Shaffer LG, Phillips MD. Successful treatment of acquired hemophilia with oral immunosuppressive therapy. Ann Intern Med 1997;127: 206–209.
63. Schulman S, Langevitz P, Livneh A, et al. Cyclosporine therapy for acquired factor VIII inhibitor in a patient with systemic lupus erythematosus. Thromb Haemost 1996;76:344–346.
64. Aggarwal A, Grewal R, Green R, et al. Rituximab for autoimmune haemophilia: a proposed treatment algorithm. Haemophilia 2005;11: 13–19.
65. Gordon EM, Al-Batniji F, Goldsmith JC. Continuous infusion of monoclonal antibody–purified factor VIII: rational approach to serious hemorrhage in patients with allo-/auto-antibodies to factor VIII. Am J Hematol 1994;45:142–145.
66. Negrier C, Goudemand J, Sultan Y, et al. Multicenter retrospective study on the utilization of FEIBA in France in patients with factor VIII and factor IX inhibitors. Thromb Haemost 1997;77:1113–1119.
67. Shapiro AD, Gilchrist GS, Hoots WK, et al. Prospective, randomised trial of two doses of rFVIIa (NovoSeven) in haemophilia patients with inhibitors undergoing surgery. Thromb Haemost 1998;80:773–778.
68. Key NG, Aledort LM, Beardsley D, et al. Home treatment of mild to moderate bleeding episodes using recombinant factor VIIa (NovoSeven) in haemophiliacs with inhibitors. Thromb Haemost 1998;80:912–918.
69. Schneiderman J, Nugent DJ, Young G. Sequential therapy with activated prothrombin complex concentrate and recombinant factor VIIa in patients with severe haemophilia and inhibitors. Haemophilia 2004;10:347–351.
70. Key NS, Christie B, Henderson N, Nelsestuen GL. Possible synergy between recombinant factor VIIa and prothrombin complex concentrate in hemophilia therapy. Thromb Haemost 2002;88:60–65.
71. Chediak J, Ashenhurst JB, Garlick I, Desser RK. Successful management of bleeding in a patient with factor V inhibitor by platelet transfusions. Blood 1980;56:835–841.
72. Edson JR, Vogt JM, Hasegawa DK. Abnormal prothrombin crossed-immunoelectrophoresis in patients with lupus inhibitors. Blood 1984; 64:807–816.
73. Bajaj SP, Rapaport SI, Fierer DS, et al. A mechanism for the hypoprothrombinemia of the acquired hypoprothrombinemia-lupus anticoagulant syndrome. Blood 1983;61:684–692.
74. Fleck RA, Rapaport SI, Rao VM. Anti-prothrombin antibodies and the lupus anticoagulant. Blood 1988;72:512–519.
75. Bajaj SP, Rapaport SI, Barclay S, Herbst KD. Acquired hypoprothrombinemia due to nonneutralizing antibodies to prothrombin: mechanism and management. Blood 1985;65:1538–1543.
76. Lee MT, Nardi MA, Hu G, et al. Transient hemorrhagic diathesis associated with an inhibitor of prothrombin with lupus anticoagulant in an 10-year-old girl: report of a case and review of the literature. Am J Hematol 1996;51:307–314.
77. Bernini JC, Buchanan GR, Ashcroft J. Hypoprothrombinemia and severe hemorrhage associated with a lupus anticoagulant. J Pediatr 1993;123:937–939.
78. Lorand L. Acquired inhibitors of fibrin stabilization: A class of hemorrhagic disorders of diverse origins. In Green D (ed). Anticoagulants: Physiologic, Pathologic, and Pharmacologic. Boca Raton, Fla., CRC Press, 1994, pp 169–191.
79. McDonagh J. Hereditary and acquired deficiencies of activated factor XIII. In Beutler E, Lichtman MA, Coller BS, Kipps TJ (eds). Williams' Hematology, 5th ed. New York, McGraw-Hill, 1995, pp 1455–1458.
80. Abbondanzo SL, Gootenberg JE, Lofts RS, McPherson RA. Intracranial hemorrhage in congenital deficiency of factor XIII. Am J Pediatr Hematol Oncol 1988;10:65–68.
81. Larsen PD, Wallace JW, Frankel LS, Crisp D. Factor XIII deficiency and intracranial hemorrhage in infancy. Pediatr Neurol 1990;6:277–278.
82. Miesbach W, Boehm M, Scharrer: Case Report: rituximab in the treatment of factor XIII inhibitor possibly caused by ciprofloxacin. Thromb Haemost 2005;93:1001–1003.
83. Baglin T. Management of warfarin (coumarin) overdose. Blood Rev 1998;12:91–98.
84. Butler AC, Tait RC. Management of oral anticoagulant-induced intracranial haemorrhage. Blood Rev 1998;12:35–44.
85. Ansell J, Hirsh J, Poller L, et al. The pharmacology and management of the vitamin K antagonists. The Seventh ACCP Conference on Antithrombotic and Thrombolytic Therapy. Chest 2004;126:204S–233S Available at www.chestjournal.org.
86. Voora D, McLeod HL, Eby C, Gage B. The pharmacogenetics of coumarin therapy. Pharmacogenomics 2005;6:503–513.
87. D'Andrea G, D'Ambrosio RL, DiPerna P, et al. A polymorphism in the *VKORC1* gene is associated with an interindividual variability in the dose-anticoagulant effect of warfarin. Blood 2005;105:645–649.
88. Roberts HR, Bingham MD. Other coagulation factor deficiencies. In Loscalzo J, Schafer AI (eds).Thrombosis and Hemorrhage, 2nd ed. Philadelphia, Williams & Wilkins, 1998, pp 773–802.
89. Wijdicks EFM, Schievink WI, Brown RD, Mullany CJ. The dilemma of discontinuation of anticoagulation therapy for patients with intracranial hemorrhage and mechanical heart valves. Neurosurgery 1998;42:769–773.
90. Deveras RAE, Kessler CM. Reversal of warfarin-induced excessive anticoagulation with recombinant human factor VIIa concentrate. Ann Intern Med 2002;137:884–888.
91. Babcock J, Hartman K, Pedersen A, et al. Rodenticide-induced coagulopathy in a young child: a case of Munchausen syndrome by proxy. Am J Pediatr Hematol Oncol 1993;15:126–130.
92. Nieuwenhuis HK, Albada J, Banga JD, Sixma JJ. Identification of risk factors for bleeding during treatment of acute venous thromboembolism with heparin or low molecular weight heparin. Blood 1991;78:2337–2343.
93. Campbell NRC, Hull RD, Brant R, et al. Aging and heparin-related bleeding. Arch Intern Med 1996;156:857–860.
94. Levine MN, Raskob G, Landefeld S, Kearon C. Hemorrhagic complications of anticoagulant treatment. Chest 1998;114:511S–523S.
95. Hirsh J, Raschke R. Heparin and low-molecular-weight heparin. The Seventh ACCP Conference on Antithrombotic and Thrombolytic Therapy. Chest 2004;126:188S–203S.
96. Levin MN, Raskob G, Beyth RJ, et al. Hemorrhagic complications of anticoagulant treatment. The Seventh ACCP Conference on Antithrombotic and Thrombolytic Therapy. Chest 2004;126:287S–310S.
97. Vandermeulen EP, Van Aken H, Vermylen J. Anticoagulants and spinal-epidural anesthesia. Anesth Analg 1994;79:1165–1177.
98. Horlocker TT, Heit JA. Low molecular weight heparin: biochemistry, pharmacology, perioperative prophylaxis regimens, and guidelines for regional anesthetic management. Anesth Analg 1997;85:874–875.

99. Horlocker TT, Wedel DJ. Spinal and epidural blockade and perioperative low molecular weight heparin: smooth sailing on the Titanic. Anesth Analg 1998;86:1153–1156.
100. Weitz JI, Hirsh J, Samama NM. New anticoagulant drugs. The Seventh ACCP Conference on Antithrombotic and Thrombolytic Therapy. Chest 2004;126:265s–286s.
101. Kuo Khm, Kovacs MJ. Fondaparinux: A potential new therapy for HIT. Hematology 2005;10:271–275.
102. Bradner J, Hallisey RK, Kuter DJ. Fondaparinux in the treatment of heparin-induced thrombocytopenia. Blood 2004;104:492a (abstract)
103. Bijsterveld N, Moons A, Boekholdt SM, et al. Ability of recombinant factor VIIa to reverse the anticoagulant effect of the pentasaccharide fondaparinux in healthy volunteers. Circulation 2002;106:2550–2554.
104. Greinacher A, Volpel H, Janssens U, et al. Recombinant hirudin (lepirudin) provides safe and effective anticoagulation in patients with heparin-induced thrombocytopenia: A prospective study. Circulation 1999;99:73–80.
105. Vanholder R, Camez A, Veys N, et al. Pharmacokinetics of recombinant hirudin in hemodialyzed end-stage renal failure patients. Thromb Haemost 1997;77:650–655.
106. Vanholder R, Camez A, Veys N, et al. Recombinant hirudin: A specific thrombin inhibiting anticoagulant for hemodialysis. Kidney Int 1994;45:1754–1759.
107. Potzsch B, Riess FC, Volpel H, et al. Recombinant hirudin as anticoagulant during open-heart surgery. Thromb Haemost 1995;73:1456a.
108. Parent F, Bridey F, Dreyfus M, et al. Treatment of severe venous thromboembolism with intravenous hirudin (HBW 023): An open pilot study. Thromb Haemost 1993;70:386–388.
109. Hein OV, Heymann C, Morgera S, et al. Protracted bleeding after hirudin anticoagulation for cardiac surgery in a patient with HIT II and chronic renal failure. Artificial Organs 2005;29:507–513.
110. Warkentin TE, Greinacher A. Heparin-induced thrombocytopenia: Recognition, treatment, and prevention The Seventh ACCP Conference on Anththrombotic and Thrombolytic Therapy. Chest 2004;126:311s–337s.
111. Swan SK, Hursting MJ. The pharmacokinetics and pharmacodynamics of argatroban: effects of age, gender, and hepatic or renal dysfunction. Pharmacotherapy 2000;20:318–329.
112. Reddy BV, Grossman EJ, Trevino SA, et al. Argatroban anticoagulation in patients with heparin-induced thrombocytopenia requiring renal replacement therapy. Ann Pharmacother 2005;39:1601–1605.
113. Lewis BE, Iaffaldano R, McKiernan TL, et al. Report of successful use of argatroban as an alternative anticoagulant during coronary stent implantation in a patient with heparin-induced thrombocytopenia and thrombosis syndrome. Cathet Cardiovasc Diagn 1996;38:206–209.
114. Bagdasarian SB, Sing I, Militello MA, et al. Argatroban dosage in critically ill patients with HIT. Blood 2004;104: 493a (abstract).
115. The EPISTENT Investigators: randomised placebo-controlled and balloon-angioplasty-controlled trial to assess safety of coronary stenting with use of platelet glycoprotein-IIb/IIIa blockade. Lancet 1998;352:87–92.
116. PRISM-Plus Study Investigators: inhibition of the platelet glycoprotein IIb/IIIa receptor with tirofiban in unstable angina and non-Q-wave myocardial infarction. NEJM 1998;338:1488–1497.
117. The RESTORE Investigators: effects of platelet glycoprotein IIb/IIIa blockade with tirofiban on adverse cardiac events in patients with unstable angina or acute myocardial infarction undergoing coronary angioplasty. Circulation 1997;96:1445–1453.
118. The PURSUIT Trial Investigators: inhibition of platelet glycoprotein IIb/IIIa with eptifibatide in patients with acute coronary syndromes. NEJM 1998;339:436–443.
119. Kleiman NS. Pharmacokinetics and pharmacodynamics of glycoprotein IIb-IIIa inhibitors. Am Heart J 1999;13:S263–S275.
120. Ferguson JJ, Kereiakes DJ, Adgey AAJ, et al. Safe use of platelet GP IIb/IIIa inhibitors. Am Heart J 1998;135:77s–89s.
121. Gammie JS, Zenati M, Kormos RL, et al. Abciximab and excessive bleeding in patients undergoing emergency cardiac operations. Ann Thorac Surg 1998;65:465–469.
122. Madan M, Berkowitz SD. Understanding thrombocytopenia and antigenicity with glycoprotein IIb-IIIA inhibitors. Am Heart J 1999;138: 317s–326s.
123. Aster RH. Immune thrombocytopenia caused by glycoprotein IIb/IIIa inhibitors. Chest 2005;127:535–595.
124. Berkowitz SD, Harrington RA, Rund MM, Tcheng JE. Acute profound thrombocytopenia after c7E3 Fab (abciximab) therapy. Circulation 1997;95:809–813.
125. Quinn MJ, Fitzgerald DJ. Ticlopidine and clopidogrel. Circulation 1999;100:1667–1672.
126. Bennett CL, Weinberg PD, Rozenberg-Ben-Dror K, et al. Thrombotic thrombocytopenic purpura associated with ticlopidine. A review of 60 cases. Ann Intern Med 1998;128:541–544.
127. Gent M, Beaumont D, Blanchard J, et al. A randomised, blinded, trial of clopidogrel versus aspirin in patients at risk of ischaemic events (CAPRIE). Lancet 1996;348:1329–1339.
128. Savcic M, Hauert J, Bachmann F, et al. Clopidogrel loading dose regimens: Kinetic profile of pharmacodynamic response in healthy subjects. Semin Thromb Hemost 1999;25(Suppl 2):15–19.
129. Cattaneo M, Gachet C. ADP receptors and clinical bleeding disorders. Arterioscler Thromb Vasc Biol 1999;19:2281–2285.

Chapter 36

Obstetric and Intrauterine Transfusion

Jeannie Callum • Jon Barrett

INTRODUCTION

Transfusion care of the pregnant woman and fetus can be extremely challenging despite the rarity of its occurrence. Pregnant women and fetuses require special considerations and properly selected blood components for transfusion. In this chapter five core aspects of obstetric and intrauterine transfusion will be reviewed, including the management and prevention of postpartum hemorrhage, prevention of RhD alloimmunization, monitoring of the severity of alloimmunization, management of alloimmunization, and neonatal alloimmune thrombocytopenia.

POSTPARTUM HEMORRHAGE

Definition

Postpartum hemorrhage can threaten the life of a healthy woman undergoing an otherwise uncomplicated vaginal delivery. It is the ultimate test of the obstetrical, anesthesia, nursing, and transfusion services. Processes should be in place in every obstetrical unit to clearly delineate the management of these women. Primary hemorrhage in the obstetric patient can be defined as any of the following within 24 hours of delivery: estimated blood loss greater than 1500 mL, 40 g/L or greater drop in the hemoglobin level, or the transfusion of 4 or more units of red blood cells.[1] Other definitions for postpartum hemorrhage have been proposed. A common definition is blood loss in excess of 500 mL after vaginal birth or greater than 1000 mL after cesarean section. The difficulty with the latter definition is illustrated by studies assessing blood loss in the postpartum period, showing that mean blood loss after vaginal and cesarean deliveries is approximately 500 mL and 1000 mL, respectively.[2,3] Clearly, the first definition more accurately identifies patients with a significant postpartum hemorrhage who are at risk for transfusion.

Incidence and Etiology

Postpartum hemorrhage is a leading cause of death in the pregnant patient worldwide, including the United States,[4] United Kingdom,[5] and France.[6] It is estimated that 125,000 women worldwide die of postpartum hemorrhage each year.[7] Causes of postpartum hemorrhage include placenta previa, uterine atony, retained placental tissue, coagulopathy, uterine inversion, uterine rupture, vaginal lacerations, and congenital bleeding disorders.

A review of 48,865 women admitted for delivery in the United Kingdom revealed 327 cases meeting the above definition (0.67%), of whom 51 (0.10%) required the transfusion of four or more units of red blood cells.[1] Risk factors for hemorrhage from this report are shown in Table 36–1. Of note, the use of both antidepressants and antiseizure medications increased the risk of hemorrhage. Use of both serotonin reuptake inhibitors[8,9] and valproate[10,11] have been associated with bleeding. Obstetrical hemorrhage was responsible for two thirds of all maternal morbidity seen in their patients. In another series, risk factors for hemorrhage included Asian race, maternal blood disorders, prior postpartum hemorrhage, history of retained placenta, multiple pregnancy, antepartum hemorrhage, genital tract lacerations, macrosomia (>4 kg), induction of labor, chorioamnionitis, stillbirth, compound fetal presentation, epidural anesthesia, prolonged first/second stage of labor, and forceps delivery after a failed vacuum extraction.[12]

Failure of the placenta to deliver spontaneously is an important contributor to postpartum hemorrhage.[13] The phase of delivery during which the placenta is removed is termed the *third stage*. If the third stage of labor is 30 minutes or longer, the risk of postpartum hemorrhage is 6 times higher than in patients whose third stage is less than 30 minutes.[14] After this initial wait time for the placenta to deliver spontaneously, the clinician usually attempts a manual extraction of the placenta to reduce the risk of postpartum hemorrhage, although studies are lacking on the efficacy of this approach. Studies have also found that a prolonged second stage of delivery in nulliparous women increases the risk of postpartum hemorrhage by an odds ratio of 1.16 (95% confidence interval [CI], 1.09–1.24) for each hour of the second stage.[15] Post-term delivery (42 weeks or greater) is associated with an increased risk of postpartum hemorrhage (odds ratio, 1.37; 95% CI, 1.28–1.46).[16] One quarter of women with HELLP syndrome (hemolysis, elevated liver enzymes, and low platelet count) require transfusion at delivery.[17]

Placenta previa is a complication of pregnancy affecting 0.6% of deliveries in one series of 93,384 deliveries.[18] Hemorrhage due to placenta previa requiring transfusion complicated 25% of deliveries in this series. Patients at greater risk of transfusion were those delivered under general anesthesia and those with a history of previous cesarean section. For those women who require emergency hysterectomy following a cesarean section, the median number of red cells transfused is 6.2 units, with women under regional anesthesia requiring less red cell transfusions (3.3 units vs 6.6 units, $p < 0.005$). A systematic review of the literature found that

Table 36–1 Risk Factors for Obstetrical Hemorrhage and Their Respective Odds Ratio*

Risk Factor	Odds Ratio	95% Confidence Interval
Manual removal of the placenta	13.12	7.72–22.30
Antidepressant therapy	10.55	2.19–50.71
Iron therapy	5.98	2.28–15.65
Anti-seizure therapy	5.75	1.28–25.72
Emergency cesarean	3.09	2.29–4.17
Underlying social issues	2.91	1.76–4.82
Previous postpartum hemorrhage	2.74	1.69–4.44
Multiple pregnancies	2.29	1.20–4.37
Age over 35 years	1.41	1.03–1.95

*Waterstone M, Bewley S, Wolfe C. Incidence and predictors of severe obstetric morbidity: case-control study. BMJ 2001;322:1089–1094.

the use of neuroaxial blockage with epidural or spinal anesthesia in elective surgery reduced the risk of transfusion.[19]

Uterine rupture is a rare complication of delivery (approximately 0.03% of deliveries), with more than 50% to 90% of cases occurring in women with a history of previous cesarean section.[20,21] Red cell transfusion is required in 25% to 55% of these women, particularly those with complete uterine rupture.[20,21]

Secondary Postpartum Hemorrhage

Secondary postpartum hemorrhage is defined as hemorrhage between 24 hours and 6 weeks after delivery of a degree to warrant obstetrical care.[22] In one series of 19,136 deliveries, 0.8% were complicated by secondary hemorrhage.[23] Contributing factors included early postpartum hemorrhage and manual removal of the placenta.[23] Seventeen percent of patients required transfusion and 64% of patients presented between day 8 and 21. Approximately 2% of women require readmission after initial discharge, with postpartum hemorrhage accounting for a quarter of these readmissions.[24]

Primary Prevention

Spontaneous delivery of the placenta, compared to manual removal, during cesarean section is associated with a reduced risk of hemorrhage and transfusion.[25–27] Sharp incision at the time of cesarean section, as compared to blunt expansion, increases the incidence of postpartum hemorrhage (13% vs. 9%) and need for a transfusion (2% vs 0.4%).[28] Oxytocic therapy used postpartum has been associated with a reduction in the risk of postpartum hemorrhage. The most commonly employed oxytocic drug is synthetic oxytocin. It may be given by intramuscular or intravenous injection either at delivery of the infant shoulder or after delivery of the placenta. Oxytocin is superior to oral misoprostol alone in the prevention of postpartum hemorrhage.[29,30] The combination of oxytocin and misoprostol may reduce the risk of postpartum hemorrhage when compared to either agent alone in the management of the third stage of labor.[31] A bolus injection of oxytocin is more effective than a dilute infusion in the prevention of blood loss.[32] However, bolus injection is rarely associated with coronary vasospasm. Misoprostol alone is no more effective than placebo in the prevention of postpartum hemorrhage.[33–34]

Efforts should be made to correct iron deficiency anemia before the third trimester to reduce likelihood of allogeneic transfusion in the event of a postpartum hemorrhage.[35]

Management

Introduction

Enquiries into maternal deaths suggest that many are avoidable and point to a phenomenon of "too little, too late."[36] Strategies to manage postpartum hemorrhage should be predefined in all obstetrical institutions to ensure rapid and consistent care. Strategies should be in place to prevent delays in pharmacologic strategies, transfusion, embolization, and surgical management. Adherence to a consistent approach to postpartum bleeding is successful in reducing the number of women with massive postpartum hemorrhage.[37]

Pharmacologic Strategies

Oxytocic drugs are the mainstay of treatment and a stepwise approach to them is recommended. The Society of Obstetricians and Gynecologists of Canada published guidelines on the use of these agents in 2005. The reader is directed to the Society's website for the details of this evidence-based guideline.[38]

Several case reports and case series in the literature examine the treatment of refractory postpartum hemorrhage with recombinant activated factor VII.[39–41] The vast majority of published cases show immediate cessation of bleeding. There are no randomized controlled trials in this setting. Randomized controlled trials of recombinant factor VIIa in liver resection,[42] upper gastrointestinal bleeding,[43] and trauma[44] did not show any reduction in transfusion requirements. Randomized clinical trials in both spontaneous intracranial hemorrhage[45] and elective prostate surgery[46] showed promising results. Only in the spontaneous intracranial hemorrhage randomized clinical trial was there a concern regarding excess thromboembolic complications. In the absence of both efficacy and safety data in this population, the current role of this agent remains unknown.

Randomized clinical trial data supports the routine use of antifibrinolytic therapy to reduce hemorrhagic complications and transfusion in cardiac surgery,[47] joint replacement surgery,[48] and liver transplant.[49] The literature in obstetrics is limited to case reports.[50] In the absence of both efficacy and safety data in this population, the current role of antifibrinolytics in the management of postpartum hemorrhage remains unknown.

Interventional Radiology

Uterine artery embolization is a technique used by interventional radiologists to control uterine bleeding from multiple causes. The procedure is usually performed with conscious sedation or less commonly with general anesthesia. The procedure can be done through either one or both femoral arteries. The uterine artery is reached via the internal iliac artery. Deux and coworkers reported a case series and a review of the literature of uterine artery embolization for the management of postpartum hemorrhage.[51] Of 108 reported attempts at embolization for postpartum hemorrhage, 97% were successful. In 52% of patients, angiography revealed arterial extravasation directing embolization. In the absence of extravasation, bilateral embolization of the uterine arteries was performed. Gelatin foam is preferred because it allows for transient devascularization and thus preservation of fertility. Gelatin foam dissolves in 1 to 3 weeks after the procedure. Complications, seen in 9% of patients, include fever, pain, vaginal abscess, uterine necrosis, and arterial perforation.[52–54] Uncomplicated pregnancy has been reported after embolization of the uterine arteries.[55,56] In one series of 28 women who underwent embolization for hemorrhage, all women who desired to get pregnant were successful and overall had six uncomplicated pregnancies.[57] Case series suggest that embolization before hysterectomy results in fewer complications, less red cell transfusions, shorter stay in intensive care, and preservation of uterine function.[58] Benefits of a primary radiology approach include the avoidance of general anesthesia, avoidance of an open surgical procedure, and the ability to identify and embolize sources of bleeding other than hypogastric arteries. One case report of two patients described arterial balloon occlusion of the internal iliac arteries for 48 hours, instead of embolization, and was successful in stopping uterine bleeding in both.[59]

Surgical Strategies

Multiple surgical strategies have been attempted to arrest ongoing bleeding, including uterine compression sutures,[60] uterine artery ligation (vaginal[61] or abdominal route[62]), and hysterectomy. Cesarean hysterectomy or postpartum hysterectomy (after vaginal delivery) complicates 0.8 per 1000 deliveries, most commonly for management of hemorrhage secondary to uterine atony and placenta accreta.[63] The median blood loss is 3500 mL, requiring a median of 7 units of red cells.[63]

Transfusion Strategies

During an obstetrical hemorrhage, red cells should be administered to maintain the patient free of signs and symptoms of inadequate tissue oxygen delivery. The hemoglobin should be maintained between 60 and 100 g/L during the resuscitation phase. Care should be taken to ensure that all fluids and blood products are warmed prior to infusion and that the appropriate blood tubing is utilized. In the majority of obstetrical hemorrhages there is little advance warning; thus, blood warmers and blood tubing should be available and accessible at all times. Where time allows, the use of other components should be dictated by the results of laboratory testing. During active bleeding the patient's hemoglobin, platelet count, prothrombin time (PT)/International Normalized Ratio (INR), activated partial thromboplastin time (aPTT), and fibrinogen should be monitored frequently to ensure adequate replacement with components. The platelet count should be maintained over 50,000/μL with platelet transfusions and the PT and aPTT should be maintained at less than 1.5 times normal with fresh frozen plasma at a dose of 15 mL/kg. Cryoprecipitate is commonly needed during an obstetrical hemorrhage due to rapid consumption of fibrinogen from disseminated intravascular coagulation. Cryoprecipitate should be administered if the fibrinogen level falls below 1.0 g/L or during a massive hemorrhage where the emergency does not allow one to wait for the results of the fibrinogen assay. The recommended dosage of cyroprecipitate is 1 U per 5 to 10 kg of body weight. Once there is evidence of cessation of bleeding, component use should be restricted to those patients who are deemed at high risk of rebleeding, because rapid restoration of laboratory parameters is seen once hemostasis is achieved.

Complications

Complications secondary to postpartum hemorrhage include Sheehan's syndrome,[64] myocardial ischemia,[65] acute renal failure, acute lung injury, and consumptive coagulopathy. Myocardial ischemia is detected in 51% of women with a postpartum hemorrhage of greater than 1000 mL in the setting of hemorrhagic shock, as determined by an elevated cardiac troponin I at 24 hours (median, 10 μg/L; range, 4 to 27 μg/L), electrocardiographic changes, and a reduction in myocardial contractility. Myocardial ischemia is seen particularly in those women with hypotension (<88/50 mmHg) and tachycardia (heart rate > 115 beats/min).[65]

PREVENTION OF RhD ALLOIMMUNIZATION

Prenatal Testing

When developing algorithms for prenatal testing, it is important to ensure that all RhD-negative women are appropriately treated with Rh immune globulin (RhIG) and all clinically important alloantibodies are detected while ensuring a cost-effective testing strategy. A sample algorithm for prenatal testing is shown in Figure 36–1. All pregnant women should be tested for the D antigen and for sensitization to the D antigen, ideally at the first-trimester visit.[66] No further D-antigen testing is required once two concordant D results are obtained during the first pregnancy. The second D-antigen testing is usually performed before the administration of RhIG at 28 weeks or at delivery. The patient's D-antigen status should be re-evaluated with each subsequent pregnancy, including in those patients who are found to be D-positive. Testing for weak expression of the D antigen is not required by the British Committee for Standards in Haematology[67] (United Kingdom), American Association of Blood Banks,[68] or the American College of Obstetricians and Gynecologists.[69] Despite economic pressures, it is unfortunate that 58% of laboratories participating in the College of American Pathologist (CAP) surveys still routinely perform weak D testing on RhD-negative patients.[70] If the decision is made to test for weak expression of the D antigen, women who test positive do not require RhIG. It is not known if women with a partial expression of the D antigen benefit from the administration of RhIG, nor is it known what dose would be required to prevent immunization.[71] Presumably, the maternal red cells would absorb the anti-D, leaving only those immunoglobulin G molecules with specificity for the epitope(s) lacking on the maternal red cells. It is uncertain whether the remaining anti-D is sufficient to prevent alloimmunization in the partial D mother. Notwithstanding, the presence of anti-D has been reported in the plasma of untreated partial D patients, some of whom

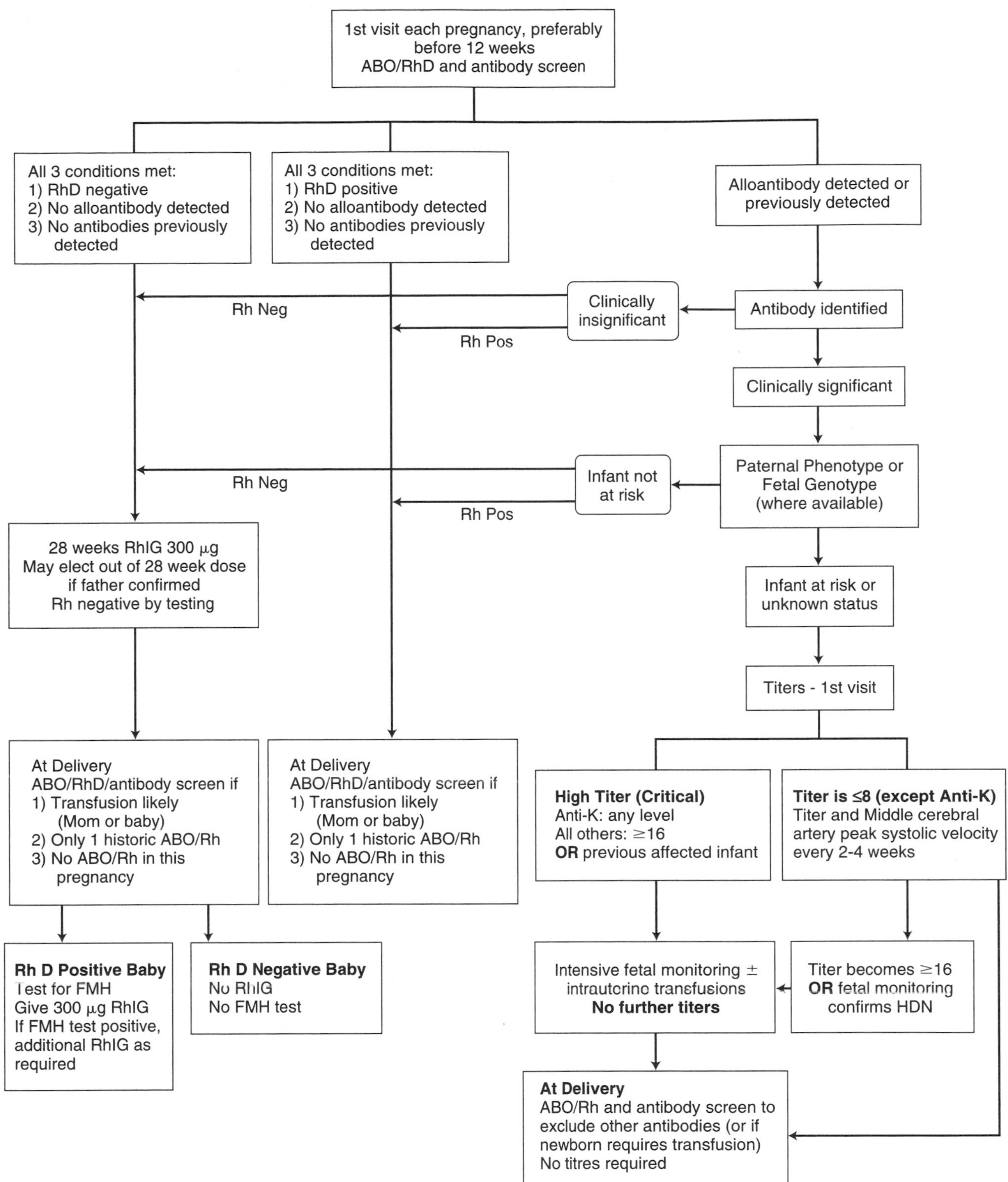

Figure 36–1 Sample algorithm for antenatal and peripartum blood bank testing.

have delivered infants with hemolytic disease of the fetus and newborn (HDFN).[72]

The risk of alloimmunization to the D antigen between the first trimester and 28 weeks' gestation is exceptionally low (0.18%)[73]; therefore, the cost effectiveness of repeat antibody screening before administration of RhIG at 28 weeks has been questioned. Two retrospective series found that routine antibody screening in the third trimester or at delivery was also of low yield (0.06% to 0.24%) and no significant neonatal sequelae resulted from the newly formed antibodies.[74,75] Thus, antibody screening can be safely restricted to those patients at delivery requiring pretransfusion testing or investigation for HDFN. Titration studies after RhIG administration to ensure adequate coverage for prevention of alloimmunization or to differentiate between active and passive anti-D are not useful nor recommended.[66] There is no data to support the need for an additional dose of RhIG in the last few weeks of pregnancy, even if the antibody screen is found to be negative.

Some clinicians recommend routine pretransfusion testing at delivery on all patients, in case there is a need for an emergency transfusion and the patient has an antibody that was not previously detected. A large retrospective study does not support this opinion.[76] This group estimated that only 1 in 11,050 patients undergoing cesarean sections would have both a new clinically significant antibody and the need for a red cell transfusion. The investigators performed the same analysis for those with vaginal deliveries and found this dual occurrence to be 1 in 61,343 deliveries. Their data supports the practice of withholding pretransfusion testing in patients undergoing vaginal delivery or cesarean section, unless significant risk factors for hemorrhage are present. In the unfortunate event of an unexpected obstetrical hemorrhage, group O, RhD-negative blood should be provided while expediting blood grouping and antibody screening.

Rh Immune Globulin Administration

A combination of an antepartum and a postpartum dose of RhIG reduces the risk of sensitization to 0.1% in clinical studies.[77] All unsensitized RhD-negative women are candidates for RhIG at 28 weeks, at delivery of an RhD-positive fetus, and in the case of spontaneous abortion, ectopic pregnancy, therapeutic abortion, amniocentesis, chorionic villus sampling, external cephalic version, abdominal trauma, antepartum hemorrhage, and other inciting events.[78] If the father of the fetus has been tested and has been shown to be RhD-negative, the woman may elect not to receive RhIG. The paternal sample should be obtained during the current pregnancy, and the result should be placed in the medical records of the pregnant partner. Beyond 20 weeks' gestation, quantification of fetomaternal hemorrhage should be performed to determine if a single dose of RhIG is adequate for prevention of immunization. Such testing must be performed at each inciting event where RhIG administration is required. After 20 weeks, the fetal blood volume exceeds 30 mL[79]; thereafter, a single dose of 300 μg may be insufficient and testing for fetomaternal hemorrhage is recommended.[68,80] Massive fetomaternal hemorrhage may occur without any foreseen cause; therefore, the need for testing should not be dictated by clinical judgment of the risk of fetomaternal hemorrhage.[81] Massive fetomaternal hemorrhage in excess of 30 mL is rare. In one series of 1131 patients tested for fetomaternal hemorrhage by hemoglobin F quantitation, 1.3% were found to have a hemorrhage of greater than 30 mL.[82] If a dose of RhIG is inadvertently not administered within the recommended 72 hours of an inciting event, the dosage should be given as soon as possible and up to 28 days postpartum.[83]

Risks of Rh Immune Globulin

Rh immune globulin is manufactured with multiple viral inactivation strategies to minimize the risk of transmitting blood-borne diseases. The safety strategies include donor selection, donor transmissible disease testing, solvent-detergent viral inactivation, and nanofiltration. Failures in the manufacturing process or donor testing could result in infectious complications. RhIG has been implicated in the transmission of hepatitis C virus in Ireland, where inadequate viral safety measures were in place.[84] In North America, there has been no evidence of viral transmission from this pooled human blood product. Of 624,939 female donors included in a U.S. study to determine the viral safety of RhIG, there were no significant differences in the prevalence of hepatitis C virus and human immunodeficiency virus between Rh-negative and Rh-positive female donors.[85] Adverse drug reactions are uncommon and may include fever and pain at the injection site. Hypersensitivity reactions are rare.[86]

Fetomaternal Hemorrhage Testing

Fetomaternal hemorrhage quantitation is usually performed by acid elution test (Kleihauer-Betke test) or hemoglobin F quantitation by flow cytometry, although other methods are available. The test is performed to determine either the appropriate dosage of RhIG in an RhD-negative mother or to diagnose and quantitate a fetomaternal hemorrhage. The Kleihauer-Betke test has numerous limitations, including low sensitivity, poor reproducibility, and a tendency to overestimate the volume of hemorrhage. An important limitation of the Kleihauer-Betke test is the inability to differentiate between maternal and fetal F cells. This is particularly a problem in the second trimester, when maternal F cells may occasionally reach 5% to 10%. If a Kleihauer-Betke test is performed during this time, this physiologic change may be mistaken for a fetomaternal hemorrhage.

Hemoglobin F quantitation by flow cytometry has been found to be simple, reliable, and more precise than the Kleihauer-Betke test.[82,87] In the 2001 CAP survey, samples representing a 20-mL and a 40-mL bleed were sent as external proficiency testing. Beyond a 30-mL fetomaternal hemorrhage, a single 300-μg dose of RhIG would be insufficient to prevent alloimmunization. For the 20-mL hemorrhage, 88% of laboratories utilizing hemoglobin F quantitation and 50% of the laboratories using the Kleihauer-Betke test correctly reported the result as less than 30 mL. For the 40 mL hemorrhage, 100% of laboratories utilizing hemoglobin F quantitation and 89% of the laboratories using Kleihauer-Betke correctly reported the result as greater than 30 mL. This data suggests that hemoglobin F quantitation may be a superior test method. No clinical management decisions should be based solely on the results of fetomaternal hemorrhage testing given the inaccuracies found in the studies and surveys described above. See Figure 36–2 for sample histograms from control and patient samples tested with the hemoglobin F quantitation method.

MONITORING OF ALLOIMMUNIZATION DURING PREGNANCY

Incidence of Alloimmunization and Hemolytic Disease of the Fetus and Newborn

Overall, approximately 6.8 per 1000 pregnancies are complicated by RhD alloimmunization.[88] In one large series, 1% of pregnancies were shown to be complicated by alloimmunization to antigens implicated in HDFN.[89] The implicated antibody in this series was anti-D in 41%, other Rh antibodies in 30%, and non-Rh antibodies in 29%. In 244 alloimmunized pregnancies, there were 3 intrauterine deaths, 3 fetuses requiring intrauterine transfusion, 10 infants requiring allogeneic transfusion after delivery, and 27 infants requiring phototherapy. Half of Rh-positive infants born to women alloimmunized to the D antigen require no treatment for HDFN.[90] In the presence of

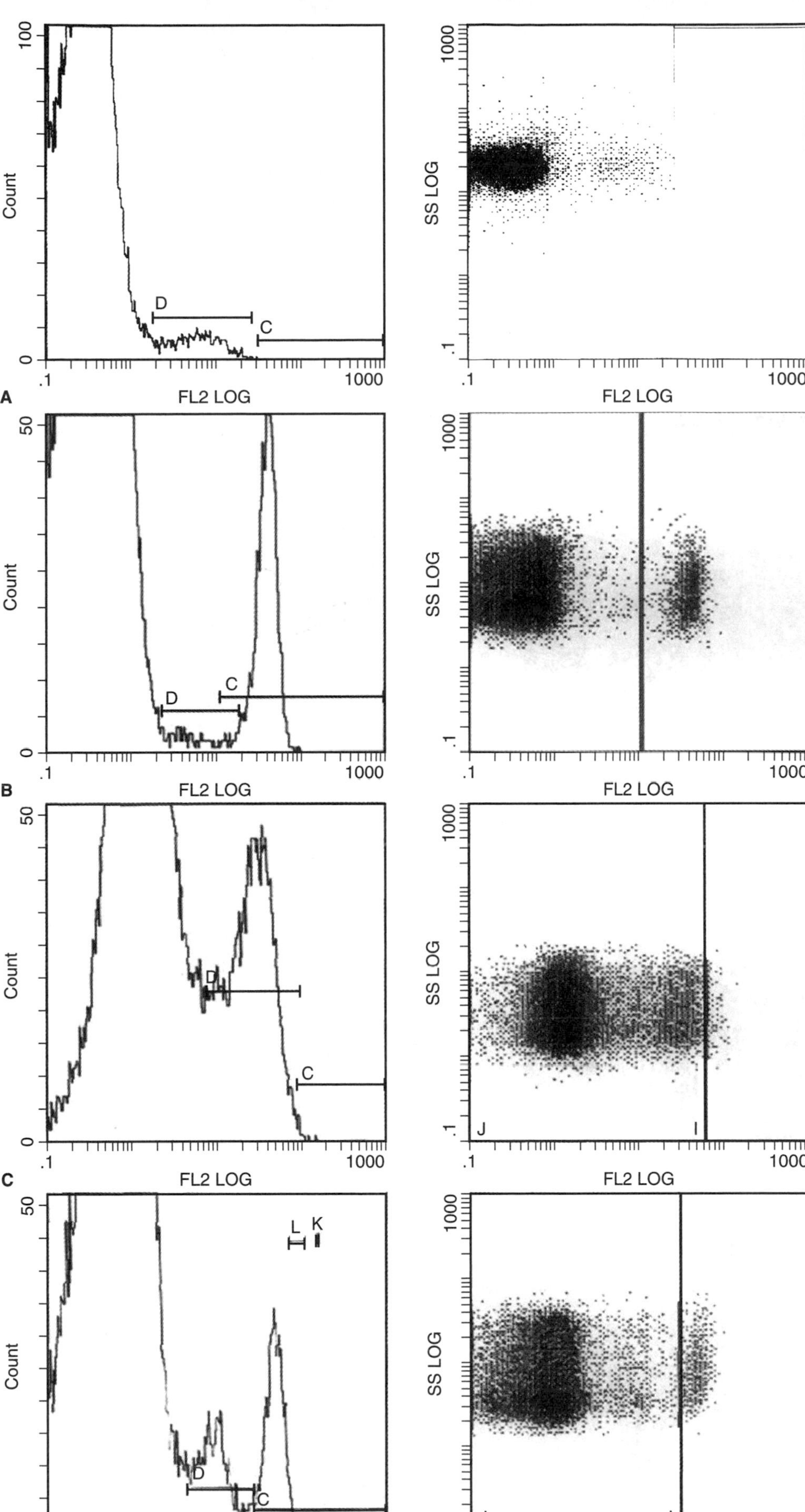

Figure 36–2 Hemoglobin F quantitation performed by flow cytometry with anti–hemogobin F in a nonpregnant control and three patients. For each sample, a quantitative histogram of fluorescence intensity (*left*) and a dot plot representation of side scatter vs. fluorescence (*right*) are shown. Panel A is a female nonpregnant control. Panel B is a patient with a massive fetomaternal hemorrhage (gate C, 7.0%). Panel C is from a woman with a suspected fetomaternal hemorrhage in her second trimester of pregnancy. No fetomaternal hemorrhage was detected, although the patient had a striking increase in maternal F cells (gate D, 15%). Panel D represents a massive fetomaternal hemorrhage (gate C, 3.9%) with a concomitant increase in maternal F cells (gate D, 3.5%). The gating was set with control samples run concurrently with the patient samples.

multiple antibodies, the presence of an anti-D is the single most significant factor predicting the risk of HDFN, with the presence of anti-D plus another antibody further increasing that risk.[91] Table 36–2 details the clinical significance of red cell alloantibodies in HDFN.

Assessing the Severity of Hemolytic Disease of the Fetus and Newborn

Introduction

The role of laboratory testing and fetal imaging is to determine whether intrauterine transfusion or early delivery is warranted in the management of an alloimmunized pregnancy. The risk of complications from such interventions must be weighed against the perceived benefits.

Antibody Titers and Cellular Assays

The role of blood bank testing is to identify the alloantibodies present, to determine their clinical significance, and to perform titrations to assist the clinicians as to when more invasive fetal monitoring is required. An excellent review on the role of titrations has been published and should be reviewed prior to setting testing algorithms.[66] Titers should be performed by the saline tube technique, with previous samples run in parallel. The use of gel technology should be avoided unless validation studies are performed within the laboratory to establish a new critical titer. The use of

Table 36–2 Potential of Blood Group Alloantibodies to Cause Hemolytic Disease of the Fetus and Newborn (HDFN)*

Blood Group System	Specificity	Severity of HDFN
ABO	A/B	Common, mild to moderate
	A_1	No
P	P_1	No
MNS	M	Rare, mild
	N	Rare, in infants born to N–U– women
	S/s	Rare, mild to severe
RH	All	Common, mild to severe
LU	All	No to mild
KEL	All	No to severe
LE	All	No
FY	Fy^a	Rare, mild to severe
	Fy^b	Rare, mild
	Fy3	Rare, mild
JK	Jk^a	Rare, mild to moderate
	Jk^b	Rare, mild
	Jk3	No to mild
DI	Most	Mild to severe; some, no data
YT	Yt^a	No
	Yt^b	No
XG	Xg^a	No
SC	Sc1, Sc2	Positive DAT, No HDFN
	Sc3, Sc4	Mild to severe
DO	All	No, or positive DAT, no HDFN
CO	Co^a	Rare, mild to severe
	Co^b	Mild
	Co3	Severe
LW	All	Rare, no to mild
CH/RG	All	No
H	H	In infants born to O_h women
XK	Kx	Not applicable
GE	Ge3	No to severe
	Others	No
CROM	All	No, or no data
KN	All	No
IN	In^a/In^b	Positive DAT, no HDFN
OK	Ok^a	No
MER2	MER2	No data
JMH	JMH	No
I	I	No
GLOB	P	No to mild
GIL	GIL	Positive DAT, no HDFN

*Guidelines for Prenatal and Perinatal Immunohematology. Bethesda, Md., AABB Press, 2005.

heterozygous cells and enhancement strategies, such as gel technology, likely explains the wide disparity in titer results seen in external proficiency testing programs. A sample algorithm is shown in Figure 36–1. The *critical titer* varies between laboratories and is approximately 8 to 32 for anti-D.[66,92] The critical titer is thought only to be of value in evaluating the first affected pregnancy.[93] The lack of correlation of titers with fetal outcomes has caused some to question whether titers have any role in the antenatal assessment of alloimmunized pregnancies.[94] A critical titer for non-D antibodies has not yet been defined, and the role of titers for non-D alloimmunization pregnancies remains unclear. Anti-Kell is a clear example of an instance where titers of 4 or less can be associated with HDFN.[95,96] Given the above limitations of titrations, once the critical titer is reached, more invasive testing such as ultrasonography, Doppler assessment of the middle cerebral artery peak systolic velocity, amniocentesis, and cordocentesis is warranted. After the titer has reached a critical level, no further titers should be performed. Titration studies are of no value after delivery. It is recommended that titrations be performed on homozygous cells for the offending antigen and when anti-D is present on R_2R_2 cells, where the expression of the D antigen is more uniform donor to donor.[66] In addition, where available, the current sample should be run in parallel with the previous sample.[97] Titrations should be performed every 2 to 4 weeks after 18 weeks' gestation. If there is a previously affected infant with HDFN, titers should not be performed and more aggressive monitoring should be adopted early in pregnancy.[98]

Cellular assays, such as the monocyte monolayer assay, the chemiluminescence test, and antibody-dependent cell-mediated cytotoxicity assay, which are sensitive to factors affecting antibody function, have been developed to improve the prediction of disease severity.[99] These assays are cumbersome and not broadly available. There are data to suggest that these cellular assays provide clinically useful information to complement serologic testing.[100]

Middle Cerebral Artery Peak Systolic Velocity and Fetal Ultrasonography

Middle cerebral artery peak systolic velocity, measured by Doppler ultrasonography, is an accurate test for detecting fetal anemia.[101,102] This technique is noninvasive and therefore presents no risk of miscarriage or preterm labor, and thus is a preferable method of screening for fetal anemia when compared to invasive alternatives. There is a reciprocal relationship between the fetal hemoglobin concentration and the velocity of cerebral blood flow. Middle cerebral artery peak systolic velocity can also be utilized to predict fetal anemia in non-Rh alloimmunized pregnancies, including anti-K alloimmunized pregnancies.[103] Intrahepatic umbilical venous maximum velocity may also correlate with middle cerebral artery peak systolic velocity and fetal anemia.[103] A threshold value for the peak systolic velocity of 1.50 multiples of the median for gestational age has a 100% sensitivity (95% CI, 86%–100%) for the detection of moderate or severe anemia in fetuses without hydrops.[102] Compared with conventional management, middle cerebral artery peak systolic velocity may have a better predictive accuracy for moderate to severe fetal anemia.[104] Management with middle cerebral artery peak systolic velocity will likely eliminate the need for amniocentesis and reduce the number of periumbilical cord blood samplings performed in red blood cell alloimmunized pregnancies. As ultrasonography evolves and improves, it is extremely likely that titers will prove to be obsolete for predicting which fetuses have significant HDFN.

Invasive Monitoring with Amniocentesis and Periumbilical Cord Blood Sampling

Serial amniocentesis with measurement of the OD450 allowed Liley to divide infants into three risk zones, see Figure 36–3.[105] The timing of repeat amniocentesis or cord blood sampling depends on the level of amniotic fluid bilirubin. Unfortunately, prior to 27 weeks' gestation its reliability

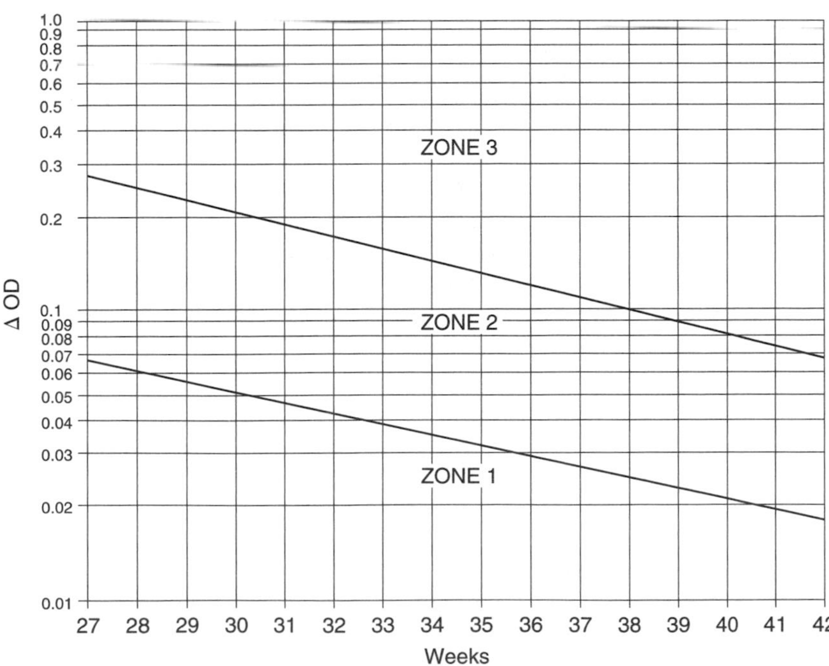

Figure 36–3 Liley graph used to plot degree of alloimmunization. (From American College of Obstetrics and Gynecology. Management of isoimmunization in pregnancy. ACOG Technical Bulletin 227. Washington, D.C., ACOG, 1996, with permission.)

is questionable[106]; the procedure itself may cause fetomaternal hemorrhage, further stimulating alloimmunization[107]; it carries the risk of procedure-related pregnancy loss of 0.6%.[108] Thus, serial middle cerebral artery peak systolic velocity, instead of amniotic fluid OD450 measurement, is used to identify fetuses in whom periumbilical cord blood sampling is required. Once an at-risk infant is identified by either middle cerebral artery peak systolic velocity or amniocentesis, cordocentesis can be used for: measurement of the fetal hemoglobin, reticulocyte count, and bilirubin; determination of blood group; and for performance of the direct antiglobulin test and, where necessary, intrauterine transfusion. Cordocentesis is associated with a risk of fetal loss of approximately 1.0% per procedure.[109,110] Cordocentesis can be complicated by infection, bleeding, fetal bradycardia, intrauterine growth retardation, and premature rupture of the membranes.[109,110]

Fetal Blood Typing

The first step in fetal blood typing is to perform paternal Rh phenotyping for Rh DCE or the offending antigen to determine whether the father is homozygous or heterozygous. If the father is homozygous, all infants will express the offending antigen; and if the father is heterozygous, half of the infants are at risk. Paternal zygosity can be assessed by serologic analysis of the major Rh antigens, and the most probable genotype can be determined by haplotype tables.[111] Alternatively, quantitative polymerase chain reaction analysis can be performed to evaluate genomic DNA for the presence of one or two copies of the RhD gene.[112]

If the fetus is at risk of expressing the antigen, fetal genotyping can be performed on cells obtained from either chorionic villus sampling or amniocentesis. Molecular genotyping is available for most clinically significant antigens; therefore, cordocentesis for fetal red cell phenotyping is not required. Noninvasive methods have been developed to obtain fetal DNA from maternal plasma. This testing is performed simultaneously with maternal and paternal genotyping. Such testing is complicated by the fact that the D-negative status can arise from multiple genetic variations.[113]

MANAGEMENT OF ALLOIMMUNIZATION DURING PREGNANCY

Intrauterine Red Cell Transfusions

Intrauterine transfusions are performed by direct infusion of allogeneic blood into the umbilical cord, the intrahepatic portion of the hepatic vein, or intraperitoneally. Red blood cells are selected to be group O, RhD-negative, Kell-negative, cytomegalovirus-seronegative, leukoreduced, irradiated, hemoglobin S–negative, and less than 72 hours old.[114,115] The unit must also be negative for the offending antigen and crossmatch-compatible with the maternal plasma. Kell-negative red cells are selected to eliminate the risk of immunizing the mother against an additional antigen that has been implicated in severe HDFN. Irradiated red blood cells are warranted to eliminate the risk of transfusion-transmitted graft-versus-host disease (GVHD), especially if maternal red cells are selected for transfusion. In the absence of compatible allogeneic blood, such as alloantibodies to high-frequency antigens, maternal blood is usually selected for transfusion. In rare situations, maternal ABO-mismatched blood is an acceptable source for intrauterine transfusion where antigen-compatible allogeneic blood is unavailable.[116]

The red cell unit should be plasma-reduced to a final hematocrit of 75% to 80%.[93] The red cells should be washed before transfusion if they are older than 7 days or of maternal origin.[117] Intrauterine transfusions become feasible around 20 weeks' gestation when safe cannulation of the umbilical cord can be performed.[118] Intrauterine red cell transfusions may be indicated for reasons other than red cell alloimmunization, including pure red cell aplasia from parvovirus B19 infection, fetomaternal hemorrhage, twin-to-twin transfusion, and hemoglobin Bart's (α-thalassemia with complete absence of all four α-globin genes).

The infant is paralyzed with a short-acting paralytic agent and then the needle is inserted into the umbilical vein under continuous ultrasound guidance. Blood samples are drawn for hematocrit and bilirubin. The amount of blood infused is based on a formula that takes into consideration the fetoplacental volume estimated by fetal weight using ultrasound, the fetal hematocrit, and the unit hematocrit (Fig. 36–4).[114] The final target hematocrit is usually 40%.[93] For severely anemic fetuses, the hematocrit should not be increased by more than fourfold at the first infusion.[119] Samples are also obtained at the completion of the transfusion for final hematocrit and for hemoglobin F quantitation to determine the ratio of transfused red blood cells to fetal red blood cells. Transfusions are repeated every 14 days or less, with the interval based on the rate of decline in the hematocrit from the previous transfusion. Severely affected fetuses may require transfusions as frequently as every 7 days. The final transfusion is performed at or before 35 weeks, with delivery planned at 37 weeks' gestation.

Fetal outcome is superior when intrauterine transfusions are begun before the onset of hydrops (mortality is 22% to 30% for hydropic and 2% to 8% for nonhydropic fetuses).[120,121] The vast majority of infants require only top-up transfusions in the neonatal period for management of their HDFN.[122] Intrauterine transfusions suppress erythropoiesis and can cause hypoproliferative anemia in the neonatal period, especially if the last transfusion occurs close to the time of delivery.[123] It is critical that infants born to alloimmunized mothers receive close follow-up so that late anemia is detected and managed appropriately.

A cohort study of 254 fetuses treated with 740 intrauterine transfusions for red cell alloimmunization between 1988 and 2001 documented the risk of fetal death from procedure-related complications at 1.6%.[124] In this series, the overall procedure-related complication rate was 3.1% (0.1% premature rupture of membranes, 0.3% infection, 2.0% emergency cesarean section, 0.9% fetal death, 0.7% neonatal death). Other known complications of intrauterine transfusion include circulatory overload, splenic rupture, and iron overload.[125–127] Bleeding from the puncture site is thought to occur more

$$\frac{\text{Desired PCV} - \text{Fetal PCV}}{\text{Donor PCV} - \text{Desired PCV}} \times \text{Fetoplacental blood volume}$$

PCV = Packed cell volume

Figure 36–4 Formula for the calculation of the volume of red blood cells required for an intrauterine transfusion. (From Rodeck CH, Dean A. Red cell allo-immunization. In Rodeck CJ, Whittle MJ (eds). Fetal Medicine: Basic Science and Clinical Practice. London, Churchill Livingstone, 1999, pp 785–804.)

frequently when thrombocytopenia and severe hydrops are present, with some physicians recommending routine platelet transfusions for infants with hydrops.[128] Transamniotic cord needling or arterial puncture is thought to increase the incidence of bleeding and both should be avoided. Infants should be closely monitored during and after the procedure. The procedure should be performed in close proximity to the operating room, so that if emergency cesarean section is required it can be performed without delay.

Despite severe fetal hemolytic disease, normal developmental outcome can be expected for children treated with intrauterine transfusions based on a study with long-term follow-up.[129] In this report, 40 children who survived severe HDFN were followed until age 62 months, and no difference was found in the global developmental quotient (101.9 +/− 9.5, compared to the mean for the normal population of 100). There was no correlation between the global developmental quotient and the severity of the HDFN (fetal hematocrit, fetal bilirubin, presence of hydrops fetalis, total number of intrauterine transfusions, duration of neonatal phototherapy, and number of neonatal exchange transfusions).

Intravenous Immunoglobulin

Intravenous immunoglobulin (IVIG) is effective in the postnatal treatment of infants affected with HDFN. In this setting, IVIG reduces the length of hospital stay, the duration of phototherapy, and the need for exchange transfusion (odds ratio, 0.28; CI, 0.17–0.47).[130] Prenatally, the reports of IVIG are limited to encouraging case reports[131] and case series[132,133]; thus, the efficacy of this therapy prenatally is unknown. Encouraging case reports have also been published on the use of plasma exchange and IVIG in the treatment of severe HDFN presenting before intrauterine transfusions are feasible.[134]

Phenobarbital Administration

The rate-limiting enzyme in bilirubin metabolism is bilirubin-UDP-glucuronosyltransferase (UGT1A1). By increasing the expression of UGT1A1, phenobarbital enhances the capacity of the neonatal liver to conjugate and eliminate bilirubin. Phenobarbital binds to a 290–base pair enhancer sequence on the gene for UGT1A1, leading to an increase in the production of this enzyme. A retrospective case-control study found prenatal administration to be effective in decreasing the need for exchange transfusion.[135] Intrauterine transfusions were continued until 35 weeks' gestation. After the last intrauterine transfusion, women were offered phenobarbital 30 mg orally three times a day for 10 days. Delivery was planned after the 10-day treatment. Of 71 women identified with HDFN, 33 were administered phenobarbital. Both the exchange transfusion rate (9% vs 52%, $p < 0.01$) and neonatal mortality rate (0% vs 24%) were reduced by the administration of phenobarbital. After adjusting for gestational age at delivery and neonatal peak total bilirubin, administration of phenobarbital decreased the relative risk of exchange transfusion (risk ratio, 0.23; 95% CI, 0.06–0.76). Halpin and colleagues also found promising results in an earlier report on phenobarbital.[136] These preliminary studies suggest that predelivery phenobarbital is an effective method to prevent exchange transfusion in documented HDFN.

Premature Delivery

Early delivery is performed in all cases of severe HDFN, usually between 35 and 37 weeks' gestation. No data exist to guide the exact timing of delivery in HDFN; however, once fetal lung maturity has been achieved and hemolysis is ongoing, delivery should be expedited.

NEONATAL ALLOIMMUNE THROMBOCYTOPENIA

Incidence

Neonatal alloimmune thrombocytopenia is a serious disorder resulting from platelet–antigen incompatibility between the mother and fetus. It is the most common cause of severe thrombocytopenia in an otherwise healthy infant.[137] Overall, 2.5% of women are HPA-1a negative, with 12% of these mothers having detectable anti-HPA-1a.[138] Thus, 1 of 350 pregnancies is alloimmunized with anti-HPA-1a. The risk of alloimmunization is highest in women who are HLA class II DRB3*0101 (DR52a).[139] The incidence of severe thrombocytopenia secondary to anti-HPA-1a is estimated at 1 in 1000 neonates.[140] The diagnosis is usually made after the discovery of unexpected neonatal thrombocytopenia or when an intracranial hemorrhage is visualized on a routine prenatal ultrasound. Approximately 10% to 20% of affected fetuses have intracranial hemorrhages, one quarter to one half of which occur in utero.[141] The initial platelet count is <20,000/μL in 50% of affected fetuses, including 46% of fetuses sampled before 24 weeks' gestation.[142] Fetuses with HPA-1a incompatibility have more severe thrombocytopenia than fetuses with other platelet–antigen incompatibilities. A history of antenatal intracranial hemorrhage in a sibling predicts a greater severity of thrombocytopenia in a subsequent fetus.[142] One report estimated a 79% risk of intracranial hemorrhage after a diagnosis of intracranial hemorrhage in a previous infant.[143] The literature strongly suggests that neonatal alloimmune thrombocytopenia is currently underdiagnosed.[144] In comparison to HDFN, where first children are rarely affected, 20% to 59% of NAIT cases occur during the first pregnancy.[141]

Etiology

HPA-1a and HPA-5b antibodies are implicated in approximately 80% and 10% of cases of neonatal alloimmune thrombocytopenia, respectively. In one series of 1162 serologically confirmed cases in the United States, the implicated antigens were HPA-1a (79%), HPA-5b (9%), HPA-1b (4%), HPA-3a (2%), and others (6%).[145] Antibody identification is performed using an enzyme-linked immunosorbent assay or monoclonal antibody immobilization of platelet antigens assay. PCR sequence-specific primer assays capable of testing for the 15 HPA allelic variants has been developed and allows for rapid and accurate HPA genotyping.[146] Alternatively, phenotyping can be performed using HPA monoclonal antibodies. Paternal genotyping is performed to determine if the chance of recurrence in a subsequent pregnancy is 100% (HPA-1a/1a) or 50% (HPA-1a/1b).

Management

Maternal Administration of Intravenous Immunoglobulin and Corticosteroids

The role of maternal IVIG, compared to IVIG plus dexamethasone, in the antenatal management of neonatal alloimmune thrombocytopenia was evaluated in a controlled trial of 54 affected pregnancies. No additional benefit was seen with the combination over IVIG alone. Overall, there was a mean platelet increase from the first to the second fetal blood sampling of 36,000/μL and from the first fetal blood sampling to birth of 69,000/μL. A total of 62% to 85% of fetuses responded.[147] In another report, 18 women who had previously delivered infants with severe alloimmune thrombocytopenia were treated with weekly 1 g/kg infusions of IVIG from the diagnosis of fetal thrombocytopenia until birth. Only three treated fetuses had platelet counts of less than 30,000/μL, compared with 16 of 20 untreated siblings.[148] If IVIG treatment fails to give a response, high-dose steroids (60 mg prednisone/day) are often added, although their efficacy is uncertain. Although the above data are limited, antenatal IVIG appears to be a promising therapy. Maternal IVIG is usually commenced when the fetal platelet count by cordocentesis is found to be less than 100,000/μL. Infants are followed for response by both cordocentesis and ultrasonography.

Intrauterine Platelet Transfusions

In the presence of persistent fetal thrombocytopenia, despite maternal IVIG therapy, frequent fetal blood sampling is required to monitor the severity of thrombocytopenia and to provide intrauterine platelet transfusion support for platelet counts of less than 50,0000 to 100,000/μL. Where required for severe thrombocytopenia, the first cordocentesis is usually performed at 22 to 24 weeks' gestation and is repeated at weekly intervals.[149] Antigen-negative, irradiated maternal platelets are recommended. The platelets should be irradiated to eliminate the risk of transfusion-transmitted GVHD. The platelets should be plasma-reduced to minimize the passive transfer of the maternal alloantibodies and resuspended in saline or compatible plasma. Pretransfusion and post-transfusion platelets counts are performed. The median drop in the platelet count after transfusion is approximately 24,000/μL per day; thus, the post-transfusion platelet count can be used to estimate the required interval between procedures.[150] The incidence of fetal loss at the time of each cordocentesis and intrauterine platelet transfusion is estimated at 0.6% to 1.2%.[149,151] Early delivery after achievement of fetal lung maturity is recommended.

Neonatal Platelet Transfusions

Often when a neonate with unexpected thrombocytopenia is suspected of having neonatal alloimmune thrombocytopenia, the management is problematic due to difficulty in obtaining compatible platelets for infusion. Where possible, plasma-depleted, irradiated maternal platelets are recommended because compatibility with maternal antibodies is assured. Maternal platelets can be collected from a unit of whole blood or by platelet apheresis. Where apheresis collection is not immediately available for the collection of maternal platelets, a unit of whole blood can be collected. Once obtained, the unit can be separated into its components in the hospital transfusion service and the autologous red cells can be transfused back to the mother. In addition, the maternal plasma must be tested for transmissible diseases, as required for all allogeneic units. The platelets are almost always required for emergency transfusion before the results of the transmissible disease testing are available. Where maternal platelets are unavailable or unsuitable, matched allogeneic platelets should be obtained. This can be complicated by the delay in obtaining compatible platelets due to the time required for laboratory confirmation of the diagnosis, the identification of compatible donors, the platelet apheresis collection, the donor transmissible disease testing, and the transport of the product to the hospital transfusion service. Several blood suppliers have evaluated the effectiveness of platelet concentrates collected from a panel of donors to maintain an "off-the-shelf" supply of HPA-1a/5b negative platelets, which would be appropriate for 90% of affected neonates.[152] The estimated cost of identifying one eligible HPA-1a/5b negative donor was £8,000, because several thousand donors must be screened to find an eligible donor. It was also suggested that HPA-1a/5b negative platelets be utilized for all neonates, thereby ensuring that most infants with neonatal alloimmune thrombocytopenia would be managed correctly from a platelet transfusion perspective and fewer units would be outdated. The ability to genotype donors on a large scale for HPA-1a/5b may be one means of generating an extensive list of eligible donors to maintain in-date stock of antigen-negative platelets by targeting these donors to enroll as apheresis platelet donors.

Neonatal Intravenous Immunoglobulin

The role of IVIG to treat thrombocytopenia after delivery has been less well-characterized but is often employed.[153] IVIG is usually administered in combination with HPA-matched platelets.

Prevention

Testing all pregnancies to identify women at risk of delivering children with neonatal alloimmune thrombocytopenia secondary to anti-HPA-1a has been studied.[154] The low rate of intracranial hemorrhage in affected pregnancies, the high complication rate from cordocentesis, the lack of certainty on the best course of treatment, and our inability to screen all pregnancies for all platelet alloantibodies have prevented the implementation of widespread population screening for this condition.[155] It is critical that all mothers delivering neonates with unexplained thrombocytopenia should be screened for antibodies implicated in neonatal alloimmune thrombocytopenia to ensure that future pregnancies are appropriately managed.

REFERENCES

1. Waterstone M, Bewley S, Wolfe C. Incidence and predictors of severe obstetric morbidity: case-control study. BMJ 2001;322:1089–1094.
2. Andolina K, Daly S, Roberts N, et al. Objective measurement of blood loss at delivery: Is it more than a guess? Am J Obstet Gynecol 1999; 180:S69.
3. Ueland K. Maternal cardiovascular dynamics. VII. Intrapartum blood volume changes. Am J Obstet Gynecol 1976;126:671–677.
4. Panchal S, Arria A, Labhsetwar S. Maternal morbidity during hospital admission for delivery: a retrospective analysis using a state-maintained database. Anesth Analg 2001;93:134–141.
5. Mousa HA, Walkinshaw S. Major postpartum haemorrhage. Curr Opin Obstet Gynecol 2001;13:595–603.

6. Goffinet F. Hémorragies de la délivrance. Gynecol Obstet Fertil 2000; 28:141–151.
7. Drife J. Management of primary postpartum hemorrhage. BJOG 1997; 104:275–277.
8. Meijer WE, Heerdink ER, Nolen WA, et al. Association of risk of abnormal bleeding with degree of serotonin reuptake inhibition by antidepressants. Arch Intern Med 2004;164:2367–2370.
9. Movig KL, Janssen MW, de Waal Malefijt J, et al. Relationship of serotonergic antidepressants and need for blood transfusion in orthopedic surgical patients. Arch Intern Med 2003;163:2354–2358.
10. Serdaroglu G, Tutuncuoglu S, Kavakli K, et al. Coagulation abnormalities and acquired von Willebrand's disease type 1 in children receiving valproic acid. J Child Neurol 2002;17:41–43.
11. Acharya S, Bussel JB. Hematologic toxicity of sodium valproate. J Pediatr Hematol Oncol 2000;22:62–65.
12. Magann EF, Evans S, Hutchinson M, et al. Postpartum hemorrhage after vaginal birth: an analysis of risk factors. South Med J 2005;98:419–422.
13. Dombrowski MP, Bottoms SF, Saleh AA, et al. Third stage of labor: analysis of duration and clinical practice. Am J Obstet Gynecol 1995; 172:1279–1284.
14. Magann EF, Evans S, Chauhan SP, et al. The length of the third stage of labor and the risk of postpartum hemorrhage. Obstet Gynecol 2005; 105:290–293.
15. Cheng YW, Hopkins LM, Caughey AB. How long is too long: does a prolonged second stage of labor in nulliparous women affect maternal and neonatal outcomes? Am J Obstet Gynecol 2004;191:933–938.
16. Olesen AW, Westergaard JG, Olsen J. Perinatal and maternal complications related to postterm delivery: a national register-based study, 1978–1993. Am J Obstet Gynecol 2003;189:222–227.
17. Haddad B, Barton JR, Livingston JC, et al. Risk factors for adverse maternal outcomes among women with HELLP (hemolysis, elevated liver enzymes, and low platelet count) syndrome. Am J Obstet Gynecol 2000;183:444–448.
18. Frederiksen Mc, Glassenberg R, Stika CS. Placenta previa: a 22-year analysis. Am J Obstet Gynecol 1999;180:1432–1437.
19. Rodgers A, walker N, Schug S, et al. Reducation of postoperative mortality and morbidity with epidural or spinal anesthesia: results from overview of randomized trials. BMJ 2000;321:1493–1497.
20. Kieser KE, Baskett TF. A 10-year population-based study of uterine rupture. Obstet Gynecol 2002;100:749–753.
21. Ofir K, Sheiner E, Levy A, et al. Uterine rupture: risk factors and pregnancy outcomes. Am J Obstet Gynecol 2003;189:1042–1046.
22. El-Refaey H, Rodeck C. Post-partum haemorrhage: definitions, medical and surgical management. A time for change. Br Med Bull 2003;67: 205–217.
23. Hoveyda F, MacKenzie IZ. Secondary postpartum haemorrhage: incidence, morbidity and current management. Br J Obstet Gynaecol 2001;108:927–930.
24. Liu S, Heaman M, Joseph KS, et al. Risk of Maternal postpartum readmission associated with mode of delivery. Obstet Gynecol 2005; 105:836–842.
25. Morales M, Ceysens G, Jastrow N, et al. Spontaneous delivery or manual removal of the placenta during caesarean section: a randomized controlled trial. Br J Obstet Gynaecol 2004;111:908–912.
26. Wilkinson C, Enkin MW. Manual removal of placenta at caesarean section. Cochrane Database Syst Rev 2, 2000;CD000130.
27. Baksu A, Kalan A, Ozkan A, et al. The effect of placental removal method and site of uterine repair on postcesarean endometritis and operative blood loss. Acta Obstet Gynecol Scand 2005;84:266–269.
28. Magann EF, Chauhan SP, Bufkin L, et al. Intra-operative haemorrhage by blunt versus sharp expansion of the uterine incision at caesarean delivery: a randomised clinical trial. BJOG 2002;109:448–452.
29. Villar J, Gülmezoglu AM, Hofmeyr GJ, et al. Systematic review of randomized controlled trials of misoprostol to prevent postpartum hemorrhage. Obstet Gynecol 2002;100:1301–1312.
30. Gülmezoglu AM, Villar J, Ngoc NTN, et al. WHO multicentre randomized trial of misoprostol in the management of the thirs stage of labour. Lancet 2001;358:689–695.
31. Çaliskan E, Dilbaz B, Meydanli MM, et al. Oral misoprostol for the third stage of labour: a randomized controlled trial. Obstet Gynecol 2003;101:921–928.
32. Davies GAL, Tessier JL, Woodman MC, et al. Maternal hemodynamics after oxytocin bolus compared with infusion in the third stage of labor: a randomized controlled trial. Obstet Gynecol 2005;105:294–299.
33. Bhullar A, Carlan SJ, Hamm J, et al. Buccal misoprostol to decrease blood loss after vaginal delivery: a randomized trial. Obstet Gynecol 2004;104:1282–1288.
34. Walraven G, Dampha Y, Bittaye B, et al. Misoprostol in the treatment of postpartum haemorrhage in addition to routine management: a placebo controlled trial. Br J Obstet Gynaecol 2004;111:1014–1017.
35. Silverman JA, Barrett J, Callum JL. The appropriateness of red blood cell transfusions in the peripartum patient. Obstet Gynecol 2004;104: 1000–1004.
36. Confidential Enquiries into Maternal Deaths. Why Mothers Die: Triennial Report 1997–1999. London, RCOG Press, 2001.
37. Rizvi F, Mackey R, Barrett T, et al. Successful reduction of massive postpartum haemorrhage by use of guidelines and staff education. Br J Obstet Gynaecol 2004;111:495–498.
38 Guidelines on use of oxytocics by the Society of Obstetricians and Gynecologists of Canada. Available at http://www.sogc.org/guidelines/public/88e%2Dcpg%2Dapril2000.pdf
39. Bouwmeester FW, Jonkhoff AR, Verheijen RHM, et al. Successful treatment of lifethreatening postpartum hemorrhage with recombinant activated factor VII. Obstet Gynecol 2003;101:1174–1176.
40. Boehlen F, Morales MA, Fontana P, et al. Prolonged treatment of massive postpartum haemorrhage with recombinant factor VIIa: case report and review of the literature. Br J Obstet Gynaecol 2004;111:284–287.
41. Ahonen J, Jokela R. Recombinant factor VIIa for life-threatening postpartum haemorrhage. Br J Anaesth 2005;94:592–595.
42. Lodge JP, Jonas S, Oussoultzoglou E, et al. Recombinant coagulation factor VIIa in major liver resection: a randomized, placebo-controlled, double-blind clinical trial. Anesthesiology 2005;102:269–275.
43. Bosch J, Thabut D, Bendtsen F, et al. Recombinant factor VIIa for upper gastrointestinal bleeding in patients with cirrhosis: a randomized, double-blind trial. Gastroenterology 2004;127:1123–1130.
44. Boffard KD, Riou B, Warren B, et al. Recombinant factor VIIa as adjunctive therapy for bleeding control in severely injured trauma patients: two parallel randomized, placebo-controlled, double-blind clinical trials. J Trauma 2005;59:8–18.
45. Mayer SA, Brun NC, Begtrup K, et al. Recombinant activated factor VII for acute intracerebral hemorrhage. NEJM 2005;352:777–785.
46. Friederich PW, Henny CP, Messelink EJ, et al. Effect of recombinant activated factor VII on perioperative blood loss in patients undergoing retropubic prostatectomy: a double-blind placebo-controlled randomised trial. Lancet 2003;361:201–205.
47. Levi M, Cromheecke ME, de Jonge E, et al. Pharmacological strategies to decrease excessive blood loss in cardiac surgery: a meta-analysis of clinically relevant endpoints. Lancet 1999;354:1940–1947.
48. Ho KM, Ismail H. Use of intravenous tranexamic acid to reduce allogeneic blood transfusion in total hip and knee arthroplasty: a meta-analysis. Anaesth Intensive Care 2003;31:529–537.
49. Boylan JF, Klinck JR, Sandler AN, et al. Tranexamic acid reduces blood loss, transfusion requirements, and coagulation factor use in primary orthotopic liver transplantation. Anesthesiology 1996;85:1043–1048.
50. Dunn CJ, Goa KL. Tranexamic acid: a review of its use in surgery and other indications. Drugs 1999;57:1005–1032.
51. Deux J-F, Bazot M, Le Blanche AF, et al. Is selective embolization of uterine arteries a safe alternative to hysterectomy in patients with postpartum hemorrhage? AJR Am J Roentgenol 2001;177:145–149.
52. Stancato-Pasik A, Mitty HA, Richard HM III, et al. Obstetric embolotherapy: effect on menses and pregnancy. Radiology 1997;204:791–793.
53. Gilbert WM, Moore TR, Resnik R, et al. Angiographic embolization in the management of hemorrhagic complications of pregnancy. Am J Obstet Gynecol 1992;166:493–497.
54. Greenwood LH, Glickman MG, Schwartz PE, et al. Obstetric and nonmalignant gynecologic bleeding: treatment with angiographic embolization. Radiology 1987;164:155–159.
55. Deux J-F, Bazot M, Le Blanche AF, et al. Is selective embolization of uterine arteries a safe alternative to hysterectomy in patients with postpartum hemorrhage? AJR Am J Roentgenol 2001;177:145–149.
56. Wang H, Garmel S. Successful term pregnancy after bilateral uterine artery embolization for post-partum hemorrhage. Obstet Gynecol 2003; 102:603–604.
57. Ornan D, White R, Pollak J, et al. Pelvic embolization for intractable postpartum hemorrhage: long-term follow-up and implications for fertility. Obstet Gynecol 2003;102:904–910.
58. Bloom AI, Verstandig A, Gielchinsky Y, et al. Arterial embolisation for persistent primary postpartum haemorrhage: before or after hysterectomy? Br J Obstet Gynaecol 2004;111:880–884,.
59. Oei SG, Kho SN, ten Broeke EDM, et al. Arterial balloon occlusion of the hypogastric arteries: a life-saving procedure for severe obstetric hemorrhage. Am J Obstet Gynecol 2001;185:1255–1256.
60. Hayman RG, Arulkumaran S, Steer PJ. Uterine compression sutures: Surgical management of postpartum hemorrhage. Obstet Gynecol 2002; 99:502–506.

61. Hebisch G, Huch A. Vaginal uterine artery ligation avoids high blood loss and puerperal hysterectomy in postpartum hemorrhage. Obstet Gynecol 2002;100:574–578.
62. Abdrabbo SA. Stepwise uterine devascularization: a novel technique for management of uncontrolled postpartum hemorrhage with preservation of the uterus. Am J Obstet Gynecol 1994;171:694–700.
63. Forna F, Miles AM, Jamieson DJ. Emergency peripartum hysterectomy: a comparison of cesarean and postpartum hysterectomy. Am J Obstet Gynecol 2004;190:1440–1444.
64. Tulandi T, Yusuf N, Posner BI. Diabetes insipidus: a postpartum complication. Obstet Gynecol 1987;70:492–495.
65. Karparti PCJ, Rossignol M, Pirot M, et al. High incidence of myocardial ischemia during postpartum hemorrhage. Anesthesiology 2004;100:30–36.
66. Judd JW, for the Scientific Section Coordinating Committee of the AABB. Practice guidelines for prenatal and perinatal immunohematology, revisited. Transfusion 2001;41:1445–1452.
67. British Committee for Standards in Haematology, Blood Transfusion Task Force. Guidelines for blood grouping and red cell antibody testing during pregnancy. Transf Med 1996;6:71–74.
68. American Association of Blood Banks. Standards for Blood Banks and Transfusion Services, 22nd ed. Bethesda, Md., AABB, 2003.
69. ACOG Practice Bulletin. Prevention of Rh D alloimmunization. Int J Gynaecol Obstet 1999;66:63–70.
70. Domen RE. Policies and procedures related to weak D phenotype testing and Rh immune globulin administration. Arch Pathol Lab Med 2000;124:1118–1121.
71. Lubenko A, Contreras M, Habash J. Should anti-Rh immunoglobulin be given D variant women? Br J Haematol 1989;72:429–433.
72. Cannon M, Pierce R, Taber EB, et al. Fatal hydrops fetalis caused by anti-D in a mother with partial D. Obstet Gynecol 2003;102: 1143–1145.
73. Bowman JM, Chown B, Lewis M, et al. Rh isoimmunization during pregnancy: antenatal prophylaxis. CMAJ 1978;118:623–627.
74. Rothenberg JM, Weirermiller B, Dirig K, et al. Is a third-trimester antibody screen in Rh+ women necessary? Am J Manag Care 1999;5: 1145–1150.
75. Heddle NM, Klama L, Frassetto R, et al. A retrospective study to determine the risk of red cell alloimmunization and transfusion during pregnancy. Transfusion 1993;23:217–220.
76. Larsen R, Titlestad K, Lillevang ST, et al. Cesarean section: is pretransfusion testing for red cell alloantibodies necessary? Acta Obstet Gynecol Scand 2005;84:448–455.
77. Pollack W, Gorman JG, Freda VJ, et al. Results of clinical trials of RhoGAM in women. Transfusion 1968;8:151–153.
78. Hartwell EA. Use of Rh immune globulin. ASCP Practice Parameter. Am J Clin Pathol 1998;110:281–292.
79. Nicolaides KH, Clewell WH, Rodeck CH. Measurement of human fetoplacental blood volume in erythroblastosis fetalis. Am J Obstet Gynecol 1987;157:50–53.
80. BCSH Blood Transfusion and General Haematology Task Forces Working Party. The estimation of fetomaternal haemorrhage. Transfus Med 1999;9:87–92.
81. Pourbabak S, Rund CR, Crookston KP. Three cases of massive fetomaternal hemorrhage presenting without clinical suspicion. Arch Pathol Lab Med 2004;128:463–465.
82. Chen JC, Davis BH, Wood B, et al. Multicenter clinical experience with flow cytometric method for fetomaternal hemorrhage detection. Cytometry 2002;50:285–290.
83. Bowman JM. Controversies in Rh prophylaxis: who needs Rh immune globulin and when should it be given? Am J Obstet Gynecol 1985;151:289–294.
84. Smith DB, Lawlor E, Power J. A second outbreak of hepatitis C virus infection from anti-D immunoglobulin in Ireland. Vox Sang 76:175–80, 1999.
85. Watanabe KK, Busch MP, Schreiber GB. Evaluation of the safety of Rh immunoglobulin by monitoring viral markers among Rh-negative female blood donors. Vox Sang 2000;78:1–6.
86. Hong F, Ruiz R, Price H. Safety profile of WinRho anti-D. Semin Hematol 1998;35:9–13.
87. Davis BH, Olsen S, Bigelow NC, et al. Detection of fetal red cells in fetomaternal hemorrhage using a fetal hemoglobin monoclonal antibody by flow cytometry. Transfusion 1998;38:749–756.
88. Martin JA, Hamilton BE, Ventura SJ, et al. Births: final data for 2000. Nat Vital Stat Rep 2002;50:1–101.
89. Howard H, Martlew V, McFadyen I, et al. Consequences for fetus and neonate of maternal red cell allo-immunisation. Arch Dis Child Fetal Neonat 1998;78:F62–F66.
90. Bowman J. The management of hemolytic disease in the fetus and newborn. Semin Perinatol 1997;21:39–44.
91. Spong CY, Porter AE, Queenan JT. Management of isoimmunization in the presence of multiple maternal antibodies. Am J Obstet Gynecol 2001;185:481–484.
92. Filbey D, Berseus O, Sandstrom B, et al. The evaluation of maternal anti-D concentrations during pregnancy. Early Hum Dev 1987;15:1–9.
93. Moise KJ. Red blood cell alloimmunization in pregnancy. Semin Hematol 2005;42:169–178.
94. van Dijk BA, Dooren MC, Overbeeke MA. Red cell antibodies in pregnancy: there is no "critical titre." Transfus Med 1995;5:199–202.
95. Fleetwood P, De Silva PM, Knight RC. Clinical significance of red cell antibody concentration in pregnancy (abstract). Brit J Haematol 1996;93(Suppl 1):13.
96. Bowman JM, Pollock JM, Manning FA, et al. Maternal Kell blood group alloimmunization. Obstet Gynecol 1992;79:239–244.
97. Vengelen-Tyler V (ed). Technical Manual, 13th ed. Bethesda, Md., American Association of Blood Banks, 1999.
98. Spinnato JA. Hemolytic disease of the fetus: a plea for restraint. Obstet Gynecol 1992;80:873–877.
99. Hadley AG. Laboratory assays for predicting the severity of haemolytic disease of the fetus and newborn. Transpl Immunol 2002;10:191–198.
100. Garner SF, Gorick BD, Lai WY, et al. Prediction of the severity of haemolytic disease of the newborn. Quantitative IgG anti-D subclass determinations explain the correlation with functional assay results. Vox Sang 1995;68:169–176.
101. Bullock R, Martin WL, Coomarasamy A, et al. Prediction of fetal anemia in pregnancies with red-cell alloimmunization: comparison of middle cerebral artery peak systolic velocity and amniotic fluid OD450. Ultrasound Obstet Gynecol 2005;25:331–334.
102. Mari G, Deter RL, Carpenter RL, et al. Noninvasive diagnosis by Doppler ultrasonography of fetal anemia due to maternal red-cell alloimmunization. Collaborative Group for Doppler Assessment of the Blood Velocity in Anemic Fetuses. NEJM 2000;342:9–14.
103. van Dongen H, Klumper FJ, Sikkel E, et al. Non-invasive tests to predict fetal anemia in Kell-alloimmunized pregnancies. Ultrasound Obstet Gynecol 2005;25:341–345.
104. Pereira L, Jenkins TM, Berghella V. Conventional management of maternal red cell alloimmunization compared with management by Doppler assessment of middle cerebral artery peak systolic velocity. Am J Obstet Gynecol 2003;189:1002–1006.
105. Liley AW. Liqour amnii analysis in the management of pregnancy complicated by Rhesus sensitization. Am J Obstet Gynecol 1961;82:1359.
106. Rahman F, Detti L, Ozcan T, et al. Can a single measurement of amniotic fluid delta optical density be safely used in the clinical management of Rhesus-alloimmunized pregnancies before 27 weeks gestation? Acta Obstet Gynecol Scand 1998;77:804–807.
107. Bowman JM, Pollock JM. Transplacental fetal hemorrhage after amniocentesis. Obstet Gynecol 1995;66:749–754.
108. Seeds JW. Diagnostic mid trimester amniocentesis: how safe? Am J Obstet Gynecol 2004;191:607–615.
109. Ghidini A, Sepulveda W, Lockwood CJ, et al. Complications of fetal blood sampling. Am J Obstet Gynecol 1993;168:1339–1344.
110. Daffos F, Capella-Pavlovsky M, Forestier F. Fetal blood sampling during pregnancy with use of a needle guided by ultrasound: a study of 606 consecutive cases. Am J Obstet Gynecol 1985;153:655–660.
111. Morrant AE. The Distribution of Human Blood Group and Other Polymorphisms, 2nd ed. London, Oxford University Press, 1975.
112. Rossa W, Chiu K, Murphy MF, et al. Determination of Rh D zygosity: Comparison of a double amplification refractory mutation system approach and a multiplex real-time quantitative PCR approach. Clin Chem 2001;47: 667–672.
113. Daniels G, Finning K, Martin P, et al. Fetal blood group genotyping from DNA from maternal plasma: an important advance in the management and prevention of haemolytic disease of the fetus and newborn. Vox Sang 2004;87:225–232.
114. Mollison PL. Blood Transfusion in Clinical Medicine, 10th ed. Oxford, UK, Blackwell Science, 1997, pp 408–409.
115. AABB Technical Manual, 14th ed. Bethesda, Md., AABB Press, 2002, pp 504–505.
116. Denomme GA, Ryan G, Seaward PG, et al. Maternal ABO-mismatched blood for intrauterine transfusion of severe hemolytic disease of the newborn due to anti-Rh17. Transfusion 2004;44:1357–1360.
117. Mintz PD. In Mintz PD (ed), Transfusion Therapy. Clinical Principles and Practice, 2nd ed. Bethesda, Md., AABB Press, 2005, pp 159–168.
118. Sampson AJ, Permezel M, Doyle LW, et al. Ultrasound guided fetal intravascular transfusions for severe erythroblastosis, 1984–1993. Aust NZ J Obstet Gynecol 2004;34:125–130.

119. Radunovic N, Lockwood CJ, Alvarez M, et al. The severely anemic and hydropic isoimmune fetus: changes in final hematocrit associated with intrauterine death. Obstet Gynecol 1992;79:390–393.
120. Schumacher B, Moise KJ. Fetal transfusion for red blood cell alloimmunization in pregnancy. Obstet Gynecol 1996;88:137–150.
121. Van Kamp IL, Klumper FJCM, Bakkum RSLA, et al. The severity of immune fetal hydrops is predictive of fetal outcome after intrauterine treatment. Am J Obstet Gynecol 2001;185:668–673.
122. Koenig JM, Ashton RD, De Vore GR, et al. Late hyporegenerative anemia in Rh hemolytic disease. J Pediatr 1989;115:315–318.
123. Saade GR, Moise KJ Jr, Belfort MA, et al. Fetal and neonatal hematologic parameters in red cell alloimmunization: predicting the need for late neonatal transfusions. Fetal Diagn Ther 1993;8:161–164.
124. Van Kamp IL, Klumper FJ, Oepkes D, et al. Complications of intrauterine intravascular transfusion for fetal anemia due to maternal red-cell alloimmunization. Am J Obstet Gynecol 2005;192:171–177.
125. Whitecar PW, Depcik-Smith ND, Strauss RA, et al. Fetal splenic rupture following transfusion. Obstet Gynecol 2001;97:824–825.
126. Sreenan C, Idikio HA, Osiovich H. Successful chelation therapy in a case of neonatal iron overload following intravascular intrauterine transfusion. J Perinatol 2000;20:509–512.
127. Welch R, Rampling MW, Anwar A, et al. Changes in hemorheology with fetal intravascular transfusion. Am J Obstet Gynecol 1994;170:726–732.
128. Harman CR. Invasive techniques in the management of alloimmune anemia. In Hartman CR (ed). Invasive Fetal Testing and Treatment. Boston, Blackwell Scientific, 1995, pp 107–191.
129. Hudon L, Moise KJ Jr, Hegemier SE, et al. Long-term neurodevelopmental outcome after intrauterine transfusion for the treatment of fetal hemolytic disease. Am J Obstet Gynecol 1998;179:858–863.
130. Gottstein R, Cooke RWI. Systematic review of intravenous immunoglobulin in haemolytic disease of the newborn. Arch Dis Child Fetal Neonatal 2003;88:F6–F10.
131. Porter TF, Silver RM, Jackson GM, et al. Intravenous immune globulin in the management of severe Rh D hemolytic disease. Obstet Gynecol Surv 1997;52:193–197.
132. Gottvall T, Selbing A. Alloimmunization during pregnancy treated with high dose intravenous immunoglobulin. Effects on fetal hemoglobin concentration and anti-D concentrations in the mother and fetus. Acta Obstet Gynecol Scand 1995;74:777–783.
133. Margulies M, Voto LS, Mathet E, et al. High-dose intravenous IgG for the treatment of severe Rhesus alloimmunization. Vox Sang 1991;61: 181–189.
134. Fernandez-Jimenez MC, Jimenez-Marco MT, Hernandez D, et al. Treatment with plasmapheresis and intravenous immunoglobulin in pregnancies complicated with anti-PP1Pk or anti-K immunization: a report of two patients. Vox Sang 2001;80:117–120.
135. Trevett TN, Dorman K, Lamvu G, et al. Antenatal maternal administration of phenobarbital for the prevention of exchange transfusion in neonates with hemolytic disease of the fetus and newborn (HDFN). Am J Obstet Gynecol 2005;192:478–482.
136. Halpin TF, Jones AR, Bishop HL, et al. Prophylaxis of neonatal hyperbilirubinemia with phenobarbital. Obstet Gynecol 1972;40:85–90.
137. Dreyfus M, Kaplan C, Verdy E, et al. Frequency of immune thrombocytopenia in newborns: a prospective study. Immune Thrombocytopenia Working Group. Blood 1997;89:4402–4406.
138. Williamson LM, Hackett G, Rennie J, et al. The natural history of fetomaternal alloimmunization to the platelet-specific antigen HPA-1a as determined by antenatal screening. Blood 1998;92:2280–2287.
139. Décary F, L'Abbé D, Tremblay L, et al. The immune response to the HPA-1a antigen: association with HLA-DRw52a. Transfus Med 1991; 1:55–59.
140. Dreyfus M, Kaplan C, Verdy E, et al. Frequency of immune thrombocytopenia in newborns: a prospective study. Immune Thrombocytopenia Working Group. Blood 1997;89:4402–4406.
141. Mueller-Eckhardt C, Kiefel V, Grubert A, et al. 348 cases of suspected neonatal alloimmune thrombocytopenia. Lancet 1989;18:363–366.
142. Bussel JB, Zabusky MR, Berkowitz RL, et al. Fetal alloimmune thrombocytopenia. NEJM 1997;337:22–26.
143. Radder CM, Brand A, Kanhai HH. Will it ever be possible to balance the risk of intracranial haemorrhage in fetal or neonatal alloimmune thrombocytopenia against the risk of treatment strategies to prevent it? Vox Sang 2003;84:318–325.
144. Davoren A, McParland P, Barnes CA, et al. Neonatal alloimmune thrombocytopenia in the Irish population: a discrepancy between observed and expected cases. J Clin Pathol 2002;55:289–292.
145. Davoren A, Curtis BR, Aster RH, et al. Human platelet antigen-specific alloantibodies implicated in 1162 cases of neonatal alloimmune thrombocytopenia. Transfusion 2004;44:1220–1225.
146. Jones DC, Bunce M, Fuggle SV, et al. Human platelet alloantigens (HPAs): PCR-SSP genotyping of a UK population for 15 HPA alleles. Eur J Immunogenet 2003;30:415–419.
147. Bussel JB, Berkowitz RL, Lynch L, et al. Antenatal management of alloimmune thrombocytopenia with intravenous gamma-globulin: a randomized trial of the addition of low-dose steroid to intravenous gamma-globulin. Am J Obstet Gynecol 1996;174:1414–1423.
148. Lynch L, Bussel JB, McFarland JG, et al. Antenatal treatment of alloimmune thrombocytopenia. Obstet Gynecol 1992;80:67–71.
149. Overton TG, Duncan KR, Jolly M, et al. Serial aggressive platelet transfusion for fetal alloimmune thrombocytopenia: platelet dynamics and perinatal outcome. Am J Obstet Gynecol 2002;186:826–831.
150. Nicolini U, Tannirandorn Y, Gonzalez P, et al. Continuing controversy in alloimmune thrombocytopenia: fetal hyperimmunoglobulinemia fails to prevent thrombocytopenia. Am J Obstet Gynecol 1990;163:1144–1146.
151. Hohlfeld P, Forestier F, Kaplan C, et al. Fetal thrombocytopenia: a retrospective survey of 5,194 fetal blood samplings. Blood 1994;84: 1851–1856.
152. Allen DL, Samol J, Benjamin S, et al. Survey of the use and clinical effectiveness of HPA-1a/5b-negative platelet concentrates in proven or suspected platelet alloimmunization. Transfus Med 2004;14:409–441.
153. Bussel JB. Alloimmune thrombocytopenia in the fetus and newborn. Semin Thromb Hemostas 2001;27:245–252.
154. Davoren A, McParland P, Crowley J, et al. Antenatal screening for human platelet antigen-1a: results of a prospective study at a large maternity hospital in Ireland. Br J Obstet Gynaecol 2003;110:492–496.
155. Bussel JB. Alloimmune thrombocytopenia in the fetus and newborn. Semin Thromb Hemostas 2001;27:245–252.

Chapter 37

Transfusion of Neonates and Pediatric Patients

Cassandra D. Josephson • Ronald G. Strauss*

The principles of transfusion support for older children and adolescents are similar to those for adults, but infants and younger children have many special needs. Therefore, administration of each component to each of these two age groups is discussed separately. Because many issues dealing with transfusion therapy in adults, as discussed in other chapters, apply to older children, the bulk of information in this chapter deals with transfusion in infants and younger children. The following types of components for transfusion will be discussed as they apply to neonates and pediatric patients: red blood cells (RBCs), platelets (PLTs), and neutrophils (granulocytes), fresh frozen plasma (FFP), and cryoprecipitate. General guidelines and recommendations are given for pediatric blood component transfusions. However, it is important that they be adapted to fit local standards of practice. In particular, terms used to describe clinical conditions, such as *severe* and *symptomatic,* must be defined by local physicians.

RED BLOOD CELL TRANSFUSIONS

Older Children and Adolescents

Red blood cells, the most frequently transfused blood component, are given to increase the oxygen-carrying capacity of the blood, the goal being to maintain satisfactory tissue oxygenation. Guidelines for RBC transfusions in older children and adolescents are similar to those for adults (Table 37–1).[1] However, transfusions may be given more stringently to children, because normal hemoglobin (Hb) levels are lower in healthy children than in adults, and most children do not have the concomitant cardiorespiratory and vascular diseases that develop with aging in adults, who then may require more aggressive RBC transfusions.[2] Therefore, children generally have greater abilities to compensate for anemia and may be transfused at lower Hb or hematocrit (Hct) levels.

In the perioperative period or after resuscitation for trauma, it is unnecessary for most children to maintain Hb levels greater than 8.0 g/dL or Hct greater than 24%, a level frequently desired for adults. There should be a compelling reason to administer any postoperative RBC transfusion, because most children (without continued bleeding) can quickly restore their RBC volume if given iron and adequate nutritional therapy.[3] As is true for adults, the most important measures in the treatment of acute hemorrhage occurring with surgery or injury are first to control the hemorrhage and restore blood volume and tissue perfusion with crystalloid and/or colloid solutions. Then, if the estimated blood loss is greater than 25% of the circulating blood volume (i.e., >17 mL/kg body weight) and the patient's condition remains unstable, RBC transfusions may be indicated.

In acutely ill children with severe cardiac or pulmonary disease, particularly in those who require assisted ventilation, it is common practice to maintain the Hb level close to the normal range at a level of 100 to 110 g/L (10 to 11 g/dL) or Hct at 30% to 33%. Although this practice seems logical, its efficacy has not been documented by controlled scientific studies in children, and it has been challenged.[3] The variability of practices in critical care settings was demonstrated by a survey administered to Canadian, French, Belgium, and Swiss pediatric intensivists regarding transfusion practices in a tertiary care pediatric setting. They were queried about patients with bronchiolitis, septic shock, trauma, and about postoperative care of a patient with tetralogy of Fallot. The pretransfusion Hb transfusion "trigger" was 7 to 13 g/dL for the majority of scenarios.[4]

Randomized prospective studies are needed to define optimal pediatric practices because liberal RBC transfusion practices in critically ill adults have been reported to have detrimental effects.[5] A similar harmful effect has been proposed in a retrospective cohort study, including 240 critically ill children (131 transfused and 109 nontransfused; mean age, 5.5 years) with mean initial Hb levels of 7.4 ± 1.4 g/dL, where the number of days of oxygen use, mechanical ventilation, vasoactive agents used, and pediatric intensive care unit and hospital lengths of stay were all significantly increased in association with RBC transfusion.[6] Hospital mortality in the transfused group was 6.9% versus 0.9% ($p = 0.43$) in the nontransfused group. However, mortality could not be adequately evaluated due to the limited number of deaths observed in the study. Overall, the investigators concluded that RBC transfusions are associated with an increase in

*This work was supported in part by National Institutes of Health Program Project Grant P01 HL46925. Transfusions of blood components are mandatory for modern management in many premature infants, children with cancer and hematologic disorders, recipients of hematopoietic progenitor cell transplants and organ allografts, and children undergoing various surgical procedures. Although transfusions can be lifesaving, they are not without risks. Accordingly, they should be given only when true benefits are likely—for example, to correct a deficiency or functional defect of a blood component that has caused or threatens to cause a clinically significant problem. Because of the extended life span of children after transfusions, it is critical to avoid post-transfusion complications that may lead to progressive morbidity and mortality and to considerable expense over the years (e.g., hepatitis).

Table 37–1 Authors' Guidelines for Transfusing Children and Adolescents*

Red Blood Cells
Hemoglobin < 13.0 g/dL (Hct < 40%) with *severe* cardiopulmonary disease
Hemoglobin < 8.0 g/dL (Hct < 24%) in the perioperative period
Hemoglobin < 8.0 g/dL (Hct < 24%) with *symptomatic* chronic anemia
Hemoglobin < 8.0 g/dL (Hct < 24%) with marrow failure
Acute loss >25% estimated blood volume
Platelets
Blood platelets < 50 × 10^9/L and *significant* bleeding
Blood platelets < 50 × 10^9/L and invasive procedure
Blood platelets < 20 × 10^9/L prophylaxis with bleeding risk factors
Blood platelets < 10 × 10^9/L prophylaxis without bleeding risk factors
Platelet dysfunction with bleeding or invasive procedure
Neutrophils
Blood neutrophils < 0.5 × 10^9/L and bacterial infection unresponsive to antibiotics
Blood neutrophils < 0.5 × 10^9/L and yeast or fungal infection progressing or appearing during treatment with antimicrobials
Neutrophil dysfunction with bacterial, yeast, or fungal infection unresponsive to antimicrobials

*Words in italics must be defined according to local practices.
Hct, hematocrit.

resource utilization in this patient population. Importantly, due to the study's retrospective nature a true cause-and-effect relationship between transfusions and adverse outcomes could not be proven. Obviously, a randomized, controlled clinical trial is essential to help clinicians make more evidence-based decisions regarding when to transfuse RBCs to critically ill children.[6]

With anemias that develop slowly, the decision to transfuse RBCs should not be based solely on the blood Hb concentration, because children with chronic anemias may be asymptomatic despite very low Hb levels. Children with iron deficiency anemia, for example, often are treated successfully with oral iron alone, even at Hb levels lower than 5.0 g/dL. Factors other than Hb concentration that must be considered in the decision to transfuse RBCs include the patient's symptoms, signs, and functional capacities; the presence or absence of cardiorespiratory and central nervous system disease; the cause and anticipated course of the underlying anemia; and use of alternative therapies such as iron or recombinant human erythropoietin (EPO) therapy, the latter of which has been demonstrated to reduce the need for RBC transfusions and to improve the overall condition of children with chronic renal insufficiency. In anemias that are likely to be permanent (e.g., thalassemia, hemoglobinopathies), the effects of anemia on growth and development (which might be ameliorated by RBC transfusions) must be balanced against the potential toxicities of repeated transfusions (e.g., iron overload).

Infants and Younger Children

Pathophysiology of the Anemia of Prematurity

All infants experience a decline in circulating RBC volume during the first weeks of life. This decline results both from physiologic factors and, in sick preterm infants, from phlebotomy blood losses for laboratory monitoring. In healthy full-term infants, the nadir Hb value rarely is lower than 9.0 g/dL at age 10 to 12 weeks. The decline is more rapid (i.e., nadir at age 4 to 6 weeks) and the blood Hb concentration falls to lower levels in infants born prematurely—to approximately 8.0 g/dL in infants with birth weights of 1.0 to 1.5 kg and to approximately 7.0 g/dL in infants with birth weights lower than 1.0 kg.[7–9] Because this postnatal drop in Hb level in full-term infants is well tolerated, it is commonly referred to as the *physiologic anemia of infancy*. However, the pronounced decline in Hb concentration that occurs in many extremely preterm infants is associated with abnormal clinical signs and the need for RBC transfusions. Therefore, the *anemia of prematurity* is not accepted to be a normal, benign event.[10,11]

Many interacting physiologic factors are responsible for the anemia of prematurity. A key reason that the Hb nadir is lower in preterm than in full-term infants is the former group's diminished plasma EPO level in response to anemia.[9,12–15] Although anemia provokes EPO production in premature infants, the plasma levels achieved in anemic infants, at any given Hct, are lower than those observed in comparably anemic older persons.[14] Erythroid progenitor cells in blood[16] and bone marrow[17] of preterm infants are quite responsive to EPO in vitro—a finding suggesting that inadequate production of EPO is the major cause of physiologic anemia, not marrow unresponsiveness.

The mechanisms responsible for the diminished EPO output by preterm neonates are only partially defined. One factor is that the primary site of EPO production in preterm infants is the liver rather than the kidneys.[18,19] Because the liver is less sensitive to anemia and tissue hypoxia, a relatively sluggish EPO response to the falling Hct occurs. The timing of the switch from liver to kidney is set at conception and is not accelerated by preterm birth. Viewed from a teleologic perspective, decreased hepatic production of EPO under in utero conditions of tissue hypoxia may be an advantage for the fetus. If this were not the case, normal levels of fetal hypoxia could trigger high levels of EPO and produce marked erythrocytosis and consequent hyperviscosity in utero. After birth, however, diminished EPO responsiveness to tissue hypoxia is disadvantageous and leads to anemia because of impaired compensation for the falling Hct.

Diminished EPO production cannot entirely explain low plasma EPO levels in preterm infants, however. Extraordinarily high plasma levels of EPO were reported in some fetuses of postconceptional age, comparable to those of neonates treated in intensive care settings,[20,21] and macrophages from human cord blood were found to produce normal quantities of EPO messenger RNA and protein.[22] These studies documented intact synthetic capability, at least under some circumstances. Therefore, additional mechanisms are likely to contribute to diminished plasma EPO levels. For example, plasma EPO levels undoubtedly are influenced by metabolism (clearance) as well as by production. Data obtained in human infants[23,24] and in neonatal monkeys[25] demonstrate that low plasma EPO levels may result from increased plasma clearance and volume of distribution and from shorter fractional elimination and mean residence times for EPO in neonates compared with adults. Therefore, accelerated catabolism may contribute to the low plasma levels—with the low plasma EPO in infants possibly representing the combined effects of decreased synthesis and increased metabolism.

Phlebotomy blood losses play a key role in the anemia of prematurity. The modern practice of neonatology requires critically ill neonates to be monitored closely with serial laboratory studies such as blood gases, electrolytes, blood counts, and cultures. Small preterm infants are the most critically ill, require the most frequent blood sampling, and suffer the greatest proportional loss of RBCs because their circulating RBC volumes are the smallest. Promising "in-line" devices that withdraw blood, measure multiple analytes, and then reinfuse the sampled blood are being investigated.[26] However, until these devices are proven effective and safe for infants, the replacement of blood losses due to phlebotomy will remain a critical factor responsible for multiple RBC transfusions in critically ill neonates.

Recommendations for RBC Transfusions during Infancy

Guidelines for transfusing RBCs to neonates are controversial, and practices vary.[7,27–29] The lack of a consistent approach stems from incomplete knowledge of the cellular and molecular biology of erythropoiesis during the perinatal period as well as incomplete understanding of the infant's compensation for anemia and the physiologic response to RBC transfusions. Generally, RBC transfusions are given to maintain the level of Hb or Hct believed to be most desirable for each neonate's clinical condition. Broad guidelines for RBC transfusions during early infancy are listed in Table 37–2.[30] These guidelines are very general, and it is important that terms used to describe clinical conditions, such as *severe* and *symptomatic,* be defined to fit local practices.

Most RBC transfusions given to infants are small in volume (10 to 15 mL/kg) and are repeated frequently to replace blood drawn for laboratory studies. There is no proven benefit to routine replacement of phlebotomy blood losses "milliliter for milliliter." Instead, RBCs should be transfused to maintain a Hct level deemed appropriate for the clinical condition of the infant. In neonates with severe respiratory disease, such as those requiring high volumes of oxygen with ventilator support, it is customary to maintain the Hct at greater than 40% (Hb concentration > 13.0 g/dL), particularly if blood is being drawn frequently for testing. This practice is based on the belief that transfused donor RBCs containing adult Hb will provide optimal oxygen delivery throughout the period of diminished pulmonary function that requires mechanical ventilation. Consistent with this rationale for ensuring optimal oxygen delivery in neonates with pulmonary failure, it seems logical—although unproven by controlled studies—to maintain the Hct at greater than 40% in infants with congenital heart disease that is severe enough to cause either cyanosis or congestive heart failure.

Definitive studies are not available to establish the optimal Hb level for infants facing major surgery. However, it seems reasonable to maintain the Hb at greater than 10.0 g/dL (Hct > 30%) because of the limited ability of the infant heart, lungs, and vasculature to compensate for anemia. Additional factors include the inferior off-loading of oxygen by neonatal RBCs that results from the diminished interaction between fetal Hb and 2,3-diphosphoglycerate and from the developmental impairment of neonatal renal, hepatic, and neurologic function. This transfusion guideline is simply a recommendation for perioperative management, not a firm indication, and it should be applied with flexibility to individual infants who are facing surgical procedures of varying complexity.

The clinical indications for RBC transfusions in preterm infants who are not critically ill but nonetheless develop moderate anemia (Hct < 24% or blood Hb concentration < 8.0 g/dL) are extremely variable.[7,29] In general, it was accepted that infants who are clinically stable despite modest anemia do not require RBC transfusions unless they exhibit significant problems that either are ascribed to the presence of anemia or are predicted to be corrected by RBC transfusions. To illustrate, proponents of RBC transfusions to treat disturbances of cardiopulmonary rhythms believe

Table 37–2 Authors' Guidelines for Transfusing Infants*

Red Blood Cells
Hemoglobin < 13.0 g/dL (Hct< 40%) with *severe* cardiopulmonary disease
Hemoglobin < 10.0 g/dL (Hct< 30%) with *moderate* cardiopulmonary disease
Hemoglobin < 10.0 g/dL (Hct< 30%) with *major* surgery
Hemoglobin < 8.0 g/dL (Hct< 24%) with *symptomatic* anemia
Acute loss > 25% estimated blood volume
Platelets
Blood platelets < 50 to < 100×10⁹/L and *significant* bleeding
Blood platelets < 50 × 10⁹/L and invasive procedure
Blood platelets < 20 × 10⁹/L prophylaxis and clinically *stable*
Blood platelets < 50 to < 100 × 10⁹/L prophylaxis and clinically *unstable*
Neutrophils
Blood neutrophils < 3 × 10⁹/L and *fulminant* sepsis during first week of life
Blood neutrophils < 1 × 10⁹/L and *fulminant* sepsis after first week of life

*Words in italics must be defined according to local practices.
Hct, hematocrit.

that a low Hct contributes to tachypnea, dyspnea, apnea, and tachycardia or bradycardia because of decreased oxygen delivery to the respiratory center of the brain. If this theory is true, transfusions of RBCs should decrease the number of apneic spells by improving oxygen delivery to the central nervous system. However, results of clinical studies have been contradictory.[7,29]

A recent study by Bell and colleagues provides evidence to the contrary.[31] In this study, 100 preterm infants, weighing from 500 to 1300 grams, were randomized to either a liberal or restrictive RBC transfusion regimen (i.e., a relatively low or high pretransfusion Hct level, respectively). The investigators found that the mean number of RBC transfusions was higher in the liberal group than the restrictive group; however, because a "single donor/unit program" was used, the number of donor exposures was not statistically significantly different. Furthermore, the most surprising finding was that those infants in the more restrictive group were more likely to have severe grades of intraparenchymal brain hemorrhage or periventricular leukomalacia as well as having increased frequency of apnea. The authors suggest that more restrictive transfusion practices may be detrimental to preterm infants and hypothesize that decreased oxygen delivery to brain tissue may be the pathophysiology of the brain injury and increased frequency of apnea—a speculation supported by another study in which high cerebral fractional oxygen extraction was found in infants with hemorrhagic parenchymal infarction as a manifestation of possible low cerebral blood flow.[31,32] Very importantly, a multicenter study of similar design with only preliminary reports to date[33] found results contradictory to Bell and colleagues. In the randomized study, 451 preterm infants were transfused according to either relatively low or high pretransfusion blood Hb concentrations. In contrast to the findings of Bell and colleagues, no difference in morbidity and mortality were found—favoring acceptance of relatively low pretransfusion blood Hb or Hct levels in clinical practice. Because the experimental design and outcomes were not identical in the two studies, there is no definitive recommendation possible for transfusion practices at this time. However, the potential for harm due to "undertransfusion," if very low pretransfusion Hb or Hct levels are accepted, must be considered when transfusion decisions are made.

Generally in practice, the decision whether to transfuse RBCs is based on the desire to maintain the Hct at a level judged to be most beneficial for the infant's clinical condition. Investigators who believe that this "clinical" approach is too imprecise have suggested the use of "physiologic" criteria for transfusions, such as RBC mass,[34] available oxygen,[35] mixed venous oxygen saturation, or measures of oxygen delivery and utilization,[36] to develop guidelines for transfusion decisions. In one study of 10 infants with severe (oxygen-dependent) bronchopulmonary dysplasia, improvement in physiologic end points (increased systemic oxygen transport and decreased oxygen use) was shown to be a consequence of small-volume RBC transfusions.[36] However, these promising but technically demanding methods are, at present, difficult to apply in the day-to-day practice of neonatology, and studies conducted directly in infants are needed. Application of data obtained from studies of animals and adult humans that correlate tissue oxygenation with the clinical effects of anemia and the need for RBC transfusions is confounded by the differences between infants and adults in Hb oxygen affinity, ability to increase cardiac output, and regional patterns of blood flow.

Another physiologic factor to be considered in the transfusion decision is the use of circulating RBC volume rather than blood Hct or Hb level.[11,34,37] Although circulating RBC volume is a potentially useful index of the blood's oxygen-carrying capacity, it cannot be predicted accurately by measurement of the Hct in infants.[38] Low circulating RBC volume identifies, better than Hb or Hct, those infants who will respond to transfusion with a decrease in cardiac output.[39] At present, circulating RBC volume measurements are not widely available. However, promising techniques using nonradioactive biotin to tag RBCs have been adapted for infant studies. Strauss and coworkers were able to demonstrate with this technique that the post-transfusion recovery and in vivo survival of donor RBCs, stored for up to 42 days, confirmed earlier studies that defined the efficacy and safety of stored allogeneic RBCs for small-volume transfusions to neonates. Specifically, no significant differences were observed between allogeneic RBCs stored on days 1 to 21 compared to days 22 to 42.[39–41]

Selecting an RBC Product to Transfuse an Infant

The RBC products usually chosen for small-volume transfusions given to infants are RBCs suspended either in citrate-phosphate-dextrose-adenine solution (CPDA) or in extended storage media (AS-1, AS-3, AS-5) at a Hct ranging from 55% to 70%. Some centers prefer to centrifuge RBC aliquots before transfusion, to prepare packed RBCs at a Hct of 80% to 90%. Most RBC transfusions are infused slowly over 2 to 4 hours at a dose of about 15 mL/kg body weight. Because of the small quantity of RBC preservative fluid infused and the slow rate of transfusion, the type of anticoagulant/preservative medium selected is believed not to pose risks for the majority of premature infants given small-volume transfusions.[42] Accordingly, the traditional use of relatively fresh RBCs (<7 days of storage) has been challenged, and it has been shown by many investigators[43–45] that donor exposure of multiply transfused infants can be diminished safely by the exclusive use of a dedicated unit of stored RBCs (i.e., 21 to 42 days after collection) for each infant.

Neonatologists who object to stored RBCs and continue to insist on transfusing infants with fresh RBCs generally raise three objections: the rise in plasma potassium (K^+) and the drop in RBC 2,3-diphosphoglycerate that occur during extended storage and the possible dangers of additives present in extended-storage media. After 42 days of storage, plasma K^+ levels in RBC units approximate 50 mEq/L (0.05 mEq/mL), a value that, at first glance, seems alarmingly high. By simple calculations, however, the dose of bioavailable K^+ transfused (i.e., ionic K^+ in the extracellular fluid) is shown to be very small. An infant weighing 1 kg who is given a 15 mL/kg transfusion of packed RBCs (Hct, 80%) will receive 3 mL of extracellular fluid, containing only 0.15 mEq of K^+, which will be infused slowly. Even if RBCs are not packed but are removed from the blood bag and directly infused at a Hct of 60%, the K^+ dose will be only 0.3 mEq. These doses are quite small compared with the usual daily K^+ requirement of 2 to 3 mEq/kg. However, this rationale does not apply to large-volume transfusions (>25 mL/kg), in which larger doses of K^+ may be harmful, especially if the infusion is rapid. Cardiac surgeons and other pediatric surgeons who may transfuse large RBC volumes expectedly or unexpectedly need to be especially cognizant of this point.

As for the second objection, 2,3-diphosphoglycerate is totally depleted from RBCs by 21 days of storage, and

Table 37–3 Formulation of Anticoagulant-Preservative Solutions Present in Blood Collection Sets

Constituent	CPDA	AS-1	AS-3	AS-5
Volume (mL)	63*	100†	100†	100†
Sodium chloride (mg)	None	900	410	877
Dextrose (mg)	2000	2200	1100	900
Adenine (mg)	17.3	27	30	30
Mannitol (mg)	None	750	None	525
Trisodium citrate (mg)	1660	None	588	None
Citric acid (mg)	206	None	42	None
Sodium phosphate (monobasic) (mg)	140	None	276	None

*Approximately 450 mL of donor blood is drawn into 63 mL of CPDA. A unit of red blood cells (hematocrit, approximately 70%) is prepared by centrifugation and removal of most plasma.

†When AS-1 or AS-5 is used, 450 mL of donor blood is first drawn into 63 mL of CPD, which is identical to CPDA except that it contains 1610 mg of dextrose per 63 mL and has no adenine. When AS-3 is used, donor blood is drawn into CP2D, which is identical to CPD except that it contains double the amount of dextrose. After centrifugation and removal of almost all plasma, red blood cells are resuspended in 100 mL of the additive solution (AS-1, AS-3, or AS-5) at a hematocrit of approximately 55% to 60%.

AS-1, AS-3, and AS-5, extended storage media; CPDA, citrate-phosphate-dextrose-adenine solution.

Data from Luban NLC, Strauss RG, Hume HA. Commentary on the safety of red blood cells preserved in extended storage media for neonatal transfusions. Transfusion 1990;30:229.

this is reflected by a decrease in the oxygen half-saturation pressure (P_{50}) from about 27 mmHg in fresh blood to 18-mmHg at the time of outdate. The last value of older transfused RBCs corresponds to the "physiologic" P_{50} obtained from the RBCs of many normal preterm infants at birth, reflecting the relatively high affinity for oxygen normally exhibited by infant RBCs. Therefore, the P_{50} of older transfused RBCs is no worse than that of RBCs produced endogenously by the infant's own bone marrow. Moreover, these older adult RBCs provide a benefit to the infant because the 2,3-diphosphoglycerate and the P_{50} of transfused RBCs (but not of endogenous infant RBCs) increase rapidly after transfusion.

Regarding the third objection, the quantity of additives present in RBCs stored in extended-storage media is believed not to be dangerous to neonates given small-volume transfusions (≤15 mL/kg).[42] A comparison of CPDA with three types of extended-storage media is presented in Table 37–3. Regardless of the type of suspending solution, the quantity of additives is quite small in the clinical setting, in which infants are given small-volume transfusions of RBCs transfused over 2 to 4 hours, and it is far lower than doses believed to be toxic (Table 37–4). Importantly, the efficacy and safety of these theoretical calculations have been confirmed by clinical experience. In addition, many investigators have reported the successful transfusion of stored, rather than fresh, RBCs for small-volume transfusions in infants.[43–46] The small-volume nature of these transfusions cannot be overemphasized. Therefore, these same rules do not apply to massive transfusion situations, which many pediatric surgeons and neonatologists may encounter knowingly or unknowingly and for which they need to be prepared accordingly. This information is especially important for surgeons and neonatologists who are recommending that the parents, relatives, or friends of their patients perform directed RBC donation. Communication between the physicians and blood bank is encouraged for many reasons: to confirm the child's blood type so type-compatible RBCs can be donated; to help with the collection center's choice of anticoagulant-preservative solution into which the units will be drawn (i.e., CPDA and/or AS units), which might differ if a massive transfusion situation seems likely; and to coordinate timing of the surgery so that tested units are in hospital inventory prior to the surgical date and time.

Recombinant Erythropoietin in the Anemia of Prematurity

Recognition of the low plasma EPO levels in preterm infants provides a rational basis for the use of recombinant human EPO as therapy for the anemia of prematurity. More than 20 controlled trials have tested several doses and treatment schedules in preterm infants, and results are mixed, making consensus impossible on the optimal role of recombinant human EPO treatment in the anemia of prematurity.[7,47,48]

Table 37–4 Constituents Infused (mg/kg) in 10 mL/kg Red Blood Cells (Hematocrit, 60%)

Additive	CPDA	AS-1	AS-3	Toxic Dose*
NaCl	0	28	5	137 mg/kg/day
Dextrose	13	86	15	240 mg/kg/hr
Adenine	0.2	0.4	0.4	15 mg/kg/dose
Citrate	12	6.5	8.4	180 mg/kg/hr
Phosphate	9	1.3	3.7	>60 mg/kg/day
Mannitol	0	22	0	360 mg/kg/day

*Actual toxic dose is difficult to predict accurately because the infusion rate usually is slow, permitting metabolism and distribution from blood into extravascular sites, and dextrose, adenine, and phosphate enter red blood cells and are somewhat sequestered. Potential toxic doses are based on Luban, Strauss, and Hume (1990).[32]

AS-1 and AS-3, extended storage media; CPDA, citrate-phosphate-dextrose-adenine solution.

Data from Luban NLC, Strauss RG, Hume HA. Commentary on the safety of red blood cells preserved in extended storage media for neonatal transfusions. Transfusion 1990;30:229.

Unquestionably, proper doses of recombinant human EPO and iron effectively stimulate erythropoiesis in preterm infants, as evidenced by increased marrow erythroid activity and blood reticulocyte counts. However, the efficacy of recombinant human EPO in substantially diminishing the number of RBC transfusions—the major goal for which it is prescribed—has not been convincingly demonstrated for all groups of preterm infants.[48] In many trials, the subjects were relatively large preterm infants and those in stable clinical condition; such infants currently receive few RBC transfusions when given only standard supportive care (i.e., not given recombinant human EPO).[27,49] Currently, even without use of recombinant human EPO, fewer than 50% of infants with birth weights greater than 1.0 kg receive RBC transfusions. Almost all infants weighing less than 1.0 kg at birth are given RBCs, and most transfusions are given during the first 3 to 4 weeks of life.[49]

To illustrate the difficulty of avoiding RBC transfusions, a multicenter, randomized North American trial, in which infants received either recombinant human EPO or placebo during a 6-week study period, reported a statistically significant difference but only modest success.[50] Although significantly fewer RBC transfusions were given to infants treated with recombinant human EPO during the study phase (1.1 transfusion vs 1.6 for placebo), all infants required multiple transfusions during the 3-week prestudy phase. Therefore, recombinant human EPO exerted only a modest effect on total RBC transfusions given throughout the entire study (4.4 for recombinant human EPO vs 5.3 for placebo) and did not resolve the problem of severe neonatal anemia.[50]

Physicians wishing to prescribe recombinant human EPO are faced with a dilemma. The relatively large or stable preterm infants who respond best to recombinant human EPO plus iron are given relatively few RBC transfusions and, accordingly, have little need for recombinant human EPO to avoid transfusions. Extremely preterm infants, who are sick and have the greatest need for RBC transfusions shortly after birth, have not consistently responded to recombinant human EPO plus iron, again questioning the efficacy of recombinant human EPO therapy.[47] However, extremely preterm infants are being evaluated in therapeutic trials of recombinant human EPO and iron, both given intravenously shortly after birth.[51,52] Although preliminary review of these promising studies suggests success in avoiding transfusions early in life, the data are limited and are insufficient to clearly establish efficacy or to detect potential toxicity. Therefore, firm guidelines for the use of recombinant human EPO in the treatment of the anemia of prematurity cannot be offered at this time.

PLATELET TRANSFUSIONS

Older Children and Adolescents

Guidelines for platelet support of children and adolescents with quantitative and qualitative platelet disorders are similar to those for adults (see Table 37–1), in whom the risk of life-threatening bleeding that occurs after injury or spontaneously can be related to the severity of thrombocytopenia (when low blood platelet counts are caused by diminished marrow production). Thrombocytopenia caused by accelerated turnover (e.g., immune thrombocytopenia) usually is not treated with platelet transfusions. Platelet transfusions should be given to patients with platelet counts lower than 50×10^9/L due to marrow failure if they are bleeding or are scheduled for an invasive procedure. Studies of patients with thrombocytopenia caused by poor marrow production indicate that spontaneous bleeding increases markedly when platelet levels fall to less than 20×10^9/L, particularly in patients who are ill with infection, anemia, or dysfunction of the liver, kidneys, or lungs. For this reason, many pediatricians recommend prophylactic platelet transfusions to maintain the platelet count at greater than 20×10^9/L in children with thrombocytopenia due to bone marrow failure. This threshold has been challenged, and some favor a platelet transfusion trigger of 5 to 10×10^9/L for patients with uncomplicated conditions. Many pediatric hematology/oncology and stem cell transplantation physicians have lowered their prophylactic platelet transfusion trigger to 10×10^9/L, extrapolating from the adult acute myeloid leukemia studies by Rebulla and colleagues in 1997 and Wandt and coworkers in 1998.[53,54] These prospective clinical trials, among others, demonstrated that nonbleeding stable thrombocytopenic patients without coexisting symptoms can be managed safely with a more restrictive platelet transfusion trigger, 10×10^9/L, and fewer platelet transfusions were given. However, those with fever, active bleeding, and/or a coagulation disorder had a higher trigger of at least 20×10^9/L.

Qualitative platelet disorders may be inherited or acquired (e.g., in advanced hepatic or renal insufficiency, after cardiopulmonary bypass procedures). In such patients, platelet transfusions are justified only if significant bleeding occurs. Because individuals with platelet dysfunction may have intermittent bleeding episodes throughout their life necessitating repeated transfusions, which may lead to alloimmunization and refractoriness, prophylactic platelet transfusions are rarely justified unless an invasive procedure is planned. In such cases, a bleeding time greater than twice the upper limit of laboratory normal may be taken as diagnostic evidence that platelet dysfunction exists, but this test is poorly predictive of hemorrhagic risk or the need to transfuse platelets. The bleeding time has been supplanted by other platelet function assays and is rarely performed anymore, especially in children. In these patients, alternative therapies, particularly subcutaneous or intranasal desmopressin acetate, should be considered to avoid platelet transfusions.

Infants and Younger Children

Pathophysiology of Neonatal Thrombocytopenia

Blood platelet counts of 150×10^9/L or greater are present in normal fetuses (=17 weeks of gestation) and neonates. Lower platelet counts indicate potential problems, and preterm infants exhibit thrombocytopenia commonly.[55,56] In one neonatal intensive care unit, 22% of infants had blood platelet counts lower than 150×10^9/L during hospitalization.[55] Although multiple pathogenic mechanisms probably are involved in these sick neonates, a predominant one is accelerated platelet destruction, as shown by shortened platelet survival time, increased platelet-associated immunoglobulin G, increased platelet volume, a normal number of megakaryocytes, and an inadequate increment in blood platelet values after platelet transfusion.[55,57] Another major mechanism contributing to neonatal thrombocytopenia is diminished platelet production, as evidenced by decreased numbers of clonogenic megakaryocyte progenitors[58,59] and relatively low levels of thrombopoietin[59,60] in response to thrombocytopenia, when compared with children and adults. Similar to the situation with EPO and the anemia of prematurity, thrombopoietin is produced by thrombocytopenic preterm infants, but at relatively low levels. Controlled clinical trials are needed to determine the possible role and potential toxicity of recombinant thrombopoietin therapy in infants.

Blood platelet counts lower than 100 × 10^9/L pose significant clinical risks for premature neonates. In one study, infants with birth weights lower than 1.5 kg and blood platelet counts lower than 100 × 10^9/L were compared with nonthrombocytopenic control infants of similar size.[56] The bleeding time was prolonged when platelet counts were lower than 100 × 10^9/L, and in many infants platelet dysfunction was suggested by bleeding times that were disproportionately long for the degree of thrombocytopenia present. Hemorrhage was more frequent in the thrombocytopenic infants, with the incidence of intracranial hemorrhage being 78% in those weighing less than 1.5 kg at birth, compared with 48% for nonthrombocytopenic infants of similar size. Moreover, the extent of hemorrhage and neurologic morbidity was greater in the group of thrombocytopenic infants.[56]

Recommendations for Platelet Transfusions during Infancy

The use of prophylactic platelet transfusions in an attempt to prevent bleeding in preterm neonates has been studied systematically.[61] However, no randomized clinical trials have been reported examining therapeutic platelet transfusions in bleeding thrombocytopenic neonates. Therefore, basic questions regarding the relative risks of different degrees of thrombocytopenia in various clinical settings during infancy remain largely unanswered. However, it seems logical to transfuse platelets to thrombocytopenic infants, and guidelines acceptable to many neonatologists are listed in Table 37–2. Two firm indications for neonatal platelet transfusions are to treat hemorrhage that has already occurred and to prevent hemorrhage from complicating an invasive procedure. Little disagreement exists regarding the use of a blood platelet count lower than 50 × 10^9/L as a "transfusion trigger" in these instances. However, platelet transfusions are given to infants by some physicians to treat bleeding that occurs at higher platelet counts (between 50 and 100 × 10^9/L) or to diminish the threat of intracranial hemorrhage in high-risk preterm infants whenever the platelet count is lower than 100 × 10^9/L.[56]

Prophylactic platelet transfusions can be given under two circumstances: to prevent bleeding when severe thrombocytopenia is present and poses a risk of spontaneous hemorrhage and to maintain the presence of a normal platelet count to prevent the infant from slipping into high-risk situations. Regarding the first circumstance, most agree that it is reasonable to give platelets to any neonate whose blood platelet count is lower than 20 × 10^9/L. There is broad acceptance that spontaneous hemorrhage is a risk with platelet counts below this level. Also, severe thrombocytopenia occurs most commonly in sick infants who, because of their illnesses, receive medications that may further compromise platelet function. Because all of these factors are pronounced in extremely preterm infants, some neonatologists favor prophylactic platelet transfusion whenever the platelet count falls to less than 50 × 10^9/L, or even 100 × 10^9/L, in critically ill infants.[56]

Regarding the second circumstance, the need to maintain a completely normal platelet count (≥150 × 10^9/L) or even higher in preterm infants without bleeding is unproven. Intracranial hemorrhage occurs commonly in sick preterm infants, and, although the etiologic role of thrombocytopenia and the therapeutic benefit of platelet transfusions have not been conclusively established in this disorder, it seems logical to presume that thrombocytopenia is a risk factor.[62] However, a randomized trial designed to address this issue—in which transfusion of platelets whenever the platelet count fell to less than 150 × 10^9/L so as to maintain the average platelet count at greater than 200 × 10^9/L was compared with transfusion of platelets only when the platelet count fell to less than 50 × 10^9/L—did not detect a difference in the incidence of intacranial hemorrhage (28% vs 26%, respectively).[61] Therefore, there is no documented benefit to transfusing "prophylactic platelets" to maintain a completely normal platelet count, compared with transfusing "therapeutic platelets" in response to thrombocytopenia when it actually occurs.

Currently, there are no alternatives to platelet transfusions to treat thrombocytopenia in neonates. Recombinant thrombopoietin (i.e., c-*mpl* ligand or megakaryocyte growth and differentiation factor) and interleukin-11 are promising agents. However, neither is recommended for use during infancy, and both have potential toxicities that might preclude their use in sick preterm infants. Clearly, they must not be prescribed at present, except in experimental settings.

Selecting a Platelet Product to Transfuse an Infant or Younger Child

The ideal goal of most platelet transfusions is to raise the platelet count to greater than 50 × 10^9/L or, for sick preterm infants, to greater than 100 × 10^9/L. This goal can be achieved by the infusion of 5 to 10 mL/kg of standard (i.e., unmodified) platelet concentrates, collected by centrifugation of fresh units of whole blood or from a plateletpheresis unit collected by automated plateletpheresis. The platelet dose should be transfused as rapidly as the overall condition permits, certainly within 2 hours. Routinely reducing the volume of platelet concentrates for infants by additional centrifugation steps is both unnecessary and unwise. Transfusion of 10 mL/kg platelet concentrate provides approximately 10 × 10^9/L platelets. Assuming that the estimated blood volume of an infant is 70 mL/kg body weight, the platelet dose of 10 mL/kg will increase the platelet count by 143 × 10^9/L. This calculated increment is consistent with the observed increment after this dose reported in clinical studies.[61] In general, 10 mL/kg is not an excessive transfusion volume, provided that the intake of other intravenous fluids, medications, and nutrients is monitored and adjusted. It is desirable that the infant and the platelet donor be of the same ABO blood group, and it is important to minimize repeated transfusions of group O platelets to group A or B recipients, because large quantities of passive anti-A or anti-B can lead to hemolysis, resulting in severe morbidity and mortality in children.[63–66]

Although proven methods exist to reduce the volume of platelet concentrates when truly warranted (i.e., when many transfusions are anticipated in which multiple doses of passive anti-A or anti-B might lead to hemolysis or when there is failure to respond to 10 mL/kg of unmodified platelet concentrate), additional processing (i.e., plasma volume reduction) should be performed with great care because of probable platelet loss, clumping, and dysfunction caused by the additional handling.

NEUTROPHIL TRANSFUSIONS

Older Children and Adolescents

Several methodologic advances—in particular, the use of recombinant granulocyte colony-stimulating factor (G-CSF) to stimulate donors—have made it possible to collect extraordinarily large numbers of normal neutrophils (polymorphonuclear neutrophils, PMNs) for transfusion into neutropenic patients who have life-threatening infections. Because larger doses of PMNs can be transfused, renewed interest has arisen in the use of PMN (granulocyte) transfusions to treat adult oncology patients and hematopoietic progenitor cell transplant recipients, in whom neutropenia complicated by severe infections persists as a significant problem despite combination antibiotic therapy, recombinant cytokines, myeloid growth factors, and use of mobilized peripheral blood progenitor cells to minimize neutropenic infections. If children are suffering significant morbidity and mortality from neutropenic infections despite modern supportive care, it is logical to explore the efficacy, potential toxicity, and cost effectiveness of tranulocyte transfusion therapy through properly designed, randomized clinical trials performed in pediatric subjects.[67]

Serious and repeated infections with bacteria, yeast, and fungi are a consequence of severe neutropenia and PMN dysfunction in some settings. In the multicenter Trial to Reduce Alloimmunization to Platelets (TRAP) study, 7% of adult patients with acute nonlymphocytic leukemia died from infection during first-remission induction therapy, despite the use of modern antibiotic therapy.[68] In another study of patients given intensive chemotherapy, some of whom also received transfusions of autologous hematopoietic stem cells, 7.6% of patients experienced systemic fungal infection.[69] Unless severe neutropenia is reversed fairly quickly in adult patients, the mortality of systemic fungal infections approaches 100%. Therefore, modern "high-dose" granulocyte transfusion therapy is considered by some experts to be very promising for adult oncology and transplantation patients.[70,71] However, contrary data suggest that, with appropriate anti-infective therapy, serious infections are rare in patients who are transplanted with adequate numbers of peripheral blood progenitor cells.[72]

Because of these controversial views, pediatricians must survey the outcome of life-threatening infections with bacteria, yeast, and fungi in children who are undergoing intense chemotherapy or hematopoietic progenitor cell transplantation in their own institutions to determine whether there is a need for therapeutic granulocyte transfusion. If infections in neutropenic children respond promptly to antibiotics plus standard supportive care and survival approaches 100%, granulocyte transfusion is unnecessary. Moreover, it should not be used if there is no apparent need, because the lack of demonstrable benefit would not outweigh the potential risks. However, if significant numbers of infected high-risk patients fail to respond to antibiotics alone, or if the intensity of therapy is compromised because it is limited by fear of neutropenia, the addition of granulocyte transfusion should be considered, along with other modifications of therapy intended to reduce infections, such as selection of different antibiotics, closer monitoring of antibiotic blood levels, and use of intravenous immunoglobulin (IVIG), G-CSF, other recombinant cytokines, and immune-modulating agents.

The role of granulocyte transfusion added to antibiotics for patients with severe neutropenia ($<0.5 \times 10^9/L$) caused by bone marrow failure is similar in adults and children (see Table 37–1). Infected neutropenic patients usually respond to antibiotics alone, provided bone marrow function recovers early in infection. Because children with newly diagnosed leukemia respond rapidly to induction chemotherapy, only rarely are they candidates for granulocyte transfusion. In contrast, infected children with sustained bone marrow failure (e.g., malignant neoplasms resistant to treatment, aplastic anemia, bone marrow transplantation) may benefit from the addition of granulocyte transfusion to antibiotic therapy. The use of granulocyte transfusion for bacterial sepsis that is unresponsive to antibiotics in patients with severe neutropenia ($<0.5 \times 10^9/L$) is supported by most controlled studies.[67,70]

Children with qualitative neutrophil defects (neutrophil dysfunction) usually have adequate numbers of blood neutrophils but are susceptible to serious infections because their cells kill pathogenic microorganisms inefficiently. Neutrophil dysfunction syndromes are rare, and no definitive studies have established the efficacy of granulocyte transfusion in these patients. However, several patients with progressive life-threatening infections have improved strikingly with the addition of granulocyte transfusion to antimicrobial therapy.[73] These disorders are chronic, and because of the risk of inducing alloimmunization, GTX is recommended only if the infections are clearly unresponsive to antimicrobial drugs.

Infants and Younger Children

Pathophysiology of Neonatal Neutropenia and Neutrophil Dysfunction

Neonates are unusually susceptible to severe bacterial infections, and several defects of neonatal body defenses have been reported as possible contributing factors. PMNs isolated from the blood of neonates exhibit both quantitative and qualitative abnormalities that may be related to the increased incidence, morbidity, and mortality of bacterial infections. Abnormalities of neonatal PMNs include absolute and relative neutropenia, diminished chemotaxis, abnormal adhesion and aggregation, defective cellular orientation and receptor capping, decreased deformability, inability to alter membrane potential during stimulation, imbalances of oxidative metabolism, and a diminished ability to withstand oxidant stress.[74] A complete discussion of neonatal PMN physiology is beyond the scope of this chapter, and only aspects that are particularly relevant to PMN transfusions and alternative therapies are reviewed here.

Neutropenia can occur during neonatal bacterial infections, particularly with fulminant sepsis. Because a physiologic neutrophilia occurs in normal neonates, it is considered quite abnormal for the absolute blood PMN count to fall below $3.0 \times 10^9/L$ during the first week of life. Although an abnormally low PMN count can occur in neonates with disorders as diverse as sepsis, asphyxia, and maternal hypertension, suspicion of severe bacterial infection must always be high whenever relative neutropenia (PMN count, $<3.0 \times 10^9/L$) occurs. The mechanisms responsible are only partially defined, but abnormalities of neonatal granulopoiesis frequently are involved. As one factor, the postmitotic marrow PMN storage pool (metamyelocytes and mature, segmented PMNs) is small. The PMN storage pool accounts for 26% to 60% of all nucleated cells in the bone marrow of normal neonates. Neonates with sepsis may exhibit a storage pool numbering less than 10% of nucleated marrow cells and are considered to have severely diminished marrow PMN reserves.[75] Second, storage pool PMNs are released at an excessively rapid and, apparently, poorly regulated rate from the marrow during stress. Third, PMN production in response to infection is decreased. The number of committed (clonogenic) PMN precursors in neonatal marrow is lower in neonates than in older patients, and a high percentage of these cells are proliferating even when studied at an apparently basal state.[75,76] Therefore, neonatal marrow is functioning at capacity and is unable to rapidly expand production to meet the increased demands of infection.[77] For this reason, it is logical to consider PMN transfusions until the marrow recovers.

Recommendations for Neutrophil Transfusions during Infancy

Because both quantitative and qualitative abnormalities of neonatal PMNs have been reported, PMN transfusions have been used to treat neonatal sepsis with or without neutropenia. Neonates exhibiting fulminant sepsis, relative neutropenia (PMN count, $<3.0 \times 10^9$/L during the first week of life or $<1.0 \times 10^9$/L thereafter), and a severely diminished PMN marrow storage pool (less than 10% of nucleated marrow cells being postmitotic PMNs) are at increased risk of death if treated only with antibiotics. Results of 11 studies[78–88] on the use of PMN transfusions to treat infected neonates, 6 of which were designed as controlled studies,[78–81,86,87] have been reported. The fact that four of the six controlled studies noted significant benefit from PMN transfusions is encouraging.[78–81] However, the controlled studies contained several experimental flaws.[89]

Because of these scientific imperfections, firm recommendations for the role of PMN transfusions in the treatment of neonatal sepsis cannot be made at this time. Guidelines for PMN transfusions are presented in Table 37–2. Although antibiotics are the key to successful treatment of neonatal sepsis, antibiotic therapy is not 100% successful, and attempts to bolster body defenses are warranted. PMN transfusions have not provided a complete answer; although they are efficacious for infants with neutropenia and fulminant sepsis,[89] only PMN transfusions obtained by automated leukapheresis have demonstrated effectiveness.[88,89] Moreover, in many instances, standard supportive care with antibiotics seems adequate. Each institution must assess its own experience with neonatal sepsis. If almost all infants survive without apparent long-term morbidity when treated only with antibiotics, PMN transfusions are unnecessary, and attention should be focused on prompt diagnosis and optimal antibiotic therapy. If the outcome of standard therapy is not optimal, alternative therapies such as PMN transfusions must be considered to improve the outlook.

Alternatives to Neonatal Neutrophil Transfusions

Not all neonatologists prescribe PMN transfusions. Their proper role has not been irrefutably established by controlled clinical trials. Moreover, the preparation of PMN concentrates by leukapheresis can be cumbersome and expensive, and the process of collecting and transfusing PMNs can pose risks for both neonates and donors. Accordingly, alternative therapies have been suggested. However, their efficacy has not been clearly established, their risks are only partially defined, and they require extensive study before they can be widely accepted. Two modalities that have been suggested are IVIG and myeloid cytokines or growth factors.

Most studies evaluating IVIG to prevent infections have found little or only modest benefit.[90–101] However, results are inconsistent. Only a few studies have suggested prophylactic benefit.[88–90] In contrast, several therapeutic studies have demonstrated a benefit from the addition of IVIG to antibiotics in the treatment of neonatal infections.[102–106] In a meta-analysis, studies of prophylactic IVIG were found to demonstrate only minimal benefit, whereas studies of therapeutic IVIG exhibited unequivocal benefit.[107] Overall, the data are insufficient to justify the routine use of IVIG in all preterm neonates to prevent or treat sepsis. However, modest "physiologic" doses (0.3 to 0.4 mg/kg) may lessen the severity of bacterial sepsis in newborns with very low birth weights, who are likely to be hypogammaglobulinemic as a result of extremely premature birth (i.e., before the major placental transport of immunoglobulin G has taken place). However, caution must be used when prescribing IVIG therapy to prevent or treat neonatal sepsis. IVIG therapy, particularly at high doses, can impair body defense mechanisms.[108–110]

To date, properly designed clinical studies of recombinant myeloid growth factors given to human neonates are limited. In a controlled study,[111] 42 neonates with presumed bacterial sepsis, recognized within the first 3 days of life, were randomly assigned to receive three doses of either G-CSF or a placebo. Although the outcome of sepsis was not reported, G-CSF induced a significant increase in the blood PMN count, an increase in the marrow PMN storage pool, and an increase in PMN membrane C3bi expression—the last being an indication of enhanced functional capability.

In a controlled study of granulocyte-macrophage colony-stimulating factor (GM-CSF) in premature neonates,[112] 20 premature neonates were randomly assigned within 72 hours after birth to receive either GM-CSF or a placebo for 7 days. GM-CSF increased the blood PMN count, the marrow PMN storage pool, and C3bi receptor expression. In addition, neonates receiving GM-CSF exhibited an increase in blood monocyte and platelet counts. The study was not designed to assess efficacy in the prevention or treatment of infections.

Two additional randomized clinical trials have been conducted to assess the efficacy of G-CSF and GM-CSF. Neither demonstrated clear clinical benefit. In the G-CSF trial, 20 infants with neutropenia and sepsis received either G-CSF (10 mg/kg/day) or placebo for 3 days.[113] Acknowledging that the number of study subjects was too small for definitive conclusions, the study authors noted that G-CSF did not significantly improve severity of illness, morbidity, or mortality. In a preliminary report of the GM-CSF trial,[114] preterm infants received either GM-CSF (8 μg/kg/day) or placebo for the first 28 days of life in an attempt to reduce the incidence of infections. Although GM-CSF was well tolerated and significantly increased blood leukocyte counts, it did not significantly decrease infection rates. Therefore, firm guidelines cannot be made at this time regarding the proper role of myeloid growth factors in the management of neonatal neutropenia or sepsis.

Clearly, there is no universally accepted role for PMN transfusions, IVIG, or myeloid growth factors in the treatment of neonatal sepsis. However, it seems reasonable to treat fulminant sepsis in neonates with neutropenia (blood PMN counts $<3 \times 10^9$/L during the first week of life or $<1 \times 10^9$/L thereafter) as follows. For infants born before 30 weeks' gestation, give one dose of 500 mg/kg of IVIG plus 5 μg/kg of G-CSF on 3 consecutive days. For infants born at 30 weeks' gestation or later, give 5 μg/kg of G-CSF on 3 consecutive days. This therapy should be adjunctive to optimal antibiotic and supportive care.

PLASMA PRODUCT TRANFUSIONS

Recommendations for use of plasma product transfusions do not need to be broken down into sections for older children and adolescents and infants and younger children because product selection is similar in each group and in adults. However, due to smaller plasma volumes in many of these individuals, certain aspects need to be emphasized. First, plasma (all types) should be ABO-compatible with the recipient's RBCs; in other words, it should not contain donor isohemagglutinins that may react with the recipient A and/or B red cell antigens. This is to prevent a "minor side" ABO incompatibility that could result in an acute hemolytic transfusion reaction, which has a higher probability of occurring in a smaller patient receiving "out-of-group" plasma.[66,115] When considering the patient's RhD status, FFP is usually not matched because it contains very low numbers of RBCs. However, when large volumes of RhD-positive FFP (>20 mL/kg) are being transfused to RhD-negative pediatric patients (or women of childbearing age), RhD immunization prevention with RhD immune globulin should be considered.

Frozen Plasma

Recommendations with regard to blood component administration and guidelines for transfusion of FFP, plasma frozen within 24 hours F24, and cryoreduced plasma have been recently published for neonates and pediatric patients.[1,116] The indications and contraindications are very similar for neonates and pediatric patients as for adults; however, dosing is in mL/kg rather than units. The dose of FFP in children is 10 to 20 mL/kg (Table 37–5). This dose will raise most coagulation factor levels by approximately 20%.[117] However, plasma frozen within 24 hours has lower levels of factor VIII and factor V and thus might not increase those factors as high as 20%.[118] Generally, this is not of clinical significance, and FFP and plasma frozen within 24 hours are used interchangeably. On the other hand, cryoreduced plasma (devoid of factor VIII, von Willebrand factor, factor XIII, and fibrinogen) was recently approved by the U.S. Food and Drug Administration for use in refractory thrombotic thrombocytopenic purpura (TTP), those patients who are unresponsive to standard therapy with FFP, as its only true indication. Some authorities advocate the use of cryoreduced plasma as a first-line therapy for TTP, an off-label use. However, in 2001 the North American TTP Group published a multicenter prospective, randomized trial comparing exchange transfusion with FFP to cryoreduced plasma for the initial treatment of TTP. They demonstrated that survival was the same in both study groups and concluded equal efficacy between FFP and cryoreduced plasma for initial therapy in TTP.[119,120]

Reference values of plasma concentrations for each coagulation factor for pediatric patients under age 6 months are lower than for children and adults with regard to vitamin K–dependent factors (factors II, VII, IX, and X) in addition to the contact factors and the vitamin K–dependent natural inhibitors of coagulation. As a result the prothrombin time and activated partial thromboplastin time are prolonged. This distinct difference should be taken into account when considering frozen plasma therapy for prolonged screening tests in children under age 6 months who are septic with disseminated intravascular coagulation and hemorrhage from surgery or trauma, because these already low factors may be depleted due to lower baseline levels initially and may warrant earlier intervention with plasma transfusion.[121] Another important point regarding frozen plasma is that it is not indicated for volume expansion nor for improving wound healing.[1,122]

Table 37-5 Guidelines for the Dosing and Transfusion of FFP/F24/CRP and Cryoprecipitate

Fresh Frozen Plasma (FFP)/Plasma Frozen in 24 hr (F24)/Cryoprecipitate Reduced Plasma (CRP)

Dosing: 10–20 mL/kg to achieve approximately 20% rise in factor levels (assuming 100% recovery)

Indications:

1. Supportive care during disseminated intravascular coagulation management
2. Replacement therapy
   a. Factor replacement when concentrates not available (e.g., antithrombin III and protein S deficiencies, and factors II, V, X, and XI deficiencies)
   b. Therapeutic plasma exchange when FFP/F24/CRP is indicated
3. Warfarin reversal in emergency situations (e.g., prior to invasive surgical procedure with active bleeding)

Cryoprecipitate

Dosing: 1–2 units/10 kg body weight to increase fibrinogen by 60–100 mg/dL (assuming 100% recovery)

Indications:

1. Hypofibrinogenemia or dysfibrinogenemia with active bleeding
2. Hypofibrinogenemia or dysfibrinogenemia prior to invasive procedure
3. Factor XIII deficiency with active bleeding or prior to invasive procedure
4. vWD and hemophilia A with active bleeding and no plasma-derived factor vWF/FVIII concentrate available and no recombinant FVIII product available, respectively
5. Uremic bleeding
6. Fibrin glue sealant preparation

Adapted from Roseff SD, Luban NLC, Manno CS. Guidelines for assessing appropriateness of pediatric transfusion. Transfusion 2002;42:1398.

CRYOPRECIPITATE

Just as with the various types of frozen plasmas available, the indications for cryoprecipitate transfusion are the same in children as in adults. Again, in children it is recommended to give ABO-compatible units; however, the RhD group need not be honored. The dose is approximately 1 to 2 pooled units for every 10 kg of body weight. Table 37–5 outlines the dosing and indications for transfusion of cryoprecipitate. In neonates and pediatric patients cryoprecipitate is mostly administered to increase fibrinogen. It is rarely transfused in the United States for von Willebrand's disease or factor VIII deficiency because safer products are recommended, such as virally inactivated and recombinant factor VIII products.[123]

REFERENCES

1. Roseff SD, Luban NLC, Manno CS. Guidelines for assessing appropriateness of pediatric transfusion. Transfusion 2002;42:1398–1413.
2. Wu WC, Rathmore SS, Wand Y, et al. Blood transfusion in elderly patients with acute myocardial infarction. NEJM 2001;345:1230–1236.
3. Bratton SL, Annich GM. Packed red blood cell transfusions for critically ill pediatric patients: when and for what conditions? J Pediatr 2003;142:95–97.
4. Laverdiere C, Gauvin F, Hebert PC, et al. Survey on transfusion practices of pediatric intensivists. Pediatr Crit Care Med 2002;3:381–382.
5. Hebert PC, Wells G, Blajchman MA, et al, and the Transfusion Requirements in Critical Care Investigators for the Canadian Critical Care Trials Group. A multicenter, randomized, controlled clinical trial of transfusion requirements in critical care. NEJM 1999;340:409–417.
6. Goodman AM, Murray PM, Kantilal PM, Luban NLC. Pediatric red blood cell transfusions increase resource use. J Pediatr 2003;142:123–127.
7. Strauss RG. Red blood cell transfusion practices in the neonate. Clin Perinatol 1995;22:641–655.
8. Strauss RG, Sacher RA, Blazina JF, et al. Commentary on small-volume red cell transfusions for neonatal patients. Transfusion 1990;30:565–570.
9. Stockman JA. Anemia of prematurity: current concepts in the issue of when to transfuse. Pediatr Clin North Am 1986;33:111–128.
10. Wardrop CA, Holland BM, Veale KE, et al. Nonphysiological anaemia of prematurity. Arch Dis Child 1978;53:855–860.
11. Holland BM, Jones JG, Wardrop CA. Lessons from the anemia of prematurity. Hematol Oncol Clin North Am 1987;1:355–366.
12. Stockman JA III, Garcia JF, Oski FA. The anemia of prematurity: factors governing the erythropoietin response. NEJM 1977;296:647–650.
13. Brown MS, Phibbs RH, Garcia JF, Dallman PR. Postnatal changes in erythropoietin levels in untransfused premature infants. J Pediatr 1983; 103:612–617.
14. Stockman JA III, Graeber JE, Clark DA, et al. Anemia of prematurity: Determinants of the erythropoietin response. J Pediatr 1984;105:786–792.
15. Brown MS, Garcia JF, Phibbs RH, Dallman PR. Decreased response of plasma immunoreactive erythropoietin to "available oxygen" in anemia of prematurity. J Pediatr 1984;105:793–798.
16. Shannon KM, Naylor GS, Torkildson JC, et al. Circulating erythroid progenitors in the anemia of prematurity. NEJM 1987;317:728–733.
17. Rhondeau SM, Christensen RD, Ross MP, et al. Responsiveness to recombinant human erythropoietin of marrow erythroid progenitors from infants with the "anemia of prematurity." J Pediatr 1988;112: 935–940.
18. Zanjani ED, Ascensao JL, McGlave PB, et al. Studies on the liver to kidney switch of erythropoietin production. J Clin Invest 1981;67:1183–1188.
19. Dame C, Fahnenstich H, Freitag P, et al. Erythropoietin mRNA expression in human fetal and neonatal tissue. Blood 1998;92:3218–3225.
20. Widness JA, Susa JB, Garcia JF, et al. Increased erythropoiesis and elevated erythropoietin in infants born to diabetic mothers and in hyperinsulinemic rhesus fetuses. J Clin Invest 1981;67:637–642.
21. Snijders RJ, Abbas A, Melby O, et al. Fetal plasma erythropoietin concentration in severe growth retardation. Am J Obstet Gynecol 1993; 168:615–619.
22. Ohls RK, Li Y, Trautman MS, Christensen RD. Erythropoietin production by macrophages from preterm infants: implications regarding the cause of the anemia in prematurity. Pediatr Res 1994;35:169–170.
23. Widness JA, Veng-Pedersen P, Peters C, et al. Erythropoietin pharmacokinetics in premature infants: developmental, nonlinearity, and treatment effects. J Appl Physiol 1996;80:140–148.
24. Ruth V, Widness JA, Clemons G, Raivio KO. Postnatal changes in serum immunoreactive erythropoietin in relation to hypoxia before and after birth. J Pediatr 1990;116:950–954.
25. George JW, Bracco CA, Shannon KM, et al. Age related difference in erythropoietic response to recombinant human erythropoietin: comparison of adults and infants rhesus monkeys. Pediatr Res 1990; 28:567–571.
26. Widness JA, Kulhavy JC, Johnson KJ, et al. Clinical Performance of an in-line point-of-care monitor in neonates. Pediatrics 2000;106: 497–504.
27. Ringer SA, Richardson DK, Sacher RA, et al. Variations in transfusion practice in neonatal intensive care. Pediatrics 1998;101:194–200.
28. Bednarek FJ, Weisberger S, Richardson DK, et al, for the SNAP II Study Group. Variations in blood transfusions among newborn intensive care units. J Pediatr 1998;133:601–607.
29. Ramasethu J, Luban NL. Red blood cell transfusions in the newborn. Semin Neonatol 1999;4:5–16.
30. Blanchette VS, Hume HA, Levy GJ, et al. Guidelines for auditing pediatric blood transfusion practices. Am J Dis Child 1991;145:787–796.
31. Bell EF, Strauss RG, Widness RG, et al. Randomized trial of liberal versus restrictive guidelines for red blood cell transfusion in preterm infants. Pediatrics 2005;115:1685–1691.
32. Kissack CM, Garr R, Wardle SP, Weindling AM. Postnatal changes in cerebral oxygen extraction in the preterm infant are associated with intraventricular hemorrhage and hemorrhagic parenchymal infarction but not periventricular leukomalacia. Pediatr Res 2004;56:111–116.
33. Heddle NM, Kirpalani H. Identifying the optimal red cell transfusion threshold for extremely low birth weight infants: the Premature In Need of Transfusion (PINT) study. Transfusion 2004;44:1A.
34. Phillips HM, Holland BM, Abdel-Moiz A, et al. Determination of red-cell mass in assessment and management of anaemia in babies needing blood transfusion. Lancet 1986;1:882–884.
35. Jones JG, Holland BM, Veale KE, Wardrop CA. "Available oxygen," a realistic expression of the ability of the blood to supply oxygen to tissues. Scand J Haematol 1979;22:77–82.
36. Alverson DC, Isken VH, Cohen RS. Effect of booster blood transfusions on oxygen utilization in infants with bronchopulmonary dysplasia. J Pediatr 1988;113:722–726.
37. Hudson IR, Cavill IA, Cooke AD, et al. Biotin labeling of red cells in the measurement of red cell volume in preterm infants. Pediatr Res 1990;28:199–202.
38. Hudson I, Cooke A, Holland B, et al. Red cell volume and cardiac output in anaemic preterm infants. Arch Dis Child 1990;65:672–675.
39. Mock DM, Lankford GL, Widness JA, et al. Measurement of circulating red blood cell volume using biotin labeled red cells: validation against ^{51}Cr labeled red cells. Transfusion 1999;39:149–155.
40. Mock DM, Lankford GL, Widness JA, et al. Measurement of red cell survival using biotin labeled red cells: Validation against ^{51}Cr labeled red cells. Transfusion 1999;39:156–162.
41. Strauss RG, Mock DM, Widness JA, et al. Posttransfusion 24-hour recovery and subsequent survival of allogeneic red blood cells in the bloodstream of newborn infants. Transfusion 2004;6:871–876.
42. Luban NLC, Strauss RG, Hume HA. Commentary on the safety of red blood cells preserved in extended storage media for neonatal transfusions. Transfusion 1990;30:229–235.
43. Liu EA, Mannio FL, Lane TA. Prospective, randomized trial of the safety and efficacy of a limited donor exposure transfusion program for premature neonates. J Pediatr 1994;125:92–96.
44. Lee DA, Slagle TA, Jackson TM, Evans CS. Reducing blood donor exposures in low birth weight infants by the use of older, unwashed packed red blood cells. J Pediatr 1995;126:280–286.
45. Wood A, Wilson N, Skacel P, et al. Reducing donor exposure in preterm infants requiring multiple blood transfusions. Arch Dis Child Fetal Neonat 1995;72:F29–F33.
46. Strauss RG, Burmeister LF, Johnson K, et al. AS-1 red blood cells for neonatal transfusions: a randomized trial assessing donor exposure and safety. Transfusion 1996;36:873–878.
47. Strauss RG. Recombinant erythropoietin for the anemia of prematurity: still a promise, not a panacea. J Pediatr 1997;131:653–655.
48. Widness JA, Strauss RG. Recombinant erythropoietin in treatment of the premature newborn. Semin Neonatol 1998;3:163.
49. Widness JA, Seward VJ, Kromer IJ, et al. Changing patterns of red blood cell transfusion in very low birthweight infants. J Pediatr 1996; 129:680–687.

50. Shannon KM, Keith JF III, Mentzer WC, et al. Recombinant human erythropoietin stimulates erythropoiesis and reduces erythrocyte transfusions in very-low-birth-weight preterm infants. Pediatrics 1995;95:1–8.
51. Ohls RK, Veerman MW, Christensen RD. Pharmacokinetics and effectiveness of recombinant erythropoietin administered to preterm infants by continuous infusion in total parenteral nutrition solution. J Pediatr 1996;128:518–523.
52. Ohls RK, Harcum J, Schibler KR, Christensen RD. The effect of erythropoietin on the transfusion requirements of preterm infants weighing 750 grams or less: a randomized, double-blind, placebo-controlled study. J Pediatr 1997;131:661–665.
53. Rebulla P, Finazzi G, Marangoni F, et al. The threshold for prophylactic platelet transfusions in adults with acute myeloid leukemia. Gruppo Italiano Malattie Ematologiche Maligne dell'Adulto. NEJM 1997;337:1870–1875.
54. Wandt H, Frank M, Ehninger G, et al. Safety and cost effectiveness of a 10×10^9/L trigger for prophylactic platelet transfusions compared with the traditional 20×10^9/L trigger: a prospective comparative trial in 105 patients with acute myeloid leukemia. Blood 1998;91:3601–3606.
55. Castle V, Andrew M, Kelton J, et al. Frequency and mechanism of neonatal thrombocytopenia. J Pediatr 1986;108:749–755.
56. Andrew M, Castle V, Saigal S, et al. Clinical impact of neonatal thrombocytopenia. J Pediatr 1987;110:457.
57. Castle V, Coates G, Kelton JG, Andrew M. ^{111}In-oxine platelet survivals in thrombocytopenic infants. Blood 1987;70:652–656.
58. Murray NA, Roberts IA. Circulating megakaryocytes and their progenitors in early thrombocytopenia in preterm neonates. Pediatr Res 1996;40:112–119.
59. Wolber E-M, Dame C, Fahnenstich H, et al. Expression of the thrombopoietin gene in human fetal and neonatal tissues. Blood 1999;94:-97–105.
60. Murray NA, Watts TL, Roberts IA. Endogenous thrombopoietin levels and effect of recombinant human thrombopoietin on megakaryocyte precursors in term and preterm babies. Pediatr Res 1998;43:148–151.
61. Andrew M, Vegh P, Caco C, et al. A randomized trial of platelet transfusions in thrombocytopenic premature infants. J Pediatr 1993;123: 285–291.
62. Lupton BA, Hill A, Whitfield MF, et al. Reduced platelet count as a risk factor for intraventricular hemorrhage. Am J Dis Child 1988;142: 1222–1224.
63. Conway LT, Scott EP. Acute hemolytic transfusion reaction due to ABO incompatible plasma in a plateletpheresis concentrate. Transfusion 1984;24:413–414.
64. Pierce RN, Reich LM, Mayer K. Hemolysis following platelet transfusions from ABO-incompatible donors. Transfusion 1985;25:60–62.
65. Valbonesi M, Deluigi MC, Lercari G, et al. Acute intravascular hemolysis in two patients transfused with dry-platelet units obtained from the same ABO incompatible donor. Int J Artif Organs 2000;23:642–646.
66. Angiolillo A, Luban NLC. Hemolysis following an out-of-group platelet transfusion in an 8-month-old with Langerhans cell histiocytosis. J Pediatr Hematol Oncol 2004;26:267–269.
67. Strauss RG. The rebirth of granulocyte transfusions: Should it involve pediatric oncology and transplant patients? Am J Pediatr Hematol Oncol 1999;21:475–478.
68. The Trial to Reduce Alloimmunization to Platelets Study Group. Leukocyte reduction and ultraviolet B irradiation of platelets to prevent alloimmunization and refractoriness to platelet transfusions. NEJM 1997;337:1861–1870.
69. Peters BG, Adkins DR, Harrison BR, et al. Antifungal effects of yeast-derived rhu-GM-CSF in patients receiving high-dose chemotherapy given with or without autologous stem cell transplantation: a retrospective analysis. Bone Marrow Transplant 1996;18:93–102.
70. Vamvakas EC, Pineda AA. Meta-analysis of clinical studies of efficacy of granulocyte transfusions in the treatment of bacterial sepsis. J Clin Apher 1996;11:1–9.
71. Adkins D, Spitzer G, Johnson M, et al. Transfusions of granulocyte-colony-stimulating factor-mobilized granulocyte components to allogeneic transplant recipients: analysis of kinetics and factors determining posttransfusion neutrophil and platelet counts. Transfusion 1997;37:737–748.
72. Kolbe K, Domkin D, Derigs HG, et al. Infectious complications during neutropenia subsequent to peripheral blood stem cell transplantation. Bone Marrow Transplant 1997;19:143–147.
73. Ikinciogullari A, Dogu F, Solaz N, et al. Granulocyte transfusions in children with chronic granulomatous disease and invasive aspergillosis. Ther Apher Dial 2005;2:137–141.
74. Rosenthal J, Cairo MS. Neonatal myelopoiesis and immunomodulation of host defenses. In Petz LD, Swisher SN, Kleinman S, et al (eds): clinical Practice of Transfusion Medicine, 3rd ed. New York, Churchill Livingstone, 1995, p 685.
75. Christensen RD, MacFarlane JL, Taylor NL, et al. Blood and marrow neutrophils during experimental group B streptococcal infection: quantification of the stem cell, proliferative, storage and circulating pools. Pediatr Res 1982;16:549–553.
76. Erdman SH, Christensen RD, Bradley PP, Rothstein G. Supply and release of storage neutrophils: A developmental study. Biol Neonate 1982;41:132–137.
77. Christensen RD, Harper TE, Rothstein G. Granulocyte-macrophage progenitor cells in term and preterm neonates. J Pediatr 1986;109: 1047–1051.
78. Christensen RD, Rothstein G, Anstall HB, Bybee B. Granulocyte transfusions in neonates with bacterial infection, neutropenia and depletion of mature marrow neutrophils. Pediatrics 1982;70:1–6.
79. Laurenti F, Ferro R, Isacchi G, et al. Polymorphonuclear leukocyte transfusion for the treatment of sepsis in the newborn infants. J Pediatr 1981;98:118–123.
80. Cairo MS, Rucker R, Bennetts GA, et al. Improved survival of newborns receiving leukocyte transfusions for sepsis. Pediatrics 1984;74: 887–892.
81. Cairo MS, Worcester C, Rucker R, et al. Role of circulating complement and polymorphonuclear leukocyte transfusion in treatment and outcome in critically ill neonates with sepsis. J Pediatr 1987;110: 935–941.
82. DeCurtis M, Romano G, Scarpato N, et al. Transfusions of polymorphonuclear leukocytes (PMN) in an infant with necrotizing enterocolitis (NEC) and a defect of phagocytosis. J Pediatr 1981;99:665–666.
83. Christensen RD, Anstall H, Rothstein G. Neutrophil transfusion in septic neutropenic neonates. Transfusion 1982;22:151–153.
84. Laing IA, Boulton FE, Hume R. Polymorphonuclear leukocyte transfusion in neonatal septicemia. Arch Dis Child 1983;58:1003–1005.
85. Laurenti F, LaGreca G, Ferro R, Bucci G. Transfusion of polymorphonuclear neutrophils in a premature infant with *Klebsiella* sepsis. Lancet 1978;2:111–112.
86. Baley JE, Stork EK, Warkentin PI, Shurin SB. Buffy coat transfusions in neutropenic neonates with presumed sepsis: a prospective, randomized trial. Pediatrics 1987;80:712–720.
87. Wheeler JC, Chauvenet AR, Johnson CA, et al. Buffy coat transfusions in neonates with sepsis and neutrophil storage pool depletion. Pediatrics 1987;79:422–425.
88. Newman RS, Waffarn F, Simmons GE, et al. Questionable value of saline prepared granulocytes in the treatment of neonatal septicemia. Transfusion 1988;28:196–197.
89. Strauss RG. Current status of granulocyte transfusions to treat neonatal sepsis. J Clin Apheresis 1989;5:25–29.
90. Haque KN, Zaidi MN, Haque SK, et al. Intravenous immunoglobulin for prevention of sepsis in preterm and low birth weight infants. Pediatr Infect Dis 1986;5:622–625.
91. Chirico G, Rondini G, Plebani A, et al. Intravenous gammaglobulin therapy for prophylaxis of infection in high-risk neonates. J Pediatr 1987;110:437–442.
92. Clapp DW, Kliegman RM, Baley JE, et al. Use of intravenously administered immune globulin to prevent nosocomial sepsis to low birth weight infants: report of a pilot study. J Pediatr 1989;115:973–978.
93. Conway SP, Ng PC, Howel D, et al. Prophylactic intravenous immunoglobulin in preterm infants: a controlled trial. Vox Sang 1990;59: 6–11.
94. Stabile A, Miceli Sopo S, Romanelli V, et al. Intravenous immunoglobulin for prophylaxis of neonatal sepsis in premature infants. Arch Dis Child 1988;63:441–443.
95. Magny JF, Bremard-Oury C, Brault D, et al. Intravenous immunoglobulin therapy for prevention in high-risk premature infants: report of a multicenter, double-blind study. Pediatrics 1991;88:437–443.
96. Baker CJ, Melish ME, Hall RT, et al. Intravenous immune globulin for the prevention of nosocomial infection in low-birth-weight neonates. The Multicenter Group for the Study of Immune Globulin in Neonates. NEJM 1992;327:213–219.
97. Bussel JB. Intravenous gammaglobulin in the prophylaxis of late sepsis in very-low-birth-weight infants: preliminary results of a randomized, double-blind, placebo-controlled trial. Rev Infect Dis 1990;12:S457–S461.
98. Fanaroff AA, Korones SB, Wright LL, et al, for the National Institute of Child Health and Human Development Neonatal Research Network. A controlled trial of intravenous immune globulin to reduce nosocomial infections in very-low-birth-weight infants. NEJM 1994;330:1107–1113.
99. van Overmeire B, Bleyaert S, van Reempts PJ, van Acker KJ: The use of intravenously administered immunoglobulins in the prevention of severe infection in very low birth weight neonates. Biol Neonate 1993;64:110–115.
100. Weisman LE, Stoll BJ, Kueser TJ, et al. Intravenous immune globulin prophylaxis of late-onset sepsis in premature neonates. J Pediatr 1994;125:922–930.

101. Christensen RD, Hardman T, Thornton J, Hill HR. A randomized, double-blind, placebo-controlled investigation of the safety of intravenous immune globulin administration to preterm neonates. J Perinatol 1989;9:126–130.
102. Sidiropoulos D, Boehme U, von Muralt G, et al. Immunoglobulin supplementation in prevention or treatment of neonatal sepsis. Pediatr Infect Dis J 1986;5:S193–S194.
103. Haque KN, Zaidi MH, Bahakim H. IgM-enriched intravenous immunoglobulin therapy in neonatal sepsis. Am J Dis Child 1988;142:1293–1296.
104. Friedman CA, Wender DG, Temple DM, Rawson JE. Intravenous gamma globulin as adjunct therapy for severe group B streptococcal disease in the newborn. Am J Perinatol 1990;7:1–4.
105. Weisman LE, Stoll BJ, Kueser TJ, et al. Intravenous immune globulin therapy for early-onset sepsis in premature neonates. J Pediatr 1992;121:434–443.
106. Haque KN, Remo C, Bahakim H. Comparison of two types of intravenous immunoglobulins in the treatment of neonatal sepsis. Clin Exp Immunol 1995;101:328–333.
107. Jenson HB, Pollock BH. Meta-analyses of the effectiveness of intravenous immune globulin for prevention and treatment of neonatal sepsis. Pediatrics 1997;99:E2.
108. Cross AS, Siegel G, Byrne WR, et al. Intravenous immune globulin impairs anti-bacterial defenses of a cyclophosphamide-treated host. Clin Exp Immunol 1989;76:159–164.
109. Weisman LE, Lorenzetti PM. High intravenous doses of human immune globulin suppress neonatal group B streptococcal immunity in rats. J Pediatr 1989;115:445–450.
110. Cross AS, Alving BM, Sadoff JC, et al. Intravenous immune globulin: A cautionary note. Lancet 1984;1:912.
111. Gillan ER, Christensen RD, Suen Y, et al. A randomized, placebo-controlled trial of recombinant human granulocyte colony-stimulating factor administration in newborn infants with presumed sepsis: significant induction of peripheral and bone marrow neutrophilia. Blood 1994;84:1427–1433.
112. Cairo MS, Christensen R, Sender LS, et al. Results of a phase I/II trial of recombinant human granulocyte-macrophage colony-stimulating factor in very low birthweight neonates: significant induction of circulatory neutrophils, monocytes, platelets, and bone marrow neutrophils. Blood 1995;86:2509–2515.
113. Schibler KR, Osborne KA, Leung LY, et al. A randomized, placebo-controlled trial of granulocyte colony-stimulating factor administration to newborn infants with neutropenia and clinical signs of early-onset sepsis. Pediatrics 1998;102:6–13.
114. Cairo MS, Agosti J, Ellis R, et al. A randomized, double-blind, placebo-controlled trial of prophylactic recombinant human granulocyte-macrophage colony-stimulating factor to reduce nosocomial infections in very low birth weight neonates. J Pediatr 1999;134:64–70.
115. Duguid JKM, Minards J, Bolton-Maggs PHB. Incompatible plasma transfusions and haemolysis in children. BMJ 1999;31:176–177.
116. Pisciotto P (ed). Pediatric Hemotherapy Data Card. Bethesda, Md., American Association of Blood Banks, 2002.
117. Hume HA, Limoges P. Perioperative blood transfusion therapy in pediatric patients. Amer J Therap 2002;9:396–403.
118. Downes KA, Wilson E, Yomtovian R, Sarode R. Serial measurements of clotting factors in thawed plasma stored for 5 days. Transfusion 2001;41:570.
119. Blackall DP, Uhl L, Spitalnik SL. Cryoprecipitate-reduced plasma: Rationale for use and efficacy in the treatment of thrombotic thrombocytopenic purpura. Transfusion 2001;41:840–844.
120. Zeigler ZR, Gryn JF, Rintels PB, et al. Cryoprecipitate poor plasma does not improve early response in primary adult thrombotic thrombocytopenic purpura (TTP). J Clin Apheresis 2001;16:19–22.
121. Goodnight SH, Hathaway WE. Disorders of Hemostasis and Thrombosis. New York, McGraw-Hill, 2001, p 31.
122. Luk C, Eckert KM, Barr RM, Chin-Yee IH. Prospective audit of the use of fresh-frozen plasma, based on Canadian Medical Association transfusion guidelines. Can Med Assoc J 2002;166:1539–1540.
123. Josephson CD, Abshire T. The new albumin-free recombinant factor VIII concentrates for treatment of hemophilia: do they represent an actual incremental improvement? Clin Adv Hematal Oncol 2004;2:441–446.

Chapter 38

Transfusion of the Hemoglobinopathy Patient

Krista L. Hillyer • James R. Eckman

SICKLE CELL DISEASE

Pathogenesis and Clinical Pathology

Eight percent of African Americans are heterozygous carriers of hemoglobin S (HbS), and 1 in every 300 has sickle cell disease (SCD). The homozygous state (HbSS), also known as *sickle cell anemia,* is the most common type of SCD in the United States; 1 in 600 African Americans has HbSS.[1,2] Compound heterozygote states, such as sickle cell hemoglobin C (HbSC) disease, together with the combination of HbS and β-thalassemia (sickle cell/β-thalassemia), account for most of the remaining African American cases of SCD.[1,2] Other types of SCD arise from the interaction of HbS with rarer hemoglobin variants; these account for a small number of SCD cases in North America.

Patients with SCD have HbS levels greater than 50% of the total hemoglobin (Hb) concentration. This abnormal sickle hemoglobin, when deoxygenated, forms polymers within the erythrocyte that distort its shape and decrease its deformability, leading to vaso-occlusive phenomena. A detailed description of the molecular pathogenesis of SCD is beyond the scope of this text; the reader is referred to Bunn[3] and Steinberg[4] for recent extensive reviews of this topic.

The vaso-occlusive events, abnormal blood rheology, complex cellular interactions, and other poorly understood factors resulting from the polymerization of HbS cause hemolytic anemia and increased susceptibility to infection, infarctive organ damage, and recurrent episodes of severe pain (Table 38–1). As a result of these complications, patients with HbSS have a reduced life span.[5] Many of the complications of SCD can be abrogated, ameliorated, or prevented by transfusion of donor red blood cells (RBCs). Because of the numerous proven clinical benefits from transfusion and the complex rheologic properties of sickle blood, there are a number of unique goals, indications, and methods for transfusion in SCD.

Goals of Transfusion Therapy

The goals of RBC transfusion in SCD patients are: to improve oxygen-carrying capacity by increasing the total Hb concentration; to decrease blood viscosity and improve blood flow by diluting RBCs containing sickle hemoglobin; and to suppress endogenous erythropoiesis by increasing tissue oxygenation.[6] The first goal is common to many clinical indications for RBC transfusion. The latter two goals for RBC transfusion are required only in individuals with hemoglobinopathies. They also provide unique potential benefits, as well as associated complications, when compared with standard methods of transfusion.

Methods of Transfusion Therapy

Unique Transfusion Considerations in Sickle Cell Disease

Several methods of RBC transfusion therapy are used for SCD patients (Table 38–2) because of the potential limitations of acute simple transfusions, including acute volume overload and reduction in blood flow from increased blood viscosity.[7] Patients with SCD have normal or increased total blood volume because plasma volume is increased in response to chronic anemia. Acute increases in total blood volume after transfusion of RBCs may increase cardiac work to the point of precipitating congestive heart failure.

Perhaps a more important consideration in SCD relates to changes in blood viscosity from the transfusion of RBCs.[8] Viscosity of deoxygenated or oxygenated sickle blood is increased, when compared with normal blood at any hematocrit (Hct).[7]

Because of the opposing effects of Hct on oxygen content and blood viscosity, the optimal Hct is approximately 40% for normal arterial blood. The optimal Hct for sickle blood is strongly dependent on oxygen tension, varying from 18% at a PO_2 of 18 mmHg to 31% for fully oxygenated arterial blood.[7]

Transfusion of normal RBCs significantly increases sickle blood viscosity when the proportion of HbS-containing cells is greater than 60%.[7] The increase in viscosity is minimal when the proportion is less than 40%.[7]

These in vitro observations translate into clinically relevant reductions in tissue oxygenation in SCD patients who are transfused to a Hct greater than 30%. This forms the rationale for the use of acute exchange transfusion in many sickle complications.[8] Chronic erythrocytapheresis is primarily used to decrease iron overload.[8]

Acute Simple Transfusion

In *simple transfusion,* normal donor RBCs are infused into the patient without removal of the patient's own RBCs. In general, acute simple transfusion is indicated when the immediate need for oxygen-carrying capacity is increased but there is no need for a dramatic decrease in the percentage of HbS in the patient's blood.[9] The volume of RBCs to be transfused can be calculated by the formula shown in Figure 38–1.

Table 38–1 **Clinical Complications of Sickle Cell Disease**

Central Nervous System
Cerebrovascular accidents
Subarachnoid hemorrhage
Meningitis
Skeletal System
Bone pain
Bony abnormalities
Delayed growth
Osteonecrosis
Dactylitis
Osteomyelitis
Cardiopulmonary System
Tachycardia
Pulmonary infarctions
Acute chest syndrome
Pulmonary fibrosis
Pulmonary hypertension
Pneumonia
Genitourinary System
Renal concentrating defect
Hematuria
Papillary necrosis
Renal tubular acidosis
Renal failure
Priapism
Hepatobiliary System
Jaundice
Hepatomegaly
Intrahepatic cholestasis
Spleen
Splenomegaly
Autosplenectomy
Eye
Retinopathy
Retinal hemorrhage
Retinal detachment
Visual loss
Skin
Leg ulcers

When transfusing patients with SCD, it is desirable to maintain the Hct at 30% or less. Once the Hct rises above 30%, oxygen delivery to the tissues may decrease, owing to increases in viscosity.[10] Because the primary goal of RBC transfusion is to rapidly improve oxygen delivery to tissues to prevent ongoing ischemia, the maximum beneficial Hct to be achieved by transfusion is 30%.

For simple transfusion, donor RBCs may be infused through an 18- to 23-gauge needle or catheter, depending on the size of the patient and the accessibility of his or her peripheral veins, using a standard blood infusion set.[11]

Chronic Simple Transfusion

Chronic simple transfusion is indicated for a variety of clinical situations in which it is desirable to increase oxygen-carrying

Table 38–2 **Methods of Transfusion for the Patient with Sickle Cell Disease**

Acute simple transfusion
Chronic simple transfusion
Erythrocytapheresis (acute and chronic)
Manual red blood cell exchange transfusion

capacity and to chronically depress the percentage of HbS in the patient's blood.[9] When a specific decrease in HbS percentage is desired, the calculation shown in Figure 38–2 estimates the dilutional effects of transfusion on HbS.

As for acute simple transfusion, the typical goal of chronic transfusion therapy is to maintain the HbS percentage at less than 30% of the total Hb concentration.[9,12] In average-size adults, maintenance of less than 30% HbS usually requires transfusion of 2 to 3 units of RBCs every 3 to 5 weeks. For children, the amount may be calculated from the formula in Figure 38–2. The total volume of RBCs to be transfused at each regular interval in a chronic simple transfusion protocol is determined by the pretransfusion level of hemoglobin A (HbA). If the HbA percentage is too low (in most cases, 70% HbA or higher is the goal), either the volume of RBCs to be transfused is increased or the time interval between transfusions is decreased.

In the case of chronic simple RBC transfusion therapy, catheters may be surgically implanted and used for multiple transfusion events. This allows for improved venous access and less patient discomfort. Peripheral veins may also be used for chronic transfusion.

Red Blood Cell Exchange Transfusion (Manual and Automated)

Donor RBCs are infused while the patient's own RBCs are removed simultaneously in the method of transfusion known as *RBC exchange therapy*. The major benefits of RBC exchange are the rapid adjustments in the patient's Hct and HbS levels. This is a critically important factor during acute sickling episodes, the major indication for RBC exchange; during certain acute ischemic episodes, the replacement of sickled RBCs with normal donor RBCs (improving oxygen delivery to ischemic tissues) must be accomplished quickly to prevent further tissue damage.[9] In addition, unlike simple transfusion, RBC exchange allows for removal of the same volume of RBCs as is replaced, decreasing the risk of iron overload associated with chronic simple transfusion.

The usual measurable end points of RBC exchange therapy are: HbA level of 70%; HbS level of 30%; and overall Hct of 30% or less.[13] The Hct is maintained at 30% or less to achieve balance of viscosity.

Red blood cell exchange transfusion is typically performed with the use of an automated apheresis instrument (erythrocytapheresis). This instrument removes the patient's blood, separates the RBCs from the platelet-rich plasma by

$$\text{Volume of replacement RBCs (mL)} = \frac{[(\text{desired \% Hct} - \text{initial \% Hct}) \times \text{TBV}]}{\text{\% Hct of replacement RBCs}}$$

Figure 38–1 Volume of red blood cells (RBCs) to be transfused to sickle cell patients using the acute simple transfusion method. Hct, hematocrit. (From Wayne AS, Kevy SV, Nathan DG. Transfusion management of sickle cell disease. Blood 1993;81:1109–1123.)

$$\% \text{ HbS desired} = \frac{[1 - (\text{transfused RBC volume} \times \text{Hct of replacement RBCs})]}{[(\text{TBV} \times \text{initial Hct}) + (\text{transfused RBC volume} \times \text{Hct of replacement RBCs})] \times (\text{initial \% HbS})}$$

Figure 38–2 Volume of red blood cells (RBCs) to be transfused to sickle cell patients using the chronic simple transfusion method. HbS, sickle hemoglobin; Hct, hematocrit; TBV, total blood volume. (From Wayne AS, Kevy SV, Nathan DG. Transfusion management of sickle cell disease. Blood 1993;81:1109–1123.)

centrifugation, returns the plasma to the patient, and discards the patient's sickled RBCs. At the same time, donor RBCs are infused, maintaining a stable blood volume throughout the procedure. In the past, RBC exchange transfusion could be performed only manually, and a variety of formulas were used to estimate the appropriate exchange volumes. Today, indications still exist for manual RBC exchange, but erythrocytapheresis is currently the most common method of RBC exchange.

The automated apheresis instrument has an internal programmable computer that precisely calculates both the volume of the patient's RBCs to be removed and the volume of the donor's RBCs to be infused. First, the patient's total blood volume and RBC volume are calculated by entering into the computer the patient's gender, height, weight, and current Hct. Next, the desired HbS percentage, the desired final Hct, and the Hct of the donor RBC preparation are entered, and the appropriate volumes for exchange are determined. However, the formula shown in Figure 38–3 provides a general, practical estimate of the number of RBC units to be used in automated RBC exchange transfusion. Having an estimate of the number of units to be exchanged before initiation of the procedure is important, because the blood bank may need extra time to procure the appropriate RBC units.

The process of erythrocytapheresis is as follows. In most cases, central venous access is established, typically in the subclavian vein or the internal jugular vein, using a hemodialysis-grade, rigid-wall, large-lumen, double-bore catheter that can withstand high flow rates. In adults and larger children with easily accessible peripheral veins, the antecubital veins may be acceptable for use, with 16- to 18-gauge needles used for blood removal and 18- to 20-gauge catheters for blood return. The apheresis instrument, after being programmed with the appropriate patient data and the desired end points for therapy, is used by a trained operator to remove the patient's RBCs and replace them with donor RBCs. Of note, it is usually desirable to replace the patient's sickled RBCs with HbS-negative (sickle trait–negative) donor RBCs in an exchange procedure, for the purposes of appropriately calculating and achieving the desired percentages of HbS and HbA.[12] However, if HbS-negative units cannot be procured in a timely manner, it is at the clinician's discretion (dependent on the severity and acuteness of patient illness) whether or not to wait for HbS-negative units to be identified.

In infants and small children, the amount of blood in the extracorporeal circuit of the automated apheresis machine represents a significant percentage of the child's total blood volume, which may lead to hypotension or a critically low Hct, or both, if the machine is primed with saline. Instead, the automated apheresis instrument should be primed with RBCs if the extracorporeal circuit represents 12% or more of the child's blood volume, the child weighs less than 20 kg, or the child is anemic or unstable.[13]

Occasionally, certain patients require manual RBC exchange transfusions. Manual RBC exchange may be necessary in infants who have very small total blood volumes and in emergencies involving children or adults, when the additional time required to establish appropriate venous access or to mobilize the apheresis team would be deleterious to the patient's health. A rapid manual partial RBC exchange may be performed by withdrawing blood from a peripheral (usually antecubital) vein and infusing RBCs via a stopcock into the same vein (or directly into a different peripheral vein), using the methods outlined in Table 38–3. The requirements that must be honored to ensure a safe and effective manual exchange transfusion are the following: marked increases in blood viscosity should be avoided; blood volume should be maintained throughout the exchange; and the exchange should be completed in the shortest length of time possible.[14] These three important factors must be evaluated and balanced, based on the unique clinical circumstances of the individual patient in need of exchange transfusion.

$$\text{Exchange RBC volume (mL)} = \text{desired \% Hct} \times \text{TBV}$$

Figure 38–3 Practical estimate of the volume of red blood cells (RBCs) to be transfused to sickle cell patients using the automated RBC exchange transfusion method. Hct, hematocrit; TBV, total blood volume. (From Wayne AS, Kevy SV, Nathan DG. Transfusion management of sickle cell disease. Blood 1993;81:1109–1123.)

SELECTION OF ANTICOAGULANT/PRESERVATIVE SOLUTIONS

In the past, when RBC units were collected primarily in citrate-phosphate-dextrose (CPD) or citrate-phosphate-dextrose-adenine (CPDA-1) solutions, these units were reported to have average hematocrits of 80% or more, and it was recommended that RBCs be "reconstituted" to the volume and Hct of whole blood (30% to 40%) by adding albumin or saline to the blood bag or syringe before manual exchange transfusion to the SCD patient.[14]

However, the current average Hct of an RBC unit is approximately 50% to 70%,[11,15] whether collected in CDPA-1 solutions or in additive systems (e.g., AS-1, AS-3) that extend the shelf life of the product. The alternating administration to an SCD patient of RBCs and saline in equal volumes (see Table 38–3) should theoretically deliver a product essentially identical to "reconstituted" whole blood.

Red blood cells containing additive solutions have more adenine and/or mannitol, in comparison with CPD or CPDA-1–preserved RBC units, depending on the type of additive solution used. Some clinicians hesitate to transfuse RBC units with additional mannitol and adenine, in response to case reports of renal toxicity and significant fluid shifts, in neonates given large volumes of these substances. In a comprehensive review of the existing literature, Strauss concluded that small-volume transfusions of RBCs stored in additive solutions administered to neonates do not lead to an increased risk of adverse events.[16] In the setting of large-volume transfusions, such as RBC exchanges, existing literature does not support or disavow the use of RBCs stored in additive solutions. Thus, many clinical protocols choose to utilize RBC units stored in

Table 38-3 Method for Rapid Manual Red Blood Cell (RBC) Exchange Transfusion in Sickle Cell Patients, Using Practical Exchange Volume Estimates, for Children and Adults.

Children

1. Calculate exchange volume, using 60 mL/kg as a practical estimate.
2. Divide the calculated exchange volume of RBCs into four equal aliquots.
3. Withdraw blood from the patient equal to one exchange aliquot.
4. Infuse saline equal to one exchange aliquot.
5. Withdraw blood from the patient equal to one exchange aliquot.
6. Transfuse a volume of RBCs equal to two exchange aliquots.
7. Repeat steps 3-6.

Adults

1. The exchange volume is 6–8 RBC units, depending on the size of the patient (an average 70-kg man requires approximately 6 RBC units).
2. Withdraw 500 mL of blood from the patient.
3. Infuse 500 mL of saline.
4. Withdraw 500 mL of blood from the patient.
5. Transfuse two units of RBCs.
6. Repeat until 6–8 RBC units have been transfused.

RBC units and saline infused in this alternating manner should theoretically deliver a blood product that is essentially "reconstituted" (within the patient) to the volume and hematocrit of whole blood (30% to 40%), because the current estimated average hematocrit of an RBC unit is 50% to 70%.[60,130] However, if a known exact percent hematocrit of the blood product to be infused is desired, RBCs may be reconstituted to the volume and hematocrit of whole blood (30% to 40%) within a blood bag or syringe, by the addition of saline or other diluents.[131] (From Reid CD, Charache S, Lubin B (eds). Management and Therapy of Sickle Cell Disease, 3rd ed. Bethesda, Md., National Institutes of Health Publication No.99-2117, 1999, p 62.)

CPDA-1 solution for large-volume transfusions in neonates, particularly if these children have liver or kidney dysfunction that would put them at risk for adverse events.

In addition, the amount of potassium transfused to neonates is of concern to clinicians, because mortality following transfusion of RBCs with high potassium levels has been reported.[17] As the shelf life of RBC units is extended, potassium is known to leak from the RBCs, although in amounts that are typically easily processed by individuals with normal kidney function. However, in large-volume and RBC exchange transfusions, many transfusion protocols for SCD patients recommend (but do not require) the use of RBC units that are 7 days old or less. This general practice of transfusing "young" RBC units to SCD patients is of practical use as well, in that younger RBCs will remain in the circulation of the patient for a longer period than will older RBCs.

Chronic Erythrocytapheresis (Automated Red Blood Cell Exchange)

Iron overload is one of the serious long-term complications of chronic transfusion in SCD patients.[18] As a result, certain investigators[19–23] have suggested that *chronic erythrocytapheresis* should be used in place of chronic simple transfusion for the prevention of complications of SCD and to decrease long-term iron accumulation in these patients.

The procedure for chronic erythrocytapheresis is the same as that for acute erythrocytapheresis. Similarly, target postpheresis HbS levels for chronic erythrocytapheresis are usually less than 30%, with desirable postpheresis hematocrits of 30% or less. Currently, chronic erythrocytapheresis is not universally used in the United States for SCD patients, although recent reports suggest that the potential benefits of this method may outweigh its risks and costs. A detailed review of the current literature regarding the role of chronic erythrocytapheresis is provided later in this chapter (see "Iron Overload").

Indications for Transfusion Therapy

RBCs may be administered to patients with SCD by simple RBC infusion or by RBC exchange, either episodically, for the relief of acute symptoms, or chronically, for the prevention of long-term complications. A summary of indications for transfusion of RBCs in SCD patients is shown in Table 38–4. These indications are characterized in the following sections as *generally indicated* or *controversial*, based on several recently published reviews of of the work of various sickle cell experts.[13,24]

Indications for Episodic Transfusion

ACUTE SYMPTOMATIC ANEMIA

Because patients with SCD are chronically anemic, they are often asymptomatic despite very low Hb levels. Biochemical and physiologic factors that decrease symptoms during chronic anemia include increased levels of 2,3-diphosphoglycerate, decreased oxygen–Hb affinity, increased plasma volume, and increased cardiac stroke volume and output.[25] Patients may become acutely symptomatic, making simple transfusion necessary, if they experience a rapid decrease in Hb, hypoxia, or acute cardiac decompensation. Acute anemia can result from bleeding, suppression of erythropoiesis by infection, sequestration, or increased hemolysis. Pulmonary or cardiac disease can cause decompensation, requiring acute transfusion to increase the Hb level above the patient's stable baseline.

APLASTIC CRISIS

Aplastic crisis, typically defined as a decrease in Hb of more than 3.0 g/dL with reticulocytopenia, is a relatively common occurrence in SCD.[26] Aplastic crisis occurs in SCD patients after marked suppression of erythropoiesis for 7 to 10 days, usually as a result of infection of RBC precursors in the bone marrow by human parvovirus B19. In a sample group of 308 children with SCD, human parvovirus B19 accounted for all cases of aplastic crisis that occurred during an 8-year observation period.[27] Because mean RBC survival time in many SCD patients is only 12 to 15 days, the acute life-threatening anemia caused by human parvovirus B19 infection necessitates immediate RBC transfusion to sustain oxygen delivery to the tissues until the bone marrow recovers. Simple RBC transfusion is usually administered slowly (1 mL/kg/hr), because these patients have expanded plasma volumes due to chronic anemia and care must be taken to avoid volume-induced congestive heart failure.[8,28] Partial exchange transfusion, performed by manually removing whole blood and returning RBCs to the patient without replacing the plasma, may be preferred if heart failure from acute volume overload is of significant concern.[9]

ACUTE CHEST SYNDROME

According to a report by the Cooperative Study of Sickle Cell Disease, acute chest syndrome occurs at least once

Table 38–4 Clinical Indications for Transfusion in Patients with Sickle Cell Disease

Type of Transfusion	Indication	Controversial Indications	Nonindications
Episodic	Acute symptomatic anemia	Acute painful episode (acute pain crisis)	Normal pregnancy
	Transient red cell aplasia ("aplastic crisis")	Acute priapism	
	Acute chest syndrome	Preparation for infusion of contrast media	
	Hyperhemolysis		
	Acute splenic sequestration		
	Acute hepatic sequestration		
	Stroke		
	Prior to surgery requiring general anesthesia		
	Prior to eye surgery		
	Acute multiorgan system failure		
	Severe infection with concurrent severe anemia		
Chronic	Prevention of recurrent strokes in children	Recurrent priapism	Leg ulcers
	Prevention of first stroke in children	"Silent" cerebral infarcts	Growth and developmental delays
	Complicated pregnancy	Neurocognitive defects	Early retinopathy
	Chronic hypoxic lung disease	Recurrent acute chest syndrome	Early renal disease
	Frequent severe pain episodes	Prevention of pulmonary hyper-tension/cor pulmonale	
	Chronic heart failure		
	Chronic renal failure		

in approximately 30% of SCD patients, and half of these patients will experience one or more recurrent episodes.[24] Acute chest syndrome is the second most common reason after infection for hospital admission among SCD patients,[29,30] and it is responsible for 25% of all deaths in this population.[31]

Transfusion therapy is vital to the treatment of acute chest syndrome early in its course,[32] and exchange transfusion has been shown to result in rapid improvement of acute chest syndrome if instituted within 48 hours after diagnosis.[33] Simple transfusion causes dramatic improvement of symptoms in children with acute chest syndrome (compared with nontransfused children) if it is begun within 24 hours after diagnosis[34]; therefore, in patients with less serious compromise, simple transfusion is preferred.[35] For those patients with either a progressive decline in arterial oxygen pressure ($Pa{O_2}$ <60 mm Hg in adults, <70 mm Hg in children) or a rapid clinical deterioration, RBC exchange transfusion is recommended.

ACUTE SPLENIC OR HEPATIC SEQUESTRATION

Acute splenic sequestration occurs in SCD patients when sickled RBCs are trapped within splenic sinusoids. As the spleen enlarges, it traps a significant proportion of the circulating RBCs, leading to increased anemia and circulatory failure.[36] The fatality rate from acute splenic sequestration approaches 10%, and approximately 50% of those who survive a first episode will experience another.[36] Immediate simple RBC transfusion has been shown to produce rapid resolution of acute splenic sequestration.[36,37] Splenic sequestration occurs in HbSS patients early in life. It occurs less frequently, but at all ages, in patients with HbSC or sickle cell/β-thalassemia.

Older patients may develop acute hepatic sequestration, which responds well to a similar transfusion strategy.[38]

ACUTE STROKE

Approximately 3.75% of patients with SCD will experience one or more cerebrovascular accidents, according to a longitudinal clinical trial published by the Cooperative Study of Sickle Cell Disease in 1998.[39] The occurrence of infarctive stroke is greatest in children and older patients, whereas the occurrence of hemorrhagic stroke is greatest in patients 20 to 29 years of age. Because the neurologic sequelae of strokes are often devastating, immediate RBC exchange transfusion is indicated upon diagnosis of stroke.[13] Dramatic recovery of neurologic function has been documented after exchange therapy in SCD patients with acute stroke.[39,40]

The stroke prevention trial in sickle cell anemia (the STOP study)[41] identified children who were at high risk for stroke based on elevated cerebral blood flow, as measured by transcranial Doppler (TCD) screening tests. The STOP study also showed that children at high risk for stroke who received intermittent simple transfusions (chronic RBC transfusions) had a 90% relative decline in stroke rates during the transfusion study period, as compared with children at risk for stroke who did not receive intermittent simple transfusions. The many informative results of the STOP study[41,42] have led to the general implementation of chronic simple RBC transfusion in children at high risk for stroke as measured by TCD (see discussion in "Indications for Chronic Transfusion").

Transfusion in the Perioperative Period

BEFORE SURGERY REQUIRING GENERAL ANESTHESIA

Hypoxia, volume depletion, hypotension, hypothermia, and acidosis are all complications of general anesthesia that can lead to intravascular sickling and vascular occlusion, resulting in high rates of morbidity and mortality among SCD patients undergoing general anesthesia.[43] In a prospective study of 717 SCD patients, including 1079 surgical procedures, those patients undergoing low-risk surgeries who received perioperative RBC transfusions had a 4.8% rate of SCD-related postoperative complications, compared with a significantly higher complication rate of 12.9% among similar patients who were not transfused.[44] For minor procedures and tonsillectomies, many patients did not receive transfusions and complication rates were very low.[44] Similarly, in a prospective trial of 364 SCD patients undergoing cholecystectomy, the most common surgical procedure among pediatric and adult SCD patients,[44] those who were not transfused perioperatively had a higher incidence of sickle cell events (32%) than transfused patients did.[45]

In a controlled, randomized trial, Vichinsky and colleagues[43] compared "aggressive" versus "conservative" transfusion regimens in the perioperative management of 604 operations in 551 patients with SCD. The aggressive transfusion regimen was designed to maintain a preoperative Hb level of 10 g/dL and an HbS level at or below 30%. The conservative transfusion regimen only maintained a preoperative Hb level of 10 g/dL, regardless of the percentage of HbS. Results showed that the frequency of serious perioperative complications was similar in the aggressive and conservative transfusion groups (31% and 35%, respectively), whereas the transfusion-related complication rates were 14% and 7%, respectively. The authors concluded that a conservative transfusion regimen is as effective in preventing perioperative complications as an aggressive transfusion regimen.

Conversely, Adams and associates[42] published a retrospective review of 92 children with SCD who underwent 130 surgical procedures using an aggressive transfusion regimen, with most RBC units phenotypically matched to recipients for Rh and Kell antigens. Major perioperative complications occurred in only 12% of surgical procedures, compared with 31% to 35% in Vichinsky's study.[43] The transfusion-related complication rate in Adams' pediatric study (8%) was similar to the rate observed in the conservative arm of Vichinsky's adult and pediatric study (7%). Although Adams suggested that the more aggressive approach with phenotypically matched blood is superior, it is difficult to directly compare the results of this small, retrospective study with those of a large, randomized, controlled clinical trial.

For adults and pediatric patients with SCD who are to undergo general anesthesia, current National Institutes of Health guidelines recommend simple transfusion to increase the preoperative Hb level to 10 g/dL, together with intraoperative or postoperative RBC replacement for blood loss,[46] a position supported by a recent Cochrane Database Review, which concluded that recommendations regarding optimal use of RBC transfusions prior to surgery cannot be adequately assessed at this time and require further study.[47]

BEFORE EYE SURGERY

The use of transfusions in patients undergoing eye surgery is controversial. Although early studies advocated the use of aggressive exchange transfusion for patients undergoing retinal or vitreous surgery, more recent studies have documented that this approach may not be necessary.[48]

Although eye surgery is typically performed under local anesthesia, the microvascular nature of the surgery and the importance of avoiding permanent damage to the eye justify the use of blood transfusion for this indication. Until further data are available, it is reasonable to follow guidelines similar to those used for transfusion of SCD patients undergoing surgical procedures performed under general anesthesia.

ACUTE MULTIORGAN FAILURE SYNDROME

Acute multiorgan failure syndrome may occur after some episodes of severe pain crisis in SCD patients and affects at least two of the following three organs: lung, liver, or kidney. Immediate initiation of RBC transfusion is recommended for the treatment of acute multiorgan failure syndrome.[13,49] Dramatic clinical improvement and rapid reversal of organ dysfunction have been observed after prompt, aggressive transfusion therapy. Simple transfusion is indicated for patients with severe anemia and rapidly falling Hb levels. Exchange transfusion is indicated for those with higher Hb levels or more severe organ failure.[49]

SEVERE INFECTION

Bacterial and malarial infections are common, life-threatening complications occurring in SCD patients worldwide. Some experts do consider it acceptable medical practice to transfuse individuals with severe anemia who have concomitantly serious infections.[13] Infection without concomitant anemia is not a widely accepted indication for transfusion in SCD patients.

Indications for Chronic Transfusion

PREVENTION OF RECURRENT STROKES IN CHILDREN

Approximately 3.75% of SCD patients will experience one or more cerebrovascular accidents, or strokes.[39] Without therapeutic intervention, strokes will recur in more than two thirds of this patient group within 2 to 3 years.[50] Chronic RBC transfusions provide a reduction of up to 90% in the risk of recurrent stroke in these SCD patients (10% risk of recurrent stroke while undergoing a chronic RBC transfusion regimen).[41,46,47,51,52]

The chronic simple transfusion regimen recommended for prevention of recurrent stroke, in the 3.75% of SCD patients who have experienced a stroke, is simple RBC transfusion every 3 to 4 weeks, with a goal of maintaining HbS at less than 30% and Hct at 30% or less.[41,46,47,51,53]

In a small group of patients in whom the desired HbS level was modified to 50% after they had been neurologically stable for 3 years, Cohen and colleagues[54] reported no increased risk of recurrent stroke with chronic transfusion maintaining a 30% HbS level. The major benefit of this modified regimen was a 31% decrease in blood requirements for simple transfusions, which reduced cost, decreased inconvenience, and mitigated the development of alloimmunization and iron overload. Although the sample size was too small to conclude that this method is absolutely effective at preventing recurrent stroke, some experts allow the HbS percentage to increase to 50% in patients who have been stable neurologically for 3 years with chronic transfusion.[13] However, the most widely used guideline is to maintain HbS levels at or below 30% for those SCD patients on a chronic simple transfusion protocol for stroke prevention.

The optimal duration of chronic transfusion for prevention of recurrent stroke is not known, although much productive and informative research has been recently published in this regard.[55] In the 1990s, Wang and coworkers[56] reported that 5 of 10 patients had recurrent strokes within 1 year after discontinuation of chronic transfusions, after a median period without recurrence (since first stroke) of 9.5 years. This rate was significantly greater than the 10% estimated risk of recurrent stroke among patients receiving chronic transfusion therapy. Therefore, most centers since that time have recommended continuation of chronic transfusion therapy indefinitely to prevent recurrent stroke.[13,54]

The Stroke Prevention Trial II (STOP-II) was begun in 2000, with the intention of determining the optimal duration of RBC transfusion therapy in SCD children at risk for first stroke based on TCD screening. This study was halted 2 years early, because the study showed that there was clear evidence of return to high risk of stroke (and stroke itself) in that group of children randomly assigned to the "stop transfusion" group. No such risk was seen in the "continue transfusion" group.[55]

Although the intention of STOP-II was to investigate the outcomes of halting transfusions in children at risk for first stroke, the results can be extrapolated to those children with SCD who have already experienced one or more strokes. Thus, for those children with SCD who have experienced one or more strokes, it is recommended that chronic transfusion protocols be continued indefinitely to prevent recurrent strokes.

PREVENTION OF FIRST STROKE IN CHILDREN

High blood flow velocity in the internal carotid and middle cerebral arteries, detected by TCD, has been found to be predictive of subsequent stroke in children with SCD.[57,58] Adams and associates[42] used TCD to identify children at high risk for stroke, randomly assigned them to receive either standard care or chronic transfusion therapy, and then compared the incidence of stroke between the two groups. There were 11 strokes in the standard-care group but only 1 stroke in the transfusion group, a 92% difference in the risk of stroke ($p < 0.001$). The authors concluded that transfusion greatly reduces the risk of first stroke in children with SCD who have abnormal TCD results.[42] Because this diagnostic method is safe and noninvasive, and the prevention of stroke in these patients can greatly reduce the morbidity and mortality of this complication, many sickle cell centers have implemented regular TCD screening and subsequent chronic transfusion in children with repeated high flow rates, in order to prevent first strokes in children with SCD.[13,24]

The Stroke Prevention Trial II was begun in the year 2000. STOP-II was a multicenter, randomized clinical trial, the intention of which was to determine the optimal duration of RBC transfusion therapy in children with SCD at risk for first stroke, based on TCD screening.[55] The hypothesis of the investigators was that regular RBC transfusions might be safely stopped following (at minimum) 30 months of transfusion therapy, for those children with SCD at high risk for stroke.

The trial was halted by the National Heart, Lung, and Blood Institute (NHLBI) 2 years early, in November 2004, after 79 patients had been enrolled, because 14 of the 41 patients in the group who stopped regular RBC transfusions after a minimum of 30 months reverted to a high risk of stroke, as measured by TCD screening. Two of these children actually suffered strokes. In contrast, of the children who were randomly assigned to the group that are continued transfusions after 30 months, none had strokes or reversions to high risk of stroke. Therefore, the NHLBI issued a clinical alert to physicians in December 2004 that stated that stopping RBC transfusions in SCD pediatric patients at high risk for stroke could not be recommended.

Thus, at this time, it is recommended that children at high risk for stroke should continue on chronic transfusion protocols indefinitely to reduce the risk of first stroke.

COMPLICATED PREGNANCY

Although normal pregnancy in SCD patients is not an indication for prophylactic transfusion,[59–61] certain complications of either the pregnancy itself or the underlying disease process are indications for simple or exchange transfusion (see Table 38–1). These include preeclampsia/eclampsia, twin pregnancy, previous perinatal mortality, acute renal failure, sepsis, bacteremia, severe anemia with reduction in Hb of more than 20% from baseline or an Hb concentration lower than 5 g/dL, acute chest syndrome, hypoxemia, anticipated surgery, and preparation for infusion of angiographic dye.[62]

For all of these indications, simple transfusion is most often used if the Hb concentration is lower than 5 g/dL and the reticulocyte count is less than 3%. If the Hb is 8 to 10 g/dL or greater, exchange transfusion is indicated, with the goal of a post-transfusion Hb concentration of 10 g/dL and a post-transfusion HbS of 50% or less.[63]

CHRONIC ORGAN FAILURE

Patients with renal failure develop progressive anemia because of the loss of erythropoietin production by the kidney.[63] Many of these patients need regular transfusions to avoid severe symptomatic anemia. Older patients with pulmonary disease causing either chronic hypoxia or cardiac disease with chronic congestive heart failure also may require chronic transfusion to prevent symptoms.[13]

FREQUENT PAIN EPISODES

Patients with frequent severe pain episodes who have a very poor quality of life or who are unable to engage in activities of normal daily living may benefit from chronic transfusion.[13] The transfusion programs used for stroke prevention will usually prevent recurrent pain episodes.[28]

Controversial Indications for Acute or Chronic Transfusion

RECURRENT ACUTE CHEST SYNDROME

Repeated episodes of acute chest syndrome in SCD patients have been associated with worsening pulmonary function and restrictive lung disease, which may lead to severe pulmonary fibrosis, pulmonary hypertension, and cor pulmonale by adulthood.[64–68] Some authors have advocated the use of chronic transfusion protocols for the prevention and management of recurrent acute chest syndrome. Hankins and colleagues placed 27 children with SCD and history of recurrent acute chest syndrome on chronic transfusion therapy, and concluded that the number of recurrent acute chest syndrome events was mitigated, but not the severity of the events.[69] Further study is needed in this area to determine the true benefits of chronic transfusion therapy for recurrent acute chest syndrome.

PREVENTION OF PULMONARY HYPERTENSION/ COR PULMONALE

As mentioned previously, pulmonary hypertension and its resultant serious complications in both the heart and lungs have been noted to be common causes of mortality in SCD patients.[65–68,70] Gladwin and colleagues prospectively studied the prevalence and prognosis of pulmonary hypertension in 195 SCD patients, using Doppler ultrasound measurement of tricuspid regurgitant jet velocity.[70] These investigators identified significant pulmonary hypertension in 32% of these 195 patients. Based on increased severity of pulmonary hypertension, as defined by regurgitant jet velocity, 17 patients were given a variety of treatments, including RBC exchange transfusion, oxygen therapy, and vasodilator therapy (i.e., inhaled nitrous oxide). Of those 17 patients judged to be most severely affected, 11 began either chronic RBC transfusion therapy or inhaled nitrous oxide; 10 patients were alive at the time the manuscript was published.

Although Gladwin and others have introduced the concepts of Doppler ultrasound diagnosis and possible chronic RBC transfusion treatment of severe pulmonary hypertension in SCD patients, more data is required before chronic transfusion therapy can be routinely recommended for prevention of cor pulmonale and pulmonary fibrosis.

PRIAPISM

Case studies have suggested improvement in some patients with acute priapism after exchange[71,72] or simple transfusion therapy.[73,74] However, no controlled trial has been performed to establish the effectiveness of transfusion therapy in comparison with hydration, analgesia, stilbestrol,[27] or hydralazine[75,76] therapies for the treatment of acute priapism. In fact, an ***a***ssociation among ***S***CD, ***p***riapism, ***e***xchange transfusion, and subsequent ***n***eurologic events has been described in several patients and has been given the eponym *ASPEN syndrome*.[77] As a result, many centers conservatively manage priapism, using hydration and analgesia, and do not transfuse until a single episode has persisted for longer than 24 to 48 hours.[75] The indications for and the preferred method of transfusion in SCD patients with priapism require further study.

ACUTE PAIN CRISES

Episodes of severe pain, also known as *pain crises,* are the most common reason for hospital admission of SCD patients. Platt and colleagues[78] showed that occurrences of pain crises have a direct correlation with Hb levels: the more severe the anemia (i.e., the lower the Hb concentration), the less frequent the occurrence of pain crises. There is no evidence that transfusion reduces the severity or duration of pain during acute pain episodes.[13]

Therefore, simple transfusion is not indicated for the treatment of acute pain crises and could actually worsen symptoms.

NORMAL PREGNANCY

A randomized, controlled trial performed by Koshy and coworkers[59] assessed the benefits of prophylactic transfusion during pregnancy in women with SCD. Pregnant patients with SCD who were prophylactically transfused were compared with similar patients who were not transfused. No significant differences in perinatal outcome or in medical or obstetric complications were identified between these two groups. The authors concluded that prophylactic transfusion of the pregnant SCD patient, a practice common at the time their study was conducted, could be omitted without harm to mother or fetus.

Therefore, normal pregnancy is not considered an indication for prophylactic RBC transfusion.

LEG ULCERS

Statistical analysis of various methods for the treatment of leg ulcers in SCD patients (including transfusion) did not detect any differences in rate of ulcer healing.[79]

Therefore, the routine use of transfusion for the treatment of leg ulcers in SCD patients is not justified, given the long- and short-term complications of transfusion therapy.

Adverse Effects of Transfusion Therapy and Strategies for Their Prevention and Management

Although transfusion is beneficial and often necessary for treatment of SCD, adverse effects resulting from transfusion of allogeneic donor blood can lead to serious long- and short-term complications in SCD patients (Table 38–5). Both immune- and nonimmune-related complications may occur. These adverse effects, as well as recommended strategies for their prevention and management, are discussed here.

Table 38–5 Common Immune and Nonimmune Adverse Effects of Transfusion Therapy in Patients with Sickle Cell Disease and Strategies for Their Prevention and Management

Adverse Effect	Management Strategy
Immune-Related	
Febrile nonhemolytic transfusion reactions	*Prevention*: Transfuse leukoreduced blood products. *Treatment*: Administer antipyretic medication.
Alloimmunization to RBC antigens and delayed hemolytic transfusion reactions	*Prevention*: Transfuse RBC units matched for antigens most commonly associated with alloimmunization. *Treatment*: Transfuse RBC units matched for antigens to which antibodies have been made; provide supportive therapy for delayed reactions.
Autoimmunization to RBC antigens	*Prevention*: None known. *Treatment*: Administer corticosteroids with or without intravenous immune globulin.
Alloimmunization to platelet- or HLA-specific antigens	*Prevention*: Transfuse leukoreduced blood products. *Treatment*: Transfuse crossmatched or HLA-matched platelet products, if proven indication.
Nonimmune-Related	
Iron overload	*Prevention*: Provide chronic erythrocytapheresis. *Treatment*: Administer deferoxamine or deferasirox.
Transfusion-transmitted infection	*Prevention*: Use the most advanced screening tests for donated blood products; do not transfuse unnecessarily.

Immune-Related Adverse Effects

FEBRILE NONHEMOLYTIC TRANSFUSION REACTIONS

White blood cells (WBCs) synthesize and release various cytokines during storage of cellular blood products that may cause fever and chills (febrile nonhemolytic transfusion reactions) in the transfusion recipient.[80] Current technologies in leukoreduction filtration reduce the leukocyte count in RBCs to less than 5×10^6 WBC/unit, mitigating the development of febrile nonhemolytic transfusion reactions in recipients of leukoreduced blood products.[80] Because SCD patients typically receive large numbers of transfusions and febrile nonhemolytic transfusion reactions occur in association with 0.5% to 1% of transfusions,[81] most experts recommend the use of leukoreduced blood products for all SCD patients. In addition, an acute infection or a pain crisis can manifest with the same symptoms (i.e., fever, chills, malaise) as a febrile nonhemolytic transfusion reaction, confounding the clinical picture and possibly delaying appropriate treatment of underlying disorders in SCD patients.

ALLOIMMUNIZATION TO RBC ANTIGENS AND DELAYED HEMOLYTIC TRANSFUSION REACTIONS

Alloimmunization to RBC antigens is a common problem in transfused SCD patients, leading both to difficulty in obtaining compatible RBC units and to the development of delayed hemolytic transfusion reactions.[82–86] Delayed hemolytic transfusion reactions are especially problematic in SCD patients, in that the symptoms of a delayed hemolytic transfusion reaction can mimic those of a pain crisis and can even lead to a pain crisis,[85] complicating both the clinical diagnosis and the subsequent appropriate treatment of these patients.

The most comprehensive study of the frequency of and risk factors associated with alloimmunization in SCD patients was performed by Vichinsky and colleagues.[87] They prospectively determined the transfusion history, RBC antigen phenotype, and alloantibody development of 107 transfused African American patients with SCD. These results were compared with those from similar studies in 51 nontransfused African American SCD patients and in 19 Caucasian patients who had undergone multiple transfusions for other forms of chronic anemia. The results showed that the average alloimmunization rate for transfused SCD patients was 30%, compared with only 5% for the multiply transfused patients with other forms of anemia ($p < 0.001$). None of the nontransfused SCD patients developed alloantibodies, and the alloimmunization rate in individual SCD patients increased exponentially with increasing numbers of transfusions. Of the 32 patients who developed alloantibodies, 17 developed multiple antibodies, and 12 of these 17 patients had more than three different alloantibodies.

After conducting an RBC phenotyping study of local blood bank donors and comparing these phenotypes with those of SCD patients and of white patients with other forms of chronic anemia, the authors suggested that the increased alloimmunization rate in SCD patients most likely resulted from RBC antigenic differences between the SCD patients (African Americans) and the blood donors (the majority of whom were Caucasian). Such antigenic differences did not exist between blood donors and the multiply transfused Caucasian patients who had other forms of chronic anemia.

Because of this documented lack of phenotypic compatibility in antigen profile between the majority of volunteer allogeneic donor RBCs and those of SCD patients, many centers have suggested that SCD patients receive RBC units matched for antigens most commonly associated with alloimmunization (Table 38–6).[83,85,87]

In Vichinsky's study, comparable to reports by other researchers,[83,86–89] 66% of all alloantibodies that formed in transfused SCD patients were directed against C, E, and K RBC antigens.[87] See Table 38–6 for a summary of the most common antigens to which antibodies are made by SCD patients.

Tahhan and coworkers[90] reported that none (0%) of 40 patients studied who received matched transfusions for C, E, K, Fy^a, JK^b, and S antigens developed alloantibodies, whereas 16 (34.8%) of 46 patients who received both matched and nonmatched transfusions became alloimmunized against one or more of these antigens.

A College of American Pathologists (CAP) study, published in 2005, surveyed 1182 laboratories to determine the extent of RBC antigen phenotyping and RBC antigen matching used in the care of nonalloimmunized SCD patients throughout North America.[91] Of the laboratories surveyed by the CAP, 63% did not routinely phenotype SCD patients any differently than other patients (ABO and RhD antigen phenotyping only). The remaining one third of the North American laboratories reported routinely performing additional RBC phenotyping for SCD patients; 75% of these centers gave units phenotypically matched for additional RBC antigens C, E, and K to SCD patients.

Protocols for phenotyping and limited RBC antigen matching differ among sickle cell centers. In many academic centers, all SCD patients undergo extensive RBC antigen phenotyping before their first transfusion, a policy supported by most experts.[86,89–91] Those SCD patients who have not yet made RBC alloantibodies routinely receive RBC units phenotypically matched for the antigens responsible for most of the alloantibodies made by SCD patients to allogeneic donor RBCs, most often C, E, and K antigens.

Once an SCD patient has made an RBC alloantibody, he or she then typically receives RBC units matched for other RBC antigens to which SCD patients are known to most frequently make antibodies. C, E, K, Fy^a, Jk^b, and S are the six most common and most clinically significant antibodies made by SCD patients (see Table 38–6).[87] These concepts are supported by most centers who do extended phenotype

Table 38–6 Average Frequencies of the Most Common Red Blood Cell Alloantibodies Made by Patients with Sickle Cell Disease

Antibody	Average Frequency (%)
E	21
K	18
C	14
Le^a	8
Fy^a	7
Jk^b	7
D	7
Le^b	7
S	6
Fy^b	5
M	4
e	2
c	2

Data from references 74–77.

antigen matching, and antigen-matched transfusion results in an alloimmunization rate of approximately 1% to 5%, a significant decrease compared with the rates observed among SCD patients transfused with RBCs not matched for these common RBC antigens.[9,83,86,87,90,92]

Limited donor pool programs offer a similar approach to preventing, or at least limiting, alloimmunization in SCD patients. This strategy combats RBC alloimmunization by transfusing RBCs only from donors who are ethnically or antigenically closely matched with the SCD patient, most often for the four RBC antigens (C, D, E, and K) to which antibodies are most commonly made. Sosler and colleagues suggested a model to reduce alloimmunization in SCD patients by using RBC units only from ethnically similar (African American) donors, based on the fact that 93% of African Americans shared the typical SCD phenotype of E, C, Fy^a, Jk^b, and K antigen-negativity, whereas only 7% of the Caucasion population had the same phenotype.[93] Ambruso and associates[92] reported that such a limited donor antigen-matching program can diminish by tenfold the incidence of alloimmunization in transfused SCD patients. However, administrative problems reported in Ambruso's study included difficulties in recruiting eligible donors from the African American community, in inventory management, and in distribution and transfusion of the matched blood, as well as increased expense of the program. Tahhan and coworkers[90] reported that the cost of operating an antigen-matching (not a limited donor) program was 1.5 to 1.8 times that of a standard transfusion protocol.

Hillyer and colleagues[94] conducted a retrospective review of the records of 85 patients who were enrolled in a limited donor pool antigen-matching program (Partners for Life, PFL) between January 1993 and August 2000 and reported that the average number of donors per PFL patient was 9.5, average number of RBC units transfused before PFL was 17.8, and the average number of RBC units transfused during participation in PFL was 39.4.

The overall alloimmunization rate for PFL patients was 7% (6 of 85 developed new RBC antibodies while enrolled in PFL). Of the 6 patients who developed new antibodies, 3 had previously identified antibodies at enrollment, and 3 had no previously identified antibodies. One patient with previously identified antibodies developed anti-V, another developed anti-Go^a, and the third developed anti-Cw and anti-Kp^a (all antigens not routinely matched for in PFL). Two of the three patients without previously formed antibodies developed anti-Fy^a (an antigen not matched for in PFL patients without previously formed alloantibodies). The other patient without previously formed antibodies developed an anti-E after being for in PFL 1.5 years with no antibody formation; however, she was known to have received nonantigen-matched RBCs at a nonparticipating institution immediately prior to her anti-E formation.

Although this limited donor pool program was successful in mitigating RBC alloimmunization (7% overall rate) for this group of patients, it was not successful in limiting the exposure of SCD patients to only this small, dedicated blood donor pool of 9 to 10 donors, due to technical difficulties in having these units available at the time they were needed by the patients. Only 6% of PFL patients received all of their RBC units from their dedicated donors. The majority (57%) received a combination of RBC units from their dedicated donors and antigen-matched RBC units from the general volunteer donor pool. The 7% alloimmunization rate for patients enrolled in the antigen-matching, dedicated donor PFL program is significantly lower than the published 30% rate observed in SCD patients who routinely received non-antigen-matched RBCs, but it is similar to rates observed in other antigen-matching programs without the dedicated donor aspect.[86,90,92,95]

Based on Hillyer's review and the fact that the program was expensive and labor intensive (with respect to recruitment, collection, inventory management, and distribution of dedicated RBC units), this limited donor pool program was changed to an antigen-matching program only, using primarily African American donors from the general volunteer donor pool. This program works well; nearly 13% of blood donors in the associated blood center self-identify as African American. In other parts of the country in which the general donor pool does not have such a high percentage of African American donors, special recruitment efforts within the African American community would need to be made to procure the required number of phenotypically similar RBC units for SCD patients.

The standard-setting association for transfusion medicine, the AABB (formerly the American Association of Blood Banks; www.aabb.org) is developing recommended guidelines for limited phenotypic matching RBC transfusion protocols for SCD patients. These guidelines are sensitive to the different approaches to limited antigen-matching protocols for SCD patients used by different centers. The recommendations will review the current literature regarding limited RBC antigen matching and its merits, suggest possible strategies for antigen-matching programs, and assist in engaging the community of physicians, nurses, transfusion medicine experts, blood banks, and blood centers in developing programs to suit the needs of their individual hospitals and patients.

AUTOIMMUNIZATION TO RBC ANTIGENS

Development of autoantibodies to RBC antigens in association with transfusions in certain SCD patients has been described.[96] In 1999, Castellino and associates[97] reported on the frequency, characteristics, and significance of erythrocyte autoantibodies in a large group of multiply transfused children with SCD.[97] The rate of warm (immunoglobulin G) RBC autoantibody formation in this group was 7.6%; 29% of patients with erythrocyte autoantibodies had clinically significant hemolysis thought to be caused by the autoantibody. All patients with clinically significant hemolysis had both immunoglobulin G and complement detected on the surface of their RBCs. There was a strong association between autoantibody formation and the presence of RBC alloantibodies: 86% of patients with autoantibodies also had one or more alloantibodies.

The phenomenon of RBC autoantibody formation in association with blood transfusion is not well understood, but several theories exist. Alloantibodies may bind to transfused cells and cause conformational changes in the RBC antigenic epitopes, leading to stimulation of autoantibody formation.[97] Alternatively, some SCD patients may simply have a predisposition to develop RBC autoantibodies, perhaps because of an overall dysfunction of their immune systems.[97,98] For example, the loss of a functional spleen in patients with SCD could lead to immune dysregulation, because some experimental evidence suggests that the spleen is important in the regulation of RBC autoantibody formation.[97,99]

Whatever the cause, physicians should be aware that a syndrome of clinically significant post-transfusion hemolysis may occur in SCD patients in which both autologous and transfused RBCs are destroyed (bystander hemolysis) and that hemolysis may be exacerbated by further transfusions.[100] Serologic findings may be negative or simply not helpful in identification of the autoantibody.[97] In most cases, corticosteroids with or without intravenous immunoglobulin are beneficial in slowing hemolysis and allowing for successful continuation of necessary transfusions.[100]

ALLOIMMUNIZATION TO HLA-SPECIFIC OR PLATELET-SPECIFIC ANTIGENS

As bone marrow/stem cell transplantation (BMT) becomes a viable option for selected patients with SCD,[101–107] alloimmunization to platelets presents more serious problems for this group. Friedman and coworkers[108] reported that 85% of SCD patients receiving 50 or more transfusions, 48% of SCD patients receiving 1 to 49 transfusions, and no non-transfused SCD patients demonstrated alloimmunization to human leukocyte antigen (HLA)-specific or platelet-specific antigens. Because platelet refractoriness is a serious complication during BMT, prevention of platelet alloimmunization appears prudent in this group of patients.

Most transfusion experts support the use of leukoreduced cellular blood products to prevent or reduce platelet alloimmunization and refractoriness in SCD patients, a practice employed for a variety of multiply transfused patient groups.[109–112]

Nonimmune-Related Adverse Effects

IRON OVERLOAD

Iron overload resulting in hemosiderosis is a serious long-term complication of chronic transfusion in SCD patients. The most informative reports regarding transfusion-associated iron overload were described in patients with thalassemia; see "Thalassemias" for a discussion of the pathophysiology of iron overload. Patients who develop iron overload may be treated with long-term chelation therapy in the form of deferoxamine; however, this therapy is expensive, and due to multiple side effects and a history of difficulty of administration of the drug, the compliance rate has been notoriously poor among patients.[113] However, with the November 2005 FDA approval of the first oral iron chelator available in the United States,[114] compliance to long-term chelation therapy may improve as a result of increased ease of use.

One potential transfusion methodology for the prevention of iron overload currently being investigated in SCD patients is chronic erythrocytapheresis. Chronic erythrocytapheresis procedures may be performed at 3- to 4-week intervals. In contrast to simple transfusions, the patient's own sickled RBCs are removed while an equal volume of normal donor RBCs is infused. The obvious potential benefit of chronic erythrocytapheresis compared with simple transfusion is the prevention of long-term iron accumulation and hemosiderosis.

Although it has not been universally implemented, chronic erythrocytapheresis appears to be clinically effective in reducing iron overload in chronically transfused SCD patients. Four investigative teams[19–22] have described their individual experiences with chronic erythrocytapheresis transfusion protocols for SCD patients. All suggested that erythrocytapheresis does limit iron accumulation in SCD patients, but three of the four groups reported that erythrocytapheresis does not obviate the need for chelation therapy in those patients with previously accumulated iron.[20–22] In general, ferritin levels decreased in patients undergoing chronic erythrocytapheresis who received concurrent chelation therapy, and they either mildly decreased or stabilized in patients who were not receiving chelation therapy. However, at-risk patients who began erythrocytapheresis without a long history of previous chronic simple transfusions maintained very low serum ferritin levels not requiring chelation therapy.[20–22]

Therefore, it appears that chronic erythrocytapheresis may be most beneficial when it is initiated early in the course of chronic transfusion therapy, before significant iron accumulation occurs. Nevertheless, chronic erythrocytapheresis does appear to stabilize or decrease serum ferritin levels in patients who have already developed significant iron overload and continue on chelation therapy.[20–22]

The primary potential problems with the chronic erythrocytapheresis transfusion protocol (compared with chronic simple transfusion protocols) are increased blood product exposure, with concomitant increased risks of alloimmunization to RBCs and platelets and of transfusion-transmitted infection, and the increased cost (i.e., increased numbers of blood products used, increased cost of phenotypically similar units, if chosen for transfusion, and the added cost of the automated procedures themselves).

The four published reports[19–22] indicated that SCD patients' blood product exposures increase in chronic erythrocytapheresis protocols, with reported increases in blood utilization rates ranging from 52% to almost 100% (i.e., one to two times more RBC units transfused than with previous simple transfusions of the same patients). However, of the combined 43 patients studied, only 1 patient developed an alloantibody[20] during the period of erythrocytapheresis treatment. Three of these centers used antigen-matched RBC units for the erythrocytapheresis procedures: Singer and associates[22] matched for C, E, and K; Hilliard and colleagues[21] for C, E, K, Fy^a, and Jk^b; and Adams and associates[20] for C, E, K, and Jk^b. When evaluating the very low alloimmunization rates that have been reported for chronic erythrocytapheresis protocols, it is important to realize that the majority of SCD patients studied received RBC units matched for at least the C, E, and K antigens.

The high cost of erythrocytapheresis is an important issue. Hilliard and colleagues[21] compared the total cost of 1 year of erythrocytapheresis ($36,085) with the total annual cost for simple transfusion ($26,058) and found an economically significant difference. They suggested that the added cost of chelation therapy ($29,480) with simple transfusion (for a total of $62,143) makes erythrocytapheresis without chelation a much less expensive alternative. However, for patients who have significant iron accumulation at the time erythrocytapheresis therapy is initiated, chelation therapy must be continued to achieve serum ferritin level reduction or stabilization.[19–21] This cost comparison provides further evidence that, if it is technically feasible, early initiation of chronic erythrocytapheresis in SCD patients before significant iron accumulation occurs may be preferable to long-term chronic simple transfusion and the resulting complications of iron overload and the need for chelation therapy.

TRANSFUSION-TRANSMITTED INFECTIONS

The risk of transmission via transfusion of most known infectious agents, particularly viruses, has become substantially reduced in the developed world since the 1990s,[115,116] largely owing to improved screening tests for donated blood products. Because the risk of contracting the most harmful transfusion-transmitted diseases in the United States and many other developed countries is quite low (e.g., an estimated 1 in 2 to 4 million chance of contracting human immunodeficiency virus [HIV] per RBC unit transfused[116]), it is a generally accepted practice that blood products should not be withheld (if an appropriate clinical indication for transfusion exists) for the sole purpose of preventing a low-risk transfusion-transmitted disease.

In developing countries, however, the same cannot be said; in some countries in Africa, such as Zambia and Botswana, HIV may affect upward of one third of the country's population.[117] However, the risks of all adverse effects of transfusion (see Table 38–5), including transfusion-transmitted disease, should be balanced against the clinical need for transfusion on a case-by-case basis.

THALASSEMIAS

Pathogenesis and Clinical Pathology

Thalassemias are among the most prevalent genetic disorders caused by a single gene, occurring in high frequency in Southeast Asia, southern China, Indonesia, India, the Middle East, Africa, and the Mediterranean basin.[118] α-thalassemias are caused by mutations that reduce the synthesis of the α-globin chain of hemoglobin, and β-thalassemias from mutations that reduce β-globin synthesis. The complex molecular genetics of these disorders is beyond the scope of this discussion and has been reviewed elsewhere.[119–121] The only definitive cure for β-thalassemia major is BMT, which has cured more than 1000 individuals with β-thalassemia major worldwide. BMT is considered in all β-thalassemia major children with a suitable donor.

By definition, chronic transfusion is required to maintain wellness in homozygous individuals and compound heterozygotes with β-thalassemia major. Individuals with β-thalassemia intermedia have complex genetics and may have severe anemia that requires episodic transfusion. Hemoglobin H disease is caused by structural or functional loss of globin synthesis from three of the normal four α-globin genes. Individuals usually are not transfusion dependent, but they may require transfusion support for complications. Compound heterozygotes with β-thalassemia and hemoglobin E disease, which is very common in individuals from East Asia, can have clinical manifestations ranging from mild microcytic anemia to severe transfusion-dependent β-thalassemia major.[122]

Clinical manifestations of severe β-thalassemias include transfusion-dependent anemia, expansion of medullary bone and extramedullary hematopoiesis, severe iron overload, increased infections, retarded growth and development, and osteopenia.[120] Anemia results from severe ineffective erythropoiesis and hemolysis. The excess α-globin chain from unbalanced globin chain synthesis leads to arrested development and accelerated intramedullary apoptosis. Erythropoietic activity may be increased tenfold, but more than 95% of the erythropoietin produced may be ineffective. Precipitated α-globin in mature erythrocytes alters membrane proteins and causes oxidant damage, shortening RBC survival time. Progressive hypersplenism further reduces RBC survival.

A primary consequence of the ineffective erythropoiesis is increased iron absorption and progressive accumulation of iron in tissues. Anemia, increased erythropoiesis, and hypersplenism also cause marked expansion of the plasma volume and blood volume. Extramedullary hematopoiesis can cause pressure symptoms from perivertebral masses. Expanded marrow activity causes skeletal changes, including osteopenia and characteristic deformities in the skull and face.[123]

Goals of Transfusion Therapy

The goals of therapy in β-thalassemia major are to increase oxygen-carrying capacity by correcting the anemia, preventing progressive hypersplenism, suppressing erythropoiesis, and reducing increased gastrointestinal absorption of iron.[120] Transfusion therapy is begun early in life to ameliorate the symptoms and signs of anemia and to support normal growth and development. Adequate transfusion reduces progression of hypersplenism, delaying the need for splenectomy.[124] Suppression of erythropoiesis prevents skeletal changes, prevents complications of extramedullary hematopoiesis, and reduces pathologic fractures and other complications from osteopenia.[125] Suppression of ineffective erythropoiesis decreases transfusion requirements by reducing blood volume[126] and suppresses the increased intestinal absorption of iron.[127]

Indications for Transfusion

Transfusion therapy is initiated in childhood when the symptoms and signs of anemia are present, including growth retardation and failure to thrive. Transfusions are occasionally initiated in β-thalassemia intermedia and hemoglobin H disease to prevent facial and skull deformity from expansion of the medullary bone space. Progressive hypersplenism may require transfusion to postpone splenectomy in β-thalassemia intermedia. Splenectomy is indicated to prevent excessive transfusion requirements.[125]

Methods of Transfusion

Simple transfusion of leukoreduced RBCs to maintain a Hb level greater than 9.5 g/dL is the standard approach to transfusion in thalassemia.[121] The older practice of maintaining higher pretransfusion Hb levels[124–126] has been associated with excessive iron loading and generally is not advocated.[120,128,129] Splenectomy is recommended when hypersplenism increases the transfusion requirement beyond 200 to 250 mL/kg/year.[124,129]

Another approach to reducing iron loading has been the use of neocytes prepared by cell separators, cell processors, or other density means.[130–137] The use of "neocyte" transfusions was shown to allow a 15% extension in transfusion interval while maintaining the same pretransfusion Hb level.[137] The costs of this approach are increased blood use, increased donor unit exposure, and an estimated fivefold increase in the cost of transfusion.[137] This approach is not presently advocated by most thalassemia experts.

Erythrocytapheresis has also been applied to thalassemia transfusion therapy. The use of automated RBC exchange, returning patient and donor "neocytes" and removing the "gerocytes," resulted in a 30% reduction in RBC transfusion requirement and a 43% increase in transfusion interval.[138,139] Further clinical trials of this approach are warranted.

Adverse Effects of Transfusion

Iron Overload

A primary consequence of the ineffective erythropoiesis is increased iron absorption and progressive accumulation of iron in tissues. Anemia, increased erythropoiesis, and hypersplenism also cause marked expansion of the plasma volume and blood volume. Extramedullary hematopoiesis can cause pressure symptoms from perivertebral masses. Expanded marrow activity causes skeletal changes, including osteopenia and characteristic changes in the skull and face.[123]

Individuals with β-thalassemia major are transfusion-dependent from early life; indeed, chronic transfusion support has markedly improved the prognosis of patients with thalassemias. Transfused children develop iron overload from increased absorption caused by ineffective erythropoiesis and iron administered during transfusion. Cardiac, hepatic, and endocrine failure results in death in the second or third decade without effective therapy to remove excess iron.

Although no ideal approach to treatment of transfusion-related iron overload exists, until recently, the treatment of choice consisted of subcutaneous infusion of deferoxamine over 8 to 12 hours, 5 to 7 days a week. This approach appeared to control iron accumulation and prevent cardiac and liver damage, thereby improving life expectancy in patients with thalassemia. However, the difficulty of administration of deferoxamine and the many side effects caused a poor compliance rate in most patients.

On November 9, 2005, the FDA announced the approval of deferasirox, the first orally absorbed iron chelator developed to treat chronic iron overload due to multiple blood transfusions available for use in the United States.[114] Deferasirox was approved through the FDA's accelerated approval program; further clinical studies from the company who makes the drug are required to maintain the drug's approval and confirm clinical benefits. Clinical trials of less than 1 year's duration showed reduction in hepatic iron concentration following once-daily (oral) deferasirox therapy in patients who had been receiving multiple transfusions. Side effects such as nausea and abdominal pain and other less common difficulties were noted.[140] However, the greater ease of administration of this drug and its apparent efficacy with typically mild side effects may markedly improve the care and treatment of patients with transfusion-dependent iron overload.[141] In other countries, such as India, different oral iron chelators have been widely used, safely and with good success, for the treatment of transfusion-dependent iron overload in patients with thalassemia.[142]

Alloimmunization to RBC Antigens

Reported rates of alloimmunization to RBC antigens in chronically transfused thalassemia patients range from 5% to 30%.[143–147] The largest of these studies followed alloimmunization rates in 973 Greek patients, primarily children, and found an alloimmunization rate of 23% in this group.[146]

Some evidence exists that thalassemia major patients who begin chronic transfusion therapy at younger ages develop fewer alloantibodies.[145,146] Michail-Merianou and colleagues reported that children who began transfusion therapy before age 12 months had a 9% alloimmunization rate; children who started chronic transfusions after age 12 months had a 39% alloimmunization rate.[145]

There are no agreed-upon hypotheses as to what specifically affects increased alloimmunization rates in thalassemia patients. Ethnic differences have been proposed, but there is little data to support this claim.[144–148] Leukoreduction has been suggested as a possible means of decreasing alloimmunization in thalassemics, but no data exists to support this hypothesis. Splenectomy has also been suggested as a trigger for increased alloimmunization to RBCs, but Singer and colleagues found that although such a trend existed in their group of patients studied, it did not reach statistical significance.[149]

Risks of alloimmunization in thalassemic patients include delay of transfusion due to difficulties in finding compatible RBC units, if patients make multiple alloantibodies; a potential for hemolytic disease of the newborn in thalassemic patients who become pregnant; and a possible relationship between RBC alloantibody development and secondary RBC autoantibody development and/or autoimmune hemolytic anemia.[149–151]

Some studies have shown that limited phenotypic RBC antigen matching reduces the rate of alloimmunization in thalassemia patients, particularly in those patients whose first transfusion occurred after age 12 months.[145,146,149] More data is required, however, before evidence-based recommendations can be made regarding the feasibility of RBC phenotypic matching for thalassemic patients.

REFERENCES

1. Heller P, Best WR, Nelson RB, et al. Clinical implications of sickle cell trait and glucose-6-phosphate dehydrogenase deficiency in hospitalized black male patients. NEJM 1979;300:1001–1005.
2. Beutler E. The sickle cell diseases and related disorders. In Beutler E, Lichtman MA, Coller BS, et al (eds). Williams Hematology, 6th ed. New York, McGraw-Hill, 2001, p 585.
3. Bunn HF. Mechanisms of disease: pathogenesis and treatment of sickle cell disease. NEJM 1997;337:762–769.
4. Steinberg MH. Management of sickle cell disease. NEJM 1999;340: 1021–1030.
5. Platt OS, Brambilla DJ, Rosse WF, et al. Mortality in sickle cell disease: life expectancy and risk factors for early death. NEJM 1994;330: 1639–1644.
6. Reed W, Vichinsky EP. New considerations in the treatment of sickle cell disease. Annu Rev Med 1998;49:461–474.
7. Schmalzer EA, Lee JO, Brown AK, et al. Viscosity of mixtures of sickle and normal red cells at varying hematocrit levels. Transfusion 1987;27:228–233.
8. Eckman JR. Techniques for blood administration in sickle cell patients. Semin Hematol 2001;38:23–29.
9. Wayne AS, Kevy SV, Nathan DG. Transfusion management of sickle cell disease. Blood 1993;81:1109–1123.
10. Sharon BI. Transfusion therapy in congenital hemolytic anemias. Hematol Oncol Clin North Am 1994;8:1053–1086.
11. Vengelen-Tyler V (ed). AABB Technical Manual, 13th ed. Bethesda, Md., American Association of Blood Banks, 1999, p 486.
12. Embury SH, Vichinsky EP. Sickle Cell Disease. In Hoffman R, Benz EJ Jr, Shattil SJ, et al (eds). Hematology: Basic Principles and Practice, 3rd ed. Philadelphia, Churchill Livingstone, 2000, p 539.
13. Ohene-Frempong K. Indications for red cell transfusion in sickle cell disease. Semin Hematol 2001;38:5–13.
14. Piomelli S, Seaman C, Ackerman K, et al. Planning an exchange transfusion in patients with sickle cell syndromes. Am J Pediatr Hematol Oncol 1990;12:268–276.
15. Hillyer KL, Hillyer CD. Packed red blood cells and related products. In Hillyer CD, Hillyer KL, Strobl FJ, et al (eds). Handbook of Transfusion Medicine. Philadelphia, Academic Press, 2001, p 29.
16. Strauss R. Data-driven blood banking practices for neonatal RBC transfusions. Transfusion 2000;40:1528–1540.
17. Hall T, Barnes A, Miller J, et al. Neonatal mortality following transfusion of red cells with high plasma potassium levels. Transfusion 1993;33:606–609.
18. Cohen A, Kron E, Brittenham G. Toxicity of transfusional iron overload in sickle cell anemia. Blood 1984;64(Suppl 1):47a.

19. Kim H, Dugan N, Silber J. Erythrocytapheresis therapy to reduce iron overload in chronically transfused patients with sickle cell disease. Blood 1994;83:1136–1142.
20. Adams D, Schultz W, Ware R, et al. Erythrocytapheresis can reduce iron overload and prevent the need for chelation in chronically transfused pediatric patients. J Pediatr Hematol Oncol 1996;18: 46–50.
21. Hilliard LM, Williams BF, Lounsbury AE, et al. Erythrocytapheresis limits iron accumulation in chronically transfused sickle cell patients. Am J Hematol 1998;59:28–35.
22. Singer ST, Quirolo K, Nishi K, et al. Erythrocytapheresis for chronically transfused children with sickle cell disease: an effective method for maintaining a low hemoglobin S level and reducing iron overload. J Clin Apheresis 1999;14:122–125.
23. Lawson SE, Oakley S, Smith NA, et al. Red cell exchange in sickle cell disease. Clin Lab Haematol 1999;21:99–102.
24. Vichinsky EP. Current issues in blood transfusion in sickle cell disease. Semin Hematol 2001;38:14–22.
25. Embury SH. The clinical pathophysiology of sickle cell disease. Ann Rev Med 1986;37:361–376.
26. Goldstein AR, Anderson MJ, Serjeant GR. Parvovirus-associated aplastic crisis in homozygous sickle cell disease. Arch Dis Child 1987; 62:585–588.
27. Serjeant GR, de Ceulaer K, Maude GH. Stilboestrol and stuttering priapism in homozygous sickle-cell disease. Lancet 1985;2:1274.
28. Vichinsky E. Transfusion. In Embury SH, Hebbel RP, Mohandas N, et al (eds). Sickle Cell Disease: Basic Principles and Clinical Practice. New York, Raven Press, 1994, pp 261–283.
29. Castro W, Brambilla DJ, Thorington B, et al. The acute chest syndrome in sickle cell disease: incidence and risk factors. Blood 1994;84: 643–649.
30. Quinn C, Rogers Z, Buchanan G. Survival of children with sickle cell disease. Blood 2004;103:4023–4027.
31. Gray J, Anionwu EN, Davies SC, et al. Patterns of mortality in sickle cell disease in the United Kingdom. J Clin Pathol 1991;44:459.
32. Dreyer ZE. Chest infections and syndromes in sickle cell disease of childhood. Semin Respir Infect 1996;11:163–172.
33. Davies SD, Luce PJ, Win AA, et al. Acute chest syndrome in sickle-cell disease. Lancet 1984;1:36–38.
34. Mallouh AA, Asha M. Beneficial effect of blood transfusion on children with sickle cell chest syndrome. Am J Dis Child 1988;142:178–182.
35. Emre U, Miller ST, Gutierez M, et al. Effect of transfusion in acute chest syndrome of sickle cell disease. J Pediatr 1995;127:901–904.
36. Emond AM, Collis R, Darvill D, et al. Acute splenic sequestration in homozygous sickle cell disease: natural history and management. J Pediatr 1985;107:201–206.
37. Seeler RA, Shwiaki MZ: Acute splenic sequestration crises (ASSC) in young children with sickle cell anemia. Clin Pediatr 1972;11:701–704.
38. Sheehy TW, Law DE, Wade BH. Exchange transfusion for sickle cell intrahepatic cholestasis. Arch Intern Med 1980;140:1364–1366.
39. Ohene-Frempong K, Weiner SJ, Sleeper LA, et al. Cerebrovascular accidents in sickle cell disease: Rates and risk factors. Blood 1998;91: 288–294.
40. Russell MO, Goldberg HI, Reis L, et al. Transfusion therapy for cerebrovascular abnormalities in sickle cell disease. JAMA 1979;242: 2317–2318.
41. Adams R, McKie V, Brambilla D, et al. Stroke prevention trial in sickle cell anemia. Control Clin Trials 1998;19:100–129.
42. Adams RJ, McKie VC, Hsu L, et al. Prevention of a first stroke by transfusions in children with sickle cell anemia and abnormal results on transcranial Doppler ultrasonography. NEJM 1998;339:5–11.
43. Vichinsky EP, Haberkern CM, Neumayr L, et al. A comparison of conservative and aggressive transfusion regimens in the perioperative management of sickle cell disease. NEJM 1995;333:206–213.
44. Koshy M, Weiner SJ, Miller ST, et al. Surgery and anesthesia in sickle cell disease. Blood 1995;86:3676–3684.
45. Haberkern CM, Neumayr LD, Orringer EP, et al. Cholecystectomy in sickle cell anemia patients: perioperative outcome of 364 cases from the National Preoperative Transfusion Study. Blood 1997;89: 1533–1542.
46. U.S. Department of Health and Human Services. National Institutes of Health. The Management of Sickle Cell Disease (ed 4). NIH Publication 02–2117. Bethesda, Md., NIH, 2002.
47. Riddington C, Williamson L. Preoperative blood transfusions for sickle cell disease. Cochrane Database Syst Rev 2001; 3:CD003149.
48. Serjeant GR. Sickle Cell Disease, 2nd ed. Oxford, Oxford Medical Publishers, 1992, p 332.
49. Hassell KL, Eckman JR, Lane PA. Acute multiorgan failure syndrome: a potentially catastrophic complication of severe sickle cell pain episodes. Am J Med 1994;96:155–162.
50. Powars D, Wilson B, Imbus C, et al. The natural history of stroke in sickle cell disease. Am J Med 1978;65:461–471.
51. Russell MO, Goldberg HI, Hodson A, et al. Effect of transfusion therapy on arteriographic abnormalities and on recurrence of stroke in sickle cell disease. Blood 1984;63:162–169.
52. Peglow CH, Adams RJ, McKie V, et al. Risk of recurrent stroke in patients with sickle cell disease treated with erythrocyte transfusion. J Pediatr 1995;126:896–899.
53. Williams J, Goff JR, Anderson HR Jr, et al. Efficacy of transfusion therapy for one to two years in patients with sickle cell disease and cerebrovascular accidents. J Pediatr 1980;96:205–209.
54. Cohen AR, Martin MB, Silber JF, et al. A modified transfusion program for prevention of stroke in sickle cell disease. Blood 1992;79:1657–1661.
55. U.S. Department of Health and Human Services. National Institutes of Health. National Heart, Lung, and Blood Institute. Clinical Alert, December 5, 2004. Available at http://www.nhlbi.nih.gov/health/prof/blood/sickle/clinical-alert-scd.htm.
56. Wang WC, Kovnar EH, Tonkin IL, et al. High risk of recurrent stroke after discontinuance of five to twelve years of transfusion therapy in patients with sickle cell disease. J Pediatr 1991;118:377–382.
57. Adams R, McKie V, Nichols F, et al. The use of transcranial ultrasonography to predict stroke in sickle cell disease. NEJM 1992;326:605–610.
58. Adams RJ, McKie VC, Carl EM, et al. Long-term stroke risk in children with sickle cell disease screened with transcranial Doppler. Ann Neurol 1997;42:699–704.
59. Koshy M, Burd L, Wallace D, et al. Prophylactic red cell transfusions in pregnant patients with sickle cell disease. NEJM 1988;319:1447–1452.
60. El-Shafei AM, Dhaliwal JK, Sandhu AK, et al. Indications for blood transfusion in pregnancy with sickle cell disease. Aust NZ J Obstet Gynaecol 1995;35:405–408.
61. Tuck SM, James CE, Brewster EM, et al. Prophylactic blood transfusion in maternal sickle cell syndromes. BJOG 1987;94:121–125.
62. Koshy M. Sickle cell disease and pregnancy. Blood Rev 1995;9: 157–164.
63. Morgan AG, Gruber CA, Serjeant GR. Erythropoietin and renal function in sickle cell disease. BMJ 1982;285:1686–1688.
64. Weil JV, Castro O, Malik AR, et al. Pathogenesis of lung disease in sickle hemoglobinopathies. Am Rev Respir Dis 1993;148:249–256.
65. Simmons B, Santhanam V, Castaner A, et al. Sickle cell heart disease: Two-dimensional echo and Doppler ultrasonographic findings in the hearts of adult patients with sickle cell anemia. Arch Intern Med 1988;148:1526–1528.
66. Sutton L, Castro O, Cross D, et al. Pulmonary hypertension in sickle cell disease. Am J Cardiol 1994;74:626–628.
67. Castro O. Systemic fat embolism and pulmonary hypertension in sickle cell disease. Hematol Oncol Clin North Am 1996;10:1289–1303.
68. Vichinsky E. Pulmonary hypertension in sickle cell disease. NEJM 2004;350:857–859.
69. Hankins J, Jeng M, Harris S, et al. Chronic transfusion therapy for children with sickle cell disease and recurrent acute chest syndrome. J Pediatr Hematol Oncol 2005;27:158–161.
70. Gladwin M, Sachdev V, Jison M, et al. Pulmonary hypertension as a risk factor for death in patients with sickle cell disease. NEJM 2004;350:886–895.
71. Rifkind S, Waisman J, Thompson R, et al. RBC exchange pheresis for priapism in sickle cell disease. JAMA 1979;242:2317–2318.
72. Walker EM, Mitchum EN, Rous SN, et al. Automated erythrocytapheresis for relief of priapism in sickle cell hemoglobinopathies. J Urol 1983;130:912–916.
73. Seeler RA. Intensive transfusion therapy for priapism in boys with sickle cell anemia. J Urol 1973;110:360–361.
74. Seeler RA. Priapism in children with sickle cell anemia. Clin Pediatr 1971;10:418–419.
75. Miller ST, Rao SP, Dunn KE, et al. Priapism in children with sickle cell disease. J Urol 1995;154:844–847.
76. Baruchel S, Rees J, Bernstein ML, et al. Relief of sickle cell priapism by hydralazine: report of a case. Am J Pediatr Hematol Oncol 1993;15:115.
77. Siegel JF, Rich MA, Brock WA. Association of sickle cell disease, priapism, exchange transfusion and neurological events: ASPEN syndrome. J Urol 1993;150:1480–1482.
78. Platt OS, Thorington BD, Brambilla DJ, et al. Pain in sickle cell disease. NEJM 1991;325:11–16.
79. Koshy M, Entsuah R, Koranda A, et al. Leg ulcers in patients with sickle cell disease. Blood 1989;74:1403–1408.

80. Miller JP, AuBuchon JP. Leukocyte-reduced and cytomegalovirus-reduced-risk blood components. In Mintz PD (ed). Transfusion Therapy: Clinical Principles and Practice. Bethesda, Md., AABB Press, 1999, p 313.
81. Stack G, Judge JV, Snyder EL. Febrile and nonimmune transfusion reactions. In Rossi EC, Simon TL, Moss GS, et al (eds). Principles of Transfusion Medicine, 2nd ed. Baltimore, Williams & Wilkins, 1996, pp 773–784.
82. Orlina AR, Unger PJ, Koshy M. Post-transfusion alloimmunization in patients with sickle cell disease. Am J Hematol 1978;5:101–106.
83. Davies SC, McWilliam AC, Hewitt PE, et al. Red cell alloimmunization in sickle cell disease. Br J Hematol 1986;63:241–245.
84. Reisner EG, Kostyo DD, Phillips G, et al. Alloantibody responses in multiply transfused sickle cell patients. Tissue Antigens 1987;30: 161–166.
85. Cox JV, Steane E, Cunningham G, et al. Risk of alloimmunization and delayed hemolytic transfusion reactions in patients with sickle cell disease. Arch Intern Med 1988;148:2485–2489.
86. Rosse WF, Gallagher D, Kinney T. Transfusion and alloimmunization in sickle cell disease. Blood 1990;76:1431–1437.
87. Vichinsky EP, Earles A, Johnson RA, et al. Alloimmunization in sickle cell anemia and transfusion of racially unmatched blood. NEJM 1990;322:1617–1621.
88. Coles SM, Klein HG, Holland PV: Alloimmunization in two multi-transfused patient populations. Transfusion 1981;21:462–466.
89. Luban NL. Variability in rates of alloimmunization in different groups of children with sickle cell disease: effect of ethnic background. Am J Pediatr Hematol Oncol 1989;11:314–319.
90. Tahhan HR, Holbrook CT, Braddy LR, et al. Antigen-matched donor blood in the transfusion management of patients with sickle cell disease. Transfusion 1994;34:562–569.
91. Osby M, Shulman I. Phenotype matching of donor red blood cell units for non-alloimmunized sickle cell disease patients: a survey of 1182 North American Laboratories. Arch Path Lab Med 2005; 129:190–193.
92. Ambruso DR, Githens JH, Alcorn R, et al. Experience with donors matched for minor blood group antigens in patients with sickle cell anemia who are receiving chronic transfusion therapy. Transfusion 1987;27:94–98.
93. Sosler S, Jilly B, Saporito C, et al. A simple, practical model for reducing alloimmunization in patients with sickle cell disease. Am J Hematol 1993;43:103–106.
94. Hillyer KL, Hare VW, Eckman JR, et al. Decreased alloimmunization rates in chronically-transfused sickle cell disease patients in a directed-donor, red blood cell antigen-matching program entitled "Partners for Life" (PFL). Blood 2001;98:2274.
95. Vichinsky EP, Luban NL, Wright E, et al. Prospective red blood cell phenotype matching in a stroke-prevention trial in sickle cell anemia: a multicenter transfusion trial. Transfusion 2001;41:1086–1092.
96. Wenz B, Gurtlinger A, Wheaton D, et al. A mimicking red blood cell autoantibody accompanying transfusion and alloimmunization. Transfusion 1982;22:147–150.
97. Castellino SM, Combs MR, Zimmerman SA, et al. Erythrocyte autoantibodies in paediatric patients with sickle cell disease receiving transfusion therapy: frequency, characteristics, and significance. Br J Haematol 1999;104:189–194.
98. Test ST, Woolworth VS: Defective regulation of complement by the sickle erythrocyte: evidence for a defect in control of membrane attack complex formation. Blood 1994;83:842–852.
99. Cox KO, Finlay-Jones JJ. Impaired regulation of erythrocyte autoantibody production after splenectomy. Br J Exp Pathol 1979;60: 466–470.
100. Cullis JO, Win N, Dudley TM, et al. Post-transplant hyperhaemolysis in a patient with sickle cell disease: use of steroids and intravenous immunoglobulin to prevent further red cell destruction. Vox Sang 1995;69:355–357.
101. Vermylen C, Cornu G. Bone marrow transplantation in sickle cell anaemia. Blood Rev 1993;7:1–3.
102. Vermylen C, Cornu G, Ferster A, et al. Haematopoietic stem cell transplantation for sickle cell anaemia: the first 50 patients transplanted in Belgium. Bone Marrow Transplant 1998;22:1–6.
103. Walters MC, Patience M, Leisenring W, et al. Bone marrow transplantation for sickle cell disease. NEJM 1996;335:369–376.
104. Platt OS, Guinan EC: Bone marrow transplantation in sickle cell anemia: the dilemma of choice. NEJM 1996;335:426–428.
105. Brichard B, Vermylen C, Ninane J, et al. Persistence of fetal hemoglobin production after successful transplantation of cord blood stem cells in a patient with sickle cell anemia. J Pediatr 1996;128:241–243.
106. Ferster A, Corazza F, Vertongen F, et al. Transplanted sickle-cell disease patients with autologous bone marrow recovery after graft failure develop increased levels of fetal haemoglobin which corrects disease severity. Br J Haematol 1995;90:804–808.
107. Souillet G. Indications and results of progenitor cell transplant in congenital haemopathies (except Fanconi anaemia). Bone Marrow Transplant 1998;21:S28–S33.
108. Friedman D, Lukas M, Jawad A, et al. Alloimmunization to platelets in heavily transfused patients with sickle cell disease. Blood 1996;88: 3216–3222.
109. Slichter SJ. Platelet transfusion therapy. Hematol Oncol Clin North Am 1990;4:291–311.
110. Sniecinski I, O'Donnell MR, Nowicki B, et al. Prevention of refractoriness and HLA-alloimmunization using filtered blood products. Blood 1988;71:1402–1407.
111. Saarinen UM, Kekomaki R, Simes MA, et al. Effective prophylaxis against platelet refractoriness in multitransfused patients by use of leukocyte-free blood components. Blood 1990;75:512–517.
112. Brand A, Claas FHJ, Voogt PJ, et al. Alloimmunization after leukocyte-depleted multiple random donor platelet transfusions. Vox Sang 1988;54:160–166.
113. Cohen AR, Martin MB: Iron chelation therapy in sickle cell disease. Semin Hematol 2001;38(Suppl 1):69–72.
114. U.S. Food and Drug Administration. FDA Approves First Oral Drug for Chronic Iron Overload. FDA News Release P05–86, November 9, 2005. Available at http://www.fda.gov/bbs/topics/news/2005/NEW01258.html.
115. Schrieber G, Busch M, Kleinman S, et al. The risk of transfusion-transmitted viral infections. NEJM 1996;334:1685–1690.
116. Stramer SL, Glynn SA, Kleinman SH, et al. Detection of HIV-1 and HCV infections among antibody-negative blood donors by nucleic acid amplification testing. NEJM 2004;351:760–768.
117. World Health Organization. Regional Office for Africa, Harare, Zimbabwe. HIV/AIDS Epidemiological Surveillance Update for the WHO African Region 2002, September 2003. Available at http://www.afro.who.int/aids/surveillance/resources/hiv_surveillance_report_2002.pdf.
118. Weatherall DJ, Clegg JB. Thalassemia: a global public health problem. Nat Med 1996;2:847–849.
119. Higgs DR. Molecular mechanisms in α thalassemia. In Steinberg MH, Forget BG, Higgs DR, et al (eds). Disorders of Hemoglobin: Genetics, Pathophysiology, and Clinical Management. Cambridge, Cambridge University Press, 2001, p 405.
120. Oliveri NF. The β-thalassemias. NEJM 1999;341:99–100.
121. Higgs DR. α-Thalassemia. Baillieres Clin Haematol 1993;6:117–150.
122. Weatherall DJ. Hemoglobin E beta-thalassemia: an increasingly common disease with some diagnostic pitfalls. J Pediatr 1998;132:765–767.
123. Rioja L, Girot R, Garabedian M, et al. Bone disease in children with homozygous beta-thalassemia. Bone Miner 1990;8:69–86.
124. Piomelli S, Graziano J. Reduction in iron overload in thalassemia. Birth Defects 1982;18:339–346.
125. Fosburg MT, Nathan DG. Treatment of Colley's anemia. Blood 1990; 76:435–444.
126. Propper R, Button L, Nathan D. New approach to the transfusion management of thalassemia. Blood 1980;55:55–60.
127. Pootrakul P, Kitcharoen K, Yansukon P, et al. The effect of erythroid hyperplasia on iron balance. Blood 1988;71:1124–1129.
128. Cazzola M, Borgna-Pignatti C, Locatelli F, et al. A moderate transfusion regimen may reduce iron loading in β-thalassemia major without producing excessive expansion of erythropoiesis. Transfusion 1997;37:135–140.
129. Olivieri NF, Brittenham GM. Iron-chelation therapy and treatment of thalassemia. Blood 1997;89:739–761.
130. Piomeli S, Seaman C, Reibman J, et al. Separation of younger red cells with improved survival in vivo: An approach to chronic transfusion therapy. Proc Natl Acad Sci USA 1978;74:3473–3478.
131. Corash L, Klein H, Deisseroth A, et al. Selective isolation of young erythrocytes for transfusion support of thalassemia major patients. Blood 1981;57:599–606.
132. Bracey AW, Klein HG, Chambers S, et al. Ex vivo selective isolation of young red blood cells using the IBM-2991 cell washer. Blood 1983;61:1068–1071.
133. Cohen AR, Schmidt JM, Martin MB, et al. Clinical trial of young red cell transfusions. J Pediatr 1984;104:865–868.
134. Marcus RE, Wonke B, Bantock HM, et al. A prospective trial of young red cells in 48 patients with transfusion-dependent thalassemia. Br J Haematol 1985;60:153–159.
135. Kevy SV, Jacobson MS, Fosburg M, et al. A new approach to neocyte transfusion: preliminary report. J Clin Apheresis 1988;4:194–197.

136. Simon TL, Sohmer P, Nelson EF. Extended survival of neocytes produced by a new system. Transfusion 1989;29:221–225.
137. Collins AF, Dias GC, Haddad S, et al. Evaluation of a new neocyte transfusion preparation vs. washed cell transfusion in patients with homozygous beta thalassemia. Transfusion 1994;34:517–520.
138. Berdoukas VA, Moorew RC. A study of the value of red cell exchange transfusions in transfusion dependent anemias. Clin Lab Haematol 1986;8:209–220.
139. Cohen AR, Porter JB. Transfusion and iron chelation therapy in thalassemia and sickle cell anemia. In Steinberg MH, Forget BG, Higgs DR, et al (eds). Disorders of Hemoglobin: Genetics, Pathophysiology, and Clinical Management. Cambridge, Cambridge University Press, 2001, p 982.
140. Capelleni MD. Iron-chelating therapy with the new oral agent ICL670 (Exjade). Best Pract Res Clin Hematol 2005;18:289–298.
141. Cunningham MJ, Nathan DG. New developments in iron chelators. Curr Opin Hematol 2005;12:129–134.
142. Naithani R, Chandra J, Sharma S: Safety of oral iron chelator deferiprone in young thalassemics. Eur J Haematol 2005;74:217–220.
143. Bhatti FA, Salamat N, Nadeem A, et al. Red cell immunization in beta-thalassemia major. J Coll Physicians Surg Pak 2004;14: 657–660.
144. Ameen R, Al-Shemmari S, Al-Humood R, et al. RBC alloimmunization and autoimmunization among transfusion-dependent Arab thalassemia patients. Transfusion 2003;43:1604–1610.
145. Michail-Merianou V, Pamphili-Panousopoulou L, Piperi-Lowes L, et al. Alloimmunization to red cell antigens in thalassemia: comparative study of usual versus better match transfusion programmes. Vox Sang 1987;52:95–98.
146. Spanos T, Karageorga M, et al. Red cell alloantibodies in patients with thalassemia. Vox Sang 1990;58:50–55.
147. Hmida S, Mojaat N, Maamar M, et al. Red cell alloantibodies in patients with haemoglobinopathies. Nouv Rev Fr Hematol 1994;36:363–366.
148. Sirchia G, Zanella A, Parravicini A, et al. Red cell alloantibodies in thalassemia major. Transfusion 1985;25:110–112.
149. Singer ST, Wu V, Mignacca R, et al. Alloimmunization and erythrocyte autoimmunization in transfusion-dependent patients of primarily Asian descent. Blood 2000;96:3369–3373.
150. Mizon P, Cossement C, Mannessier L, et al. Severe hemolysis relation to an association of erythrocye allo- and autoantibodies in thalassemia patients. Transfusion Clin Biol 1996:3;257–261.
151. Kruatrachue M, Sirisinha S, Pacharee P, et al. An association between thalassemia and autoimmune hemolytic anemia (AIHA). Scand J Haematol 1980;25:259–263.

Chapter 39

Transfusion to Bone Marrow or Solid Organ Transplant Recipients

Richard M. Kaufman • Steven R. Sloan

HEMATOPOIETIC STEM CELL TRANSPLANTATION

Kinetics of Engraftment and Blood Product Support

In a standard hematopoietic stem cell transplant (HSCT), the recipient's bone marrow is ablated using chemotherapy and irradiation. Between the time of stem cell infusion and engraftment/hematologic recovery, red cell and platelet transfusions are critical to sustain the recipient. Although the HSCT patient's blood component needs may be substantial, the indications for transfusion are essentially the same as for other clinical settings. However, a number of blood bank considerations specifically apply to the HSCT situation.

Three sources of hematopoietic stem cells are presently in use for clinical transplantation: bone marrow, mobilized peripheral blood stem cells, and umbilical cord blood. The cellular composition of these three products differs considerably.[1,2] Clinically, the single most important factor seems to be the dose of CD34+ cells contained in each product type. Peripheral blood stem cell products contain about three times more CD34+ cells than bone marrow–derived products, and 10 times more CD34+ cells than umbilical cord blood (Table 39–1). Peripheral blood stem cells grafts also contain 5 to 10 times more mature T cells than bone marrow. Umbilical cord blood contains far fewer CD34+ cells and T cells than either peripheral blood stem cells or bone marrow. Several randomized studies directly comparing peripheral blood stem cells to bone marrow have all shown that hematologic recovery occurs faster in recipients of peripheral blood stem cells than in recipients of bone marrow. The median number of days to a platelet count grater than 20,000/L is about 13 for peripheral blood stem cells recipients versus about 19 days for bone marrow recipients.[3–8] The more rapid engraftment of peripheral blood stem cells products has been primarily attributed to their higher CD34+ cell content. As would be expected, faster engraftment rates have been associated with decreased blood component requirements.[9,10] Umbilical cord blood grafts contain significantly fewer CD34+ cells, so recipients of these grafts predictably demonstrate slower hematologic recovery (median of 50 days to exceed 20,000/L platelets).[1]

Although peripheral blood is now by far the most commonly used source of stem cells for transplantation, interest in umbilical cord blood transplants has increased in recent years. Only about 30% of patients requiring HSCT have a human leukocyte antigen (HLA)-matched related donor, and 50% to 80% of the remaining transplant candidates will find an unrelated matched donor.[11] For patients lacking a matched donor, umbilical cord blood transplantation may represent a critical therapeutic option because HLA matching is not as important for umbilical cord blood transplants as it is for other sources of HSCT. This is especially true in cases where transplantation is needed urgently and there is insufficient time available to do a search for a matched unrelated donor. Relative to bone marrow and peripheral blood stem cells, umbilical cord blood contains higher numbers of primitive long-term culture-initiating cells and has superior engraftment in SCID mice.[12] Umbilical cord blood appears to require less stringent HLA matching than bone marrow or peripheral blood stem cell products and is associated with a lower incidence of graft-versus-host disease (GVHD). The major disadvantage of umbilical cord blood is the low number of CD34+ cells. This is a particular problem in the adult transplant setting, given the larger size of adult versus pediatric recipients. The low CD34+ cell content is associated with a higher rate of graft failure as well as slower hematologic recovery.[13–15] Despite this key limitation, umbilical cord blood transplants have been used increasingly for adult patients. One approach is to transplant two (or more) umbilical cord blood products simultaneously. Double-unit grafts appear to facilitate engraftment and hematologic recovery. One graft eventually predominates and generates 100% of the recipient's hematopoietic cells. It has been hypothesized that the nonsustained graft helps the predominating unit engraft via as-yet undefined immunologic mechanisms.[16]

In addition to CD34+ cell dose, a number of clinical factors may affect both the rate of hematologic recovery and transfusion requirements after HSCT. More rapid platelet recovery has been associated with a higher pretransplant platelet count, and with HLA-identical sibling donor transplants. Factors that have been associated with slower platelet recovery include the presence of fever, GVHD, hepatic veno-occlusive disease, previous radiation treatment, and the use of post-transplant granulocyte colony-stimulating factor or granulocyte-macrophage colony-stimulating factor.[17] The administration of recombinant human erythropoietin (EPO) has been shown to accelerate red blood cell (RBC) recovery and decrease RBC product requirements among allogeneic HSCT patients.[18–21] Finally, the conditioning regimen used also affects hematologic recovery. In particular, recipients of nonmyeloablative HSCT (known as *reduced intensity conditioning* or

Table 39–1 **Composition of Unmanipulated Allogeneic Stem Cell Products**

Product	Median CD34+ Cell Dose × 10^6/kg	Median T-Cell Dose × 10^8/kg
Bone marrow	1.4	0.3
Peripheral blood	4.2	1.8
Cord blood	0.12	0.05

Data from Schmitz N, Barrett J. Optimizing engraftment—source and dose of stem cells. Semin Hematol 2002;39:3–14.

mini-transplants) typically have significantly decreased transfusion requirements relative to patients undergoing traditional myeloablative conditioning.[22,23]

ABO

Unlike blood transfusion, the ABO system is not a barrier to HSCT. Up to 40% of allogeneic HSCTs involve donor–recipient pairs that are ABO-mismatched.[24] Such mismatches are classified as major (recipient has ABO antibody against donor RBCs), minor (donor has ABO antibody against recipient RBCs), or major-minor (ABO mismatch in both directions). Examples of these mismatches and potential clinical consequences are summarized in Table 39–2. Although HLA compatibility has critical consequences for stem cell transplantation, most published studies currently indicate that ABO compatibility has no significant effect on overall rates of survival, disease recurrence, graft failure, or GVHD.[25–32]

Major ABO Mismatch: Immunohematologic Consequences

The recipient of a major ABO incompatible HSCT (e.g., group A donor → group O recipient) is at risk for several different hemolytic complications. First, red cells contaminating the graft may be immediately destroyed by preformed ABO antibody in the recipient. This risk is lower for recipients of peripheral blood stem cells, because these products contain far fewer red cells than are found in bone marrow grafts.[24] To prevent acute hemolysis, stem cell products may be depleted of RBCs. Typically, processing yields products containing less than 10 mL of incompatible RBCs, which effectively prevents most acute hemolytic reactions. Plasma exchange has been rarely used to lower the recipient's ABO antibody titer.

A second potential adverse consequence of major ABO-mismatched HSCT is delayed red cell recovery post-transplantation. This is a form of pure red-cell aplasia (PRCA) that results from recipient plasma cells continuing to produce antibody against donor ABO antigen, despite cytoreductive therapy. On histologic examination, the bone marrow is characteristically devoid of erythroid precursors, and reticulocytopenia is observed in the peripheral blood. A persistently elevated ABO antibody titer is usually seen. In some cases, patients remain red cell transfusion dependent for months to years, until the anti-ABO antibody titer drops to a low level.[33–42] Of note, although red cell *reconstitution* is delayed in these cases, red cell *engraftment* is not. Using in vitro colony assays, the presence of early erythroid progenitors can be demonstrated in the recipient's bone marrow at the same time point after transplant that myeloid progenitors are detected.[43] Early erythroid progenitors do not express ABO antigens and survive normally. On differentiation, the erythroid precursors begin expressing ABO antigens; at which point they are targeted for destruction within the bone marrow by host ABO antibodies. Proposed risk factors for the development of PRCA include high initial host antidonor antibody levels,[39] the use of cyclosporine A for GVHD prophylaxis,[34] and the use of nonmyeloablative conditioning regimens.[34,44,45] The optimal management strategy for PRCA is currently unclear. Various investigators have reported success with high-dose EPO,[46–48] plasma exchange,[24,42] immunoabsorption,[49] rituximab,[38] donor lymphocyte infusion,[50] discontinuation of cyclosporine and antithymocyte globulin.[51,52] In very rare cases, erythroid maturation gets beyond the precursor stage and mature donor-type red cells leave the bone marrow—only to be cleared by persistent recipient ABO antibodies.[53,54] This situation occurs far less often than PRCA.

Minor ABO Mismatch: Immunohematologic Consequences

Minor ABO-incompatible HSCT (e.g., group O donor→ group A recipient) can lead to immediate hemolysis from passively transfused donor ABO antibody and delayed hemolysis (known as the *passenger lymphocyte syndrome*). Minor ABO incompatibility does not appear to affect overall rates of graft rejection, GVHD, or patient survival.[26,27,55,56] Depletion of donor plasma in the graft generally eliminates the problem of immediate hemolysis caused by passively

Table 39–2 **ABO-Mismatched Stem Cell Transplantation**

ABO Mismatch Type	Example	Physiology	Potential Complications
Major	A donor → O recipient	Recipient has antibody against donor RBCs	*Immediate:* Hemolysis of RBCs in graft *Delayed:* Pure red cell aplasia *Delayed:* Hemolysis of RBCs produced by graft (very rare)
Minor	O donor → A recipient	Donor has antibody against recipient RBCs	*Immediate:* Hemolysis from passively transfused antibody *Delayed:* Donor lymphocyte syndrome/ hemolysis
Major-minor	A donor → B recipient	Both of the above	All of the above

transfused ABO antibody. The more serious potential problem is the passenger lymphocyte syndrome. In this syndrome, mature donor lymphocytes are transfused into the host along with the stem cell graft. The donor lymphocytes produce anti-ABO antibodies that bind to and cause hemolysis of circulating host RBCs. This complication typically occurs 1 to 3 weeks after the transplant and is heralded by a positive direct antiglobulin test (DAT) and a fall in hematocrit. Hemolysis may be massive.[57] In some cases, hemolysis becomes clinically apparent 1 to 2 days before the causative antibody is detectable in the recipient's plasma (i.e., before the DAT turns positive).[53,58] Currently, the standard practice is to transfuse either group O or donor group RBCs and to monitor the patient closely for clinical and laboratory evidence of hemolysis. Red cell exchange transfusion has been performed in this setting, but is usually unnecessary.

Blood product selection for ABO-mismatched HSCT is detailed in Table 39–3. During the period between transplant and engraftment, the blood bank should provide RBCs that are compatible with the plasma of both donor and recipient and platelets/plasma that are compatible with both donor and recipient RBCs. These transfusion restrictions are begun on day 0 of HSCT, or earlier if feasible. Because these patients are immunocompromised and therefore at risk for transfusion-associated GVHD, it is critically important to irradiate all cellular blood components.

ABO antigens are widely expressed on endothelial tissues; thus, HSCT recipients may be considered ABO chimeras even after full RBC recovery. For example, a type A recipient of a type O transplant will eventually convert to having 100% type O (donor-type) red cells—but the patient's plasma will usually lack the anti-A normally seen in a type O individual.

Non-ABO Antibodies

In principle, donor lymphocytes may make an antibody in response to any recipient red cell antigen; conversely, recipient lymphocytes may make an antibody against any donor red cell antigen. In practice, however, clinically significant hemolysis caused by non-ABO RBC antibodies (e.g., Rh system antibodies) occurs only rarely in the post-HSCT setting.[59–61] Ting and colleagues[62] observed the formation of non-ABO antibodies in 13 of 150 patients (8.7%) after bone marrow transplantation. de la Rubia[63] reported a 3.7% rate of non-ABO antibody formation in 217 stem transplant recipients. The rate of clinically significant hemolysis seems to be lower still: in a review of 427 stem cell transplants, Young and colleagues[60] found an approximately 1% incidence of alloimmune hemolysis caused by non-ABO antibodies. When such hemolysis does occur though, it may be severe.[64] Red cell antigen systems that have been implicated in post-transplantation hemolysis include Rh, Kell, Kidd, MNS, and Lewis.[59] Because clinically significant hemolysis caused by non-ABO antibodies is seen so rarely, it is not considered necessary to give antigen-negative red cell units unless the patient forms the corresponding antibody.

Prophylactic Platelet Transfusions

A period of thrombocytopenia is expected between the time of myeloablation and stem cell engraftment. In this setting, the vast majority of platelet transfusions given are administered to nonbleeding patients as prophylaxis, rather than to treat active bleeding. For many years, a platelet count of 20,000/μL was used as a standard transfusion trigger.[65,66] Later, it was demonstrated that prophylactic platelet transfusions can safely be provided using lower thresholds, with considerable savings in both product inventory and cost. In an observational study of leukemia patients, Gmur and colleagues[67] reported that a platelet transfusion trigger of 5,000/μL could safely be used for patients without fever or bleeding (a 10,000/μL trigger was used for patients with such comorbidities). Later, two randomized, controlled trials of patients with acute leukemia directly compared the use of a 10,000/μL versus 20,000/μL trigger.[68,69] Both of these studies, as well as a third nonrandomized prospective study,[70] showed no increased bleeding risk when a 10,000/μL trigger was used. Of note, all of these trials included provisions for transfusing patients at higher platelet counts if specified risk factors for bleeding (e.g., fever) were present. Few studies have directly examined platelet transfusion triggers in the specific setting of HSCT. Nevertheless, the 10,000/μL trigger has been widely applied to the HSCT patient population, and it appears to be safe for patients lacking associated clinical

Table 39–3 Product Selection for ABO-Mismatched HSCT: Peritransplant Period

Recipient	Donor	RBC	PLT 1st Choice	PLT Next Choice*	FFP
A	B	O	AB	A, B, O	AB
	O	O	A, AB	B, O	A, AB
	AB	A, O	AB	A, B, O	AB
B	A	O	AB	B, A, O	AB
	O	O	B, AB	A, O	B, AB
	AB	B, O	AB	B, A, O	AB
O	A	O	A, AB	B, O	A, AB
	B	O	B, AB	A, O	B, AB
	AB	O	AB	A, B, O	AB
AB	A	A, O	AB	A, B, O	AB
	B	B, O	AB	B, A, O	AB
	O	O	AB	A, B, O	AB

*Volume reduction recommended for "next choice" platelets.
All cellular products must be irradiated.
FFP; fresh frozen plasma; PLT, platelets; RBC, red blood cells.

factors (e.g., infection, GVHD).[71,72] Often, these clinical factors are more important determinants of bleeding risk than the platelet count alone. Approximately two thirds of bleeding events after HSCT occur in patients with platelet counts above 20,000/μL.[17,73]

Alloimmunization and Platelet Refractoriness

Platelet refractoriness may be defined as an inappropriately low platelet increment following repeated platelet transfusions. Several nonimmune factors can cause platelet refractoriness, including fever, sepsis, disseminated intravascular coagulation, medications, bleeding, splenomegaly, hepatic veno-occlusive disease, and GVHD. In a subset of cases, platelet refractoriness is caused by alloimmunization. Platelets express HLA class I antigens, ABO antigens,[74] and several platelet-specific antigens. Any of these molecules could potentially serve as an immune stimulus in a transfusion recipient. Antibodies directed against HLA molecules are responsible for most cases of immune-mediated platelet refractoriness. Notably, less than half of all platelet-refractory patients have demonstrable antiplatelet or anti-HLA antibodies.[75,76] Platelet counts obtained at 10 minutes and 1 hour post-transfusion that repeatedly fail to demonstrate an adequate corrected count increment usually indicate an immune mechanism of platelet destruction.[77] If the 10 minute and 1 hour post-transfusion platelet count shows a reasonable increment but the platelet count falls back to baseline by 18 to 24 hours, a nonimmune mechanism of refractoriness may be presumed. HLA antibody screening (*percent reactive antibody*, or PRA) provides valuable supporting evidence that allosensitization has occurred.[78,79] A patient with a PRA greater than 70% may be considered to be *severely immunized*[80] and a good candidate for HLA-matched platelets.

Although they express HLA class I antigens, platelets themselves are fairly weak immunogens. It has been shown that contaminating leukocytes in platelet products are primarily responsible for stimulating HLA antibody formation in platelet transfusion recipients.[81–84] Thus, removal of white cells from blood products helps prevent alloimmunization and platelet refractoriness. The definitive study showing this was the Trial to Reduce Alloimmunization to Platelets (TRAP study),[84] which compared alloimmunization rates in 530 newly diagnosed acute myelogenous leukemia patients randomized to receive either unmodified, pooled platelet concentrates (control); filtered, pooled platelet concentrates (F-PC); filtered single-donor apheresis platelets (F-AP); or UVB-irradiated pooled platelet concentrates (UVB-PC). Anti-HLA antibodies were detected in 45% of controls, compared with 17% to 21% of patients receiving modified platelets. Of the control group patients, 13% became platelet-refractory, versus only 3% in the F-PC group, 4% in the F-AP group, and 5% in the UVB-PC group.

Once platelet refractoriness has been demonstrated, several strategies may help in obtaining therapeutic platelet increments in vivo. A trial of ABO-matched, fresh (1 to 2 days old) platelets may be helpful.[85] In cases of immune-mediated refractoriness, a trial of HLA-matched platelets,[78,86–88] antigen-negative platelets,[89] or crossmatched platelets[90–92] should be considered. Due to the high degree of polymorphism of the HLA loci, it is often not possible to find perfect HLA-A and HLA-B locus matches, leading to the use of platelets mismatched at one or more loci. Grade A (HLA identical) or BU (partially homozygous) matched platelets provide the highest probability of a successful response.[87]

SOLID-ORGAN TRANSPLANTATION

The total number of organ transplants performed in the United States has been gradually increasing over the past several years. Indeed, between 2000 and 2004, the total number of transplants performed in the United States increased by 16%, to 27,036 per year. During this time period, the numbers of kidney and liver transplants increased while the number of heart transplants remained stable (United Network of Organ Sharing, www.unos.org). The blood transfusion requirements for a transplant depend on several factors, including the type of organ being transplanted, the clinical condition of the patient, the experience of the transplant center, and use of antifibrinolytic agents such as aprotinin.

Blood Product Support

Liver Transplants

Although liver transplants often require substantial transfusion of blood components, the transfusion needs of these patients has declined as centers have gained experience.[93] The transfusion requirements can vary significantly and depend on the medical center and on the complexity of the case and the patient's condition.[94,95] Red cells are transfused in 80% to 90% of cases, and the median number of RBC units required ranges from 4 to 12, depending on the center.[93,96–98]

Although not all patients undergoing liver transplantation require platelet transfusions, some patients with liver failure develop thrombocytopenia that can be compounded by blood loss during surgery. Platelets are transfused in about 55% of cases,[93] and the median number of platelets transfused is about 10 whole blood–derived platelet units.[93,96–98]

Plasma transfusions are also used to support about 75% of liver transplants.[93] Patients with more severe coagulopathies and greater blood loss during surgery are more likely to require plasma transfusions.[94,95] The use of plasma transfusions varies greatly between institutions,[93] with the median number of units of plasma used ranging from 0 to 19.[93,96–98] Additionally, some institutions use cryoprecipitate for some of their liver transplants.[97,98]

Heart Transplants

Although heart transplant patients do not usually have a coagulopathy or thrombocytopenia prior to surgery, they invariably require blood component support because of the blood volume diverted to the cardiopulmonary bypass circuit and because platelets are damaged when flowing through bypass circuits. There is significant variability in product usage between institutions, with these patients using a median of 3 to 9 units of red cells, 3 to 10 units of plasma, and 0 to 13 units of platelets.[96,99,100]

Lung Transplants and Heart-Lung Transplants

Transfusion support for single or double lung transplants differs significantly, because double lung transplants require cardiopulmonary bypass. Single lung transplants have been reported to require a mean of 1.7 units of red cells, 1.5 units of platelets, 1.3 units of plasma, and 0.8 units of cryoprecipitate[101]; double lung transplants or heart-lung transplants require 6.4

to 13.3 units of red cells, 3 to 13.6 units of platelets, 4 to 8 units of plasma, and 0 to 15.8 units of cryoprecipitate.[100–102] One report found that the use of aprotinin was able to reduce the use of red cell and whole blood units from a mean of 13.3 to 7, the use of plasma units from a mean of 6.1 to 2, and to eliminate the use of platelets or cryoprecipitate.[102]

Other Solid Organ Transplants

Small bowel transplants are relatively uncommon. They can require a median of 7 units of red cells, 3 units of plasma, and 8 units of platelets.[96] The far more common kidney transplants usually only require 0 to 2 units of red cells.[96]

ABO

Overview

Endothelial cells express ABO antigens.[103,104] Hence, the potential exists for antibody-mediated rejection when a transplanted vascular organ expresses ABO antigens that are absent in the patient (i.e., there is a major ABO mismatch). However, because the supply of organs is severely limited and organs are sometimes needed emergently or are provided by living related donors, a variety of centers have attempted to perform ABO mismatched organ transplants using a variety of strategies. Overall, success has been mixed. Currently, although 70% to 80% of ABO-compatible hearts, livers, or cadaveric kidneys survive 1 year, only 50% to 60% of ABO-incompatible transplants survive at least 1 year, even though those patients often undergo intensive immunosuppression.[105]

Results from many reports of transplanting ABO-mismatched organs need to be viewed with caution because of the paucity of controlled studies. Even without special protocols, the results of ABO-incompatible organ transplants are variable; whereas some transplanted organs are rapidly rejected, others survive for long periods of time. Also, in addition to ABO issues, transplant results are affected by the medical status of patients prior to transplant and by the immunosuppressive treatments used to prevent or treat rejection.

One strategy to breach the ABO barrier is to limit the transplants to those in whom only low levels of the ABO antigen are expressed. Specifically, some transplanters have limited ABO-incompatible transplants to those in which the donor types as an A_2 and the recipient lacks the A antigen entirely.[106,107]

Another strategy for performing ABO-incompatible transplants is to limit the transplants to patients whose immune system is less likely to reject the ABO-incompatible organ. One way to identify such patients may be to limit ABO-incompatible transplants to patients with low titers of the relevant isohemagglutinin. Another set of patients that may not reject ABO-incompatible organs is very young children with immature immune systems. Isohemagluttinins are usually absent in the first few months of life and the titers usually remain low in the first year of life.[108]

A third strategy for performing ABO-incompatible solid organ transplants is to suppress the immune system with some combination of drugs, plasmapheresis, and splenectomy.

ABO Compatibility in Liver Transplants

In comparison to other vascular organs, the liver is thought to be less susceptible to humoral rejection, possibly because the Kupffer cells may be able to remove antigen–antibody complexes.[109] Indeed, HLA matching is not usually performed for liver allografts.[110,111] Early studies suggested that ABO barriers could be ignored because patients rarely developed hyperacute rejection.[112] However, additional experience revealed that ABO-incompatible liver allografts can undergo ABO-mediated hyperacute rejection[113,114] and the allografts have a significantly diminished survival. For instance, one group reported a 30% 2-year graft survival rate for ABO-incompatible livers compared with a 76% to 80% 2-year graft survival rate for ABO-compatible liver allografts.[115] Other centers have also found a significant decrease in 1-year or 2-year survival of ABO-incompatible liver allografts.[105,116]

ABO-incompatible liver transplants appear to be safer in young children. In patients less than 1 year old, the 5-year survival following an ABO-incompatible liver transplant was 76% at one Japanese center.[117] Similar results have been seen in an American hospital with 81% of ABO-incompatible allografts surviving long-term following transplants into children who were less than 3 years old.[118]

One report suggests that group A_2 livers can be safely transplanted into blood group O patients.[119] However, further work is needed in this area because this report only included 6 patients who suffered nine episodes of rejection that responded to standard treatment.

Plasmapheresis has been used by some groups to remove incompatible isohemagglutinins either before or after transplant.[105,120,121] However, there is no evidence that plasmapheresis improves survival of the graft or the patient since the patients generally received intensive immunosuppressive treatments and graft survival rates were usually no better than 60%. Additionally, plasmapheresis may be associated with increased septic complications in these patients.[122]

ABO Compatibility in Heart and Lung Transplants

ABO compatibility is a requirement for heart transplants in adults. Five of eight cases of unintentional transplants of ABO-incompatible hearts resulted in hyperacute rejection.[123] An unintentional transplant of an ABO-incompatible heart and lung also resulted in hyperacute rejection,[124] whereas an unintentional ABO-incompatible lung transplant was able to be sustained for at least 3 years through the addition of antigen-specific immunoadsorption, anti-CD20 monoclonal antibody, and recombinant soluble complement receptor type 1 to an immunosuppressive regimen of cyclophosphamide, antithymocyte globulin, cyclosporine, mycophenolate mofetil, and prednisone.[125]

Increasing evidence demonstrates that infants can be transplanted successfully with ABO-incompatible hearts. This finding was ariginally reported in 2001 by West and colleagues[126]; experience in almost 50 patients at several medical centers has shown that many young infants can be safely transplanted with ABO-incompatible hearts.[127]

Although most ABO-incompatible heart transplants have been performed in infants too young to produce isohemagglutinins, the blood banks supporting such transplants have implemented special procedures. Starting prior to a possible ABO-incompatible transplant, patients are usually provided with blood components lacking isohemagglutinins (i.e., AB plasma and washed cellular blood components). Even with these precautions, a patient's plasma may contain incompatible isohemagglutinins that were passively transfused, of maternal origin, or were produced by the infant's own immune system. Such isohemagglutinins are usually removed immediately prior to the transplant either by plasmapheresis or by whole blood exchange as the patient is placed on cardiopulmonary bypass for surgery. Incompatible anti-A and/or anti-B antibodies that are detected after the transplant may be removed by plasmapheresis.

Although the mean age of patients that have been successfully transplanted with incompatible hearts is 117 days,[127] patients as old as 14 months have received transplants.[128] However, experience with patients older than age 8 months is limited; one patient who received a transplant at age 9 months developed rejection mediated by an isohemagglutinin that was successfully treated with rituximab.[128]

ABO Compatibility in Renal Transplants

Early experiences demonstrated that transplantation of an ABO-incompatible kidney could lead to hyperacute or acute rejection; the 1-year survival of such transplanted kidneys was only 4%.[129–133] However, many attempts have been made to transplant ABO-incompatible kidneys because the wait list for cadaveric kidneys is very long and many patients are offered ABO-incompatible kidneys from family members. This has been of particular importance in Japan where traditionally very few cadaveric kidneys have been made available for transplant.

Many reports suggest that the safest ABO-incompatible renal transplants are ones in which the kidney is from a donor whose cells express the A_2 antigen and the recipient is of blood group O or B with low titers of anti-A antibodies. An early report of A_2-incompatible transplants using the standard immunosuppression of the time found limited success with 12 of 20 such grafts surviving long-term and 8 of the grafts being lost within 1 month.[134] Subsequent work suggested that patients with an immunoglobulin M titer of <64 against A_2 red blood cells were less likely to reject an A_2 kidney than patients with higher anti-A_2 titers.[135] Some American transplant programs currently transplant kidneys in which the A_2 antigen confers major incompatibility. These programs have restricted the transplants to patients whose initial anti-A antibody titer is ≤4 or ≤8, which in some cases had been reduced by pretransplant plasmapheresis.[135–139] Even with these protocols occasional cases of acute rejection have occurred. However, these centers have reported at least 90% 1-year and 85% 5-year survival of the grafts, which is similar to graft survival rates that these centers have achieved with ABO-compatible transplants.[138,139]

Starting in the 1980s, some centers tried transplanting kidneys with major ABO incompatibility with the recipients, based on expression of A_1 and/or B antigens on the renal allografts. Several of these centers modeled their immunosuppressive treatment protocols on the approach used by a Belgian group that included pretransplant antibody removal by plasmapheresis or immunoadsorption, steroids, azathioprine, cyclosporine or tacrolimus, antilymphocyte globulin, and splenectomy.[140] In some of these series patients also received pretransplant infusion of the relevant A and/or B substance.[141] In most cases in which the transplanted kidneys survived, incompatible isohemagglutinins returned to the patient's plasma and the kidney continued to express the ABO antigen.[141–143]

At least 309 ABO-incompatible renal transplants have been reported with a combined 1-year graft survival rate of 83%,[130] which is equivalent to the survival rate seen with ABO compatible grafts in the multicenter Collaborative Transplant Study.[105] However, data from these selected reports must be considered cautiously; long-term analysis of the original patients reveals that 23 of 31 ABO-incompatible renal transplants from living related donors have survived at least 15 years, which is a long-term survival rate equivalent to that seen with ABO-compatible renal transplants at that center.[141] The specific immunosuppressive treatment is especially important in ABO-incompatible transplants, with one report finding that the addition of mycophenolate mofetil allowed ABO-incompatible kidneys to survive as long as ABO-compatible transplants.[144]

Several centers have continued to perform transplants using this or similar approaches. In some of these protocols, patients only receive transplants if plasmapheresis can reduce the anti-A/B antibody titer to no more that 4:1 or 8:1 before the transplant. Recent studies demonstrate that pretransplant removal of anti-A/B antibodies is necessary for successful transplants of ABO-incompatible kidneys (other than A_2 kidneys).[145,146] Some studies also suggest that splenectomy is unnecessary for ABO-incompatible renal transplants, especially if patients are treated with newer potent immunosuppressive treatments that can modify B-cell responses, such as rituximab, mycophenolate mofetil, or intravenous immunoglobulin (IVIG).[141,145,147–151]

Non-ABO Antibodies

Although transplanted organs can induce alloantibodies to erythrocyte antigens,[152] such antibodies have little impact on graft survival. Early studies suggested that renal allografts survived longer if the Lewis type of the kidney donor matched the type of the patient.[153] However, this has not been seen in more recent studies. It is now accepted that kidneys can be safely transplanted into patients with preexisting anti–red cell antibodies such as anti-RhD.[154–156]

Pretransplant Transfusion for Kidneys to Increase Survival

Starting in 1973, studies have shown that blood transfusions prior to renal transplantation prolong survival and reduce rejection of renal allografts.[96,157] The beneficial effect of pretransplant transfusion had only been seen for kidney transplants. Then, new immunosuppressive drugs such as cyclosporine were developed and it was unclear whether transfusions conferred any additional benefit to patients who were receiving these drugs.[96,158] Because it had also become clear that transfusions can transmit infectious diseases and induce alloimmunization, the practice of pretransplant transfusion to prolong the survival of renal allografts was largely abandoned.

Several recent studies have found that even with the use of immunosuppressive drugs such as cyclosporine or tacrolimus, pretransplant transfusion may still decrease the risk of rejection of the renal allograft.[159–162] In the pediatric setting, this benefit was observed in patients receiving one to five transfusions, but was not seen in patients receiving more than five transfusions.[161] Despite these studies, most centers are not currently using transfusions for this purpose.

Passenger Lymphocyte Syndrome

Donor B lymphocytes contained in solid organ allografts can sometimes produce anti-erythrocyte antibodies, resulting in a condition known as the *passenger lymphocyte syndrome.*

Typically, the antibodies are detected 1 to 2 weeks after the transplant as a positive DAT.[96] Elution reveals anti-A and/or anti-B. These patients may develop hemolysis, which can be severe in rare cases. Although at least one death has been attributed to this hemolysis, most patients recover and the antibody usually disappears in about 1 month.[96,163]

Most cases of passenger lymphocyte syndrome involve antibodies to ABO antigens. As reported by Ramsey's extensive analysis of the literature,[163] the observed rate of ABO antibodies and hemolysis from passenger lymphocyte syndrome is lowest in kidney transplant patients (17% and 9%, respectively), intermediate in liver transplant patients (40% and 29%, respectively), and highest in heart-lung transplant patients (both 70%). Notably, most of these reports were prior to the advent of cyclosporine or tacrolimus. In kidney transplant patients, cyclosporine increases the incidence of passenger lymphocyte syndrome so that 30% of patients develop antibodies and 17% develop hemolysis.

No risk factors for passenger lymphocyte syndrome have been proven. It has been hypothesized that passenger lymphocyte syndrome is more likely when the donor has a high-titer antibody or when the recipient is a nonsecretor or is of the A_2 subtype.[163,164] Although it is possible that these donor and recipient characteristics are risk factors for passenger lymphocyte syndrome, no large studies have been performed, and individual case reports demonstrate that secretors and non-A_2 patients can develop passenger lymphocyte syndrome. The only prophylactic treatment that has been shown to reduce the incidence of passenger lymphocyte syndrome in renal transplant patients is post-transplant irradiation of the graft.[163,165]

Passenger lymphocyte syndrome resulting in hemolysis has rarely been caused by non-ABO antibodies including anti-RhD, anti-Rh^e, anti-Rh^c, anti-Rh^E and anti-Jk^a antibodies[163,166–168] Case reports suggest that passenger lymphocyte syndrome involving these antibodies only occurs when the donor is alloimmunized to the antigen prior to donating the organ.

Plasmapheresis to Prevent or Treat Anti-HLA Antibody-Mediated Rejection of Transplanted Organs

No randomized, controlled prospective trials have analyzed the efficacy of plasmapheresis in preventing or treating anti-HLA antibody-mediated rejection of transplanted solid organs. However, several transplant centers incorporate plasmapheresis into their treatment protocols based on success from case reports, case series, and retrospective analyses of local data. Plasmapheresis in this setting has been used for cardiac and renal transplants, and very rarely with hepatic transplants.

Patients who have significant levels of anti-HLA antibodies at the time of cardiac transplant have reduced long-term survival,[169] and patients with antibodies that react against the heart donor's HLA antigens appear to have a very high mortality rate.[170] If patients with anti-HLA antibodies are treated by plasmapheresis followed by IVIG immediately before transplant, patient and cardiac allograft survival rates improve to levels comparable to those of patients without pre-existing anti-HLA antibodies.[171,172] Alternatively, some institutions have had success performing multiple plasma exchanges on alloimmunized patients awaiting heart transplants.

Several centers have also reported success with treating acute humoral rejection of cardiac allografts with an immunosuppressive regimen that includes plasmapheresis.[173–179] In some cases in which the rejection failed to respond to multiple pharmacologic interventions, there was significant clinical improvement following plasmapheresis.[175]

Plasmapheresis has also been used to remove anti-HLA antibodies prior to renal transplants. This approach has been used with apparent success in renal transplant patients receiving either living donor allografts[180,181] or cadaveric allografts.[182] Plasmapheresis combined with other immunosuppressive therapy such as IVIG has also been used to successfully treat acute humoral rejection of renal allografts.[178,179,183,184]

Plasmapheresis for primary allograft nonfunction after liver transplantation has been attempted with mixed results.[185,186]

TRANSFUSION-RELATED COMPLICATIONS IN IMMUNOCOMPROMISED PATIENTS

Cytomegalovirus Infection

Cytomegalovirus (CMV) is a member of the herpesvirus group, which includes the herpes simplex viruses 1 and 2, Epstein-Barr virus, and varicella-zoster virus. CMV is capable of infecting a variety of cell types, including mature white blood cells and their progenitors. In the immunocompromised host, CMV infection can lead to significant morbidity and mortality. Allogeneic HSCT patients in particular are at risk to develop serious manifestations of CMV disease, which include pneumonitis, gastroenteritis, hepatitis, encephalitis, and retinitis. CMV disease is much less commonly seen in the autologous HSCT setting.[187] Because of the risk of transfusion-transmitted CMV disease in transplant recipients, "CMV safe" blood products should be provided to CMV-negative transplant recipients.

Serologic screening of blood products is currently the most effective means of reducing the risk of transfusion-transmitted CMV. The rare cases of transfusion-transmitted CMV disease still observed in large part reflect donations made in the preseroconversion window period.[188] Because the seroprevalence of CMV ranges in different communities from 40% to 80%, it is logistically difficult for blood banks to maintain an inventory of CMV-seronegative components.[189] Several studies have demonstrated that leukoreduction can be used as an alternative to serologic screening to provide blood that is "CMV safe."[187,190–195] Although unquestionably efficacious, leukoreduction appears to be slightly inferior to providing seronegative products for the prevention of CMV transmission.[190,196,197] Overall, although transfusion-transmitted CMV remains a problem in the HSCT and solid-organ transplant population, the transmission rates seen using either seronegative or leukoreduced products are far lower than in the past, due in large part to improvements in both surveillance and preemptive therapy.[198]

Transfusion-Associated Graft-versus-Host Disease

Transfusion-associated GVHD (TA-GVHD) is a devastating complication of transfusion that primarily affects immunocompromised patients, including hematopoietic stem cell and solid organ transplant recipients. TA-GVHD occurs when immunocompetent lymphocytes in a blood product proliferate in the transfusion recipient. The donor lymphocytes attack host organs, including bone marrow, skin, liver, and intestines. TA-GVHD usually becomes clinically apparent 7 to 10 days after transfusion. Patients usually present with fever, skin rash, elevated results on liver function tests, and gastrointestinal symptoms. Severe pancytopenia is often observed. In classical GVHD, the bone marrow is typically spared, because donor and recipient bone marrow are selected to be HLA-compatible. In contrast, TA-GVHD involves immune rejection of host marrow cells, and as a result generally carries a worse prognosis than classical GVHD. TA-GVHD is almost always fatal within 4 weeks of transfusion, with most deaths attributable to bleeding or infection resulting from marrow failure.

No effective therapy for TA-GVHD currently exists, but it is prevented by gamma-irradiation of blood products before transfusion. TA-GVHD was previously reported to occur following blood product irradiation to 1500 rads,[199] and other studies indicated that irradiation to 2000 rads is needed to reduce mitogen-responsive lymphocytes by 5 to 6 logs.[200] Irradiated blood products are now required to receive 2500 rads (25 Gy) to the center of the container, with a minimum dose of 1500 rads (15Gy) to any other point.[201] Cellular blood products are required to be irradiated in the following situations: recipients identified to be at risk for TA-GVHD, donations made by blood relatives of the recipient, and donors selected to be HLA-matched with the recipient.[202]

REFERENCES

1. Schmitz N, Barrett J. Optimizing engraftment—source and dose of stem cells. Semin Hematol 2002;39:3–14.
2. Singhal S, Powles R, Kulkarni S, et al. Comparison of marrow and blood cell yields from the same donors in a double-blind, randomized study of allogeneic marrow vs blood stem cell transplantation. Bone Marrow Transplant 2000;25:501–505.
3. Bensinger WI, Martin PJ, Storer B, et al. Transplantation of bone marrow as compared with peripheral-blood cells from HLA-identical relatives in patients with hematologic cancers. NEJM 2001;344:175–181.
4. Blaise D, Kuentz M, Fortanier C, et al. Randomized trial of bone marrow versus lenograstim-primed blood cell allogeneic transplantation in patients with early-stage leukemia: a report from the Societe Francaise de Greffe de Moelle. J Clin Oncol 2000;18:537–546.
5. Heldal D, Tjonnfjord G, Brinch L, et al. A randomised study of allogeneic transplantation with stem cells from blood or bone marrow. Bone Marrow Transplant 2000;25:1129–1136.
6. Powles R, Mehta J, Kulkarni S, et al. Allogeneic blood and bone marrow stem cell transplantation in haematological malignant diseases: a randomised trial. Lancet 2000;355:1231–1237.
7. Schmitz N, Linch DC, Dreger P, et al. Randomised trial of filgrastim-mobilised peripheral blood progenitor cell transplantation versus autologous bone marrow transplantation in lymphoma patients. Lancet 1996;347:353–357.
8. Vigorito AC, Azevedo WM, Marques JF, et al. A randomised, prospective comparison of allogeneic bone marrow and peripheral blood progenitor cell transplantation in the treatment of haematological malignancies. Bone Marrow Transplant 1998;22:1145–1151.
9. Kiss JE, Rybka WB, Winkelstein A, et al. Relationship of CD34+ cell dose to early and late hematopoiesis following autologous peripheral blood stem cell transplantation. Bone Marrow Transplant 1997;19:303–310.
10. Haas R, Mohle R, Fruhauf S, et al. Patient characteristics associated with successful mobilizing and autografting of peripheral blood progenitor cells in malignant lymphoma. Blood 1994;83:3787–3794.
11. Lane TA. Umbilical cord blood grafts for hematopoietic transplantation in adults: a cup half empty or half full? Transfusion 2005;45:1027–1034.
12. Wang JC, Doedens M, Dick JE. Primitive human hematopoietic cells are enriched in cord blood compared with adult bone marrow or mobilized peripheral blood as measured by the quantitative in vivo SCID-repopulating cell assay. Blood 1997;89:3919–3924.
13. Rubinstein P, Carrier C, Scaradavou A, et al. Outcomes among 562 recipients of placental-blood transplants from unrelated donors. NEJM 1998;339:1565–1577.
14. Benito AI, Diaz MA, Gonzalez-Vicent M, et al. Hematopoietic stem cell transplantation using umbilical cord blood progenitors: review of current clinical results. Bone Marrow Transplant 2004;33:675–690.
15. Rocha V, Sanz G, Gluckman E. Umbilical cord blood transplantation. Curr Opin Hematol 2004;11:375–385.
16. Barker JN, Weisdorf DJ, DeFor TE, et al. Transplantation of 2 partially HLA-matched umbilical cord blood units to enhance engraftment in adults with hematologic malignancy. Blood 2005;105:1343–1347.
17. Bernstein SH, Nademanee AP, Vose JM, et al. A multicenter study of platelet recovery and utilization in patients after myeloablative therapy and hematopoietic stem cell transplantation. Blood 1998;91: 3509–3517.
18. Klaesson S, Ringden O, Ljungman P, et al. Reduced blood transfusions requirements after allogeneic bone marrow transplantation: results of a randomised, double-blind study with high-dose erythropoietin. Bone Marrow Transplant 1994;13:397–402.
19. Link H, Boogaerts MA, Fauser AA, et al. A controlled trial of recombinant human erythropoietin after bone marrow transplantation. Blood 1994;84:3327–3335.
20. Biggs JC, Atkinson KA, Booker V, et al. Prospective randomised double-blind trial of the in vivo use of recombinant human erythropoietin in bone marrow transplantation from HLA-identical sibling donors. The Australian Bone Marrow Transplant Study Group. Bone Marrow Transplant 1995;15:129–134.
21. Miller CB, Lazarus HM. Erythropoietin in stem cell transplantation. Bone Marrow Transplant 2001;27:1011–1016.
22. Weissinger F, Sandmaier BM, Maloney DG, et al. Decreased transfusion requirements for patients receiving nonmyeloablative compared with conventional peripheral blood stem cell transplants from HLA-identical siblings. Blood 2001;98:3584–3588.
23. Ruiz-Arguelles GJ, Morales-Toquero A, Lopez-Martinez B, et al. Bloodless (transfusion-free) hematopoietic stem cell transplants: the Mexican experience. Bone Marrow Transplant 2005;36:715–720.
24. Rowley SD. Hematopoietic stem cell transplantation between red cell incompatible donor-recipient pairs. Bone Marrow Transplant 2001;28: 315–321.
25. Buckner CD, Clift RA, Sanders JE, et al. ABO-incompatible marrow transplants. Transplantation 1978;26:233–238.
26. Mielcarek M, Leisenring W, Torok-Storb B, et al. Graft-versus-host disease and donor-directed hemagglutinin titers after ABO-mismatched related and unrelated marrow allografts: evidence for a graft-versus-plasma cell effect. Blood 2000;96:1150–1156.
27. Mielcarek M, Torok-Storb B, Storb R. ABO incompatibility and relapse risk in patients undergoing allogeneic marrow transplantation for acute myeloid leukemia. Bone Marrow Transplant 2002;30:547–548.
28. Kim JG, Sohn SK, Kim DH, et al. Impact of ABO incompatibility on outcome after allogeneic peripheral blood stem cell transplantation. Bone Marrow Transplant 2005;35:489–495.
29. Goldman J, Liesveld J, Nichols D, et al. ABO incompatibility between donor and recipient and clinical outcomes in allogeneic stem cell transplantation. Leuk Res 2003;27:489–491.
30. Klumpp TR. Immunohematologic complications of bone marrow transplantation. Bone Marrow Transplant 1991;8:159–170.
31. Worel N, Kalhs P, Keil F, et al. ABO mismatch increases transplant-related morbidity and mortality in patients given nonmyeloablative allogeneic HPC transplantation. Transfusion 2003;43:1153–1161.
32. Canals C, Muniz-Diaz E, Martinez C, et al. Impact of ABO incompatibility on allogeneic peripheral blood progenitor cell transplantation after reduced intensity conditioning. Transfusion 2004;44:1603–1611.
33. Griffith LM, McCoy JP Jr, Bolan CD, et al. Persistence of recipient plasma cells and anti-donor isohaemagglutinins in patients with delayed donor erythropoiesis after major ABO incompatible non-myeloablative haematopoietic cell transplantation. Br J Haematol 2005; 128:668–675.
34. Bolan CD, Leitman SF, Griffith LM, et al. Delayed donor red cell chimerism and pure red cell aplasia following major ABO-incompatible nonmyeloablative hematopoietic stem cell transplantation. Blood 2001;98:1687–1694.
35. Gmur JP, Burger J, Schaffner A, et al. Pure red cell aplasia of long duration complicating major ABO-incompatible bone marrow transplantation. Blood 1990;75:290–295.
36. Bensinger WI, Buckner CD, Thomas ED, et al. ABO-incompatible marrow transplants. Transplantation 1982;33:427–429.

37. Lee JH, Choi SJ, Kim S, et al. Changes of isoagglutinin titres after ABO-incompatible allogeneic stem cell transplantation. Br J Haematol 2003;120:702–710.
38. Maschan AA, Skorobogatova EV, Balashov DN, et al. Successful treatment of pure red cell aplasia with a single dose of rituximab in a child after major ABO incompatible peripheral blood allogeneic stem cell transplantation for acquired aplastic anemia. Bone Marrow Transplant 2002;30:405–407.
39. Lee JH, Lee KH, Kim S, et al. Anti-A isoagglutinin as a risk factor for the development of pure red cell aplasia after major ABO-incompatible allogeneic bone marrow transplantation. Bone Marrow Transplant 2000;25:179–184.
40. Damodar S, George B, Mammen J, et al. Pretransplant reduction of isohaemagglutinin titres by donor group plasma infusion does not reduce the incidence of pure red cell aplasia in major ABO-mismatched transplants. Bone Marrow Transplant 2005;36:233–235.
41. Bar BM, Van Dijk BA, Schattenberg A, et al. Erythrocyte repopulation after major ABO incompatible transplantation with lymphocyte-depleted bone marrow. Bone Marrow Transplant 1995;16:793–799.
42. Benjamin RJ, Connors JM, McGurk S, et al. Prolonged erythroid aplasia after major ABO-mismatched transplantation for chronic myelogenous leukemia. Biol Blood Marrow Transplant 1998;4: 151–156.
43. Maciej Zaucha J, Mielcarek M, Takatu A, et al. Engraftment of early erythroid progenitors is not delayed after nonmyeloablative major ABO-incompatible haematopoietic stem cell transplantation. Br J Haematol 2002;119:740–750.
44. Veelken H, Wasch R, Behringer D, et al. Pure red cell aplasia after allogeneic stem cell transplantation with reduced conditioning. Bone Marrow Transplant 2000;26:911–915.
45. Peggs KS, Morris EC, Kottaridis PD, et al. Outcome of major ABO-incompatible nonmyeloablative hematopoietic stem cell transplantation may be influenced by conditioning regimen. Blood 2002;99: 4642–4643.
46. Santamaria A, Sureda A, Martino R, et al. Successful treatment of pure red cell aplasia after major ABO-incompatible T cell-depleted bone marrow transplantation with erythropoietin. Bone Marrow Transplant 1997;20:1105–1107.
47. Paltiel O, Cournoyer D, Rybka W. Pure red cell aplasia following ABO-incompatible bone marrow transplantation: response to erythropoietin. Transfusion 1993;33:418–421.
48. Heyll A, Aul C, Runde V, et al. Treatment of pure red cell aplasia after major ABO-incompatible bone marrow transplantation with recombinant erythropoietin. Blood 1991;77:906.
49. Rabitsch W, Knobl P, Prinz E, et al. Prolonged red cell aplasia after major ABO-incompatible allogeneic hematopoietic stem cell transplantation: Removal of persisting isohemagglutinins with Ig-Therasorb immunoadsorption. Bone Marrow Transplant 2003;32:1015–1019.
50. Verholen F, Stalder M, Helg C, et al. Resistant pure red cell aplasia after allogeneic stem cell transplantation with major ABO mismatch treated by escalating dose donor leukocyte infusion. Eur J Haematol 2004;73: 441–446.
51. Bierman PJ, Warkentin P, Hutchins MR, et al. Pure red cell aplasia following ABO mismatched marrow transplantation for chronic lymphocytic leukemia: response to antithymocyte globulin. Leuk Lymphoma 1993;9:169–171.
52. Labar B, Bogdanic V, Nemet D, et al. Antilymphocyte globulin for treatment of pure red cell aplasia after major ABO incompatible marrow transplant. Bone Marrow Transplant 1992;10:471–472.
53. Petz LD, Garratty G. Immune Hemolytic Anemias, 2nd ed. Philadelphia, Churchill Livingstone, 2004.
54. Lopez J, Steegmann JL, Perez G, et al. Erythropoietin in the treatment of delayed immune hemolysis of a major ABO-incompatible bone marrow transplant. Am J Hematol 1994;45:237–239.
55. Buckner CD, Clift RA, Sanders JE, et al. ABO-incompatible marrow transplants. Transplantation 1978;26:233.
56. Lasky LC, Warkentin PI, Kersey JH, et al. Hemotherapy in patients undergoing blood group incompatible bone marrow transplantation. Transfusion 1983;23:277–285.
57. Bolan CD, Childs RW, Procter JL, et al. Massive immune haemolysis after allogeneic peripheral blood stem cell transplantation with minor ABO incompatibility. Br J Haematol 2001;112:787–795.
58. Hows J, Beddow K, Gordon-Smith E, et al. Donor-derived red blood cell antibodies and immune hemolysis after allogeneic bone marrow transplantation. Blood 1986;67:177–181.
59. Franchini M, Gandini G, Aprili G. Non-ABO red blood cell alloantibodies following allogeneic hematopoietic stem cell transplantation. Bone Marrow Transplant 2004;33:1169–1172.
60. Young PP, Goodnough LT, Westervelt P, et al. Immune hemolysis involving non-ABO/RhD alloantibodies following hematopoietic stem cell transplantation. Bone Marrow Transplant 2001;27:1305–1310.
61. Zupanska B, Zaucha JM, Michalewska B, et al. Multiple red cell alloantibodies, including anti-Dib, after allogeneic ABO-matched peripheral blood progenitor cell transplantation. Transfusion 2005;45:16–20.
62. Ting A, Pun A, Dodds AJ, et al. Red cell alloantibodies produced after bone marrow transplantation. Transfusion 1987;27:145–147.
63. de La Rubia J, Arriaga F, Andreu R, et al. Development of non-ABO RBC alloantibodies in patients undergoing allogeneic HPC transplantation. Is ABO incompatibility a predisposing factor? Transfusion 2001;41:106–110.
64. Leo A, Mytilineos J, Voso MT, et al. Passenger lymphocyte syndrome with severe hemolytic anemia due to an anti-Jk[a] after allogeneic PBPC transplantation. Transfusion 2000;40:632–636.
65. Platelet transfusion therapy. National Institutes of Health Consensus Conference. Transfus Med Rev 1987;1:195–200.
66. Beutler E. Platelet transfusions: The 20,000/μL trigger. Blood 1993;81: 1411–1413.
67. Gmur J, Burger J, Schanz U, et al. Safety of stringent prophylactic platelet transfusion policy for patients with acute leukaemia. Lancet 1991; 338:1223–1226.
68. Heckman KD, Weiner GJ, Davis CS, et al. Randomized study of prophylactic platelet transfusion threshold during induction therapy for adult acute leukemia: 10,000/μL versus 20,000/μL. J Clin Oncol 1997;15:1143–1149.
69. Rebulla P, Finazzi G, Marangoni F, et al. The threshold for prophylactic platelet transfusions in adults with acute myeloid leukemia. Gruppo Italiano Malattie Ematologiche Maligne dell'Adulto. NEJM 1997;337:1870–1875.
70. Wandt H, Frank M, Ehninger G, et al. Safety and cost effectiveness of a 10×10^9/L trigger for prophylactic platelet transfusions compared with the traditional 20×10^9/L trigger: a prospective comparative trial in 105 patients with acute myeloid leukemia. Blood 1998;91:3601–3606.
71. Gil-Fernandez JJ, Alegre A, Fernandez-Villalta MJ, et al. Clinical results of a stringent policy on prophylactic platelet transfusion: nonrandomized comparative analysis in 190 bone marrow transplant patients from a single institution. Bone Marrow Transplant 1996;18:931–935.
72. Schiffer CA, Anderson KC, Bennett CL, et al. Platelet transfusion for patients with cancer: clinical practice guidelines of the American Society of Clinical Oncology. J Clin Oncol 2001;19:1519–1538.
73. Nevo S, Enger C, Hartley E, et al. Acute bleeding and thrombocytopenia after bone marrow transplantation. Bone Marrow Transplant 2001; 27:65–72.
74. Cooling LL, Kelly K, Barton J, et al. Determinants of ABH expression on human blood platelets. Blood 2005;105:3356–3364.
75. Doughty HA, Murphy MF, Metcalfe P, et al. Relative importance of immune and nonimmune causes of platelet refractoriness. Vox Sang 1994;66:200–205.
76. Yankee RA, Graffs KS, Dowling R, et al. Selection of unrelated compatible platelet donors by lymphocyte HLA matching. NEJM 1973;288:760.
77. Daly PA, Schiffer CA, Aisner J, et al. Platelet transfusion therapy. One-hour posttransfusion increments are valuable in predicting the need for HLA-matched preparations. JAMA 1980;243:435–438.
78. Duquesnoy RJ, Filip DJ, Rodey GE, et al. Successful transfusion of platelets "mismatched" for HLA antigens to alloimmunized thrombocytopenic patients. Am J Hematol 1977;2:219–226.
79. Lee EJ, Schiffer CA. Serial measurement of lymphocytotoxic antibody and response to nonmatched platelet transfusions in alloimmunized patients. Blood 1987;70:1727–1729.
80. Nance ST, Hsu S, Vassallo RR, et al. Review: Platelet matching for alloimmunized patients—room for improvement. Immunohematol 2004;20:80–88.
81. Oksanen K, Kekomaki R, Ruutu T, et al. Prevention of alloimmunization in patients with acute leukemia by use of white cell-reduced blood components—a randomized trial. Transfusion 1991;31:588–594.
82. Saarinen UM, Kekomaki R, Siimes MA, et al. Effective prophylaxsis against platelet refractoriness in multitransfused patients by use of leukocyte-free components. Blood 1990;75:512.
83. van Marwijk Kooy M, van Prooijen HC, Moes M, et al. Use of leukocyte depleted platelet concentrates for the prevention of refractoriness and primary HLA alloimmunization: a prosective, randomized trial. Blood 1991;77:201.
84. The Trial to Reduce Alloimmunization to Platelets Study Group. Leukocyte reduction and ultraviolet B irradiation of platelets to prevent alloimmunization and refractoriness to platelet transfusions. NEJM 1997;337:1861–1869.

85. Friedberg RC, Donnelly SF, Boyd JC, et al. Clinical and blood bank factors in the management of platelet refractoriness and alloimmunization. Blood 1993;81:3428–3434.
86. Yankee RA, Grumet FC, Rogentine GN. Platelet transfusion: the selection of compatible platelet donors for refractory patients by lymphocyte HL-A typing. NEJM 1969;281:1208–1212.
87. Moroff G, Garratty G, Heal JM, et al. Selection of platelets for refractory patients by HLA matching and prospective crossmatching. Transfusion 1992;32:633–640.
88. Murphy MF, Brozovic B, Murphy W, et al. Guidelines for platelet transfusions. British Committee for Standards in Haematology, Working Party of the Blood Transfusion Task Force. Transfus Med 1992;2:311–318.
89. Petz LD, Garratty G, Calhoun L, et al. Selecting donors of platelets for refractory patients on the basis of HLA antibody specificity. Transfusion 2000;40:1446–1456.
90. Rachel JM, Summers TC, Sinor LT, et al. Use of a solid phase red blood cell adherence method for pretransfusion platelet compatibility testing. Am J Clin Pathol 1988;90:63–68.
91. von dem Borne AE, Ouwehand WH, Kuijpers RW. Theoretic and practical aspects of platelet crossmatching. Transfus Med Rev 1990;4: 265–278.
92. Gelb AB, Leavitt AD. Crossmatch-compatible platelets improve corrected count increments in patients who are refractory to randomly selected platelets. Transfusion 1997;37:624–630.
93. Ozier Y, Pessione F, Samain E, et al. Institutional variability in transfusion practice for liver transplantation. Anesthesia and Analgesia 2003;97:671–679.
94. Findlay JY, Rettke SR. Poor prediction of blood transfusion requirements in adult liver transplantations from preoperative variables. J Clin Anesth 2000;12:319–323.
95. Steib A, Freys G, Lehmann C, et al. Intraoperative blood losses and transfusion requirements during adult liver transplantation remain difficult to predict. Can J Anaesth 2001;48:1075–1079.
96. Triulzi DJ. Specialized transfusion support for solid organ transplantation. Curr Opin Hematol 2002;9:527–532.
97. Laine E, Steadman R, Calhoun L, et al. Comparison of RBCs and FFP with whole blood during liver transplant surgery. Transfusion 2003;43:322–327.
98. McNicol PL, Liu G, Harley ID, et al. Blood loss and transfusion requirements in liver transplantation: experience with the first 75 cases. Anaes Intensive Care 1994;22:666–671.
99. Danielson CF, Filo RS, O'Donnell JA, et al. Institutional variation in hemotherapy for solid organ transplantation. Transfusion 1996; 36:263–267.
100. Hunt BJ, Sack D, Amin S, et al. The perioperative use of blood components during heart and heart-lung transplantation. Transfusion 1992; 32:57–62.
101. Triulzi DJ, Griffith BP. Blood usage in lung transplantation. Transfusion 1998;38:12–15.
102. Peterson KL, DeCampli WM, Feeley TW, et al. Blood loss and transfusion requirements in cystic fibrosis patients undergoing heart-lung or lung transplantation. J Cardiothorac Vasc Anesth 1995;9:59–62.
103. Westhoff CM, Reid ME. ABO and related antigens. In Roush KS (ed). Blood Banking and Transfusion Medicine: Basic Principles and Practice. Philadelphia, Churchill Livingstone, 2003, pp 21–30.
104. Oriol R. Tissular expression of ABH and Lewis antigens in humans and animals: expected value of different animal models in the study of ABO-incompatible organ transplants. Transplant Proc 1987;19:4416–4420.
105. Wu A, Buhler LH, Cooper DKC. ABO-incompatible organ and bone marrow transplantation: current status. Transpl Int 2003;16:291–299.
106. Rydberg L. ABO incompatibility in solid organ transplantation. Transfus Med 2001;11:325–342.
107. Fishbein TM, Emre S, Guy SR, et al. Safe transplantation of blood type A2 livers to blood type O recipients. Transplantation 1999;67: 1071–1073.
108. Fong SW, Qaqundah BY, Taylor WF. Developmental patterns of ABO isoagglutinins in normal children correlated with the effects of age, sex, and maternal isoagglutinins. Transfusion 1974;14:551–559.
109. Wardle EN. Kupffer cells and their function. Liver 1987;7:63–75.
110. Gordon RD, Fung JJ, Iwatsuki S, et al. Immunological factors influencing liver graft survival. Gastroenterol Clin North Am 1988;17:53–59.
111. Poli F, Scalamogna M, Aniasi A, et al. A retrospective evaluation of HLA-A, B and -DRB1 matching in liver transplantation. Transpl Int 1998;11(Suppl 1):S347–S349.
112. Starzl TE, Ishikawa M, Putnam CW, et al. Progress in and deterrents to orthotopic liver transplantation, with special reference to survival, resistance to hyperacute rejection, and biliary duct reconstruction. Transplant Proc 1974;6:129–139.
113. Demetris AJ, Jaffe R, Tzakis A, et al. Antibody-mediated rejection of human orthotopic liver allografts. A study of liver transplantation across ABO blood group barriers. Am J Pathol 1988;132:489–502.
114. Rego J, Prevost F, Rumeau JL, et al. Hyperacute rejection after ABO-incompatible orthotopic liver transplantation. Transplant Proc 1987; 19:4589–4590.
115. Gugenheim J, Samuel D, Reynes M, et al. Liver transplantation across ABO blood group barriers. Lancet 1990;336:519–523.
116. Reding R, Veyckemans F, de Ville de Goyet J, et al. ABO-incompatible orthotopic liver allografting in urgent indications. Surg Gynecol Obstet 1992;174:59–64.
117. Egawa H, Oike F, Buhler L, et al. Impact of recipient age on outcome of ABO-incompatible living-donor liver transplantation. Transplantation 2004;77:403–411.
118. Varela-Fascinetto G, Treacy SJ, Lillehei CW, et al. Long-term results in pediatric ABO-incompatible liver transplantation. Transplant Proc 1999;31:467–468.
119. Fishbein TM, Emre S, Guy SR, et al. Safe transplantation of blood type A2 livers to blood type O recipients. Transplantation 1999;67:1071–1073.
120. Mor E, Skerrett D, Manzarbeitia C, et al. Successful use of an enhanced immunosuppressive protocol with plasmapheresis for ABO-incompatible mismatched grafts in liver transplant recipients. Transplantation 1995;59:986–990.
121. Tanaka A, Tanaka K, Kitai T, et al. Living related liver transplantation across ABO blood groups. Transplantation 1994;58:548–553.
122. Farges O, Kalil AN, Samuel D, et al. The use of ABO-incompatible grafts in liver transplantation: a life-saving procedure in highly selected patients. Transplantation 1995;59:1124–1133.
123. Cooper DK. Clinical survey of heart transplantation between ABO blood group-incompatible recipients and donors. J Heart Transplant 1990;9:376–381.
124. Campion EW. A death at Duke. NEJM 2003;348:1083–1084.
125. Pierson RN 3rd, Loyd JE, Goodwin A, et al. Successful management of an ABO-mismatched lung allograft using antigen-specific immunoadsorption, complement inhibition, and immunomodulatory therapy. Transplantation 2002;74:79–84.
126. West LJ, Pollock-BarZiv SM, Dipchand AI, et al. ABO-incompatible heart transplantation in infants. NEJM 2001;344:793–800.
127. West LJ, Pollock-BarZiv SM, Ang A, et al. ABO-incompatible infant heart transplantation: The World Experience. J Heart Lung Transplant 2005;24:S63–S64.
128. Fan XH, Ang A, BarZiv SMP, et al. Donor-specific B-cell tolerance after ABO-incompatible infant heart transplantation. Nature Med 2004;10:1227–1233.
129. Cook DJ, Graver B, Terasaki PI. ABO incompatibility in cadaver donor kidney allografts. Transplant Proc 1987;19:4549–4552.
130. Rydberg L. ABO-incompatibility in solid organ transplantation. Transfus Med 2001;11:325–342.
131. Starzl T, Marchioro T, Holmes J, et al. Renal homografts in patients with major donor–recipient blood group incompatibilities. Surgery 1964;55:195–200.
132. Murray J, Merill J, Damin G, et al. Study on transplantation immunity after total body iradiation: clinical and experimental investigation. Surgery 1960;48:272–284.
133. Hume D, Merill J, Miler B, et al. Experiences with renal allotransplantation in the human: report of nine cases. J Clin Invest 1955;34: 372–382.
134. Rydberg L, Breimer ME, Samuelsson BE, et al. Blood group ABO-incompatible (A_2 to O) kidney transplantation in human subjects: a clinical, serologic, and biochemical approach. Transplant Proc 1987;19:4528–4537.
135. Welsh KI, van Dam M, Koffman CG, et al. Transplantation of blood group A2 kidneys into O or B recipients: the effect of pretransplant anti-A titers on graft survival. Transplant Proc 1987;19:4565–4567.
136. Alkhunaizi AM, de Mattos AM, Barry JM, et al. Renal transplantation across the ABO barrier using A2 kidneys. Transplantation 1999; 67:1319–1324.
137. Nelson PW, Landreneau MD, Luger AM, et al. Ten-year experience in transplantation of A2 kidneys into B and O recipients. Transplantation 1998;65:256–260.
138. Nelson PW, Shield CF 3rd, Muruve NA, et al. Increased access to transplantation for blood group B cadaveric waiting list candidates by using A2 kidneys: time for a new national system? Am J Transplant 2002;2:94–99.
139. Norman DJ, Prather JC, Alkhunaizi AM, et al. Use of A_2 kidneys for B and O kidney transplant recipients: report of a series of patients transplanted at a single center spanning a decade. Transplant Proc 2001;33:3327–3330.
140. Alexandre GP, Squifflet JP, De Bruyere M, et al. Present experiences in a series of 26 ABO-incompatible living donor renal allografts. Transplant Proc 1987;19:4538–4542.

141. Squifflet J-P, De Meyer M, Malaise J, et al. Lessons learned from ABO-incompatible living donor kidney transplantation: 20 years later. Exper Clin Transplant 2004;2:208–213.
142. Bach FH, Ferran C, Hechenleitner P, et al. Accommodation of vascularized xenografts: expression of "protective genes" by donor endothelial cells in a host Th2 cytokine environment. Nat Med 1997;3:196–204.
143. Reding R, Squifflet JP, Latinne D, et al. Early postoperative monitoring of natural anti-A and anti-B isoantibodies in ABO-incompatible living donor renal allografts. Transplant Proc 1987;19:1989–1990.
144. Tanabe K, Tokumoto T, Ishida H, et al. ABO-incompatible renal transplantation at Tokyo Women's Medical University. In Checka JM, Terasaki P (eds). Clinical Transplants 2003. Los Angeles, UCLA Immunogenetics Center, 2004, pp 175–181.
145. Ishida H, Koyama I, Sawada T, et al. Anti-AB titer changes in patients with ABO incompatibility after living related kidney transplantations: survey of 101 cases to determine whether splenectomies are necessary for successful transplantation. Transplantation 2000;70:681–685.
146. Shimmura H, Tanabe K, Ishikawa N, et al. Role of anti-A/B antibody titers in results of ABO-incompatible kidney transplantation. Transplantation 2000;70:1331–1335.
147. Warren DS, Simpkins CE, Cooper M, et al. Modulating alloimmune responses with plasmapheresis and IVIG. Current Drug Target 2005;5:215–222.
148. Tanabe K, Tokumoto T, Ishida H, et al. Excellent outcome of ABO-incompatible living kidney transplantation under pretransplantation immunosuppression with tacrolimus, mycophenolate mofetil, and steroid. Transplant Proc 2004;36:2175–2177.
149. Mannami M, Mitsuhata N. Improved outcomes after ABO-incompatible living-donor kidney transplantation after 4 weeks of treatment with mycophenolate mofetil. Transplantation 2005;79:1756–1758.
150. Sonnenday CJ, Warren DS, Cooper M, et al. Plasmapheresis, CMV hyperimmune globulin, and anti-CD20 allow ABO-incompatible renal transplantation without splenectomy. Am J Transplant 2004;4: 1315–1322.
151. Tyden G, Kumlien G, Fehrman I. Successful ABO-incompatible kidney transplantations without splenectomy using antigen-specific immunoadsorption and rituximab. Transplantation 2003;76:730–731.
152. Cummins D, Contreras M, Amin S, et al. Red cell alloantibody development associated with heart and lung transplantation. Transplantation 1995:59:1432–1435.
153. Lenhard V, Hansen B, Roelcke D, et al. Influence of Lewis and other blood group systems in kidney transplantation. Proc Eur Dialysis Transplant Assoc 1983;19:432–437.
154. White AG, Kumar MS, Abouna GM. HLA, MLR, P and Lewis antigens and living donor renal transplantation in a single centre in the Middle East. Tissue Antigens 1986;27:279–284.
155. Etheredge EE, Bettonville P, Sicard GA, et al. Anti-erythrocyte antibodies, leukocytotoxins and human renal allograft survival. Tissue Antigens 1982;19:205–212.
156. Bryan CF, Mitchell SI, Lin HM, et al. Influence of the RhD blood group system on graft survival in renal transplantation. Transplantation 1998;65:588–592.
157. Opelz G, Sengar DP, Mickey MR, et al. Effect of blood transfusions on subsequent kidney transplants. Transplant Proc 1973;5:253–259.
158. Egidi MF, Scott DH, Corry RJ. The effect of transfusions on renal allograft survival in the cyclosporine era: a single center report. Clinical Transplant 1993;7:240–244.
159. Reinsmoen NL, Matas AJ, Donaldson L, et al. Impact of transfusions and acute rejection on posttransplantation donor antigen-specific responses in two study populations. Cooperative Clinical Trial in Transplantation Research Group. Transplantation 1999;67:697–702.
160. Higgins RM, Raymond NT, Krishnan NS, et al. Acute rejection after renal transplantation is reduced by approximately 50% by prior therapeutic blood transfusions, even in tacrolimus-treated patients. Transplantation 2004;77:469–471.
161. Chavers BM, Sullivan EK, Tejani A, et al. Pretransplant blood transfusion and renal allograft outcome: a report of the North American Pediatric Renal Transplant Cooperative Study. Pediatr Transplant 1997;1:22–28.
162. Galvao MM, Peixinho ZF, Mendes NF, et al. Stored blood—an effective immunosuppressive method for transplantation of kidneys from unrelated donors. An 11-year follow-up. Braz J Medical Biol R 1997;30:727–734.
163. Ramsey G. Red cell antibodies arising from solid organ transplants. Transfusion 1991;31:76–86.
164. Sternberg AJ, Lee G, Croxton T, et al. Severe haemolysis after an ABO unmatched kidney transplant—a nonsecretor transplanted from a donor with high anti-A titre. Transfusion Med 2000;10:87–89.
165. Ishida H, Tanabe K, Tokumoto T, et al. The evaluation of graft irradiation as a method of preventing hemolysis after ABO-mismatched renal transplantation. Transplant Int 2002;15:421–424.
166. Hareuveni M, Merchav H, Austerlitz N, et al. Donor anti-Jk^a causing hemolysis in a liver transplant recipient. Transfusion 2002;42:363–367.
167. Fung MK, Sheikh H, Eghtesad B, et al. Severe hemolysis resulting from D incompatibility in a case of ABO-identical liver transplant. Transfusion 2004;44:1635–1639.
168. Larrea L, delaRubia J, Arriaga F, et al. Severe hemolytic anemia due to anti-E after renal transplantation. Transplantation 1997;64:550–551.
169. Loh E, Bergin JD, Couper GS, et al. Role of panel-reactive antibody cross-reactivity in predicting survival after orthotopic heart transplantation. J Heart Lung Transplant 1994;13:194–201.
170. Singh G, Thompson M, Griffith B, et al. Histocompatibility in cardiac transplantation with particular reference to immunopathology of positive serologic crossmatch. Clin Immunol Immunopathol 1983; 28:56–66.
171. Pisani BA, Mullen GM, Malinowska K, et al. Plasmapheresis with intravenous immunoglobulin G is effective in patients with elevated panel reactive antibody prior to cardiac transplantation. J Heart Lung Transplant 1999;18:701–706.
172. Robinson JA, Radvany RM, Mullen MG, et al. Plasmapheresis followed by intravenous immunoglobulin in presensitized patients awaiting thoracic organ transplantation. Therap Apheresis 1997;1:147–151.
173. McOmber D, Ibrahim J, Lublin DM, et al. Non-ischemic left ventricular dysfunction after pediatric cardiac transplantation: treatment with plasmapheresis and OKT3. J Heart Lung Transplant 2004;23:552–557.
174. Grauhan O, Knosalla C, Ewert R, et al. Plasmapheresis and cyclophosphamide in the treatment of humoral rejection after heart transplantation. J Heart Lung Transplant 2001;20:316–321.
175. Berglin E, Kjellstrām C, Mantovani V, et al. Plasmapheresis as a rescue therapy to resolve cardiac rejection with vasculitis and severe heart failure. A report of five cases. Transplant Int 1995;8:382–387.
176. Malafa M, Mancini MC, Myles JL, et al. Successful treatment of acute humoral rejection in a heart transplant patient. J Heart Lung Transplant 1992;11:486–491.
177. Partanen J, Nieminen MS, Krogerus L, et al. Heart transplant rejection treated with plasmapheresis. J Heart Lung Transplant 1992;11:301–305.
178. Takemoto SK, Zeevi A, Feng S, et al. National conference to assess antibody-mediated rejection in solid organ transplantation. Am J Transplant 2004;4:1033–1041.
179. Jordan SC, Vo AA, Tyan D, et al. Current approaches to treatment of antibody-mediated rejection. Pediatr Transplant 2005;9:408–415.
180. Thielke J, DeChristopher PJ, Sankary H, et al. Highly successful living donor kidney transplantation after conversion to negative of a previously positive flow-cytometry cross-match by pretransplant plasmapheresis. Transplant Proc 2005;37:643–644.
181. Sonnenday CJ, Ratner LE, Zachary AA, et al. Preemptive therapy with plasmapheresis/intravenous immunoglobulin allows successful live donor renal transplantation in patients with a positive cross-match. Transplant Proc 2002;34:1614–1616.
182. Alarabi A, Backman U, Wikstrom B, et al. Plasmapheresis in HLA-immunosensitized patients prior to kidney transplantation. Int J Artificial Organs 1997;20:51–56.
183. White NB, Greenstein SM, Cantafio AW, et al. Successful rescue therapy with plasmapheresis and intravenous immunoglobulin for acute humoral renal transplant rejection. Transplantation 2004;78:772–774.
184. Montgomery RA, Zachary AA, Racusen LC, et al. Plasmapheresis and intravenous immune globulin provides effective rescue therapy for refractory humoral rejection and allows kidneys to be successfully transplanted into cross-match-positive recipients. Transplantation 2000;70:887–895.
185. Mandal AK, King KE, Humphreys SL, et al. Plasmapheresis: an effective therapy for primary allograft nonfunction after liver transplantation. Transplantation 2000;70:216–220.
186. Skerrett D, Mor E, Curtiss S, et al. Plasmapheresis in primary dysfunction of hepatic transplants. J Clin Apher 1996;11:10–13.
187. Wingard JR, Chen DYH, Burns WH, et al. Cytomegalovirus infection after autologous bone marrow transplantation with comparison to infection after allogeneic bone marrow transplantation. Blood 1988;71:1432.
188. American Association of Blood Banks. Leukocyte reduction for the prevention of transfusion-transmitted cytomegalovirus (TT-CMV). AABB Bulletin 1997;2:1.
189. Roback JD. CMV and blood transfusions. Rev Med Virol 2002;12: 211–219.
190. Bowden RA, Slichter SJ, Sayers M, et al. A comparison of filtered leukocyte-reduced and cytomegalovirus (CMV)-seronegative blood

products for the prevention of transfusion-associated CMV infection after marrow transplant. Blood 1995;86:3598.

191. Bowden RA, Slichter SJ, Sayers MH, et al. Use of leukocyte-depleted platelets and cytomegalovirus-seronegative red blood cells for prevention of primary cytomegalovirus infection after marrow transplant. Blood 1991;78:246–250.

192. De Witte T, Schattenberg A, Van Djik BA, et al. Prevention of primary cytomegalovirus infection after allogeneic bone marrow transplantation by using leukocyte-poor blood products from cytomegalovirus-unscreened blood bank donors. Transplantation 1990;50:964.

193. Gilbert GL, Hayes K, Hudson IL, et al. Prevention of transfusion-aquired cytomegalovirus infection in infants by blood filtration to remove leukocytes. Lancet 1989;1:1228.

194. Miller WJ, McCullough J, Balfour HH Jr, et al. Prevention of cytomegalovirus infection following bone marrow transplantation: a randomized trial of blood product screening. Bone Marrow Transplant 1991;7:227–234.

195. Lang DJ, Ebert PA, Rodgers BM, et al. Reduction of postperfusion cytomegalovirus infections following the use of leukocyte depleted blood. Transfusion 1977;17:391.

196. Nichols WG, Price TH, Gooley T, et al. Transfusion-transmitted cytomegalovirus infection after receipt of leukoreduced blood products. Blood 2003;101:4195–4200.

197. Vamvakas EC. Is white blood cell reduction equivalent to antibody screening in preventing transmission of cytomegalovirus by transfusion? A review of the literature and meta-analysis. Transfus Med Rev 2005;19:181–199.

198. Zaia JA. Prevention and management of CMV-related problems after hematopoietic stem cell transplantation. Bone Marrow Transplant 2002;29:633–638.

199. Lowenthal RN, Challis DR, Griffiths AE, et al. Transfusion-associated graft-versus-host disease: report of an occurence following the administration of irradiated blood. Transfusion 1993;33:524.

200. Pelszynski MM, Moroff G, Luban N, et al. Effect of gamma irradiation of red blood cell units on T-cell inactivation as assessed by limiting dilution analysis: Implications for preventing transfusion-associated graft-versus-host disease. Blood 1994;83:1683.

201. U.S. Food and Drug Administration. FDA memorandum to registered blood establishments: recommendations reguarding license amendments and proceedures for gamma irradiation of blood products. Washington, D.C., July 22, 1993.

202. Menitove JE (ed). Standards for Blood Banks and Transfusion Services, 21st ed. Bethesda, Md., American Association of Blood Banks, 2002.

Chapter 40

Transfusion of the Platelet-Refractory Patient

Thomas S. Kickler

Platelet transfusion therapy has improved over the past 2 decades with new methods for collection, storage, and processing of platelets. With the development of aggressive forms of chemotherapy, organ transplantation, and new strategies to treat aplastic anemia and related bone marrow failure disorders, the clinician relies heavily on the availability of platelet transfusions. Consequently, practitioners of platelet transfusion therapy must know how to use platelet transfusions effectively so that resources are not wasted. This chapter describes the use of platelet transfusions in a variety of medical conditions, especially in patients requiring multiple platelet transfusions. Because refractoriness to platelet transfusions is a serious problem, methods to circumvent or prevent it are also described.

INDICATIONS FOR PLATELET TRANSFUSIONS

In patients with thrombocytopenia, the risk of hemorrhage increases progressively once the platelet count drops below 100,000/μL.[1–3] Many studies have attempted to define the bleeding time or platelet count necessary to achieve hemostasis in surgical patients, with conflicting results.[3–7] Some generalities do exist, however. With normally functioning platelets, most major surgery can be performed safely if the count is maintained in the range of 50,000 to 75,000/mL. A higher range may be necessary for longer and more technically difficult procedures involving extensive incisions or exposure of large surface areas. Performance of surgery on the central nervous system should be done only with platelet counts greater than 100,000/μL.[3] Table 40–1 shows general guidelines for the transfusion of platelets in different clinical situations.

In amegakaryocytic thrombocytopenia, platelet transfusions are given prophylactically or therapeutically and for the performance of invasive procedures. There is considerable interest in trying to define the lowest safe platelet concentration, so that fewer donor exposures occur and limited blood resources are conserved. Physicians have been generally aware that hemorrhage is more common during the most severe stages of thrombocytopenia. A study of 92 consecutive patients treated for acute leukemia between 1956 and 1959 at the National Cancer Institute led to the current prophylactic guidelines. Platelet counts lower than 100,000/μL were associated with an increased risk of bleeding. Patients with platelet counts of 5,000/μL or less manifested gross hemorrhage on approximately one third of days at risk. A platelet count of 20,000/μL or less was associated with moderate bleeding manifestations such as epistaxis and petechiae. Based on these studies, a prophylactic platelet transfusion strategy, using a platelet count of 20,000/μL as the transfusion trigger, has been commonly employed.[8]

More recently, in a randomized study of prophylactic platelet transfusion, Rebulla and coworkers[5] showed that giving transfusions only when the platelet count dips below 10,000/μL can decrease platelet use with only a small adverse effect on bleeding and no effect on mortality. It therefore appears that, with amegakaryocytic thrombocytopenia, prophylactic transfusions should be given if the count falls below 5000/μL. At values between 5000 and 10,000/μL, transfusion may be withheld if the patient is stable and if no other conditions make spontaneous bleeding likely.[5] Such conditions include blast crisis, rapidly falling platelet count, anticoagulation with heparin for disseminated intravascular coagulation (DIC), drugs that affect platelet function, uremia, and recent invasive procedures, including spinal taps or placement of central venous catheters.[9]

PLATELET TRANSFUSION REFRACTORINESS

Failure to achieve an expected increment with a platelet transfusion is called *platelet transfusion refractoriness*. Refractoriness may be caused by an immune or a nonimmune condition. Clinically, one can assess the response to a platelet transfusion by measuring the increment in platelet count 1 to 18 hours after the transfusion. The post-transfusion platelet response should be calculated on the basis of the patient's body surface area in square meters and corrected for the number of platelets transfused. The corrected platelet count increment (CCI) is calculated by the following formula:

$$\mathrm{CCI} = \frac{\begin{bmatrix}\text{body}\\ \text{surface}\\ \text{area (m}^2\text{)}\end{bmatrix} \times \begin{bmatrix}\text{platelet}\\ \text{count}\\ \text{increment}\end{bmatrix} \times 10^{11}}{\text{number of platelets transfused}}$$

In general, a successful CCI should be greater than 7500 within 10 to 60 minutes after a transfusion and greater than 4500 if measured 18 to 24 hours after transfusion. It has been suggested that the CCI determined 1 hour after platelet transfusion is a useful indirect measure to document alloimmunization.[2] However, human leukocyte antigen (HLA) antibodies are only one of many factors that influence the CCI at 1 hour. Furthermore, even if platelet antibodies are present, excellent 1-hour CCIs may be achieved.[10] This latter phenomenon may be seen after platelets with weak expression of HLA-B locus antigens are given.[2,3,9]

Table 40–1 Platelet Transfusion Guidelines

Platelet products: The benefits of pooled platelets or single-donor platelets are similar; the two products can be used interchangeably. Single-donor platelets from selected donors are used when histocompatible platelet transfusion (i.e., HLA-A and HLA-B antigen matched) are needed.

Prophylactic Platelet Transfusion Thresholds:

Acute leukemia: For adult patients a threshold of 10,000/μL is recommended. Transfusion at higher levels may be necessary in the newborn or in patients with hemorrhage, high fever, hyperleukocytosis, rapid fall in platelet count, or coagulation abnormalities.

Hematopoietic stem cell transplantation: Same as for acute leukemia, with similar exceptions.

Chronic stable severe thrombocytopenia: Many patients can be observed without prophylactic transfusion, reserving transfusion for episodes of hemorrhage or during times of active treatment.

Solid tumors: Evidence supports the benefit of prophylactic transfusion at a threshold of 10,000/μL or less. A threshold of 20,000/μL should be considered for patients receiving aggressive therapy for bladder cancer, as well as for those with demonstrated necrotic tumors.

Surgical or invasive procedures: A platelet count of 40 to 50,000/μL is sufficient to perform major invasive procedures safely, in the absence of associated coagulation abnormalities. Certain procedures, such as bone marrow aspiration/biopsy, can be performed safely with counts <20,000/μL; lumbar puncture in children is safe at platelet counts >10,000/μL.

Immunologic Basis of Platelet Transfusion Refractoriness

Soon after the introduction of prophylactic platelet transfusions, it became apparent that serial transfusion results in decreasing effectiveness in many patients.[10] Through the work of Yankee and others,[11] it is now recognized that transfusion failures result from the induction of alloantibodies to HLA and other antigens. Yankee and coworkers[11] were able to show that most cases of platelet refractoriness could be reversed by the use of platelet transfusions phenotypically matched at the HLA-A and HLA-B loci. It was also recognized that the development of HLA antibodies, as measured by lymphocytotoxic activity, correlated with the development of the immune refractory state.[12] It is now well recognized that the alloimmune response to HLA-A and HLA-B locus antigens is the major cause of post-transfusion alloimmune transfusion failure.

Antibodies to the human platelet-specific antigens (HPAs) only rarely cause platelet transfusion refractoriness. In a large series of patients who received platelet transfusions, only 2% had detectable antibodies to HPAs. Most of these antibodies were found in patients who were also alloimmunized to HLA class I antigens. If HLA-identical platelet transfusions fail, antibodies to the HPAs should be considered. Antibody specificity to the HPAs can be identified by enzyme-linked antiglobulin assay and isolated platelet glycoproteins of different phenotypes.[13,14] In general, few donor centers have a donor population typed for the HPAs, except for those in the HPA-1 system. The recent introduction of DNA-based typing for HPAs permits accurate typing of donors and even thrombocytopenic patients, because lymphocyte-derived DNA is used.[15]

Detection of Antibodies in Platelet Transfusion Refractoriness

Specific identification of alloimmunization can be done by measurement of HLA antibodies using lymphocytotoxicity testing.[16] Serial lymphocytotoxic antibody measurements are helpful in the management of alloimmunization. Some patients have decreases or a loss of lymphocytotoxic antibody, either permanently or transiently, and can be successfully transfused with platelet concentrates.[17] It should be noted that some patients have antibodies to HLA class I and yet do not have platelet transfusion failures. Commercially available solid-phase enzyme-linked immunoassays that detect the presence of immunoglobulin G anti-HLA antibodies with the use of purified HLA antigens prepared from platelet concentrates are available.[18]

HLA Alloantigens and Antibodies

Understanding the HLA system is important so that compatible platelet transfusions may be selected for alloimmunized patients.[19] Only HLA-A and HLA-B antigens have been shown to be important in causing immune-mediated platelet transfusion refractoriness. Two broad types of HLA antibodies are made in response to platelet transfusions. The first type recognizes epitopes unique to a particular HLA allele, referred to as *antibodies to private specificities.* Antibodies to HLA-A2 and HLA-B12 fall into this group. The second type of HLA antibody recognizes more than one gene product. These antibodies recognize structural similarities between gene products (cross-reactive epitopes) or identical epitopes present on gene products of different alleles and are referred to as *antibodies to public epitopes.* Traditionally, HLA serology has placed the greatest emphasis on classification of the private antigens. Recently, more importance has been placed on the clinical importance of public HLA specificities. The best known examples of public specificities are HLA-Bw4 and HLA-Bw6. These antigens are encoded by a diallelic system and are associated with two different groups of HLA-B class I antigens. Other public antigens carried by HLA-B class I antigens have been divided into four cross-reactive groups: HLA-B5, HLA-B7, HLA-B8, and HLA-B12. The observation that the specificity of HLA antibodies in multiply transfused individuals is usually against public epitopes suggests that matching for these public antigens is important. With improved serologic approaches to the identification of specificities to class I HLA antigens, selection of platelets for transfusion may be simplified by relying on public specificities.

CLINICAL FEATURES OF ALLOIMMUNE REFRACTORINESS

In a series reported by Dutcher and colleagues,[20] 42% of 114 patients developed lymphocytotoxic antibody within the first 8 weeks after transfusion. Approximately one fourth of these patients developed antibody within 1 week, suggesting the presence of an anamnestic response, and 75% of responders appeared to have a de novo response. Of those patients who manifested lymphocytotoxic antibody, 17 ultimately lost antibody despite further transfusions. Of those initial patients who did not respond by developing lymphocytotoxic antibody in the first 8 weeks, 92% remained unresponsive despite continued transfusion therapy. Therefore, the development of an alloimmune response after transfusion seems to be an early event in therapy. Responsiveness or nonresponsiveness to HLA antigens develops during the first weeks of therapy, and this pattern is apparently maintained throughout subsequent therapy.[20]

Antiplatelet Glycoprotein Antibodies

In addition to the phenotypic differences that arise because of polymorphisms in platelet glycoproteins, patients may form antibodies to the entire platelet glycoprotein molecule. For example, individuals who have the Bernard-Soulier syndrome may become immunized to glycoprotein Ib, and those with Glanzmann thrombasthenia may become immunized to glycoprotein IIb/IIIa. Patients who lack these important membrane glycoproteins and require platelet transfusions may become immunized to normal platelets. This results in transfusion refractoriness and significantly complicates the transfusion management of qualitative platelet disorders.[21]

ABO Blood Group Antigens

Platelets have ABO antigens on their surface; some are intrinsically present, and some are adsorbed from the plasma. Although platelets are usually regarded as having only weak expression of A and B antigens, some donors have strong A or B antigen expression that may result in refractoriness to isolated units. The importance of platelet ABO antigens in platelet recovery was clearly demonstrated in 1965 by Aster.[22] After group A platelets were transfused to group O volunteers, the average recovery was 19%, whereas after transfusion with ABO-compatible platelets it was 63%, similar to recovery after autologous platelets. In general, however, less striking differences are seen in practice: increments are only about 20% lower for transfusion with ABO-incompatible compared with ABO-compatible units.[22–25]

Nonimmune Refractoriness

Platelet transfusions may not result in an increment if the stored platelets are defective. This result should be relatively uncommon, given the close scrutiny devoted to quality control of blood products. However, one should remember to consider freshness of a given platelet transfusion as the cause of a single instance of platelet transfusion failure.[2]

Coagulopathy

Disseminated intravascular coagulation has classically been associated with platelet refractoriness. This syndrome is associated with bacterial sepsis, which is common in transfused patients, and with acute progranulocytic leukemia. The quantitative role of DIC in the platelet refractory state has not been well characterized.[2,3]

Splenic Sequestration

Splenomegaly has been shown to be a major cause of platelet transfusion failure. Normally some 30% of a patient's platelet mass is contained within the spleen. With increases in splenic size, up to 90% of circulating platelets can be sequestered in this organ. Characteristically, splenic sequestration is associated with a reduced 1-hour platelet recovery but normal survival.[2,3]

Fever and Infection

Studies by several groups have implicated both fever and infection as a cause for decreased platelet survival. One study noted that platelet transfusion requirements were increased by 50% in febrile patients. This increase may be greater in patients with major infections, particularly DIC.[26,27]

Other Factors

Platelet refractoriness has been reported with a number of medications. Amphotericin in particular has been implicated in decreasing platelet recovery and survival. Similarly, vancomycin has been reported to be a major cause of platelet refractoriness, as have antithymocyte globulin, granulocyte-macrophage colony-stimulating factor, granulocyte colony-stimulating factor, and other interferons. In view of the large number of drugs cancer patients characteristically receive, it would not be surprising if a number of additional agents were implicated in accelerated platelet destruction.[2,26,27]

MANAGEMENT OF THE ALLOIMMUNIZED PATIENT

Because alloimmunization to HLA antigens accounts for the majority of cases of alloimmune platelet transfusion refractoriness, platelets can be selected on the basis of HLA matching.[2,3] Depending on the HLA type of an individual, there may be little difficulty in locating platelets that are identical. In some patients with unusual HLA types, such as in diverse ethnic groups, HLA matching may be more difficult.

Kickler and coworkers[28] studied the effectiveness of HLA matching as the sole method of platelet selection for alloimmunized patients. Of 50 HLA-identical platelet transfusions, 20% were unsuccessful. Of transfusions selected on the basis of crossreactivities without regard to matching of public specificities, 41% (23 of 56) were failures. One third of those transfusions in which one or two antigen-mismatched platelets were used were failures. These observations indicated that matching of platelets on the basis of HLA private antigens is frequently unreliable as a sole criterion. On the other hand, even if patients are alloimmunized, they may receive mismatched platelets and have successful transfusions.[28]

For these reasons, refining the selection process of platelets for alloimmunized patients has been the subject of much investigation. Table 40–2 outlines a practical approach to selection of platelets for the alloimmunized patient that takes into account the importance of HLA matching and platelet compatibility testing. Numerous investigators have evaluated the usefulness of crossmatching a recipient's platelets with those of potential donors. This approach can be readily followed because pheresis platelets are stored for 5 days. By analyzing aliquots of platelets taken from integrally attached tubing segments, compatible platelets can be found in the inventory of stored platelets. Compatible donors may be found even if a patient is broadly alloimmunized.[29,30]

Because providing crossmatched platelets may be difficult or impractical given frequent transfusions and the need to crossmatch against a large number of potential donors, there is much interest in developing methods of pretransfusion

Table 40–2 **Non–Antibody-Specific Approach to Selection of Platelets for Alloimmunized Patients**

Determine human leukocyte antigen (HLA) phenotype and ABO type of the recipient.
Screen patient's serum for lymphocytotoxic antibody or antibodies to human platelet antigens if there is a history of failing HLA-identical platelets.
Select from the donor pool those units with the most compatible HLA antigens and, if possible, ABO systems; alternatively, crossmatch available platelet units without regard to patient or donor HLA type.
Crossmatch the recipient's serum with selected potential donors and select the most compatible unit.

testing, similar to those used to select compatible red blood cells. These procedures are well known to transfusion services and involve phenotyping of donors and recipients and identification of the specificity of antibodies present in a patient's serum. Specifically for platelets, HLA phenotyping of donors and recipients, and identification of the HLA antibody specificities are required. Petz and coworkers[29] extensively evaluated this approach, and it appears to be highly reliable and successful in identifying donors who would ordinarily be excluded if only exact HLA matches were considered. These investigators coined the phrase *antibody specificity prediction* (ASP) method to describe these procedures.

Petz and coworkers[29] reported data on the utility of ASP for 1621 platelet transfusions in 114 persons with platelet transfusion refractoriness. They compared the effectiveness of platelets selected by the ASP method with that of platelets selected on the basis of HLA matching or crossmatching or, if selected components were not available, on a random basis. They concluded that the ASP method was as effective as HLA matching or crossmatching, and that all three methods were superior to the random selection of platelets. Further, in a file of HLA-matched donors, many more potential donors were identifiable by the ASP method than by HLA matching, which makes the acquisition of compatible platelets for alloimmunized refractory patients much more feasible. This approach appears to be logistically simple on a regional basis when the testing is offered by blood centers, and it promises to harmonize the selection of platelets with the selection process used for red blood cell transfusions.

Management of Platelet Transfusion Refractoriness and Bleeding

A variety of approaches have been attempted when no compatible platelets can be found for a patient who is alloimmunized and continues to bleed or may be undergoing invasive procedures.[2,31] Therapeutic modalities have included splenectomy, corticosteroids, plasmapheresis, administration of intravenous immunoglobulin (IVIG), and repeated platelet transfusions. Except for IVIG, there is little evidence that any of these treatments work.

Kickler and coworkers[32] performed a randomized, placebo-controlled clinical trial investigating the use of IVIG in alloimmunized thrombocytopenic patients. In this trial, IVIG was administered at a dose of 400 mg/kg for 5 days. An incompatible platelet transfusion from the same donor was used before and after the administration of IVIG or placebo. Although platelet recovery in 1 to 6 hours was satisfactory in five of seven patients after IVIG treatment, 24-hour survival was not improved in most of them. It could not be excluded that this poor 24-hour survival result was due to nonimmune causes of shortened platelet survival. None of the placebo group (five patients) achieved a satisfactory 1-hour CCI. By *t*-test, the post-treatment mean 1-hour CCI values were significantly greater in those who received IVIG than in the control group.[32]

If all conventional methods fail to increase the platelet count to hemostatic levels, the only remaining alternative that has been tried is continuous transfusion of platelets (massive transfusion). It has been argued that, although the platelet count is not increased, transfused platelets still exert some effect, permitting platelet plug formation or maintenance of endothelial integrity. These arguments are based on clinical observations. In one well-established animal model of alloimmune thrombocytopenia, if the platelet count did not increase above 60,000/μL, capillary leakage or bleeding still persisted.[2,3]

Other Approaches

In uncontrolled studies and in small controlled studies, the antifibrinolytic agents aminocaproic acid and tranexamic acid have been used.[31] The results have been mixed in terms of reduction of microvascular hemorrhage and reduction of platelet transfusion requirements. The differing results probably are related to the small number of patients studied. Immunosuppressive agents, splenectomy, and plasma exchange have not been proven effective.[2,3]

PREVENTION OF ALLOIMMUNIZATION

Reduction of Donor Exposures

Several studies have shown a direct relationship between the number of platelet transfusions and alloimmunization.[33,34] Others have not documented a dose–response relationship.[2] The reasons for these contradictory conclusions are not clear. In part, clinical differences in the study populations, such as the multiparous state of transfusion recipients, may be the main explanation. Another problem in the literature has been the definition of alloimmunization, including the laboratory end point and the method used to measure HLA antibodies. For a primary immune response, 2 to 3 weeks may be required. If sera are not collected over a sufficient interval, an antibody response may not be measured. Alternatively, some patients may lose antibody by the time of testing, contributing to negative responses. The published data are also consistent with the hypothesis that the alloimmune response has a threshold effect. Over a low range of exposure, there may be a dose–response effect. With larger numbers of exposures, further alloimmunization may not develop if tolerance has been established.

Preventive Measures

Results of early animal studies showed that depletion of contaminating leukocytes from donor blood components was effective in preventing alloantibody response to the major histocompatibility complex (MHC).[33] Other approaches, such as inactivation of donor leukocytes by ultraviolet irradiation, provided further evidence of the important role of donor leukocytes in eliciting immune responses to class I MHC antigens. With the development of highly efficient methods to remove leukocytes from blood products, a number of clinical trials were instituted. In general, if fewer than 1 $\times 10^6$ contaminating leukocytes remained, alloimmunization was reduced by 30% to 50%. Many of these studies in thrombocytopenic patients also showed some success in the use of leukocyte-poor blood components to prevent HLA alloimmunization or platelet transfusion refractoriness. However, the results obtained from a variety of clinical trials have been inconclusive and not reproducible, perhaps because of variability in blood product preparation and heterogeneity in the patient populations studied.

Because of the confusing data, a large multicenter clinical trial was done in the United States. This Trial to Reduce Alloimmunization to Platelets (TRAP) tested the efficacy of transfusion with platelets modified by leukocyte reduction or ultraviolet irradiation or with leukocyte-depleted, single-donor platelets.[34] The results obtained with these modified platelet products were compared with transfusion of platelet concentrates. All patients received leukocyte-depleted red blood cells. A total of 534 patients with acute myeloid leukemia were studied during an 8-week period for the development of platelet alloantibodies. Of patients in the control group, 45% developed HLA antibodies compared with 22% of those in the ultraviolet-irradiated group, 18% in the filtered platelet concentrate group, and 17% in the filtered apheresis group. All three types of treated platelets were associated with a significant reduction in the development of HLA antibodies and alloimmune platelet refractoriness compared with the control group. These maneuvers were effective even though 26% of the patients had received previous transfusions of nontreated blood products. Importantly, none of the treatment maneuvers reduced the rate of alloimmunization to HPAs (6% to 10%). Therefore, this large study documented the usefulness of either leukocyte removal or inactivation by ultraviolet irradiation in the chronically transfused platelet recipient. The use of platelet concentrates derived from whole blood did not increase the risk of alloimmunization compared with single-donor platelets. Several other studies have confirmed these findings.[35]

REFERENCES

1. Kickler TS. The platelet transfusion refractory state: Transfusion practices and clinical management. In Kurtz SR, Brubaker DB (eds). Clinical Decisions in Platelet Therapy. Bethesda, Md., American Association of Blood Banks, 1992, pp 87–104.
2. Benson K: Criteria for diagnosing refractoriness to platelet transfusions. In Kickler TS, Herman JH (eds). Current Issues in Platelet Transfusion Therapy and Platelet Alloimmunity. Bethesda, Md., American Association of Blood Banks, 1999, pp 33–63.
3. Freidburg RC, Gaupp B: Platelet indications, considerations, and specific clinical settings. In Kickler TS, Herman JH (eds). Current Issues in Platelet Transfusion Therapy and Platelet Alloimmunity. Bethesda, Md., American Association of Blood Banks, 1999, p 1.
4. Hersh EM, Mbodey GP, Nies BA, et al. Causes of death in acute leukemia: a 10-year study of 414 patients. JAMA 1965;193:99–103.
5. Rebulla P, Finazzi G, Marangoni F, et al. A multicenter randomized study of the threshold for prophylactic platelet transfusions in adults with acute leukemia. NEJM 1997;337:1870–1875.
6. Higby DJ. The prophylactic treatment of thrombocytopenic leukemic patients. Transfusion 1974;14:440–446.
7. Roy AJ, Jaffe N, Djerassi I. Prophylactic platelet transfusions. Transfusion 1973;13:283–290.
8. Gaydos LA, Freirich EJ, Mantel N. The quantitative relation between platelet count and hemorrhage in acute leukemia. NEJM 1962;266:905–909.
9. National Institutes of Health. Consensus conference: platelet transfusion therapy. JAMA 1987;257:1777–1780.
10. Bishop JF, Matthews JP, Yuen K, et al. The definition of refractoriness to platelet transfusion. Transfus Med 1992;2:35–41.
11. Yankee RA, Grumet D, Rogentine GN. Platelet selection by HLA matching. NEJM 1973;288:760–767.
12. Hogge DE, Dutcher JP, Aisner J, Schiffer CA. Lymphocytotoxic antibody is a predictor of response to random donor platelet transfusion. Am J Hematol 1983;14:363–369.
13. Kickler TS, Kennedy SD, Braine HG. Alloimmunization to platelet specific antigens on glycoprotein IIB/IIIA and IB/IX in multitransfused thrombocytopenic patients. Transfusion 1990;30:622–625.
14. Kiefel V, Santoso S, Weisheit M, Mueller-Eckhardt C. Monoclonal antibody-specific immobilization of platelet antigens (MAIPA): a new tool for the identification of platelet-reactive antibodies. Blood 1987;70:1722–1726.
15. Kim HO, Jing Y, Kickler TS, et al. Immunogenetic studies on the genotypic differences in platelet antigens. Transfusion 1995;35:863–867.
16. Fuller TC, Cosimi AB, Russell PS. Use of an antiglobulin-ATG reagent for detection of low levels of alloantibody: improvement of allograft survival in presensitized recipients. Transplant Proc 1978;10:463–468.
17. Lee EJ, Schiffer CA. Serial measurement of lymphocytotoxic antibody and response to nonmatched platelet transfusions in alloimmunized patients. Blood 1987;70:1727–1729.
18. Kao KJ, Scornik JC, Small S. Enzyme linked immunoassay for anti-HLA antibodies: an alternative to panel studies by lymphocytotoxicity. Transplantation 1993;55:192–196.
19. Rodey GE. Class I antigens: HLA A, B, C and cross reactive groups. In Moulds J (ed). Scientific and Technical Aspects of the Major Histocompatibility Complex. Arlington, Va., American Association of Blood Banks, 1989, p 23.
20. Dutcher JP, Schiffer CA, Aisner J, Wiernik PH. Long-term followup of patients with leukemia receiving platelet transfusions: identification of a large group of patients who do not become alloimmunized. Blood 1981;58:1007–1011.
21. Shulman NR, Marder VJ, Hiller MC, Collier EM. Platelet and leucocyte isoantigens and their antibodies: Serologic, physiologic, and clinical studies. Prog Hematol 1964;4:222–304.
22. Aster RH. Effect of anticoagulant and ABO incompatibility on recovery of transfused human platelets. Blood 1965;26:732–743.
23. Dunstan RA, Simpson MB, Knowles RW, Rosse WF. The origin of ABH antigens on human platelets. Blood 1985;65:615.
24. Ogasawara K, Ueki J, Takenaka M, Furihata K. Study on the expression of ABH antigens on platelets. Blood 1993;82:993–999.
25. Heal JM, Masel D, Rowe JM, Blumberg N. Circulating immune complexes involving the ABO system after platelet transfusion. Br J Haematol 1993;85:566.
26. Bishop JF, McGrath K, Wolf MM, et al. Clinical factors influencing the efficacy of pooled platelet transfusions. Blood 1988;71:383–387.
27. Klingemann H-G, Self S, Banaji M, et al. Refractoriness to random donor platelet transfusions in patients with aplastic anemia: a multivariate analysis of data from 264 cases. Br J Haematol 1987;66:115–121.
28. Kickler TS, Braine HG, Ness PM. The predictive value of platelet crossmatching. Transfusion 1985;25:385–389.
29. Petz LD, Garratty G, Calhoun L, et al. Selecting donors of platelets for refractory patients on the basis of HLA antibody specificity. Transfusion 2000;40:1446–1456.
30. Rachel JM, Summers TC, Sinor LT, Plapp FV. Use of a solid phase red blood cell adherence method for pretransfusion platelet compatibility testing. Am J Clin Pathol 1989;90:63–68.
31. Sarkodee-Adoo CB, Heyman MR. Alternative management strategies in alloimmunized thrombocytopenic patients. In Kickler TS, Herman JH (eds). Current Issues in Platelet Transfusion Therapy and Platelet Alloimmunity. Bethesda, Md., American Association of Blood Banks, 1999, pp 135–160.
32. Kickler TS, Ness PM, Herman JH, et al. A randomized double-blinded study on the effectiveness of high dose gammaglobulin in ameliorating platelet transfusion refractoriness. Blood 1990;75:313–316.
33. Semple J, Freedman J. The basic immunology of platelet induced alloimmunization. In Kickler TS, Herman JH (eds). Current Issues in

Platelet Transfusion Therapy and Platelet Alloimmunity. Bethesda, Md., American Association of Blood Banks, 1999, pp 77–101.

34. The Trial to Reduce Alloimmunization to Platelets (TRAP) Study Group. Leukocyte reduction and ultraviolet B irradiation of platelets to prevent alloimmunization and refractoriness to platelet transfusions. NEJM 1997;337:1861–1869.

35. Kao KJ. A critical analysis of clinical trials to prevent platelet alloimmunization. In Kickler TS, Herman JH (eds). Current Issues in Platelet Transfusion Therapy and Platelet Alloimmunity. Bethesda, Md., American Association of Blood Banks, 1999, pp 103–134.

Chapter 41

Autoimmune Hemolytic Anemias

Leslie E. Silberstein • Melody J. Cunningham

SPECTRUM OF AUTOIMMUNE HEMOLYTIC SYNDROMES

Autoimmune hemolytic anemias refer to a spectrum of disorders in which autoantibodies against antigens on the erythrocyte membrane cause shortened survival of native as well as transfused red blood cells (RBCs). Three categories of antierythrocyte autoantibodies exhibit distinctive serologic properties and result in characteristic clinical disorders (Table 41–1). Immunoglobulin G (IgG) warm autoantibodies attach to erythrocytes at 37°C, IgM cold autoantibodies clump RBCs at cold temperatures, and IgG Donath-Landsteiner antibodies bind to RBC membranes in the cold and cause hemolysis at 37°C; in this chapter, the associated clinical entities are referred to as *warm autoimmune hemolytic anemia* (AIHA), *cold agglutinin disease*, and *paroxysmal cold hemoglobinuria* (PCH), respectively. All of these antibodies are capable of simply attaching to the RBC membrane without having any pathologic effect or inducing fulminant hemolysis.[1] The antibodies may be idiopathic or may develop secondary to another disease process or in response to exposure to a drug.

Historical Background

The first recognized form of hemolytic anemia was PCH, probably because its clinical manifestation, the passage of black urine after exposure to cold, is so striking. Reports of apparent cold-induced hematuria began to appear in medical literature in the mid-1800s. By 1884, the association of PCH with syphilis was noted. In 1904, Donath and Landsteiner determined that an autolysin fixed to the patient's RBCs in the cold and that a heat-labile serum factor lysed the erythrocytes at 37°C.

The first report of cold agglutinin disease appeared in 1918, but the fact that cold agglutinating serum antibodies were found in healthy individuals initially obscured the significance of cold autolysins. In 1937, these cold-reactive antibodies were discovered to occur in much higher, thus pathologic, levels in affected patients. Dameshek and Schwartz established the first experimental model of immune hemolytic anemia, inducing hemolysis by injection of heterologous antierythrocyte antibodies into guinea pigs. Yet the idea of an "autoimmune" form of hemolytic anemia was resisted for several reasons, punctuated by the difficulty in making the diagnosis.

The antiglobulin test, designed to detect nonagglutinating anti-erythrocyte antibodies, was introduced into clinical medicine by Coombs and associates[2] in 1945. Within 1 year, this test was used to diagnose autoimmune hemolytic anemia.[3] In 1954, autoimmune hemolytic anemia in dogs was reported,[4] and in 1958, the first easily bred animal model of the disease, the NZB mouse, was described.[5] This last discovery was a turning point in the development of a scientific basis for the study of autoimmunization.

WARM AUTOIMMUNE HEMOLYTIC ANEMIA

Epidemiology in Children and Adults

The incidence of AIHA is estimated to be approximately 1 in 100,000 adults and less than 0.2 in 100,000 children. The disorder is less common than immune thrombocytopenia.[6] In

Table 41–1 Characteristics of Autoimmune Hemolytic Anemia (AIHA)

Characteristic	Type of AIHA		
	Warm-Reactive	Cold Agglutinin Disease	Paroxysmal Cold Hemoglobinuria
Antibody isotype	IgG Rare IgA, IgM	IgM	IgG
Direct antiglobulin test result	IgG Rare C3	C3	C3
Antigen specificity	Multiple, primarily Rh	I/I, Pr	P
Hemolysis	Primarily extravascular	Primarily extravascular	Intravascular
Common disease associations	B-cell neoplasia, lymphoproliferative, collagen-vascular	Viral, neoplastic	Tertiary syphilis, viral

Ig, immunoglobulin.

teenagers and adults, AIHA is more common in women than in men. In children, boys are somewhat more affected than girls. AIHA occurs at all ages but more commonly in midlife. In pediatric cases, the mortality is less than 10% and primarily occurs in adolescents with a chronic refractory course.[7]

Approximately half of cases of AIHA are idiopathic. In children, AIHA in patients younger than age 2 and older than age 12 is more likely to have a chronic unremitting course.[8] Some cases are induced by drugs, and others occur concomitantly with another autoimmune disease or malignancy. A substantial proportion of cases develop in patients with systemic lupus erythematosus (SLE), B-cell lymphomas, or chronic lymphocytic leukemia (CLL). A number of other diseases have also been complicated by AIHA, but only as unusual exceptions.[9] Treatment of the underlying process can often resolve the AIHA. In other instances, presumably by affecting T cells more than B cells, drugs induce a disturbance in immunoregulatory T cells and trigger the onset of hemolytic anemia.[10,11]

As more diseases, malignant and nonmalignant, are treated with bone marrow transplantation (BMT) and peripheral blood stem cell transplantation (PBST), the numbers of cases of post-transplant autoimmune hemolysis are expected to increase. An overall 2.6% incidence was reported in a recent study in post-BMT patients. A 5% incidence was found in those patients surviving 6 months.[12] The timing of development of post-BMT AIHA appears to depend on the antibody mediating the hemolysis, possibly because IgM reconstitutes earlier than IgG. In this clinical setting, three distinct mechanisms can mediate the hemolysis. Investigations to determine the etiology of hemolysis will appropriately direct therapy, expected duration, and prevention.[13] The three possibilities are true autoimmune hemolysis, immune hemolysis mediated by passenger lymphocytes, and immune hemolysis in the setting of chimerism and major blood group mismatch[13] (Table 41-2).

Pathophysiology

Attachment of autoantibody to the surface of the RBC may lead to intravascular or extravascular hemolysis. The pathologic effect is determined by the class or subclass as well as the avidity of the antibody attached and the extent to which complement is activated. IgA, IgM, IgG1, and IgG3 can all fix complement, although IgA is a rare cause of AIHA.[14] If complement is activated through the C5 to C9 membrane attack complex, intravascular hemolysis occurs.[15] The RBCs coated with simply antibody or complement component C3b are phagocytized by macrophages and destroyed extravascularly in the spleen or liver, respectively. Cells coated with IgG are destroyed primarily in the spleen; those with IgM, in the liver.[16]

The interaction of macrophages with RBCs coated with IgG or C3b (or both) occurs through receptors specific for the Fc portion of IgG (especially IgG1 and IgG3) and for C3b.[17,18] The presence on the erythrocyte membrane of both IgG and C3b accelerates immune clearance,[19–21] suggesting that the Fc and C3b macrophage receptors act synergistically.

Red Blood Cell Injury

The opsonized RBC may be phagocytosed and destroyed entirely by macrophages. Alternatively, proteolytic enzymes may digest part of the membrane surface, producing spherocytes. The spherocytes are less deformable and consequently are hemolyzed in the spleen. The predominant mechanism of destruction of erythrocytes coated with IgG with or without C3b occurs extravascularly in AIHA. The amount of immune clearance is also mediated by the entire reticuloendothelial system; thus, viral or bacterial infections may exacerbate hemolysis.[22] In vitro assays of the ability of blood monocytes from patients with viral infections to phagocytose immunoglobulin-coated RBCs have shown marked deviations from normal.[23,24]

Clinical Findings

The clinical findings in AIHA are variable. They are determined by the rate of hemolysis and by the abilities of the body to process breakdown products and of the bone marrow to mount a reticulocytosis. Some of the signs are associated with hyperdynamic circulation secondary to anemia and a concomitant decrease in oxygen-carrying capacity. They include hepatomegaly and, in more severe cases, pulmonary edema, lethargy, and obtundation. Splenomegaly can also occur

Table 41–2 Post-Transplant Immune Hemolysis

Immune Hemolysis	AIHA	Passenger Lymphocyte	ABO Rh Mismatch
Mediated By	Donor lymphocytes	Donor memory B cells in solid organ or stem cells	Recipient Ab
Directed Against	Donor RBCs	Recipient RBCs	Donor RBCs
Cause	T-cell dysfunction; immunomodulatory medications	GVHD-like reaction with production of Ab	Preformed Ab or Ab formed in response to donor tissue
Onset	2–25 months post-transplant	5–17 days	Acute; timing depends on preformed or newly formed Abs
Duration	Variable, depending on response to therapy	Usually resolves in 3 months	
Treatment Options	Same as idiopathic AIHA	Compatible RBC transfusions; plasma or RBC exchange	Compatible RBC transfusion; immunosuppression
Prevention	None known	Prophylactic donor-compatible RBC transfusions	Removal of recipient Ab by plasma exchange or donor RBC purge

AIHA, autoimmune hemolytic anemia; GVHD, graft-versus-host disease; RBC, red blood cells.

from an increase in white pulp. Other signs and symptoms, such as jaundice, fever, and renal insufficiency, are caused by the breakdown products and subsequent vasoconstriction. It has now been demonstrated that decreased renal perfusion, not injury due to free hemoglobin, is the mechanism leading to renal insufficiency.

Autoimmune hemolytic anemia may have a fulminant presentation, with rapid onset of profound anemia, or may develop gradually, with concomitant physiologic compensation. Occasionally, unsuspected AIHA is diagnosed through a positive direct antiglobulin test (DAT) result in an anemic patient who has been referred for transfusion. The presence of lymphadenopathy, fever, hypertension, renal failure, rash, petechiae, or ecchymoses necessitates careful investigation for an underlying malignancy or collagen vascular disease.

Laboratory Evaluation

Direct and Indirect Antiglobulin Tests

It can be difficult to distinguish AIHA from other forms of hemolytic anemia on the basis of laboratory data. The positive result of a DAT, also known as the *Coombs' test*, is considered pathognomonic of immune-mediated hemolysis. The test detects the presence of IgG or complement bound to the RBC membrane (Fig. 41–1). Severe disease usually produces a strong DAT response, but this finding does not always correlate with the degree of hemolysis.[1] The indirect antiglobulin test (IAT; indirect Coombs' test), which detects the presence of antibodies in the patient's serum, usually has a positive result in AIHA (Fig. 41–2).

A positive DAT result is occasionally noted in a healthy person without anemia or evidence of hemolysis.[25] Conversely, patients with known AIHA may have a negative DAT result; this latter finding can be caused infrequently by laboratory error or by the presence of IgA, IgM, or low-affinity IgG autoantibodies.[26]

More commonly, the test is not sensitive enough to detect small numbers of erythrocyte-bound IgG molecules; this occurs most often in AIHA associated with lymphoma or CLL. If the DAT result is positive, specific reagents are required to identify the erythrocyte-bound protein.

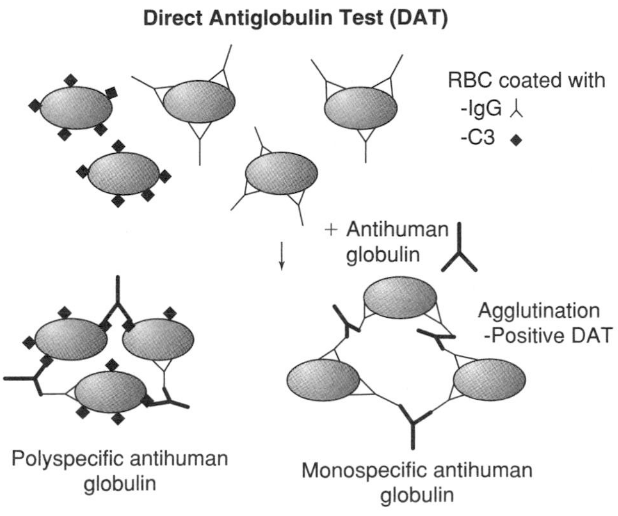

Direct Antiglobulin Test (DAT)

RBC coated with
-IgG
-C3

+ Antihuman globulin

Agglutination -Positive DAT

Polyspecific antihuman globulin

Monospecific antihuman globulin

Figure 41–1 Direct antiglobulin test (DAT). C3, complement component 3; IgG, immunoglobulin G; RBC, red blood cell.

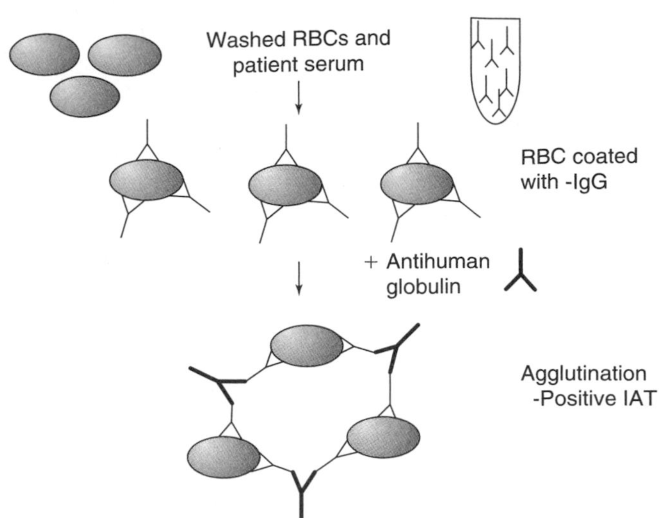

Figure 41–2 Indirect antiglobulin test (IAT). IgG, immunoglobulin G; RBC, red blood cell.

In approximately 80% of patients with AIHA, the autoantibodies are present in serum as well as on RBC membranes.[27] IAT detects the presence of these serum antibodies in the patient's serum. These may be autoantibodies in a patient with AIHA or they may be alloantibodies induced by blood transfusion or maternal-fetal incompatibility. Alloantibodies, present only in the serum, have specificity for RBC antigens not present on the patient's erythrocytes. The DAT result is therefore negative in alloimmunization as long as the patient has not recently been transfused with RBCs that have the target antigen. In the setting of a recent transfusion, the alloantibodies may bind to recently transfused RBCs, yielding a positive DAT result.

Other Supportive Laboratory Investigations

It is difficult to distinguish intravascular from extravascular hemolysis. The hemoglobin, hematocrit, lactate dehydrogenase (LDH), bilirubin, and haptoglobin values are similarly affected in both types of hemolysis. A significant urine hemosiderin level can indicate intravascular hemolysis yet often appears too late to be a helpful clinical tool. An unchanged hemoglobin or hematocrit value obtained within 4 hours after a transfusion of RBCs is an indicator of intravascular hemolysis. The intravascular destruction occurs so rapidly that no evidence of transfusion is reflected in the laboratory values. Intravascular hemolysis is important to recognize, because the patient may require greater supportive care to treat the anemia and consequent organ injury from intravascular hemolysis.

Like clinical symptoms, laboratory findings reflect the intensity of the hemolytic process as well as the ability of the body to process the RBC breakdown products and of the bone marrow to respond to the anemia. In fulminant cases, with an RBC life span of less than 5 days, the anemia is severe and erythropoiesis increases eight- to tenfold. As a result, the reticulocyte count rises, sometimes to levels greater than 40% of RBCs. If the regenerative capacity of the bone marrow lags only slightly behind the rate of RBC destruction, a mild anemia with an elevated reticulocyte count results. Between these extremes are many variations. Inspection of the blood smear in a typical case reveals polychromatophilia, spherocytes, a few fragmented RBCs, nucleated RBCs, and, occasionally, erythrophagocytosis. Examination of the bone marrow, which is rarely indicated, shows erythroid hyperplasia, often with megaloblastoid features. Occasionally, RBC autoantibodies or parvovirus B19[28] cause reticulocytopenia and dyserythropoiesis, thereby contributing to the severity of anemia.[29]

Patients with severe hemolytic anemia and markedly increased erythropoiesis occasionally experience folate deficiency and frank megaloblastosis. The growth of hematopoietic tissue in the bone marrow also leads to moderate increases in the white blood cell and platelet counts. The absence of reticulocytosis does not exclude the diagnosis of AIHA but portends a serious prognosis.[30–33] In addition, reticulocytopenia may represent excessive apoptosis of erythroblasts.[30,31,33,34] Presumably as a result of destruction of young erythrocytes by the autoantibody, the reticulocytopenia aggravates the severity of the anemia and increases the need for RBC transfusions.

Therapy

General Principles

The severity of AIHA may range from indolent to life threatening. The impetus to initiate treatment, as well as the determination about whether the treatment required is immediate transfusion or an attempt to modulate the immune system's production of autoantibody, must be based on a thorough appraisal of symptoms and the extent of the clinical compromise.

Rapidly developing anemia with a hematocrit less than 20% requires urgent management. In less aggressive forms of the disease, however, it may be prudent to allow physiologically compensated anemia rather than to institute treatment. The management of AIHA depends in part on whether the disease is primary or is secondary to such disorders as a B-cell malignancy or SLE.[35,36] This, too, demands a careful assessment before any treatment begins. In some cases of AIHA secondary to lymphoma or CLL, the pathogenic autoantibody (usually monoclonal) is secreted by the neoplastic B cells. Combination chemotherapy or irradiation of the underlying malignancy often brings the hemolytic anemia under control.[37–39]

In other cases, however, the autoantibodies (usually polyclonal) do not originate from the B-cell neoplasm but probably result from abnormal immune regulation instigated by the neoplastic B cells. Treatment of the latter type of secondary AIHA with immunosuppressive agents may improve the anemia but may also trigger an exacerbation.[40] Multiple chemotherapeutic agents and immunosuppressive medications interfere with T-cell function and can thus trigger autoimmune processes in general and AIHA specifically. Fludarabine and cladribine given as therapy for CLL have been demonstrated to precipitate autoimmune processes by interfering with the balance of T- and B-cell functions.[11]

The ultimate goal of therapy is control of the B-cell populations that secrete pathogenic autoantibodies. However, so little is known about such cells[41,42] that the currently available therapy is, by default, nonspecific and often aimed at reducing RBC clearance by macrophages. The desired therapeutic effect is eradication of the abnormal hemolytic process, not reversal of the serologic abnormalities. Indeed, DAT results often remain positive in the presence of a hematologic response.

BOX 41–1 *Transfusion Therapy and Autoimmune Hemolysis*

There are times when a patient requires transfusion of incompatible RBCs or when transfusion must occur before completion of the blood bank evaluation. Autoimmune hemolytic anemia always complicates and prolongs the blood bank evaluation, which may take up to 24 to 48 hours to complete. It is imperative, however, that the patient receive RBCs expeditiously, *even though they are crossmatch-incompatible*, if the hematocrit is not stabilized or cardiac or cerebral function is compromised. In these situations, the patient should be very closely monitored and should receive the smallest volume of blood necessary to alleviate the life-threatening symptoms.

Transfusion

Some cases of AIHA may be life threatening and may necessitate transfusion with RBCs (Box 41–1). It is important to recognize that, in the majority of cases, the patient receives crossmatch-incompatible blood.[43–46] The presence of autoantibodies complicates and prolongs the evaluation performed by the blood bank. In situations of fulminant hemolysis, transfusion of incompatible blood or transfusion performed on an emergency basis before completion of the evaluation may be imperative and lifesaving. Severe anemia may cause high-output cardiac failure and subsequent pulmonary edema, somnolence, and even obtundation, which require immediate intervention with RBC transfusion. The hemoglobin level at which these symptoms occur varies according to the rate of fall of the hemoglobin level, the capacity for cardiac compensation, and other underlying clinical features. Occasionally (1% to 2% of cases), relative specificity of the autoantibodies can be demonstrated. This specificity usually occurs within the Rh system, and RBCs lacking the corresponding Rh antigen survive better in vivo than those that express the antigen.[47–50] Specificities of IgG autoantibodies for multiple other blood groups have been described.[51]

In addition, the blood bank must look for alloantibodies that may be masked by the autoantibodies. Alloantibodies, usually with specificity for the Rh or Kell blood group systems, occur in approximately 30% of patients with AIHA who have a history of blood group immunization by maternal-fetal incompatibility or previous transfusions.[52–54] The nonspecific serum autoantibodies that react with nearly all normal RBCs must be removed to ensure that no concomitant alloantibodies are present. An adsorption test is performed, using either the patient's cells or cells of known phenotype to absorb the autoantibodies from the serum—a process known as *autologous adsorption* or *heterologous adsorption*, respectively.

These tests are not performed by all laboratories and should not be required before transfusion of a patient in need. However, standard antibody detection and identification tests with both the patient's serum and an eluate prepared from the patient's cells should be performed whenever possible. Titration of the eluate and the serum against RBCs of various Rh phenotypes can indicate an autoantibody specificity (or preference) within the Rh system. Any such specificity should be respected in the selection of donor units.[55,56]

Red blood cell substitutes have been transfused in a few situations of severe hemolytic anemia and have demonstrated benefit to the patients.[57,58] Further investigation of these substitutes is necessary to determine their efficacy and safety. They could potentially be of benefit in the short-term emergent situation when the presence of underlying alloantibodies cannot be ruled out or when the hemolysis is so brisk that transfusion of least incompatible cells does not result in any increase in hemoglobin and thus in oxygen-carrying capacity.[59]

Corticosteroids

Corticosteroids are the first line of treatment for most patients with symptomatic, unstable AIHA, either idiopathic or secondary. The clinical response to prednisone results primarily from its ability to disable macrophages from clearing IgG- or C3b-coated erythrocytes. Corticosteroids interfere with both the expression and function of macrophage Fc receptors. This interference is probably the earliest, and perhaps even the primary, mechanism in the ability of steroids to diminish the immune clearance of blood cells.[60–63] Prednisone can also reduce autoantibody production, but only after several weeks of therapy.

The side effects of corticosteroids often preclude the long-term use of high-dose therapy. The cushingoid features that develop can lead to noncompliance, especially in adolescents. The associated osteoporosis and immunosuppression as well as the risk of gastric bleeding may warrant discontinuation of therapy.

Splenectomy

Splenectomy has been used as therapy for AIHA for many years.[64] Indications for splenectomy include failure to respond to prednisone, need for prednisone dosages higher than 10 to 20 mg/day, and intractable corticosteroid side effects. The procedure can be highly effective, presumably through removal of the major reticuloendothelial site of RBC destruction; an animal model demonstrated that IgG-coated RBCs are removed almost exclusively by the spleen.[60] In addition, the procedure eliminates many phagocytosing macrophages and autoantibody-producing B cells.

In most young adults with chronic AIHA, the question of splenectomy arises almost inevitably. However, in an elderly patient with a stable but incomplete remission, maintenance therapy with prednisone at a dose of 10 mg/day for an indefinite period may be the better alternative. There is a slight risk that overwhelming sepsis by encapsulated organisms may develop immediately and up to 25 years after splenectomy.[65] The risk is higher in children, especially those younger than age 6, so a conservative approach to splenectomy is prudent in this age group. The risk of overwhelming sepsis is lessened by immunization with pneumococcal and meningococcal vaccines, which are optimally administered at least 2 weeks preoperatively, and by the prompt use of antibiotics for febrile illness.[66] The *Haemophilus influenzae* series of vaccines should also be completed in children before splenectomy.

The response to splenectomy does not correlate with the age of the patient, the presence or absence of an underlying B-cell disorder, the strength of the antiglobulin test result, prior response to prednisone, or the pattern of sequestration of chromium 51 (^{51}Cr)-labeled RBCs. Between 50% and 60% of patients with classic AIHA have a good to excellent initial response to splenectomy. They will need less than 15 mg/day of prednisone to maintain an adequate level of hemoglobin.[67] Information regarding the clinical implications of an accessory spleen in AIHA is meager. Faced with such a rare finding in a patient with relapse, many hematologists would recommend its removal. The role of splenectomy in patients with mixed IgG, IgM, or mixed cold- and warm-reactive IgG antibodies is unclear.

Rituximab Therapy

Rituximab, a chimeric anti-CD20 monoclonal antibody with a well-established, favorable safety profile, has possibilities for widespread clinical application in autoimmune disease in general and AIHA specifically.[68,69] Rituximab induces cell death through complement-dependent lysis, antibody-dependent cellular toxicity, and cellular apoptosis.[68] Although plasma cells, fully differentiated B cells, are CD20-negative, the response rates of patients with AIHA and thrombocytopenia suggest that earlier CD20-positive B cells are producing antibody or that other as-yet not clearly delineated effects of rituximab are effecting the disease remission. Reports that rituximab induces remission in patients with idiopathic thrombocytopenic purpura within 1 week of first infusion suggest that the mechanism of action may involve more than elimination of B cells.[69]

The efficacy and safety of rituximab have been demonstrated in multiple large trials in adult patients with non-Hodgkin's lymphomas.[69] Infusion-related side effects, including fever, respiratory distress, and hypotension, are reported to occur in a small population of lymphoma patients.[69–71] No side effects have precluded completion of planned therapy in patients with autoimmune disease.[72] The occurrence and severity of side effects seem to be related to B-cell level and, thus, tumor burden.[70] It is anticipated and has been demonstrated that the side effect profile will be even more favorable in patients with autoimmune disease who have a lower level of B cells.[73]

No large, prospective trials have studied the efficacy and safety of rituximab in patients with warm AIHA. However, the results of multiple case reports, case series, pilot studies, and small therapeutic trials indicate that rituximab warrants further study in patients with autoimmune disease and have prompted some experts in the field to attempt a trial of rituximab prior to splenectomy in warm AIHA. The literature reveals successful use of anti-CD20 treatment in multiple autoimmune diseases.[6,7,74–79]

Rituximab Therapy: Mechanism(s) of Action

Rituximab's mechanism of action appears to be multifaceted, complex, and incompletely understood. It is known that it induces cell death through complement-dependent lysis; antibody-dependent cellular toxicity; antibody-dependent phagocytosis mediated by Fc, complement, and phosphatidylserine receptors; direct antibody effects of CD20 ligation leading to inhibition of proliferation, apoptosis, and sensitization to chemotherapy; and induction of active immunity.[68] Although plasma cells are CD20-negative, the response rate of patients with AIHA and thrombocytopenia suggest that earlier, CD20-positive B cells are producing antibody or that other as-yet not clearly delineated mechanisms are effecting disease remission. Reports that rituximab induces remission in patients with AIHA within 1 to 3 weeks of first infusion suggest that the mechanism of action may involve more than elimination of B cells. Table 41-3 summarizes the case reports and small case series of patients with AIHA treated with rituximab.

Table 41–3 Summary of Studies and Case Report Data for Rituximab for AIHA

Number of Patients/ Disease	Rituximab Dose	Dosing Schedule	% Response	Previous Regimens*	Splenectomy	Follow-up Period
15 pediatric/idiopathic[79]	375 mg/m^2	Weekly × 2–4	87 (13/15)	Two or more S, C, I, CyA, Az	2/15	7–28 months
1 pediatric/SLE,[78] idiopathic[158]	375 mg/m^2	Weekly × 2	100 (2/2)	S, C, I, CyA	0/2	5–7 months
6 pediatric/idiopathic[77]	375 mg/m^2	Weekly × 4 Weekly × 12 (2pt)	100 (6/6)	S, I, Ph, CyA, Az	2/6	15–22 months
4 pediatric/idiopathic[159]	375 mg/m^2	Weekly × 4–6	100 (4/4)	S, V, CyA, Az, I, C, T	2/4	3–14 months
1 pediatric/idiopathic[160]	375 mg/m^2	Weekly × 4 then repeat	100 (1/1)	S, I, C, CyA, ATG, Ph, Az	Yes	19 months
3–1 CAD, 2 WAIHA[161]	375 mg/m^2	Weekly × 4	33 (1/3)	S, C, Az	0/4	96 months
6 adult/5 lymphoma; 1 idiopathic[123]	375 mg/m^2	Weekly × 4	17 (1/6) PR in 4/6	3 untreated S, C, Cl, Chl	1/6	6–14 months
1 pediatric/Hurler's post-BMT[162]	375 mg/m^2	Weekly × 3	100 (1/1)	I, S, CyA	0/1	21 months
1 pediatric post-BMT/ β-thalassemia,[163] WAS[164]	375 mg/m^2	Weekly × 2 Weekly × 4	100 (2/2)	S, I	0/2	3–12 months
1 adult/idiopathic CAD+ WAIHA3	375 mg/m^2	Weekly × 4, then 1 month later Weekly × 4	100 (1/1)	S × 2 long tapers	No	7 months
9 adult/CAD +/– lymphoma/CLL[165–172]	375 mg/m^2	Weekly × 4	100 (9/9)	S, CyA, Chl, Az, C, MM, CHOP for lymphoma	1/9	9–36 months
6 adults/CAD[173]	375 mg/m^2	Weekly × 4	1 CR, 4 PR, 1 NR	S, Chl, C, Cl	1/6	6–14 months
8 adult/CLL[174]	375 mg/m^2	Q 4 weeks Given w/ C and D	100 (8/8)	S, F, C, Chl	0/8	7–23 months
27 adults/CAD {123}	375 mg/m^2	Weekly × 4 +/– IFN	ICR, 19 PR	S, C, MP	Not reported	2–42 months

*Regimens: ATG, antithymocyte globulin; Az, azathioprine; C, cyclophosphamide; Ch l, chlorambucil; Cl, cladribine; CyA, cyclosporine; I, intravenous immune globulin; IFN, interferon; MM, mycophenolate mofetil; MP, mercaptopurine; Ph, plasmapheresis; S, corticosteroids; T, tacrolimus; V, vincristine.

Intravenous Immune Globulin

Intravenous immune globulin (IVIG) has been found effective in the management of selected cases of AIHA. The soluble IgG in the material may lengthen the life span of IgG-coated RBCs by saturating Fc receptors on macrophages. In a study of patients who had AIHA associated with lymphoproliferative disorders, a long-term benefit was observed with a maintenance dosage schedule of intravenous IgG every 21 days. A decrease in antiglobulin titer was found in these patients, suggesting a mechanism other than blockade of Fc receptors by intravenous IgG.[80] The mechanism of action of IVIG has been further elucidated by Samuelsson and colleagues.[81] They investigated the mechanism of protection in a murine model of immune thrombocytopenia that may have relevance to mechanism of action in other autoimmune diseases. Their model demonstrated that the inhibitory Fc receptor FcγRIIB was necessary for IVIG to confer protection against platelet destruction.[81] This finding suggests that modulation of inhibitory signals in macrophages could possibly be involved in autoimmunity and could be investigated as therapeutic targets in other autoimmune diseases, such as AIHA.

Immunosuppressive Therapy

Most experience with immunosuppressive drugs in the treatment of AIHA has been with alkylating agents (cyclophosphamide and chlorambucil) and thiopurines (azathioprine and mercaptopurine).[82] The basis for the clinical use of these drugs is their inhibitory effect on the immune system, possibly affecting both B cells and T cells.[83,84]

Cyclophosphamide and azathioprine, like prednisone, can induce numerous side effects. The early side effects include bone marrow suppression and impairment of the immune response (particularly T cell–mediated immunity) that occur concomitantly with therapy. After sustained administration, cyclophosphamide may damage ovarian function, inhibit spermatogenesis,[85–88] and cause bladder fibrosis.[89] Acute myeloid leukemia can develop years after administration of this drug.[83] By contrast, the prolonged use of azathioprine has not been associated with a statistically significant increase in malignant diseases. All of these considerations mandate careful monitoring of any patient treated with either cyclophosphamide or azathioprine.

Cyclosporine, a powerful T-cell modulator, has been used alone and in combination to elicit successful and sometimes durable remission in patients with AIHA and Evans's syndrome.[90] Cyclosporine and other immunosuppressive agents are discussed here and have been reported in the literature. However, their long-term use is not recommended, because the benefits do not usually offset the side effects inherent in the prolonged use of these agents.

Plasma Exchange

Because a single-volume plasma exchange replaces only about 60% of the patient's plasma volume, its therapeutic advantage lies in the removal of plasma antibodies to IgG, IgM, or both, which mediate the hemolysis. Unfortunately, continuous antibody production and the large extravascular distribution of IgG limit the long-term efficacy of plasma exchange in IgG-mediated AIHA. On cessation of therapy, the rate of return to pretreatment levels of autoantibody depends on the rate of autoantibody production.[91] However, there are some reports that this modality is efficacious in IgG-mediated disease.[92] Occasional dramatic responses have been reported in patients being prepared for surgery or when plasma exchange was used as a temporizing measure after initiation of immunosuppressive therapy.[92,93] This therapy is reserved for patients in critical condition whose AIHA is unresponsive to transfusion because of rapid destruction and clearance of the RBCs.

COLD AGGLUTININ DISEASE

Cold agglutinin disease refers to a group of disorders caused by anti-erythrocyte autoantibodies (e.g., cold agglutinins) that preferentially bind RBCs at cold temperatures (4°C to 18°C) and may or may not induce hemolysis. Virtually all sera from healthy individuals contain low-titer cold agglutinins, which are regarded as benign or harmless RBC autoantibodies and are considered polyclonal. Similarly, cold agglutinins that arise after certain infections are also polyclonal and usually benign; in rare cases, a transient form of cold agglutinin disease ensues. By contrast, monoclonal cold agglutinins are generally pathogenic and are derived from clonal B-cell expansions (as in idiopathic or chronic cold agglutinin disease), which may be a prelude to frank lymphoma.

Chronic Cold Agglutinin Disease

The most common type of cold agglutinin disease, a chronic form characterized principally by a stable anemia of moderate severity and attacks of acrocyanosis precipitated by exposure to cold, constitutes about one third of all cases of immune hemolytic anemia. Cold agglutinins cause the cardinal abnormalities of the disease. The acrocyanosis stems from intra-arteriolar agglutination of erythrocytes in the relatively cool tips of the fingers, feet, ear lobes, and nose. The occurrence of this hemolytic anemia depends on the capacity of the cold agglutinins to initiate activation of the complement cascade on the surface of the RBC. Most patients with chronic cold agglutinin disease are in the fifth to eighth decade of life and have a B-cell neoplasm or lymphoma, Waldenström macroglobulinemia, or CLL. The cold agglutinin in cases secondary to such diseases is monoclonal, almost always IgMκ, and may show up as a monoclonal band in the γ region of the serum protein electrophoretic pattern. In the absence of a B-cell neoplasm, the spleen and lymph nodes are rarely enlarged; therefore, the finding of splenic and lymph node enlargement warrants a search for the neoplasm.

Transient Cold Agglutinin Disease

A second type of cold agglutinin disease, usually acute and always self-limited, occurs as a rare complication of several infectious diseases, most notably *Mycoplasma pneumoniae* infection and infectious mononucleosis. Patients with this form of cold agglutinin disease are therefore much younger than those with chronic cold agglutinin disease. The onset is abrupt, occurring as the infection wanes, and the anemia can be severe. Cold agglutinin titers are moderately elevated, and the cold agglutinins are polyclonal. Often, these polyclonal cold agglutinins coincide with high-titer warm-reactive IgG RBC autoantibodies.

ANTIGENIC TARGETS OF COLD AGGLUTININ DISEASE

The antigenic specificity of cold agglutinins is usually identified from their degree of reactivity with RBCs from adults (blood group I) and from cord blood (blood group i). The cold-reactive autoantibody produced after some cases of *M. pneumoniae* infection has anti-I specificity,[94] whereas the antibody in infectious mononucleosis frequently, but not always, has anti-i specificity.[95,96] Additional specificities have been identified by tests with rare adult RBCs that lack the I-antigen or with enzyme-treated erythrocytes. Rarely, cold agglutinins are specific for the A blood group antigen.[46]

Laboratory Evaluation

The usual laboratory findings in hemolytic anemia (i.e., anemia, reticulocytosis, polychromatophilia, spherocytosis, erythroid hyperplasia in the bone marrow, and elevations in serum bilirubin and LDH levels) are generally not striking in chronic cold agglutinin disease. Hemagglutination may be visible to the unaided eye in blood drawn from a patient with cold agglutinin disease and can interfere with automated blood counts. The anemia is often mild and stable, because the C3b inactivator in serum limits the extent of cold agglutinin–induced complement activation on the erythrocyte membrane. Exposure to cold may greatly augment the binding of cold agglutinins, however, exceeding the restraints of the inactivator system. That occurrence can lead to a sudden drop in hematocrit value, with complement-mediated intravascular hemolysis and renal failure.

In a distinctive subset of patients with aggressive cold agglutinin disease, the cold agglutinin titer is relatively low but the autoantibody has a high thermal amplitude. Recognition that a patient has this variant of cold agglutinin disease is important because it may respond to prednisone,[62] whereas high-titer cold agglutinin disease usually does not.

In typical cases of chronic cold agglutinin disease, the cold agglutinin titer is very high (>1:10^5 and occasionally >1:10^6). The antibodies are most reactive in the cold, and hemagglutination disappears as the temperature rises toward 37° C. In some cases, however, the antibody is reactive at relatively high temperatures and occasionally even at 37° C. The reactivity of the cold agglutinin at high temperatures (i.e., its thermal amplitudes), not the titer of the antibody, most accurately predicts the severity of the disease. The DAT result is positive because of erythrocyte-bound C3d, but results of tests with anti-IgG reagents are negative. The result of the IAT, which is conducted at 37° C, is negative. In addition to monoclonal IgM cold agglutinins, IgG-IgM mixed cold agglutinins have been reported.[97–99] Besides the usual high titers of IgM cold agglutinins, some patients with cold agglutinin disease have low titers of IgG and IgA cold agglutinins.

Cold agglutinins are not cryoglobulins. The latter are most often monoclonal IgM immunoglobulins that, in the cold, either self-associate and precipitate from solution (type I cryoglobulinemia) or precipitate as complexes with polyclonal IgG molecules (type II cryoglobulinemia, often due to a monoclonal IgM rheumatoid factor). Type III cryoglobulins consist of a mixture of polyclonal IgM and polyclonal IgG immunoglobulins. The clinical manifestations of the cryoglobulinemic syndromes are highly variable: type I and type II cryoglobulinemias occur in B-cell neoplasms (Waldenström macroglobulinemia, multiple myeloma, lymphoma, and CLL); type II and type III cryoglobulinemias can produce a picture of immune complex–mediated vasculitis, with vascular purpura, arthritis, and nephritis as the dominant complications. In occasional patients, the cryoglobulin can also be a cold agglutinin.[100–103]

Pathophysiology

The pathogenic IgM autoantibody in cold agglutinin disease is highly efficient in activating the classic complement pathway on the erythrocyte membrane.[36,104] However, the thermal dependency of the antibody constrains its pathogenic effects. The autoantibody rapidly elutes off RBCs at 37°C, the temperature of the visceral circulation, but in the cool peripheral circulation of the hands and feet, the cold agglutinin remains on the erythrocyte membrane for at least a few seconds. That amount of time is sufficient to activate the complement cascade to the stage of C3b, which adheres to the RBC after it reenters the central circulation. In the hepatic circulation, C3b-positive RBCs encounter macrophages with receptors specific for C3b[19,105,106]; however, C3b sensitization is only a weak signal for the activation of phagocytosis—the hepatic clearance of C3b-coated RBCs requires 500 to 800 C3b molecules per RBC. As a result, many C3b-positive RBCs escape unharmed into the systemic circulation, where they come under the influence of the regulatory proteins of the complement system. The C3b inactivator system degrades C3b into C3dg, C3d, or both. The result is a cohort of erythrocytes coated with C3d but not with the IgM autoantibody.[107] Macrophages bind to C3d with even lower avidity than to C3b, thus the C3d-positive erythrocytes tend to have near-normal survival in vivo despite a heavy coating with that degradation product of C3.[108,109] It is important to recognize that if transfusion is necessary, the transfused cells will not have the protection conferred by C3d and therefore may be rapidly lysed.[109]

These limits on the pathogenicity of cold agglutinins account for the subdued hematologic picture in most patients with cold agglutinin disease. If, however, the regulatory C3b inactivator proteins are impaired, limiting cleavage of RBC-bound C3b, or if the production of IgM autoantibodies with a high thermal amplitude is impaired, permitting completion of the complement cascade in the visceral circulation, severe extravascular hemolysis can occur. Several patients with high titers of IgA cold agglutinins have been reported. Such cases are not associated with cold agglutinin disease, which may relate to the lack of complement activation by IgA antibodies.[109–118]

Therapy

Chronic Cold Agglutinin Disease

Therapy for the cold agglutinin syndromes depends on the gravity of the symptoms, the serologic characteristics of the autoantibody, and any underlying disease. In the idiopathic, or primary, form of chronic cold agglutinin disease, prolonged survival and spontaneous remissions and exacerbations are not unusual. The anemia is generally mild, and the simple measure of avoiding exposure to cold temperatures can avoid exacerbations, especially if the cold agglutinin responsible has a low thermal amplitude. Prednisone has been beneficial in rare cases in which there are relatively low titers of cold agglutinins of a high thermal amplitude or an IgG cold-reactive antibody is produced. However, prednisone is not useful therapy in most patients with primary IgM-induced cold agglutinin disease, and its administration should not be undertaken lightly, given the chronicity of the disease.[119,120] Plasma exchange may help as a temporary measure in acute situations.[93] Splenectomy is usually ineffective because the liver is the dominant site of sequestration of RBCs heavily sensitized with C3b. However, rare cases in patients with enlarged spleens have responded to splenectomy; in some of these patients, a localized splenic lymphoma was found, whereas in others, only lymphoid hyperplasia was evident.

It is essential to seek evidence of a B-cell neoplasm before therapy for chronic cold agglutinin disease is initiated. Oral alkylating agents (chlorambucil or cyclophosphamide) help many patients with the secondary form of cold agglutinin disease because of their effect on the B-cell neoplasm, but only occasionally do they benefit patients with the primary form of the disease.[121,122] When cold agglutinin disease is part of an established B-cell malignancy, the severity of hemolysis often waxes and wanes in parallel with the activity of the neoplasm.

Patients with IgM-mediated hemolysis can be dramatically helped with plasma exchange. Because of its large size, the antibody is located primarily in the intravascular space and is efficiently removed by plasma exchange. Some patients with Waldenström macroglobulinemia are maintained over the long term with this therapy.

A recent publication of a prospective, phase II study of patients with primary cold agglutinin disease reported a 54% response rate in 27 patients treated with 37 courses of rituximab. Some of the patients who did not respond to the first course of four weekly doses of rituximab were treated with a combination of rituximab and interferon-α. Of the responses, one patient achieved complete remission and 19 partial remission. The complete remission was sustained at 42 months, although all but one of the patients with partial remission relapsed at a mean of 11 months.[123]

Transient Cold Agglutinin Disease

Transient cold agglutinin disease is a rare form that is always self-limited. Supportive measures, including transfusions and avoidance of cold, may suffice to tide the patient over the episode of hemolysis. Corticosteroids are usually not helpful, and splenectomy is almost never indicated.

PAROXYSMAL COLD HEMOGLOBINURIA

Clinical Features

Paroxysmal cold hemoglobinuria was historically associated with tertiary syphilis, which is rarely seen today. PCH is now more commonly seen primarily in children after a viral or, much less commonly, bacterial illness.[124] Most commonly, the viral etiology is not known but is associated with an upper respiratory tract infection. However, case reports in both adults and children have reported an association of PCH with varicella.

Although the Donath-Landsteiner antibody often occurs in tertiary or congenital syphilis, it generally does not cause hemolytic disease in this situation. On exposure to cold, an occasional patient experiences paroxysms of hemoglobinuria and constitutional symptoms (fever, back pain, leg pain, abdominal cramps, and rigors) followed by hemoglobinuria. In contrast, the postviral form of PCH[125–127] is characterized by constitutional symptoms with fulminant intravascular hemolysis and its associated signs of hemoglobinemia, hemoglobinuria, jaundice, severe anemia, and sometimes renal failure. The disease is self-limited, usually lasting 2 to 3 weeks, although it can be life threatening because of the severity of the hemolysis and consequent anemia.

Laboratory Evaluation

The IgG antibody responsible for PCH is found in the patient's serum through incubation of normal erythrocytes, fresh normal serum as a source of complement, and the patient's serum, first at 4°C and then at 37°C, with appropriate controls. The Donath-Landsteiner antibody fixes the first two components of complement in the cold and completes the cascade on warming to 37°C.[128] The DAT result is almost always negative, but occasionally weak reactions for erythrocyte-bound complement are manifested. The IAT result is negative. Most Donath-Landsteiner antibodies have specificity for the P blood group system,[129,130] but other specificities have been described.[131–133] The diagnosis depends on recognition of the clinical picture, because tests for the Donath-Landsteiner antibody are not routinely performed.

Therapy

No specific treatment for PCH has been found. Unlike the effectiveness of steroids in most IgG-mediated autoimmune diseases, prednisone is not useful for PCH. The best approach consists of supportive care, transfusions to alleviate symptoms, and avoidance of cold temperatures. The patient should be kept in a warm room, and transfusions should be given through a blood warmer.

DRUG-ASSOCIATED IMMUNE HEMOLYTIC ANEMIA

Drug-associated immune hemolytic anemia can be either induced by or dependent on a drug. Four distinct mechanisms are associated with the disorder. The first involves any drug that can bind to the RBC membrane. The patient then makes antibodies against the drug (e.g., penicillin), which combine with the erythrocyte-bound drug, opsonizing and preparing the RBC for destruction. Discontinuation of the drug brings the hemolytic anemia to a rapid halt, because the antibodies have no specificity for antigens on the RBC membrane. Clues to the diagnosis are the appropriate clinical setting, a positive DAT result, a negative IAT result, and failure of antibodies eluted from the patient's RBCs to bind to normal erythrocytes. The diagnosis is established when both the eluate and the patient's serum contain antibodies directed against the drug-coated cells. In the case of penicillin,[134] hemolytic anemia occurs only when large amounts are administered; in patients treated with lower doses, a positive DAT result without hemolytic anemia is not unusual, because the production of low-avidity IgG antipenicillin antibodies is a common event.

The second mechanism involves immune complexes. The offending drug, or drug metabolite, binds to a plasma protein, forming an immunogenic conjugate. If the patient develops an antibody to the conjugate, it is usually IgM. This antibody then binds to the immunogenic conjugate, forming an immune complex that adheres to RBCs. The resulting clinical picture consists of intravascular hemolysis and concomitant hemoglobinemia, hemoglobinuria, and even renal failure through efficient activation of complement on the erythrocyte membrane. This chain of events accounts for most reported examples of drug-induced immune hemolytic anemia. Reports concerning the nonsteroidal drug diclofenac have shown that autoimmune hemolytic anemia is induced by sensitization to the glucuronide conjugate of the drug.[135] Serologic findings in erythrocyte-bound immune complexes are similar to those of the first mechanism, except that the DAT reveals only complement bound to the RBC; the IgM antibody is presumed to be no longer present after complement activation. The patient's serum reacts with RBCs (lacking antidrug antibody) in the presence of the offending drug, and the eluate from the patient's RBCs generally does not react with normal erythrocytes.

The third mechanism involves in vivo sensitization to drugs through the formation of immunogenic drug–RBC complexes. In these cases, the specificity of the drug-induced antibodies is contributed to not only by the drug (or its metabolites), but also by defined RBC antigens, particularly those of the Rh and I/i systems.[136]

The fourth mechanism of drug-associated immune hemolytic anemia involves the induction of authentic autoantibodies against RBCs by a drug; methyldopa is the classic example.[137] In as many as 20% of patients treated with methyldopa, the DAT result turns positive, but few demonstrate hemolytic anemia. The DAT result may take several months to a year or more after the start of drug therapy to become positive. In patients with hemolytic anemia, discontinuation of the drug results in only gradual cessation of the hemolytic anemia and disappearance of the autoantibody, because the drug itself is not required for the hemolytic process, only for the initiation of antibody production. Curiously, the autoantibody is usually specific for antigens of the Rh system. The serologic findings are indistinguishable from those in primary AIHA; they consist of a positive DAT result, usually a positive IAT result, and an eluate that reacts with normal erythrocytes. Patients taking methyldopa often have other antibodies in addition to the RBC autoantibodies. The mechanism by which methyldopa induces autoantibodies is unknown, but it may involve effects on immunoregulatory T cells.

Drug-induced immune hemolytic anemia was commonly seen when penicillin was administered in large doses (i.e., >20 million U/day) and when methyldopa was widely used in the treatment of hypertension.[138,139] However, the disease is unusual in present-day clinical practice.[140] Numerous drugs can induce hemolytic anemia.

ANIMAL MODELS OF AUTOIMMUNE HEMOLYTIC ANEMIA

Insights into Pathogenesis and Therapeutic Targets

NZB Mice

The inbred NZB mouse is genetically programmed to develop AIHA at around age 6 to 8 months (the life span of a normal mouse is approximately 2 years). Anti-erythrocyte autoantibodies begin to appear at around age 3 months; by age 9 months, the DAT result is positive in 60% to 80% of animals. Typical signs of hemolytic anemia develop—reticulocytosis, spherocytosis, a shortened RBC survival time, and splenomegaly.[141]

Okamoto and colleagues[142] developed a transgenic murine model of AIHA. The symptoms in this model range from unaffected to severe anemia. The B1 subpopulation has been demonstrated to mediate the AIHA.[143] They are activated in both T cell–dependent and T cell–independent ways.[144] These cells are unique from B2, the more prevalent B cells, in several ways. B1 cells preferentially locate in the peritoneal and pleural cavities, produce 50% of the natural serum IgM, and escape clonal deletion in these immunoprivileged sites. Interleukin-10 influences T cell–dependent proliferation of B1 cells and continuous administration of anti-interleukin-10 monoclonal antibody depletes B1 but not B2 cells in murine models. The influence of this Th2 cytokine on the behavior of the B1 cells in vivo[145] suggests possible avenues for treatments.

Origins of Anti-erythrocyte Autoantibodies

The vast improvement in our understanding of what prevents autoimmunization has not yet informed us of the mechanism that causes autoimmunization. Very little is known of the origins of warm-reactive IgG anti-erythrocyte autoantibodies, despite the availability of a thoroughly investigated, spontaneous animal model of the disease (the NZB mouse) and stocks of pathogenic autoantibodies, which are readily obtained from patients with the disease. A major impediment to advances in our understanding of how autoimmune hemolytic anemia originates is that the autoantigens are for the most part unknown. Even in those cases in which blood group specificity of the autoantibodies has been identified, the relevant structures have not been elucidated. Leddy and associates[146] have succeeded in identifying four proteins on the RBC membrane that bind to anti-erythrocyte autoantibodies; they are the band 3 anion transporter, glycophorin A, and two polypeptides, probably related to the Rh family of antigens. Various combinations of those four autoantibody specificities were found in a group of 20 patients with AIHA.

The association of AIHA with SLE and with immune thrombocytopenia (Evans's syndrome), the induction of the disease by drugs that seem to perturb immune regulation, and the graft-versus-host model of AIHA all suggest that, at least in some cases, there is antigen-independent activation of clones of B cells with the capacity to produce IgG anti-RBC autoantibodies. Such polyclonal B-cell activation may account for the production of anti-erythrocyte autoantibodies in patients with acquired immunodeficiency syndrome (AIDS).[94,147] Hypergammaglobulinemia and other signs of nonspecific activation of B cells are prominent in human immunodeficiency virus infection.[148]

The immunologic basis of AIHA in patients with CLL or a B-cell lymphoma is equally obscure.[149] In CLL, the autoantibodies are IgG and often polyclonal,[150] whereas the malignant CD5+ B cells of that disease generally produce only IgM antibodies that are monoclonal. It is therefore likely that B cells other than those constituting the leukemia produce the autoantibodies. The large mass of CD5+ B cells in CLL might induce nonneoplastic CD5− B cells to produce IgG autoantibodies, perhaps through a disturbance of immunoregulatory idiotypic networks. The demonstration of the simultaneous presence of autoantibodies and anti-idiotypic antibodies on RBCs in AIHA[151] suggests that such networks may indeed have a role in the disease.

In contrast to the antigens that incite warm-reactive autoantibodies, the structures of the autoantigens of cold agglutinin disease, the I/i system, are known[152]; this knowledge has clarified our thinking about the immunology of this group of disorders. There is little reason to doubt that the very high levels of monoclonal cold agglutinins found in some patients with B-cell neoplasms are produced by the malignant cells. The demonstration that an idiotypic marker on monoclonal cold agglutinins could be detected not only on the patients' neoplastic B cells, but also on 3% to 10% of normal B cells[153] supports the view that these autoantibodies are part of the normal immune repertoire; malignant transformation of a cold agglutinin–producing B cell results in a lymphoma complicated by chronic cold agglutinin disease.

The basis of the association of PCH with syphilis may be antigenic mimicry, in which structural similarities between a microbial antigen and a self-antigen trigger an autoantibody response. In the case of PCH, the infecting organism, *Treponema pallidum*, should possess two antigenic determinants (epitopes), one recognized by T cells (the foreign epitope) and the other by self-reactive B cells (the mimicking epitope). Donath-Landsteiner antibodies would be produced only by syphilitic patients whose class II major histocompatibility complex glycoproteins could present the foreign epitope in an immunogenic form to T cells. A similar mechanism could apply to postinfectious acute cold agglutinin disease, in which a crossreaction involving antigenic determinants of *M. pneumoniae* and the I blood group substance has been incriminated.[154]

Structural analyses of monoclonal anti-I and anti-i autoantibodies from patients with B-cell neoplasms are beginning to yield important clues about the origins of chronic cold agglutinin disease. A striking observation is the repetitive use of the same immunoglobulin V_H gene, V_{H4-34}, in monoclonal IgM cold agglutinins, regardless of the anti-I or anti-i specificity of the autoantibody.[155,156] In each case, the V_{H4-34} heavy chain gene had a different CDR3 (complementarity-determining region 3); the light chains of cold agglutinins with anti-I or anti-i specificity differed as well. The V_{H4-34} genes of these cold agglutinins contained few or no somatic mutations of the type that would lead to amino acid substitutions (replacement mutations). This finding, together with the variations in their CDR3 and in the light chains, implies that the V_{H4-34} germline gene segment itself encodes a binding site for the I and i antigens. In contrast to the heavy chain gene, the light chain genes of the cold agglutinins do contain replacement mutations, especially in their hypervariable regions.[156]

It appears from these results that the germline V_{H4-34} heavy chain encodes the dominant specificity of monoclonal cold agglutinins, the somatic mutations of the light chain genes of the cold agglutinins are the result of an immune response, and the V_H CDR3 and the light chain confer fine specificity (e.g., for I or i) on the cold agglutinin and influence its affinity. These data make a convincing case that monoclonal cold agglutinins arise as the result of an immune response, perhaps an autoimmune response to an autoantigen on erythrocytes. The results of these molecular studies of cold agglutinins complement other evidence favoring a role for antigen-mediated clonal selection in some types of B-cell neoplasms.

In contrast to monoclonal cold agglutinins associated with chronic cold agglutinin disease, the naturally occurring IgM cold agglutinins that are present in low titers in normal serum are not restricted to the V_{H4-34} gene segment. They are associated with different genes of the V_{H3} family as well as the V_{H4-34} gene.[156] It therefore appears that B-cell neoplasia is an important but not exclusive element in the association between V_{H4-34} and cold agglutinins. The correlation with lymphomas has additional interest, because V_{H4-34} has been independently linked to B-cell lymphomas that do not secrete cold agglutinins.[157]

PERSPECTIVE

In previous years, there have been many debates concerning the factors that contribute to the severity of AIHA. Previous studies have focused to a large extent on the humoral aspect of the autoimmune response. The antibodies were easily available from peripheral blood, allowing for many serologic investigations. However, none of the serologic parameters by itself—the quantity of serum RBC autoantibodies, titer, thermal amplitude, or allotype—has proved useful in predicting severity of the disease in patients. This fact is perhaps not surprising, because RBC clearance in both cold and warm AIHA occurs predominantly extravascularly through the actions of macrophages rather than intravascularly through antibody-mediated complement lysis. Also, membrane receptors on macrophages, such as FcγIIRB and SIRPα (signal regulation protein-α), have been identified that have the ability to modulate RBC clearance and, thus, severity of hemolysis. Therefore, it is possible that the activity of these receptors may vary among patients as well, contributing to the severity of disease expression. Moreover, these macrophage receptors may prove to be viable targets for the development of more specific immunotherapy than the methods currently used (i.e., corticosteroid therapy and IVIG). Another potentially exciting therapeutic approach is targeting of the humoral immune response, either through direct targeting of the B cells, such as with anti-CD20 antibody, or through interference with the interactions between B and T lymphocytes, such as with costimulatory molecule blockade (e.g., anti-CD40 antibody).

REFERENCES

1. Sloan S, Silberstein LE. Transfusion: in the face of autoantibodies. In Reid M, Nance SJ (ed). Red Cell Transfusion: A Practical Guide. Totowa, N.J., Humana Press, 1998.
2. Coombs R, Mourant AE, Race RR. A new test for the detection of weak and incomplete Rh agglutinins. Br J Exp Pathol 1945;26:255.
3. Boorman K, Dodd BE, Loutit JF. Hemolytic icterus (acholuric jaundice): congenital and acquired. Lancet 1946;1:812.
4. Lewis R, Henry WB, Thornton GW, et al. A syndrome of autoimmune hemolytic anemia and thrombocytopenia in dogs. Proc J Am Vet Med Assoc 1963;1:140.
5. Bielschowsky M, Helyer BJ, Howie JB. Spontaneous hemolytic anemia in mice of the NZB/Bl strain. Proc Univ Otago Med Sch 1959; 37:9.
6. Petschner F, Walter UA, Schmitt-Graff A, et al. "Catastrophic systemic lupus erythematosus" with Rosai-Dorfman sinus histiocytosis. Successful treatment with anti-CD20/rutuximab. Dtsch Med Wochenschr 2001;126:998–1001.
7. Stasi R, Pagano A, Stipa E, et al. Rituximab chimeric anti-CD20 monoclonal antibody treatment for adults with chronic idiopathic thrombocytopenic purpura. Blood 2001;98:952–957.
8. Sackey K. Hemolytic anemia: part 1. Pediatr Rev 1999;20:152–159.
9. Pirofsky B. Autoimmunization and the Autoimmune Hemolytic Anemias. Baltimore, Williams & Wilkins, 1969.
10. Myint H, Copplestone JA, Orchard J, et al. Fludarabine-related autoimmune haemolytic anaemia in patients with chronic lymphocytic leukaemia. Br J Haematol 1995; 91:341–344.

11. Robak T, Blasinska-Morawiec M, Krykowski E, et al. Autoimmune haemolytic anaemia in patients with chronic lymphocytic leukaemia treated with 2-chlorodeoxyadenosine (cladribine). Eur J Haematol 1997;58:109–113.
12. Drobyski WR, Potluri J, Sauer D, et al. Autoimmune hemolytic anemia following T cell-depleted allogeneic bone marrow transplantation. Bone Marrow Transplant 1996;17:1093–1099
13. Sokol RJ, Stamps R, Booker DJ, et al. Posttransplant immune-mediated hemolysis. Transfusion 2002;42:198–204.
14. Beckers EA, van Guvdener C, Overbeeke MA, et al. Intravascular hemolysis by IgA red cell autoantibodies. Neth J Med 2001;58:204–207.
15. Janeway C, Travers P, Walport M, Capra JD (eds). In Immunobiology: the Immune System in Health and Disease, 4th ed. New York, Garland Publishing, 1999.
16. Domen RE. An overview of immune hemolytic anemias. Cleve Clin J Med 1998;65:89–99.
17. Huber H, Polley MJ, Linscott WD, et al. Human monocytes: distinct receptor sites for the third component of complement and for immunoglobulin G. Science 1968;162:1281–1283.
18. LoBuglio AF, Cotran RS, Jandl JH. Red cells coated with immunoglobulin G: binding and sphering by mononuclear cells in man. Science 1967;158:1582–1585.
19. Fleer A, van der Meulen FW, Linthout E, et al. Destruction of IgG-sensitized erythrocytes by human blood monocytes: modulation of inhibition by IgG. Br J Haematol 1978;39:425–436.
20. Schreiber AD, Frank MM. Role of antibody and complement in the immune clearance and destruction of erythrocytes. I. In vivo effects of IgG and IgM complement-fixing sites. J Clin Invest 1972;51:575–582.
21. Schreiber AD, Frank MM. Role of antibody and complement in the immune clearance and destruction of erythrocytes. II. Molecular nature of IgG and IgM complement-fixing sites and effects of their interaction with serum. J Clin Invest 1972;51:583–589.
22. Meite M, Leonard S, Idrissi ME, et al. Exacerbation of autoantibody-mediated hemolytic anemia by viral infection. J Virol 2000;74: 6045–6049.
23. Brown DL, Lachmann PJ, Dacie JV. The in vivo behaviour of complement-coated red cells: studies in C6-deficient, C3-depleted and normal rabbits. Clin Exp Immunol 1970;7:401–421.
24. Munn LR, Chaplin H Jr. Rosette formation by sensitized human red cells—effects of source of peripheral leukocyte monolayers. Vox Sang 1977;33:129–142.
25. Gorst DW, Rawlinson VI, Merry AH, et al. Positive direct antiglobulin test in normal individuals. Vox Sang 1980;38:99–105.
26. Unger LJ. A method for detecting Rho antibodies in extremely low titer. J Lab Clin Med 1951;37:825–837.
27. Issitt PD, et al. Anti-Wrb and other autoantibodies responsible for positive direct antiglobulin tests in 150 individuals. Br J Haematol 1976;34:5–18.
28. Smith MA, Shah NS, Lobel JS. Parvovirus B19 infection associated with reticulocytopenia and chronic autoimmune hemolytic anemia. Am J Pediatr Hematol Oncol 1989;11:167–169.
29. Roush GR, Rosenthal NS, Gerson SL, et al. An unusual case of autoimmune hemolytic anemia with reticulocytopenia, erythroid dysplasia, and an IgG2 autoanti-U. Transfusion 1996;36:575–580.
30. Conley CL, Lippman SM, Ness P. Autoimmune hemolytic anemia with reticulocytopenia. A medical emergency. JAMA 1980;244:1688–1690
31. Conley CL, Lippman SM, Ness PM, et al. Autoimmune hemolytic anemia with reticulocytopenia and erythroid marrow. NEJM 1982;306:281–286
32. Crosby WH, Rappaport H. Reticulocytopenia in autoimmune hemolytic anemia. Blood 1956;11:929–236.
33. Mangan KF, Besa EC, Shadduck RK, et al. Demonstration of two distinct antibodies in autoimmune hemolytic anemia with reticulocytopenia and red cell aplasia. Exp Hematol 1984;12:788–793.
34. Van De Loosdrecht AA, Hendriks DW, Blom NR, et al. Excessive apoptosis of bone marrow erythroblasts in a patient with autoimmune haemolytic anaemia with reticulocytopenia. Br J Haematol 2000;108:313–315.
35. Frank M. NIH conference. Pathophysiology of immune hemolytic anemia. Ann Intern Med 1977;87:210–222.
36. Pruzanski W, Shumak KH. Biologic activity of cold-reacting autoantibodies (first of two parts). NEJM 1977;297:538–542.
37. Crisp D, Pruzanski W. B-cell neoplasms with homogeneous cold-reacting antibodies (cold agglutinins). Am J Med 1982;72:915–922.
38. Silberstein LE, Goldman J, Kant JA, et al. Comparative biochemical and genetic characterization of clonally related human B-cell lines secreting pathogenic anti-Pr2 cold agglutinins. Arch Biochem Biophys 1988;264:244–252.
39. Silberstein LE, Robertson GA, Harris AC, et al. Etiologic aspects of cold agglutinin disease: evidence for cytogenetically defined clones of lymphoid cells and the demonstration that an anti-Pr cold autoantibody is derived from a chromosomally aberrant B cell clone. Blood 1986;67:1705–1709.
40. Rosenthal MC, Pisciotta AV, Komninos ZD, et al. The auto-immune hemolytic anemia of malignant lymphocytic disease. Blood 1955;10: 197–227
41. Hamblin TJ, Oscier DG, Young BJ. Autoimmunity in chronic lymphocytic leukaemia. J Clin Pathol 1986;39:713–716.
42. Sikora K, Krikorian J, Levy R. Monoclonal immunoglobulin rescue from a patient with chronic lymphocytic leukemia and autoimmune hemolytic anemia. Blood 1979;54:513–518.
43. Petz LD. Transfusing the patient with autoimmune hemolytic anemia. Clin Lab Med 1982;2:193–210.
44. Plapp FV, Beck ML. Transfusion support in the management of immune haemolytic disorders. Clin Haematol 1984;13:167–183.
45. Rosenfield RE, Jagathambal. Transfusion therapy for autoimmune hemolytic anemia. Semin Hematol 1976;13:311–321.
46. Sokol RJ, Hewitt S, Booker DJ, et al. Patients with red cell autoantibodies: selection of blood for transfusion. Clin Lab Haematol 1988;10:257–264.
47. Dacie JV, Cutbush M. Specificity of auto-antibodies in acquired haemolytic anaemia. J Clin Pathol 1954;7:18–21.
48. Hogman C, Killander J, Sjolin S. A case of idiopathic auto-immune haemolytic anaemia due to anti-e. Acta Paediatr 1960;49:270–280.
49. Sachs V. Anti-C as a sole autoantibody in autoimmune hemolytic anemia. Transfusion 1985;25:587–588.
50. Weiner W, Battey DA, Cleghorn TE, et al. Serological findings in a case of haemolytic anaemia, with some general observations on the pathogenesis of this syndrome. BMJ 1953;2:125–128.
51. Issitt P, Anstee DJ. In Montgomery (ed). Applied Blood Group Serology, 4th ed. Durham, N.C., Scientific Publications, 1998.
52. James P, Rowe GP, Tozzo GG. Elucidation of alloantibodies in autoimmune haemolytic anaemia. Vox Sang 1988;54:167–171.
53. Laine ML, Beattie KM. Frequency of alloantibodies accompanying autoantibodies. Transfusion 1985;25:545–546.
54. Wallhermfechtel MA, Pohl BA, Chaplin H. Alloimmunization in patients with warm autoantibodies. A retrospective study employing three donor alloabsorptions to aid in antibody detection. Transfusion 1984;24:482–485
55. Mollison PL. Measurement of survival and destruction of red cells in haemolytic syndromes. Br Med Bull 1959;15:59–67.
56. Petz L, Garratty G (ed). Acquired Immune Hemolytic Anemias. New York, Churchill Livingstone, 1980.
57. Gould SA, Rosen AL, Sehgal LR, et al. Fluosol-DA as a red-cell substitute in acute anemia. NEJM 1986;314:1653–1656.
58. Mullon J, Giacoppe G, Clagett C, et al. Transfusions of polymerized bovine hemoglobin in a patient with severe autoimmune hemolytic anemia. NEJM 2000;342: 1638–1643.
59. Klein HG. The prospects for red-cell substitutes. NEJM 2000;342: 1666–1668.
60. Atkinson JP, Schreiber AD, Frank MM. Effects of corticosteroids and splenectomy on the immune clearance and destruction of erythrocytes. J Clin Invest 1973;52:1509–1517
61. Fries LF, Brickman CM, Frank MM. Monocyte receptors for the Fc portion of IgG increase in number in autoimmune hemolytic anemia and other hemolytic states and are decreased by glucocorticoid therapy. J Immunol 1983;131:1240–1245.
62. Schreiber AD. Clinical immunology of the corticosteroids. Prog Clin Immunol 1977;3:103–114.
63. Schreiber AD, Parsons J, McDermott P, et al. Effect of corticosteroids on the human monocyte IgG and complement receptors. J Clin Invest 1975;56:1189–1197.
64. Collins PW, Newland AC. Treatment modalities of autoimmune blood disorders. Semin Hematol 1992;29:64–74.
65. Schwartz SI, Bernard RP, Adams JT, et al. Splenectomy for hematologic disorders. Arch Surg 1970;101:338–247.
66. Committee on Infectious Disease. American Academy of Pediatrics: Red Book: report of the Committee on Infectious Diseases, 24th ed. Elk Grove Village, Ill., American Academy of Pediatrics, 1997.
67. Parker A, MacPherson AI, Richmond J. Value of radiochromium investigation in autoimmune haemolytic anemia. BMJ 1977;6055:208.
68. Gopal AK, Press OW. Clinical applications of anti-CD20 antibodies. J Lab Clin Med 1999;134:445–450.
69. Grillo-Lopez AJ, White CA, Varns C, et al. Overview of the clinical development of rituximab: first monoclonal antibody approved for the treatment of lymphoma. Semin Oncol 1999;26:66–73.
70. Dillman RO. Infusion reactions associated with the therapeutic use of monoclonal antibodies in the treatment of malignancy. Cancer Metastasis Rev 1999;18:465–471.
71. Dillman RO. Monoclonal antibodies in the treatment of malignancy: Basic concepts and recent developments. Cancer Invest 2001;19:833–841.

72. Waldmann T, Levy R, Coller BS. Emerging therapies: spectrum of applications of monoclonal antibody therapy. In Hematology (Am Soc Hematol Educ Program). 2000;394.
73. Hagberg H, Holmbom E. Risk factors for side effects during first infusion of rituximab-definition of a low risk group. Med Oncol 2000; 17:218–221.
74. Berentsen S, Tjonnfjord GE, Brudevold R, et al. Favourable response to therapy with the anti-CD20 monoclonal antibody rituximab in primary chronic cold agglutinin disease. Br J Haematol 2001;115:79–83.
75. Borradori L, Lombardi T, Samson J, et al. Anti-CD20 monoclonal antibody (rituximab) for refractory erosive stomatitis secondary to CD20+ follicular lymphoma-associated paraneoplastic pemphigus. Arch Dermatol 2001;137:269–272.
76. Heizmann M, Itin P, Wernli M, et al. Successful treatment of paraneoplastic pemphigus in follicular NHL with rituximab: report of a case and review of treatment for paraneoplastic pemphigus in NHL and CLL. Am J Hematol 2001;66:142–144.
77. Quartier P, Brethon B, Philippet P, et al. Treatment of childhood autoimmune haemolytic anaemia with rituximab. Lancet 2001;358: 1511–1513.
78. Zecca M, De Stefano P, Nobili B, Locatelli F. Anti-CD20 monoclonal antibody for the treatment of severe, immune-mediated, pure red cell aplasia and hemolytic anemia. Blood 2001;97:3995–3997.
79. Zecca M, Nobili B, Ramenghi U, et al. Rituximab for the treatment of refractory autoimmune hemolytic anemia in children. Blood 2003;101:3857–3861.
80. Besa EC. Rapid transient reversal of anemia and long-term effects of maintenance intravenous immunoglobulin for autoimmune hemolytic anemia in patients with lymphoproliferative disorders. Am J Med 1988;84:691–698.
81. Samuelsson A, Towers TL, Ravetch JV. Anti-inflammatory activity of IVIG mediated through the inhibitory Fc receptor. Science 2001; 291:484–486.
82. Murphy S, LoBuglio AF. Drug therapy of autoimmune hemolytic anemia. Semin Hematol 1976;13:323–334.
83. Fauci AS, Dale DC, Wolff SM. Cyclophosphamide and lymphocyte subpopulations in Wegener's granulomatosis. Arthritis Rheum 1974; 17:355–361.
84. Steinberg A. Cytotoxic drugs in treatment of nonmalignant diseases. Ann Intern Med 1972;76:619–642.
85. Fahey JL. Cancer in the immunosuppressed patient. Ann Intern Med 1971;75:310–312.
86. Floersheim GL. A comparative study of the effects of anti-tumour and immunosuppressive drugs on antibody-forming and erythropoietic cells. Clin Exp Immunol 1970;6:861–870.
87. Miller JJ 3rd, Williams GF, Leissring JC. Multiple late complications of therapy with cyclophosphamide, including ovarian destruction. Am J Med 1971;50:530–535.
88. Qureshi M, Pennington JH, Goldsmith HJ, Cox PE. Cyclophophamide. Lancet 1972;7790:1290.
89. Johnson WW, Meadows DC. Urinary-bladder fibrosis and telangiectasia associated with long-term cyclophosphamide therapy. NEJM 1971;284:290–294.
90. Emilia G, et al. Long-term salvage treatment by cyclosporin in refractory autoimmune haematological disorders. Br J Haematol 1996; 93:341–344.
91. Orlin JB, Berkman EM. Partial plasma exchange using albumin replacement: removal and recovery of normal plasma constituents. Blood 1980;56:1055–1059.
92. Silberstein LE, Berkman EM. Plasma exchange in autoimmune hemolytic anemia (AIHA). J Clin Apher 1983;1:238–242.
93. Kutti J, Wadenvik H, Safai-Kutti S, et al. Successful treatment of refractory autoimmune haemolytic anaemia by plasmapheresis. Scand J Haematol 1984;32:149–152.
94. Rapoport AP, Rowe JM, McMican A. Life-threatening autoimmune hemolytic anemia in a patient with the acquired immune deficiency syndrome. Transfusion 1988;28:190–191.
95. Capra JD, Dowling P, Cook S, et al. An incomplete cold-reactive gamma G antibody with i specificity in infectious mononucleosis. Vox Sang 1969;16:10–17.
96. Rosenfield RE, Schmidt PJ, Calvo RC, et al. Anti-i, a frequent cold agglutinin in infectious mononucleosis. Vox Sang 1965;10:631–634.
97. Silberstein, LE, Shoenfeld Y, Schwartz RS, et al. A combination of IgG and IgM autoantibodies in chronic cold agglutinin disease: Immunologic studies and response to splenectomy. Vox Sang 1985;48: 105–109.
98. Szymanski IO, Teno R, Rybak ME. Hemolytic anemia due to a mixture of low-titer IgG lambda and IgM lambda agglutinins reacting optimally at 22°C. Vox Sang 1986;51:112–116.
99. Tschirhart DL, Kunkel L, Shulman IA. Immune hemolytic anemia associated with biclonal cold autoagglutinins. Vox Sang 1990;59:222–226.
100. Deutsch HF. Properties and modifications of a cryomacroglobulin possessing cold agglutinin activity. Biopolymers 1969;7:21–37.
101. Kuenn JW, Weber R, Teague PO, et al. Cryopathic gangrene with an IgM lambda cryoprecipitating cold agglutinin. Cancer 1978;42: 1826–1833.
102. Tsai CM, Zopf DA, Yu RK, et al. A Waldenström macroglobulin that is both a cold agglutinin and a cryoglobulin because it binds *N*-acetylneuraminosyl residues. Proc Natl Acad Sci USA 1977;74:4591–4594.
103. Umlas J, Kaufman M, MacQueston C, et al. A cryoglobulin with cold agglutinin and erythroid stem cell suppressant properties. Transfusion 1991;31:361–364.
104. Ruddy S, Gigli I, Austen KF. The complement system of man. I. NEJM 1972;287:489–495.
105. Borsos T, Rapp HJ. Complement fixation on cell surfaces by 19S and 7S antibodies. Science 1965;150:505–506.
106. Konig AL, Kather H, Roelcke D. Autoimmune hemolytic anemia by coexisting anti-I and anti-Fl cold agglutinins. Blut 1984;49:363–368.
107. Sokol RJ, Booker DJ, Stamps R. The pathology of autoimmune haemolytic anaemia. J Clin Pathol 1992;45:1047–1052.
108. Abramson N, Gelfand EW, Jandl JH, et al. The interaction between human monocytes and red cells. Specificity for IgG subclasses and IgG fragments. J Exp Med 1970;132:1207–1215.
109. Atkinson JP, Frank MM. Studies on the in vivo effects of antibody. Interaction of IgM antibody and complement in the immune clearance and destruction of erythrocytes in man. J Clin Invest 1974;54:339–348.
110. Ambrus M, Bajtain G. A case of an IgG-type cold agglutinin disease. Haematologia 1969;3:225.
111. Angevine CD, Andersen BR, Barnett EV. A cold agglutinin of the IgA class. J Immunol 1966;96:578–586.
112. Dellagi K, Brouet JC, Schenmetzler C, et al. Chronic hemolytic anemia due to a monoclonal IgG cold agglutinin with anti-Pr specificity. Blood 1981;57:189–191.
113. Garratty G, Petz LD, Brodsky I, et al. An IgA high-titer cold agglutinin with an unusual blood group specificity within the Pr complex. Vox Sang 1973;25:32–38.
114. Moore J, Chaplin H Jr. Autoimmune hemolytic anemia associated with an IgG cold incomplete antibody. Vox Sang 1973;24:236.
115. Pruzanski W, Cowan DH, Parr DM. Clinical and immunochemical studies of IgM cold agglutinins with λ type light chains. Clin Immunol Immunopathol 1974;2:234–245.
116. Shulman IA, et al. Autoimmune hemolytic anemia with both cold and warm autoantibodies. JAMA 1985;253:1746–1748.
117. Silberstein LE, Berkman EM, Schreiber AD. Cold hemagglutinin disease associated with IgG cold-reactive antibody. Ann Intern Med 1987;106:238–242.
118. Tonthat H, et al. A new case of monoclonal IgAκ cold agglutinin with anti-Pr1d specificity in a patient with persistent HB antigen cirrhosis. Vox Sang 1976;30:464–468.
119. Andrzejewski C Jr, Gault E, Briggs M, et al. Benefit of a 37°C extracorporeal circuit in plasma exchange therapy for selected cases with cold agglutinin disease. J Clin Apher 1988;4:13–17.
120. Park JV, Weiss CI. Cardiopulmonary bypass and myocardial protection: management problems in cardiac surgical patients with cold autoimmune disease. Anesth Analg 1988;67:75–78.
121. Hippe E, Jensen KB, Olesen H, et al. Chlorambucil treatment of patients with cold agglutinin syndrome. Blood 1970;35:68–72.
122. Schubothe H. The cold hemagglutinin disease. Semin Hematol 1966;3: 27–47.
123. Berentsen S, Ulvestad E, Gjersten BT, et al. Rituximab for primary chronic cold agglutinin disease: a prospective study of 37 courses of therapy in 27 patients. Blood 2004;103:2925–2928.
124. Godder K, Pati AR, Abhyankar SH, et al. De novo chronic graft-versus-host disease presenting as hemolytic anemia following partially mismatched related donor bone marrow transplant. Bone Marrow Transplant 1997;19:813–817.
125. Gottsche B, Salama A, Mueller-Eckhardt C. Donath-Landsteiner autoimmune hemolytic anemia in children. A study of 22 cases. Vox Sang 1990;58:281–286.
126. Heddle NM. Acute paroxysmal cold hemoglobinuria. Transfus Med Rev 1989;3:219–229.
127. Nordhagen R, Stensvold K, Winsnes A, et al. Paroxysmal cold haemoglobinuria. The most frequent acute autoimmune haemolytic anaemia in children? Acta Paediatr Scand 1984;73:258–262.
128. Hinz D, Picken MD, Lepow IH. Studies on immune human hemolysis II: the Donath-Landsteiner reaction as a model system for studying the mechanism of action of complement and the role of C1 and C1 esterase. J Exp Med 1961;113:193.

129. Levine P, Celano MJ, Falkowski F. The specificity of the antibody in paroxysmal cold hemoglobinuria (PCH). Transfusion 1963;3: 278–280.
130. Worlledge SM, Rousso C. Studies on the serology of paroxysmal cold haemoglobinuria (PGH), with special reference to its relationship with the P blood group system. Vox Sang 1965;10:293–298.
131. Engelfriet CP, Borne AV, Moes M, et al. Serological studies in autoimmune haemolytic anaemia. Bibl Haematol 1968;29:473–478.
132. Judd WJ, Wilkinson SL, Issitt PD, et al. Donath-Landsteiner hemolytic anemia due to an anti-Pr-like biphasic hemolysin. Transfusion 1986;26:423–425.
133. Weiner W, Gordon EG, Rowe D. A Donath-Landsteiner antibody (non-syphilitic type). Vox Sang 1964;9:684–697.
134. Petz LD, Fudenberg HH. Coombs-positive hemolytic anemia caused by penicillin administration. NEJM 1966;274:171–178.
135. Bougie D, Johnson ST, Weitekamp LA, et al. Sensitivity to a metabolite of diclofenac as a cause of acute immune hemolytic anemia. Blood 1997;90:407–413.
136. Salama A, Mueller-Eckhardt C. On the mechanisms of sensitization and attachment of antibodies to RBC in drug-induced immune hemolytic anemia. Blood 1987;69:1006–1010.
137. Carstairs K, Breckenridge A, Dollery CT, Worlledge SM. Incidence of a positive direct Coombs test in patients on alpha-methyldopa. Lancet 1966;7455:133.
138. Petz LD. Drug-induced immune haemolytic anaemia. Clin Haematol 1980;9:455–482.
139. Worlledge SM. Immune drug-induced hemolytic anemias. Semin Hematol 1973;10:327–344.
140. Danielson DA, Douglas SW III, Herzog P, et al. Drug-induced blood disorders. JAMA 1984;252: 3257–3260.
141. Theofilopoulos AN, Dixon FJ. Murine models of systemic lupus erythematosus. Adv Immunol 1985;37:269–390.
142. Okamoto M, Murakami M, Shimizu A, et al. A transgenic model of autoimmune hemolytic anemia. J Exp Med 1992;175:71–79.
143. Sakiyama T, Ikuta K, Nisitani S, et al. Requirement of IL-5 for induction of autoimmune hemolytic anemia in anti-red blood cell autoantibody transgenic mice. Int Immunol 1999;11:995–1000.
144. Nisitani S, Honjo T. Breakage of B cell tolerance and autoantibody production in anti-erythrocyte transgenic mice. Int Rev Immunol 1999;18:259–270.
145. Nisitani S, Sakiyama T, Honjo T. Involvement of IL-10 in induction of autoimmune hemolytic anemia in anti-erythrocyte Ig transgenic mice. Int Immunol 1998;10:1039–1047.
146. Leddy JP, Falany JL, Kissel GE, et al. Erythrocyte membrane proteins reactive with human (warm-reacting) anti-red cell autoantibodies. J Clin Invest 1993;91: 1672–1680.
147. Bloy C, Blanchard D, Lambin P, et al. Human monoclonal antibody against Rh(D) antigen: partial characterization of the Rh(D) polypeptide from human erythrocytes. Blood 1987;69:1491–1497.
148. Lane HC, Masur H, Edgar LC, et al. Abnormalities of B-cell activation and immunoregulation in patients with the acquired immunodeficiency syndrome. NEJM 1983;309:453–458.
149. Kipps TJ, Carson DA. Autoantibodies in chronic lymphocytic leukemia and related systemic autoimmune diseases. Blood 1993;81:2475–2487.
150. Leddy JP, Bakemeier RF. Structural aspects of human erythrocyte autoantibodies. I. L chain types and electrophoretic dispersion. J Exp Med 1965;121:1–17.
151. Masouredis SP, Branks MJ, Victoria EJ. Antiidiotypic IgG crossreactive with Rh alloantibodies in red cell autoimmunity. Blood 1987;70: 710–715.
152. Hakomori S. Blood group ABH and Ii antigens of human erythrocytes: Chemistry, polymorphism, and their developmental change. Semin Hematol 1981;18:39–62.
153. Stevenson FK, Smith GJ, North J, et al. Identification of normal B-cell counterparts of neoplastic cells which secrete cold agglutinins of anti-I and anti-i specificity. Br J Haematol 1989;72:9–15.
154. Costea N, Yakulis VJ, Heller P. Inhibition of cold agglutinins (anti-I) by *M. pneumoniae* antigens. Proc Soc Exp Biol Med 1972;139:476–479.
155. Pascual V, Victor K, Lelsz D, et al. Nucleotide sequence analysis of the V regions of two IgM cold agglutinins. Evidence that the VH_{4-21} gene segment is responsible for the major cross-reactive idiotype. J Immunol 1991;146:4385–4391.
156. Silberstein LE, Jefferies LC, Goldman J, et al. Variable region gene analysis of pathologic human autoantibodies to the related i and I red blood cell antigens. Blood 1991;78:2372–2386.
157. Stevenson FK, Spellerberg MB, Treasure J, et al. Differential usage of an Ig heavy chain variable region gene by human B-cell tumors. Blood 1993;82:224–230.
158. Perrotta S, Locatelli F, La Manna A, et al. Anti-CD20 monoclonal anti body (rituximab) for life-threatening autoimmune haemolytic anaemia in a patient with systemic lupus erythematosus. Br J Haematol 2002;116:465–467.
159. Motto DG, Williams JA, Boxer LA. Rituximab for refractory childhood autoimmune hemolytic anemia. Isr Med Assoc J 2002;4:1006–1008.
160. McMahon C, Babu L, Hodgson A, et al. Childhood refractory autoimmune haemolytic anaemia: is there a role for anti-CD20 therapy (rituximab)? Br J Haematol 2002;117:480–483.
161. Zaja F, Iacona I, Masolini P, et al. B-cell depletion with rituximab as treatment for immune hemolytic anemia and chronic thrombocytopenia. Haematologica 2002;87:189–195.
162. Corti P, Bonanomi S, Vallinoto C, et al. Rituximab for immune hemolytic anemia following T- and B-cell-depleted hematopoietic stem cell transplantation. Acta Haematol 2003;109:43–45.
163. Hongeng S, Tardtong P, Worapongpaiboon S, et al. Successful treatment of refractory autoimmune haemolytic anaemia in a post-unrelated bone marrow transplant paediatric patient with rituximab. Bone Marrow Transplant 2002;29:871–872.
164. Ship A, May W, Lucas K. Anti-CD20 monoclonal antibody therapy for autoimmune hemolytic anemia following T cell-depleted, haplo-identical stem cell transplantation. Bone Marrow Transplant 2002;29: 365–366.
165. Lee EJ, Kueck B. Rituxan in the treatment of cold agglutinin disease. Blood 1998;92:3490–3491.
166. Layios N, Van Den NE, Jost E, et al. Remission of severe cold agglutinin disease after rituximab therapy. Leukemia 2001;15:187–188.
167. Zaja F, Russo D, Fuga G, et al. Rituximab in a case of cold agglutinin disease. Br J Haematol 2001;115:232–233.
168. Bauduer F. Rituximab: A very efficient therapy in cold agglutinins and refractory autoimmune haemolytic anaemia associated with CD20-positive, low-grade non-Hodgkin's lymphoma. Br J Haematol 2001;112:1085–1086.
169. Chemnitz J, Draube A, Diehl V, Wolf J. Successful treatment of steroid and cyclophosphamide-resistant hemolysis in chronic lymphocytic leukemia with rituximab. Am J Hematol 2002;69:232–233.
170. Pulik M, Genet P, Lionnet F, Touahri T. Treatment of primary chronic cold agglutinin disease with rituximab: maintenance therapy may improve the results. Br J Haematol 2002;117:998–999.
171. Engelhardt M, Jakob A, Ruter B, et al. Severe cold hemagglutinin disease (CHD) successfully treated with rituximab. Blood 2002;100:1922–1923.
172. Gharib M, Poynton C. Complete, long-term remission of refractory idiopathic cold haemagglutinin disease after Mabthera. Br J Haematol 2002;117:248–249.
173. Berentsen S, Tjonnfjord GE, Brudevold R, et al. Favourable response to therapy with the anti-CD20 monoclonal antibody rituximab in primary chronic cold agglutinin disease. Br J Haematol 2001; 115:79–83.
174. Gupta N, Kavuru S, Patel D, et al. Rituximab-based chemotherapy for steroid-refractory autoimmune hemolytic anemia of chronic lymphocytic leukemia. Leukemia 2002;16:2092–2095.

Chapter 42

Transfusion in Economically Restricted and Developing Countries

Audrey N. Schuetz • Kenneth A. Clark

Until the human immunodeficiency virus (HIV) pandemic in the 1980s, transfusion services in many economically restricted countries remained poorly developed, primarily due to economic constraints. With the institution of HIV testing in 1985 in the United States and in other developed countries, economically restricted countries were encouraged to place a stronger focus on transfusion safety practices. Although transfusion safety has improved somewhat over the past few decades, many economically restricted countries continue to struggle with inadequate resources and infrastructure that hinder establishment of a safer blood supply. According to the World Health Organization (WHO), only 20% of the worldwide supply of safe and screened blood is available to people living in economically restricted countries, where approximately 80% of the world's population resides.[1,2]

Enforcement of a successful transfusion service depends on several levels of commitment, from the government administration to the staff delivering the blood. Optimally, blood transfusion services consist of education, recruitment and adequate selection of safe blood donors; collection, processing, and storage of blood products; performance of serologic and other tests on the products before transfusion at the collection facility; and, finally, transportation and subsequent release of the blood to patients with appropriate need for transfusion.

Commitment of governments to a well-developed and organized blood transfusion service is the first key to sustainable and successful blood transfusion systems. Many economically restricted countries are faced with a high disease burden but lack the infrastructure to address the problem. Various organizational structures of blood services are described in this chapter, as is the commitment of the WHO to worldwide blood safety.

A second key to optimizing blood transfusion services includes selection of safe blood donors by recruitment of nonremunerated (*nonpaid or voluntary*) individuals. In the developed world, donor screening focuses on excluding individuals who carry a higher "risk" of infectious disease than the general population; such individuals include intravenous drug users, men who have sex with men, and commercial sex workers. In economically restricted countries, such as Africa, where heterosexual transmission has accounted for as much as 80% of all HIV infections, such focused donor screening is less effective.[3,4] A strategy employed by economically restricted countries to select safe blood donors involves predonation laboratory testing of blood with rapid diagnostic tests.

In the third place, proper laboratory testing of donated blood and adequate record keeping present challenges to blood centers with financial and logistical restrictions. Testing and storage of blood is limited by the lack of reliable sources of electricity and refrigeration, as well as by the cost of machinery, reagents, and testing kits.

Finally, transfusion safety relies on appropriate blood administration to recipients. Given the difficulties in donor screening and laboratory testing of blood, consideration must be given to balancing the risk of exposure to a transfusion-transmitted infection versus the risk of no transfusion. Furthermore, because children comprise the largest proportion of transfusion recipients in certain regions and pregnancy- or malaria-associated anemia also rank among the highest indications for transfusion in many economically restricted countries, the morbidity and mortality associated with a transfusion-transmitted infection may be potentially high among certain populations.

Although two decades have passed since relatively simple HIV tests became available to screen blood donors and products, the lack of economic and political resources has compromised the blood supply in many areas of the world. The overwhelming challenges are evident when faced with the fact that approximately 10% of all acquired immunodeficiency syndrome (AIDS) cases in certain areas of the world are transfusion associated.[5,6] However, improvements have already begun; Zimbabwe was the third country in the world to routinely test donated blood for HIV.[7] Various organizations are currently gathering data on methods to improve governmental infrastructure, to understand disease epidemiology, and to adjust current transfusion practices and attitudes toward blood safety in economically restricted countries.

GOVERNMENTAL ORGANIZATION OF BLOOD SERVICES

Development and organization of blood transfusion services in economically restricted countries has not only lagged behind blood services in developed countries but has also lagged behind other parts of the health care system as well.[8] The sustainability of high-quality transfusion systems in economically restricted countries is best achieved with national oversight and a national commitment to safe blood transfusion as part of the health care system. The WHO claims that a well-organized blood transfusion service is a prerequisite

Table 42–1 Key Organizational Elements of a National Blood Transfusion Service

Formalization of government commitment and support
Establishment of a national blood policy or plan
Establishment of legal authority through legal or regulatory framework
Establishment of a responsible organization to oversee and implement the national blood transfusion service
Appointment of a national blood service medical director, a quality manager, and appropriate advisory groups
Development of financial and budgetary systems to ensure sustainability of the national transfusion service
Establishment of a national quality system[9]

for the safe and effective use of blood products while emphasizing government commitment as a strategic priority.[9,10] The WHO also recommends that governments establish blood transfusion services as a separate entity with an adequate budget, effective management, and trained staff.[9,11]

The key organizational elements of a national blood transfusion service in an economically restricted country, as suggested by the WHO, are listed in Table 42–1. Organization of blood services varies considerably throughout the world with regard to geographic regions and availability of resources. The organizational structure of blood services is outlined in Table 42–2.

Several types of organizational blood banking structures operate worldwide. Hospital-based systems predominate in economically restricted countries; centralized or regionalized blood transfusion systems operate largely in developed countries.[12,14,15] In sub-Saharan Africa, where blood services are predominantly hospital-based, blood transfusion systems are moving toward a more centralized or regionalized approach in countries such as South Africa, Uganda, Kenya, Zimbabwe, and Togo.[16] In addition, some northern African countries bordering the Mediterranean Sea have made considerable progress toward centralization. Centralized blood collection systems are more advantageous than small hospital-based systems, because they have a greater number of highly trained specialists with the ability to handle a larger number of blood units.[17] In contrast, blood programs in economically restricted areas of South and Central America are largely decentralized, some to a high degree. For example, Argentina has more than 1000 blood banks.[18–20] A similar situation exists in economically restricted areas of Southeast Asia, where there is extensive decentralization of the blood system.[18]

Blood services in economically restricted countries, just as in more developed countries, should be defined by a legal framework that states the national blood policy and describes the processes governing the collection, processing, and transfusion of blood.[21–23] A variety of organizations collect and process the blood in economically restricted countries, typically including the ministries of health, social security systems, the armed forces, private organizations, and nongovernmental organizations. Blood transfusion services, which oversee the delivery of blood products to patients, are usually operated by health care facilities, such as hospitals.[19]

The WHO recommends that governments of economically restricted countries take responsibility to ensure a safe and adequate blood supply. Indicating the need for national support of blood transfusion programs, the 58th World Health Assembly (WHA) passed resolution WHA58.13 in May 2005, urging member states to support full implementation of well-organized, nationally coordinated, and sustainable blood programs with appropriate regulatory systems.[24] In particular, the resolution advocated government commitment and support for national blood programs with quality management systems, by means of a legal framework and a national blood safety policy and plan. Many economically restricted countries have made significant organizational advances in the past decade, but improvements are still required.

BLOOD DONOR RECRUITMENT, SELECTION, AND SCREENING

In 1975, the WHA adopted Resolution WHA28.72, which required its members to promote the development of national transfusion services based on the use of voluntary, nonpaid blood donors.[2,25] Replacement donors are recruited from among the family or relatives of hospitalized patients who require blood transfusions. A number of studies have shown that voluntary donors often have a lower prevalence and incidence of infectious transfusion-transmitted diseases than do family/replacement donors and paid donors.[17,26–33] In Kenya, a study comparing volunteer donors from mobile blood units with donors recruited by family members showed that HIV seroprevalence among voluntary donors was significantly lower than among family-recruited donors (1.7% and 9.1%, respectively; odds ratio, 5.9).[34] Information collected in the Global Database on Blood Safety has repeatedly shown the importance of recruiting voluntary blood donors.[35]

Blood centers in sub-Saharan Africa routinely rely on family/replacement or paid donors for a significant percentage of their blood collection needs, often due to shortages in supply of donor blood in the blood banks. A lack of resources to train personnel and to provide transport for mobile blood campaigns contributes to blood shortages as well. From 50% to 70% of donations are collected from family/replacement and paid donors worldwide, often in countries with relatively high prevalence of HIV, hepatitis B virus (HBV),

Table 42–2 Organizational Structure of Blood Services

Centralized	One national blood center operates the blood services for the country, with or without regional blood centers.
Regionalized	The country is divided into regions of varying degrees of autonomy, with different mechanisms to achieve national coordination.
Hospital-based	Each hospital operates its own blood collection and processing system, with or without national control.
Combination of above	There may be a national blood transfusion system, but hospitals may find the national coverage unsatisfactory and choose to operate their own systems.[12,13]

and hepatitis C virus (HCV) infection.[25,36,37] A blood bank in Armenia reported that 12% of the 1010 units of whole blood collected in 2004 were drawn from paid donors, and 88% were drawn from patient relatives (JB Gorlin, personal communication, November 17, 2005).

Although the WHA resolution has not been fully adopted in many economically restricted countries despite its implementation more than a quarter-century ago, progress has been made. By the year 2000, 39 of the 192 WHA member states had achieved 100% voluntary, nonremunerated blood donation.[24] Approximately 40% of the 30.2 million blood donations performed in 1999 in economically restricted countries were obtained from low-risk voluntary donors. One of the blood banks in Armenia has, for the first time, organized blood drives and collected 172 units of blood from volunteer donors, including medical students (JB Gorlin, personal communication, November 17, 2005).

To emphasize these problems, the WHA reiterated the call for encouraging voluntary blood donations in resolution WHA58.13.[24] Some countries have reported that elimination of paid donors has paralleled a decline in the seroprevalence of HIV in individuals who present for blood donation.[20,38–40] Although recruitment of voluntary blood donors is costly and difficult, marketing strategies aimed at increasing the proportion of repeat voluntary donors have met success in countries such as Venezuela, Nicaragua, and Cuba.[41,42]

Donor Selection

Despite inherent difficulties in selecting donors in areas of high prevalence of infectious diseases, donor recruiters in economically restricted countries have attempted to identify effective risk factor deferral criteria using medical history, demographic information, and social history.[43–54] In sub-Saharan Africa, age has been used as a surrogate marker for infectious risk. Although the age for peak seroprevalence of HIV varies in different regions in sub-Saharan Africa, peak seroprevalence of HIV is typically age 15 to 29 in women and age 25 to 39 in men.[55] Therefore, recruitment of donors has shifted to secondary school students and older adults in such areas of the world.

Another potential surrogate marker for donor infectious risk is demographic status. In general, HIV prevalence is lower in rural populations than in urban centers.[56] However, recruitment of rural donors can be difficult and is more expensive due to limited transportation infrastructure and potentially lower levels of nutritional health, which result in higher rates of anemia.[30]

One study reported that blood donor self-deferral can reduce the risk of HIV transmission through blood transfusion.[57] Self-deferred donors demonstrated significantly higher rates of HIV, HBV, and HCV as compared to general donors.

In an effort to circumvent the problem of identifying a suitable low-risk donor population by risk-deferral screening, donor recruitment activity often focuses on secondary schools, selected businesses, churches, and repeat-donor clubs. For example, in Zimbabwe, attempts have been made to collect blood only from individuals with a recent prior blood donation history and to establish repeat-donor groups.[37]

Because funding and resources for mobile donor recruitment are limited, blood centers are often forced to rely on family/replacement donors to fill the available blood deficit.

Predonation Testing

Worldwide, prospective blood donors are screened for transfusion-transmissible diseases. In addition, adequate hematocrit should also be assessed. The high prevalence of anemia often contributes to a dearth of eligible blood donors, such as at a transfusion center in Nigeria, where 75% of donors were rejected for anemia alone.[58]

In certain countries, blood services and hospitals test donors for HIV and other infectious disease markers by rapid test methods before donation. Proponents of predonation testing argue that the advantages of pretesting in areas of high prevalence of HIV, HBV, and HCV, such as in sub-Saharan Africa, outweigh the disadvantages. Advantages of pretesting include:

1. Savings on the cost of blood collection bags and waste disposal
2. Savings on the cost of the equipment and supplies needed for postdonation enzyme immunoassay testing
3. Fewer units of stored blood to include only screen-negative units
4. The ability to quickly inform deferred donors of their test results in regions where mail and telephone communication is poor and the likelihood of repeat donation is low[59,60]

Collection centers in populations with high infectious disease prevalence may find predonation testing strategies attractive from a cost- and resource-savings perspective.

High prevalence of infectious diseases in donors not only compounds the risk to the recipient, but also increases the overall cost of the transfusion product. Because blood collection bags represent as much as one third of the blood bank budget, money is wasted on bags thrown away due to infected donors.[35] Rates of donor deferral after laboratory screening, based on a positive infectious disease result in the donor, may exceed 10%. Positive HBV surface antigen (HBsAg) tests on donor units accounted for more than half of the discarded units in one Ghanaian study.[60] The decrease in cost associated with predonation screening may be significant when transfusion-transmitted infection prevalence among donors reaches 15% to 20%.[59] Well-organized blood safety programs that depend mainly on voluntary, nonremunerated blood donors should expect discard rates of less than 10%, even in areas with high infectious disease prevalence.

Even though prescreening donor units may be economical, it poses a challenge when used to prescreen for HIV or hepatitis, particularly in sub-Saharan Africa.[61–63] Most often performed in blood collection sites in small rural hospitals and clinics, predonation testing may be troublesome due to the lack of qualified staff, organized recruitment system for volunteer donors, or quality management system. In many countries, low-skilled technicians may perform donor prescreening with rapid tests and may not have the skills to perform more complex tests for follow-up or to guarantee that the other basic operations and functions of a proper transfusion service are carried out.[59] Counseling and physician referral of positive donors may not routinely take place; when performed, counseling may be inadequate due to insufficiently trained staff.

Caution must be exercised while practicing predonation testing, because blood transfusion centers have the potential to become test sites for persons who simply wish to know their HIV status.[64] Voluntary counseling and testing (VCT) centers in many economically restricted countries with high HIV prevalence enable persons to discover their HIV status and provide them with counseling and prevention advice. Blood centers that prescreen donors may themselves be at risk of becoming alternative VCT centers. Some persons may choose to be tested at blood transfusion centers, rather than at VCT centers, due to a lower perceived stigma in visiting a blood collection center. Blood centers that prescreen donors may attract persons who primarily wish to know their HIV status and, by inference, have high-risk behaviors. If an error occurs in the testing procedures and an infected person is overlooked, blood donations from such individuals could compromise the safety of the blood supply. For this reason, efforts should be made to separate the process of blood donation from determination of infection status.

Another disadvantage of the predonation testing process is the disqualification of many donors at the donation site. In areas of high HIV prevalence, the public may be suspicious that any deferral is due to a positive HIV test result. Therefore, the donor or public may consider any deferral, even for a low hemoglobin value, as synonymous with HIV positivity. The stigma attached to this label is well known and significant.[59]

Most importantly, adoption of the practice of predonation testing by itself does not address the larger obligation of blood centers to establish a reliable donor recruitment system. Because clinicians may transfuse blood from prescreened donors very soon after collection, sometimes without the support of additional postdonation testing, a safe pool of volunteer donors is important. In many economically restricted countries, few organized blood donor recruitment systems with networks of repeat donors exist.

Rather than accepting high-risk donors as the norm, an organized blood donation system should attempt to develop strong programs of donor recruitment and selection, with strong quality management. The optimal blood donation practice would only allow blood collection facilities with a sufficient scale of operation and with sufficient numbers of qualified staff to properly collect blood from a network of low-risk blood donors. The development of a pool of safe and reliable donors should be a primary goal for blood transfusion safety programs in economically restricted countries.

INFECTIOUS DISEASE TESTING OF BLOOD

In the practice of transfusion safety, laboratory testing of donated blood provides the link between choice of a suitable blood donor and appropriate transfusion to the recipient. Regional epidemiologic data guide the choice of infectious disease testing. Globally, the major mode of HIV transmission is sexual, and HIV tests have become the cornerstone of testing in many economically restricted countries. HIV, HCV, and HBV are 10 to 100 times more prevalent in Tanzania, for example, than in many developed countries.[65] Blood banks in Latin America screen for the parasite *Trypanosoma cruzi*, the etiologic agent of Chagas disease, which infects an estimated 18 to 24 million people in Latin America.[66]

The choice of screening assays by the blood bank or laboratory depends not only on the region's infectious disease epidemiology, but also on the quality and types of assays available. Financial and logistical limitations may also limit the choice of an assay. A detailed description of infectious disease blood screening assays is offered elsewhere in this textbook (see Chapters 14 and 43–48). Here we present an overview of some screening methods practiced in economically restricted countries.

Rates of Infectious Disease Screening

Despite differences in disease epidemiology and financial resources between countries, the WHO strategy for laboratory screening of blood recommends HIV, HBV, and syphilis screening of all donated blood and, when appropriate, screening for HCV, malaria, and Chagas disease.[25] Yet, according to the WHO's Global Database on Blood Safety, less than 60% of economically restricted countries screen all their blood for HIV and even fewer countries screen for HBV or HCV.[25] Among the 75 million donations per year worldwide, 30 million are collected in economically restricted countries, where only 43% of the blood supply is screened for HIV, HBV, HCV, syphilis, and Chagas disease.[67] Based on those figures, approximately 12.9 million donations (17% of annual blood donations worldwide) are potentially infectious for HIV, HBV, HCV, syphilis, and/or *T. cruzi*. The WHO estimates that in 2002, 90% of blood donations in Africa were screened for HIV, whereas only 40% were screened for HCV.[68] In sub-Saharan Africa, only one half of the blood supply is currently screened for HBV.[69] Brazilian blood banks report low rates of screening for HTLV and HBV core antibody, ranging from 17% to 60%.[70,71]

Although the WHO standard has not yet been reached, much progress has been made. By 1998, the number of blood donors in Uruguay with Chagas disease was negligible, in part due to 100% compulsory blood screening.[72] Reports of blood donor screening in Latin America show that greater than 95% of the blood units are tested for HIV, HCV, and HBV; Costa Rica, Mexico, and Panama report the lowest numbers of units screened for *T. cruzi*.[20,22,38,73] However, some Latin American countries, such as Colombia and some areas of Argentina, report low rates of screening.[74,75] According to the Pan American Health Organization (PAHO), the countries of Latin America and the Caribbean collected approximately 6 million units of blood in 1999, of which approximately 99% underwent screening for HIV and HBV and 94% for HCV.[38] In 2001, despite an increase of 14% in the number of units collected as compared to 1999, greater than 99.9% screening coverage for HIV, HBV, and HCV continued in Latin America and the Caribbean.[38] A 1994 study in India claimed that only 25% to 75% of blood donations were being screened for HIV.[76] However, by 2000, a nationwide study of 604 blood banks in India reported 95% screening coverage for HIV, 94% for syphilis, 87% for HBV, 67% for malaria, and 6% for HCV.[77] Accurate data on rates of blood bank screening are difficult to obtain and vary according to region but are nonetheless important in assessing safety of donated blood.

Infectious Disease Screening Tests

In general, screening tests for HIV antibodies, HBsAg, and HCV are performed with enzyme immunoassay (EIA) test kits. Polymerase chain reaction testing and HIV p24 antigen testing are usually not affordable, nor are they logistically appropriate for use in most economically restricted countries.

Although most countries screen their blood supply for antibodies to HIV-1 and HIV-2, some regions are exploring other diagnostic methods. Rapid HIV testing may be an adjunct to predonation screening or a field alternative to technical laboratory testing. The HIVCHEK rapid test, an instrument-free, single-unit system that can be stored at ambient temperature, was judged suitable for use in underequipped transfusion centers when tested in the Democratic Republic of Congo.[61] Nucleic acid amplification testing (NAT), which effectively identifies infectious donations in the preseroconversion window period, was compared to the traditional HIV antibody test and the p24 antigen test in South Africa, an area where HIV-1 infection is endemic.[78] In the South Africa study, researchers found that implementation of NAT in addition to HIV antibody screening allowed discovery of only an additional 17 to 23 HIV-positive donations per year if p24 antigen testing were eliminated from the screening regimen. The cost-benefit ratio of introducing an expensive technology, such as NAT, in an economically restricted country merits further assessment.

The high HIV prevalence in the general population in some economically restricted countries increases the probability of false-negative tests. Although the EIA tests most commonly used for antibody screening are highly sensitive, window period donation incurs residual risks of infection. Researchers estimate that the rate of transfusion-associated transmission of HIV due to window period donation in South Africa ranges from 1:25,641 to 1:90,909 tested units, which is 10 times greater than the rate of laboratory false negatives.[78] Two of the three probable transfusion-transmitted HIV cases that were reported to the hemovigilance program in 2003 in South Africa occurred during the window period of infectivity.[79]

Some countries across the globe have reported an increase in the prevalence of infectious disease markers, which could be due in part to an improvement in the sensitivity of screening markers. In Thailand, the prevalence of HIV in the supply of donated blood rose from 0.0065% in 1987 to 0.95% in 1993.[80] A review of blood donor screening results in India from 1996 to 2001 showed an increase in the prevalence of HIV from 0.16% in 1996 to 0.3% in 2002.[81]

See Table 42–3 for prevalence data on infectious disease markers in selected studies. The prevalence of serologic markers for HIV, HBV, HCV, and *T. cruzi* in many Latin American countries was extensively reviewed by the PAHO.[20] Refer to the PAHO article by Schmunis and Cruz for a complete review of seroprevalence rates among blood donors in Latin America.

Hepatitis C virus presents a significant public health problem, with major associated morbidity and mortality in both developed and economically restricted areas of the world. In Korea, where mortality due to liver cancer ranks high worldwide, the prevalence of anti-HCV among Koreans older than age 40 was 1.29%, with blood transfusion as the strongest risk factor for transmission of HCV.[102]

Investigators from a major hospital in Ghana, where the prevalence of HBV in blood donors was 8% to 15%, compared three HBV screening assays (HBsAg latex agglutination, HBsAg dipstick, and HBsAg enzyme immunoassay) in blood donors.[69] The latex agglutination and dipstick assays, which are used in Africa due to their low cost and flexibility, had low sensitivities of 54% and 71%, respectively, but they continue to be used in many areas of the world.

Table 42–3 Percentage Prevalence of Infectious Diseases among Blood Donors in Selected Countries

Location	HIV	HCV	HBV	Syphilis	HTLV	*T. cruzi*	Reference No.
Cameroon	7.9†	4.8†	10.7†	9.1†	1.6†		82
Ghana			8–15*				69
Ivory Coast	2.1						83
Kenya	6–9.3	0					84,85
Nigeria			1.6				86
Tanzania	8.7	8.0	11–20	12.7	0		45
Zambia	15.9						87
India	0.86			0.95			88
	0.3	0.4	0.99	0.1–0.7			81
		0.25–0.9*	1.7–2.2*				89
China		1.1	3.1				90
	9.1–17						91,92
					0.2		93
Thailand	0.9						80
					0		94
	2.2†						95
		1.4†					96
Armenia		3–6	1–2				Gorlin§
Georgia		6.9–7.8‡					97,98
Saudi Arabia	0	0.4	1.5		0		99
Turkey		0.2	1.5				100
Bolivia	0.04	0.3	0.6			9.9	20
Chile	0.03	0.1	0.07			0.5	20
Colombia	0.5	1.1	0.62			0.1	20
Guatemala	0.5	0.8	1.1			1.0	20
Venezuela					0.1		101

† Voluntary donors.
* Majority replacement donors.
‡ 100% paid or replacement donors.
§ JB Gorlin, personal communication, November 17, 2005.

In contrast to developed countries, economically restricted countries continue to rely on syphilis testing as a means of disease screening. Both the reagin tests, such as the Venereal Disease Research Laboratory (VDRL) test, and the treponemal tests, such as the *Treponema pallidum* hemagglutination assay (TPHA-FTA ABS), detect syphilis antibodies. Some countries with a low prevalence of syphilis use TPHA-FTA ABS, because its sensitivity and specificity are higher than those of the reagin tests.[103,104] Yet, the TPHA-FTA ABS costs more and is more complex than the reagin tests. In countries with high syphilis prevalence, the VDRL test may be more appropriate in diagnosing the infectious phase of syphilis. In Thailand, at a clinic for laborers, HIV-1 seropositivity correlated positively with positive TPHA-FTA ABS results, with an odds ratio of 1.8 ($p = 0.015$).[105] Such findings support the continued use of syphilis screening as both a marker for other diseases and as a means of disease diagnosis in economically restricted countries.

Antibody testing for HTLV-I, the etiologic agent of adult T-cell leukemia, is generally not performed in economically restricted countries. HTLV-I is endemic in southwest Japan, the Caribbean, Central and South America, sub-Saharan Africa, Papua New Guinea, Australia, the Solomon Islands, and western Asia but is not a required test in many of these regions.[106,107]

Screening for Chagas disease in endemic areas of Latin America is performed using EIA methods to detect *T. cruzi* antibodies. The main serologic methods for identification of *T. cruzi* antibodies are the indirect hemagglutination assay, the indirect immunofluorescence assay, and the enzyme-linked immunosorbent assay (ELISA). The indirect hemagglutination assay, although easy to perform and widely used, is the least sensitive of the three tests.[108,109] Blood centers in Brazil most often use the ELISA, according to a series of external quality control assessments of blood bank laboratories performed in 1999 and 2000.[108] The use of two different screening methods, most often the combination of an ELISA test and an indirect hemagglutination test, minimizes the risk of false negatives.[108,110] The indirect immunofluorescence assay is less commonly used.

Although recommended in malaria-endemic areas, malaria screening in very high prevalence areas, such as sub-Saharan Africa, is neither practical nor effective, because the majority of donors and recipients would test positive. In areas of low malaria prevalence, such as Southeast Asia, malaria screening with Geimsa-stained blood films is common but not universal.

Cytomegalovirus (CMV) antibody testing also is not routinely performed in the economically restricted world, and very few studies are available on its use. In a recent study in India, none of the 200 voluntary blood donors in Delhi tested positive for CMV immunoglobulin M (IgM) antibody, but 95% were positive for CMV IgG antibody.[111] Testing of donors would be superfluous, because very few seronegative blood units would be available for transfusion.

Very few studies on human herpes virus-8 (HHV-8) have been performed in economically restricted countries. HHV-8 antibodies among 306 blood donors in South Africa were present in 2% to 10% of individuals, with increasing prevalence with age.[112] Because the seropositivity for HHV-8 was relatively high in these blood donors, screening for this herpesvirus may be useful, given the association between HHV-8 and Kaposi sarcoma.

Finally, although hundreds of cases of human infection with *Babesia* spp. have been reported in the United States, only a few cases have been described in China, Egypt, Mexico, South Africa, and Taiwan, currently indicating a low need for *Babesia* screening in economically restricted countries.[113]

Other potential laboratory surrogate markers for infectious disease risk have been examined in economically restricted countries, such as serum alanine aminotransferase (ALT) levels, yet they have met with limited success. Studies of serum ALT in Indian blood donors have shown no correlation with viral seropositivity of HBV, HCV, HIV, or CMV.[114]

Transfusion-Associated Infectious Risks

Transfusion-transmitted infections are among the largest risks of receiving a blood transfusion in economically restricted countries. Among the infectious diseases, HIV has one of the most serious adverse consequences. In contrast to data from the United States, where significantly less than 1% of HIV infections are estimated to be transfusion transmitted, data from economically restricted countries show that 5% to 10% of new and existing HIV infections are due to blood transfusion.[31,115–117]

Although estimates on transfusion-transmitted HIV proved difficult to gather during the early stages of the AIDS epidemic, as many as 25% of HIV-infected children and women in Africa are believed to have acquired HIV from blood transfusions.[118–120] McFarland and colleagues estimate that in sub-Saharan Africa alone, 25% of pediatric AIDS cases, 20% of adult female AIDS cases, and 10% of all other AIDS cases may be associated with transfusion.[121] Blood transfusions in sub-Saharan Africa rank third among modes of HIV transmission, most notably affecting children under age 5.[122,123] In the Caribbean, 1.1% of AIDS cases are due to blood transfusion.[124] In Brazilian blood donors, a history of blood transfusion is thought to be the etiology in 15% of HCV-positive cases.[125] Transfusion before 1992 is considered to be the major route of transmission for HCV in Japan.[126]

The risk of receiving HIV-positive blood in Africa ranges from less than 1% to more than 20% per unit of blood, depending on the country studied.[6] In a 2001 survey of 1482 blood units in six government hospitals in Kenya, 31 (~2%) units tested HIV-positive on follow-up at the reference laboratory, of which 14 had tested negative by the hospital and were not removed from the blood supply.[34] HIV test results for 1290 donor–recipient pairs showed that 26 of the 31 HIV-positive donations had been given to individuals who were HIV-negative before transfusion. As a result, the estimated HIV transmission rate was 2% in these hospitals. In 1985 in Kinshasa, Democratic Republic of Congo, 561 HIV-positive blood units were transfused to children in one pediatric hospital ward.[127]

Studies continue to show unacceptably high rates of HIV transmission from blood transfusion. In a pediatric tertiary care center in India, 33 of the 285 HIV-positive children were infected through blood transfusion from 1994 to 2001.[128] A study in rural China in a region with a large percentage of paid donors showed that 1% of the 115 HIV-positive residents obtained infection through blood transfusion.[129] Finally, in a consecutive survey of 222 women at prenatal and pediatric clinics who had received transfusions between 1980 and 1985 in Kigali, Rwanda, HIV seroprevalence was

45%, compared to 28% in nontransfused women presenting to the clinics.[130]

The probability of seroconversion from transfusion with a single HIV-positive unit of blood is 90%.[131] The risk of HIV from a screened unit of blood in Ivory Coast in 1992 was two to three times greater than the risk of acquiring HIV from a seropositive needlestick exposure.[132,133] Approximately 142 to 276 units of potentially infected blood units were transfused annually in the early 1990s in the Ivory Coast, despite routine testing.

Paid plasma donors are becoming an increasingly recognized reservoir of infection in the blood bank community. Paid donors typically become infected at plasmapheresis centers through unsafe practices, such as the use of nonsterile needles, sharing of intravenous lines, and injection of donors with blood to hyperimmunize them for anti-Rh_o and serum typing production.[134,135] Unlicensed plasmapheresis centers began appearing in the 1990s in China, where poor peasants in communities with few risk factors for HIV began selling their plasma at unsanitary centers and became subsequently infected.[90,136] Some of these centers directly contributed to spread of disease in donors through the pooling of blood from donors of the same ABO type before returning the red cells to each donor. High rates of HIV seropositivity have been discovered among repeat blood donors, especially paid donors.[137,138] At one illegal plasma collection site discovered in central China between 1998 and 1999, 71 of the 96 paid donors were positive for HIV.[139] At another site, 50% and 100% of all donors tested positive for syphilis and HCV, respectively, and the entire group of 142 tested samples were positive for HIV.[90]

Multifaceted approaches to curb the use of unscreened or unsafe blood are needed. In response to the high use of unscreened blood for transfusion in Nigeria, the government instituted a law to regulate blood transfusions by requiring blood banks to register their blood donors, with fines and imprisonment for offenders.[140]

Hemovigilance data systems throughout the world are incomplete, particularly in economically restricted countries. More data on infectious disease prevalence are needed to assess effectiveness of screening procedures and guide further laboratory testing.

Logistics and Finances of Laboratory Screening

Although basic compatibility testing is performed in economically restricted countries, many blood banks run only ABO grouping and Rh typing in lieu of crossmatching. More extensive testing, such as additional alloantibody or autoantibody identification, extends beyond the current capabilities of blood banks in economically restricted countries due to limited technical expertise and a lack of automation, reagents, and adequate training.

Logistical problems often challenge laboratories in economically restricted countries. Laboratories may lack a standardized reporting system for results or have poor record keeping. Educational systems for blood bank personnel are also lacking. The cold chain for laboratory support may be compromised, with lack of a standard refrigerator, often with inadequate storage space for blood components. One researcher emphasizes the logistical problems by pointing out that:

> [a]lthough Tanzania's health policy is that all blood should be screened anonymously for infections which can be transmitted on transfusion, health experts say that a lack of systematic and comprehensive blood-screening support programme has undermined this goal. There is no screening for other infections, because the health ministry does not routinely supply test kits to hospitals due to financial constraints.[45]

Small blood banks may exist as unregulated commercial operations without quality control.[141]

Innovative answers to logistical problems in economically restricted countries are needed. One such example is the development of the slide Polybrene method for pretransfusion compatibility testing, in response to the lack of centrifuges in some areas.[142] Simple to use, the slide Polybrene can be performed by personnel with minimal training.

During an attempt to simulate suboptimal storage conditions in economically restricted countries, researchers tested blood units for HIV with inappropriately stored or expired rapid antibody assays in Zambia.[143] The sensitivity and specificity of the tests were 11% to 18% lower than the manufacturer's claim, with a risk of contracting HIV through transfusion at least six times higher than expected.

Blood screening for infectious diseases proves cost effective, especially in areas with large numbers of HIV-positive individuals.[27,61,144] Supplies and equipment comprise the majority of cost in blood transfusion.[145] To prevent one case of HIV in Africa, measures to improve blood transfusion safety may cost from $US 20 to $US 1000.[146] One study reported that savings exceeded costs by a factor of 2.7 to 3.5 in a region of Zambia with an HIV seroprevalence among donors of 16%.[87] A Tanzanian study showed that safe transfusion practices can be assured at an annual cost of $US 0.07 per capita.[147] One method of recovering the cost of screening blood involves charging all inpatients a fee that covers the screening costs on admission.[13] Charging all patients rather than only those patients who received blood by transfusion is easier to institute and does not lay the cost burden on the women and children who require the majority of transfusions.

Poor funding and lack of government support also lead to suboptimal practices. In a survey of 62 hospitals in the Democratic Republic of Congo in 1991, only 29% regularly received HIV testing kits due to lack of funding.[148] As a result, 28% of the blood units transfused during the study period were not screened for HIV. Logistic and economic issues should be better understood to assess the feasibility of laboratory testing in economically restricted countries.

BLOOD USAGE

Clinicians must weigh several factors when administering blood products, including the recipient's underlying need for transfusion, infectious contamination risks, and other noninfectious risks of transfusion. Despite the considerations that should be made in deciding to transfuse, blood transfusions continue to be performed unnecessarily in some instances.

Transfusion Recipient Populations

Transfusion recipient populations in economically restricted countries differ from those in more industrialized countries. Blood recipients in developed countries generally include cancer or transplant patients, adults undergoing surgery, and hemophiliacs. In economically restricted countries, recipients typically include children, pregnant women, sickle cell disease patients, victims of trauma, and persons with hemoglobinopathies, severe parasitic infections, and nutritional anemia.

In many areas of the world, children comprise a large percentage of those receiving transfusions. Between 19% and 67% of hospitalized children in Africa receive transfusions.[67,118,119,127,149,150] In Uganda, 65% of all transfusions are performed on children under age 5, the majority of whom suffer from malaria and other infections, malnutrition, and sickle cell disease.[151] Often, the youngest children require the majority of transfusions, due in part to the length of time required for children to develop immunity to certain pathogens, specifically malaria. A study conducted among six government hospitals in Kenya found that 58% of transfusions were requested for children age 10 or younger, and 37% for children under age 2.[34] Pediatric transfusions were primarily administered for malaria (49%), but were also administered for surgery (14%) and chronic anemia (11%). Finally, a retrospective study of blood usage in Mozambique showed that the pediatric department ordered nearly half of the blood used for transfusion, primarily for management of anemia.[152]

A second population group that receives a large proportion of transfusions in economically restricted countries is pregnant women. In sub-Saharan Africa, pregnant women often suffer from anemia due to malaria, iron and folate deficiency, or sickle cell trait or disease, which may be compounded by malnutrition or other health problems such as hookworm infestation.[153] Tanzanian studies show that pregnant women receive 8% to 11% of all transfusions.[154,155]

Patients with sickle cell disease are another large population sector requiring multiple transfusions. Most of the world's population with sickle cell disease resides in Africa, with the remainder in the Middle East or India.[156,157] Other areas of the world have reported significant numbers of sickle cell disease as well. Since implementation of neonatal sickle cell screening in 2000, one case of sickle cell disease per 1196 births in Brazil has been diagnosed.[158] Insufficient transfusion facilities unfortunately hinder the application of long-term transfusion protocols for these patients.

Finally, thalassemia patients comprise another major population group that receives a large proportion of blood transfusions in economically restricted countries. Thalassemia is an important public health problem in Southeast Asia, Africa, India, and the Middle East. Adequate data on the transfusion needs of people with thalassemia are not generally available from economically restricted countries. A small study of 330 multiply transfused patients with thalassemia in rural Bengal, India, diagnosed 3 (approximately 1%) HIV-positive patients who had received over 10 transfusions each.[159]

Appropriate Uses of Blood Transfusion

In deciding whether to transfuse, the clinician weighs the risks of obtaining potentially infected blood against the risk of the patient's not receiving blood. Often, blood is requested emergently and may not be properly screened. As shown in Table 42–4, a high number of blood transfusions are deemed inappropriate in many countries. The authors of one Tanzanian study found no difference in mortality between transfused and nontransfused anemic children, unless the child showed signs of cardiac failure, acute hemorrhage, or pneumonia.[163] However, the subjects were only followed for 8 weeks in this study, which did not take into account morbidity associated with transfusion-transmitted infections. In another decision analysis, African children with severe malarial anemia showed no transfusion benefit when the chance of survival without transfusion was greater than 95%.[164]

Researchers have attempted to quantify the risks and benefits of transfusions to certain patient populations in order to provide blood banks with precise guidelines of whom to transfuse.[165–171] Implementation of such guidelines has proven practical as well as effective. For instance, an observational study showed that Kenyan children benefited from transfusion under the following circumstances: when the hemoglobin level is less than 5.0 g/dL and when they are transfused within 48 hours of admission.[118,172]

The effect of implementing the above consensus guidelines on appropriate use of blood transfusions in Tanzania was examined, and it was found that the proportion of avoidable

Table 42–4 Avoidable Blood Transfusions in Selected Countries

		No. (%) Transfused			
Country	**Patient Group**	**Total**	**Avoidable**	**Year of Study**	**Reference No.**
Tanzania	Total patients	1029 (100)	334 (39)	1992	154
	Operated patients	191 (19)	26 (24)		
	Pregnant, no blood loss	52 (5)	5 (10)		
	Pregnant, acute blood loss	57 (6)	0 (0)		
	Children < 5 years	520 (51)	257 (52)		
	Children 5–15 years	43 (4)	10 (25)		
	Adults	166 (16)	36 (25)		
Kenya	Children < 15 years	83 (47)	39 (47)	1993	119
Ghana	Total patients	277 (25)	46 (17)	1991	160
	Surgical		(75)		
Tanzania	Total patients		(27–44)	1992	161
	Children < 5 years		(34–56)		
Zaire	Children		(13)	1990	149
	Adults		(21)		
Tanzania	Total patients		(35–40)	1994	162

transfusions decreased from 52% to 33% in the pediatric population after strict supervision by senior medical staff and adequate education through regular clinic meetings.[162] Physician education programs and a monitoring system to ensure adherence to established guidelines are needed to reduce waste of blood.

Blood Component Therapy

The WHO rarely recommends use of whole blood for transfusions, suggesting that at least 90% of collected units should be separated into components.[22] However, in many rural hospitals, whole blood still meets much of the transfusion need. Although some areas of Latin America follow WHO guidelines, few African countries have either the need to separate blood into components or the technology. In Mozambique, few plasma and platelet components are ordered, which may be due to poor clinician knowledge of component therapy.[152] A national survey of 604 blood banks in India found that only 21% of blood banks prepare blood-derived components; however, some component therapy does appear to be appropriately used.[77,173] The use of component therapy in other areas of the world is increasing, as reported in China, where components comprised approximately 40% of transfusions in 2000, as compared to 20% in 1996.[90] Peru's National Blood Banking Program reports that 80% of the blood is now fractionated.[174]

Alternatives to Allogeneic Blood Transfusion

Although autologous blood has been shown to decrease the need for allogeneic transfusions, it is infrequently used in economically restricted countries.[155] In a teaching hospital in Delhi, India, despite the fact that 68% of doctors reported a knowledge of autologous blood transfusion, only 22% considered autologous blood for their patients.[175] Of over 11,000 patients transfused in the Delhi teaching hospital, only 0.49% received autologous blood transfusions. Autologous blood is difficult to order before scheduled surgery in countries where many transfusions may be performed on an urgent or emergent basis.[176] Also, because autologous blood should be stored in a separate refrigerator from allogeneic blood, limited storage space augments the problem. One Nigerian hospital started an autologous blood donation program in response to rising HIV seropositivity in paid donors.[177] The researchers found that autologous blood transfusion was significantly less expensive than allogeneic, mainly due to less infectious disease morbidity in autologous blood recipients.

Quality Assurance

The WHO guidelines for quality assurance laboratory conditions should be followed in economically restricted countries whenever financial and logistic constraints allow. Laboratory infectious disease testing should be supervised, and adequate training should be provided. Protocols must be developed for procedures, reagents, techniques, equipment use, maintenance, and personnel. Performance evaluation programs should also be periodically offered.

Yet, quality assurance programs are often inadequate. Despite implementation of performance evaluations for immunohematology and serologic infectious disease testing, only a portion of blood banks typically participate.[20] In fact, when surveyed, only one third of central African hospital blood banks reported following standard practice protocols for documentation of HIV results.[148]

In summary, the laboratory testing guidelines suggested by the WHO and the PAHO are generally geared toward highly industrialized countries with low disease prevalence and adequate financial resources; the guidelines prove difficult to adhere to in economically restricted countries, which not only often face large logistic and financial constraints, but also operate in different infectious disease settings. We have reviewed the major challenges faced by many countries, including the lack of enough blood for patients, lack of reagents for screening, faulty equipment, and lack of continuing education for staff.

Innovative solutions are thus required to resolve the difficulties faced in these countries. One such solution is the option of predonation infectious disease screening of blood donors for relevant infections, aimed at decreasing blood bag waste. Although current predonation screening tests are not optimal, one can argue that suboptimal screening in many of these countries offers a better temporary solution than no screening at all. The selection of low-risk blood donors by screening, with the exclusion of paid or replacement donors, has also proven invaluable. Untested or suspect donor blood should be quarantined to prevent crossover into the blood supply. Another promising pretransfusion compatibility screening method aimed at circumventing the lack of centrifuges is the slide Polybrene method. Long-distance education programs would also prove helpful, especially to clinicians and blood banks, in an effort to promote appropriate clinical use of blood in avoiding unnecessary transfusions.

As epidemiologic studies continue gathering data on infectious disease trends in regions, certain population groups, such as the paid plasma donors with high infectious disease prevalence discovered in the 1990s, will continue to be regulated. Finally, each country's government must be dedicated to regulation and oversight of their blood banks, in an effort to optimize safety of their blood supply.

REFERENCES

1. Dhingra N, Lloyd SE, Fordham J, et al. Challenges in global blood safety. World Hosp Health Serv 2004;40:45–52.
2. Dhingra N. Blood safety in the developing world and WHO initiatives. Vox Sang 2002;83(Suppl 1):173–177.
3. Chin J, Sato PA, Mann JM. Projections of HIV infections and AIDS cases to the year 2000. Bull WHO 1990;68:1–11.
4. Implications of HIV variability for transmission: scientific and policy issues. Expert Group of the Joint United Nations Programme on HIV/AIDS. AIDS 11:UNAIDS1-UNAIDS15, 1997.
5. Shrestha P. Transmission of HIV through blood or blood products in the Eastern Mediterranean Region. East Mediterr Health J 1996;2:283–289.
6. Heymann SJ, Brewer TF. The problem of transfusion-associated acquired immunodeficiency syndrome in Africa: a quantitative approach. Am J Infect Control 1992;20:256–262.
7. Steinberg J. AIDS prevention is thicker than blood. Zimbabwe. Available at http://www.oxfam.org.uk/what_we_do/issues/gender/links/index.htm. Links 9:3,1992. Accessed October 11, 2005.
8. Kasili EG. Blood transfusion services in a developing country: the concept and problems of organization. East Afr Med J 1981;58:81–83.
9. World Health Organization. Aide-Memoire for National Transfusion Programmes. Blood Safety Unit. Geneva, World Health Organization, 2002. Available at http://www.who.int/gb/ebwha/pdf_files/WHA58/WHA58_13-en.pdf. Accessed October 11, 2005.

10. Emmanuel JC. Blood transfusion systems in economically restricted countries. Vox Sang 1994;67(Suppl 3):267–269.
11. Williamson LM. Using haemovigilance data to set blood safety priorities. Vox Sang 2002;83(Suppl 1):65–69.
12. Koistinen J. Organization of blood transfusion services in developing countries. Vox Sang 1994;67(Suppl 3):247–249.
13. Hensher M, Jefferys E. Financing blood transfusion services in sub-Saharan Africa: a role for user fees? Health Policy Plan 2000;15: 287–295.
14. Faber JC. Worldwide overview of existing haemovigilance systems. Transfus Apheresis Sci 2004;31:99–110.
15. Martinez MC. Management of scarce resources in blood services in developing countries. Vox Sang 2002;83(Suppl 1):137–140.
16. Sodahlon YK, Segbena AY, Prince-David M, et al. Blood transfusion safety in a limited resources setting: the elaboration of a rational National Blood Policy in Togo. Sante 2004;14:115–120.
17. Fraser B. Seeking a safer blood supply. Lancet 2005;365:559–560.
18. Faber JC. Haemovigilance around the world. Vox Sang 2002;83 (Suppl 1):71–76.
19. Cruz JR. Basic components of a national blood system. Rev Panam Salud Publica 2003;13:79–84.
20. Schmunis GA, Cruz JR. Safety of the blood supply in Latin America. Clin Microbiol Rev 2005;18:12–29.
21. Emmanuel J. Establishment and organization of a blood transfusion service. Vox Sang 1994;67(Suppl 5):4–7.
22. Cruz JR, Perez-Rosales MD. Availability, safety, and quality of blood for transfusion in the Americas. Rev Panam Salud Publica 2003;13: 103–110.
23. Sullivan P. Developing an administrative plan for transfusion medicine: a global perspective. Transfusion 2005;45(4 Suppl):224S–240S.
24. World Health Organization.Blood Safety: Proposal to Establish World Blood Donor Day. Geneva, World Health Organization, 2005. Available at http://www.who.int/gb/ebwha/pdf_files/WHA58/WHA58_13-en.pdf. Accessed October 19, 2005.
25. World Health Organization. Global Database on Blood Safety, Summary Report 1998–1999. Geneva, World Health Organization, 2001.
26. Nanu A, Sharma SP, Chatterjee K, et al. Markers for transfusion-transmissible infections in north Indian voluntary and replacement blood donors: prevalence and trends 1989–1996. Vox Sang 1997;73:70–73.
27. Lackritz EM. Prevention of HIV transmission by blood transfusion in the developing world: achievements and continuing challenges. AIDS 1998;12(Suppl A):S81–S86.
28. Garg S, Mathur DR, Garg DK. Comparison of seropositivity of HIV, HBV, HCV, and syphilis in replacement and voluntary blood donors in western India. Indian J Pathol Microbiol 2001;44:409–412.
29. Rukundo H, Tumwesigye N, Wakwe VC. Screening for HIV 1 through the regional blood transfusion service in southwest Uganda: the Mbarara experience. Health Transit Rev 1997;7(Suppl):101–104.
30. Jacobs B, Berege ZA, Schalula PJ, et al. Secondary school students: a safer blood donor population in an urban area with high HIV prevalence in east Africa. East Afr Med J 1994;71:720–723.
31. McFarland W, Mvere D, Shandera W, et al. Epidemiology and prevention of transfusion-associated human immunodeficiency virus transmission in sub-Saharan Africa. Vox Sang 1997;72:85–92.
32. Durosinmi MA, Mabayoje VO, Akinola NO, et al. A retrospective study of prevalence antibody to HIV in blood donors at Ile-Ife, Nigeria. Niger Postgrad Med J 2003;10:220–223.
33. Zhang L, Chen Z, Cao Y, et al. Molecular characterization of human immunodeficiency virus type 1 and hepatitis C virus in paid donors and injection drug users in China. J Virol 2004;78:13591–13599.
34. Moore A, Herrera G, Nyamongo J, et al. Estimated risk of HIV transmission by blood transfusion in Kenya. Lancet 2001;358:657–660.
35. Beal R. Transfusion science and practice in developing countries: "…a high frequency of empty shelves…." [editorial]. Transfusion 1993;33: 276–278.
36. Shreedhar J. AIDS in India. Harv AIDS Rev Fall 1995:2–9.
37. Dodd RY. Notes on global blood safety. Blood Ther Med 2003;4:2–4.
38. Cruz JR. Blood services in the region of the Americas. Rev Panam Salud Publica 2003;13:77–78.
39. Mundee Y, Kamtorn N, Chaiyaphruk S, et al. Infectious disease markers in blood donors in northern Thailand. Transfusion 1995;35:264–267.
40. Chattopadhya D, Riley LW, Kumari S. Behavioural risk factors for acquisition of HIV infection and knowledge about AIDS among male professional blood donors in Delhi. Bull WHO 1991;69:319–323.
41. Goncalez T, Sabino EC, Chamone DF. Trends in the profile of blood donors at a large blood center in the city of Sao Paulo, Brazil. Rev Panam Salud Publica 2003;13:144–148.
42. Gutierrez MG, de Tejada ES, Cruz JR. [A study of sociocultural factors related to voluntary blood donation in the Americas]. [Spanish] Rev Panam Salud Publica 2003;13:85–90.
43. Sawanpanyalert P, Uthaivoravit W, Yanai H, et al. Donation deferral criteria for human immunodeficiency virus positivity among blood donors in northern Thailand. Transfusion 1996;36:242–249.
44. Kitayaporn D, Bejrachandra S, Chongkolwatana V, et al. Potential deferral criteria predictive of human immunodeficiency virus positivity among blood donors in Thailand. Transfusion 1994;34:152–157.
45. Matee MI, Lyamuya EF, Mbena EC, et al. Prevalence of transfusion-associated viral infections and syphilis among blood donors in Muhimbili Medical Centre, Dar es Salaam, Tanzania. East Afr Med J 1999;76:167–171.
46. McFarland W, Mvere D, Shamu R, et al. Risk factors for HIV seropositivity among first-time blood donors in Zimbabwe. Transfusion 1998;38:279–284.
47. Chikwem JO, Mohammed I, Okara GC, et al. Prevalence of transmissible blood infections among blood donors at the University of Maiducuri Teaching Hospital, Maiduguri, Nigeria. East Afr Med J 1997;74:213–216.
48. Mathai J, Sulochana PV, Satyabhama S, et al. Profile of transfusion transmissible infections and associated risk factors among blood donors of Kerala. Indian J Pathol Microbiol 2002;45:319–322.
49. Choudhury N, Singh P, Chandra H. AIDS awareness in blood donors in north India. Transfus Med 1995;5:267–271.
50. Chattopadhya D, Aggarwal RK, Baveja UK, et al. Evaluation of epidemiological and serological predictors of human immunodeficiency virus type-1 (HIV-1) infection among high risk professional blood donors with Western blot indeterminate results. J Clin Virol 1998;11:39–49.
51. Van de Perre P, Carael M, Nzaramba D, et al. Risk factors for HIV seropositivity in selected urban-based Rwandese adults. AIDS 1987;1: 207–211.
52. Galel SA, Lifson JD, Engleman EG. Prevention of AIDS transmission through screening of the blood supply. Annu Rev Immunol 1995;13:201–227.
53. McFarland W, Mvere D, Katzenstein D. Risk factors for prevalent and incident HIV infection in a cohort of volunteer blood donors in Harare, Zimbabwe: implications for blood safety. AIDS 1997;11(Suppl 1): S97–S102.
54. Dodd RY. Current estimates of transfusion safety worldwide. Dev Biol (Basel) 2005;120:3–10.
55. Fleming AF. HIV and blood transfusion in sub-Saharan Africa. Transfus Sci 1997;18:167–179.
56. Barongo LR, Borgdorff MW, Mosha FF, et al. The epidemiology of HIV-1 infection in urban areas, roadside settlements and rural villages in Mwanza Region, Tanzania. AIDS 1992;6:521–528.
57. Urwijitaroon Y, Barusrux S, Romphruk A, et al. Reducing the risk of HIV transmission through blood transfusion by donor self-deferral. Southeast Asian J Trop Med Public Health 1996;27:452–456.
58. Adediran IA, Fesogun RB, Oyekunle AA. Haematological parameters in prospective Nigerian blood donors rejected on account of anaemia and/or microfilaria infestation. Niger J Med 2005;14:45–50.
59. Clark KA, Kataaha P, Mwangi J, et al. Predonation testing of potential blood donors in resource-restricted settings [editorial]. Transfusion 2005;45:130–132.
60. Owusu-Ofori S, Temple J, Sarkodie F, et al. Predonation screening of blood donors with rapid tests: implementation and efficacy of a novel approach to blood safety in resource-poor settings. Transfusion 2005;45:133–140.
61. Laleman G, Magazani K, Perriens JH, et al. Prevention of blood-borne HIV transmission using a decentralized approach in Shaba, Zaire. AIDS 1992;6:1353–1358.
62. Owusu-Ofori S, Temple J, Sarkodie F, et al. Predonation testing of potential blood donors in resource-restricted settings. Transfusion 2005;45:1542–1543.
63. Gorlin JB. Predonation testing of potential blood donors in resource-restricted settings. Tranfusion 2005;45:1541–1542.
64. Lau JT, Thomas J, Lin CK. HIV-related behaviours among voluntary blood donors in Hong Kong. AIDS Care 2002;14:481–492.
65. Gorlin JB. Strengthening blood transfusion services and blood safety in Tanzania: CDC and Department of Health and Human Services RFP. Reference H75/CCH523411–01, 2004.
66. Schmunis GA. American trypanosomiasis as a public health problem. Chagas' disease and the nervous system. PAHO Sci Pub 1994;547:3–29.
67. Bianco C. International aspects of blood services. In Simon TL, Dzik WH, Snyder EL, et al (eds). Rossi's Principles of Transfusion Medicine, 3rd ed. Philadelphia, Lippincott Williams & Wilkins, 2002, pp 953–957.

68. Tapko JB. Regional strategy: Priority interventions for improving blood safety in the African region. Meeting of the International Consortium for Blood Safety and Liaised Organizations and Institutions, 2003 Feb 15–17, Atlanta. Cited in Clark KA, Kataaha P, Mwangi J, et al. Predonation testing of potential blood donors in resource-restricted settings [editorial]. Transfusion 2005;45:130–132.
69. Allain J-P, Candotti D, Soldan K, et al. The risk of hepatitis B virus infection by transfusion in Kumasi, Ghana. Blood 2003;101: 2419–2425.
70. Saez-Alquezar A, Otani MM, Sabino EC, et al. [External serology quality control programs developed in Latin America with the support of PAHO from 1997 through 2000]. [Spanish] Rev Panam Salud Publica 2003;13:91–102.
71. Periago MR. Promoting quality blood services in the region of the Americas. Rev Panam Salud Publica 2003;13:73–74.
72. Uruguay declared free of Chagas disease transmission. TDR News 1998;56:6.
73. Schmunis GA, Zicker F, Cruz JR, et al. Safety of blood supply for infectious diseases in Latin American countries, 1994–1997. Am J Trop Med Hyg 2001;65:924–930.
74. Oknaian S, Remesar M, Ferraro L, et al. [External performance evaluation of screening in blood banks in Argentina: results and strategies for improvement]. [Spanish] Rev Panam Salud Publica 2003;13: 149–153.
75. Duran MB, Guzman MA. [External evaluation of serology results in blood banks in Colombia]. [Spanish] Rev Panam Salud Publica 2003;13:138–143.
76. Jain MK, John TJ, Keusch GT. A review of human immunodeficiency virus infection in India. J AIDS 1994;7:1185–1194.
77. Kapoor D, Saxena R, Sood B, et al. Blood transfusion practices in India: results of a national survey. Indian J Gastroenterol 2000;19:64–67.
78. Sitas F, Fleming AF, Morris J. Residual risk of transmission of HIV through blood transfusion in South Africa. S Afr Med J 1994;84:142–144.
79. South African National Blood Service. Haemovigilance Annual Report: Blood Transfusion South Africa, 2003. Available at http://www.sanbs.org.za/medical/haemovigilance.htm. Accessed October 18, 2005.
80. Isarangkura P, Chiewsilp P, Tanprasert S, et al. Transmission of HIV infection by seronegative blood in Thailand. J Med Assoc Thai 1993;76 (Suppl 2):106–113.
81. Sharma RR, Cheema R, Vajpayee M, et al. Prevalence of markers of transfusion transmissible diseases in voluntary and replacement blood donors. Natl Med J India 2004;17:19–21.
82. Mbanya DN, Takam D, Ndumbe PM. Serological findings amongst first-time blood donors in Yaounde, Cameroon: is safe donation a reality or a myth? Transfus Med 2003;13:267–273.
83. Minga AK, Huet C, Coulibaly I, et al. [Profile of HIV infected patients among blood donors in Abidjan, Cote d'Ivoire 1992–1999]. [French] Bull Soc Pathol Exot 2005;98:123–126.
84. CDC finds Kenya's blood stocks unsafe. AIDS Anal Afr 1995;5:2.
85. Karuru JW, Lule GN, Joshi M, et al. Prevalence of HCV and HIV/HCV co-infection among volunteer blood donors and VCT clients. East Afr Med J 2005;82:166–169.
86. Ejele OA, Ojule AC. The prevalence of hepatitis B surface antigen (HBsAg) among prospective blood donors and patients in Port Harcourt, Nigeria. Niger J Med 2004;13:336–338.
87. Foster S, Buve A. Benefits of HIV screening of blood transfusions in Zambia. Lancet 1995;346:225–227.
88. Gupta N, Kaur A. Study of prevalence and correlation between HIV and syphilis among blood donors in a teaching hospital in Ludhiana, India. Indian J Med Sci 2002;56:161–164.
89. Singh B, Verma M, Verma K. Markers for transfusion-associated hepatitis in North Indian blood donors: Prevalence and trends. Jpn J Infect Dis 2004;57:49–51.
90. Shan H, Wang JX, Ren FR, et al. Blood banking in China. Lancet 2002;360:1770–1775.
91. Yan JY, Zheng XW, Zhang XF, et al. The survey of prevalence of HIV infection among paid blood donors in one county of China. Chin J Epidemiol (Chin) 2000;21:10–12. Cited in Wang L, Zheng XW, Qian HZ, et al. Epidemiological study on human immunodeficiency virus infection among children in a former paid plasma donating community in China. Chin Med J 2005;118:720–724.
92. Zheng XW, Wang Z, Xi J, et al. Epidemiologic study of HIV infections among paid blood donors in a county of China. Chin J Epidemiol (Chin) 2000;21:352–255. Cited in Wang L, Zheng XW, Qian HZ, et al. Epidemiological study on human immunodeficiency virus infection among children in a former paid plasma donating community in China. Chin Med J 2005;118:720–724.
93. Cao F, Ji Y, Huang R, et al. Prevalence of antibodies to HTLV-I/II in blood donors and risk populations in South China [letter]. Vox Sang 1998;75:154.
94. Urwijitaroon Y, Barusrux S, Puapairoj C, et al. Seroepidemiology of HTLV-I infection in northeast Thailand: a 4-year surveillance. J Med Assoc Thai 1997;80(Suppl 1):S102–S105.
95. Nantachit N, Robison V, Wongthanee A, et al. Temporal trends in the prevalence of HIV and other transfusion-transmissible infections among blood donors in northern Thailand, 1990 through 2001. Transfusion 2003;43:730–735.
96. Wiwanitkit V. Anti HCV seroprevalence among the voluntary blood donors in Thailand. Hematol 2005;10:431–433.
97. Zaller N, Nelson KE, Aladashvili M, et al. Risk factors for hepatitis C virus infection among blood donors in Georgia. Eur J Epidemiol 2004;19:547–553.
98. Butsashvili M, Tsertsvadze T, McNutt LA, et al. Prevalence of hepatitis B, hepatitis C, syphilis and HIV in Georgian blood donors. Eur J Epidemiol 2001;17:693–695.
99. El-Hazmi MM. Prevalence of HBV, HCV, HIV-1,2 and HTLV-I/II infections among blood donors in a teaching hospital in the Central region of Saudi Arabia. Saudi Med J 2004;25:26–33.
100. Sakarya S, Oncu S, Ozturk B, et al. Effect of preventive applications on prevalence of hepatitis B virus and hepatitis C virus infections in West Turkey. Saudi Med J 2004;25:1070–1072.
101. Leon G, Quiros AM, Lopez JL, et al. [Seropositivity for human T-lymphotropic virus types I and II among donors at the Municipal Blood Bank of Caracas and associated risk factors]. [Spanish] Rev Panam Salud Publica 2003;13:117–124.
102. Shin HR. Epidemiology of hepatitis C virus in Korea. Intervirology 2006;49:18–22.
103. De Schryver A, Meheus A. Syphilis and blood transfusion: a global perspective. Transfusion 1990;30:844–847.
104. International Forum. Does it make sense for blood transfusion services to continue the time-honored syphilis screening with cardiolipin antigen? Vox Sang 1981; 41:183–192.
105. Suwanagool S, Sonjai A, Ratanasuwan W, et al. Risk factors for HIV infection among Thai laborers during 1992–1993. J Med Assoc Thai 1993;76:663–671.
106. Weber T, Hunsmann G, Stevens W, et al. Human retroviruses. Baillieres Clin Haematol 1992;5:273–314.
107. Sandler SG, Yu H, Rassai N. Risks of blood transfusion and their prevention. Clin Adv Hematol Oncol 2003;1:307–313.
108. Saez-Alquezar A, Murta M, Marques W, et al. [The results of an external quality control program for serological screening for antibodies against *Trypanosoma cruzi* in blood donors in Brazil]. [Spanish] Rev Panam Salud Publica 2003;13:129–137.
109. Wendel S. Transfusion-transmitted Chagas' disease. Curr Opin Hematology 1998;5:406–411.
110. Pirard M, Iihoshi N, Boelaert M, et al. The validity of serologic tests for *Trypanosoma cruzi* and the effectiveness of transfusional screening strategies in a hyperendemic region. Transfusion 2005;45: 554–561.
111. Kothari A, Ramachandran VG, Gupta P, et al. Seroprevalence of cytomegalovirus among voluntary blood donors in Delhi, India. J Health Popul Nutr 2002;20:348–351.
112. Stein L, Carrara H, Norman R, et al. Antibodies against human herpesvirus 8 in South African renal transplant recipients and blood donors. Transpl Infect Dis 2004;6:69–73.
113. Gorenflot A, Moubri K, Precigout E, et al. Human babesiosis. Ann Trop Med Parasitol 1998;92:489–501.
114. Choudhury N, Ramesh V, Saraswat S, et al. Effectiveness of mandatory transmissible diseases screening in Indian blood donors. Indian J Med Res 1995;101:229–232.
115. HIV/AIDS Surveillance Report. Centers for Disease Control, June 1994, p 7. Cited in McFarland W, Mvere D, Shandera W, et al. Epidemiology and prevention of transfusion-associated human immunodeficiency virus transmission in sub-Saharan Africa. Vox Sang 1997;72:85–92.
116. World Health Organization. Current and Future Dimensions of the HIV/AIDS Pandemic: A Capsule Summary. WHO [WHO/GPA/SF1/90.2] Geneva, World Health Organization, 1990. Cited in Lackritz EM. Prevention of HIV transmission by blood transfusion in the developing world: Achievements and continuing challenges. AIDS 1998;12(Suppl A):S81–S86.
117. Beal RW, Bontinck M, Fransen L (eds). Safe blood in developing countries. Brussels, EEC AIDS Task Force, 1992, pp 11–12. Cited in Lackritz EM. Prevention of HIV transmission by blood transfusion in the

developing world: Achievements and continuing challenges. AIDS 1998;12(Suppl A):S81–S86.
118. Lackritz EM, Campbell CC, Ruebush TK II, et al. Effect of blood transfusion on survival among children in a Kenyan hospital. Lancet 1992;340:524–528.
119. Lackritz EM, Ruebush II TK, Zucker JR, et al. Blood transfusion practices and blood-banking services in a Kenyan hospital. AIDS 1993;7: 995–999.
120. Torrey BB, Mulligan M, Way PO. Blood Donors and AIDS in Africa: The Gift Relationship Revisited. Staff paper no. 53. Washington, D.C., U.S. Bureau of the Census Center for International Research, 1990. Cited in Heymann SJ, Brewer TF. The problem of transfusion-associated acquired immunodeficiency syndrome in Africa: a quantitative approach. Am J Infect Control 1992;20:256–262.
121. McFarland W, Kahn JG, Katzenstein DA, et al. Deferral of blood donors with risk factors for HIV saves lives and money in Zimbabwe. J AIDS Hum Retrovirol 1995;9:183–192.
122. UNAIDS. Position Paper on Modes of Transmission of HIV, with Particular Reference to Sub-Saharan Africa and Unsafe Injection. World Health Organization. September 30, 2004. Available at http://www.commissionforafrica.org/english/report/background/shisana_and_letlape_background.pdf. Accessed July 15,2005.
123. Chin J, Mann JM. Global surveillance and forecasting of AIDS. Bull WHO 1989;67:1–7.
124. Narain J. Caribbean. AIDS Action 1990;10:7.
125. Silva GF, Nishimura NF, Coelho KI, et al. Grading and staging chronic hepatitis C and its relation to genotypes and epidemiological factors in Brazilian blood donors. Braz J Infect Dis 2005;9:142–149.
126. Fujino Y, Mizoue T, Tokui N, et al. A prospective study of blood transfusion history and liver cancer in a high-endemic area of Japan. Transfus Med 2002;12:297–302.
127. Greenberg AE, Nguyen-Dinh P, Mann JM, et al. The association between malaria, blood transfusions, and HIV seropositivity in pediatric population in Kinshasa, Zaire. JAMA 1988;259:545–549.
128. Merchant RH, Oswal JS, Bhagwat RV, et al. Clinical profile of HIV infection. Indian Pediatr 2001;38:239–246.
129. Cheng H, Qian X, Cao GH, et al. [Study on the seropositive prevalence of human immunodeficiency virus in a village residents living in rural region of central China]. [Chinese] Chung Hua Liu Hsing Ping Hsueh Tsa Chih 2004;25:317–321.
130. Allen S, Van de Perre P, Serufilira A, et al. Human immunodeficiency virus and malaria in a representative sample of childbearing women in Kigali, Rwanda. J Infect Dis 1991;164:67–71.
131. Donegan E, Stuart M, Niland JC, et al. Infection with human immunodeficiency virus type 1 (HIV-1) among recipients of antibody-positive blood donations. Ann Intern Med 1990;113:733–739.
132. Savarit D, De Cock KM, Schutz R, et al. Risk of HIV infection from transfusion with blood negative for HIV antibody in a west African city. BMJ 1992;305:498–502.
133. Marcus R. Surveillance of health care workers exposed to blood from patients infected with the human immunodeficiency virus. NEJM 1988;319:1118–1123.
134. Volkow P, Marin Lopez A, Torres I. Plasma trade and the HIV epidemic. Lancet 1997;349:327–328.
135. Volkow P, del Rio C. Paid donation and plasma trade: unrecognized forces that drive the AIDS epidemic in developing countries. Int J STD AIDS 2005;16:5–8.
136. Wang L, Zheng XW, Qian HZ, et al. Epidemiological study on human immunodeficiency virus infection among children in a former paid plasma donating community in China. Chin Med J 2005;118:720–724.
137. Ji Y, Qu D, Jia G, et al. Study of HIV antibody screening for blood donors by a pooling serum method. Vox Sang 1995;9:255–256.
138. Ji Y, Zhang Y, Jia G, et al. An HIV antibody positive plasma donor detected at the early stage of HIV infection in China. Transfus Med 1996;6:291–292.
139. Shan H, Wang JX, Ren FR, et al. Blood banking in China. Lancet 2002;360:1770–1775.
140. Raufu A. Rising HIV infection through blood transfusion worries Nigerian health experts. AIDS Anal Afr 2000;11:15.
141. Okpara R. Transmission of HIV through blood transfusion. Afr Health 1992;14:15–17.
142. Lin M. Compatibility testing without a centrifuge: the slide Polybrene method. Transfusion 2004;44:410–413.
143. Consten EC, van der Meer JT, de Wolf F, et al. Risk of iatrogenic human immunodeficiency virus infection through transfusion of blood tested by inappropriately stored or expired rapid antibody tests in a Zambian hospital. Transfusion 1997;37:930–934.
144. Over M, Piot P. Human immunodeficiency virus infection and other sexually transmitted diseases in developing countries: public health importance and priorities for resource allocation. J Infect Dis 1996;174(Suppl 2):S162–S175.
145. Lema RA. Quality control in haematology and blood transfusion in sub-Saharan region of Africa. East Afr Med J 1993;70(4 Suppl): 21–22.
146. Creese A, Floyd K, Alban A, et al. Cost-effectiveness of HIV/AIDS interventions in Africa: a systematic review of the evidence. Lancet 2002;359:1635–1642.
147. Jacobs B, Mercer A. Feasibility of hospital-based blood banking: A Tanzanian case study. Health Policy Plan 1999;14:354–362.
148. N'tita I, Mulanga K, Dulat C, et al. Risk of transfusion-associated HIV transmission in Kinshasa, Zaire. AIDS 1991;5:437–439.
149. Jager H, N'Galy B, Perriens J, et al. Prevention of transfusion-associated HIV transmission in Kinshasa, Zaire: HIV screening is not enough. AIDS 1990;4:571–574.
150. Coulter JB. HIV infection in African children. Ann Trop Paediatr 1993;13:205–215.
151. Ndugwa CM, Friesen H. Uganda: Paediatric AIDS. AIDS Action 1998;5:5.
152. Barradas T, Schwalbach T, Novoa A. Blood and blood products usage in Maputo. Cent Afr J Med 1994;40:56–60.
153. Jager H, Jersild C, Emmanuel JC. Safe blood transfusions in Africa. AIDS 1991;5(Suppl 1):S163–S168.
154. Gumodoka B, Vos J, Kigadye F, et al. Blood transfusion practices in Mwanza Region, Tanzania. AIDS 1993;7:387–392.
155. Vos J, Gumodoka B, Ng'weshemi JZ, et al. Are some blood transfusions avoidable? A hospital record analysis in Mwanza Region, Tanzania. Trop Geogr Med 1993;45:301–303.
156. World Health Organization. Global Database on Blood Safety, Summary Report, 1998–1999. Geneva, World Health Organization, 2001.
157. Diagne I, Diagne-Gueye ND, Signate-Sy H, et al. [Management of children with sickle cell disease in Africa: Experience in a cohort of children at the Royal Albert Hospital in Dakar]. [French] Med Trop 2003;63:513–520.
158. Lobo CL, Bueno LM, Moura P, et al. [Neonatal screening for hemoglobinopathies in Rio de Janeiro, Brazil]. [Spanish] Rev Panam Salud Publica 2003;13:154–159.
159. Sur D, Chakraborty AK, Mukhopadhyay SP. Dr. P.C. Sen Memorial Award Paper. A study of HIV infection in thalassaemia patients of rural Bengal. Indian J Public Health 1998;42:81–87.
160. Addo-Yobo EO, Lovel H. How well are hospitals preventing iatrogenic HIV? A study of the appropriateness of blood transfusions in three hospitals in Ashanti region, Ghana. Trop Doct 1991;21:162–164.
161. Dolmans WM, Klokke AH, Van Asten H, et al. Prevention of HIV transmission through blood transfusion in Tanzania. Trop Geogr Med 1992;44:285.
162. Vos J, Gumodoka B, van Asten HA, et al. Changes in blood transfusion practices after the introduction of consensus guidelines in Mwanza region, Tanzania. AIDS 1994;8:1135–1140.
163. Holzer BR, Egger M, Teuscher T, et al. Childhood anemia in Africa: To transfuse or not transfuse? Acta Trop 1993;55:47–51.
164. Obonyo CO, Steyerberg EW, Oloo AJ, et al. Blood transfusions for severe malaria-related anemia in Africa: a decision analysis. Am J Trop Med Hyg 1998;59:808–812.
165. Simon TL, Alverson DC, AuBuchon J, et al. Practice parameter for the use of red blood cell transfusions. Arch Pathol Lab Med 1998;122: 130–138.
166. Stehling L, Luban NLC, Anderson KC, et al. Guidelines for blood utilization review. Transfusion 1994;34:438–448.
167. Ryder RW: Difficulties associated with providing an HIV-free blood supply in tropical Africa. AIDS 1992;6:1395–1397.
168. Wake DJ, Cutting WA. Blood transfusion in developing countries: Problems, priorities and practicalities. Trop Doct 1998;28:4–8.
169. English M, Ahmed M, Ngando C, et al. Blood transfusion for severe anaemia in children in a Kenyan hospital. Lancet 2002;359: 494–495.
170. Salazar M. [Guidelines for the transfusion of blood and its components]. [Spanish] Rev Panam Salud Publica 2003;13:183–190.
171. Fang CT, Field SP, Busch MP, et al. Human immunodeficiency virus-1 and hepatitis C virus RNA among South African blood donors: estimation of residual transfusion risk and yield of nucleic acid testing. Vox Sang 2003;85:9–19.
172. Lackritz EM, Hightower AW, Zucker JR, et al. Longitudinal evaluation of severely anemic children in Kenya: the effect of transfusion on mortality and hematologic recovery. AIDS 1997;11:1487–1494.

173. Chaudhary R, Singh H, Verma A, et al. Evaluation of fresh frozen plasma usage at a tertiary care hospital in North India. ANZ J Surg 2005;75:573–576.
174. Ribera Salcedo JF, Roca Valencia O. [Peru's experience with a national blood banking program]. [Spanish] Rev Panam Salud Publica 2003;13: 165–171.
175. Dhingra-Kumar N, Sikka M, Madan N, et al. Evaluation of awareness and utilization of an autologous blood transfusion programme. Transfus Med 1997;7:197–202.
176. Cruz JR. Seeking a safer blood supply. Lancet 2005;365:1463–1464.
177. Nnodu OE, Odunkuwe N, Odunubi O, et al. Cost effectiveness of autologous blood transfusion—a developing country hospital's perspective. West Afr J Med 2003;22:10–12.

B. Complications of Transfusion

i. Infectious Complications

Chapter 43

Hepatitis A, B, and Non-A, Non-B, Non-C Viruses

Roger Y. Dodd

INTRODUCTION

Hepatitis was recognized as an adverse consequence of transfusion almost from the outset of transfusion therapy. In fact, viral hepatitis was originally classified either as *infectious* or *serum* hepatitis according to its predominant transmission mode. We now realize that infectious hepatitis was almost entirely accounted for by hepatitis A virus (HAV), whereas serum hepatitis was most likely due to infection with hepatitis B and C viruses. Other hepatitis viruses have been recognized, including hepatitis D virus (previously delta virus) and hepatitis E virus. Additional viruses have also been identified in the context of hepatitis, although they do not appear to be primary causative agents of the disease; included in this group are the hepatitis G virus and the TTV/SEN-V complex.

HEPATITIS A

Hepatitis A is usually a relatively mild disease, and there are no reports of chronic infection or disease. The mortality rate is 0.2% or less. Although symptoms may be severe, most cases are inapparent, as the seroprevalence rates may range from 5% to 74% of subsets of the U.S. population, depending on age. The incubation period averages 25 to 30 days, with a range of approximately 15 to 45 days. When symptoms are present, there may be a short prodromal phase lasting 2 to 10 days, involving fever, chills, malaise, and arthralgias. During this phase, the alanine aminotransaminase (ALT) levels rise; they peak during the appearance of the more definitive symptoms of hepatitis, namely anorexia, nausea and vomiting, and epigastric tenderness. Laboratory diagnosis is normally based on evaluation of serum ALT levels plus the use of an immunoassay for anti-HAV immunoglobulin M (IgM).

The virus is typically transmitted by the fecal-oral route. High levels of virus are shed in the feces during the prodromal stage. Food-borne outbreaks are relatively common, and the source is usually an infected food handler. Uncooked shellfish from contaminated waters are also a common source of infection. Infection is often transmitted among diapered infants in day care and in hospital nursery settings. Immune serum globulin preparations have been used prophylactically and are quite effective. However, a vaccine for HAV is now available and is recommended for those at significant risk of exposure.

The HAV is a picornavirus, classified in the genus *Hepatovirus*. As such, it is a nonenveloped virus, approximately 27 nm in diameter. It was first recognized in the 1970s on immunoelectron microscopy of fecal samples. Unlike other hepatitis viruses, HAV can be readily grown in tissue culture.[1]

Transfusion-transmitted HAV is uncommon, with approximately 25 cases reported in the literature, and a risk estimated as considerably less than 1 case per million transfused component units. Interestingly, some of the reported cases did involve young children, and there were secondary cases as a result of transmission in the nursery.[2–6] The low frequency of transfusion-transmitted HAV is usually attributed to the rather short period of viremia before the appearance of symptoms. Bower and colleagues[7] have reported, however, that HAV RNA could be detected in the blood an average of 17 days before and 79 days after the peak of serum ALT. Such findings do not necessarily correlate with infectivity. A recently published study used molecular methods to unequivocally link transfusion-transmitted HAV infection from a unit drawn 3 days before the donor's clinical presentation.[8] The relatively recent introduction of testing for HAV RNA in plasma destined for further manufacture has provided an opportunity for assessment of the prevalence of HAV viremia among routine blood donors. At least in the American Red Cross donor base, the frequency of such viremia has proven to be on the order of 1 per 2.3 million donations (data from the American Red Cross, personal communication from Susan L. Stramer).

In the United States, individuals with a history of viral hepatitis are not permitted to give blood unless they had the disease before age 11. This practice recognizes the fact that almost all hepatitis occurring before this age is due to HAV, which would not offer any risk of transmission. There are no other specific measures in place to prevent transfusion-transmitted HAV infection. However, it is usual to withdraw blood products if it is learned that the donors were recently exposed to HAV (e.g., through a known food-borne outbreak). One such outbeak occurred in 2003[9] and was the source of significant concern, resulting in donor deferral for a period of 1 year after potential exposure. Another issue has been the extent to which HAV may be transmitted in crowded unhygienic conditions, such as those occasionally attendant on sheltering individuals during disasters. Although this was a potential concern during the hurricane disasters in 2005, no outbreak of hepatitis A was seen.

There has also been concern about transmission of HAV via some specific lots of antihemophilic factor products.[10–13] Whether the contamination derived from the plasma donors or was introduced elsewhere in the processing is unclear. However, it was clear that the solvent-detergent process failed to inactivate the contaminating virus, a finding that is not unexpected for a nonenveloped virus. As a result of these events, additional inactivation steps are used, and manufacturing pools are monitored for HAV RNA. Additionally, it is recommended that certain recipients of plasma products (including solvent-detergent–treated plasma) should receive the hepatitis A vaccine.

HEPATITIS B

Overview

Hepatitis B is the prototypic transfusion-transmitted disease. Until the early 1970s, it was considered the only form of parenterally transmitted hepatitis. Exposure to hepatitis B virus (HBV) may result in a prolonged but asymptomatic infection with the potential for high titers of circulating virus, even in the presence of a vigorous immune response. Indeed, a number of lines of evidence, including early studies of human transmission, animal inoculation, and nucleic acid amplification testing (NAT), show that such titers may reach 10^9 to 10^{10} virions per milliliter.[14]

The essentially serendipitous discovery by Blumberg and associates[15,16] of "Australia antigen" (hepatitis B surface antigen [HBsAg]) and its subsequent linkage to one form of viral hepatitis can be considered the first seminal event in the development of modern blood donor screening procedures and policies. Not only was HBsAg clearly associated with what was then known as hepatitis B, but some studies had also established that blood that was positive for the antigen clearly transmitted hepatitis B to recipients.[17]

Test methods became available around 1969 but were not uniformly adopted until about 1970 or 1971. The very first test to be implemented was Ouchterlony agar gel diffusion (AGD), which used human or animal antibodies to detect the antigen in donor serum. It is important to recognize, however, that the actual level of HBsAg in a highly infectious sample was extraordinarily high—tens to hundreds of micrograms per milliliter. The AGD test was soon replaced by directed immunoprecipitation systems, such as counterimmunoelectrophoresis, or rheophoresis, in which an electrical potential or evaporative buffer flow forced the antibodies and antigen together, thus increasing the speed and sensitivity of the test. The tests were, however, highly subjective. Some alternative methods, such as reversed passive hemagglutination, were also developed and achieved a limited degree of implementation. A historical footnote is that AGD was (retrospectively) defined as a *first-generation test,* and the agglutination and directed immunoprecipitation tests were defined as *second-generation.*

Ling and Overby,[18] working at Abbott Laboratories, soon developed a tube-based, solid-phase radioimmunoassay (RIA) for the detection of HBsAg. This method clearly had greatly improved analytical sensitivity (i.e., ≈1 ng/mL) relative to second-generation tests and was formally defined as a *third-generation test.* It was not long before the Bureau of Biologics (the 1970s equivalent of the U.S. Food and Drug Administration) published a notice in the *Federal Register,* indicating that licensure of this third-generation test was imminent and "advising" blood establishments to "become familiar" with it.

At the time of implementation of the RIA, a solution to the problem of post-transfusion hepatitis was widely anticipated. Previously, it had been recognized that second-generation tests did not eliminate all post-transfusion hepatitis—indeed, there was only about a 20% decline in reporting rates. However, by what turned out to be a coincidence, RIA generated about fivefold more reactive results than did the second-generation tests. However, it soon became apparent that most of the additional "detections" represented false-positive results. This finding was a disappointment, but it led directly to the introduction of additional confirmatory tests and an enhanced perception of the rights of the donor to be properly informed about the significance of screening test results. After a relatively short time, RIA was replaced by the enzyme immunoassay (EIA). Subsequent developments have included chemiluminescent immunoassays with analytic sensitivity of approximately 0.08 ng/mL. Additionally, NAT for HBV DNA has been developed and has seen limited use for blood donor screening since around the year 2000.

Clinical Aspects

The clinical outcomes of hepatitis B vary in terms of severity, from asymptomatic to fatal, and in terms of chronicity, from acute to lifelong. There do not seem to be any very clear predictors of the severity of disease, other than the presence of detectable levels of the viral e antigen (HBeAg) in the circulation of an infected individual. However, it is clear that the likelihood of chronic infection is very much a function of the age of the patient at the time of infection. Chronic infection is common among persons who were infected in infancy, but the frequency is reduced to 5% or fewer of persons who were infected in adolescence or adulthood.[14]

Hepatitis B differs little from other viral hepatitides in its clinical manifestations, although such manifestations may often be somewhat more severe than those of hepatitis A or C. The incubation period is about 8 to 12 weeks, although it may extend to 6 months or longer, particularly if hepatitis B immune globulin has been used for postexposure prophylaxis. The majority of infections appear to be asymptomatic, although up to 30% of infected adults experience some level of jaundice. Hepatitis B may be fulminant and leads to death in about 0.5% to 1% of cases. As previously pointed out, a variable proportion of infections, irrespective of the occurrence of acute disease, resolve without further clinical symptoms with the development of essentially lifelong immunity, as indicated by the development and maintenance of detectable levels of antibodies to HBsAg (anti-HBs). However, it should be noted that such individuals may continue to harbor virus in the liver, as demonstrated by the occurrence of hepatitis B in transplanted livers from anti-HBs–positive donors.[19]

Chronic hepatitis B may be asymptomatic, but there is a wide range of symptomatic outcomes, up to and including fatal disease. As with other chronic hepatitis viruses, a proportion of patients may eventually demonstrate cirrhosis. In addition, chronic hepatitis B infection may result in the development of primary hepatocellular carcinoma, probably as a direct result of viral integration into the host cell genome. Unlike with hepatitis C, liver cancer induced by HBV may occur in the absence of cirrhosis.

There are also a number of extrahepatic manifestations of HBV infection, including rashes, arthritis, vasculitis, and glomerulonephritis.[14] Most are related to the formation of immune complexes involving HBsAg.

Treatment

There is no established treatment for acute hepatitis B, but therapies are approved for chronic disease. Currently, a 4- to 6-month course of interferon alfa-2b (5 to 10 million units, three times per week) is recommended. Improvement, as evidenced by HBe seroconversion, normalization of ALT, and sustained loss of HBV DNA in the circulation, may be seen in 20% to 30% of treated patients, although only about 10% lose HBsAg expression. Similar results are seen after a 12-month course of lamivudine, and response rates improve with more prolonged therapy.[20] Subsequently, more detailed recommendations have been published, establishing a variety of regimens for differing presentations of hepatitis B.[21] In general, in addition to interferon, lamivudine and adefovir are recommended for a year or more. Indicators of effective treatment include loss of detectable HBeAg and/or normalization of ALT levels. Pegylated interferon and lamivudine combination therapy seems most effective for HBeAg-positive patients.[22] Similarly prolonged treatment with adefovir appears to be effective for HBeAg-negative cases.[23]

Epidemiology

Hepatitis B virus is transmitted parenterally. Key risk factors for HBV include injection drug use; sexual exposure (both male-to-male and heterosexual); other parenteral exposures to blood and body fluids, including nonsterile tattooing and body piercing, as well as more subtle exposure via minor skin abrasion; and familial exposure. There is also geographic risk related to residence in areas of high prevalence. Transmission occurs readily, as a consequence of the high titers of infectious virus found during acute and chronic infection. In addition, infection may be transmitted from a viremic woman to her infant during birth.

In countries such as the United States, which have relatively low prevalence and incidence rates for HBV, most infection occurs horizontally between adults. Because adult infection generally has an acute outcome, opportunities for secondary transmission tend to be limited. Some behavior patterns, however, such as sharing of needles during injection drug use or frequent sexual contact with many partners, do result in a very high incidence of HBV infection. In areas with a high prevalence of chronic infection, both horizontal and perinatal patterns of infection occur, and the latter frequently leads to chronic infection and a prolonged carrier state. Thus, high prevalence rates are maintained; such a situation is seen in parts of the Far East, for example.

The overall prevalence of serologic evidence of HBV infection in the United States is approximately 5.6%, as indicated by measurements of HBsAg and antibodies to hepatitis B core antigen (anti-HBc).[24] However, infection rates are much higher among groups engaging in risky behaviors, such as male-to-male sex and injection drug use. The national prevalence of active infection, as defined by the presence of HBsAg is much lower, however—0.1% or less. In contrast, some parts of the world have seroprevalence rates of 50% or greater, with correspondingly high rates of active infection. Within the United States, the prevalence and incidence of HBV markers among blood donors are much lower than those seen in the overall population, reflecting the efficacy of measures used for donor selection.[25] Indeed, many of the donor screening questions in current use derived from efforts to minimize the transmission of hepatitis B. Additionally, questions used to reduce the risk of transmission of human immunodeficiency virus (HIV) are also likely to have had a significant impact on the number of infected donors.

There is no question that HBV vaccination policies are having an impact on the incidence (and ultimately the prevalence) of HBV infection. Widespread vaccination of infants offers the promise of interrupting maternal-child transmission of the virus and thus reducing the frequency of chronic infection and its sequelae. In the United States, there has been a clear decline in the frequency of reported cases of HBV infection,[26] which has been reflected in the continuing decrease in the frequency of HBV marker rates (particularly anti-Hc) among U.S. blood donors.

Virology

The human hepatitis B virus is the prototype of a small group of unusual DNA viruses known as the Hepadnaviridae. They have a lipid envelope and a small, partially double-stranded DNA genome, the full-length section of which has approximately 3200 bases, encoding four overlapping reading frames. DNA replicates in the hepatocyte nucleus by means of a unique mechanism involving a viral DNA polymerase and an RNA intermediate that is reverse transcribed. The transcription system does not have any inherent error-correction mechanism, so there is a much higher than usual frequency of nucleic acid substitution and thus mutation during viral replication. The virus itself is approximately 42 nm in diameter. The outer envelope is lipoprotein, antigenic, and known as HBsAg. The virus-specific antigen is termed "a," and there are a variety of antigenic subtypes, broadly and simplistically defined as two pairs of mutually exclusive alleles: d,y and w,r. The w determinant has itself been further characterized into four subspecificities. The major significance of these antigenic subtypes has been their use in epidemiologic studies.

Assessment of genome sequence variation of the virus has led to the recognition of six genotypes, A through F, on the basis of sequence variations of 8% or more. There is no systematic relationship between genotypes and antigenic subtypes. Genotyping may supplant antigenic subtyping for definition of the molecular epidemiology of HBV infection. Additionally, genotypes are more likely to reflect variations in the biology of different viral isolates.

Perhaps the most intriguing characteristic of HBV is that active HBV infection leads to copious overproduction of HBsAg, which is released into the circulation as self-assembled spheres and tubules, 22 nm in diameter. As already mentioned, HBsAg was first recognized (as Australia antigen) by Blumberg and associates.[15,16] The subsequent finding that

HBsAg is associated with hepatitis B led directly to blood donor testing for the antigen in the early 1970s and indirectly to the recognition of other hepatitis viruses.

The inner capsid of the virus has a different immunologic specificity and is known as the *hepatitis B core antigen.* This antigen was first recognized on immunoelectron microscopy of detergent-treated samples of virus-containing blood.[27] The core antigen is not normally detectable in serum or plasma, because it is located within the virus. It may, however, be detected in the nuclei of liver cells with active viral replication. Also coded by the gene for the core antigen is a smaller polypeptide sequence, masked in the full-length transcript, that includes a separate antigenic specificity termed *HBeAg.* This smaller peptide can be found free in the circulation during active infection.[28]

Laboratory investigations have clearly demonstrated the sequence of appearance of plasma markers of HBV infection.[29] Some 25 days after exposure to the virus, HBV DNA may be detected at low levels (hundreds or thousands of copies per milliliter). About 25 days later, these levels rise significantly, and at the same time, HBsAg becomes detectable by relatively insensitive techniques such as EIA. Generally, this period coincides with the appearance of symptoms of hepatitis and elevated liver function markers. About 4 to 8 weeks after the initial appearance of HBsAg, anti-HBc may be detected in the circulation.

A specific test for IgM anti-HBc is available and is extremely useful for diagnosis of HBV infection. With use of the available tests, IgM antibody may be detectable for 3 to 6 months. The IgG antibody persists over many years, whether or not the infection is frankly chronic. In the event of self-limited infection, HBsAg may be detected for about 6 to 12 weeks, but its level declines as anti-HBs becomes detectable. The presence of anti-HBs is usually taken to signal resolution of infection and the absence of infectious virus in the circulation. However, as pointed out previously, virus may persist in the liver.

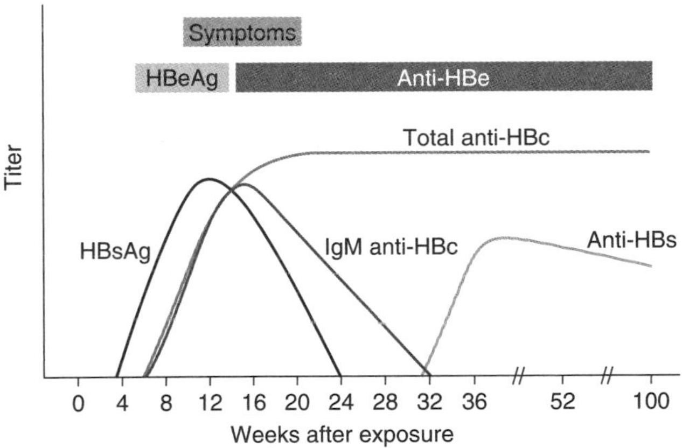

Figure 43–1 Typical serologic course of acute hepatitis B virus infection with recovery. Serologic markers of hepatitis B virus (HBV) infection vary, depending on whether the infection is acute or chronic. The first serologic marker to appear after acute infection is hepatitis B surface antigen (HBsAg), which can be detected as early as 1 or 2 weeks and as late as 11 or 12 weeks (mode, 30–60 days) after exposure to HBV. In persons who recover, HBsAg is no longer detectable in serum after an average of about 3 months. Hepatitis B e antigen (HBeAg) is generally detectable in patients with acute infection; the presence of HBeAg in serum correlates with higher titers of HBV and greater infectivity. A diagnosis of acute HBV infection can be made on the basis of the detection of immunoglobulin M (IgM) class antibody to hepatitis B core antigen (IgM anti-HBc) in serum; IgM anti-HBc is generally detectable at the time of clinical onset and declines to subdetectable levels with 6 months. IgG anti-HBc persists indefinitely as a marker of past infection. Anti-HBs becomes detectable during convalescence after the disappearance of HBsAg in patients who do not experience chronic infection. The presence of anti-HBs after acute infection generally indicates recovery and immunity from re-infection. (Courtesy of Centers for Disease Control and Prevention; from a publicly available slide set.)

Diagnostic Testing and Donor Screening

The primary diagnosis of hepatitis relies on cinical symptoms and the results of liver function tests. However, such tests do not permit differentiation of the etiology, and serologic testing is required. During the course of infection, a variety of patterns of expression of different markers is seen. To some extent, it is possible to define the stage of infection on the basis of these patterns.[14,28] The simplest situation is in acute infection (or the early stages of an infection that becomes chronic), in which the most reliable diagnostic marker is IgM anti-HBc. Figures 43–1 and 43–2 illustrate the patterns of marker expression in acute self-limited infection and chronic infection, respectively. Table 43–1 summarizes the interpretation of differing patterns of expression of key diagnostic markers.

In the United States, all whole blood donations are tested for HBsAg and for anti-HBc to reduce the risk of transmission of HBV. Interestingly, testing for anti-HBc was initially introduced in 1986 as a surrogate test for infectivity for non-A, non-B hepatitis. In the face of sensitive tests for hepatitis C virus (HCV), there is now no such surrogate value for anti-HBc testing. In fact, the actual benefit of anti-HBc testing in prevention of HBV infection is unclear, although it has been shown that, among voluntary donations that are anti-HBc positive but HBsAg-negative, somewhat fewer than 1% have detectable HBV DNA.[30] Many years ago, anti-HBc testing was also thought to be beneficial in detecting infectious samples during a window when HBsAg was no longer detectable and effective levels of anti-HBs had not developed. This window is no longer apparent with HBsAg tests at their current levels of sensitivity.

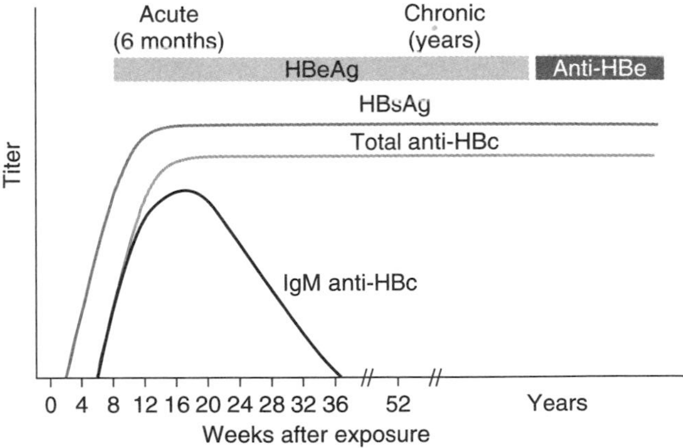

Figure 43–2 Typical serologic course of progression to chronic hepatitis B virus infection. In patients with chronic hepatitis B virus (HBV) infection, both hepatitis B surface antigen (HBsAg) and immunoglobulin G (IgG) antibody to hepatitis B core antigen (anti-HBc) remain persistently detectable, generally for life. Hepatitis B e antigen (HBeAg) is variably present in these patients. The presence of HBsAg for 6 months or longer generally indicates chronic infection. In addition, a negative test result for IgM anti-HBc together with a positive test for HBsAg in a single serum specimen usually indicates that an individual has chronic HBV infection. (Courtesy of Centers for Disease Control and Prevention; from a publicly available slide set.)

Table 43–1 Interpretation of Results of Hepatitis B Test Panel

Tests	Results	Interpretation
HBsAg Anti-HBc Anti-HBs	Negative Negative Negative	Susceptible
HBsAg Anti-HBc Anti-HBs	Negative Positive Positive	Immune because of natural infection
HBsAg Anti-HBc Anti-HBs	Negative Negative Positive	Immune because of hepatitis B vaccination
HBsAg Anti-HBc IgM anti-HBc Anti-HBs	Positive Positive Positive Negative	Acutely infected
HBsAg Anti-HBc IgM anti-HBc Anti-HBs	Positive Positive Negative Negative	Chronically infected
HBsAg Anti-HBc Anti-HBs	Negative Positive Negative	Four interpretations possible*

*The patient (1) may be recovering from acute HBV infection; (2) may be distantly immune (the test is not sensitive enough to detect very low levels of anti-HBs in serum); (3) may be susceptible with a false-positive anti-HBc test result; or (4) may have an undetectable level of HBsAg in serum, so is actually a carrier.

Anti-HBc, antibody to hepatitis B core antigen; anti-HBs, antibody to hepatitis B surface antigen; HBsAg, hepatitis B surface antigen; Ig, immunoglobulin. Courtesy of Centers for Disease Control and Prevention.

Estimates of the residual risk of HBV transmission are surprisingly high; in 1996, Schreiber and colleagues[31] suggested a figure of 1:63,000 donations. Some researchers express concern that this figure may be inappropriately high, on the basis of questions about the underlying assumptions and the absence of observed post-transfusion hepatitis B. In fact, in 2001, even with the same assumptions made by Schreiber,[31] the risk of HBV transmission was estimated to have at least halved as a result of the decreased incidence of HBV among U.S. donors. The most recent estimate of the residual risk of post-transfusion HBV infection is 1:205,000 among repeat donations or 1:144,000 among all donations, in the absence of NAT.[32,33] However, such estimates inherently depend on a number of assumptions and extrapolations, and the frequency of observed cases of post-transfusion hepatitis B is insufficient to support this estimate. Additionally, it seems likely that many of the cases of post-transfusion hepatitis that are reported are not, in fact due to transfusion transmission, as recently shown by Alter and her associates (presented at the Advisory Committee on Blood Safety and Availability, August 26 to 27, 2004; see http://www.hhs.gov/bloodsafety/presentations/MiriamAlter.pdf). She found that only one of 49 cases of supposed post-transfusion hepatitis could be unequivocally linked to transfusion of an infectious unit. On the other hand, there is little in the way of organized lookback for hepatitis B, at least in the United States, but data from Japan clearly show that window-period HBV infection may occur.

Nucleic acid amplification testing for HBV is available and has been implemented in a number of countries around the world. As of late 2005, one test had been licensed for use in the United States, and clinical trials have been completed for another, in a triplex format that includes HIV and HCV testing.[34] However, it is clear that the current minipool approach will not have any significant benefits, because NAT has essentially the same sensitivity as the newest of the serologic tests for HBsAg.[35] Nevertheless, clinical trials of one of the U.S. tests did generate a measurable yield of about 1:250,000 HBV DNA-positive, seronegative donations, even in a pooled testing format. Such NAT for HBV DNA has been implemented in some European locations (where anti-HBc testing is not performed) and by some manufacturers of pooled plasma products.[36] The potential added value of single-unit (i.e., nonpooled) NAT for HBV DNA has not been well-defined, although it will certainly prevent cases of post-transfusion HBV infection. Perhaps the greatest value of HBV NAT will be in regions where testing for anti-HBc is not used, because it could detect those samples that are positive for anti-HBc and viremic for HBV. However, such samples generally have a low level of DNA, and a sensitive test will be needed.

Mutants and Vaccines

A number of mutants of HBV have been recognized, and there is evidence that the representation of such mutants is increasing. Perhaps of greatest concern for transfusion medicine are those mutants that do not express HBsAg.[37–39] This group includes those described as *escape mutants*—a term signifying an ability to evade the protective effects of HBV vaccines (which are currently based on HBsAg). However, infection with these mutants still provokes the formation of detectable levels of anti-HBc, so that most such infections would be detected, at least in the United States and other countries where anti-HBc testing of donations is routine.

Currently available hepatitis B vaccines prepared from recombinant antigens are safe and effective and are recommended for universal use in infants. It is to be expected that consistent use of these vaccines will eventually lead to significant reduction in HBV infection rates and thus to a decline in the prevalence of chronic infection. Current vaccines provoke only anti-HBs and so do not interfere with routine blood donation testing. However, it should be noted that HBsAg itself may be detectable in the circulation for a few days after inoculation. Although there is no need to defer a recent vaccine recipient for safety reasons, it is wise to avoid collection of blood from such a person for about 7 days after vaccination. Otherwise, there is a risk that the donor will be confirmed positive for HBsAg and will thus be deferred. Finally, although the risk of transmission of HBV by blood components has almost been eliminated and although there should be no cases from manufactured plasma products as a result of careful donor management and viral inactivation of the final product, chronic users of blood and blood products should certainly receive the HBV vaccine.

HEPATITIS D

Hepatitis D is caused by a small satellite virus, originally termed the *delta virus*, that can replicate only in the presence of HBV infection. The virus is an RNA virus and, almost unique among animal viruses, has a circular genome. It encodes a single peptide, originally observed in infected hepatocytes and termed *delta antigen*. The infectious form of HDV is coated with HBsAg. Co-infection with HBV and HDV results in a more serious disease than does HBV infection alone. In truth, HDV has little current relevance to transfusion safety, because measures designed to detect infectivity for HBV also detect all individuals co-infected with HDV.[40,41]

HEPATITIS E

Hepatitis E virus (HEV) causes an epidemic form of hepatitis that is self-limited.[42,43] The disease is somewhat similar to hepatitis A, although it is much more severe in pregnancy. Transmission is by the fecal-oral route and is most often water-borne. The virus is related to the calicivirus group and, as such, is a nonenveloped virus that has an RNA genome. Although there is some evidence (based largely on seroprevalence studies) that HEV is present in the United States, it is found predominantly in tropical countries. Indeed, most cases identified in the United States appear to have resulted from infections that occurred in countries where HEV is endemic. HEV infection is self-limited and acute, and it has generally been thought that there is little risk of transmission by transfusion. Until recently, no cases of transfusion-associated HEV infection have been reported.[44] However, a number of recent cases of such transmission have been reported from nonendemic areas, emphasizing that acute infections are also transmissible by transfusion, as long as there is an asymptomatic viremic phase.[45,46] This has, of course, been abundantly illustrated by the example of West Nile virus in the United States.[47]

HEPATITIS G VIRUS/GBV-C

The vast majority of cases of post-transfusion hepatitis have been shown to be caused by HBV or HCV. Nevertheless, there continue to be some residual cases of hepatitis associated with transfusion. For example, in Alter's continuing studies at the National Institutes of Health, approximately 12% of cases of non-A, non-B hepatitis could not be attributed to either HBV or HCV. These residual cases appear to be mild and self-limited, and some may not even have an infectious etiology. Such cases have, however, led to a continuing search for additional hepatitis viruses. The first of such putative hepatitis viruses was identified by two separate groups in the late 1990s. In one case, scientists at Abbott Laboratories looked for genomic sequences related to those of an existing isolate known as the *GB virus* (GBV), which had previously been associated with hepatitis in a physician. Three viruses were identified, one of which (termed GBV-C) was found among a number of human sources.[48] Working in parallel, but using a different approach, scientists at Gene-Labs isolated viral RNA sequences and characterized a virus they termed *hepatitis G virus* (HGV).[49] It is generally accepted that these two isolates were, in fact, representatives of essentially the same virus group, which is now known as HGV.

HGV, like HCV, appears to be closely related to the Flavivirus group. It is found among a relatively high proportion of the normal population, as exemplified by blood donors. Its presence has been demonstrated both by seroprevalence studies, in which the frequency of antibodies is 3% to 15%, and more interestingly by detection of viral RNA in the plasma of 1% to 3% of normal subjects.[50] Perhaps not surprisingly, the virus is readily transmissible by transfusion and is found at high prevalence among individuals who have undergone multiple transfusions. However, it has not proved possible to demonstrate that infection with HGV is associated with hepatitis or even with signs of mild liver disease, such as elevated ALT levels. Indeed, HGV appears to be a virus that is currently in search of a disease. The term *hepatitis* in its name may be a misnomer, attributable only to the fact that the virus was found in association with hepatitis in the first place. It is also important to recognize that the worldwide distribution of HGV clearly shows that it is not a new virus but rather one that has coexisted with humans for many centuries.

There have, however, been some intriguing observations that clearly suggest that HGV/GBV-C may have an impact on the course of HIV disease. For example, studies have shown lower mortality among co-infected individuals relative to those with HIV only.[51,52] The mechanism for this effect is unclear, but it may be due to the effects of infection on the levels of a number of chemokines.[53]

TTV AND SEN-V

Curiously, another pair of viruses were separately identified among individuals with hepatitis and were also shown to be poorly, if at all, associated with hepatitis. These viruses were also found to cause prolonged viremia and, in some cases, turned out to be present in up to 90% of the population. Like HGV, they were readily transmitted by transfusion. Both viruses were thought to be representatives of the circovirus group: small, nonenveloped viruses with a circular DNA genome. This group of viruses had not previously been described among humans.

Workers in Japan used representational difference analysis to isolate DNA sequences from three patients with unexplained post-transfusion hepatitis. The sequence was established as viral, and the virus was named *TTV*, reflecting the initials of the patient from whom it was isolated.[54] A considerable amount of research has revealed some of the key features of this agent.[55] It is a small virus with a covalently closed, circular DNA genome of approximately 3800 bases. The virus is thought to be nonenveloped and is most closely related to the circoviruses, which are responsible for a number of diseases in plants and a handful of mammalian and avian disease states. The classification of TTV is currently incomplete, and proposals have been made to place it in at least two genera. What has become apparent is that TTV is a member of an extremely diverse group of viruses, as demonstrated by considerable variation in genomic sequence.

Epidemiologic studies have confirmed that TTV is a widely distributed virus and have clearly established that it is transmissible by transfusion. Interestingly, it also appears to be transmitted by the vertical, fecal-oral, and perhaps other routes.

A key issue is the clinical significance of this group of viruses. Although the original source of the virus and its apparent association with ALT elevations implied that TTV was indeed a hepatitis virus, this identification no longer seems tenable. Indeed, there are far more infections without ALT elevations than with such evidence of liver disease. Even in clear, transfusion-associated transmission of TTV, the recipients did not manifest ALT elevations in any pattern that could be associated with the infection. Thus, at this stage, there is little evidence that this virus expresses any pathogenic potential. However, it is certainly too early to conclude that this entire group of viruses is without any clinical significance.

After the recognition of TTV, the search for hepatitis viruses continued, and Primi and colleagues[56,57] used degenerate primers derived from TTV to probe samples from selected patients. An isolate was identified and named *SEN-V* (after the initials of the source patient, an HIV-infected injection drug user). Eventually, at least eight different strains were isolated, termed A through H. The SEN group has been shown to be one branch of the TTV group, seeming to share its epidemiologic characteristics. Although two of the strains (D and H) have been associated with evidence of transfusion-associated hepatitis, a causal relationship has not been established.[56,57]

Thus, attempts to define the etiologic agent(s) of non-A through E hepatitis do not appear to have been successful to date. The availability of powerful genomic techniques has certainly led to the recognition of previously undescribed viruses, but it has not been possible to associate any particular disease with these remarkably widespread viruses. No doubt other such orphan viruses will be identified. However, it will be important to avoid an automatic assumption of causality when such viruses are isolated from patients with any given disease state. It may also be important to question whether all residual transfusion-associated hepatitides do indeed have an infectious etiology.

REFERENCES

1. Cuthbert JA. Hepatitis A: Old and new. Clin Microbiol Rev 2001;14:38–58.
2. Hollinger FB, Khan NC, Oefinger PE, et al. Posttransfusion hepatitis type A. JAMA 1983;250:2313–2317.
3. Azimi PH, Roberto RR, Guralnick J, et al. Transfusion-acquired hepatitis A in a premature infant with secondary nosocomial spread in an intensive care nursery. Am J Dis Child 1986;140:23–27.
4. Giacoia GP, Kasprisin DO. Transfusion-acquired hepatitis A. South Med J 1989;82:1357–1360.
5. Lee KK, Vargo LR, Le CT, Fernando L. Transfusion-acquired hepatitis A outbreak from fresh frozen plasma in a neonatal intensive care unit. Pediatr Infect Dis 3 1992;11:122–123.
6. Mosley JW, Nowicki MI, Kasper CK, et al. Hepatitis A virus transmission by blood products in the United States. Vox Sang 1994;67(Suppl)1:24–28.
7. Bower WA, Nainan OV, Han XH, Margolis HS. Duration of viremia in hepatitis A virus infection. J Infect Dis 2000;182:12–17.
8. Gowland P, Fontana S, Niederhauser C, Taleghani BM. Molecular and serologic tracing of a transfusion-transmitted hepatitis A virus. Transfusion 2004;44:1555–1561.
9. CDC. Hepatitis A outbreak associated with green onions at a restaurant—Monaca, Pennsylvania, 2003. MMWR Morb Mortal Wkly Rep 2003;52:1155–1157.
10. Soucie JM, Robertson BH, Bell BP, et al. Hepatitis A virus infections associated with clotting factor concentrate in the United States. Transfusion 1998;38:573–579.
11. Mannucci PM, Gdovin S, Gringeri A, et al. Transmission of hepatitis A to patients with hemophilia by factor VIII concentrates treated with organic solvent and detergent to inactivate viruses. Ann Intern Med 1994;120:1–7.
12. Johnson Z, Thornton L, Tobin A, et al. An outbreak of hepatitis A among Irish haemophiliacs. Int J Epidemiol 1995;24:821–828.
13. Lawlor E, Graham S, Davidson F, et al. Hepatitis A transmission by factor IX concentrates. Vox Sang 1996;71:126–128.
14. Lee WM. Hepatitis B virus infection. NEJM 1997;337:1733–1745.
15. Blumberg BS, Alter HJ, Visnich S. A "new" antigen in leukemia sera. JAMA 1965;191:541–546.
16. Blumberg BS, Gerstley BJS, Hungerford DA, et al. A serum antigen (Australia antigen) in Down's syndrome, leukemia and hepatitis. Ann Intern Med 1967;66:924.
17. Gocke DJ, Greenberg HB, Kavey NB. Correlation of Australia antigen with posttransfusion hepatitis. JAMA 1970;212:877–879.
18. Ling CM, Overby LR. Prevalence of hepatitis B virus antigen as revealed by direct radioimmune assay with 125-1-antibody. J Immunol 1972;109:834–841.
19. Dodson SF, Issa S, Araya V, et al. Infectivity of hepatic allografts with antibodies to hepatitis B virus. Transplantation 1997;64:1582–1584.
20. Lin OS, Keeffe EB. Current treatment strategies for chronic hepatitis B and C. Annu Rev Med 2001;52:29–49.
21. Lok ASF, McMahon BJ. Chronic hepatitis B: update of recommendations. Hepatology 2004;39:1–5.
22. Lau GKK, Piravisuth T, Luo KX, et al. Peg-interferon alfa-2a, lamivudine, and the combination for HBeAg-positive chronic hepatitis B. NEJM 2005;352:2682–2695.
23. Hadziyannis SJ, Tassopoulos NC, Heathcote EJ, et al. Long-term therapy with adefovir dipivoxil for HBeAg-negative chronic hepatitis B. NEJM 2005;352:2673–2681.
24. McQuillan GM, Coleman PJ, Kruszon-Moran D, et al. Prevalence of hepatitis B virus infection in the United States: The National Health and Nutrition Examination Surveys, 1976 through 1994. Am J Public Health 1999;89:14–18.
25. Dodd RY. Germs, gels, and genomes: A personal recollection of 30 years in blood safety testing. In Stramer SL (ed): Blood Safety in the New Millenium. Bethesda, Md., American Association of Blood Banks, 2001, pp 97–122.
26. CDC. Hepatitis Surveillance Report No. 60. Atlanta: U.S. Department of Health and Human Services, Centers for Disease Control and Prevention, 2005.
27. Almeida JD, Rubenstein D, Stott EJ. New antigen–antibody system in Australia-antigen positive hepatitis. Lancet 1971;2:1225–1227.
28. Mahoney FJ. Update on diagnosis, management, and prevention of hepatitis B virus infection. Clin Microbiol Rev 1999;12:351–366.
29. Busch MP. HIV, HBV and HCV: new developments related to transfusion safety. Vox Sang 2000;78:253–256.
30. Kleinman SH, Kuhns MC, Todd DS, et al. Frequency of HBV DNA detection in U.S. blood donors testing positive for the presence of anti-HBc: implications for transfusion transmission and donor screening. Transfusion 2003;43:696–704.
31. Schreiber GB, Busch MP, Kleinman SH, Korelitz JJ. The risk of transfusion-transmitted viral infections. NEJM 1996;334:1685–1690.
32. Dodd RY, Notari EP, Stramer SL. Current prevalence and incidence of infectious disease markers and estimated window-period risk in the American Red Cross blood donor population. Transfusion 2002;42:975–979.
33. Dodd RY. Current safety of the blood supply in the United States. Int J Hematol 2004;80:301–305.
34. Stramer SL. Pooled hepatitis B virus DNA testing by nucleic acid amplification: Implementation or not. Transfusion 2005;44:1242–1246.
35. Biswas R, Tabor E, Hsia CC, et al. Comparative sensitivity of HBV NATs and HBsAg assays for detection of acute HBV infection. Transfusion 2003;43:788–798.
36. Roth WK, Weber M, Seifried E. Feasibility and efficacy of routine PCR screening of blood donations for hepatitis C virus, hepatitis B virus, and HIV-1 in a bloodbank setting. Lancet 1999;353:359–363.
37. Blum HE. Hepatitis B virus: Significance of naturally occurring mutants. Intervirology 1993;35:40–50.
38. Hsu HY, Chang MH, Liaw SH, et al. Changes of hepatitis B surface antigen variants in carrier children before and after universal vaccination in Taiwan. Hepatology 1999;30:1312–1317.
39. Jongerius IM, Wester M, Cuypers HTM, et al. New hepatitis B virus mutant form in a blood donor that is undetectable in several hepatitis B surface antigen screening assays. Transfusion 1998;38:56–59.
40. Lai MMC. The molecular biology of hepatitis delta virus. Annu Rev Biochem 1995;64:259–286.
41. Liaw YF, Tsai SL, Sheen IS, et al. Clinical and virological course of chronic hepatitis B virus infection with hepatitis C and D virus markers. Am J Gastroenterol 1998;93:354–359.
42. Purcell RH. The discovery of the hepatitis viruses. Gastroenterology 1993;104:955–963.
43. Thomas DL, Yarbough PO, Vlahov D, et al. Seroreactivity to hepatitis E virus in areas where the disease is not endemic. J Clin Microbiol 1997;35:1244–1247.
44. Mateos ML, Camarero C, Lasa E, et al. Hepatitis E virus: Relevance in blood donors and other risk groups. Vox Sang 1998;75:267–269.
45. Matsubayashi K, Nagaoka Y, Sakata H, et al. Transfusion-transmitted hepatitis E caused by apparently indigenous hepatitis E virus strain in Hokkaido, Japan. Transfusion 2004;44:934–940.
46. Boxall EH, Herborn A, Kochethu G, et al. Transfusion transmitted hepatitis E in a "non endemic" country. Transfus Med 2006;16:79–83.

47. Pealer LN, Marfin AA, Petersen LR, et al. Transmission of West Nile virus through blood transfusion in the United States in 2002. NEJM 2003;349:1236–1245.
48. Leary TP, Muerhoff AS, Simons JN, et al. Sequence and genomic organization of GBV-C. A novel member of the Flaviviridae associated with human non-A-E hepatitis. J Med Virol 1996;48:60–67.
49. Linnen J, Wages J Jr, Zhang-Keck ZY, et al. Molecular cloning and disease association of hepatitis G virus: a transfusion transmissible agent. Science 1996;271:505–508.
50. Allain JP. Emerging viral infections relevant to transfusion medicine. Blood Rev 2000;14:173–181.
51. Tillmann HL, Heiken H, Knapik-Botor A, et al. Infection with GB virus C and reduced mortality among HIV-infected patients. NEJM 2001;345:715–724.
52. Xiang J, Wunschmann S, Diekema DJ, et al. Effect of coinfection with GB virus C on survival among patients with HIV infection. NEJM 2001;345:707–714.
53. Xiang J, George SL, Wunschmann S, et al. Inhibition of HIV-1 replication by GB virus C infection through increases in RANTES, MIP-1α, MIP-1β, and SDF-1. Lancet 2004;363:2040–2046.
54. Nishizawa T, Okamoto H, Konishi K, et al. A novel DNA virus (TTV) associated with elevated transaminase levels in posttransfusion hepatitis of unknown etiology. Biochem Biophys Res Commun 1997;241:92–97.
55. Bendinelli M, Pistello M, Maggi F, et al. Molecular properties, biology, and clinical implications of Tf virus, a recently identified widespread infectious agent of humans. Clin Microbiol Rev 2001;14:98–113.
56. Umemura T, Yeo AE, Sottini A, et al. SEN virus infection and its relationship to transfusion-associated hepatitis. Hepatology 2001;33:1303–1311.
57. Tanaka Y, Primi D, Wang RY, et al. Genomic and molecular evolutionary analysis of a newly identified infectious agent (SEN virus) and its relationship to the TT virus family. J Infect Dis 2001;183:359–367.

Chapter 44

Hepatitis C

Roger Y. Dodd

INTRODUCTION

For many years, hepatitis C was the most common infectious complication of blood transfusion in the United States. Indeed, a number of studies in the 1970s showed that more than 10% of blood recipients had biochemical evidence of what was then termed *non-A, non-B hepatitis* (NANBH).[1,2] Subsequently, almost all of these cases were shown to be due to infection with the hepatitis C virus (HCV). Fortunately, the implementation of increasingly sensitive tests for HCV infection has now reduced the incidence of post-transfusion hepatitis C infection to levels that are essentially undetectable by direct study; by early 2001, the risk was estimated at about 1 infection per 1.4 million component units.[3]

THE DISEASE

The symptoms of acute hepatitis C do not differ significantly from those of other viral hepatitides, although they may be somewhat less severe than those of hepatitis B. The incubation period is 7 to 8 weeks, but a wide range has been noted. It has been estimated that about 25% of acute cases may be accompanied by symptoms that, in some cases, may be quite mild. When present, symptoms include fatigue, anorexia, abdominal pain, and weight loss. A proportion (perhaps 20% to 30%) of patients with acute hepatitis C may become jaundiced. Symptoms may last for up to 10 weeks. Alanine aminotransferase (ALT) levels are elevated during the acute phase; such elevations tend to be moderate (i.e., around 300 to 400 IU/L) but may be quite high (up to 2000 IU/L). Acute disease is rarely fatal, with mortality rates of 1% or less.

Approximately 20% of acute infections resolve. The remaining 80% (whether symptomatic or not) become chronic. The natural history of chronic HCV infection is not completely understood. Such chronic infections may last for the lifetime of the patient, although there is growing evidence that 26% to 45% of these cases may eventually resolve, as shown by the disappearance of detectable HCV RNA in the circulation and in some instances by the eventual loss of detectable antibody.[4] Many infected individuals may remain completely asymptomatic for several years (perhaps even their whole lives), but a good number have histologic evidence of liver disease, including hepatitis, fibrosis, and cirrhosis. In some cases, hepatocellular carcinoma develops.

Alter and Seeff[4] have published a framework representing the outcome of HCV infection that is based on a large number of published studies. They conclude that 20% of infected individuals resolve the acute infection. Of the remaining 80% who become chronically infected, 30% demonstrate a stable chronic hepatitis with a favorable outcome. Another 30% have severe, progressive hepatitis, and the remaining 40% may have some variable progression. Prospective studies have shown, however, that chronic symptomatic hepatitis may take an average of 10 to 14 years (and, frequently, much longer) to develop, whereas cirrhosis may take an average of 21 years and hepatocellular carcinoma almost 30 years. Although life-threatening outcomes may be uncommon or considerably delayed, it is still true that the consequences of HCV infection are the leading indicator for liver transplantation in the developed world.

From the perspective of transfusion medicine, this pattern of disease has two important consequences. First, although the immediate consequences of post-transfusion hepatitis C may seem to be largely trivial, the long-term outcomes cannot be ignored. Second, the preponderance of asymptomatic, chronic infection leads to a relatively large population of individuals who are at risk of transmitting the infection via blood donation.

TREATMENT

In 1997, a National Institutes of Health Consensus Development Conference gave recommendations for treatment of chronic hepatitis C, applicable to individuals with significant histologic findings on biopsy, presence of HCV antibody, elevated ALT, and detectable levels of HCV RNA.[5] In brief, such patients should initially be treated with 3 million units of interferon alfa three times a week for 12 months. In the absence of any response (i.e., normalization of ALT and loss of detectable HCV RNA), this therapy should be discontinued after 3 months and the patient should be considered for combination therapy with interferon and ribavirin. Overall, about 50% of patients show temporary improvement with this regimen, but ultimately, only about 25% of all patients show definitive resolution of disease. A subsequent Consensus Development Conference in 2002 updated these recommendations, emphasizing the value of combination therapy.

These treatment recommendations have been updated by Liang and colleagues[6] on the basis of experience with combination therapies. In fact, a review of two studies revealed that a sustained response to interferon alone was observed in 29% of patients after treatment for either 24 or 48 weeks.[6] However, among those receiving combination therapy (interferon plus ribavirin), 33% showed a sustained response at 24 weeks, and 41% showed such a response after 48 weeks of therapy. It was also noted that treatment for more than 24 weeks was unnecessary in patients with HCV subtypes

2 and 3, because of the greater responsiveness of these subtypes to treatment. A number of studies have indicated that pegylated interferon is more effective than the standard product; it is now the preferred version, particularly for treatment of recurrent disease.[7,8] Detailed recommendations for diagnosis, management, and treatment of hepatitis C have recently been published by the American Association for the Study of Liver Diseases.[9] Current therapeutic approaches result in a sustained response in 42% to 82% of patients with chronic disease, depending on the viral genotype.

EPIDEMIOLOGY

Hepatitis C virus is globally distributed and, with a few notable exceptions, the seroprevalence rate is remarkably constant from one region to another, usually on the order of 1% to 2%.[10] Although some countries or localities have startlingly high rates, these may be due to cultural factors, including the use of traditional medicine practices; in Egypt, for example, numerous infections were attributed to a program involving injections for control of schistosomiasis.[11] In the United States, the overall seroprevalence rate has been estimated at 1.8%, and 65% of persons infected with HCV are age 30 to 49.[12]

Transmission of HCV is primarily confined to parenteral routes. In the United States, it is clear that many of the currently identified infections are a result of previous exposure via illegal injection of drugs. In addition, many infections are believed to have resulted from blood transfusions given before the availability of sensitive tests.[13] Other epidemiologic associations are the use of clotting factor concentrates before the implementation of effective viral inactivation in 1987, exposure in a health care setting, household exposure, multiple sexual partners, and low socioeconomic level.[14]

There has been considerable speculation about the natural transmission routes of HCV, which have presumably been responsible for maintaining the baseline viral prevalence levels over centuries or even millennia. Some evidence exists for sexual and perinatal transmission, but in both cases, it seems likely that transmission may occur only during early acute infection. HCV infection does not show the strong association with male-to-male sex that has been seen for hepatitis B and human immunodeficiency viruses (HIVs).

The incidence of new HCV infections has declined by 80% or more since 1989. Clearly, there has been a major reduction in transfusion transmission of the virus, and the majority of new infections (about 60%) are attributable to injection drug use. Even though incidence is declining, it is anticipated that the burden of HCV disease will continue to rise over the foreseeable future because of the large number of chronically infected individuals.[10,15]

Studies on the epidemiology of HCV infection among blood donors are of significant importance in the context of strategies for donor selection and questioning. Conry-Cantilena and associates[16] studied a population of 481 blood donors who were found to be reactive in screening tests for anti-HCV. Among the 241 with positive strip immunoassay (SIA) results, 27% had a history of transfusion, 68% had used cocaine intranasally, 42% had a history of intravenous drug use, and 53% reported a history of sexual promiscuity; ear-piercing among men was also significantly associated with a positive test result. Many of these risk factors were confounded. Nonetheless, these observations prompted the institution of donor questions regarding intranasal cocaine use; a formal requirement for this question was subsequently eliminated, however.

It is of interest to note that, in a study performed in blood donors who tested positive for HCV RNA but negative for HCV antibody, 29.2% reported recent intravenous drug use. A history of recent incarceration was independently associated with nucleic acid amplification test (NAT) positivity.[17] The prevalence of HCV infection in current injection drug users is estimated to be 79%, although this rate does appear to be declining.[10] Donor history questioning can certainly be improved, but it is unclear how to obtain more accurate information on previous illicit drug exposures, whether they be recent or many years ago. Fortunately, individuals with past histories do not contribute to window period risk.

VIROLOGY

The hepatitis C virus was first recognized in 1989 as the principal etiologic agent of NANBH. A small RNA genome segment was isolated from a presumptive viral pellet prepared from the plasma of an experimentally infected chimpanzee. When the encoded peptide was expressed in bacteria through the use of a lambda phage vector, it was reactive with antibodies present in convalescent serum from a patient with NANBH.[18] This RNA fragment, termed *5-1-1,* was used as a basis for the eventual sequencing of the entire genome of the virus. The 5-1-1 sequence was also used to develop the capture reagent (the c100-3 peptide) incorporated into the initial version of an HCV antibody enzyme immunoassay (EIA). This peptide represents a portion of the NS3 region of the HCV genome.[19] Subsequently, additional peptides have been expressed and incorporated into improved versions of the HCV antibody test.

The virus itself is an enveloped, single-strand RNA virus now classified as a separate genus (*Hepacivirus*) within the Flaviviridae. It has a positive-strand genome of barely less than 10,000 bases. The functional organization of the genome has been well-defined.[20]

Recently, there has been notable success in establishing a laboratory culture system for the virus, in which a replicative form of the viral genome has been used to infect cells in vitro. Virus produced from such systems has been shown to be infectious for chimpanzees.[21,22] These culture systems offer considerable promise for the further study of the virus.

Hepatitis C virus is characterized by considerable genetic variability, expressed at three levels: genotype, subtype, and isolate. There are six major genotypes of HCV, designated by the Arabic numerals 1 to 6. The RNA sequence varies between genotypes by some 25% to 35%, and this level of differentiation has probably emerged over periods of 500 to 2000 years. Subtypes within a genotype, designated by lowercase letters (a, b, etc.), represent RNA sequence variation of 15% to 25% that evolved over about 300 years. Individual isolates within a subtype may vary by 5% to 10% in RNA sequence.[23–27] Overall, these studies indicate that the frequency of major subtypes in the United States is as follows: 1a, 42.6%; 1b, 29.2%; 2a, 2.7%; 2b, 8.1%; 3a, 4.7%.

Additionally, there are hypervariable regions in the genome, and many quasispecies of HCV are likely to develop in an individual patient over time. In general, any variation below the level of subtype is unlikely to be reliable enough to differentiate sources of infection. The distribution of HCV subtypes may change with geography. It has been suggested that the clinical outcome of HCV infection and the response to treatment may vary with subtype. Genotypes 2 and 3 are more responsive to treatment than the more common subtypes 1a and 1b.[5,9,28,29]

The sequence of events after infection with HCV has been well-characterized at the level of viral markers in the circulation. Antibodies may be detected by version 3.0 tests an average of 70 days after exposure, although this period may be quite variable.[30,31] However, some 40 to 60 days prior to the appearance of such antibodies, HCV RNA may be detected in the plasma. The HCV RNA levels rise rapidly (over a few days) to 10^5 to 10^7 copies/mL. This level is generally maintained at least until significant levels of antibody are expressed. It is now apparent that a soluble viral core antigen is also present and can be detected once the RNA levels exceed about 50,000 copies/mL.[32,33] Elevated levels of ALT are frequently observed a few days before antibodies are detectable, but always after the steep rise in RNA levels. Interestingly, there is growing evidence that there may be occasional low levels of viral RNA in the circulation during the early eclipse phase, after infection and prior to the steep rise to peak levels of RNA.[5,29]

The implementation of widespread NAT for HCV RNA has been shown to detect a meaningful number of RNA-positive, anti-HCV–negative donations. Stramer and colleagues[34] reviewed the results of the first 3 years of testing in the United States. Among almost 40 million donations tested by the Chiron/Gen-Probe or Roche assays in small pools of plasma samples (16 and 24 samples per pool, respectively), 170 RNA-positive, anti-HCV nonreactive samples were identified. This reflected an overall rate of 1 in every 230,000 donations. Although there was no significant difference in the rates from the two different HCV RNA tests, the rate amongst donations tested by the more sensitive test for anti-HCV was 1 in 270,000. Within the Red Cross system, the rate was 1:251,000 for the first 3 years of HCV NAT, increasing to 1:221,000 in the following 2 years. The increase was not statistically signficant. Overall, of 156 evaluable cases, 51 would have been excluded as donors as a result of other test results, primarily ALT elevations, which occurred among 46 of the 51.[34] Thus, in retrospect, ALT testing probably did have a modest impact on blood safety, but at significant cost in terms of blood supply. These data, along with other information showing that donor ALT levels were of little or no demonstrable value for interdicting other supposed transfusion-transmitted hepatitides, led to its elimination for blood component testing.

In Stramer's study, RNA-positive donors were entered into follow-up investigations. It was found that 75 of 90 enrolled donors seroconverted, as detected in samples collected a median of 35 days post-donation. The majority of those who failed to seronconvert had only been followed for 12 to 58 days. In a more comprehensive study of 67 RNA-positive donors, 7 failed to complete follow up, 2 had abortive infections, and 3 did not seroconvert after periods of 1.5 to 3 years. It is of interest to note that the median time to observed follow-up is approximately 50% of the supposed window period, although 35 days is probably something of an overestimate because of the sampling intervals in the study.[34]

Once antibodies are detectable, RNA levels may decrease or become variable. In the evaluation of samples from blood donors, HCV RNA is detected in about 80% of samples that are reactive on a version 3.0 EIA and confirmed reactive on the version 3.0 SIA.[35] The frequency of RNA detection declines with the strength of the antibody response (as defined by the number and intensity of bands on the SIA).[36] It seems likely that the antibody-positive, RNA-negative samples actually represent resolved infections. In some cases, antibodies may eventually decline to undetectable levels.

There is a vigorous humoral and cytotoxic immune response to HCV, but in most cases, it is clearly unable to eliminate the virus. The mechanisms underlying the ability of the virus to escape the immune response are not well understood. The infecting virus often generates a wide variety of quasispecies; further, the representation of these variant forms changes rapidly over time.[20,37] Yet it appears that these changes may contribute only in part to viral persistence.

SEROLOGIC TESTS FOR HCV INFECTION

Two licensed EIA tests for HCV antibodies are currently available in the United States. Although both use recombinant viral antigens as the solid-phase capture reagent, they differ in their physical format and in the number and nature of viral antigens used (Table 44–1). The test manufactured by Ortho Clinical Diagnostics uses a microplate solid phase and has been designated as a 3.0 version by the manufacturer. The peptides that are coated onto the microplate well are known as c22-3 from the C (core) region, c200 from the NS3-NS4 regions, and an NS-5 peptide. The test manufactured by Abbott Laboratories uses a polystyrene bead solid phase and is designated as a version 2.0 test. The capture reagents for this test are c22-3, and c33 and c100-3 (both from the NS3/NS4 region). Both test procedures use an antiglobulin conjugate to detect the analyte antibodies. The performance characteristics of the tests, representing the manufacturers' claims (see Table 44–1), have been validated by extensive clinical trials, and the tests have been licensed as biologics by the U.S. Food and Drug Administration (FDA). Other tests on fully

Table 44–1 Enzyme Immunoassay Tests for Anti-HCV: Components and Performance Characteristics

Version of Test (manufacturer)	Peptides	Sensitivity*	Specificity*
1.0 (Ortho Clinical Diagnostics)	C100	81%	>99.4%
2.0 (Abbott Laboratories)	HC34 (c22), HC31 (c33), c100	85.7%†	99.83%
3.0 (Ortho Clinical Diagnostics)	c22, c200‡, NS-5	88.1%†	99.95%

*Based on manufacturers' claims in product inserts.
†Based on a diagnosis of chronic non-A, non-B hepatitis—ALT elevated >6 months, HBsAg negative.
‡Includes c33 and c100 sequences.

automated platforms are available elsewhere in the world and are soon expected to be licensed in the United States. Most diagnostic reagents are defined as devices, but those that are used in the preparation of blood and blood products are required to meet the more stringent biologics requirements, because blood itself is defined as a biologic.

The sensitivity of these tests was defined in trials using patients diagnosed with NANBH. Because this diagnosis is not specific, the significance of the sensitivity figures is unclear. Of more importance now, at least in the context of blood donor screening, is the ability of the test method to detect infection at the earliest possible time during the seroconversion period. Studies of seroconversion panels suggest that currently available tests detect antibodies, on average, 70 to 80 days after exposure to the source of infection and 40 to 60 days after the initial detection of HCV RNA in the plasma. In addition, it should be noted that earlier versions of the EIA tests clearly failed to detect some infected individuals.[38] This is not surprising, because only a very limited number of viral epitopes were included in the capture reagent. Current tests for anti-HCV are whole-antibody assays. No tests are yet available for specific detection of immunoglobulin M anti-HCV.

Although these EIA tests have high sensitivity and specificity, there is a possibility that some reactive test results are nonspecific. When the EIA is used to screen blood donors, its actual positive predictive value is 70% to 80%.[36] Consequently, it is recommended that all asymptomatic individuals who test as reactive on EIA repeatedly should be further tested with an additional, more specific procedure. Currently, only one such immunologic method is licensed and available in the United States. This is a strip immunoblot assay (RIBA 3.0) that is constructed by application of recombinant or synthetic viral peptides representing c22, c33, c100, 5-1-1, and NS5 regions to nitrocellulose strips in a fixed pattern. The c-100 and 5-1-1 peptides are present in the same band on the strip. The expression carrier protein for the recombinant viral antigens is also applied (superoxide dismutase, SOD), as are strong and weak positive controls. Patient or donor samples are added to the strips and, after washing, adherent antibodies are detected by an appropriate enzyme-conjugated antiglobulin and visualization reaction. The number and intensity of bands are scored, and the result is interpreted as follows:

- *Positive:* Two or more bands with an intensity equal to, or greater than, that of the weak positive control band, plus nonreactive SOD band.
- *Negative:* No band with a greater intensity than the weak positive control.
- *Indeterminate:* Only one band reactive or any pattern in association with a reactive SOD band.

Table 44–2 summarizes the results of testing a large number of volunteer blood donations with HCV EIA and SIAs.

Unlike the situation with HIV, there does not seem to be a common pattern for the sequence of appearance of reactive bands in the blot during seroconversion with HCV. However, a number of studies have defined the relationship between particular bands, or band patterns, and the likelihood that a sample will also contain detectable HCV RNA. For example, Dow and colleagues[35] reviewed data from 177 blood donor specimens that were reactive on EIA and tested positive on the version 3.0 SIA. Among 82 samples with four positive bands, 69 (84.1%) were RNA-positive. Of the 54 samples with three positive bands, 40 (74.1%) were RNA-positive, whereas only 14 (34.1%) of the 41 samples with two positive bands were RNA-positive. Among the samples with indeterminate SIA results, the frequencies of RNA-positive results were 3 of 154 for c22, 1 of 220 for c33, 1 of 191 for c100, and 0 of 380 for NS5.[35] Thus, a few of the indeterminate patterns may be associated with the presence of RNA and, therefore, of active HCV infection. Similar data were published by Dodd and Stramer.[36]

TESTS FOR HCV RNA

Tests for HCV RNA serve an important role in diagnosis and patient management.[9,39] A variety of procedures is available, all of which depend on nucleic acid amplification, with one exception. The reverse transcriptase polymerase chain reaction (RT-PCR) is perhaps the most familiar. Viral RNA is reverse-transcribed to DNA, and two primers are used to define a sequence for repetitive amplification using a temperature-resistant DNA polymerase and a temperature-cycling protocol. A variety of methods may be used to detect the resulting amplified sequence, including visualization in gels, hybridization with labeled probes, and detection of amplicons in real time. Both qualitative and quantitative procedures are available.[5,40,41] In most cases, a conserved segment of the 5′ untranslated region of the genome is selected for amplification. PCR-based assays are available commercially (e.g., Roche Molecular Systems) as well as from independent reference laboratories; alternatively, they may be developed in-house with the use of standard technologies.

Table 44–2 Results of Testing 19.2 Million Blood Donations with HCV 3.0 EIA and Version 3.0 SIA and Percentage of RNA-Positive Samples among Subgroups of SIA-Positive Subjects

	Number of Subjects with SIA Finding (% RNA+)		
	Positive (% RNA+)	Indeterminate	Negative
HCV EIA RR	19,541	4898	6241
N = 30,680			
SIA			
>2 bands	17,139 (82%)*	NA	NA
2 bands only	2402 (42%)†	NA	NA

*Sample of 200 tested.
†2347 tested.
EIA, enzyme immunoassay; HCV, hepatitis C virus; NA, not applicable; RR, repeatedly reactive; SIA, Strip immunoblot assay.
Data courtesy of Susan L. Stramer, Ph.D.(personal communication).

Another technique, known as nucleic acid sequence–based amplification (NASBA; a proprietary technology from Organon-Technika),[42] and the very similar transcription-mediated amplification (TMA; a proprietary technology from Gen-Probe Inc.) can be performed without temperature cycling. Two enzymes are used to produce an RNA amplicon, which can be detected by a variety of methods, including the hybridization protection assay. It should be noted that Chiron owns patent rights to the HCV genomic sequence used for amplification.

Sample collection, stability, and preparation for amplification are all important and must be properly controlled. HCV RNA is quite labile, and it is preferable, if not essential, to collect specimens in EDTA. Samples should be maintained at refrigerated temperatures and tested with minimal delay. A number of different methods may be used to prepare the RNA for testing, including conventional extraction from ultracentrifugal pellets, extraction on silica, and probe-capture techniques.

Finally, in a method known as the branched-chain DNA assay (B-DNA), a probe is labeled with a large branched DNA molecule that carries many copies of the detection label. This method does not amplify the target nucleic acid; rather, it provides a system in which numerous label molecules may be associated with a single target sequence. As might be expected, this technique is not as sensitive as amplification. However, the lack of sensitivity can be exploited to differentiate those patients with high levels of circulating RNA.[43,44]

Within the United States, almost all blood donations have been tested for HCV RNA since 1999.[34] Two methods are in use, RT-PCR(Roche) and TMA (Chiron/Gen-Probe). To date, all such testing has been performed on small pools of plasma samples, with current pool sizes of 24 for the Roche procedure and 16 for the Chiron/Gen-Probe method. Both tests have been licensed for routine use by the FDA and both have an analytical sensitivity of 12 or fewer copies of RNA/mL by probit analysis and a 95% detection level of 30 to 60 copies/mL. The overall sensitivity of the testing is, of course, proportionately reduced in pooled testing.

A number of methods are available for the determination of genotype and subtype. Not all methods are able to discriminate every genotype or subtype, however. Available methods may be broadly separated into those that depend on immunologic differentiation and those that directly detect variation in nucleic acid sequences. In the former case, specific peptides derived from the NS4 region are used to probe for antibodies in the specimen. Nucleic acid–based techniques include sequencing amplicons from selected genomic areas, PCR using genome-specific primers, DNA-enzyme immunoassay (DEIA), restriction fragment length polymorphism (RFLP) analysis of amplicons, and differential hybridization of amplicons with specific probes. Two of these approaches are commercially available (GEN-ETI-K DEIA kit and INNO-LiPA HCVI and HCV II). The reader is referred elsewhere for further details.[23,45]

Relatively little information is available about the impact of HCV genotype on the sensitivity of diagnostic tests, and some data suggest little variation in the analytic sensitivity of NAT.[46] However, a recent publication reviewing the performance characteristics of numerous blood screening assays for HCV antibodies suggests that most tests are not seriously impacted by genotype variations (El-Nageh, in press).

DIAGNOSTIC ALGORITHM

The Centers for Disease Control and Prevention (CDC) has published an algorithm for diagnostic testing for HCV among asymptomatic individuals (Fig. 44–1).[14] This algorithm is somewhat different from that recommended for blood donor screening, in that it explicitly permits the use of NAT to confirm a repeatedly reactive EIA result. However, NAT-negative samples must be further evaluated by an SIA. This algorithm also provides useful guidance in the context of treatment, but a more comprehensive guide to treatment was published in 2004.[9] Given that blood donors are now routinely evaluated by NAT for HCV RNA, it is hoped that these results may be incorporated into the notification and management of seropositive donors.[37,45]

IMPACT OF BLOOD DONOR SCREENING AND TESTING FOR HCV

Results of Testing

In 2001, the frequency of positive results among first-time blood donations as defined by RIBA was 0.3%, which is about one fifth of the national prevalence rate of 1800 per 100,000. The incidence of new infections in the donor population is 1.9 new infections per 100,000 person-years; the corresponding national incidence figure is 13.4 per 100,000 person-years.[47] Thus, the donor rate is about one fifth of the national rate. These differences are attributable, at least in part, to the procedures used to recruit safer populations for donation and to the measures used to question presenting donors about their medical and behavioral histories. However, it should be

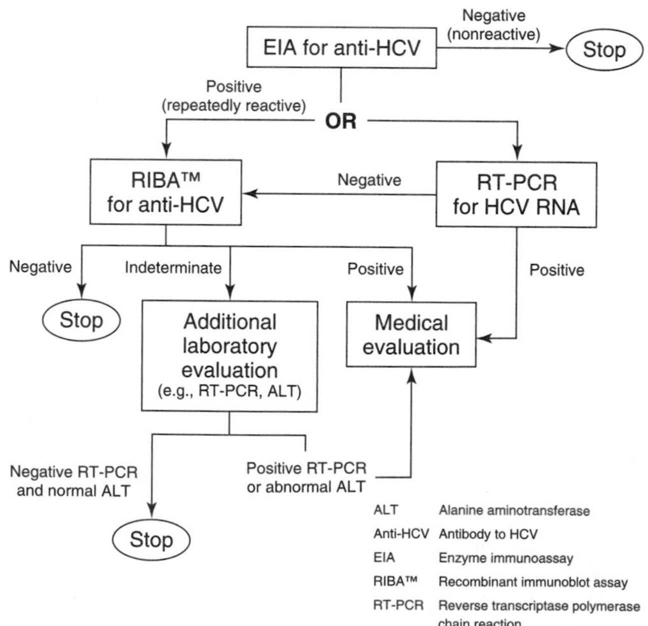

Figure 44–1 Algorithm for hepatitis C virus (HCV) testing among asymptomatic individuals. (From Centers for Disease Control and Prevention: Recommendations for prevention and control of hepatitis C virus (HCV) infection and HCV-related chronic disease. MMWR Morb Mortal Wkly Rep 1998;487[RR-19]:1–39.)

noted that only a very few donors are actually deferred on the basis of their response to risk questions, in part because donors do not always provide complete answers[48] but also perhaps because potential donors make a conscious decision to avoid giving blood so as not to have to answer the questions.

Risk of Post-transfusion HCV Infection

It is clear from a number of published studies that donor screening and testing measures have had a profound impact on the incidence of post-transfusion hepatitis C. Indeed, prospective studies have not demonstrated any infections since the implementation of the so-called multi-antigen tests for antibodies to HCV. But there is also substantial evidence for the efficacy of a variety of screening approaches used even before this time. The essentially complete elimination of commercial donation of whole blood had a major effect on reducing the frequency of post-transfusion hepatitis. It is also believed that a further reduction was seen as a result of more stringent donor questioning to reduce the risk of transmission of HIV and acquired immunodeficiency syndrome (AIDS), although subsequent information implies that the major effect would have come from a reduction in the number of injection drug users.

The first study to clearly demonstrate the impact of testing measures on hepatitis C infection was published by Nelson and colleagues.[49] They evaluated samples from a large population of patients undergoing cardiac surgery, using the first-generation test for anti-HCV. These researchers found that the risk of infection was 0.45% per unit prior to the implementation of any testing. After implementation of testing for ALT and anti-HBc, the rate of infection dropped to 0.19%. Finally, once the version 1.0 EIA test was implemented, the rate dropped to 1 per 3300 units (0.03%), a reduction of 84%.[49] A subsequent reevaluation using the more sensitive version 2.0 test on the blood recipients suggested that the actual risk was closer to 1:1700.[50] Once the version 2.0 test was introduced for blood donor screening, however, the frequency of residual infection declined profoundly. As pointed out previously, cases of hepatitis C were no longer observed in prospective studies, and risk estimates then had to be developed on the basis of the length of the window period (as determined from post-transfusion infections) and the incidence of new infections within the donor population. In a landmark publication in 1996, Schreiber and colleagues estimated the residual risk of HCV infection at 1 per 103,000 donations, based on a window period of 82 days and an incidence rate of 4.84 per 100,000 person-years.[51] Subsequent evaluations account for a 12- to 13-day reduction in the window period attendant on the implementation of the version 3.0 EIA and an overall decline in the incidence of HCV infection to 2.09 per 100,000 person-years. The latter figure translated to a residual risk of 1:276,000 repeat donations. The addition of HCV NAT was estimated to markedly reduce this risk to 1:1.935 million repeat donations. In the same paper, it was observed, on the basis of the results of NAT, that the incidence of HCV infections was 2.4 times higher among first-time donors.[52] Allowing for a 23% frequency of first-time donors in the Red Cross system, this translated to an overall risk of 1:1.39 million donations.[3] The relative stability of the detection rates for HCV RNA and the lack of change in prevalence rates for HCV antibody[53] suggest that this risk is not changing significantly, at least through the end of 2003.

It is interesting to speculate about the higher incidence of infections among first-time donors, but there are no definitive data. One possibility is that there are more test-seekers among people presenting to donate for the first time, although this is not necessarily supported by published data on interviews of RNA NAT-positive donors, because both first-time and repeat donors were found to be positive and to acknowledge risk factors for infection.[17] It is also possible that the process of giving blood has an educational impact and that individuals who learn about risk factors for blood-borne infections defer themselves from future donation.

Finally, it should be noted that there are cases in which HCV has been transmitted by blood units that have been fully tested for HCV, even after the implementation of NAT.[54] Such cases have usually been detected as a result of lookback and are too few to offer any quantitative estimate of residual risk. Window-period theory would strongly suggest that such cases would occur, and this is supported by the detection of HCV RNA in window-period samples, using ultrasensitive test methods. It is of interest to speculate on the minimal infectious dose of HCV. Busch has developed models based on the conservative assumption that it is as low as one genome equivalent per 20 mL of plasma. Using this assumption and back-calculating, the theoretical window period from the observed doubling rate of HCV plasma RNA during early infection has led to estimates that are largely compatible with currently accepted window period estimates.[55]

LOOKBACK

A positive test result for HCV antibodies does not provide any information about the duration of infection, even if accompanied by a positive finding for HCV RNA. Consequently, if a blood donor is found to be HCV antibody positive, it is possible that prior donations from that individual were infectious for HCV. This could occur by two broad mechanisms. First, a previous donation could have been made in the infectious but seronegative window period. Second, the prior donations could have been collected at a time when a less sensitive test was in use or even before testing was initiated. Accordingly, a focused lookback program has been initiated to locate, notify, test, and, if appropriate, treat recipients of such potentially infectious prior donations. Studies in Canada and elsewhere suggest that up to 70% of such recipients may indeed have been infected.[56,57] However, in the United States, the effort appears to have been less productive.

A team from the CDC reported that an estimated 98,484 blood components were identified as potentially infectious.[58] Of these, 85% had been transfused. This interim study found that lookback had been completed for 80% of the transfused products; 69% of the recipients had died. Of those living, 78% were successfully notified that they had received a potentially infectious blood component. It was estimated that, of recipients notified, 49.5% were tested for anti-HCV; of those, 18.9% were seropositive, but 32% of these individuals were already aware that they were seropositive. Thus, at the time of publication of the study, it was estimated just over 1000 individuals were newly notified of unexpected HCV infection; this estimate translated to a national figure of 1520, on the assumption that the lookback process was to be completed. The figure represents fewer than 1% of all individuals who may have been infected as a result of transfusion.[58] It should be noted that this component of the lookback program was restricted only to donations that were identified as a result of testing with multi-antigen tests (i.e., versions 2.0 or 3.0). It is likely that, as lookback is extended to cover donors initially identified by the version 1.0 test, the proportional yield will be greater, but the efficiency of the process will certainly be affected by availability of required records.

On the other hand, the essential completion of achievable lookback affecting recipients of blood donated prior to the implementation of testing means that almost all available cases now represent lookback from incident cases of HCV infection. The yield of this aspect of lookback is now extremely low, and such yield will be further reduced as the impact of NAT is manifested. The ethical imperatives for lookback continue, but the public health benefits of this process are becoming vanishingly small.

COMMENT AND SUMMARY

In its way, the history of hepatitis C has been as remarkable as that of HIV and AIDS. In retrospect, hepatitis C was the blood-borne agent most commonly transmitted by transfusion in the United States, right up until the early 1990s. The legacy of this problem will be seen for many years, as the long-term health consequences of HCV infection become manifest. The almost complete elimination of the problem of transfusion-transmitted HCV is the result of many years of dedicated study of an intractable problem. There were no simple solutions; the virus was refractory to laboratory study, and there was a truly frustrating inability to identify any serologic markers of infection. Indeed, only at the very end of the 20th century was a naturally occurring, circulating viral antigen recognized and then only in the few weeks preceding seroconversion.

As with HIV, the first laboratory approach to abrogating transfusion-transmitted HCV infection was the development of serologic tests. In the case of HCV, however, this development was achieved through the combination of years of study of the disease, development of animal models, and the painstaking application of new recombinant technology. It is fitting that Harvey Alter and Michael Houghton received the 2000 Lasker award for this work, but hundreds of others contributed over many years.

Serologic and nucleic acid testing have essentially eliminated the risk of transfusion-transmitted HCV. Plasma derivatives are prepared from highly tested starting material and are further treated with advanced inactivation procedures. It is of interest to note, however, that whereas the early tests removed a substantial fraction of antibody-positive units, they failed to identify all infectious units, probably leading to the unexpected occurrence of HCV in recipients of some immunoglobulin products.

Despite the success of testing for HCV, there continue to be barriers to other aspects of management of this virus. As with many viral diseases, treatment options for HCV are limited and incomplete. More baffling, however, are the difficulties inherent in understanding and manipulating the interactions between the immune system and HCV. Development of an effective vaccine seems to be a particularly elusive goal.

REFERENCES

1. Aach RD, Szmuness W, Mosley JW, et al. Serum alanine aminotransferase of donors in relation to the risk of non-A, non-B hepatitis in recipients. The Transfusion-Transmitted Viruses Study. NEJM 1981;304:989–994.
2. Alter HJ, Purcell RH, Holland PV, et al. Donor transaminase and recipient hepatitis: Impact on blood transfusion services. JAMA 1981;246: 630–634.
3. Dodd RY. Current safety of the blood supply in the United States. Int J Hematol 2004;80:301–305.
4. Alter HJ, Seeff LB. Recovery, persistence, and sequelae in HCV infection: a perspective on long-term outcome. Semin Liver Dis 2001;20:17–35.
5. Management of Hepatitis C. NIH Consensus Statement 1997;15:1–41.
6. Liang TJ, Rehermann B, Seeff LB, Hoofnagle JH. Pathogenesis, natural history, treatment, and prevention of hepatitis C. Ann Intern Med 2000; 132:296–305.
7. Carrat F, Bani-Sadr F, Pol S, Rosenthal E, et al. Pegylated interferon alfa-2b vs standard interferon alfa-2b, plus ribavirin, for chronic hepatitis C in HIV-infected patients: A randomized controlled trial. JAMA 2004;292:2839–2848.
8. Jacobson IM, Gonzalez SA, Ahmed F, et al. A randomized trial of pegylated interferon alpha-2b plus ribavirin in the retreatment of chronic hepatitis C. Am J Gastroenterol 2005;100:2453–2462.
9. Strader DB, Wright T, Thomas DL, Seeff LB. Diagnosis, management and treatment of hepatitis C. Hepatology 2004;39:1147–1171.
10. Shepard CW, Finelli L, Alter MJ. Global epidemiology of hepatitis C virus infection. Lancet Infect Dis 2005;5:558–567.
11. Frank C, Mohamed MK, Strickland GT, et al. The role of parenteral antischistosomal therapy in the spread of hepatitis C virus in Egypt. Lancet 2000;355:887–891.
12. Alter MJ, Kruszon-Moran D, Nainan OV, et al. The prevalence of hepatitis C virus infection in the United States, 1988 through 1994. NEJM 1999;341:556–562.
13. Alter MJ. Hepatitis C virus infection in the United States. J Hepatol 1999;31:88–91.
14. CDC. Recommendations for prevention and control of hepatitis C virus (HCV) infection and HCV-related chronic disease. MMWR Morb Mortal Wkly Rep 1998;47 (RR-19):1–39.
15. Alter MJ. Epidemiology of hepatitis C and lookback. Hematology 1999;1999:418–421.
16. Conry-Cantilena C, VanRaden M, Gibble J, et al. Routes of infection, viremia, and liver disease in blood donors found to have hepatitis C virus infection. NEJM 1996;334:1691–1696.
17. Orton SL, Stramer SL, Dodd RY, Alter MJ. Risk factors for HCV infection among blood donors confirmed to be positive for the presence of HCV RNA and not reactive for the presence of anti-HCV. Transfusion 2004;44:275–281.
18. Choo Q-L, Kuo G, Weiner AJ, et al. Isolation of a cDNA clone derived from a blood-borne non-A, non-B viral hepatitis genome. Science 1989;244:359–362.
19. Kuo G, Choo Q-L, Alter HJ, et al. An assay for circulating antibodies to a major etiologic virus of human non-A, non-B hepatitis. Science 1989;244:362–364.
20. Simmonds P. Genetic diversity and evolution of hepatitis C virus—15 years on. J Gen Virol 2004;85:3173–3188.
21. Wakita T, Pietschmann T, Kato T, et al. Production of infectious hepatitis C virus in tissue culture from a cloned viral genome. Nat Med 2005;11:791–796.
22. Zhong J, Gastaminza P, Cheng G, et al. Robust hepatitis C virus infection in vitro. Proc Natl Acad Sci USA 2005;102:9739–9740.
23. Lau JYN, Mizokami M, Kolberg JA, et al. Application of six hepatitis C virus genotyping systems to sera from chronic hepatitis C patients in the United States. J Infect Dis 1995;171:281–289.
24. Simmonds P, Holmes EC, Cha T-A, et al. Classification of hepatitis C virus into six major genotypes and a series of subtypes by phylogenetic analysis of the NS-5 region. J Gen Virol 1993;74:2391–2399.
25. McOmish F, Yap PL, Dow BC, et al. Geographical distribution of hepatitis C virus genotypes in blood donors: an international collaborative survey. J Clin Microbiol 1994;32:884–892.
26. Simmonds P, Alberti A, Alter HJ, et al. A proposed system for the nomenclature of hepatitis C viral genotypes. Hepatology 1994;19: 1321–1324.
27. Zein NN, Persing DH. Hepatitis C genotypes: Current trends and future implications. Mayo Clin Proc 1996;71:458–462.
28. Martin P. Hepatitis C genotypes: the key to pathogenicity. Ann Intern Med 1995;122:227–228.
29. Cooreman MP, Schoondermark-Van de Ven EME. Hepatitis C virus: Biological and clinical consequences of genetic heterogeneity. Scand J Gastroenterol 1996;31(Suppl 218):106–115.

30. Busch MP, Korelitz JJ, Kleinman SH, et al. Declining value of alanine aminotransferase in screening of blood donors to prevent posttransfusion hepatitis B and C virus infection. Transfusion 1995;35:903–910.
31. Busch MP. HIV, HBV and HCV: New developments related to transfusion safety. Vox Sang 2000;78:253–256.
32. Couroucé AM, Le Marrec N, Bouchardeau F, et al. Efficacy of HCV core antigen detection during the preseroconversion period. Transfusion 2000;40:1198–1202.
33. Tanaka E, Ohue C, Aoyagi K, et al. Evaluation of a new enzyme immunoassay for hepatitis C virus (HCV) core antigen with clinical sensitivity approximating that of genomic amplification of HCV RNA. Hepatology 2000;32:388–393.
34. Stramer SL, Glynn SA, Kleinman SH, et al. Detection of HIV-1 and HCV infections among antibody-negative blood donors by nucleic acid-amplification testing. NEJM 2004;351:760–768.
35. Dow BC, Buchanan I, Munro H, et al. Relevance of RIBA-3 supplementary test to HCV PCR positivity and genotypes for HCV confirmation of blood donors. J Med Virol 1996;49:132–136.
36. Dodd RY, Stramer SL. Indeterminate results in blood donor testing: What you don't know can hurt you. Transfus Med Rev 2000;14:151–160.
37. Farci P, Shimoda A, Coiana A, et al. The outcome of acute hepatitis C predicted by the evolution of the viral quasispecies. Science 2000;288: 339–344.
38. Alter MJ, Margolis HS, Krawczynski K, et al. The natural history of community-acquired hepatitis C in the United States. NEJM 1992;327: 1899–1905.
39. Gretch DR, Dela Rosa C, Carithers RL Jr, et al. Assessment of hepatitis C viremia using molecular amplification technologies: correlations and clinical implications. Ann Intern Med 1995;123:321–329.
40. Lunel F, Mariotti M, Cresta P, et al. Comparative study of conventional and novel strategies for the detection of hepatitis C virus RNA in serum: Amplicor, branched-DNA, NASBA and in-house PCR. J Virol Methods 1995;54:159–171.
41. Hawkins A, Davidson F, Simmonds P. Comparison of plasma virus loads among individuals infected with hepatitis C virus (HCV) genotypes 1, 2, and 3 by Quantiplex HCV RNA assay versions 1 and 2, Roche monitor assay, and an in-house limiting dilution method. J Clin Microbiol 1997;35:187–192.
42. Damen M, Sillekens P, Sjerps M, et al. Stability of hepatitis C virus RNA during specimen handling and storage prior to NASBA amplification. J Virol Methods 1998;72:175–184.
43. Sangiovanni A, Morales R, Spinzi GC, et al. Interferon alfa treatment of HCV RNA carriers with persistently normal transaminase levels: a pilot randomized controlled study. Hepatology 1998;27:853–856.
44. Halfon P, Khiri H, Gerolami V, et al. Impact of various handling and storage conditions on quantitative detection of hepatitis C virus RNA. J Hepatol 1996;25:307–311.
45. Lau JYN, Davis GL, Prescott LE, et al. Distribution of hepatits C virus genotypes determined by line probe assay in patients with chronic hepatitis C seen at tertiary referral centers in the United States. Ann Intern Med 1996;124:868–876.
46. Forman MS, Valsamakis A: Increased sensitivity of the Roche COBAS AMPLICOR HCV test, version 2.0, using modified extraction techniques. J Mol Diagn 2004;6:225–230.
47. Dodd RY. Current estimates of transfusion safety worldwide. In Vyas GN, Williams AE (eds). Advances in Transfusion Safety. Basel, Karger, 2005, pp 3–10.
48. Williams AE, Thomson RA, Schreiber GB, et al. Estimates of infectious disease risk factors in US blood donors. JAMA 1997;277:967–972.
49. Donahue JG, Murioz A, Ness PM, et al. The declining risk of post-transfusion hepatitis C virus infection. NEJM 1992;327:369–373.
50. Nelson KE, Ahmed F, Ness P, Donahue JG. The incidence of post-transfusion hepatitis: Reply. NEJM 1993;328:1280–1281.
51. Schreiber GB, Busch MP, Kleinman SH, et al. The risk of transfusion-transmitted viral infections. NEJM 1996;336:1685–1690.
52. Dodd RY, Notari EP, Stramer SL. Current prevalence and incidence of infectious disease markers and estimated window-period risk in the American Red Cross blood donor population. Transfusion 2002;42:975–979.
53. Zou S, Notari EP, Stramer SL, et al. Patterns of age- and sex-specific prevalence of major blood-borne infections in United States blood donors, 1995 to 2002: American Red Cross blood donor study. Transfusion 2004;44:1640–1647.
54. Schüttler CG, Caspari G, Jursch CA, Willems WR, Schaefer S. Hepatitis C virus transmission by a blood donation negative in nucleic acid amplification tests for viral RNA. Lancet 2000;355:41–42.
55. Busch MP, Glynn SA, Stramer SL, et al. A new strategy for estimating risks of transfusion-transmitted viral infections based on rates of detection of recently infected donors. Transfusion 2005;45:254–264.
56. Long A, Spurll G, Demers H, Goldman M. Targeted hepatitis C lookback: Quebec, Canada. Transfusion 1999;39:194–200.
57. Christensen PB, Groenboek K, Krarup HB, Danish HVL. Transfusion-acquired hepatitis C: the Danish lookback experience. Transfusion 1999;39:188–193.
58. Culver DH, Alter MJ, Mullan RJ, Margolis HS. Evaluation of the effectiveness of targeted lookback for HCV infection in the United States—interim results. Transfusion 2000;40:1176–1181.

Chapter 45

HIV, HTLV, and Other Retroviruses

Eberhard W. Fiebig • Edward L. Murphy • Michael P. Busch

This chapter provides a general overview of retroviruses, with emphasis on those aspects of human retrovirus epidemiology, pathophysiology, and detection of greatest relevance to specialists in transfusion medicine. The four major known pathogenic human retroviruses—human immunodeficiency virus types 1 and 2 (HIV-1 and HIV-2) and human T-cell lymphotropic virus types 1 and 2 (HTLV-1 and HTLV-2) are considered in detail. Strategies to further reduce the risk of retrovirus transfusion transmission are addressed.

DEFINITION, LIFE CYCLE, AND DISTRIBUTION OF RETROVIRUSES

Retroviruses were among the first viruses described in the scientific literature. They constitute a major class of membrane-coated, diploid, single-stranded RNA viruses with wide distribution in nature; examples exist in genera ranging from insects to reptiles to virtually all mammals.[1] The human retroviruses HIV and HTLV belong to the lentivirus and oncornavirus groups of the retrovirus family, respectively.[2] Characteristic features of retroviruses are a distinct genomic organization, the presence of viral particle (virion)-associated reverse transcriptase, and a unique replication cycle (Fig. 45–1).

The first step of infection is attachment of virus particles to the cell membrane. In the case of HIV, which has tropism for T cells and macrophages, virus glycoprotein 120 (gp120) attaches to CD4 molecules expressed on the surface of these cells. Efficient infection also requires engagement of viral proteins with chemokine coreceptors, identified as CCR5 on macrophages and CXCR4 on T cells.[3] After entry into a host cell, typically by fusion of the virion and host cell membranes, the reverse transcriptase enzyme copies viral RNA into complementary double-stranded DNA (cDNA). Virion-associated integrase then mediates integration of this cDNA into random sites in the host cell's genome, forming integrated viral cDNAs termed *proviruses.* Subsequent transcription, processing, and translation of viral genes are mediated principally by host cell enzymes, although both viral and host cell regulatory gene products influence the level and pattern of viral gene expression and replication. The classic retrovirus life cycle is completed when nascent particles associate and bud from the plasma membrane to form progeny virions, which can then infect other cells and other organisms.

Retroviruses can also spread horizontally, by fusion of infected and uninfected cells, or vertically, by replication of integrated viral DNA along with cellular DNA during mitosis or meiosis. Indeed, integrated proviruses have evolved that are passed congenitally through the germline; these so-called *endogenous retroviral elements* (as contrasted with vertically transmitted exogenous retroviruses) are present in many species, including humans, and in some species account for up to 10% of total genomic DNA.[2]

Disease manifestations of retroviruses are highly variable. Many animal species harbor exogenous or endogenous retroviruses that appear to be benign and may in fact be beneficial in restricting infection by related pathogenic retroviruses. On the other hand, retroviruses became the focus of intense research in the 1960s and 1970s because of their capacity to induce malignancies in a wide range of species. The demonstration that certain retroviruses (termed *acute RNA tumor viruses*) rapidly transform target cells in vitro and induce tumors within days to weeks of inoculation into animals greatly facilitated experimental investigation of viral carcinogenesis.[4] Studies of the molecular differences between these acute retroviruses and genetically related *slow viruses* (which failed to transform cells in vitro and only occasionally caused tumors many months after inoculation) led to the discovery of viral oncogenes, which were responsible for tumorigenesis. This achievement was followed by the revolutionary discovery that these viral oncogenes had in fact arisen by recombination events between slow viruses and key cellular genes termed *proto-oncogenes.*[4] Thus, investigation of retrovirus-induced cancers in animals led to unparalleled insights into normal cell biology and disease pathogenesis in humans. Retroviruses have also attracted interest from researchers who explore nonpathogenic strains as vehicles for therapeutic gene transfer.

DISCOVERY OF HUMAN RETROVIRUSES

The first report of successful isolation and characterization of a bona fide human retrovirus (later termed *HTLV-1*) occurred in 1980 and involved a patient with a rare type of leukemia (now called *adult T-cell leukemia/lymphoma* [ATL]).[5] Subsequently, HTLV-1 was also identified as the cause of a rare neurologic condition known as *HTLV-associated myelopathy/tropical spastic paraparesis* (HAM/TSP).[6] A second, closely related human retrovirus (HTLV-2) was isolated in 1982 from a patient with a somewhat more common type of leukemia (hairy cell leukemia)[7]; further surveys failed to show a relationship between HTLV-2 and hairy cell leukemia, but established the virus as a causative agent of HAM/TSP.[6,8] Both HTLV-1 and HTLV-2 are thought to be derived from simian T-lymphotropic retroviruses transmitted to humans over the past hundreds to thousands of years.

The full pathogenic potential of human retroviruses was not realized until HIV was established as the cause of

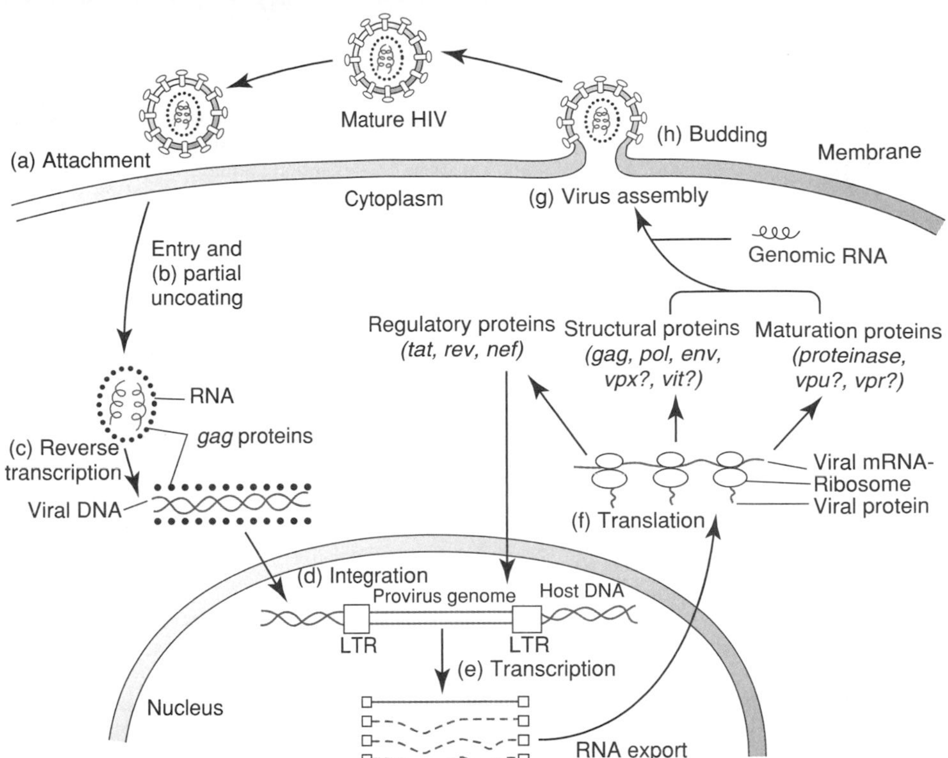

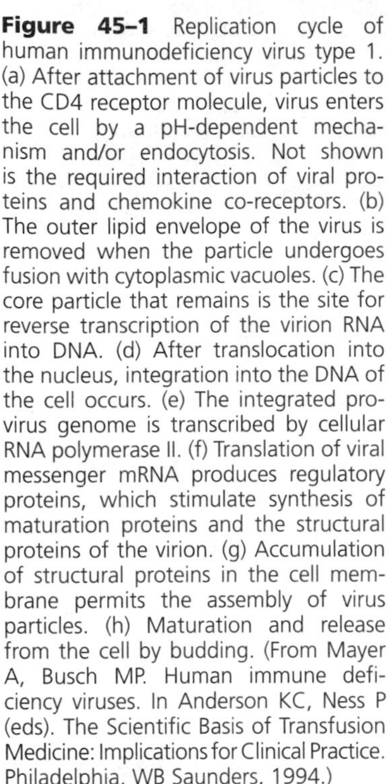
Figure 45–1 Replication cycle of human immunodeficiency virus type 1. (a) After attachment of virus particles to the CD4 receptor molecule, virus enters the cell by a pH-dependent mechanism and/or endocytosis. Not shown is the required interaction of viral proteins and chemokine co-receptors. (b) The outer lipid envelope of the virus is removed when the particle undergoes fusion with cytoplasmic vacuoles. (c) The core particle that remains is the site for reverse transcription of the virion RNA into DNA. (d) After translocation into the nucleus, integration into the DNA of the cell occurs. (e) The integrated provirus genome is transcribed by cellular RNA polymerase II. (f) Translation of viral messenger mRNA produces regulatory proteins, which stimulate synthesis of maturation proteins and the structural proteins of the virion. (g) Accumulation of structural proteins in the cell membrane permits the assembly of virus particles. (h) Maturation and release from the cell by budding. (From Mayer A, Busch MP. Human immune deficiency viruses. In Anderson KC, Ness P (eds). The Scientific Basis of Transfusion Medicine: Implications for Clinical Practice. Philadelphia, WB Saunders, 1994.)

AIDS in 1984. It is now thought that the virus originated in nonhuman primate species and was introduced into native people of the central African rain forest.[9] There may have been multiple introductions of the virus into humans dating back several centuries (based on phylogenetic *molecular clock* analyses); so far, however, the earliest documented evidence of HIV infection in humans comes from a blood sample collected in 1959.[10] Sub-Saharan Africa remains the area worst affected by the epidemic today, with an estimated 60% of the global caseload.[11] According to World Health Organization figures, 4.1 million people were newly infected in 2005, raising the projected number of infected people to a staggering 38.6 million worldwide.[11]

HUMAN IMMUNODEFICIENCY VIRUS

Genomic Organization and Virion Structure

The organization of the HIV RNA genome is shown in Figure 45–2. The products of the *gag*, *pol*, and *env* genes that are shared among all retroviruses give rise to the structural elements of the virion, which is shown in Figure 45–3. Similar to other lentiviruses, HIV contains at least six additional genes, which encode for regulatory proteins and virulence factors that appear to play an important role in pathogenicity. Detection of specific antibodies against viral proteins or identification of viral nucleic acid sequences in infected hosts provides the basis for screening and supplemental assays used in blood donor eligibility testing.

HIV Diversity: HIV-1 Subtypes and HIV-2

Extensive genetic diversity is a hallmark of HIV and other lentiviruses. A contributing factor is the high error rate during reverse transcription, which has been attributed to the negligible proofreading exonuclease activity of the reverse transcriptase.[12] Nucleotide misincorporations may occur at an astonishingly high rate of 5 to 10 per HIV genome per replication cycle, a phenomenon known as *hypermutation.* Insertions, deletions, and intergenic recombination add to the trend toward genetic diversification.[13] Within an HIV-1–infected individual, a swarm of "quasispecies," or HIV variants, develops over time,[14] and dual and multiple infections with recombination between the infecting HIV-1 strains have been reported.[15,16]

On the basis of relatedness of genomic sequences, the HIV-1 family is divided into main (M), outlier (O), and non-M, non-O (N) groups, with 11 distinct subtypes or clades (A through K) recognized within group M.[17] Of note is the currently almost exclusive prevalence of clade B strains in the United States and, to a lesser degree, Europe; other clades are more predominant in South America and Asia. The greatest genetic diversity of HIV-1 strains is found in central Africa, in keeping with this area's role as the presumed point of origin of the pandemic. The worldwide distribution of HIV-1 and -2 subgroups and clades is depicted in Figure 45–4. A recent survey of 292 U.S. blood donors detected by anti-HIV-1/HIV-2 screening in the late 1990s identified only 7 (2.3%) non-B subtypes, which nonetheless reflects a trend toward increasing diversity relative to earlier periods (e.g., 3 [0.8%] of 383 donors from 1993 through 1996).[18] This is a concern because the seroconversion window period from beginning of infectiousness to detectability of anti-HIV is prolonged with non-B strains when testing is performed with assays in routine use for blood donor screening in the United States, which are optimized for subtype B detection.[18]

Group O viral strains are most common in Cameroon and surrounding West African countries, where an estimated 1% to 2% of HIV infections are caused by these viral strains.[19,20]

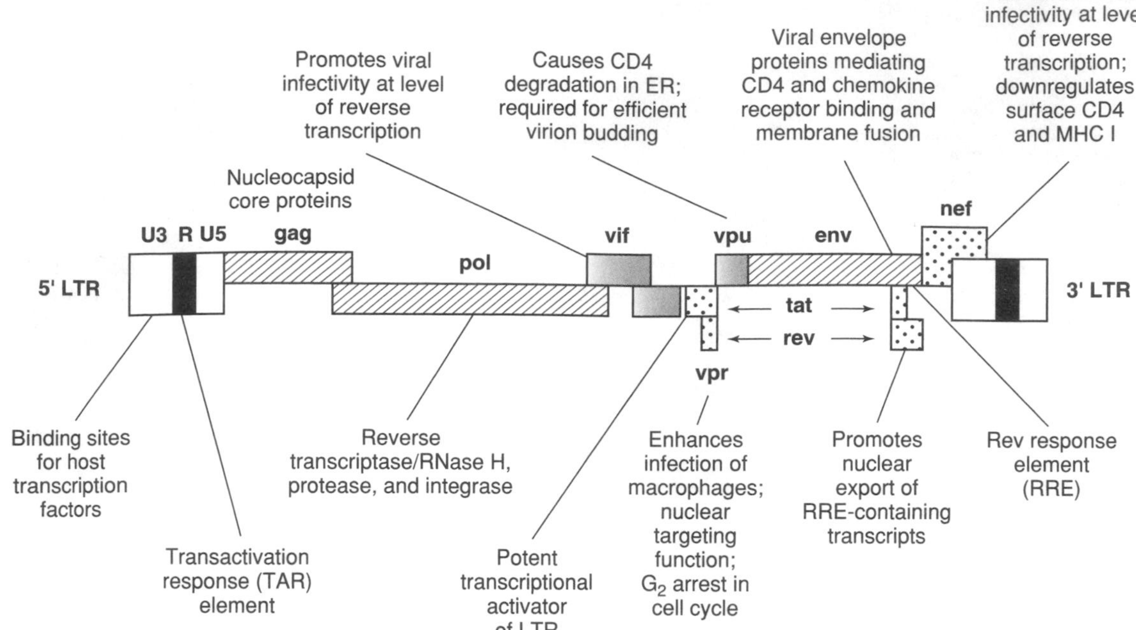

Figure 45–2 Genomic structure of HIV-1. The nine known genes of HIV-1 are shown, and their recognized primary functions are summarized. The 5' and 3' long terminal repeats (LTRs) containing regulatory sequences recognized by various host transcription factors are also depicted, and the positions of the Tat and Rev RNA response elements—transactivation response (TAR) element and Rev response element (RRE)—are indicated. ER, endoplasmic reticulum; MHC I, major histocompatibility complex class I. (Reproduced with permission from Geleziunas R, Greene WC. Molecular insights into HIV-1 infection and pathogenesis. In Sande MA, Volberding PA (eds). The Medical Management of AIDS, 6th ed. Philadelphia, WB Saunders, 1999, p 24.)

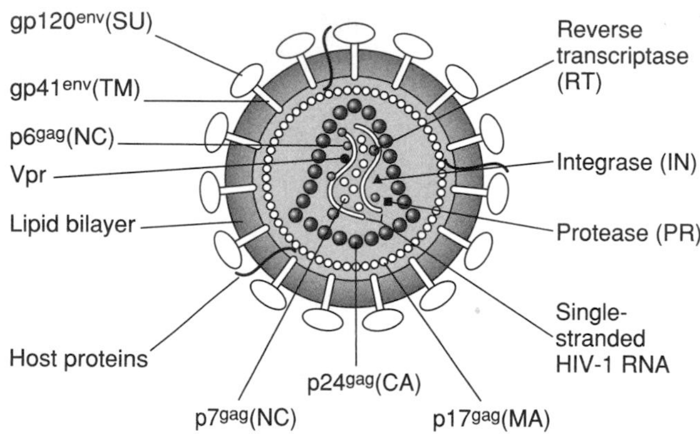

Figure 45–3 Schematic of the HIV-1 virion. Each of the virion proteins making up the envelope (gp120env and gp41env) and inner core (p24gag, p17gag, p7gag, and p6gag) is identified. In addition, the diploid RNA genome is shown associated with reverse transcriptase (RT), an RNA- and DNA-dependent DNA polymerase. Integrase (IN) and protease (PR) are also found in the mature HIV-1 virion. The auxiliary protein Vpr is incorporated into the HIV-1 virion through an interaction with the p6gag protein, which comprises the carboxyl terminus of the p55gag precursor protein. CA, capsid protein; MA, matrix protein; NC, nucleocapsid protein; SU, surface protein; TM, transmembrane protein. (Reproduced with permission from Geleziunas R, Greene WC. Molecular insights into HIV-1 infection and pathogenesis. In Sande MA, Volberding PA (eds). The Medical Management of AIDS, 6th ed. Philadelphia, WB Saunders, 1999, p 25.)

Outside this geographic area, group O isolates have rarely been seen. The current risk of HIV-1 group O infection in the United States is very low. Only two such infections have been reported; both involved immigrants from West Africa who had never donated blood or plasma. Furthermore, surveillance testing for HIV-1 divergent strains did not detect any group O viral isolates among 1072 serum samples from high- and low-risk population groups in the United States and Puerto Rico.[21] Nonetheless, concern arose in the mid-1990s when studies demonstrated that some group O isolates were not reliably detected by a number of HIV-1 and HIV-1/HIV-2 combination assays,[22] including some that are used for blood donor screening.[23] Antibody assays employing synthetic peptides or recombinant antigens on the solid phase, and those using the so-called *third-generation antigen-sandwich format,* were especially prone to false-negative results. Since then, test manufacturers have moved quickly to enhance their assays' sensitivity to unusual variants such as subtype O. As an added precaution, the U.S. Food and Drug Administration (FDA) continues to recommend permanent deferral of blood and plasma donors who were born, resided, or traveled in West Africa since 1977 or had sexual contact with someone identified by these criteria.[24]

HIV-2, discovered in 1985 in several countries in West Africa,[25] was initially called HTLV-4 and lymphadenopathy-associated virus type 2. Although still primarily concentrated in West Africa, HIV-2 has now spread throughout Western Europe, where a substantial number of infected blood donors have been detected, and cases of transfusion transmission have been documented.[26] HIV-2 is transmitted in the same manner as HIV-1 (i.e., by sexual contact, intravenous drug use, and, at a lower rate than for HIV-l, from mother to child) and causes progressive immunodeficiency, with susceptibility to an array of opportunistic infections similar to those seen with HIV-1. Rates of disease progression and secondary viral transmission appear to be lower, however, in persons infected with HIV-2 than in those infected with HIV-1, possibly owing to lower viral burden in HIV-2 infection.[27,28]

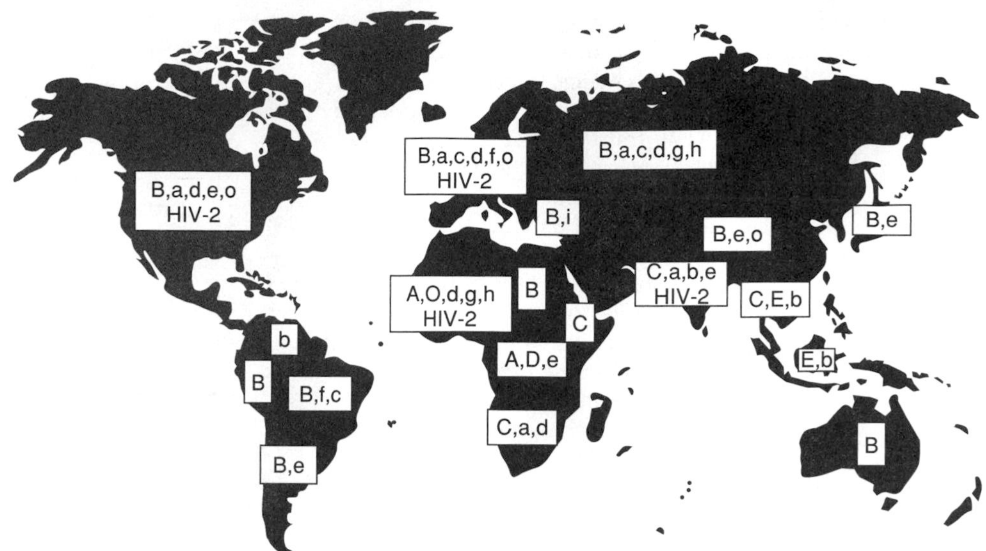

Figure 45–4 Distribution of human immunodeficiency virus (HIV) throughout the world according to the prevalence of its types and subtypes (clades). The distribution of HIV-1 clades is indicated by letters A to I (more prevalent in capital letters). Clades of HIV-2 are not shown separated. (Reproduced with permission from Diaz RS, Busch MP. Human immunodeficiency viruses. In Anderson KC, Ness PM (eds). Scientific Basis of Transfusion Medicine: Implications for Clinical Practice, 2nd ed. Philadelphia, WB Saunders, 2000, p 508.)

HIV-l and HIV-2 are highly (>50%) homologous at the nucleic acid sequence level, and they crossreact immunologically to a great extent (particularly the core and polymerase antigens). For this reason, up to 90% of sera from HIV-2–infected persons have been found to test positive with FDA-licensed anti-HIV-1 assays, with variable reactivity on HIV-1 Western blot analysis.[29,30] This crossreactivity undoubtedly prevented transfusion transmission of HIV-2 by blood screened for anti-HIV-1 in areas where the type 2 virus was present before implementation of combination HIV-1/HIV-2 screening tests. This high-level crossreactivity has also facilitated surveillance for HIV-2 in regions where it was rare or absent.[31,32] From 1987, when the first case of HIV-2 infection was diagnosed in the United States, to 1998, a total of 79 persons with HIV-2 infections were documented, of which approximately two thirds had been born in West Africa.[33]

Combination HIV-l/HIV-2 assays were developed in the late 1980s,[34–36] and mandatory implementation of either a combination test or a separate anti-HIV-2 test in the donor screening setting was required by the FDA effective June 1, 1992.[37] From the implementation of HIV-2 screening in 1992 through 1996, three prospective U.S. blood donors were found to be HIV-2 positive at the time of attempted donation.[38] One was a U.S.-born woman without identifiable risks for HIV infection; the other two were men, born in France and Liberia, West Africa respectively, who had resided for years in West Africa. These three cases of HIV-2 infection were detected from screening of more than 50 million whole blood donations, indicating that the prevalence of HIV-2 is very low (less than 1 in 15 million screened donations). A more recent study identified a single HIV-2–infected donor among 7.2 million donations at 18 U.S. blood centers from 1997 through mid-2000.[18] As of 2001, no cases of HIV-2–infected transfusion recipients had been reported in the United States.

Clinical HIV-1 Disease

In approximately 60% of acute HIV infections newly infected persons experience a nonspecific flulike illness, usually within 2 to 4 weeks of exposure.[39] This *retroviral syndrome* coincides with appearance of antibody to HIV antigens and is thought to represent a reaction of the immune system to the rapidly proliferating virus. In most cases signs and symptoms of acute HIV disease subside within weeks to a few months, giving way to a clinically silent period that can last several years. The lack of clinical symptoms during this stage of the disease is deceptive, however, because viremia persists in untreated infection and the number of CD4+ lymphocytes, the primary target of HIV, is gradually declining.[40] Paralleling the loss of CD4+ lymphocytes are clinical disease manifestations, such as opportunistic infections, numerous conditions related to suppression and dysfunction of the immune system, direct viral effects on multiple organ systems, and ultimately death after a median survival of 8 to 10 years from exposure. Although it appeared initially that disease manifestations and clinical course of transfusion-transmitted HIV infection follows a more rapid course than HIV infection due to other routes of transmission, subsequent analysis did not confirm this impression.[40]

Also not confirmed were concerns that allogeneic transfusions—via immune stimulation by donor leukocytes—may result in accelerated disease progression and shortened survival in HIV-infected transfusion recipients. The Viral Activation by Transfusion Study (VATS), a large multicenter U.S. clinical trial, specifically addressed this issue and found no evidence of significant activation of HIV replication or accelerated disease progression in HIV-1–infected recipients of either leukoreduced or nonleukoreduced transfusions.[41]

Widespread availability of potent antiretroviral therapy in western countries since the late 1990s has changed the course of HIV disease to that of a manageable chronic condition with reduction in opportunistic infections and other HIV-related complications and has markedly prolonged survival. Unfortunately, current treatment regimens are not capable of eradicating HIV from cell- and tissue-based sanctuaries throughout the body, and therapy-related side effects and development of resistant viral strains add to the problems of managing HIV-infected patients.[42]

Efficiency of HIV Transmission by Blood and Blood Products and Transmission Risk Prior to Blood Donor Screening

Human immunodeficiency virus is sensitive to drying[43] but survives refrigeration of blood and freezing of plasma. Virus present in the bloodstream of an undetected infected donor is therefore readily passed on by transfusion. Data from the Transfusion Safety Study (TSS), which traced and enrolled recipients of retrospectively identified HIV-1–seropositive units,[44,45] demonstrated HIV transmission in 111 of 124 (89.5%) enrolled recipients.[45] Neither characteristics of the donor's infection nor inherent recipient susceptibility factors significantly influenced transmission of HIV-1 by transfusions.[46] Variables that have been identified to correlate with likelihood of HIV-1 transmission are the type of blood component transfused and its duration of storage.[46,47] Washed red blood cell (RBC) units and RBC units stored more than 26 days had lower transmission rates than other components. This observation, as well as experimental evidence,[48] suggests that component manipulations that reduce the number of viable leukocytes, free virus, or both may reduce but not eliminate infectiousness.

With regard to recipients of clotting factor concentrates, an average of approximately 50% of hemophiliacs treated with factor VIII in the early 1980s experienced seroconversion.[49,50] However, the rate of seroconversion to anti-HIV-l positivity in hemophiliacs who were treated with very high doses of factor VIII (>500,000 units) approached 100%.[49] This finding indicates that, perhaps with the rare exception of persons lacking HIV-1 co-receptors required for infection,[51] virtually no one is resistant to HIV-1 infection, given a large enough inoculum and repeated exposures.

Given the high efficiency of HIV transmission by intravenous administration of infected blood and blood products, it is not surprising that the majority of HIV transmissions in the United States occurred before discovery of the virus and institution of blood donor screening. A principal lesson learned from the HIV-1 epidemic is how an infectious agent with a prolonged interval between infection and manifestation of clinical disease can spread silently within a population (and its blood donor base) for years before recognition.[52] In the United States, this early phase was localized primarily to homosexual and bisexual men, groups who were eligible blood donors at the time. Although we know now that the virus began to spread at an exponential rate in these men in the late 1970s, it was not until 1981 that clusters of Kaposi sarcoma and *Pneumocystis* pneumonia were first recognized among homosexual men in New York and Los Angeles. In late 1982, descriptions of AIDS-like illnesses in hemophiliacs and recipients of blood components first appeared.[53,54] With these reports, a blood-borne infectious etiology for AIDS became probable, and efforts were initiated to exclude from blood donation persons with symptoms of or risk factors associated with AIDS.[55] Approximately a year later, HIV-1 was discovered,[56] an event soon followed by development of diagnostic anti-HIV-1 tests, which were licensed for donor screening in March 1985.

Epidemiologic evidence showed that the risk of transfusion-associated HIV-1 infection in the San Francisco Bay Area, one of the epicenters of the early HIV epidemic in the United States, rose rapidly from its first occurrence in 1978 to a peak risk of approximately 1.1% per transfused unit in late 1982 (Fig. 45–5). Beginning in early 1983 and continuing through implementation of anti-HIV-1 screening, there was a marked, progressive decline in risk as a result of diminishing numbers of blood donations from at-risk or infected individuals. This decline was directly attributable to growing awareness of the infectious nature of AIDS in the homosexual community and to implementation and refinement of

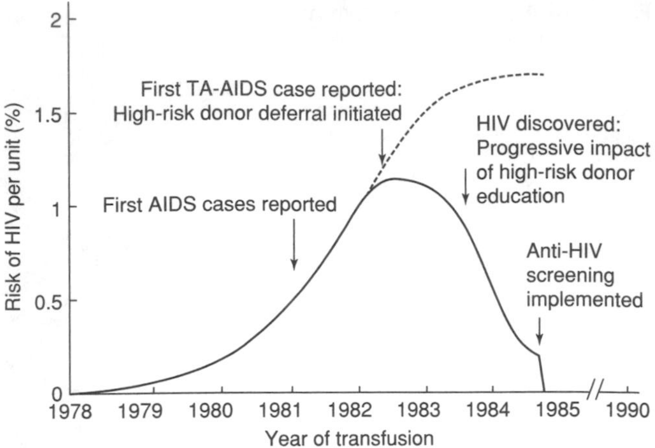

Figure 45–5 Risk of human immunodeficiency virus (HIV-1) infections from transfusions in San Francisco before anti-HIV screening. *Solid line* represents estimated risk of recipient infection per unit transfused. *Dashed line* indicates what the risk would have been if high-risk donor deferral measures had not been implemented. The risk in the United States as a whole probably trailed that in San Francisco by approximately 1 year, and the peak risk was of lower magnitude. (Modified from Busch MP, Young MJ, et al. Risk of human immunodeficiency virus (HIV) transmission by blood transfusions prior to the implementation of HIV-1 antibody screening. Transfusion 1991;31:4-11.)

donor education and deferral measures by blood banks.[57,58] In fact, it was estimated that approximately 90% of high-risk men in San Francisco who were donors between 1980 and 1982 deferred themselves from blood donation before implementation of the anti-HIV-1 test in early 1985.[57] These data demonstrate the effectiveness of donor education and self-deferral measures. Despite successful interventions like these, it has been estimated that more than 12,000 transfusion recipients in the United States were infected with HIV from transfusions administered before implementation of blood donor screening for HIV infection.[59]

Hemophiliacs, who are exquisitely vulnerable to transfusion-transmitted diseases because of exposure to factor concentrates derived from plasma pooled from thousands of blood donors, were hit especially hard by the early epidemic of transfusion-transmitted AIDS.[50] Incidence and prevalence data from 1978 through 1990 for 16 hemophiliac cohorts in the United States and Europe show that infections began in 1978, peaked in October 1982 at 22 infections per 100 person-years at risk, and declined to 4 per 100 person-years by July 1984. Few new infections occurred among hemophiliacs after 1986, but by that time, 50% of subjects in the combined cohort were infected. The decline in incidence from the infection peak in late 1982 coincided with health interventions introduced to reduce transmission, including recommendations for reduction in use of factor concentrates in 1982, voluntary donor deferral in 1983, and the availability of heat-treated factor VIII in 1984 and of HIV-1 screening in 1985.

Blood Donor Testing for HIV-1 and HIV-2 Antibody

The development of a sensitive and specific test for antibodies to HIV that was suitable for diagnosis (with confirmation by immunoblot analysis) and large-scale screening[60] represented a major breakthrough in combating the evolving pandemic in the early 1980s. Mandatory screening of all blood, plasma, and platelet donor samples for HIV with the antibody test began in the United States shortly after the assay became commercially available in March 1985.[61] Initial testing for antibodies to HIV-1 and HIV-2 is performed on serum or plasma from *pilot* tubes collected at the time of donation. If the initial test result is reactive, duplicate retesting is performed. If results of one or both second tests are reactive, the unit is designated *repeat reactive* and discarded. A process is also initiated to identify and quarantine all in-date components from any prior donations from that donor and to notify recipients who received blood components from prior donations.[62] Developments in test methodology have occurred at a rapid rate, and blood banks have implemented improved assays as soon as possible after FDA licensure. The evolution of antibody assays has been achieved through improvements in the antigens on the solid phase and in assay formats. From crude viral lysates, production moved to viral lysate assays spiked with purified HIV-1 antigens, and then on to the use of cloned (recombinant DNA [rDNA]-derived) and synthetic peptide antigens. Although concerns have been raised about the sensitivity of rDNA-derived and peptide antigen-based enzyme immunoassays (EIAs) to immunologically variant strains,[22,23] these assays have been "engineered" to include highly selected antigenic regions of HIV-1 and HIV-2 that maximize sensitivity to infected subjects from around the world. Consequently, rDNA-derived and synthetic peptide antigen-based assays are now in wide use in U.S. and non-U.S. blood banks.

Test manufacturers have also developed new assay formats with greater capacity to detect low-titer immunoglobulin M (IgM) antibody produced during early seroconversion. For example, the recombinant "antigen sandwich" EIA format allows use of lower dilutions of donor sera and detects IgM with better sensitivity.[34–36] The progressive introduction of assays with increased sensitivity to early infection has led to significant narrowing of the seroconversion window period and concomitant reductions in the HIV transmission risk associated with receiving screened blood.[63,64] The realization that HIV-1 subgroup and variant strains may not be reliably detected by current HIV-1/HIV-2 assays has led to demands by the FDA and efforts by kit manufacturers to reengineer standard assay formats to improve detection of unusual viral strains without compromising their sensitivity to main group HIV-1/HIV-2 strains.[65]

Testing for HIV Antigen

Testing of blood donor samples for HIV-1 antigens (in practice p24 antigen) was implemented in the United States in 1996 in addition to HIV antibody testing. This decision was based on studies showing that HIV-1 antigen appears in blood early in the course of infection, approximately 1 week before antibody is detectable. Transmission of HIV has been reported from transfusion of seronegative blood that was later shown to contain p24 antigen; the donors subsequently showed seroconversion.[66] Mathematical models, constructed with findings from geographic areas with very high incidence of new HIV infections, suggested that routine antigen testing would detect 1 antigen-positive/antibody-negative donation in every 1.6 million tested.[67] In reality, this projection was not achieved. Only seven donations from infected window-phase (p24 antigen-positive/anti-HIV-negative) volunteer donors were intercepted on the basis of p24 antigen testing alone in the first 5 years of screening, for an observed yield of 1 in 10 million donations.[68] A possible explanation for the underperformance of HIV-1 antigen testing in detecting HIV-1 antibody-negative window period infections is that prospective blood donors in the early phase of HIV-1 infection who have HIV-1 antigen only may be experiencing symptoms from acute retroviral infection that deter them from blood donation or result in their rejection during the predonation history and physical examination. After licensing of several nucleic acid amplification testing (NAT) assays suitable for blood and source plasma donor screening beginning in September 2001, the FDA allowed discontinuation of HIV-1 p24 antigen testing for blood donor samples screened by a licensed NAT assay.[69] In practice, this has resulted in virtual disappearance of p24 antigen testing from blood donor screening algorithms in the United States. However, antigen/antibody combination tests are employed in many developing countries where NAT screening is not feasible.

Nucleic Acid Testing

Detection of genomic HIV RNA sequences in plasma by NAT represents the most sensitive method for identification of newly infected persons who have not yet developed antibody to the virus (i.e., are in the preseroconversion window period of the infection).[70,71] An unrecognized new HIV infection in a healthy-appearing blood donor is by far the greatest single risk factor for transmission of the virus via transfusion,[72] development of suitable NAT assays for large-scale blood donor screening in the late 1990s was an important milestone toward the ultimate goal of complete prevention of HIV transmission from screened blood units. NAT assays began to be used in Europe for regional blood donor screening in 1997.[73] In the United States, routine testing of blood donor samples with combination NAT assays for HIV and hepatitis C virus (HCV) began in the spring of 1999 in the form of large-scale clinical trials conducted under investigational new drug (IND) applications to the FDA. Despite the research aspect, NAT quickly became the standard of practice, and by July 2001 essentially the entire U.S. blood supply was screened for HIV (and HCV) with the new technology. NAT is currently performed on pools of 16 to 24 blood donor samples, known as *minipool NAT*. The pooling strategy lowers the sensitivity of the test but allows faster turnaround times, which is critically important for on-time release of cellular blood components. In 3 years of practical experience in the United States from March 1999 to April 2002, HIV NAT detected 10 HIV-1 RNA-positive, HIV-1 EIA-negative, p24 antigen-negative donors out of 37 million donations tested (approximately 1 in 4 million) and missed no p24 antigen-positive, HIV-1 EIA-negative donations.[70] These results are consistent with a modest reduction in the infectious window period of HIV, averaging approximately 10 to 12 days against a sensitive HIV-1 antibody and 3 days against p24 antigen testing. Rare, unfortunate cases of HIV transmission from minipool NAT-screened units have occurred, demonstrating the potential infectiousness of such units.[62,74–77] The two NAT test systems for blood donor screening were licensed by the FDA in 2002, allowing facilities that incorporated licensed HIV NAT systems to discontinue HIV-1 antigen testing.

Supplemental Testing

Because of the exquisite sensitivity of HIV EIAs used in blood donor screening and the low pretest probability of HIV infection among low-risk blood donors, the majority of positive screening results are false positive, despite the excellent specificity of the tests. Supplemental assays are therefore essential to confirm positive screening results before donor counseling. Supplemental testing must use FDA-licensed reagents and must rule out both HIV-1 and HIV-2 infection.[37] Although combination HIV-1/HIV-2 supplemental assays using rDNA-derived or synthetic peptide antigens that appear to accurately detect and discriminate anti-HIV-1 and anti-HIV-2 have been developed,[78] they have never been approved by the FDA. Therefore, current confirmatory algorithms in U.S. blood banks employ HIV-1 viral lysate-based Western blots or immunofluorescence assays, in combination with a licensed anti-HIV-2 EIA and an unlicensed HIV-2 supplemental assay.[37] Interpretive criteria for Western blots have evolved over time as tests have improved and our understanding of the meaning of various banding patterns has grown. For currently licensed assays, a positive interpretation requires antibody reactivity to two of the following three HIV antigens: p24 (the major gag protein), gp41 (transmembrane env protein), and gp120/160 (external env protein/env precursor protein). Although these criteria are generally accurate, it is clear that some donors who show antibody reactivity only to the envelope glycoproteins are not infected with HIV-1, resulting in false-positive classifications by Western blots.[79] It is important, therefore, that all initial positive Western blot results are confirmed by testing of a separate follow-up sample, both to rule out specimen mix-up or testing errors and to discriminate nonspecific patterns from early seroconversion. A *negative* test result by Western blot is, by definition, the absence of any bands. Any other pattern of reactivity that does not meet criteria for a positive result is classified as *indeterminate.* Only a very small proportion of donors who test indeterminate on Western blot are infected with HIV-1.[80] Holodniy and Busch[81] provide a detailed discussion of interpretive criteria and review of developments in HIV supplemental test technology.

Because HIV NAT testing results are now routinely available on essentially all U.S. blood donations, this information can provide valuable additional clues regarding the infectious status of a donor with inconclusive serologic HIV test results. Donors with true positive repeat reactive HIV EIA results are expected to be reactive on minipool NAT testing[82]; a negative NAT test result thus suggests a false-positive HIV EIA result. It should be noted, however, that NAT has not been approved for supplemental HIV testing and is not yet incorporated in official confirmatory testing algorithms.

Recipients of prior donations from donors with confirmed positive antibody or NAT results are traced in a process called *lookback.*[62,83] Seronegative donors whose supplemental test results are negative (or persistently indeterminate and NAT-negative) are eligible for possible reentry into the donor pool according to an FDA-specified protocol,[37] although in practice, logistical and legal considerations have generally prevented reinstatement of such donors.

Risk of Infection from Screened Donations

Implementation of anti-HIV-1 screening in 1985 resulted in a marked decline of virus transmission by transfusion over the first several years of screening.[84,85] However, initial hopes that the newly developed antibody test would lead to eradication of HIV transmission by blood donor screening were not fulfilled.

In the late 1980s, well-documented cases of HIV-1 transmission from screened blood transfusions were reported,[86] and 14 of 106 (13%) cases initially reported as due to infections from screened blood transfusions could be confirmed. It was therefore clear that a small number of transmissions continued, despite screening with antibody tests. After adjusting for uninvestigated cases, and assuming an equal distribution of infections from 1986 through 1991, investigators from the Centers for Disease Control and Prevention (CDC) estimated that during that period, approximately five transfusion-associated AIDS cases due to infections from anti-HIV-screened blood transfusions had occurred per year.[87]

In the United States, two prospective studies estimated the risk of HIV transmission from antibody-screened donations at approximately 1 in 60,000 units between 1985 and 1991.[88,89] These studies were discontinued in 1992 because of their high cost. Since then, an alternative approach has been developed for estimating the risk of HIV infection from transfusions, now known as the *incidence-window period model.*[67] It is based on the premise that the risk of viral transmission by blood transfusion in a given geographic area is primarily a function of the *incidence rate*—that is, the number of newly infected blood donors per person-years of observation—and the length of the *window period*—defined as the time from infectiousness to antibody seroconversion. This concept of a window period can also be applied to other HIV tests, such as p24 antigen test, HIV-1 RNA NAT, Western blot, and "detuned" HIV-1 antibody assays, where results with a sensitive antibody test are compared with a modified less sensitive assay to discriminate recent from well-established infections.[90]

Sequential emergence of assay reactivity allows classification of primary HIV-1 infection into distinct laboratory stages (Fig. 45–6).[82] Determination of the length of window periods associated with HIV-1 assays enables estimation of residual risk of HIV-1 transmission from repeat donors and, with some adjustments, from first-time donors. Window period estimates for HIV-1 antibody tests in use in the United States dropped from a median of 45 days (95% confidence interval, 34–55 days) for the overall period from 1985 to 1990 to approximately 22 to 25 days after routine introduction in 1992 of new format anti-HIV-1/HIV-2 combination tests, which detect HIV-specific IgM antibody 10 to 15 days earlier than previously available assays.[63] By combining the 25-day window period estimate with data on the frequency of HIV seroconversions in large U.S. donor populations, two independent studies derived point estimates for the risk for HIV transmission during the period 1992 through 1995 as 1:450,000[91] and 1:495,000.[92] Introduction of HIV-1 antigen screening in 1995 further reduced the risk, but because fewer than expected HIV-1 antigen-positive HIV-1/2 antibody-negative units were intercepted once the test was introduced, the test's contribution to risk reduction seems to have been rather limited. In contrast, incorporation of minipool NAT into routine blood donor screening[93] was able to reduce the risk of HIV transmission to approximately 1 in 2 million blood component units transfused.[70] Multiplying the per-unit risk estimates by approximately 20 million components transfused to 5 million recipients per year in the United States leads to the expectation that fewer than 10 recipients per year are transfused with HIV-1-infected blood. The risk of HIV-2 transmission has been estimated at less than 1 in 15 million,[38] with other rare subtypes (e.g., HIV-1 subtype O)[22] being of even lesser concern. These combined risks are more than 10,000-fold lower than the risk existing at the peak of the transfusion-associated AIDS epidemic between 1982 and 1984.[57]

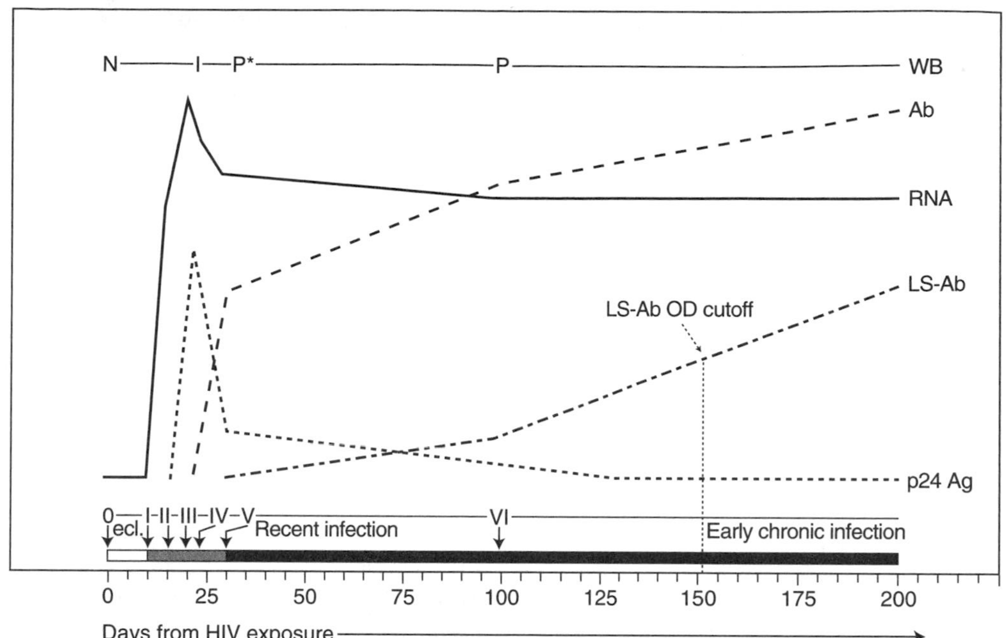

Figure 45–6 Schematic, semi-quantitative display of the progression of HIV markers (from top to bottom: WB, western blot; Ab, HIV antibody; RNA, HIV RNA; LS-Ab, HIV antibody determined by sensitive/less sensitive EIA testing strategy[90]; p24 Ag, HIV p24 antigen), from time of exposure (day 0) through the first 200 days of infection. As each of the markers appears in the bloodstream, the infection is assigned a new stage from 0, characterized by undetectable viral markers in blood samples, except for perhaps low-level viral blips[96]; through stage I (definitive HIV RNA viremia), stage II (p24 antigenemia), stage III (HIV EIA Ab reactive), stage IV (WB indeterminate, "I"), stage V (WB positive without p31 band, "P*"), and stage VI (WB positive, "P" with p31 band). Stages I–VI were derived from analysis of 435 serial samples from 51 plasma donors with new HIV-1 infection.[82] Incorporation of LS Ab EIA testing would allow further characterization of stage VI samples as representing recent vs. early chronic infection, i.e., infection that occurred within vs. beyond approximately 6 months from Ab seroconversion by an IgM-sensitive EIA.[90] The standardized optical density (OD) cutoff for the LS Ab EIA may be varied with recommended cutoffs from 0.5–1.0. Shown in the figure are the results for an OD cutoff of 0.75, as chosen in the original publication.[90] Cutoffs of 0.5 and 1.0 would result in average demarcations of recent from early chronic infection at 124 and 186 days, respectively. (Reproduced with permission from Fiebig EW et al. Dynamics of HIV viremia and antibody seroconversion in plasma donors: Implications for diagnosis and staging of primary HIV infection. AIDS 2003;17:1871–1879.)

Investigators have frequently used calculations based on the incidence-window period model to project the risk of transmission of HIV and other viruses by transfusion in different geographic areas and at various periods of the epidemic. Experience over time has confirmed the validity of the approach, and the risk projections derived from the model are generally accepted as meaningful and reliable estimates of the true risk.[94,95] Decreasing projections of the magnitude of risk in the same population over time reflect removal of high-risk donors and improvements in blood donor screening. Recently, widespread use of NAT assays in blood donor screening led to application of a new strategy for estimating risk of HIV transmission based on rates of detection of recently infected donors.[72] The method takes into account the expected increase of viral genomic equivalents (viral load) in blood donor samples during the initial phase of viral replication before appearance of HIV antibodies.[72,82] By back-extrapolation of the viral load from a reference point such as appearance of p24 antigen or detection of HIV infection by minipool NAT to a minimal viral concentration that is thought to be infective (e.g., 1 viral copy per 20 mL plasma), the window period between the infectious threshold and the reference point can be projected. By substituting the reference point with a theoretical threshold such as assay sensitivity of a new NAT, the window period for that assay can be estimated. A practical application of the new method is the projection of risk reduction for transfusion transmission of HIV by testing individual donor samples rather than minipools of 16 to 24 samples. The result suggests a rather modest decrease in risk, from approximately 1 per 2 million component units transfused with MP-NAT, to 1 in 3 to 4 million units with ID-NAT,[82] at considerably higher cost and potentially delayed availability of transfusable cellular blood components. Not addressed by the novel strategy of estimating residual transmission risk of HIV based on viral replication dynamics is the finding of low-level (estimated 1 to 10 copies/mL) viral "blips" in the 2- to 3-week long period between infection and ramp-up phase of viremia, sometimes referred to as the *eclipse phase* of HIV infection (see Fig. 45–6). Such "blips" have been observed at intervals of approximately 1 to 3 weeks before HIV ramp-up viremia in 6 of 15 plasma donors with newly acquired HIV infection.[96] The added risk from blood donations during the eclipse phase is unknown, but might contribute slightly to the overall risk estimate associated with current NAT blood donor screening.[96]

HUMAN T-CELL LYMPHOTROPIC VIRUS

Although eclipsed by concerns about HIV, HTLV is nonetheless relevant to the safety of blood transfusion. Both HTLV-1 and HTLV-2 are transmitted by blood transfusion, cause chronic retroviral infection of humans, and are associated with serious disease outcomes. Serologic testing for HTLV-1 in U.S. blood donors has been in place since 1988. This policy has led to the unexpected discovery that at least half of blood donors testing positive for HTLV-1 are in fact infected with HTLV-2, for which disease outcomes are less well described.[97–99]

Virology

Both HTLV-1 and HTLV-2 are human retroviruses of the oncornavirus class. As previously mentioned, the first report of HTLV-1 discovery was published in 1980 and that of HTLV-2 in 1982.[5,7] With RNA genomes of approximately 8000 nucleotides in length, the genetic organizations of HTLV-1 and HTLV-2 are similar to those of other retroviruses (Fig. 45–7).[100,101] The HTLV genome contains *gag* regions coding for viral core proteins, *pol* regions coding for viral reverse transcriptase, protease and integrase *env* regions coding for the viral envelope proteins, and finally the *tax* or *px* region (analogous to the HIV *tat* gene), which is responsible for transcriptional regulation of HTLV-1 and HTLV-2. HTLV-1 and HTLV-2 have approximately 60% nucleotide sequence homology. Many of their viral proteins crossreact serologically, although peptides eliciting specific immune responses and allowing differential serologic diagnosis of HTLV-1 versus HTLV-2 have been discovered.

HTLV-1 predominantly infects CD4+ T lymphocytes, whereas HTLV-2 has a broader tropism with preference for CD8+ lymphocytes and, to a lesser degree, CD4+ lymphocytes, B lymphocytes, and macrophages.[102,103] Neither virus has high levels of cell-free viremia, perhaps accounting for lower transmissibility than either hepatitis B virus or HIV. Also in contrast to HIV, there is relatively little active replication of HTLV-1 and HTLV-2 in infected humans. Instead, most expansion of the pool of infected lymphocytes appears to occur by lymphocytic division and the proliferation of clones of infected lymphocytes.[104] Corollaries of these observations are that descriptions of HTLV viral load refer to measurements of proviral DNA in the cellular compartment. There has been only one report of measurable HTLV RNA in cell-free plasma[105]; however, further research will be necessary to exclude the possibility of a significant viremia in cell-free plasma.

Epidemiology and Modes of Transmission

HTLV-1 is endemic in sub-Saharan Africa; the Caribbean region and parts of South America, including Colombia, Peru, and Brazil as a result of the slave trade; southwestern Japan; and parts of Melanesia and Australia.[106] HTLV-1 has also been reported from Iran, India, and Taiwan as well as in countries containing significant immigrant populations from the main endemic areas. Given the high HTLV-1 prevalence in southwestern Japan, the absence of HTLV-1 infection in mainland China and in Korea as well as other parts of Southeast Asia poses an epidemiologic puzzle. Molecular epidemiologic studies have indicated the presence of at least two viral subtypes in Africa; a cosmopolitan subtype found in Africa, Japan, the Caribbean, and other more recent foci of HTLV-1 infection; and a distantly related Melanesian subtype.[107]

HTLV-2 has also been found to be endemic in a number of Amerindian tribes throughout South, Central, and North America.[108–110] Not all tribes are infected, and tribes with the least intermingling with Western settlers, such as the Kayapo of Brazil, appear to have the highest prevalence rate.[108] The other endemic focus of HTLV-2 infection appears to be among Pygmies in sub-Saharan Africa, again in tribes having relatively little contact with European settlers.[111] HTLV-2 infection is also prevalent among injection drug users and their sexual partners in the United States, Brazil, and Europe.[112] Given the relative recency of injection drug use behavior, there appears to have been an epidemic spread of HTLV-2 over the past 40 or 50 years as a result of the introduction of endemic HTLV-2 into the injection drug use population and subsequent spread through sharing of contaminated needles.[113]

In endemic populations, both HTLV-1 and HTLV-2 show age-specific seroprevalence rates that rise steadily with age, from 1% or less among infected children to 5% to 10% of older individuals.[113–116] Female seroprevalence is generally greater than male seroprevalence, presumably owing to more efficient sexual transmission from males to females than vice versa.

In one large study of blood donors in the United States in the 1990s, HTLV-1 seroprevalence was approximately 10 per

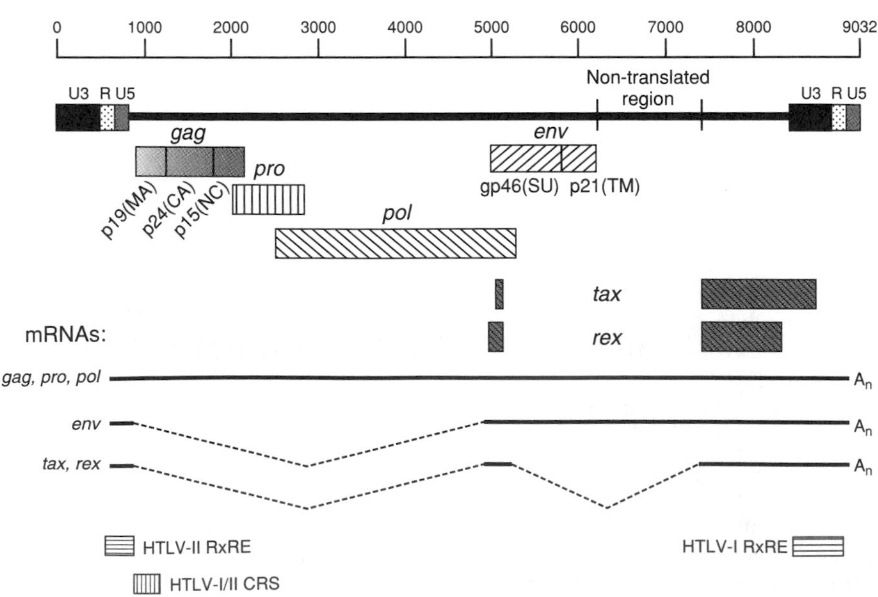

Figure 45–7 Structure and organization of the HTLV genome. The HTLV provirus genome is shown at the top of the figure. Positions of known genes are indicated. Sizes and positions of the proteins encoded by the provirus are shown beneath the provirus. The structure of the three messenger RNA species produced are shown at the bottom of the figure. (Reproduced with permission from Fields BN, Knipe DM, Howley PM (eds). Fields Virology, 3rd ed. Philadelphia, Lippincott-Raven, 1996, p 1850.)

100,000 overall, rising steadily with age, and was twice as prevalent in females as in males.[113] In contrast, HTLV-2 was found among the same U.S. blood donors at a rate of 20 per 100,000 overall.[113] Other studies of U.S. donors have shown similar overall prevalence, but a more equal ratio of HTLV-2 to HTLV-1.[114] Although there is at least a twofold female excess of infection, the age prevalence curve peaks in persons aged 30 to 49 and falls in older individuals (Fig. 45–8). This apparent birth cohort effect is consistent with the hypothesis of an epidemic of HTLV-2 transmitted by injection drug use and secondary sexual transmission beginning in the late 1960s and 1970s.[113]

HTLV-1 and HTLV-2 have similar modes of transmission. Mother-to-child transmission is important for both viruses, and between 20% and 30% of infants born to infected mothers become infected themselves.[117] In contrast to HIV, however, the great majority of such transmission appears to occur by means of breast-feeding. Public health intervention studies in Japan have documented a decrease in the transmission rate from 30% to 3% when infected mothers substituted bottle-feeding for breast-feeding.[117]

Sexual transmission also occurs for both HTLV-1 and HTLV-2, presumably by means of infected lymphocytes or other cells contained in seminal fluid.[118,119] The earlier impression that transmission from males to females is more efficient than vice versa and that HTLV-1 is more readily transmitted than HTLV-2 may not be true.[120] The most important factors determining whether transmission will occur between HTLV-serodiscordant couples (i.e., one seropositive and one seronegative for HTLV) are the total duration of the sexual relationship and the HTLV proviral load in the male.[121] The frequency or type of sexual activities performed appears to have little effect on the risk of transmission, although the predominant behavior in this study was heterosexual vaginal intercourse. The CDC recommends prevention of sexual transmission through the use of condoms by HTLV-serodiscordant couples as well as by HTLV-seropositive single individuals with multiple sexual partners.[121]

HTLV-1 and HTLV-2 are also transmitted efficiently by the sharing of contaminated needles or other parenteral exposures, leading to high seroprevalence among injection drug users.[112,122] Data on transmission by blood transfusion are provided in more detail later. There is no data supporting the casual transmission of HTLV-1 or HTLV-2 within households or between individuals who do not have any of the preceding risk factors for transmission.

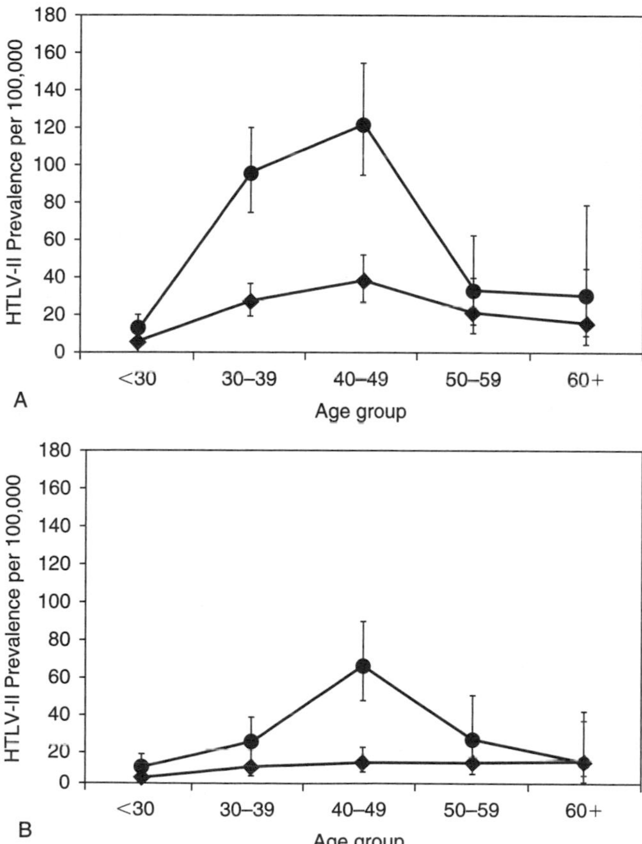

Figure 45–8 Age-specific seroprevalence of human T-cell lymphotropic virus type 2 among female **(A)** and male **(B)** blood donors in five U.S. cities participating in the multicenter Retrovirus Epidemiology Donor Study, stratified by two western *(solid circle)* and 3 eastern or central *(solid diamond)* blood centers. Seroprevalence is expressed per 100,000 donors.

Disease Outcomes

Soon after its discovery, HTLV-1 was associated with a CD4+ T-lymphocytic lymphoma, ATL.[123,124] This lymphoma, which has a leukemic phase in one fourth to one third of infected individuals, is also associated with hypercalcemia, skin lesions, and hepatosplenomegaly.[125] Atypical malignant lymphocytes with convoluted nuclei, referred to as *flower cells,* are seen in a high number of patients with leukemic-phase ATL and may also be seen in low numbers in asymptomatic persons who are seropositive for HTLV-1.[126,127] The prognostic implications of having flower cells are not well defined, although individuals with either very high HTLV proviral loads or with relatively high numbers of circulating flower cells appear to be predisposed to a higher risk of ATL.[128] An individual infected with HTLV-1 at birth has an estimated 4% lifetime risk of ATL, and the risk is presumably lower for those infected sexually as adults.[129] There are two case reports of ATL occurring after apparent transfusion-related HTLV-1 infection.[130] Chemotherapy is often less effective for ATL than for other lymphomas and leukemia, and a high mortality is associated with this hematologic malignancy.[131,132]

Although both HTLV-1 and HTLV-2 are known to cause spontaneous lymphocytic proliferation in vitro,[133–135] HTLV-2 does not appear to cause hematologic malignancy. Even though HTLV-2 was initially isolated from two cases of atypical T-lymphocytic hairy cell leukemia, subsequent epidemiologic studies of hairy cell leukemia have not revealed an association with HTLV-2 infection.[136–139] Similarly, initial case reports of mycosis fungoides and large granular cell leukemia among HTLV-2-infected persons have not led to confirmed associations after further investigation.[140–142]

The other major disease association of both HTLV-1 and HTLV-2 is HAM/TSP. Initially described by Gessain and colleagues[143] in Martinique, the association with HAM/TSP was soon confirmed by investigators in Japan and others.[144–147] HAM/TSP is a slowly progressive myelopathy characterized by spastic paraparesis of the lower extremity, hyperreflexia, bowel and bladder symptomatology, and relative sparing of both upper extremity strength and cognitive function.[148]

The disease course is slow but progressive, with 10 years often elapsing between the first signs and severe paraplegia necessitating the use of a wheelchair. There is no definitive treatment for HAM/TSP, although the use of systemic steroids, immunosuppression with azathioprine, and the use of the androgenic agent danazol have had transient success.[148] Clinical trials are planned to evaluate the efficiency of various treatment regimens.

A cohort study has estimated the risk of HAM/TSP to be about 2% in HTLV-1–positive persons.[149] Sexual acquisition of HTLV-1 may be a risk factor for HAM/TSP[150]; however, the incubation period may be shortest after transfusion-acquired infection.[151–153] Cases of typical HAM/TSP have been reported in HTLV-2–infected humans, although the risk appears to be slightly less than or equal to that with HTLV-1.[149] In contrast to some initial reports, there is no association of either HTLV-1 or HTLV-2 and classic multiple sclerosis.[154–156] Likewise, the implication of HTLV-1 and HTLV-2 in other neurologic syndromes is controversial, because individuals infected with HTLV-2 may have genetic or environmental factors that also cause neurologic disease.[157]

Other immunologic diseases and phenomena have been reported in relation to HTLV-1 and HTLV-2. HTLV-1 has been associated with lymphocytic pneumonitis and uveitis.[158,159] HTLV-1–positive cases of polymyositis have also been reported, and both HTLV-1 and HTLV-2 may be associated with a higher incidence of arthritis.[159–161] Of particular interest, a cohort study has shown that HTLV-1, and particularly HTLV-2, may be associated with a higher incidence of other infections, including pneumonia, acute bronchitis, and urinary tract infection.[162] This finding is consistent with the association of HTLV-1 and infective dermatitis in children.[163] The mechanism of these disease associations has not yet been described and may be due to either subclinical immune dysfunction or increased inflammation. It is not clear whether either HTLV-1 or HTLV-2 contributes to an increased incidence of other types of malignancy; a study in Japan has reported an increased risk of "viral-associated" malignancy such as hepatoma.[164] However, a study in the United States showed no increase of any nonhematologic malignancy with HTLV-1 or HTLV-2.[162] Intriguingly, infection with HTLV-2 but not HTLV-1 was found recently to be associated with increased mortality in blood donors.[165] In another recent study on the impact of co-infection with HTLV-1/2 in HIV-infected patients, co-infection with HTLV-2 was associated with a higher rate of clinical complications but paradoxically also with longer survival and delayed progression to AIDS.[166] However, a well-designed meta-analysis, which accounted for date of HIV infection, showed no effect of HTLV-2 co-infection on HIV disease progression.[167]

Transfusion-Related Transmission

Soon after its discovery, HTLV-1 was shown to be transmitted by blood transfusion, with transmission efficiency in Japan of at least 50%.[168,169] A cohort study in Jamaica in the late 1980s demonstrated a 25% to 30% risk of HTLV-1 infection after transfusion of one unit of HTLV-1-infected blood, with a 50-day mean latency period between the implicated transfusion and the development of de novo anti-HTLV antibodies.[170] Results of the TSS in the United States, with data from the mid-1980s, showed a much lower rate of transmission, only 10% to 20% for HTLV-1 and HTLV-2.[171] Differences between these transmission rates may be due to the requirement that HTLV-infected, viable lymphocytes must be present in the transfused unit for it to be classified as infected. A significant inverse correlation between the duration of refrigerated storage (presumably related to lymphocyte viability) and the risk of HTLV transmission was demonstrated in the TSS. Although such data were not reported, it is conceivable that blood unit storage times were shorter in the Japanese and Jamaican studies than in the U.S. study, and therefore viable infected lymphocytes were more frequently transfused.

A later study of recipients of large-volume transfusions in the United States showed estimated risks of HTLV transmission to be 12 per 100,000 units before and 1.4 per 100,000 units after the 1988 institution of universal screening for HTLV antibodies.[88] The screening was introduced in that year after consideration of early data on HTLV-1 prevalence in blood donors, its transfusion transmissibility, and diseases associated with the infection.[114] Studies estimating the current risk of HTLV-1 by blood transfusion, similar to those of other low-frequency agents, are hindered by the large sample sizes required to measure low-frequency events. Nonetheless, the Retrovirus Epidemiology Study and the American Red Cross (ARC) have measured the incidence of HTLV-1 and HTLV-2 infection among serial blood donors and have used these data, along with estimates of the window period between infection and the development of antibodies, to model the residual risk of HTLV-1 infection. The most recent published projections, based on voluntary donations to the ARC system from 2000 to 2001, estimated a residual risk of approximately 1 per 3 million transfused units for HTLV-1, which is lower than the current risk of HIV and hepatitis B or C infection, and evidence of further dramatic risk reduction since the early 1990s.

The risk of transmission of HTLV-1 by cell-free plasma is controversial. The Jamaican study showed no episodes of transfusion transmission in individuals receiving only plasma transfusions,[170] and laboratory studies have shown that cell-free transmission of HTLV-1 is difficult. A report on the detection by RT-PCR of HTLV-1 viral RNA in cell-free plasma is of concern, if its findings can be replicated.[105] Nonetheless, transfusion of blood products containing residual leukocytes appears to carry a higher risk of HTLV transmission than transfusion of products free of leukocytes.[90]

Also of note in regard to transfusion safety is the definite association between HTLV-2 infection and previous injection drug use or sexual relations with an injection drug user. Because injection drug users are more effectively screened out of the blood donor population, the typical HTLV-2-infected individual is a middle-aged woman who reports remote sexual exposure to an injection drug user. These data highlight the need to continue refining behavioral screening criteria, including consideration of banning donors who admit any prior sexual contact with injection drug users.[172]

Laboratory Diagnosis

Screening for HTLV-1 and HTLV-2, analogous to HIV screening, is generally performed with EIAs. The earliest assays included only HTLV-1 native viral proteins. It soon became apparent, however, that these assays were deficient in the native HTLV envelope proteins because of the viral purification process used to produce the proteins. This problem led to the subsequent addition of recombinant envelope proteins to the EIA antigen mix to improve the test's sensitivity. Because HTLV-1 and HTLV-2 have 60% nucleotide sequence homology, there is significant cross-reaction of HTLV-2 with HTLV-1 EIAs.[101] However, because 10% to 15% of HTLV-2 infections were missed by earlier HTLV-1 EIAs,[173] subsequent EIAs utilized a recombinant transmembrane envelope glycoprotein, rgp21, that had greater sensitivity for both HTLV-2 and HTLV-1, and later generations of EIAs use recombinant proteins from both HTLV-2 and HTLV-1. Thus, the FDA has permitted the labeling of single assays for the combined detection of HTLV-1 and HTLV-2.

Supplemental testing for HTLV-1 and HTLV-2 has continued to be more problematic. The earliest and most common supplemental test is the Western blot. Because of a deficiency in viral envelope protein, however, Western blots using only HTLV-1 native viral proteins are relatively nonspecific and may also be insensitive to HTLV-2. Western blots supplemented with rgp21, which have greater sensitivity to HTLV-2 because of its crossreactivity with rgp21, soon became available. However, false-positive reactivity to rgp21 in combination with nonspecific reactivity with the *gag* p19 or p24 bands occasionally led to false-positive Western blot interpretations.[174] Radioimmunoprecipitation has been used in research laboratories over the years to more specifically confirm the presence of antibodies to envelope proteins of HTLV-1 and HTLV-2. However, this assay is very labor intensive and so is not suitable for use as a routine supplemental test in blood banks.

Second-generation Western blots have been developed that contain native HTLV-1 proteins supplemented with a refined version of rgp21, to decrease nonspecific reactions, in addition to recombinant peptides specific to both HTLV-1 (rgp46-I) and HTLV-2 (rgp46-II).[175,176] In the research setting, these assays have proved to be both sensitive and specific for the diagnosis of HTLV-1 and HTLV-2. Because of the presence of the type-specific epitopes, they allow the differentiation of HTLV-1 from HTLV-2 infection in the great majority of cases.[177,178] HTLV type-specific peptides are also available in the EIA format; however, these tests should be used for typing specimens that have already been confirmed by other supplemental assays.[177–179] This issue is important, because counseling of the infected donor should be specific to the disease outcomes to be expected with either HTLV-1 or HTLV-2, and risk factor profiles have been shown to be specific to either HTLV-1 or HTLV-2.[122]

Few of the HTLV supplemental tests described have been licensed by the FDA, however, so they have been used only under provisions for research. Thus, the counseling of infected donors based on the results of such tests has carried potential regulatory risks. In addition, because of the complexity of some of these supplemental assays, proficiency of the laboratories performing them depended on the local expertise and the volume of supplemental testing performed. This situation has led the FDA to ban the use of nonlicensed supplemental assays in the diagnosis of blood donors who test positive on the HTLV EIA. Although the regulatory reasons for this decision are understandable, it has significantly reduced the specificity of the diagnosis of HTLV-infected blood donors, because only 10% to 25% of EIA-positive blood donors are in fact seropositive for HTLV-1 or HTLV-2, and donors with indeterminate EIA results are unlikely to be infected with HTLV in the absence of definite risk factors.[180] The lack of accurate licensed supplemental tests means that a large number of HTLV EIA-positive donors are falsely being informed that they are potentially seropositive for HTLV. Thus, there is an urgent need for the development of licensed supplemental assays that would differentiate HTLV-1 and HTLV-2 infections.

Less clear is the need for improving the sensitivity of HTLV blood donor screening by implementing NAT-based HTLV testing. Lower incidence rates of infection than seen for the other major transfusion-transmitted viruses, at least partial protection of blood recipients from HTLV transmission by widespread use of leukoreduced cellular blood components, and low disease penetrance in the 5% range argue against such a proposition, especially if cost effectiveness is considered. On the other hand, tolerance of even a low risk of retroviral infection has not been acceptable in a political environment that demands zero risk. Before large-scale blood donor screening with HTLV NAT assays could be introduced, however, technical issues would also have to addressed. Current NAT systems do not have the capacity to extract cell-associated nucleic acids, so detection of HTLVs (and other cell-associated pathogens, including parasites) by NAT will have to await a new generation of high-throughput screening systems.

ADDITIONAL RETROVIRUSES

Besides HIVs and HTLVs, there may be additional human retroviruses that have not as yet been discovered. It is also now well established that retroviruses from other species can be transmitted to humans and subsequently pose a risk to the blood supply. These concerns led some to call for active surveillance for new and emerging retroviruses with potential relevance for transfusion safety. Indeed two new HTLV variants, tentatively named HTLV-3 and HTLV-4, have been isolated from a few human Pygmies and Bantu living in remote areas of sub-Saharan Africa.[181,182] Because the infected humans hunted and butchered monkeys or kept them as pets, the authors suggest that recent cross-species transmission may have occurred.

Interestingly, it is known that 5% to 10% of the genomes of humans and many other species is comprised of endogenous retroviral sequences. The origin and functions of human endogenous retroviral (HERV) sequences remain unclear, although it is generally believed that these sequences represent relics of ancestral retroviral infections that have been conserved through evolution for functional properties, including protection from exogenous retroviral infection. To date there is no convincing evidence that HERVs are associated with any disease or that they can be transmitted horizontally by blood transfusion or other routes. However, there is concern that endogenous retroviruses in the genomes of other species could be activated into exogenous retroviruses and be transmitted to humans.[183,184] This was highlighted recently by demonstration of in vitro transmission of porcine endogenous retrovirus sequences to human cells.[183] The potential of cross-species infection is of particular concern with animal-derived blood constituents (e.g., porcine-derived clotting factors, bovine albumin, equine immunoglobulins) or organs in xenotransplantation protocols. Reassuringly, recent studies to examine the issue of whether endogenous retroviruses from other species may have infected humans exposed to blood products or organs from these species have failed to document any cases of infection using sensitive serologic and molecular assays.[184,185]

A further concern that has been raised regarding cross-species transmission of exogenous retroviruses is the potential that such transmissions could result in accelerated transmission patterns and increased pathogenicity with humans, similar to what likely happened with SIV/HIV. For example, a clinical syndrome called idiopathic (HIV-negative) CD-4 lymphocytopenia, described in the early 1990s, was speculated to result from a novel retrovirus infection. However, subsequent studies both in high-risk and blood donor populations failed to confirm a retroviral or other infectious etiology, with the exception of a subset of cases due to group O HIV-1.[186] There has also been speculation over the years that donors with indeterminate seroreactivity for HIV or HTLV may harbor crossreactive primate or ungulate retroviruses.[187] However, most studies that have probed samples from donors with indeterminate test results have failed to identify evidence for infection based on type-specific serologic or PCR analyses.[187]

Over the past several years novel assays have been developed that allow for investigation of donor and other specimens for evidence of unknown retroviruses. These include amplified reverse transcriptase assays (Amp-RT), also called *product-enhanced RT assays* (PERT), and generic PCR assays that target conserved regions of polymerase and *gag* genes that are common among highly divergent retroviral families. Continued application of these tools to samples from blood donor–recipient repositories, both in developed and developing countries, will be important to reassure the public that additional retroviral agents do not pose a risk to blood safety.

APPROACHES FOR FURTHER REDUCING THE RISK OF RETROVIRAL TRANSMISSION BY TRANSFUSIONS

Twenty years of blood donor screening for HIV and HTLV, including utilization of sensitive NAT technology for HIV RNA detection since the late 1990s, have greatly contributed to improved blood safety with regard to retroviral transmission in high-income nations that can afford and support the required infrastructure for sophisticated blood screening programs. Yet, despite the now exceedingly small likelihood of becoming infected with HIV or HTLV from a screened blood transfusion, there continues to be the call for and expectation of a blood supply that is risk free in regard to HIV and other infectious disease transmission.

Principal avenues that are actively being pursued in the effort to eliminate transfusion-transmitted retroviral infections are the selection of the safest possible donor populations, continuing improvements in blood donor testing, and introduction of safe, effective, and affordable viral inactivation methods into transfusion practice.

Because of the disproportionate impact of the HIV epidemic on poor urban racial minorities and the known higher prevalence of HIV among minority donors, some have argued for what has been termed *demographic recruitment.* However, this concept fails to recognize the critical need for a genetically diverse donor base to support the transfusion needs of a similarly diverse recipient population. Others have proposed expanding or modifying the risk factor interview process by, for example, adding questions on recent heterosexual activity, using cartoon depictions of risk behaviors to improve understanding by less-educated donors, and implementing computer-based interview strategies to enhance confidentiality.[188] Convincing data to support these proposals have not been generated, however.[189] Risk factor profiles of seropositive donors have changed over time. For example, Petersen and associates[190] compared HIV risk factors among 508 seropositive donors identified at 20 blood centers between May 1988 and August 1989 with those of 472 seropositive donors identified from January 1990 through May 1991. The overall rate of seropositive donations declined slightly over time (from 0.021% to 0.018%), primarily as a result of a decrease in infected donations by homosexual and bisexual men. In contrast, the rate of infected donations by persons probably exposed through heterosexual contact remained stable. Toward the end of the observation period, 56% of infected female donors and 12% of infected male donors had seropositive heterosexual partners; another 41% of infected female donors and 29% of infected heterosexual male donors were probably infected by heterosexual contact (on the basis of serologic studies for sexually transmitted disease markers), even though specific infected sex partners could not be identified. These researchers rejected the option of deferring donors on the basis of recent or lifetime number of heterosexual partners, because numeric cutoffs that would identify only half of the seropositive heterosexual donors would also result in a loss of 7% to 13% of all donations. This study illustrates the significant tradeoffs required to maintain an adequate as well as safe blood supply.

Incentives for blood donors pose a similar dilemma. Paid blood donors have long been identified as having a higher risk for transmissible viral diseases, and a volunteer-only blood donor system is considered a cornerstone in ensuring blood safety.[191] Nonmonetary incentives are widely used to attract volunteer donors, however, and surveys have shown that some of these incentives may also entice high-risk donors to give blood.[192]

Since implementation of NAT testing in the so-called *mini-pool format,* strategies to further improve blood donor screening for HIV focus on introduction of individual donation (ID) testing. As studies have shown, however, the expected additional risk reduction from ID-NAT testing would be modest,[72] and complete elimination of transmission risk is unlikely to be achieved by blood screening alone.

An added layer of safety is provided by viral inactivation technology, which has been used for almost 2 decades in the manufacturing of plasma derivatives and almost as long for treatment of pooled plasma in many European countries.[193] Various methods are being used, with solvent-detergent treatment being the most common principle employed.[194] Effectiveness of the solvent-detergent method is very high for lipid-enveloped viruses, including HIV and HTLV, but the procedure does not reliably inactivate nonenveloped viruses.[195] The safety of the solvent-detergent treatment process for fresh frozen plasma came under further scrutiny by the finding of preferential inactivation of antithrombotic proteins in treated plasma that could result in a prothrombotic state in large-volume recipients. Reports of venous thrombotic events (VTE) in patients receiving exchange transfusions with solvent-detergent–treated fresh frozen plasma,[196,197] and several fatalities associated with VTEs in liver transplant patients who received solvent-detergent–treated fresh frozen plasma, contributed to the discontinuation of use of the product in the United States, although it is still available in Europe.[195]

Newer chemical, photodynamic, and photochemical methods capable of inactivating a wide range of pathogens, including known transfusion-transmissible viruses, bacteria, and parasites, have been developed. These work with single-donation platelets and fresh frozen plasma components, thereby avoiding the risks associated with pooling of blood components.[193] One photochemical inactivation system was licensed in Europe in early 2002; however, licensing in the United States has been delayed for now. Systems of pathogen inactivation of red cell products are at an earlier stage of development and clinical study and are therefore further away from possible implementation.[195] An impediment to the introduction of any new viral inactivation method for blood components is the concern that these methods may themselves pose adverse consequences for transfusion recipients, potentially offsetting the benefits of the new treatment method in comparison with existing strategies. Pathogen inactivation methods are discussed in more detail in Chapter 27 .

An ongoing struggle is the prevention of transfusion-transmitted retroviral and other infections in low-income and developing nations. Burgeoning prevalence and incidence rates as well as lack of resources make effective blood donor screening in these areas a challenge that has only been partially met. It is hoped that blood safety in developing countries can be improved gradually through establishment of sufficiently funded national and regional programs that incorporate establishment of donor recruitment networks and high-quality screening capacity.[198]

REFERENCES

1. Zanotto PM, Gibbs MJ, Gould EA, Holmes EC. A reevaluation of the higher taxonomy of viruses based on RNA polymerases. J Virol 1996;70:6083–6096.
2. Levy J. HIV and the Pathogenesis of AIDS. Washington, D.C., ASM Press, 1998.
3. Rowland-Jones SL. Timeline: AIDS pathogenesis: What have two decades of HIV research taught us? Nat Rev Immunol 2003;3:343–348.
4. Bishop JM. The molecular genetics of cancer. Science 1987;235: 305–311.
5. Poiesz BJ, Ruscetti FW, Cazdar AF, et al. Detection and isolation of type C retrovirus particles from fresh and cultured lymphocytes of a patient with cutaneous T-cell lymphoma. Proc Natl Acad Sci USA 1980;77:7415–7419
6. Blattner WA (ed). Human Retrovirology: HTLV. New York, Raven Press, 1990.
7. Kalyanaraman VS, Sarngadharan MG, Robert-Guroff M, et al. A new subtype of human T-cell leukemia virus (HTLV-II) associated with a T-cell variant of hairy cell leukemia. Science 1982;218:571–573.
8. Rosenblatt JD, Chen IS, Golde DW. HTLV-II and human lymphoproliferative disorders. Clin Lab Med 1988;8:85–95.
9. Gao F, Bailes E, Robertson DL, et al. Origin of HIV-1 in the chimpanzee *Pantroglodytes troglodytes*. Nature 1999;397:436–444.
10. Zhu T, Korber BT, Nahmias AJ, et al. An African HIV-1 sequence from 1959 and implications for the origin of the epidemic. Nature 1998;391: 594–597.
11. UNAIDS. Joint United Nations Programme on HIV/AIDS. 2006 Report on the Global AIDS Epidemic: Executive Summary. UNAIDS, Geneva, Switzerland, May 2006. Available at http://www.unaids.org/en/publications. Accessed June 30, 2006.
12. Roberts JD, Bebenek K, Kunkel TA. The accuracy of reverse transcriptase from HIV-1. Science 1988;242:1171–1174.
13. Vartanian J-P, Meyerhans A, Asjo B, et al. Selection, recombination, and G-A hypermutation of HIV-1 genomes. J Virol 1991;65:1779–1788.
14. Zhu T, Mo H, Wang N, et al. Genotypic and phenotypic characterization of HIV-1 in patients with primary infection. Science 1993;261: 1179–1181.
15. Zhu T, Wang N, Carr A, et al. Evidence for coinfection by multiple strains of human immunodeficiency virus type 1 subtype B in an acute seroconverter. J Virol 1995;69:1324–1327.
16. Diaz R, Sabino EC, Mayer A, et al. Dual human immunodeficiency virus type 1 infection and recombination in a dually-exposed transfusion recipient. J Virol 1995;69:3273–3281.
17. Perrin L, Kaiser L, Yerly S. Travel and the spread of HIV-1 genetic variants. Lancet Infect Dis 2003;3:22–27.
18. Delwart EL, Orton S, Parekh B, et al. Two percent of HIV-positive U.S. blood donors are infected with non-subtype-B strains. AIDS Res Hum Retrovir 2003;19:1065–1070.
19. Nkengasong JN, Janssens W, Heyndrickx L, et al. Genotypic subtypes of HIV-1 in Cameroon. AIDS 1994;8:1405–1412.
20. Peeters M, Gueye A, Mboup S, et al. Geographical distribution of HIV-1 group O viruses in Africa. AIDS 1997;11:493–498.
21. Pau CP, Hu HDJ, Spruill C, et al. Surveillance for human immunodeficiency virus type 1 group O infections in the United States. Transfusion 1996;36:398–400.
22. Loussert-Ajaka I, Ly TD, Chaix ML, et al. HIV-1/HIV-2 seronegativity in HIV-1 subtype O infected patients. Lancet 1994;343:1393–1394.
23. Schable C, Zekeng L, Pau CP, et al. Sensitivity of United States HIV antibody tests for detection of HIV-1 group O infections. Lancet 1994;344:1333–1334.
24. U.S. Food and Drug Administration. Interim Recommendations For Deferral of Donors at Increased Risk for HIV-1 Group O Infection. Rockville, Md., Center for Biologics Evaluation and Research (CBER), 1996.
25. Clavel F, Guetard D, Brun-Vezinet F, et al. Isolation of a new human retrovirus from West African patients with AIDS. Science 1986;233: 343–346.
26. O'Brien TR, George JR, Holmberg SD. Human immunodeficiency virus type 2 infection in the United States: epidemiology, diagnosis, and public health implications. JAMA 1992;267:2775–2779.
27. Marlink R, Kanki P, Thior I, et al. Reduced rate of disease development after HIV-2 infections as compared to HIV-1. Science 1994;265: 1587–1590.
28. Poulsen AG, Aaby P, Larsen O, et al. 9-year HIV-2-associated mortality in an urban community in Bissau, West Africa. Lancet 1997;349:911–914.
29. George JR, Rayfield MA, Phillips S, et al. Efficacies of U.S. Food and Drug Administration licensed HIV-1-screening enzyme immunoassays for detecting antibodies to HIV-2. AIDS 1990;4:321–326.
30. de Cock KM, Porter A, Kouadio J, et al. Cross-reactivity on Western blots in HIV-1 and HIV-2 infection. AIDS 1991;5:859–863.
31. Busch MP, Petersen L, Schable C, Perkins HA. Monitoring blood donors for HIV-2 infection by testing anti-HIV-1 reactive sera. Transfusion 1990;30:184–187.
32. Centers for Disease Control. Surveillance for HIV-2 infection in blood donors—United States, 1987–1989. MMWR Morb Mortal Wkly Rep 1990;39:829.
33. Centers for Disease Control and Prevention. Human Immunodeficiency Virus Type 2, updated October 1998. Available at http://www.cdc.gov/hiv/pubs/facts/hiv2.htm. Accessed July 7, 2005.
34. Parry JV, McAlpine L, Avillez MF. Sensitivity of six commercial enzyme immunoassay kits that detect both anti-HIV-l and anti-HIV-2. AIDS 1990;4:355–360.
35. Gallarda JL, Henrard DR, Liu D, et al. Early detection of antibody to HIV-1 using an antigen conjugate immunoassay correlates with the presence of IgM antibody. J Clin Microbiol 1992;30:2379–2384.
36. Zaaijer HL, v Exel-Oehlers P, Kraaijeveld T, et al. Early detection of antibodies to HIV-1 by third-generation assays. Lancet 1992;340:770–772.
37. U.S. Food and Drug Administration. Revised Recommendations for the Prevention of Human Immunodeficiency Virus (HIV) Transmission by Blood and Blood Products. Rockville, Md., Center for Biologics Evaluation and Research (CBER), 1992.
38. Sullivan MT, Guido EA, Metler RP, et al. Identification and characterization of an HIV-2 antibody-positive blood donor in the United States. Transfusion 1998;38:189–193.
39. Kahn JO, Walker BD. Acute human immunodeficiency virus type 1 infection. NEJM 1998;339:33–39.
40. Operskalski EA, Busch MP, Mosley JW, Stram DO. Comparative rates of disease progression among persons infected with the same or different HIV-1 strains. The Transfusion Safety Study Group. J Acquir Immune Defic Syndr Hum Retrovirol 1997;15:145–150.
41. Collier AC, Kalish LA, Busch MP, et al. Leukocyte-reduced red blood cell transfusions in patients with anemia and human immunodeficiency virus infection: the Viral Activation Transfusion Study: A randomized controlled trial. JAMA 2001;285:1592–1601.
42. Wood E, Hogg RS, Harrigan PR, et al. When to initiate antiretroviral therapy in HIV-1-infected adults: a review for clinicians and patients. Lancet Infect Dis 2005;5:407–414.
43. Tjotta E, Hungnes O, Grinde B. Survival of HIV-1 activity after disinfection, temperature and pH changes, or drying. J Med Virol 1991;35: 223–227.
44. Kleinman SH, Niland JC, Azen SP, et al, and the Transfusion Safety Study Group.Prevalence of antibodies to human immunodeficiency virus type 1 among blood donors prior to screening: the Transfusion Safety Study/NHLBI donor repository. Transfusion 1989;29:572–580.
45. Donegan E, Stuart M, Niland JC, et al, and the Transfusion Safety Study Group. Infection with human immunodeficiency virus type I

(HIV-1) among recipients of antibody-positive blood donations. Ann Intern Med 1990;113:733–739.
46. Busch MP, Operskalski EA, Mosley JW, et al. Factors influencing human immunodeficiency virus type 1 transmission by blood transfusion. Transfusion Safety Study Group. J Infect Dis 1996;174:26–33.
47. Donegan E, Lenes BA, Tomasulo RA, Mosley JW, and the Transfusion Safety Study Group. Transmission of HIV-l by components type and duration of shelf storage before transfusion. Transfusion 1990;30: 851–852.
48. Rawal BD, Busch MP, Endow R, et al. Reduction of human immunodeficiency virus-infected cells from donor blood by leukocyte filtration. Transfusion 1989;26:460–462.
49. Kim HC, Nahum K, Raska K Jr, et al. Natural history of acquired immunodeficiency syndrome in hemophilic patients. Am J Hematol 1987;24:168–176.
50. Kroner BL, Rosenberg PS, Aledort LM, et al, for the Multicenter Hemophilia Cohort Study. HIV-1 infection incidence among persons with hemophilia in the United States and western Europe, 1978–1990. J AIDS Hum Retrovirol 1994;7:279–286.
51. O'Brien SJ, Moore JP. The effect of genetic variation in chemokines and their receptors on HIV transmission and progression to AIDS. Immunol Rev 2000;177:99–111.
52. Kilbourne ED. New viral diseases: a real and potential problem without boundaries. JAMA 1990;264:68–70.
53. Centers for Disease Control. Update on acquired immune deficiency syndrome (AIDS) among patients with hemophilia A. MMWR Morb Mortal Wkly Rep 1982;31:844.
54. Centers for Disease Control and Prevention. Possible transfusion-associated acquired immune deficiency syndrome (AIDS)—California. MMWR Morb Mortal Wkly Rep 1982;31: 652.
55. American Association of Blood Banks (AABB), Council of Community Blood Centers (CCBC), American Red Cross (ARC). Joint statement on acquired immune deficiency syndrome (AIDS) related to transfusion. Transfusion 1983;23:87–88.
56. Gallo RC. Historical essay. The early years of HIV/AIDS. Science 2002; 298:1728–1730.
57. Busch MP, Young MJ, Samson SM, et al, and the Transfusion Safety Study Group: risk of human immunodeficiency virus transmission by blood transfusions prior to the implementation of HIV antibody screening in the San Francisco Bay Area. Transfusion 1991;31:4–11.
58. Perkins HA, Samson S, Busch MP. How well has self-exclusion worked? Transfusion 1988;28:601–602.
59. Centers for Disease Control and Prevention. Human immunodeficiency virus infection in transfusion recipients and their family members. MMWR Morb Mortal Wkly Rep 1987;36:137–114.
60. Sarngadharan MG, Popovic M, Bruch L, et al. Antibodies reactive with human T-lymphotropic retroviruses (HTLV-III) in the serum of patients with AIDS. Science 1984;224:506–508.
61. Code of Federal Regulations 610.40. Title 21. Food and Drug Administration. U.S. Department of Health and Human Services, National Archives and Records Administration, 2005.
62. U.S. Food and Drug Administration. Current good manufacturing practices for blood and blood components: notification of consignees receiving blood and blood components at increased risk for transmitting HIV infection. Fed Regist 1996;61:47413–47423.
63. Busch MP, Lee LLL, Satten GA, et al. Time course of detection of viral and serological markers preceding HTLV- I seroconversion: Implications for blood and tissue donor screening. Transfusion 1995;35:91–97.
64. Lindback S, Thorstensson R, Karlsson AC, et al. Diagnosis of primary HIV-1 infection and duration of follow-up after HIV exposure. Karolinska Institute Primary HIV Infection Study Group. AIDS 2000;14:2333–2339.
65. Dorn J, Masciotra S, Yang C, et al. Analysis of genetic variability within the immunodominant epitopes of envelope gp41 from human immunodeficiency virus type 1 (HIV-1) group M and its impact on HIV-1 antibody detection. J Clin Microbiol 2000;38:773–780.
66. U.S. Food and Drug Administration. Memorandum: Recommendation for Donor Screening With A Licensed Test for HIV-1 Antigen. Rockville, Md., Center for Biologics Evaluation and Research (CBER), 1995.
67. Kleinman S, Busch MP, Korelitz JJ, Schreiber GB. The incidence/window period model and its use to assess the risk of transfusion-transmitted human immunodeficiency virus and hepatitis C virus infection. Transfus Med Rev 1997;11:155–172.
68. Busch MP, Stramer SL. The efficiency of HIV p24 antigen screening of US blood donors: Projections versus reality. Presentation at Satellite symposium Sensitivity and Validity of HIV Screening Methods, Joint Congress of the International Society of Blood Transfusion and the German Society for Transfusion Medicine and Immunohematology, Frankfurt, Oct. 1997. Infusionther Transfusionmed 1998; 25:5–8.
69. U.S. Department of Health and Human Services. FDA, Center for Biologics Evaluation and Research. Guidance for Industry. Use of Nucleic Acid Tests on Pooled and Individual Samples from Donors of Whole Blood and Blood Components (Including Source Plasma and Source Leukocytes) to Adequately and Appropriately Reduce the Risk of Transmission of HIV-1 and HCV. Rockville, Md., Center for Biologics Evaluation and Research (CBER), 2004.
70. Stramer SL, Glynn SA, Kleinman SH, et al. Detection of HIV-1 and HCV infections among antibody-negative blood donors by nucleic acid-amplification testing. NEJM 2004;351:760–768.
71. Pilcher CD, Fiscus SA, Nguyen TQ, et al. Detection of acute infections during HIV testing in North Carolina. NEJM 2005;352:1873–1883.
72. Busch MP, Glynn SA, Stramer SL, et al. A new strategy for estimating risks of transfusion-transmitted viral infections based on rates of detection of recently infected donors. Transfusion 2005;45:254–264.
73. Roth WK, Weber M, Buhr S, et al. Yield of HCV and HIV-1 NAT after screening of 3.6 million blood donations in central Europe. Transfusion 2002;42:862–868.
74. Ling AE, Robbins KE, Brown TM, et al. Failure of routine HIV-1 tests in a case involving transmission with preseroconversion blood components during the infectious window period. JAMA 2000; 284:210–214.
75. Dreier J, Gotting C, Wolff C, et al. Recent experience with human immunodeficiency virus transmission by cellular blood products in Germany: antibody screening is not sufficient to prevent transmission. Vox Sang 2002;82:80–83.
76. Stramer SL, Chambers L, Page PL, et al. Third reported US case of breakthrough HIV transmission from NAT screened blood. (Abstract) Transfusion 2003;43(9 Suppl):40a–41a.
77. Delwart E, Kalmin N, Jones T, et al. First case of HIV transmission by an RNA screened blood donation. Vox Sang 2004;86:171–177.
78. Phelps R, Robbins K, Liberti T, et al. Window-period human immunodeficiency virus transmission to two recipients by an adolescent blood donor. Transfusion 2004;44:929–933.
79. Kleinman S, Busch MP, Hall L, et al for the Retrovirus Epidemiology Donor Study. False-positive HIV-1 test results in a low-risk screening setting of voluntary blood donation. JAMA 1998;280:1080–1085.
80. Busch MP, Kleinman SH, Williams AE, et al, and the Retrovirus Epidemiology Donor Study (REDS). Frequency of human immunodeficiency virus (HIV) infection among contemporary anti-HIV-1 and anti-HIV-1/anti-HIV-2 supplemental test-indeterminate blood donors. Transfusion 1996;36:37–44.
81. Holodniy M, Busch MP. Establishing the diagnosis of HIV infection. In Dolin R, Masur H, Saag MS (eds). AIDS Therapy, 2nd ed. New York,Churchill Livingstone (Elsevier), 2002, pp 3–20.
82. Fiebig EW, Wright DJ, Rawal BD, et al. Dynamics of HIV viremia and antibody seroconversion in plasma donors: implications for diagnosis and staging of primary HIV infection. AIDS 2003;17:1871–1879.
83. Busch MP. Let's look at human immunodeficiency virus lookback before leaping into hepatitis C virus lookback! Transfusion 1991;31:655–661.
84. Leitman SF, Klein HG, Melpolder JJ, et al. Clinical implications of positive tests for antibodies to human immunodeficiency virus type I in asymptomatic blood donors. NEJM 1989;321:917–924.
85. Busch MP, Operskalski EA, Mosley JW, et al, and the Transfusion Safety Study Group. Epidemiologic background and long-term course of disease in human immunodeficiency virus type 1-infected blood donors identified before routine laboratory screening. Transfusion 1994;34: 858–864.
86. Ward JW, Holmberg SD, Allen JR, et al. Transmission of human immunodeficiency virus (HIV) by blood transfusions screened as negative for HIV antibody. NEJM 1988;318:473–478.
87. Selik RM, Ward JW, Buehler JW. Trends in transfusion-associated acquired immune deficiency syndrome in the United States, 1982 through 1991. Transfusion 1993;33:890–893.
88. Nelson KE, Donahue JG, Munoz A, et al. Transmission of retroviruses from seronegative donors by transfusion during cardiac surgery: A multicenter study of HIV-1 and HTLV-I/II infections. Ann Intern Med 1992;117:554–559.
89. Busch MP, Eble BE, Khayam-Bashi H, et al. Evaluation of screened blood donations for human immunodeficiency virus type I infection by culture and DNA amplification of pooled cells. NEJM 1991;325:1–5.
90. Janssen RS, Satten GA, Stramer SL, et al. New testing strategy to detect early HIV-1 infection for use in incidence estimates and for clinical and prevention purposes. JAMA 1998;280:42–48.

91. Lackritz EM, Satten GA, Aberle-Grasse J, et al. Estimated risk of transmission of the human immunodeficiency virus by screened blood in the United States. NEJM 1995;333:1721–1725.
92. Schreiber GB, Busch MP, Kleinman SH, Korelitz JJ. The risk of transfusion-transmitted viral infections. The Retrovirus Epidemiology Donor Study. NEJM 1996;334:1685–1690.
93. Busch MP, Kleinman SH, Jackson B, et al. Committee report. Nucleic acid amplification testing of blood donors for transfusion-transmitted infectious diseases: Report of the Interorganizational Task Force on Nucleic Acid Amplification Testing of Blood Donors. Transfusion 2000;40:143–159.
94. Glynn SA, Kleinman SH, Wright DJ, et al. International application of the incidence rate/window period model. Transfusion 2002;42: 966–972.
95. Coste J, Reesink HW, Engelfriet CP, Laperche S, et al. ISBT International Forum: Implementation of Donor Screening for Infectious Agents Transmitted by Blood by Nucleic Acid Technology: Update through 2003. Vox Sang 2005;88:289–303.
96. Fiebig EW, Heldebrant CM, Smith RI, et al. Intermittent low-level viremia in very early primary HIV-1 infection. J AIDS 2005;39:133–137.
97. Lee HH, Swanson P, Rosenblatt JD, et al. Relative prevalence and risk factors of HTLV-I and HTLV-II infection in US blood donors. Lancet 1991;337:1435–1439.
98. Taylor PE, Stevens CE, Pindyck J, et al. Human T-cell lymphotropic virus in volunteer blood donors. Transfusion 1990;30:783–786.
99. Eble BE, Busch MP, Guiltinan A, et al. Determination of human T-lymphotropic virus type by PCR and correlation with risk factors in northern California blood donors. J Infect Dis 1993;167:954–957. Erratum in: J Infect Dis 1993;168:262.
100. Cann AJ, Chen ISY. Human T-cell leukemia virus types I and II. In Fields BN, Knipe DM (eds). Virology. New York, Raven Press, 1990.
101. Hall WW, Ishak R, Zhu SW, et al. Human T lymphotropic virus type II (HTLVII): Epidemiology, molecular properties, and clinical features of infection. J AIDS Hum Retrovirol 1996;13(Suppl 1):s204–s214.
102. Lal RB, Owen SM, Rudolph DL, et al. In vivo cellular tropism of human T lymphotropic virus type II is not restricted to CD8+ cells. Virology 1995;210:441–447.
103. Casoli C, Cimarelli A, Bertazzoni U. Cellular tropism of human T cell leukemia virus type II is enlarged to B lymphocytes in patients with high proviral load. Virology 1995;206:1126–1128.
104. Wattel E, Vartanian JP, Pannetier C, Wain-Hobson S: Clonal expansion of human T cell leukemia virus type I infected cells in asymptomatic and symptomatic carriers without malignancy. J Virol 1995;69:2863–2868.
105. Rios M, Pombo de Oliveira MS, Correa RB, et al. HTLV-I viremia in infected individuals with and without disease [abstract ME 19]. Presented at the Eighth International Conference on Human Retrovirology: HTLV, Rio de Janeiro, June 9–13, 1997.
106. Manns A, Hisada M, La Grenade L. Human T lymphotropic virus type I infection. Lancet 1999;353:1951–1958.
107. Gessain A, Mahieux R, de The G. Genetic variability and molecular epidemiology of human and simian T cell leukemia/lymphoma virus type I. J AIDS Hum Retrovirol 1996;13(Suppl 1):s132–s145.
108. Black FL, Biggar RJ, Neel JV, et al. Endemic transmission of HTLV type II among Kayapo Indians of Brazil. AIDS Res Hum Retrovir 1994;10: 1165–1171.
109. Reeves WC, Cutler JR, Gracia F, et al. Human T cell lymphotropic virus infection in Guayami Indians from Panama. Am J Trop Med Hyg 1990;43:410–418.
110. Hjelle B, Mills R, Swenson S, et al. Incidence of hairy cell leukemia, mycosis fungoides, and chronic lymphocytic leukemia in first known HTLV-II-endemic population. J Infect Dis 1991;163:435–440.
111. Gessain A, Mauclere P, Froment A, et al. Isolation and molecular characterization of a human T-cell lymphotropic virus type II (HTLV-II), subtype B, from a healthy Pygmy living in a remote area of Cameroon: An ancient origin for HTLV-II in Africa. Proc Natl Acad Sci USA 1995;92: 4041–4045.
112. Khabbaz RF, Onorato IM, Cannon RO, et al. Seroprevalence of HTLV-I and HTLV-II among intravenous drug users and persons in clinics for sexually transmitted diseases. NEJM 1992;326:375–380.
113. Murphy EL, Watanabe K, Nass CC, et al. Evidence among blood donors for a 30-year old epidemic of HTLV-II infection in the United States. J Infect Dis 1999;180:1777–1783.
114. Williams AE, Fang CT, Slamon DJ, et al. Seroprevalence and epidemiological correlates of HTLV-I infection in U.S. blood donors. Science 1988;240:643–646. Erratum in: Science 1989;244:757.
115. Murphy EL, Figueroa JP, Gibbs WN, et al. Human T-lymphotropic virus type I (HTLV-I) seroprevalence in Jamaica. I: Demographic determinants. Am J Epidemiol 1991;133:1114–1124.
116. Vitek CR, Gracia FI, Giusti R, et al. Evidence for sexual and mother to child transmission of human T lymphotropic virus type II among Guayami Indians, Panama. J Infect Dis 1995;171:1022–1026.
117. Hino S, Katamine S, Miyata H, et al. Primary prevention of HTLV1 in Japan. Leukemia 1997;11(Suppl 3):57–59.
118. Murphy EL, Figueroa JP, Gibbs WN, et al. Sexual transmission of human T-lymphotropic virus type I. Ann Intern Med 1989;111:555–560.
119. Kaplan J, Khabbaz RF, Murphy EL, et al, and the Retrovirus Epidemiology Donor Study Group.Male to female transmission of human T lymphotropic virus types I and II: association with viral load. J AIDS Hum Retrovirol 1996;12:193–201.
120. Roucoux DF, Wang B, Smith D, et al. A prospective study of sexual transmission of human T lymphotropic virus (HTLV)-I and HTLV-II. J Infect Dis 2005;191:1490–1497.
121. Centers for Disease Control and Prevention (CDC) and the U.S. PHS Working Group. Guidelines for counseling persons infected with human T-lymphotropic virus type I (HTLV-l) and type II (HTLV-II). Ann Intern Med 1993;118:448–454.
122. Feigal E, Murphy EL, Vranizan K, et al. HTLV-I/II in intravenous drug users in San Francisco: Risk factors associated with seropositivity. J Infect Dis 1991;164:36–42.
123. Hinuma YK, Nagata K, Hanoaka M, et al. Adult T-cell leukemia: Antigen in an ATL cell line and detection of antibodies to the antigen in human sera. Proc Natl Acad Sci USA 1981;78:6476–6480.
124. Hinuma YK, Komoda H, Chosa T, et al. Antibodies to adult T-cell leukemia-virus-associated antigens (ATLA) in sera from patients with ATL and controls in Japan: A nationwide seroepidemiologic study. Int J Cancer 1982;29:631–635.
125. Bunn PA Jr, Schechter GP, Jaffe E, et al. Clinical course of retrovirus-associated adult T-cell lymphoma in the United States. NEJM 1983;309:257–264.
126. Seiki M, Eddy R, Shows TB, Yoshida M. Non-specific integration of the HTLV provirus into adult T-cell leukemia cells. Nature 1984;309: 640–642.
127. Kinoshita K, Amagasaki T, Ikeda S, et al. Preleukemic state of adult T cell leukemia: Abnormal T lymphocytosis induced by human adult T cell leukemia-lymphoma virus. Blood 1985;66:120–127.
128. Tachibana N, Okayama A, Ishihara S, et al. High HTLV-I proviral DNA level associated with abnormal lymphocytes in peripheral blood from asymptomatic carriers. Int J Cancer 1992;51:593–595.
129. Murphy EL, Hanchard B, Figueroa JP, et al. Modeling the risk of adult T-cell leukemia/lymphoma in persons infected with human T-lymphotropic virus type I. Int J Cancer 1989;43:250–253.
130. Chen Y-C, Wang C-H, Su I-J, et al. Infection of human T-cell leukemia virus type I and development of human T-cell leukemia/lymphoma in patients with hematologic neoplasms: a possible linkage to blood transfusion. Blood 1989;74:388–394.
131. Prince H, Kleinman S, Doyle M, et al. Spontaneous lymphocyte proliferation in vitro characterizes both HTLV-I and HTLV-II infection. J AIDS Hum Retrovirol 1990;3:1199–1200.
132. Wiktor SZ, Jacobson S, Weiss SH, et al. Spontaneous lymphocyte proliferation in HTLV-II infection. Lancet 1991;337:327–328.
133. Portis T, Harding JC, Ratner L. The contribution of NF-kappa B activity to spontaneous proliferation and resistance to apoptosis in human T-cell leukemia virus type 1 Tax-induced tumors. Blood 2001; 98:1200–1208.
134. Lal RB, Rudolph DL, Dezzutti CS, et al. Costimulatory effects of T cell proliferation during infection with human T lymphotropic virus types I and II are mediated through CD80 and CD86 ligands. J Immunol. 1996;157:1288–1296.
135. Prince HE, York J, Owen SM, Lal RB. Spontaneous proliferation of memory (CD45RO+) and naive (CD45RO−) subsets of CD4 cells and CD8 cells in human T lymphotropic virus (HTLV) infection: distinctive patterns for HTLV-I versus HTLV-II. Clin Exp Immunol 1995;102: 256–261.
136. Rosenblatt JD, Giorgi JV, Golde DW, et al. Integrated human T-cell leukemia virus II genome in CD8+ T cells from a patient with "atypical" hairy cell leukemia: Evidence for distinct T and B cell lymphoproliferative disorders. Blood 1988;71:363–369.
137. Rosenblatt JD, Gasson JC, Glaspy J, et al. Relationship between human T-cell leukemia virus-II and atypical hairy cell leukemia: a serologic study of hairy cell leukemia patients. Leukemia 1987;1:397–401.
138. Lion T, Razvi N, Golomb HM, Brownstein RH. B-lymphotropic hairy cells contain no HTLV-II DNA sequences. Blood 1988;7 2:1428–1430.
139. Katayama I, Maruyama K, Fukushima T, et al. Cross-reacting antibodies to human T cell leukemia virus-I and -II in Japanese patients with hairy cell leukemia. Leukemia 1987;1:401–404.

140. Zucker-Franklin D, Coutavas EE, Rush MG, Zouzias DC. Detection of human T-lymphotropic virus-like particles in cultures of peripheral blood lymphocytes from patients with mycosis fungoides. Proc Natl Acad Sci USA 1991;88:7630–7634.
141. Busch MP, Murphy EL, Nemo G: More on HTLV tax and mycosis fungoides. NEJM 1993;329:2035–2036.
142. Loughran TP Jr, Coyle T, Sherman MP, et al. Detection of human T cell leukemia/lymphoma virus, type II, in a patient with large granular lymphocyte leukemia. Blood 1992;80:1116–1119.
143. Gessain A, Vernant JC, Sonan T, et al. Antibodies to human T-lymphotropic virus type-I in patients with tropical spastic paraparesis. Lancet 1985;2(8452):407–410.
144. Osame M, Usuku K, Izumo S, et al. HTLV-I associated myelopathy, a new clinical entity. Lancet 1986;1(8488):1031–1032.
145. Maloney EM, Cleghorn FR, Morgan OS, et al. Incidence of HTLV-I associated myelopathy/tropical spastic paraparesis (HAM/TSP) in Jamaica and Trinidad. J AIDS Hum Retrovirol 1998;17:167–170.
146. Jacobson S, Raine CS, Mingioli ES, McFarlin DE. Isolation of an HTLV-l-like retrovirus from patients with tropical spastic paraparesis. Nature 1988;331:540–543.
147. Bhagavati S, Ehrlich G, Kula R, et al. Detection of human T-cell lymphoma/leukemia virus type 1 DNA and antigen in spinal fluid and blood of patients of chronic progressive myelopathy. NEJM 1988;318:1141–1147.
148. Gessain A, Gout O. Chronic myelopathy associated with human T-lymphotropic virus type I (HTLV-I). Ann Intern Med 1992;117:933–946.
149. Murphy EL, Fridey J, Smith JW, et al. HTLV associated myelopathy in a cohort of HTLV-I and HTLV-II infected blood donors. The REDS Investigators. Neurology 1997;48:315–320.
150. Kramer A, Maloney EM, Morgan OSC, et al. Risk factors and cofactors for HAM/TSP in Jamaica. Am J Epidemiol 1995;142:1212–1220.
151. Gout O, Baulac M, Gessain A, et al. Rapid development of myelopathy after HTLV-I infection acquired by transfusion during cardiac transplantation. NEJM 1990;322:383–388.
152. Kurosawa M, Machii T, Kitani T, et al. HTLV-I associated myelopathy (HAM) after blood transfusion in a patient with CD2+ hairy cell leukemia. Am J Clin Pathol 1991;95:72–76.
153. Osame M, Janssen R, Kubota H, et al. Nationwide survey of HTLV-I-associated myelopathy in Japan: association with blood transfusion. Ann Neurol 1990;28:50–56.
154. Reddy EP, Sandberg-Wollheim M, Mettus R, et al. Amplification and molecular cloning of HTLV-I sequences from DNA of multiple sclerosis patients. Science 1989; 243:529–533. Erratum in: Science 1989; 246:246.
155. Madden DL, Mundon FK, Tzan NR, et al. Serologic studies of MD patients, controls, and patients with other neurologic diseases: antibodies to HTLV-I, II, III. Neurology 1988;38:81–84.
156. Richardson JH, Wucherpfennig KW, Endo N, et al. PCR analysis of DNA from multiple sclerosis patients for the presence of HTLV-I. Science 1989;246:821–824.
157. Hjelle B, Appenzeller O, Mills R, et al. Chronic neurodegenerative disease associated with HTLV-II infection. Lancet 1992;339:645–646.
158. Sugimoto M, Nakashima H, Watanabe S, et al. T-lymphocyte alveolitis in HTLV-I-associated myelopathy. Lancet 1987;2(8569):1220.
159. Mochizuki M, Watanabe T, Yamaguchi K, et al. HTLV-I uveitis: a distinct clinical entity caused by HTLVI. Jpn J Cancer Res 1992;83:236–239.
160. Morgan OS, Rodgers-Johnson P, Mora C, Char G. HTLV-I and polymyositis in Jamaica. Lancet 1989;2(8673):1184–1187.
161. Kitajima I, Maruyama I, Maruyama Y, et al. Polyarthritis in human T lymphotropic virus type I-associated myelopathy. Arthritis Rheum 1989;32:1342–1344.
162. Murphy EL, Glynn SA, Fridey J, et al. Increased incidence of infectious diseases and neurologic abnormalities during prospective follow-up of HTLV-II and -I infected blood donors. Arch Intern Med 1999;159:1485–1491.
163. LaGrenade L, Hanchard B, Fletcher V, et al. Infective dermatitis of Jamaican children: a marker for HTLV-I infection. Lancet 1990;336:1345–1347.
164. Stuver SO, Okayama A, Tachibana N, et al. HCV infection and liver cancer mortality in a Japanese population with HTLV-I. Int J Cancer 1996;67:35–37.
165. Orland JR, Wang B, Wright DJ, et al. Increased mortality associated with HTLV-II infection in blood donors: a prospective cohort study. Retrovirology 2004;1:4–12. Available at http://www.retrovirology.com/content/1/1/4.
166. Beilke MA, Theall KP, O'Brien M, et al. Clinical outcomes and disease progression among patients coinfected with HIV and human T lymphotropic virus types 1 and 2. Clin Infect Dis 2004;39:256–263.
167. Hershow RC, Galai N, Fukuda K, et al. An international collaborative study of the effects of coinfection with human T-lymphotropic virus type II on human immunodeficiency virus type 1 disease progression in injection drug users. J Infect Dis 1996;174:309–317.
168. Okochi K, Sato H, Hinuma Y. A retrospective study on transmission of adult T cell leukemia virus by blood transfusion: seroconversion in recipients. Vox Sang 1984;46:245–253.
169. Kamihira S, Nakasima S, Oyakawa Y, et al. Transmission of human T-cell lymphotropic virus type I by blood transfusion before and after mass screening of sera from seropositive donors. Vox Sang 1987;52:43–44.
170. Manns A, Wilks RJ, Murphy EL, et al. A prospective study of transmission by transfusion of HTLV-I and risk factors associated with seroconversion. Int J Cancer 1992;51:886–891.
171. Donegan E, Lee H, Operskalski EA, et al. Transfusion transmission of retroviruses: human T-lymphotropic viruses types I and II compared with human immunodeficiency virus type 1. Transfusion 1994;34:478–483.
172. Kleinman S: Donor selection and screening procedures. In Nance SJ (ed). Blood Safety: Current Challenges. Bethesda, Md., American Association of Blood Banks, 1992, pp 169–200.
173. Hjelle B, Wilson C, Cyrus S, et al. Human T-cell leukemia virus type II infection frequently goes undetected in contemporary U.S. blood donors. Blood 1993;81:1641–1644.
174. Kleinman S, Kaplan J, Khabbaz, et al. Evaluation of a p21e-spiked Western blot (Immunoblot) in confirming human t-cell lymphotropic virus type I and II infection in volunteer blood donors. J Clin Microbiol 1994;32:603–607.
175. Lal RB, Brodine S, Kuzura J, et al. Sensitivity and specificity of a recombinant transmembrane glycoprotein (rgp21)-spiked Western immunoblot for serologic confirmation of human T-cell lymphotropic virus type I and type II infection. J Clin Microbiol 1992;30:296–299.
176. Brodine SK, Kaime EM, Roberts C, et al. Simultaneous confirmation and differentiation of human T-lymphotropic virus types I and II infection by modified Western blot containing recombinant envelope glycoproteins. Transfusion 1993;33:925–929.
177. Lal RB, Heneine W, Rudolph DL, et al. Synthetic peptide-based immunoassays for distinguishing between human T-cell lymphotropic virus type I and type II infections in seropositive individuals. J Clin Microbiol 1991;29:2253–2258.
178. Lal RB, Rudolph DL, Lairmore MD, et al. Serologic discrimination of human T cell lymphotropic virus infection by using a synthetic peptide-based enzyme immunoassay. J Infect Dis 1991;163:41–46.
179. Viscidi RP, Hill PM, Li S, et al. Diagnosis and differentiation of HTLV-I and HTLV-II infection by enzyme immunoassays using synthetic peptides. J AIDS Hum Retrovirol 1991;4:1190–1198.
180. Busch MP, Laycock M, Kleinman SH, et al. Accuracy of supplementary serological testing for human T-lymphotropic virus (HTLV) types I and II in US blood donors. The Retrovirus Epidemiology Donor Study. Blood 1994;83:1143–1148.
181. Calattini S, Chevalier SA, Duprez R, et al. Discovery of a new human T-cell lymphotropic virus (HTLV-3) in Central Africa. Retrovirology 2005;2:30.
182. Wolfe ND, Heneine W, Carr JK, et al. Emergence of unique primate T-lymphotropic viruses among central African bushmeat hunters. Proc Natl Acad Sci USA 2005;102:7994–7999.
183. Patience C, Takeuchi Y, Weiss RA. Infection of human cells by an endogenous retrovirus of pigs. Nat Med 1997;3:282–286.
184. Heneine W, Tibell A, Switzer WM, et al. No evidence of infection with porcine endogenous retrovirus in recipients of porcine islet-cell xenografts. Lancet 1998;352:695–699.
185. Heneine W, Switzer WM, Soucie JM, et al. Evidence of porcine endogenous retroviruses in porcine factor VIII and evaluation of transmission to recipients with hemophilia. J Infect Dis 2001;183:648–652.
186. Busch MP, Holland PV. Idiopathic CD4+ T-lymphocytopenia (ICL) and the safety of blood transfusions: What do we know and what should we do? Transfusion 1992;32:800–804.
187. Busch MP, Switzer WM, Murphy EL, et al. Absence of evidence of infection with divergent primate T-lymphotropic viruses in United States blood donors who have seroindeterminate HTLV test results. Transfusion 2000;40:443–449.
188. Mayo DJ, Rose AM, Matchett SE, et al. Screening potential blood donors at risk for human immunodeficiency virus. Transfusion 1991;31:466–474.
189. Johnson ES, Doll LS, Satten GA, et al. Direct oral questions to blood donors: the impact on screening for human immunodeficiency virus. Transfusion 1994;34:769–774.
190. Petersen LR, Doll LS, White CR, et al. Heterosexually acquired human immunodeficiency virus infection and the United States blood supply:

considerations for screening of potential blood donors. HIV Blood Donor Study Group. Transfusion 1993;33:552–557.
191. Eastlund T: Monetary blood donation incentives and the risk of transfusion-transmitted infection. Transfusion 1998;38:874–882.
192. Munsterman KA, Grindon AJ, Sullivan J, et al. Assessment of motivations for return donation among deferred blood donors. Amer Red Cross ARCNET Study Group. Transfusion 1998;38:45–50.
193. Council of Europe. Expert Committee in Blood Transfusion. Study Group on Pathogen Inactivation of Labile Blood Components. Pathogen inactivation of labile blood products. Transfus Med 2001;11:149–175.
194. Klein HG, Dodd RY, Dzik WH, et al. Current status of solvent/detergent-treated frozen plasma. Transfusion 1998;38:102–107.
195. Allain JP, Bianco C, Blajchman MA, et al. Protecting the blood supply from emerging pathogens: the role of pathogen inactivation. Transfus Med Rev 2005;19:110–126.
196. Flamholz R, Jeon HR, Baron JM, et al. Study of three patients with thrombotic thrombocytopenic purpura exchanged with solvent/detergent-treated plasma: Is its decreased protein S activity clinically related to their development of deep venous thromboses? J Clin Apher 2000; 15:169–172.
197. Yarranton H, Cohen H, Pavord SR, et al. Venous thromboembolism associated with the management of acute thrombotic thrombocytopenic purpura. Br J Haematol 2003;121:778–785.
198. Clark KA, Kataaha P, Mwangi J, et al. Predonation testing of potential blood donors in resource-restricted settings. Transfusion 2005;45: 130–132.

Chapter 46

Human Herpesvirus Infections

John D. Roback

INTRODUCTION

The Herpesviridae is a family of approximately 100 viruses with common structural features. Each virus has a linear 120- to 230-kb double-stranded DNA genome maintained in a toroidal conformation and surrounded by an icosadeltahedral nucleocapsid. The 100 nm diameter capsid, composed of 162 capsomeres, is encompassed by a dense tegument or matrix and an outer trilaminar lipid envelope that contains proteins of both viral and host cell origins.[1] Herpesviruses share a number of biologic characteristics as well, including expression of viral enzymes that participate in DNA synthesis and nucleic acid metabolism, confinement of viral DNA synthesis and packaging to the host cell nucleus, destruction of the infected cell during active viral replication, and capacity to remain in a latent state indefinitely.[1]

Of the herpesviruses, eight are known to infect humans (Table 46–1). Members of the human herpesvirus (HHV) family are categorized into three subfamilies based on biologic properties including cell tropism, genome structure, and sequences of conserved open reading frames (ORFs). Most have a commonly employed name, such as cytomegalovirus (CMV); each is also known by an accompanying HHV designation, according to guidelines from the International Committee on Taxonomy of Viruses (e.g., CMV is HHV-5).[2] This chapter focuses primarily on CMV, the herpesvirus with most clinical relevance to transfusion medicine, along with discussion of other leukocytotropic herpesviruses (Epstein-Barr virus [EBV], HHV-6, HHV-7, and HHV-8) that may contaminate blood components.

CYTOMEGALOVIRUS (HHV-5)

Molecular and Cellular Virology of CMV

Viral Structure

CMV was the first identified betaherpesvirus and remains the prototype of this group. The CMV virion contains a linear double-stranded DNA genome of approximately 230 kbp in length, the largest of the herpesviruses.[3,4] The genome is divided into unique long (UL) and unique short (US) segments, each flanked by a pair of inverted repeat regions.[4] The UL and US segments can each independently invert with respect to one another, yielding four different genomic isomers. After infection, the termini of the linear genome are joined to produce a circular, or concatemeric, replicative form.[5] Circularized CMV genomes have also been identified in latently infected peripheral blood CD14+ leukocytes.[6] At least 200 ORFs have been identified within the CMV genome, many of which encode viral proteins of still unknown function.[4] After translation, viral proteins may undergo modifications, including phosphorylation, glycosylation, and cleavage. Mature virions range from 150 to 200 nm in diameter[7] and contain approximately 30 viral proteins distributed in the capsid, tegument, and envelope. Recently, viral RNA transcripts have also been identified packaged with viral DNA in mature virions.[8] This appears to be a relatively nonspecific process, mediated by viral proteins, including the tegument protein pp28, because cellular RNA transcripts are also incorporated into the virions.[9,10] The function of these packaged RNA transcripts is unclear, but they may allow viral protein translation to begin immediately on infection.[8] Additionally, in analogy with structural studies of retroviruses,[11] packaged RNA transcripts may also be important to the integrity of the viral particles.

Biology of Infection

VIRAL–CELLULAR INTERACTIONS

CMV can infect a range of cell types, including those of endothelial, epithelial, mesenchymal, hematopoietic, and neuronal lineages, frequently causing characteristic cellular enlargement (cytomegalia).[4,12] Infection appears to involve three sequential steps: viral attachment to the target cell, fusion of the viral and cellular membranes, and penetration of the viral capsid into the cell. Each step may require interactions between multiple viral coat proteins and cellular membrane proteins, the latter serving the role of viral receptors. The observation that the CMV genome contains at least 54 ORFs that encode putative viral membrane glycoproteins[13] hints at the potential complexity of these processes.

Viral attachment, the formation of a low-affinity dissociable viral–cellular interaction, involves interactions between viral proteins and cell surface receptors. One receptor class consists of ubiquitously expressed cell surface heparan sulfate proteoglycans, which appear to interact with the viral glycoprotein M/N (gM/gN) and/or gB envelope complexes and are required but not sufficient for infection.[14–18] The viral gB complex (sometimes called gcI, UL55, or gp130/55) is a disulfide-linked complex composed of 120- to 130-kDa and 55- to 60-kDa viral glycoproteins. The most abundant component in the viral envelope, gB is also a prominent target of neutralizing antibodies produced during natural infection.[15] gB binds to multiple cellular receptors. The epidermal growth factor receptor (EGFR) appears to be one member of this group of receptors.[19] Viral gB stably docks with EGFR and can displace EGF from its binding site. CMV infection leads to EGFR phosphorylation, Akt activation, and calcium mobilization. Furthermore, cell lines that did not express

Table 46–1 Human Herpesviruses

Subfamily	HHV Designation	Common Name
Alphaherpesvirinae	HHV-1	Herpes simplex-I (HSV-1)
	HHV-2	Herpes simplex-2 (HSV-2)
	HHV-3	Varicella-zoster virus (VZV)
Betaherpesvirinae	HHV-5	Cytomegalovirus (CMV)
	HHV-6A, -6B	—
	HHV-7	—
Gammaherpesvirinae	HHV-4	Epstein-Barr virus (EBV)
	HHV-8	Kaposi's sarcoma-associated herpesvirus (KSHV)

EGFR were resistant to CMV infection.[19] Because hematopoietic target cells do not express EGFR, other unidentified docking receptors for gB are probably involved. gB also activates Toll-like receptors, conserved cellular membrane proteins involved in initiating antipathogen responses.[20]

Although attachment complexes are initially dissociable, they can be stabilized by membrane fusion. After attachment, interactions between gB and its receptors may initiate fusion. In addition, the viral protein complex gp86 (gcIII, UL75:UL115, or gH:gL) appears to be involved in these processes.[21] Evidence indicates that gp86 is composed of the viral gH and gL proteins, as well as a third component not yet identified.[22] The cell membrane receptor for gp86 has been identified as a 92.5-kD constitutively phosphorylated glycoprotein.[23,24] Binding of gB and gp86 to the target cell initiates signaling processes that may be important to CMV infection. Interactions between gB and its cellular receptor(s) activates signal transduction through the interferon-response pathway, leading to induction of the interferon-responsive genes *OAS* and *ISG54*,[25] and binding of gp86 to the cellular 92.5-kD protein can alter intracellular calcium concentration.[26]

After fusion, the viral capsid penetrates into the host cell and releases viral DNA. The molecules mediating these processes have not been identified. Additional proteins have also been hypothesized to mediate viral infection. For example, cellular human leukocyte antigen (HLA) class I proteins may promote viral attachment through interactions with β_2-microglobulin attached to the virion membrane.[27]

VIRAL LIFE CYCLE

Active and Latent Infections After the steps of viral attachment, fusion, and penetration, active infection occurs if the target cell is permissive for the complete sequence of viral gene expression, viral genome replication, and production of progeny virions. During active infection, viral genes are expressed in coordinated waves. Three distinct kinetic classes of viral genes have been identified: immediate early (α), followed by delayed early (β) and then late (γ).[4] α-Class gene transcription is controlled by a combination of constitutively expressed host cell proteins and viral proteins present in the infecting virion. Thus, α genes can be transcribed in the presence of pharmacologic inhibitors of protein synthesis. Viral α proteins, in turn, are required for expression of viral genes of the β and γ classes.[28–30] The β protein products perform viral DNA replication and metabolic functions; the γ genes encode structural proteins required for assembly of progeny virions. Finally, mature virions are transported through the Golgi apparatus and are released from infected cells by exocytosis,[31] eventually resulting in host cell destruction.

Cytomegalovirus may also assume a latent state when it infects target cells that are not permissive for viral replication. Latency, the presence of viral DNA in an infected cell in the absence of active viral replication, may persist indefinitely because the host cell is not destroyed by the virus. The latent CMV genome retains the capacity to reactivate viral gene expression, produce infectious virions, and enter lytic growth at a later time. Studies with human and murine CMV have demonstrated that latency can be established in hematopoietic cells, primarily those of the granulocyte-monocyte lineage, as well as in endothelial cells.[32–38] The possibility of CMV latency in other cell types has not been excluded. The molecular mechanisms regulating CMV latency and reactivation from latency have not been completely elucidated. In the herpesvirus EBV, a clearly defined set of viral proteins have been identified that control latency and reactivation.[39] Similarly, CMV latency-associated transcripts (LATs) have been detected in 0.01% to 0.001% of sorted CD33+ lineage-committed hematopoietic progenitors from the peripheral blood of naturally infected individuals.[36,40] CMV LATs are transcribed from the viral IE gene locus and encode immunogenic viral proteins that are targets of naturally arising antibodies in CMV-seropositive individuals.[32,40,41] The function of LATs is currently unknown. Circularization of the CMV genome is associated with latency in CD14+ peripheral blood monocytes in CMV-seropositive individuals,[6] a phenomenon also seen during latent infections with other herpesviruses.[42–44] The possibility of persistent viral infections, an intermediate state between active and latent infection in which low levels of virus are produced, remains a topic of considerable debate.[45,46]

Viral Genes Important to Pathogenesis In addition to viral proteins that control expression of viral genes and virion assembly and provide structural support for the viral particle, CMV also encodes proteins that favor viral replication at the expense of host cell metabolism and disrupt the host's ability to combat viral infection. For example, CMV infection alters the expression, accumulation, and activity of the cellular tumor suppressor proteins, cyclins, and cyclin-associated kinases. These alterations in the cellcycle machinery act to simultaneously promote progression toward the G_1/S transition but prevent cellular DNA synthesis and cell division, resulting in cell-cycle arrest and cellular aneuploidy. It has been hypothesized that in the arrested state cellular DNA synthesis would be blocked but the cellular milieu would contain abundant nucleotides and other metabolic precursors that could support viral replication.[47–50] One viral protein involved in this process is the immediate-early IE1

72-kDa protein, which complexes with the cellular Rb-related protein p107 and blocks its ability to repress E2F-responsive promoters.[51] The IE1-mediated derepression at the level of E2F, in turn, allows expression of cellular genes that promote cell-cycle progression.[51] CMV infection also activates cyclin-dependent kinase 2 (CDK2), a cellular protein that controls progression through the G_1 and S phases of the cell cycle. The importance of CDK2 to viral replication was illustrated by blocking CDK2 activity with either a dominant-negative mutant or the pharmacologic inhibitor roscovitine. In both cases, inhibition of CDK2 activity prevented CMV replication and production of progeny virus.[50]

Cytomegalovirus has also developed mechanisms to interfere with antiviral immune function (reviewed in Hengel and colleagues[52] and Reddehase[53]). The UL37 ORF of CMV encodes vMIA, an anti-apoptotic protein that localizes to the mitochondria and protects infected cells from immune-mediated apoptosis by blocking the effects of Fas, tumor necrosis factor receptor-1 (TNFR-1), and granzyme B.[54] Monocytes are a prominent site of CMV latency, and monocyte-derived macrophages can support active CMV replication. During differentiation to macrophages, CMV in monocytes displays delayed replication kinetics and viral particles are retained in the Golgi apparatus, which may facilitate immune evasion until sufficient progeny virions have been produced.[55] In contrast, in patients with compromised antiviral immunity, CMV can replicate with rapid kinetics, displaying viral doubling times approaching 24 hours.[56]

Despite sophisticated viral mechanisms of immune evasion, clinical and experimental evidence demonstrates that the competent immune system can effectively suppress viral replication. For example, the murine CMV gp40 and gp48 glycoproteins (ORFs *m152* and *m06*, respectively) can decrease expression of cellular class I major histocompatibility complex (MHC) proteins during infection of fibroblasts and thus decrease CMV antigen presentation to CD8+ T cells. However, the significance of these mechanisms during natural infection are unclear because CMV infection does not disrupt class I MHC expression and antigen presentation in macrophages, the professional antigen-presenting cell most important in initiating the anti-CMV immune response.[57] Furthermore, although human CMV has also evolved mechanisms to interfere with antigen presentation by infected cells,[58,59] the immune system circumvents these obstacles by utilizing structural proteins in the infecting viral particle as immunodominant epitopes for an immune response.[60,61] Thus, the immune response can be initiated before expression of antiviral proteins that halt antigen presentation by the infected cell. CMV has also developed strategies to interfere with interferon-γ (IFN- γ) signals that normally upregulate MHC expression during viral infection.[62] Interestingly, downregulation of class I MHC cell surface expression by CMV should lead to destruction of the infected cells by host natural killer (NK) cells.[63] However, expression of the viral class I MHC homologue m144 by murine CMV decreases the susceptibility of the infected cell to NK-mediated lysis.[64]

CMV Infection, Immune Response, and Diagnosis

Transmission, Prevalence, and Epidemiology

During CMV infection, active viral replication results in shedding of infectious virions into plasma and bodily fluids, including saliva, tears, breast milk, urine, stool, and semen. Community-acquired CMV infection is usually the result of close contact with a person shedding CMV. The incidence of community-acquired CMV infection varies with the study population. For example, the yearly CMV seroconversion rate in health care workers has been estimated at 0.6% to 3.3%,[65] similar to rates of 2.0% to 6.3% reported in middle-class women during and between pregnancies.[66] In contrast, rates as high as 13% per year have been observed in adolescents.[67] In blood donors, the CMV seroconversion rate is estimated at approximately 1% per year.[68] Most studies have shown that 50% to 80% of the population is CMV seropositive,[4] although the incidence can be higher in some urban populations and lower in some groups of blood donors.[69]

Most individuals contracting community-acquired CMV infection are immunocompetent, and the infection is often asymptomatic. However, a mild self-limited infectious mononucleosis syndrome can occur, with symptoms that include fever, malaise, hepatosplenomegaly, and a rash.[70] CMV can be isolated from bodily secretions during the symptomatic phase. The infected individual mounts both a humoral and cell-mediated immune response and viral symptoms rapidly resolve, leading to a complete recovery. However, despite effective control of CMV infection by the competent host immune system, the virus is not completely eliminated but instead becomes latent.

Transplacental transmission of CMV to a developing fetus is an important viral cause of birth defects.[71,72] Fetal infection occurs in 40% to 50% of cases in which a seronegative mother contracts a primary CMV infection during pregnancy.[73,74] CMV disease occurs in 5% to 15% of the infected infants, presenting most often with intrauterine growth retardation, deafness, mental retardation, blindness, and thrombocytopenic bleeding.[72,73] However, when mothers are seropositive before pregnancy, maternal antiviral immunity can limit congenital CMV infection and disease. For example, in one study of seropositive mothers the rate of vertical transmission was approximately 1%.[73] Furthermore, no cases of symptomatic CMV infections were seen in 27 congenitally infected infants born to seropositive mothers.[73]

Cytomegalovirus can also be transmitted by blood transfusion or transplantation of hematopoietic stem cells and solid organs from infected donors. When the recipients are immunocompromised, CMV transmission through these mechanisms can produce serious clinical consequences. Prevention of CMV infection is an important concern in transfusion medicine.

CMV Infection of Peripheral Blood and Marrow Cells

CELL TROPISM

From the perspective of transfusion medicine, the most important target cells of CMV infection are peripheral blood leukocytes and their progenitors. Under appropriate conditions, these cell types can either harbor latent CMV or allow active viral replication, and thus are well-suited to mediate transfusion-transmitted CMV infection.

CMV infection of bone marrow hematopoietic progenitor cells likely occurs during primary infection[75] (Fig. 46–1). Most evidence suggests that these cells restrict viral replication but support viral latency,[32,33] although some studies have shown low levels of CMV replication in bone marrow–derived cells in culture.[75,76] CMV DNA has been identified

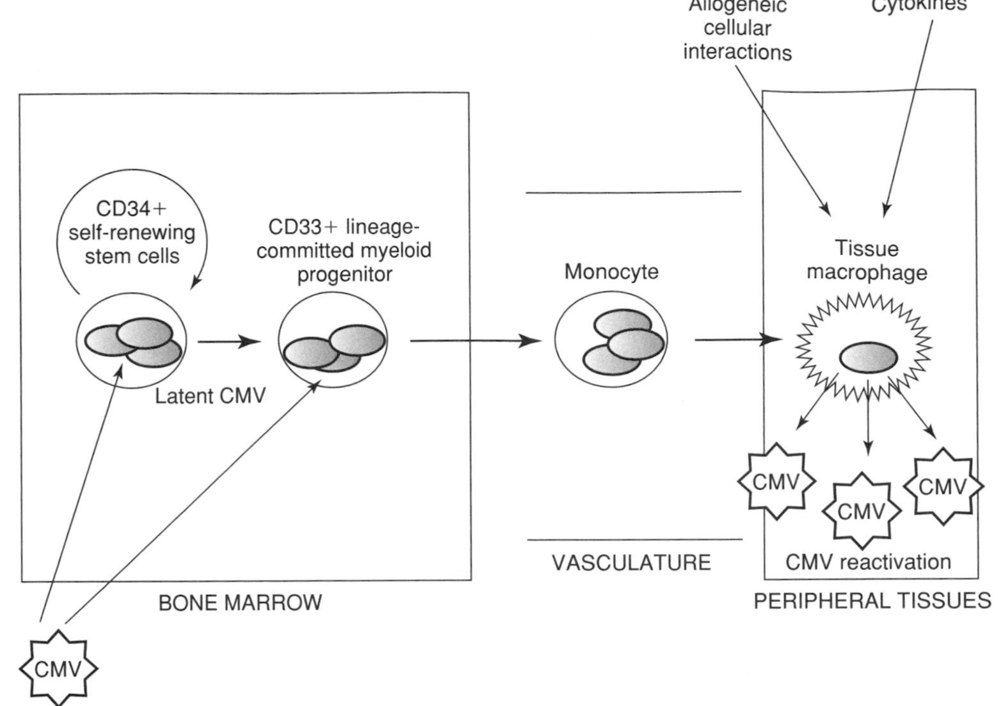

Figure 46–1 Hypothetical model integrating long-term latency of cytomegalovirus (CMV) in the hematopoietic compartment with transmission of CMV by blood transfusion and hematopoietic stem cell transplantation. CMV infects CD34+ multipotent progenitors during primary infection, and latently infected cells retain the viral genome during self-renewal. Committed progenitors in the marrow may also be directly infected with CMV. Either cell type may transmit CMV to a seronegative transplant recipient. CMV remains latent as CD33+ progenitors differentiate into circulating peripheral blood monocytes. Latently infected monocytes subsequently differentiate into tissue macrophages, either in the original host or after transfusion into a recipient. The allogeneic or cytokine-mediated signals monocytes encounter during differentiation render them permissive to CMV reactivation and viral replication. See text for detailed discussion.

by polymerase chain reaction (PCR) in sorted multipotent CD34+ progenitor cells from the bone marrow of seropositive, and in some cases seronegative, donors.[33,36,77,78] Because of their capacity for self-renewal, latently infected hematopoietic progenitor cells represent a potential long-term reservoir of latent virus. In fact, when CMV-infected CD34+ cells are grown in suspension cultures, transfer of CMV DNA to progeny cells during mitosis has been demonstrated.[34] CMV DNA has also been identified in myeloid-lineage-committed CD33+ progenitor cells in the marrow or mobilized into the peripheral blood by granulocyte-macrophage colony-stimulating factor. Lineage-committed progenitors appear to be latently infected, as indicated by the presence of CMV LATs in 0.01% to 0.001% of sorted CD33+CD14+ or CD33+CD15+ bone marrow cells from seropositive donors.[36] These findings support a model for latency in which early hematopoietic progenitor cells are latently infected during primary CMV infection and thereafter serve as viral reservoirs. Furthermore, latently infected marrow progenitor cells are a likely vector for transmission of CMV infection by hematopoietic stem cell transplantation.

As CD33+ progenitors continue to differentiate they enter the peripheral blood. Monocytes appear to retain latent virus, but as they differentiate into macrophages CMV replication with production of progeny virus has been observed[35,79] (see Fig. 46–1). Cells of the monocytic lineage have been hypothesized to mediate transfusion-transmitted CMV, but the prevalence of latently infected monocytes in the peripheral blood appears to be low. It has been estimated that 0.004% to 0.01% of peripheral blood mononuclear cells (PBMCs) mobilized by granulocyte colony-stimulating factor[38] and 0.01% to 0.12% of PBMCs from healthy seropositive blood donors[35] contain CMV DNA, with a range of 2 to 13 viral genomes per infected cell.[38] Because approximately 5% of PBMCs are monocytes, latently infected monocytes may comprise only 1 to 25 of every million peripheral blood white blood cells (WBCs). The low numbers of latently infected leukocytes in transfused blood components may contribute to the variable incidence of transfusion-transmitted CMV observed clinically.

Cytomegalovirus is also found associated with other cell types in the peripheral blood and marrow. In immunocompromised patients with CMV infections, polymorphonuclear leukocytes (PMNs) phagocytose and contain large amounts of virus.[80] Although PMNs do not appear to support the complete viral replication cycle, they can retain CMV in a viable and infectious form under experimental circumstances.[81] CMV can also productively infect megakaryocytic precursors and mature megakaryocytes.[82] Plasma free virus appears to be less stable than intracellular virus, and the presence of free virus in plasma is usually transient.[83] For example, in one study of recently infected adolescents, only a minority (25% to 40%) had plasma viremia, which was rarely identified more than 4 months after seroconversion.[67] Based on the available evidence, these other peripheral blood sources of CMV are unlikely to be as important as latently infected monocytes to the pathogenesis of transfusion-transmitted CMV.

VIRAL LOADS

Quantitation of peripheral blood CMV load is clinically useful in immunocompromised patients, where viral loads can reach 10^8 copies per milliliter of plasma or greater,[84] and correlate with the severity of viral disease.[85–90] For example, in liver transplant recipients a 50% probability of CMV disease was associated with a viral load of $10^{5.1}$ genomes/mL of blood, and a 90% probability with $10^{5.5}$ genomes/mL.[87] Infectious virus can also be cultured readily from the blood of immunocompromised patients with active infections.[91]

In contrast, the peripheral blood viral load in CMV-infected but otherwise healthy individuals is much lower and rarely quantitated. For example, in a series of published studies CMV could be cultured from only 2 of over 1500 buffy coat samples from healthy blood donors.[70,92,93] Nonetheless, a consideration of CMV loads in healthy individuals who are potential blood donors is useful in understanding the biology of transfusion-transmitted CMV (Fig. 46–2). WBC-associated viremia is often detectable for 6 months after infection,[67,94] in contrast to plasma free virus, which often disappears by 4 months. In recently seroconverted adolescents, 75% to 80% of WBC samples were positive for CMV DNA by PCR within the first 4 months of infection, compared with 25% to 40% of plasma samples within this same period.[67] A study of 98 seroconverting blood donors likewise identified a low frequency of transient plasma viremia.[83] In recently infected pregnant women, WBC-associated CMV DNA was detected in 100% of samples during the first month of infection using PCR and in 90% of samples during the second month of infection. None of the samples were positive after 6 months of infection.[94] WBC-associated viral load decreased substantially during early infection. During the first month 60% of positive samples had viral loads of more than 10 CMV genome-equivalents (GE)/10^5 WBCs (range of 10 to 398), whereas only 3.3% of positive samples during the second month of infection had more than 10 GE/10^5 WBCs.[94] Thus, shortly after infection of the immunocompetent host, the patient's viral load peaks. The subsequent decline in viral load correlates with the development of host anti-CMV immunity.

Host Immune Response

HUMORAL IMMUNITY

CMV infection initiates both a humoral and cellular immune response in the host, although anti-CMV antibodies exert limited control over CMV infection and disease. Antibody expression is typical of other humoral responses, with transient anti-CMV IgM synthesis followed by persistent expression of antiviral immunoglobulin G (IgG) (see Fig. 46–2). In a study of recently infected adolescents, anti-CMV antibodies were usually detectable by 6 to 8 weeks postinfection, a time of high peripheral blood viral loads.[67] However, despite the fact that anti-CMV, anti-gB, as well as viral neutralizing antibodies could be detected during the humoral response, they were insufficient to produce a precipitous decline in CMV DNA in either the plasma (free virus) or WBCs. Plasma and WBC-associated viral DNA were present in 25% to 40% and 75% to 80% of individuals, respectively, during the first 16 weeks of infection, and could still be detected in some individuals at 48 weeks of infection. Development of an antibody response likewise failed to immediately suppress viral shedding because CMV could be isolated from 59% of urine specimens during the first 80 weeks of infection.[67] Consistent with these observations, infectious virus has also been identified in saliva and cervical secretions of remotely infected seropositive individuals.[95,96] These findings indicate that anti-CMV antibodies, including those with neutralizing activities in vitro, may not completely prevent viral infectivity in vivo.

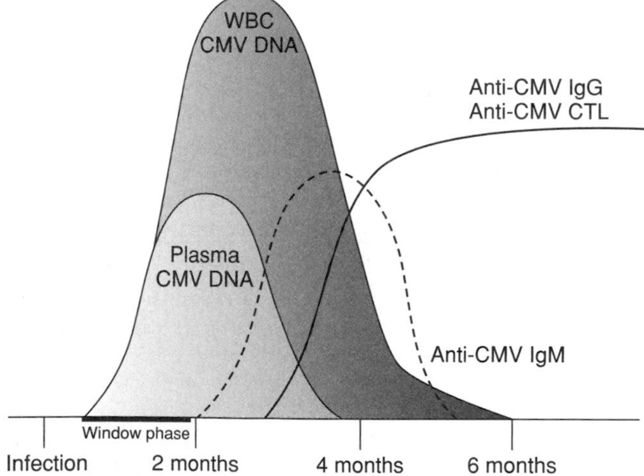

Figure 46–2 Temporal relationships between detection of plasma and white blood cell (WBC)-associated cytomegalovirus (CMV) DNA and the development of an immune response after primary infection. CMV DNA can be detected by polymerase chain reaction in both the plasma and WBC peripheral blood compartments during the first month of infection, and subsequently declines to undetectable levels over 4 to 6 months. The curves are not meant to be quantitative, but rather to illustrate that WBC-associated virus is more frequently detectable than plasma CMV during primary infection and also persists for a longer time. A humoral response is usually detectable by 8 weeks postinfection, and persists indefinitely, along with a cytotoxic T-lymphocyte response. The window phase represents the period between the initial presence of CMV in the peripheral blood and the first serologic evidence of CMV infection. Seronegative blood components obtained from donors in the window phase may explain some episodes of breakthrough transfusion-transmitted CMV in patients transfused exclusively with seronegative blood. See text for detailed discussion.

Nonetheless, anti-CMV antibodies can protect against sequelae of CMV infections in some circumstances. In a study of neonatal CMV infection, 10 of 10 (50%) infants born to seronegative mothers who subsequently contracted transfusion-transmitted CMV developed serious or fatal CMV disease. In contrast, 32 infants born to seropositive mothers contracted CMV infections, but none developed CMV disease, suggesting that passively acquired maternal CMV antibodies abrogated disease severity.[97] Therapeutic administration of antiviral antibodies, such as those present in intravenous immunoglobulin (IVIg) preparations, can also be efficacious in altering CMV disease course in some circumstances.[98]

Although anti-CMV antibodies generated during natural infection display a spectrum of specificities, among the more important targets is viral gB. Radioimmunoprecipitation assays using recombinant gB demonstrated the presence of anti-gB antibodies in the serum of all 48 seropositive donors tested.[99] Furthermore, the anti-gB antibodies were a significant component of the CMV-neutralizing activity in the serum samples. When anti-gB antibodies were absorbed with recombinant gB protein, viral neutralizing titer in the serum was reduced an average of 48%.[99] Similarly, other studies have demonstrated that 40% to 88% of serum CMV-neutralizing activity in naturally infected donors is directed against gB.[100,101] These results lend support for the use of recombinant gB as a subunit CMV vaccine.

CELLULAR IMMUNE RESPONSE

Cellular immune responses play an important role in the control of CMV infection. In bone marrow transplant (BMT) recipients, a patient population at high risk for CMV infection, development of a class I HLA-restricted CD8+ cytotoxic T-lymphocyte (CTL) response to CMV was significantly associated with the effective control of CMV infections.[102–106] In a study of 58 allogeneic BMT recipients with low or absent anti-CMV CTL activity at enrollment, 43 developed CMV infections, which were lethal in 12 of the patients.[102] Detectable anti-CMV CTL activity developed in all survivors of CMV infection, but in only 2 of the 12 patients who succumbed to CMV disease. NK cell activity was also depressed in the patients with fatal CMV infection but not in those who controlled their infections.[102,103] In another study, 10 of 20 recipients of allogeneic BMT developed CMV-specific CTL activity by 3 months post-transplantation. Six of the 10 patients who failed to develop anti-CMV CTL activity died of CMV pneumonitis, and all 10 patients with a detectable CMV CTL response were protected.[104] Similar conclusions regarding the protective effects of CMV CTLs were reached with CMV-seropositive patients who underwent autologous peripheral blood stem cell or bone marrow transplantation. In these patients, whose preexisting CMV-specific CTLs were suppressed by the preparative regimen, the reappearance of anti-CMV CTL activity was positively correlated with control of CMV infections ($p = 0.002$).[105] The investigators also noted that a CD4 T-helper cell response to CMV always preceded the reappearance of anti-CMV CTLs, and appeared to be obligatory for the CTL response.[105,106]

Using a murine model, investigators specifically depleted CD4+ and CD8+ T cells from the animals before experimental CMV infection to determine the contribution of each subset to antiviral immunity. These studies showed that CMV-primed CD8+ CTLs were capable of controlling CMV infections in the absence of CD4+ cells, except in salivary glands.[107,108] Furthermore, the mice deficient in CD4+ cells did not make high levels of anti-CMV antibodies, indicating that when the antiviral CTL response is intact a humoral response is unnecessary for effective control of CMV infection.[107] In the murine model, NK cells are also important for control of acute CMV infection.[64,109] IFN-γ production appears to be one of the principal mechanisms through which CD8+ and NK cells exert this effect.[109–114] The observation that cellular immunity plays a critical role in controlling CMV infection has led to successful early-stage clinical trials in which CMV-immune CTLs were adoptively transferred into immunocompromised BMT recipients.[115]

Laboratory Diagnosis of CMV Infection

Accurate detection of CMV infection enables the identification of transfusion recipients at risk for CMV infection, as well as blood donors whose components are potentially infectious. Furthermore, quantitation of the degree of viral replication is important for guiding appropriate use of antiviral therapies, such as ganciclovir, cidofovir, and foscarnet, in immunocompromised patients. The standard approach for identifying a previously infected individual is through detection of anti-CMV antibodies (Table 46–2). Serologic assays have been developed in multiple configurations, including indirect hemagglutination, complement fixation, solid phase fluorescence immunoassay, enzyme immunoassay (EIA), latex or particle agglutination, and solid phase red cell adherence, although the first three of these techniques are no longer frequently used.[116–120] These assays detect anti-CMV antibodies of the IgG, and in some cases IgM and IgA, classes. Direct comparisons of the sensitivities and specificities of the latter four methodologies are difficult to perform owing to the lack of good standards. Some EIAs have stated sensitivities and specificities of approximately 99% and because of their objective readouts may have advantages over techniques such as latex agglutination. However, anti-CMV antibodies may not be detected by serology until 6 to 8 weeks after primary infection,[67] and serology cannot accurately identify or quantitate the extent of active CMV infection. Although viral culture can be used for these purposes, conventional tube cultures can require 2 weeks or more to yield results, and the more recently implemented shell vial methodology may still require 24 to 48 hours to detect the presence of infectious CMV.[121,122] Furthermore, these assays are only quantitative in a limiting-dilution format, which is labor intensive and not suited to routine clinical use.

The CMV antigenemia assay (which uses immunostaining to identify and quantitate peripheral blood leukocytes that contain CMV proteins) and CMV PCR have solved some of these problems.[123–127] The antigenemia assay can be used for both viral diagnosis and surveillance. Significantly, this methodology is sensitive enough for early quantitative detection of CMV infections, allowing the institution of preemptive (presymptomatic) antiviral therapies.[128,129] Qualitative PCR allows even earlier detection of CMV infection than does antigenemia.[86,130–132] However, due to its sensitivity, in some earlier studies PCR displayed poor positive predictive value for identifying patients at risk for CMV disease because some patients with low but detectable viral loads did not develop disease.[86,129,131] The recent introduction of quantitative PCR assays for CMV may provide a more rapid, sensitive, and specific predictor of patients at risk for CMV disease.[133] For example, the results obtained with a moderately sensitive (400 copies of CMV DNA/mL) quantitative CMV PCR assay strongly correlated with results from the antigenemia method and with development of CMV disease.[134] Advantages of the PCR method included reduced turnaround time, smaller sample requirements (200 µL plasma versus 3 to 5 mL blood), simplified specimen processing, improved stability of specimens before processing, and ability to test samples from patients with leukopenia.

Table 46–2 Routine Diagnostic Laboratory Methods for CMV

Method	Rapid	Quantitative	Detects Active Infection	Detects Latent Infection	Differentiates Active from Latent Infection
Serology	++	No	Yes	Yes	No
Culture	No	No	Yes	No	Yes
Antigenemia	+	Yes	Yes	No	Yes
PCR	++	Yes*	Yes	Yes	Yes*

++, < 6 hours turnaround time.
+, < 24 hours turnaround time.
*Depending on assay; see text for details.
PCR, polymerase chain reaction.

Turnaround time for PCR testing may be reduced even further by adopting assays to the real-time format.[84] Alternative nucleic acid testing methodologies, such as nucleic acid sequence-based amplification of CMV IE mRNA, may also be useful in CMV diagnosis.[135,136]

Transfusion-Transmitted CMV Infections

Background

By the mid-1960s, a number of investigators had described an illness with clinical similarities to infectious mononucleosis occurring in patients who were exposed to blood products during cardiopulmonary bypass for open-heart surgery.[137,138] Patients typically presented with fever, splenomegaly, and atypical lymphocytosis within 3 to 8 weeks of surgery, but had a negative heterophile antibody test and did not experience exudative pharyngitis or lymphadenopathy. Klemola and Kaariainen subsequently demonstrated an increase in the titer of complement-fixing anti-CMV antibodies concurrent with the illness, suggesting that the etiology was CMV infection acquired from transfused blood products.[139,140] Further support for this hypothesis was provided by culturing CMV shed into the urine or blood of patients experiencing what was then called *cytomegalovirus mononucleosis.*[141] In the ensuing years, the disease has come to be known as *transfusion-transmitted cytomegalovirus infection* and has been described in a wide variety of clinical circumstances, although it is of most significance in immunocompromised transfusion recipients.[142–147] In most cases the diagnosis of transfusion-transmitted CMV is correlative: evidence of primary CMV infection in a previously seronegative patient who received a cellular blood component (red cells, platelets, or granulocytes) that was neither CMV-seronegative nor filtered. However, in at least one instance unequivocal molecular evidence for transfusion-transmitted CMV was provided by demonstrating identical restriction endonuclease digestion patterns of CMV isolates from a seropositive blood donor and from the neonates who were transfused with his blood component and subsequently developed CMV infection.[148]

Transfusion can lead to active CMV infection in the recipient by three mechanisms. The term *transfusion-transmitted CMV* is used to describe a primary CMV infection occurring in a seronegative recipient transfused with an infectious blood component. In contrast, *reactivated CMV infection* can occur when a seropositive transfusion recipient experiences reactivation of their latent CMV infection after blood transfusion from a seronegative donor. The mechanism underlying reactivated CMV infection likely involves immunomodulatory interactions between MHC mismatched leukocytes of the donor and recipient. Consistent with this mechanism, studies indicate that the incidence of CMV reactivation is independent of donor serostatus and component storage time, but increases with the volume of blood transfused.[149,150] Finally, *CMV superinfection* (second-strain infection) occurs when a seropositive recipient contracts a new strain of CMV from an infectious blood component. The diagnosis of both reactivation and superinfection is based on a fourfold or greater rise in the titer of anti-CMV antibodies and/or renewed viral shedding in secretions of seropositive transfusion recipients.[70] Although reactivation and superinfection can be distinguished from one another by restriction endonuclease genotyping of CMV strains,[151] this analysis has no significant clinical implications. These three mechanisms of transfusion-associated CMV infection appear to occur with similar frequencies. A review of five early studies of transfused CMV-seropositive patients calculated a 26% cumulative incidence of CMV reactivation or superinfection (66 of 252 patients), compared to a 31% incidence (99 of 323) of transfusion-transmitted CMV in seronegative recipients reported in seven contemporary studies (reviewed in Adler[70]). Nonetheless, the clinical significance of transfusion-transmitted CMV overshadows that of CMV reactivation and superinfection because transfusion-transmitted CMV results in a primary infection against which the recipient has no preexisting immunologic memory. In contrast, CMV reactivation and superinfection are unlikely to cause morbidity in the transfusion recipient.[152] Finally, it should be noted that although most cases of suspected transfusion-transmitted CMV result from the transfused component,[153,154] a minority of cases may result from community-acquired CMV infection occurring in temporal proximity to the transfusion.

Patients at Risk and Incidence

Although transfusion-transmitted CMV produces a primary CMV infection, in the immunocompetent transfusion recipient it is of no more clinical significance than community-acquired CMV infection. Furthermore, the risk of transfusion-transmitted CMV is very low in these patients. Early studies showed that 1.2% or fewer of immunocompetent patients experienced transfusion-transmitted CMV.[155,156] In a more recent study of 76 seronegative children with malignancies, there were no cases of transfusion-transmitted CMV in patients who received either seronegative or unscreened units, resulting in a calculated risk of less than 1 in 698 donor exposures in this population.[157] It should be noted that for reasons unrelated to study design, some of the units transfused in this study were washed or filtered. Follow-up of these children revealed that 2 of 76 subsequently developed community-acquired CMV infections (1.7% per patient-year), demonstrating the relatively greater incidence of community-acquired CMV infections than transfusion-transmitted CMV in this immunocompetent population. Furthermore, even in one early study where 32% of nonimmunosuppressed patients undergoing tumor resection developed transfusion-transmitted CMV, there was no evidence of CMV disease.[149] Thus, at present there are no compelling reasons to provide nonimmunosuppressed seronegative transfusion recipients with special components for the purposes of preventing transfusion-transmitted CMV.

In contrast, transfusion-transmitted CMV can be an important cause of morbidity and mortality in immunocompromised patients (Table 46–3). Most studies suggest that 13% to 37% of these patients will contract CMV from transfusion of unscreened and unfiltered cellular blood components.[97,158–161] The most well-established patient groups at risk for transfusion-transmitted CMV include premature low-birth-weight infants (<1250 to 1500 grams) born to seronegative mothers, seronegative recipients of seronegative allogeneic or autologous BMT, seronegative recipients of seronegative solid organ transplants, and seronegative patients with AIDS.[145,147,162] In these patients, the first manifestations of transfusion-transmitted CMV are often a viral syndrome, characterized by a flulike illness, including fever, chills, malaise, leukopenia, thrombocytopenia, and mild abnormalities

Table 46–3 Patients at Risk for Transfusion-Transmitted CMV

Category A: Clear morbidity and mortality from transfusion-transmitted CMV; CMV-safe components proven efficacious in decreasing incidence of transfusion-transmitted CMV, and should be used for all transfusions.
• Low-birth-weight infants (<1500 grams) of seronegative mothers
• Seronegative recipients of autologous or seronegative allogeneic bone marrow transplantation
• Seronegative recipients of seronegative solid organ transplants, excluding renal and cardiac
Category B: Identified risk of morbidity and mortality from transfusion-transmitted CMV; benefit of CMV-safe products is possible or likely, but not proven; consider using CMV-safe components when availability allows.
• Seronegative pregnant women requiring antepartum blood transfusion or intrauterine transfusion
• Seropositive women requiring intrauterine transfusion
• Low-birth-weight infants or seronegative immunosuppressed patients requiring granulocyte transfusions
• Seronegative HIV-infected patients
• Children born to HIV-infected mothers
• Low-birth-weight infants of seropositive mothers
• Seronegative patients who may be candidates for bone marrow transplantation
Category C: Morbidity and mortality of transfusion-transmitted CMV low or poorly documented, but likely greater than Category D; consider CMV-safe products on a case-by-case basis.
• Infants with birthweight > 1500 grams, born to seronegative mothers
• Neonates receiving ECMO or extensive transfusion support (e.g., exchange transfusions)
• Seronegative recipients of seronegative renal or cardiac transplantation
• Seronegative patients receiving chemotherapy
• Seronegative patients experiencing major trauma or splenectomy
Category D: Low morbidity and mortality of transfusion-transmitted CMV; CMV-safe components not indicated.
• Infants with birthweight > 1500 grams, born to seropositive mothers
• All other transfusion recipients not listed above

Modified with permission from Preiksaitis JK. The cytomegalovirus-"safe" blood product: Is leukoreduction equivalent to antibody screening? Transfus Med Rev 2000;14(2):112–136.

in liver function tests. The illness can progress to disseminated tissue-invasive CMV disease, including CMV hepatitis, retinitis, interstitial pneumonitis, encephalitis, and gastroenteritis, including esophagitis.[163] Progression to disease is more likely in patients with elevated viral loads. CMV infections are also associated with, and may predispose to, other complications in immunocompromised patients, including graft-versus-host disease (GVHD) in allogeneic marrow transplant recipients,[164–166] accelerated solid organ graft rejection,[167,168] and other opportunistic infections, including invasive fungal disease.[163,169]

Seronegative infants transfused with unscreened blood products had a 13.5% incidence of transfusion-transmitted CMV.[97] When greater than 50 mL of packed red cells were transfused, the incidence of transfusion-transmitted CMV increased to 24%. Of the infants who acquired transfusion-transmitted CMV, five (50%) developed serious symptoms or fatal disease, all of them weighing less than 1200 grams.[97] In other studies, seronegative neonates weighing less than 1250 to 1500 grams also experienced a high incidence of transfusion-transmitted CMV (reviewed in Preiksaitis[170]), likely due to their immature immune systems. It should be noted, however, that low-birth-weight infants born to seropositive mothers can also be at risk for lethal CMV infection, despite the transfer of humoral immunity.[171]

Marrow transplant recipients are at significant risk of morbidity and mortality from CMV infections. Up to one third of those patients who contract CMV infection can develop CMV pneumonitis, a frequently fatal complication.[172] In seropositive marrow recipients, CMV infection is usually due to viral reactivation, making CMV seropositivity the most important risk factor for CMV infection and disease.[172–175] CMV infection also occurs frequently in seronegative recipients of seropositive marrow.[158–160] However, in seronegative recipients of seronegative marrow or autologous transplants, transfusion is the primary mechanism for CMV infection.[158–160] Solid-organ transplant recipients are also susceptible to CMV infection and disease. In contrast to marrow transplantation, the most important source of CMV infection is the donor organ, with transfusion-transmitted CMV being less significant.[144,176–179] In seronegative recipients of seronegative organs, transfusion of unscreened blood products has been associated with an incidence of CMV ranging from 0 to 33%, with a cumulative incidence of approximately 9% (reviewed in Roback[147] and Preiksaitis[170]). Among organ transplant recipients, those receiving heart, heart-lung, liver, and pancreas transplants usually require numerous transfusions and thus have an increased risk of transfusion-transmitted CMV. Early studies showed that even in heavily transfused organ transplant recipients, the use of seronegative blood products could effectively prevent transfusion-transmitted CMV.[180–182]

In addition to these patient populations with well-defined susceptibility to transfusion-transmitted CMV, there are other groups that may be susceptible and may also benefit from transfusion of CMV-safe blood components (see Table 46–3). For example, it is well-documented that primary CMV infection during pregnancy carries high risks of congenital fetal infection. Although there is no direct evidence that primary maternal infection resulting from transfusion-transmitted CMV can in turn lead to fetal infection,[68,156] it is prudent to provide CMV-safe blood components to pregnant women who are seronegative. Because of the high incidence of CMV reactivation and infection in seropositive marrow recipients, 69% in one study,[172] transfusion-transmitted CMV is not a significant concern in these patients. However, special components may be considered for seronegative patients who are candidates for BMT, including immunosuppressed oncology patients, to prevent infection before transplant.

Blood Components Implicated in Transfusion-Transmitted CMV

Most evidence suggests that the primary vector for transfusion-transmitted CMV is the CMV-infected leukocyte (Table 46–4). Transfusion-transmitted CMV has not been observed in patients receiving blood components that are free of WBCs, arguing that plasma free virus is not significantly involved in the pathogenesis of transfusion-transmitted CMV.[183] For example, there was no evidence of transfusion-transmitted CMV in a group of 21 immunosuppressed seronegative recipients of seronegative BMT undergoing total plasma exchange, although they were exposed to an average of 47.6 +/− 19.5 units of unscreened fresh frozen plasma (FFP).[184] The absence of CMV after transfusion of FFP may be due to the scarcity of plasma free virus in healthy seropositive donors, as well as neutralization of virus by anti-CMV antibodies.

In contrast, there is an abundance of evidence that transfusion-transmitted CMV can be mediated by WBCs in blood components and that the incidence of transfusion-transmitted CMV correlates with the WBC load. For example, multiple studies have demonstrated transfusion-transmitted CMV after granulocyte transfusions, most often by seropositive granulocyte preparations transfused to seronegative recipients.[154,172,185] Red blood cell and platelet transfusions are also known to transmit CMV infections[97] (see Table 46–4).

Comparison of data over the past 4 decades reveals a correlation between decreased usage of fresh blood since the 1960s and a decline in the incidence of transfusion-transmitted CMV produced by unscreened units over the same period.[186] Most early evidence suggested that fresh blood (donated within 24 hours) from seropositive donors was more infectious than stored blood.[145,155] For example, in the initial descriptions, transfusion-transmitted CMV typically occurred following open-heart surgery in which the patient was exposed to fresh whole blood.[138–140] In nonimmunosuppressed seronegative transfusion recipients, 6 of 7 patients who seroconverted were transfused with fresh whole blood. In contrast, among 585 patients who did not seroconvert, only 53 had received fresh blood ($p < 0.001$).[155] Similar findings were made in a pediatric study where transfusion-transmitted CMV occurred in 13 of 15 children (87%) who received fresh blood (<24 hours old) as compared to 1 of 6 children (17%; $p = 0.01$) receiving blood more than 24 hours old.[161] In the same study, none of the children receiving only CMV-seronegative blood developed CMV, compared to the 36% rate of CMV in children receiving unscreened blood.[161] Overall, the infection rate with transfusion of fresh blood has been documented at 10% to 59% (reviewed in Lee and coworkers[161]). A decline in infectivity with storage has also been shown experimentally. When naturally infected blood obtained from AIDS patients with CMV viremia was refrigerated under standard conditions, CMV infectivity was rapidly lost during the first 5 days of storage.[187] However, not all studies have demonstrated an effect of product storage interval on the incidence of transfusion-transmitted CMV.[70,149,153,188]

It is also useful to consider the percentage of donated blood components that can transmit CMV infection. In a review of 10 studies published between 1968 and 1988, including data from 2806 patients, Ho calculated the changing risk of contracting transfusion-transmitted CMV over this period.[186] The risk per unit of unscreened and unfiltered blood was calculated at 11% to 12% in 1968 to 1970, and remained at greater than 1% per unit until the early 1980s. However, the risk subsequently fell to 0.4% or less by 1988.[186] Possible reasons for changes in the epidemiology of transfusion-transmitted CMV include decreasing use of fresh blood, improved tools for CMV serologic screening of blood donors and recipients, implementation of improved protocols to screen for other viral infections, and exclusion of blood from homosexual men starting in the mid-1980s.[186] The risk of transfusion-transmitted CMV also varies with different groups of transfusion recipients. In studies where recipients were immunosuppressed, 2.5% to 12% of unscreened blood components were estimated to be infectious.[70,97,144] Adler estimated that although 5% of all units were capable of producing CMV infection, 15% of seropositive units were potentially infectious.[189] In nonimmunosuppressed patients, in contrast, the risk may be as low as 0.14% of randomly selected units, or 0.38% of seropositive units.

Pathobiology of Transfusion-Transmitted CMV Infections

Clinical evidence for the involvement of leukocytes in transfusion-transmitted CMV include the observations that CMV is transmitted with high frequency by granulocyte transfusions from seropositive donors,[154] whereas the incidence of transfusion-transmitted CMV can be attenuated by removing leukocytes from blood components.[146,190] Furthermore, these WBCs are in almost all cases latently infected. When more than 1500 buffy coat samples from healthy blood donors were subject to viral culture in multiple studies, only 2 samples (both seropositive) grew infectious CMV.[70,92,93] These results demonstrate that when WBC-associated CMV is present, it is nearly always in the latent state. Experimental studies have indicated that WBCs of the monocyte lineage are

Table 46–4 Component-associated Risk of Transfusion-Transmitted CMV

Blood Component	Transfusion-Transmitted CMV Risk?	Processing to Abrogate Transfusion-Transmitted CMV
Red cells	Yes	Screening, filtration, frozen-deglycerolized
Platelets	Yes	Screening, filtration
Granulocytes	Yes	Screening
Fresh frozen plasma	No	n/a
Cryoprecipitate	No*	n/a
Clotting factors	No	n/a

*Not specifically tested, but other plasma-derived components have not been shown to be infectious for CMV.
n/a, not applicable.

the most likely to carry latent CMV in seropositive donors,[36] and thus are likely to be of most importance for transfusion-transmitted CMV (see Fig. 46–1). Circulating latently infected monocytes must be able to support viral reactivation from latency to mediate transfusion-transmitted CMV. Cultured monocytes can be differentiated in vitro into multinucleated giant cells by exposure to allogeneic cells. The degree of differentiation has been positively correlated with levels of CMV replication.[191] Latently infected monocytes and CD33+ bone marrow cells became permissive for CMV reactivation and viral replication after exposure to T-cell conditioned medium and hydrocortisone[192] or the combination of IFN-γ, tumor necrosis factor α, and interleukin-4, respectively[36] (see Fig. 46–1). When monocytes from healthy seropositive donors were grown in a mitogen-stimulated culture system containing allogeneic adherent mononuclear cells, the resulting differentiated monocyte-derived macrophages initiated production of infectious CMV.[35] These studies demonstrate that naturally infected peripheral blood monocytes contain latent CMV and that exposure to allogeneic cells or appropriate cytokine milieus such as would be encountered in transfusion recipients renders them permissive to viral reactivation with production of infectious CMV[36] (see Fig. 46–1).

There may also be additional factors, including recipient-related mechanisms, that modulate the incidence and severity of transfusion-transmitted CMV.[68] For example, as compared to immunologically competent transfusion recipients, immunocompromised patients have higher rates of transfusion-transmitted CMV and CMV diseases, including retinitis, esophagitis, and interstitial pneumonitis.[72,146] Even among immunocompromised patients there are factors that can affect the recipient's susceptibility to CMV infection and disease. In recipients of cadaveric renal transplants who were at risk for CMV infection, the immunosuppressive regimen employed significantly influenced survival.[193] The development of GVHD affects the incidence of CMV infection and disease in BMT recipients.[172,173] In a study of 181 recipients of allogeneic BMT, CMV infections occurred in 34 of 81 who developed acute GVHD as compared to 20 of 100 who did not ($p < 0.001$). Of the 34 patients who developed both CMV infection and GVHD, diagnosis of GVHD preceded the onset of CMV infection by a mean of 33.7 days, suggesting that GVHD predisposed to CMV infection.[175] A comparison of seronegative recipients of either autologous or seronegative allogeneic BMT showed that both groups had similar rates of transfusion-transmitted CMV, but the incidence of CMV interstitial pneumonitis was significantly greater following allogeneic transplantation, particularly if the allogeneic recipients developed GVHD.[164–166] Preiksaitis has recently suggested that the following factors may also predispose to transfusion-transmitted CMV: sequential transfusion over a long period of time as compared to large transfusion volumes given at one time, the use of HLA-matched donors, repetitive transfusions from the same donor, and the degree of immunosuppression and cytokine expression profile in the host.[68] However, the biologic variables potentially affecting transfusion-transmitted CMV are difficult to dissect in the clinical setting and will likely be more amenable to investigation in experimental models. For example, a murine model of transfusion-transmitted CMV has been developed in which the incidence of transfusion-transmitted CMV is affected by viral load and MHC mismatches between blood donor and recipient.[194,195]

Prevention of Transfusion-Transmitted CMV

The incidence of transfusion-transmitted CMV, as well as that of other untoward effects of transfusion, can be reduced by limiting transfusions to appropriate, clinically indicated circumstances. However, when transfusions are necessary, the most common approaches to decrease the risk of transfusion-transmitted CMV are the use of CMV-seronegative or filtered components (see Table 46–4). Nonetheless, it is clear that there remains a small residual risk of transfusion-transmitted CMV associated with the use of either type of component.[190]

SERONEGATIVE BLOOD COMPONENTS

Multiple studies, including prospective randomized, controlled trials, have demonstrated that exclusive use of CMV-seronegative units for transfusion can decrease the incidence of transfusion-transmitted CMV, as compared to use of unscreened units.[97,155,158,160,161,196] An early study of newborn infants demonstrated that none of 90 seronegative infants transfused with seronegative components contracted CMV infections, as compared to 13.5% of seronegative infants receiving transfusions from seropositive donors.[97] The exclusive use of seronegative units in immunocompromised adult seronegative recipients of allogeneic seronegative BMTs also decreased the incidence of CMV and severity of resulting CMV disease as compared to the use of unscreened blood products.[160] However, the use of seronegative units was only beneficial in seronegative recipients of seronegative donor marrow. Seronegative recipients of seropositive marrow transplants had a 46% incidence of CMV infection when transfused with unscreened blood, which was not significantly different from the 32% incidence when these patients received seronegative blood products.[160] The absence of a beneficial effect of seronegative transfusions for seronegative recipients of seropositive marrow was also observed in another study.[158] In nonimmunosuppressed seronegative patients, transfusion of seronegative blood components can also prevent transfusion-transmitted CMV,[155] although there are few indications for use of seronegative blood in this population. Based on these and other data, seronegative units remain the gold standard for the prevention of CMV in susceptible transfusion recipients (see Table 46–4).

Despite exclusive use of seronegative units for transfusion, up to 4% of susceptible recipients have acquired CMV.[158,160,190] False-negative donor serology may have contributed to some of these cases of breakthrough transfusion-transmitted CMV, particularly in studies using earlier generation serology assays.[157,196] Even sensitive and specific assays that detect anti-CMV antibodies of IgG, IgM, and in some cases IgA classes can show significant disagreement when applied to samples from blood donors.[69] Alternatively, some donors may have been in the 6- to 8-week *window-phase* following primary CMV infection, during which anti-CMV antibodies cannot be detected reliably[67] (see Fig. 46–2). During this period there are high peripheral blood viral loads,[67] suggesting that transfusions from these "seronegative" donors may be infectious. Detection of anti-CMV antibodies of the IgM class early during the course of infection appears to be important for preventing transfusion-transmitted CMV.[197] In one study, patients who received components with detectable IgM anti-CMV antibodies had a CMV infection rate of 8.4% (7 of 83 recipients) compared to a rate of 0.3% (1 of 280 patients; $p < 0.001$) in those who received blood without IgM anti-CMV.[198] Interestingly, in this study only 1 of 163 neonates who received seropositive, but IgM-negative, blood developed CMV.[198] However, other investigators have found that screening for IgM anti-CMV antibodies had poor sensitivity and specificity for identifying infectious blood components.[68]

FILTERED BLOOD COMPONENTS

The seroprevalence rate for CMV ranges from 40% to 80% in the United States.[4,69,72] The difficulties in maintaining a sufficient inventory of CMV seronegative blood components motivated efforts to identify alternative strategies to provide CMV-safe components for susceptible patients. Because WBCs latently infected with CMV are the primary vector for transfusion-transmitted CMV, removal of WBCs from components was an attractive approach to mitigate transfusion-transmitted CMV. Current third-generation filtration technology can produce a 3 to 4 $\log_{10}$ reduction in monocytes and other leukocytes in blood components.[199] Alternatively, platelets and red cells can be prepared from donors by apheresis procedures, resulting in process-leukoreduced components with 10^5 to 10^6 residual leukocytes, depending on instrumentation and separation technique.[200] This level of leukoreduction has been shown to significantly reduce the incidence of transfusion-transmitted CMV in multiple studies.[146,159,201–204] In the largest prospective, randomized, controlled clinical trial to address this issue to date, Bowden and colleagues randomized 502 seronegative recipients of autologous or seronegative allogeneic BMT to receive either unscreened blood products filter-leukoreduced at the bedside or CMV-seronegative components.[190] Between 21 and 100 days post-transplantation, the predefined window phase for identifying transfusion-transmitted CMV, the probabilities of developing CMV infection were similar in patients receiving filtered units (2.4%) and those receiving seronegative components (1.3%; $p = 1.00$). The probabilities of developing CMV disease were also similar in these two groups (2.4% vs 0%, respectively; $p = 1.00$). Based on an intention-to-treat analysis, the authors concluded that seronegative and filtered units carried equivalent risks of transfusion-transmitted CMV. The interpretation of this study was complicated by an analysis of all data from days 0 to 100 that showed a statistically greater progression to CMV disease in the group receiving filtered components as compared to those receiving seronegative components (2.4% vs 0%, respectively; $p = 0.03$). In fact, five of six patients who contracted CMV from filtered units developed CMV disease that progressed to fatal CMV pneumonia, whereas none of four patients infected with CMV from seronegative components developed CMV disease ($p = 0.005$ by Fisher's exact test).[190,205] The biologic basis for this difference remains unexplained,[205,206] leaving open the possibility that there are differences between filtered and seronegative units with respect to the risk of transfusion-transmitted CMV. However, it should be noted that this study utilized bedside filtration, which is unlikely to produce the degree and reproducibility of leukoreduction achievable with prestorage filtration methods. A more recent large retrospective study also showed an increased incidence of transfusion-transmitted CMV in patients who received leukoreduced products.[207] Weekly surveillance for the presence of CMV viremia was performed on a cohort of 807 CMV-seronegative stem cell transplant recipients, demonstrating a significant increase in the incidence of transfusion-transmitted CMV when seronegative units were partially replaced by filtered blood components. In particular, the use of filtered red blood cell units was positively associated with an increase in CMV infection.[207] In a recent review, Preiksaitis provided a detailed discussion of the theoretical and observed differences between the use of CMV-seronegative units and filtered units.[68]

OTHER COMMON COMPONENT PROCESSING METHODOLOGIES

In seronegative neonates, the exclusive use of frozen-deglycerolized red cells markedly reduces the incidence of transfusion-transmitted CMV, providing a third option along with seronegative and filtered components for patients at risk for CMV.[146,208,209] However, given the labor-intensive nature of preparing frozen-deglycerolized red cells, this approach is rarely used. In contrast, it is unclear whether washing of components can adequately decrease the incidence of transfusion-transmitted CMV. In one study of seronegative neonates, transfusion of washed red cells from seropositive donors was associated with a 1.3% incidence of transfusion-transmitted CMV,[210] below the historical incidence of 13% to 37%.[97,158–160] However, in another study transfusion of washed red cells resulted in an 11.1% incidence of CMV in seronegative neonates.[211] Given these conflicting data, together with the logistics of washing blood components, this procedure cannot be recommended for preparation of CMV-safe blood components. Likewise, standard gamma-irradiation protocols used to prevent transfusion-associated GVHD are not effective at abrogating transfusion-transmitted CMV.

IMMUNOGLOBULIN PREPARATIONS AND ANTIVIRAL DRUGS

The efficacy of passively acquired maternal anti-CMV antibodies to abrogate CMV infection and disease in neonates suggested that CMV immunoglobulin preparations may be useful in immunocompromised adults. In an early randomized trial of prophylactic hyperimmune CMV IVIg, BMT recipients receiving IVIg were protected against CMV infection ($p = 0.009$), interstitial pneumonia, and CMV mortality ($p = 0.014$) as compared to the control group.[212] Other studies have produced similar findings.[213] A meta-analysis derived from 12 published clinical trials of prophylactic IVIg in BMT patients confirmed that passive CMV antibodies could significantly reduce fatal CMV infection (95% confidence interval (CI), 0.23–0.99), CMV pneumonitis (CI, 0.42–0.89), non-CMV interstitial pneumonia (CI, 0.35–0.95), and total CMV mortality (CI, 0.55–0.99).[98] However, the efficacy of IVIg in preventing transfusion-transmitted CMV is more difficult to assess. For example, when seronegative study patients were transfused with seronegative blood, the current standard of care, there was no significant effect of IVIg on CMV infection and disease.[158] Furthermore, intramuscular CMV immune globulin was ineffective in preventing transfusion-transmitted CMV in seronegative patients who received seropositive granulocyte infusions.[214]

In allogeneic marrow transplantation, ganciclovir can provide effective prophylaxis against CMV disease.[215,216] However, ganciclovir can also cause untoward effects, including marrow suppression with neutropenia, delayed reconstitution of cellular immunity predisposing to opportunistic infections, and outgrowth of resistant viral mutants.[217–219] Even limited use of ganciclovir has caused severe neutropenia in 33% (10 of 30) of treated patients, 7 of whom subsequently developed opportunistic infections.[220] Furthermore, despite adequate control of CMV infections in these patients, they experienced increased mortality due to other infectious complications, including *Aspergillus fumigatus, Streptococcus pneumoniae*, and *Pneumocystis carinii* pneumonia.[220] In a randomized, placebo-controlled trial of prophylactic ganciclovir in marrow transplant recipients, ganciclovir usage lead to delayed recovery of anti-CMV CTL activity, which may predispose patients to late-onset CMV disease.[106] Up to 15% of BMT recipients develop late CMV disease after discontinuation of ganciclovir prophylaxis,[215] and the mortality of late-onset disease approaches 70%.[106] Prolonged ganciclovir therapy can also lead to selection of drug-resistant CMV mutants. In one study, 38% (5 of 13) of AIDS patients treated with ganciclovir longer than 3 months shed resistant mutants.[221] Children receiving T cell–depleted marrow transplants also appear to be at increased risk for developing ganciclovir-resistant mutants, as well as strains resistant to the antiviral compounds foscarnet and cidofovir.[222] These concerns underscore the importance of preventing CMV transmission, rather than treating resulting CMV infections and disease.[223] Furthermore, when compared to the proven efficacy of seronegative or filtered units to decrease the incidence of transfusion-transmitted CMV, the use of IVIg and/or antiviral agents would be more expensive and possibly not as effective, and thus these interventions cannot be recommended for abrogation of transfusion-transmitted CMV.

NAT-SCREENED COMPONENTS

With standard serologic assays, both uninfected donors and those in the window phase of a CMV infection test as seronegative. Some window phase donors have high plasma and WBC-associated viral loads, and thus although seronegative their blood may be infectious on transfusion.[67,94] Blood components from most CMV-seropositive donors do not produce transfusion-transmitted CMV, but serologic testing is unable to distinguish these from infectious seropositive units. Filter leukoreduction decreases the incidence of transfusion-transmitted CMV but immunocompromised patients who acquire CMV from filtered blood can develop significant CMV-associated disease.[190] Thus, neither serologic screening nor leukoreduction produces a blood supply that is completely CMV-safe. In analogy with NAT screening for human immunodeficiency virus (HIV) and hepatitis C, NAT screening for CMV DNA may identify blood components that can produce transfusion-transmitted CMV and may serve as a useful adjunct to serology and filtration.

Because most seropositive donors are remotely infected (>6 months), they are likely to have peripheral blood viral loads near or below the limits of detection of even sensitive NAT assays. Assays sufficiently sensitive to detect these low viral loads may be subject to problems, including nonspecific amplification of background DNA. For this reason, it is not surprising that several studies investigating the presence of CMV DNA in healthy blood donors have yielded conflicting results. Some investigators have identified CMV DNA in WBCs or isolated monocytes from both seropositive and seronegative donors.[224–226] In a study of 270 healthy blood donors in Sweden, the use of nested PCR demonstrated CMV DNA in peripheral blood mononuclear cells from 14% of seronegative donors using both UL123 and UL32 PCR assays, although the CMV DNA detection rate increased to 55% if monocyte-enriched samples from seronegative donors were assayed.[227] These investigators also identified CMV DNA in 100% of seropositive donors. In contrast, other investigators have been unable or only rarely able to identify CMV by PCR in peripheral blood from seropositive or seronegative donors.[83,94,126,127,130,228–230] These latter findings appear more consistent with the clinical experience that seronegative blood components only rarely transmit CMV infections to transfusion recipients, and that only 0.4% to 12% of seropositive blood units appear capable of CMV transmission.[155,156,180] The variability of the results in these prior studies demonstrate that technical hurdles remain prior to implementation of CMV NAT for testing of the blood supply.

To identify CMV PCR assays with appropriate performance characteristics for screening healthy blood donors, a multicenter trial was undertaken to determine the sensitivity, specificity, and reproducibility of seven previously described assays.[231] In practice, the DNA yield from 250,000 WBCs (approximately 2 μg of DNA) is the maximum tolerated input for most PCR assays. Based on estimates that 0.004% to 0.12% of PBMCs are latently infected,[35,38] it was predicted that an average of 4 to 120 latently infected cells would be present per 250,000 WBCs (PBMCs typically comprise 40% of WBCs). Given the reported presence of 2 to 13 viral genomes per latently infected cell,[38] it was hypothesized that PCR assays used in donor screening should be sufficiently sensitive to detect 8 to 1560 CMV genome equivalents (GE) in 250,000 WBCs. Five of the examined assays displayed sufficient sensitivity for donor screening based on consistent detection of a minimum of 25 CMV GE in analytical controls constructed to contain from 1 to 100 CMV GE in background DNA from 250,000 cells.[231] Of these five assays, two detected CMV DNA in a subset of 20 pedigreed CMV seronegative samples. However, these results were found to be inconsistent when the seronegative samples were reanalyzed. The other three sensitive assays did not detect CMV DNA in the seronegative samples, and two of these were selected for further study. These assays, a nested PCR directed at the CMV UL93 ORF and the Roche Monitor assay, were used to screen 1000 blood samples from healthy donors.[69] Of the 416 seropositive donor samples, 2 (0.5%) tested positive for CMV DNA with both assays, and 7 other samples tested positive with only one assay and did not confirm on retesting. When the two positive samples were subjected to limiting dilution analysis they were found to have viral loads of 1 to 10 copies per 250,000 WBCs, demonstrating that CMV DNA loads in healthy blood donors are at or below the limits of detection of even sensitive PCR assays. Six of the seronegative samples tested positive with only one assay and were not confirmed on repeat testing. These results suggest that only a small percentage of seropositive samples from healthy blood donors have viral loads that are reproducibly detectable by extremely sensitive PCR assays, potentially limiting the use of PCR to prevent transfusion-transmitted CMV. It should be noted that the minimal viral load required for transfusion-transmitted CMV has not been determined, and it must be assumed at present that any CMV-seropositive or CMV DNA-positive unit is potentially infectious.

VIRAL INACTIVATION, CMV VACCINATION, AND ADOPTIVE IMMUNOTHERAPY TO DECREASE THE INCIDENCE OF TT-CMV

As opposed to current approaches such as the use of seronegative and filtered components, the application of pathogen inactivation technology to cellular blood components carries the potential for completely preventing transfusion-transmitted CMV, as well as eliminating the transmission of other infectious agents. The psoralen derivative 8-methoxypsoralen (8-MOP), when exposed to ultraviolet light, can inactivate a spectrum of both gram-positive and gram-negative organisms that can contaminate platelet components, including *Staphylococcus aureus*, *Staphylococcus epidermidis*, *Escherichia coli*, *Yersinia enterocolitica*, *Salmonella choleraesuis*, *Serratia marcescens*, and *Pseudomonas aeruginosa*.[232–234] Bacterial concentrations of 10^4 to 10^7 CFU/mL can be inactivated, which compares favorably with estimated bacterial concentrations of 10 to 10^3 CFU/mL in naturally infected units.[235] In vitro platelet function was not adversely affected by 8-MOP treatment. Similar results were obtained with another psoralen derivative, S-59, which could efficiently inactivate more than 10^6 plaque-forming units per milliliter of HIV, duck hepatitis B virus, and bovine diarrhea virus (a model for HCV) in experimentally infected platelet components.[236–238] S-59 also effectively prevented transfusion-transmitted CMV in a murine transfusion model.[195] Viral inactivation technology has entered clinical trials and is the subject of Chapter 27 in this volume.

Given the limited risk of transfusion-associated CMV disease in seropositive recipients, vaccination of seronegative patients prior to immunosuppression may mitigate the risks of CMV in this population. Use of an attenuated Towne CMV strain as a live virus vaccine in 237 renal transplant recipients demonstrated that vaccinated seronegative recipients of seropositive grafts had similar rates of infection to unvaccinated controls but experienced less severe disease. Furthermore, the survival of cadaveric renal grafts at 36 months was improved by vaccination compared with the control group ($p = 0.04$).[239] Although there were no episodes of Towne CMV reactivation following latency in these immunosuppressed patients, this possibility must be considered when evaluating the safety of this approach. The use of recombinant CMV proteins as subunit vaccines represents a potentially safer method of vaccination. In experimental settings, recombinant gB protein can induce protective immunity,[101] and anti-gB antibodies in naturally infected donors comprise a large component of the CMV-neutralizing activity in seropositive donor serum.[99,101]

Recovery of CMV-specific CTLs following marrow transplantation provides protection from CMV infection and disease.[102–104,106] However, at 40 days post-transplantation, 65% of marrow transplant recipients had deficient CD8+ CTL responses in one study.[104] In immunocompromised patients who cannot mount an effective CTL response, passive transfer of CTLs is an attractive approach to augment cellular immunity. However, early attempts to restore cellular immunity through administration of unselected donor Tcells to marrow recipients was associated with GVHD.[240–242] In an alternative approach, CD3+,CD8+,CD4− CMV-specific CTLs were cloned from CMV-seropositive marrow donors, expanded in culture, and then infused into marrow recipients.[243] Each recipient received four infusions, 1 week apart, in escalating doses. Importantly, the CMV antigen-specific CTLs did not produce GVHD or other morbidity in the recipient.[243] Further studies demonstrated that transferred clones could persist and retain anti-CMV cytotoxic activity for at least 12 weeks following infusion.[244] However, CTL activity declined if recipient anti-CMV CD4+ T cells were not generated. There was no evidence of CMV viremia or disease in any patient receiving CTL therapy.[244] Although adoptive cellular immunotherapy is an attractive approach for prophylaxis of immunocompromised patients, the currently used methods for deriving and expanding donor CTL clones is lengthy, labor-intensive, and costly. However, as this technology improves and becomes more commonplace, transfusion medicine physicians will likely play a significant role in the procurement, processing, and administration of CTL components. For example, studies in a murine model have demonstrated that a rapid and simple method using psoralen-treated MHC-mismatched donor lymphocytes is highly efficacious at clearing CMV infections without causing GVHD following bone marrow transplantation.[245]

RECOMMENDATIONS

The exclusive use of CMV-seronegative blood components for the transfusion of seronegative immunocompromised patients susceptible to transfusion-transmitted CMV remains the standard of care (see Table 46–4). If seronegative units are not available, the evidence suggests that filtered, unscreened components are an acceptable substitute. Although the AABB guidelines state that seronegative and leukoreduced units are equivalent for prevention of transfusion-transmitted CMV,[246] other panels that have reviewed this issue disagree. For example, Swiss clinical practice recommendations consider seronegative units to be the gold standard for prevention of transfusion-transmitted CMV and conclude that leukoreduced units have not yet been proven equivalent for this purpose.[247] A Canadian consensus conference reached similar conclusions when the majority of the panel agreed that seronegative blood components should continue to be provided to at-risk patients despite implementation of universal leukoreduction in Canada.[248] The use of frozen-deglycerolized red cells is also an acceptable alternative to seronegative units, but their preparation is expensive and labor intensive. In contrast, washed red cell and platelet components cannot be considered CMV-safe. The use of IVIg and ganciclovir or other antiviral drugs, are unlikely to be clinically efficacious or cost-effective approaches to preventing transfusion-transmitted CMV.

At the present time, there is no compelling scientific argument for the implementation of CMV NAT screening to prevent transfusion-transmitted CMV. Using the most sensitive and reproducible PCR tests currently available, only about 0.2% of blood donations are found to contain CMV DNA. Furthermore, there are no studies to correlate the risk of transfusion-transmitted CMV with the presence of CMV DNA, although such an association is theoretically attractive. Nonetheless, the potential of CMV NAT to detect seronegative window phase donations, as well as components that retain a residual CMV load postfiltration, remains an interesting possibility to be evaluated. However, implementation of CMV vaccination or virus-inactivated cellular blood components in the future is likely to render the above issues moot.

EPSTEIN-BARR VIRUS (EBV, HHV-4)

The genome of EBV, a gammaherpesvirus, is 172 kbp in length. Two genetically distinguishable types of EBV exist, EBV-1 and EBV-2, as well a number of variants resulting from genomic recombination. In immunocompetent patients primary infection with EBV results in a spectrum of clinical sequelae ranging from an asymptomatic infection to heterophile-positive infectious mononucleosis.[39,249] EBV can also cause lymphomagenesis, as can the other human gammaherpesvirus HHV-8. EBV is an etiologic agent in endemic Burkitt's lymphoma, AIDS-related lymphoma, post-transplant lymphoproliferative disease (PTLD) and nasopharyngeal carcinoma.[249] After immune-mediated resolution of acute infection, EBV is not completely eliminated but rather achieves a lifelong latent state. The EBV genome is episomal in latently infected B cells, which probably represent the true EBV reservoir in the latently infected host. One in 10^5 to 10^6 B cells is estimated to be latently infected after primary infection. Latent EBV in B cells may undergo sporadic reactivation with subsequent release of infectious progeny virus. Eleven viral gene products are known to be expressed during latent infection, including nuclear antigens (EBNA 1, 2, 3A, 3B, 3C, LP), membrane proteins (LMP 1, 2A, 2B), and noncoding nuclear RNAs (EBER 1, 2).[39] These latent gene products disrupt B-cell regulatory mechanisms, leading to the characteristic polyclonal B-cell lymphoproliferation seen in infectious mononucleosis.

Epstein-Barr virus is transmitted by close contact, and the majority of the adult population (>95%) has been infected with EBV, based on serologic investigations. Seropositive individuals are at risk for reactivation of latent EBV infection if they become immunocompromised (e.g., in the setting of pharmacologic immunosuppression for organ or marrow transplantation).[249] However, the most significant EBV-associated risk is that of primary EBV infection occurring during immunosuppression for transplantation. Primary infection can be community acquired or can result from blood transfusion or transplantation from an EBV-seropositive donor.[249] An important clinical example is pediatric orthotopic liver transplantation, where EBV-associated PTLD has been identified in 10% to 20% of patients immunosuppressed with tacrolimus.[250–252] PTLD encompasses a range of disorders from benign polyclonal B-cell lymphoid hyperplasia to malignant high-grade non-Hodgkin's lymphoma. In pediatric orthotopic liver transplantation, PTLD is a cause of significant morbidity, including graft loss,[253] as well as mortality rates of up to 20%.[254]

Transmission of EBV by blood transfusion can present in a similar manner to classic infectious mononucleosis. As with transfusion-transmitted CMV, viral genotyping has been used to document transfusion-transmitted EBV from a blood donor to a recipient, who subsequently developed EBV-driven PTLD.[255] In most cases of transfusion-transmitted EBV the blood donor has been found to be in the incubation period for infectious mononucleosis with high B-cell viral loads.[256] Although the use of EBV-seronegative blood components may reduce the incidence of transfusion-transmitted EBV, they are difficult to obtain given the high seroprevalence of EBV (Table 46–5). Because EBV is highly B-cell associated and B cells are efficiently removed by blood filtration,[199] exclusive use of leukoreduced cellular blood components for transfusion is likely to decrease the probability of transfusion-transmitted EBV infections in at-risk seronegative patients. This possibility has, however, not been subject to controlled clinical trials.

HUMAN HERPESVIRUS 6 (HHV-6)

HHV-6 was first identified in lymphocytes from AIDS patients with lymphoproliferative diseases and was originally named *human B-cell lymphotropic virus.*[257] However, the primary tropism of HHV-6 is now recognized to be CD4+ T lymphocytes, although it can also infect CD8+ T cells, NK cells, monocytes, macrophages, and megakaryocytes. The linear double-stranded DNA genome of HHV-6 consists of a 143 kb unique segment flanked by 8 to 13 kb terminal direct repeats. Overall, there is 66% sequence similarity between HHV-6 and CMV, the prototypical betaherpesvirus,[258] and greater than 90% sequence similarity between the two HHV-6 variants, HHV-6A and HHV-6B.

Human herpesvirus-6B is the principal etiologic agent of the childhood illness roseola infantum (sixth disease), which presents with a fever of 2 to 5 days' duration followed by a maculopapular skin rash (exanthem subitum) and rapid defervescence.[259] Serologic investigations have demonstrated that HHV-6 is endemic, with 70% or more of children infected by age 1,[260] and over 90% of the population displaying evidence of community-acquired infection during infancy. HHV-6, like other herpesviruses, can persist in a latent state, possibly within PBMCs. In addition to roseola infantum, in immunocompetent individuals there is a weak association between HHV-6 infection and diseases that include heterophile-negative mononucleosis, hepatitis, multiple sclerosis, chronic fatigue syndrome, hemophagocytic syndrome, encephalitis, Rosai-Dorfman disease, Kawasaki disease, Kikuchi lymphadenitis, sarcoidosis, a variety of lymphoproliferative disorders, and rare cases of anemia and granulocytopenia.[261] However, significant problems are rare in immunocompetent individuals. In contrast, immunocompromised patients can experience HHV-6–related complications, including fever, leukopenia, graft rejection,

Table 46–5 Transfusion Transmission of WBC-Associated Human Herpesviruses

Virus	Seronegative Recipients	Morbidity following Transfusion Transmission	Special Components for Susceptible Recipients	
			Seronegative	Filtered
CMV	20%–60%	Yes	Acceptable	Acceptable
EBV	<5%	Rare	n/a	?
HHV-6	<5%	Not documented	n/a	?
HHV-7	<5%	Not documented	n/a	?
HHV-8	70%–95%	Not documented	n/a	?

n/a, not routinely available.
?, No clinical evidence for reduction in the risk of transfusion transmission, but possibly effective because viruses are WBC-associated.

interstitial pneumonitis, encephalitis, and marrow suppression.[262–265] Fatal HHV-6 encephalitis has been documented after BMT.[266]

HHV-6 transmission by marrow and solid organ transplantation has been demonstrated.[263,267] However, while PCR analysis of PBMCs showed HHV-6 DNA in up to 90% of blood donors,[268] HHV-6 transmission by blood transfusion has not been definitively documented (see Table 46–5). In analogy with EBV, another highly seroprevalent WBC-associated human herpesvirus, seronegative units are not generally available for transfusion of susceptible recipients. Although filtered components are hypothesized to reduce the risk of transfusion-transmitted HHV-6, clinical efficacy has not been shown.

HUMAN HERPESVIRUS 7 (HHV-7)

Along with HHV-6A, HHV-7 is the only other human herpesvirus with primary tropism for T lymphocytes. HHV-6 and HHV-7 are closely related betaherpesviruses, with an overall 40% sequence similarity. The HHV-7 genome consists of a long unique segment of 133 kb, flanked by single direct repeats of 6 kb on each end.[269] HHV-7, which was originally isolated in 1990 from CD4+ T lymphocytes of a healthy individual,[270] displays much more restricted tropism than HHV-6. In culture HHV-7 can only infect activated CD4+ T cells and the CD4+ cell line SupT1,[271] although in vivo HHV-7 also infects cells of the salivary glands.[272] Infections occur slightly later in life than with HHV-6, but most children are seropositive by age 5. Although a causative role for HHV-7 in pityriasis rosea and a minority of cases of exanthem subitum has been suggested,[273–275] the spectrum of diseases attributable to this virus is still unclear. Because HHV-7 infects CD4+ T cells and viral DNA has been identified in WBCs from 66% of German blood donors,[276] HHV-7 may be transmissible by blood transfusion. The same considerations regarding transfusion transmission of HHV-6 apply to this virus (see Table 46–5).

HUMAN HERPESVIRUS 8 (HHV-8; KAPOSI'S SARCOMA HERPESVIRUS)

HHV-8, a gammaherpesvirus, was originally isolated from Kaposi's sarcoma (KS) skin lesions using representational difference analysis.[277] The HHV-8 genome is approximately 170 kb in size and encodes an estimated 81 ORFs.[278,279] Sequence analysis revealed that HHV-8 is closely related to herpesvirus saimiri and the other human gammaherpesvirus, EBV.[277] As with EBV, HHV-8 can cause uncontrolled proliferation of infected cells. In addition to KS, HHV-8 is also associated with primary effusion lymphoma and multicentric Castleman's disease in patients with POEMS syndrome (polyneuropathy, organomegaly, endocrinopathy, M protein, skin changes).[280–282] There is still significant debate concerning the role of HHV-8 in the pathogenesis of multiple myeloma and monoclonal gammopathy of undetermined significance (MGUS).[283,284] If HHV-8 is present in multiple myeloma lesions, it is generally agreed that it is not in the malignant plasma cells, but rather in a subset of surrounding stromal cells. The case has been made that HHV-8 has not yet fulfilled Koch's postulates or Hill's epidemiologic criteria for causality of multiple myeloma.[284]

Human herpesvirus-8 is primarily transmitted through sexual contact, and infection is rare before puberty. The seroprevalence of HHV-8 has been intensely investigated. In most studies, 1% to 11% of the healthy adults in Western countries had detectable anti–HHV-8 antibodies.[285–288] However, when HHV-8 lytic antigens were used as serologic targets, up to 25% of the general population, 90% of HIV-infected homosexual men, and almost all KS patients had detectable antibodies.[289] HHV-8 can be transmitted by infected renal allografts transplanted into seronegative recipients.[290] However, the same study argued against frequent transmission by blood products because no episodes of HHV-8 seroconversion were documented among seronegative recipients of seronegative transplants who received blood transfusions. Nonetheless, HHV-8 DNA has been identified in PBMCs of 55% of patients with KS[291] and in the blood of some renal transplant patients.[292] An HHV-8 seroprevalence of 35% to 82% has been reported in healthy non–HIV-infected individuals in central Africa.[286,287,289] Approximately 22% of apparently healthy central African blood donors had low levels of WBC-associated HHV-8 DNA, compared to about 0 to 2% in healthy Europeans.[291,293,294] Furthermore, there is an association of HHV-8 infection and intravenous drug use in women, independent of sexual activity, which also argues for the possibility of blood-borne transmission.[295]

Recent studies lend support to the possibility that HHV-8 is transfusion-transmitted, albeit at low rates. In Uganda, HHV-8 seropositivity positively correlated with number of transfusions, with a calculated 2.6% risk of infection per transfused blood component.[296] Using archived samples from Frequency of Agents Communicable by Transfusion study (FACTS), a repository created before the widespread use of leukoreduction, 2 HHV-8 seroconversions were identified among 284 seronegative transfusion recipients (risk per component, 0.082%).[297] Although the current risk of transmitting HHV-8 by blood transfusion is unclear, the clinical issues associated with providing HHV-8 "safe" blood components are more similar to those associated with CMV than with EBV, HHV-6, or HHV-7 (see Table 46–5). Thus, it may be possible to provide either HHV-8 seronegative units or filtered components to abrogate the risk of transfusion-transmitted HHV-8. However, further investigations will be necessary to validate the efficacy and usefulness of these approaches.

REFERENCES

1. Roizman B. Herpesviridae. In Fields BN, Knipe DM, Howley PM, et al (eds). Fields Virology, 3rd ed. Philadelphia, Lippincott-Raven, 1996, pp 2221–2230.
2. Roizmann B, Desrosiers RC, Fleckenstein B, et al. The family Herpesviridae: an update. The Herpesvirus Study Group of the International Committee on Taxonomy of Viruses. Arch Virol 1992;123:425–449.
3. Mach M, Stamminger T, Jahn G. Human cytomegalovirus: recent aspects from molecular biology. J Gen Virol 1989;70:3117–3146.
4. Mocarski ES. Cytomegalovirus and their replication. In Fields BN, Knipe DM, Howley PM, et al (eds). Fields Virology, 3rd ed. Philadelphia, Lippincott-Raven, 1996, pp 2447–2492.
5. LaFemina RL, Hayward GS. Replicative forms of human cytomegalovirus DNA with joined termini are found in permissively infected human cells but not in non-permissive Balb/c-3T3 mouse cells. J Gen Virol 1983;64:373–389.
6. Bolovan-Fritts CA, Mocarski ES, Wiedeman JA. Peripheral blood CD14+ cells from healthy subjects carry a circular conformation of latent cytomegalovirus genome. Blood 1999;93:394–398.
7. Wright HTJ, Goodheart CR, Lielausis A. Human cytomegalovirus. Morphology by negative staining. Virology 1964;23:419–424.

8. Bresnahan WA, Shenk T. A subset of viral transcripts packaged within human cytomegalovirus particles. Science 2000;288:2373–2376.
9. Greijer AE, Dekkers CA, Middeldorp JM. Human cytomegalovirus virions differentially incorporate viral and host cell RNA during the assembly process. J Virol 2000;74:9078–9082.
10. Terhune SS, Schroer J, Shenk T. RNAs are packaged into human cytomegalovirus virions in proportion to their intracellular concentration. J Virol 2004;78:10390–10398.
11. Wang SW, Aldovini A. RNA incorporation is critical for retroviral particle integrity after cell membrane assembly of Gag complexes. J Virol 2002;76:11853–11865.
12. Fish KN, Soderberg-Naucler C, Mills LK, et al. Human cytomegalovirus persistently infects aortic endothelial cells. J Virol 1998;72:5661–5668.
13. Chee MS, Bankier AT, et al. Analysis of the protein-coding content of the sequence of human cytomegalovirus strain AD169. Curr Top Microbiol Immunol 1990;154:125–169.
14. Compton T. Receptors and immune sensors: the complex entry path of human cytomegalovirus. Trends Cell Biol 2004;14:5–8.
15. Pietropaolo RL, Compton T. Direct interaction between human cytomegalovirus glycoprotein B and cellular annexin II. J Virol 1997; 71:9803–9807.
16. Wright JF, Kurosky A, Wasi S. An endothelial cell-surface form of annexin II binds human cytomegalovirus. Biochem Biophys Res Commun 1994;198:983–989.
17. Compton T, Nowlin DM, Cooper NR. Initiation of human cytomegalovirus infection requires initial interaction with cell surface heparan sulfate. Virology 1993;193:834–841.
18. Boyle KA, Compton T. Receptor-binding properties of a soluble form of human cytomegalovirus glycoprotein B. J Virol 1998;72:1826–1833.
19. Wang X, Huong SM, Chiu ML, et al. Epidermal growth factor receptor is a cellular receptor for human cytomegalovirus. Nature 2003;424: 456–461.
20. Compton T, Kurt-Jones EA, Boehme KW, et al. Human cytomegalovirus activates inflammatory cytokine responses via CD14 and Toll-like receptor 2. J Virol 2003;77:4588–4596.
21. Keay S, Baldwin B. Anti-idiotype antibodies that mimic gp86 of human cytomegalovirus inhibit viral fusion but not attachment. J Virol 1991;65:5124–5128.
22. Huber MT, Compton T. Characterization of a novel third member of the human cytomegalovirus glycoprotein H–glycoprotein L complex. J Virol 1997;71:5391–5398.
23. Keay S, Merigan TC, Rasmussen L. Identification of cell surface receptors for the 86-kilodalton glycoprotein of human cytomegalovirus. Proc Natl Acad Sci USA 1989;86:10100–10103.
24. Keay S, Baldwin B. The human fibroblast receptor for gp86 of human cytomegalovirus is a phosphorylated glycoprotein. J Virol 1992;66: 4834–4838.
25. Boyle KA, Pietropaolo RL, Compton T. Engagement of the cellular receptor for glycoprotein B of human cytomegalovirus activates the interferon-responsive pathway. Mol Cell Biol 1999;19:3607–3613.
26. Keay S, Baldwin BR, Smith MW, Wasserman SS, Goldman WF. Increases in [Ca^{2+}]i mediated by the 92.5-kDa putative cell membrane receptor for HCMV gp86. Am J Physiol 1995;269:C11–C21.
27. Grundy JE, McKeating JA, Griffiths PD. Cytomegalovirus strain AD169 binds β_2 microglobulin in vitro after release from cells. J Gen Virol 1987;68:777–784.
28. Pizzorno MC, O'Hare P, Sha L, et al. Trans-activation and autoregulation of gene expression by the immediate-early region 2 gene products of human cytomegalovirus. J Virol 1988;62:1167–1179.
29. Stenberg RM, Depto AS, Fortney J, Nelson JA. Regulated expression of early and late RNAs and proteins from the human cytomegalovirus immediate-early gene region. J Virol 1989;63:2699–2708.
30. Malone CL, Vesole DH, Stinski MF. Transactivation of a human cytomegalovirus early promoter by gene products from the immediate-early gene IE2 and augmentation by IE1: mutational analysis of the viral proteins. J Virol 1990;64:1498–1506.
31. Kari B, Radeke R, Gehrz R. Processing of human cytomegalovirus envelope glycoproteins in and egress of cytomegalovirus from human astrocytoma cells. J Gen Virol 1992;73:253–260.
32. Kondo K, Kaneshima H, Mocarski ES. Human cytomegalovirus latent infection of granulocyte-macrophage progenitors. Proc Natl Acad Sci USA 1994;91:11879–11883.
33. Mendelson M, Monard S, Sissons P, Sinclair J. Detection of endogenous human cytomegalovirus in CD34+ bone marrow progenitors. J Gen Virol 1996;77:3099–3102.
34. Zhuravskaya T, Maciejewski JP, Netski DM, et al. Spread of human cytomegalovirus (HCMV) after infection of human hematopoietic progenitor cells: model of HCMV latency. Blood 1997;90:2482–2491.
35. Soderberg-Naucler C, Fish KN, Nelson JA. Reactivation of latent human cytomegalovirus by allogeneic stimulation of blood cells from healthy donors. Cell 1997;91:119–126.
36. Hahn G, Jores R, Mocarski ES. Cytomegalovirus remains latent in a common precursor of dendritic and myeloid cells. Proc Natl Acad Sci USA 1998;95:3937–3942.
37. Koffron AJ, Hummel M, Patterson BK, et al. Cellular localization of latent murine cytomegalovirus. J Virol 1998;72:95–103.
38. Slobedman B, Mocarski ES. Quantitative analysis of latent human cytomegalovirus. J Virol 1999;73:4806–4812.
39. Rickinson AB, Kieff E. Epstein-Barr virus. In Fields BN, Knipe DM, Howley PM, et al (eds). Fields Virology, 3rd ed. Philadelphia, Lippincott-Raven, 1996, pp 2397–2446.
40. Kondo K, Xu J, Mocarski ES. Human cytomegalovirus latent gene expression in granulocyte-macrophage progenitors in culture and in seropositive individuals. Proc Natl Acad Sci USA 1996;93:11137–11142.
41. Kondo K, Mocarski ES. Cytomegalovirus latency and latency-specific transcription in hematopoietic progenitors. Scand J Infect Dis Suppl 1995;99:63–67.
42. Adams A, Lindahl T. Epstein-Barr virus genomes with properties of circular DNA molecules in carrier cells. Proc Natl Acad Sci USA 1975; 72:1477–1481.
43. Gardella T, Medveczky P, Sairenji T, Mulder C. Detection of circular and linear herpesvirus DNA molecules in mammalian cells by gel electrophoresis. J Virol 1984;50:248–254.
44. Decker LL, Shankar P, Khan G, et al.The Kaposi sarcoma-associated herpesvirus (KSHV) is present as an intact latent genome in KS tissue but replicates in the peripheral blood mononuclear cells of KS patients. J Exp Med 1996;184:283–288.
45. Garcia-Blanco MA, Cullen BR. Molecular basis of latency in pathogenic human viruses. Science 1991;254:815–820.
46. Yu Y, Henry SC, Xu F, Hamilton JD. Expression of a murine cytomegalovirus early-late protein in "latently" infected mice. J Infect Dis 1995;172:371–379.
47. Jault FM, Jault JM, Ruchti F, et al. Cytomegalovirus infection induces high levels of cyclins, phosphorylated Rb, and p53, leading to cell cycle arrest. J Virol 1995;69:6697–6704.
48. Dittmer D, Mocarski ES. Human cytomegalovirus infection inhibits G_1/S transition. J Virol 1997;71:1629–1634.
49. Salvant BS, Fortunato EA, Spector DH. Cell cycle dysregulation by human cytomegalovirus: Influence of the cell cycle phase at the time of infection and effects on cyclin transcription. J Virol 1998;72:3729–3741.
50. Bresnahan WA, Boldogh I, Chi P, et al. Inhibition of cellular Cdk2 activity blocks human cytomegalovirus replication. Virology 1997;231: 239–247.
51. Poma EE, Kowalik TF, Zhu L, et al. The human cytomegalovirus IE1-72 protein interacts with the cellular p107 protein and relieves p107-mediated transcriptional repression of an E2F-responsive promoter. J Virol 1996;70:7867–7877.
52. Hengel H, Brune W, Koszinowski UH. Immune evasion by cytomegalovirus—survival strategies of a highly adapted opportunist. Trends Microbiol 1998;6:190–197.
53. Reddehase MJ. Antigens and immunoevasins: opponents in cytomegalovirus immune surveillance. Nature Rev Immunol 2002;2:831–844.
54. Goldmacher VS, Bartle LM, Skaletskaya A, et al. A cytomegalovirus-encoded mitochondria-localized inhibitor of apoptosis structurally unrelated to Bcl-2. Proc Natl Acad Sci USA 1999;96:12536–12541.
55. Fish KN, Britt W, Nelson JA. A novel mechanism for persistence of human cytomegalovirus in macrophages. J Virol 1996;70:1855–1862.
56. Emery VC, Cope AV, Bowen EF, Gor D, Griffiths PD. The dynamics of human cytomegalovirus replication in vivo. J Exp Med 1999;190: 177–182.
57. Hengel H, Reusch U, Geginat G, et al. Macrophages escape inhibition of major histocompatibility complex class I-dependent antigen presentation by cytomegalovirus. J Virol 2000;74:7861–7868.
58. Beersma MF, Bijlmakers MJ, Ploegh HL. Human cytomegalovirus down-regulates HLA class I expression by reducing the stability of class I H chains. J Immunol 1993;151:4455–4464.
59. Wiertz EJ, Mukherjee S, Ploegh HL. Viruses use stealth technology to escape from the host immune system. Mol Med Today 1997;3:116–123.
60. Riddell SR, Rabin M, Geballe AP, et al. Class I MHC-restricted cytotoxic T lymphocyte recognition of cells infected with human cytomegalovirus does not require endogenous viral gene expression. J Immunol 1991;146:2795–2804.
61. Riddell SR, Walter BA, Gilbert MJ, Greenberg PD. Selective reconstitution of CD8+ cytotoxic T lymphocyte responses in immunodeficient bone marrow transplant recipients by the adoptive transfer of T cell clones. Bone Marrow Transplant 1994;14:S78–S84.

62. Heise MT, Connick M, Virgin HW. Murine cytomegalovirus inhibits interferon gamma-induced antigen presentation to CD4 T cells by macrophages via regulation of expression of major histocompatibility complex class II-associated genes. J Exp Med 1998;187:1037–1046.
63. Hoglund P, Sundback J, Olsson-Alheim MY, et al. Host MHC class I gene control of NK-cell specificity in the mouse. Immunol Rev 1997; 155:11–28.
64. Farrell HE, Vally H, Lynch DM, et al. Inhibition of natural killer cells by a cytomegalovirus MHC class I homologue in vivo [see comments]. Nature 1997;386:510–514.
65. Dworsky ME, Welch K, Cassady G, Stagno S. Occupational risk for primary cytomegalovirus infection among pediatric health-care workers. NEJM 1983;309:950–953.
66. Stagno S, Cloud GA. Working parents: the impact of day care and breast-feeding on cytomegalovirus infections in offspring. Proc Natl Acad Sci USA 1994;91:2384–2389.
67. Zanghellini F, Boppana SB, Emery VC, et al. Asymptomatic primary cytomegalovirus infection: Virologic and immunologic features. J Infect Dis 1999;180:702–707.
68. Preiksaitis JK. The cytomegalovirus-"safe" blood product: Is leukoreduction equivalent to antibody screening? Transfus Med Rev 2000;14: 112–136.
69. Roback JD, Drew WL, Laycock ME, et al. CMV DNA is rarely detected in healthy blood donors using validated PCR assays [comment]. Transfusion 2003;43:314–321.
70. Adler SP. Transfusion-associated cytomegalovirus infections. Rev Infect Dis 1983;5:977–993.
71. Stagno S, Pass RF, Cloud G, et al. Primary cytomegalovirus infection in pregnancy. Incidence, transmission to fetus, and clinical outcome. JAMA 1986;256:1904–1908.
72. Britt WJ, Alford CA. Cytomegalovirus. In Fields BN, Knipe DM, Howley PM, et al (eds). Fields Virology, 3rd ed. Philadelphia, Lippincott-Raven, 1996, pp 2493–2523.
73. Stagno S, Pass RF, Dworsky ME, et al. Congenital cytomegalovirus infection: the relative importance of primary and recurrent maternal infection. NEJM 1982;306:945–949.
74. Alford CA, Stagno S, Pass RF, Britt WJ. Congenital and perinatal cytomegalovirus infections. Rev Infect Dis 1990;12(Suppl 7):S745–S753.
75. Reiser H, Kuhn J, Doerr HW, et al. Human cytomegalovirus replicates in primary human bone marrow cells. J Gen Virol 1986;67:2595–2604.
76. Maciejewski JP, Bruening EE, Donahue RE, et al. Infection of hematopoietic progenitor cells by human cytomegalovirus. Blood 1992;80:170–178.
77. von Laer D, Meyer-Koenig U, Serr A, et al. Detection of cytomegalovirus DNA in CD34+ cells from blood and bone marrow. Blood 1995;86: 4086–4090.
78. Sindre H, Tjoonnfjord GE, Rollag H, et al. Human cytomegalovirus suppression of and latency in early hematopoietic progenitor cells. Blood 1996;88:4526–4533.
79. Soderberg-Naucler C, Fish KN, Nelson JA. Interferon-γ and tumor necrosis factor-α specifically induce formation of cytomegalovirus-permissive monocyte-derived macrophages that are refractory to the antiviral activity of these cytokines. J Clin Invest 1997;100:3154–3163.
80. Gerna G, Zipeto D, Percivalle E, et al. Human cytomegalovirus infection of the major leukocyte subpopulations and evidence for initial viral replication in polymorphonuclear leukocytes from viremic patients. J Infect Dis 1992;166:1236–1244.
81. Revello MG, Percivalle E, Arbustini E, et al. In vitro generation of human cytomegalovirus pp65 antigenemia, viremia, and leukoDNAemia. J Clin Invest 1998;101:2686–2692.
82. Crapnell K, Zanjani ED, Chaudhuri A, et al. In vitro infection of megakaryocytes and their precursors by human cytomegalovirus. Blood 2000;95:487–493.
83. Drew WL, Tegtmeier G, Alter HJ, et al. Frequency and duration of plasma CMV viremia in seroconverting blood donors and recipients [comment]. Transfusion 2003;43:309–313.
84. Schaade L, Kockelkorn P, Ritter K, Kleines M. Detection of cytomegalovirus DNA in human specimens by LightCycler PCR. J Clin Microbiol 2000;38:4006–4009.
85. Stagno S, Reynolds DW, Tsiantos A, et al. Comparative serial virologic and serologic studies of symptomatic and subclinical congenitally and natally acquired cytomegalovirus infections. J Infect Dis 1975;132:568–577.
86. Gerna G, Zipeto D, Parea M, et al. Monitoring of human cytomegalovirus infections and ganciclovir treatment in heart transplant recipients by determination of viremia, antigenemia, and DNAemia. J Infect Dis 1991;164:488–498.
87. Cope AV, Sabin C, Burroughs A, et al. Interrelationships among quantity of human cytomegalovirus (HCMV) DNA in blood, donor-recipient serostatus, and administration of methylprednisolone as risk factors for HCMV disease following liver transplantation. J Infect Dis 1997; 176:1484–1490.
88. Spector SA, Wong R, Hsia K, et al. Plasma cytomegalovirus (CMV) DNA load predicts CMV disease and survival in AIDS patients. J Clin Invest 1998;101:497–502.
89. Gor D, Sabin C, Prentice HG, et al. Longitudinal fluctuations in cytomegalovirus load in bone marrow transplant patients: Relationship between peak virus load, donor/recipient serostatus, acute GVHD and CMV disease. Bone Marrow Transplant 1998;21:597–605.
90. Hassan-Walker AF, Kidd IM, Sabin C, et al. Quantity of human cytomegalovirus (CMV) DNAemia as a risk factor for CMV disease in renal allograft recipients: relationship with donor/recipient CMV serostatus, receipt of augmented methylprednisolone and antithymocyte globulin (ATG). J Med Virol 1999;58:182–187.
91. Cox F, Hughes WT. Cytomegaloviremia in children with acute lymphocytic leukemia. J Pediatr 1975;87:190–194.
92. Diosi P, Moldovan E, Tomescu N. Latent cytomegalovirus infection in blood donors. BMJ 1969;4:660–662.
93. Jordan MC. Latent infection and the elusive cytomegalovirus. Rev Infect Dis 1983;5:205–215.
94. Revello MG, Zavattoni M, Sarasini A, et al. Human cytomegalovirus in blood of immunocompetent persons during primary infection: prognostic implications for pregnancy. J Infect Dis 1998;177:1170–1175.
95. Tamura T, Chiba S, Chiba Y, Nakao T. Virus excretion and neutralizing antibody response in saliva in human cytomegalovirus infection. Infect Immun 1980;29:842–845.
96. Waner JL, Hopkins DR, Weller TH, Allred EN. Cervical excretion cytomegalovirus: correlation with secretory and humoral antibody. J Infect Dis 1977;136:805–809.
97. Yeager AS, Grumet FC, Hafleigh EB, et al. Prevention of transfusion-acquired cytomegalovirus infections in newborn infants. J Pediatr 1981;98:281–287.
98. Bass EB, Powe NR, Goodman SN, et al. Efficacy of immune globulin in preventing complications of bone marrow transplantation: a meta-analysis. Bone Marrow Transplant 1993;12:273–282.
99. Marshall GS, Rabalais GP, Stout GG, Waldeyer SL. Antibodies to recombinant-derived glycoprotein B after natural human cytomegalovirus infection correlate with neutralizing activity. J Infect Dis 1992;165:381–384.
100. Britt WJ, Vugler L, Butfiloski EJ, Stephens EB. Cell surface expression of human cytomegalovirus (HCMV) gp55–116 (gB): use of HCMV-recombinant vaccinia virus-infected cells in analysis of the human neutralizing antibody response. J Virol 1990;64:1079–1085.
101. Gonczol E, deTaisne C, Hirka G, et al. High expression of human cytomegalovirus (HCMV)-gB protein in cells infected with a vaccinia-gB recombinant: the importance of the gB protein in HCMV immunity. Vaccine 1991;9:631–637.
102. Quinnan GV, Kirmani N, Rook AH, et al. Cytotoxic T cells in cytomegalovirus infection: HLA-restricted T- lymphocyte and non-T-lymphocyte cytotoxic responses correlate with recovery from cytomegalovirus infection in bone-marrow-transplant recipients. NEJM 1982;307:7–13.
103. Quinnan GV, Burns WH, Kirmani N, et al. HLA-restricted cytotoxic T lymphocytes are an early immune response and important defense mechanism in cytomegalovirus infections. Rev Infect Dis 1984;6:156–163.
104. Reusser P, Riddell SR, Meyers JD, Greenberg PD. Cytotoxic T-lymphocyte response to cytomegalovirus after human allogeneic bone marrow transplantation: Pattern of recovery and correlation with cytomegalovirus infection and disease. Blood 1991;78:1373–1380.
105. Reusser P, Attenhofer R, Hebart H, et al. Cytomegalovirus-specific T-cell immunity in recipients of autologous peripheral blood stem cell or bone marrow transplants. Blood 1997;89:3873–3879.
106. Li CR, Greenberg PD, Gilbert MJ, et al. Recovery of HLA-restricted cytomegalovirus (CMV)-specific T-cell responses after allogeneic bone marrow transplant: correlation with CMV disease and effect of ganciclovir prophylaxis. Blood 1994;83:1971–1979.
107. Jonjic S, Mutter W, Weiland F, et al. Site-restricted persistent cytomegalovirus infection after selective long-term depletion of CD4+ T lymphocytes. J Exp Med 1989;169:1199–1212.
108. Steffens HP, Kurz S, Holtappels R, Reddehase MJ. Preemptive CD8 T-cell immunotherapy of acute cytomegalovirus infection prevents lethal disease, limits the burden of latent viral genomes, and reduces the risk of virus recurrence. J Virol 1998;72:1797–1804.
109. Orange JS, Wang B, Terhorst C, Biron CA. Requirement for natural killer cell-produced interferon γ in defense against murine cytomegalovirus infection and enhancement of this defense pathway by interleukin-12 administration. J Exp Med 1995;182:1045–1056.

110. Orange JS, Biron CA. Characterization of early IL-12, IFN-αβ, and TNF effects on antiviral state and NK cell responses during murine cytomegalovirus infection. J Immunol 1996;156:4746–4756.
111. Welsh RM, Brubaker JO, Vargas-Cortes M, O'Donnell CL. Natural killer (NK) cell response to virus infections in mice with severe combined immunodeficiency. The stimulation of NK cells and the NK cell-dependent control of virus infections occur independently of T and B cell function. J Exp Med 1991;173:1053–1063.
112. Presti RM, Pollock JL, Dal Canto AJ, et al. Interferon gamma regulates acute and latent murine cytomegalovirus infection and chronic disease of the great vessels. J Exp Med 1998;188:577–588.
113. Fennie EH, Lie YS, Low MA, et al. Reduced mortality in murine cytomegalovirus infected mice following prophylactic murine interferon-gamma treatment. Antiviral Res 1988;10:27–39.
114. Hengel H, Lucin P, Jonjic S, et al. Restoration of cytomegalovirus antigen presentation by gamma interferon combats viral escape. J Virol 1994;68:289–297.
115. Riddell SR, Greenberg PD. Principles for adoptive T cell therapy of human viral diseases. Annu Rev Immunol 1995;13:545–586.
116. Phipps PH, Gregoire L, Rossier E, Perry E. Comparison of five methods of cytomegalovirus antibody screening of blood donors. J Clin Microbiol 1983;18:1296–1300.
117. Adler SP, McVoy M, Biro VG, et al. Detection of cytomegalovirus antibody with latex agglutination. J Clin Microbiol 1985;22:68–70.
118. Beckwith DG, Halstead DC, Alpaugh K, et al. Comparison of a latex agglutination test with five other methods for determining the presence of antibody against cytomegalovirus. J Clin Microbiol 1985;21:328–331.
119. McHugh TM, Casavant CH, Wilber JC, Stites DP. Comparison of six methods for the detection of antibody to cytomegalovirus. J Clin Microbiol 1985;22:1014–1019.
120. Taswell HF, Reisner RK, Rabe DE, et al. Comparison of three methods for detecting antibody to cytomegalovirus. Transfusion 1986;26:285–289.
121. Gleaves CA, Smith TF, Shuster EA, Pearson GR. Comparison of standard tube and shell vial cell culture techniques for the detection of cytomegalovirus in clinical specimens. J Clin Microbiol 1985;21:217–221.
122. Brumback BG, Bolejack SN, Morris MV, et al. Comparison of culture and the antigenemia assay for detection of cytomegalovirus in blood specimens submitted to a reference laboratory. J Clin Microbiol 1997;35:1819–1821.
123. van der Bij W, Schirm J, Torensma R, et al. Comparison between viremia and antigenemia for detection of cytomegalovirus in blood. J Clin Microbiol 1988;26:2531–2535.
124. van der Bij W, van Son WJ, van der Berg AP, et al. Cytomegalovirus (CMV) antigenemia: rapid diagnosis and relationship with CMV-associated clinical syndromes in renal allograft recipients. Transplant Proc 1989;21:2061–2064.
125. van der Bij W, Torensma R, van Son WJ, et al. Rapid immunodiagnosis of active cytomegalovirus infection by monoclonal antibody staining of blood leucocytes. J Med Virol 1988;25:179–188.
126. Jiwa NM, Van Gemert GW, Raap AK, et al. Rapid detection of human cytomegalovirus DNA in peripheral blood leukocytes of viremic transplant recipients by the polymerase chain reaction. Transplantation 1989;48:72–76.
127. Cassol SA, Poon MC, Pal R, et al. Primer-mediated enzymatic amplification of cytomegalovirus (CMV) DNA. Application to the early diagnosis of CMV infection in marrow transplant recipients. J Clin Invest 1989;83:1109–1115.
128. Mazzulli T, Rubin RH, Ferraro MJ, et al. Cytomegalovirus antigenemia: clinical correlations in transplant recipients and in persons with AIDS. J Clin Microbiol 1993;31:2824–2827.
129. Tanabe K, Tokumoto T, Ishikawa N, et al. Comparative study of cytomegalovirus (CMV) antigenemia assay, polymerase chain reaction, serology, and shell vial assay in the early diagnosis and monitoring of CMV infection after renal transplantation. Transplantation 1997;64:1721–1725.
130. Nolte FS, Emmens RK, Thurmond C, et al. Early detection of human cytomegalovirus viremia in bone marrow transplant recipients by DNA amplification. J Clin Microbiol 1995;33:1263–1266.
131. Barber L, Egan JJ, Lomax J, et al. Comparative study of three PCR assays with antigenaemia and serology for the diagnosis of HCMV infection in thoracic transplant recipients. J Med Virol 1996;49:137–144.
132. Abecassis MM, Koffron AJ, Kaplan B, et al. The role of PCR in the diagnosis and management of CMV in solid organ recipients: what is the predictive value for the development of disease and should PCR be used to guide antiviral therapy? Transplantation 1997;63:275–279.
133. Ferreira-Gonzalez A, Fisher RA, Weymouth LA, et al. Clinical utility of a quantitative polymerase chain reaction for diagnosis of cytomegalovirus disease in solid organ transplant patients. Transplantation 1999;68:991–996.
134. Caliendo AM, St George K, Kao SY, et al. Comparison of quantitative cytomegalovirus (CMV) PCR in plasma and CMV antigenemia assay: clinical utility of the prototype AMPLICOR CMV MONITOR test in transplant recipients. J Clin Microbiol 2000;38:2122–2127.
135. Gerna G, Baldanti F, Lilleri D, et al. Human cytomegalovirus immediate-early mRNA detection by nucleic acid sequence-based amplification as a new parameter for preemptive therapy in bone marrow transplant recipients. J Clin Microbiol 2000;38:1845–1853.
136. Witt DJ, Kemper M, Stead A, et al. Analytical performance and clinical utility of a nucleic acid sequence-based amplification assay for detection of cytomegalovirus infection [In Process Citation]. J Clin Microbiol 2000;38:3994–2999.
137. Kreel I, Zaroff LI, Canter JW, et al. A syndrome following total body perfusion. Surg Gynecol Obstet 1960;111:317–321.
138. Smith D. A syndrome resembling infectious mononucleosis after open-heart surgery. BMJ 1964;1:945–948.
139. Klemola E, Kaariainen L. Cytomegalovirus as a possible cause of a disease resembling infectious mononucleosis. BMJ 1965;5470:1099–1102.
140. Kaariainen L, Klemola E, Paloheimo J. Rise of cytomegalovirus antibodies in an infectious-mononucleosis-like syndrome after transfusion. BMJ 1966;5498:1270–1272.
141. Lamb SG, Stern H. Cytomegalovirus mononucleosis with jaundice as presenting sign. Lancet 1966;2:1003–1006.
142. Nankervis GA, Kuman ML. Diseases produced by cytomegaloviruses. Med Clin North Am 1978;62:1021–1035.
143. Sandler SG, Grumet FC. Posttransfusion cytomegalovirus infections. Pediatrics 1982;69:650–653.
144. Tegtmeier GE. Transfusion-transmitted cytomegalovirus infections: Significance and control. Vox Sang 1986;51:22–30.
145. Sayers MH, Anderson KC, Goodnough LT, et al. Reducing the risk for transfusion-transmitted cytomegalovirus infection. Ann Intern Med 1992;116:55–62.
146. Hillyer CD, Emmens RK, Zago-Novaretti M, Berkman EM. Methods for the reduction of transfusion-transmitted cytomegalovirus infection: filtration versus the use of seronegative donor units. Transfusion 1994;34:929–934.
147. Roback JD. CMV and blood transfusions. Rev Med Virol 2002;12:211–219.
148. Tolpin MD, Stewart JA, Warren D, et al. Transfusion transmission of cytomegalovirus confirmed by restriction endonuclease analysis. J Pediatr 1985;107:953–956.
149. Stevens DP, Barker LF, Ketcham AS, Meyer HM Jr. Asymptomatic cytomegalovirus infection following blood transfusion in tumor surgery. JAMA 1970;211:1341–1344.
150. Adler SP, Baggett J, McVoy M. Transfusion-associated cytomegalovirus infections in seropositive cardiac surgery patients. Lancet 1985;2:743–747.
151. Huang ES, Huong SM, Tegtmeier GE, Alford C. Cytomegalovirus: Genetic variation of viral genomes. Ann NY Acad Sci 1980;354:332–346.
152. Adler SP, McVoy MM. Cytomegalovirus infections in seropositive patients after transfusion. The effect of red cell storage and volume. Transfusion 1989;29:667–671.
153. Prince AM, Szmuness W, Millian SJ, David DS. A serologic study of cytomegalovirus infections associated with blood transfusions. NEJM 1971;284:1125–1131.
154. Winston DJ, Ho WG, Howell CL, et al. Cytomegalovirus infections associated with leukocyte transfusions. Ann Intern Med 1980;93:671–675.
155. Wilhelm JA, Matter L, Schopfer K. The risk of transmitting cytomegalovirus to patients receiving blood transfusions. J Infect Dis 1986;154:169–171.
156. Preiksaitis JK, Brown L, McKenzie M. The risk of cytomegalovirus infection in seronegative transfusion recipients not receiving exogenous immunosuppression. J Infect Dis 1988;157:523–529.
157. Preiksaitis JK, Desai S, Vaudry W, et al. Transfusion- and community-acquired cytomegalovirus infection in children with malignant disease: a prospective study. Transfusion 1997;37:941–946.
158. Bowden RA, Sayers M, Flournoy N, et al. Cytomegalovirus immune globulin and seronegative blood products to prevent primary cytomegalovirus infection after marrow transplantation. NEJM 1986;314:1006–1010.
159. Bowden RA, Slichter SJ, Sayers MH, et al. Use of leukocyte-depleted platelets and cytomegalovirus-seronegative red blood cells for prevention of primary cytomegalovirus infection after marrow transplant. Blood 1991;78:246–250.
160. Miller WJ, McCullough J, Balfour HH Jr, et al. Prevention of cytomegalovirus infection following bone marrow transplantation:

a randomized trial of blood product screening. Bone Marrow Transplant 1991;7:227–234.
161. Lee PI, Chang MH, Hwu WL, et al. Transfusion-acquired cytomegalovirus infection in children in a hyperendemic area. J Med Virol 1992;36:49–53.
162. Hillyer CD, Lankford (Hillyer) KV, Roback JD, et al. Transfusion of the HIV-seropositive patient: immunomodulation, viral reactivation, and limiting exposure to EBV (HHV-4), CMV (HHV-5), and HHV-6, 7, and 8 [see comment]. Transfus Med Rev 1999;13:1–17.
163. Avery RK. Prevention and treatment of cytomegalovirus infection and disease in heart transplant recipients. Curr Opin Cardiol 1998;13: 122–129.
164. Applebaum FR, Meyers JD, Fefer A, et al. Nonbacterial nonfungal pneumonia following marrow transplantation in 100 identical twins. Transplantation 1982;33:265–268.
165. Santos GW, Hess AD, Vogelsang GB. Graft-versus-host reactions and disease. Immunol Rev 1985;88:169–192.
166. Wingard JR, Chen DY, Burns WH, et al. Cytomegalovirus infection after autologous bone marrow transplantation with comparison to infection after allogeneic bone marrow transplantation. Blood 1988;71:1432–1437.
167. Carlquist JF, Shelby J, Shao YL, et al. Accelerated rejection of murine cardiac allografts by murine cytomegalovirus-infected recipients. Lack of haplotype specificity. J Clin Invest 1993;91:2602–2608.
168. Evans PC, Soin A, Wreghitt TG, et al. An association between cytomegalovirus infection and chronic rejection after liver transplantation. Transplantation 2000;69:30–35.
169. George MJ, Snydman DR, Werner BG, et al. The independent role of cytomegalovirus as a risk factor for invasive fungal disease in orthotopic liver transplant recipients. Am J Med 1997;103:106–113.
170. Preiksaitis JK. Indications for the use of cytomegalovirus-seronegative blood products. Transfus Med Rev 1991;5:1–17.
171. de Cates CR, Roberton NR, Walker JR. Fatal acquired cytomegalovirus infection in a neonate with maternal antibody. J Infect 1988;17: 235–239.
172. Meyers JD, Flournoy N, Thomas ED. Risk factors for cytomegalovirus infection after human marrow transplantation. J Infect Dis 1986;153: 478–488.
173. Wingard JR, Piantadosi S, Burns WH, et al. Cytomegalovirus infections in bone marrow transplant recipients given intensive cytoreductive therapy. Rev Infect Dis 1990;12(Suppl 7):S793–S804.
174. Pillay D, Webster A, Prentice HG, Griffiths PD. Risk factors for viral reactivation following bone marrow transplantation. Ann Hematol 1992;64(Suppl):A148–A151.
175. Miller W, Flynn P, McCullough J, et al. Cytomegalovirus infection after bone marrow transplantation: an association with acute graft-v-host disease. Blood 1986;67:1162–1167.
176. Glenn J. Cytomegalovirus infections following renal transplantation. Rev Infect Dis 1981;3:1151–1178.
177. Chou SW. Acquisition of donor strains of cytomegalovirus by renal-transplant recipients. NEJM 1986;314:1418–1423.
178. Chou S, Kim DY, Norman DJ. Transmission of cytomegalovirus by pretransplant leukocyte transfusions in renal transplant candidates. J Infect Dis 1987;155:565–567.
179. Grundy JE, Lui SF, Super M, et al. Symptomatic cytomegalovirus infection in seropositive kidney recipients: reinfection with donor virus rather than reactivation of recipient virus. Lancet 1988;2:132–135.
180. Hillyer CD, Snydman DR, Berkman EM. The risk of cytomegalovirus infection in solid organ and bone marrow transplant recipients: transfusion of blood products. Transfusion 1990;30:659–666.
181. Kurtz JB, Thompson JF, Ting A, et al. The problem of cytomegalovirus infection in renal allograft recipients. Q J Med 1984;53:341–349.
182. Tegtmeier GE. Cytomegalovirus infection as a complication of blood transfusion. Semin Liver Dis 1986;6:82–95.
183. Adler SP. Data that suggest that FFP does not transmit CMV [letter]. Transfusion 1988;28:604.
184. Bowden R, Sayers M. The risk of transmitting cytomegalovirus infection by fresh frozen plasma. Transfusion 1990;30:762–763.
185. Hersman J, Meyers JD, Thomas ED, et al. The effect of granulocyte transfusions on the incidence of cytomegalovirus infection after allogeneic marrow transplantation. Ann Intern Med 1982;96:149–152.
186. Ho M. Epidemiology of cytomegalovirus infections. Rev Infect Dis 1990;12(Suppl 7):S701–S710.
187. Dworkin RJ, Drew WL, Miner RC, et al. Survival of cytomegalovirus in viremic blood under blood bank storage conditions. J Infect Dis 1990;161:1310–1311.
188. Tegtmeier GE. Posttransfusion cytomegalovirus infections. Arch Pathol Lab Med 1989;113:236–245.
189. Adler SP, Chandrika T, Lawrence L, Baggett J. Cytomegalovirus infections in neonates acquired by blood transfusions. Pediatr Infect Dis 1983;2:114–118.
190. Bowden RA, Slichter SJ, Sayers M, et al. A comparison of filtered leukocyte-reduced and cytomegalovirus (CMV) seronegative blood products for the prevention of transfusion-associated CMV infection after marrow transplant. Blood 1995;86:3598–3603.
191. Ibanez CE, Schrier R, Ghazal P, et al. Human cytomegalovirus productively infects primary differentiated macrophages. J Virol 1991; 65:6581–6588.
192. Lathey JL, Spector SA. Unrestricted replication of human cytomegalovirus in hydrocortisone-treated macrophages. J Virol 1991;65:6371–6375.
193. Rubin RH, Tolkoff-Rubin NE, Oliver D, et al. Multicenter seroepidemiologic study of the impact of cytomegalovirus infection on renal transplantation. Transplantation 1985;40:243–249.
194. Cheung KS, Lang DJ. Transmission and activation of cytomegalovirus with blood transfusion: a mouse model. J Infect Dis 1977;135:841–845.
195. Jordan CT, Saakadze N, Newman JL, et al. Photochemical treatment of platelet concentrates with amotosalen hydrochloride and ultraviolet A light inactivates free and latent cytomegalovirus in a murine transfusion model. Transfusion 2004;44:1159–1165.
196. Bowden RA, Sayers M, Gleaves CA, et al. Cytomegalovirus-seronegative blood components for the prevention of primary cytomegalovirus infection after marrow transplantation. Considerations for blood banks. Transfusion 1987;27:478–81.
197. Beneke JS, Tegtmeier GE, Alter HJ, et al. Relation of titers of antibodies to CMV in blood donors to the transmission of cytomegalovirus infection. J Infect Dis 1984;150:883–888.
198. Lamberson HV, McMillian JA, Weiner LB, et al. Prevention of transfusion-associated cytomegalovirus (CMV) infection in neonates by screening blood donors for IgM to CMV. J Infect Dis 1988;157:820–823.
199. Roback JD, Bray RA, Hillyer CD. Longitudinal monitoring of WBC subsets in packed RBC units after filtration: implications for transfusion transmission of infections. Transfusion 2000;40:500–506.
200. Sweeney JD, Holme S, Stromberg RR, Heaton WA. In vitro and in vivo effects of prestorage filtration of apheresis platelets. Transfusion 1995;35:125–130.
201. Verdonck LF, de Graan-Hentzen YC, Dekker AW, et al. Cytomegalovirus seronegative platelets and leukocyte-poor red blood cells from random donors can prevent primary cytomegalovirus infection after bone marrow transplantation. Bone Marrow Transplant 1987;2:73–78.
202. Gilbert GL, Hayes K, Hudson IL, James J. Prevention of transfusion-acquired cytomegalovirus infection in infants by blood filtration to remove leucocytes. Neonatal Cytomegalovirus Infection Study Group [see comments]. Lancet 1989;1:1228–1231.
203. de Graan-Hentzen YC, Gratama JW, Mudde GC, et al. Prevention of primary cytomegalovirus infection in patients with hematologic malignancies by intensive white cell depletion of blood products. Transfusion 1989;29:757–760.
204. De Witte T, Schattenberg A, Van Dijk BA, et al. Prevention of primary cytomegalovirus infection after allogeneic bone marrow transplantation by using leukocyte-poor random blood products from cytomegalovirus-unscreened blood-bank donors. Transplantation 1990;50:964–968.
205. Landaw EM, Kanter M, Petz LD. Safety of filtered leukocyte-reduced blood products for prevention of transfusion-associated cytomegalovirus infection (letter). Blood 1996;87:4910.
206. Bowden RA, Slichter S, Sayers M. Safety of filtered leukocyte-reduced blood products for prevention of transfusion-associated cytomegalovirus infection (response). Blood 1996;87:4910–4911.
207. Nichols WG, Price TH, Gooley T, et al. Transfusion-transmitted cytomegalovirus infection after receipt of leukoreduced blood products. Blood 2003;101:4195–4200.
208. Brady MT, Milam JD, Anderson DC, et al. Use of deglycerolized red blood cells to prevent posttransfusion infection with cytomegalovirus in neonates. J Infect Dis 1984;150:334–339.
209. Taylor BJ, Jacobs RF, Baker RL, et al. Frozen deglycerolyzed blood prevents transfusion-acquired cytomegalovirus infections in neonates. Pediatr Infect Dis 1986;5:188–191.
210. Luban NL, Williams AE, MacDonald MG, et al. Low incidence of acquired cytomegalovirus infection in neonates transfused with washed red blood cells. Am J Dis Child 1987;141:416–419.
211. Demmler GJ, Brady MT, Bijou H, et al. Posttransfusion cytomegalovirus infection in neonates: role of saline-washed red blood cells. J Pediatr 1986;108:762–765.
212. Condie RM, O'Reilly RJ. Prevention of cytomegalovirus infection by prophylaxis with an intravenous, hyperimmune, native, unmodified cytomegalovirus globulin. Randomized trial in bone marrow transplant recipients. Am J Med 1984;76:134–141.

213. Winston DJ, Ho WG, Lin CH, et al. Intravenous immune globulin for prevention of cytomegalovirus infection and interstitial pneumonia after bone marrow transplantation. Ann Intern Med 1987;106:12–18.
214. Meyers JD, Leszczynski J, Zaia JA, et al. Prevention of cytomegalovirus infection by cytomegalovirus immune globulin after marrow transplantation. Ann Intern Med 1983;98:442–446.
215. Goodrich JM, Mori M, Gleaves CA, et al. Early treatment with ganciclovir to prevent cytomegalovirus disease after allogeneic bone marrow transplantation. NEJM 1991;325:1601–1607.
216. Boeckh M, Gooley TA, Bowden RA. Effect of high-dose acyclovir on survival in allogeneic marrow transplant recipients who received ganciclovir at engraftment or for cytomegalovirus pp65 antigenemia. J Infect Dis 1998;178:1153–1157.
217. Goodrich JM, Bowden RA, Fisher L, et al. Ganciclovir prophylaxis to prevent cytomegalovirus disease after allogeneic marrow transplant. Ann Intern Med 1993;118:173–178.
218. Winston DJ, Ho WG, Bartoni K, et al. Ganciclovir prophylaxis of cytomegalovirus infection and disease in allogeneic bone marrow transplant recipients. Results of a placebo-controlled, double-blind trial. Ann Intern Med 1993;118:179–184.
219. Prentice HG, Kho P. Clinical strategies for the management of cytomegalovirus infection and disease in allogeneic bone marrow transplant. Bone Marrow Transplant 1997;19:135–142.
220. Broers AE, van Der Holt R, van Esser JW, et al. Increased transplant-related morbidity and mortality in CMV-seropositive patients despite highly effective prevention of CMV disease after allogeneic T-cell-depleted stem cell transplantation. Blood 2000;95:2240–2245.
221. Drew WL, Miner RC, Busch DF, et al. Prevalence of resistance in patients receiving ganciclovir for serious cytomegalovirus infection. J Infect Dis 1991;163:716–719.
222. Eckle T, Prix L, Jahn G, et al. Drug-resistant human cytomegalovirus infection in children after allogeneic stem cell transplantation may have different clinical outcomes. Blood 2000;96:3286–3289.
223. Erice A, Chou S, Biron KK, et al. Progressive disease due to ganciclovir-resistant cytomegalovirus in immunocompromised patients. NEJM 1989;320:289–293.
224. Stanier P, Taylor DL, Kitchen AD, et al. Persistence of cytomegalovirus in mononuclear cells in peripheral blood from blood donors [see comments]. BMJ 1989;299:897–898.
225. Bevan IS, Daw RA, Day PJ, et al. Polymerase chain reaction for detection of human cytomegalovirus infection in a blood donor population. Br J Haematol 1991;78:94–99.
226. Taylor-Wiedeman J, Sissons JG, Borysiewicz LK, Sinclair JH. Monocytes are a major site of persistence of human cytomegalovirus in peripheral blood mononuclear cells. J Gen Virol 1991;72:2059–2064.
227. Larsson S, Soderberg-Naucler C, Wang FZ, Moller E. Cytomegalovirus DNA can be detected in peripheral blood mononuclear cells from all seropositive and most seronegative healthy blood donors over time. Transfusion 1998;38:271–278.
228. Rowley AH, Wolinsky SM, Sambol SP, et al. Rapid detection of cytomegalovirus DNA and RNA in blood of renal transplant patients by in vitro enzymatic amplification. Transplantation 1991;51:1028–1033.
229. Bitsch A, Kirchner H, Dupke R, Bein G. Failure to detect human cytomegalovirus DNA in peripheral blood leukocytes of healthy blood donors by the polymerase chain reaction [see comments]. Transfusion 1992;32:612–617.
230. Smith KL, Kulski JK, Cobain T, Dunstan RA. Detection of cytomegalovirus in blood donors by the polymerase chain reaction. Transfusion 1993;33:497–503.
231. Roback JD, Hillyer CD, Drew WL, Laycock ME, et al. Multicenter evaluation of PCR methods for detecting CMV DNA in blood donors. Transfusion 2001;41:1249–1257.
232. Lin L, Wiesehahn GP, Morel PA, Corash L. Use of 8-methoxypsoralen and long-wavelength ultraviolet radiation for decontamination of platelet concentrates. Blood 1989;74:517–525.
233. Corash L, Lin L, Wiesehahn G. Use of 8-methoxypsoralen and long wavelength ultraviolet radiation for decontamination of platelet concentrates. Blood Cells 1992;18:57–74.
234. Corash L. Inactivation of viruses, bacteria, protozoa, and leukocytes in platelet concentrates: current research perspectives. Transfus Med Rev 1999;13:18–30.
235. Lin L, Londe H, Janda JM, et al. Photochemical inactivation of pathogenic bacteria in human platelet concentrates. Blood 1994;83:2698–2706.
236. Lin L. Inactivation of cytomegalovirus in platelet concentrates using Helinx technology. Semin Hematol 2001;38:27–33.
237. Lin L, Cook DN, Wiesehahn GP, et al. Photochemical inactivation of viruses and bacteria in platelet concentrates by use of a novel psoralen and long-wavelength ultraviolet light. Transfusion 1997;37:423–435.
238. Corash L. Pathogen reduction technology: methods, status of clinical trials, and future prospects. Curr Hematol Rep 2003;2:495–502.
239. Plotkin SA, Starr SE, Friedman HM, et al. Effect of Towne live virus vaccine on cytomegalovirus disease after renal transplant. A controlled trial [see comments]. Ann Intern Med 1991;114:525–531.
240. Storb R, Doney KC, Thomas ED, et al. Marrow transplantation with or without donor buffy coat cells for 65 transfused aplastic anemia patients. Blood 1982;59:236–246.
241. Kolb HJ, Mittermuller J, Clemm C, et al. Donor leukocyte transfusions for treatment of recurrent chronic myelogenous leukemia in marrow transplant patients. Blood 1990;76:2462–2465.
242. Papadopoulos EB, Ladanyi M, Emanuel D, et al. Infusions of donor leukocytes to treat Epstein-Barr virus-associated lymphoproliferative disorders after allogeneic bone marrow transplantation [see comments]. NEJM 1994;330:1185–1191.
243. Riddell SR, Watanabe KS, Goodrich JM, et al. Restoration of viral immunity in immunodeficient humans by the adoptive transfer of T cell clones [see comments]. Science 1992;257:238–241.
244. Walter EA, Greenberg PD, Gilbert MJ, et al. Reconstitution of cellular immunity against cytomegalovirus in recipients of allogeneic bone marrow by transfer of T-cell clones from the donor [see comments]. NEJM 1995;333:1038–1044.
245. Roback JD, Hossain MS, Lezhava L, et al. Allogeneic T-cells treated with amotosalen prevent lethal cytomegalovirus disease without producing graft-versus-host disease following bone marrow transplantation. J Immun 2003;171:6023–6031.
246. Smith DMJ. Leukocyte reduction for the prevention of transfusion-transmitted cytomegalovirus (TT-CMV). Bulletin #97–2. Bethesda, Md. American Association of Blood Banks, 1997, pp 10–11.
247. Zwicky C, Tissot JD, Mazouni ZT, et al. [Prevention of post-transfusion cytomegalovirus infection: recommendations for clinical practice]. Schweiz Med Wochenschr 1999;129:1061–1066.
248. Blajchman MA, Goldman M, Freedman JJ, Sher GD. Proceedings of a consensus conference: prevention of post-transfusion CMV in the era of universal leukoreduction. Transfus Med Rev 2001;15:1–20.
249. Griffin BE, Xue SA. Epstein-Barr virus infections and their association with human malignancies: some key questions. Ann Med 1998;30:249–259.
250. Thomas JA, Crawford DH, Burke M. Clinicopathologic implications of Epstein-Barr virus related B cell lymphoma in immunocompromised patients. J Clin Pathol 1995;48:287–290.
251. Reding R, Wallemacq PE, Lamy ME, et al. Conversion from cyclosporine to FK506 for salvage of immunocompromised pediatric liver allografts. Efficacy, toxicity, and dose regimen in 23 children. Transplantation 1994;57:93–100.
252. Sokal EM, Antunes H, Beguin C, et al. Early signs and risk factors for the increased incidence of Epstein-Barr virus-related posttransplant lymphoproliferative diseases in pediatric liver transplant recipients treated with tacrolimus. Transplantation 1997;64:1438–1442.
253. Green M, Cacciarelli TV, Mazariegos GV, et al. Serial measurement of Epstein-Barr viral load in peripheral blood in pediatric liver transplant recipients during treatment for posttransplant lymphoproliferative disease. Transplantation 1998;66:1641–1644.
254. McDiarmid S, Goss J, Seu P, et al. One hundred children treated with tacrolimus after primary orthotopic liver transplantation. Transplant Proc 1998;30:1397–1398.
255. Alfieri C, Tanner J, Carpentier L, et al. Epstein-Barr virus transmission from a blood donor to an organ transplant recipient with recovery of the same virus strain from the recipient's blood and oropharynx. Blood 1996;87:812–817.
256. Walsh JH, Gerber P, Purcell RH. Viral etiology of the postperfusion syndrome. Am Heart J 1970;80:146.
257. Salahuddin SZ, Ablashi DV, Markham PD, et al. Isolation of a new virus, HBLV, in patients with lymphoproliferative disorders. Science 1986;234:596–601.
258. Lawrence GL, Chee M, Craxton MA, et al. Human herpesvirus 6 is closely related to human cytomegalovirus. J Virol 1990;64:287–299.
259. Yamanishi K, Okuno T, Shiraki K, et al. Identification of human herpesvirus-6 as a causal agent for exanthem subitum [see comments]. Lancet 1988;1:1065–1067.
260. Farr TJ, Harnett GB, Pietroboni GR, Bucens MR. The distribution of antibodies to HHV-6 compared with other herpesviruses in young children. Epidemiol Infect 1990;105:603–607.
261. Braun DK, Dominguez G, Pellett PE. Human herpesvirus 6. Clin Microbiol Rev 1997;10:521–567.
262. Kadakia MP, Rybka WB, Stewart JA, et al. Human herpesvirus 6: Infection and disease following autologous and allogeneic bone marrow transplantation. Blood 1996;87:5341–5354.

263. Lau YL, Peiris M, Chan GC, et al. Primary human herpes virus 6 infection transmitted from donor to recipient through bone marrow infusion. Bone Marrow Transplant 1998;21:1063–1066.
264. Singh N, Carrigan DR. Human herpesvirus-6 in transplantation: an emerging pathogen. Ann Intern Med 1996;124:1065–1071.
265. Wang FZ, Dahl H, Linde A, et al. Lymphotropic herpesviruses in allogeneic bone marrow transplantation. Blood 1996;88:3615–3620.
266. Drobyski WR, Knox KK, Majewski D, Carrigan DR. Brief report: Fatal encephalitis due to variant B human herpesvirus-6 infection in a bone marrow-transplant recipient. NEJM 1994;330:1356–1360.
267. Ward KN, Gray JJ, Efstathiou S. Brief report: primary human herpesvirus 6 infection in a patient following liver transplantation from a seropositive donor. J Med Virol 1989;28:69–72.
268. Cuende JI, Ruiz J, Civeira MP, Prieto J. High prevalence of HHV-6 DNA in peripheral blood mononuclear cells of healthy individuals detected by nested-PCR. J Med Virol 1994;43:115–118.
269. Nicholas J. Determination and analysis of the complete nucleotide sequence of human herpesvirus. J Virol 1996;70:5975–5989.
270. Frenkel N, Schirmer EC, Wyatt LS, et al. Isolation of a new herpesvirus from human CD4+ T cells.7]. Proc Natl Acad Sci USA 1990;87: 748–752. Erratum in: 1990;87:7797.
271. Black JB, Burns DA, Goldsmith CS, et al. Biologic properties of human herpesvirus 7 strain SB. Virus Res 1997;52:25–41.
272. Black JB, Inoue N, Kite-Powell K, et al. Frequent isolation of human herpesvirus 7 from saliva. Virus Res 1993;29:91–98.
273. Tanaka K, Kondo T, Torigoe S, et al. Human herpesvirus 7: another causal agent for roseola (exanthem subitum). J Pediatr 1994;125:1–5.
274. Drago F, Ranieri E, Malaguti F, et al. Human herpesvirus 7 in patients with pityriasis rosea. Electron microscopy investigations and polymerase chain reaction in mononuclear cells, plasma and skin [see comments]. Dermatology 1997;195:374–378.
275. Drago F, Ranieri E, Malaguti F, et al. Human herpesvirus 7 in pityriasis rosea [letter]. Lancet 1997;349:1367–1368.
276. Wilborn F, Schmidt CA, Lorenz F, et al. Human herpesvirus type 7 in blood donors: detection by the polymerase chain reaction. J Med Virol 1995;47:65–69.
277. Chang Y, Cesarman E, Pessin MS, et al. Identification of herpesvirus-like DNA sequences in AIDS-associated Kaposi's sarcoma [see comments]. Science 1994;266:1865–1869.
278. Renne R, Lagunoff M, Zhong W, Ganem D. The size and conformation of Kaposi's sarcoma-associated herpesvirus (human herpesvirus 8) DNA in infected cells and virions. J Virol 1996;70:8151–8154.
279. Russo JJ, Bohenzky RA, Chien MC, et al. Nucleotide sequence of the Kaposi sarcoma-associated herpesvirus (HHV8). Proc Natl Acad Sci USA 1996;93:14862–14867.
280. Cesarman E, Chang Y, Moore PS, et al. Kaposi's sarcoma-associated herpesvirus-like DNA sequences in AIDS-related body-cavity-based lymphomas [see comments]. NEJM 1995;332:1186–1191.
281. Knowles DM, Cesarman E. The Kaposi's sarcoma-associated herpesvirus (human herpesvirus-8) in Kaposi's sarcoma, malignant lymphoma, and other diseases. Ann Oncol 1997;8:123–129.
282. Belec L, Mohamed AS, Authier FJ, et al. Human herpesvirus 8 infection in patients with POEMS syndrome-associated multicentric Castleman's disease. Blood 1999;93:3643–3653.
283. Berenson JR, Vescio RA. HHV-8 is present in multiple myeloma patients. Blood 1999;93:3157–3159.
284. Tarte K, Chang Y, Klein B. Kaposi's sarcoma-associated herpesvirus and multiple myeloma: lack of criteria for causality. Blood 1999;93: 3159–3164.
285. Kedes DH, Operskalski E, Busch M, et al. The seroepidemiology of human herpesvirus 8 (Kaposi's sarcoma-associated herpesvirus): distribution of infection in KS risk groups and evidence for sexual transmission [see comments] Nat Med 1996;2:918–924. Erratum in: 1996;2:1041.
286. Gao SJ, Kingsley L, Li M, et al. KSHV antibodies among Americans, Italians and Ugandans with and without Kaposi's sarcoma [see comments]. Nat Med 1996;2:925–928.
287. Simpson GR, Schulz TF, Whitby D, et al. Prevalence of Kaposi's sarcoma associated herpesvirus infection measured by antibodies to recombinant capsid protein and latent immunofluorescence antigen. Lancet 1996;348:1133–1138.
288. Chatlynne LG, Lapps W, Handy M, et al. Detection and titration of human herpesvirus-8-specific antibodies in sera from blood donors, acquired immunodeficiency syndrome patients, and Kaposi's sarcoma patients using a whole virus enzyme-linked immunosorbent assay. Blood 1998;92:53–58.
289. Lennette ET, Blackbourn DJ, Levy JA. Antibodies to human herpesvirus type 8 in the general population and in Kaposi's sarcoma patients [see comments]. Lancet 1996;348:858–861.
290. Regamey N, Tamm M, Wernli M, et al. Transmission of human herpesvirus 8 infection from renal-transplant donors to recipients [see comments]. NEJM 1998;339:1358–1363.
291. Whitby D, Howard MR, Tenant-Flowers M, et al. Detection of Kaposi sarcoma associated herpesvirus in peripheral blood of HIV-infected individuals and progression to Kaposi's sarcoma [see comments]. Lancet 1995;346:799–802.
292. Hudnall SD, Rady PL, Tyring SK, Fish JC. Serologic and molecular evidence of human herpesvirus 8 activation in renal transplant recipients. J Infect Dis 1998;178:1791–1794.
293. Belec L, Cancre N, Hallouin MC, et al. High prevalence in Central Africa of blood donors who are potentially infectious for human herpesvirus 8. Transfusion 1998;38:771–775.
294. De Milito A, Venturi G, Catucci M, et al. Lack of evidence of HHV-8 DNA in blood cells from heart transplant recipients. Blood 1997;89: 1837–1838.
295. Cannon MJ, Dollard SC, Smith DK, et al; for Group HIVERS. Blood-borne and sexual transmission of human herpesvirus 8 in women with or at risk for human immunodeficiency virus infection. NEJM 2001;344:637–643.
296. Mbulaiteye SM, Biggar RJ, Bakaki PM, et al. Human herpesvirus 8 infection and transfusion history in children with sickle-cell disease in Uganda. J Natl Cancer Inst 2003;95:1330–1335.
297. Dollard SC, Nelson KE, Ness PM, et al. Possible transmission of human herpesvirus-8 by blood transfusion in a historical United States cohort [see comment]. Transfusion 2005;45:500–503.

Chapter 47

Bacterial Infections: Bacterial Contamination, Testing, and Post-Transfusion Complications

Sandra M. Ramírez-Arcos • Mindy Goldman • Morris A. Blajchman

Bacterial contamination of blood components has been recognized as the oldest and most prevalent current transfusion-associated infectious risk.[1–3] Although the risk of acquiring transfusion-transmitted viral infections has decreased substantially over the past 20 years, cases of life-threatening reactions resulting from bacterial contamination continue to be reported.[2–8] Prospective studies have indicated that the range of clinical severity is very wide and that mild reactions are often misidentified as febrile nonhemolytic transfusion reactions.[3,9–16] Although severe reactions are relatively uncommon, bacterial contamination of blood products is currently the major microbiologic cause of transfusion-associated morbidity and mortality, with platelets being the blood product most susceptible to bacterial contaminants.[2,3] Because platelet components are stored at room temperature, they offer the most favorable medium for bacterial growth; thus, bacterial contamination has been the limiting factor in decreasing the permissible length of platelet storage. Although they are most common with platelet components, reactions associated with contaminated red blood cells (RBCs), plasma, cryoprecipitate, and albumin have also been reported.[2,17–20] Moreover, bacterial contamination remains one of the residual complications of autologous transfusions.[21–24]

Many methods have been developed to detect bacterial contamination in blood products, each with differing sensitivity and specificity. These methods range from simple visual inspection to sophisticated molecular methods.[25,26] Changes in every step of blood component preparation, from donor screening to phlebotomy procedures, pretransfusion bacterial detection, as well as improved component production and storage, have been proposed to decrease the frequency of bacterial contamination. In several countries, routine pretransfusion culture of platelets has been implemented, in some cases to permit extended storage of up to 7 days before transfusion.[3] Finally, methods of photochemical inactivation of bacteria are under active development, which may eliminate the problem of bacterial contamination in the future.[3,27,28]

PRESENTATION AND PREVALENCE

Red Blood Cells

Sepsis associated with the transfusion of bacterially contaminated RBCs is regarded as a very rare event, with a prevalence of significant clinical outcomes of 1 in 250,000.[3] This low prevalence is due to poor viability of most bacteria in whole blood or RBCs stored at 1°C to 6°C. However, psychrophilic pathogenic gram-negative bacteria such as *Yersinia enterocolitica* retain viability and replicate under RBC storage conditions. Infections caused by such bacteria are associated with a mortality rate of approximately 70%.[2,7,8,19] Septic reactions are characterized by temperatures higher than 38.5°C, rigors, and hypotension beginning during the transfusion. Nausea, vomiting, dyspnea, and diarrhea occur in a significant number of cases; septic shock, oliguria, and disseminated intravascular coagulation are also frequent complications.[29] Anesthetized patients may present with hypotension, oliguria, and excessive bleeding. The acute reactions are thought to be caused by the concomitant infusion of bacterial endotoxin followed by the massive release by the recipient of cytokines (e.g., tumor necrosis factor-α) that are important mediators of the pathogenesis of shock.[30,31] In most reported transfusion-associated septic reactions, the RBCs had been stored for longer than 21 days and therefore likely carried a high bacterial and endotoxin load.[29]

There have been few prospective studies examining the frequency of bacterial contamination in patients receiving RBC transfusions. In two consecutive studies done at the Dana Farber Cancer Institute, cultures of RBCs and recipients involved in transfusion reactions demonstrated a possible contamination rate of 1 in 38,465 units transfused, for a rate of 2.6 per 100,000 transfusions.[11,14]

Although RBCs are not routinely screened for bacterial contamination, bacterial testing of whole blood-derived platelets (WBDPs) increases the microbiologic safety of RBC components in an indirect way, because most RBC units associated with contaminated WBDP units will generally not be transfused. In some European countries, 100% of WBDP units are screened for bacterial contamination, resulting in a significant decrease in transfusion of contaminated units.[32] There is some evidence that approximately 40% of RBC and plasma units associated with bacterially contaminated WBDPs test positive when screened.[3]

Apheresis Platelets and Platelet Concentrates

Because platelets are stored at 22 ± 2°C, they provide a hospitable culture medium for a wide variety of bacteria; therefore, bacterial contamination poses *the* major microbiologic cause of adverse transfusion reactions to platelet components.

Clinical sequelae of transfusing bacterially contaminated platelets are variable and may be acute or delayed, depending on the severity of the recipient's medical condition, the type and concentration of the contaminant bacteria, and the timing of transfusion.[2] Because only the most severe reactions are likely to be recognized and reported, case reports represent the severe end of the clinical spectrum of transfusion reactions associated with bacterial contamination. Prospective studies demonstrate that the majority of recipients of contaminated platelet transfusions develop either no symptoms, or fever and chills with no clinical sequelae.[9,11–14] These reactions may be clinically indistinguishable from febrile nonhemolytic transfusion reactions.[33,34] Despite the introduction of routine bacteriologic screening, many platelet units are released into inventory and transfused without any reaction, and are then found to be contaminated.[3]

Reports on the prevalence of bacterial contamination in platelets are variable due to the use of different methods for bacterial detection. It is estimated that 1 in 1000 to 1 in 3000 platelet units are bacterially contaminated.[2,3,35] Clinical sepsis due to the transfusion of bacterially contaminated platelets occurs in approximately 1 in 25,000 transfusions, and a fatality is expected in approximately 1 in 60,000 transfusions.[3,35] Fatality rates vary in different countries, most likely due to the presence or absence of adequate hemoviligance systems and an environment of active reporting.

Fresh Frozen Plasma and Cryoprecipitate

Because plasma and plasma derivatives are stored frozen, they are less likely to contain clinically significant numbers of bacteria at the time of transfusion. However, there are reports of patients who developed wound infections, endocarditis, or septicemia several days after receiving cryoprecipitate or plasma that were thawed in bacterially contaminated water baths.[36,37] As indicated, approximately 40% of the co-components of contaminated platelet units, including plasma, have been also found to be contaminated.[3]

Peripheral Blood Stem Cells

It has been found that the incidence of bacterial contamination of untreated peripheral blood stem cells ranged from 0.23% to 4.5%, increasing by an additional 1% after cryopreservation.[1,38,39] The organisms usually implicated are part of the normal skin flora, including coagulase-negative staphylococci, *Propionibacterium acnes*, and α-hemolytic streptococci, although in some cases bacteria of potential clinical significance such as *Staphylococcus aureus* and *Enterobacter cloacae* can be isolated.[1,38,39] No adverse clinical sequelae from the infusion of culture-positive collections have been reported, probably because most recipients were receiving prophylactic antibiotic treatment at the time of the stem cell infusion.[38,39]

Determinants of Clinical Severity

The clinical consequences of transfusing bacterially contaminated blood components range from minimal or no reaction to fatal septic shock and death. The bacterial and recipient characteristics known to influence the clinical severity of a transfusion-associated infection include: the bacterial species present in the blood component, with gram-negative bacteria the cause of the most severe reactions due to endotoxin production; the concentration and growth rate of the bacterial contaminant; and recipient characteristics such as underlying disease, status of the immune system, and ongoing treatment with antimicrobial therapy.[29,35]

BACTERIA IMPLICATED

Red Blood Cell Concentrates

Yersinia enterocolitica is responsible for approximately 56% of the reported cases of RBC-associated sepsis, with a case-fatality rate of approximately 60%.[7,8,40–42] This pathogen is usually acquired by the ingestion of contaminated foods, producing mild symptoms such as abdominal pain and diarrhea. The frequency of *Y. enterocolitica*–associated RBC septic reactions varies markedly in different geographic locations and in different time periods. For example, the incidence of transfusion-transmitted *Yersinia* infections in New Zealand is 80 times higher than in other countries, including the United States.[1]

Because *Y. enterocolitica* lacks siderophores, growth is enhanced in an iron-rich environment such as stored RBCs. This has been noted particularly for *Y. enterocolitica* serotype O:3, whose growth rate is proportional to the availability of iron in the environment and which renders it the most common *Yersinia* pathogenic type.[1,43] Data from spiking experiments with *Y. enterocolitica* show that a lag phase of approximately 2 weeks is followed by exponential growth. A concentration of 10^9 organisms per millimeter is usually reached after 4 weeks of RBC storage, with a parallel rise in endotoxin level.[44]

A changing trend in the bacterial species that contaminate RBCs has been noted in the past few years.[2] Other RBC contaminant species include *Serratia* spp., *Pseudomonas* spp., *Enterobacter* spp., *Campylobacter* spp., and *Escherichia coli*, which also have the potential to cause endotoxic shock in recipients.[1] *Serratia liquefaciens* has been increasingly recognized as the cause of transfusion-associated sepsis with a high mortality rate.[2,45] *Pseudomonas aeruginosa* and other *Pseudomonas* spp. have also been involved in sepsis transmitted by RBC transfusions.[2,19,44] The plant pathogen *Pantoeae agglomerans* (previously known as *Enterobacter agglomerans*) has been implicated in two fatal post-transfusion sepsis cases.[47]

There have been four reports of septic shock related to the contamination of autologous RBC units; all four patients survived.[21–24] In retrospect, in the three cases involving *Y. enterocolitica*, the donors had experienced gastrointestinal symptoms in the days before or after their autologous donation.[21,22,24] In the one case involving *Serratia liquefaciens*, an infected toe ulcer may have been the source of a transient bacteremia at the time of the implicated autologous blood donation.[23]

Apheresis Platelets and Platelet Concentrates

In both case reports and prospective studies, the majority of organisms isolated in platelet-associated bacteremic episodes are part of the normal skin flora.[9–17] *Staphylococcus aureus*, coagulase-negative staphylococci, aerobic and anaerobic diphtheroid bacilli, streptococci, and gram-positive bacilli are the most frequently isolated organisms.[1] On rare occasions, gram-positive bacteria such as *Streptococcus bovis* that are neither part of the normal skin flora nor environmental contaminants have been implicated in infections resulting from transfused platelets.[48,49]

Although most fatal cases of the bacterial contamination of platelets involve gram-negative organisms,[2,3,20] fatalities due to transfusion of platelets contaminated with gram-positive bacteria have been reported in North America and in Europe. Coagulase-negative *Staphylococcus lugdunensis* was recently involved in a fatal bacterial infection associated with the transfusion of a platelet unit.[50] The U.S. Food and Drug Administration (FDA) reported that in the United States, from 1976 to 1998, 41% of the transfusion-associated septic fatalities were caused by gram-positive organisms, including 10% of the fatal outcomes caused by coagulase-negative staphylococci.[20] A combined summary of the data issued by the United Kingdom (UK) Serious Hazard of Transfusion (SHOT) hemoviligance program, the French BACTHEM study, and the U.S. Bacterial Contamination of blood (BaCon) study showed that 12% of fatalities were due to transfusion of platelets contaminated with gram-positive normal skin flora; 8% of these bacteria were coagulase-negative staphylococci.[20]

Transfused microorganisms have also been involved in delayed post-transfusion illnesses. Seven patients who received contaminated platelet units containing *Salmonella* did not develop symptoms until 5 to 12 days after transfusion. All units had been obtained from the same donor, who had an occult chronic osteomyelitis.[51] Although not always possible, bacterial infections caused by contaminated platelets can be discovered in retrospect. During the investigation of two sepsis cases due to RBCs contaminated with *S. liquefaciens*, it was discovered that the associated platelet units had also been the cause of fatal sepsis and bacteremia in the recipients.[45]

Fresh Frozen Plasma and Cryoprecipitate

Burkholderia cepacia (previously known as *P. cepacia*) and *Pseudomonas aeruginosa* are environmental organisms that grow optimally at 30°C. They have been isolated from cryoprecipitate and plasma thawed in contaminated water baths.[36,37] *Enterobacter cloacae* has also been implicated as a contaminant of human albumin that caused septicemia in two patients. Cracked glass bottles were the suspected cause of this contamination.[52]

INTRACELLULAR BACTERIA: RICKETTSIAS AND SPIROCHETES

Rickettsias such as *Rickettsia rickettsii*, *Ehrlichia equi* and *Ehrlichia chaffeensis*, and *Orientia tsutsugamushi* are obligate intracellular bacterial parasites transmitted by insects or ticks. These bacteria are the etiologic agents of Rocky Mountain spotted fever, ehrlichiosis, and scrub typhus, respectively, and may theoretically be transmitted by transfusion. However, there are no reports of adverse transfusion reactions in recipients who have received blood units from rickettsia-infected donors.[53,54] Similarly, recipients of blood components from donors subsequently diagnosed as having Lyme disease, which is caused by the tick-borne spirochete *Borrelia burgdorferi*, have not demonstrated any signs or symptoms of the disease.[55–61]

SOURCES OF CONTAMINATION

Possible mechanisms of blood component contamination, listed in Table 47–1, involve the blood donor, the collection procedure, the collection pack, and the various blood processing procedures. It is recognized that in most cases the source of the bacterial contamination cannot be determined.

Donor Bacteremia

Obviously, most bacteremic people are symptomatic and would not be accepted as blood donors. In many countries, including Canada and the United States, the donor temperature must be no higher than 37.5°C. However, donors in an asymptomatic incubation period or in the recovery phase from a bacterial-associated upper respiratory tract infection or gastroenteritis have been linked to episodes of bacterial contamination.[2,9,19] In cases of transfusion-

Table 47–1 Sources of Bacterial Contamination and Control Mechanisms

Source of Contamination	Implicated Bacteria (Reference)	Control Measures
Transient asymptomatic donor bacteremia	*Yersinia enterocolitica*[1,7,8,40–43] *Streptococcus bovis*[48,49] *Staphylococcus aureus*[3] *Salmonella enterica*[65] *Treponema pallidum*[19]	Donor screening Pretransfusion detection
Blood collection	*Staphylococcus epidermidis, Staphylococcus aureus*[2,3,20] *Clostridium perfringens*[6] *Enterobacter cloacae*[3,66,67] *Serratia marcescens*[66,67] *Pseudomonas fluorescens*[68]	Improved skin disinfection Initial aliquot diversion Increased collection of apheresis platelets
Collection packs	*Serratia marcescens*[2,69–72] *Burkholderia cepacia*[73] *Enterobacter cloacae*[55]	Improved quality control
Blood processing procedures	*Burkholderia cepacia, Pseudomonas aeruginosa*[36,37,59]	Improved quality control

associated *Y. enterocolitica* septicemia reported to the U.S. Centers for Disease Control and Prevention (CDC), approximately 75% of donors recalled having diarrhea in the days preceding or following their donation.[8,43] In addition, most of these donors had high antibody titers against *Y. enterocolitica* indicating a recent infection.[2,43] Gastrointestinal symptoms were also noted retrospectively in the *Y. enterocolitica* cases in autologous donors discussed previously.[21,22,24]

Streptococcus bovis can also be transiently present in the bloodstream of asymptomatic donors who have underlying colonic problems. Investigation of a fatal transfusion-associated reaction due to platelets contaminated with this organism revealed that the donor did not present with any symptom of illness at the time of donation; however, the donor had undergone removal of a benign colonic polyp 2 months before the donation.[48] Recently, a second case of an asymptomatic donor carrying *S. bovis* in her bloodstream was reported. It was subsequently found that the woman had a colonic adenocarcinoma, which was removed without complications.[49]

A Canadian case illustrates a *S. aureus* septicemia in a patient who had been transfused with a pool of five platelet units. The donor of one of these units felt ill 3 days after his blood donation and went into septic shock with blood cultures positive for *S. aureus*. Soon after the donor's admission to the hospital, a family member informed the attending physician that he had donated blood 4 days earlier. The *S. aureus* isolates from both the donor and the recipient were found to be identical on antibiotic sensitivity testing profiles and gene mapping, indicating that they were probably from the same source. Had the blood donor not presented with a septic episode subsequent to donation, the link between the fatal septicemia and the blood transfusion would not have been made in this recipient.[3]

Similarly, donors infected with *Treponema pallidum* can be asymptomatic and have a negative nonspecific serologic test for syphilis during periods of spirochetemia. The spirochete is inactivated after several days of storage at 4°C, but rare cases of transmission have been reported with blood stored for less than 24 hours.[19]

Isolated cases of bacterial contamination also have been linked to donors with intermittent, low-grade bacteremia associated with chronic infection or transient bacteremia after dental repair.[19,51]

Blood Collection

The majority of organisms isolated from contaminated platelet components are part of the normal skin flora and are thought to enter into the venesection needle during venipuncture.[19,62] Organisms such as *Staphylococcus epidermidis*, *S. aureus*, and *Bacillus* spp. are frequent contaminants in blood culture studies. It has been postulated that, despite adequate surface disinfection, viable bacteria remain in the deeper layers of the skin, especially skin associated with a scarred phlebotomy site.[19,63] It has also been shown that *S. aureus* and *S. epidermidis* can adhere firmly to human hair despite skin disinfection.[64]

The donor's skin may also be the source of unusual pathogens. A fatal platelet transfusion reaction due to *Clostridium perfringens* was linked to a donor who had frequently changed his children's diapers.[6] Arm swab cultures from this donor revealed the presence of *C. perfringens* and other bacteria that are normal components of fecal flora, such as *E. coli* and *Enterococcus faecalis*.

A rare case of a donor who had a pet boa was linked to two transfusion-associated sepsis events in recipients of platelets contaminated with *Salmonella enterica*. The same bacterium was isolated from the recipient's blood cultures, the platelet components, and a stool sample from the boa but not from the blood donor. It is possible that the bacterium was present on the donor's skin at the time of the platelet donations.[65]

Contaminated vacuum tubes used for specimen collection after donation and nonsterile intravenous solutions used during apheresis procedures were implicated in episodes of *Serratia marcescens* and *E. cloacae* sepsis, respectively.[66,67]

Unusual practices during collection could also result in the contamination of blood products. Chaffin[68] described how a cool cloth contaminated with *Pseudomonas fluorescens*, which was placed over the sterile gauze of a donor with low pain tolerance, led to heavy contamination of an RBC unit that was transfused, causing a near-fatal transfusion reaction.

Blood Bag and Container Damage or Defect

In June 1991, six patients in Denmark and Sweden developed *S. marcescens* septicemia after transfusion of RBCs (five patients) or platelets (one patient). At least five more cases with milder symptoms were subsequently diagnosed.[69,70] All of the episodes were related to blood bags produced in a plant in Belgium. The same ribotype of *S. marcescens* was isolated from each recipient, the implicated products, 0.3% to 1.5% of blood units collected during this time period, and the dust in the factory. It was hypothesized that *S. marcescens* had contaminated the exterior of the blood bags, which were put into a clean but not sterile outer plastic package. *S. marcescens* grows well at 4°C and 22°C, even under poor nutritional conditions, and may use the plasticizer leaking out of the blood bag as a carbon source. After massive contamination of the exterior of the blood bag, the bacteria probably entered the unit at the time of blood donation, either through suction into the needle or contamination of the phlebotomist's hands and subsequently of the donor's skin.[71] In 1995, the National Blood Authority in England withdrew 7000 blood bags because of faulty seals in some of the bags.[72] At least one case of post-transfusion *Serratia* septicemia may have been caused by the faulty bags.

In 1973, a cluster of cases of *B. cepacia* was traced to low-frequency contamination of a lot of albumin vials in the United States.[73] In 1996, several cases of *E. cloacae* septicemia in the United States were related to damage to albumin vials during transport in the manufacturing facility, which resulted in cracks. This led to the recall of 10 lots of albumin and 1 lot of factor VIII by the manufacturer.[52]

Blood Processing

Contamination of plasma or cryoprecipitate on thawing in heavily contaminated water baths has been reported to lead to *B. cepacia* or *P. aeruginosa* bacteremia, endocarditis, or mediastinal wound infection.[37,38,59] Contamination can occur as a result of microscopic cracks in the bags or entry of bath water into the packs at the time of pooling. Although bacterial contamination may theoretically occur during platelet pooling, cases of sepsis associated with platelet pool contaminations has always been traced to a constituent unit. Because of the short time frame between pooling and transfusion used in North America, the introduction of small numbers of bacteria most likely would be of little clinical consequence. However, if a sterile connecting device is used to weld tubing of platelet or RBC units before more lengthy storage, care must be taken to ensure that the connections are intact.

BACTERIOLOGIC SURVEILLANCE OF CELLULAR BLOOD PRODUCTS

Bacteriologic surveillance is part of hemovigilance in several countries. Surveillance may involve culturing of a certain number of products as part of quality assurance, culturing of platelet components as part of the routine donor testing, culturing of recipients and of the remaining blood products of all recipients who experience transfusion reactions, and reporting of such transfusion reactions to a central registry. Data obtained from studies conducted in several countries revealed that the current prevalence of bacterial contamination in platelets and RBCs is approximately 1 in 3000.[3]

In the United States, the BaCon study was conducted from 1998 to 2000 by the AABB, the American Red Cross, the CDC, and the Department of Defense. The results of this study revealed a sepsis rate of 1 in 100,000 for apheresis and whole blood–derived platelets and 1 in 5 million for RBCs. The fatality rate was 1 in 500,000 for platelets and 1 in 10 million for RBCs.[74] Because of very stringent case definitions and under-reporting, this study most likely underestimated the true frequency of septic reactions. From 2001 to 2003, 14.1% of transfusion-associated deaths reported to the FDA were due to bacterial contamination.[3]

French law requires the reporting of all transfusion reactions to the Agence Française du Sang.[75] Designated personnel in each hospital are responsible for submitting standardized reports, and the reactions are graded according to severity and possible etiology. Of the 12,058 moderate and severe reactions reported in 1996 and 1997, 405 (1.3%) were thought to be caused by bacterial contamination, as were 5 (15%) of the 33 fatal reactions for which transfusion-related causality could be clearly established. From 1994 to mid-1997, the estimated frequency of a bacteria-associated transfusion reaction was 1 in 60,000 transfused components, with 1 in 185,000 components resulting in a severe reaction and 1 in 700,000 resulting in a lethal reaction. Four reactions occurred in association with autologous RBC transfusions.[75,76] The French BACTHEM case-control study was started in 1996 to determine risk factors and sources of contamination in cases of transfusion reactions caused by bacteria.[77] This study documented a fatality rate of 1 in 140,000 due to transfusion of bacterially contaminated platelets.[78]

In the UK, the SHOT voluntary reporting system was initiated in late 1996 to compile reports of severe transfusion reactions.[79] The last SHOT report, issued in 2004, showed that from 1995 to 2003, 29 cases of bacterial infections and 7 deaths were due to the transfusion of bacterially contaminated blood products[80]; 25 platelet units and 4 RBC units were implicated in these reactions.

In Canada, 39 (11.3%) out of the 344 adverse transfusion reactions reported from April 2001 to December 2003 to The Transfusion Transmitted Injuries Surveillance System were deemed possibly due to bacterially contaminated blood products[81]; 15 units of RBCs, 18 platelet units, and 6 fresh frozen plasma units were implicated in these reactions. From 2001 to 2003, 4576 adverse transfusion reactions were reported to The Quebec Hemoviligance System[82]; 46 of these cases were deemed potentially due to bacterially contaminated blood products, although only 7 cases were confirmed (same bacterium isolated from the blood product and from blood of the recipient). Of the 7 confirmed cases, 5 involved platelets and 2 involved RBCs. One fatality was reported with one of the RBC units.

APPROACHES TO REDUCE TRANSFUSION-ASSOCIATED SEPTIC REACTIONS

Measures proposed to prevent transfusion-associated bacterial sepsis include donor screening, skin disinfection, initial aliquot diversion, and pretransfusion bacterial detection.

Donor Screening

Screening of donors to detect possible transient bacteremia is performed worldwide. Donors may be questioned about the occurrence of fevers as well as dental or medical procedures in the hours or days before donation. Retrospective questioning of donors of RBC units contaminated with *Y. enterocolitica* often reveals symptoms of gastroenteritis that occurred during the month preceding donation. However, several studies have demonstrated that the addition of questions about such symptoms would lead to unacceptable donor loss and the exclusion of many healthy blood donors.[28,83,84]

Donors who develop symptoms indicative of infection in the week after donation may be asked to notify the transfusion service. However, it has been shown that it is very likely that blood donors who develop these symptoms after donation are rarely infectious.[85] Donors may be asked about tick bites in areas where Lyme disease is endemic. However, because there have been no reported cases of Lyme disease transmission from asymptomatic donors, an AABB Advisory Group concluded that the addition of a specific question about tick bites was not necessary.[86]

Improved Skin Disinfection

Complete skin sterilization is not possible because bacteria residing in the sebaceous glands and hair follicles of the dermal connective tissue layer below the epidermis may be inaccessible to disinfectants.[2,20] Improvements in skin surface disinfection have, however, led to significantly lower blood product contamination rates. Factors affecting skin disinfection include the type and concentration of the antiseptic(s) applied, the use of single versus multiple antiseptics, one- or two-stage antiseptic application, the method of application (i.e., scrub, swab, ampule, applicator), the contact time between the antiseptic and the skin, and the expertise of the phlebotomist.[20] Data obtained from several studies suggest that superior disinfection results are associated with the use of a two-stage method, the use of a kit containing a sponge scrub followed by an ampule, and the use of tincture of iodine and alcohol instead of povidone-iodine.[20]

The AABB Technical Manual recommends the use of a two-stage method involving an initial 30-second scrub with a 0.7% iodophor solution followed by application of a 10% iodophor compound. The solution should be allowed to dry for 30 seconds after application. In Canada, a two-stage skin disinfection method has also been implemented involving a 70% isopropyl alcohol scrub followed by the application of a 2% iodine tincture solution.[20,87] Chlorhexidine or double isopropyl alcohol is used for blood donors who give a history of allergic reactions to iodine.[2,20] In the UK, skin surface cultures after donor arm disinfection are monitored as part of quality control.[88]

Diversion of the First Aliquot of Donor Blood

Bacteria that are part of normal skin flora may be introduced into the blood bag in association with a skin core that enters the collection needle at the time of venisection.[2,19,20,62] This possibility was first proposed in 1991 by Goldman and Blajchman.[19] The removal of the first 10 to 42 mL of donor blood has been shown to significantly decrease the bacterial load in the collection bag.[2,20] Several manufacturers have developed blood collection sets with a Y configuration that permit the diversion of up to 42 mL of blood. These sets are designed so that backflow into the main bag is prevented. Samples contained in the satellite bag are then used for blood grouping and infectious disease testing.[20] Initial aliquot diversion is used for all collections in several countries, including France, the Netherlands, and Canada, but it is not mandatory in the United States.

Pretransfusion Detection

The ideal test for the detection of bacteria in blood components does not currently exist. Several methods have been designed to detect bacterial contamination in blood products, including automated bacterial culture, visual inspection of platelets before issue, monitoring of alteration in metabolic parameters during storage, direct staining for bacteria, nucleic acid amplification testing for bacterial DNA, bacterial ribosomal assays, and endotoxin or peptidoglycan detection.[26] Table 47–2 summarizes the pretransfusion detection methods that are available; they can be used either soon after blood collection or just prior to a transfusion.

Because bacteria can replicate in blood components, bacterial detection is more complex than detection of other infectious agents, whose concentration does not increase after blood collection.[89] Several factors should be considered when selecting a bacterial screening method, including timing of the test (i.e., by the blood supplier or in the hospital before transfusion), the methodology to be used for sample collection, the volume of sample needed for testing, the time required to perform the test, and whether a quarantine time is necessary for the blood product while testing is being performed.[89]

Low bacterial concentrations soon after collection require a very sensitive screening method when testing is performed by the blood supplier. Although the minimum inoculum size necessary for bacterial proliferation varies in different studies with different organisms, for many strains a very small inoculum, such as 1 colony-forming unit (CFU)/mL, may be sufficient for bacterial growth. In platelet inoculation experiments, there is usually a lag phase, followed by exponential growth, to reach a maximum concentration of 10^8 to 10^9 CFU/mL on day 2 to day 5, depending on the organism.[90] Because of bacterial proliferation during storage, less sensitive methods may be used when screening is performed shortly before transfusion.

Screening Methods Used by Blood Suppliers

Two culture systems have been licensed in Europe and North America to detect bacterial contamination in platelets, the BacT/ALERT system and the Pall Bacterial Detection System. The Scansystem, a more rapid method using solid phase laser cytometry, has been approved for use both in Europe and the United States. Another more rapid method that has been approved for use in Europe is based on the use of dielectrophoresis.

BacT/ALERT System

The BacT/ALERT system uses liquid media with a sensor at the bottom of the culture bottles that changes color when CO_2 is produced as a result of bacterial growth. The bottles are inoculated with 4 to 10 mL of platelet samples, incubated at 37°C for 1 to 7 days, and are automatically examined every 10 minutes by computer software that records the color change in the sensor. This system is not completely closed because the bottles are inoculated with needles.[91] The BacT/ALERT system is highly sensitive, with levels of detection of 1 to 10 CFU/mL.[91–93] Table 47–3 shows the results of routine platelet screening by several blood suppliers in Europe and North America using this system.[3,94–100]

The BacT/ALERT system has been used for bacterial testing of both apheresis platelets and WBPD concentrates prepared by the buffy-coat method. However, detection of bacterial contamination in WBDPs produced by the platelet-rich plasma method is problematic because prestorage pooling of these platelets is not permitted in some countries (e.g., Canada), and culturing individual units is costly and signifi-

Table 47–2 Methods Used for Detection of Bacterial Contamination in Platelets

Time of Sampling	Method	Volume Used (mL)	Detection Time (hours)	Sensitivity (CFU/mL)	Specificity
Soon after blood collection	BacT/ALERT system	4–10	6–30	1–10	>90%
	Pall system	6	24–30	100–500	>90%
	Enhanced Pall system	6	24–30	1–5	>90%
	Scansystem	3	1–2	$>10^3$	>90%
	Dielectrophoresis		<1	10^3–10^5	UND
Prior to transfusion	Microscopic examination	<1	<1	$>10^6$	>90%
	Multireagent strip testing	1–2	Minutes	$>10^7$	Low
	Swirling	na	Seconds	10^7–10^8	Low

na, not applicable; UND, undetermined.

Table 47–3 Results of Routine Platelet Screening with the BacT/ALERT 3D System

Center/ Country	Plts*	Time of Testing (hr)†	Sample Volume (mL)	No. (rate) of Results Initial Positive	True Positive	False Positive‡	False Negative	Units Tested	Collection Period	Reference
American Red Cross, Washington, DC/US	A	>24		50 (1/1440)	13 (1/5538)	23 (1/3130)	unknown	72,000	Mar-May 2004	94
Puget Sound Blood Center, Seattle, WA/US	A	>24	4		5 (1/2000)	11 (1/909)	unknown	10,000	June 2003–	95
New York Blood Center, NY/US	A	24	4	15	5 (1/4981)	10 (1/2490)	unknown	24,909	Oct 2003– Apr 2004	96
American Red Cross, Dedham, MA/US	A	>24			1 (1/6255)	5 (1/1245)	unknown	6,225	Mar and Apr 2004	97
Community Blood Center, Kansas City, MO/US	A	24	4		2 (1/3657)	4 (1/1828)	unknown	7,315	Sep 2003– Apr 2004	98
Red-Cross Flanders/Belgium	A	22	7	237 (1/135)	181 (1/176)	41 (1/780)	1 (1/31,998)	31,998	1999–2002	3
	B	22	7	793 (1/95)	622 (1/121)	140 (1/541)		75,829	1999–2002	3
Copenhagen Blood Transfusion Service Center/ Denmark	B	§	8–10	50 (1/443)	34 (1/651)	16 (1/1385)	‖	22,165	Jan 2002 –2004	3
Sanquin Blood Bank/The Netherlands	B	16–24	7.5		295 (1/131)		2 (1/19,332)	38,664	Oct 2001– Apr 2004	3
Department of Immunology and Transfusion Medicine/Norway	B	24	5–10	88 (1/419)	12 (1/3074)	14 (1/2635)	#	36,896	May 1998– May 2004	100
Héma Québec/ Canada	A	>24	4–6	11 (1/1213)	3 (1/4450)	8 (1/1668)	1 (1/13,351)	13,351	2002–Aug 2004	99
Canadian Blood Services (CBS)/Canada	A	>24	4–6	28 (1/843)		28 (1/843)	1 (1/23,617)	23,617	Mar 2004– May 2005	CBS database

*Plt, platelets; A, apheresis platelets; B, buffy coat-derived platelets.
†Time of testing after blood collection.
‡False-positive cultures include cultures that were not confirmed on reculture and false signals of the BacT/ALERT system.
§ Immediately after platelet production.
‖ Screening of 2472 buffy-coat platelets on day 3 of storage revealed 6 false negatives (1/412).[3]
Screening of 1061 outdated platelets yielded 2 false negatives (1/531).[100]

cantly reduces the platelet unit content. The Hong Kong Red Cross developed a pooled culture method that involves stripping of five platelet segments, which are disinfected before collecting a sample of pooled platelets that is inoculated into a BacT/ALERT culture bottle.[101,102] This method was modified, validated, and adopted by one Canadian Blood Services Center.[103] An adaptation to the Hong Kong method using sterile docking has also been reported.[104] Similarly, the BacT/ALERT system has been validated for the detection of bacteria in WBDPs in a pooled format by Brecher and colleagues.[92]

Because the initial inoculum of bacteria is probably very small (<10 microorganisms/mL), even a very sensitive technique will miss some contaminated units. This has been demonstrated by several reports of false-negative results in platelet units tested by the BacT/ALERT system, including one case each of *Salmonella* and *S. marcescens* in Canada, a case of *S. lugdunensis* in the United States,[50] and two cases of *Bacillus cereus* in the Netherlands,[105] all of which resulted in severe or fatal reactions.

To evaluate the incidence of false negatives using the BacT/ALERT system, the Copenhagen Blood Transfusion Service Center conducted a trial with 946 buffy-coat–derived platelet units. Bacterial cultures were performed immediately after platelet production and repeated after 7 or more days of storage. This study reported that 0.63% of units that were negative on initial culture were positive during the later second screening, most of them contaminated with coagulase-negative staphylococci.[3] A similar study was conducted in Norway, from 2002 to 2004. Two out of 1061 outdated platelets were contaminated with *Bacillus* spp. and *S. epidermidis,* which were missed in the initial bacterial cultures.[100] Likewise, during the implementation of bacterial testing of pooled platelets at the Hong Kong Red Cross, it was shown that BacT/ALERT cultures missed initial positive cultures in units contaminated with *P. acnes* and coagulase-negative staphylococci.[102] These studies demonstrate that the BacT/ALERT system may not be sufficiently sensitive to pick up low levels of bacterial contamination.

Most centers are routinely testing for aerobic bacteria, because the majority of clinically significant organisms belong to this group. However, there are reports of transfusion reactions due to the presence of *P. acnes*.[32] It is also true that some bacteria commonly found as platelet contaminants (e.g., some *Streptococcus* spp.) can grow better in anaerobic culture media. The question of whether it is worthwhile to also implement anaerobic bacterial cultures is subject to ongoing debate.

Recently, the FDA cleared Gambro BCT's apheresis platelet technology for routine storage and transfusion for up to 7 days when bacterial testing is done using the BacT/ALERT system as a release test. Based on a pilot study that was conducted from March to October 2004, a standardized sampling and testing protocol has been described by Gambro BCT. To implement transfusion of 7-day platelets, blood centers need to follow the optimized protocol and obtain proper FDA approvals to use the BacT/ALERT system as a release test.[106] This approach will likely reduce platelet outdating, ensuring a more adequate platelet supply. It has been shown that platelets stored for up to 7 days retain acceptable in vitro functionality.[107] In vivo effectiveness of these platelets has also been demonstrated in an autologous transfusion model using healthy volunteers.

The Pall Bacterial Detection System (BDS)

This culture method uses the decrease in oxygen concentration as an indicator of bacterial growth in platelets. Approximately 6 mL of platelet samples are passed through the filter of this closed system to remove remaining leukocytes and platelets and allow 50% of bacteria to pass with the plasma into an incubation bag. After 24 to 30 hours of incubation, the oxygen concentration of this bag is measured with an oximeter. A decrease in the percent of oxygen to 19.5% or less is indicative of bacterial growth.[91] This system detects gram-positive and gram-negative bacteria at the levels of 100 to 500 CFU/mL with a sensitivity of 96.5%.[108] Recently, an enhanced Pall detection system (eBDS) has been developed, which does not have the platelet-retaining filter, allowing for improved bacterial recovery and sensitivity.[109]

The U.S. Blood Centers of the Pacific have implemented bacterial detection of platelets using the Pall BDS system. Out of 15,823 screened units, 1 containing coagulase-negative staphylococci was missed by this system and transfused, causing a moderate febrile transfusion reaction in the recipient.[110]

The Pall eBDS system has also been validated for bacterial detection in leukoreduced RBCs. In a study of this system, 270 RBC units were spiked with eight bacteria to final concentrations of 10 and 100 CFU/mL before storage at 4°C for up to 6 weeks. Samples were taken weekly and evaluated by the Pall system. The only bacterium that exponentially increased in concentration over the 6-week period of this study was *Y. enterocolitica*. *P. aeruginosa* and *S. epidermidis* did not increase in concentration but survived at a constant concentration during the whole study. The other bacterial species studied slowly decreased over the course of the study. Nonetheless, the results of this study suggest that the Pall eBDS system may be suitable for bacterial detection in RBCs.[111]

Scansystem

The Scansystem method involves testing a leukoreduced platelet sample that is mixed with a solution containing both a platelet aggregation agent and a DNA labeling dye. After 40 minutes of incubation, the mixture is passed through a filter that retains the aggregated platelets. The flowthrough solution containing bacteria is then further incubated for 20 minutes before filtration through a 0.4-μm black membrane that captures the fluorescently labeled bacteria. The black membrane is then placed on the analyzer (solid phase cytometer), which uses a laser light to detect any fluorescent signals. Positive signals on the membrane are manually confirmed using a microscope. Results are obtained within 90 minutes of sample processing.[91,112,113] The Scansystem has been used for the bacterial screening of platelets at the Belgium Red Cross (La Louvière Blood Center, Belgium) since March 2005, at the Kuwait City Blood Bank since June 2005, and at the German Red Cross (Munster Blood Bank, Munster, Germany) since 2004 (Agnès Bouyé, Marketing Director, HEMOSYSTEM, personal communication).

The Scansystem has been recently modified for bacterial detection in RBCs. This method involves the agglutination and removal of RBCs from the sample followed by bacteria labeling and final recovery on a black membrane for analysis using the cytometer. The entire test can also be completed in 90 minutes and has been shown to be very sensitive for detecting gram-positive and gram-negative bacteria at levels of 1 to 10 CFU/mL.[114]

Dielectrophoresis

Dielectrophoresis is based on the observation that cells placed in nonuniform electric fields move toward electrodes, as determined by their dielectric properties. Bacteria are released from the electrodes when the electric field is discontinued. Levels of bacteria detected by this system vary between 10^3 and 10^5 CFU/mL.[91]

Screening Methods for Use Prior to Transfusion

The number of bacteria in blood components associated with severe transfusion reactions is usually greater than 10^6 CFU/mL. Therefore, a less sensitive technique may be adequate to detect clinically significant contamination in the hospital transfusion service immediately before transfusion. However, such a test would have to be rapid to avoid delaying product issue. Also, it should not require specialized equipment or specially trained personnel. In addition, the test should be specific to avoid blood wastage or delays in product issue. Unfortunately, screening methods currently used shortly before transfusion are typically subjective, nonsensitive, and/or complex and time consuming.

Microscopic Examination

Microscopic observation of platelet smears using Gram staining, acridine orange, or fluorophores usually yield positive results at bacterial concentrations greater than 10^6 CFU/mL.[91] However, such methods require specific reagents, complex equipment, and/or skilled personnel. Because some hospital laboratories have Wright staining equipment, they can perform an initial identification of bacterial contamination, which can be followed by Gram classification.[91]

Multireagent Strip Testing

Because most bacteria metabolize glucose, thereby producing acid that causes a decrease in pH, diminished pH and glucose levels can be expected in platelet units contaminated with bacteria. Several studies have investigated the use of multireagent strips for the rapid detection of decreased pH and glucose levels as indicators of bacterial contamination in platelets. The sensitivity of this method is very low, with levels of detection on the order of 10^7 to 10^8 CFU/mL of bacteria. Because the tested parameters may change due to multiple factors (e.g., presence of certain anticoagulants, increase in pH after glucose exhaustion), a major disadvantage of this method is its low specificity, which may result in platelet wasting.[91] The use of a pH meter to measure pH has also proven to be inaccurate, with many false positives causing product wasting, especially in units with high WBC and platelet content.[115]

Visual Examination

Bacterial proliferation in RBC units causes decreased oxygen and glucose concentrations, which in turn leads to RBC hemolysis. Darkening of RBC units due to hemolysis has been used as a screening method for bacterial contamination, although sensitivity is relatively poor.

Due to their discoid morphology, platelets reflect light and produce a "streaming" phenomenon (swirling). Bacterial contamination of platelets causes a decrease in pH, resulting in the loss of the swirling effect. Swirling loss is nonspecific, because it is often associated with conditions other than the presence of bacteria.

These visual inspection methods are very subjective and have very low sensitivity, which means that low levels of clinically significant bacteria would usually be missed. The low specificity of these techniques is also problematic; it has been reported that RBCs and platelets that are close to the end of their shelf life present darkening and decreased swirling, respectively, in spite of not being contaminated with bacteria.[91]

Screening Methods under Development

Several systems for the detection of bacterial contaminants in blood components are under development. Due to their high rapidity, sensitivity, and specificity, molecular methods such as nonamplified chemiluminiscence-linked rRNA probes or PCR-based methods[89] are very attractive. However, bacterial contamination of laboratory reagents and materials, as well as common bacterial sequences found in human blood, complicate the use of these techniques. Recent studies have shown promising results using reverse transcriptase PCR methods that minimize the risk of amplifying genetic material from dead bacterial cells.[116,117]

Rapid-detection systems that are under development include the BUG's BEADS system, which uses magnetic beads coupled with PCR; an enzyme immunoassay to detect peptidoglycan; and an immunoassay developed by Verax Biomedical. All of these systems have a sensitivity of greater than 10^3 CFU/mL.[2,118]

One important factor to consider when optimizing molecular techniques is that due to their complexity, it would be difficult to implement such technology in a wide range of blood centers or transfusion services.

Limitation of Component Storage

Most severe septic transfusion reactions occur with RBCs stored for longer than 21 days and platelet concentrates stored for longer than 3 days. In 1986, the FDA reduced the platelet storage time from 7 to 5 days because of concern about the increasing number of case reports of platelet-associated sepsis occurring with concentrates transfused after 5, 6, or 7 days of storage.[119]

Apheresis Platelets versus Random Platelet Concentrates

Apheresis platelets have a lower risk of being contaminated than pooled platelets since they are collected from a single donor. A 12-year prospective study conducted by Ness and Campbell-Lee[120] showed that the incidence of septic platelet transfusion reactions decreased from 1 in 4818 to 1 in 15,098 when the use of single-donor apheresis platelets increased from 51.7% to 99.4% in their institution. The authors also observed that the rate of septic reactions was five times higher in recipients of pooled platelets than in recipients of single-donor platelets. These septic events were clinically serious; 4 out of 23 cases (17.4%) were fatal.

Leukocyte Reduction

Phagocytes may be important in the elimination of viable bacteria present in blood components during the first few hours after venipuncture.[121] In the case of organisms such as *Y. enterocolitica*, the bacteria may already be present in the phagocytes in the donor's blood; with bacteria introduced from the donor's skin, phagocytosis may occur during initial storage, particularly if there is a room temperature hold for several hours before refrigeration. Bacteria may then either be released back into the blood component as the leukocytes disintegrate during storage, or they may be eliminated by prestorage leukodepletion. Several spiking experiments have demonstrated reduced bacterial growth of *Y. enterocolitica* in contaminated RBC units that were leukoreduced in the hours after controlled contamination.[122,123] Data on the efficacy of leukoreduction in preventing growth of other bacterial strains in RBC or platelet concentrates have been less conclusive.[122]

Temperature and Time of Storage before Component Preparation

There is marked variability among countries with regard to the time and temperature of whole blood storage before component preparation. Time and temperature of storage may influence bacterial growth, extent of phagocytosis, and the occurrence of complement-mediated killing. The few studies done on this subject have come to varying conclusions, possibly because of confounding variables such as differences in component preparation methods and leukoreduction.[124–126]

Lowering Component Storage Temperature

Platelet storage at room temperature maintains platelet hemostatic efficacy, but this temperature provides a hospitable culture medium for many bacteria. The development of various storage solutions that putatively permit retention of platelet function at 4°C could considerably decrease bacterial growth in platelets. For example, glycolysation of platelets with uridine diphosphate-galactose prior to chilling prevents platelet early sequestration, a typical drawback of cold-stored platelets.[127] Another recent approach was the addition of a solution of trehalose and phosphate to platelets, which experimentally appears to be effective in protecting platelet structure and function during cryopreservation.[128] Investigators have also found that the proliferation of *Y. enterocolitica* in RBCs may be decreased by storage at 0°C.[129] This interesting approach needs further evaluation.

Water Bath Disinfection

Water baths used for thawing plasma and cryoprecipitate should be emptied and disinfected weekly, to prevent the heavy growth of organisms such as *B. cepacia* and *P. aeruginosa.* Plasma and cryoprecipitate units should also be kept dry during thawing by use of a plastic overwrap.[59]

Photochemical Treatment (PCT) to Achieve Pathogen Inactivation

The best studied methodology for pathogen inactivation of platelets is use of the combination of the psoralen amotosalen HCl with long-wavelength ultraviolet light (UVA).[130] After being subjected to large phase III clinical trials in Europe and the United States, the commercial product based on this methodology, INTERCEPT Blood System for Platelets, has been introduced on a limited scale in some blood centers in Europe (Belgium, Italy, Norway, Portugal, Spain, and Sweden).[3]

Another PCT methodology combines riboflavin and UVA illumination. Using a light dose of 6.2 J/mL, this method can inactivate from 4 to 6 logs of *S. epidermidis* and *E. coli* without disrupting in vitro platelet functionality.[27] This process has not yet been studied in randomized, controlled clinical trials.

In addition to the inactivation of bacteria, both of these PCT approaches have been shown to inactivate other blood-borne pathogens in platelet concentrates, making these systems potentially very attractive to ensure blood safety. Nevertheless, before the worldwide implementation of a pathogen inactivation method, it has to be shown to be safe, efficacious, and cost effective.[3,27,28]

PREFERRED APPROACH

Hospital Transfusion Service

A high index of suspicion is necessary to correctly diagnose a transfusion-associated septic reaction. If a septic reaction is suspected, the blood product transfusion should be stopped and an intravenous line for venous access should be left in place. The blood bag should be returned to the blood bank and inspected for evidence of color change, hemolysis, clots, or bag defects. A Gram stain should be done on the remaining blood component, although this test may be negative in one third of cases due to insensitivity of the technique. Aerobic and anaerobic cultures of the remaining product should also be performed. Nutrient broth may be introduced into the blood bag if very little product remains for culture. Blood cultures also should be taken from the recipient. Symptoms are often nonspecific, so, in the case of a severe reaction, serologic investigation to rule out an acute hemolytic reaction due to an immunologic incompatibility should also be done.

For patients suspected of having a transfusion-associated septic reaction, broad-spectrum antibiotic coverage should be initiated even before culture results are obtained. Aggressive supportive care with intravenous fluids and vasopressors may be necessary if septic shock occurs.

Ideally, the diagnosis is firmly established when the same organism is isolated from both the blood component and the patient. In some studies, microbial identity has been determined with the use of antibiotic susceptibility tests and fingerprinting methods. Laboratory diagnosis can be difficult, because cultures from a recipient who is taking antibiotics may be negative, and cultures of the remaining blood component may be positive due to post-transfusion contamination. The detection of an unusual pathogen in a transfusion recipient should prompt a search for a possible contaminated blood component. Clustering of cases of septicemia with unusual organisms should initiate a search for contaminated blood components or another iatrogenic cause (e.g., contaminated saline solutions). Finally, the blood supplier should be informed as soon as possible about the suspected transfusion-associated septic reaction.

The AABB issued a document in February 2005 to alert clinicians of the risk of septic transfusion reactions due to bacterially contaminated platelet units.[131] This document outlines procedures for the management of patients receiving platelet transfusions and the management of donors referred for follow-up after a donated platelet unit has been found positive for bacterial contamination. In all cases, the AABB urges that clinicians collaborate with hospital transfusion service, blood collection center, and health department when notification is necessary. It is important to note that a survey of infectious diseases consultants, conducted by the Infectious Diseases Society of America in 2004, showed that only 36% of respondents were aware of transfusion-associated septic reactions.[50] It is therefore essential that clinicians are educated to recognize, notify, and appropriately manage patients suspected of receiving blood components with bacterial contamination.

Blood Supplier

When informed of a possible septic transfusion reaction, the transfusion service should recall and culture the other components from the same donation. If a defect is found in the bag or a cluster of cases has been reported, quarantine and investigation of other products from the same lot may be necessary. In the case of an organism that is not part of the normal skin flora, the donor should be contacted and asked about the development of infections before or shortly after blood donation.

In October 2004, the AABB issued Bulletin No.04–07 to provide guidelines for the follow-up of initial positive tests for possible bacterially contaminated platelet units.[132] This document strongly recommends that all blood centers have standardized definitions when referring to the bacterial testing of platelets. Similarly, AABB bulletin No.05–02 was issued in January 2005 as guidance for managing platelet donors with positive or abnormal results on bacterial detection testing.[133] According to this bulletin, donor notification of an initially positive result is indicated if the donor is suspected to be infected with pathogenic bacteria. Donor referral should be based on medical judgment once confirmatory results are obtained and the microorganism identified is considered to be dangerous for either the donor and/or the recipient.

Transfusion services should encourage the hospitals they serve to report septic transfusion reactions, and they in turn should report such reactions to national registries. Estimates of the frequency of such reactions are an important part of transfusion medicine hemovigilance, in order to continue to improve the safety of the blood supply.

REFERENCES

1. Yomtovian R, Palavecino E. Bacterial contamination of blood components—history and epidemiology. In Brecher ME (ed). Bacterial and Parasitic Contamination of Blood Components. Bethesda, Md., American Association of Blood Banks, 2003, pp 1–30.
2. Brecher ME, Hay SN. Bacterial contamination of blood components. Clin Microbiol Rev 2005;18:195–204.
3. Blajchman MA, Beckers EAM, Dickmeiss E, et al. Bacterial detection of platelets: Current problems and possible resolutions. Transfus Med Rev 2005;19:259–272.
4. Kleinman S, Chan P, Robillard P. Risks associated with transfusion of cellular blood components in Canada. Transfus Med Rev 2003;17: 120–162.
5. Boulton FE, Chapman ST, Walsh TH. Fatal reaction to transfusion of red-cell concentrate contaminated with *Serratia liquefaciens.* Transfus Med 1998;8:15–18.
6. McDonald CP, Hartley S, Orchard K, et al. Fatal *Clostridium perfringens* sepsis from a pooled platelet transfusion. Transfus Med 1998;8:19–22.
7. Theakston EP, Morris AJ, Streat SJ, et al. Transfusion-transmitted *Yersinia enterocolitica* infection in New Zealand. Aust NZ J Med 1997;127:62–67.
8. Centers for Disease Control and Prevention. Red blood cell transfusions contaminated with *Yersinia enterocolitica*—United States, 1991–1996, and initiation of a national study to detect bacteria-associated transfusion reactions. MMWR Morb Mortal Wkly Rep 1997;46:553–555.
9. Morrow JF, Braine HG, Kickler TS, et al. Septic reactions to platelet transfusions. JAMA 1991;266:555–558.
10. Blajchman MA, Ali AM. Bacteria in the blood supply: an overlooked issue in transfusion medicine. In Nance SJ (ed). Blood Safety: Current Challenges. Bethesda, Md., American Association of Blood Banks, 1992, pp 213–228.
11. Barrett BB, Anderson JW, Anderson KC. Strategies for the avoidance of bacterial contamination of blood components. Transfusion 1993;33:228–233.
12. Yomtovian R, Lazarus HM, Goodnough LT, et al. A prospective microbiologic surveillance program to detect and prevent the transfusion of bacterially contaminated platelets. Transfusion 1993;33:902–909.
13. Chiu EKW, Yuen KY, Lie AKW, et al. A prospective study on symptomatic bacteremia from platelet transfusion and its management. Transfusion 1994;34:950–965.
14. Dzieczkowski JS, Barrett BB, Nester D, et al. Characterization of reactions after exclusive transfusion of white cell-reduced cellular blood components. Transfusion 1995;35:20–25.
15. Blajchman MA, Ali A, Lyn P, et al. A prospective study to determine the frequency of bacterial contamination in random donor platelet concentrates [Abstract]. Blood 1994;84S:529a.
16. Leiby DA, Kerr KL, Compos JM, et al. A prospective analysis of microbial contaminants in outdated random-donor platelets from multiple sites. Transfusion 1997;37:259–263.
17. Blajchman MA, Ali A, Lyn P, et al. Bacterial surveillance of platelet concentrates: Quantitation of bacterial load [Abstract]. Transfusion 1997;37(Suppl):74S.
18. Liu H, Yuen K, Cheng T, et al. Reduction of platelet transfusion-associated sepsis by short-term bacterial culture. Vox Sang 1999;77:1–5.
19. Goldman M, Blajchman MA. Blood product-associated bacterial sepsis. Transfus Med Rev 1991;5:73–83.
20. Goldman M, Lee J-H, Blajchman M. Skin antisepsis and initial aliquot diversion. In Brecher ME (ed). Bacterial and Parasitic Contamination of Blood Components. Bethesda, Md., American Association of Blood Banks, 2003, pp 31–56.
21. Richards C, Kolins J, Trindale CD. Autologous transfusion-transmitted *Yersinia enterocolitica* [Letter]. JAMA 1992;268:1541–1542.
22. Sire JM, Michelet C, Mesnard R, et al. Septic shock due to *Yersinia enterocolitica* after autologous transfusion [Letter]. Clin Infect Dis 1993;17:954–955.
23. Duncan KL, Ransley J, Elterman M. Transfusion-transmitted *Serratia liquefaciens* from an autologous blood unit [Letter]. Transfusion 1994;34:738–739.
24. Haditsch M, Binder L, Gabriel C, et al. *Yersinia enterocolitica* septicemia in autologous blood transfusion. Transfusion 1994;34:907–909.
25. Mitchell KMT, Brecher ME. Approaches to the detection of bacterial contamination in cellular blood products. Transfus Med Rev 1999;13:132–144.
26. Blajchman MA, Goldman M, Baeza F. Improving the bacteriological safety of platelet transfusions. Transfus Med Rev 2004;18:11–24.
27. Perez-Pujol A, Tonda R, Lozano B et al. Effects of a new pathogen-reduction technology (Mirasol PRT) on functional aspects of platelet concentrates. Transfusion 2005;45:911–919.
28. Allain JP, Bianco C, Blajchman MA et al. Protecting the blood supply from emerging pathogens: the role of pathogen inactivation. Transfus Med Rev 2005;19:110–126.
29. Goldman M, Blajchman MA. Bacterial contamination. In Popovsky M (ed). Transfusion Reactions, 2nd ed. Bethesda, Md., American Association of Blood Banks, 2001, pp 129–154.
30. McAllister SK, Bland LA, Arduino MJ, et al. Patient cytokine response in transfusion-associated sepsis. Infect Immun 1994;62:2126–2128.
31. Schwalbe B, Späth-Schwalbe E. Endotoxin concentrations and cytokine responses in a patient with fatal transfusion-associated sepsis [Letter]. Transfusion 1998;38:703–705.
32. de Korte D. Implementation of a screening system for bacterial detection. In Brecher ME (ed). Bacterial and Parasitic Contamination of Blood Components. Bethesda, Md., American Association of Blood Banks, 2003, pp 83–105.
33. Olsen KE, Sandler SG. Febrile neutropenia contributes to underreporting of potential septic platelet transfusion reactions [Letter]. Vox Sang 1996;70:118.
34. Zaza S, Tokars JI, Yomtovian R, et al. Bacterial contamination of platelets at a university hospital: Increased identification due to intensified surveillance. Infect Control Hosp Epidemiol 1994;15:82–87.
35. Hillyer CD, Josephson CD, Blajchman MA, et al. Bacterial contamination of blood components: Risks, strategies, and regulation. Joint ASH and AABB educational session in transfusion medicine. Hematology 2003:575–589.
36. Rhame FS, McCullough J. Follow-up on nosocomial *Pseudomonas cepacia* infection. MMWR Morb Mortal Wkly Rep 1979;28:409.
37. Casewell MW, Slater NGP, Cooper JE. Operating theatre water-baths as a cause of *Pseudomonas* septicaemia. J Hosp Infect 1981;2:237–240.
38. Attarian H, Bensinger WI, Buckner CD, et al. Microbial contamination of peripheral blood stem cell collections. Bone Marrow Transplant 1996;17:699–702.
39. Kamble R, Pant S, Selby GB, et al. Microbial contamination of hematopoietic progenitor cell grafts-incidence, clinical outcome, and cost-effectiveness: an analysis of 735 grafts. Transfusion 2005;45:874–878.
40. Aber RC. Transfusion-associated *Yersinia enterocolitica.* Transfusion 1990;30:193–195.
41. Mitchell R, Barr A. Transfusing *Yersinia enterocolitica* [Letter]. BMJ 1992;305:1095–1096.
42. Beresford AM. Transfusion reaction due to *Yersinia enterocolitica* and review of other reported cases. Pathology 1995;27:133–135.
43. Leclercq A, Martin L, Vergnes ML, et al. Fatal *Yersinia enterocolitica* biotype 4 serovar O:3 sepsis after red blood cell transfusion. Transfusion 2005;45:814–818.
44. Arduino MJ, Bland LA, Tipple MA, et al. Growth and endotoxin production of *Yersinia enterocolitica* and *Enterobacter agglomerans* in packed erythrocytes. J Clin Microbiol 1989;27:1483–1485.
45. Roth VR, Arduino MJ, Nobiletti SC, et al. Transfusion-related sepsis due to *Serratia liquefaciens* in the United States. Transfusion 2000;40: 931–935.
46. Shimbun Y. 80 likely contracted diseases via tainted blood since April. The Daily Yomiuri. Available at http://www.yomiuri.co.jp/newse/20040812wo32.htm. Accessed Sept. 30, 2005.
47. Benfell C. Unusual bacteria blamed for blood transfusion death. Circulator 2004;Fall:2. Available at http://chapters.redcross.org/ca/norcal/phys/pdf/Circulator_Oct2004.pdf. Accessed Sept. 30, 2005.
48. Chang AH, Kirsch CM, Mobashery N, et al. *Streptococcus bovis* septic shock due to contaminated transfused platelets. Am J Hematol 2004;77:282–286.
49. Haimowitz MD, Hernandez LA, Herron RM Jr. A blood donor with bacteremia. Lancet 2005;365:1596.
50. Arendt A, Carmean J, Koch E, et al. Fatal bacteria infections associated with platelet transfusions—United States, 2004. MMWR Morb Mortal Wkly Rep 2005;54:168–170.
51. Rhame FS, Root RK, MacLowry JD, et al. *Salmonella* septicemia from platelet transfusions: study of an outbreak traced to a hematogeneous carrier of *Salmonella choleraesius.* Ann Intern Med 1973;78:633–641.
52. Wang SA, Tokars JI, Bianchine PJ, et al. *Enterobacter cloacae* bloodstream infections traced to contaminated human albumin. Clin Infect Dis 2000;30:35–40.
53. Arguin PM, Singleton J, Rotz LD et al. An investigation into the possibility of transmission of tick-borne pathogens via blood transfusion. Transfusion 1999;39:828–833.

54. Casleton BG, Salata K, Dasch GA, et al. Recovery and viability of *Orientia tsutsugamushi* from packed red cells and the danger of acquiring scrub typhus from blood transfusion. Transfusion 1998;38:680–689.
55. Badon SJ, Fister RD, Cable RG. Survival of *Borrelia burgdorferi* in blood products. Transfusion 1989;29:581–583.
56. Goodman JL, Bradley JF, Ross AE, et al. Bloodstream invasion in early Lyme disease: Results from a prospective, controlled, blinded study using the polymerase chain reaction. Am J Med 1995;99:6–12.
57. Aoki SK, Holland PV. Lyme disease: another transfusion risk? Transfusion 1989;29:646–650.
58. Centers for Disease Control and Prevention. Lyme disease—United States, 1996. MMWR Morb Mortal Wkly Rep 1997;46:531–535.
59. Halkier-Sorensen L, Kragballe K, Nedergaard St, et al. Lack of transmission of *Borrelia burgdorferi* by blood transfusion [Letter]. Lancet 1990;1:550.
60. Cable R, Krause P, Badon S, et al. Acute blood donor co-infection with *Babesia microti* [Abstract]. Transfusion 1993;33(Suppl):50S.
61. Gerber MA, Shapiro ED, Krause PJ, et al. The risk of acquiring Lyme disease or babesiosis from a blood transfusion. J Infect Dis 1994;170:231–234.
62. Gibson T, Norris W. Skin fragments removed by injection needles. Lancet 1958;2:983–985.
63. Anderson KC, Lew MA, Gorgone BC, et al. Transfusion-related sepsis after prolonged platelet storage. Am J Med 1986;81:405–411.
64. Mase K, Hasegawa T, Horii T, et al. Firm adherence of *Staphylococcus aureus* and *Staphylococcus epidermidis* to human hair and effect of detergent treatment. Microbiol Immunol 2000;44:653–656.
65. Jafari M, Forsberg J, Gilcher RO, et al. *Salmonella* sepsis caused by a platelet transfusion from a donor with a pet snake. NEJM 2002; 347:1075–1078.
66. Blajchman MA, Thornley JH, Richardson H, et al. Platelet transfusion-induced *Serratia marcescens* sepsis due to vacuum tube contamination. Transfusion 1979;19:39–44.
67. Kosmin M. Bacteremia during leukapheresis [Letter]. Transfusion 1980;20:115.
68. Chaffin DJ. *Pseudomonas fluorescens*-related septic transfusion reaction resulting from contaminated cold cloths. [Abstract]. Transfusion 2002;42(Suppl):41S.
69. Heltberg O, Skov F, Gerner-Smidt P, et al. Nosocomial epidemic of *Serratia marcescens* septicemia ascribed to contaminated blood transfusion bags. Transfusion 1993;33:221–227.
70. Högman CF, Fritz H, Sandberg L. Posttransfusion *Serratia marcescens* septicemia [Editorial]. Transfusion 1993;33:189–191.
71. Högman CF, Engstrand L. Serious bacterial complications from blood components: How do they occur? Transfus Med 1998;8:1–3.
72. Dyer O. Blood authority investigates faulty blood bags. BMJ 1995;311:145.
73. Steere AC, Terrey JH, Mackel DC, et al. *Pseudomonas* species bacteremia caused by contaminated normal human serum albumin. J Infect Dis 1977;135:729–735.
74. Kuehnert MJ, Roth VR, Haley NR, et al. Transfusion-transmitted bacterial infection in the United States, 1998 through 2000. Transfusion 2001;41:1493–1499.
75. Noel L, Debeir J, Cosson A. The French haemovigilance system. Vox Sang 1998;74(Suppl 2):441–445.
76. Perez P, Ngombet R, Debeir J, et al. Les incidents transfusionnels par contamination bactérienne: synthèse de la littérature et des données d'hémovigilance. Transfus Clin Biol 1998;5:203–210.
77. Noël L, Audurier A. Contaminations bactériennes des produits sanguins labiles [Abstract]. Transfus Clin Biol 1998;5(Suppl 1):256S.
78. Perez P, Salmi LR, Follea G, et al. Determinants of transfusion-associated bacterial contamination: results of the French BACTHEM case-control study. Transfusion 2001;41:862–871.
79. Williamson LW, Love EM. Reporting serious hazards of transfusion: The SHOT program. Transfus Med Rev 1998;12:28–35.
80. Serious Hazards of Transfusion (SHOT). Summary of annual report 2003. Available at http://www.shotuk.org/SHOT%20Report%202003.pdf. Accessed Sept. 30, 2005.
81. MacDonald N.Transfusion and risk infection in Canada: Update 2005. Paediatr Child Health 2005;10:149–153.
82. Robillard P, Nawej KI. Four-year trends in the incidence of bacterial contaminations in the Quebec hemovigilance system. [Abstract]. Transfusion 2004;44(Suppl):19A.
83. Grossman BJ, Kollins P, Lau PM, et al. Screening blood donors for gastrointestinal illness: a strategy to eliminate carriers of *Yersinia enterocolitica*. Transfusion 1991;31:500–501.
84. Ness PM, Perkins HA. Transient bacteremia after dental procedures and other minor manipulations. Transfusion 1980;20:82–85.
85. Goldman M, Long A, Roy G, et al. Incidence of positive bacterial cultures after donor call-back [Letter]. Transfusion 1996;36:1035.
86. AABB News Briefs 1989;12:1–4.
87. Goldman M, Roy G, Fréchette N, et al. Evaluation of donor skin disinfection methods. Transfusion 1997;37:309–312.
88. Kitchen AD, Howe PHJ. Donor arm swabbing: how clean is clean? [Abstract]. Transfus Med 1995;5(Suppl):50.
89. Goldman M. Challenges in developing a bacterial detection system. Vox Sang 2002;83(Suppl 1):125–127.
90. Wagner SJ, Moroff G, Katz AJ, Friedman LI. Comparison of bacteria growth in single and pooled platelet concentrates after deliberate inoculation and storage. Transfusion 1995;35:298–302.
91. Brumit MC, Hay SN, Brecher ME. Bacteria detection. In Brecher ME (ed). Bacterial and Parasitic Contamination of Blood Components. Bethesda, Md., American Association of Blood Banks, 2003, pp 57–81.
92. Brecher ME, Hay SN, Rothenberg SJ. Validation of BacT/ALERT plastic culture bottles for use in testing of whole-blood-derived leukoreduced platelet-rich-plasma-derived platelets. Transfusion 2004;44: 1174–1178.
93. Brecher ME, Heath DG, Hay SN, et al. Evaluation of a new generation of culture bottle using an automated bacterial culture system for detecting nine common contaminating organisms found in platelet components. Transfusion 2002;42:774–779.
94. Chambers LA. Initial results of culturing apheresis platelets to detect bacterial contamination [Abstract]. Transfusion 2004;44(Suppl):19A.
95. Fayed R, Taylor C, Linauts S. Evaluation of BacT/ALERT 3D signature in a blood bank setting, one-year anniversary. [Abstract]. Transfusion 2004;44(Suppl):52A.
96. Jacobson JL, Strauss DL, O'Brien TC, et al. Quality control testing using the BacT/ALERT on apheresis platelet collections to reduce the risk of transfusion-transmitted bacterial sepsis [Abstract]. Transfusion 2004;44(Suppl):20A.
97. Rios JA, Norton J, Benjamin RJ. Bacterial testing of platelets pheresis using BacT/ALERT [Abstract]. Transfusion 2004;44(Suppl):52A.
98. Peck KB, Horn KD, Tegtmeier GE, et al. Bacterial testing of platelets pheresis using BacT/ALERT [Abstract]. Transfusion 2004;44 (Suppl):53A.
99. Goldman M, Delage G. Culturing of apheresis platelets-CBS and Héma-Québec experience. 2005 Joint Conference of the CSTM, CBS, and Héma-Québec. 21–24 April 2005, Banff, AB, Canada.
100. Larsen CP, Ezligini F, Hermansen NO, et al. Six years' experience of using the BacT/ALERT system to screen all platelet concentrates, and additional testing of outdated platelet concentrates to estimate the frequency of false-negative results. Vox Sang 2005;88:93–97.
101. Liu HW, Yuen KY, Cheng TS, et al. Reduction of platelet transfusion-associated sepsis by short-term bacterial culture. Vox Sang 1999;77:1–5.
102. Lee CK, Ho PL, Lee KY, et al. Estimation of bacterial risk in extending the shelf life of PLT concentrates from 5 to 7 days. Transfusion 2003;43:1047–1052.
103. Ramirez-Arcos S, Goldman M. Evaluation of pooled cultures for bacterial detection in whole blood-derived platelets. Transfusion 2005;45:1275–1279.
104. Malone T, Williams D, Leparc GF. Routine bacterial culture of apheresis and whole blood-derived platelets: regional blood centre experience. [Abstract]. Transfusion 2004;44(Suppl):170A.
105. te Boekhorst PA, Beckers EA, Vos MC, et al. Clinical significance of bacteriologic screening in platelet concentrates. Transfusion 2005;45:514–519.
106. FDA Center for Biologics Evaluation and Research, March 2005. Available at http://www.fda.gov/cber/510ksumm/k040086s.htm. Accessed Sept. 30, 2005.
107. Rock G, Neurath D, Cober N, et al. Seven-day storage of random donor PLT concentrates. Transfusion 2003;43:1374–1377.
108. Ortolano GA, Freundlich LF, Holme S, et al. Detection of bacteria in WBC-reduced PLT concentrates using percent oxygen as a marker for bacteria growth. Transfusion 2003;43:1276–1285.
109. Holme S, McAlister MB, Ortolano GA, et al. Enhancement of a culture-based bacterial detection system (eBDS) for platelet products based on measurement of oxygen consumption. Transfusion 2005;45:984–993.
110. Nguyen K-A T, Yamamoto T, Svoboda R, et al. Clinical performance of the Pall BDS bacterial detection system: one year's experience in a blood center setting [Abstract]. Transfusion 2004;44(Suppl):20A.
111. Yu JC, Chong C, Cortus MA, et al. Bacteria growth in leukoreduced AS-3 red cell concentrates (RCC) and detection with PALL Ebds [Abstract]. Transfusion 2004;44(Suppl):45A.
112. Jacobs MR, Bajaksouzian S, Windau A, et al. Evaluation of the Scansystem method for detection of bacterially contaminated platelets. Transfusion 2005;45:265–269.

113. McDonald CP, Colvin J, Robbins S, et al. Use of a solid-phase fluorescent cytometric technique for the detection of bacteria in platelet concentrates. Transfus Med 2005;15:175–183.
114. Ribault S, Faucon A, Grave L, et al. Detection of bacteria in red blood cell concentrates by the Scansystem method. J Clin Microbiol 2005;43:2251–2255.
115. Yazer MH, Triulzi DJ. Use of a pH meter for bacterial screening of whole blood platelets. Transfusion 2005;45:1133–1137.
116. Dreier J, Stormer M, Kleesiek K. Two novel real-time reverse transcriptase PCR assays for rapid detection of bacterial contamination in platelet concentrates. J Clin Microbiol 2004;42:4759–4764.
117. Mohammadi T, Pietersz RN, Vandenbroucke-Grauls CM. Detection of bacteria in platelet concentrates: comparison of broad-range real-time 16S rDNA polymerase chain reaction and automated culturing. Transfusion 2005;45:731–736.
118. Engen T, Refseth U, Kleveland E, et al. Evaluation of a novel method for detection of bacterial contamination of platelet concentrates. [Abstract]. ASM General Meeting, New Orleans, La., 2004.
119. Yomtovian R. Bacterial contaminaton of blood: Lessons from the past and road map for the future. Transfusion 2004;44:450–460.
120. Ness PM, Campbell-Lee SA. Single donor versus pooled random donor platelet concentrates. Curr Opin Hematol 2001;8:392–396.
121. Högman CF, Gong J, Eriksson L, et al. White cells protect donor blood against bacterial contamination. Transfusion 1991;31:620–626.
122. Goldman M, Delage G. The role of leukodepletion in the control of transfusion-transmitted disease. Transfus Med Rev 1995;9:9–19.
123. Heal JM, Cohen HJ. Do white cells in stored blood component reduce the likelihood of posttransfusion bacterial sepsis? [Editorial]. Transfusion 1991;31:581–583.
124. Reesink HW, Hanfland P, Hertfelder H, et al. International forum: what is the optimal storage temperature for whole blood prior to preparation of blood components? Vox Sang 1993;65:320–327.
125. Pietersz RNI, Reesink HW, Dekker MA, et al. Elimination of *Yersinia enterocolitica* by a 20h hold of whole blood and removal of leukocytes by filtration [Abstract]. Transfusion 1992;32(Suppl):66S.
126. Wagner S, Moroff G, Katz A, Friedman L. Bacterial levels in components, prepared from deliberately inoculated whole blood held for 8 and 24 hours at room temperature [Abstract]. Transfusion 1994;34(Suppl):9S.
127. Hoffmeister KM, Josefsson EC, Isaac NA, et al. Glycosylation restores survival of chilled blood platelets. Science 2003;301:1457.
128. Nie Y, de Pablo JJ, Palecek SP. Platelet cryopreservation using a trehalose and phosphate formulation. Biotechnol Bioeng 2005;92:79–90.
129. Bradley RM, Gander RM, Patel SK, et al. Inhibitory effect of 0°C storage on the proliferation of *Yersinia enterocolitica* in donated blood. Transfusion 1997;37:691–695.
130. Lin L, Dikeman R, Molini B, et al. Photochemical treatment of platelet concentrates with amotosalen and long-wavelength ultraviolet light inactivates a broad spectrum of pathogenic bacteria. Transfusion 2004;44:1496–1504.
131. AABB. Bacterial contamination of platelets: Summary for clinicians on potential management issues related to transfusion recipients and blood donors. Available at http://www.aabb.org/Pressroom/In_the_News/bactcontplat022305.htm. Accessed Sept. 30, 2005.
132. AABB. Bulletin #04–07. Available at http://www.aabb.org/members_only/archives/association_bulletins/ab04-7.htm. Accessed Sept. 30, 2005.
133. AABB. Bulletin #05–02. Available at hhtp://www.aabb.org/Members_Only/Archives/Association_Bulletins/ab05-2.htm. Accessed Sept. 30, 2005.

Chapter 48

Other Viral, Bacterial, Parasitic and Prion-Based Infectious Complications

Jay E. Menitove • Gary E. Tegtmeier

INTRODUCTION

During the last decade of the 20th century, diagnostic advancements dramatically reduced the transmission of human immunodeficiency virus (HIV), hepatitis C virus (HCV), and hepatitis B virus (HBV) by transfusion. However, simultaneously, the emergence of additional pathogens as potential blood contaminants gained attention. Some of these agents represented newly discovered entities (e.g., severe acute respiratory syndrome [SARS-CoA]). Others were known sources of transfusion complications that expanded into the United States (e.g., Chagas disease). Additionally, some agents demonstrated species jumping from animal hosts to humans (e.g., variant Creutzfeldt-Jakob disease [VCJD], Asian influenza, and West Nile virus). Increasing globalization through commerce, travel, and social interaction requires that many infectious agents, once thought exotic or of remote significance, must be considered as potential blood-component contaminants.[1,2] Alternatively, new information may reduce some concerns. For example, porcine endogenous retrovirus (PERV), previously linked to humans undergoing xenotransplantation, currently appears less threatening.[3]

This chapter addresses agents endemic to the United States and those emerging in other parts of the world that have been transmitted or are theoretically capable of transmission by transfusion, and approaches to reduce the associated risks.

BABESIA

Babesiosis, a zoonosis caused by the rodent-borne piroplasm protozoan, *Babesia microti*, is transmitted by *Ixodes scapularis*, the deer or black-legged tick. *I. scapularis* also transmits the agents of Lyme disease and human granulocyte ehrlichiosis (discussed later).[4–10]

The white-footed mouse (*Peromyscus leucopus*) is the natural reservoir for *B. microti*; once infected, a mouse remains parasitemic indefinitely. *I. scapularis* transmits the piroplasm most frequently during the nymphal stage when the tick is 1.5 mm long. Tick bites, at this stage, often go unnoticed despite the 48- to 72-hour feeding time during which infection occurs.[11] *B. microti* is the agent most frequently associated with clinical illness; MO1-type, WA1-type, and CA1-type also cause clinical disease.[12,13] Endemic areas include coastal and island areas of New England and New York as well as parts of California, Washington, Missouri, Wisconsin, and Minnesota.[6,7,9,12,13] Ticks coinfected with *B. microti* and *Borrelia burgdorferi* (the agent of Lyme disease) transmit *B. microti* less frequently than *B. burgdorferi* because the tick is a less competent host for *B. microti*. The intraerythrocytic localization of *B. microti*, however, favors transfusion transmission of this agent over that of *B. burgdorferi*.[6]

In humans, circulating *B. microti* DNA persists, on average, for 82 days in asymptomatic patients and in those not given specific treatment. Co-infection with Lyme disease does not alter the duration of parasitemia. Parasites circulate for only 16 days in persons who are treated with clindamycin and quinine; alternative antibiotic regimens include atovaquone and azithromycin.[13] Silent *Babesia* infections occur commonly. Some infected individuals develop a chronic carrier state lasing months to years. In others, recrudescence occurs spontaneously or after splenectomy or immunosuppression.[11,14] The parasite retains infectivity in red blood cell (RBC) components at refrigerated or frozen temperatures and in the residual RBCs contained in platelet concentrates stored at room temperature.[5,8]

To date, more than 50 post-transfusion cases involving *B. microti* and other *Babesia* species have been reported.[5,6,9,12,15] Several reports involve donors who transmitted infections through multiple donations given up to 6 months apart.[11,16] The overall risk of acquiring transfusion-associated babesiosis is low, but varies regionally. In Connecticut, 1.9% of seronegative donors became seropositive on a subsequent donation. In another study, 0.9% of donors in endemic and nonendemic areas of Connecticut had confirmatory indirect immunofluorescence assay (IFA)-positive test results for *Babesia* infection; the prevalence rates peaked in July when 1.2% of donors were seropositive.[15] This represents a relatively high potential threat in an endemic area because 8 of 51 recipients became seropositive after receiving blood from IFA-positive blood donors.[17]

Asplenia, older age, immunodeficiency, organ transplantation, and liver disease increase the risk of severe *Babesia* illness. In acute symptomatic cases, fatigue, malaise, weakness, and fever occur in more than 90% of the patients. Shaking chills, diaphoresis, nausea, anorexia, headaches, and myalgia occur frequently. Heart murmurs, hepatomegaly, and splenomegaly are found in 10% to 20% of patients; jaundice occurs less frequently. Renal failure, disseminated intravascular coagulation, and adult respiratory distress syndrome have been reported.[13] The average hemoglobin concentration was 11.3 g/dL in a review of hospitalized patients with community-acquired babesiosis.[4]

Examination of blood smears for intraerythrocytic ring forms and maltese cross–like tetrads (including more than two parasites per cell, contorted shapes, vacuoles, and budding),[18] antibabesial antibody assays, and polymerase chain reaction (PCR) assays for babesial DNA provide laboratory evidence of infection.[4,14] (Fig. 48–1)

Most transfusion-associated babesia cases involve RBC transfusions, although frozen-deglycerolized RBC and platelet units have been implemented.[5,8,13] Transfusion-acquired cases have an incubation period of 2 to 6.5 weeks.[4,6,8,13,15] Blood-collection agencies ask all prospective donors whether they have ever had babesiosis. Those answering affirmatively are deferred. However, donors are not asked about a recent history of tick bites or geographic residence because of the low predictive value associated with these questions. For example, 0.4% of donors in Connecticut reporting tick bites were seropositive for babesiosis antibodies compared with 0.3% in those not reporting tick bites.[9] Serologic or PCR testing is impractical at this time. The absence of specific interventions to interdict donors capable of transmitting *Babesia* infections relegates clinical awareness and prompt antibiotic therapy as the primary modality for treating this infrequent complication of transfusion therapy.

LYME DISEASE

The *Borrelia burgdorferi* spirochete causes Lyme disease, a tick-borne zoonosis present in mice, squirrels, and other small animals. More than 20,000 human Lyme disease cases occur annually in the United States, although none has been associated with transfusion. Endemic areas include the northeastern, mid-Atlantic, and upper north-central regions of the United States.[10,19]

Ixodes scapularis, the black legged deer tick, transmits *B. burgdorferi* in the northeastern and north-central parts of the United States. *I. pacificus,* the western black-legged tick, transmits the infection along the Pacific Coast. The ticks feed predominantly in the late spring and early summer during their nymphal stage, and Lyme disease usually results from bites of infected nymphs. Deer do not become infected but rather transport and maintain the ticks.[10]

Patients with Lyme disease typically present with a characteristic erythema migrans rash accompanied by fever, malaise, headaches, myalgia, arthralgia, or Bell's palsy. The rash occurs 3 to 30 days after a tick bite. *B. burgdorferi* spirochetes disseminate from the entry site via cutaneous, lymphatic, and blood-borne routes. In one study, spirochetes were isolated from the blood of 44% of patients with symptomatic Lyme disease.[20] *B. burgdorferi* has also been isolated from erythema migrans lesions.

The diagnosis of Lyme disease is based primarily on characteristic symptoms, physical examination findings, and a history of possible tick exposure.[10,20–23] Serologic tests, including enzyme-linked immunoassays and IFA tests, become positive 4 to 6 weeks after infection. Western blot testing is used to confirm the results of reactive screening tests. Treatment with antibiotics clears the infection, but additional treatment to relieve symptoms is prescribed when arthritis persists after two antibiotic courses and for post–Lyme disease syndrome.[20–23]

Despite documentation that the spirochete survives routine RBC and frozen plasma storage, testing blood donors is not under consideration because no reports exist of transfusion-associated Lyme disease.[10] Of note, transfusion of RBCs or platelets collected during peak deer tick activity to 155 patients undergoing cardiothoracic surgery resulted in no serologic or clinical evidence of Lyme disease.[5] Individuals with a history of Lyme disease are accepted as blood donors provided they have been treated and are asymptomatic 12 months after the last dose of antibiotics.

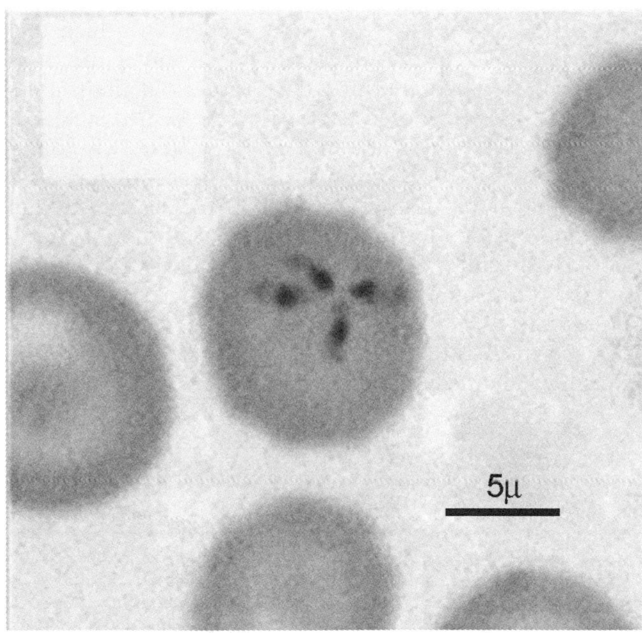

Figure 48–1 *Babesia microti* parasites infect up to 5% of red cells. Although more common in infections with *B. gibsoni* (WA-1) than *B. microti,* tetrad or Maltese cross structures are pathognomonic for *Babesia* infections. They result from budding with four nucleated intraerythrocytic merozoites remaining attached to each other after division. (From Pantanowitz L, Monahan-Earley R, Dvorak A, et al. Morphologic hallmarks of *Babesia*. Transfusion 2002;42:1389.)

TRANSFUSION TRANSMISSION OF OTHER TICK-BORNE PATHOGENS

The rickettsial agents human monocytic ehrlichiosis (HME) and human granulocytic ehrlichiosis (HGE) are intracellular organisms that survive in stored blood and cause mild to severe illnesses.[10] *Ehrlichia chaffeensis* causes HME and is transmitted to humans through the bite of the Lone Star tick (*Amblyomma americanum*) previously infected by contact with deer or possibly dogs.[9,10] Most of the reported cases have occurred in the south-central and southeastern United States.

Anaplasma phagocytophila causes HGE and is related closely to species infecting horses (*Ehrlichia equi)* or ruminants (*Ehrlichia phagocytophila*). This illness occurs predominantly in the northeastern, upper midwestern, and northwestern areas of the United States and is transmitted to humans by *I. scapularis* or *I. pacificus* ticks.[5,9,24–26] Fifty percent of ticks examined in one study in Connecticut were infected with the HGE agent, but none was infected with *E. chaffeensis.*[27]

Patients with HME and HGE present similarly, with fever, headache, myalgia, thrombocytopenia, leukopenia, and elevated liver enzyme concentrations. A rash occurs in one third of patients with HME but in fewer patients with HGE. Membrane-bound intracytoplasmic ehrlichia aggregates, or morulae, are present in monocytes. Complications include respiratory distress, renal failure, neurologic disorders, and disseminated intravascular coagulation. Septicemia, vasculitis, and thrombotic thrombocytopenic purpura should be considered in the differential diagnosis.[5,10,24,25] Doxycycline is the treatment of choice.

Because ehrlichia are present in blood, transfusion transmission must be considered. One case of transfusion-associated HGE occurred 9 days after an RBC transfusion donated by an asymptomatic donor who had been exposed to extensive deer ticks 2 months previously. The infected RBCs were stored for 30 days before transfusion.[28] An in vitro study suggested that leukocyte reduction may not be completely effective at preventing *E. chaffeensis* transmission because some pathogens are found in the cell free plasma fraction.[29]

An extensive epidemiologic study in Arkansas involving military trainee blood donors who had been exposed to tick bites and unknowingly infected with the agents of ehrlichiosis and Rocky Mountain spotted fever (RMSF) found no clinical illness among the recipients of RBCs and platelets donated by these soldiers. However, possible seroconversion to RMSF occurred in one of the recipients.[30]

A single case report has been published of clinical illness associated with transfusion-transmitted RMSF infection. The donor developed symptoms of RMSF 3 days after donation and died 6 days later. The recipient, who developed fever and headache 6 days after receiving the implicated *Rickettsia rickettsii*–infected transfusion, was notified about the donor's illness and was treated effectively.[10]

Other tick-borne agents implicated in transfusion-associated cases include Colorado tick fever virus and tick-borne encephalitis virus.[10] Although the risk of transfusion transmission of these agents is low, clinical suspicion is important as a mechanism for determining infection by these organisms.

MALARIA

Etiology, Life Cycle, Diagnosis

Malaria is a protozoan disease caused by four species of the genus *Plasmodium: P. falciparum, P. vivax, P. ovale,* and *P. malariae* (Table 48–1). These protozoa are transmitted to humans by the bite of an infected female mosquito of the genus *Anopheles.* Infection of the human host, absent treatment, results in a chronic intraerythrocytic infection that can be transmitted by blood transfusion.

The two-host life cycle of the malaria parasite is diagrammed in Figure 48–2.

Although the signs and symptoms of malaria are variable, most patients are febrile, and many also manifest headache, chills, sweating, nausea, vomiting, diarrhea, back pain, myalgia, and cough. A diagnosis of malaria should be considered for any patient with these symptoms who has a history of travel to a malaria-endemic area or recent blood transfusion. Given the periodic reports of local mosquito-borne transmission, malaria should also be considered in the differential diagnosis of patients who have fever of unknown origin regardless of their travel history.

Malaria is diagnosed microscopically by finding intraerythrocytic parasites on Giemsa-stained peripheral blood smears. Properly prepared thick and thin smears must be examined by trained laboratory personnel to make an accurate laboratory diagnosis. Patients with negative smears suspected of having malaria should have additional smears examined daily for 3 days. PCR can be a useful adjunct in cases in which serial testing of smears yields negative results.

Epidemiology

Malaria is a huge global public health problem with an estimated annual incidence of 300 to 500 million cases and 3 million deaths per year.[31] Malaria-endemic areas include parts of Africa, Asia, Central America, Hispaniola, North America, Oceania, and South America.

During the early part of the 20th century, specifically 1914, an estimated 600,000 cases of malaria occurred in the continental United States, but since the 1940s, improved socioeconomic conditions, water management, vector control, and case management have prevented endemic malaria transmission.[32] Ongoing malaria surveillance in the United States by the Centers for Disease Control and Prevention (CDC) continues to identify cases in immigrants and in residents and travelers to areas of the world where malaria transmission still occurs. Additionally, each year, a few cases are reported that might represent local mosquito-borne transmission.[33] For example, seven cases of locally acquired, mosquito-transmitted *P. vivax* malaria were reported in Palm Beach County, Florida. Multilocus genotyping of the ribosomal RNA of the isolates from the seven patients revealed that they were infected by the same strain.[34] Congenital infections and transfusion-acquired infections round out the sources of malaria cases diagnosed each year in the United States.

Of 1337 cases of malaria in the United States with onset of symptoms in 2002, one was due to transmission of *P. malariae* by blood transfusion.[35] Of 1278 cases reported in 2003, one was due to transmission of *P. falciparum* after a blood transfusion.[36] The overwhelming majority of reported cases in both years were imported (i.e., acquired outside the United States).

Data from 1979 through 1986 showed that cases were more frequently identified in foreign civilians than in U.S. civilians.

Table 48–1 Transfusion-transmitted Malaria in the United States 1963–2004*

	Plasmodium falciparum	*Plasmodium vivax*	*Plasmodium ovale*	*Plasmodium malariae*
Transfusion-associated cases, 1963–2004 (% of total)	34 (36%)	25 (27%)	5 (5%)	26 (28%)
Average incubation period (days)	17 (range, 8–36)	20 (range, 11–42)	24 (range, 18–30)	51 (range, 8–90)
Relapse	No (manifests clinically within 1 yr)	Yes (usually within 3 yr)	Yes (usually within 3 yr)	Yes (prolonged)

*Three cases were due to mixed infections. The etiologies of two cases were unknown.

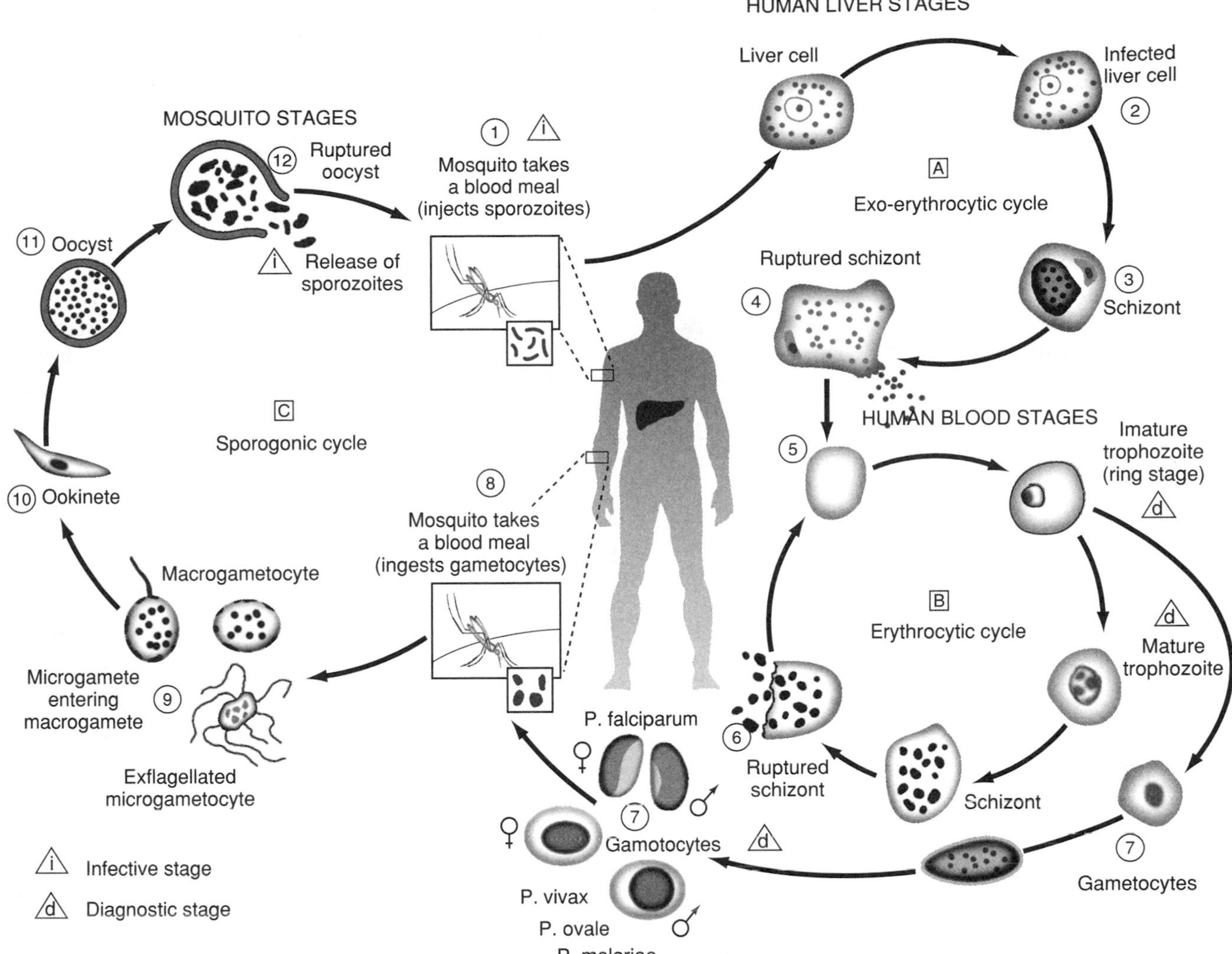

Figure 48–2 The malaria parasite life cycle involves two hosts. During a blood meal, a malaria-infected female *Anopheles* mosquito inoculates sporozoites into the human host. Sporozoites infect liver cells and mature into schizonts, which rupture and release merozoites. (Of note, in *Plasmodium vivax* and *P. ovale,* a dormant stage [hypnozoites] can persist in the liver and cause relapses by invading the bloodstream weeks, or even years later.) After this initial replication in the liver (exo-erythrocytic schizogony), the parasites undergo asexual multiplication in the erythrocytes (erythrocytic schizogony). Merozoites infect red blood cells. The ring-stage trophozoites mature into schizonts, which rupture, releasing merozoites. Some parasites differentiate into sexual erythrocytic stages (gametocytes). Blood-stage parasites are responsible for the clinical manifestations of the disease. The gametocytes, male (microgametocytes) and female (macrogametocytes), are ingested by an *Anopheles* mosquito during a blood meal. The parasites' multiplication in the mosquito is known as the sporogonic cycle. While in the mosquito's stomach, the microgametes penetrate the macrogametes, generating zygotes. The zygotes in turn become motile and elongated (ookinetes) and invade the midgut wall of the mosquito where they develop into oocysts. The oocysts grow, rupture, and release sporozoites, which make their way to the mosquito's salivary glands. Inoculation of the sporozoites into a new human host perpetuates the malaria life cycle. (Figure and legend are taken from the Centers for Disease Control and Prevention [CDC] website http://www.cdc.gov/malaria/biology/life_cycle.htm.)

However, since 1997, the situation has reversed. Cases in United States civilians are now reported at 2.5 to 3 times the number in foreign civilians, most likely due to increased travel by U.S. civilians to endemic areas and decreased immigration since 2001.[36] From 75% to 90% of the cases among U.S. civilian travelers occurs in persons who failed to take prophylactic drugs, had not taken CDC-recommended drugs, or were noncompliant with a recommended drug.

Mosquitoes of the genus *Anopheles*, with few exceptions, feed between dusk and dawn. The exceptions are daytime feedings in densely shaded woodlands or dark interiors of houses or shelters. Therefore, travelers who visit malarial areas during bright daylight hours are at little or no risk for acquiring malaria if they return to a nonmalarial area before dusk.

Transmission by Transfusion and Risk Reduction

Transfusion-transmitted malaria occurs at an estimated rate of 0.25 cases per 1 million blood units collected.[37] Because of this low incidence and the lack of a laboratory test approved by the U.S. Food and Drug Administration (FDA), prevention of transfusion-transmitted malaria continues to depend solely on the donor-deferral guidelines established by the FDA and most recently updated in 1994.[38] Currently, prospective donors who are residents of countries where malaria is not endemic but who have traveled to a malaria-endemic area are temporarily deferred until 1 year after their departure from the endemic area if they have remained free of symptoms suggestive of malaria. Immigrants, refugees, citizens, and residents of malaria-endemic areas are deferred for 3 years after their departure from the endemic area if they have remained free of symptoms suggestive of malaria. Prospective donors who were diagnosed and treated for malaria are deferred for 3 years after becoming asymptomatic.

Between 1996 and 1998, three cases of post-transfusion malaria due to *P. falciparum*, two of which were fatal,[39] were diagnosed in the United States, prompting a review by the CDC of all cases of transfusion-transmitted malaria reported between 1963 and 1999[40] (see Table 48-1, which has been updated to include reported cases in 2002 and 2003[35,36]). In total, 95 cases (2.5 per year) were reported through 2003. Thirty-four (36%) cases were caused by *P. falciparum*, 25 (27%) by *P. vivax*, 26 (28%) by *P. malariae*, 5 (5%) by *P. ovale*, 3 (3%) by mixed species, and 2 (2%) by an undetermined species. *P. falciparum* cases increased in frequency over the period 1990 to 2003, accounting for 11 (73%) of 15 cases during that interval, compared with 15 (24%) of 62 cases reported between 1970 and 1989. Of 10 (11%) fatal cases overall, 6 were associated with *P. falciparum*, 2 with *P. vivax*, and 2 with *P. malariae*.

The incubation period in these cases ranged from 8 to 90 days, with *P. falciparum* having the shortest time (mean, 17 days; range, 8 to 36 days) and *P. malariae* having the longest (mean, 51 days; range, 8 to 90 days). The period between onset of symptoms and the time of diagnosis ranged from 1 to 180 days, with a median of 10 days. Ninety-four percent of the cases were associated with transfusion of whole blood or RBCs; 6% were platelet-associated.

Implicated donors were defined as having met one or more of the following criteria (1) a blood smear that demonstrated malaria parasites, (2) a positive result on malaria serology, and (3) being the only donor. Ninety-three donors were implicated in the 95 cases. The median number of donors per case was seven (range, 1 to 192). Donors were overwhelmingly male (90%) and ranged in age from 19 to 59 years (median, 27 years). Foreign-born donors accounted for 60% (64% of those from Africa); 40% were born in the United States.

Of 60 donors implicated in the cases for which epidemiologic follow-up was complete, serology was the most effective tool for identifying transmitting donors (73%); only 10% were identified by a positive blood smear. Serology and blood smear were both positive in 15%, and 3% were implicated as the only donor to a case.

Analysis of all cases using current donor deferral guidelines revealed that 23 (24%) cases occurred despite proper application of the guidelines. When reviewed against the guidelines in place at the time they occurred, 3 cases could not be evaluated because their dates of onset were before 1970 when guidelines were vague; 18 of the remaining 20 cases would still have occurred, but 2 would have been prevented if then-current guidelines had been applied properly. Not surprisingly, most (65%) of the cases that occurred despite following guidelines were caused by *P. malariae*.

The continued occurrence of cases in the face of current history questions highlights the reality that malaria risk from transfusion, although low, cannot be fully prevented by questioning of donors. Although the deferral guidelines currently in place are based on the biology of the four species of *Plasmodia* that cause malaria, they represent a balance struck between maximizing safety and minimizing donor loss. *P. vivax* and *P. ovale*, species that give rise to relapsing infections, rarely persist longer than 3 years.[42] However, some infections do persist, and individuals with these prolonged infections will transmit malaria if their blood is transfused. Likewise, disease caused by *P. falciparum*, a nonrelapsing species, manifests within 1 year after departure from a malarious area 99% of the time, but a report of falciparum malaria occurring 13 years after departure from a malarious area has been published.[41] The well-known ability of *P. malariae* to persist asymptomatically for decades in some individuals further highlights the difficulty of eradicating the risk of post-transfusion malaria through questioning of donors.[42]

The AABB has advocated the use of uniform donor screening questions to elicit malaria risk from prospective donors, including questions that inquire about a history of malaria and about the prospective donor's travel history within the past 3 years. A "yes" answer to travel outside the United States and Canada triggers further inquiry to pinpoint travel destinations in malarious areas.

The FDA is in the process of revising its guidelines for deferral of blood donors because of risk of malaria. However, it is unclear when the agency will issue the new guidelines. The proposed guidelines were discussed at the FDA's Blood Products Advisory Committee meeting in June 1999.[46] In addition to retaining the provisions for donor deferral outlined in the FDA memo of July 26, 1994,[38] the revised guidelines recommend adding the following question sequence to the donor history form: (1) "Were you born in the United States?" If yes, ask: (2) "In the past 3 years, have you been outside the United States or Canada?" If the answer to (1) is no, ask: (3) "When did you arrive in the United States, and, since your arrival, have you traveled outside the United States or Canada?" If the answer to question (2) or the second question in (3) is yes, follow-up questions will be asked of the donor to determine when and which country or countries were visited. The impetus for revision of the guidelines includes the increased number of imported malaria cases in the United States, the large number of postdonation events related to malaria reported to the FDA, and the recognition that eliciting an accurate donor history is the only currently available defense against transfusion-transmitted malaria.

From time to time, proposals to test donors for evidence of malaria have been advanced, but no FDA-approved tests or policies for screening donors are currently in place. Selective screening of high-risk donors has been suggested as an alternative to universal screening.[43] Blood-smear diagnosis is both impractical and insensitive as a donor-screening technique. The IFA test is useful diagnostically but is unsuitable for large-scale donor screening, although it could be used to test high-risk donors and to determine their suitability.[43] Although antibody assays detect most individuals with parasitemia, they also are positive in treated persons who are no longer parasitemic.[44] Hence, noninfectious donors would also be deferred if selective antibody screening were implemented. PCR is a promising approach that may have the required sensitivity and specificity, but it is currently not standardized and not available outside research laboratories.[45]

CHAGAS DISEASE

Life Cycle

American trypanosomiasis, or Chagas disease, is a zoonosis caused by the hemoflagellate protozoan parasite *Trypanosoma cruzi*. The life cycle of *T. cruzi* involves transmission from insect vectors to mammalian hosts including humans. *T. cruzi* infects humans when triatomid (reduviid) or kissing bugs ingest a blood meal from the host and deposit infected feces into the wound or when contaminated feces contact the mucosal surface of the eye or mouth. Hematogenous spread occurs subsequently. In addition, *T. cruzi* crosses the placenta and can cause congenital disease[47–51] (Fig. 48–3).

Clinical Course

Acute Chagas disease is associated with fever, facial edema, generalized lymphadenopathy, and hepatosplenomegaly. Symptomatic myocarditis and meningioencephalitis can occur, and fulminant illness can develop in immunologically immature children or immunocompromised adults. However, in more than 95% of patients, the illness is mild and symptoms resolve in 4 to 6 weeks. If untreated, hosts then enter an indeterminate phase. Ten percent to 30% of patients progress from the indeterminate asymptomatic phase to a chronic symptomatic phase associated with cardiac enlargement, apical aneurysms, mural thrombi, megaesophagus, or megacolon, appearing years to decades after infection.[48–51]

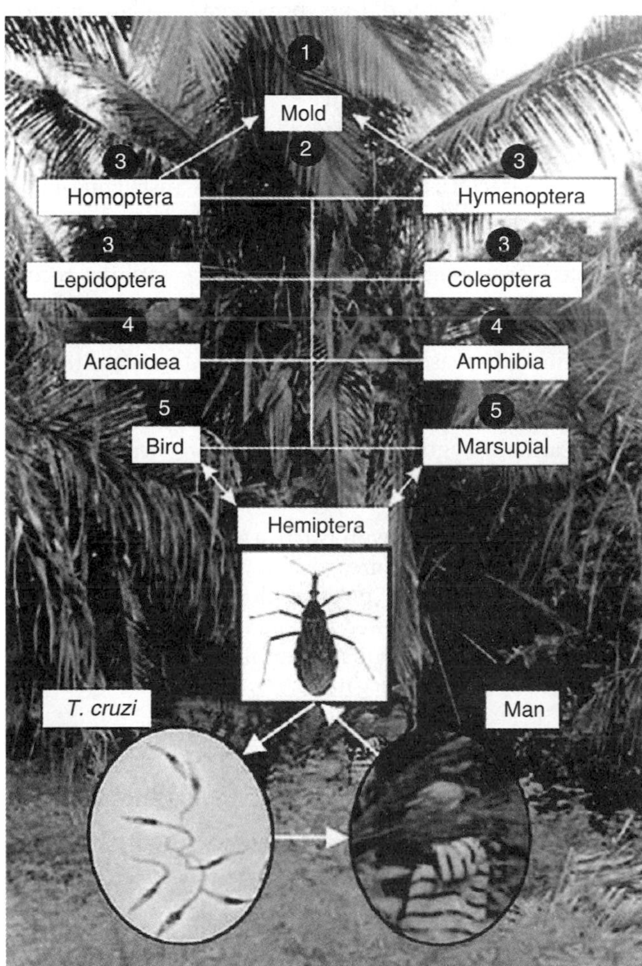

Figure 48–3 Triatomia bugs (Reduvidae), infected with *Trypanosoma cruzi*, reside in palm-tree frond clefts. Whereas birds are refractory to *T. cruzi* infections, marsupials and other residents of palm trees serve as reservoirs of infection. During the wet season when birds and mammals are scarce, triatomine bugs seek humans as a source of feeding, thereby spreading infection. (From Teixera ARL, Monteiro PS, Rebelo JM, et al. Emerging Chagas disease: Trophic network and cycle of transmission of *Trypanosoma cruzi* from palm trees in the Amazon. Emerg Infect Dis 2002;7:100–112).

Epidemiology

An estimated 16 to 18 million people are infected in South America, Central America, and Mexico, where Chagas disease is endemic and, historically, triatomid insects reside in cracks of rural and suburban houses with adobe walls. In the United States, an estimated 25,000 to 100,000 persons and 1 in 25,000 blood donors may be infected with *T. cruzi*.[48] Almost all are immigrants from Central and South America. Chagas disease is responsible for 50,000 deaths worldwide annually.[53]

Lifelong low-grade parasitemia persists in approximately 50% of those infected, and up to 63% of seropositive blood donors have parasitemia.[52] This presents a risk of transfusion transmission and of vertical transmission to infants. Between 12% and 48% of recipients of parasitemic blood become infected.

Transmission by Transfusion

Estimates of risk for transfusion-associated Chagas disease are related to immigration patterns from endemic regions. During the mid-1980s, 4.9% of 205 Nicaraguan and Salvadorian immigrants living in Washington, D.C., had serologic evidence of *T. cruzi* infection. Parasites were isolated from half.[54] In the early 1990s, 0.11% of a selected blood-donor population in California and the U.S. southwest was seropositive for *T. cruzi* antibodies. At least 50% of these donors were of Hispanic origin.[55] During the mid-1990s, 39.5% of donors at a hospital in Los Angeles responded affirmatively to questions inquiring about birth in Chagas disease–endemic areas or residing in dwellings constructed of palm leaf–thatched roofs or walls made of mud,[56] and 0.5% tested positive for *T. cruzi* antibodies. In a study conducted in the mid-to-late 1990s involving more than 1.1 million blood donors, 1 in 7500 in Los Angeles and 1 in 9000 in Miami were *T. cruzi* seropositive.[52]

Although a correlation exists between the percentage of immigrants from endemic areas and the percentage of blood donors with serologic evidence of *T. cruzi* infection, investigators have also identified seropositive blood donors who were born in the United States.[57] Congenital transmission may explain infection in these individuals. In addition, autochthonous transmission has been reported in the United States,[58] and an infestation of triatomines has been reported in Texas.[59]

Since 1989, seven cases of transfusion-associated Chagas disease have occurred in the United States and Canada.[61–65] Symptoms developed approximately 2 to 3 months after transfusion. In at least six of the cases, platelets were the implicated blood component; however, in the seventh case, the implicated unit was not identified.[63] Centrifugation may sediment *T. cruzi* into the platelet layer during component preparation, accounting for the association with platelet transfusions. Whereas room-temperature storage of platelets may favor parasite survival, *T. cruzi* has been shown to survive in refrigerated RBCs and whole blood for at least 18 to 21 days.[51] In six of the North American transfusion-associated cases, a donor emigrating from a *T. cruzi*–endemic region (Bolivia, Mexico, Paraguay, Chile) was identified. Four of the donors emigrated between 16 and 33 years before the implicated donation. Given this small number of cases, transfusion transmission of Chagas disease may be inefficient. In a study of 18 patients receiving blood from blood donors subsequently found to be *T. cruzi* seropositive, none of the recipients became seropositive after transfusion. However, only two received platelet transfusions.[52] A report of Chagas disease also has been reported after transplantation involving an organ donor who emigrated from Central America appeared in 2002.[60] The recipient of a kidney and pancreas died of acute Chagas myocarditis 5 months after transplant. The recipients of the other kidney and the liver were both also infected with *T. cruzi.*

Transfusion Risk Reduction

Interventions to reduce the risk of transfusion-transmitted Chagas disease include questioning donors about geographic location of birth, extended stay or transfusion in areas endemic for Chagas disease, and serologic testing.[51,66,67] Donor history questions may be only 75% effective.[51] At least one candidate serologic screening assay has undergone clinical trials in the United States and is currently under review at the FDA. The U.S. FDA has indicated that it will require testing for Chagas disease if an appropriate screening assay achieves licensure. This decision reflects the reported transfusion- and organ transplant–associated cases and the concern that up to 600 transmissions may occur annually in the United States.[52] Leukocyte reduction by filtration is modestly effective, reducing *T. cruzii* transmission by 50% to 70% in a mouse transfusion model.[68]

SYPHILIS

Serologic testing of blood donations for syphilis was instituted in 1938 and required by regulation in 1958. No cases of transfusion-associated syphilis have occurred in the United States since 1966.[69] Multiple factors—improved donor selection, uniform serologic testing, lack of spirochete viability in blood stored at refrigerated temperatures, and widespread antibiotic use—apparently contribute to the current absence of transfusion-transmitted syphilis cases.[69-71] In 1978, the AABB Standards Committee deleted the requirement for syphilis testing, and an FDA advisory panel proposed eliminating the requirement for serologic syphilis testing in 1985. However, these changes were not made because of the belief that such testing might identify those at risk of transmitting the HIV. Subsequently, observational data did not support this assumption. Nonetheless, a National Institutes of Health Consensus Statement, issued in January 1995, recommended continuation of syphilis testing because its role in preventing transfusion-transmitted syphilis was not "understood."[70] A lack of complete laboratory data also supports test retention. Although spirochetes survive 96 to 120 hours at refrigerated temperatures,[72,73] viability at room temperature (e.g., in platelet concentrates) has not been studied. Furthermore, loss of viability during storage is an incomplete protection mechanism.

No single optimal laboratory test exists for syphilis. The infectious agent, *Treponema pallidum*, is an anaerobic organism that cannot be cultured in vitro.[73] During treponema infection, nontreponemal and treponemal antibodies are produced. The nontreponemal antibodies (reagin antibodies) react against phospholipid isolated from beef heart or cardiolipin. These antibodies are detected by the Venereal Disease Research Laboratory (VDRL), rapid plasma reagin (RPR), and other tests in response to the interaction of infected host tissue with *T. pallidum*. They parallel the pathologic course but have no relation to immunity. Treponema-specific antibodies have a higher serologic sensitivity in the early stages of syphilis but are less effective indicators of disease activity. During the first 3 weeks after primary infection, the VDRL is positive in 30% of cases, and the fluorescent treponemal antibody-absorption (FTA-ABS) test is positive in 50%. Other treponemal antibody tests, often used to confirm nontreponemal tests, include *T. pallidum* particle aggregation (TP-PA) and recombinant antigen tests. An automated test for treponemal antibodies, PK (TM) treponema pallidum (PK-TP), performed on the Olympus PK 7200, is widely used.[74–76] Reaction patterns characterized by positive RPR or PK-TP tests and negative FTA-ABS reactions (so-called false-positive reactions) may be caused by hepatitis, mononucleosis, viral pneumonia, chickenpox, measles, immunizations, pregnancy, or laboratory error. Persistent false-positive reactions have been reported in patients with rheumatoid arthritis, cirrhosis, ulcerative colitis, vasculitis, and older age.[74–76] Among PK-TP– and FTA-ABS–positive blood donors, approximately half give a prior history of a treated syphilis infection.[75] A history of lupus, rheumatoid arthritis, and diabetes did not provide an explanation for nonconfirmed PK-TP results.

The typical first sign of syphilis, a chancre, appears 3 to 90 days (average, 21 days) after exposure. The exact timing of spirochetemia and *T. pallidum* dissemination from the chancre and of seroconversion is not known. Secondary syphilis, characterized by a disseminated rash and spirochetemia, occurs 6 to 8 weeks after infection. Serologic tests are almost universally positive. If patients remain untreated, recurrent fulminant secondary syphilis recurs within 2 years in approximately 20%. Subsequently, patients become immune to reinfection and become noninfectious. VDRL titers decrease over time. Unless patients are treated in the primary stage, treponemal antibodies persist in both treated and untreated patients. Tertiary syphilis develops after a variable length of time. Reactivation is clinically and serologically noticeable via anticardiolipin and treponemal antibody detection.[72,74,76]

Currently, donations with reactive syphilis screening tests are unsuitable unless nonreactive in a confirmatory test. If the confirmatory test is positive, donors are deferred for 1 year; they are then allowed to donate again, provided that they have undergone adequate treatment for syphilis, and a nontreponemal assay is negative.[76]

HUMAN PARVOVIRUS

Clinical Findings and Epidemiology

Human parvovirus B19 was discovered serendipitously in human plasma during blood-donor screening for hepatitis B surface antigen in 1975. Initially, parvovirus was linked causally with transient aplastic crises in patients with sickle cell anemia and subsequently in patients with other inherited hemolytic diseases, as a result of severe reticulocytopenia and anemia. B19 was later found to be the etiologic agent of fifth disease or erythema infectiosum, a common childhood illness that manifests as an erythematous rash.[77,78] The rash occurs less often in infected adults than children. Fever and nonspecific symptoms precede the rash and arthralgia, both of which probably result from immune complex deposition in the skin and other organs. Hepatitis, myocarditis, vasculitis, and the gloves-and-socks syndrome have also been linked to B19 infection (Fig. 48–4).

B19 infects only humans, and transmission occurs most commonly via the respiratory route. In addition, transplacental transmission of parvovirus B19 occurs in 30% of women infected during pregnancy. In women infected during weeks 9 to 20 of pregnancy, hydrops fetalis and fetal death occur in approximately 11%.[79] The virus is highly tropic for erythroid progenitor cells, gaining access to cells through the blood group P antigen, or globoside, which has been identified as the virus receptor.[77,78,80] The viral genome consists of single-stranded DNA that codes for three proteins. The nonstructural protein, NS1, is cytopathic to host cells. Viral protein 1 and viral protein 2 code for α-helical loops that appear on the capsid surface. Neutralizing antibodies recognize VP1. The nonenveloped virus consists of symmetric particles 25 mm in diameter.

B19 infection is ubiquitous in human populations and is already prevalent in pediatric age groups. Seroprevalence studies show antibody frequencies of 50% in high school–age children and up to 90% in older adults.[77,78] Epidemics and sporadic infections may occur at any time of year, with major outbreaks of erythema infectiosum occurring every 3 to 6 years. Persistent parvovirus infection, including pure RBC aplasia, occurs in those not developing neutralizing antibodies to VP1. The virus circulates at high titer, greater than 10^{12} genome copies per milliliter.[77,78] Patients receiving cytotoxic chemotherapy, immunosuppressive drugs, organ transplant recipients, and patients with immunodeficiency and the acquired immunodeficiency syndrome (AIDS) are at higher risk of developing chronic infections. The therapeutic approach for persistent parvovirus infection involves discontinuing immunosuppressive therapy, administering intravenous immunoglobulin (IVIG) preparations, instituting antiviral therapy for AIDS patients, and giving repeated courses of IVIG as needed.[77,78]

Transmission by Transfusion

The transient 1- to 2-week, high-titer viremia accompanying acute asymptomatic B19 infection allows virus transmission by blood, blood derivatives, and organ transplantation.[77,78,81] The infrequent recognition of transfusion-associated cases reflects the short viremic phase and the high frequency of immunity among transfusion recipients.

In contrast to recipients of blood transfusions, almost all recipients of plasma-derived factor VIII and IX concentrate are at risk for B19. Parvovirus circulates in the blood of approximately 1 in 800 plasma donors.[90] Fourteen percent had titers between 10^4 and 10^7 genome equivalents per milliliter, and 1 in 13,000 had greater than 10^7 genome equivalent per milliliter. Not surprisingly, in plasma derivatives

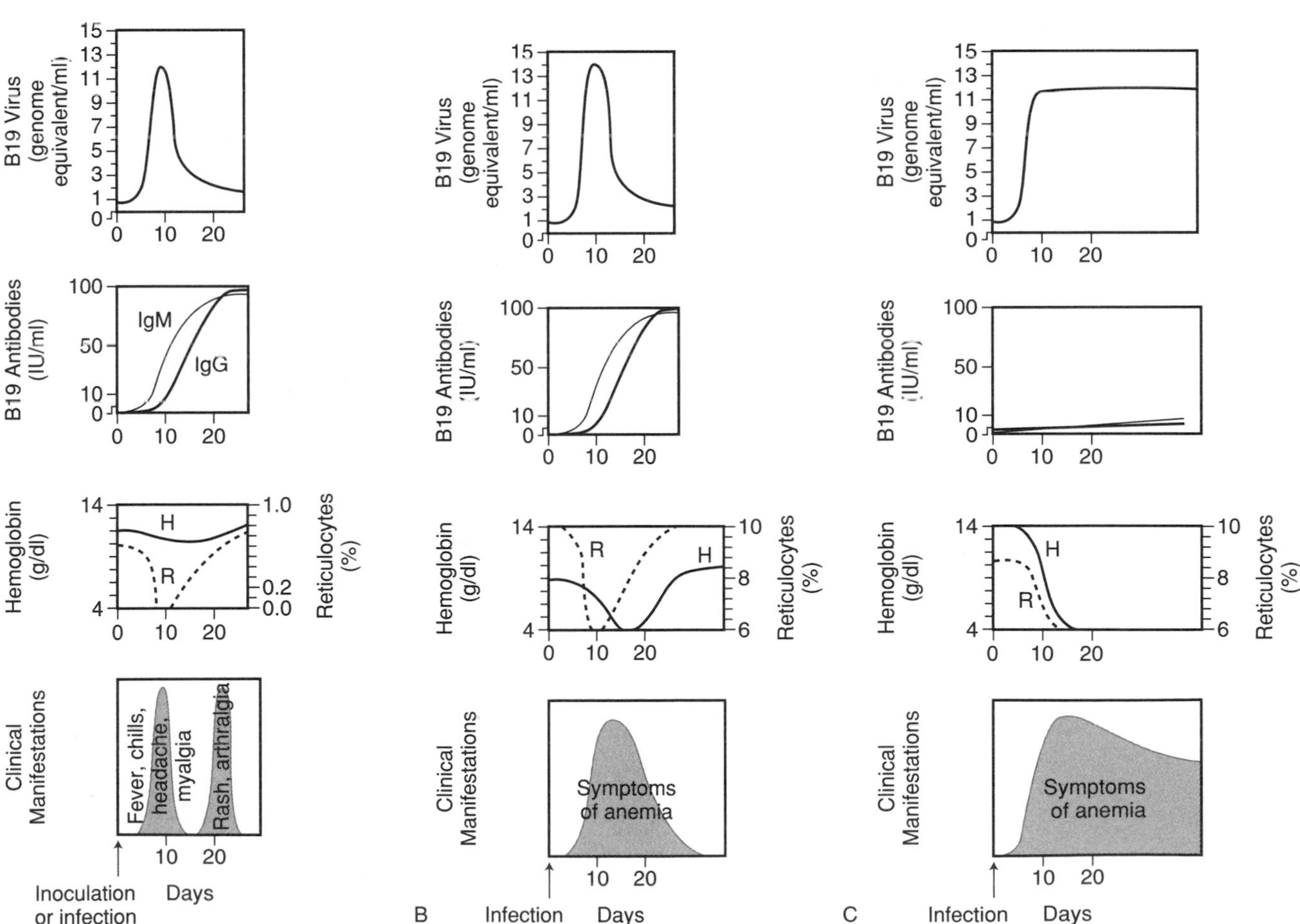

Figure 48–4 Parvovirus B19 infection: The viral titer progression, antibody response, hemoglobin and reticulocyte levels, and symptom complex vary among those with transient infections (**A**), patients with transient aplastic crisis (**B**), and patients developing red cell aplasia (persistent infection) (**C**). (From Young NS, Brown KE. Mechanisms of disease: Parvovirus B19. N Engl J Med 2004;350:586–597.)

prepared from large-scale plasma pools, PCR testing detects parvovirus B19 in most lots. In observational studies, recipients of solvent/detergent–treated plasma seroconverted after infusion of products with high-titer parvovirus DNA, $10^{7.5}$ to $10^{8.5}$ genome copies per milliliter, suggesting that the presence of anti-B19 antibodies was not protective against large viral loads. Seroconversion did not occur among recipients of lots with viral titers between $10^{0.5}$ and $10^{3.5}$ genome copies per milliliter.[78] The virus is resistant to viral-inactivation steps such as solvent/detergent treatment and heat after lyophilization or in the vapor stage. Heat may reduce infectivity if applied in the liquid state. Children receiving plasma-derived factor VIII concentrates were at least 1.9- to 7.6-fold more likely to be B19 seropositive than were those receiving no product or recombinant-derived anti-hemophilic factor.[87] Parvovirus seemingly becomes concentrated in the plasma fraction used in factor VIII preparations. Despite the high frequency of parvovirus exposure, long-term sequelae appear subtle.[82,87] For example, parvovirus B19–seropositive hemophilic children had an 8-degree loss in joint range of motion, a 0.48% difference, compared with seronegative children. Unlike factors VIII and IX, albumin has not transmitted parvovirus B19.[82–88] One report implicated parvovirus transmission by IVIG based on detection of viral DNA by PCR.[89] However, no documentation showed the same viral genotype in the recipient and the immunoglobulin preparation.

Measures to Reduce Transfusion Transmission

In light of these data, in 1999, regulatory agencies and manufacturers of plasma derivatives sought to reduce B19 DNA levels below 10^4 genome copies per milliliter in plasma pools containing 1000 to 3300 plasma donations. However, subsequent reports showed that parvovirus transmission occurred in a recipient of solvent/detergent–treated antihemophilic factor containing 1.3×10^3 genome equivalents per milliliter[83] and a recipient of a dry-heat–treated factor VIII product containing 4×10^3 genome equivalents per milliliter.[85] In these cases, smaller plasma batches with high viral loads were combined to form larger pools used in manufacturing the antihemophilic factor concentrates.

Currently, manufacturers conduct "in-process" testing to eliminate plasma donors with high-titer B19 levels. For example, "recovered plasma" (plasma obtained from whole-blood donations) that is intended for fractionation into plasma derivatives undergoes B19 DNA testing via nucleic acid amplification testing (NAT) assays on aliquots from pooled samples. Subpool analyses are performed to determine which of the samples contained the high-titer donor. These high-titer units, approximately 1 per 10,000 donations, are withheld from product manufacture. Because the infection is transient and a carrier states does not exist, the infected donor is not identified specifically or permanently deferred. Because whole-blood donations rarely transmit parvovirus infections, testing of single unit RBCs, platelets, or plasma for parvovirus B19 is not under consideration in the United States.

CREUTZFELDT-JAKOB DISEASE

Transmissible spongiform encephalopathies (TSEs) occurring in humans include kuru, CJD, Gerstmann-Sträussler-Scheinker disease (a phenotypic variant of CJD), fatal familial insomnia, and variant CJD (vCJD). TSEs occurring in animals include scrapie (sheep and goats), wasting disease of deer and elk, transmissible mink encephalopathy, and bovine spongiform encephalopathy.[91–93]

The TSE infectious agents are classified as prions, or proteinaceous infectious particles that lack nucleic acid. TSEs resist inactivating agents such as alcohol, formalin, ionizing and ultraviolet irradiation, proteases, and nucleases but are disrupted by autoclaving, phenols, detergents, and extremes in pH that affect proteins. The normal host membrane prion protein PrP (designated PrP^c), whose function is unknown, is protease sensitive, soluble, and has a high α-helix content. All prion diseases appear to involve conformational modification of PrP^c to a protease-resistant altered isoform that forms amyloid fibrils (designated PrP^{sc}). The conversion of PrP^c to PrP^{sc} results in refolding of a portion of the α-helical and coil structure of PrP^c into β-sheets. Neuronal loss and vacuolization leads to a spongioform appearance in the brain cortex and deep nuclei.

CJD occurs at an incidence of 0.5 to 1.5 cases per 1 million population worldwide. This rate has increased slightly over the past decade presumably on the basis of improved diagnostic accuracy and greater numbers of older individuals.[92,94] Fewer than 300 cases per year are reported in the United States. Sporadic CJD, causing approximately 85% of CJD cases, occurs in persons 40 to 80 years of age (average age at onset is 60 years) and is manifested by disordered sleep and decreased appetite, behavioral or cognitive changes or focal signs such as visual loss, cerebellar ataxia, asplasia, and motor deficits.[91] The mean survival time is 5 months. The mode of infection for sporadic CJD is uncertain. Approximately 10% to 15% of CJD cases occur in patients with a family history of CJD, suggesting an autosomal dominant inheritance pattern and mutations in the *PRMP* gene that codes for the prion protein. More than 50 mutations in this gene, located on the short arm of chromosome 20, have been identified, but 4 point mutations at codons 102, 178, 200, and 210 occur in 95% of familial cases.[91] Approximately 1% of CJD cases involve iatrogenic transmission. For example, CJD was transmitted by a corneal transplant from a patient with undiagnosed CJD, whereas stereotactic electroencephalographic silver electrodes previously implanted in a patient with CJD subsequently resulted in two iatrogenic CJD cases.[91,92] More than 130 young adults have died 5 to 30 years after receiving intramuscular human growth hormone injections prepared from cadaveric pituitary glands from donors with unsuspected CJD.[91,95] Cadaveric dura mater grafting with a commercial product prepared by batch processing resulted in at least 100 CJD cases worldwide, some occurring 18 years after graft placement.[91,96] In sporadic and iatrogenic cases of CJD, a polymorphism involving codon 129 in the PrP gene appears to affect susceptibility. Normally 37% of the population are methionine/methionine homozygous, and 11% are valine/valine homozygous at codon 129. The remaining 52% are heterozygous. Homozygous individuals represent almost 90% of sporadic and iatrogenic CJD cases.[96,100] Those homozygous for methionine are at risk for fatal familial insomnia, whereas those homozygous for valine are at risk of clinical CJD.[91]

In experiments involving mice infected with a strain of Gerstmann-Sträussler-Scheinker disease, blood-component infection was demonstrated.[97] In contrast, no evidence of transfusion-associated CJD was documented in case-control studies involving more than 600 patients with CJD or in recipients of blood from persons who subsequently developed CJD.[98–100] Examination of brain tissue from deceased hemophilia patients showed no evidence of CJD.[91,101,102] No transfusion-associated CJD cases have been reported to date. Nonetheless, the occurrence of iatrogenic cases and the theoretical risk of CJD transmission by blood led the FDA to issue a recommendation to defer donors if they have one or more blood relatives with CJD or if they have received human pituitary–derived growth hormone injections or a dura mater transplant. All in-date products from donors with these risk factors must be quarantined and destroyed, and the previous recipients of blood from implicated donors, with the exception of those who have only one family member with CJD, must be notified.[92]

VARIANT CREUTZFELDT-JAKOB DISEASE

In the spring of 1985, several dairy cows in the United Kingdom displayed aggressive behavior, ataxia, and falling. These "mad cows" were found to have spongiform lesions in brain tissue resembling scrapie that was subsequently termed *bovine spongiform encephalopathy* (BSE). More than 180,000 cattle succumbed to BSE, but almost 1 million may have been infected. Because the mean incubation period for BSE is 5 years and most cows were slaughtered between 2 and 3 years of age, most cattle did not manifest disease.[91–93] Approximately 50,000 BSE-infected cattle entered the food chain before the first BSE case was recognized in 1986. Subsequently, the onset of the BSE epidemic was traced to a meat-and-bone cattle feed made from sheep, cattle, and pig offal. The rendering process presumably resulted in the feeding of scrapie-infected material to cows. Use of sheep offal or other tissues from ruminant animals as feed for other ruminant animals was banned in 1989. The annual incidence of clinical cases in cattle peaked in 1992. After March 1996, only animals younger than 30 months were eligible for food preparation.[93]

Surveillance for human CJD cases heightened in the United Kingdom after recognition of the BSE epidemic. Ten of 207 CJD patients in 1994 and 1995 had unusual neuropathologic changes.[103,104] They had predominantly psychiatric and sensory symptoms, ataxia, dementia, and myoclonus. All were younger than 45 years, a distinctly unusual characteristic for CJD. Electroencephalographic features were not typical of CJD, and florid PrP plaques were seen on neuropathologic examination. Median survival time was 14 months, in contrast to 4 months for CJD. These cases were considered a new variant of CJD (vCJD). The median incubation period for food-borne vCJD is 13 years.[105] Extensive investigations using animal models provided evidence that the same prion strain causes BSE and vCJD.[106] Ingestion of British beef, therefore, was identified as a risk factor for BSE.[107]

As of June 2006, 159 cases of vCJD have been reported in the United Kingdom, 17 in France, 4 in Ireland, 1 each in Portugal, Spain, Italy, the Netherlands, Saudi Arabia, Japan, and Canada, and 2 in the United States. The latter three plus one Irish patient were thought to result from exposure in the United Kingdom. The Japanese patient spent only 24 days in the United Kingdom. All patients tested were homozygous for methionine at PrP codon 129. By 2000, the incidence of human vCJD cases peaked, suggesting that clinical manifestations among methionine/methionine homozygotes may be less than anticipated after extensive exposure to cattle with subclinical disease.[105,108,109]

Concern about transfusion transmission of vCJD increased because PrP^{sc} is found consistently in the lymphoreticular system of vCJD patients, the possibility that circulating prions transfer the infection from the gut to the brain, and eventually because of animal studies.[105,108,109] In animal model experiments, sheep were fed aliquots of brain obtained from BSE-infected cattle. Subsequently, the sheep underwent phlebotomy at periodic intervals. Among 24 sheep receiving blood from iatrogenically infected donor sheep, 2 given blood from donors in the preclinical BSE phase developed BSE, and 2 receiving blood from clinically affected sheep showed clinical signs of BSE. Among 21 sheep transfused with blood from natural scrapie-infected animals, 4 demonstrated clinical signs of scrapie.[110,111]

An active investigation to determine whether transfusion associated-vCJD transmission occurs in humans began in the United Kingdom in 1997 by identifying vCJD patients who donated blood before illness. Eventually, 48 recipients of blood from 15 donors with vCJD were identified. Three of the 48 recipients, to date, have evidence of vCJD. One, at age 62 years, received non–leukocyte-reduced RBCs from a 24-year-old donor who developed vCJD 3.5 years after the blood donation. The transfusion recipient developed vCJD 6.5 years after transfusion.[112] The second patient received a transfusion of non–leukocyte-reduced RBCs in 1999.[113] The donor developed vCJD 18 months later. The asymptomatic recipient died of a ruptured abdominal aortic aneurysm 5 years after transfusion. At autopsy, protease-resistant prions were present in the spleen and cervical lymph nodes. Prions were not detected in the brain. The recipient, found to be heterozygous (methionine/valine at codon 129), did not have clinical vCJD, raising concern that the incubation period may be longer in codon 129 heterozygotes. In animal studies, a primary challenge with vCJD prions resulted in a significantly reduced transmission rate in mice with valine at codon 129 compared with that in animals homozygous for methionine.[114] Additional data are needed to confirm whether the incubation period varies among methionine homozygous and heterozygous individuals. The third case developed vCJD approximately 8 years after receiving non-leukocyte-reduced red cells from a person who developed vCJD 20 months postdonation.[114a]

The U.K. National Blood Service also determined that approximately 100 people donated blood to four patients who subsequently showed clinical signs of vCJD. These donors were notified that they may be at higher risk of developing vCJD despite the uncertainty of whether the patients contracted vCJD through food or blood transfusion. In addition, UK authorities notified recipients of factor XI concentrates that donors of these components developed vCJD after donation on the ethical tenet of transparency. The United Kingdom currently imports plasma from the United States for patients younger than 16 years and uses apheresis-derived platelets in these patients to reduce donor exposures.[94,116]

The identification of presumed transfusion-associated vCJD cases appears to validate the steps taken in response to the precautionary principle to decrease the risk of transmitting vCJD by transfusion.[92] Donors who visited or resided in the United Kingdom for a cumulative period of 3 months or longer between 1980 and 1996 are deferred indefinitely. Donors who spent 5 years or more in Europe before 1980 and the present are also deferred. In addition, donors are indefinitely deferred if they injected bovine insulin after 1980, received transfusions in the United Kingdom and France between 1980 and the present, or served in the military on bases in Europe for 6 months or more between 1980 and 1996. This geography-based donor-deferral protocol evolved in various phases beginning in 1999. Approximately 3.5% of potential donors in the United States have been deferred as a result of this policy.[117] The impact was higher in Canada.[118] In-date blood components and plasma intended for derivative production from these donors must be recalled, quarantined, and destroyed. Ongoing surveillance of vCJD cases, which increased after identification of a Texas cow with BSE, is currently being conducted, including a recommendation to notify the CDC about all patients younger than 55 years who are diagnosed with CJD.[115]

In addition to geographic exclusion policies, other strategies for preventing vCJD transmission include removal of the infectious agent and testing. In the United Kingdom, all blood components undergo leukocyte reduction by filtration, based on observations that prions associate with leukocytes. Leukocyte reduction, however, is only partially effective, removing only 42% of total prion infectivity.[120] Filters that specifically remove prions and laboratory tests that detect infectious prions are currently being developed and evaluated. The latter, if implemented, will be accompanied by significant ethical concerns.[119]

LEISHMANIASIS

Visceral forms of leishmaniasis result from infection with *Leishmania donovani* or *Leishmania infantum*. Cutaneous lesions occur in persons infected with *Leishmania braziliensis* or *Leishmania tropica*, the cause of Old World cutaneous leishmaniasis. However, at least eight soldiers returning from eastern Saudi Arabia after Operation Desert Storm developed visceral leishmaniasis that was attributed to *L. tropica*.[121,122]

The leishmania organisms, transmitted primarily by bites from infected sand flies, are endemic in the tropical and subtropical regions of the Sudan, Eastern India, Bangladesh, Nepal, Brazil, and the Mediterranean.[123]

After transmission by sand fly bite, parasites reside intracellularly in monocytes, which circulate before taking up residence in internal organs. In the most severe manifestation of visceral leishmaniasis, kala-azar, patients have marked hepatosplenomegaly, pancytopenia, hypergammaglobulinemia, and cachexia. The incubation period is approximately 6 months.[123] Anti–*L. donovani* antibodies form shortly after infection. In studies conducted in Brazil, 21 seropositive asymptomatic blood donors were found to have positive PCR results for *L. donovani*, demonstrating the ongoing potential of transfusion transmission in endemic areas.[124]

At least 10 transfusion-associated cases of leishmaniasis attributed to *L. donovani* have been reported in endemic regions. Most of those infected were young children or neonates. A probable case of platelet transfusion–transmitted *Leishmania* was reported recently.[125] Transfusion-transmission also appears to occur in dogs receiving transfusions of RBCs from seropositive dog-blood donors.[126]

Veterans of Operation Desert Storm who served in the Persian Gulf region between August 1990 and December 1992 were deferred from blood donation for 1 year, after the report of *L. tropica*–related viscerotropic leishmaniasis. The patients had nonspecific clinical manifestations, including prolonged fever, malaise, abdominal pain, and intermittent diarrhea, which occurred up to 7 months after they returned to the United States.[121] *L. tropica* was found in the bone marrow of seven patients and in a lymph node in one patient. Intracellular amastigotes were seen in the peripheral blood of the one patient in whom this was studied.[127] After reports of hundreds of cases of cutaneous leishmaniasis and two cases of visceral leishmaniasis in troops involved in the Iraq war, a similar 1-year deferral after departure from Iraq was instituted in October 2003.[127] *L. tropica* within human monocytes survives in blood stored at 1° C to 6° C, in frozen RBCs, and in platelet concentrates stored at room temperature. However, *L. tropica* has not been detected in relatively cell-free fresh frozen plasma. Animal studies demonstrate transmission by contaminated blood.[126]

No cases of transfusion-transmitted leishmaniasis have been reported in the United States to date. For this reason, surveillance and targeted donor deferral appear to be appropriate. Use of leukocyte filters to reduce *Leishmania* transmission is under investigation.[128]

TOXOPLASMOSIS

Toxoplasma gondii is a ubiquitous parasite whose usual host is the domestic cat. Infection sometimes results in lymphadenopathy, malaise, fever, headache, sore throat, splenomegaly, hepatomegaly, and rash. Retinopathy and lethal infections occur in immunocompromised hosts.

Transfusion transmission was reported in 1971. However, the cases occurred among leukemia patients given granulocyte transfusions obtained from other leukemic patients. Another case report suggested that a patient undergoing chemotherapy for a leukemic relapse 3 years after receiving an allogeneic marrow transplant developed toxoplasma pneumonitis. A person with serologic evidence of recent toxoplasma infection donated one of the units of blood transfused to the patient.[130] In addition, a 52-year-old woman with drug-induced thrombocytopenia developed toxoplasma retinochoroiditis, presumably related to a platelet transfusion.[130] A case further emphasizing the importance of nontraditional routes of infection in immunocompromised patients involved a renal transplant recipient who developed toxoplasmosis.[131] The infection was presumably transmitted by a kidney obtained from a seropositive organ donor.

DENGUE

Dengue, transmitted by *Aedes* mosquitoes, has infected at least 77 U.S. travelers to Caribbean islands (including Puerto Rico and the U.S. Virgin Islands), Pacific islands, Asia, Central America, Africa, and Hawaii between 2001 and 2004.[132,133] The incubation period is 3 to 14 days. Infections cause either no symptoms, mild illness, or severe disease including hemorrhagic manifestations and shock.[134] Transmission by bone marrow transplantation and several reports of transmission after needle-stick injuries involving symptomatic patients raise the possibility of transfusion transmission by asymptomatic travelers returning from endemic areas.[135–137]

SIMIAN FOAMY VIRUS

More than 70% of nonhuman primates in zoos or in animal research facilities are infected with simian foamy virus (SFV), an endogenous, cell-associated retrovirus found in New and Old World primates.[138] Surveillance studies indicate that approximately 5% of zoo and biomedical research personnel working with chimpanzees and baboons are infected with SFV. Evaluation of archival samples documented infection for 8 to 26 years (median, 22 years). All subjects remained healthy, and each of three spouses undergoing testing for SFV were nonreactive. In addition, 1% of bush hunters in central Africa and 1% of those exposed to free-ranging nonhuman primates in Asia tested positive for SFV.[139,140] Presumably, those infected were inoculated through exposure to saliva from bites or close contact through exposure to body fluids.

Only limited information is available about transfusion transmission. One occupationally exposed SFV-infected individual donated blood 6 times during an interval when SFV test results, conducted retrospectively, were positive. None of the tested recipients of RBCs, leukocyte-reduced RBCs, or platelets was SFV positive. Three of these blood components were stored for less than 8 days.[141]

LYMPHOCYTIC CHORIOMENINGITIS VIRUS

Infections with lymphocytic choriomenigitis virus (LCMV), a rodent-borne arenavirus, usually cause mild, self-limited illness or aseptic meningitis in nonimmunosuppressed patients. Human infections typically follow exposures to body fluids or infected animal excretions. Vertical transmission occurs, but LCMV is not considered to be communicable from person to person. LCMV has been transmitted to four organ transplant recipients via an asymptomatic organ donor who had a cerebrovascular accident and subsequent brain death.[142] The donor apparently became infected by exposure to a pet hamster. Within 3 weeks of transplantation, the recipients of the liver, lungs, and two kidneys developed fever, rash, or diarrhea; three of the four recipients died. A previous case also involving four transplant recipients was unrecognized until this case was reported. Transfusion transmission has not been reported but is a possibility, given transmission by solid-organ transplantation.

H5N1 AVIAN INFLUENZA VIRUS

The avian influenza A/H5N1 virus has spread epidemically among birds and poultry since emerging in Hong Kong in 1997.[143] Since that time, more than 100 million birds and poultry have died or been culled to prevent epidemic progression via bird migration in Cambodia, China, Indonesia, Japan, Laos, South Korea, Thailand, Vietnam, Malaysia, Turkey, Romania, and Russia. Transmission to humans via contact with infected poultry or contaminated surfaces has resulted in more than 60 deaths.

To date, human-to-human transmission has occurred infrequently.[144] However, concern exists that mutations, reassortments, or recombinant rearrangements of the virus with pathogenic human influenza viruses could produce a virus capable of jumping the species barrier and causing a worldwide pandemic. Influenza viremia is infrequent, although highly pathogenic avian influenza can be transmitted via blood.[145] Although transfusion transmission is a theoretical risk, a more likely impact would be large-scale donor illness and blood shortages.

SEVERE ACUTE RESPIRATORY SYNDROME

SARS, caused by a novel enveloped RNA coronavirus, infected more than 1800 patients in 17 countries in February and March 2003.[146] This highly contagious illness dominated worldwide public health attention, resulting in rapid identification, travel advisories, patient quarantine, and eventual eradication of the epidemic.[147] The 2-week asymptomatic incubation period fostered spread of the virus through close person-to-person contact and raised the possibility of blood-borne infection. For this reason, the U.S. FDA issued a guidance document in April 2003 requiring blood-collection agencies to defer anyone from donating blood for at least 14 days after possible exposure to SARS.[148] Those with a suspected SARS illness were deferred for at least 28 days after recovery. Notices were posted in blood centers apprising donors about SARS-affected areas, and donors were asked about recent travel history. Those traveling to affected areas, including transit in an airport at these locations, were deferred from blood donation. The epidemic subsided within months. No reports of transfusion-associated SARS exist.

WEST NILE VIRUS

West Nile Virus (WNV) is a mosquito-borne, lipid-enveloped, RNA virus in the Japanese encephalitis flaviridae complex. The viral genome codes for capsid, membrane, envelope, and nonstructural proteins.[149]

The virus, transmitted from bird to bird by mosquito vectors, infects humans as incidental hosts. The virus was identified in the West Nile district of Uganda in 1937. Outbreaks occurred subsequently in the Mid-East, South Africa, and Europe. The first North American cases were recorded in New York City in 1999.[150–153] WNV infections in humans have occurred predominantly between June through October, peaking in August through late September and remitting during the winter. Starting in July 2000, WNV cases were reported in Mid-Atlantic states. In July 2001, 66 cases occurred in the eastern one third of the United States. In 2002 the epidemic spread to the Midwest and eastern Plains states; 4156 cases were reported including 2946 with meningoencephalitis. In 2003, further western spread saw the majority of cases in the Plains states of Nebraska, Colorado, North and South Dakota, and Wyoming; 9862 cases were reported, including 2775 with neuroinvasive complications. In 2004, the epidemic spread farther westward to include Arizona and southern California. WNV activity was reported in 47 states, involving 2470 reports. WNV cases in 2005 progressed farther down the West Coast; 2435 cases were reported through October 2005.[154] In addition, 372 viremic blood donors were identified.

WNV activity in birds and mosquitos occurs throughout the year, especially in warmer regions. The virus becomes detectable in blood 1 to 3 days after a mosquito bite, followed by an increase in viral loads. However, peak titers are relatively low (median of 3500 copies per milliliter) compared with HIV and HCV (10^5 to 10^7 per milliliter). RNA levels decrease markedly 7 to 10 days after infection when immunoglobulin M (IgM) antibodies, and subsequently IgG anitibodies, appear. IgM antibodies persist for more than 398 days in approximately two thirds of those infected.[155] The mean duration of viremia is 6 days. However, WNV RNA was detected up to 104 days after infection in one blood donor.[157–162] (Fig. 48–5)

Approximately 80% of persons infected with WNV remain asymptomatic. The 20% with symptomatic infections report abdominal pain, chills, fever, generalized weakness, headache, joint pain, muscle weakness and pain, new macular rash on the trunk and extremities, new difficulty thinking, painful eyes, and swollen glands.[163] One in 150 infected persons develops meningitis, encephalitis, or asymmetric flaccid paralysis. Fatal outcomes occur in 4% to 14% of those with severe disease.

WNV transmission in four recipients of organ donations was reported in 2002.[163] The organ donor, in turn, received blood transfusions from 63 donors, one of whom subsequently was found to be WNV infected. A sample from the organ donor subsequently tested WNV RNA positive, but WNV IgM negative. Initial reports of transmission by blood transfusion in 2002 eventually resulted in confirmation of 23 cases of transfusion-associated WNV infection.[162] The interval between transfusion and symptom onset was 10 days (median interval range, 2 to 21 days). Nine of 14 implicated blood donors reported WNV-associated symptoms before donation.

After intense collaboration among U.S. public health authorities, test manufacturers, and blood-collection agencies, NAT for WNV RNA was implemented before the 2003 WNV season. As a direct result of testing, more than 1000 donors were found to be WNV RNA positive in 2003, preventing WNV transmission to approximately 1500 recipients of RBCs and components prepared from these donations.[156,157,159] During the summer months, approximately 1 per 7000 units was WNV RNA positive. In high WNV endemic areas, 1 in approximately 150 donors was WNV viremic. In 2003, six transfusion-associated WNV cases were reported.[158] All of the implicated donors had extremely low-level viremia that escaped detection by routine testing in minipools containing aliquots from 6 to 16 donations. Testing of individual samples in high-incidence areas increases test sensitivity by approximately 7% and was introduced in 2004 when incident cases exceeded preestablished thresholds (approximately 1 WNV-positive donor per 1000 donations). Only one confirmed transmission occurred in 2004. Among the 30 confirmed transfusion cases, all implicated donations were WNV IgM antibody negative.[164,165]

A second transplant-associated incident involving three of four organ recipients who developed WNV infection after transplant was reported in 2005.[166] Of note, the organ donor (infected through mosquito bites) was WNV RNA positive and IgM antibody positive. This report raises concern that organ-transplant recipients and other heavily immunosuppressed patients are at extremely high risk for severe WNV complications and that the virus remains viable in organ/tissue reservoirs despite a humoral immune response.

Overall, the rapid implementation of WNV testing within months of the initial transplant and transfusion-associated cases resulted in dramatic reduction of further transfusion-transmitted cases. Assuming that RNA-positive, IgM antibody–positive donors do not transmit WNV through blood transfusion, the residual risk of transfusion-associated WNV after implementation of NAT is approximately 1 per 350,000 donations.[164,165]

RABIES

In June 2004, the CDC confirmed the diagnosis of rabies in recipients of a liver and two kidneys from an organ donor subsequently found infected with rabies via a bat bite. The recipients developed tremors, myoclonic jerks, altered mental status, or anorexia 21 to 27 days after transplant. All died. It is unlikely that these transplant-related cases portend a risk for transfusion-transmission, in that exposure to infected neuronal tissue appears to be the vector in these cases. The rabies virus is not transmitted hematologically, and contact with blood, urine or feces is not considered an exposure risk.[167]

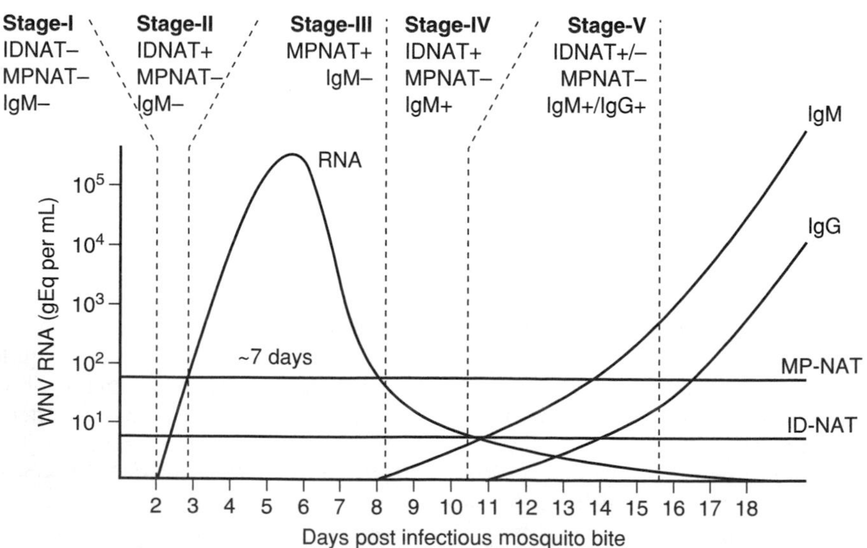

Figure 48–5 West Nile virus (WNV) RNA circulates at relatively low levels for 7 to 10 days after the bite of an infected mosquito. Minipool nucleic acid testing (MP-NAT) detects 43 to 309 viral copies per milliliter within a few days of infection. In contrast, individual donation NAT (ID-NAT) detects 3.4 to 29 copies per milliliter and reduces the window period between infection and test detection. All transfusion-associated WNV cases have occurred in the NAT-positive/IgM antibody–negative stages. (From Busch MP. West Nile virus window period. Transfusion 2005;45:cover figure.)

REFERENCES

1. Fauci AS. Emerging infectious diseases: a clear and present danger to humanity. JAMA 2004;292:187–188.
2. Busch MP, Kleinman SH, Nemo GJ. Current and emerging infectious risks of blood transfusions. JAMA 2003;289:959–962.
3. Zhang L, Yu P, Bu H, et al. Porcine endogenous retrovirus transmission from pig cell line to mouse tissues but not human cells in nude mice. Transplant Proc 2005;37:493–495.
4. White DJ, Talarico J, Chang HG, et al. Human babesiosis in New York State: review of 139 hospitalized cases and analysis of prognostic factors. Arch Intern Med 1998;158:2149–2154.
5. McQuiston JH, Childs JE, Chamberland ME, et al. Transmission of tick-borne agents of disease by blood transfusion: a review of known and potential risks in the United States. Transfusion 2000;40:274–284.
6. Linden JV, Wong SJ, Chu FK, et al. Transfusion-associated transmission of babesiosis in New York State. Transfusion 2000;40:285–289.
7. Krause PJ, Telford SR, Ryan R, et al. Geographical and temporal distribution of babesial infection in Connecticut. J Clin Microbiol 1991; 29:1–4.
8. Popovsky MA. Transfusion-transmitted babesiosis. Transfusion 1991;31:296–298.
9. Leiby DA, Chung AP, Cable RG, et al. Relationship between tick bites and the seroprevalence of *Babesia microti* and *Anaplasma phagocytophila* (previously *Ehrlichia* sp.) in blood donors. Transfusion 2002; 42:1585–1591.
10. Leiby D, Gill J. Transfusion-transmitted tick-borne infections: a cornucopia of threats. Trans Med Rev 2004;18:293–306.
11. Herwaldt BL, Neitzel DR, Gorlin JB, et al. Transmission of *Babesia micoti* in Minnesota through four blood donations from the same donor over a 6-month period. Transfusion 2002;42:1154–1158.
12. Kjemtrup AM, Lee B, Fritz CL, et al. Investigation of transfusion transmission of a WA1-type babesial parasite to a premature infant in California. Transfusion 2002;42:1482–1487.
13. Lux JZ, Weiss D, Linden JV, et al. Transfusion-associated babesiosis after heart transplant. Emerg Infect Dis 2003;9:116–119.
14. Krause PJ, Spielman A, Telford SR, et al. Persistent parasitemia after acute babesiosis. N Engl J Med 1998;339:160–165.
15. Leiby DA, Chung APS, Gill JE, et al. Demonstrable parasitemia among Connecticut blood donors with antibodies to *Babesia microti.* Transfusion 2005;45:1804–1810.
16. Dobroszycki J, Herwaldt BL, Boctor F, et al. A cluster of transfusion-associated babesiosis cases traced to an asymptomatic donor. JAMA 1999;281:927–930.
17. Cable RG, Johnson ST, Gill JE, et al. Reduced prevalence of donor *Babesia microti* parasitemia following initiation of a research antibody testing program. Transfusion 2005;45:16A–17A.
18. Pantanowitz L, Monahan-Earley R, Dvorak A, et al. Morphologic hallmarks of *Babesia.* Transfusion 2002;42:1389.
19. CDC. Lyme Disease: United States 2001–2002. MMWR Morb Mortal Wkly Rep 2004;53:365–367.
20. Wormser GP, McKenna D, Carlin J, et al. Brief communication: Hematogenous dissemination in early Lyme disease. Ann Intern Med 2005;142:751–755.
21. Steere AC, Sikand VK. The presenting manifestations of Lyme disease and the outcomes of treatment [Letter]. N Engl J Med 2003;348: 2472–2474.
22. Stanek G, Strle F. Lyme borreliosis. Lancet 2003;362:1639–1647.
23. Hayes EB, Piesman J. How can we prevent Lyme disease? N Engl J Med 2003;348:2424–2430.
24. McQuiston JH, Paddock CD, Holman RC, et al. The human ehrlichioses in the United States. Emerg Infect Dis 1999;5:635–642.
25. Goodman JL. Ehrlichiosis: Ticks, dogs, and doxycycline. N Engl J Med 1999;341:195–197.
26. Spencer BR, Johnson S, Nguyen ML, et al. Longitudinal study of exposure to human granulocyte ehrlichiosis in healthy blood donors. Transfusion 2005;45:16A.
27. Magnarelli L, Ijdo J, Anderson J, et al. Human exposure to a granulocytic *Ehrlichia* and other tick-borne agents in Connecticut. J Clin Microbiol 1998;36:2823–2827.
28. Eastlund T, Persing D, Mathieson D, et al. Human granulocyte ehrlichiosis after red cell transfusion. Transfusion 1999;93:117S.
29. McKechnie DB, Slater KS, Childs JE, et al. Survival of *Ehrlichia chaffeensis* in refrigerated, ADSOL-treated RBCs. Transfusion 2000;40: 1041–1047.
30. Arguin PM, Singleton J, Rotz LD, et al. An investigation into the possibility of transmission of tick-borne pathogens via blood transfusion. Transfusion 1999;39:828–833.
31. World Health Organization. World malaria situation in 1993. Wkly Epidemiol Rec 1996;71:17–24.
32. Pan American Health Organization. Report for Registration of Malaria Eradication from the United States of America. Washington, D.C., Pan American Health Organization, 1969.
33. Zucker JR. Changing patterns of autochthonous malaria transmission in the United States: a review of recent outbreaks. Emerg Infect Dis 1996;2:37–43.
34. CDC. Local transmission of *Plasmodium vivax* malaria: Palm Beach County, Florida. MMWR Morb Mortal Wkly Rep 2003;52:908–911.
35. Shah S, Filler S, Causer LM, et al. Malaria surveillance: United States, 2002; CDC Surveillance Summaries (April 30, 2004). MMWR Morb Mortal Wkly Rep 2004;53:SS–1.
36. Eliades MJ, Shah S, Ngugen-Dinh P, et al. Malaria surveillance: United States, 2003; CDC Surveillance Summaries (June 3, 2005). MMWR Morb Mortal Wkly Rep 2005;54:SS–2.
37. Guerrero IC, Weniger BC, Schultz MG. Transfusion malaria in the United States, 1972–1981. Ann Intern Med 1983;99:221–226.
38. Zoon K. Recommendations for Deferral of Donors for Malaria Risk: Letter to All Registered Blood Establishments. Rockville, Md., U.S. Department of Health and Human Services, Food and Drug Administration, July 24, 1994.
39. Transfusion-transmitted malaria: Missouri and Pennsylvania, 1996–1998. MMWR Morb Mortal Wkly Rep 1999;48:253–256.
40. Mungai M, Tegtmeier G, Chamberland M, et al. Transfusion-transmitted malaria in the U.S., 1963–1998. N Engl J Med 2001;344:1973–1978.
41. Besson PP, Robert JF, Reviron J, et al. Á propos de deux observations du paludisme transfusionnel. [Two cases of transfusional malaria.] Rev Fr Transfus Immunohématol 1976;19:369–373.
42. Shulman IA. Parasitic infections and their impact on blood donor selection and testing. Arch Pathol Lab Med 1994;118:366–370.
43. Brasseur P, Bonneau J-C. Le paludisme transfusionnel: risque, prévention et coût: Rev Fr Transfus Hématol 1981;24:597–608.
44. Sulzer AJ, Wilson M. The indirect fluorescent antibody test for the detection of occult malaria in blood donors. Bull WHO 1971;45:375–379.
45. Kachur SP, Bloland PB. Malaria. In Wallace RB (ed): Maxcy-Rosenau-Last Textbook of Public Health and Preventive Medicine, 14th ed. Norwalk, Appleton & Lange, 1998, pp 313–326.
46. U.S. Department of Health and Human Services, Food and Drug Administration. Center for Biologics Evaluation and Research. Proceedings of the Blood Products Advisory Committee, 63rd meeting, Washington, DC, June 18, 1999.
47. Teixera ARL, Monteiro PS, Rebelo JM, et al. Emerging Chagas disease: Trophic network and cycle of transmission of *Trypanosoma cruzi* from palm trees in the Amazon. Emerg Infect Dis 2002;7:100–112.
48. Leiby DA. Threats to blood safety posed by emerging protozoan pathogens. Vox Sang 2004;87:120–122.
49. Kirchhoff LV. American trypanosomiasis (Chagas' disease): a tropical disease now in the United States. N Engl J Med 1993;329:639–644.
50. Moraes-Souza H, Bordin JO. Strategies for prevention of transfusion-associated Chagas' disease. Transfus Med Rev 1996;10:161–170.
51. Shulman IR. Intervention strategies to reduce the risk of transfusion-transmitted *Trypanosoma cruzi* infection in the United States. Transfus Med Rev 1999;13:227–234.
52. Leiby DA, Herron RM, Read EJ, et al. *Trypanosoma cruzi* in Los Angeles and Miami blood donors: impact of evolving donor demographics on seroprevalence and implications for transfusion transmission. Transfusion 2002;42:549–555.
54. Kirchhoff LV, Gam AA, Gilliam FC. American trypanosomiasis (Chagas' disease) in Central American immigrants. Am J Med 1987; 82:915–920.
55. Brashear RJ, Winkler MA, Schur JD, et al. Detection of antibodies to *Trypanosoma cruzi* among blood donors in the southwestern and western United States, I: evaluation of the sensitivity and specificity of an enzyme immunoassay for detecting antibodies to *T. cruzi.* Transfusion 1995; 35:213–218.
56. Shulman IA, Appleman MD, Saxena S, et al. Specific antibodies to *Trypanosoma cruzi* among blood donors in Los Angeles, California. Transfusion 1997;37:727–731.
57. Leiby DA, Fucci MH, Stumpf RJ. *Trypanosoma cruzi* in low-to moderate-risk blood donor population: seroprevalence and possible congenital transmission. Transfusion 1999;39:310–315.
58. Herwaldt BL, Grijalva MJ, Newsome AL, et al. Use of polymerase chain reaction to diagnose the fifth reported US case of autochthonous transmission of *Trypanosoma cruzi,* in Tennessee, 1998. J Infect Dis 2000;181:395–399.
59. Beard CB, Pye G, Steurer FJ. Chagas disease in a domestic transmission cycle in southern Texas, USA. Emerg Infect Dis 2003;9:103–105.

60. CDC. Chagas disease after organ transplantation: United States, 2001. MMWR Morb Mortal Wkly Rep 2002;51:210–212.
61. Nickerson P, Orr P, Schroeder ML, et al. Transfusion-associated *Trypanosoma cruzi* infection in a non-endemic area. Ann Intern Med 1989;111:851–853.
62. Grant IH, Gold JWM, Wittner M, et al. Transfusion-associated acute Chagas' disease acquired in the United States. Ann Intern Med 1989;111:849–851.
63. Cimo PL, Luper WE, Scouros MA. Transfusion-associated Chagas' disease in Texas: report of case. J Tex Med 1993;89:48–50.
64. Leiby DA, Lenes BA, Tibbals MA, et al. Prospective evaluation of a patient with *Trypanosoma cruzi* infection transmitted by transfusion. N Engl J Med 1999;341:1237–1239.
65. Lane DJ, Sher G, Ward B, et al. Investigation of the second case of transfusion transmitted Chagas disease in Canada. Blood 2000;96:60a(S).
66. Appleman MD, Shulman IA, Saxena S, et al. Use of a questionnaire to identify potential blood donors at risk for infection with *Trypanosoma cruzi*. Transfusion 1993;33:61–64.
67. Galel SA, Kirchhoff LV. Risk factors for *Trypanosoma cruzi* infection in California blood donors. Transfusion 1996;36:227–231.
68. Moraes-Souza H, Bordin JO, Bardossy L, et al. Prevention of transfusion-associated Chagas' disease: Efficacy of white cell-reduction filters in removing *Trypanosoma cruzi* from infected blood. Transfusion 1995;35:723–726.
69. Schmidt PJ. Syphilis, a disease of direct transfusion. Transfusion 2001; 41:1069–1071.
70. Infectious Disease Testing for Blood Transfusions. NIH Consensus Statement. Online 1995 Jan 9–11;13(1):1–29.
71. Herrera GA, Lackritz RS, Janssen VP, et al. Serologic test for syphilis as a surrogate marker for human immunodeficiency virus infection among United States blood donors. Transfusion 1997;37:836–840.
72. Cable RG. Evaluation of syphilis testing of blood donors. Transfus Med Rev 1996;10:296–302.
73. Greenwalt TJ, Rios JA. To test or not to test for syphilis: a global problem. Transfusion 2001;41:976.
74. Aberle J, Grasse SL, Notari OE, et al. Predictive value of past and current screening tests for syphilis in blood donors: changing from a rapid plasma reagin test to an automated specific treponemal test for screening. Transfusion 1999;39:206–211.
75. Orton SL, Dodd RY, Williams AE. Absence of risk factors for false-positive test results in blood donors with a reactive test result in an automated treponemal test (PK-TP) for syphilis. Transfusion 2001;41:744–750.
76. FDA-CBER. Guidance for industry: revised recommendations for donor and product management based on screening tests for syphilis. June 2003.www.fda.gov/cber/guidance.htm
77. Young NS, Brown KE. Mechanisms of disease: Parvovirus B19. N Engl J Med 2004;350:586–597.
78. Brown KE, Young NS, Barbosa LH, et al. Parvovirus B19: Implications for transfusion medicine: Summary of a workshop. Transfusion 2001;41:130–135.
79. Enders M, Weidner A, Zoellner I, et al. Fetal morbidity and mortality after acute human parvovirus B19 infection in pregnancy: prospective evaluation of 1018 cases. Prenat Diagn 2004;24:513–518.
80. Brown KE, Anderson SM, Young NS. Erythrocyte P antigen-cellular receptor for B19 virus. Science 1993;262:114–117.
81. Azzi A, Morfini M, Mannucci PM. The transfusion-associated transmission of parvovirus B19. Transfus Med Rev 1999;13:194–204.
82. Ragni MV, Koch WC, Jordan JA. Parvovirus B19 infection in patients with hemophilia. Transfusion 1996;36:238–241.
83. Wu C, Mason B, Jong J, et al. Parvovirus B19 transmission by a high-purity factor VIII concentrate. Transfusion 2005;45:1003–1010.
84. Just B, Lefevre H. Detection of parvovirus B19 DNA in solvent-detergent plasma. Vox Sang 2002;83:167.
85. Blümel J, Schmidt I, Effenberger W, et al. Parvovirus B19 transmission by heat-treated clotting factor concentrates. Transfusion 2002;42:1473–1481.
86. Gaboulaud V, Parquet A, Tahiri C, et al. Prevalence of IgG antibodies to human parvovirus B19 in haemophilia children treated with recombinant factor (F)VIII only or with at least one plasma-derived FVIII or FIX concentrate: results from the French haemophilia cohort. Br J Haematol 2002;116:383–389.
87. Soucie JM, Siwak EB, Hooper WC, et al. Human parvovirus B19 in young male patients with hemophilia A: associations with treatment product exposure and joint range-of-motion limitation. Transfusion 2004;44:1179–1185.
88. Blümel J, Schmidt I, Willkommen H, et al. Inactivation of parvovirus B19 during pasteurization of human serum albumin. Transfusion 2002;42:1011–1018.
89. Hayakawa F, Imada K, Towatari M, et al. Life threatening human parvovirus B19 infection transmitted by intravenous immune globulin. Br J Haematol 2002;118:1187–1189.
90. Weimer T, Streichert S, Watson C, et al. High-titer screening PCR: a successful strategy for reducing the parvovirus B19 load in plasma pools for fractionation. Transfusion 2001;41:1500–1504.
91. Johnson R. Prion disease. Lancet Neurol 2005;4:635–642.
92. FDA-CBER. Guidance for Industry: revised preventative measures to reduce the possible risk of transmission of Creutzfeldt-Jacob disease (CJD) and variant Creutzfeldt-Jacob disease (vCJD) by blood and blood products. January 2002.www.fda.gov/cber/guidance.htm.
93. Collinge J. Variant Creutzfeldt-Jacob disease. Lancet 1999;354: 317–323.
94. Creutzfeldt-Jakob disease surveillance in the UK: Twelfth Annual Report 2003. www.cjd.ed.ac.uk/twelfth/rep2003.htm
95. Huillard d'Aignaux J, Costagliola D, Maccario J, et al. Incubation period of Creutzfeldt-Jacob disease in human growth hormone recipients in France. Neurology 1999;53:1197–1201.
96. Centers for Disease Control and Prevention. Creutzfeldt-Jacob disease associated with cadaveric dura mater grafts: Japan, January 1979–May 1996. MMWR Morb Mortal Wkly Rep 1997;46:1066–1069.
97. Cervenakova L, Yakovleva O, McKenzie C, et al. Similar levels of infectivity in the blood of mice infected with human-derived vCJD and GSS strains of transmissible spongiform encephalopathy. Transfusion 2003;43:1687–1764.
98. Sullivan MT, Schonberger LB, Kessler D, et al. Creutzfeldt-Jakob Disease (CJD) investigational look-back study. Transfusion 1997; 37:2S.
99. Collins S, Law MG, Fletcher A, et al. Surgical treatment and risk of sporadic Creutzfeldt-Jacob disease: a case-control study. Lancet 1999; 353:693–697.
100. Wientjens DPWM, Davanipour Z, Hofman A, et al. Risk factors for Creutzfeldt-Jacob disease: a reanalysis of case-control studies. Neurology 1996;46:1287–1291.
101. Evatt B, Austin H, Barnhart E, et al. Surveillance for Creutzfeldt-Jacob disease among persons with hemophilia. Transfusion 1998;38: 817–820.
102. Lee CA, Ironside JW, Bell JE, et al. Retrospective neuropathological review of prion disease in UK haemophilic patients. Thromb Haemost 1998;80:909–911.
103. Will RG, Ironside JW, Zeidler M, et al. A new variant of Creutzfeldt-Jacob disease in the UK. Lancet 1996;347:921–925.
104. Zeidler M, Stewart GE, Barraclogh CR, et al. New variant Creutzfeldt-Jacob disease: Neurological features and diagnostic tests. Lancet 1997;350:903–907.
105. Belay ED, Sejvar JJ, Shieh WJ, et al. Variant Creutzfeldt-Jakob disease death, United States. Emerg Infect Dis 2005;11:1351–1354.
106. Hill AF, Desbruslais M, Joiner S, et al. The same prion strain causes vCJD and BSE. Nature 1997;389:448–450.
107. Bons N, Mestre-Frances N, Belli P, et al. Natural and experimental oral infection of nonhuman primates by bovine spongiform encephalopathy agents. Proc Natl Acad Sci USA 1999;96:4046–4051.
108. http://www.cjd.ed.ac.uk/figures.htm.
109. Houston F, Foster JD, Chong A, et al. Transmission of BSE by blood transfusion in sheep. Lancet 2000;356:999–1000.
110. Hunter N, Foster J, Chong A, et al. Transmission of prion diseases by blood transfusion. J Gen Virol 2002;83:2897–2905.
111. Llewelyn CA, Hewitt PE, Knight RS, et al. Possible transmission of variant Creutzfeldt-Jakob disease by blood transfusion. Lancet 2004;363:417–421.
112. Peden AH, Head MW, Ritchie DL, et al. Preclinical vCJD after blood transfusion in a PRNP codon 129 heterozygous patient. Lancet 2004;364:527–529.
113. Wadsworth JDF, Asante EA, Desbruslais M, et al. Human prion protein with valine 129 prevents expression of variant CJD phenotype. Science 2004;306:1793–1796.
114. Donnelly CA. Bovine spongiform encephalopathy in the United States: an epidemiologist's view. N Engl J Med 2004;350:539–542.
114a. CDR Weekly 2006;16(6), Feb.9.
115. UK National Blood Service notifies 110 donors of vCJD risk, implements new blood component safeguards. ABC Newsl 2005;28:1–4.
116. Murphy EL, Connor D, McEvoy P, et al. Estimating blood donor loss due to the variant CJD travel deferral. Transfusion 2004;44: 645–650.
117. O'Brien SF, Chiavetta JA, Goldman M, et al. Predictive ability of sequential surveys in determining donor loss from increasingly stringent variant Creutzfeldt-Jakob disease deferral policies. Transfusion 2006;46:461-468.

118. McCullough J, Anderson D, Brookie D, et al. Consensus conference on vCJD screening of blood donors: report of the panel. Transfusion 2004;44:675–683.
119. Gregori L, McCombie N, Plamer D, et al. Effectiveness of leucoreduction for removal of infectivity of transmissible spongiform encephalopathies from blood. Lancet 2004;264:529–531.
120. Magaill AJ, Grögal M, Gasser RA, et al. Visceral infection caused by *Leishmania tropica* in veterans of Operation Desert Storm. N Engl J Med 1993;328:1383–1387.
121. Fichoux YL, Quaranta JF, Aufeuvre JP, et al. Occurrence of *Leishmania infantum* parasitemia in asymptomatic blood donors living in an area of endemicity in Southern France. J Clin Microbiol 1999;37: 1953–1957.
122. CDC. Viscerotropic leishmaniasis in persons returning from Operation Desert Storm 1990–1991. MMWR Morb Mortal Wkly Rep 1992;41:63–65.
123. Otero AC, da Silva VO, Luz KG, et al. Short report: occurrence of *Leishmania donovani* DNA in donated blood from seroreactive Brazilian blood donors. Am J Trop Med Hyg 2000;2:128–131.
124. Mathur P, Samantaray JC. The first probable case of platelet transfusion-transmitted visceral leishmaniasis. Transfus Med 2004;14:319–321.
125. Giger U, Oakley DA, Owens SD, et al. *Leishmania donovani* transmission by packed RBC transfusion to anemic dogs in the United States. Transfusion 2002;42:381–383.
126. Grogl M, Daugirda JL, Hoover DL, et al. Survivability and infectivity of viscerotropic *Leishmania tropica* from Operation Desert Storm participants in human blood products maintained under blood bank conditions. Am J Trop Med Hyg 1993;49:308–315.
127. AABB. Deferral for risk of leishmaniasis exposure. Assoc Bull 2003;03:14.
128. Cardo LJ, Salata JM, Harman RW, et al. The use of leukodepletion filters at collection to reduce the risk of transfusion transmission of *Leishmania donovani infantum* and *Leishmania major*. Transfusion 2005;45:30a.
129. Saad R, Vincent JF, Cimon B, et al. Pulmonary toxoplasmosis after allogeneic bone marrow transplantation: case report and review. Bone Marrow Transplant 1996;18:211–212.
130. Nelson JC, Kauffmann JH, Ciavarella D, et al. Acquired toxoplasmic retinochoroiditis after platelet transfusions. Ann Ophthalmol 1989; 21:253–254.
131. Wulf MWH, van Creval R, Portier R. Toxoplasmosis after renal transplantation: implications of a missed diagnosis. J Clin Microbiol 2005; 43:3544–3547.
132. CDC. Travel-associated dengue infections: United States 2001–2004. MMWR Morb Mortal Wkly Rep 2004;54:556–558.
133. Wilder-Smith A, Schwartz E. Dengue in travelers. N Engl J Med 2005;353:924–932.
134. Rigau-Perez JG, Vorndam AV, Clark CG. The dengue and dengue hemorrhagic fever epidemic in Puerto Rico, 1994–1995. Am J Trop Med Hyg 2001;64:67–74.
135. Wagner D, de With K, Huzly D, et al. Nosocomial acquisition of dengue. Emerg Infect Dis 2004;10:1872–1873.
136. Chen LH, Wilson ME. Nosocomial dengue by mucocutaneous transmission [Letter]. Emerg Infect Dis 2005;11:775.
137. Nemes Z, Kiss G, Madrassi E, et al. Nosocomial dengue by mucocutaneous transmission [Letter]. Emerg Infect Dis 2005;11:1880–1881.
138. Switzer WM, Bhullar V, Shanmugam, et al. Frequent simian foamy virus infection in persons occupationally exposed to nonhuman primates. J Virol 2004;78:2780–2789.
139. Wolfe ND, Switzer WM, Carr JK, et al. Naturally acquired simian retrovirus infections in central African hunters. Lancet 2004;363:932–937.
140. Jones-Engel L, Engel G, Schillaci A, et al. Primate-to-human retroviral transmission in Asia. Emerg Infect Dis 2005;11:1028–1035.
141. Boneva RS, Grindon AJ, Orton SL, et al. Simian foamy virus infection in a blood donor. Transfusion 2002;42:886–891.
142. CDC: Lymphocytic choriomeningitis virus infection in organ transplant recipients: Massachusetts, Rhode Island, 2005. MMWR Morb Mortal Wkly Rep 2005;54:537–539.
143. The World Health Organization Global Influenza Program Surveillance Network. Evolution of H5N1 avian influenza viruses in Asia. Emerg Infect Dis 2005;11:1515–1521.
144. Ungchusak K, Auewarakul P, Dowell SF, et al. Probable person-to-person transmission of Avian influenza A (H5N1). N Engl J Med 2005; 352:333–340.
145. Webby RJ, Webster RG. Are we ready for pandemic influenza? Science 2003;302:1519–1522.
146. Ksiazek TG, Erdman D, Goldsmith CS. A novel coronavirus associated with severe acute respiratory syndrome. N Engl J Med 2003;348: 1953–1966.
147. Gerberding JL. Faster but fast enough? Responding to the epidemic of severe acute respiratory syndrome. N Engl J Med 2003;348: 2030–2031.
148. CDC. Update: Outbreak of severe acute respiratory syndrome worldwide 2003. MMWR Morb Mortal Wkly Rep 2003;52:241–247.
149. Hayes EB, Sejar JJ, Zaki SR, et al. Virology, pathology, and clinical manifestations of West Nile virus disease. Emerg Infect Dis 2005;11:1174–1179.
150. Peterson LR, Hayes EB. Westward ho? The spread of West Nile virus. N Engl J Med 2004;351:2257–2259.
151. Hayes EB, Komar N, Nasci RS, et al. Epidemiology and transmission dynamics of West Nile virus disease. Emerg Infect Dis 2005;11:8.
152. FDA-CBER. Guidance for industry: assessing donor suitability and blood and blood product safety in cases of known or suspected West Nile virus infection. www.fda.gov/cber/guidelines.htm.
153. Biggerstaff BJ, Peterson LR. Estimated risk of West Nile virus transmission through blood transfusion during an epidemic in Queens, New York City. Transfusion 2002;42:1019–1026.
154. West Nile Virus Surveillance: Reported to CDC as of November 1, 2005. www.cdc.gov/ncidod/dvbid/westnile/surv&control.htm.
155. Busch MP. West Nile virus window period. Transfusion 2005;45:cover figure.
156. Stramer SL, Fand CT, Foster GA, et al. West Nile virus among blood donors in the United States, 2003 and 2004. N Engl J Med 2005;353:451–459.
157. Busch MP, Caglioti S, Robertson EF, et al. Screening the blood supply for West Nile virus RNA by nucleic amplification testing. N Engl J Med 2005;353:460–467.
158. Montgomery S, Brown J, Kuehnert M, et al. Transfusion-associated transmission of West Nile virus, United States.
159. Kleinman S, Glynn SA, Busch M, et al. The 2003 West Nile virus United States epidemic: the America's Blood Centers Experience. Transfusion 2005;45:469–479.
160. Tobler LH, Bianco C, Glynn SA, et al. Detection of West Nile virus RNA and antibody in frozen plasma components from a voluntary market withdrawal during the 2002 peak epidemic. Transfusion 2005;45:480–486.
161. Busch MP, Tobler LH, Saldanha J, et al. Analytical and clinical sensitivity of West Nile virus RNA screening and supplemental assays available in 2003. Transfusion 2005;45:492–499.
162. Pealer LN, Marfin AA, Peterson LR, et al. Transmission of West Nile virus through blood transfusion in the United States in 2002. N Engl J Med 2003;349:1236–1245.
163. CDC. West Nile virus activity: United States, September 26–October 2, 2002, and investigations of West Nile virus infections in recipients of blood transfusion and organ tranplantation. MMWR Morb Mortal Wkly Rep 2002;51:884,895.
164. Epstein J. Insights on donor screening for West Nile virus. Transfusion 2005;45:460–462.
165. Peterson LR, Epstein JS. Problem solved? West Nile virus and transfusion safety. N Engl J Med 2005;353:516–517.
166. CDC. West Nile virus infections in organ transplant recipients: New York and Pennsylvania, August-September, 2005. MMWR Morb Mortal Wkly Rep 2005;54:1–3.
167. CDC. Investigation of rabies infections in organ and transplant recipients: Alabama, Arkansas, Oklahoma, and Texas, 2004. MMWR Morb Mortal Wkly Rep 2004;53:586–589.

ii. Noninfectious Complications

Chapter 49

Hemolytic Transfusion Reactions: Acute and Delayed

R. Sue Shirey • Karen E. King • Paul M. Ness

ACUTE HEMOLYTIC TRANSFUSION REACTIONS

The most feared adverse reaction to blood transfusion is an acute hemolytic transfusion reaction (AHTR). These reactions most commonly occur when red cells (RBCs) are transfused to a patient with a preexisting antibody that is capable of destroying incompatible RBCs through intravascular hemolysis. These reactions can produce hypotension and shock, often accompanied by acute renal failure and disseminated intravascular coagulation (DIC), and have a high mortality rate. Because of the devastating nature of the most severe cases of AHTR, blood centers and transfusion services have developed standard operating procedures to avoid these consequences. Clinicians are taught to be suspicious of AHTRs and to initiate treatment rapidly in the hope of preventing the many complications and sequelae.

Definition and Incidence

An AHTR features rapid destruction of RBCs immediately after a transfusion, but a hemolytic reaction occurring within 24 hours of the inciting transfusion is generally considered to be an AHTR.[1] AHTRs produce serologic abnormalities and clinical events, but most reports do not distinguish how the cases were identified, and the literature has not developed a consensus case definition. Most reported reactions occur with RBCs, but AHTR reactions due to RBC antibodies contained in the plasma of other blood components (platelets or plasma-derived products) have historically and more recently been recognized as producing AHTRs.[2]

The incidence of AHTR in clinical practice has never been precisely determined. Historic studies have estimated their occurrence to be from 1 in 10,000 to 1 in 50,000 transfused blood components.[3,4] Other information has been gleaned from reports to the Food and Drug Administration (FDA) on transfusion fatalities, but these numbers clearly misrepresent the totality of AHTR reactions.[5,6] Any transfusion-medicine veteran knows of many cases or near misses from quality assurance activities or medical/legal cases that are never reported. The growing use of hemovigilance reporting around the world may provide better data in the future. As an example, a report from Canada documented 11 cases of AHTR from 138,605 units of RBC administered in 2000.[7] Because these reactions occurred in hospitals where transfusion safety officers were already in place, it is likely that the incidence is higher in sites where hemovigilance activities have not been initiated.

It is logical that reaction severity will correlate with the amount of incompatible blood that is administered. Published reports document death rates of 25% when less than 1 L of RBCs was given, with mortality increasing to 44% when infusions of greater than 1 L were transfused.[8] Conversely, small aliquots of blood have caused major reactions,[6] and whole units of RBCs that were ABO incompatible caused no sequelae.

Pathophysiology

Transfusion of RBCs that are incompatible with antibodies in the patient's plasma most commonly initiates AHTR. Less commonly, antibodies can be transfused from the donor that will destroy the patient's incompatible RBCs. The antibodies that cause AHTR are most commonly within the ABO system, where high-titer naturally occurring antibodies react with the dense ABO antigen sites on RBCs, producing hemolysis. Anti-A is the most common culprit, because it has a higher titer in most group O individuals, and transfusion errors involving administration of group A blood to group O individuals are statistically most probable. Although ABO antibodies account for the majority of fatal cases of AHTR, other antibodies in the Kell, Rh, Kidd, and Duffy systems can be equally severe in some cases.[3]

The initiating events of an AHTR involve the binding of antibody to incompatible RBCs and the subsequent destruction of the RBCs by intravascular hemolysis. These events activate the complement system, the release of hemoglobin from the RBCs, and the presence of residual RBC stroma in the circulation. Although AHTR is typically considered a classic example of intravascular hemolysis, most likely some elements of extravascular hemolysis occur as well with clearance of some damaged red cells by the reticuloendothelial system.

Immune hemolysis with complement activation generates the major complications of AHTR through a series of activated complement components, anaphylotoxins, and other immune mediators such as cytokines and vasoactive amines.[1] These events cause hypotension, vasoconstriction and renal ischemia, and the activation of the coagulation system of platelets and clotting factors. When complement is fully activated and RBC stroma and enzymes are released into the vascular space, hypotension results from the actions of anaphylotoxins and mast cell degranulation, with release of histamine and serotonin. Hypotension and renal failure are also facilitated by the activity of cytokines and interleukins produced as a result of immune hemolysis.[9] The kallikrein system and bradykinin are also activated, causing vasodilation with increased capillary permeability, adding to the clinical picture of shock with renal failure, along with elements of adult respiratory distress syndrome.[10] The massive release of proinflammatory molecules such as tumor necrosis factor (TNF)-α, interleukin (IL)-1, and IL-8 activate neutrophils and monocytes, enhancing the clinical picture of shock, renal failure, and pulmonary compromise.[11,12]

These catastrophic events have profound effects on platelets and the coagulation system as well. Platelets are activated by the immune hemolytic reaction, releasing additional serotonin and histamine, which furthers the vasoconstrictive events. Platelet phospholipid (platelet factor 3) is also released, with procoagulant effects on coagulation.[13,14] As a result, the intrinsic coagulation system is activated with the presence of bioactive thrombin, the consumption of fibrinogen, and the initiation of fibrinolysis. These procoagulant forces produce microthrombi, exacerbating renal damage, and diminished platelets and coagulation factors in many patients produce the clinical picture of DIC and hemostatic compromise.

Most of the evolving picture of the pathophysiology of AHTR has been extracted from clinical case reports and descriptions. Much of this picture was well described in an early review by Goldfinger[15] in 1977. This seminal review was updated with a more comprehensive picture of the implications of the systemic inflammatory response in AHTR later by Capon and Goldfinger[16] formulating a model for the consideration of therapy. The pathophysiology of AHTR has also been studied in animals in recent years by Davenport,[12,13] with the identification of important clinical roles of immune mediators such as IL-1 and monocyte chemoattractant protein. We hope that animal models will provide insights into potential therapies because clinical trials of newer agents will be difficult to perform in the sporadic cases that occur in multiple locations.

Clinical Picture

No consistent clinical picture of AHTR exists, with reactions being described in all settings where transfusion therapy is being administered. Most commonly, an alert patient might complain of chills, and the vital signs that are monitored with transfusion therapy will detect hypotension and fever. Pain at the infusion site, flank pain, a general feeling of being unwell, and anxiety with a feeling of impending doom have also been described. In patients who are unconscious or in surgery, vital-sign changes and the onset of unexplained bleeding due to DIC or the observation of hemoglobinuria in catheterized patients may be the only warning. Because the presentation of AHTR is nonspecific, it is critical that all patients undergoing transfusion therapy be closely observed with careful monitoring of vital signs and that any untoward complication be evaluated immediately as a suspected transfusion reaction. A list of common signs and symptoms of AHTR is found in Table 49–1, although the list is by no means exhaustive.

Table 49–1 Signs and Symptoms of Acute Hemolytic Transfusion Reactions

Fever	Nausea and vomiting
Chills	Dyspnea
Rigors	Hypotension
Anxiety, feeling of doom	Hemoglobinuria
Facial flushing	Oliguria/anuria
Chest and abdominal pain	Pain at the infusion site
Flank and back pain	Diffuse bleeding

Differential Diagnosis

Because patients receiving transfusion therapy can develop a clinical picture of hemolysis from many sources, it is important to distinguish an AHTR from acute hemolysis of other causes. Probably the most common cause of hemolysis in transfused patients is the improper storage of RBCs, leading to hemolysis of the unit; these events can occur if the blood is affected by thermal injury, subjected to mechanical trauma from constricted access lines or pressurized infusions, inappropriately mixed with hypotonic solutions or drugs, or contaminated by bacteria. These forms of nonimmune hemolysis can be avoided by careful attention to routinely available transfusion protocols for the storage and administration of blood components.

Some patients with congenital or acquired forms of hemolytic anemia may be incorrectly assumed to have had an AHTR. Acute hemolysis in congenital hemolytic anemias such as hereditary spherocytosis, sickle cell anemia, or RBC enzyme deficiency states can occasionally be misidentified as an AHTR. Other conditions in critically ill patients can confuse transfusing clinicians, such as a coexistent microangiopathic hemolytic anemia, a patient with thrombotic thrombocytopenic purpura (TTP)/hemolytic-uremic syndrome (HUS), or patients with mechanical fragmentation of RBCs due to heart valves or other implanted circulatory devices.

Confirmation of the Diagnosis

The initial suspicion of an AHTR should prompt discontinuation of the ongoing transfusion and an initial laboratory investigation (Table 49–2) including observation of the post-transfusion plasma for hemolysis and the performance of a direct antiglobulin test. Visual inspection of the plasma is subject to many causes of false-positive results, including the enumerated sources of nonimmune hemolysis, the presence of another hemolytic state, or an improperly drawn blood sample. The direct antiglobulin test also is subject to false-positive results. If either of these screening tests is positive, however, particularly in the presence of a compelling clinical story, further testing should be initiated in the transfusion service. Administration sets and blood bags should be examined, and the pretransfusion testing of the patient should be repeated. It is critically important in these cases to affirm the identity of the patient, to assure that the pretransfusion specimen was actually from the patient who encountered the reaction, to affirm that other patients are not involved in an identification error, and to withhold further transfusions unless urgently required until the presence or absence of an AHTR has been confirmed.

Table 49–2 Laboratory Investigations for Acute Hemolytic Transfusion Reactions

Blood product	Confirm ABO, Rh Confirm other antigen types, if indicated
Blood bank laboratory	Direct antiglobulin test Confirm ABO, Rh, antibody screen and identification Post-transfusion hemolysis check
Clinical laboratory	Complete blood count Platelet count Urinalysis for hemoglobin Serum bilirubin Creatinine, urine quantitation Coagulation profile DIC evaluation

DIC, disseminated intravascular coagulation.

The treating physician may want to order additional laboratory tests to confirm the clinical suspicion of an AHTR or to provide additional tests to facilitate therapy and monitor the patient's status. These tests might include a complete blood count including platelets, coagulation screening, serum chemistries including creatinine, and tests to confirm hemolysis, such as haptoglobin, lactic dehydrogenase, and bilirubin. In complicated cases, a visual inspection of the post-transfusion blood smear also can be helpful.

The laboratory may also be required to perform a more definitive evaluation for DIC in confirmed cases.

Therapy

The first element of therapy of an AHTR is to stop the infusion of the suspected incompatible blood.[16] It also is critical to maintain intravenous access for the patient, so the intravenous line should not be removed or sent to the laboratory for evaluation. In a suspected reaction, emergency measures may precede definitive confirmation. The early management should include careful monitoring of the vital signs, maintenance of the blood pressure and blood volume, and transfer of the patient to the appropriate acute care setting (most likely an intensive care unit [ICU]) for aggressive management, if required (Table 49–3). An intensive care specialist or a nephrologist or both should be consulted because dialysis therapy may be required. If AHTR due to ABO compatibility is confirmed, a pulmonary artery catheter may be critical for monitoring. Aggressive fluid replacement is subsequently administered, and vasopressors, such as dopamine, are commonly used in an attempt to mitigate renal complications. Diuretics such as furosemide are commonly administered to maintain urine output along with fluid support.[17] If renal failure ensues, however, dialysis should be initiated promptly.

In the event that bleeding ensues or the laboratory confirms that DIC has developed, supportive therapy with platelet concentrates and plasma products may become important. The use of heparin has been advocated to prevent or reduce the complications of DIC but may be difficult in the face of surgical bleeding.[18] The use of protein C concentrates to interrupt DIC should also be considered, although clinical trial support is obviously lacking.[19]

The classic clinical descriptions of AHTR did not include the respiratory failure that can occur and is now more commonly recognized. Pulmonary function should be carefully monitored, with oxygen therapy and ventilator support initiated early by the intensive care specialists. Whether specific inflammatory inhibitors that have been studied for other chronic inflammatory states (inhibitors of IL-1 or TNF) would be useful is not known, but their use in severe situations appears justifiable.

PREVENTION

The basic procedures used by blood banks for pretransfusion testing and management of transfusion practices are designed to eliminate AHTR. The most important cornerstone is the proper identification of the blood recipient and the collection of a carefully identified blood sample from the recipient for pretransfusion testing. Blood banking procedures are often deemed to be unnecessarily rigid by clinicians, but they must be enforced to lessen AHTR and other preventable transfusion consequences. The most effective systems require identification of the patient at the bedside and creating a unique identifier based on the personal identification by the phlebotomist. Barrier systems also prevent transfusion without the precise identification of the recipient.[20] Computer technology is being adapted to make sample and recipient matching more rigorous in the hope of preventing transfusion errors and transfusion reactions.[21] Another trend that should reduce transfusion reactions such as AHTR is the development of quality assurance systems (hemovigilance) that monitor transfusion practices, investigate transfusion reactions, reinforce training of physicians and nurses about transfusion care, and help to develop improved systems in hospitals to lessen transfusion risks.

Once a sample is obtained in the blood bank, blood bank procedures are designed to detect ABO discrepancies and alloantibodies that can cause immune hemolysis and AHTR. Procedures are designed to be very sensitive so that antibodies will not be missed, but some highly sensitive procedures produce a problem with a high incidence of false-positive

Table 49–3 Therapy for Acute Hemolytic Transfusion Reactions

General Considerations	Prevent Renal Complications	Pulmonary Complications	Management of DIC
Establish venous access	Maintain blood pressure and urine output	Monitor pulmonary function	Consider heparin
Monitor vital signs	Diuretics	Oxygen therapy	Platelet transfusions
ICU transfer	Dopamine	Ventilator support	Plasma for coagulopathy
Pulmonary artery catheter	Dialysis		Protein C

DIC, disseminated intravascular coagulation; ICU, intensive care unit.

results due to clinically insignificant antibodies or other contaminating substances. In the case of AHTR, in which the culprit is most commonly a sampling problem en route to the laboratory, increased sensitivity in testing is unlikely to offer any real progress.

Another common teaching by transfusion professionals is to avoid unnecessary transfusions, in part to reduce the fear that they may cause adverse consequences such as AHTR. Most hospitals have reduced their transfusion trigger for RBCs[22] largely to handle concerns about infectious complications, so transfusion avoidance is not likely to reduce the rate of AHTR significantly.

Because safe blood transfusion continues to depend on well-trained practitioners to obtain samples and administer blood products, it seems unlikely that enhanced training programs will ever totally eliminate this significant problem that is largely caused by human error. Technologic developments that might better handle this problem should be encouraged. The evolving capability to create universal group O blood by enzymatically removing A and B blood group antigens from RBC might be a technologic solution to the serious problem of AHTR.[23]

DELAYED HEMOLYTIC TRANSFUSION REACTIONS

In contrast to AHTR, in which clinical symptoms occur immediately or within 24 hours of transfusion, *delayed* hemolytic transfusion reactions (DHTRs) are generally not recognized until 3 to 10 days after transfusion of blood that appeared to be serologically compatible.[24–26] DHTRs commonly occur in patients who have been immunized to foreign blood group antigens during previous transfusions and/or pregnancies, but the antibody decreases over time and is not detected in subsequent pretransfusion testing. An anamnestic response is stimulated by the transfusion of seemingly compatible blood, causing increased production of antibody that sensitizes the antigen-positive donor RBCs leading to intravascular and/or extravascular hemolysis. Although the clinical symptoms associated with DHTRs are generally milder than those observed in AHTRs, DHTRs with severe hemolysis leading to disseminated intravascular hemolysis and acute renal failure have been reported.[27–30] Because a time delay occurs between transfusion and the appearance of clinical sequelae in these cases, clinicians may not suspect DHTR.[30] Often it is the blood bank or transfusion service that initiates the investigation of DHTR, prompted by the serologic findings observed in post-transfusion testing.[30]

Definition and Incidence

Mollison[24] defined DHTR as accelerated destruction of transfused red cells that begins only when sufficient antibody has been produced as a result of an immune response induced by the transfusion. Since the first case of DHTR attributed to Boorman and colleagues[31] was reported in 1946, numerous cases have been described in the literature.[32–37] Although exceptions are found,[38–42] most DHTRs share these characteristics:

1. DHTRs generally occur in patients who have been alloimmunized to RBC antigens by previous transfusions or pregnancies.
2. Because the titer has decreased below detectable levels, the implicated antibody is not detected in pretransfusion antibody screening or compatibility testing.
3. DHTR is usually suspected 3 to 10 days after transfusion, when clinical symptoms associated with hemolysis are observed and/or serologic findings consistent with DHTR are noted (Table 49–4).
4. The clinical symptoms most frequently associated with DHTR include unexplained decreases in hemoglobin and hematocrit, fever, and jaundice.
5. The hallmark serologic findings in DHTR are the development of a positive direct antiglobulin test (DAT) and/or a positive antibody screening test in post-transfusion testing because of the presence of RBC antibodies that were not detected in pretransfusion testing.
6. Antibodies directed against Rh (CEce) and Kidd (Jk^a, Jk^b) system antigens are the antibodies most commonly implicated in DHTR; however, numerous other specificities have been described.

The frequencies of DHTR reported in early studies vary widely.[29,36] In the first series conducted at the Mayo Clinic from 1964 to 1973, the incidence of DHTR was reported as 1 DHTR per 11,650 RBC units transfused, with 22 (96%) of the 23 cases having clinical manifestations of hemolysis, and 3 deaths attributed to DHTR.[29] In the second series from 1974 to 1977, the incidence of DHTR had increased to 1 DHTR per 4000 RBC units transfused, and only 24 (65%) of 37 had clinical evidence of hemolysis; the remaining 13 (35%) demonstrated serologic findings consistent with a DHTR, but no clinical or laboratory evidence of hemolysis was associated with transfusion.[36] This

Table 49–4 Time Line of DHTR

Time (days)	Event	Explanation
0	Pretransfusion tests negative	Antibody titer below detectable levels
1	Red cell transfusion	
3–10	Clinical signs of hemolysis may appear	Accelerated destruction of transfused donor RBC
10–21	Post-transfusion sample: Positive DAT and positive antibody screen due to newly detected antibody	Antibody titer increases; sensitizes donor red cells
>21	DAT may become negative	In vivo removal of antibody-sensitized donor red cells from the circulation
>21 to 300 days	DAT may persist as positive; eluates may demonstrate alloantibody specificity or panagglutination	Alloantibody binding nonspecifically to autologous RBC, or development of warm autoantibodies

DAT, direct antiglobulin test; DHTR, Delayed hemolytic transfusion reaction; RBC, red blood cell.

trend of increased frequency, but decreased clinical significance, appears to be related, in part, to the manner in which DHTRs were defined. If the frequency of DHTR is determined on the basis of clinical reporting alone, then the incidence would be far lower than the true rate, because the signs and symptoms of hemolysis are nonspecific and may be difficult to distinguish from the complicated medical course of multitransfused patients.[26,27] If DHTR is defined by post-transfusion serologic testing, then the frequency is likely to increase, and the clinical findings may diminish, because correlation between serologic results and clinical hemolysis is often poor.[30]

The definition of DHTR was clarified by Ness and colleagues[30] in 1990, when the authors introduced the term delayed *serologic* transfusion reaction (DSTR) to describe cases with serologic evidence of DHTR (i.e., the development of a positive post-transfusion DAT result and a newly identified alloantibody in eluate studies or plasma studies or both), but no clinical evidence of hemolysis. The authors strictly defined DHTR as a subset of DSTR in which clinical evidence of hemolysis was attributable to a transfusion reaction. In their series at the Johns Hopkins Hospital, only 6 (18%) of 34 consecutive patients identified with serologic findings consistent with DHTR had clinical evidence of hemolysis associated with transfusion and could be defined as DHTR by strict definition. Twenty-eight (82%) of the 34 DSTR cases had no clinical evidence of hemolysis, as determined by retrospective chart review. The ratio of DHTR to DSTR can be expressed as 18:82 (Table 49–5). The combined frequency of DSTR and DHTR was calculated as 1:1605 (0.06%) RBC units transfused. The frequency of true DHTR was only 1 case per 9094 units (0.01%) transfused.

By using the same definitions as prescribed by Ness and colleagues,[30] the Mayo Clinic reported a combined frequency of DHTR/DSTR as 1 per 1899 allogeneic RBC units transfused with a DHTR/DSTR ratio of 36:64 when patients were evaluated for clinical hemolysis concurrent with the detection of positive post-transfusion serology.[43] The most recent study from the Mayo Clinic spanning the years 1993 to 1998 indicates a decline in DHTR and a concomitant increase in DSTR, which the authors attributed to the implementation of a more-sensitive antibody screening method and a decrease in the average length of hospital stay for inpatients.[44] Interestingly, their current rates of observed reactions and the DHTR/DSTR ratio are very similar to those reported by Ness and colleagues[30] in 1990 (see Table 49–5).

Diagnosis

The blood bank plays an important role in recognizing and reporting potential cases of DHTR. The clinician may submit a post-transfusion sample with a request for RBC transfusions, not suspecting that the patient's decreased hemoglobin and hematocrit are due to DHTR. Generally, positive antibody screening tests on the post-transfusion sample trigger antibody-identification studies and investigation of DHTR. The laboratory investigation of DHTR is outlined in Table 49–6. The serologic findings in classic cases of DHTR include the development of a post-transfusion positive DAT that may have a mixed-field appearance because of the presence of IgG antibody–sensitized donor RBCs interspersed with DAT-negative autologous RBCs and the presence of a newly identified alloantibody in the red cell eluate or plasma studies or both approximately 3 to 10 days (or usually by 20 days) after the index transfusion (see Table 49–4).[26] If the patient's transfusion history and post-transfusion serologic findings are consistent with DHTR, then the patient should be evaluated for clinical and laboratory evidence of hemolysis associated with RBC transfusions (see Table 49–6). The patient's physician should be notified, and a transfusion reaction report should be generated so that the findings become a part of the patient's medical records.

Serologic Complexities of DHTR

Diagnostic Difficulties

For many years, it was generally accepted that in DHTR, the sensitized donor red cells would be removed from the circulation within approximately 14 days (or no later than 21 days) after the putatively responsible transfusion (see Table 49–4).[26] Therefore, DAT and eluate studies should become negative coinciding with the in vivo destruction of transfused donor RBCs that provoked the immune response. It is now clear from long-term studies of DHTR that it is not uncommon for DAT to persist as positive because of IgG antibody or complement sensitization or both of RBCs for many weeks or months after the transfusion reaction, long after the transfused, antigen-positive donor RBCs would be expected to be removed from the circulation.[30,45] In addition, these long-term studies showed that eluates prepared from samples drawn more than 6 months after DHTR, when all the transfused donor RBCs would have been removed from circulation, may still demonstrate the alloantibody responsible for the reaction. Several theories are proposed to explain these remarkable phenomena.[26,45] Salama and Mueller-Eckhardt[45] suggested that alloantibody binds nonspecifically in vivo to antigen-negative autologous red cells and activates complement via the classic pathway in all DHTRs. Thus DAT may remain positive long after the removal of transfused donor RBCs because of nonspecific sensitization of autologous RBCs with alloantibody or complement or both during DHTR.[45–48] Although the mechanisms remain unclear and a subject of contention, the persistence of a positive DAT and reactive eluates after DHTR does not generally appear to correlate with in vivo hemolysis.[26,30] The practical application of these long-term

Table 49–5 Incidence of Delayed Hemolytic Transfusion Reaction and Delayed Serologic Transfusion Reaction

Series	Incidence*	DHTR/DSTR
Ness et al[30] Johns Hopkins Hospital (Jan 1986–Aug 1987)	1:1605	18:82
Vamvakas et al[43] Mayo Clinic (1980–1992)	1:1899	36:64
Pineda et al[44] Mayo Clinic (1993–1998)	1:1300	19:81

*Incidence expressed as DHTR/DSTR per number of red cell units transfused.

Table 49–6 Outline for Laboratory Investigation of Suspected DHTR

1. **Initial Serologic Investigation**
   Post-transfusion sample tests
   Antibody identification studies: Initiated as a result of positive antibody screening tests (and/or positive DAT results) on the post-transfusion sample
   DAT profile: (DAT with polyspecific and monospecific anti-IgG and anti-C3 antiglobulin reagents)
   Eluate studies: Performed if DAT positive due to IgG sensitization of RBC and history of recent RBC transfusions
2. **Supplemental Serologic Tests**
   Retrieve pretransfusion sample (if available): Perform DAT and repeat antibody screening tests
   Retrieve retained segments from transfused RBC donor units: Phenotype for antigen corresponding to identified antibody
3. **Review Serologic Findings and Transfusion History**
   Results evaluated by transfusion medicine attending physician
4. **Generate Suspected Transfusion Reaction Report**
   The transfusion medicine attending physician assesses the patient for clinical signs and symptoms of DHTR and notifies the patient's physician

studies of DHTR is the recognition that serology consistent with DHTR may persist long after the reaction has occurred and the patient has recovered. Consequently, serologic findings alone can be misleading and difficult to interpret. The investigation of DHTR must consider not only the serologic findings, but also the temporal relation of antigen-positive RBC transfusions to the serologic test results, coupled with a clinical evaluation and laboratory assessment of the patient for evidence of hemolysis associated with RBC transfusions.

DHTR and Autoantibody

Many anecdotal cases of allo- and autoimmunization occurring concurrently have appeared in the literature over the past 40 years.[49–59] For example, Lalezari and colleagues[55] described a patient who had DHTR due to allo-anti-D and subsequently developed autoantibodies. The post-transfusion DAT remained positive for 6 months after DHTR, and eluates demonstrated panagglutination consistent with the presence of warm autoantibodies having a broad specificity. Worlledge[54] noted as early as 1978 that alloimmunization can lead to autoimmunization and that even immunized recipients who are given compatible blood may subsequently develop a positive DAT because of autoantibodies. It is not surprising that long-term studies by Ness and associates[30] found that the development of warm autoantibodies after DHTR was relatively common. Approximately one third of patients with DHTR who were followed for more than 25 days after DHTR had persistence of a positive DAT due to warm autoantibodies with broad specificity (i.e., eluate panagglutinin) (see Table 49–4). The frequency of autoantibody development after DHTR may be even higher, because autoantibodies can mimic alloantibody specificities.[58,59] It is possible that DHTR cases with apparent alloantibody recovered in long-term eluate studies may actually represent cases of warm autoantibodies mimicking alloantibody specificities.[30,45] Although the postreaction autoantibodies appeared to be clinically benign in the cases followed by Ness and colleagues,[30] some reports indicate that DHTRs have evolved into the production of pathologic warm autoantibodies leading to severe autoimmune hemolytic anemia.[49–53]

Severe DHTR

Fortunately, the clinical symptoms in most DHTRs generally resolve within 2 to 3 weeks of the index transfusion without medical intervention other than transfusion support with appropriate antigen-negative blood transfusions. However, severe DHTR with life-threatening anemia has been reported and occurs most often in alloimmunized patients with sickle cell disease (SCD).[60,61] Because patients with SCD have a high alloimmunization rate ranging from 17.6% to 36%, they are at greater risk for DHTR.[62–67] Frequencies of DHTR in SCD range from 4% to 22%[63,66,69,70] compared with the frequency of true, clinical DHTR in all transfused patients of only 0.04% (one DHTR per 2537 transfused patients)[71] to 0.1% (one DHTR per 854 transfused patients).[30]

The diagnosis of DHTR in patients with SCD may be difficult. Patients may have symptoms that are misdiagnosed as sickle cell pain crisis, and delays in initiating appropriate treatment could lead to significant morbidity or even death.[72–77] Confusion can be avoided by making certain that an accurate transfusion history is obtained on admission and that a sample is sent to the transfusion service for processing in the event that blood transfusions are required.

The causes of severe DHTR in SCD are unclear and controversial. Explanations for the profound anemia observed in severe DHTR include bystander hemolysis, sickle cell hemolytic transfusion reaction syndrome, and hyperhemolysis.[60,61,78,79]

Bystander hemolysis has been defined as the immune destruction of autologous RBCs that may occur during DHTR. The mechanism(s) of bystander hemolysis is unclear. One theory has proposed that activation of complement could occur when alloantibodies react with transfused antigen-positive donor RBCs, leading to destruction of allogeneic and "innocent bystander" autologous red cells.[80–82] Bystander hemolysis is difficult to document but may be suspected when post-transfusion reaction hemoglobin and hematocrit are less than the pretransfusion values, suggesting that simultaneous destruction of transfused donor RBCs and autologous RBCs may be present. The phenomenon of bystander hemolysis in DHTRs has been reported in patients without SCD.[80–82] However, bystander hemolysis may actually be more prevalent in patients with SCD, because sickle cells have a regulatory defect in the formation of the complement membrane attack complex, causing the cells to be more susceptible to complement-mediated hemolysis.[83] Garratty[71] suggested that complement activation in these cases may be triggered not only by antibody reacting with transfused RBC antigens, but also by antibody reacting with other foreign antigens (e.g., human leukocyte antigen [HLA], plasma proteins). Thus the mechanism of bystander hemolysis during DHTRs in patients with

SCD may be similar to that of paroxysmal nocturnal hemoglobinuria (PNH), in which immune complex formation may result in hemolysis of "innocent" autologous RBCs.[82]

One well-documented case of bystander hemolysis was reported by King and coworkers[60] in a study in which they monitored five patients who had DHTR after preoperative exchange transfusions. By monitoring the hemoglobin A (transfused allogeneic donor RBCs) and hemoglobin S (autologous sickle cells) levels, the authors showed that in one of the cases, a substantial loss of autologous RBCs occurred (i.e., bystander hemolysis), as well as loss of allogeneic RBCs during DHTR.

Petz and colleagues[61] reported five cases of hemolytic transfusion reactions in SCD in which the severe anemia appeared to be due to the destruction of transfused donor RBCs coincident with suppression of erythropoiesis. The authors defined these cases as "the sickle cell hemolytic transfusion reaction syndrome," in which reticulocytopenia coupled with the hemolysis of transfused donor RBCs caused life-threatening anemia. In their series, none of the patients appeared to have accelerated autologous RBC destruction (i.e., bystander hemolysis).

Hyperhemolysis is a term that has been used to describe severe DHTR in SCD in which the ongoing hemolysis of autologous cells seems to be accelerated during the course of a hemolytic reaction.[78,79] Win and associates[78] suggested that the accelerated destruction of autologous cells that may occur in DHTR could be due to hyperactive macrophages that readily sequester both mature RBCs and reticulocytes. Interestingly, Darabi and Dzik[84] recently reported hyperhemolysis after DHTR due to anti-K1 in a patient without SCD.

Treatment of Severe DHTR

Regardless of the mechanisms that may be involved, it is important to recognize that severe DHTR in patients with SCD is not an infrequent finding and may mimic a painful crisis.[72–77] Effective treatment requires prompt diagnosis and conservative transfusion support with appropriate antigen-negative RBCs. Steroid therapy and intravenous immune globulin infusions have been successfully used for the treatment of the most severe cases.[78,79] Some have suggested administration of recombinant erythropoietin, depending on the patient's reticulocyte count.[85]

Prevention of DHTRs

The frequency of DHTRs has diminished with implementation of improved pretransfusion antibody-screening methods.[44] The current challenge is to find a rapid, automated antibody-screening method that is sufficiently sensitive to detect most clinically important antibodies, but not so highly sensitive that clinically benign, unwanted antibodies are detected.[86] Because antibody titers may decline below detectable levels, it is important that clinically significant antibodies be well documented in the transfusion service and medical records, and it may be helpful to provide patients with personal identification cards listing the antibodies and transfusion requirements.[87,88] It must be emphasized that patients diagnosed with DSTRs are at risk for severe DHTR with future transfusions and must receive donor blood negative for the antigen(s) corresponding to the implicated alloantibodies.[26,30]

The high rate of alloimmunization and the high risk of DHTRs in SCD appears to be due, at least in part, to the disparity in antigen frequencies between the African American recipient and white donor population.[63] For example, 73% of African Americans are C negative and may develop anti-C antibodies when transfused with blood from white donors, because 70% of whites are C positive. Therefore, increasing African American donations, particularly if the donations could be linked to patients with SCD requiring transfusion support, might be of benefit.

It is generally accepted that patients with SCD should be extensively phenotyped (e.g., Rh antigens [CEce], K1, MNSs, Fy^a, Fy^b, Jk^a, Jk^b) so that antibodies the patients may potentially produce can be easily discerned.[89–91] Having the extensive or complete phenotype on file is particularly advantageous in resolving complex antibody problems that are frequently presented by multitransfused patients with SCD. DNA typing for RBC antigens is now available and can be used in cases in which phenotyping is precluded by recent RBC transfusions or by scarcity of rare antisera.[92,93]

Prophylactic antigen matching of donor RBCs with the recipient's complete phenotype has been advocated for patients with SCD in an effort to reduce the rate of alloimmunization and severe DHTR.[89,90,94] Various transfusion protocols that differ in the number of antigens that are considered for prophylactic matching have been examined by Castro and colleagues[94]

Ness[91] has proposed that prophylactic antigen matching should be considered only when the patient has developed one or more RBC alloantibodies, thereby indicating that the patient is a "responder" and may be at greater risk for further alloimmunization and DHTRs with subsequent RBC transfusions. This protocol is particularly appealing because it avoids unnecessary prophylactic antigen matching of donor blood for the approximately 70% of patients with SCD who do not become alloimmunized even after multiple transfusions.

Prophylactic antigen matching may prevent some cases of DHTR, but even protocols that call for extensive prophylactic antigen matching cannot prevent severe hemolytic transfusion reactions due to unusual alloantibody specificities or the development of pathologic warm autoantibodies.[60,95–97]

FUTURE DIRECTIONS

The development of blood substitutes for transfusion and/or exchange transfusion in SCD seems to offer the most hope for preventing severe DHTR and for circumventing difficulties in providing compatible blood for patients with complex antibody problems.[98,99]

With the rapidly growing sophistication of DNA technology, we may be able to distinguish "responders" from "nonresponders" by genotyping, so that special transfusion protocols could be applied more appropriately. Automated technology for rapid genotyping of blood donors is already under study and may permit the provision of genotype-matched donor blood to recipients in the near future.[100]

REFERENCES

1. Davenport RD. Hemolytic transfusion reactions. In Popovsky MA (ed). Transfusion Reactions, 2nd ed. Bethesda, Md, American Association of Blood Banks, 2001, p 1.
2. Josephson CD, Mullis NC, Van Demark C, et al. Significant numbers of apheresis-derived group O platelet units have "high-titer" anti-A/A,B: Implications for transfusion policy. Transfusion 2004;44:805–808.

3. Pineda AA, Brzica SM Jr, Taswell HF. Hemolytic transfusion reactions: recent experience in a large blood bank. Mayo Clin Proc 1978;53:378.
4. Lichtiger B, Perry-Thorton E. Hemolytic transfusion reactions in oncology patients: experience in a large cancer center. J Clin Oncol 1984;25:438.
5. Honig CL, Bove JR. Transfusion associated fatalities: review of Bureau of Biologics reports 1976–1978. Transfusion 1980;20:653.
6. Sazama K. Reports of 355 transfusion-associated deaths, 1976 through 1985. Transfusion 1990;30:583.
7. Robillard P, Itaj NK, Corriveau P. ABO incompatible transfusions, acute and delayed hemolytic transfusion reactions in the Quebec hemovigilance system-year 2000. Transfusion 2002;42:(Suppl): 25S.
8. Bluemle LW Jr. Hemolytic transfusion reactions causing acute renal failure: serologic and clinical considerations. Postgrad Med 1965; 38:484.
9. Davenport RD, Strieter RM, Kunkel SL. Red cell ABO incompatibility and production of tumour necrosis factor-alpha. Br J Haematol 1991;79:525.
10. Morat HZ, DiLorenzo NL. Activation of plasma kinin system by antigen-antibody aggregates. I: Generation of permeability factor in guinea pig serum. Lab Invest 1968;19:187.
11. Davenport RD, Strieter RM, Standiford TJ, et al. Interleukin-8 production in red blood cell incompatibility. Blood 1990;76:2439.
12. Davenport RD, Burdick MD, Streiter RM, et al. Monocyte chemoattractant protein production in red cell incompatibility. Transfusion 1994;34:16.
13. Pfueller SL, Luscher EF. Studies of the mechanisms of human platelet release reaction induced by immunologic stimuli. I: Complement-dependent and complement-independent reactions. J Immunol 1974;112:1201.
14. Davenport RD, Polak TJ, Schmouder RE, et al. Endothelial cell procoagulant activity inducted by red cell incompatibility. Transfusion 1994;34:943.
15. Goldfinger D. Acute hemolytic transfusion reactions: a fresh look at pathogenesis and considerations regarding therapy. Transfusion 1974;27:171.
16. Capon SM, Goldfinger D. Acute hemolytic transfusion reaction, a paradigm of the systemic inflammatory response: new insights into pathophysiology and treatment. Transfusion 1995;35:513.
17. Capon SM, Sacher RA. Hemolytic transfusion reactions: a review of mechanisms, sequelae, and management. J Intensive Care Med 1989;4:100 111.
18. Rock RC, Bove JR, Nemerson Y. Heparin treatment of intravascular coagulation accompanying hemolytic transfusion reactions. Transfusion 1969;9:57.
19. Rivard GE, David M, Farrell C, et al. Treatment of purpura fulminans in meningococcemia with protein C concentrate. J Pediatr 1995; 126:646.
20. Mercuriali F, Inghilleri F, Colotti MT, et al. One year use of the Bloodloc system in an orthopedic institute. Transfus Clin Biol 1994;1:227.
21. Dzik W. Emily Cooley Lecture 2002: Transfusion safety in the hospital. Transfusion 1003;43:11290.
22. Carson JL, Hill S, Carless P, et al. Transfusion triggers: a systematic review of the literature. Transfus Med Rev 2002;16:187.
23. Lenny LL, Hurst R, Goldstein J, et al. Transfusions to group O subjects of 2 units of red cells enzymatically converted from group B to group O. Transfusion 1999;34:209.
24. Mollison PL. Antibody-mediated destruction of red cells. Clin Immunol Newsl 1985;6:700–703.
25. Mollison PL. Blood Transfusion in Clinical Medicine, 9th ed. Oxford, Blackwell Scientific, 1993, pp 434–542.
26. Shirey RS, Ness PM. New concepts of delayed hemolytic transfusion reactions. In Nance SJ (ed). Clinical and Basic Science Aspects of Immunohematology. Arlington, Va., American Association of Blood Banks, 1991, pp 179–197.
27. Solanki D, McCurdy PR. Delayed hemolytic transfusion reactions: an often missed entity. JAMA 1978;239:729–731.
28. Holland PV, Wallerstein RO. Delayed hemolytic transfusion reaction with acute renal failure. JAMA 1968;204:1007–1008.
29. Pineda AA, Taswell HF, Brzica SM Jr. Delayed hemolytic transfusion reaction: An immunologic hazard of blood transfusion. Transfusion 1978;18:1–7.
30. Ness PM, Shirey RS, Thoman SK, et al. The differentiation of delayed serologic and delayed hemolytic transfusion reactions: incidence, long-term serologic findings and clinical significance. Transfusion 1990;30:688–693.
31. Boorman KE, Dodd BE, Loutit JF, et al. Some results of transfusion of blood to recipients with "cold" agglutinins. Br Med J 1946;i:751.
32. Rauner RA, Tanaka KR. Hemolytic transfusion reactions associated with the Kidd system antibody (Jk^a). N Engl J Med 1967;276:1486.
33. Kurtides ES, Salkin MS, Widen AL. Hemolytic reaction due to anti-Jkb. JAMA 1966;197:816.
34. Fudenberg H, Allen FJ Jr. Transfusion reactions in the absence of demonstrable incompatibility. N Engl J Med 1957;256:1180–1184.
35. Walker PC, Jennings ER, Monroe C. Hemolytic transfusion reactions after the administration of apparently compatible blood. Am J Clin Pathol 1965;44:193–197.
36. Moore SB, Taswell HF, Pineda AA, et al. Delayed hemolytic transfusion reactions: Evidence of the need for an improved pretransfusion compatibility test. Am J Clin Pathol 1980;74:94–97.
37. Taswell HF, Pineda AA, Moore SB: Hemolytic transfusion reactions: Frequency and clinical and laboratory aspects. In Bell CA (ed). A Seminar on Immune-mediated Red Cell Destruction. Washington, D.C., American Association of Blood Banks, 1981, pp 71–92.
38. Taddie SJ, Barrasso C, Ness PM. A delayed transfusion reaction caused by anti-K6. Transfusion 1982;22:68–69.
39. Patten E, Reddi CR, Riglin H, et al. Delayed hemolytic transfusion reaction caused by a primary immune response. Transfusion 1982;22: 248–250.
40. Davey RJ, Gustafson M, Holland PV. Accelerated immune red cell destruction in the absence of serologically detectable alloantibodies. Transfusion 1983;23:40–44.
41. Baldwin ML, Barrasso C, Ness PM, et al. A clinically significant erythrocyte antibody detectable only by 51R survival studies. Transfusion 1983;23:40–44.
42. Kim HH, Park TS, Oh SH, et al. Delayed hemolytic transfusion reactions due to anti-Fy^b caused by a primary immune response: a case study and review of the literature. Immunohematology 2004;20: 384–386.
43. Vamvakas EC, Pineda AA, Lreisner R, et al. The differentiation of delayed hemolytic and delayed serologic transfusion reactions: incidence and predictors of hemolysis. Transfusion 1995;35:16–32.
44. Pineda AA, Vamvakas EC, Gorden LD, et al. Trends in the incidence of delayed hemolytic and delayed serologic transfusion reactions. Transfusion 1999;10:1097–1103.
45. Salama A, Mueller-Eckhardt C. Delayed hemolytic transfusion reactions: evidence for complement activation involving allogeneic and autologous red cells. Transfusion 1984;24:188–193.
46. Chaplin H Jr. The implication of red cell-bound complement and delayed hemolytic transfusion reactions [Editorial]. Transfusion 1984; 24:185–187.
47. Salama H, Mueller-Eckhardt C. Binding of fluid phase C3b to nonsensitized bystander human red cells: A model for in vivo effects of complement activation on blood cells. Transfusion 1985;25:528–534.
48. Devine DV. Complement. In Anderson KC, Ness PM (eds). Scientific Basis of Transfusion Medicine: Implications for Clinical Practice, 2nd ed. Philadelphia, WB Saunders, 2000, pp 107–119.
49. Sosler SD, Perkins JT, Saporito C, et al. Severe autoimmune hemolytic anemia induced by transfusion in two alloimmunized patients with sickle cell disease [Abstract]. Transfusion 1989;29(Suppl):495.
50. Chaplin H Jr, Zarkowsky HS. Combined sickle cell disease and autoimmune hemolytic anemia [Abstract]. Arch Intern Med 1981;141:1091.
51. Reed W, Walker P, Haddix T, et al. Acute anemic events in sickle cell disease. Transfusion 2000;40:267–273.
52. Castellino SM, Combs MR, Zimmerman MA, et al. Erythrocyte autoantibodies in pediatric patients with sickle cell disease receiving transfusion therapy: frequency, characteristics and significance. Br J Haematol 1999;104:189–194.
53. Chan D, Poole GD, Binney M, et al. Severe intravascular hemolysis due to autoantibodies stimulated by blood transfusion. Immunohematology 1996;12:80–83.
54. Worlledge SM. The interpretation of a positive direct antiglobulin test. Br J Haematol 1978;39:157–162.
55. Lalezari P, Talleyrand NP, Wenz B, et al. Development of direct antiglobulin reaction accompanying alloimmunization in a patient with Rh(d) (D, category III) phenotype. Vox Sang 1975;28:19–24.
56. Cook IA. Primary rhesus immunization of male volunteers. Br J Haematol 1971;20:369–375.
57. Beard MEJ, Pemberton J, Blagdon J, et al. Rh immunization following incompatible blood transfusion and a possible long-term complication of anti-D immunoglobulin therapy. J Med Genet 1971;8:317–320.
58. Issitt PD, Zellner DC, Rolih SD, et al. Autoantibodies mimicking alloantibodies. Transfusion 1977;17:531–538.
59. Issitt PD, Pavone BG. Critical re-examination of the specificity of auto-anti-Rh antibodies in patients with a positive direct antiglobulin test. Br J Haematol 1978;38:63–74.

60. King KE, Shirey RS, Lankiewicz MW, et al. Delayed hemolytic transfusion reactions in sickle cell disease. Transfusion 1997;37:376–381.
61. Petz LD, Calhoun L, Shulman IA, et al. The sickle cell hemolytic transfusion reaction syndrome. Transfusion 1997;37:382–392.
62. Shirey RS, King KE. Alloimmunization to blood group antigens. In Anderson KC, Ness PM (eds). Scientific Basis of Transfusion Medicine: Implications for Clinical Practice, 2nd ed. Philadelphia, WB Saunders, 2000, pp 393–400.
63. Vichinsky EP, Earles PNP, Johnson RA, et al. Alloimmunization in sickle cell anemia and transfusion of racially unmatched blood. N Engl J Med 1990;322:1617–1621.
64. Rosse WF, Gallagher D, Kinney TR, et al. Cooperative study of sickle cell disease: transfusion and alloimmunization in sickle cell disease. Blood 1990;76:1431–1437.
65. Orlina AR, Unger PJ, Koshy M. Post-transfusion alloimmunization in patients with sickle cell disease. Am J Hematol 1978;5:101–106.
66. Cox JV, Steane E, Cunningham G, et al. Risk of alloimmunization and delayed hemolytic transfusion reactions in patients with sickle cell disease. Arch Intern Med 1988;148:2485–2489.
67. Ambruso DR, Githens JH, Alcorn R, et al. Experience with donors matched for minor blood group antigens in patients with sickle cell anemia who are receiving chronic transfusion therapy. Transfusion 1987;27:94–98.
68. Rosse WF, Telen M, Ware RE. Transfusion Support for Patients with Sickle Cell Disease. Bethesda, Md., AABB Press, 1998, pp 73–92.
69. Koshy M, Burd L, Wallace D, et al. Prophylactic red cell transfusions in pregnant patients with sickle cell disease: a randomized cooperative study. N Engl J Med 1988;319:1447–1452.
70. Diamond WJ, Brown Fl Jr, Bitterman P, et al. Delayed hemolytic transfusion reaction presenting as sickle-cell crisis. Ann Intern Med 1980;93:231–234.
71. Garratty G. Severe reactions associated with transfusion of patients with sickle cell disease [Editorial]. Transfusion 1997;37:357–361.
72. Heddle NM, Sortar RL, O'Hoski P, et al. A prospective study to determine the frequency and clinical significance of alloimmunization post-transfusion. Br J Haematol 1995;91:1000–1005.
73. Rao KR, Patel AR. Delayed hemolytic transfusion reactions in sickle cell anemia. South Med J 1989;9:1034–1036.
74. Kalyanaraman M, Heidemann SM, Sarnaik AP, et al. Anti-s antibody-associated delayed hemolytic transfusion reaction in patients with sickle cell anemia. J Pediatr Hematol Oncol 1999;21:10–13.
75. Fabron JA, Moreira JG, Bordin JO. Delayed hemolytic transfusion reaction presenting as a painful crisis in a patient with sickle cell anemia. Rev Paul Med 1999;117:385–389.
76. Milner PF, Squires JE, Larison PJ, et al. Posttransfusion crises in sickle cell anemia: role of delayed hemolytic reactions to transfusion. South Med J 1985;78:1462–1469.
77. Petz LD, Garratty G. Acquired Immune Hemolytic Anemia, 2nd ed. New York, Churchill Livingstone, 2004, pp 547–549.
78. Win N, Doughty H, Telfer P, et al. Hyperhemolytic transfusion reaction in sickle cell disease. Transfusion 2001;41:323–328.
79. Cullis JO, Win N, Dudley JM, et al. Post-transfusion hyperhaemolysis in a patient with sickle cell disease: use of steroids and intravenous immunoglobulin to prevent further red cell destruction. Vox Sang 1995;69:355–357.
80. Polesky HF, Bove JR. A fatal hemolytic transfusion reaction with acute autohemolysis. Transfusion 1964;4:285–292.
81. Wiener AS. Hemolytic reactions following transfusions of blood of the homologous group. II: Further observations on the role of property Rh, particularly in cases without demonstrable iso-antibodies. Arch Pathol 1941;32:227–250.
82. Petz LD. The expanding boundaries of transfusion medicine. In Nance LST (ed). Clinical and Basic Science Aspects of Immunohematology. Arlington, American Association of Blood Banks, 1991, pp 73–113.
83. Test ST, Woolworth VS. Defective regulation of complement by the sickle erythrocyte: evidence for a defect in control of membrane attack complex formation. Blood 1994;83:842–852.
84. Darabi K, Dzik S. Hyperhemolysis syndrome in anemia of chronic disease. Transfusion 2005;45:1930–1933.
85. Telen MJ, Coombs M. Management of massive delayed hemolytic transfusion reactions in patients with sickle cell disease [Abstract]. Transfusion 1999;36(Suppl):97S.
86. Bunker ML, Thomas Cl, Geyer SJ. Optimizing pretransfusion antibody detection and identification: a parallel, blinded comparison of tube PEG, solid-phase, and automated methods. Transfusion 2001;41:621–626.
87. Taswell HF, Pineda AA, Moore SB. Hemolytic transfusion reactions: Frequency and clinical and laboratory aspects. In Bell CA (ed). A Seminar on Immune-mediated Red Cell Destruction. Washington, D.C., American Association of Blood Banks, 1981, pp 71–92.
88. Schonewille H, Haak HL, van Zijl AM. RBC antibody persistence. Transfusion 2000;40:1127–1131.
89. Tahhan HR, Holbrook CT, Braddy LR, et al. Antigen matched donor blood in the transfusion management of patients with sickle cell disease. Transfusion 1994;34:562–569.
90. Vichinsky EP, Luban NLC, Wright E, et al. Prospective RBC phenotype matching in a stroke prevention trial in sickle cell anemia: a multicenter transfusion trial. Transfusion 2001;41:1086–1092.
91. Ness PM. To match or not to match: The question for chronically transfused patients with sickle cell anemia [Editorial]. Transfusion 1994;34:558–560.
92. Storry JR, Westhoff CM, Charles-Pierre D, et al. DNA analysis for donor screening of Dombrock blood group antigens. Immunohematology 2003;19:33–36.
93. Hult A, Hellberg A, Wester ES, et al. Blood group genotype analysis for the quality improvement of reagent test cells. Vox Sang 2005;88:465–470.
94. Castro O, Sandler SG, Houston-Yu P, et al. Predicting the effect of transfusing only phenotype-matched RBCs to patients with sickle cell disease: Theoretical and practical considerations. Transfusion 2002;42:684–690.
95. Strupp A, Cash K, Uehlinger J. Difficulties in identifying antibodies in the Dombrock blood group system in multiply alloimmunized patients. Transfusion 1998;38:1022–1025.
96. Campbell SA, Shirey RS, King KE, et al. An acute hemolytic transfusion reaction due to anti-IH in a patient with sickle cell disease. Transfusion 2000;40:828–831.
97. Callahan DL, Kennedy MS, Ranalli MA, et al. Delayed hemolytic transfusion reaction caused by Jk(b) antibody detected by only solid phase technique [Abstract]. Transfusion 2000;40(Suppl):113S.
98. Lanskron S, Moliterno AR, Norris EJ, et al. Polymerized human Hb use in acute chest syndrome: a case report. Transfusion 2002;42:1422–1427.
99. Winslow RM. Red cell substitutes. In Anderson KC, Ness PM (eds). Scientific Basis of Transfusion Medicine: Implications for Clinical Practice, 2nd ed. Philadelphia, WB Saunders, 2000, pp 588–598.
100. Beiboer SHW, Wieringa-Jelsma T, VanWijk M. Rapid genotyping of blood group antigens by multiplex polymerase chain reaction and DNA microarray hybridation. Transfusion 2005;45:667–679.

Chapter 50

Febrile, Allergic, and Other Noninfectious Transfusion Reactions

Nancy Heddle • Kathryn E. Webert

The transfusion of blood and blood products can be associated with a number of different noninfectious complications. The frequency of these events is variable, depending on the type of blood product being transfused and the patient population requiring the product. It is useful to categorize these types of reactions as acute (occurring during or within 8 hours of the transfusion) or delayed (presenting a week or two after transfusion), as this will facilitate the differential diagnosis and identification of these adverse events. The challenge for physicians and health care providers when these reactions occur is, first, to recognize that the reaction may be transfusion associated, and second, to use the clinical signs, symptoms, and situation to identify systematically the differential diagnosis, the reaction type, and the cause so that appropriate treatment and prevention strategies can be used. These challenges are complicated by the fact that many of the clinical signs and symptoms are common to several different types of reactions and that comorbidities may complicate the recognition of these events. In this chapter, the immediate and delayed noninfectious complications to transfusion are summarized in terms of their definition, manifestation, prevalence, pathophysiology (when known), diagnosis, treatment, and prevention. An approach is presented to illustrate how this information can be used to work systematically through the complex clinical presentation, generate a differential diagnosis, and identify the cause of the event.

ACUTE NONINFECTIOUS TRANSFUSION REACTIONS

Most of the acute noninfectious reactions occur during a transfusion or within a few hours of the transfusion; however, in some situations, signs and symptoms may not present until 6 to 8 hours after transfusion.[1] As the interval between the transfusion and presentation of symptoms increases, it becomes less likely that the reaction will be recognized as transfusion related; hence it is important for physicians to be aware not only of reactions with early presentation but also of those reactions with delayed onset. The noninfectious reactions in the acute category include febrile nonhemolytic, allergic, anaphylactic, transfusion-related acute lung injury (TRALI), hypotensive, transfusion-associated circulatory overload (TACO), hemolytic reactions (immediate and delayed), and a variety of metabolic complications (Tables 50–1 and 50–2). Hemolytic reactions, TRALI, and bacterial

Table 50–1 Summary of the Signs and Symptoms Typically Observed with Different Types of Acute Reactions to Blood and Blood Products

	Types of Symptoms					
	Cutaneous	Inflammatory	Pain	Respiratory	Cardiovascular	GI
Reaction Type	Pruritis Urticaria Erythema Flushing	Fever Chills Shakes Cold Feeling Rigors	Headache Chest Back Abdominal Site of Infusion	Hoarseness Stridor Lump in Throat Wheezing Chest Tightness Substernal Pain Dyspnea Cyanosis	Hypotension Loss of Consciousness Shock Tachycardia Cardiac Arrhythmias Cardiac Arrest	Nausea Vomiting Abdominal Cramps Diarrhea
Hemolytic		X	X	X	X	X
Allergic (mild)	X					
Allergic (anaphylactic)	X			X	X	X
FNHTR		X	x			x
TRALI		X		X	X	
Bacterial sepsis		X	X	X	X	X
Hypotensive	x			x	X	x
Circulatory overload (TACO)			x	X	X (hypertension)	

X, typical symptoms; x, symptoms sometimes observed; GI, gastrointestinal; FHNTR, febrile nonhemolytic transfusion reaction; TRALI, transfusion-related acute lung injury.

Table 50–2 **Summary of the Incidence, Etiology, Treatment, and Prevention of Noninfectious Transfusion Reactions**

Type of Acute Reaction	Incidence (per 100 transfusions)[6]	Incidence (per 100,000 transfusions*)[6] or incidence (per 100,000 patients**)	Etiology	Treatment	Prevention
Acute hemolytic reactions		*Red cells: 1.1–9.0	1. Pre-existing antibody in the patient's plasma binds to an incompatible antigen on the transfused red cells causing destruction. 2. Antibody in donor plasma binds to the patient's red cells causing hemolysis	Stop the transfusion. Notify transfusion service. Send appropriate samples to investigate. Provide supportive care including intravenous fluids. Maintain urine output. Treat DIC and shock as required.	Follow SOPs (clinical areas and laboratory) to ensure appropriate sample, patient and product identification. Ensure all staff are educated to the importance of these procedures.
Delayed hemolytic transfusion reaction (DHTR)		*Red cells: 0.7–24.9	Patient is alloimmunized (sometimes primary but usually secondary) by the transfusion and the antibody binds to the transfused red cells causing destruction.	Supportive care, if required. No specific treatment usually indicated.	Blood for future transfusions should be antigen negative.
Delayed serologic transfusion reaction (DSTR)		*Red cells: 28.9–68.4	Can be caused by active or passive antibody binding to the red cells and causing a positive DAT. No clinical signs of hemolysis.	No treatment required. Observe patient to ensure that delayed hemolysis does not occur.	Future transfusions should be with antigen-negative blood
Febrile nonhemolytic reactions (FNHTRs)	Red cells: 0.07–6.8 Platelets: 0.13–37.5		Red cells: Most reactions are due to a white cell antibody in the patient's plasma that interacts with leukocytes in the red cell product. Platelets: Storage generated proinflammatory cytokines cause of reactions; white cell antigen/antibody interactions cause about 9% of reactions.	Discontinue transfusion. Antipyretics. Supportive care.	Premedication with antipyretics. Leukoreduced blood products (must be prestorage LR for preventing platelet reactions. Other options include fresher products, plasma reduced, or washed cellular products.
Mild Allergic	Red cells: 0.02–1.07 Platelets: 0.06–7.6 All components: 3.0		Soluble antigens in the donor plasma react with IgE bound to mast cells causing histamine release.	Temporarily stop the infusion keeping line open with saline. Administer antihistamines. If urticaria abates, transfusion may be restarted.	Pretransfusion medication with antihistamine.

Anaphylactic		*Red cells: 0.3–4.3 *Apheresis platelets: 7.7 *Platelet pools: 62.5 *All components: 2.1	Patient is IgA deficient and has IgG antibodies to IgA. Other possible mechanisms: antibodies to other serum proteins absent in the patient; transfused allergens; passive transfer of IgE; mast cell activation by anaphylactoxins.	Discontinue transfusion; antihistamine administration. Subcutaneous, intramuscular, or intravenous epinephrine if needed. Supportive care.	Depends on the reaction severity and etiology. Anaphylactoid reactions may be prevented by antihistamine use. Anaphylactic reactions may require avoidance of all plasma containing products if reaction is due to anti-IgA or stringent washed cellular products.
TRALI	Red cells: 1–11 Platelets: 1–46 Not specified: 7–36		Multiple causes: passive transfusion on leukocyte antibody in the donor plasma. Storage generated lipids in the blood product (two-hit model). Other mechanisms not yet understood.	Supportive care only. No specific therapy indicated.	Removal of donors with potent leukocyte antibodies from the donor pool. Transfusion of fresher blood products or washed blood products may have a lower risk of causing these reactions.
Transfusion-associated circulatory overload (TACO)		**All products: 16.8–8000*	Infusion of too much fluid into the circulation in a short time. Patients with cardiovascular disease at greater risk.	Stop the transfusion. Diuretics and supplemental oxygen therapy.	Recognize patients at high risk for TACO. Administer transfusion slowly (split units if necessary). Use of diuretics.
Transfusion-transmitted bacterial infection (TTBI)† Deaths from TTBI		*Platelet pools: 1.1–47.5† *Apheresis: 1.0–7.5 *Red cells: 0.02–1.5 *Platelet pools: 0.2–6.3 *Apheresis: 0.2–1.5 *Red cells: 0–1.0	Bacteria in the blood product release endotoxin or once in the patient's circulation cause infection.	Stop the transfusion. Provide aggressive supportive therapy including broad-spectrum antibiotics.	Inspect all blood products for visual evidence of contamination before infusion; employ measures at the blood center and transfusion service to decrease risk.
Hypotensive reactions	Unknown		Mediated by kinins generated by activation of the contact system. Patients on ACE inhibitors appear to be more susceptible.	Stop the transfusion.	Avoid the use of negatively charged bedside leukoreduction filters.
Post-transfusion purpura	Unknown		Recipient has alloantibody directed against an antigen on the donor's platelets. Patient's own platelets are also destroyed: mechanism not clearly understood.	IVIG infusions are the first-line therapy. Plasmapheresis may also be effective. Patients may respond to antigen-negative platelets if bleeding.	Future transfusions should consist of platelets negative for the antigen to which the antibody is directed (i.e., HPA-1a negative).

*The higher rate was observed in elderly patients (mean age, 67 years) undergoing hip or knee surgery.

† One study from Hong Kong reported the risk of TTBI with platelet pools to be 280/100,000 transfusions; however, all other reports have ranged between 1.1 and 47.5.

contamination are summarized in Chapters 41, 43, and 50, respectively; further clinical details on these complications are not presented. However, these two complications are included in the practical approach to classify acute transfusion reactions described at the end of this chapter.

FEBRILE NONHEMOLYTIC TRANSFUSION REACTIONS

Definition/Manifestations/Prevalence

Febrile nonhemolytic transfusion reactions (FNHTRs) have traditionally been defined as a temperature increase of at least 1° C with or without chills, a cold sensation, or discomfort, occurring during or within a few hours of the transfusion.[1] However, increasing recognition exists that this traditional definition should be modified. Although the name implies that fever is always present, this may not be the case. A recent study has shown that, frequently, the symptoms of chills, cold sensation, and discomfort may occur in the absence of fever.[2] It is not uncommon that the temperature increase is suppressed by the use of antipyretic premedication. Studies performed at our center have shown that FNHTR characterized by chills, cold, and/or discomfort can occur without fever in about 85% of reactions. Severe reactions can be characterized by rigors and, rarely, headache, nausea, and vomiting.[2]

The frequency of FNHTRs varies depending on the type and age of the blood product being transfused, the patient population, and differences in the recording of symptoms by nursing staff and whether premedications are given.[3–5] The reported incidence of FNHTR with red cell products ranges from 0.07 to 6.8 reactions per 100 red cell units transfused.[6] The use of prestorage leukoreduced red cells appears to result in an absolute risk reduction ranging from 0.14% to 0.22%.[7–9] FNHTRs appear to be more common when platelets are transfused; however, the incidence reported in the literature is extremely variable, ranging from 0.19 to 37.5 per 100 platelet transfusions.[6] Historically, FNHTRs have been the most commonly encountered reaction, accounting for approximately 43% to 75% of all transfusion reactions reported at some centers.[10,11] However, centers that use prestorage leukoreduced blood products have seen a dramatic decrease in the frequency of these events, especially those reactions associated with platelet transfusions.[2,7,12]

Pathophysiology

At least two mechanisms seem to result in the clinical manifestations of FNHTR. The first mechanism involves the presence of a white cell alloantibody in the patient's plasma that interacts with white cells in the blood product.[13–15] Both granulocyte[14,16–20] and human leukocyte antigen (HLA) antibodies[18,20] have been implicated in these reactions. This antigen-antibody interaction causes release of endotoxins that act on the hypothalamus, resulting in fever and the other symptoms typical of FNHTR. This mechanism appears to be the primary cause of FNHTR after the transfusion of red cells but accounts for only approximately 9% of platelet reactions.[21] The second mechanism involves the generation of leukocyte-derived cytokines during storage of the product. A variety of cytokines have been detected in stored blood products; however, the proinflammatory cytokines (interleukin [IL]-1, IL-6, IL-8, and tumor necrosis factor [TNF]-α) are likely to be the predominant cause of FNHTR.[21–29] The release and/or production of cytokines during storage occurs mainly at warmer temperatures; hence this mechanism accounts for approximately 90% of the reactions to platelets that are not prestorage leukoreduced, as this product is stored at room temperature but is unlikely to be the cause of red cell reactions, as cytokine production/release is inhibited by the 4° C storage.[30] Therefore, poststorage leukoreduction will be effective at preventing FNHTR to red cells, which are mainly due to white cells in the product, but will have minimal impact on platelet reactions. In contrast, prestorage leukoreduction of both of these products is an effective method for prevention of FNHTR due to both red cells and platelets.[2,7–9] Although this approach has been shown to be effective for preventing most reactions, residual reactions still occur (0.2% for red cells and 1.0% with platelets), suggesting that other minor mechanisms may also play a role.[2] The exact cause of these residual reactions is unknown; however, possible mechanisms that have been suggested include platelet-derived substances such as CD154 (CD40 ligand).[31,32] It has also been postulated that some febrile reactions may represent immune responses to infused substances, such as IL-6, which has been found to be elevated in patients who experience an FNHTR.[33,34]

Diagnosis and Treatment

The diagnosis of FNHTR is one of exclusion. Other causes of fever must be excluded, including other acute transfusion reactions that manifest with fever and clinical comorbidities and/or medications (Fig. 50–1). Sometimes the timing of the reaction may be helpful in the differential diagnosis. FNHTRs tend to be dependent on the dose or concentration of leukocytes and/or cytokines infused and therefore appear toward the end of the transfusion.[1,2,12] It is atypical for this type of reaction to occur during the initial stage of the transfusion. Clinical experience has also suggested that the rate of infusion is another important variable that may contribute to these events.[35]

Treatment of these reactions consists of the administration of an antipyretic such as acetaminophen. Severe shaking chills (rigors) may necessitate meperidine administration. These symptoms resolve with or without treatment and do not typically lead to additional or long-term adverse sequelae. The decision to stop the transfusion requires clinical judgment based on the severity of the symptoms, the type of product being transfused, the timing of the symptoms in relation to the amount of product infused, and the history and clinical state of the patient.[5]

Prevention

The approach for preventing FNHTR differs slightly depending on whether the product is red cells or platelets. For red cell reactions, the first line of prevention would include either poststorage or prestorage leukoreduction. If reactions still occur to leukoreduced products, other approaches that may be effective include the transfusion of fresher blood products and or washed blood products. To prevent FNHTR to platelet transfusions, prestorage leukoreduction has been shown to be the most effective method. For patients who still react to the prestorage leukoreduced product, other options include removing the residual plasma from the platelet product, washing the product, or selecting fresher products

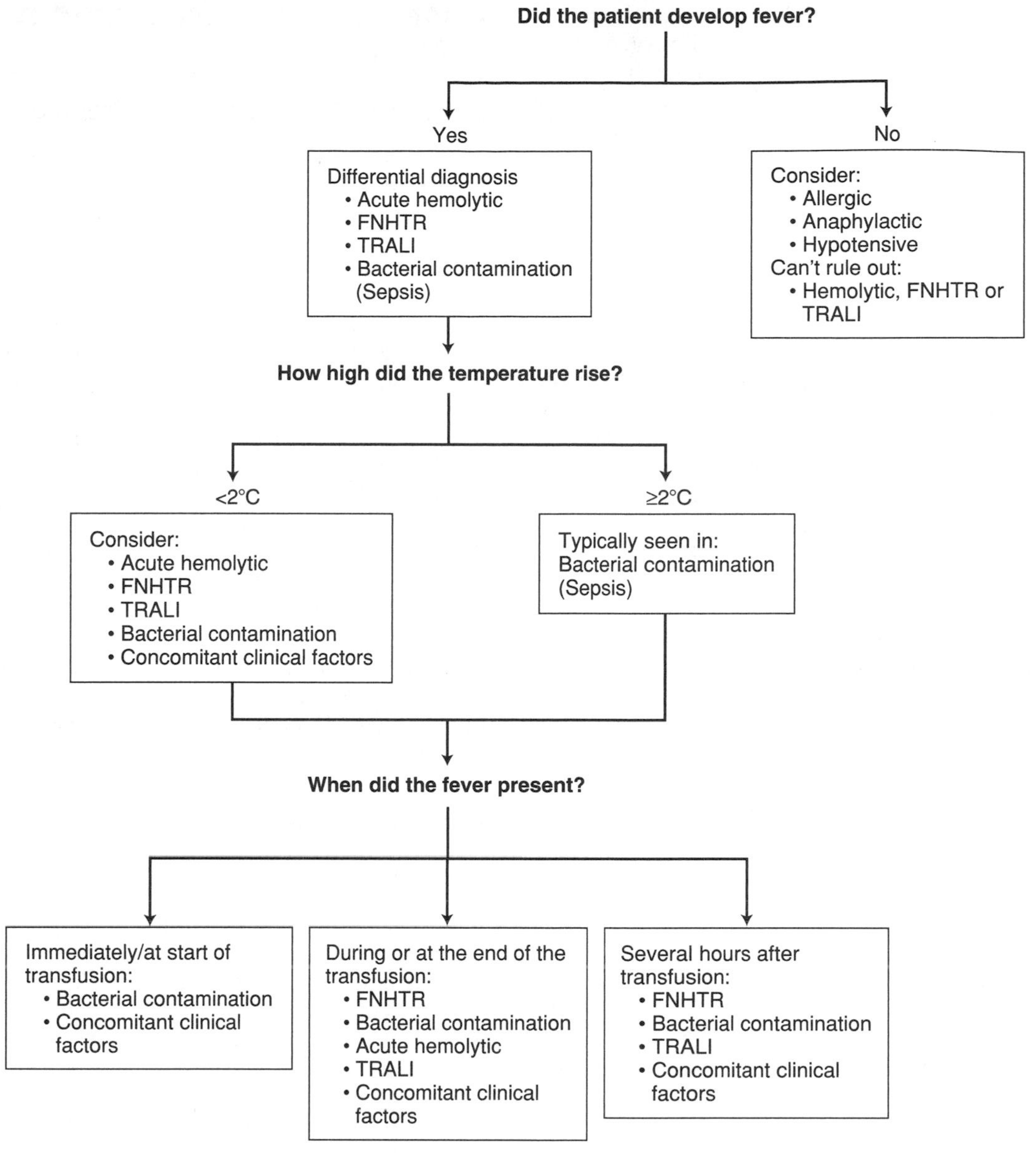

Figure 50–1 Algorithm to assist with the differential diagnosis of acute transfusion reactions associated with fever.

for transfusion.[5] Pretransfusion antipyretic administration may be effective in some patients for preventing recurrent FNHTR. One concern about this strategy is that fever associated with other types of reactions (hemolytic transfusion reactions and reactions to bacterially contaminated products) may be masked. In the past, microaggregate filtration was postulated as a method to reduce the granulocyte concentration, and therefore FNHTR, in red blood cell units.[36,37] However, this did not become common practice and is not generally recommended.

ALLERGIC REACTIONS

Allergic transfusion reactions may be grouped into three categories by severity; however, the categories can have overlapping presentations: (1) uncomplicated allergic reactions, (2) anaphylactoid reactions, and (3) anaphylactic reactions. At the mild end of the spectrum, uncomplicated allergic reactions consist of only cutaneous manifestations. At the severe end of the spectrum are anaphylactic reactions characterized by severe hypotension with a high likelihood of morbidity or mortality due to shock. The term *anaphylactoid* has been used to characterize reactions that are moderate in severity involving cutaneous symptoms as well as some degree of hypotension, stridor, wheezing, dyspnea, chest pain, or tachycardia. As the etiology of the mild allergic reactions is different from that of anaphylactoid and anaphylactic reactions, they are discussed as separate entities.

MILD ALLERGIC REACTIONS

Definition/Manifestations/Prevalence

Mild allergic reactions are characterized by a localized or confluent red raised itching rash (urticaria) in the absence of fever. For a reaction to be classified as uncomplicated urticaria, no additional symptoms must be present, such as asthma-like attacks, coughing, difficulty in breathing, or other symptoms associated with anaphylactoid or anaphylactic reactions.[38,39] Very few well-designed prospective studies provide information on the incidence of mild allergic reactions. One would anticipate that the incidence would vary depending on the type of blood product, the amount of plasma in the product, and patient population being transfused (see Pathophysiology later). Several studies have reported that mild allergic reactions occur with approximately 3% of all blood products transfused.[40–42] The reported frequency of reactions to platelet transfusions has varied from 0.02% to 7.6%.[2,43–47]

Pathophysiology

These reactions presumably occur as a result of cutaneous hypersensitivity in which the recipient has been previously sensitized to soluble allergens found in the donor unit.[38] The soluble antigen in the donor plasma is bound to immunoglobulin E (IgE) on mast cells, which causes the release of histamine and the cutaneous symptoms typically observed. It is important to note that most allergic reactions appear as a spectrum and that reactions that begin as urticaria may develop into anaphylactoid or anaphylactic reactions, although this is rare.

A recent report suggests that allergic reactions can also occur as delayed events. In this case report, the patient developed urticaria and shortness of breath several days after a plasma transfusion while eating peanut butter. The patient had no known peanut allergies, and serologic investigations demonstrated a potent antibody specific for peanuts in the donor's plasma. Although this case is unusual, it illustrates the importance of considering the transfusion history for patients who experience these types of events.[48]

Diagnosis

Diagnosis of skin-restricted allergy is straightforward and requires recognition of a rash with associated itching but without additional symptoms. As soluble plasma antigens are the cause of these reactions, the reactions tend to be dose dependent, occurring later in the transfusion. The rash resolves when the transfusion is stopped and/or an antihistamine is given.

Treatment

Treatment for uncomplicated urticaria requires temporary discontinuation of the blood-product infusion and administration of an antihistamine. If the symptoms resolve, the transfusion may be resumed, and a formal transfusion reaction assessment is not required. If the symptoms do not resolve or if they progress during treatment or on continuance of the transfusion, the transfusion should be stopped and a new unit obtained.[38]

Prevention

Premedication with an antihistamine will prevent urticarial reactions in most patients who have a history of allergic reactions. If premedication is not effective or if repeated reactions of increasing severity occur, washed cellular products may be beneficial. As donor leukocytes are not involved in the etiology of these reactions, leukoreduction has no role in the prevention of these events. This has been demonstrated in a large observational study of more than 47,000 red cell transfusions, in which the frequency of mild allergic reactions was 0.04% before universal leukoreduction, and 0.06% after implementation of universal leukoreduction.[49]

ANAPHYLAXIS/ANAPHYLACTOID REACTIONS

Definition/Manifestations/Prevalence

Anaphylactic transfusion reactions are severe systemic reactions characterized by hypotension, bronchospasm or dyspnea, nausea, vomiting, diarrhea, and urticaria.[38,50–55] The most serious symptoms include lower airway obstruction, laryngeal edema, and hypotension. Typically, these reactions appear after a small volume (<10 mL) of product has been infused.[1,38] Most reactions occur in patients who are IgA deficient and who have IgG alloantibodies to IgA detectable in their plasma.[52] Although IgA deficiency is not uncommon (1 in 700 individuals), anaphylactic reactions are relatively rare, occurring in of 1 in 20,000 to 1 in 47,000 (0.002% to 0.005%) products transfused,[41] a rate considerably less than the sector of the population thought to be at risk (0.08%).[56] Canadian data suggest that these reactions occur even less frequently, with an incidence of incidence of 0.00013% per unit transfused.[6] Between 1976 and 1985, three deaths were attributed to transfusion-associated anaphylaxis in the United States.[57]

Anaphylactoid reactions are generally less severe than anaphylaxis. Severe and even fatal reactions, however, have been reported in patients with detectable levels of IgA and concurrent specific anti-IgA.[41,50,57–59]

Pathophysiology

Anaphylactic reactions are most commonly due to preformed, class-specific, recipient anti-IgA to infused donor IgA proteins in patients with IgA deficiency.[41] However, other case reports have linked anaphylactic reaction to HLA-associated antibodies in platelet transfusion,[60] anti-C4 in a C4-deficient patient,[61] and antihaptoglobin in an ahaptoglobinemic patient.[62] One study involving 32,376 random blood donors found an IgA deficiency incidence of 0.26% (1 in 372).[56] IgA deficiency with associated anti-IgA in the same study was found to occur at a rate of 0.08% (1 in 1200).[56] From this, one may infer that the incidence of anti-IgA in IgA-deficient donors is approximately 31% (0.26/0.08).

Anaphylactoid reactions are typically associated with subclass, allotypic, or specific anti-IgA in patients who have demonstrable and often normal levels of IgA.[41,50,56,58,59] It is difficult to identify patients who may have a specific anti-IgA because that would involve a seemingly infinite number of specific IgA proteins. These types of reactions may also be due to other transfused products found in donor units, such as peanut allergen transfused to patients who may have peanut allergy.

Diagnosis

Anaphylaxis/anaphylactoid reactions should be recognized immediately when a patient has the symptoms just described. When anaphylaxis related to blood transfusion is suspected, administration of any additional plasma-containing blood product should be avoided, if possible, until an appropriate diagnostic evaluation can be performed. Differential diagnosis of transfusion-related anaphylaxis includes hypotensive reactions occurring in patients taking angiotensin-converting enzyme (ACE) inhibitors, TRALI (Chapter 43), and other events unrelated to transfusion, including myocardial infarction or pulmonary embolus.[38] When anaphylaxis occurs in association with blood transfusion, IgA deficiency with concomitant anti-IgA must be investigated. For a firm diagnosis, this requires demonstration of recipient anti-IgA.[41,50,52–54,59,63,64]

The initial investigation may include nephelometry for the detection of IgA. Demonstration of IgA by this method effectively negates a diagnosis of anaphylaxis related to anti-IgA. If IgA is not detected, additional studies should be performed because some patients have IgA levels that are below the limit of detection by nephelometry. To detect anti-IgA in these cases, passive hemagglutination assays (PHAs) utilizing IgA-coated red blood cells are performed. Most often, the IgA used to coat these red blood cells is from patients with multiple myeloma whose monoclonal protein is IgA.[41,50,52–54,56,58,59,63–65]

Treatment

In addition to immediate discontinuation of product infusion, treatment of anaphylaxis includes prompt administration of epinephrine, which will quickly reverse the action of histamine. Other supportive care may include vasopressors and airway support. Intravenous steroids and an H_1-receptor antagonist can be given to reduce the risk of protracted anaphylaxis.[38,39]

Prevention

Prevention of anaphylactic reactions in patients who are determined to be IgA deficient with anti-IgA antibodies requires avoidance of transfusion with plasma-containing IgA. Cellular products can be washed to remove the residual plasma containing IgA, or products can be collected from donors who are known to be IgA deficient.[56] When red cells are required, autologous donation and frozen blood may also be feasible options. Most often, IgA-deficient donors are identified by screening immunodiffusion methods[66] followed by a confirmatory passive hemagglutination inhibition assay (PHIA).[56,59,65,67] This assay differs from PHA by the addition of a known amount of reagent anti-IgA and the observation of inhibition of agglutination, which is due to the presence of donor IgA; that is, no agglutination inhibition would be observed in donors who lacked IgA.[51,56,65,68] It is important to use a sensitive method such as PHIA to confirm IgA deficiency in donors. Case reports show that some patients found to be at risk for IgA-deficient anaphylactic reaction were transfused with presumptive IgA-deficient plasma containing products that led to anaphylactic reactions. Retesting of these products by more sensitive methods showed that they contained low levels of IgA.[56]

HYPOTENSIVE REACTIONS

Definition/Manifestation/Prevalence

Hypotension is a relatively rare complication of blood transfusion that is typically seen in TRALI, sepsis due to bacterial contamination, and anaphylactic transfusion reactions. In addition to these transfusion-related complications, another type of reaction characterized by acute hypotension within the first few minutes of a transfusion has been described. These hypotensive reactions are first seen with a decrease in systolic or diastolic blood pressure of at least 30 mm Hg occurring within 10 minutes of starting the transfusion and are distinguishable from other adverse events with hypotension as they resolve rapidly once the transfusion is stopped. Some patients may also have facial flushing, abdominal pain and nausea, loss of consciousness, respiratory distress, and shock.[69] The initial reports of these reactions all occurred in patients taking ACE inhibitors who were transfused blood products through a bedside leukoreduction filter[69–71]; however, the reactions may not always be related to the use of these filters.[72] The overall frequency of these events is not currently known, as reports in the literature have been individual case reports or case series.

Pathophysiology

Hypotensive transfusion reactions are thought to be mediated by bradykinin and des-Arg-bradykinin, which are two vasoactive kinins that are generated by the activation of the contact system. Activated factor XII converts prekallikrein to kallikrein, which cleaves high-molecular-weight kininogen and releases bradykinin. This vasodilatory nonapeptide causes hypotension and edema by activating B2-kinin receptors on the vascular endothelium.[73,74] Bradykinin is rapidly inactivated by ACE; however, if a patient is taking an ACE inhibitor, this inactivation process will be impaired. The original reports of hypotensive reactions occurred with negatively charged bedside leukoreduction filters, which have been demonstrated to result in kinin activation and accumulation. If the patient was taking an ACE inhibitor, kinin inactivation was impaired, and acute hypotension occurred.[75] Other reports documented that these reactions could also occur when positively charged bedside filters were used.[76] We have recently postulated that other factors may contribute to these hypotensive reactions after investigating two patients undergoing radical prostatectomy who were transfused blood by using standard blood filters and a warming device. Possible contributing factors may include activation of the contact system by using the blood warmer; release of prostate specific human glandular kallikrein (hK2) and hK3 (prostate specific antigen) during surgery, which can cause bradykinin generation; and/or an inherent defect in the patient's ability to degrade kinins.[72] Several pathways and factors may contribute to the hypotensive reactions, and further studies will be required to improve our understanding of these adverse events.

Treatment

Hypotensive reactions should be treated by immediately stopping the infusion of the blood product transfusion and by providing the patient with supportive care. Typically, the symptoms resolve quickly once these measures have been taken, as indicated by the two case reports by Arnold and colleagues.[72]

Prevention

Most hypotensive reactions can be prevented by avoiding the use of bedside leukoreduction filters. In 1999, the U.S. Food and Drug Administration (FDA) warned consumers about the risk of hypotensive reactions with bedside leukoreduction filters and recommended the use of prestorage leukoreduction as a safe alternative.[71] Some physicians have also suggested that ACE inhibitor therapy should be temporarily discontinued just before surgery; however, no clinical data suggest that this is a beneficial and risk-free alternative for preventing hypotensive reactions.

CIRCULATORY OVERLOAD

Definition/Manifestation/Prevalence

TACO appears as acute respiratory distress that begins during or shortly after the administration of a blood product. Symptoms and signs of TACO include dyspnea that worsens as pulmonary edema progresses, orthopnea, chest tightness, cough, tachycardia, hypertension, and widened pulse pressure. TACO generally occurs near the end of administration of the transfusion or within 6 hours of completion. The frequency of circulatory overload varies depending on the patient population being transfused and the blood product being given; however, it has been estimated to occur in about 1% of transfusions and is often unrecognized.[77] Patients at higher risk for TACO include elderly patients, patients of small stature, patients with compromised cardiac function, and small children.

Pathophysiology

It is difficult to overload the circulatory system if a patient has normal cardiac function; however, patients with congestive heart failure or other heart and pulmonary diseases are susceptible to this complication when transfusions are given. Infants are also at increased risk of circulatory overload. The intravascular volume may be overtaxed by either an inappropriate rate of transfusion or an inappropriate volume of transfusion in addition to other infused substances. When cardiac output cannot be maintained, pulmonary edema can occur. The problem can also be magnified in a patient with renal failure.

Diagnosis

The physical examination will reveal the patient to have an elevated jugular venous pulse. Auscultation of the chest will suggest pulmonary congestion with rales and crackles. The cardiovascular examination may reveal the presence of an S3 gallop. Findings suggestive of TACO on radiographic examination of the chest include pulmonary vascular redistribution, alveolar and interstitial edema, Kerley B-lines, cardiomegaly, and pleural effusions.

The measurement of an elevated brain natriuretic peptide (BNP) has recently been proposed as a useful adjunct marker in confirming volume overload as a cause of dyspnea.[78] BNP is a polypeptide secreted from the cardiac ventricles. It is increased in heart failure and fluid overload by ventricular cells in response to increased filling pressures.[79] BNP causes natriuresis and diuresis, vasodilation, and inhibits the renin-angiotensin aldosterone system.[80,81] Zhou and colleagues.[78] demonstrated the use of BNP in patients with suspected TACO to have a sensitivity of 81% and a specificity of 87%. Furthermore, plasma BNP measurement was approved by the FDA as an aid in the diagnosis of heart failure, and it is recommended that measurement of BNP levels should be part of the diagnostic approach to patients with suspected heart failure.

Treatment

Treatment includes the cessation or reduction of the rate of blood-product infusion, the placement of the patient in a sitting position, diuretics, and other supportive therapy such as supplemental oxygen.

Prevention/Recurrence

In general, blood products may routinely be transfused at a rate of 2.0 to 2.5 mL/kg/hr. However, in patients with a previous history of TACO or who are thought to be at an increased risk of TACO (i.e., the elderly, those with poor cardiac function, small infants), this rate should be decreased to approximately 1 mL/kg/hr. When a red cell or plasma product cannot be infused within the 4-hour period specified in safety standards, the product may be split into two parts, with one part being stored at a cold temperature while the other part is slowly infused. Patients considered to be at risk for TACO should be monitored closely during and after the transfusion for signs and symptoms of TACO. Pretransfusion and intratransfusion therapy with diuretics may also be beneficial in patients with any degree of cardiac or renal failure. These medications should never be added directly to the blood product or infused through the same line as the blood product. If a rapid transfusion is required, procedures such as isovolemic exchange transfusion have been described in the literature and may decrease the risk of TACO.[82]

OTHER ACUTE REACTIONS

Metabolic Complications

A number of metabolic complications can occur when blood products are infused. These complications are most commonly observed in neonatal patients or in circumstances in which rapid, large-volume infusions occur. Such metabolic complications include effects of citrate toxicity (hypocalcemia), hyperkalemia, and hypothermia.

Citrate Toxicity

Sodium citrate is the anticoagulant used during blood collection. The final citrate concentration in blood components is highest in plasma products. Normally the liver rapidly metabolizes transfused citrate; however, during massive transfusion, the capacity of the liver for citrate clearance may be exceeded.[83] The citrate forms a complex with calcium, resulting in decreased ionized calcium and a hypocalcemic state. Although transient hypocalcemia is usually well tolerated, nerve cell membranes can be affected, causing perioral or acral paresthesia. Clinical manifestations may include lightheadness, shivers, twitching, and tremors. Severe hypocalcemia can cause continuous muscle contractions and, if not corrected, can progress to tetany with spasms in multiple muscle groups.[84] It is important to recognize early symptoms of hypocalcemia so treatment can be initiated. Oral administration of calcium in antacid tablets and /or milk is commonly used for mild citrate toxicity. If symptoms progress, the infusion may have to be stopped or the flow rate decreased, or parenteral Ca^{2+} supplementation given.[84]

Hyperkalemia

When red cell products are stored, potassium leaks from the cells, increasing the plasma potassium concentration. During massive transfusion, transient hyperkalemia can occur; however, the cause is probably multifactorial, being related to the patient's acid-base balance, the ionized calcium concentration, the rate of the infusion, and the potassium level in the product.[85–89] In most cases, hyperkalemia can be reversed by correcting the underlying acid-base imbalance and slowing the rate of infusion.

Hypothermia

As red cell and plasma products are stored at cold temperatures, their rapid infusion may contribute to hypothermia, especially in patients with major trauma who may already be susceptible to hypothermia, depending on the nature and extent of the injuries.[90] Hypothermia results in a number of metabolic impairments including a decrease in the rate of citrate and lactate metabolism, increased oxygen affinity of hemoglobin, and increased red cell potassium release.[91–95] In addition, the decreased core body temperature may affect cardiac function with associated morbidity and mortality. Hypothermia can be minimized by warming the blood products before transfusion by using an approved blood-warming device.[96–98]

Red-Eye Syndrome

Other transfusion reactions that have been attributed to leukoreduction filters include ocular reactions, the so-called red-eye syndrome.[99] In all reports of red-eye syndrome, the patient exhibited bilateral conjunctival injection or hemorrhage, which occurred within 1 day of transfusion and had an average duration of approximately 5 days. Other features of the reaction were eye pain, headache, periorbital edema, arthralgias, nausea, dyspnea, and rash.[99] These reactions were predominantly linked to a specific leukoreduction filter, which has since been taken off the market.

DELAYED NONINFECTIOUS TRANSFUSION REACTIONS

Post-Transfusion Purpura

Definition/Manifestations/Prevalence

Post-transfusion purpura (PTP) was initially described approximately 50 years ago.[100–102] It is a rare but serious complication of transfusion. PTP manifests as sudden and severe thrombocytopenia (platelet count $<10 \times 10^9$/L) and purpura occurring within 5 to 10 days (range, 1–24 days) of red cells, plasma, or platelet transfusions.[103] Fevers and chills may occur during the implicated transfusion. The risk of PTP is unknown, but approximately 300 cases are reported in the literature.

Pathophysiology

PTP is generally thought to be caused by recipient alloantibodies directed against donor platelet antigens that the recipient lacks. The alloantibodies are IgG immunoglobulins.[104,105] The most common platelet alloantibody identified in patients with PTP occurs in patients who are homozygous for human platelet-specific alloantigen 1b (HPA-1b) and is directed against HPA-1a, although antibodies of other specificities have been identified.[106–114]

The platelet destruction that occurs includes the transfused platelets as well as the autologous platelets, leading to a profound thrombocytopenia. The mechanism causing the destruction of the autologous platelets is poorly understood. A number of theories have been proposed to explain the clearance of the antigen-negative platelets in the presence of anti–HPA-1a antibodies. The mechanisms proposed include (1) the nonspecific absorption of alloantigen-alloantibody immune complexes to the recipient's own platelets, with subsequent clearance mediated by complement or by the reticuloendothelial system (also known as the innocent-bystander effect)[115]; (2) the binding to autologous platelets of soluble or microparticle-associated alloantigen derived from the destruction of transfused blood product, thus making the recipient platelets a target for the alloantibodies; or (3) the presence of pseudo-specific alloantibodies that are produced in the early phase of the anamnestic response and can bind to determinants on autologous platelets, leading to their destruction.[116,117]

Female patients are approximately 5 times more likely to develop PTP after transfusion than are male patients, because of sensitization during previous pregnancies.[104] Because prior transfusion can also be the initial immunizing event, previously transfused male patients may also develop PTP. Approximately 3% of the white population are homozygous for the HPA-1b antigen and are therefore potentially at risk for PTP, if they are alloimmunized against HPA-1a.[118] However, fewer than 30% of these patients are able to form anti–HPA-1a.The development of such alloantibodies is highly associated with the presence of maternal HLA-DRw52a (HLA-DRB3*0101).[119]

Treatment

The usual treatment for this reaction is intravenous immunoglobulin (IVIG) at a dose of 1 g/kg for 2 days. The mechanism of action of IVIG is not well understood but may involve reticuloendothelial blockade or nonspecific antibody adherence to the target antigen that blocks access by specific antibody. Case reports have suggested that treatment with IVIG may shorten the duration of thrombocytopenia.[108,120–125] If a poor response to IVIG occurs, plasmapheresis may be used to reduce the antibody and possibly soluble antigen titers.[126,127] Corticosteroids, to depress immune system responsiveness, have also been used in the treatment of this disease, but they are no longer generally used because IVIG with or without plasmapheresis is effective therapy. In patients who are bleeding, the transfusion of antigen-negative platelets may provide a good increment of the platelet count and clinical hemostasis.[128,129] In general, routine allogeneic platelet transfusion is not recommended because it may exacerbate the reaction process and does not typically increase the platelet count.

PTP is a serious disorder, with fatal bleeding, usually intracranial or gastrointestinal hemorrhage, occurring in approximately 10% to 20% of patients. If PTP does not lead to death resulting from hemorrhage, it is a self-limited disease, with recovery typically occurring within 4 to 5 days of therapy. Recovery may be hastened by the use of antigen-negative platelets if the specificity of the antibody has been determined and antigen-negative platelets are available.[130,131]

Prevention/Recurrence

Little has been published about the recurrence or prevention of PTP. In general, it is recommended to avoid antigen-positive red blood cell and platelet transfusions in patients in whom PTP has previously occurred. The use of washed or filtered random red cells has been demonstrated to be effective by some authors[131,132]; however, this practice is not supported by all experts. An additional important consideration is that female patients with a history of PTP are potentially at risk for the delivery of an infant with neonatal alloimmune thrombocytopenia and should be counseled appropriately. Family members should also be counseled.

Iron Overload

Definition/Manifestations/Prevalence

Iron overload is an uncommon complication of transfusion that occurs after long periods in patients who receive red cell transfusions for chronic disease, such as sickle cell anemia and thalassemia.

Pathophysiology

Each unit of red cells contains approximately 200 to 250 mg of iron. The excess iron is initially stored in the patient's macrophages. As iron stores increase, the iron is stored in the liver parenchymal cells, myocardium, and endocrine organs. Chronic iron overload leads to liver dysfunction, heart failure, skin pigmentation, and endocrine disorders such as diabetes mellitus. The toxic manifestations of excess iron stores depend on such factors as (1) the amount of excess iron, (2) the rate of iron accumulation, (3) the ascorbate level, (4) alcohol use, and (5) viral hepatitis infection.[133,134]

Diagnosis

The iron content of different organs may be estimated or measured directly. The serum ferritin, although commonly performed, is a poor measure of total body iron, as it is affected by other variables, such as inflammation. Hepatic storage iron has been demonstrated to correlate with total body iron stores.[135] Liver iron can be measured after liver biopsy or by supraconducting quantum interface device (SQUID) or by magnetic resonance imaging (MRI). Patients with liver iron levels greater than 15 mg of iron per gram of liver are at increased risk for hepatic fibrosis and other complications.[136] Cardiac iron may be indirectly measured by using MRI. Other measures of iron status include the measurement of non–transferrin-bound iron and urine iron excretion. Patients with iron overload should also have the function of potentially affected organs assessed: the heart, liver, and endocrine glands.

Treatment

Transfusion-related iron overload is fatal in patients who are dependent on red cell transfusion, unless these patients are treated with agents that chelate the iron and promote its excretion. Therefore, the goal of iron chelation therapy is to decrease the iron deposition in tissues to levels that will not cause iron-mediated toxicity. Treatment with these agents is usually begun after 10 to 20 transfusions have been given.[137] Desferoxamine (DFO) is the most widely available chelating agent administered subcutaneously or intravenously. Regular chelation therapy with DFO has been associated with decreased hepatic fibrosis, decreased risk of cardiac disease, and decreased risk of endocrine dysfunction.[136,138–140] Because of the inconvenience, expense, and difficulty of treating patients with subcutaneous or intravenous infusion, oral chelating agents are being developed and tested. These agents include deferiprone and deferasirox (ICL 670).

Other Delayed Noninfectious Complications

Transfusion-associated graft-versus-host disease, transfusion-induced refractoriness to platelet transfusion, and other transfusion-related immunomodulations also occur and are discussed in detail in Chapters 44 and 45.

INVESTIGATION OF ACUTE REACTIONS

Most publications dealing with the management of acute transfusion reactions recommend that the transfusion of the blood product should always be stopped when signs and symptoms of a reaction are present while an assessment and transfusion-reaction investigation is performed. This approach is based on many years of experience and observation indicating a direct correlation between the severity of some reactions and the volume of the blood product transfused. Indeed this correlation is true for acute hemolytic transfusion reactions. However, some types of patients may frequently be spiking a temperature because they have sepsis, or may be known to react to almost every transfusion that is given, and stopping and investigating a transfusion every time mild symptoms are observed may not be practical or clinically justified. To provide a single algorithm on when to stop and when to continue a transfusion is not a practical solution because of the many factors that must be incorporated into the decision-making process. This decision requires clinical judgment, and the best way to ensure effective clinical decision making is for all health care professionals to be familiar with the types of reactions that occur and how these reactions appear, and to use a logical approach that balances risk, benefit, and resource utilization. In this section, some of the factors that can assist in the clinical management of transfusion reactions are described.

1. Cutaneous symptoms only: General agreement exists that when mild cutaneous signs and symptoms occur during transfusion with no other clinical manifestations, a transfusion-reaction investigation is not required. Depending on the discomfort experienced by the patient, the transfusion may have to be temporarily stopped and an antihistamine administered. Slowing the rate of infusion may also be of clinical benefit.
2. Did the patient develop fever? Fever is a commonly encountered symptom that can be present with several different types of acute reactions (hemolytic, TRALI, bacterial sepsis) (see Fig. 50–1). The absence of fever when cutaneous symptoms are present is characteristic (and diagnostic) of allergic reactions. However, it is important to remember that more than one type of reaction can occur simultaneously; hence fever and cutaneous symptoms sometimes both occur and should alert one to consider multiple events.
3. How high did the temperature rise? Most transfusion-associated fevers result in a modest increase in temperature (<2° C). A temperature increase above 2° C has been frequently reported in cases where blood products contaminated with bacteria have been transfused; hence bacterial contamination of the blood product should always be considered (and ruled out) when a dramatic increase in temperature occurs.
4. What is the temporal association between the fever and the amount of blood transfused? Noting whether

the fever occurs early or late in the transfusion can also be helpful to identify the type of reaction.

5. Is hypotension present, and when did it present? Hypotension does not occur with mild allergic reactions or with FNHTR. When hypotension is present, the differential diagnosis should include acute hemolytic reactions, anaphylaxis, bacterial contamination, TRALI, hypotensive reactions, or concomitant clinical factors associated with the patient's illness. Hypotension will be seen very early in the transfusion (after 5 to 10 mL of product) when it is related to anaphylaxis or hypotensive reactions, whereas the symptoms associated with acute hemolysis usually require 50 to 100 mL of blood to be infused. Hypotension associated with bacterial contamination and TRALI may occur during the transfusion or up to several hours after transfusion.
6. Did the patient complain of pain? The spectrum of transfusion-related pain can include headache, abdominal pain, flank or back pain, or pain at the site of the infusion. Headaches typically occur in FNHTR, whereas abdominal and back pain are more typically noted with acute hemolytic reactions and the infusion of bacterially contaminated product.

The questions summarized in this section can be used as a guide to assist with establishing a differential diagnosis and to identify systematically the most probable cause of the adverse event. Although these questions will be helpful, many other factors must also be considered, including the patient's clinical condition and diagnosis, a history of previous reactions, the type and age of the blood product being transfused, and medications.

When a transfusion-related adverse event is suspected and clinical findings warrant further investigation, the following approach should be used:

Stop the transfusion, keeping the administration line open with saline.

Provide supportive therapy to the patient if required.

Perform a bedside clerical check to ensure that the right product is being transfused to the right patient.

Document all signs and symptoms on a transfusion-reaction form and notify the Transfusion Service that a reaction has occurred.

If the decision is made to proceed with a serologic investigation to rule out an acute hemolytic reaction, a blood sample should be collected and sent to the laboratory for investigation. In most situations, the laboratory can perform three basic tests/procedures that will indicate whether a reaction has occurred: a clerical check of laboratory records, visual examination of the patient's plasma for free hemoglobin, and a direct antiglobulin test. If all three of these procedures are negative or show no discrepancy, then it is unlikely that the reaction is due to acute hemolysis; however, if the clinical manifestations support a diagnosis of hemolysis, then further serologic investigations may be warranted. All reactions must be documented in the patient's chart. In all cases in which the transfusion is thought to cause or contribute to death, appropriate notifications should be made. In the United States, the FDA must be notified by phone within 24 hours after discovery, and this must followed up with a written report within 7 days (21 CFR 606.170). Specific requirements vary by country.

If the decision is made to continue the transfusion, the patient should be closely monitored for signs and symptoms suggestive of a more severe transfusion reaction. If these occur, the transfusion should be stopped immediately.

CONCLUSION

This chapter has provided an overview of acute and delayed noninfectious complications of blood transfusion. When reactions occur, all clinical signs and symptoms must be documented, and, based on these observations, a differential diagnosis should be established. When working through the differential diagnosis, it is helpful to consider the presence or absence of fever and when it occurred, and whether hypotension, pain, or cutaneous signs and symptoms were present. Laboratory tests to rule out acute hemolytic reactions or to identify contaminated blood products are readily available in most hospitals; however, the other types of acute noninfectious transfusion reactions are typically based on a clinical diagnosis. For some types of reactions, confirmatory laboratory tests are possible; however, this usually involves the referral of samples to a specialized reference laboratory and a delay of days to weeks before results are available. For this reason, it is important that health care professionals be familiar with how acute and delayed noninfectious transfusion reactions occur to ensure an accurate clinical diagnosis that will facilitate effective treatment and optimal methods for preventing future reactions.

REFERENCES

1. AABB. Technical Manual, 14th ed. Bethesda, Md., American Association of Blood Banks, 2002, p 1.
2. Heddle NM, Blajchman MA, Meyer RM, et al. A randomized controlled trial comparing the frequency of acute reactions to plasma-removed platelets and prestorage WBC-reduced platelets. Transfusion 2002;42:556–566.
3. Heddle NM, Klama LN, Griffith L, et al. A prospective study to identify the risk factors associated with acute reactions to platelet and red cell transfusions. Transfusion 1993;33:794–797.
4. Muylle L, Wouters E, De Bock R, et al. Reactions to platelet transfusion: the effect of the storage time of the concentrate. Transfus Med 1992;2:289–293.
5. Heddle NM, Kelton JG. Febrile nonhemolytic transfusion reactions. In Popovsky MA (ed), Transfusion Reactions, 2nd ed. Bethesda, Md. AABB Press, 2001, pp 45–82.
6. Kleinman S, Chan P, Robillard P. Risks associated with transfusion of cellular blood components in Canada. Transfus Med Rev 2003;17:120–162.
7. Yazer MH, Podlosky L, Clarke G, et al. The effect of prestorage WBC reduction on the rates of febrile nonhemolytic transfusion reactions to platelet concentrates and RBC. Transfusion 2004;44:10–15.
8. Paglino JC, Pomper GJ, Fisch GS, et al. Reduction of febrile but not allergic reactions to RBCs and platelets after conversion to universal prestorage leukoreduction. Transfusion 2004;44:16–24.
9. King KE, Shirey RS, Thoman SK, et al. Universal leukoreduction decreases the incidence of febrile nonhemolytic transfusion reactions to RBCs. Transfusion 2004;44:25–29.
10. Baker RJ, Moinichen SL, Nyhus LM. Transfusion reaction: a reappraisal of surgical incidence and significance. Proc Inst Med Chic 1969;27:214–215.
11. Ahrons S, Kissmeyer-Nielsen F. Serological investigations of 1,358 transfusion reactions in 74,000 transfusions. Dan Med Bull 1968; 15:259–262.
12. Heddle NM. Pathophysiology of febrile nonhemolytic transfusion reactions. Curr Opin Hematol 1999;6:420–426.
13. Brittingham TE, Chaplin H. Febrile transfusion reactions caused by sensitivity to donor leukocytes and platelets. JAMA 1957;167: 819–825.

14. de Rie MA, van der Plas-van Dalen CM, Engelfriet CP, et al. The serology of febrile transfusion reactions. Vox Sang 1985;49:126–134.
15. Perkins HA, Payne R, Ferguson J, et al. Nonhemolytic febrile transfusion reactions: quantitative effects of blood components with emphasis on isoantigenic incompatibility of leukocytes. Vox Sang 1966;11:578–600.
16. Greenwalt TJ, Gajewski M, McKenna JL. A new method for preparing buffy coat-poor blood. Transfusion 1962;2:221–229.
17. Ward HN. Pulmonary infiltrates associated with leukoagglutinin transfusion reactions. Ann Intern Med 1970;73:689–694.
18. Heinrich D, Mueller-Eckhardt C, Stier W. The specificity of leukocyte and platelet alloantibodies in sera of patients with nonhemolytic transfusion reactions: absorptions and elution studies. Vox Sang 1973;25:442–456.
19. Wolf CF, Canale VC. Fatal pulmonary hypersensitivity reaction to HL-A incompatible blood transfusion: report of a case and review of the literature. Transfusion 1976;16:135–140.
20. Decary F, Ferner P, Giavedoni L, et al. An investigation of nonhemolytic transfusion reactions. Vox Sang 1984;46:277–285.
21. Heddle NM, Klama L, Singer J, et al. The role of the plasma from platelet concentrates in transfusion reactions. N Engl J Med 1994;331: 625–628.
22. Muylle L, Peetermans ME. Effect of prestorage leukocyte removal on the cytokine levels in stored platelet concentrates. Vox Sang 1994; 66:14–17.
23. Stack G, Snyder EL. Cytokine generation in stored platelet concentrates. Transfusion 1994;34:20–25.
24. Aye MT, Palmer DS, Giulivi A, et al. Effect of filtration of platelet concentrates on the accumulation of cytokines and platelet release factors during storage. Transfusion 1995;35:117–124.
25. Kluter H, Muller-Steinhardt M, Danzer S, et al. Cytokines in platelet concentrates prepared from pooled buffy coats. Vox Sang 1995;69:38–43.
26. Flegel WA, Wiesneth M, Stampe D, et al. Low cytokine contamination in buffy coat-derived platelet concentrates without filtration. Transfusion 1995;35:917–920.
27. Snyder EL. The role of cytokines and adhesive molecules in febrile nonhemolytic transfusion reactions. Immunol Invest 1995;24:333–339.
28. Klinger MH, Wilhelm D, Bubel S, et al. Immunocytochemical localization of the chemokines RANTES and MIP-1 alpha within human platelets and their release during storage. Int Arch Allergy Immunol 1995;107:541–546.
29. Bubel S, Wilhelm D, Entelmann M, et al. Chemokines in stored platelet concentrates. Transfusion 1996;36:445–449.
30. Heddle N, Tan M, Klama L, et al. Factors affecting cytokine production in platelet concentrates. Transfusion 1994;34(suppl):67S.
31. Phipps RP, Kaufman J, Blumberg N. Platelet derived CD154 (CD40 ligand) and febrile responses to transfusion. Lancet 2001;23: 2023–2024.
32. Blumberg N, Phipps RP, Kaufman J, et al. The causes and treatment of reactions to platelet transfusions. Transfusion 2003;43:291–292.
33. Boyle L, McLesky S, Freter C, et al. High circulating interleukin-6 levels associated with acute transfusion reaction: Cause or effect? Blood 1991;78(Suppl):355a.
34. Sacher RA, Boyle L, Freter CE. High circulating interleukin 6 levels associated with acute transfusion reaction: cause or effect? Transfusion 1993;33:962–963.
35. Couban S, Carruthers J, Andreou P, et al. Platelet transfusions in children: Results of a randomized, prospective, crossover trial of plasma removal and a prospective audit of WBC reduction. Transfusion 2002;42:753–758.
36. Wenz B, Gurtlinger KF, O'Toole AM, et al. Preparation of granulocyte-poor red blood cells by microaggregate filtration: a simplified method to minimize febrile transfusion reactions. Vox Sang 1980;39:282–287.
37. Wenz B. Microaggregate blood filtration and the febrile transfusion reaction: A comparative study. Transfusion 1983;23:95–98.
38. Vamvakas EC, Pineda A. Allergic and anaphylactic reactions. In Popovsky MA (ed). Transfusion Reactions, 2nd ed. Bethesda, Md AABB Press, 2001, pp 83–120.
39. Perrotta PL, Snyder EL. Non-infectious complications of transfusion therapy. Blood Rev 2001;15:69–83.
40. Stephen CR, Martin RC, Bourgeois-Gavardin M. Antihistaminic drugs in treatment of nonhemolytic transfusion reactions. JAMA 1955;158:525–529.
41. Pineda AA, Taswell HF. Transfusion reactions associated with anti-IgA antibodies: report of four cases and review of the literature. Transfusion 1975;15:10–15.
42. Kevy SV, Schmidt PJ, McGinniss MH, et al. Febrile, nonhemolytic transfusion reactions and the limited role of leukoagglutinins in their etiology. Transfusion 1962;2:7–16.
43. Dzieczkowski JS, Barrett BB, Nester D, et al. Characterization of reactions after exclusive transfusion of white cell-reduced cellular blood components. Transfusion 1995;35:20–25.
44. Federowicz I, Barrett BB, Andersen JW, et al. Characterization of reactions after transfusion of cellular blood components that are white cell reduced before storage. Transfusion 1996;36:21–28.
45. Sarkodee-Adoo CB, Kendall JM, Sridhara R, et al. The relationship between the duration of platelet storage and the development of transfusion reactions. Transfusion 1998;38:229–235.
46. Tanz WS. Reevaluation of transfusion reaction rates associated with leukocyte-reduced red blood cells. Transfusion 2001;41:7S.
47. Robillard P, Karl I. Incidence of adverse transfusion reactions in the Quebec hemovigilance system. Vox Sang 2002;83(Suppl):120.
48. Arnold DM, Lo GK, Blajchman MA, et al. Passive transfer of peanut hypersensitivity by plasma transfusion. Transfus Med (in press); abstract.
49. Uhlmann EJ, Isgriggs E, Wallhermfechtel M, et al. Prestorage universal WBC reduction of RBC units does not affect the incidence of transfusion reactions. Transfusion 2001;41:997–1000.
50. Vyas GN, Perkins HA, Fudenberg HH. Anaphylactoid transfusion reactions associated with anti-IgA. Lancet 1968;2:312–315.
51. Vyas GN, Fudenberg HH. Isoimmune anti-IgA causing anaphylactoid transfusion reactions. N Engl J Med 1969;280:1073–1074.
52. Schmidt AP, Taswell HF, Gleich GJ. Anaphylactic transfusion reactions associated with anti-IgA antibody. N Engl J Med 1969;280: 188–193.
53. Miller WV, Holland PV, Sugarbaker E, et al. Anaphylactic reactions to IgA: A difficult transfusion problem. Am J Clin Pathol 1970;54:618–621.
54. Leikola J, Koistinen J, Lehtinen M, et al. IgA-induced anaphylactic transfusion reactions: A report of four cases. Blood 1973;42:111–119.
55. Koistinen J. Selective IgA deficiency in blood donors. Vox Sang 1975;29:192–202.
56. Sandler SG, Eckrich R, Malamut D, et al. Hemagglutination assays for the diagnosis and prevention of IgA anaphylactic transfusion reactions. Blood 1994;84:2031–2035.
57. Sazama K. Reports of 355 transfusion-associated deaths: 1976 through 1985. Transfusion 1990;30:583–590.
58. Strauss RA, Gloster ES, Schanfield MS, et al. Anaphylactic transfusion reaction associated with a possible anti-A2m(1). Clin Lab Haematol 1983;5:371–377.
59. Vyas GN, Holmdahl L, Perkins HA, et al. Serologic specificity of hun anti-IgA and its significance in transfusion. Blood 1969;34:573–581.
60. Take H, Tamura J, Sawamura M, et al. Severe anaphylactic transfusion reaction associated with HLA-incompatible platelets. Br J Haematol 1993;83:673–674.
61. Lambin P, Le Pennec PY, Hauptmann G, et al. Adverse transfusion reactions associated with a precipitating anti-C4 antibody of anti-Rodgers specificity. Vox Sang 1984;47:242–249.
62. Morishita K, Shimada E, Watanabe Y, et al. Anaphylactic transfusion reactions associated with anti-haptoglobin in a patient with ahaptoglobinemia. Transfusion 2000;40:120–121.
63. Wells JV, Buckley RH, Schanfield MS, et al. Anaphylactic reactions to plasma infusions in patients with hypogammaglobulinemia and anti-IgA antibodies. Clin Immunol Immunopathol 1977;8:265–271.
64. Koistinen J, Heikkila M, Leikola J. Gammaglobulin treatment and anti-IgA antibodies in IgA-deficient patients. BMJ 1978;2:923–924.
65. Eckrich RJ, Mallory DM, Sandler SG. Laboratory tests to exclude IgA deficiency in the investigation of suspected anti-IgA transfusion reactions. Transfusion 1993;33:488–492.
66. Ochterlony O. Diffusion in gel methods of immunological analysis. Prog Allergy 1958;5:1.
67. Holt PD, Tandy NP, Anstee DJ. Screening of blood donors for IgA deficiency: A study of the donor population of south-west England. J Clin Pathol 1977;30:1007–1010.
68. Fudenberg HH, Koistinen J. Manual of Clinical Immunology, 2nd ed. Washington, D.C., American Society for Microbiology, 1980, p 767.
69. Hume HA, Popovsky MA, Benson K, et al. Hypotensive reactions: A previously uncharacterized complication of platelet transfusion? Transfusion 1996;36:904–909.
70. Sweeney JD, Dupuis M, Mega AP. Hypotensive reactions to red cells filtered at the bedside, but not to those filtered before storage, in patients taking ACE inhibitors. Transfusion 1998;38:410–411.
71. Gauvin F, Toledano B, Hume HA, et al. Hypotensive reaction associated with platelet transfusion through leukocyte reduction filter. J Intensive Care Med 2000;15:329–332.

72. Arnold DM, Molinaro G, Warkentin TE, et al. Hypotensive transfusion reactions can occur with blood products that are leukoreduced before storage. Transfusion 2004;44:1361–1366.
73. Takahashi TA, Abe H, Fujihara M, et al. Quality of platelet components: the role of suspension medium and leukocyte depletion. Transfus Clin Biol 1994;1:481–487.
74. Abe H, Ikebuchi K, Shimbo M, et al. Hypotensive reactions with a white cell-reduction filter: activation of kallikrein-kinin cascade in a patient. Transfusion 1998;38:411–412.
75. Mair B, Leparc GF. Hypotensive reactions associated with platelet transfusions and angiotensin-converting enzyme inhibitors. Vox Sang 1998;74:27–30.
76. Belloni M, Alghisi A, Bettini C, et al. Hypotensive reactions associated with white cell-reduced apheresis platelet concentrates in patients not receiving ACE inhibitors. Transfusion 1998;38:412–415.
77. Popovsky MA, Audet AM, Andrzejewski C Jr. Transfusion-associated circulatory overload in orthopedic surgery patients: a multi-institutional study. Immunohematology 1996;12:87–89.
78. Zhou L, Giacherio D, Cooling L, et al. Use of B-natriuretic peptide as a diagnostic marker in the differential diagnosis of transfusion-associated circulatory overload. Transfusion 2005;45:1056–1063.
79. Kinnunen P, Vuolteenaho O, Ruskoaho H. Mechanisms of atrial and brain natriuretic peptide release from rat ventricular myocardium: Effect of stretching. Endocrinology 1993;132:1961–1970.
80. Stein BC, Levin RI. Natriuretic peptides: physiology, therapeutic potential, and risk stratification in ischemic heart disease. Am Heart J 1998;135:914–923.
81. Holmes SJ, Espiner EA, Richards AM, et al. Renal, endocrine, and hemodynamic effects of human brain natriuretic peptide in normal man. J Clin Endocrinol Metab 1993;76:91–96.
82. McLeod BC, Reed S, Viernes A, et al. Rapid red cell transfusion by apheresis. J Clin Apheresis 1994;9:142–146.
83. Dzik WH, Kirkley SA. Citrate toxicity during massive blood transfusion. Transfus Med Rev 1988;2:76–94.
84. Strauss RG, McLeod BC. Complications of therapeutic apheresis. In Popovsky MA (ed), Transfusion Reactions, 2nd ed. Bethesda, Md. AABB Press, 2001, p 315.
85. Wilson RF, Binkley LE, Sabo FM Jr, et al. Electrolyte and acid-base changes with massive blood transfusions. Am Surg 1992;58:535–544.
86. Jameson LC, Popic PM, Harms BA. Hyperkalemic death during use of a high-capacity fluid warmer for massive transfusion. Anesthesiology 1990;73:1050–1052.
87. Carvalho B, Quiney NF. "Near-miss" hyperkalemic cardiac arrest associated with rapid blood transfusion. Anaesthesia 1999;54:1094–1096.
88. Buntain SG, Pabari M. Massive transfusion and hyperkalaemic cardiac arrest in craniofacial surgery in a child. Anaesth Intensive Care 1999;27:530–533.
89. Murthy BV. Hyperkalaemia and rapid blood transfusion. Anaesthesia 2000;55:398.
90. Cosgriff N, Moore EE, Sauaia A, et al. Predicting life-threatening coagulopathy in the massively transfused trauma patient: hypothermia and acidoses revisited. J Trauma 1997;42:857–861.
91. Kruskall MS, Mintz PD, Bergin JJ, et al. Transfusion therapy in emergency medicine. Ann Emerg Med 1988;17:327–335.
92. Roher MJ, Natale AM. Effect of hypothermia on the coagulation cascade. Crit Care Med 1992;20:1402–1405.
93. Gubler KD, Gentilello LM, Hassantash SA, et al. The impact of hypothermia on dilutional coagulopathy. J Trauma 1994;36:847–851.
94. Michelson AD, MacGregor H, Barnard MR, et al. Reversible inhibition of human platelet activation by hypothermia in vivo and in vitro. Thromb Haemost 1994;71:633–640.
95. Michelson AD, Barnard MR, Khuri SF, et al. The effects of aspirin and hypothermia on platelet function in vivo. Br J Haematol 1999;104:64–68.
96. Eddy VA, Morris JA Jr, Cullinane DC. Hypothermia, coagulopathy, and acidosis. Surg Clin North Am 2000;80:845–854.
97. Pappas CG, Paddock H, Goyette P, et al. In-line microwave blood warming of in-date human packed red blood cells. Crit Care Med 1995;23:1243–1250.
98. Herron DM, Grabowy R, Connolly R, et al. The limits of bloodwarming: Maximally heating blood with an inline microwave bloodwarmer. J Trauma 1997;43:219–226.
99. Adverse ocular reactions following transfusion—United States, 1997–1998. MMWR Morb Mortal Weekly Report. 1998;47:49–50.
100. Shulman R, Aster RH, Leitner A, et al. Immunoreactions involving platelets, V: Post-transfusion purpura due to a complement-fixing antibody against a genetically controlled platelet antigen: a proposed mechanism for thrombocytopenia and its relevance in "autoimmunity." Natl Inst Arthritis Metabol Dis 1961;21:1597–1618.
101. Zucker MB, Ley AB, Borelli J, et al. Thrombocytopenia with a circulating platelet agglutinin, platelet agglutinin, platelet lysin and clot retraction inhibitor. Blood 1959;14:148–161.
102. Van Loghem JJ, Dorfmeijer H, Van HM, Schreuder F. Serological and genetical studies on a platelet antigen (Zw). Vox Sang 1959;4:161–169.
103. McFarland JG. Posttransfusion purpura. In Popovsky MA (ed), Transfusion Reactions, 2nd ed. Bethesda, Md. AABB, 2001, p 187.
104. Taaning E, Svejgaard A. Post-transfusion purpura: A survey of 12 Danish cases with special reference to immunoglobulin G subclasses of the platelet antibodies. Transfus Med 1994;4:1–8.
105. Morrison FS, Mollison PL. Post-transfusion purpura. N Engl J Med 1966;275:243–248.
106. Vogelsang G, Kickler TS, Bell WR. Post-transfusion purpura: a report of five patients and a review of the pathogenesis and management. Am J Hematol 1993;21:259–267.
107. Ertel K, Al-Tawil M, Santoso S, et al. Relevance of the HPA-15 (Gov) polymorphism on CD109 in alloimmune thrombocytopenic syndromes. Transfusion 2005;45:366–373.
108. Ziman A, Klapper E, Pepkowitz S, et al. A second case of post-transfusion purpura caused by HPA-5a antibodies: successful treatment with intravenous immunoglobulin. Vox Sang 2002;83:165–166.
109. Anolik JH, Blumberg N, Snider J, et al. Posttransfusion purpura secondary to an alloantibody reactive with HPA-5a (Br[b]). Transfusion 2001;41:633–636.
110. Christie DJ, Pulkrabek S, Putnam JL, et al. Posttransfusion purpura due to an alloantibody reactive with glycoprotein Ia/IIa (anti-HPA-5b). Blood 1995;77:2785–2789.
111. Kiefel V, Santoso S, Glockner WM, et al. Posttransfusion purpura associated with an anti-Bak. Vox Sang 1989;56:93–97.
112. Kickler TS, Herman JH, Furihata K, et al. Identification of Bakb, a new platelet-specific antigen associated with posttransfusion purpura. Blood 1988;71:894–898.
113. de Waal LP, van Dalen CM, Engelfriet CP, et al. Alloimmunization against the platelet-specific Zwa antigen, resulting in neonatal alloimmune thrombocytopenia or posttransfusion purpura, is associated with the supertypic DRw52 antigen including DR3 and DRw6. Hum Immunol 1986;17:45–53.
114. Davoren A, Curtis BR, Aster RH, et al. Human platelet antigen-specific alloantibodies implicated in 1162 cases of neonatal alloimmune thrombocytopenia. Transfusion 2004;44:1220–1225.
115. Lubenow N, Eichler P, Albrecht D, et al. Very low platelet counts in post-transfusion purpura falsely diagnosed as heparin-induced thrombocytopenia: report of four cases and review of literature. Thromb Res 2000;100:115–125.
116. Warkentin TE, Smith JW. The alloimmune thrombocytopenic syndromes. Transfus Med Rev 1997;11:296–307.
117. Santoso S, Kiefel V. Human platelet alloantigens. Wien Klin Wochenschr 2001;113:806–813.
118. Murphy MF, Williamson LM, Urbaniak SJ. Antenatal screening for fetomaternal alloimmune thrombocytopenia: should we be doing it? Vox Sang 2002;83(Suppl 1):409–416.
119. L'Abbe D, Tremblay L, Filion M, et al. Alloimmunization to platelet antigen HPA-1a (PIA1) is strongly associated with both HLA-DRB3*0101 and HLA-DQB1*0201. Hum Immunol 1992;34:107–114.
120. Glud TK, Rosthoj S, Jensen MK, et al. High-dose intravenous immunoglobulin for post-transfusion purpura. Scand J Haematol 1983;31:495–500.
121. Salama A, Mueller-Eckhardt C, Kiefel V. Effect of intravenous immunoglobulin in immune thrombocytopenia. Lancet 1983;2:193–195.
122. Becker T, Panzer S, Maas D, et al. High-dose intravenous immunoglobulin for post-transfusion purpura. Br J Haematol 1985;61:149–155.
123. Berney SI, Metcalfe P, Wathen NC, et al. Post-transfusion purpura responding to high dose intravenous IgG: further observations on pathogenesis. Br J Haematol 1985;61:627–632.
124. Hamblin TJ, Naorose Abidi SM, Nee PA, et al. Successful treatment of post-transfusion purpura with high dose immunoglobulins after lack of response to plasma exchange. Vox Sang 1985;49:164–167.
125. Mueller-Eckhardt C, Kuenzlen E, Thilo-Korner D, et al. High-dose intravenous immunoglobulin for post-transfusion purpura. N Engl J Med 1983;308:287.
126. McLeod BC, Strauss RG, Ciavarella D, et al. Management of hematological disorders and cancer. J Clin Apheresis 1993;8:211–230.
127. Mueller-Eckhardt C, Kiefel V. High-dose IgG for post-transfusion purpura, revisited. Blut 1988;57:163–167.
128. Win N, Peterkin MA, Watson WH. The therapeutic value of HPA-1a-negative platelet transfusion in post-transfusion purpura complicated by life-threatening haemorrhage. Vox Sang 1995;69:138–139.

129. Loren AW, Abrams CS. Efficacy of HPA-1a (PlA1)-negative platelets in a patient with post-transfusion purpura. Am J Hematol 2004;76:258–262.
130. Brecher ME, Moore SB, Letendre L. Posttransfusion purpura: The therapeutic value of PlA1-negative platelets. Transfusion 1990;30:433–435.
131. Win N, Matthey F, Slater GP. Blood components: transfusion support in post-transfusion purpura due to HPA-1a immunization. Vox Sang 1996;71:191–193.
132. Gabriel A, Lassnigg A, Kurz M, et al. Post-transfusion purpura due to HPA-1a immunization in a male patient: response to subsequent multiple HPA-1a-incompatible red-cell transfusions. Transfus Med 1995;5:131–134.
133. Merson L, Olivier N. Orally active iron chelators. Blood Rev 2002;16:127–134.
134. Olivieri NF, Brittenham GM. Iron-chelating therapy and the treatment of thalassemia. Blood 1997;89:739–761.
135. Angelucci E, Muretto P, Nicolucci A, et al. Effects of iron overload and hepatitis C virus positivity in determining progression of liver fibrosis in thalassemia following bone marrow transplantation. Blood 2002;100:17–21.
136. Brittenham GM, Griffith PM, Nienhuis AW, et al. Efficacy of deferoxamine in preventing complications of iron overload in patients with thalassemia major. N Engl J Med 1994;331:567–573.
137. Hoffbrand AV, Cohen A, Hershko C. Role of deferiprone in chelation therapy for transfusional iron overload. Blood 2003;102:17–24.
138. Gabutti V, Piga A. Results of long-term iron-chelating therapy. Acta Haematol 1996;95:26–36.
139. Olivieri NF, Nathan DG, MacMillan JH, et al. Survival in medically treated patients with homozygous beta-thalassemia. N Engl J Med 1994;331:574–578.
140. Olivieri NF. The beta-thalassemias. N Engl J Med 1999;341:99–109.

Chapter 51

Transfusion-Related Acute Lung Injury

Kathryn E. Webert • Steven H. Kleinman • Morris A. Blajchman

Transfusion-related acute lung injury (TRALI) is a complication of allogeneic blood transfusion, typically manifested by shortness of breath due to noncardiogenic pulmonary edema, fever, and hypotension. The first description of noncardiogenic pulmonary edema after an allogeneic blood transfusion was reported in 1951, and TRALI was recognized as a distinct clinical entity in the 1980s.[1,2] TRALI has been recognized increasingly as an important cause of transfusion-associated mortality. The United States Food and Drug Administration (FDA) recently observed TRALI to be the leading cause of transfusion-related deaths reported to the agency in 2003.[3] The Serious Hazards of Transfusion (SHOT) Annual Report for 2003 reported that, in Great Britain, TRALI was the second highest cause of transfusion-related morbidity and mortality and the major cause of transfusion-associated mortality.[4] The French Haemovigilance System found TRALI to be responsible for 25% of transfusion-associated fatalities in 2003.[5] Clearly, TRALI represents an important clinical syndrome with the potential for serious recipient adverse outcomes. However, much about the pathogenesis, treatment, and prevention of TRALI is poorly understood or still quite controversial or both.

DEFINITION

The need for a common definition of TRALI has been identified as a priority by the TRALI Working Group convened by the National Heart, Lung, and Blood Institute (NHLBI) of the National Institutes of Health (NIH), the Canadian Consensus Conference (Towards an Understanding of TRALI) sponsored by Canadian Blood Services and Héma-Québec, and authors of recent reviews.[6–12] A universally accepted case definition is crucial for the accurate diagnosis of TRALI, the collection of accurate and reliable epidemiologic data, and the comparison of TRALI reports between centers and countries. Furthermore, the lack of a uniform TRALI definition makes the interpretation of existing data about TRALI problematic because of variations of the TRALI definition used in the reported studies.

The NHLBI Working Group definition of TRALI is "new acute lung injury (ALI) that develops with a clear temporal relationship to transfusion, in patients without or with alternate risk factors for ALI."[9] The NHLBI group used the definition for ALI developed by the North American-European Consensus Conference in 1994 (Table 51–1).[13] Strengths of this definition are that it provides objective criteria for the diagnosis of TRALI and includes consideration of TRALI in patients with risk factors for ALI or acute respiratory distress syndrome (ARDS).[8]

A Canadian Consensus Conference on TRALI, held in Toronto, Canada, in April 2004, was entitled "Towards and Understanding of TRALI," with the goal of providing recommendations about several outstanding issues including the lack of a common definition of TRALI.[7,8] After considering information presented by expert panelists, and a review of relevant literature and deliberation, the following definition of TRALI was proposed by the panel: "a new episode of ALI that occurs during or within 6 hours of a completed transfusion which is not temporally related to a competing etiology for ALI" (Table 51–2).[7] In the development of this definition, TRALI was considered to be a clinical syndrome rather than a disease of a single etiology. Furthermore, the diagnosis of TRALI was considered to be a clinical and radiographic diagnosis, not dependent on the results of laboratory testing or any specific pathophysiologic mechanism.

The Canadian definition represented an adaptation of that suggested by the United States NHLBI Working Group on TRALI.[9] Two main differences between the definitions are first that, in the Canadian definition, the ALI criteria for hypoxemia were expanded to include other clinical evidence of hypoxemia for the purposes of patient care and surveillance studies when pulse oximetry measurements on room air are not available. Second, because of the uncertainty of the relation of ALI to transfusion in instances in which other risk factors for ALI (other than massive transfusion) are present (Table 51–3), the Canadian Consensus Panel recommended the use of the term *possible TRALI*. This was considered important to be able to include the uncertainty of the relationship of the ALI to the transfusion event in possible TRALI, the need to categorize such cases separately in surveillance systems to permit accurate comparisons across systems, the ability to selectively target research protocols to TRALI or possible TRALI cases, and the possible adoption of differing approaches to donor investigation in TRALI versus possible TRALI cases.[7]

The NHLBI Working Group also recognized these problematic cases (e.g., cases of ALI in recipients with recognized ALI risk factors other than massive transfusion) but recommended that critical care experts make the assessment of whether a case of ALI in such a patient is TRALI before reporting it to the blood bank. The NHLBI Working Group recognized that some of these cases would be difficult to classify accurately and proposed the classification of indeterminate for these cases.[9]

Both definitions have limitations, including the exclusion of mild TRALI cases whose clinical symptoms fall short of the case definition, cases in which symptoms develop after 6 hours (which occur rarely), and cases in which TRALI coexists with cardiogenic pulmonary edema.

Table 51–1 Criteria for Diagnosing Acute Lung Injury (ALI). Proposed by the North American-European Consensus Conference on Acute Respiratory Distress Syndrome and Modified by the NHLBI TRALI Working Group

Acute onset
No evidence of circulatory overload
  Pulmonary artery occlusion pressure: <18 mmHg when measured; or
  Lack of clinical evidence of left atrial hypertension
Bilateral infiltrates on frontal chest radiograph
Hypoxemia
  Ratio of $Pao_2/Fio_2 \leq 300$ mm Hg regardless of positive end-expiratory pressure level; or
  Oxygen saturation of ≤90% on room air

Modified from Toy P, Popovsky MA, Abraham E, et al. Transfusion-related acute lung injury: Definition and review. Crit Care Med 33:721–726, 2005; Bernard GR, Artigas A, Brigham KL, et al. Report of the American-European Consensus conference on acute respiratory distress syndrome: definitions, mechanisms, relevant outcomes, and clinical trial coordination. Consensus Committee. J Crit Care 1994;9:72–81.

Table 51–2 Canadian Consensus Conference Criteria for TRALI and Possible TRALI

Criteria for *TRALI*
a. ALI
   i. Acute onset
   ii. Hypoxemia
      In research setting
         Ratio of $Pao_2/Fio_2 \leq 300$; or
         $Spo_2 < 90\%$ on room air
      In a nonresearch setting
         Ratio of $Pao_2/Fio_2 \leq 300$ or
         $Spo_2 < 90\%$ on room air; or
         Other clinical evidence of hypoxemia
   iii. Bilateral infiltrates on frontal chest radiograph
   iv. No evidence of left atrial hypertension (i.e., circulatory overload)
b. No pre-existing ALI before transfusion
c. During or within 6 hr of transfusion and
d. No temporal relation to an alternative risk factor for ALI.

Criteria for *possible TRALI*
1. ALI (see above)
2. No pre-existing ALI before transfusion
3. During or within 6 hr of transfusion and
4. A clear temporal relation to an alternative risk factor for ALI

Modified from Kleinman S, Caulfield T, Chan P, et al. Toward an understanding of transfusion-related acute lung injury: Statement of a consensus panel. Transfusion 2004;44:1774–1789.

It was acknowledged by the Canadian TRALI Consensus Panel that its definition of TRALI represented the start to the development of an international consensus definition and would evolve as more data became available from additional surveillance, epidemiologic studies, pathologic evaluations, and research.[7]

EPIDEMIOLOGY

The incidence of TRALI is not well defined but has been estimated to occur between 0.014% and 0.08% per allogeneic blood product unit transfused or 0.04% to 0.16% per patient transfused.[14–18] Furthermore, the incidence rates for various blood products vary widely, with estimates ranging from 1 in 432 to 1 in 88,000 per unit of whole blood platelets, 1 in 1224 per unit of apheresis platelets, 1 in 4000 to 1 in 557,000 per unit of red blood cells (RBCs), and 1 in 7896 to 1 in 74,000 per unit of fresh frozen plasma (FFP) transfused.[7,8,18,19]

In the United Kingdom for the year 2003, 36 cases of TRALI were reported. This represents an increase from the 26 cases reported from October 2001 until September 2002 and an increase from an average of 14 cases per year for the years 1996 through 2000.[4] This trend most likely indicates increasing awareness of the condition. However, it is generally agreed that TRALI is still underdiagnosed and under-reported and that the true incidence of TRALI may be higher than current estimates.[18,20,21] This is likely due in part to a lack of recognition of the condition, in that TRALI can be easily confused with other diagnoses such as ARDS, fluid overload, and congestive heart failure.[21] Furthermore, because TRALI often occurs in patients in poor clinical condition, the respiratory distress of TRALI may be attributed to the underlying clinical condition and not to the allogeneic transfusion.

The risk factors that contribute to the development of TRALI are unknown. Cases of TRALI have occurred in all age groups and appear to be distributed evenly among male and female patients.[8,17,22] Most TRALI patients have no history of transfusion reactions, and no specific diagnoses are clearly associated with increased risk for TRALI.[17] It has been suggested that certain clinical conditions are associated with an increased risk. These include thrombotic thrombocytopenic purpura (TTP), organ transplantation, hematologic malignancy, and various cardiac diseases.[23–27] Although many TRALI cases appear to occur in patients in poor clinical condition at the time of the administration of implicated transfusion,[28] TRALI has been documented to occur in otherwise healthy subjects.[21,29]

Most blood components, including whole blood, RBCs, platelets, FFP, cryoprecipitate, intravenous immunoglobulin (IVIG), allogeneic bone marrow, autologous RBCs, and granulocyte concentrates have been implicated in the

Table 51–3 Risk Factors for Acute Lung Injury (ALI)

Direct lung injury
  Aspiration
  Pneumonia
  Toxic inhalation
  Lung contusion
  Near drowning
Indirect lung injury
  Severe sepsis
  Shock
  Multiple trauma
  Burn injury
  Acute pancreatitis
  Cardiopulmonary bypass
  Drug overdose

Note: Although massive transfusion (i.e., one blood volume in a 12- to 24-hr period) is also a recognized risk factor for ALI, it has been excluded from this list because ALI occurring within 6 hr of any transfusion (including massive transfusion) is considered to be TRALI.
Modified from Kleinman S, Caulfield T, Chan P, et al. Toward an understanding of transfusion-related acute lung injury: Statement of a consensus panel. Transfusion 2004;44:1774–1789.

pathogenesis of TRALI.[17,22,30–35] FFP is the most frequently implicated blood product.[22] In most reported cases of TRALI, the implicated blood product usually has contained more than 60 mL of plasma; however, cases of TRALI have occurred after the transfusion of products containing less than 60 mL of plasma, such as cryoprecipitate and platelet concentrates.[20] The severity of TRALI appears not to be related to the type of blood product transfused. The relation to antibody specificity has not been well studied, but several case reports suggest that antibodies against one specific neutrophil antigen, HNA-3a (5b), may be more prone to cause severe TRALI reactions.[36] It has been claimed that TRALI incidence may be increased with the administration of older components. However, the only evidence to support this claim is a study by Silliman and colleagues,[18] in which implicated whole blood–derived platelet units were only slightly older than nonimplicated units (4.5 + 0.2 days vs. 4.2 + 0.1 days; $P = 0.014$).

CLINICAL PRESENTATION AND LABORATORY INVESTIGATIONS

TRALI is clinically indistinguishable from acute lung injury due to a variety of causes.[16] The clinical manifestations of TRALI typically begin within 6 hours of a transfusion, and most cases occur during or within 2 hours of transfusion.[14] The symptoms and signs of TRALI typically include acute respiratory distress, severe hypoxemia, hypotension, and fever (Table 51–4). The hypotension is frequently unresponsive to the administration of intravenous fluids.[20] Less typically, hypertension may be present. The physical examination is usually consistent with noncardiogenic pulmonary edema. Rales and diminished breath sounds are usually present without other evidence of fluid overload (normal jugular venous pressure or absent third heart sound or both). Radiographic investigations typically reveal bilateral pulmonary infiltrates consistent with pulmonary edema. The infiltrates are usually both alveolar and interstitial and involve both lung fields; however, initially the radiographic pattern may be that of a patchy infiltrate.[20] It has been noted that a discrepancy may exist between the severity of the radiographic findings and the auscultatory findings.[14,37] The pulmonary wedge pressure is almost invariably normal.

Because the diagnosis of ALI can be difficult, when a case of TRALI is reported from the hospital ward to the blood bank, it is important for the blood bank medical director to communicate with the attending physician to determine whether that case has a high probability of increased left atrial pressure. If so, the pulmonary edema is more likely cardiogenic pulmonary edema, rather than ALI.

Table 51–4 Symptoms Associated with Transplant-Associated Acute Long Injury

Symptom/Sign	Relative Frequency
Dyspnea, respiratory distress	Very common
Hypoxia	Very common
Pulmonary edema	Very common
Fever (1°C to 2°C increase)	Very common
Tachycardia	Common
Hypotension	Common
Cyanosis	Common
Hypertension	Rare

With the current proposed definitions of TRALI, milder acute lung injury caused by transfusion will not be diagnosed as TRALI. However, data indicate that such cases do exist, but do not meet the proposed definition of TRALI.[20] For example, in a look-back investigation, approximately half of the symptomatic cases identified retrospectively involved findings of dyspnea and hypoxia without evidence of pulmonary edema.[15] The European Hemovigilance Network has proposed classifying such cases as *transfusion-associated dyspnea* to ensure that such cases are tabulated in transfusion-surveillance systems.

Patient laboratory findings of TRALI may include transient leucopenia, neutropenia, monocytopenia, and hypocomplementemia.[8,38] Additional laboratory studies performed on donor blood or the transfused blood component may elicit data that are useful to help classify the mechanism of TRALI (e.g., leukoagglutinating or leukocytotoxic antibodies or both in the donor, high levels of active lipids in the donor plasma, and neutrophil-priming activity in the blood component or post-transfusion donor and patient plasma).[8] These laboratory findings should not be used to make the diagnosis of TRALI, which is currently a clinical and radiographic diagnosis.

PATHOPHYSIOLOGY OF TRALI

The exact pathophysiologic mechanisms of TRALI have not been clearly elucidated. Both immunologic and nonimmunologic mechanisms have been suggested. It is likely that the mechanism of TRALI pathogenesis may vary from patient to patient, representing a spectrum including immunologic mechanisms, nonimmunologic mechanisms, or a combination of both. Regardless of the initiating mechanism, it appears that biologically active molecules (for example, cytokines and antibodies) affect (activate) leukocytes, leading to pulmonary endothelial cell injury and pulmonary edema, which appears to be the common final pathophysiologic pathway in the pathogenesis of TRALI.

Immunologic Mechanisms

Most investigators have postulated that TRALI is an antibody-mediated event.[15,21,39] In the first reported large case series of 36 cases of TRALI, 89% of donors had HLA or leukoagglutinating alloantibodies, with antibody/antigen concordance between donor and recipient demonstrated in 59% of cases.[14]

The alloantibodies thought to be responsible for TRALI have been identified as antineutrophil or anti-human leukocyte antigen (anti-HLA) class I or class II antibodies.[14,15,21,26,40–49] The mechanism of TRALI caused by HLA class II antibodies may differ from that associated with neutrophil and HLA class I antibodies in that resting neutrophils do not express HLA class II antigens. Occasional reports of TRALI have been associated with antilymphocyte, antimonocyte, or anti-immunoglobulin alloantibodies.[15,21,50–54] The specific neutrophil alloantigens that have been implicated in TRALI episodes include HNA-1a (NA1); HNA-1b (NA2); HNA-3a (5b); and HNA-2a (NB1).[29,40,55–59]

The pathogenic alloantibodies are typically of donor origin[21,39] but in fewer than 10% of cases, the alloantibodies may be of recipient origin directed against donor-specific leukocyte alloantigens.[21,40] Blood donors most commonly implicated in TRALI are multiparous women in whom maternal alloantibody formation occurred after exposure to paternally derived alloantigens on the fetal white blood cells entering the maternal circulation during pregnancy. Donors who had previously been transfused may also have formed such alloantibodies.

The immunologic mechanism postulates that donor alloantibodies in the transfused blood product interact with the recipient's leukocyte (usually neutrophil) antigens, leading to activation of the complement cascade, mobilization of cytokines, or priming of neutrophils. Although the initiating antigen-antibody interaction is generally thought to involve neutrophil alloantigens, the initial interaction may also occur between antibodies and monocyte or endothelial cell alloantigens.[15] This antigen-antibody interaction could also lead to the production of activated complement components, such as C5a, possibly resulting in pulmonary leukostasis and activation of white blood cells.[60] Alternately, antibody-antigen complexes may activate neutrophils through one of the Fc receptors (CD16, CD32, CD64). The activation of neutrophils then could result in the production of inflammatory mediators to cause increased vascular permeability,[39] leading to capillary leak and pulmonary tissue damage.[14,61] Some experimental evidence supports this hypothesis. For example, the infusion of leukoagglutinating antibodies in humans has been shown to cause the localization of granulocytes in the pulmonary circulation.[62] Furthermore, in animal models, these alloantibodies have been demonstrated to cause acute pulmonary edema in the presence of a complement source.[63] The sequestration of neutrophils has been demonstrated to occur only in the lungs; however, it is possible that accumulations of granulocytes also occur in other organs; but no clinical evidence exists that other organs are damaged in patients with TRALI.

The ability of transfused HLA alloantibodies to induce TRALI reactions was elegantly illustrated in a case report of a patient who had previously undergone a single lung transplant.[64] The patient developed TRALI after the transfusion of a unit of packed RBCs, which was subsequently demonstrated to contain antibodies to HLA-B44. The lung injury occurred only in the patient's transplanted lung, which expressed the HLA-B44 antigen on endothelial cells, and not in the native lung, which was HLA-B44 negative.

Nonimmunologic Mechanisms

Antigranulocyte or anti-HLA antibodies or both have been reported to be present in the majority of TRALI cases, in up to 89% of cases in one case series.[17] However, in at least 15% of typical cases of TRALI, antibodies are not detected in either the recipient or the donor.[65] Some investigators have found this latter number to be much higher.[18,28] For example, in a recent prospective study by Silliman and colleagues[18] an anti-HLA or antigranulocyte antibody was found in the donor plasma in only 25% of TRALI cases, and only 3.6% of TRALI cases had an antibody with definable specificity. Furthermore, in the same study, control cases without a diagnosis of TRALI were just as likely to have been transfused an allogeneic blood component from a donor with an antileukocyte antibody as were those patients who developed TRALI.[18] This may be explained either (1) by the fact that the responsible antibodies were of an unknown specificity; (2) that the antibodies were sequestered within immune complexes fixed to pulmonary tissue and were therefore not detectable in the circulation; (3) the antibodies were HLA class I but were not complement binding or present in a low titer and were missed by the standard lymphocytotoxicity assays[57]; or (4) that some other factor was involved.[66] The authors concluded that their findings were consistent with an alternate hypothesis—that the pathogenesis of TRALI may be non–antibody mediated. Suggested mechanisms postulated by these investigators include the generation of biologically active lipids, or the interleukins (IL)-6 or -8, present in increased concentrations in stored cellular blood products.[18,66,67]

Two-Event Model

It has been hypothesized that many TRALI cases are the result of two insults, the first related to the underlying clinical condition of the patient, and the second, to the infusion of biologic response modifiers within the blood component transfused.[18,54] Severe TRALI is clinically very similar to ARDS, and it has been demonstrated in animal models that the development of ARDS requires at least two pulmonary insults.[68,69] Similarly, it has been hypothesized that two events are required to produce clinical evidence of TRALI: the first being a predisposing clinical condition, such as surgery, trauma, or severe infection, and the second being the transfusion of biologically active lipids, cytokines, or leukoagglutinating alloantibodies in the blood product transfused.[28] This mechanism postulates that the first event results in activation of the pulmonary endothelium, which causes a release of cytokines and an increase in the number of adhesion molecules expressed on the endothelial cell surface.[1] As a result, neutrophils are primed for their subsequent attraction and adherence to the endothelial surface. The second event then results in neutrophil activation and release of substances leading to pulmonary damage as well as capillary leakage.[1,69,70]

Cytokines that may be involved in the pathogenesis of TRALI include tumor necrosis factor (TNF)-α, IL-1, IL-6, and IL-8.[18,39] Silliman and colleagues[18,28,71–74] have demonstrated that the occurrence of TRALI is associated with the transfusion of certain types of lipids with neutrophil-priming activity. These lipids have been identified mainly as lysophosphatidyl cholines, demonstrated to accumulate in cellular blood products with prolonged storage.[18] It is unlikely, however, that such biologically active lipids are responsible for all cases of TRALI, as they have not been demonstrated to be in FFP, even though the transfusion of FFP has been linked to many cases of TRALI.[15,43,47]

Animal Models of TRALI

Information about the pathogenesis of TRALI has been obtained through studies in animal models of TRALI or acute lung injury. These models are described in greater detail in a recent review.[75]

The first animal model of TRALI was described by Seeger and associates.[76] In this model, ex vivo isolated rabbit lungs were perfused with albumin buffer with HNA-3a–positive human granulocytes added. The presence of an antibody with HNA-3a specificity, with rabbit plasma as a complement source, caused severe pulmonary edema within 3 to 6 hours associated with increased lung vascular permeability. No pulmonary edema occurred in the absence of anti–HNA-3a antibody, HNA-3a–positive neutrophils, or rabbit plasma. Vascular permeability was also not increased when

HNA-3a–negative neutrophils were used. These experiments corroborated the role of leukoagglutinating antibodies in initiating neutrophil-dependent lung injury and suggested that concomitant complement activation played a role in its pathogenesis.

Sachs and colleagues[77] recently published studies using a similar ex vivo rat lung model of TRALI. Their experiments demonstrated that the induction of TRALI by antileukocyte antibodies was dependent on the density of the cognate antigen. However, the induction of TRALI did not require the addition of complement. Furthermore, the anti–HNA-2a antibodies used in this model did not induce leukoagglutination. The authors thus concluded that TRALI does not necessarily require either the leukoagglutinating properties of the antibody or the presence of complement proteins. The authors hypothesized that antibody-mediated neutrophil activation and the subsequent release of reactive oxygen species represent key events in the pathophysiologic cascade that leads to some cases of immune TRALI.

Silliman and colleagues[73] also described an ex vivo two-event model of TRALI. In this model, rats were pretreated with endotoxin in vivo. Isolated lungs were then perfused with saline, fresh human plasma, stored human plasma, lipid extracts from stored human plasma, or purified lysophosphatidyl cholines. Lungs pretreated with endotoxin developed significant pulmonary edema when perfused with stored plasma, lipid extracts, or lysophosphatidylcholines. Similar results were obtained in subsequent studies when the lungs were perfused with plasma from stored platelet concentrates.[78] This model demonstrated that biologically active lipids, which may be produced during the storage of blood products, can cause acute lung injury in a two-step fashion.

DIAGNOSIS OF TRALI

No rapid or conclusive test exists with which to diagnose TRALI. The initial diagnosis of TRALI should be suspected if a blood-product recipient has appropriate clinical findings (acute onset of hypoxemia, as demonstrated by a ratio of Pao_2/Fio_2 less than 300 mm Hg or an oxygen saturation less than or equal to 90% on room air with no evidence of circulatory overload) within 6 hours of a transfusion, together with the exclusion of other causes of pulmonary edema. The clinical findings should be corroborated with a radiograph of the chest demonstrating bilateral infiltrates. It is particularly important to exclude pulmonary edema secondary to cardiac causes, or volume overload, as these latter conditions are managed very differently from TRALI. It has been suggested that the determination of brain-derived natriuretic peptide (BNP) levels may help to differentiate TRALI and the volume overload observed in congestive heart failure (CHF), as elevated levels of BNP are highly predictive of CHF.[79] This interesting hypothesis requires further study and confirmation.

After the urgent management of the TRALI patient, laboratory investigations may be performed to gather information to support the antibody-mediated mechanism of TRALI. In the majority of cases in most published series, the donor plasma has been found to contain anti-HLA or antineutrophil antibodies or both.[17] Rarely, the recipient may be shown to have antibodies reactive with antigens on donor neutrophils.[17,42] As the diagnosis of TRALI in the past has typically required the presence of recipient-specific antibodies in the donor plasma, TRALI cases not associated with alloantibodies may have been underdiagnosed. Although not required for the diagnosis of TRALI, investigation of associated donors for the presence of anti-HLA class I and class II and antineutrophil antibodies may be performed to guide donor management.

TREATMENT

The treatment of TRALI is primarily supportive. The patient's hemodynamic status should be maintained. Ventilatory supportive care may be required, which may include oxygenation, intubation, and even mechanical ventilation.[17,66] In the original case series, all patients with TRALI required supplemental oxygen, and more than 70% of patients required mechanical ventilation.[8] Vasopressor medications may be necessary to treat the hypotension as TRALI patients are usually unresponsive to the infusion of fluids. Diuretics should not be used.[20] Treatments that have been suggested, but which have no established direct benefit, include the use of corticosteroids, prostaglandin E_1, anti-endotoxin antibodies, nonsteroidal anti-inflammatory medications, anti-TNF antibodies, pentoxiphylline, and surfactant.[21,80] However, practices and recommendations among transfusion medicine experts vary. A recent case report describes the successful use of extracorporeal membrane oxygenation (ECMO) for the treatment of TRALI in a 4-year-old patient undergoing elective cardiac surgery.[81] The authors recommended that, where facilities exist, ECMO or cardiopulmonary bypass should be considered in the management of severe TRALI when conventional treatment is proving insufficient. It is important to point out that if TRALI is suspected during the transfusion of a blood product, the transfusion should be immediately discontinued.

PROGNOSIS

TRALI patients generally improve clinically within 48 to 96 hours of onset.[17] Usually a resolution of the pulmonary infiltrates, as assessed by chest radiographs, occurs within 1 to 4 days.[17,30] However, in approximately 20% of patients, the hypoxemia and pulmonary infiltrates may persist for longer than 7 days. In those patients who recover rapidly, no long-term sequelae are found.[17]

Despite the usually excellent prognosis, it should be noted that TRALI can be a serious condition. TRALI is fatal in 5% to 10% of reported cases.[14,17,21,82] It is one of the top three causes of transfusion-related mortality.[3,8,27,83] TRALI has been suspected or confirmed in more than 10% of fatalities related to transfusion reported to the FDA from 1997 to 2000 and more than 13% of the fatalities reported to the FDA in 2003.[22] The SHOT Annual Report for 2003 found that TRALI was the major cause of transfusion-associated mortality in Great Britain over a 6-year period.[4] In France, TRALI was reported to have been responsible for 25% of transfusion-associated fatalities in 2003.[5]

EVALUATION OF DONORS ASSOCIATED WITH TRALI

In 2005, the AABB issued a TRALI-related interim standard (Standard 5.4.2.1) to supplement Standards for Blood Banks and Transfusion Services (23rd edition).[84] The standard states that "donors implicated in TRALI or associated with multiple events of TRALI shall be evaluated regarding their continued eligibility to donate."[85] As per the recommendations of the Canadian Consensus Conference, "associated" and "implicated" donors were defined as follows:

- A donor is *associated* with a TRALI reaction if one of his or her blood components was transfused during the 6 hours preceding the first clinical manifestation of TRALI.
- An associated donor is *implicated* in TRALI only if found to have antibodies to an HLA class I or II antigen or HNA and either that antibody has specificity for an antigen present on the recipient's leukocytes or a positive reaction is demonstrated between donor serum and recipient leukocytes (i.e., a positive crossmatch).

In cases of suspected TRALI, all allogeneic blood components transfused to the patient within 6 hours of the reaction should be examined.[17] Samples of donor plasma should be tested for HLA-I and -II and neutrophil antibodies. It has been suggested that one may increase efficiency by checking donors at greatest risk of having antibodies first, for example, women with three or more pregnancies. However, in one series of cases reported to the FDA, some male donors were found to be positive for anti-HLA antibodies. This suggests that, if sequential donor testing is performed, male donors should be tested if no implicated female donors are identified.[22] Other proposed strategies to increase efficiency of testing include (1) the sequential testing of donors beginning with the testing of donors whose components were administered closest to the onset of the TRALI reaction; and (2) the sequential testing of donors of plasma, platelets, cryoprecipitate, and RBCs, in that order. These strategies may decrease the need to test all donors associated with a TRALI case, as donor testing may be discontinued once an implicated donor has been identified. It should be noted that using any one of these approaches to donor testing will not eliminate the need for the testing of all donors.

If an antibody is found, its specificity should be determined, and it should be determined whether it reacts with the recipient's leukocyte (HNA and HLA) antigens either by performing antigen typing of the recipient's cells or by crossmatching donor sera with recipient cells. The clinical diagnosis of TRALI is strongly supported if concordance is found. However, even if the antibody is not reactive against the recipient's leukocytes, the presence of such alloantibodies is considered by some to be strong presumptive evidence of TRALI, as up to 40% of cases do not actually show concordance.[17] The method of diagnosis described here will result only in the identification of donors in cases of TRALI caused by the antibody-mediated mechanism but will be negative in many cases of TRALI.[18] Ideally, consideration should be given to the investigation of the implicated products or post-transfusion recipient specimens or both for neutrophil-priming agents in addition to testing donors for alloantibodies. However, currently, the testing for neutrophil priming is not readily available and at this time involves testing the respiratory burst to a specific stimulus.

MANAGEMENT OF FUTURE TRANSFUSIONS IN PATIENTS WITH A HISTORY OF TRALI

As mentioned previously, in a minority of TRALI cases, an implicated alloantibody is found in the recipient. Therefore, the possibility exists that an individual who has had TRALI in the past is at increased risk for a second (recurrent) TRALI reaction with subsequent transfusions. The care of these recipients has not been well addressed in the literature. As with any patient, the judicious use of allogeneic blood products is mandatory. It is reasonable to monitor closely patients with a history of TRALI during and after the subsequent transfusion of allogeneic blood products. It has been suggested that repeated TRALI reactions in these patients may be prevented by leukoreduction of any cellular components transfused to a TRALI patient; however, no evidence supports or refutes this practice.[20]

PREVENTION OF TRALI

Because of the multiple etiologies proposed for TRALI and the previously variable criteria for diagnosis, clear recommendations for the prevention of TRALI do not presently exist.[59] Various suggestions have been made and are discussed.

Deferral of All Implicated Donors

A general consensus exists that blood donors with demonstrable antibodies, who have been implicated in TRALI reactions, should be permanently deferred.[7,8] This is a reasonable approach, as at least two studies have suggested that donors with a leukocyte alloantibody who are implicated in a case of TRALI may represent a future transfusion hazard.[26,86] In the first study, the authors investigated all donations made by an implicated donor with alloantibodies to the HNA-3a antigen in the preceding 2 years.[82] Of the 36 patient charts evaluated, 36% of recipients had symptoms suggestive that a transfusion reaction had occurred. In the second look-back study, 15% of all donations of a donor with high-titer, leukocytotoxic class I HLA alloantibodies implicated in TRALI in a 3-year period were associated with a recorded transfusion reaction.[26] In contrast to these two studies, a look-back study performed by Win and colleagues[87] demonstrated that infusion of blood products containing leukocyte antibodies that appeared to have caused TRALI in some patients did not necessarily result in TRALI in other recipients. When the transfusion records of 43 blood components collected from six donors with alloantibodies implicated in cases of TRALI were reviewed, no documentation of transfusion reactions was found in any of the recipients of previous blood products from these donors. Similarly, Toy and associates[88] examined the records of patients who received blood components from a donor subsequently implicated in a TRALI reaction and found to have multiple HLA antibodies directed at both class I (A1, A2, A23, A24, A28, B35, Bw4) and class II (DR4, DR7, DR11, DR12, and DQ5) antigens.[88] Among the 103 patients reviewed, only one had evidence of a reaction that met criteria for TRALI, but on further review, this patient was diagnosed as having diffuse alveolar hemorrhage secondary to a stem cell transplant. Of the 55 recipients who had HLA-typing results available, none developed TRALI, even though 54 (98%) of the recipients had at least one corresponding antigen. The results of the latter two studies indicate that the deferral of all implicated donors will result in the deferral of some donors with antibodies with common specificities that may not have caused the TRALI reaction in the first instance.[7]

It is less clear what should be done with donors who are found to have antibody that does not correspond to a recipient antigen. Some authorities would recommend deferring such donors; however, as many blood donors with anti-HLA antibodies are never implicated in TRALI reactions, this approach is probably not necessary. A third possible outcome of a donor investigation is that none of the donors is found to have HLA or neutrophil alloantibodies. This is the case in at least 15% of TRALI cases in the literature.[18,31,39] No evidence exists that these antibody-negative donors are associated with an increased risk of future episodes of TRALI. The TRALI Consensus Panel and the AABB have suggested that it would be reasonable for such individuals to continue to donate.[7,85]

Rather than deferring donors whose blood products were implicated in TRALI, another option would be to use the blood products as frozen deglycerolized or washed RBCs from these donors only in special circumstances (i.e., rare donors).

Deferral of All Multiparous Women

The suggestion that all multiparous women should be deferred from donating blood is controversial. Donors implicated in TRALI reactions are often multiparous women or women who have had at least three live births.[20] In female blood donors, the frequency of anti-HLA antibodies has been demonstrated to increase with the number of pregnancies, ranging from 7.8% in nulliparous women to 26.3% in women who have had three or more pregnancies.[89] A recent study of female platelet donors demonstrated 12.9% to be positive for either HLA class I or class II antibodies.[48]

To investigate the clinical and immunologic outcomes after the transfusion of plasma from multiparous donors, Palfi and colleagues[90] performed a prospective randomized study. Patients in the intensive care unit receiving plasma were randomized to receive 1 unit of plasma from a multiparous donor and 1 unit of control plasma in a random order. The transfusion of plasma from multiparous donors was found to be associated with significantly lower oxygen saturation and higher TNF-α concentrations in the recipients compared with that seen in recipients after transfusion of control plasma. Furthermore, the mean arterial pressure increased after the transfusion of control plasma but did not change after the infusion of multiparous donor plasma. Finally, five post-transfusion reactions were observed in 100 patients, in four cases after the transfusion of plasma from multiparous donors, and in one after the transfusion of control plasma. These investigators concluded that plasma from multiparous blood donors may impair respiratory function in critically ill patients and should not be used in such patients. Clearly, further studies are required to evaluate the clinical effects of plasma from multiparous donors in other patient groups.

As TRALI is a serious, potentially fatal, condition whose frequency could be diminished by the deferral of multiparous donors, this approach has been debated.[17] However, the deferral of multiparous donors would result in a substantial reduction in the donor pool. For example, approximately one third of apheresis donors in a representative hospital apheresis program in the United States would be affected by such a policy.[89] Furthermore, it has been estimated that the use of this strategy by America's Blood Centers (ABC) members and the American Red Cross would result in the loss of 550,000 donations annually in the United States.[91] Thus as some have argued, because TRALI is a rare condition, it may be reasonable to use a more moderate approach with the deferral of only donors actually implicated in TRALI cases.[2,66] This issue is further complicated by the fact that recent prospective studies have not identified antileukocyte antibodies as a major pathogenic mechanism of TRALI.[18]

Use of Plasma from Multiparous Women Only for Fractionation

Some investigators have suggested that blood from multiparous donors who have not been screened for leukocyte alloantibodies should not be used as whole blood, FFP, or single-donor apheresis platelets.[8,17] It is uncertain whether blood products that do not contain significant amounts of plasma (such as RBCs stored in protein-poor solutions and cryoprecipitate) should be used. The transfusion of a small volume of plasma would, theoretically, carry a reduced risk of an alloantibody-mediated reaction,[17] and TRALI has been reported infrequently after the transfusion of these products.[54,92] It is generally agreed that such donors could serve as a safe source of plasma for fractionation, and as a source of frozen-deglycerolized RBCs or washed RBCs.[17] To decrease the risk of TRALI, in 2003, the National Blood Services in the United Kingdom decided not to use plasma from female donors (regardless of parity for logistic considerations) for FFP production. Since the implementation of this policy in England, more that 90% of the FFP available is now derived from male donors.[8] The potential efficacy of this initiative in reducing TRALI risk likely will be not be evaluable for several years.

Screening of All Donors (or Just Multiparous Women) for Antineutrophil and Anti-HLA Antibodies

At least one blood bank has used a preventive strategy that involves the screening of all donors for leukocyte antibodies. Those donors that are identified as having leukocyte alloantibodies are excluded from donating, or their blood is only used for blood products that do not contain significant amounts of plasma or that are fractionated.[21] This approach has been questioned, as HLA antibodies are present in many donors; most do not cause TRALI reactions.[60] In a recent study, HLA alloantibodies were found to be present in 22% of blood components tested.[93] Furthermore, this screening method would not prevent cases of TRALI caused by nonimmunologic mechanisms or those associated with alloantibodies in the recipient.

Use of Prestorage Leukoreduced Red Blood Cells

The use of leukoreduced blood components may result in decreased risk of TRALI.[94] This theory is based on the fact that animal experiments have demonstrated complement activation to have a role in initiating TRALI[63] and that leukoreduction prevents complement-mediated hemolysis in transfused patients with paroxysmal nocturnal hemoglobinuria. Further clinical data are required to confirm whether this intervention actually decreases the risk of TRALI.

Use of Younger Blood Products

One group of investigators has suggested that, in contrast to the generally accepted theories, the role of antileukocyte antibodies in the pathogenesis of TRALI is minor and that biologically active lipids and cytokines with neutrophil-priming activity may play a greater role.[18] If this is the case, the majority of cases of TRALI will not be prevented by excluding donors with anti-HLA antibodies. Preventive measures would also need to include measures to decrease the amount of neutrophil-priming agents in blood components. As biologically active lipids accumulate in blood products with storage, it has been suggested that the administration of fresh cellular components would reduce the risk of TRALI by preventing exposure of recipient neutrophils to neutrophil-priming agents.[8,18,90] However, it has been demonstrated that units of blood components implicated in TRALI have higher lipid priming activity than control units of similar storage age.[18] This finding suggests that factors other than the age of the blood product contribute to the risk of TRALI and that further study is needed before age of blood components can be used to mitigate the risk of TRALI.[66]

Appropriate Utilization of Blood Products

A simple way of decreasing the frequency of TRALI reactions is to ensure that blood products are used only when clinically indicated. Reduction of blood product utilization, by using evidence-based criteria for transfusion, may be a safe and appropriate strategy to decrease the incidence of TRALI.[7,95]

Use of Solvent/Detergent Plasma

To date, solvent/detergent (SD) plasma transfusion has not been implicated in TRALI cases. However, it is unclear whether countries that use a large amount of SD plasma have sufficiently sensitive transfusion-surveillance systems to detect these cases should they occur. It has been hypothesized that the use of SD plasma instead of FFP may decrease the risk of TRALI as a result of the plasma-pooling process, decreasing the titer of responsible antibodies.[7] However, it is also theoretically possible that an antibody could cause TRALI despite its dilution by pooling.

Other Possible Interventions

Reports have been published of TRALI occurring in children as a result of directed donations from their mothers.[96–98] As mothers may have developed alloantibodies to antigens on fetal leukocytes during the pregnancy, this, theoretically, represents a situation potentially associated with an increased risk of TRALI. TRALI should be recognized as a potential, serious consequence of directed maternal blood donation.[39]

CONCLUSIONS

TRALI is a complex clinical syndrome that probably does not represent a single pathogenic entity. The ability to define and accurately diagnose TRALI has been hampered by our poor understanding of the pathophysiologic mechanisms of TRALI. Thus the recent recognition that TRALI likely represents a spectrum of clinical presentations and the creation of a standardized TRALI definition represent potential progress in our awareness of this perplexing syndrome. Many unanswered questions and controversial issues are related to our knowledge of TRALI. Many of these issues were addressed by the recent Canadian Consensus Conference.[7,8] However, despite the outstanding job that was done by presenters at the conference and by the Consensus Conference Panel, some issues still remain unresolved.

Traditionally, the definition of TRALI has required the presence of donor leukocyte antibodies reactive against the recipient's leukocytes. However, as our understanding of TRALI has grown, it has become increasingly recognized that not all cases of TRALI are associated with antileukocyte antibodies. It has been hypothesized that such cases may involve antibodies against other antigens, antibodies of recipient origin, or pathophysiologic mechanisms of TRALI not previously recognized.[18]

One of the most urgent needs for the transfusion medicine community is to achieve consensus on a classification for TRALI. In the interest of initiating such discussions, a proposed pathophysiological classification of TRALI is shown in Table 51–5. In this classification, TRALI is classified by the pathogenic mechanism identified. It is recognized that overlap may occur, with both immunologic and nonimmunologic mechanisms occurring in the same episode of TRALI.

Finally, although TRALI is becoming increasingly well recognized by hematologists and transfusionists, it is necessary to educate physicians in all medical specialties and other health care personnel to recognize promptly and to respond appropriately to the signs and symptoms of TRALI.

Table 51–5 Proposed Classification of TRALI Based on Putative Pathogenic Mechanisms

The pathogenesis of transplant-associated acute lung injury (TRALI) reactions is complex and likely varies from patient to patient, thus representing a spectrum including immunologic mechanisms, nonimmunologic mechanisms, or a combination of both. Thus the categories listed below are not mutually exclusive. Many TRALI episodes thus may fall into two or more categories within this proposed classification.

- A. Immunologic mechanism indicated
  - 1. Donor alloantibodies detected
    - a. Concordance demonstrated (reactive against recipient antigens)
    - b. Concordance not demonstrated (not reactive against recipient antigens)
  - 2. Recipient alloantibodies detected
    - a. Concordance demonstrated (reactive against donor antigens)
    - b. Concordance not demonstrated (not reactive against donor antigens)
- B. Nonimmunologic mechanism indicated
  - 3. Predisposing clinical condition in the patient
    - a. Surgery
    - b. Trauma
    - c. Severe infection
    - d. Thrombotic thrombocytopenic purpura
    - e. Other
  - 4. Nonimmune biologic response modifiers (BRMs) present in donor product
    - a. Biologically active lipids
    - b. Cytokines
  - Other BRMs

REFERENCES

1. Silliman CC. Transfusion-related acute lung injury. Transfus Med Rev 1999;13:177–186.
2. Kopko PM, Holland PV. Transfusion-related acute lung injury. Br J Haematol 1999;105:322–329.
3. Blood Products Advisory Committee, 80th Meeting. Department of Health and Human Services, Food and Drug Administration, Center for Biologics Evaluation and Research. July 22, 2004. Available at http:/www.fed.gov/ohrms/dockets/ac/04/transcripts/2004-405t1.doc. Accessed April 29, 2005.
4. Stainsby D, Williamson L, Jones H, et al. 6 Years of SHOT reporting: Its influence on UK blood safety. Transfus Apheresis Sci 2004;31:123–131.
5. Rebibo D, Hauser L, Slimani A, et al. The French Haemovigilance System: Organization and results for 2003. Transfus Apheresis Sci 2004;31: 145–153.
6. Webert KE, Blajchman MA. Transfusion-related acute lung injury. Transfus Med Rev 2004;17:252–262.
7. Kleinman S, Caulfield T, Chan P, et al. Toward an understanding of transfusion-related acute lung injury: Statement of a consensus panel. Transfusion 2004;44:1774–1789.
8. Goldman M, Webert KE, Arnold DM, et al. Proceedings of a consensus conference: towards an understanding of TRALI. Transfus Med Rev 2005;19:2–31.
9. Toy P, Popovsky MA, Abraham E, et al. Transfusion-related acute lung injury: definition and review. Crit Care Med 2005;33:721–726.
10. Williamson LM. Transfusion hazard reporting: powerful data, but do we know how best to use it? Transfusion 2002;42:1249–1252.
11. Bux J. Transfusion-related acute lung injury (TRALI): a serious adverse event of blood transfusion. Vox Sang 2005;89:1–10.
12. Gajic O, Moore SB. Transfusion-related acute lung injury. Mayo Clin Proc 2005;80:766–770.
13. Bernard GR, Artigas A, Brigham KL, et al. Report of the American-European Consensus conference on acute respiratory distress syndrome: definitions, mechanisms, relevant outcomes, and clinical trial coordination: Consensus Committee. J Crit Care 1994;9:72–81.
14. Popovsky MA, Moore SB. Diagnostic and pathogenetic considerations in transfusion-related acute lung injury. Transfusion 1985;25:573–577.
15. Kopko PM, Popovsky MA, MacKenzie MR, et al. LA class II antibodies in transfusion-related acute lung injury. Transfusion 2001;41:1244–1248.
16. Weber JG, Warner MA, Moore SB. What is the incidence of perioperative transfusion-related acute lung injury? Anesthesiology 1995;82:789.
17. Popovsky MA, Chaplin HC Jr, Moore SB. Transfusion-related acute lung injury: a neglected, serious complication of hemotherapy. Transfusion 1992;32:589–592.
18. Silliman CC, Boshkov LK, Mehdizadehkashi Z, et al. Transfusion-related acute lung injury: epidemiology and a prospective analysis of etiologic factors. Blood 2003;101:454–462.
19. Wallis JP, Lubenko A, Wells AW, et al. Single hospital experience of TRALI. Transfusion 2003;43:1053–1059.
20. Popovsky MA. Transfusion-related acute lung injury (TRALI). In Popovsky MA (ed). Transfusion Reactions. Bethesda, Md., AABB Press, 2001, pp 155–170.
21. Engelfriet CP, Reesink HW, Brand A, et al. Transfusion-related acute lung injury (TRALI). Vox Sang 2001;81:269–283.
22. Holness L, Knippen MA, Simmons L, et al. Fatalities caused by TRALI. Transfus Med Rev 2004;18:184–188.
23. Boshkov L, Silliman C, Clarke G, et al. Transfusion related acute lung injury (TRALI) following platelet transfusion: a study of possible etiologic factors. Blood 1995;86:1403.
24. Yost CS, Matthay MA, Gropper MA. Etiology of acute pulmonary edema during liver transplantation: a series of cases with analysis of the edema fluid. Chest 2001;119:219–223.
25. Distenfeld A. Transfusion-related acute lung injury. JAMA 2002; 288:316.
26. Cooling L. Transfusion-related acute lung injury. JAMA 2002;288: 315–316.
27. Stainsby D, Cohen H, Jones H, et al. Serious Hazards of Transfusion (SHOT) Annual Report 2003. Manchester, U.K., Serious Hazards of Transfusion Office, Manchester Blood Office, 2004.
28. Silliman CC, Paterson AJ, Dickey WO, et al. The association of biologically active lipids with the development of transfusion-related acute lung injury: a retrospective study. Transfusion 1997;37:719–726.
29. Lucas G, Rogers S, Evans R, et al. Transfusion-related acute lung injury associated with interdonor incompatibility for the neutrophil-specific antigen HNA-1a. Vox Sang 2000;79:112–115.
30. Popovsky MA. Transfusion-related acute lung injury. Transfusion 1995;35:180–181.
31. Popovsky MA. Transfusion-related acute lung injury. Curr Opin Hematol 2000;7:402–407.
32. Rizk A, Gorson KC, Kenney L, et al. Transfusion-related acute lung injury after the infusion of IVIG. Transfusion 2001;41:264–268.
33. Urahama N, Tanosaki R, Masahiro K, et al. TRALI after the infusion of marrow cells in a patient with acute lymphoblastic leukemia. Transfusion 2003;43:1553–1557.
34. Covin RB, Ambruso DR, England KM, et al. Hypotension and acute pulmonary insufficiency following transfusion of autologous red blood cells during surgery: a case report and review of the literature. Transfus Med 2004;14:375–383.
35. Sachs UJ, Bux J. TRALI after the transfusion of cross-match-positive granulocytes. Transfusion 2003;43:1683–1686.
36. Davoren A, Curtis BR, Shulman IA, et al. TRALI due to granulocyte-agglutinating human neutrophil antigen-3a (5b) alloantibodies in donor plasma: a report of 2 fatalities. Transfusion 2003;43:641–645.
37. Ward HN. Pulmonary infiltrates associated with leukoagglutinin transfusion reactions. Ann Intern Med 1970;73:689–694.
38. Nakagawa M, Toy P. Acute and transient decrease in neutrophil count in transfusion related acute lung injury: cases at one hospital. Transfusion 2004;44:1689–1694.
39. Popovsky MA, Davenport RD. Transfusion-related acute lung injury: femme fatale? Transfusion 2001;41:312–315.
40. Bux J, Becker F, Seeger W, et al. Transfusion-related acute lung injury due to HLA-A2-specific antibodies in recipient and NB1-specific antibodies in donor blood. Br J Haematol 1996;93:707–713.
41. Andrews AT, Zmijewski CM, Bowman HS, et al. Transfusion reaction with pulmonary infiltration associated with HLA-specific leukocyte antibodies. Am J Clin Pathol 1976;66:483–487.
42. Popovsky MA, Abel MD, Moore SB. Transfusion-related acute lung injury associated with passive transfer of antileukocyte antibodies. Am Rev Respir Dis 1983;128:185–189.
43. Eastlund T, McGrath PC, Britten A, et al. Fatal pulmonary transfusion reaction to plasma containing donor HLA antibody. Vox Sang 1989;57:63–66.
44. Florell SR, Velasco SE, Fine PG. Perioperative recognition, management, and pathologic diagnosis of transfusion-related acute lung injury. Anesthesiology 1994;81:508–510.
45. Virchis AE, Contreras M, Navarrete C, et al. Transfusion-related acute lung injury (TRALI) due to inter-donor incompatibility. Blood 1996;88:2114.
46. Dry SM, Bechard KM, Milford EL, et al. The pathology of transfusion-related acute lung injury. Am J Clin Pathol 1999;112:216–221.
47. Varela M, Mas A, Nogues N, et al. TRALI associated with HLA class II antibodies. Transfusion 2002;42:1102.
48. Kao GS, Wood IG, Dorfman DM, et al. Investigations into the role of anti-HLA class II antibodies in TRALI. Transfusion 2003;43:185–191.
49. Win N, Brown C, Navarrete C. TRALI associated with HLA class II antibodies. Transfusion 2003;43:545–546.
50. Flesch BK, Neppert J. Transfusion-related acute lung injury caused by human leucocyte antigen class II antibody. Br J Haematol 2002;116: 673–676.
51. Dooren MC, Ouwehand WH, Verhoeven AJ, et al. Adult respiratory distress syndrome after experimental intravenous gamma-globulin concentrate and monocyte-reactive IgG antibodies. Lancet 1998;352:1601–1602.
52. Paglieroni TG, Kopko PM, Popovsky MA, et al. Monocyte antibody associated with transfusion related acute lung injury (TRALI). Blood 2001;98:57A.
53. Saigo K, Sugimoto T, Tone K, et al. Transfusion-related acute lung injury in a patient with acute myelogenous leukaemia having anti-IgA2m1 antibody. J Intern Med Res 1999;27:96–100.
54. Van Buren NL, Stroncek DF, Clay ME, et al. Transfusion-related acute lung injury caused by an NB2 granulocyte-specific antibody in a patient with thrombotic thrombocytopenic purpura. Transfusion 1990;30: 42–45.
55. Nordhagen R, Conradi M, Dromtorp SM. Pulmonary reaction associated with transfusion of plasma containing anti-5b. Vox Sang 1986; 51:102–107.
56. Zupanska B, Uhrynowska M, Konopka L. Transfusion-related acute lung injury due to granulocyte-agglutinating antibody in a patient with paroxysmal nocturnal hemoglobinuria. Transfusion 1999;39:944–947.
57. Yomtovian R, Kline W, Press C, et al. Severe pulmonary hypersensitivity associated with passive transfusion of a neutrophil-specific antibody. Lancet 1984;1:244–246.
58. Santamaria A, Moya F, Martinez C, et al. Transfusion-related acute lung injury associated with an NA1-specific antigranulocyte antibody. Haematologica 1998;83:951–952.

59. Leger R, Palm S, Wulf H, et al. Transfusion-related lung injury with leukopenic reaction caused by fresh frozen plasma containing anti-NB1. Anesthesiology 1999;91:1529–1532.
60. Clay ME, Stroncek DF. Granulocyte immunology. In Anderson KC, Ness PM (eds.). Scientific Basis of Transfusion Medicine: Implications for Clinical Practice. Philadelphia, WB Saunders, 2000, pp 180–206.
61. Carilli AD, Ramanamurty MV, Chang YS, et al. Noncardiogenic pulmonary edema following blood transfusion. Chest 1978;74:310–312.
62. McCullough J, Clay M, Hurd D, et al. Effect of leukocyte antibodies and HLA matching on the intravascular recovery, survival, and tissue localization of 111-indium granulocytes. Blood 1986;67:522–528.
63. Seeger W, Schneider U, Kreusler B, et al. Reproduction of transfusion-related acute lung injury in an ex vivo lung model. Blood 1990;76: 1438–1444.
64. Dykes A, Smallwood D, Kotsimbos T, et al. Transfusion-related acute lung injury (TRALI) in a patient with a single lung transplant. Br J Haematol 2000;109:674–676.
65. Engelfriet CP, Reesink HW. Transfusion-related acute lung injury (TRALI). Vox Sang 2001;81:269–270.
66. Lenahan SE, Domen RE, Silliman CC, et al. Transfusion-related acute lung injury secondary to biologically active mediators. Arch Pathol Lab Med 2001;125:523–526.
67. Silliman CC, Thurman GW, Ambruso DR. Stored blood components contain agents that prime the neutrophil NADPH oxidase through the platelet-activating-factor receptor. Vox Sang 1992;63:133–136.
68. Salzer WL, McCall CE. Primed stimulation of isolated perfused rabbit lung by endotoxin and platelet activating factor induces enhanced production of thromboxane and lung injury. J Clin Invest 1990;85: 1135–1143.
69. Rabinovici R, Esser KM, Lysko PG, et al. Priming by platelet-activating factor of endotoxin-induced lung injury and cardiovascular shock. Circ Res 1991;69:12–25.
70. Downey GP, Doherty DE, Schwab B III, et al. Retention of leukocytes in capillaries: role of cell size and deformability. J Appl Physiol 1990;69:1767–1778.
71. Silliman CC, Clay KL, Thurman GW, et al. Partial characterization of lipids that develop during the routine storage of blood and prime the neutrophil NADPH oxidase. J Lab Clin Med 1994;124:684–694.
72. Silliman CC, Dickey WO, Paterson AJ, et al. Analysis of the priming activity of lipids generated during routine storage of platelet concentrates. Transfusion 1996;36:133–139.
73. Silliman CC, Voelkel NF, Allard JD, et al. Plasma and lipids from stored packed red blood cells cause acute lung injury in an animal model. J Clin Invest 1998;101:1458–1467.
74. Hashim SW, Kay HR, Hammond GL, et al. Noncardiogenic pulmonary edema after cardiopulmonary bypass: an anaphylactic reaction to fresh frozen plasma. Am J Surg 1984;147:560–564.
75. Silliman CC, Kelher M. The role of endothelial activation in the pathogenesis of transfusion-related acute lung injury. Transfusion 2005;45:109S–116S.
76. Seeger W, Schneider U, Kreusler B, et al. Reproduction of transfusion-related acute lung injury in an ex vivo lung model. Blood 1990;76: 1438–1444.
77. Sachs UJH, Hattar K, Weissman N, et al. Antibody-induced neutrophil activation as a trigger for transfusion-related acute lung injury in an ex vivo rat lung model. Blood. Epub ahead of print October 6, 2005. DOI 10.1182/blood 2005–04–1744.
78. Silliman CC, Bjornsen AJ, Wyman TH, et al. Plasma and lipids from stored platelets cause acute lung injury in an animal model. Transfusion 2003;43:633–640.
79. Burgher AH, Aslan D, Laudi N, et al. Use of brain natriuretic peptide to evaluate transfusion-related acute lung injury. Transfusion 2004; 44:1533–1534.
80. Wu TJ, Teng RJ, Tsou Yau KI. Transfusion-related acute lung injury treated with surfactant in a neonate. Eur J Pediatr 1996;155:589–591.
81. Nouraei SM, Wallis JP, Bolton D, et al. Management of transfusion-related acute lung injury with extracorporeal cardiopulmonary support in a four-year-old child. Br J Anaesth 2003;91:292–294.
82. Wolf CF, Canale VC. Fatal pulmonary hypersensitivity reaction to HLA-incompatible blood transfusion: report of a case and review of the literature. Transfusion 1976;16:135–140.
83. Zoon KC. Transfusion related acute lung injury. CBER letter. 2005. hyyp://www.fda.gov/cber/ltr/trali101901.htm. Accessed June 1, 2005.
84. Menitove J (ed). Standards for Blood Banks and Transfusion Services, 23rd ed. Bethesda, Md., American Association of Blood Banks, 2005.
85. Mintz PD, Lipton KS. AABB Association Bulletin 05–09, Transfusion-related acute lung injury. Bethesda, Md., American Association of Blood Banks, August 11, 2005.
86. Kopko PM, Marshall CS, MacKenzie MR, et al. Transfusion-related acute lung injury: report of a clinical look-back investigation. JAMA 2002;287:1968–1971.
87. Win N, Ranasinghe E, Lucas G. Transfusion-related acute lung injury: a 5-year look-back study. Transfus Med 2002;12:387–389.
88. Toy P, Hollis-Perry KM, Jun J, Nakagawa M. Recipients of blood from a donor with multiple HLA antibodies: a look-back study of transfusion-related acute lung injury. Transfusion 2004;44:1683–1688.
89. Densmore TL, Goodnough LT, Ali S, et al. Prevalence of HLA sensitization in female apheresis donors. Transfusion 1999;39:103–106.
90. Palfi M, Berg S, Ernerudh J, et al. A randomized controlled trial of transfusion-related acute lung injury: is plasma from multiparous blood donors dangerous? Transfusion 2001;41:317–322.
91. Fitzpatrick GM. Transfusion related acute lung injury (TRALI): statement before the Food and Drug Administrations' Blood Products Advisory Committee. ABC Statements. July 22, 2004. Available at http://www.americasblood.org/index.cfm?fuseaction=Display.showpage&pageID=294. 7–22–0004. Accessed April 20, 2005.
92. Reese EP Jr, McCullough JJ, Craddock PR. An adverse pulmonary reaction to cryoprecipitate in a hemophiliac. Transfusion 1975;15:583–588.
93. Bray RA, Harris SB, Josephson CD, et al. Unappreciated risk factors for transplant patients: HLA antibodies in blood components. Hum Immunol 2004;65:240–244.
94. Win N, Montgomery J, Sage D, et al. Recurrent transfusion-related acute lung injury. Transfusion 2001;41:1421–1425.
95. Wallis JP, Dzik S. Is fresh frozen plasma overtransfused in the United States? Transfusion 2004;44:1674–1675.
96. Campbell DA Jr, Swartz RD, Waskerwitz JA, et al. Leukoagglutination with interstitial pulmonary edema: a complication of donor-specific transfusion. Transplantation 1982;34:300–301.
97. Goeken NE, Schulak JA, Nghiem DD, et al. Transfusion reactions in donor-specific blood transfusion patients resulting from transfused maternal antibody. Transplantation 1984;38:306–307.
98. Yang X, Ahmed S, Chandrasekaran V. Transfusion-related acute lung injury resulting from designated blood transfusion between mother and child: a report of two cases. Am J Clin Pathol 2004;121:590–592.

Chapter 52
Transfusion-Related Immunomodulation

Neil Blumberg • Joanna M. Heal

INTRODUCTION

In recent years, a more conservative approach to blood transfusion has begun to become the rule rather than the exception in clinical medicine. To a significant degree, this is the result of clinical outcomes research demonstrating that patients receiving traditional allogeneic transfusions (nonleukoreduced, nonautologous red cells) have dramatically higher rates of morbidity and mortality than do similar patients not receiving transfusions. When patients receiving a traditional therapy are shown to do much worse than those not receiving the therapy, an understandable controversy and growing reluctance exist to use that therapy. To an unknown but probably substantial degree, these inferior clinical outcomes are mediated by a complex phenomenon that has been termed *transfusion-related immunomodulation* or TRIM. Paradoxically, TRIM is now known to involve both downregulated cellular immunity and upregulated, inappropriate inflammatory responses.

Transfusion has long been known to affect the immune system. Humoral immunization to red cell alloantigens after transfusion was recognized as a cause of hemolytic disease of the newborn and hemolytic transfusion reactions in the early 20th century. Over the last 20 years, it has become apparent that transfusion also produces clinically significant immunomodulatory effects on cellular immunity.[1,2] Modulation of cellular immunity by allogeneic transfusion may be of importance equal to or greater than that of humoral allosensitization in certain clinical settings, specifically oncology, surgery, and critical care.[1,2] Unfortunately, recent reviews of transfusion immunology often fail to address this subject because of its contentious nature, and, perhaps, a reluctance to challenge long-standing clinical practices that have been in use for most of a century.[1–7]

The insight that transfusions modulate cellular immunity originated with observations in the late 1960s and early 1970s that blood transfusions reduced the rejection rate for cadaveric renal allografts.[8] A decade later, the controversial observation was made that transfusion at the time of cancer surgery is associated with increased tumor recurrence.[9,10] Tartter and colleagues[11] also reported that the incidence of postoperative infections increased in a dose-dependent fashion after perioperative transfusions. Viral infection and autoimmune disorders may be modulated by transfusion,[1] and a modest but reproducible benefit of transfusions is found in women with repetitive spontaneous abortion during pregnancy.[12] Finally, animal models[13,14] and some, but not all, randomized clinical trials[15–18] demonstrate that leukoreduction and autologous transfusion[19] can reduce the immunomodulatory effects of transfusion and minimize resulting morbidity and mortality. Many detailed reviews of TRIM have been published, and the reader is referred to these for summaries of the historical literature.[1,3–7]

TRANSFUSION AND HUMORAL ALLOSENSITIZATION

It has long been known that transfusion or pregnancy can cause formation of clinically significant antibodies to cellular and plasma components of allogeneic blood. Most blood-transfusion research in the first part of the 20th century was focused on techniques for detecting antibody formation and avoiding transfusion of incompatible red cells. Until the late 1960s and early 1970s, the accepted paradigm was that transfusion stimulated the recipient's immune system to make humoral immune responses, and that this was virtually the only immunologic complication of transfusions. Two decades later, it became clear that some antigens, when given intravenously in high dose, can promote a type 2 (primarily humoral) immune response while downregulating type 1 (primarily cellular) responses.[20–22] Approximately 1% to 5% of individuals receiving ABO and Rh(D) identical transfusions or who become pregnant with an Rh-compatible fetus will mount a humoral immune response to red cell alloantigens. About 50% of patients transfused with cellular blood components or who become pregnant will mount a humoral immune response to human leukocyte antigen (HLA)-A,B antigens present on white blood cells (WBCs). Interestingly, in experimental models when antigens are administered at higher doses, in the absence of costimulatory inflammatory "danger" signals, immune tolerance rather than immunization can occur.[23]

By 1990, leukoreduction was found to abrogate post-transfusion humoral responses to white cell antigens (primarily antibodies to HLA class I). Filtering out most (at least 99.9%) of the donor white cells before transfusion is effective at preventing 90% or more of HLA antibody sensitizations in patients undergoing myeloablative chemotherapy and transfusion.[24] Because HLA antibody formation is the primary mechanism of alloimmune platelet transfusion refractoriness, as platelets carry class I antigens, the incidence of unresponsiveness to platelet transfusions due to allosensitization decreased by an order of magnitude, from approximately 50% to 5% or less, after the introduction of filtered, white cell–reduced transfusions.[25] It is possible that leukocyte removal by filtration also decreases the allosensitization rate to red cell alloantigens.[26] One plausible mechanism is that white cell removal decreases the type 2 immune stimulus that accompanies transfusion of allogeneic white cells. Purified red cells and platelets are known to be less immunogenic than allogeneic white cells. In the absence of allogeneic WBCs, purified red cell components in particular may be less likely to provide inflammatory mediators and co-stimulatory molecules that activate the recipient's immune system.

TRANSFUSION AND SOLID ORGAN TRANSPLANTATION

More than half a century ago, Billingham, Brent, and Medawar[27] demonstrated that administration of allogeneic antigen to fetal animals resulted in immunologic tolerance. The science, if not the clinical art, of solid organ transplantation had begun. The initial evidence that blood transfusions affect recipient immunity beyond humoral alloimmunity came from clinical observations in patients receiving cadaveric renal allografts.[8,28] During the early history of renal transplantation, acute graft rejection during surgery was observed in alloimmunized recipients. This phenomenon was associated with prior transfusions, which, in the pre-erythropoietin era, were the only treatment for the anemia of renal failure. Some investigators were modestly successful at reducing alloimmunization in these patients through leukoreduction before transfusion. At that time, the sole available method of achieving leukoreduction was the use of washed or previously cryopreserved red cells, which were leukocyte reduced by about 80% to 90%, as well as plasma and platelet reduced. However, other investigators made a startling finding, which was received with substantial skepticism. They observed that transfused patients actually experienced overall improved renal allograft survival compared with nontransfused patients. This effect was later shown to be dependent on the transfusion dose and was not observed in those patients receiving leukocyte and plasma reduced blood transfusions (Fig. 52–1).[8,28]

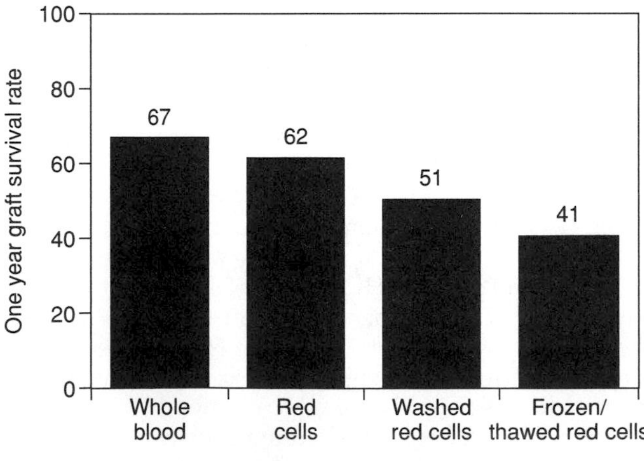

Figure 52–1 One-year kidney allograft survival in recipients of 1–5 units of allogeneic blood of the type listed is shown as a percentage of total patients with transplants. Transfusions with reduced content of allogeneic white cells, platelets, and stored supernatant plasma are associated with inferior 1-year graft-survival rates. (Data from the UCLA registry. Horimi T, Terasaki PI, Chia D, Sasaki N. Factors influencing the paradoxical effect of transfusions on kidney transplants. Transplantation 1983;35:320–323.)

Animal models supported the critical role of allogeneic white cells in mediating this "tolerogenic" result, whereas other studies[29] suggested that a similar effect could be mediated by platelet transfusions. This is of particular interest in light of recent findings that platelets and platelet-derived CD40L can stimulate secretion of prostaglandin E_2 (PGE_2) and other downregulators of cellular immunity.[30,31] Blood transfusions also appear to decrease rejection rates after heart[32] and liver[33] transplants. Donor-specific transfusions are remarkably effective at preventing rejection in animal models but are infrequently used for patients now that immunosuppressive drugs are highly effective at abrogating allograft rejection. A recent report found that the number of acute rejection episodes was inversely related to the number of blood transfusions in cardiac transplant recipients, most of whom received nonleukoreduced transfusions.[34]

TRANSFUSION AND AUTOIMMUNE DISEASES

Transfusion appears to affect favorably some autoimmune diseases thought to be mediated by cellular immunity. These include Crohn's disease (regional enteritis)[35] and rheumatoid arthritis.[36] In Crohn's disease, patients with larger sections of inflamed bowel and more-severe disease are more likely to be transfused during surgery for removal of diseased small bowel. Despite these higher risk factors for poor outcomes, transfused patients are actually less likely, or no more likely to have recurrences of their Crohn's disease than are non-transfused patients who have less-extensive and aggressive disease.[37] One potential explanation for these findings is a downregulation of the type 1 inflammatory process by allogeneic transfusion.

Similarly, rheumatoid arthritis is thought to be mediated in part by type 1 immunity and inflammation. In pilot studies, disease activity has been favorably influenced by transfusion of allogeneic white cells[38] or whole blood.[36]

TRANSFUSION AND REPETITIVE SPONTANEOUS ABORTION

One of the earliest observations regarding TRIM was that paternal or other unrelated blood transfusions improve the likelihood that women with repetitive spontaneous abortions will carry a pregnancy to term.[12] The clinical benefit is modest, and varied transfusion preparations yield different degrees of efficacy, but the effect is reproducible. This observation, although not of major clinical significance, is particularly intriguing, as successful pregnancy, similar to allogeneic TRIM, results in type 2 immune deviation, with increased expression of cytokines such as interleukin (IL)-4, IL-5, and IL-10.[39,40] Pregnancy is characterized by slightly increased risks from intracellular infectious organisms and tumors, presumably because of the mildly impaired type 1 immune defenses needed for optimal immune surveillance. One potential mechanism for the beneficial effects of transfusion in this setting is that allogeneic transfusions may downregulate pathologic type 1 immune responses that contribute to spontaneous abortion.[40]

Another parallel between the immunology of transfusion and pregnancy is the high frequency of alloimmunization and humoral immune responses, precisely as would be expected in clinical settings in which type 2 immune deviation is present. Relevant to this hypothesis, red cell transfusions that are leukocyte reduced may be less likely to result in alloimmunization, not only to WBC antigens, but to red cell alloantigens as well.[26] Leukoreduced transfusions may provoke less type 2 immune deviation than do unmodified transfusions.

TRANSFUSION AND CANCER RECURRENCE

The allograft tolerizing effects of blood transfusion, by analogy with the drugs used to prevent rejection, was termed an *immunosuppressive* effect.[41] Could this effect, beneficial in organ transplant recipients and patients with autoimmune disease or repetitive spontaneous abortions, lead to unfavorable outcomes in clinical situations in which intact recipient cellular immunity is needed? Would patients undergoing surgery or those with cancer experience negative outcomes from "transfusion immunosuppression?"

In the late 1970s, a group from Newcastle, England, observed that animals with tumors had more rapid tumor growth if transfused with allogeneic as opposed to syngeneic blood.[42] The clinical analogy would be the use of allogeneic (homologous) versus autologous transfusions. In 1982, Burrows and Tartter[9] reported that patients in a colorectal cancer trial had earlier and more frequent recurrences of their cancers if they were transfused at the initial surgical resection. Similar observations were made for most other surgically treatable tumors, although about one third of the studies did not achieve statistical significance despite uniformly poorer outcomes in the transfused patients.[43,44]

One possible explanation for the association between allogeneic transfusion and earlier tumor recurrence is simply that the need for transfusion is confounded by size or aggressiveness of the tumor. Patients who require transfusions may do so because they tend to have larger, more aggressive, and difficult-to-resect tumors. This confounding certainly explains some of the association. However, a number of studies observed that even in patients closely matched for prognostic factors, transfused patients had more frequent or earlier cancer recurrences.[45,46] In addition, transfusion practice is quite variable in almost all clinical settings, due to a lack of accepted, uniform criteria for commencing transfusion therapy. Although transfusion therapy is not given randomly, neither is it given in consistent fashion driven by evidence-based transfusion triggers. Thus it would have been surprising if the two- to threefold difference seen in tumor recurrence is completely due to confounding. In epidemiologic investigations, two- to threefold differences in outcomes usually prove to be causal relations, at least to some extent.[47,48]

When these observations appeared in the 1980s, the hypothesis that the immune system was involved in cancer outcome was falling out of favor. Failures of immune-based therapies in patients, such as interferon and bacille Calmette-Guérin (BCG) vaccination, which had efficacy in animal models, were largely responsible.[49,50] Also, immune responses to human tumors were rarely demonstrable. The possibility that "successful" tumors can evade and/or repress host immune responses had not yet been proposed or proven.[51,52] Thus the initial observations of a relation between perioperative transfusion and cancer recurrence were met with intense skepticism, much as was the case for the initial studies of the allograft-enhancing effects of blood transfusions.

Nonetheless, several investigative findings suggest that the association between blood transfusion and cancer recurrence is causal. First, as in the renal transplant data, the type of transfusion affects the likelihood of recurrence. Whole blood transfusions are associated with greater cancer recurrence rates than are equivalent numbers of red cell transfusions (which are partially depleted of plasma, white cells, and platelets) (Figs. 52–2 and 52–3).[53–55]

Second, two animal models demonstrated that removal of allogeneic leukocytes reduced the number of lung metastases seen after transfusions.[13] Third, autologous transfusions reduced the recurrence rate in patients undergoing colorectal cancer resection, as compared with patients receiving allogeneic transfusions, in one randomized trial[56] but not in another.[57] The single study that examined leukocyte reduction of transfusions as a means of reducing adverse immunomodulatory effects showed no benefit,[58] and that was supported by results of another recent report.[59]

Regrettably, few trials of leukocyte reduction, washing, autologous transfusions, or bloodless medicine and surgery techniques have been published in oncologic surgery. These are extraordinarily challenging and expensive trials to perform because they require adherence to complex protocols, large numbers of patients, and, in particular, long-term follow-up. The one existing trial of washed, leukocyte-reduced transfusions in patients with cancer demonstrated a possible benefit in younger adults with acute leukemia.[60] However, this was a small pilot study, and clear-cut benefit was seen only in subgroup analysis, increasing the chances of selection bias and confounding.

Fortunately, a trend exists toward decreasing use of transfusions in cancer surgery,[17] largely due to the concerns about

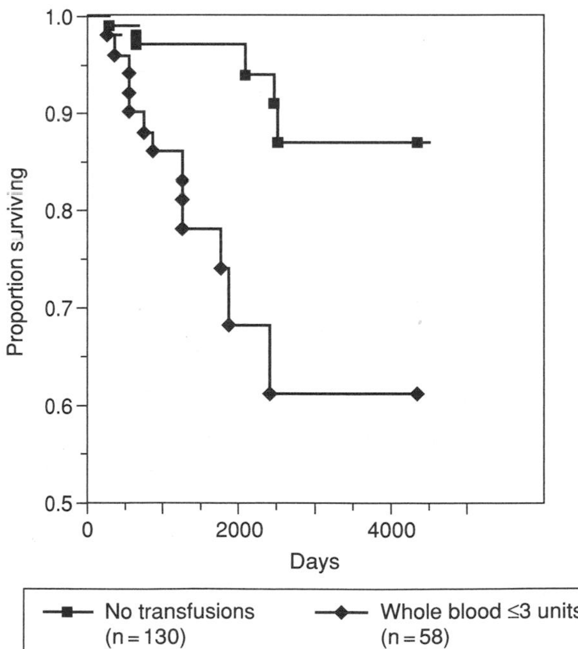

Figure 52–2 Kaplan-Meier plot of the proportion of patients remaining alive after initial surgical treatment for colorectal, cervical, or prostate cancer who received either no transfusions or ≤3 units of blood, at least one of which was whole blood. The two curves are statistically significantly different ($P < 0.001$), with the nontransfused patients having estimated mortality at 5 years of <15%, as compared with almost 40% in those receiving whole blood transfusions.[53,54]

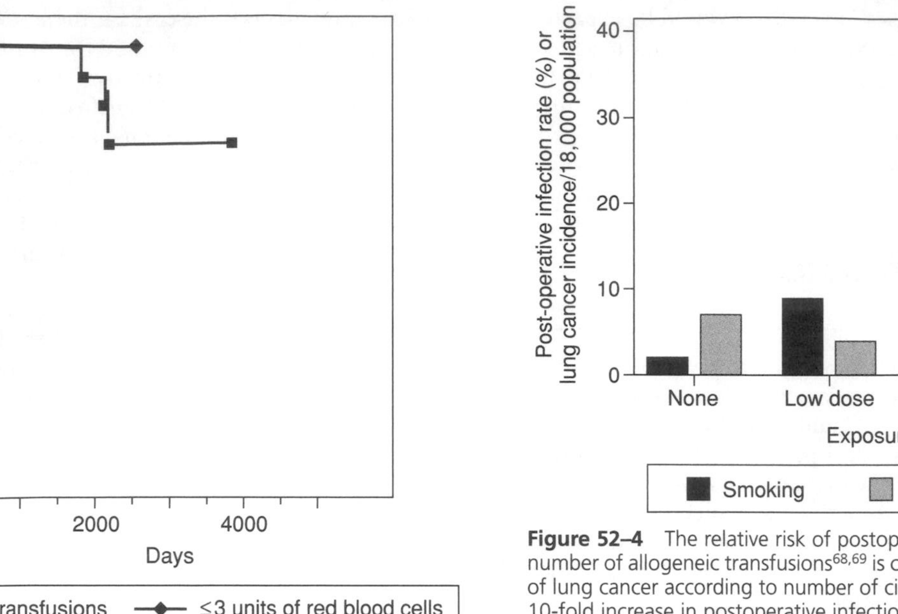

Figure 52–3 Kaplan-Meier plot of the proportion of patients remaining alive after initial surgical treatment for colorectal, cervical, or prostate cancer who received either no transfusions or ≤3 units of red cell concentrates. The two curves are not statistically significantly different.[53,54]

Figure 52–4 The relative risk of postoperative infection according to number of allogeneic transfusions[68,69] is compared with the relative risk of lung cancer according to number of cigarettes smoked.[154] The 5- to 10-fold increase in postoperative infections with increasing number of allogeneic transfusions, seen in many studies, which is in part abrogated by leukoreduced or autologous transfusions, provides prima facie evidence for a cause-and-effect relation according to Hill's principles of causation (including dose relation, size of the effect, underlying plausible mechanism, consistency across studies, and benefits of reducing the exposure).[47,48]

transfusion-transmitted human immunodeficiency virus (HIV) and hepatitis C. It is unknown whether this change in practice has contributed to decreases in recurrence rates in patients with surgically resectable tumors. With the implementation of universal leukoreduction of transfusions throughout much of the developed world, the possibility exists for before and after studies of cancer recurrence, but none has yet been published. When a 5- to 10-year follow-up period is available for patients treated after the introduction of universal leukoreduction, it may be possible to determine whether leukoreduced transfusions are less immunomodulatory in cancer surgery patients than unmodified transfusions. Our speculation is that both leukocyte reduced and washed transfusions may be needed to maximally benefit transfused cancer patients.

TRANSFUSION, POSTOPERATIVE INFECTION, AND MULTIORGAN FAILURE

Transfusions are associated with a dramatically increased risk of postoperative bacterial infection, as first reported by Paul Tartter[11,61] 20 years ago. Preoperative, intraoperative, or postoperative transfusion leads to a severalfold increase in the proportion of patients who develop an infection. This association has been confirmed in many other studies[62] and cannot be explained by confounding variables related to transfusion such as anemia, blood loss during surgery, duration of surgery, or hypotension. The quantitative strength of the association is striking. Patients who are transfused with more than 10 units of allogeneic blood experience a 5- to 10-fold increase in their likelihood of developing a postoperative infection.[63] This effect is observed in diverse surgical settings, and among studied causal relations is second in magnitude only to the association between smoking and lung cancer (Fig. 52–4). Thus the association between transfusions and postoperative infections is extremely unlikely to be explained by the bias and confounding that are limitations of most observational studies.[47,48]

It has been suggested that the effects of multiple confounding factors and a surrogacy role for transfusions might explain this association.[64] This hypothesis is quite improbable because of the extraordinarily variable and unsystematic way in which transfusion decisions are made.[65] A dose-dependent 5- to 10-fold increase in postoperative infections after allogeneic transfusion solely accounted for by confounding is extremely remote and would be unprecedented in clinical epidemiology.[47,48]

One limitation of published studies is that infection is often defined solely as culture-proven infections. This greatly underestimates the incidence of infectious morbidity, given the insensitivity of most culture techniques. This is particularly the case in surgical patients, who invariably receive prophylactic antibiotic therapy. It is preferable also to estimate infections by multiple surrogate measures including days of antibiotic treatment, length of hospital stay, and signs, laboratory tests, and symptoms of infection. Less comprehensive approaches are likely to underestimate infectious morbidity significantly. As discussed previously in this chapter, one additional body of evidence that contradicts the "transfusion as a surrogate marker for confounding variables" hypothesis is that perioperative transfusions are associated with better rather than worse clinical outcomes in patients receiving renal allografts[28] or in those with inflammatory bowel disease.[35] Were transfusion to be acting purely as a surrogate measure of clinically unfavorable comorbidities, these clinically favorable associations would not exist. To the contrary, as is discussed further, these altered outcomes support a common immunologic mechanism for both improved and poorer clinical outcomes in different clinical settings. Although some analyses that included many unrelated confounders did not find a significant association between transfusion and infection,[66] these types of analyses are neither statistically nor scientifically sound.[67] Only confounders directly and causally linked to both transfusion and infection are appropriately included in statistical models. Introduction of multiple, causally unrelated, and irrelevant variables can lead to erroneous acceptance of the null hypothesis.

A number of animal models confirm that the association of allogeneic transfusion with postoperative infection is most likely cause and effect. Alexander and colleagues[14] demonstrated in mice that allogeneic white cells were more potent in mediating this effect than were red cells or plasma. Our group and many others observed that the association between transfusion and postoperative infection is not seen in patients receiving autologous blood, supporting an immunologic mechanism for the effect (Fig. 52–5).[68,69]

The best evidence for a causal relation between allogeneic transfusion and an increased risk of postoperative infection comes from randomized clinical trials of leukoreduced allogeneic transfusions versus unmodified blood transfusions, as well as studies of autologous versus allogeneic transfusions. These studies, discussed in detail further on in this chapter, demonstrate beyond a reasonable doubt that the incidence of postoperative infection, and probably that of multiorgan failure, in transfused surgical patients can be reduced by use of leukoreduced blood transfusions[15–18,58,70–73] or the use of autologous techniques.[19] In general, a 10% absolute reduction in postoperative infection incidence is possible by using leukoreduced transfusions compared with unmodified red cells. This means that for every 10 patients treated with leukoreduced transfusions, one less postoperative infection will occur as compared with patients treated with nonleukoreduced transfusions. Recent evidence from our own center suggests that leukoreduction of blood transfusions may also reduce

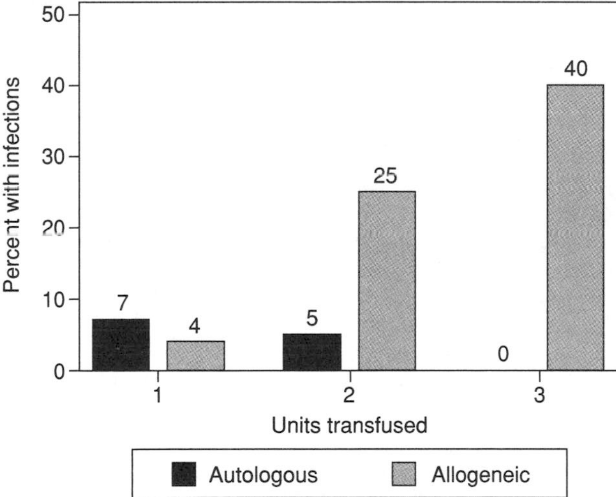

Figure 52–5 Patients undergoing posterior or anterior, cervical or lumbar spinal fusion, or primary hip replacement surgery, without malignancy, autoimmune diseases, or diabetes were grouped according to whether they had received only autologous blood or only allogeneic (homologous) blood. The proportion with culture-proven or clinically evident infections, grouped according to number of units of blood transfused, is shown. The differences between autologous and homologous recipients are statistically significant at doses of 2 or 3 units, but not for 1 unit of blood. This dose-response relation also was evident when days of antibiotics and length of hospital stay were measured. Infections were predominantly away from the wound site: two thirds were cellulitis, urinary tract, or pulmonary. Data are pooled from two studies.[68,69] (Reprinted from Anderson KE, Ness PM [eds]. Scientific Basis of Transfusion Medicine. Elsevier, 2000, p 437, with permission.)

the incidence of indwelling vascular-access catheter sepsis in a variety of nonsurgical settings by perhaps 30% to 40%.[74]

The association between transfusion and postoperative infection is also reflected in observations of a dose-dependent increase in multiorgan failure in transfused surgical patients.[75–77] Multiorgan failure is often initiated by infection in seriously ill patients. This association is not explained by confounding factors and has been detected in randomized clinical trials as well. Multiorgan failure and death after cardiac surgery appears to be reduced in patients receiving leukoreduced transfusions.[18]

Platelet transfusions also have been associated with a five-fold increase in postoperative deaths after cardiac surgery, after adjustment for other risk factors.[78] Such a large effect is unlikely to be explained primarily by confounding.[47,48] The association between platelet transfusion and mortality may be partially abrogated in patients receiving postoperative aspirin.[79] Whether the association between platelet transfusion and mortality is mediated by a predisposition to infection due to immunomodulatory effects of transfusions,[18,80] a prothrombotic effect of storage activated platelets being transfused,[81–83] exacerbation of inflammatory responses from transfused platelet CD40L and sCD40L,[30] other bioactive molecules or cells, or other mechanisms, will require further investigation.

Wound healing may also be impaired after allogeneic transfusions.[84–86] Both randomized trials and before-and-after studies suggest that leukoreduction of transfusions may reduce the risk of postoperative multiorgan failure[18] and improve wound healing.[87] It is unknown whether storage time of transfused blood influences these complications, but this seems possible.[88–90] Recent evidence suggests that postoperative morbidity and death due to immunologic mechanisms may also be increased by transfusion of ABO-mismatched blood components containing incompatible antigen or antibody.[91–93]

TRANSFUSION AND ANTIVIRAL IMMUNITY

Given the association between transfusion and postoperative bacterial infection, it was hypothesized that allogeneic transfusions might also impair host resistance to viral infection. Epidemiologic evidence suggests that transfusion accelerates the appearance of clinical manifestations of HIV-1[94] and cytomegalovirus (CMV) infection.[95] However, in end-stage HIV-1 infection, a randomized trial of leukoreduced transfusions failed to identify any immunomodulatory effects that promote viral replication or shorten survival.[96] With regard to this last trial, it has become evident in TRIM studies that multicenter studies, which typically involve small numbers of patients at large numbers of hospitals, may be less able than single-center studies to detect improved outcomes because of substantial variations in clinical practices that influence infection or survival.

Viral infections play a role in lymphoma in both animal models and humans, and prior allogeneic transfusion has been associated with the development of non-Hodgkin's lymphoma, specifically the B-cell variants.[97] Not all studies have found this association. If the association is causal, it is unclear whether viral transmission or TRIM is primarily responsible, but either or both mechanisms could be involved. TRIM drives B-cell proliferation and maturation through promotion of type 2 (Th2) immunity and downregulates type 1 (Th1) immune functions that are thought to be relevant in antiviral immunity and tumor surveillance (Fig. 52–6). Thus although the hypothesized potential of transfusion to impair host defenses to viral infection is plausible, in that transfusion downregulates natural killer cell and macrophage/monocyte cytocidal functions and promotes Th2 immune deviation, no definitive conclusions are possible, given the modest data at hand.

MECHANISMS OF TRANSFUSION IMMUNOMODULATION

Transfusion involves intravenous infusion of large doses of blood cells, proteins, lipids, and other blood constituents diluted with preservative anticoagulant solution, as well as the breakdown products that result from storage lesions. The only natural circumstances in which the immune system is exposed to such high doses of intravenous antigen are self-antigens and pregnancy.[40,98] The immune system has evolved to respond to these two situations with unresponsiveness or tolerance and to provide defense against dangerous foreign antigens that are non-self.[23] Pathogens are microorganisms, present in small quantities, at mucosal or skin locations, or altered self (i.e., cancer cells in small numbers), largely in organs. It stands to reason that large quantities of intravenous antigen containing both self and non-self determinants leads to unresponsiveness rather than allosensitization. In particular, this appears to be the case when the clinical setting is that of decreased host immune function (e.g., the immaturity of fetal life, surgical stress).

The classic investigations of Medawar and colleagues[27] proved that exposure to foreign antigens during fetal life can produce tolerance to skin grafts from the tissue donor. Felton[99] reported that when pneumococcal antigen was administered at high doses, animals have reduced capabilities for subsequent humoral immune responses to antigen administered by routes and in doses that otherwise cause sensitization ("immune paralysis"). In 1951, Snell and Kaliss[100] demonstrated that infusions of tissue extracts from allogeneic murine donors before tumor implantation led to accelerated tumor growth. Even serum transfusion before implantation led to the death of most of the mice from tumor progression. Saline-transfused control animals uniformly rejected the implanted tumor and survived. Interestingly, of all the tissue extracts transfused, infusions of lyophilized red cells were the only ones that failed to enhance tumor growth.

Whereas most studies have focused on the role of transfused allogeneic white cells and their secreted mediators or breakdown products,[101] clinical data suggest that stored supernatant plasma may also be immunomodulatory.[94] In addition, recent investigations confirm that platelets are a source of immunomodulatory mediators, such as vascular endothelial growth factor (VEGF), soluble CD40L, and transforming growth factor-β1 (TGF-β1).[30,31,102–105] In addition to platelet components, platelet-derived mediators such as soluble CD40L are also present at high concentrations in nonleukoreduced red cell concentrates and whole blood.

Allogeneic transfusions in animals result in diminished mixed lymphocyte culture reactivity, diminished antigen processing by macrophages, upregulation of both suppressor/regulatory cells and humoral immunosuppressive mediators, impaired cell killing, and production of anti-idiotypic antibodies that are immunomodulatory in vitro.[106,107] These findings indicate that impaired or dysregulated cellular immunity is likely a key mechanism underlying TRIM. Many investigations report that the presence or absence of allogeneic WBCs in the transfusion is critical to observing immunomodulatory effects, but plasma, red cells, and even purified, soluble class I

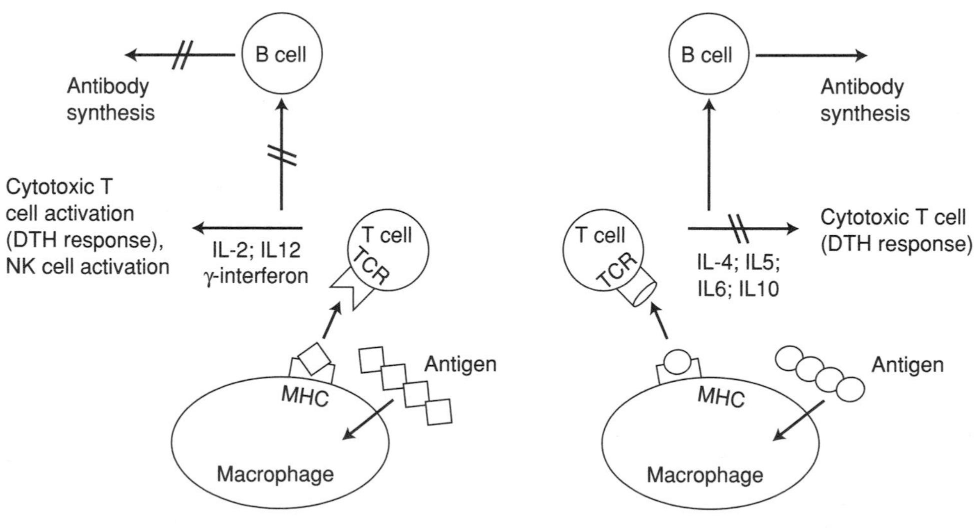

Figure 52–6 A schematic view of how alloantigens are processed by macrophages and presented to T cells is shown, with emphasis on the distinction between responses that primarily involve Th1(type 1) or Th2 (type 2) cytokines. Similarly, type 1 or type 2 deviated dendritic cells, macrophages, and CD8 cytotoxic lymphocytes have been identified. Allogeneic transfusions appear to promote primarily type 2 cytokine secretion patterns with reciprocal downregulation of type 1 cytokine secretion. Many cellular immune functions are downregulated by immune deviation, including cytotoxic T cell and NK functions.[98,155] DTH, delayed-type hypersensitivity; TCR, T-cell antigen receptor; MHC, major histocompatibility complex; NK, natural killer; IL, interleukin. Reprinted from Anderson KE, Ness PM [eds.]. Scientific Basis of Transfusion Medicine. Elsevier, 2000, p 429, with permission.)

histocompatibility antigens or peptide fragments of class I molecules[108,109] can have similar effects. The simultaneous presence of alloantigen and key mediators probably accounts for many of the clinically observed TRIM results, because autologous or syngeneic blood does not generally mediate these effects.

TRIM in the allotransplant setting is mediated at least in part by the effects of increased PGE_2 and decreased IL-2 production. Inhibition of PGE_2 secretion by indomethacin or anti-PGE_2 antibody abrogates the transfusion allograft enhancement effect.[110] In another animal model, administration of exogenous IL-2 reversed the blood-transfusion tolerance induction for renal allografts.[111] Allogeneic transfusions also impair the ability of murine and human mononuclear cells to secrete IL-2 in response to a variety of in vitro stimuli.[22,112] Table 52–1 lists some of the immunologic alterations that have been consistently described in transfused animals and patients.[98,106,107]

Several mechanisms appear to play a role common to many or even most of these clinical settings. One model for transfusion immunomodulation is depicted in Figure 52–6.[20–22,98,112–115] Immune deviation involving increased secretion of type 2 (Th2) cytokines (e.g., IL-10, IL-4) and decreased secretion of type 1 (Th1) cytokines (e.g., γ-interferon, IL-2) is one proposed mechanism by which transfusion immunomodulates recipient immune responses to allogeneic organs, tumors, and the fetus. Effective immune responses against tumors and organ allografts are thought to be primarily Th1 in nature,[116] as is rejection of the fetus as an allograft.[39] Although this scheme no doubt oversimplifies the intricate biology of such processes, clinical and animal studies demonstrate that allogeneic transfusions alter cellular immunity by promoting immune responses with increased production of IL-10, IL-4, and TGF-β. These mediators downregulate natural killer (NK) and T-effector cell functions, as well as phagocytic cell functions and generally function as anti-inflammatory mediators. NK and T cells are critical to maintaining antitumor, anti-allograft, and antimicrobial immunity. Thus, their dysregulation after allogeneic transfusion provides one plausible unifying mechanism to explain a variety of seemingly unrelated clinical outcomes.

To complicate the clinical picture, surgery alone, absent transfusion, causes immune deviation toward type 2 cytokine secretion. This effect likely accounts in part for the reduction in delayed-type hypersensitivity responses seen for the first week or two after surgery.[117–119] Whether this altered immunity is due to surgical trauma, anesthesia, or other drugs is not entirely understood. These immune effects are additive with the effects of transfusion in the clinical setting, and impairments of cellular immunity can last for days to weeks. From both immunologic and clinical standpoints, it is of interest that immune dysregulation is not seen or is seen to a lesser degree in patients receiving only autologous blood,[115,118,120] or leukocyte-depleted transfusions.[15,16,121]

Finally, evidence indicates that infusion of apoptotic allogeneic WBCs facilitates type 2 immune deviation,[122] organ allograft acceptance,[123,124] and multiorgan failure[122] in experimental animals. Apoptotic WBCs and platelets, as well as red cells, accumulate during blood storage and are selectively removed by leukocyte-reduction filters.[125] Thus, infusion of storage-damaged apoptotic allogeneic cells may provide one mechanism by which T cell, macrophage, and dendritic cell immunity is biased toward type 2 cytokine secretion, and explain why leukocyte reduction reduces adverse immunologic and clinical effects.[126]

Immune deviation, greater in intensity but similar in principle to that seen in pregnancy, is not the only event that occurs with allogeneic transfusion. However, it is the only current hypothesis that could account for a broad range of seemingly contradictory clinical findings that range from reduced spontaneous abortion, allograft rejection, and autoimmune disease, to increased postoperative infection and cancer recurrence (Table 52–2). In summary, TRIM is a pleiotropic phenomenon. It is extremely unlikely that any single mechanism fully accounts for the effects of transfusion on organ transplants, postoperative infection, cancer recurrence, pregnancy, and autoimmune diseases.

Table 52–1 Allogeneic Transfusion Effects on Immune Function

1. Decreased Th1 and increased Th2 cytokine production in vitro
2. Reduced responses in mixed lymphocyte culture
3. Decreased proliferative response to mitogens or soluble antigens in vitro; impaired delayed-type hypersensitivity skin responses
4. Increased CD8 T-cell number or suppressor function in vitro
5. Decreased natural killer cell number and activity in vitro
6. Decreased CD4 helper T cells number
7. Decreased monocyte/macrophage function in vitro and in vivo
8. Enhanced production of anti-idiotypic antibodies suppressive of mixed lymphocyte response in vitro
9. Decreased cell-mediated cytotoxicity (LAK) against target cells in vitro
10. Humoral alloimmunization to cell-associated and soluble antigens

Data from Blumberg N, Heal JM. The transfusion immunomodulation theory: The Th1/Th2 paradigm and an analogy with pregnancy as a unifying mechanism. Semin Hematol 1996;33:429–440; Blumberg N, Heal JM. Transfusion and recipient immune function. Arch Pathol Lab Med 1989;113:246–253; Blumberg N, Heal JM. Effects of transfusion on immune function: Cancer recurrence and infection. Arch Pathol Lab Med 1994;118:371–379.

METHODS TO MITIGATE TRANSFUSION IMMUNOMODULATION AND REDUCE MORBIDITY AND MORTALITY

Reducing the damaging effects of transfusion immunomodulation is not straightforward, as the underlying mechanisms have not been entirely elucidated. For example, it is not certain whether transfused cells and molecules other than allogeneic WBCs cause significant changes in clinical outcomes. However, this seems probable. Supernatants from

Table 52–2 Th1 Processes Downregulated by Allogeneic Transfusions

Allograft rejection
Tumor rejection
Rejection of the fetus as an allograft
Inflammation of Crohn's disease and rheumatoid arthritis
Inflammation of type 1 diabetes (in animals)
Antibacterial and antiviral immunity

stored platelet concentrates contain significant amounts of immunomodulatory mediators such as TGF-β1 and sCD40L, which are potential causes for some observed associations. Platelets express surface CD40L, which has been linked in preliminary work to acute lung injury.[83,127] Storage-damaged apoptotic red cells express phosphatidyl serine, which could interact with receptors on endothelial or other immunocompetent cells. Transfusion components stored under variable conditions for various periods may have differing immunomodulatory effects. Clinical data suggest that transfused whole blood has more potent immunomodulatory effects than do red cell concentrates. Whether this is attributable to variations in platelet or WBC content, supernatant plasma, or other variables is not known. Differences in leukocyte-reduction methods may yield sufficiently varied numbers of residual platelets in the transfused component that this accounts for some of the inconsistency of the results reported in randomized trials.

Despite these caveats and uncertainties, three well-established methods are known for mitigating the immunomodulatory complications of transfusion. The first is entirely avoiding transfusion via bloodless medicine and surgery practices.[128] The second is avoiding or reducing allogeneic transfusions by use of autologous transfusion, hemodilution, and blood salvage.[19] The third is administering only leukoreduced (also platelet-reduced) red cell transfusions by using high-efficiency WBC adherence filters.[15–18,58,70–73,129]

Two randomized trials of autologous predeposit versus allogeneic transfusions have produced opposite results. Heiss and colleagues[56,118] reported reduced infections and cancer recurrences in patients receiving autologous transfusions, whereas Busch and colleagues[57] found no benefit. Both these studies are limited by the most significant problem in studies of autologous or leukoreduced transfusions, which is a high protocol-violation rate. A high percentage of patients in these studies received no transfusions or the wrong types of transfusions because of insufficient availability of autologous or leukoreduced blood. When patients with protocol violations were removed from the database, the benefits of reduced cancer recurrence were much clearer in the study of Heiss and colleagues. Another caveat for both of these studies is that the control arms were buffy coat depleted (60% to 80% leukoreduced) allogeneic red cells. This partial leukoreduction of the control transfusions minimizes the opportunity for detecting a benefit because allogeneic WBCs/platelets are important mediators of TRIM.

In addition, a potentially important difference may be that the Heiss study[56,118] was a single-center study, whereas the Busch study included multiple centers.[57] Most single-center trials of leukocyte depletion or autologous transfusion have demonstrated reductions in morbidity or mortality compared with unmodified allogeneic transfusion recipients. Most multicenter trials have failed to find such benefits. The variability introduced by small numbers of patients treated by many diverse clinical protocols may have obscured potential benefits. Such variations from center to center have been shown to account for the variability in postoperative infection rates in Israeli medical centers.[130] It is interesting that an initial multicenter study by investigators in Leiden failed to find a benefit to leukoreduced transfusions in colorectal cancer surgery,[58] but a subsequent single-center study from the same investigators found beneficial effects of leukoreduced transfusions on morbidity and mortality after cardiac surgery.[18] Variation in infection-control and surgical techniques, such as time of administration of prophylactic antibiotics, significantly affects infection rates, and these uncontrolled variables may confound studies of transfusion interventions.

One large randomized trial found that leukoreduced transfusions benefited neither mortality, morbidity, length of stay, nor hospital costs.[131] These data did support the probability that leukocyte reduction was cost neutral. This study had a number of limitations. Many patients were included who might not be seriously affected by TRIM. Outpatients with anemia of chronic disease, medical inpatients with modest blood loss or hypoproliferative anemias, and other subgroups may affect the power of a large study to detect a benefit in those who are more seriously at risk, such as surgical and critical care patients. Second, as in other studies with high protocol-violation rates, more than one in eight patients in the leukoreduced arm of this study actually received nonleukoreduced blood. Third, the proportion of patients with protocol violations was significantly greater in the leukoreduced arm of the study than in the control arm. A likely explanation for this failure of randomization is that when supplies of leukoreduced blood ran short, technical staff switched patients to the nonleukoreduced protocol. As TRIM is dose dependent, this effectively removed from the leukoreduced arm of the study the heavily transfused patients most likely to benefit. This study thus cannot definitively address whether leukoreduction reduces morbidity and mortality in surgical and critical care patients, which are the settings in which the largest clinical and cost benefits may be observed.[132]

Over the last decade, a number of "meta-analyses" of randomized trials of leukoreduced transfusions to reduce postoperative infections have been published, claiming to demonstrate that leukoreduction is of little or no benefit in reducing postoperative infection.[66,133–139] However, these studies have methodologic problems. One error is failing to calculate a summary odds ratio for the effects of leukoreduced transfusions. Without a summary odds ratio, the single number representing the cumulative results of the published clinical trials, no meta-analysis is produced, but only a review containing the authors' opinions. The rationale for not calculating a summary estimate was the presence of statistically significant heterogeneity in the published original studies. Statistical heterogeneity is not a valid scientific rationale for failing to calculate a summary odds ratio, but rather is an indication for use of a random effects meta-analysis, and for further exploration of the data to investigate the sources of heterogeneity.[140]

Even more scientifically questionable is that these analyses include many nontransfused patients. Nontransfused patients compose as many as three fourths of the patients in some clinical trials in the published graphs. Nontransfused patients cannot provide answers to the question of whether TRIM has clinically significant effects, nor whether leukoreduction can reduce such effects. Most seriously, some meta-analyses do not represent the actual data from the original studies. For some of the clinical trials, the meta-analyses used data that represent "imputed" outcomes created by the authors of the review.[66,133–139]

The original authors of the studies analyzed only the patients who actually received transfusions because these are the only relevant patients for assessing whether leukoreduction has any benefits. Retrospectively to create an "intention to treat" analysis including the nontransfused patients, the meta-analysts divided in half the number of nontransfused patients and infections reported in these nontransfused patients. They then added these infections and nontransfused patients back to the actual reported data on transfused patients, as originally published. It is a violation of the scientific method to include nontransfused patients in a study of leukoreduced transfusion outcomes, whether using actual or fictional data. Estimates from properly performed meta-analyses that restrict the analysis to actual data from about 3000 patients who were transfused in eight randomized trials recently demonstrated beyond reasonable doubt that leukoreduction decreases the odds of postoperative infections in transfused surgical patients by about 40% to 50% compared with unmodified red cells, whole blood, or buffy coat–poor red cells.[129,141] This corresponds to an absolute risk reduction of 10%, yielding a number to treat of 10. For every 10 surgical patients receiving leukoreduced, instead of unmodified, transfusions, one patient will be protected from developing a postoperative infection that otherwise would have occurred (Fig. 52–7). This figure probably understates the benefits of leukoreduced transfusions because protocol violation rates of up to 11% occurred in the leukoreduced arm of these studies.

A number of implementation trials of universal leukoreduction have been reported.[142–148] These have yielded variable results, perhaps not surprisingly, when derived from before-and-after studies of infection incidence, length of stay, and other variables heavily influenced by possible temporal changes in case mix, other clinical interventions, and the confounding effects of multi-institutional observational studies. Five of the seven studies reported reductions in mortality, morbidity, and/or costs,[144–148] and three of the studies reported patient cohorts with no apparent clinical benefit.[142,143,146] None has demonstrated significant increases in morbidity, mortality, or costs with institution of universal leukoreduction, suggesting that, at worst, leukoreduction is cost neutral and causes no harm, whereas at best it can reduce morbidity, mortality, and costs significantly.

These benefits of leukoreduced transfusions are not minor public health concerns.[74,149] Depending on the percentage of the epidemiologic association that is causal, the number of TRIM–associated deaths could be as many as tens of thousands per year, far exceeding those due to other transfusion complications.[132] The opportunity to improve care involves not only morbidity and mortality averted, but also significant cost savings. Investigators in Rochester, New York, and Aarhus, Denmark, have estimated these savings at $1000 to $2000 per leukoreduced or autologous unit transfused instead of an allogeneic unit.[144,150,151] By extrapolating from these data, the estimated savings to the United States health system from universal leukocyte reduction of allogeneic transfusions to surgical patients could be as much as $6 to $12 billion per year, or 1% to 2% of the national health budget at that time.[152]

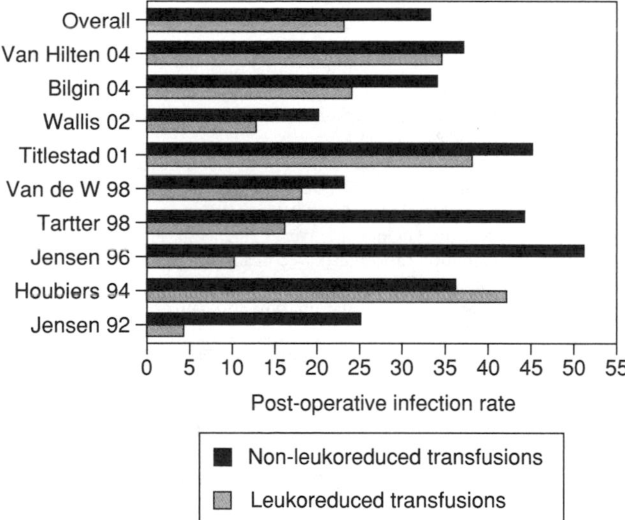

Figure 52–7 The postoperative infection rates observed in nine randomized trials of leukoreduced versus unmodified transfusions in colorectal or cardiac surgery are shown according to randomization arm (intention to treat). Six of the nine studies found statistically significant reductions in postoperative infections with leukoreduced transfusions, and in eight of nine studies, the infection rate was lower in the leukoreduced arm of the study. Nontransfused patients are excluded from these data, but patients with protocol violations (range, 0–11%) remain in the arm to which they were originally randomized. Overall, the infection rate in 1637 patients randomized to receive leukoreduced transfusions was 23%, as compared with 33% in the 1456 patients randomized to receive whole-blood, buffy-coat-poor, or unmodified red cell concentrates (equivalent to a 36% decrease in relative risk with leukoreduced transfusions; $P = .005$ in a random-effects model meta-analysis performed by Drs. Gary Lyman, Hongkun Wang, and Hongwei Zhao of the University of Rochester; unpublished data).

SUMMARY

Transfusions of allogeneic blood to animals or patients are immunomodulatory. Transfusions alter cellular adaptive immunity, innate immunity, and lead to both favorable and unfavorable reduced or increased inflammatory responses, depending on the clinical setting. Transfused patients are more likely to accept renal allografts. Whole-blood recipients have better allograft survival but higher colorectal cancer recurrence rates than patients receiving red cells alone. Allogeneic transfusion recipients are more likely to develop postoperative infections than are recipients of identical amounts of autologous transfusion. Recipients of leukocyte-reduced transfusions are less likely to develop postoperative infections than are recipients of unmodified red cells.

These observations are compatible with the finding that allogeneic transfusions lead to decreased type 1 and increased type 2 cytokine secretion in animal models and medical and surgical patients. Thus, immune deviation provides an initial concept in formulating a unifying theory of transfusion immunology, which can account for such diverse outcomes as the formation of alloantibodies (primarily a type 2 response), allergic reactions (also type 2 in origin), and downregulation of cellular immunity (a type 1 process).

The single explanation that best fits these varied clinical and laboratory observations is that allogeneic transfusions mediate clinically significant immunomodulation by modifying existing normal or abnormal immune responses.

REFERENCES

1. Blumberg N, Heal JM.Transfusion immunomodulation. In Anderson KC, Ness PM (eds). Scientific Basis of Transfusion Medicine, 2nd ed. Philadelphia, WB Saunders, 2000, pp 427–443.
2. Blumberg N, Heal JM. Immunomodulation by blood transfusion: an evolving scientific and clinical challenge. Am J Med 1996;101:399–408.
3. Tartter PI. Immunologic effects of blood transfusion. Immunol Invest 1995;24:277–288.

4. Brand A. Immunological aspects of blood transfusions [Review]. Blood Rev 2000;14:130–144.
5. Nielsen HJ. Detrimental effects of perioperative blood transfusion. Br J Surg 1995;82:582–587.
6. Lee JH, Klein HG. From leukocyte reduction to leukocyte transfusion: the immunological effects of transfused leukocytes [Review]. Baillieres Best Pract Clin Haematol 2001;13:585–600.
7. Blumberg N. Deleterious clinical effects of transfusion immunomodulation: Proven beyond a reasonable doubt. Transfusion 2005;45(2 Suppl):33S–39S; discussion 9S–40S.
8. Opelz G, Sengar DPS, Mickey MR, et al. Effect of blood transfusions on subsequent kidney transplants. Transplant Proc 1973;5:253–259.
9. Burrows L, Tartter P. Effect of blood transfusions on colonic malignancy recurrence rate [Letter]. Lancet 1982;2:662–670.
10. Blumberg N, Agarwal M, Chuang C. Relation between recurrence of cancer of the colon and blood transfusion. BMJ 1985;290:1037–1039.
11. Tartter PI, Driefuss RM, Malon AM, et al. Relationship of postoperative septic complications and blood transfusions in patients with Crohn's disease. Am J Surg 1988;155:43–47.
12. Mowbray JF, Liddell H, Underwood JL, et al. Controlled trial of treatment of recurrent spontaneous abortion by immunisation with paternal cells. Lancet 1985;1:941–943.
13. Blajchman MA, Bardossy L, Carmen R, et al. Allogeneic blood transfusion-induced enhancement of tumor growth: two animal models showing amelioration by leukodepletion and passive transfer using spleen cells. Blood 1993;81:1880–1882.
14. Gianotti L, Pyles T, Alexander JW, et al. Identification of the blood component responsible for increased susceptibility to gut-derived infection. Transfusion 1993;33:458–465.
15. Jensen LS, Andersen AJ, Christiansen PM, et al. Postoperative infection and natural killer cell function following blood transfusion in patients undergoing elective colorectal surgery. Br J Surg 1992;79:513–516.
16. Jensen LS, Kissmeyer-Nielsen P, Wolff B, Qvist N. Randomised comparison of leucocyte-depleted versus buffy-coat-poor blood transfusion and complications after colorectal surgery. Lancet 1996;348: 841–845.
17. Tartter PI, Mohandas K, Azar P, et al. Randomized trial comparing packed red cell blood transfusion with and without leukocyte depletion for gastrointestinal surgery. Am J Surg 1998;176:462–466.
18. van de Watering LMG, Hermans J, Houbiers JGA, et al. Beneficial effects of leukocyte depletion of transfused blood on postoperative complications in patients undergoing cardiac surgery: a randomized clinical trial. Circulation 1998;97:562–568.
19. Vanderlinde ES, Heal JM, Blumberg N. Autologous transfusion. BMJ 2002;324:772–775.
20. Kirkley SA, Cowles J, Pellegrini VD Jr, et al. Cytokine secretion after allogeneic or autologous blood transfusion. Lancet 1995;345:527.
21. Kirkley SA, Cowles J, Pellegrini VD Jr, et al. Blood transfusion and total joint replacement surgery: T helper 2 (Th2) cytokine secretion and clinical outcome. Transfus Med 1998;8:195–204.
22. Babcock GF, Alexander JW. The effects of blood transfusion on cytokine production by TH1 and TH2 lymphocytes in the mouse. Transplantation 1996;61:465–468.
23. Matzinger P. Tolerance, danger, and the extended family [Review]. Annu Rev Immunol 1994;12:991–1045.
24. Leukocyte reduction and ultraviolet B irradiation of platelets to prevent alloimmunization and refractoriness to platelet transfusions: The Trial to Reduce Alloimmunization to Platelets study group. N Engl J Med 1997;337:1861–1869.
25. Blumberg N, Heal JM, Kirkley SA, et al: Leukodepleted-ABO-identical blood components in the treatment of hematologic malignancies: a cost analysis. Am J Hematol 1995;48:108–115.
26. Blumberg N, Heal JM, Gettings KF. WBC reduction of RBC transfusions is associated with a decreased incidence of RBC alloimmunization. Transfusion 2003;43:945-952.
27. Billingham RE, Brent K, Medawar PB: Actively acquired tolerance of foreign cells. Nature 1953;172:603–606.
28. Opelz G, Terasaki PI. Poor kidney-transplant survival in recipients with frozen-blood transfusions or no transfusions. Lancet 1974;2: 696–698.
29. Borleffs JC, Neuhaus P, van Rood JJ, Balner H. Platelet transfusions improve kidney allograft survival in rhesus monkeys without inducing cytotoxic antibodies. Lancet 1982;1:1117–1118.
30. Phipps RP, Kaufman J, Blumberg N. Platelet derived CD154 (CD40 ligand) and febrile responses to transfusion. Lancet 2001;357: 2023–2024.
31. Blumberg N, Phipps RP, Kaufman J, Heal JM. The causes and treatment of reactions to platelet transfusions. Transfusion 2003;43:291–292.
32. Vandermast BJ, Balk AHMM. Effect of HLA-DR-shared blood transfusion on the clinical outcome of heart transplantation. Transplantation 1997;63:1514–1519.
33. Ishii E, Sumimoto R, Yamaguchi A. A role for MHC antigens in donor-specific blood transfusion for the inhibition of liver allograft rejection in the rat. Transplantation 1992;54:750–752.
34. Fernandez FG, Jaramillo A, Ewald G, et al. Blood transfusions decrease the incidence of acute rejection in cardiac allograft recipients. J Heart Lung Transplant 2005;24(7 Suppl):S255–S261.
35. Williams JG, Hughes LE. Effect of perioperative blood transfusion on recurrence of Crohn's disease. Lancet 1989;2:131–133.
36. van der Horst-Bruinsma IE, Huizinga TWJ, Lagaay EM, et al. The influence of a partially HLA-matched blood transfusion on the disease activity of rheumatoid arthritis. Rheumatology 1999;38:53–58.
37. Scott ADN, Ritchie JK, Phillips RKS. Blood transfusion and recurrent Crohn's disease. Br J Surg 1991;78:455–458.
38. Smith JB, Fort JG. Treatment of rheumatoid arthritis by immunization with mononuclear white blood cells: results of a preliminary trial. J Rheumatol 1996;23:220–225.
39. Raghupathy R, Makhseed M, Azizieh F, et al. Cytokine production by maternal lymphocytes during normal human pregnancy and in unexplained recurrent spontaneous abortion. Hum Reprod 2000;15:713–718.
40. Wegmann TG, Lin H, Guilbert L, Mosmann TR. Bidirectional cytokine interactions in the maternal-fetal relationship: is successful pregnancy a T_H2 phenomenon? Immunol Today 1993;14:353–356.
41. Biology of transfusion-induced immunosuppression: proceedings of a symposium, Snowbird, Utah, January 20–23, 1988. Transplant Proc 1988;20:1065–1208.
42. Francis DM, Shenton BK. Blood transfusion and tumour growth: evidence from laboratory animals. Lancet 1981;2:871.
43. Tartter PI. Does blood transfusion predispose to cancer recurrence? Am J Clin Oncol 1989;12:169–172.
44. Blumberg N, Heal JM. Transfusion and host defenses against cancer recurrence and infection. Transfusion 1989;29:236–245.
45. McGehee RP, Dodson MK, Moore JL, et al. Effect of blood transfusion in patients with gynecologic malignancy. Int J Gynecol Obstet 1994;46:45–52.
46. Little AG, Wu H-S, Ferguson MK, et al. Perioperative blood transfusion adversely affects prognosis of patients with stage I non-small-cell lung cancer. Am J Surg 1990;160:630–633.
47. Newman TB, Browner WS, Hulley SB. Enhancing causal inference in observational studies. In Hulley SB, Cummings SR (eds). Designing Clinical Research. Baltimore, Williams & Wilkins, 1988, pp 98–109.
48. Elwood JM. Causal Relationships in Medicine. Oxford, Oxford University Press, 1988.
49. Osanto S, Jansen R, Naipal AM, et al. In vivo effects of combination treatment with recombinant interferon-gamma and -alpha in metastatic melanoma. Int J Cancer 1989;43:1001–1006.
50. Bakker W, Nijhuis-Heddes JM, Wever AM, et al. Postoperative intrapleural BCG in lung cancer: lack of efficacy and possible enhancement of tumour growth. Thorax 1981;36:870–874.
51. Balkwill F, Mantovani A. Inflammation and cancer: back to Virchow? Lancet 2001;357:539–545.
52. Ohm JE, Carbone DP. Immune dysfunction in cancer patients. Oncology 2002;16(Suppl):11–18.
53. Blumberg N, Heal JM, Murphy P, et al. Association between transfusion of whole blood and recurrence of cancer. BMJ 1986;293:530–533.
54. Blumberg N, Heal JM, Chuang C, et al. Further evidence supporting a cause and effect relationship between blood transfusion and cancer recurrence. Ann Surg 1988;207:410–415.
55. Blumberg N, Chuang-Stein C, Heal JM. The relationship of blood transfusion, tumor staging, and cancer recurrence. Transfusion 1990; 30:291–294.
56. Heiss MM, Mempel W, Delanoff C, et al. Blood transfusion-modulated tumor recurrence: first results of a randomized study of autologous versus allogeneic blood transfusion in colorectal cancer surgery. J Clin Oncol 1994;12:1859–1867.
57. Busch ORC, Hop WCJ, Hoynck van Papendrecht MAW, et al. Blood transfusions and prognosis in colorectal cancer. N Engl J Med 1993; 328:1372–1376.
58. Houbiers JGA, Brand A, Van de Watering LMG, et al. Randomised controlled trial comparing transfusion of leucocyte-depleted or buffy-coat-depleted blood in surgery for colorectal cancer. Lancet 1994;344:573–578.
59. Jensen LS, Puho E, Pedersen L, et al. Long-term survival after colorectal surgery associated with buffy-coat-poor and leucocyte-depleted blood transfusion: a follow-up study. Lancet 2005;365:681–682.

60. Blumberg N, Heal JM, Rowe JM. A randomized trial of washed red blood cell and platelet transfusions in adult acute leukemia. BMC Blood Disord 2004;4:6.
61. Tartter PI, Quintero S, Barron DM. Perioperative blood transfusion associated with infectious complications after colorectal cancer operations. Am J Surg 1986;152:479–482.
62. Triulzi DJ, Blumberg N, Heal JM. Association of transfusion with postoperative bacterial infection. CRC Crit Rev Clin Lab Sci 1990;28:95–107.
63. Jensen LS, Andersen A, Fristrup SC, et al. Comparison of one dose *versus* three doses of prophylactic antibiotics, and the influence of blood transfusion, on infectious complications in acute and elective colorectal surgery. Br J Surg 1990;77:513–518.
64. Vamvakas EC, Carven JH. Transfusion of white-cell-containing allogeneic blood components and postoperative wound infection: effect of confounding factors. Transfus Med 1998;8:29–36.
65. Goodnough LT, Johnston MFM, Toy PTCY, Grp TMAA. The variability of transfusion practice in coronary artery bypass surgery. JAMA 1991;265:86–90.
66. Vamvakas EC, Carven JH. Transfusion of white-cell-containing allogeneic blood components and postoperative wound infection: effect of confounding factors. Transfus Med 1998;8:29–36.
67. Concato J, Horwitz RI. Beyond randomised versus observational studies. Lancet 2004;363:1660–1661.
68. Triulzi DJ, Vanek K, Ryan DH, Blumberg N. A clinical and immunologic study of blood transfusion and postoperative bacterial infection in spinal surgery. Transfusion 1992;32:517–524.
69. Murphy P, Heal JM, Blumberg N. Infection or suspected infection after hip replacement surgery with autologous or homologous blood transfusions. Transfusion 1991;31:212–217.
70. Titlestad IL, Ebbesen LS, Ainsworth AP, et al. Leukocyte-depletion of blood components does not significantly reduce the risk of infectious complications: results of a double-blinded, randomized study. Int J Colorect Dis 2001;16:147–153.
71. Bilgin YM, van de Watering LMG, Lorinser JE, et al. The effects of prestorage leukocyte-depletion of erythrocyte concentrates in cardiac surgery: a double-blind randomized clinical trial. Blood 2001; 98:828a.
72. Bilgin YM, van de Watering LM, Eijsman L, et al. Double-blind, randomized controlled trial on the effect of leukocyte-depleted erythrocyte transfusions in cardiac valve surgery. Circulation 2004;109: 2755–2760.
73. van Hilten JA, van de Watering LM, van Bockel JH, et al. Effects of transfusion with red cells filtered to remove leucocytes: randomised controlled trial in patients undergoing major surgery. BMJ 2004; 328:1281.
74. Blumberg N, Fine L, Gettings KF, Heal JM. Decreased sepsis related to indwelling venous access devices coincident with implementation of universal leukoreduction of blood transfusions. Transfusion 2005;45:1632–1639.
75. Maetani S, Nishikawa T, Tobe T, Hirakawa A. Role of blood transfusion in organ system failure following major abdominal surgery. Ann Surg 1986;203:275–281.
76. Zallen G, Offner PJ, Moore EE, et al. Age of transfused blood is an independent risk factor for postinjury multiple organ failure. Am J Surg 1999;178:570–572.
77. Moore FA, Moore EE, Sauaia A. Blood transfusion: an independent risk factor for postinjury multiple organ failure. Arch Surg 1997;132:620–625.
78. Spiess BD, Royston D, Levy JH, et al. Platelet transfusions during coronary artery bypass graft surgery are associated with serious adverse outcomes. Transfusion 2004;44:1143–1148.
79. Mangano DT. Aspirin and mortality from coronary bypass surgery. N Engl J Med 2002;347:1309–1317.
80. Rios JA, Korones DN, Heal JM, Blumberg N. WBC-reduced blood transfusions and clinical outcome in children with acute lymphoid leukemia. Transfusion 2001;41:873–877.
81. Cook D, Crowther M, Meade M, et al. Deep venous thrombosis in medical-surgical critically ill patients: prevalence, incidence, and risk factors. Crit Care Med 2005;33:1565–1571.
82. Vanderlinde E, Kaufman J, Phipps R, Blumberg N. CD40 Ligand accumulation during storage of human platelet concentrates: implications for transfusion complications. Blood 2001;98:112b.
83. Blumberg N, Boshkov LK, Silliman CC, et al. CD40 ligand (CD154) as a cofactor in the development of transfusion related acute lung injury. Blood 2004;104:237a–238a.
84. Tadros T, Wobbes T, Hendriks T. Blood transfusion impairs the healing of experimental intestinal anastomoses. Ann Surg 1992;215:276–281.
85. Chmell MJ, Schwartz HS. Analysis of variables affecting wound healing after musculoskeletal sarcoma resections. J Surg Oncol 1996;61:185–189.
86. Golub R, Golub RW, Cantu R, Stein HD. A multivariate analysis of factors contributing to leakage of intestinal anastomoses. J Am Coll Surg 1997;184:364–372.
87. Apostolidis SA, Michalopoulos AA, Hytiroglou PM, et al. Prevention of blood-transfusion-induced impairment of anastomotic healing by leucocyte depletion in rats. Eur J Surg 2000;166:562–567.
88. Vamvakas EC, Carven JH. Transfusion and postoperative pneumonia in coronary artery bypass graft surgery: effect of the length of storage of transfused red cells. Transfusion 1999;39:701–710.
89. Biffl WL, Moore EE, Offner PJ, et al. Plasma from aged stored red blood cells delays neutrophil apoptosis and primes for cytotoxicity: abrogation by poststorage washing but not prestorage leukoreduction. J Trauma 2001;50:426–431.
90. Mynster T. Blood transfusion-induced immunomodulation: is storage time important? Dan Med Bull 2003;50:368–384.
91. Blumberg N, Heal JM, Hicks GL, Risher WH. Association of ABO-mismatched platelet transfusions with morbidity and mortality in cardiac surgery. Transfusion 2001;41:790–793.
92. Blumberg N, Heal JM. ABO-mismatched platelet transfusions and clinical outcomes after cardiac surgery. Transfusion 2002;42:1527–1528; author reply 8–9.
93. Heal JM, Liesveld JL, Phillips GL, Blumberg N. What would Karl Landsteiner do? The ABO blood group and stem cell transplantation. Bone Marrow Transplant 2005;12:307–308.
94. Blumberg N, Heal JM. Evidence for plasma-mediated immunomodulation: transfusions of plasma-rich blood components are associated with a greater risk of acquired immunodeficiency syndrome than transfusions of red blood cells alone. Transplant Proc 1988;20: 1138–1142.
95. Preiksaitis JK, Brown L, McKenzie M. The risk of cytomegalovirus infection in seronegative transfusion recipients not receiving exogenous immunosuppression. J Infect Dis 1988;157:523–529.
96. Collier AC, Kalish LA, Busch MP, et al. Leukocyte-reduced red blood cell transfusions in patients with anemia and human immunodeficiency virus infection: The Viral Activation Transfusion Study: A randomized controlled trial. JAMA 2001;285:592–601.
97. Cerhan JR, Wallace RB, Dick F, et al. Blood transfusions and risk of non-Hodgkin's lymphoma subtypes and chronic lymphocytic leukemia. Cancer Epidemiol Biomarkers Prevent 2001;10:361–368.
98. Blumberg N, Heal JM. The transfusion immunomodulation theory: the Th1/Th2 paradigm and an analogy with pregnancy as a unifying mechanism. Semin Hematol 1996;33:329–340.
99. Felton LD. The significance of antigen in animal tissues. J Immunol 1949;61:107–117.
100. Kaliss N, Snell GD. The effects of injections of lyophilized normal and neoplastic mouse tissues on the growth of tumor homoiotransplants in mice. Cancer Res 1951;11:122–126.
101. Ghio M, Contini P, Mazzei C, et al. Soluble HLA class I, HLA class II, and Fas ligand in blood components: a possible key to explain the immunomodulatory effects of allogeneic blood transfusions. Blood 1999;93:1770–1777.
102. Assoian RK, Komoriya A, Meyers CA, et al: Transforming growth factor-beta in human platelets: identification of a major storage site, purification, and characterization. J Biol Chem 1983;258:7155–7160.
103. Henn V, Slupsky JR, Grafe M, et al. CD40 ligand on activated platelets triggers an inflammatory reaction of endothelial cells. Nature 1998; 391:591–594.
104. Banks RE, Forbes MA, Kinsey SE, et al. Release of the angiogenic cytokine vascular endothelial growth factor (VEGF) from platelets: significance for VEGF measurements and cancer biology. Br J Cancer 1998;77:956–964.
105. Ghio M, Ottonello L, Contini P, et al. Transforming growth factor-beta1 in supernatants from stored red blood cells inhibits neutrophil locomotion. Blood 2003;102:1100–1107.
106. Blumberg N, Heal JM. Transfusion and recipient immune function. Arch Pathol Lab Med 1989;113:246–253.
107. Blumberg N, Heal JM. Effects of transfusion on immune function: cancer recurrence and infection. Arch Pathol Lab Med 1994;118: 371–379.
108. Krensky AM, Clayberger C. Immunologic tolerance: tailored antigen. Transplant Proc 1996;28:2075–2077.
109. Buelow R, Burlingham WJ, Clayberger C. Immunomodulation by soluble HLA class I. Transplantation 1995;59:649–654.
110. Shelby J, Marushack MM, Nelson EW. Prostaglandin production and suppressor cell induction in transfusion-induced immune suppression. Transplantation 1987;43:113–116.
111. Dallman MJ, Wood KJ, Morris PJ. Recombinant interleukin-2 (IL-2) can reverse the blood transfusion effect. Transplant Proc 1989;21:1165–1167.

112. Kalechman Y, Gafter U, Sobelman D, Sredni B. The effect of a single whole-blood transfusion on cytokine secretion. J Clin Immunol 1990; 10:99–105.
113. Wood ML, Gottschalk R, Monaco AP. Effect of blood transfusion on IL-2 production. Transplantation 1988;45:930–935.
114. Gafter U, Kalechman Y, Sredni B. Blood transfusion enhances production of T-helper-2 cytokines and transforming growth factor β in humans. Clin Sci 1996;91:519–523.
115. Heiss MM, Fasolmerten K, Allgayer H, et al. Influence of autologous blood transfusion on natural killer and lymphokine-activated killer cell activities in cancer surgery. Vox Sang 1997;73:237–245.
116. Romagnani S. T-cell subsets (Th1 versus Th2) [Review]. Ann Allergy Asthma Immunol 2000;85:9–18.
117. Nielsen HJ, Hammer JH, Moesgaard F, Kehlet H. Comparison of the effects of SAG-M and whole-blood transfusions on postoperative suppression of delayed hypersensitivity. J Clin Cardiol 1991;34: 146–150.
118. Heiss MM, Mempel W, Jauch K-W, et al. Beneficial effect of autologous blood transfusion on infectious complications after colorectal cancer surgery. Lancet 1993;342:1328–1333.
119. Decker D, Schöndorf M, Bidlingmaier F, et al. Surgical stress induces a shift in the type-1/type-2 T-helper cell balance, suggesting down-regulation of cell-mediated and up-regulation of antibody-mediated immunity commensurate to the trauma. Surgery 1996;119:316–325.
120. Heiss MM, Fraunberger P, Delanoff C, et al. Modulation of immune response by blood transfusion: evidence for a differential effect of allogeneic and autologous blood in colorectal cancer surgery. Shock 1997;8:402–408.
121. Jensen LS, Hokland M, Nielsen HJ. A randomized controlled study of the effect of bedside leucocyte depletion on the immunosuppressive effect of whole blood transfusion in patients undergoing elective colorectal surgery. Br J Surg 1996;83:973–977.
122. Hotchkiss RS, Chang KC, Grayson MH, et al. Adoptive transfer of apoptotic splenocytes worsens survival, whereas adoptive transfer of necrotic splenocytes improves survival in sepsis. Proc Natl Acad Sci USA 2003;100:6724–6729.
123. Mincheff M. Changes in donor leukocytes during blood storage: implications on post-transfusion immunomodulation and transfusion-associated GVHD. Vox Sang 1998;74(Suppl 2):189–200.
124. Steinman RM, Turley S, Mellman I, Inaba K. The induction of tolerance by dendritic cells that have captured apoptotic cells. J Exp Med 2000;191:411–416.
125. Bratosin D, Estaquier J, Ameisen JC, Montreuil J. Molecular and cellular mechanisms of erythrocyte programmed cell death: impact on blood transfusion. Vox Sang 2002;83(Suppl 1):307–310.
126. Dzik S, Mincheff M, Puppo F. Apoptosis, transforming growth factor-beta, and the immunosuppressive effect of transfusion. Transfusion 2002;42:1221–1223.
127. Silliman CC, Ambruso DR, Boshkov LK. Transfusion-related acute lung injury. Blood 2005;105:2266–2273.
128. Goodnough LT, Shander A, Spence R. Bloodless medicine: clinical care without allogeneic blood transfusion. Transfusion 2003;43:668–676.
129. Blumberg N, Zhao H, Messing S, et al. Misapplication of the intention to treat principle in clinical trials and meta-analyses of leukoreduced blood transfusions in surgical patients. Blood 2003;102:562a.
130. Simchen E, Zucker D, Siegman IY, Galai N. Method for separating patient and procedural factors while analyzing interdepartmental differences in rates of surgical infections: the Israeli study of surgical infection in abdominal operations. J Clin Epidemiol 1996;49:1003–1007.
131. Dzik WH, Anderson JK, O'Neill EM, et al. A prospective, randomized clinical trial of universal WBC reduction. Transfusion 2002;42:1114–1122.
132. Blumberg N. Allogeneic transfusion and infection: economic and clinical implications. Semin Hematol 1997;34(3 Suppl 2):34–40.
133. Vamvakas EC. Transfusion-associated cancer recurrence and postoperative infection: meta-analysis of randomized, controlled clinical trials. Transfusion 1996;36:175–186.
134. Vamvakas EC. Transfusion-associated cancer recurrence and postoperative infection: meta-analysis of randomized, controlled clinical trials. Transfusion 1996;36:175–186.
135. Vamvakas EC, Blajchman MA. Prestorage versus poststorage white cell reduction for the prevention of the deleterious immunomodulatory effects of allogeneic blood transfusion [Review]. Transfus Med Rev 2000;14:23–33.
136. Vamvakas EC, Blajchman MA. Prestorage versus poststorage white cell reduction for the prevention of the deleterious immunomodulatory effects of allogeneic blood transfusion. Transfus Med Rev 2000;14:23–33.
137. Vamvakas EC, Blajchman MA. Deleterious clinical effects of transfusion-associated immunomodulation: fact or fiction? [Review]. Blood 2001;97:1180–1195.
138. Vamvakas EC, Blajchman MA. Universal WBC reduction: the case for and against [Review]. Transfusion 2001;41:691–712.
139. Vamvakas EC. Meta-analysis of randomized controlled trials investigating the risk of postoperative infection in association with white blood cell-containing allogeneic blood transfusion: the effects of the type of transfused red blood cell product and surgical setting. Transfus Med Rev 2002;16:304–314.
140. Petitti DB. Approaches to heterogeneity in meta-analysis. Stat Med 2001;20:3625–3633.
141. Fergusson D, Khanna MP, Tinmouth A, Hebert PC. Transfusion of leukoreduced red blood cells may decrease postoperative infections: two meta-analyses of randomized controlled trials. Can J Anaesth 2004;51:417–424.
142. Baron JF, Gourdin M, Bertrand M, et al. The effect of universal leukodepletion of packed red blood cells on postoperative infections in high-risk patients undergoing abdominal aortic surgery. Anesth Analg 2002;94:529–537.
143. Volkova N, Klapper E, Pepkowitz SH, et al. A case-control study of the impact of WBC reduction on the cost of hospital care for patients undergoing coronary artery bypass graft surgery. Transfusion 2002;42:123–126.
144. Blumberg N, Heal JM, Cowles JW, et al. Leukocyte-reduced transfusions in cardiac surgery results of an implementation trial. Am J Clin Pathol 2002;118:376–381.
145. Fung MK, Rao N, Rice J, et al. Leukoreduction in the setting of open heart surgery: A prospective cohort-controlled study. Transfusion 2004;44:30–35.
146. Llewelyn CA, Taylor RS, Todd AA, et al. The effect of universal leukoreduction on postoperative infections and length of hospital stay in elective orthopedic and cardiac surgery. Transfusion 2004;44:489–500.
147. Fergusson D, Hebert PC, Lee SK, et al. Clinical outcomes following institution of universal leukoreduction of blood transfusions for premature infants. JAMA 2003;289:1950–1956.
148. Hebert PC, Fergusson D, Blajchman MA, et al. Clinical outcomes following institution of the Canadian universal leukoreduction program for red blood cell transfusions. JAMA 2003;289:1941–1949.
149. Blumberg N, Heal JM. Mortality risks, costs, and decision making in transfusion medicine. Am J Clin Pathol 2000;114:934–937.
150. Jensen LS, Grunnet N, Hanberg-Sorensen F, Jorgensen J. Cost-effectiveness of blood transfusion and white cell reduction in elective colorectal surgery. Transfusion 1995;35:719–722.
151. Blumberg N, Kirkley SA, Heal JM. A cost analysis of autologous and allogeneic transfusions in hip-replacement surgery. Am J Surg 1996;171:324–330.
152. Blumberg N, Heal JM. Blood transfusion immunomodulation: the silent epidemic. Arch Pathol Lab Med 1998;122:117–119.
153. Horimi T, Terasaki PI, Chia D, Sasaki N. Factors influencing the paradoxical effect of transfusions on kidney transplants. Transplantation 1983;35:320–323.
154. Doll R, Peto R. Mortality in relation to smoking: 20 years' observations on male British doctors. BMJ 1976;2:1525–1536.
155. Mosmann TR, Sad S. The expanding universe of T-cell subsets: Th1, Th2 and more. Immunol Today 1996;17:138–146.

Chapter 53

Post-Transfusion Engraftment Syndromes: Microchimerism and TA-GVHD

William Reed • Eberhard W. Fiebig • Tzong-Hae Lee • Michael P. Busch

INTRODUCTION

Microchimerism (MC), defined as the stable presence of a minority of non-self cells in a host, and graft-versus-host disease (GVHD), a disorder marked by attack and destruction of recipient cells by engrafted donor immune cells, may be viewed as related conditions that differ dramatically in clinical significance. MC is an expected outcome after transplantation, may be observed under certain conditions after transfusion,[1–8] and is regularly present during pregnancy as a result of bidirectional trafficking of viable cells between fetus and mother.[9,10] Microchimerism has been viewed by some as a welcome sign of stable graft acceptance in solid organ transplant recipients and during pregnancy[11,12] and consequently has attracted attention as a model for investigating immune mechanisms of tolerance.[13,14] Maternal MC also offers an exciting new venue for fetal diagnosis.[15–18] In and of itself, MC after blood transfusion is not a threat to recipients, although no detailed clinical evaluation has yet been conducted of patients with transfusion-associated (TA)-MC. Given that approximately 10% of patients transfused for severe traumatic injury develop long-term TA-MC,[19–21] this is an important area for future research. GVHD, conversely, is a common complication in transplant patients[22–24] and poses a rare but very serious threat to transfusion recipients.[25,26]

In this chapter, we review the discovery and current status of our understanding of MC, with a focus on recent findings related to TA-MC. We also provide a concise review of transfusion-associated GVHD (TA-GVHD). The disease process and clinical presentation of TA-GVHD is also covered briefly to highlight the similarities and differences with TA-GVHD. A number of recent reviews specifically address basic science and clinical issues of GVHD in the transplant setting in greater detail for the interested reader.[24,27,28]

MICROCHIMERISM

A chimera is a creature that harbors cells or tissues derived from another individual. In Greek mythology, the chimera was a beast with a lion's head and foreparts, a goat's body, and a serpent's tail. Medical research on chimerism can be traced to Ray Owen, who was born on a Wisconsin dairy farm in 1915. After studying agriculture and animal husbandry at the University of Wisconsin, he joined the faculty in the Department of Genetics and turned his attention to the study of bovine blood groups. Owen was fascinated by Lillie's observations,[29] published in 1916, that "demonstrated union of the circulatory systems between twin bovine embryos of the opposite sex." Lillie had shown that hormones from a male fetus could enter the circulation of its female twin, producing developmental abnormalities of the reproductive system in the female twin. This "modified" female twin is called a *freemartin* and is an early example illustrating the effect of hormones on sexual development.

Owen examined 80 pairs of bovine twins for patterns of twinning, placental vascular anastomosis, and blood-group antigens.[30] Finding that the majority of twin pairs displayed identical blood-group patterns, Owen reasoned that neither chance nor monozygotic twinning could explain the blood-group concordance. Rather, the exchange of erythroid progenitor cells through the same vascular anastomoses that carried Lillie's hormones was likely to be responsible. This remarkable insight, attributable more to Owen's powers of observation than to available technology, changed biology[31] and introduced the notion of blood cell chimerism that was recognized by Dunsford and colleagues[32] in their early description of a human blood-group chimera.

At the tissue level, chimerism can occur with solid-organ transplantation or, in the research setting, when a portion of an animal embryo is grafted to another species during the early stages of development. This method has been used extensively to investigate the developmental biology of the nervous system.[33] In humans, organ transplant recipients are tissue chimeras and, because lymphoid tissue often accompanies a solid-organ graft, passenger leukocytes may be "co-transplanted" and go on to establish their lineage within the recipient.[11] If the tissue of interest is blood, chimerism of its cellular elements, hematopoietic chimerism, occurs readily when stem cells are transplanted. Hematopoietic chimerism is said to be complete when essentially all of the recipient's hematopoietic cells are replaced with cells derived from the donor; chimerism is said to be partial (or mixed) when a substantial proportion of donor cells is present along with those of the recipient. MC is said to exist when only a small proportion (<2.5%) of hematopoietic cells within a recipient are derived from the donor, although these terms are often used imprecisely in the literature.

MC has been demonstrated during pregnancy and is expected after stem cell transplantation. More recently, stable MC has also been demonstrated years after both blood transfusion and normal pregnancy. In each of these settings, MC has become established in the absence of any overt manipulation of host immunity. Because of these observations, which we explore in detail, a new conceptual relation is beginning to emerge to describe the relation between transfusion and transplantation, where transfusion is construed broadly to mean exposure to the viable mononuclear cells of another individual. This relation acknowledges a potential overlap between transfusion and transplantation. Despite this progress, no large scale formal study has used uniform sample collection and analytic methods of the prevalence and magnitude of MC in healthy populations as a function of specific allogeneic exposures. Table 53–1 illustrates this point by presenting a range of highly variable results for measured MC in various nonexposed populations. These types of data will be a critical base from which to advance our understanding of MC in the future.

Neither the conditions that permit stable MC in the setting of transfusion nor the biologic consequences of MC are yet understood. In some cases, MC appears to be an incidental finding in otherwise healthy individuals. In other cases, MC has been found in association with significant disease processes, including GVHD and adult-onset systemic sclerosis. In still other circumstances, chimerism may be a deliberate therapeutic strategy in transplantation or adoptive immunotherapy. Taken together, these data suggest a complex relation among allogeneic exposures, host immune factors, the development of MC, and the potential consequences of MC, either pathologic or therapeutic. We review methods for detection of blood cell MC before going on to discuss clinical studies that describe the presence of MC in various circumstances of health and disease, including blood transfusion.

Microchimerism Detection Methods

Karyotype, Microscopy, and Transfer Factor

Early studies of MC used karyotype analysis to identify allogeneic material.[5] This technique is convincing when it yields a positive result but is relatively insensitive and depends on laborious analysis of numerous individual cells and on male-female differences. The morphologic state of lymphocytes and the rate at which they take up thymidine have also been used to study transfusion-associated MC.[8] These important early studies by Schechter[4] first showed that transfused leukocytes caused lymphocyte activation in the recipient, and subsequent studies provided evidence that donor cells actually participate in the proliferative response. In 1969, Mohr and colleagues[34] reported on six patients who were shown to lack tuberculin sensitivity but received transfusions from donors with known sensitivity. When these investigators showed that each recipient transiently acquired the donor's tuberculin sensitivity after transfusion, great interest developed in "transfer factor." Transfer factor proved elusive to isolate or characterize but was suspected to be passenger leukocytes. Despite attempts to pursue these intriguing observations, detailed investigation would have to await the development of sensitive molecular methods, most often the polymerase chain reaction (PCR).

Polymerase Chain Reaction and Other Nucleic Acid–Based Detection Methods

Although PCR has extraordinary sensitivity derived from its ability to amplify a specific genetic sequence exponentially, the detection of a minor population of nucleic acid species against a highly similar genetic background present in vast excess is a technical problem for MC studies and requires unique PCR strategies to solve it. Several aspects of PCR methodology influence the detection of minor leukocyte populations. These features, summarized and annotated in Table 53–2, include the total input amount of nucleic acid in the assay, the degree and character of sequence differences distinguishing the minor and major nucleic acid population, whether the PCR strategy involves recognition of this sequence difference at the primer level or through probe specificity, preparation of isolated leukocytes or total DNA for analysis, whether quantitation is attempted, what methods are used for detection of amplified products, and finally, whether the reaction products are observed at each cycle (real-time or kinetic PCR) or only after the reaction is complete (end-point PCR).

We and others[35,36] have noted the possibility that primers that do not recognize the minor population as unique may be consumed early in the reaction through amplification of closely related sequences in the major population, which vastly outnumber the minor population sought; this would be expected to produce a false-negative MC assay. Thus, in our experience, the use of allele-specific primer pairs that recognize at least a two- to three-base-pair difference in the minor population is a superior approach and can usually be optimized for MC detection at levels as low as one chimeric cell per million host cells. Alternatively, a single-nucleotide polymorphism (SNP) can be used as an allogeneic target for detection of MC by PCR, but the detection sensitivity is reduced. Amplification strategies with less primer specificity

Table 53–1 Comparison of Reported MC Prevalence among Unexposed Healthy Populations

Lambert NC, et al[152]	Y-chr study of 26F SSC and 23 healthy never pregnant	15% of SSC+ MC+ 13% of healthy, never-pregnant women MC+
Yan Z, et al[153]	Quant Y-chr study of MC in healthy women and women with RA "without" sons	71 rheumatoid arthritis: 18% Y-chr pos 49 healthy: 24% y-chr pos Never pregnant, *n* = 48, 10% MC+ Daughters only, *n* = 26, 8% MC+ Spontaneous abortion, *n* = 23, 22% MC+ Induced abortion, *n* = 23, 57% MC+
Adams KM, et al[51]	Study of male DNA in female donor apheresis and CD34+ enriched products	29 GCSF-mobilized female HSC donors, 34% positive for Y-chromosome
Lee T-H, et al[84] Lee T-H, et al[3] Lee TH, et al[19]	Pretransfusion samples from 3 studies involving approximately 29 trauma and orthopedic patients. Both Y-chromosome and HLA methods	6 orthopedic: all negative (1995) 10 trauma non-LR: all negative (1999) 13 LR trauma: all negative (2005)

Table 53–2 Polymerase Chain Reaction Strategies and Assay Characteristics Influencing the Detection of Minor Leukocyte Populations (Microchimerism)

Characteristic	Options for Assay Development		
Degree of genetic difference between major and minor populations	Single-nucleotide polymorphism	Two- to four-base-pair difference	Wholly unique allogeneic sequence (e.g., X vs Y chromosome)
Primer specificity	Allele specific	Group specific	Locus specific
Observation of reaction	End reaction	End reaction labeled probe	Continuous by kinetic PCR (with or without specific hybridization probe)
Detection of amplified product	Sizing gel	Hybridization of amplified product using specific probe	DNA melting probe
Quantitation	None	Autoradiography standard dilutions	Cycle number by kinetic method

for the minor population are likely to be much less sensitive to the presence of MC because of nonspecific amplification of related host sequences. This principle is illustrated with the analysis of ex vivo cell mixtures in Table 53–3.[36]

Real-time PCR is a powerful strategy in which the accumulation of amplified product is observed at each amplification cycle rather than at the reaction's termination. This is accomplished by fluorometric quantitation of amplified product at the completion of each cycle. The detection chemistry may include direct intercalation of dyes such as ethidium bromide or SyBr green into accumulating double-stranded amplicons. Alternatively, TaqMan[37] or molecular beacon probes[38] can be used in detection. The advantages of real-time PCR techniques include ready quantitation of target sequence, because the copy number in the target analyte is directly related to the cycle number at which the reaction becomes positive. Real-time PCR assays based on dye intercalation, when properly validated, can achieve sensitivity and specificity the same as or better than labeled probe-based systems, at much lower cost.[39–41] However, probe-based systems offer the advantage of simultaneous detection of multiple target sequences, including internal control host sequences, if multiplexed PCR assays are optimized. Potential disadvantages of real-time PCR include the need for relatively expensive equipment and proprietary reagents. Furthermore, if probe hybridization is not used, the reaction product's precise identity may be less certain, although this can be addressed through proper assay validation, analysis of melting curves to confirm size of amplicons, and sequencing of reaction products where needed. Nested PCR methods have also been applied in analyses of MC.[42,43] Although the possibility for amplicon contamination with this method has led some groups to avoid it, nested PCR may provide some absolute advantage in sensitivity. Recent development of PCR assays based on insertion-deletion (InDel) polymorphisms[44] has provided an excellent new tool for chimerism analysis, both in the post-transplant setting and in the analysis of low-level chimerism in the research setting.[44a]

Nonamplification nucleic acid–detection methods such as fluorescence in situ hybridization (FISH) have also been applied to the detection of MC. The limited range of sensitivity of FISH derives from the need to analyze individual cells laboriously, making this method more suitable for detection of higher-level MC, such as in the post-transplantation setting. FISH has been valuable as an independent method to confirm MC demonstrated by PCR, and to study pathogenetic mechanisms by characterizing phenotypes of MC cells and interactions between donor and host cells in tissues. Microsatellite markers and analysis of variable-number tandem repeats (VNTRs) have also been widely used in chimerism analyses, but, like FISH, are generally suited to analysis of higher-level (mixed) chimerism encountered in the stem cell transplantation setting.[45]

Table 53–3 Proportion of Chimeric Cell Populations Detected in Ex Vivo Cell Mixtures as a Function of Amplification Strategy

Amplification strategy	Percentage Allogeneic (Chimeric) Cell Composition			
	10%	1%	0.1%	0.01%
Locus specific	17/18	0/16	0/18	1/17
Group specific	21/21	21/21	21/21	16/21
Allele specific	12/12	21/21	21/21	21/21

Rare Event Analysis and Stochastic Detection

When the minor leukocyte population sought is present only at extremely low levels, detection of MC may become stochastic; that is, allogeneic material may or may not be present in the limited sample volume processed for analysis in a single PCR reaction. Attempts to amplify much more than 10 μg of DNA in a single reaction predictably lead to PCR inhibition. To approach this problem of stochastic detection, larger volumes of blood must be analyzed in multiple parallel aliquots under identical reaction conditions. Such enhanced input assay methods are probably necessary to give meaning to a negative result in the study of rare events,[46] such as very low level MC.

Clinical Studies of Microchimerism

Microchimerism in Hematopoietic Stem Cell Products

Hematopoietic stem cell (HSC) products include bone marrow, cord blood, and mobilized peripheral blood. It has long been known that an increased risk for GVHD exists when the donor is a parous woman. As cord blood began to be used for clinical transplant, concern was raised that maternal cells in the product could include immunocompetent T lymphocytes that might increase the risk for GVHD in recipients. Although studies have documented maternal cells in cord blood–derived stem cell products,[47–50] these MC cells do not seem to play an important role in GVHD after cord blood transplantation. Recently, Adams[51] reported that in a study of 29 growth factor–mobilized peripheral blood mononuclear cell (G-PBMC) products from female donors, 34% were positive for male DNA, including CD34$^+$-enriched fractions, presumably derived from male fetuses during previous pregnancies. Although more study is needed, the authors suggested that these chimeric cells may contribute to the incidence of GVHD after transplant with marrow or mobilized peripheral blood from parous female donors.

Bidirectional Microchimerism at the Maternal-Fetal Interface

During pregnancy, exchange of blood across the placenta occurs in both directions. We review several key clinical studies of MC at the maternal-fetal interface.

Lo and associates[10] were the first to document the bidirectional nature of this phenomenon in an analysis of 66 mother-child pairs studied at the time of parturition. The investigators used PCR assays targeting several common polymorphisms, including Y chromosome, β-globin variants, and glutathione S-transferase genotypes. They found fetal cells in the maternal peripheral blood in 26 of 51 informative cases. Maternal cells were detectable in the corresponding placental blood in 16 of 38 informative cases. The authors found no obvious pattern to the directionality of cell trafficking, although relatively few of the cases were informative in both directions, and the genetic markers used did not include human leukocyte antigen (HLA) alleles, so maternal-fetal histocompatibility, a factor thought by some to be potentially important in determining cell persistence, could not be examined.

Bianchi and colleagues[9] studied 32 pregnant women and 8 nonpregnant control women who had given birth to a male fetus 6 months to 27 years earlier. Flow sorting was applied to these samples to isolate leukocyte subpopulations, including a stem-cell progenitor fraction; these were then analyzed for Y chromosome–specific sequences by using nested and non-nested PCR techniques. Thirteen of 19 currently pregnant women were positive for male DNA in the sorted CD34+ fraction, whereas 4 of 13 nonpregnant women were also positive. Because the latter women had a history of either male pregnancy or termination of pregnancy of unknown gender, the positive results were interpreted to indicate that male cells can persist as long as 27 years postpartum in some pregnant females. This study, although quite convincing overall, suffered from the absence of control samples from prepubertal females.

Lo and coworkers[52–54] in Hong Kong have extensively studied the presence of fetal DNA in maternal plasma and serum. Studying 43 pregnant women who delivered male infants, they found Y chromosome–specific DNA in 24 (80%) of 30 maternal plasma samples and in 21 (70%) of 30 serum samples, whereas no positive results occurred among non-pregnant control women or among women carrying female fetuses. These and other findings led Lo's group to approach the clinical problem of determining the Rh D genotype of a fetus carried by an Rh-negative mother through analysis of circulating DNA in the maternal plasma.[55] Among 42 women in the second or third trimester, they obtained perfect concordance for Rh type compared with serologic postnatal Rh typing. Among the 15 first-trimester women, Rh typing was concordant in 13, with two Rh-positive fetuses yielding false-negative PCR results. A recent clinical study by Brojer and others.[56,57] involving 255 Rh D–negative pregnant women found that 90% of samples were suitable for analysis (based on presence of fetal DNA by using a non–Rh D marker) and that prenatal typing had a 99.6% predictive value. Quantitative study by our group of the time course of fetal DNA in the maternal circulation during pregnancy demonstrated that much more fetal DNA exists in the plasma than in the leukocyte compartment, and that copy number increases to its highest levels during the third trimester before decreasing precipitately at parturition.[58] Whether this plasma DNA is derived from trophoblasts, fetal leukocytes, or parenchymal tissues is not known.

Because plasma DNA from a pregnant woman contains a mixture of maternal and fetal DNA, many groups have pursued the isolation of fetal cells from the maternal circulation as a more definitive source for fetal DNA. Trophoblastic cells are uniquely fetal in origin but have proved difficult to isolate reliably because of the paucity of specific cell surface markers for sorting; another consideration is that 1% of pregnancies display chorionic mosaicism in which the placenta, but not the fetus, manifests cytogenetic abnormalities. Leukocyte fractions of fetal origin may be isolated from the maternal circulation, but the occasional persistence of cells in the CD34+ progenitor population from a prior pregnancy raises concern about the possibility of an erroneous result. The fetal nucleated erythrocyte has drawn attention as perhaps the cell best suited for prenatal diagnosis. These cells enter the maternal circulation in relatively high numbers (~1000:1 compared with fetal leukocytes) early in pregnancy, carry a full complement of fetal genomic DNA, and should not persist from prior pregnancies. These cells are just beginning to be isolated and studied systematically for their potential value in prenatal diagnosis.[59,60] Analysis of fetal RNA in maternal plasma also has opened the possibility of profiling fetal gene expression noninvasively.[61] Circulating DNA and RNA have also been investigated widely as markers for certain cancers that produce high levels of tumor-derived nucleic acids in the circulation or other body fluids.[62]

Fetal Microchimerism and Autoimmune Diseases

A report from France in 1998 examined archival skin biopsy material from 10 women with a skin rash, polymorphous eruption of pregnancy (PEP), who later gave birth to male infants.[59] Male DNA could be demonstrated in the skin of 6 of the 10 women with PEP but in none of an extensive set of control subjects. Investigators used microdissection techniques to separate dermis from epidermis and were able to show that both were positive for fetal DNA, strongly arguing that the PCR signal did not originate from trapped circulating blood cells; having no blood vessels, the epidermis' only cellular source is the dermis. Although a PEP rash typically regresses after parturition, this elegant study provided a precedent for the idea that chimeric fetal cells may infiltrate maternal tissue and cause a pathologic reaction.

The clear similarities between clinical features of chronic GVHD and adult-onset systemic scleroderma have long led to speculation that the conditions may be related. Although the etiology of scleroderma remains unknown, application of molecular analyses is providing a convincing case that male cells are often present in the circulation and skin lesions of adult females with scleroderma. Although these allogeneic cells exist at very low levels, they have been found more often and in greater number among scleroderma cases than among control subjects.

Nelson and colleagues[63] described their findings in a study of 40 women, all of whom had given birth to at least one male infant. They studied 17 scleroderma patients, 16 healthy controls, and 7 sisters of the scleroderma patients. Histocompatibility between mother and fetus was assessed for an additional 21 patients, 32 controls, and their combined total of 105 offspring. Processing large volumes of whole blood for stochastic detection, these workers found a mean of 0.38 male genomic equivalents per 16 mL of whole blood among controls compared with 11.1 among women with scleroderma ($P = 0.0007$). In analyzing the histocompatibility data, they found that DR compatibility between mother and fetus was significantly more prevalent among scleroderma mother-child pairs than among control pairs, suggesting that DR compatibility facilitated MC while not providing an absolute requirement. They concluded that MC may be involved in the pathogenesis of scleroderma.

Artlett and colleagues[64] used a nonquantitative Y chromosome PCR to study peripheral blood and paraffin-embedded skin biopsy material from 69 women with systemic scleroderma. Thirty-two (46%) of the peripheral blood samples had demonstrable Y chromosome sequences compared with only 1 (4%) of 25 in normal women. FISH was used as an independent technique to confirm the PCR findings. Nucleated cells displaying a Y chromosome signal on FISH were demonstrable in all skin biopsy material found by PCR to contain Y chromosome sequences. The authors concluded that fetal antimaternal GVHD reactions may be involved in the pathogenesis of scleroderma for some female patients.

To follow up their earlier findings, Nelson's group used Y chromosome PCR to study subpopulations of peripheral blood lymphocytes highly enriched for CD3, CD19, CD14, and CD56/16 by flow-cytometric sorting.[65] Allogeneic cells were present in 12 of 20 women with scleroderma and 16 of 48 healthy control women ($P = 0.046$). No significant differences between immunophenotypic subsets were observed. The authors concluded that the finding of persistent, presumably fetal cells in these women suggested the existence of specific immunoregulatory pathways that allowed persistence while preventing effector function.

Blood transfusion has been identified, in some studies, as a significant risk factor for the development of rheumatoid arthritis,[66] and several groups have speculated that MC from pregnancy or transfusion may play a role in other "autoimmune" diseases, including rheumatoid arthritis and multiple sclerosis.[67] Much work remains to be done in the area of MC and autoimmune disease before a definitive causal relation is established, however. If MC cells are reproducibly present and etiologically involved, it is important to elucidate the mechanism by which so few allogeneic cells contribute to the pathogenesis of complex autoimmune disorders. Such work could lead to novel therapeutic strategies to suppress MC-mediated pathologic conditions.

The converse of fetal cells establishing MC in the mother occurs when maternal cells may cross the placenta to establish MC in the fetus and newborn. Many fewer data are available in this area. Evidence of maternal MC persisting to adult life has been published.[68] A few very small studies have examined the presence of maternal cells in aborted fetuses.[69,70] Recently, maternal cells have been associated with autoimmune syndromes in the newborn and children.[71–74] Much more work is needed in this interesting area and should be possible with improvements to the FISH technique and the availability of PCR assays for MC, such as InDel, which are not restricted to Y-chromosome or class II HLA and are not linked to the immune-response genes.

Microchimerism Associated with Solid Organ Transplantation and Stability of Pregnancy

In solid organ transplantation, MC has been attributed to engraftment of donor hematopoietic stem cells that reside in the transplanted organ.[11] After surgery, the donor cells migrate from the transplanted organ to recipient tissues throughout the body and also enter the circulation, where they may be detected as a minor cell population. In the transplant setting, establishment of MC has been viewed by some as a welcome sign of successful transplantation and a predictor of stable engraftment of the transplanted organ,[11] although others have questioned the validity of this assumption.[75] Fetal cell MC in maternal blood and tissues may similarly play a role in the establishment of immunologic tolerance that is required for successful pregnancy.[10,11,59] These observations have led to large-scale clinical evaluations of protocols in which allogeneic peripheral blood or bone marrow–derived cells are infused into patients undergoing solid organ transplantation[76,77] and into women with recurrent spontaneous abortions[78,79] in an effort to induce tolerance or reverse alloimmunization. Interest is found in development of strategies for establishing MC and immunologic tolerance to facilitate novel therapies with genetically modified allogeneic cells.[80] It has even been suggested that fetal progenitor cells may participate in the repair of injured maternal tissues.[81]

Transfusion-Associated Microchimerism

Studies by Schechter and coworkers[4,8] first demonstrated that transfusion of fresh blood is associated with transient appearance of donor leukocytes in recipients (detected by karyotype analyses) with associated recipient immune activation. In their seminal article, they[8] reported the transient appearance (days 3 to 7 after transfusion) of activated, proliferating lymphocytes in the circulation of recipients of fresh whole blood (but not frozen-deglycerolized blood). In a follow-up study, they[4] used karyotype analysis to show that, whereas the majority of proliferating lymphocytes were recipient cells, occasional donor lymphocytes were also detectable at the time of peak activation. On the basis of these data, they hypothesized that transfusion of blood containing viable donor lymphocytes results in a two-way proliferation reaction, representing an attempted GVH reaction by donor cells and graft rejection by recipient cells. Adams and colleagues[6] were among the first to deploy molecular methods for detection of donor leukocytes after transfusion. They studied 20 female patients undergoing major surgical procedures to monitor prospectively the presence of male donor leukocytes by using Y chromosome–specific PCR. The assays were nonquantitative analyses of total extracted DNA and demonstrated male sex–determining region Y (SRY) sequences up to 6 days after transfusion. A Dutch group reported a retrospective study of 21 renal transplant recipients by using samples archived from donor-specific transfusions given before renal transplantation. They analyzed the presence of donor DNA by using nested PCR based on HLA-DRB1 polymorphisms, and found that in some patients, especially those receiving blood from a partially HLA-matched donor, donor leukocytes could be detected up to 8 weeks after transfusion.[7] Hutchinson[5,82] studied the persistence of leukocytes transfused to 14 neonates from their maternal donors and compared the results with those in 48 neonates transfused with banked blood whose donors were also sex discordant. By using karyotype to identify donor cells, this group found that maternal donor cells persisted for ≥2 years in 4 of the 14 neonates, whereas no donor cells were detectable in those receiving banked blood. It remained unclear whether histocompatibility or freshness of the transfused product contributed to these observations. In 2000, Vietor and colleagues[83] reported on 10 recipients of sex-mismatched intrauterine transfusion (IUT) of unmodified red blood cells (RBCs) up to 25 years earlier. Although all of the recipients were in good general health and none had evidence of TA-MC by sex chromosome in situ hybridization, 6 of 7 had evidence of TA-MC by Y-chromosome PCR. The authors concluded that IUT could result in persistence of donor cells for ≥20 years, but this was not associated with signs of immunologic aberration.

After the work of Schechter and coworkers cited earlier,[4,8] our group used quantitative allele-specific PCR methods developed specifically for the detection of TA-MC to characterize more precisely the kinetics of donor leukocyte persistence in transfused adult women undergoing elective orthopedic surgery.[84] Each patient had received fresh unmodified packed RBCs from a male donor; both Y chromosome and class II allele-specific PCR assays were used to detect and quantitate donor leukocytes. We demonstrated a 1000-fold expansion of allogeneic donor leukocytes in the recipient's circulation 3 to 5 days after transfusion.[84] The allogeneic cells were cleared from the circulation within 2 weeks. The finding was also corroborated in a canine transfusion model[85] by irradiation of the transfused blood, which abrogated the donor leukocyte expansion phase.

Building on these findings, our group has now documented high-level and long-lasting leukocyte MC among selected victims of traumatic injury who received a large number of fresh units of blood during their resuscitation.[3] Whereas very low levels of chimeric cells were observed in scleroderma patients or after transfusions in patients having elective surgery, in these trauma patients, 3% to 4% of peripheral blood leukocytes were of donor origin, and the donor cells persisted at high levels for as long as 2 years after transfusion. Analysis of lymphocyte subsets from these recipients by using immunomagnetic bead enrichment showed that both lymphoid and myeloid lineages were represented. In some cases, HLA typing of the donor combined with MC assays based on class II polymorphisms showed a single donor to be the sole source of the chimeric leukocytes. Figure 53–1 illustrates the transient expansion of donor leukocytes in elective orthopedic surgery patients versus the long-term high-level multilineage TA-MC, which becomes established in some trauma patients after transfusion.

In a more recent study of 45 transfused trauma patients, half had detectable, though low-level, TA-MC at hospital discharge, whether or not they had received exclusively leukoreduced blood products.[20] Immunologic characterization of these patients at hospital admission showed broad

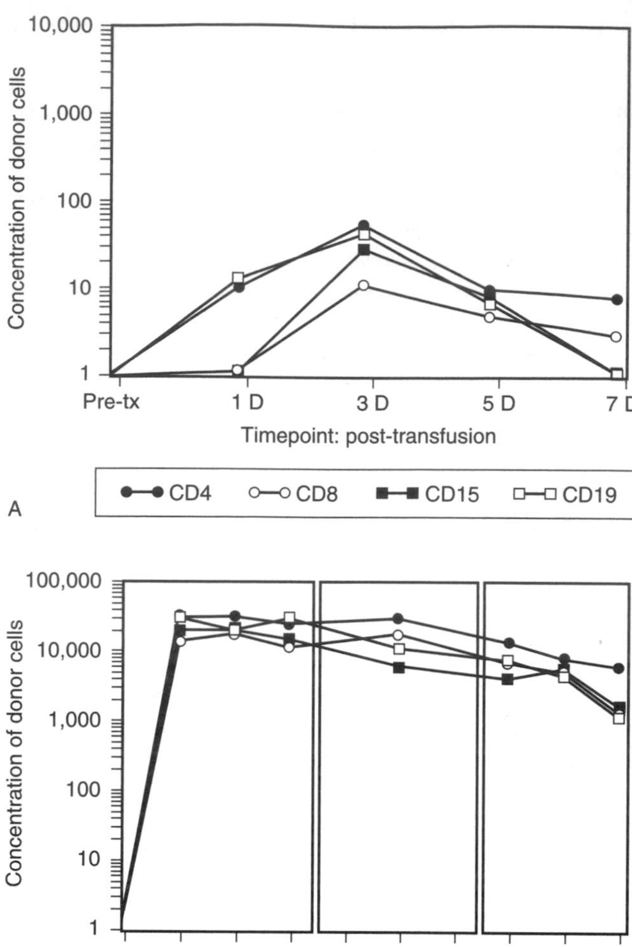

Figure 53–1 Representative survival kinetics of donor leukocyte subpopulations (including CD4, CD8, CD15, and CD19) after transfusion of female patients for (**A**) elective surgery and (**B**) severe trauma. Frozen whole blood samples were subjected to enrichment of CD4+, CD8+, CD15+, and CD19+ leukocytes subpopulations, followed by amplification, hybridization, and quantitation by using human Y chromosome–specific primers and probe. *Y*-axis: Concentration of donor cells per milliliter of recipient blood. *X*-axis: Time points when recipient blood samples were collected. (Data from Lee TH, Paglieroni T, Ohto H, et al. Survival of donor leukocyte subpopulations in immunocompetent transfusion recipients: Frequent long-term microchimerism in severe trauma patients. Blood 1999;93:3127–3139.)

diminution of donor lymphocyte response to mitogen in all trauma patients compared with controls. Among transfusion recipients who went on to develop TA-MC, lymphocyte responsiveness was initially at lower levels and recovered less by the time of hospital discharge than among transfused patients who did not develop TA-MC. Here again, leukoreduction had no measurable effect on patient's lymphocyte responsiveness.[21] In a comprehensive recall of 646 of the 656 blood donors for these patients, mixed lymphocyte reactions (MLRs) were studied in both directions between the patients' pretransfusion lymphocytes and lymphocytes from each blood donor. For each patient who went on to become chimeric, a single donor could be identified whose lymphocytes showed bidirectional hyporesponsiveness with the patient who received that donor's unit. Although the microchimeric donor could not be definitively identified from the limited data available in these studies, in each case, the low-resolution HLA type of the implicated donor matched the DR type of the chimeric cells detected by PCR targeting HLA-DR alleles, suggesting strongly that the hyporesponsive donor was the source of the chimeric cells. Finally, when a subset of these patients was followed over the long term, five of the patients with low-level chimerism demonstrated subsequent evolution to high-level chimerism, apparently attributable to the same single donor.[19] The time course of TA-MC for these patients together with the multidonor MLR data are shown in Figure 53–2.

To date, no disease state has been convincingly associated with TA-MC, although it is important to remember that the modest number of patients in whom this phenomenon has been described have not been systematically examined for either clinical or laboratory stigmata of autoimmunity or other subtle health abnormalities. Sjögren's syndrome and vitiligo were reported in a woman with post-transfusion MC, and evidence has also been presented that chimeric donor cells may participate in tumor formation in both the maternal-fetal setting[86] and in the setting of kidney transplantation, where XY cytokeratin-positive cells representing male keratinocytes could be found in tumor cell nests among females transplanted with male kidneys who developed malignant and benign tumors.[87] Clearly, much remains to be learned about the basic biology and possible health effects of MC.

Murine Model of TA-MC

To pursue a more-detailed understanding of the immunologic mechanisms of TA-MC, which is difficult to study in the human population, transfusion models have been developed with both immunologically intact recipient animals and animals with specific knockouts of key immune system genes. Immunologically normal mice show clearance of donor leukocytes that is much slower than that in humans or dogs[88] and is dependent on intact $CD8^+$ T cells and alloantibody responses.[89] For both syngeneic and allogeneic transfusions, complete clearance of transfused donor cells occurs by 8 to 10 weeks in immunocompetent mice, with diminished persistence proportional to the duration of storage of the transfused blood at 4° C before infusion. Allogeneic donor WBC clearance appears to be biphasic, suggesting that both MHC-dependent and MHC-independent mechanisms may be involved.[90] With respect to the potential for transfer of lymphocyte function by transfusion, sensitivity to 1-chloro-2-4-dinitrobenzene (DNCB) could also be transferred, albeit transiently, by transfusion of fresh blood from a sensitized donor to a naive recipient.[90]

Recently, these observations have been extended by using murine transfusion experiments in which the recipients were represented by a series of specific immunologic knockouts representing functional lymphocyte defects, including depletion of T, B, and natural killer (NK) cells, as well as defects in macrophage function and in expression of MHC class II molecules.[91] Findings from these experiments are summarized in Figure 53–3. The data indicate that for long-term TA-MC to become established in the murine setting, higher degrees of recipient immunocompromise are required, with increasing MHC disparity between donor and recipient. Of note, knockout mice that develop donor microchimerism had persistence of all lymphocyte immunophenotypes and evidence of functional immunity derived from the donors, suggesting therapeutic potential for TA-MC.

GRAFT-VERSUS-HOST DISEASE

The current concept of GVH reactions was formulated in the 1950s when it was recognized that spleen cell transplants in irradiated mice initially resulted in recovery of the animals from radiation injury and marrow aplasia but led to fatal "secondary disease" and "runting syndrome," characterized by wasting, diarrhea, skin lesions, and liver abnormalities.[92] In the 1960s, the term GVHD was coined, and Simonsen[93] and later Billingham[94] defined minimum criteria for the condition: (1) presence of immunocompetent cells in the graft, capable of reacting against the recipient; (2) major histocompatibility differences between donor and recipient; and (3) inability of the recipient to reject donor cells. With the exception of the second criterion, which has been revised to include inappropriate recognition of self-antigens (i.e., autoimmunity),[95,96] Billingham's criteria remain the basis for our understanding of the disease process in GVH reactions. Extensive research efforts have since clarified the mechanisms and conditions that lead to GVHD, although mechanistic details and causal relations of the multifactorial process are still incompletely understood.[96–98]

Clinical GVHD was first described by Shimoda[99] in 1955 as "postoperative erythroderma" in a case report of what was later identified as TA-GVHD. The first accounts of recognized TA-GVHD were published in the mid-1960s by Hathaway and associates.[100,101] Subsequently, TA-GVHD was described in immunosuppressed patients[102] and later also in immunocompetent transfusion recipients who were recognized as being at risk because of a relatedness in HLA antigens to the blood donor.[103,104] TA-GVHD remains a rare but distinct threat to at-risk recipients because of its severe course and resistance to therapy. Recognition of susceptible recipients who can be protected by gamma-irradiation of blood before transfusion is essential.

GVHD after transplantation was first recognized in 1959 in a report of "secondary-like disease" afflicting leukemia patients who had received bone marrow transplants.[92] We now recognize acute GVHD and chronic GVHD as clinically distinct entities in transplant patients, although some overlap may occur between the two conditions.[27,28] GVHD is most common in bone marrow transplant recipients but also occurs in recipients of solid organ transplants, particularly liver transplants.[105,106] Disease severity is extremely variable, but both acute and chronic GVHD after transplantation are reasonably responsive to a variety of immunosuppressive and immunomodulatory therapy protocols that have been developed.[24]

Pathophysiology

The simplified model of pathogenesis that has emerged since the pioneering studies of GVHD in the 1950s suggests that immunocompetent donor lymphocytes that are not cleared because of a compromised host immune system go on to proliferate in the recipient. This is followed by attack and destruction of host tissues in target organs, including liver, intestines, skin, and, perhaps, lung.[96] Supporting the validity of this model in TA-GVHD is a positive correlation between the number of transfused viable donor lymphocytes and the degree of immunosuppression in the host on the one side and the likelihood of occurrence and severity of TA-GVHD on the other.[92] The threshold dose of lymphocytes to incite TA-GVHD in humans is not precisely known, but case reports

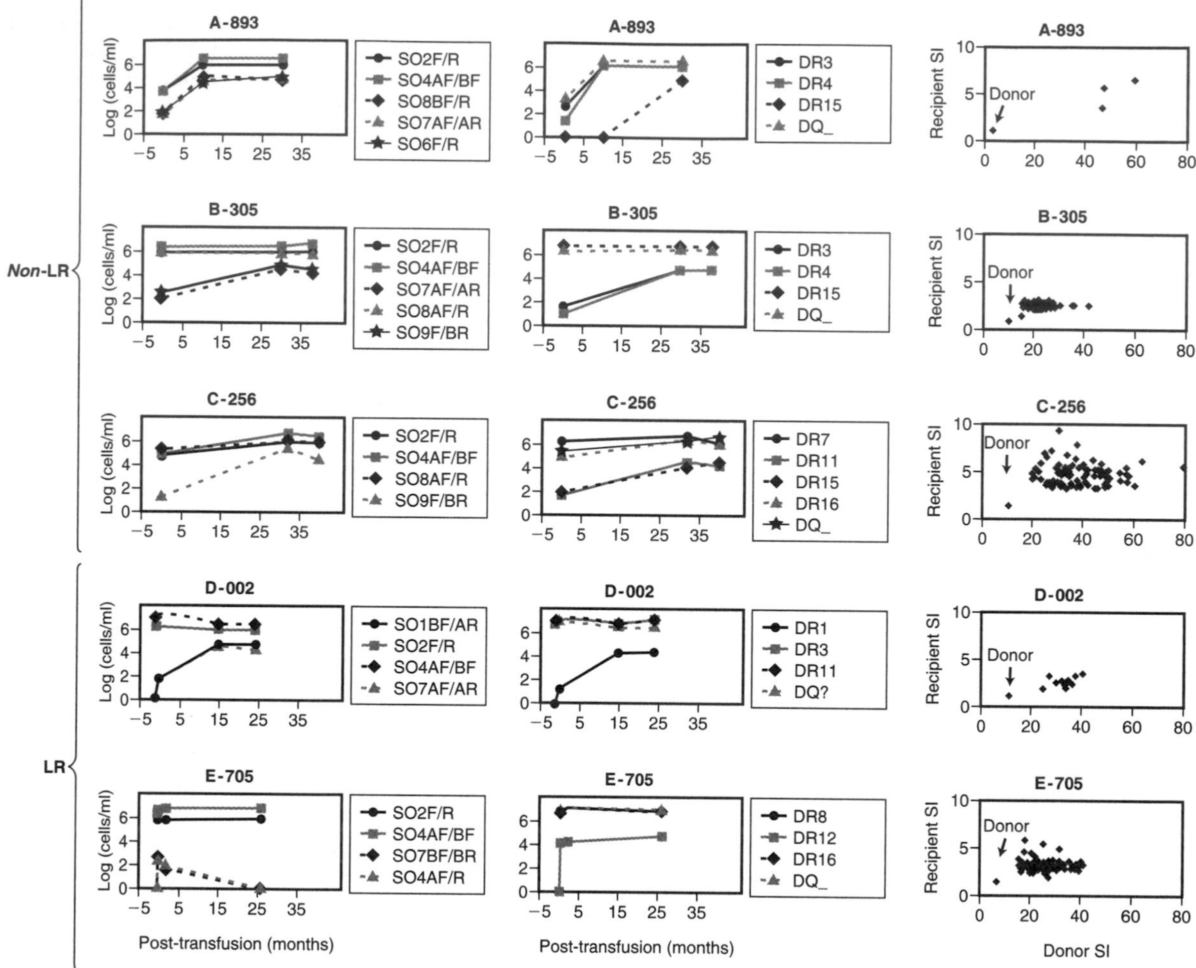

Figure 53–2 Donor leukocyte and mixed lymphocyte reaction (MLR) results of the five patients with long-term microchimerism (MC). The quantitative degree of MC (log-scale) over time in each of the patients with long-term MC is plotted in the first two columns, for InDel and HLA-DR, respectively. The concentration of the major and minor alleles, as well as HLA-DQa, a measure of genomic DNA, input per reaction, is plotted against time. The *Y*-axis is concentration (in number of target sequence per milliliter of total whole blood), and the *X*-axis is time (in months). The first three subjects received non-LR blood products, whereas the last two received exclusively LR blood products. The third column represents the corresponding donor-versus-recipient MLR for each of the five subjects. Microchimerism, indicated by an *arrow* corresponding to the implicated donor, was observed when the donor and the recipient stimulation indices were mutually low. (Data from Lee TH, Paglieroni T, Utter GH, et al. High-level long-term white blood cell microchimerism after transfusion of leukoreduced blood components to patients resuscitated after severe traumatic injury. Transfusion 2005;45:1280–1290.)

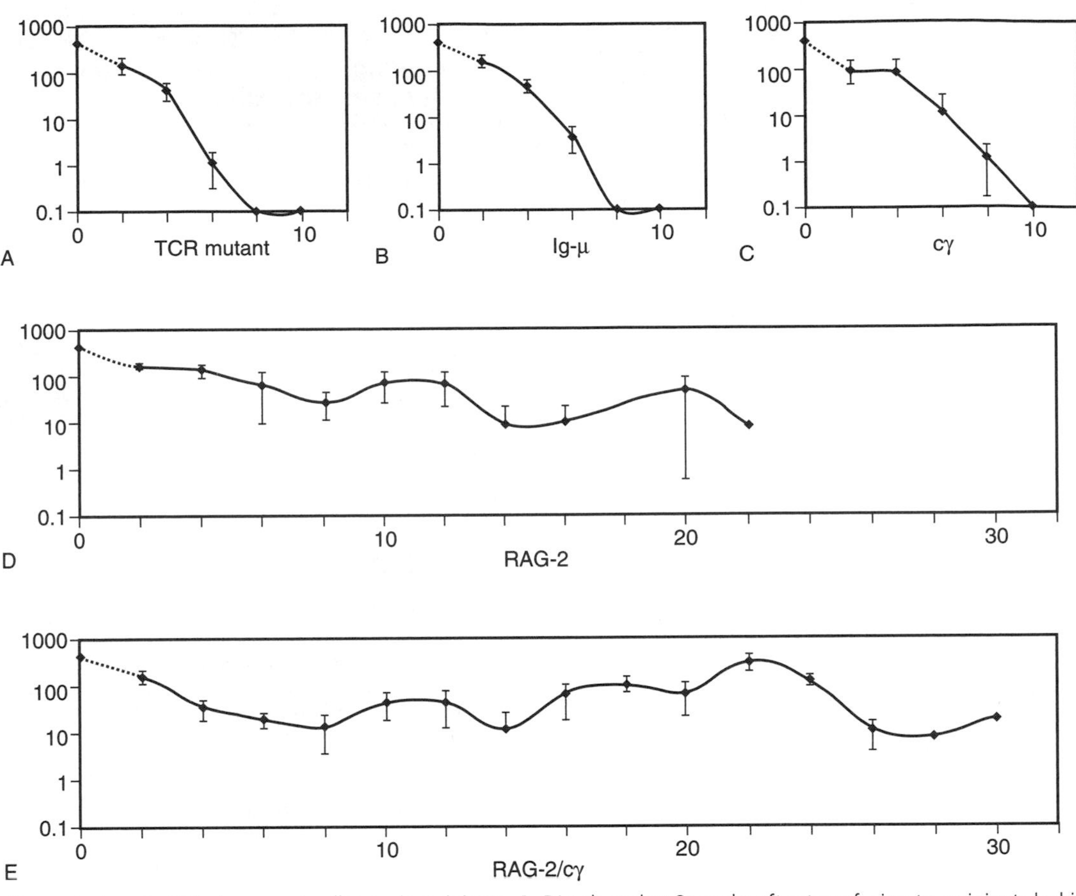

Figure 53–3 Donor leukocyte (DL) clearance in allogeneic recipients. **A,** DLs cleared at 8 weeks after transfusion to recipients lacking functional T cells. **B,** DLs cleared at 8 weeks after transfusion to recipients lacking mature B cells. **C,** DLs cleared at 10 weeks after transfusion to recipients with defective common-g receptor (receptors for cytokines [i.e., interleukin-2, IL-4, IL-7, IL-9 and IL-15]). These recipients lack natural killer (NK) cells but produce a small number of B and T cells. **D,** Proliferation of DLs after 22 weeks after transfusion to mice lacking mature B and T cells. **E,** Proliferation of DLs at 30 weeks after transfusion to recipients lacking B, T, and NK cells. (Data from Lee TH, Wen L, Montalvo L, et al. Minimum conditions of major histocompatibility complex compatibility and recipient immune compromise required to establish donor white blood cell persistence in a murine transfusion model. Transfusion 2005;45:301–314.)

suggest that leukoreduction by current filtration (usually to $<5–6 \times 10^6$ WBCs per 300 mL of blood component) is not sufficient to prevent the disease.[107–109]

Occurrence of TA-GVHD in immunocompetent recipients has been explained by a so-called one-way HLA match in which the donor cells are homozygous for an HLA type for which the recipient is heterozygous.[104] As a consequence, the recipient immune cells do not recognize the donor cells as foreign and fail to mount an immune response that would normally clear the donor cells. The latter, however, respond to the mismatched haplotype and incite the GVH reaction, which proceeds as aggressively as in immunocompromised patients.

Refinements in the basic model suggest a complex interaction of recipient and host immune cells and emphasize the notion that the latter is not a mere passive bystander but participates in and maintains the GVH reaction through dysregulated cell activation and cytokine release. Recipient T-helper subset 1 (Th1) cytokines interleukin-2 (IL-2) and interferon-β and proinflammatory cytokines IL-1 and tumor necrosis factor-β (TNF-β) appear to promote the deleterious effects of GVH, whereas Th2 cytokines IL-4 and IL-10 are thought to have a downregulating effect.[97]

New insights have also been achieved into the roles of lymphocyte subpopulations in the pathophysiology of GVHD. A mouse model provided evidence that T-cell subsets play opposite roles in the disease process, with recipient CD8 cells providing protection, whereas recipient CD4 cells promote a GVH response.[110,111] According to the authors, patients with impaired CD8 and NK cell function are at increased risk for TA-GVHD, especially if they receive HLA haploidentical blood. Interestingly, this hypothesis provides one explanation for the clinical observation that human immunodeficiency virus (HIV)-infected persons do not develop GVHD after allogeneic transfusions despite impaired cellular immunity. In these patients, CD4 counts decrease early, but CD8 counts remain high until late in the disease course. Infection of infused donor CD4 cells by HIV, followed by attack on the infected cells by cytolytic CD8 cells, may provide an additional explanation for the apparent absence of GVHD in patients with acquired immunodeficiency syndrome (AIDS).[112] Demonstration of rapid disappearance of donor leukocytes (from transfused cellular blood components) in late-stage AIDS patients has confirmed the notion that HIV infection is not associated with an increased risk of TA-GVHD, despite profound cellular immunodeficiency.[113] The precise role of recipient T-cell subsets in susceptibility to GVH reactions remains controversial, however, with others maintaining that reactive recipient CD8 cells are required for the development of GVHD.[114]

With regard to the effector cells that cause tissue damage in GVHD, evidence from studies of patients with TA-GVHD suggests that donor T cells participating in the disease process are clonally restricted in expression of T-cell–receptor repertoires[115] and are composed of a variety of CD4- and CD8-positive clones that may cause tissue damage through different mechanisms, including direct and indirect cytotoxicity.[116] The latter finding may explain the often characteristically sparse lymphocytic infiltrate of target tissues in GVHD. Indirect cell lysis may occur through an apoptosis-inducing mechanism or through cytokine release (TNF-β, IL-1) followed by attraction of platelets and neutrophils, causing cell damage by release of free radicals and elastases.

Clinical Presentation

Patients with TA-GVHD typically are first seen within 7 to 10 days of the transfusion with fever, a characteristic reddish raised rash spreading from trunk or face to the extremities, evidence of hepatitis, watery diarrhea, and nonspecific signs including anorexia, nausea, and vomiting.[25,117] The diarrhea may be profuse, and the skin lesions may progress to bullous lesions and generalized erythroderma. The development of pancytopenia caused by immune destruction of host marrow cells distinguishes TA-GVHD from GVHD after hematopoietic stem cell transplantation and is the usual cause of death of hemorrhage and overwhelming infection. Most patients die within 1 to 3 weeks after the onset of clinical symptoms.[103] In neonates, symptoms appear later, approximately a month after transfusion, and the disease tends to run a more prolonged course with survival for up to 3 months.[117] The naive T-cell population in infants and a different cytokine milieu favoring interferon-β over IL-2 may be responsible for the delayed response. Few patients survive TA-GVHD, although spontaneous recovery or development of a chronic form of GVHD has been reported.[117–119]

Epidemiology

TA-GVHD is rare in unselected U.S. transfusion recipients and has been almost exclusively observed in immunocompromised patients.[120] A list of specific immune-deficient states that have been associated with either clear, probable, or no specific risk for the complication is shown in Table 53–4. A special situation is treatment with purine analogs, particularly fludarabine. The drug induces profound, long-lasting lymphopenia, involving both T and B cells, and has been associated with at least 10 published cases of TA-GVHD. In 7 of the 10 cases, fludarabine was given for treatment of chronic lymphocytic leukemia (CLL), which resulted in listing this clinical constellation as one that clearly carries risk. However, occurrence of TA-GVHD in two patients with other hematologic conditions (acute myeloid leukemia and B-cell lymphoma) and a third recent case in a patient with lupus nephritis, suggests that fludarabine treatment in itself or in combination with alkylating agents confers risk independent of an association with CLL.[121]

Conversely, the potential for TA-GVHD in patients with no or only mild immunodeficiency is demonstrated by more than 200 documented cases in Japan,[103] where incidence rates as high as 1 in 660 patients undergoing cardiovascular surgery were reported.[122] Greater genetic homogeneity of the Japanese population and frequent use of unirradiated fresh whole blood from related donors in the past were thought to be the primary reasons for the surprisingly frequent occurrence of TA-GVHD in this country.[123,124] After adoption of and adherence to strict guidelines for prevention of the condition (including universal irradiation of cellular blood components), the number of new cases in Japan has decreased dramatically.[125]

Table 53–4 Patient Groups at Risk for Developing Transfusion-Associated Graft-versus-Host Disease

Clear Risk
Patients with selected immunodeficiencies
Congenital immunodeficiencies
Hodgkin's disease
Chronic lymphocytic leukemia (CLL) treated with fludarabine*
Newborns with erythroblastosis fetalis
Recipients of intrauterine transfusions
Recipients of hematopoietic stem cell transplants
Recipients of blood products donated by relatives
Recipients of human leukocyte antigen (HLA)–selected (matched) platelets or platelets known to be homozygous
Probable Risk
Patients with other hematologic malignancies
Patients with solid tumors treated with cytotoxic agents
Recipient-donor pairs from genetically homogeneous populations
Premature and possibly full-term neonates
No Defined Risk
Patients with acquired immunodeficiency syndrome (AIDS)
Patients taking immunosuppressive medications.

*Treatment with fludarabine (and perhaps other purine analogs) in itself, particularly in conjunction with alkylating agents, may be a clear risk, independent of combination with CLL. See discussion in Epidemiology section.

Data from Webb IK, Anderson KC. Transfusion-associated graft-versus-host disease. In Anderson KC, Ness PM (eds). Scientific Basis of Transfusion Medicine, 2nd ed. Philadelphia, WB Saunders, 2000, pp 420–426.

Reports of relatively high rates of TA-GVHD have also come from other geographic areas with genetically homogeneous populations.[126] Estimates of the risk of TA-GVHD based on genetic similarities in HLA haplotype frequencies between random blood donor-recipient pairs yielded a potential rate of 1 in 17,700 to 1 in 39,000 among whites in the United States; the risk in Japan was projected to be 1 in 1600 to 1 in 7900. Directed donations between parents and children increase the risk of histocompatibility from 10- to 20-fold.[127,128]

Diagnosis

Given the rarity of the disease, the diagnosis of TA-GVHD may be missed and is often not made until late in the course or postmortem unless a high degree of suspicion exists.[128] Other diagnoses such as drug reaction or infections are usually considered first. Routine laboratory studies are not helpful for an etiologic diagnosis. Histologic findings on skin, liver, or intestinal biopsies may suggest the diagnosis of TA-GVHD but are not pathognomonic. The only definitive method of diagnosis is the identification of donor-derived lymphocytes in the circulation or tissues of the affected patient. This may be accomplished by detailed HLA typing, cytogenetic analysis, or studies of genomic markers capable of reliably identifying donor and recipient cells.[124,129,130] For female recipients, detection of Y-chromosome regions by

PCR has been used to confirm TA-GVHD by documenting circulating male cells.[129,131] In seeking donor-derived genotypes to support the diagnosis of TA-GVHD, it is critical to consider the PCR amplification strategy; a strategy with limited primer specificity or inadequate sensitivity could result in a false-negative chimerism assay, as discussed earlier in this chapter (see Table 53–3).[36]

Therapy

Immunosuppressive therapy with corticosteroids, antithymocyte globulin, cyclophosphamide, methotrexate, and cyclosporine, alone or in combination, which is usually able to influence TA-GVHD,[27,28] is generally ineffective in TA-GVHD.[26,97,131] Hematopoietic stem cell transplantation has been attempted successfully in rare instances,[132] and infusion of leftover autologous hematopoietic progenitor cells has resulted in recovery in a single reported case.[133]

Because of the small number of case reports in which treatment resulted in recovery,[118,134] and uncertainty about whether a milder form of the disease contributed to the success, consensus treatment guidelines have not been formulated.

Prevention

Gamma-irradiation of blood components containing viable lymphocytes is virtually 100% effective in preventing TA-GVHD, although rare failures have been reported with irradiation doses considered suboptimal today.[135–137] Irradiation prophylaxis is recommended for all whole blood, RBC, platelet, and granulocyte units transfused to patients at risk.[138] Irradiation prevents proliferation of lymphocytes through crosslinkage of DNA.[139] The required dose is 25 Gy to the mid-plane of the blood container with a minimum of 15 Gy to any point of the irradiated field.[138] The Food and Drug Administration further mandated that the maximum dose not exceed 50 Gy.[131] In this dosage range, irradiation is considered safe, with unlikely harm to the recipient of the treated component.

Adverse effects of irradiation on therapeutic blood components include a moderate decrease in survival of RBCs[140] and leakage of potassium from intracellular stores.[141,142] The allowable storage period for irradiated RBC units has therefore been reduced to 28 days,[138] and caution is advised in administering stored irradiated RBC units to recipients at risk for ill effects of hyperkalemia.[143] These include primarily neonates and premature infants with renal failure or those who receive large-volume transfusions, especially if administered through central venous catheters, or treatment with extracorporeal membrane oxygenation through central venous catheters. Platelets do not appear to be affected by the recommended radiation dose during routine 5-day blood-bank storage,[144,145] and no reduction in storage time is necessary. Frozen thawed RBC units, fresh frozen plasma (FFP), and cryoprecipitate are widely viewed as "acellular" blood components, and no documented cases of TA-GVHD after administration of these components have been reported[131]; irradiation is therefore not currently recommended. TA-GVHD has, however, occurred after transfusion of fresh liquid plasma that had never been frozen,[146] and some believe that FFP may contain sufficient viable lymphocytes to be of concern.[147,148] This issue is currently under investigation. The reader is referred to Chapter 28 for a more detailed discussion of technical, procedural, and regulatory aspects of blood component irradiation.

Experimental methods of lymphocyte inactivation for TA-GVHD prophylaxis include ultraviolet B (UVB) irradiation[149] and photochemical treatment with UVA-activated psoralens.[150] The latter approach, which has been developed for pathogen inactivation in platelet and plasma units and is being evaluated in clinical trials, may be at least equally effective in preventing lymphocyte response to immunologic stimulation and proliferation.[150,151]

Patients at Risk Who Should Receive Transfusion-Associated GVHD Prophylaxis

Because TA-GVHD may occur in immunocompetent individuals, any transfusion recipient may be considered at risk, and identification of defined risk groups may provide a false sense of security to those not included in the at-risk groups. However, unless all blood components are routinely irradiated, the categorization of patients who are at particular risk on the basis of experience is useful and practically important. Table 53–3 categorizes patient groups according to risk level for developing TA-GVHD. Irradiation of cellular blood components is mandatory for patient groups with clear risk; for others, irradiation may be considered, but no universal consensus has been reached.[138]

SUMMARY

Microchimerism has been recently described in association with a number of specific allogenic exposures including pregnancy, twinning, transplantation, and blood transfusion. Despite the research reports reviewed here, the prevalence and magnitude of MC in healthy populations and the precise relation between MC and specific allogeneic exposures, such as pregnancy and transfusion, has not yet been studied systematically. In the setting of traumatic injury, leukocytes from a single blood donor may persist months to years at a level that increases over time to as much as 3% to 4% of the recipient's total circulating leukocytes. This TA-MC phenomenon may affect 50% of patients transfused for traumatic injury if measured at hospital discharge. In long-term follow-up, limited data suggest that 1 in 5 of these patients will go on to develop high-level, persistent TA-MC. It is important for future research to determine whether persistent TA-MC occurs in other clinical settings where tissue injury is prominent, the immunologic mechanisms involved, the extent of hematopoetic and immunologic engraftment, and, perhaps most important, whether it represents a harmful or beneficial consequence of blood transfusions. The latter question is especially relevant, as viable donor lymphocytes from transfused cellular blood components may on rare occasions cause an almost uniformly fatal TA-GVHD. Unlike GVHD associated with transplantation of organs or hematopoietic stem cells, which tends to be associated with a more manageable acute and/or chronic course, donor lymphocytes in TA-GVHD prominently attack recipient bone marrow stem cells, resulting in cytopenias and a rapidly lethal course. As TA-GVHD is rare, it may be overlooked. Diagnosis is based on demonstrating infiltrating donor-derived lymphocytes in recipient tissues. Treatment has rarely been successful, emphasizing the importance of prophylaxis. Gamma-irradiation of cellular blood components that render donor lymphocytes incapable of proliferation remains the only reliable and widely available method for prevention. Although some donor/recipient constellations are clearly associated with higher risk of TA-GVHD, it is difficult to identify all recipients who may be predisposed to TA-GVHD and who therefore should receive irradiated blood components. It is hoped that further research in donor-recipient factors that allow and promote microchimerism and GVHD will provide critical insight into better care of transplant patients and increased safety of transfusion recipients.

REFERENCES

1. Adams KM, Nelson JL. Microchimerism: an investigative frontier in autoimmunity and transplantation. JAMA 2004;291:1127–1131.
2. Nelson JL. Microchimerism in human health and disease. Autoimmunity 2003;36:5–9.
3. Lee TH, Paglieroni T, Ohto H, et al. Survival of donor leukocyte subpopulations in immunocompetent transfusion recipients: frequent long-term microchimerism in severe trauma patients. Blood 1999;93:3127–3139.
4. Schechter GP, Whang-Peng J, McFarland W. Circulation of donor lymphocytes after blood transfusion in man. Blood 1977;49:651–656.
5. Hutchinson DL, Turner JH, Schlesinger ER. Persistence of donor cells in neonates after fetal and exchange transfusion. Am J Obstet Gynecol 1971;109:281–284.
6. Adams PT, Davenport RD, Reardon DA, Roth MS. Detection of circulating donor white blood cells in patients receiving multiple transfusions. Blood 1992;80:551–555.
7. Vervoordeldonk SF, Doumaid K, Remmerswaal EB, et al. Long-term detection of microchimaerism in peripheral blood after pretransplantation blood transfusion. Br J Haematol 1998;102:1004–1009.
8. Schechter G, Soehnlen F, McFarland W. Lymphocyte response to blood transfusion in man. N Engl J Med 1972;287:1169–1173.
9. Bianchi DW, Zickwolf GK, Weil GJ, et al. Male fetal progenitor cells persist in maternal blood for as long as 27 years postpartum. Proc Natl Acad Sci USA 1996;93:705–708.
10. Lo YM, Lo ES, Watson N, et al. Two-way cell traffic between mother and fetus: biologic and clinical implications. Blood 1996;88:4390–4395.
11. Starzl T, Demetris A, Murase N, et al. Cell migration, chimerism and graft acceptance. Lancet 1992;339:1579–1582.
12. Starzl T. Clinical and basic scientific implications of cell migration and microchimerism after organ transplantation. Artif Organs 1997;21:1154–1155.
13. Ko S, Deiwick A, Dinkel A, et al. Functional relevance of donor-derived hematopoietic microchimerism only for induction but not for maintenance of allograft acceptance. Transplant Proc 1999;31:920–921.
14. Ko S, Deiwick A, Jager M, et al. The functional relevance of passenger leukocytes and microchimerism for heart allograft acceptance in the rat. Nat Med 1999;5:1292–1297.
15. Lo Y. Fetal RhD genotyping from maternal plasma. Ann Med 1999;31:308–312.
16. Tang N, Leung T, Zhang J, et al. Detection of fetal-derived paternally inherited X-chromosome polymorphisms in maternal plasma. Clin Chem 1999;45:2033–2035.
17. Lo YM. Application of PCR for fetal cell detection. Early Hum Dev 1996;47(Suppl):s73–s77.
18. Lo YM. Non-invasive prenatal diagnosis using fetal cells in maternal blood. J Clin Pathol 1994;47:1060–1065.
19. Lee TH, Paglieroni T, Utter GH, et al. High-level long-term white blood cell microchimerism after transfusion of leukoreduced blood components to patients resuscitated after severe traumatic injury. Transfusion 2005;45:1280–1290.
20. Utter GH, Owings JT, Lee TH, et al. Blood transfusion is associated with donor leukocyte microchimerism in trauma patients. J Trauma 2004;57:702–707, discussion 707–708.
21. Utter GH, Owings JT, Lee TH, et al. Microchimerism in transfused trauma patients is associated with diminished donor-specific lymphocyte response. J Trauma 2005;58:925–931, discussion 931–932.
22. Dey B, Sykes M, Spitzer T. Outcomes of recipients of both bone marrow and solid organ transplants. Medicine (Baltimore) 1998;77:355–369.
23. Wagner N, Quinones V. Allogeneic peripheral blood stem cell transplantation: Clinical overview and nursing implications. Oncol Nurs Forum 1998;25:1049–1055; quiz 1056–1057.
24. Klingebiel T, Schlegel P. GVHD: Overview on pathophysiology, incidence, clinical and biological features. Bone Marrow Transplant 1998;21(Suppl 2):s45–s49.
25. Rososhansky S, Badonnel MC, Hiestand LL, et al. Transfusion-associated graft-versus-host disease in an immunocompetent patient following cardiac surgery. Vox Sang 1999;76:59–63.
26. Webb IK, Anderson KC. Transfusion-associated graft-versus-host disease. In Anderson KC, Ness PM (eds). Scientific Basis of Transfusion Medicine, 2nd ed. Philadelphia, WB Saunders, 2000, pp 420–426.
27. Parkman R. Chronic graft-versus-host disease. Curr Opin Hematol 1998;5:22–25.
28. Flowers M, Kansu E, Sullivan K. Pathophysiology and treatment of graft-versus-host disease. Hematol Oncol Clin North Am 1999;13:1091–1112, viii–ix.
29. Lillie FR. The theory of the free-martin. Science 1916;43:611–613.
30. Owen R. Immunogenetic consequences of vascular anastomoses between bovine twins. Science 1945;28:400–401.
31. Burlingham WJ, Muller D. Chimerism and tolerance. Hum Immunol 1997;52:73–74.
32. Dunsford I, Bowley C, Hutchinson A, et al. A human blood group chimera. Br Med J 1953;81:ii.
33. Teillet MA, Ziller C, Le Douarin NM. Quail-chick chimeras. Methods Mol Biol 1999;97:305–318.
34. Mohr J, Killebrew L, Muchmore H, et al. Transfer of delayed hypersensitivity: The role of blood transfusions in humans. JAMA 1969;207:517–519.
35. Dzik S. The power of primers [Editorial]. Transfusion 1998;38: 118–121.
36. Reed WF, Lee TL, Trachtenberg E, et al. Detection of microchimerism by PCR is a function of amplification strategy. Transfusion 2001;41:39–44.
37. Moody A, Sellers S, Bumstead N. Measuring infectious bursal disease virus RNA in blood by multiplex real-time quantitative RT-PCR. J Virol Methods 2000;85:55–64.
38. Marras S, Kramer F, Tyagi S. Multiplex detection of single-nucleotide variations using molecular beacons. Genet Anal 1999;14:151–156.
39. Maeda H, Fujimoto C, Haruki Y, et al. Quantitative real-time PCR using TaqMan and SYBR green for *Actinobacillus actinomycetemcomitans, Porphyromonas gingivalis, Prevotella intermedia,* tetQ gene and total bacteria. FEMS Immunol Med Microbiol 2003;39:81–86.
40. Malinen E, Kassinen A, Rinttila T, Palva A. Comparison of real-time PCR with SYBR Green I or 5 -nuclease assays and dot-blot hybridization with rDNA-targeted oligonucleotide probes in quantification of selected faecal bacteria. Microbiology 2003;149:269–277.
41. Schmittgen TD, Zakrajsek BA, Mills AG, et al. Quantitative reverse transcription-polymerase chain reaction to study mRNA decay: Comparison of endpoint and real-time methods. Anal Biochem 2000; 285:194–204.
42. Carter AS, Bunce M, Cerundolo L, et al. Detection of microchimerism after allogeneic blood transfusion using nested polymerase chain reaction amplification with sequence-specific primers (PCR-SSP): a cautionary tale. Blood 1998;92:683–689.
43. Carter AS, Cerundolo L, Bunce M, et al. Nested polymerase chain reaction with sequence-specific primers typing for HLA-A, -B, and -C alleles: detection of microchimerism in DR-matched individuals. Blood 1999;94:1471–1477.
44. Alizadeh M, Bernard M, Danic B, et al. Quantitative assessment of hematopoietic chimerism after bone marrow transplantation by real-time quantitative polymerase chain reaction. Blood 2002;99: 4618–4625.
44a. Lee T-H, Chafets D, Wen L, et al. Enhanced ascertainment of microchimerism using real-time quantitative PCR amplification of insertion/deletion polymorphisms. Transfusion 2006 (in press).
45. Van Deerlin V, Leonard D. Bone marrow engraftment analysis after allogeneic bone marrow transplantation. Clin Lab Med 2000;20:197–225.
46. Dzik S. Principles of counting low numbers of leukocytes in leukoreduced blood components. Transfus Med Rev 1997;11:44–55.
47. Abecasis M, Machado A, Boavida G, et al. Haploidentical cord blood transplant contaminated with maternal T cells in a patient with advanced leukaemia. Bone Marrow Transplant 1996;17:891–895.
48. Poli F, Sirchia S, Scalamogna M, et al. Detection of maternal DNA in human cord blood stored for allotransplantation by a highly sensitive chemiluminescent method. J Hemather 1997;6:581–585.
49. Scaradavou A, Carrier C, Mollen N, et al. Detection of maternal DNA in placental/umbilical cord blood by locus-specific amplification of the noninherited maternal HLA gene. Blood 1996;88:1494–1500.
50. Socie G, Gluckman E, Carosella E, et al. Search for maternal cells in human umbilical cord blood by polymerase chain reaction by amplification of two minisatellite sequences. Blood 1994;83:340–344.

51. Adams K, Lambert N, Heimfeld S, et al. Male DNA in female donor apheresis and CD34-enriched products. Blood 2003;102:3845–3847.
52. Lo YD, Corbetta N, Chamberlain PF, et al. Presence of fetal DNA in maternal plasma and serum. Lancet 1997;350:485–487.
53. Lo Y. Detection of minority nucleic acid populations by PCR: a review. J Pathol 1994;174:1.
54. Lo Y, Tein M, Lau T, et al. Quantitative analysis of fetal DNA in maternal plasma and serum: Implications for non-invasive prenatal diagnosis. Am J Hum Genet 1998;62:768–775.
55. Lo Y, Hjelm N, Fidler C, et al. Prenatal diagnosis of fetal RhD status by molecular analysis of maternal plasma. N Engl J Med 1998;339: 1734–1738.
56. Brojer E, Zupanska B, Guz K, et al. Noninvasive determination of fetal RHD status by examination of cell-free DNA in maternal plasma. Transfusion 2005;45:1473–1480.
57. Lo Y. Recent advances in fetal nucleic acids in maternal plasma. J Histochem Cytochem 2005;53:293–296.
58. Ariga H, Ohto H, Busch MP, et al. Kinetics of fetal cellular and cell-free DNA in the maternal circulation during and after pregnancy: Implications for noninvasive prenatal diagnosis. Transfusion 2001;41:1524–1530.
59. Bianchi DW. Current knowledge about fetal blood cells in the maternal circulation. J Perinat Med 1998;26:175–185.
60. Aractingi S, Berkane N, Bertheau P, et al. Fetal DNA in skin of polymorphic eruptions of pregnancy. Lancet 1998;352:1898–1901.
61. Larrabee P, Johnson K, Lai C, et al. Global gene expression analysis of the living human fetus using cell-free messenger RNA in amniotic fluid. JAMA 2005;293:836–842.
62. Tong Y, Lo Y. Diagnostic developments including cell-free (circulating) nucleic acids. Clin Chim Acta 2006;363:187–196.
63. Nelson JL, Furst DE, Maloney S, et al. Microchimerism and HLA-compatible relationships of pregnancy in scleroderma. Lancet 1998; 351:559–562.
64. Artlett CM, Smith JB, Jimenez SA. Identification of fetal DNA and cells in skin lesions from women with systemic sclerosis. N Engl J Med 1998;338:1186–1191.
65. Evans P, Lambert N, Maloney S, et al. Long-term fetal microchimerism in peripheral blood mononuclear cell subsets in healthy women and women with scleroderma. Blood 1999;93:2033–2037.
66. Symmons D, Bankhead C, Harrison B, et al. Blood transfusion, smoking and obesity as risk factors for the development of rheumatoid arthritis: Results from a primary-based incident case-control study in Norfolk, England. Arthritis Rheumatol 1997;40:1955–1961.
67. Willer CJ, Sadovnick AD, Ebers GC. Microchimerism in autoimmunity and transplantation: potential relevance to multiple sclerosis. J Neuroimmunol 2002;126:126–133.
68. Maloney S, Smith A, Furst DE, et al. Microchimerism of maternal origin persists into adult life. J Clin Invest 1999;104:41–47.
69. Lambert NC, Erickson TD, Yan Z, et al. Quantification of maternal microchimerism by HLA-specific real-time polymerase chain reaction: Studies of healthy women and women with scleroderma. Arthritis Rheum 2004;50:906–914.
70. Srivatsa B, Srivatsa S, Johnson KL, Bianchi DW. Maternal cell microchimerism in newborn tissues. J Pediatr 2003;142:31–35.
71. Artlett CM, Miller FW, Rider LG. Persistent maternally derived peripheral microchimerism is associated with the juvenile idiopathic inflammatory myopathies. Rheumatology (Oxford). 2001;40:1279–1284.
72. Artlett CM, Ramos R, Jiminez SA, et al. Chimeric cells of maternal origin in juvenile idiopathic inflammatory myopathies: Childhood Myositis Heterogeneity Collaborative Group. Lancet 2000;356:2155–2156.
73. Stevens AM. Foreign cells in polymyositis: could stem cell transplantation and pregnancy-derived chimerism lead to the same disease? Curr Rheumatol Rep 2003;5:437–444.
74. Stevens AM, Hermes HM, Rutledge JC, et al. Myocardial-tissue-specific phenotype of maternal microchimerism in neonatal lupus congenital heart block. Lancet 2003;362:1617–1623.
75. Elwood ET, Larsen CP, Maurer DH, et al. Microchimerism and rejection in clinical transplantation. Lancet 1997;349:1358–1360.
76. Opelz G, Terasaki P. Improvement of kidney allograft survival with increased number of blood transfusions. N Engl J Med 1978;299: 799–803.
77. Opelz G, Vanrenterghem Y, Kirste G, et al. Prospective evaluation of pretransplant blood transfusions in cadaver kidney recipients. Transplantation 1997;63:964–967.
78. Ober C, Karrison T, Odem RR, et al. Mononuclear-cell immunisation in prevention of recurrent miscarriages: a randomised trial. Lancet 1999;354:365–369.
79. Recurrent Miscarriage Immunotherapy Trialist Group. Worldwide collaborative observational study and meta-analysis on allogeneic leukocyte immunotherapy for recurrent spontaneous abortion. Am J Reprod Immunol 1994;32:55–72.
80. Hillyer CD, Klein HG. Immunotherapy and gene transfer in the treatment of the oncology patient: role of transfusion medicine. Transfus Med Rev 1996;10:1–14.
81. Khosrotehrani K, Johnson KL, Cha DH, et al. Transfer of fetal cells with multilineage potential to maternal tissue. JAMA 2004;292:75–80.
82. Hutchinson D, Maxwell N, Turner J. Advantages of use of maternal erythrocytes for fetal transfusion. Am J Obstet Gynecol 1967;99:702–708.
83. Vietor HE, Hallensleben E, van Bree SP, et al. Survival of donor cells 25 years after intrauterine transfusion. Blood 2000;95:2709–2714.
84. Lee T-H, Donegan E, Slichter S, Busch M. Transient increase in circulating donor leukocytes after allogeneic transfusion in immunocompetent recipients compatible with donor cell proliferation. Blood 1995;85:1207–1214.
85. Slichter S, Deeg H, Kennedy M. Prevention of platelet alloimmunization in dogs with systemic cyclosporine and by UV-irradiation of cyclosporine-loading in donor platelets. Blood 1987;69:414–418.
86. Osada S, Horibe K, Oiwa K, et al. A case of infantile acute monocytic leukemia caused by vertical transmission of the mother's leukemic cells. Cancer Markers 1990;65:1146–1149.
87. Aractingi S, Kanitakis J, Euvrard S, et al. Skin carcinoma arising from donor cells in a kidney transplant recipient. Cancer Res 2005;65: 1755–1760.
88. Goodarzi M, Lee T-H, Pallavicini M, et al. Unusual kinetics of white cell clearance in transfused mice. Transfusion 1994;35:145–149.
89. Fast LD. Recipient elimination of allogeneic lymphoid cells: Donor CD4(+) cells are effective alloantigen-presenting cells. Blood 2000;96:1144–1149.
90. Lee TH, Reed W, Mangawang-Montalvo L, et al. Donor WBCs can persist and transiently mediate immunologic function in a murine transfusion model: effects of irradiation, storage, and histocompatibility. Transfusion 2001;41:637–642.
91. Lee TH, Wen L, Montalvo L, et al. Minimum conditions of major histocompatibility complex compatibility and recipient immune compromise required to establish donor white blood cell persistence in a murine transfusion model. Transfusion 2005;45:301–314.
92. Brubaker DB. Transfusion-associated graft-versus-host disease. In Anderson KC, Ness PM (eds). Scientific Basis of Transfusion Medicine: Implications for Clinical Practice. Philadelphia, WB Saunders, 1994, pp 544–579.
93. Simonsen M. Graft versus host reactions: their natural history, and applicability as tools of research. Prog Allergy 1962;6:349–467.
94. Billingham RE. The biology of graft-versus-host reactions. Harvey Lect 1966;62:21–78.
95. de Arriba F, Corral J, Ayala F, et al. Autoaggression syndrome resembling acute graft-versus-host disease grade IV after autologous peripheral blood stem cell transplantation for breast cancer. Bone Marrow Transplant 1999;23:621–624.
96. Vogelsang GB, Hess AD. Graft-versus-host disease: New directions for a persistent problem. Blood 1994;84:2061–2067.
97. Ferrara JL, Levy R, Chao NJ. Pathophysiologic mechanisms of acute graft-vs.-host disease. Biol Blood Marrow Transplant 1999;5: 347–356.
98. Orlin JB, Ellis MH. Transfusion-associated graft-versus-host disease. Curr Opin Hematol 1997;4:442–448.
99. Shimoda T. The case report of post-operative erythroderma. Geka 1955;17:487.
100. Hathaway WE, Brangle RW, Nelson TL, et al. Aplastic anemia and alymphocytosis in an infant with hypogammaglobulinemia: graft-versus-host reaction? J Pediatr 1966;68:713–722.
101. Hathaway WE, Fulginiti VA, Pierce CW, et al. Graft-vs-host reaction following a single blood transfusion. JAMA 1967;201:1015–1020.
102. Brubaker DB. Human posttransfusion graft-versus-host disease. Vox Sang 1983;45:401–420.
103. Ohto H, Anderson KC. Survey of transfusion-associated graft-versus-host disease in immunocompetent recipients. Transfus Med Rev 1996;10: 31–43.
104. Thaler M, Shamiss A, Orgad S, et al The role of blood from HLA-homozygous donors in fatal transfusion-associated graft-versus-host disease after open-heart surgery. N Engl J Med 1989;321:25–28.
105. Schmuth M, Vogel W, Weinlich G, et al. Cutaneous lesions as the presenting sign of acute graft-versus-host disease following liver transplantation. Br J Dermatol 1999;141:901–904.
106. Jamieson NV, Joysey V, Friend PJ, et al. Graft-versus-host disease in solid organ transplantation. Transplant Int 1991;4:67–71.
107. Akahoshi M, Takanashi M, Masuda M, et al. A case of transfusion-associated graft-versus-host disease not prevented by white cell-reduction filters. Transfusion 1992;32:169–172.

108. Hayashi H, Nishiuchi T, Tamura H, Takeda K. Transfusion-associated graft-versus-host disease caused by leukocyte-filtered stored blood. Anesthesiology 1993;79:1419–1421.
109. Heim MU, Munker R, Sauer H, et al. [Graft versus host disease with fatal outcome after administration of filtered erythrocyte concentrates]. Beitr Infusion Ther 1992;30:178–181.
110. Fast LD, Valeri CR, Crowley JP. Immune responses to major histocompatibility complex homozygous lymphoid cells in murine F1 hybrid recipients: implications for transfusion-associated graft-versus-host disease. Blood 1995;86:3090–3096.
111. Fast LD. Recipient CD8+ cells are responsible for the rapid elimination of allogeneic donor lymphoid cells. J Immunol 1996;157:4805–4810.
112. Ammann AJ. Hypothesis: absence of graft-versus-host disease in AIDS is a consequence of HIV-1 infection of CD4+ T cells. J Acquir Immune Defic Syndr 1993;6:1224–1227.
113. Kruskall MS, Lee TH, Assmann SF, et al. Survival of transfused donor white blood cells in HIV-infected recipients. Blood 2001;98:272–279.
114. Habeshaw JA, Dalgleish AG, Hounsell EF. Absence of GVH diseases in AIDS. J Acquir Immune Defic Syndr 1994;7:1287–1289.
115. Wang L, Tadohoro K, Tokunaga K, et al. Restricted use of T-cell receptor V beta genes in posttransfusion graft-versus-host disease. Transfusion 1997;37:1184–1191.
116. Nishimura M, Uchida S, Mitsunaga S, et al. Characterization of T-cell clones derived from peripheral blood lymphocytes of a patient with transfusion-associated graft-versus-host disease: fas-mediated killing by CD4+ and CD8+ cytotoxic T-cell clones and tumor necrosis factor beta production by CD4+ T-cell clones. Blood 1997;89:1440–1445.
117. Ohto H, Anderson KC. Posttransfusion graft-versus-host disease in Japanese newborns. Transfusion 1996;36:117–123.
118. Cohen D, Weinstein H, Mihm M, Yankee R. Nonfatal graft-versus-host disease occurring after transfusion with leukocytes and platelets obtained from normal donors. Blood 1979;53:1053–1057.
119. Mori S, Matsushita H, Ozaki K, et al. Spontaneous resolution of transfusion-associated graft-versus-host disease. Transfusion 1995;35:431–435.
120. Vogelsang GB. Transfusion-associated graft-versus-host disease in nonimmunocompromised hosts. Transfusion 1990;30:101–103.
121. Leitman SF, Tisdale JF, Bolan CD, et al. Transfusion-associated GVHD after fludarabine therapy in a patient with systemic lupus erythematosus. Transfusion 2003;43:1667–1671.
122. Juji T, Takahashi K, Shibata Y, et al. Post-transfusion graft-versus-host disease in immunocompetent patients after cardiac surgery in Japan. N Engl J Med 1989;6321:56.
123. Takahashi K, Juji T, Miyamoto M, et al. Analysis of risk factors for post-transfusion graft-versus-host disease in Japan: Japanese Red Cross PT-GVHD Study Group. Lancet 1994;343:700–702.
124. Wang L, Juji T, Tokunaga K, et al. Brief report: polymorphic microsatellite markers for the diagnosis of graft-versus-host disease. N Engl J Med 1994;330:398–401.
125. Asai T, Inaba S, Ohto H, et al. Guidelines for irradiation of blood and blood components to prevent post-transfusion graft-vs.-host disease in Japan. Transfus Med 2000;10:315–320.
126. Aoun E, Shamseddine A, Chehal A, et al. Transfusion-associated GVHD: 10 years' experience at the American University of Beirut-Medical Center. Transfusion 2003;43:1672–1676.
127. Wagner FF, Flegel WA. Transfusion-associated graft-versus-host disease: Risk due to homozygous HLA haplotypes. Transfusion 1995;35:284–291.
128. Shivdasani RA, Anderson KC. Transfusion-associated graft-versus-host disease: scratching the surface [Editorial; comment]. Transfusion 1993;33:696–697.
129. Hayakawa S, Chishima F, Sakata H, et al. A rapid molecular diagnosis of posttransfusion graft-versus-host disease by polymerase chain reaction. Transfusion 1993;33:413–417.
130. Kunstmann E, Bocker T, Roewer L, et al. Diagnosis of transfusion-associated graft-versus-host disease by genetic fingerprinting and polymerase chain reaction. Transfusion 1992;32:766–770.
131. Gorlin J, Mintz P. Transfusion-associated graft-versus-host disease. In Mintz P (ed). Transfusion Therapy: Clinical Principles and Practice. Bethesda, Md., AABB Press, 1999, pp 341–357.
132. Yasukawa M, Shinozaki F, Hato T, et al. Successful treatment of transfusion-associated graft-versus-host disease. Br J Haematol 1994;86:831–836.
133. Hutchinson K, Kopko PM, Muto KN, et al. Early diagnosis and successful treatment of a patient with transfusion-associated GVHD with autologous peripheral blood progenitor cell transplantation. Transfusion 2002;42:1567–1572.
134. Prince M, Szer J, van der Weyden MB, et al. Transfusion associated graft-versus-host disease after cardiac surgery: response to antithymocyte-globulin and corticosteroid therapy. Aust N Z J Med 1991;21:43–46.
135. Sproul AM, Chalmers EA, Mills KI, et al. Third party mediated graft rejection despite irradiation of blood products. Br J Haematol 1992;80:251–252.
136. Lowenthal RM, Challis DR, Griffiths AE, et al. Transfusion-associated graft-versus-host disease: report of an occurrence following the administration of irradiated blood. Transfusion 1993;33:524–529.
137. Drobyski W, Thibodeau S, Truitt RL, et al. Third-party-mediated graft rejection and graft-versus-host disease after T-cell-depleted bone marrow transplantation, as demonstrated by hypervariable DNA probes and HLA-DR polymorphism. Blood 1989;74:2285–2294.
138. AABB. Section 5.17 Selection of compatible blood and components in special circumstances. In Klein HGC, Program Committee (ed). Standards for Blood Centers and Transfusion Services, 23rd ed. Bethesda, Md., American Association of Blood Banks, 2004, pp 43–44.
139. Baskaeva IO. The formation of DNA protien cross-links in response to gamma radiation, UV irradiation and chemical agents. Radiobiologiia 1992;32:673–684.
140. Davey RJ, McCoy NC, Yu M, et al. The effect of prestorage irradiation on posttransfusion red cell survival. Transfusion 1992;32:525–528.
141. Arseniev L, Schumann G, Andres J. Kinetics of extracellular potassium concentration in irradiated red blood cells. Infusion Ther Transfusion Med 1994;21:322–324.
142. Moroff G, Holme S, AuBuchon JP, et al. Viability and in vitro properties of AS-1 red cells after gamma irradiation. Transfusion 1999;39:128–134.
143. Strauss RG. Routinely washing irradiated red cells before transfusion seems unwarranted. Transfusion 1990;30:675–677.
144. Duguid JK, Carr R, Jenkins JA, et al. Clinical evaluation of the effects of storage time and irradiation on transfused platelets. Vox Sang 1991;60:151–154.
145. Rock G, Adams GA, Labow RS. The effects of irradiation on platelet function. Transfusion 1988;28:451–455.
146. Park BH, Biggar WD, Good RA. Minnesota experience in bone-marrow transplantation in man, 1968 to June 1973. Transplant Proc 1974;6:379–383.
147. Willis JI, Lown JA, Simpson MC, Erber WN. White cells in fresh-frozen plasma: evaluation of a new white cell-reduction filter. Transfusion 1998;38:645–649.
148. Gresens CJ, Paglieroni T, Moss CB, et al. T cells in fresh frozen plasma are viable and can respond to mitogen, superantigen and allogeneic monocytes. Transfusion 1999;39(Suppl):99s.
149. van Prooijen HC, Aarts-Riemens MI, Grijzenhout MA, van Weelden H. Ultraviolet irradiation modulates MHC-alloreactive cytotoxic T-cell precursors involved in the onset of graft-versus-host disease. Br J Haematol 1992;81:73–76.
150. Grass JA, Wafa T, Reames A, et al. Prevention of transfusion-associated graft-versus-host disease by photochemical treatment. Blood 1999;93:3140–3147.
151. Fiebig E, Hirschkorn DF, Maino VC, et al. Assessment of donor T-cell function in cellular blood components by the CD69 induction assay: effects of storage, gamma radiation, and photochemical treatment. Transfusion 2000;40:761–770.
152. Lambert N, Pang J, Yan Z, et al. Male microchimerism in women with systemic sclerosis and healthy women who have never given birth to a son. Ann Rheum Dis 2005;64:845–848.
153. Yan Z, Lambert N, Guthrie K, et al. Male microchimerism in women without sons: quantitative assessment and correlation with pregnancy history. Am J Med 2005;118:899–906.

C. Therapeutic Apheresis

Chapter 54

Therapeutic Apheresis: Basic Principles and Practical Aspects

Peter A. Millward • Nicholas Bandarenko • Mark E. Brecher

INTRODUCTION

The age-old notion of "bad blood," which was the basis of blood letting, ultimately evolved to the more sophisticated blood-separation techniques of today. Apheresis, a word of Latin derivation (from the word *aphaeresis*, a withdrawal),[1] emerged in the early 20th century. In 1914 at Johns Hopkins Hospital, Roundtree, Abel, and Turner used "plasmapheresis" to mitigate symptoms after bilateral nephrectomy in dogs. Although these experiments were associated with deaths (due to apparent overbleeding and hemorrhage), the improvement in the clinical condition of the animals successfully treated was "marked." The term *apheresis* has since been generalized to refer to the separation of blood into its components, removal of one component, and return of the remainder. Thus *leukapheresis* means the removal of leukocytes, and *erythrocytapheresis* means the removal of erythrocytes. Alternative terminology such as plasma exchange and erythrocyte exchange are frequently used interchangeably for plasmapheresis and erythrocytapheresis. Some authors have suggested that the term *plasma exchange* be reserved for low-volume procedures involving no more than 500 to 600 mL of plasma, and *plasmapheresis*, for large-volume procedures, but these terms are frequently used interchangeably.

In the 1950s, therapeutic application of these techniques emerged for the treatment of patients with hyperviscosity syndromes.[2–6] An acceleration in the interest and development of apheresis applications had to await the arrival of automated cell separators in the 1970s.[7,8] The past 3 decades are testimony to major advances in apheresis including equipment, automation, plastics, microprocessors, and separation techniques. Today, apheresis has become standard of care for a diversity of diseases. These are summarized in Table 54–1. The relative frequency of therapeutic apheresis procedures by type is illustrated in Figure 54–1.

It is intriguing that, even today, requests for therapeutic apheresis inevitably arise out of desperation or ignorance in diseases and conditions when therapeutic options have been exhausted. However, apheresis procedures are not without risk or cost. One must be judicious in their application and strive to do no harm. Objective evidence provided by published clinical and basic research provides the rationale for therapeutic apheresis. Nevertheless, we must be cognizant that clinical situations do arise in which little or no literature is available to provide guidance. Under such circumstances, a reasoned collegial approach, weighing the potential risks and benefits for the patient, is mandatory, along with a full, informed consent.

MODELING OF APHERESIS KINETICS

Volume Exchanged

The choice of a volume of blood to be exchanged is based on the kinetic modeling of apheresis. Kinetic modeling of apheresis exchange is generally based on an isolated one-compartment intravascular model. This model assumes that the component removed is neither synthesized nor degraded substantially during the procedure, that it remains within the intravascular compartment, and that instantaneous mixing occurs. In the short term, these assumptions work relatively well when applied to solutes that are located predominantly in the intravascular compartment, such as immunoglobulin M (IgM) and red blood cells (RBCs); they work less well for proteins such as IgG, which are predominantly extravascular in distribution. The intravascular distribution of IgG, IgA, IgM, albumin, and fibrinogen is approximately 45%, 42%, 76%, 40%, and 80%, respectively.[10]

For continuous-flow plasma exchange, the removal of plasma or solute can be described by the same differential equation that applies to isovolemic hemodilution:

$$\frac{dS}{dV_{ex}} = \frac{-S}{\mathrm{PV}}$$

where S is the solute concentration, V_{ex} is the volume exchanged, and PV is the plasma volume. This equation can be integrated to yield:

$$V_{ex} = \mathrm{PV} \times \ln (S_i/S_f)$$

where S_i is the initial solute concentration and S_f is the final solute concentration.

This equation can be modified to yield:

$$\text{Fraction remaining} = S_f/S_i = e^{-Vex/PV}$$

For intermittent flow, if the replacement is given after the removal of the plasma, after N repetitions of plasma removal, the remaining fraction of the plasma (and the analyte in question) is given by the following equation:

$$\text{Fraction remaining} = [(\text{PV} - \text{volume removed}) / \text{PV}]^N$$

If the replacement is given before the removal of the plasma, after N repetitions of plasma removal, the remaining fraction

Table 54–1 Role of Apheresis and Treatment Categories

Disorder	Procedure	Category
ABO-mismatched marrow transplant	RBC removal (marrow)	I
	TPE (recipient)	II
Acute central nervous system inflammatory demyelinating disease	TPE	II
Acute inflammatory demyelinating polyradiculoneuropathy (Guillan-Barré)	TPE	I
AIDS (symptoms of immunodeficiency)	TPE	IV
Amyotropic lateral sclerosis	TPE	IV
Antiglomerular basement membrane antibody disease (Goodpasture's)	TPE	I
Aplastic anemia or pure red cell aplasia	TPE	III
Autoimmune hemolytic anemia	TPE	III
Chronic inflammatory demyelinating polyradiculoneuropathy (CIDP)	TPE	I
Coagulation factor inhibitors	TPE	II
Cryoglobulinemia (with or without) polyneuropathy	TPE	II
Cutaneous T-cell lymphoma	Photopheresis	I
	Leukapheresis	III
Demyelinating polyneuropathy with IgG and IgA	TPE	I
	Immunoadsorption	III
Drug overdose and poisoning (protein bound)	TPE	II
Eaton-Lambert myasthenia syndrome	TPE	II
Erythrocytosis or polycythemia vera	Phlebotomy	I
	Erythrocytapheresis	II
Heart transplant rejection	TPE	III
	Photopheresis	III
Hemolytic disease of the newborn (HDN)	TPE	III
Hemolytic uremic syndrome	TPE	III
Hepatic failure (fulminant/acute)	TPE	III
Homozygous familial hypercholesterolemia	Selective adsorption	I
	TPE	II
Idiopathic thrombocytopenia purpura (ITP)	Immunoadsorption	II
Inclusion-body myositis	TPE	III
	Leukapheresis	IV
Leukocytosis and thrombocytosis	Cytapheresis	I
Lupus nephritis	TPE	IV
Malaria or babesiosis	RBC exchange	III
Multiple myeloma with polyneuropathy	TPE	III
Multiple sclerosis		
Relapsing	TPE	III
Progressive	TPE	III
	Lymphocytopheresis	III
Myasthenia gravis	TPE	I
Myeloma, paraproteins, or hyperviscosity	TPE	II
Myeloma or acute renal failure	TPE	II
Platelet alloimmunization and refractoriness	TPE	III
	Immunoadsorption	III
Paraneoplastic neurologic syndromes	TPE	III
	Immunoadsorption	III
Phytanic acid storage disease (Refsum's)	TPE	I
POEMS syndrome	TPE	III
Polymyositis or dermatomyositis	TPE	III
	Leukapheresis	IV
Polyneuropathy with IgM (with or without Waldenström's)	TPE	II
	Immunoadsorption	III
Post-transfusion purpura	TPE	I
Systemic amyloidosis (AL)	TPE	IV
PANDAS	TPE	II
Psoriasis	TPE	IV
Rapidly progressive glomerulonephritis	TPE	II
Rasmussen's encephalitis	TPE	III
Raynaud's phenomenon	TPE	III
Renal transplant		
Rejection	TPE	IV
Sensitization	TPE	III
Recurrent focal glomerulosclerosis	TPE	III
Rheumatoid arthritis (RA)	TPE	IV
	Immunoadsorption	II
	Lymphoplasmapheresis	II

Table 54–1 Role of Apheresis and Treatment Categories (*Continued*)

Disorder	Procedure	Category
Scleroderma or progressive systemic sclerosis	TPE	III
Sickle cell disease	RBC exchange	I
Stiff-man syndrome	TPE	III
Sydenham's chorea	TPE	II
Systemic lupus erythematosus (SLE)	TPE	III
Thrombotic thrombocytopenic purpura	TPE	I
Vasculitis	TPE	III

Category I, standard acceptable therapy; Category II, sufficient evidence to suggest efficacy, usually as adjunctive therapy; Category III, inconclusive evidence of efficacy or uncertain risk-benefit ratio; Category IV, lack of efficacy in controlled trials.

Modified from Smith JW, Weinstein R, Hillyer K. Therapeutic apheresis: a summary of current indication categories endorsed by the AABB and the American Society for Apheresis. Transfusion 2003;43:820–822.

of the plasma (and the analyte in question) is given by the equation:

$$\text{Fraction remaining} = [\text{PV}/(\text{PV} + \text{volume removed})]^N$$

Because of the initial hemodilution that occurs if the replacement is given before the removal of the plasma, for each cycle of plasma removal, the fraction remaining is less than if the replacement had been given only after each repetition of plasma removal.

A comparison of continuous versus intermittent-flow plasma exchange is illustrated in Figure 54–2.

Calculations for RBC exchanges, although somewhat more complicated, can be achieved in a similar manner. In this case, total blood volume is substituted for plasma volume, and the solute of interest is either the hemoglobin concentration or the hematocrit. For example, continuous-flow apheresis can be used for a sickle cell patient who has a total blood volume (TBV) of 5 L and a hematocrit of 32%. If it is assumed that the patient has 100% hemoglobin S and the therapeutic goal is to decrease the percentage of hemoglobin S to 30% while maintaining the patient's hematocrit at 32%, the amount of blood that must be processed would be given by

$$V_{ex} = 5000\text{ mL} \times \ln(100\%/30\%) = 6020\text{ mL}$$

The volume of RBCs needed for replacement to maintain the patient's hematocrit at 32% throughout the procedure would be

$$6020\text{ mL} \times 0.32 = 1926\text{ mL}$$

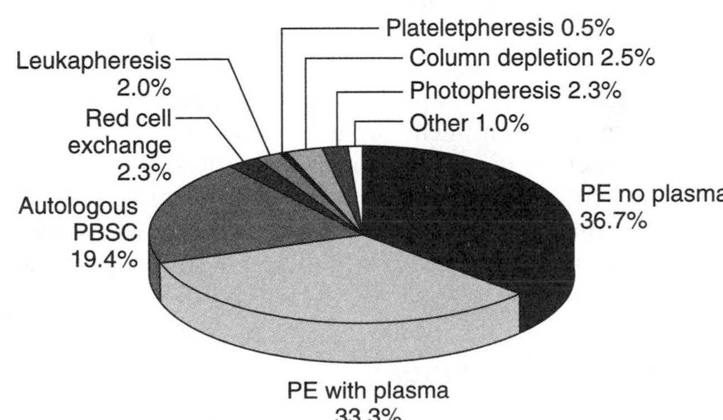

Figure 54–1 Relative frequency of therapeutic procedures by type, based on data from 18 institutions in the United States encompassing 3421 procedures. (Data from McLeod BC, Sniecinski I, Ciavarella D, et al. Frequency of immediate adverse effects associated with therapeutic apheresis. Transfusion 1999;39:282–288.)

If it is assumed that a typical allogeneic unit contains 200 mL of RBCs or RBC mass, then 10 units (1926 RBC mL/200 mL per unit = 9.6 units) would be needed.

An alternate approach takes into account that a 70% removal involves the processing of 1.2 times the RBC volume and dividing by the typical allogeneic unit RBC volume. In this case, it would be (5000 mL × 0.32 × 1.2)/200 = 9.6 units.

Timing

The timing of exchanges is generally chosen based on a balancing of the need to allow the solute or cell of interest to re-equilibrate into the vascular space and the desire to minimize the risk of bleeding with dilutional coagulopathy.

Efficiency of Immunoglobulin Removal

In the case of IgG, in which only 45% of the IgG lies within the intravascular space, a 1 plasma volume exchange would be expected to remove 63.2% of the intravascular IgG but only 28.4% of the total body IgG. Re-equilibration of the intravascular IgG with extravascular IgG typically occurs within 2 days and results in a substantial increase in the intravascular IgG level. For example, a patient with an IgG level of 10 g/L would

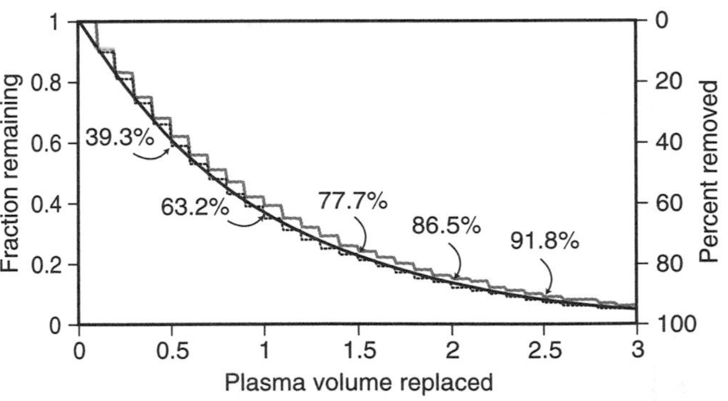

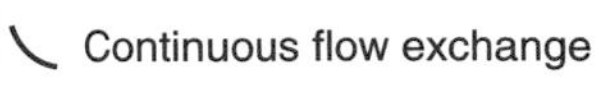

Figure 54–2 Theoretic fraction of solute remaining after plasma exchange for continuous and discontinuous flow separation.

Table 54–2 **Demonstration of the Apheresis Kinetics for Six Plasma Exchanges with a Theoretical Initial Intravascular IgG Level of 10 g/L in a Patient with a Blood Volume of 5 L, a Hematocrit of 40%, Receiving 1 Plasma Volume Exchange**

	Plasma IgG (g/L)	Intravascular IgG (g)	Extravascular IgG (g)	Total body IgG (g)
Preprocedure	10	30	36.67	66.67
1st 1PV TPE	3.68	11.04	36.67	47.71
1st Re-equilibration	7.16	21.47	26.24	47.71
2nd 1PV TPE	2.63	7.90	26.24	34.14
2nd Re-equilibration	5.12	15.36	18.78	34.14
3rd 1PV TPE	1.88	5.65	18.78	24.43
3rd Re-equilibration	3.66	10.99	13.44	24.43
4th 1PV TPE	1.35	4.05	13.44	17.48
4th Re-equilibration	2.62	7.87	9.62	17.48
5th 1PV TPE	0.97	2.90	9.62	12.51
5th Re-equilibration	1.88	5.63	6.88	12.51
6th 1PV TPE	0.69	2.07	6.88	8.95
6th Re-equilibration	1.34	4.03	4.92	8.95

have the intravascular IgG level reduced to 3.68 g/L, but after equilibration, this level would be expected to increase to 7.16 g/L (Table 54–2). Increasing the volume of plasma exchanged from 1 plasma volume to 1.5 plasma volumes is associated with only a modest increase in IgG removal (Fig. 54–3). Frequently, an overall 70% to 85% reduction of IgG is chosen as a goal of serial TPE therapy. A short-term reduction of 70% in the titer of anti-acetylcholine receptor in myasthenia gravis patients is generally associated with clinical improvement.[11]

To achieve a 70% to 85% reduction in intravascular IgG (after re-equilibration and ignoring synthesis and catabolism), one would in theory require four 1 plasma volume exchanges. Turnover of IgG is relatively slow, with an approximate half-life of 21 days, but rapid rebound frequently occurs, and sustained reductions of IgG cannot be achieved unless plasma exchange therapy is combined with immunosuppression. In practice, a 70% to 85% reduction in IgG can frequently be achieved with 5 to 6 plasma exchanges over 14 days *when combined with immunosuppression.* Despite the more-rapid synthesis of IgM (half-life of 5 to 6 days), comparable reductions of IgM are seen with

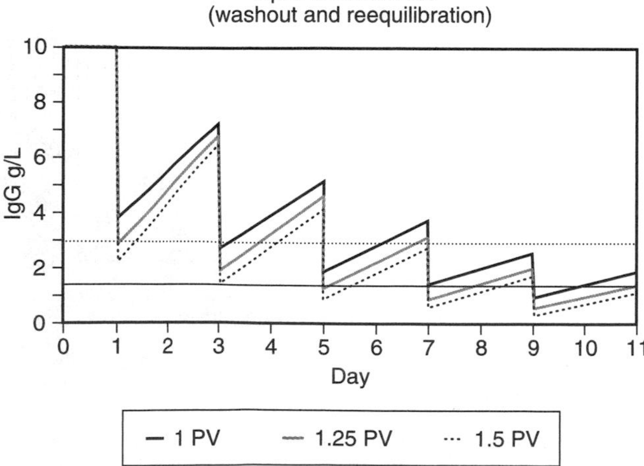

Figure 54–3 Theoretic reduction of immunoglobulin G (IgG) after plasma exchange of 1, 1.25, and 1.5 plasma volumes and after re-equilibration of total body IgG. The *solid line* indicates an 85% reduction, and the *dashed line*, a 70% reduction. The absolute reduction in IgG is reduced with each subsequent exchange. Calculations assume no degradation or synthesis of IgG and re-equilibration of IgG at 2 days.

the same number of exchanges, and rapid total body depletion of IgM (versus IgG) can be more effectively achieved because of the predominant intravascular distribution of IgM.

Reductions of IgG beyond 70% to 85% are difficult to achieve as the absolute reduction in IgG with each subsequent plasma exchange is reduced (see Fig. 54–3). For six successive 1 plasma volume exchanges, the decrease in IgG (immediately before to after procedure) in a patient with an initial IgG level of 10 g/L would be 6.3, 4.5, 3.2, 2.3, 1.7, and 1.2 g/L, respectively (see Table 54–2).

Thus the number of exchanges performed takes into account both the diminishing efficiency of removal associated with serial exchanges and the level that is generally associated with clinical efficacy.

OVERVIEW OF TECHNOLOGY

Current apheresis instrumentation involves the separation of blood components, segregation of the component being targeted by using on-line automated technology, and delivery of the remaining components back to the individual donor or patient. The use of temporary anticoagulation (with citrate alone or in combination with heparin) and disposable sterile plastic tubing sets enable these basic steps to be accomplished by a variety of instruments, which typically accommodate flow rates of 30 to 150 mL/min from either central or peripheral venous access.[12] Variations in the design of apheresis separators affects their efficiency of collection and removal and influences their suitability for specific donor or therapeutic applications. Currently licensed automated apheresis equipment separates blood components by either centrifugation or filtration and can operate with either continuous or intermittent flow. Table 54–3 summarizes the current technology.

Differential Centrifugation

Because of differences in density, anticoagulated whole blood separates into components when centrifuged. Mature RBCs have the greatest relative density, followed by neocytes, granulocytes, mononuclear cells (including lymphocytes, peripheral blood progenitor cells), and then platelets

Table 54–3 Summary of Current Apheresis Technology

Manufacturer	Instrument	Type	Flow	Access	Donor/ Therapeutic	Procedure/ Products
Haemonetics	V-50	C, bowl	I		D, T	PL
	PCS/PCS-2	C, bowl	I		D	PL
	MCS/MCS Plus	C, bowl	I		D, T	PL, PLT, Gran, RBCs, PBSCs
Gambro BCT (COBE)	Spectra	C, channel	*C*	1,2	D, T	PL, PLT, Gran, PBSC, TPE, RBCEx, cytoreduction
	Trima/Trima Accel	C, channel	*C*	1,2	D	PLT, PL, RBCs
Baxter	CS3000 Plus	C, bags	*C*	1,2	D, T	PL, PLT, Gran (mononuclear cells, PBSCs, TPE), RBCEx
	Amicus	C, bags	*C*	1,2	D	PL, PLT (future PBSCs and possibly RBCs)
	Alyx	C, bags	I	1	D	RBCs
	Autopheresis-C	SM	I	1	D	PL
Fresenius	AC104	C, channel	*C*	1,2	D, T	PL, PLT, Gran, PBSCs
Therakos (Johnson & Johnson)	UVAR II/XTS (photopheresis)	C, bowl	I	1,2	T	Photopheresis

C, centrifuge; SM, spinning membrane; I, intermittent; *C*, continuous; 1, single needle; 2, dual needle; D, donor; T, therapeutic; PL, plasma; PLT, platelets; Gran, granulocytes; RBC, red blood cells; PBSCs, peripheral blood stem cells; TPE, therapeutic plasma exchange; RBCEx, red blood cell exchange.

and finally plasma. Whole blood pumped into the apheresis separator enters a rotating bowl, chamber, tubular rotor, or a belt-shaped channel. Once equilibrium is reached, the desired fraction can be selectively removed. An optical sensor may aid in maintaining the interface between components, and all systems have a mechanism to prevent twisting of the tubing that feeds the separation chamber.

With intermittent flow (discontinuous flow), whole blood is processed in batches (refer to Fig. 54–4). With each cycle, the centrifuge device is filled; separation occurs until the dense component fills the separation container. Then processing is interrupted to empty the device. Haemonetics, Inc. (Braintree, MA) manufactures the most widely used currently licensed intermittent-flow centrifugation devices. These separators are useful for collection of plasma, platelets, leukocytes, or RBCs by a single or double venous access.

The Latham bowl is the centrifuge chamber in Haemonetics models: V50, MCS, and MCS Plus. This conical chamber has a stationary stem joined to the rotating bowl by a rotating seal. Blood enters the bottom (stationary stem) and rises between two conical surfaces. The centrifugal forces cause a vertical interface between RBCs (outside layer) and plasma (inside layer). Plasma, being of lower density, eventually exits the top of the bowl as the RBC layer widens. Ultimately, the RBCs will fill the entire bowl, necessitating interruption of processing to empty the bowl (see Fig. 54–4). The development of a surge technique has enabled greater purity of platelet and mononuclear cell products. This process involves blocking the flow of whole blood into the Latham bowl when an optical sensor detects the buffy coat. Then plasma from a reservoir bag is flushed rapidly into the still rotating bowl. The plasma flows through the cellular layers, thereby floating off platelets initially, followed by lymphocytes.

The plasmapheresis bowl for use with Haemonetics models V50 and PCS-2 is exclusively for collection of plasma. A cylindrical modification of the Latham bowl, it operates on the same principle.

Continuous-flow separators enable removal of components of different densities without interruption of processing. Equipment presently licensed includes apheresis separators manufactured by COBE/Gambro (Lakewood, Colo.), Fenwal (Baxter Biotech, Deerfield, Ill.), and Fresenius (Fresenius AG, Bad Hamburg, Germany).

The COBE/Gambro Spectra uses continuous-flow technology and is capable of double- or single-needle plateletpheresis (converts to intermittent flow for single-needle procedures) and double-needle leukapheresis as well as therapeutic procedures. The separation chamber is a belt-shaped channel with a lariat-like configuration to prevent twisting of the afferent and efferent lines. The system lacks a rotating seal. The plasma/buffy coat/RBC interface is automatically controlled by a microprocessor. Different software is used depending on the type of procedure (e.g., plasma exchange, granulocyte collection, or plateletpheresis). For plateletpheresis, a dual-stage channel maximizes product quality, including minimal contamination of leukocytes.

Like the COBE/Gambro Spectra, the Baxter CS3000 Plus is a seal-less system that relies on continuous-flow technology and is largely automated with numerous preprogrammed procedures. A closed system of plastic bags serves as the collection and separation chambers. Pressure plates, which are specific to the procedure being performed, affect the shape of these chambers, allowing a single tubing set to accommodate several different procedures. The addition of a novel platelet chamber, the TNX-6 separation chamber, has decreased leukocyte content of platelet products collected with this system.

Baxter's Amicus is a continuous-flow cell separator that is more portable, efficient, and operator friendly. Its novel features include ease of loading the disposable tubing kit and the unique drive mechanism for its centrifuge. The separation and collection containers resemble a belt around a spool and are uniquely configured to promote collection of small

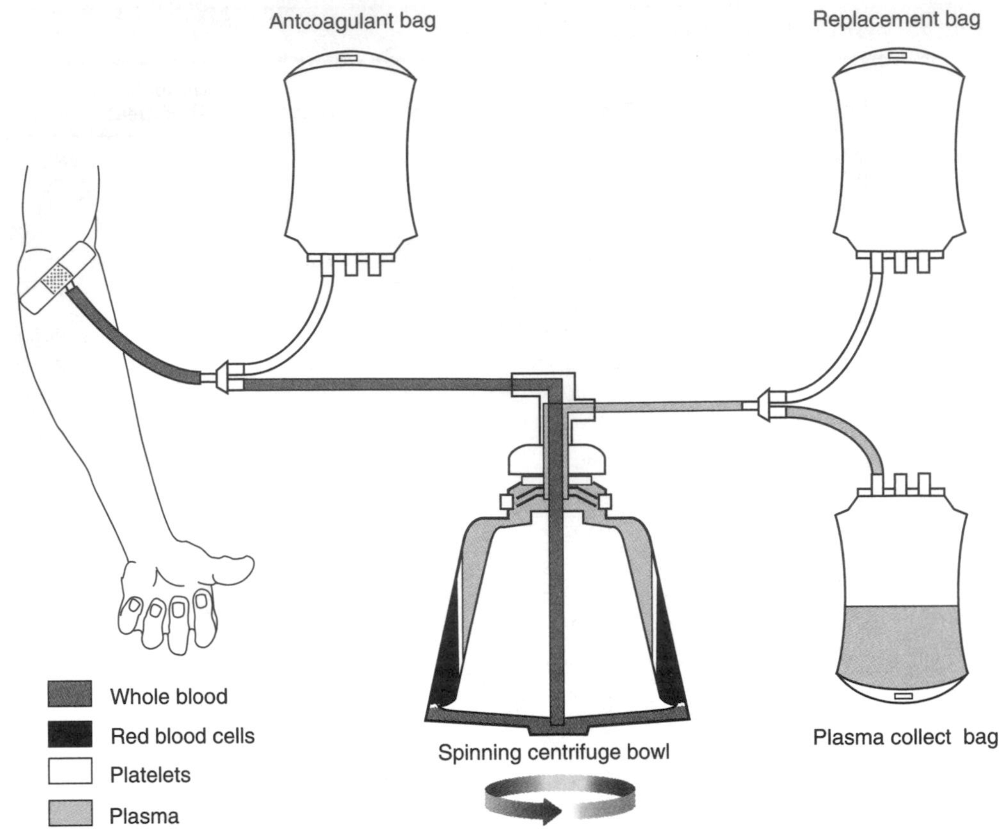

Figure 54–4 Example of an intermittent-flow apheresis procedure. Depicted is simplified representation of a plasma exchange. Whole blood enters the Latham bowl through a central channel and is dispersed at the bottom of the bowl. The blood is then forced to the periphery of the bowl and rises between two concentric conical surfaces. The centrifugal force causes the plasma, platelet-rich plasma, and red blood cells to form vertical layers. As more whole blood enters the bowl, the lighter plasma is forced up through an effluent tube and directed to the plasma collect bag. When the bowl is filled with red blood cells, the centrifuge is stopped and the pumps reversed, causing the red blood cells to be reinfused to the patient.

to large platelets, to concentrate RBCs, and to minimize mononuclear cell contamination of platelet products.

The Fresenius AS104 blood separator is another continuous-flow device using seal-less centrifugation. It offers multiple preprogrammed options as well as customized programming. For plateletpheresis, a dual-stage channel is used. A single-stage channel is used for granulocyte collections. The device also is capable of therapeutic plasmapheresis. Plasma collection as a by-product of plateletpheresis is a practical option; however, two-unit plasmapheresis collections are limited by the cost of disposable software. The AS104 does have the advantage of very low extracorporeal volume with two-needle procedures.

Filtration

Membrane-based blood separators rely on the differences in the actual size of particles rather than their density. In order of increasing size are platelets (3 μm), RBCs (7 μm), lymphocytes (10 μm), and granulocytes (13 μm). Separation of plasma from cellular elements becomes very practical because of the smaller size of instrumentation, lower extracorporeal volume, and the removal of all cellular debris, compared with centrifugal systems.

The two basic types of filtration separators are as follows: The hollow-fiber systems consist of a bundle of narrow hollow fibers with perforations along their surfaces. These are contained within a larger cylinder. As whole blood enters, the plasma will pass through the pores along the fibers, leaving a more concentrated cell suspension to exit the fibers; plasma can be collected via a side port. In the flat-plate membrane system, whole blood passes between two membranes, and plasma escapes through pores, to be collected separately from the cellular elements.

Filtration and centrifugation may be combined. Centrifugation can force plasma to separate from cellular elements via pores. Central placement of the filtration device moves the cellular elements away from the filter pores for improved efficiency. An example of this technology is the Fenwal Autopheresis-C. Originally used for plasma collection, by increasing pore size, this device can also be used to harvest platelets, although limited in efficacy. This is a discontinuous device requiring a single needle to access the donor.

Filtration techniques have been developed to attempt selective removal of a plasma constituent. If the undesirable or pathologic component is of large size, filtration of the separated plasma may afford reasonable removal. Addition of a second column with smaller pore sizes can be used. The arrangement of two or more columns in series is *cascade filtration.* Removal of low-density lipoproteins in familial hypercholesterolemia is an example of this application.[13]

Affinity Adsorption Apheresis

Affinity adsorption apheresis involves the selective extraction of immunologic or nonimmunologic substances from the circulation by means of a column, with the benefit of returning nonextracted proteins (e.g., clotting factors) to the patient. The column contains a sorbent or ligand attached to a carrier to which patient plasma is exposed while in the extracorporeal circuit. The most commonly used column is the staphylococcus protein A column, in which staph protein A as the ligand is attached to silica as the carrier (e.g., the Prosorba column; Cypres Inc., Seattle, Wash). These columns adsorb immune complexes and immunoglobulins via their Fc portion (with greatest affinity for IgG subclasses 1, 2, and 4, and lower affinity for IgG3, IgM, and IgA).[14] The majority of patients tolerate affinity apheresis without complications, although several reports have associated significant toxicity and at least one fatality with use of the staph protein A column.[15–19] It is approved for clinical use in the United States for treatment of idiopathic thrombocytopenia purpura, and, more recently, for refractory rheumatoid arthritis.

The Adacolumn (Japan Immunoresearch Laboratories Co., Ltd, Gunma, Japan) is a new adsorptive-type extracorporeal leukapheresis device. This device comprises a single-use, direct blood perfusion–type apheresis column. This column contains cellulose acetate beads in a saline solution, which have a selective affinity for granulocytes and monocytes/macrophages. As blood passes through the column, granulocytes and monocytes/macrophages bind to the beads, but other cellular elements, such as lymphocytes, platelets, or RBCs, are not significantly adsorbed. The selective removal of granulocytes and monocytes/macrophages has demonstrated clinical improvement in patients with inflammatory bowel disease, specifically, severe active ulcerative colitis, and possibly refractory Crohn's disease.[20–23] In Japan, the Adacolumn is approved for the treatment of active ulcerative colitis, but in the United States, this device is currently in phase III trials. The Cellsorba (Asahi Medical Co., Tokyo, Japan) is another selective apheresis device that uses filtration technology to remove leukocytes for management of similar diseases.

Photopheresis

An alternative approach to immunomodulation and tumor cell therapy is the use of extracorporeal photopheresis, also known as extracorporeal photochemotherapy (ECP). Photopheresis is a leukapheresis procedure in which the buffy coat is exposed to 8-methoxypsoralen (8-MOP) and ultraviolet A (UVA) radiation and reinfused into the patient.[24–26] 8-MOP is a photoreactive agent that will irreversibly crosslink DNA when exposed to UVA radiation. 8-MOP can be entered into this system by oral ingestion (in vivo) or by instilling it into the collection bag (vide infra). Because only 10% to 15% of the body's lymphocytes are manipulated during this procedure, the immune response is not secondary to direct cytotoxicity of the 8-MOP and UVA irradiation on the abnormal T cells or tumor cells.[27] The exact mechanism evoking a clinical response is still unclear. T cells isolated from the peripheral blood after photopheresis demonstrate increased apoptosis, and macrophages and dendritic cells exhibit the ability to phagocytose these apoptotic T cells.[28] It is surmised that photopheresis enhances the immune response against pathologic proliferating T-cell clones.[29–31]

Photopheresis has been FDA approved for cutaneous T-cell lymphoma (CTCL) since 1988.[32] A typical photopheresis course consists of two procedures on consecutive days every 4 weeks.[27] Several studies have also reported on its use in the management of nonmalignant immune-related conditions such as organ transplant rejection, graft-versus-host disease (acute and chronic), and autoimmune disorders.[32,33–35]

HEMAPHERESIS "DOSE" OR GOAL

The required volume of blood to be processed to achieve a treatment goal is based on the patient's TBV, PV, or RBC volume. Because the efficacy of the collection of the component being removed decreases with increasing volumes processed (see earlier discussion), it may be necessary to process several TBVs to reach a specific therapeutic goal. Patients being treated with plasma exchange typically have one PV removed per exchange. In contrast, with cytapheresis, multiple blood volumes may have to be processed to achieve a therapeutic end point. For example, patients requiring RBC exchange for sickle cell disease or malaria may require an exchange 1 to 2.5 times TBV to reach a therapeutic goal of 90% hemoglobin A or to reduce the parasitic load to less than 5%. Similarly, leukocytoreduction, used to treat patients with hyperleukocytosis, may require the processing of 1.5 to 2 times the TBV to reduce the leukocyte count by 50%.

Extracorporeal Blood Volume Assessment and Treatment Dose Calculation

To assess the patient's ability to tolerate the extracorporeal circuit and determine the "treatment dose," the patient's TBV, RBC volume, and PV must first be calculated. In general, two methods are commonly used to calculate TBV. One approach uses gender and weight, and the second uses the additional variable of height. Although both methods overestimate the TBV in obese patients and underestimate it in very muscular patients, they do provide a reasonable approximation of the TBV (Table 54–4). The patient's RBC volume and PV are calculated based on the TBV and the patient's current hematocrit.

The total extracorporeal volume is the amount of cells and plasma that is needed to displace the saline used for priming the lines (manufacturers generally provide this volume). The RBC extracorporeal volume is the RBC volume required to fill the bowl or channel and all the tubing, which is proportional to the patient's hematocrit. The lower the hematocrit, the more whole blood must be processed before RBCs are returned to the patient. Therefore the fraction of RBCs that is extracorporeal can greatly exceed the fraction of extracorporeal "blood." For example, the total volume of the extracorporeal circuit may be 10% of the TBV, but more than 10% of the packed RBC volume may be contained in the extracorporeal circuit. The extracorporeal volume also varies depending on the system (continuous vs. intermittent flow), type of procedure, and ancillary equipment such as blood warmers or single-needle devices.

Table 54–4 Calculation of Total Blood Volume

Rule of Fives[36]	**Blood Volume (mL/kg of body weight)**			
Patient Habitus	**Obese**	**Thin**	**Normal**	**Muscular**
Male	60	65	70	75
Female	55	60	65	70
Infant/child	—	—	80/70	—
Nadler's Formula (for adults)[37]				
Male	(0.006012 × height in inches³)/(14.6 × weight in pounds) + 604			
Female	(0.005835 × height in inches³)/(15 × weight in pounds) + 183			

Management of Extracorporeal Volume

The general standard of care is for neither the total extracorporeal blood volume nor the extracorporeal RBC volume to exceed 15% of the patient's total blood volume or RBC volume, respectively. If the total extracorporeal volume is 15% to 20% but the extracorporeal red RBC volume is less than 15% (i.e., in a patient with a high hematocrit), a saline bolus or colloid prime may be needed to prevent hypotension secondary to intravascular hypovolemia.

If the extracorporeal total volume is less than 15% but the patient has a low hematocrit, the extracorporeal RBC volume may exceed 15%. The patient should be carefully monitored for signs of hypoxia. If the patient has a history of cardiac or pulmonary problems or is symptomatic (short of breath, tachycardic, or requiring oxygen), priming of the extracorporeal circuit with RBCs should be considered. For asymptomatic patients, both adults and children, one approach is to calculate the intraprocedure hematocrit:

Intraprocedure hematocrit =

[(Initial RBC volume–extracorporeal RBC volume)/TBV] × 100

This formula assumes that the patient is maintained in an isovolemic state during the procedure. If the intraprocedure hematocrit is equal to or greater than 24% in an asymptomatic patient, the patient typically will not require transfusion. Asymptomatic patients with chronic anemia may be able to tolerate even lower hematocrits.

CHOICE OF REPLACEMENT SOLUTIONS FOR PLASMA EXCHANGE

In the 1970s, after the introduction of cell separators for plasma exchange, it was common practice to replace plasma removed with stored allogeneic plasma. Complications with viral contamination (particularly hepatitis) and citrate toxicity led to the search for a safer alternative. Because large amounts of plasma protein that provided colloidal osmotic pressure were being removed, it seemed reasonable to replace the removed human plasma protein with human-derived plasma protein in the form of 5% albumin (which is >96% pure albumin) or plasma protein fraction (>83% pure albumin). These replacement solutions largely resolved the problems of disease transmission and citrate toxicity. Subsequently, the introduction of partial saline replacement was integrated into replacement regimens.[38,39]

In recent years, market recalls (due to Creutzfeldt-Jakob disease or bacterial contamination) and increased demand have compromised the availability of albumin and purified protein fraction. Decreased availability, increasing costs, recognition of drug interactions with albumin (i.e., angiotensin-converting enzyme [ACE] inhibitors), and a fear of disease transmission led several groups to the use of colloidal starches (hydroxethyl starches, also known as HES) as partial or full replacement for plasma during plasma exchange.[40–45] One regimen currently in use includes 3% Hespan (6% Hespan diluted 1:1 with normal saline) at 110% replacement initially, followed by a final liter of replacement with 5% albumin at 100% replacement.[43] An alternative approach used 10% pentastarch for the first half of the colloid replacement, followed by 5% albumin.[45] In some cases, 25% albumin is diluted to 5% albumin for use as replacement. Hemolysis has occurred when hypotonic solutions have been used as a diluent; 25% albumin should be diluted with normal saline.[46–48]

In specific clinical settings, patients may require replacement of a specific plasma protein (such as von Willebrand factor metalloprotease in thrombocytopenic thrombotic purpura) or clotting factors in patients at increased risk for bleeding (e.g., Goodpasture syndrome with pulmonary hemorrhage). In such cases, plasma or modified plasma (e.g., solvent/detergent-treated plasma, cryoreduced plasma supernatant) may be indicated as full or partial replacement.

Supplementation of replacement solutions (saline, colloidal starches, and albumin) with calcium can reduce the incidence of hypocalcemia secondary to citrate toxicity. In one study, the incidence of citrate toxicity was reduced from 35.6% to 8.6% with a constant calcium gluconate infusion.[49] Possible regimens include the addition of 10% calcium gluconate (10 mL per liter of return fluid) or the addition of calcium chloride ($CaCl_2$, 200 mg per liter of return fluid).[7,48] Most patients tolerate hypocalcemia without major adverse effects. However, patients with fulminant liver failure require close monitoring of ionized calcium levels to avoid severe hypocalcemia.

VASCULAR ACCESS

Apheresis procedures require high blood flow rates. Such flow rates can typically be achieved with peripheral venous access with one to two large-bore needles (16 to 18 gauge). However, the absence of peripheral access or an inability to augment venous return by fist clenching (in patients who are unconscious, confused, or uncooperative and in those who have significant muscle weakness or are easily fatigued) often necessitate the placement of central catheters.[12] Routine central catheters are flexible and are designed for positive pressure; such "soft-walled" catheters collapse under the negative pressure exerted by the cell separators during blood withdrawal. Therefore, more-rigid, specifically designed apheresis or dialysis catheters are required for apheresis procedures. Central catheters are not without risk, and much of the morbidity associated with apheresis procedures is catheter related. Catheters can be associated with infection (line or catheter sepsis), bleeding, pneumothorax or hemothorax (if placed in the chest), and air emboli. Before the placement of a central catheter, decisions must be made regarding the optimal location of the catheter for a given patient. For example, femoral catheters are relatively easy to place but are associated with increased risk of infection. Such placement may be appropriate for a patient who requires a catheter for a brief period, whereas a subclavian or tunneled catheter may be more appropriate for prolonged access.

ANTICOAGULANTS

Citrate, heparin, or a combination of citrate and heparin is used during apheresis to prevent coagulation in the extracorporeal circuit. To determine the anticoagulant of choice, the patient should be carefully evaluated for the ability to tolerate citrate versus heparin anticoagulation. Other considerations include an assessment of how the patient will tolerate an increased intravascular volume, the type and length of the procedure, the type and volume of replacement fluid, the type of vascular access, and the inlet blood flow.

Citrate prevents coagulation by binding ionized calcium, which is required for multiple steps in the coagulation cascade. A healthy liver metabolizes citrate as quickly as it is infused at typical rates. If the infusion rate exceeds hepatic metabolism, transient hypocalcemia can occur. Low calcium levels may induce mild paresthesias (perioral, distal extremities), or progress to gastrointestinal symptoms, hypotension, and, in most extreme situations, cardiac dysrhythmias or seizures. The patient in liver failure is at greatest risk. In such clinical settings, management of the patient requires frequent monitoring of ionized calcium, the possible addition of a calcium drip, a decreased citrate infusion rate, or both.

Citrate is available in three forms: ACD-A, ACD-B, and a concentrate of trisodium citrate. ACD-A is the most widely used form; it is a 3% citrate solution that may be administered at a ratio of whole blood to anticoagulant (WB/ACD ratio) of 9:1 to 14:1. ACD-B is a 2% citrate solution that is usually administered at a ratio of 6:1 or 9:1. ACD-B is used primarily with systems that have a fixed WB/ACD ratio to reduce the risk of citrate toxicity. Trisodium citrate is used with leukapheresis. Between 30 and 40 mL of trisodium citrate concentrate (46.7%) is mixed with 500 mL of a sedimenting agent (HES or Pentastarch) during leukapheresis, permitting the anticoagulant pump to titrate the sedimenting agent as well as the anticoagulant. Trisodium citrate can also be diluted with normal saline to make a solution similar to ACD. Trisodium citrate should never be administered undiluted.[50]

Heparin, unlike citrate, is not rapidly metabolized (half-life of 90 minutes) and results in systemic anticoagulation. This can be particularly problematic during plasmapheresis with nonplasma replacement (e.g., 5% albumin or hetastarch) because of the removal of plasma-associated clotting factors. Heparin may be used alone or in combination with ACD-A or ACD-B. When a combination is used, less heparin and a lower volume of ACD-A are required for effective anticoagulation. Such combinations therefore decrease the incidence of citrate toxicity, minimize the systemic anticoagulation caused by heparin alone, and reduce the total fluid volume of the procedure. Use of heparin alone may result in platelet aggregation during cytapheresis procedures.

DRUG CLEARANCE

On rare occasions, plasma exchange is used to assist in the treatment of acute drug toxicity when other modalities such as gastric lavage, dialysis, hemoperfusion, and forced diuresis have been ineffective. Drugs that are lipophilic and highly protein bound, with long half-lives and small volumes of distribution, are most effectively removed. Plasma exchange has been used to improve drug clearance with barbiturates, theophylline, vincristine, cisplatin, digoxin antidigoxin-antibody complexes (in the presence of renal failure), paraquat, quinidine, tricyclic antidepressants, acetaminophen, and phenytoin.

More commonly, one encounters the question of the effect of plasma exchange on therapeutic drug dosing. In general, drugs that are most affected have a small volume of distribution and are extensively protein bound (similar to drugs that are treated with plasma exchange in acute toxicity). Drug kinetics in the context of plasma exchange has not been extensively studied. The limited data suggest that supplemental dosing of prednisone, digoxin, cyclosporine, ceftriaxone, ceftazidime, valproic acid, and phenobarbital after plasma exchange is not necessary.[51,52] In contrast, dosing of certain drugs such as salicylates and tobramycin should be supplemented, and phenytoin, in which there are conflicting reports of clearance, requires careful patient monitoring. In general, removal of a drug is likely to be increased during the distribution phase after administration. Therefore, it would seem prudent that when possible, drug doses should be administered after a plasma exchange and not immediately before the exchange.

EFFECT ON CLOTTING AFTER PLASMA EXCHANGE

Therapeutic plasma exchange is generally associated with the rapid (and repeated) removal of large quantities of plasma and its associated coagulant proteins.[9,42,43,53–55] When coagulant protein–deficient replacement fluids such as albumin, saline, and colloidal starches are used, an acute decrease in clotting factor activity, varying from 40% to 70% of baseline, can be observed immediately after the exchange. This is usually associated with a small prolongation in measured prothrombin time (PT) and activated partial thromboplastin time (aPTT), although such values frequently remain within the normal range. Fibrinogen, having a volume of distribution that is almost exclusively intravascular, is the clotting factor most depleted. Levels of clotting factors usually return to normal within 1 to 2 days after an exchange. The consensus is that, in the absence of an underlying hemostatic defect or liver disease, use of clotting factor–free replacement solutions is appropriate.

An unintentional consequence of plasma removal is a reduction in circulating platelets. Mean reduction of platelets after a plasma exchange has been variably reported to range from 9.4% to 52.6%.[7,43,56–58] This wide range probably reflects differences in the amount of PV processed, the cell separators used, and the settings used. Larger volumes processed and low-speed settings (decreased centrifugal force) are associated with greater platelet loss.[59] Despite mean decreases in platelet counts of 52.6% after 1.6 PVs exchanged, Sultan and colleagues[53] found that the platelets (as well as all clotting factors measured, with the exception of antithrombin [AT III]) had almost reached or even exceeded their initial values after 48 to 96 hours (just before the next plasma exchange). We have also observed normal platelet counts 48 hours after 1 PV (just before the next plasma exchange).

In a hemostatically compromised patient or if large-volume daily exchanges are performed, hemostatic parameters should be monitored, and the replacement supplemented with plasma or platelets, as clinically indicated.

ADVERSE REACTIONS

Adverse reactions associated with therapeutic apheresis are uncommon. A 1995 survey conducted by the American Association of Blood Banks Hemapheresis Committee involving 18 centers and 3429 procedures, reported 242 adverse invents involving 163 procedures (4.75% of all procedures, 6.87% of first-time procedures, and 4.28% of repeated procedures).[8] Mild reactions were not reported in this study. The types of reactions reported were as follows: transfusion reactions, 1.6%; citrate-related nausea and vomiting, 1.2%; hypotension, 1.0%; vasovagal nausea and vomiting, 0.5%; diaphoresis, 0.5%; tachycardia, 0.4%; respiratory distress, 0.3%; tetany or seizure, 0.2% (associated with fresh frozen plasma replacement); and chills or rigors, 0.2%. Three deaths, attributed to primary disease, were reported in this study. Although deaths have occurred in patients being treated with therapeutic apheresis, most have occurred in critically ill patients and were not thought to be secondary to the apheresis procedures. Mortality rates are largely a function of the patient population treated. For example, estimates of the mortality of patients with thrombotic thrombocytopenia purpura range from 10% to 20%.[60,61] Overall, estimated mortality rates of 1 per 1000 to 3 per 10,000 procedures more accurately reflect the underlying disease of the patient than the risk of the procedure.[8,62]

Adverse reactions or complications that occur in the setting of therapeutic apheresis may be caused by the procedure (anticoagulant, replacement fluids), by an underlying condition (anemia; renal, cardiac, hepatic disease; sepsis; dehydration), or adjunctive therapy (vasopressors, antihypertensives, diuretics). Before therapy is initiated, the patient should be carefully evaluated for risk factors, and a care plan should be developed to minimize risk.

Although the following reactions may occur outside the setting of apheresis, the use of citrate anticoagulation, the large volume, and the rapid infusion of a variety of replacement solutions predispose the apheresis subject to the following adverse events. Mild hypocalcemia or citrate reaction (characterized by tingling, oral paresthesias, or chest discomfort) is the most commonly encountered adverse reaction. Such reactions are usually mild and easily managed by slowing the infusion rate, changing the WB/ACD ratio, or giving oral calcium. More severe reactions may be treated or prevented by administering intravenous calcium. Calcium chloride may be added to the replacement fluid (200 mg per liter of 5% albumin or 3% to 6% HES) or given at a very slow rate intravenously (200 mg, diluted to ≥20 mg/mL, infused over 2 minutes) when replacing with fresh frozen plasma.

Allergic-type reactions, ranging from mild urticaria to anaphylaxis, are associated with the use of replacement fluids, including plasma, HES, and albumin. Premedication with antihistamines may prevent allergic reactions in most patients, but some patients develop mild to severe reactions even with premedication. In this group of patients, multiple strategies may be required. In addition to premedication with antihistamines such as $histamine_1$ antagonists (e.g., diphenhydramine), use of a $histamine_2$ blocker (e.g., hydroxyzine, cimetidine), and a continuous antihistamine drip may be effective in preventing breakthrough reactions.

Atypical allergic or anaphylactoid reactions have been described, respectively, with ethylene oxide gas sterilization of tubing sets and with drug interactions between ACE inhibitors and albumin. Ethylene oxide reactions are usually characterized by periorbital edema with chemosis and tearing.[63] Double priming of the tubing is useful in the prevention of the recurrence of such a reaction. ACE inhibitor reactions are associated with albumin infusion during therapeutic plasma exchange.[40] It is thought that the symptoms are caused by rapid infusion of low levels of prekallikrein activator (a metabolite of clotting factor XII) found in the albumin product, which activates prekallikrein to bradykinin, a naturally occurring vasoactive peptide. Metabolism of bradykinin is inhibited by the ACE inhibitor, leading to an accumulation of bradykinin. The patient may experience mild to severe facial flushing, hypotension, and a feeling of doom. ACE inhibitor therapy should be discontinued 24 to 48 hours before the start of therapeutic plasma exchange (TPE). If the patient's condition is such that the procedure cannot be delayed for 24 to 48 hours, a colloidal starch such as HES may be used for replacement.

CONCLUSION

The field of apheresis continues to evolve in both the technology and the understanding of how we can affect the pathophysiology of disease with apheresis. Careful assessment of the patient and expertise in therapeutic apheresis is essential to optimize therapy and minimize adverse consequences. Subsequent chapters explore in depth the use of therapeutic apheresis for both cellular and plasma therapy.

REFERENCES

1. Abel J. Rowntree LG, Turner BB: Plasma removal with return of corpuscles (plasmaphaeresis). J Pharmacol Exp Ther 1914;5:625–647.
2. Adams WS, Bland WH, Bassett SH. A method of human plasmapheresis. Proc Soc Exp Biol Med 1952;80:377–379.
3. Skoog WA, Adams WA. Plasmapheresis in a case of Waldenstrom's macroglobulinemia. Clin Res 1959;7:96.
4. Schwab PJ, Fahey JL. Treatment of Waldenstrom's macroglobulinemia by plasmapheresis. N Engl J Med 1969;263:574–579.
5. Solomon A, Fahey JL. Plasmapheresis therapy in macroglobulinaemia. Ann Intern Med 1963;58:789–800.
6. Reynolds WA. Late report of the first case of plasmapheresis for Waldenstrom's macroglobulinemia. JAMA 1981;245:606–607.
7. Owen HG, Brecher ME. Management of the therapeutic apheresis patient. In McLeod BC, Price TH, Drew MJ (eds). Apheresis: Principles and Practice. Bethesda, Md., American Association of Blood Banks, 1997, pp 223–249.
8. McLeod BC, Sniecinski I, Ciavarella D, et al. Frequency of immediate adverse effects associated with therapeutic apheresis. Transfusion 1999;39:282–288.
9. Smith JW, Weinstein R, Hillyer K. Therapeutic apheresis: a summary of current indication categories endorsed by the AABB and the American Society for Apheresis. Transfusion 2003;43:820–822.
10. McCullough J, Chopek M. Therapeutic plasma exchange. Lab Med 1981;12:745–753.
11. Dau PC. Plasmapheresis therapy in myasthenia gravis. Muscle Nerve 1980;3:468–482.
12. Hodgson WJB, Mercan S. Hemapheresis listening post: optimal venous access. Transfusion Sci 1991;12:274.
13. Leitman SF, Smith JW, Gregg RE. Homozygous hypercholesterolemia: selective removal of low density lipoproteins by secondary membrane filtration. Transfusion 1989;29:341.
14. Pineda AA. Immunoaffinity apheresis columns: clinical application and therapeutic mechanisms of action. In Sacher RA, Brubaker DB, Kasprisin DO, McCarthy LJ (eds). Cellular and Humoral Immunotherapy and Apheresis. Arlington, Va., American Association of Blood Banks, 1991, p 31.
15. Belak M, Widder RA, Brunner R, et al. Immunoadsorption with protein A Sepharose or silica. Lancet 1994;343:792–793.
16. Garey DC, Perry E, Jackson B. Fatal pulmonary reaction with staph protein A immune adsorption for pure red cell aplasia. Transfusion 1988;28:245a.
17. Snyder HW Jr, Cochran SK, Balint JP Jr, et al. Experience with protein A-immunoadsorption in treatment-resistant adult immune thrombocytopenic purpura. Blood 1992;79:2237–2245.
18. Smith RE, Gottschall JL, Pisciotta AV. Life-threatening reaction to staphylococcal protein A immunomodulation. J Clin Apheresis 1992;7:4–5.
19. Young JB, Ayus JC, Miller LK, et al. Cardiopulmonary toxicity in patients with breast carcinoma during plasma perfusion over immobilized protein A. Am J Med 1983;75:278–288.
20. Shimoyama T, Sawada K, Hiwatashi N, et al: Safety and efficacy of granulocyte and monocyte apheresis in patients with active ulcerative colitis: a multicenter study. J Clin Apheresis 2001;16:1–9, 2001.
21. Rembacken BJ, Newbould HE, Richards SJ, et al: Granulocyte apheresis in inflammatory bowel disease: possible mechanisms of effect. Ther Apheresis 1998;2:93–96.

22. Naganuma M, Funakoshi S, Sakuraba A, et al. Granulocytapheresis is useful as an alternative therapy in patients with steroid-refractory or -dependent ulcerative colitis. Inflamm Bowel Dis 2004;10:251–257.
23. Fukuda Y, Matsui T, Suzuki Y, et al. Adsorptive granulocytes and monocyte apheresis for refractory Crohn's disease: an open multicenter prospective study. J Gastroenterol 2004;39:1158–1164.
24. Edelson R, Berger C, Gasparro F, et al. Treatment of cutaneous T-cell lymphoma by extracorporeal photochemotherapy: preliminary results. N Engl J Med 1987;316:297–303.
25. Gollnick HP, Owsianowski M, Ramaker J, et al. Extracorporeal photopheresis: a new approach for the treatment of cutaneous T cell lymphomas. Cancer Res 1995;139:409–415.
26. Armus S, Keyes B, Cahill C, et al. Photopheresis for the treatment of cutaneous T-cell lymphoma. J Am Acad Dermatol 1990;23:898–902.
27. Christensen I, Heald P. Photopheresis in the 1990s. J Clin Apheresis 1991; 6:216–220.
28. Lamioni A, Parisi F, Isacchi G, et al. The immunological effects of extracorporeal photopheresis unraveled: induction of tolerogenic dendritic cells in vitro and regulatory T cells in vivo. Transplantation 2005;79: 846–850.
29. Zic J, Arzubiaga C, Salhany KE, et al. Extracorporeal photopheresis for the treatment of cutaneous T-cell lymphoma. J Am Acad Dermatol 1992; 27:729–736.
30. Stevens SR, Bowen GM, Duvic M, et al. Effectiveness of photopheresis in Sezary syndrome. Arch Dermatol 1999;135:995–997.
31. van Iperen HP, Beijersbergen van Henegouwen GM. Clinical and mechanistic aspects of photopheresis. J Photochem Photobiol B 1997;39: 99–109.
32. Zic JA, Miller JL, Stricklin GP, King LE. The North American experience with photopheresis. Ther Apheresis 1990;3:50–62.
33. Kumlien G, Genberg H, Shanwell A, Tyden G. Photopheresis for the treatment of refractory renal graft rejection. Transplantation 2005; 79:123–125.
34. Dall'Amico R, Messina C. Extracorporeal photochemotherapy for the treatment of graft-versus-host disease. Ther Apheresis 2002;6:296–304.
35. Foss FM, DiVenuti GM, Chin K, et al. Prospective study of extracorporeal photopheresis in steroid-refractory or steroid-resistant extensive chronic graft-versus-host disease: analysis of response and survival incorporating prognostic factors. Bone Marrow Transplant 2005;35:1187–1193.
36. Gilcher RO. Apheresis: Principles and practices. In Rossi EC, Simon TL, Moss GS, Gould SA (eds). Principles of Transfusion Medicine, 2nd ed. Baltimore, Md., Williams & Wilkins, 1996, pp 537–545.
37. Nadler SB, Hidalgo JU, Bloch T. Prediction of blood volume in normal human adults. Surgery 1962;51:224.
38. Lasky LC, Finnerty EP, Glenis L, et al. Protein and colloid osmotic pressure changes with albumin and/or saline replacement during plasma exchange. Transfusion 1984;24:256–259.
39. McLeod BC, Sassetti RJ, Stefoski D, Davis FA. Partial plasma protein replacement in therapeutic plasma exchange. J Clin Apheresis 1983;1:115–118.
40. Owen HG, Brecher ME. Atypical reactions associated with ACE inhibitors and apheresis. Transfusion 1994;34:891–894.
41. Brecher ME, Owen HG. Washout kinetics of colloidal starch as a partial or full replacement for plasma exchange. J Clin Apheresis 1996;11:123–126.
42. Owen HG, Brecher ME. Partial colloid replacement for therapeutic plasma exchange. J Clin Apheresis 1997;12:87–92.
43. Brecher ME, Owen HG, Bandarenko N. Alternatives to albumin: starch replacement for plasma exchange. J Clin Apheresis 1997;12:146–153.
44. Owen HG, Brecher ME, Howard JF, Bandarenko N. Minimizing hypovolemic reactions with 3% hetastarch replacement during therapeutic plasma exchange [Abstract]. J Clin Apheresis 1999;14:91.
45. Gross AG, Weinstein R. Pentastarch as partial replacement fluid for therapeutic plasma exchange: Effect on plasma proteins, adverse events during treatment, and serum ionized calcium. J Clin Apheresis 1999;14:114–121.
46. Steinmuller DR. A dangerous error in the dilution of 25 percent albumin [Letter]. N Engl J Med 1998;338:1226–1227.
47. Pierce LR, Gaines A, Varricchio F, Epstein J. Hemolysis and renal failure associated with the inappropriate use of sterile water to dilute human albumin 25%. N Engl J Med 1998;338:1226–1227.
48. Pierce LR, Gaines A, Finlayson JS, et al. Hemolysis and acute renal failure due to the administration of albumin diluted in sterile water [Letter]. Transfusion 1999;39:110–111.
49. Weinstein R. Prevention of citrate reactions during therapeutic plasma exchange by constant infusion of calcium gluconate with the return fluid. J Clin Apheresis 1996;11:204–210.
50. FDA issues warning on tricitrasol dialysis catheter anticoagulant, April 14, 2000. Available at http://www.fda.gov/bbs/topics/ANSWERS/ANS01009.html.
51. Pramodini BK B, Woo MW. A review of the effects of plasmapheresis on drug clearance. Pharmacotherapy 1997;17:684–695.
52. Stigelman WH, Henry DH, Talbert RL, Townsend RJ. Removal of prednisone and prednisolone by plasma exchange. Clin Pharm 1984;3: 402–407.
53. Sultan Y, Bussel A, Maisonneuve P, et al. Potential danger of thrombosis after plasma exchange in the treatment of patients with immune disease. Transfusion 1979;19:558–593.
54. Simon TL. Coagulation disorders with plasma exchange. Plasma Ther Transfus Technol 1982;3:147–153.
55. Domen RE, Kennedy MS, Jones LL, Senhauser DA. Hemostatic imbalances produced by plasma exchange. Transfusion 1984;24:336–339.
56. Orlin JB, Berkman EM. Partial plasma exchange using albumin replacement: Removal and recovery of normal plasma constituents. Blood 1980;56:1055–1059.
57. Wood L, Jacobs P. The effect of serial therapeutic plasmapheresis on platelet count, coagulation factors, plasma immunoglobulin and complement levels. J Clin Apheresis 1986;3:124–128.
58. Flaum MA, Cueo RA, Appelbaum FR, et al. The hemostatic imbalance of plasma-exchange transfusion. Blood 1979;54:694–702.
59. Owen HG, Koo A, McAteer M, Brecher ME. Evaluation of platelet loss during TPE on the COBE SPECTRA. J Clin Apheresis 1997;12:28.
60. Bandarenko N, Brecher ME, Unites States Thrombotic Thrombocytopenic Purpura Apheresis Study Group (US TTP ASG). Multicenter survey and retrospective analysis of current efficacy of therapeutic plasma exchange. J Clin Apheresis 1998;13:133–141.
61. Brailey L, Brecher ME, Bandarenko N. Thrombotic thrombocytopenia purpura. Ther Apheresis 1999;3:20–24.
62. Huestis DW. Complications of therapeutic apheresis. In Valbonesi M, Pineda AA, Bigs JC (eds). Therapeutic Hemapheresis. Milan, Wichtig Editore, 1986, pp 179–186.
63. Leitman SF, Boltansky H, Alter HJ, et al. Allergic reactions in healthy plateletpheresis donors caused by sensitization to ethylene oxide gas. N Engl J Med 1986;315:1192–1196.

Chapter 55
Therapeutic Plasma Exchange

Bruce C. McLeod

Like many true stories, the history of therapeutic plasma exchange (TPE) is sprinkled with serendipity. TPE arose from the ideas and efforts of a number of people who had no intention of treating patients and was helped along by others who were not interested in a device for exchanging plasma. After a long period of inadvertent stage setting, TPE emerged over a fairly short interval as a credible therapy and has become an important treatment for a number of diseases.

Seminal credit is usually given to Abel and colleagues,[1] who, in pursuing higher yields of antisera for serotherapy, devised manual plasmapheresis in 1914 to obtain more plasma from immunized horses without exsanguinating them. Skoog and Adams[2] and Schwab and Fahey[3] later applied this technique to patients with the hyperviscosity syndrome. Recognition should also be extended to Dr. Edwin Cohn and his associates[4] (especially his engineering consultant, Alan Latham[5]), who, in the 1950s, adapted for blood-component donation the concept of continuous-flow centrifugation invented 60-odd years earlier for the dairy industry by Carl Gustav Patrick De Laval.[6] Nor should one forget to mention Dr. Emil Freireich, George Judson, and others at the National Cancer Institute, who, in the 1960s, constructed a centrifugal blood cell separator to remove white blood cells from patients with chronic myelogenous leukemia.[7] Further refinement of concepts originating with these workers led eventually to the commercial availability of several semiautomated blood-separator instruments for clinical use.

RATIONALE FOR THERAPEUTIC PLASMA EXCHANGE

In the 1960s and early 1970s, the notion of treating a patient with a large-scale plasma exchange carried out with such an instrument began to take hold, first in Rh-sensitized women[8–10] and patients with systemic lupus erythematosus (SLE)[11,12] and then in other illnesses. The common threads linking these disorders were the beliefs that a circulating macromolecule was a crucial pathogenetic factor and that meaningful clinical improvement could be brought about by removing the material.

TPE has often been likened to the practice of bloodletting to remove evil humors. The notion of therapeutic removal is a sound one that has changed little since medieval times; however, the concept of an evil humor has been refined. Three subtypes of molecules are candidates for therapeutic removal: (1) molecules that are troublesome because of their binding specificity: these are always antibodies and usually autoantibodies; (2) molecules that confer troublesome physical properties on the plasma and hence on the blood, such as hyperviscosity or cold insolubility: these are also usually antibodies, although they are often in immune complexes; and (3) molecules that have a nonimmune toxicity, such as low-density lipoproteins (LDLs). An important therapeutic effect arising from removal is more easily envisioned for large molecules having a relatively long half-life in the circulation and a corresponding low synthetic rate. The majority of successfully treated disorders are due to pathogenic immunoglobulin G (IgG), which has these properties. It has been hypothesized at various times that removal of complement or coagulation proteins, or both, or mediators of inflammation derived from them or secreted by inflammatory cells might contribute to a therapeutic effect. Such mechanisms are unlikely to be of clinical importance because the candidate molecules have relatively short half-lives or rapid synthetic rates, and no such effect has been proven.

TPE can also be used in a fourth way, not foreseen by medieval barbers or 19th-century physicians, and that is to achieve relatively high levels of a normal plasma constituent that is not available in a concentrated form. These four distinct rationales for TPE are summarized in Table 55–1.

GENERAL PRINCIPLES OF THERAPEUTIC PLASMA EXCHANGE

Mathematical Principles

Patients sometimes liken TPE to an oil change, and it is instructive to consider why this analogy is misleading. A 5-L oil exchange that is nearly 100% efficient can be performed on an automobile engine in 10 minutes because the engine is not running during the exchange. By contrast, limitations are imposed on the rate and efficiency of TPE by the need to keep the heart pumping and the blood stream nearly full throughout the procedure. These requirements dictate that only a small proportion of the total blood volume be extracorporeal at any given moment. TPE must therefore proceed gradually, either continuously or in small increments.

Consequently, as an exchange progresses, an increasing proportion of the material removed is not the patient's plasma but replacement fluid infused earlier in the procedure. In such a process, the behavior of an entirely intravascular substance that is absent in the replacement medium is described by the formula

$$y_x = y_0 e^{-x}$$

where y_0 is the starting concentration of the substance, e is the base natural logarithm, and y_x is the concentration of the substance after x patient plasma volumes have been

Table 55–1 Rationales for Therapeutic Plasma Exchange

Goal of TPE Therapy	Example
Remove antibody with harmful specificity	Autoantibody
Remove protein (usually antibody) with harmful physical property	Hyperviscosity
Remove nonantibody toxin	Low-density lipoprotein
Correct deficiency of plasma factor	Thrombotic thrombocytopenic purpura

exchanged. If y_0 is assigned a normalized value of 1.0, a plot of the function yields the smooth asymptotic middle curve in Figure 55–1, which describes a continuous exchange. The flanking curves, which describe small incremental discontinuous exchanges, are similar.[13] Experimental work has shown that this formula is also predictive of exchange outcomes for macromolecules such as LDL[14] and IgG[15] that have a substantial extravascular reservoir, if equilibration between the intravascular and extravascular compartments is slow relative to the rate of removal.

As noted earlier, the molecule targeted for removal in many patients is an IgG antibody. Because slightly more than half of IgG is extravascular[13] and removal of intravascular IgG becomes progressively less efficient with larger exchange volumes, most practitioners choose to limit an exchange to 1 to 1.5 patient plasma volumes, which removes 60% to 75% of intravascular material and limits side effects associated with depletion of normal plasma components.

Equilibration with extravascular sources over 1 to 2 days increases the intravascular IgG level, and further removal by exchange can then be undertaken more advantageously. The effects of a series of TPEs on intravascular, extravascular, and total IgG are shown schematically in Figure 55–2. For reasons given subsequently, human serum albumin is the most common replacement fluid in TPE. In these cases, all plasma constituents except albumin are removed but not replaced, and removal in an individual exchange is almost completely nonselective.[15] However, because most other plasma constituents are resynthesized much more rapidly than IgG, a series of such exchanges results in fairly selective lowering of IgG levels over a course of exchanges,[16] as shown in Figure 55–3.

Regulation of IgG Metabolism

Because reduction of IgG levels is a frequent goal of TPE, it is worthwhile to consider certain details of IgG metabolism. The catabolic rates for IgG1, IgG2, and IgG4, which constitute about 90% of total IgG, are proportional to total IgG level. Accordingly, their half-lives are inversely proportional to concentration.[17–20] This observation has long been attributed to the existence of a saturable receptor that protects IgG from catabolic pathways.[21] This receptor has been characterized and shown to be identical to the FcRn receptor in neonatal intestinal epithelium.[22]

Synthetic rates for IgG are difficult to measure in humans. Certain animal experiments concerning levels of specific antibody fostered the belief that the synthetic rate for IgG is variable and exhibits negative feedback, such that synthesis increases when IgG or specific antibody levels, or both, are lower.[23] By contrast, Junghans[24] has shown that knockout mice genetically deficient for the FcRn receptor, which rapidly catabolize IgG, have the same IgG synthetic rate as normal mice despite maintaining very low IgG levels. This observation argues against any feedback regulation of IgG synthesis and suggests that the generalized hypogammaglobulinemia induced by TPE would not produce any rebound increase in IgG synthesis.

Intravenous immunoglobulin (IVIG) therapy has been reported effective in a number of antibody-mediated diseases

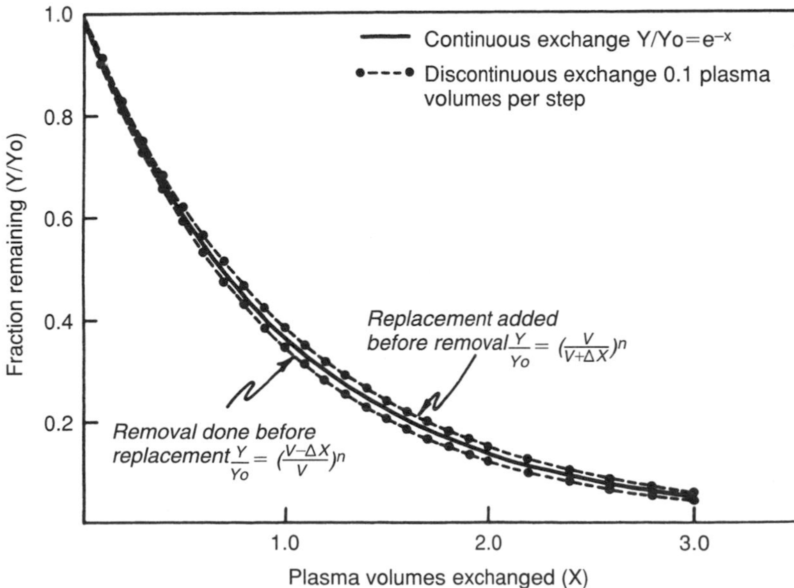

Figure 55–1 Calculated fraction of intravascular substance remaining during a plasma exchange, assuming no equilibration with extravascular material. (From Chopek M, McCullough J. Protein and biochemical changes during plasma exchange. In Berkman EM, Umlas J [eds]. Therapeutic Hemapheresis. Washington, D.C., American Association of Blood Banks, 1980, p 17.)

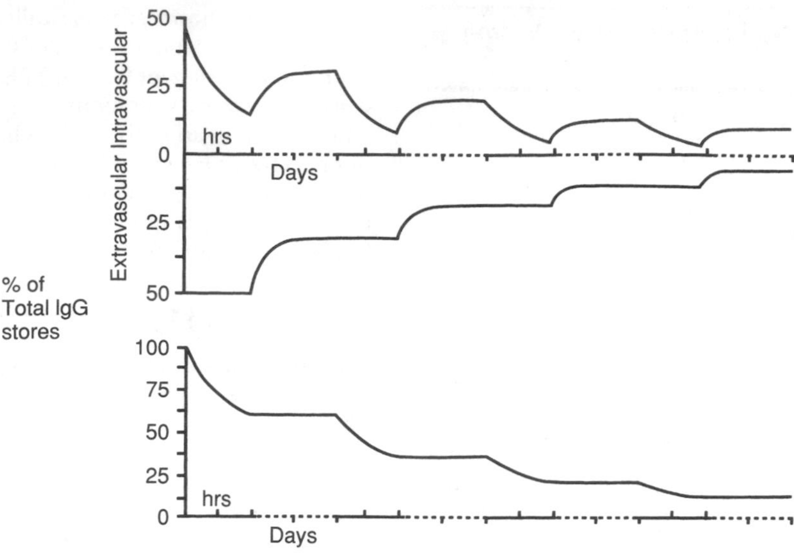

Figure 55–2 Computer-generated curve estimating amounts of intravascular and extravascular immunoglobulin G (IgG) (upper curves) and total immunoglobulin G (IgG; lower curve) during a course of four 1-plasma-volume therapeutic plasma exchanges with an IgG-free replacement medium. Published formulas were used for rates of removal during exchanges and reequilibration after exchanges.[13] No correction was made for continuing synthesis.

in which TPE has also been used. Yu and Lennon[25] have proposed that the beneficial action of IVIG is to compete with endogenous IgG antibodies for FcRn receptors and thereby promote increased catabolism of the latter, including pathogenic antibodies. In this view, the therapeutic effects of IVIG and TPE are essentially the same; that is, both lower harmful autoantibody levels. TPE lowers levels quickly but may be followed by slower catabolism, whereas IVIG presumably has a slower onset of action but promotes rapid catabolism.

Replacement Fluids

Saline replacement alone can suffice when only 500 to 1000 mL of plasma is removed in a manual plasmapheresis, but colloid must be given in a multiliter plasma exchange. Available colloid replacement fluids are listed in Table 55–2, which also summarizes their relative advantages and disadvantages. The standard replacement medium for most indications is 5% human serum albumin in normal saline; however, substitution of 25% to 50% of the volume removed with saline is well tolerated in certain groups of patients.[16,26] Although it is a pooled product, albumin is considered preferable to plasma as a source of replacement colloid because (1) it can be pasteurized under conditions that inactivate known blood-borne infectious agents, (2) it can be given without regard to blood type, and (3) it does not require thawing or other preparation before use. Adverse reactions to albumin are infrequent.[27] Albumin exchanges produce temporary deficiencies of other plasma proteins, such as coagulation factors; however, these are usually subclinical and are rapidly corrected by reequilibration and resynthesis.[15,28]

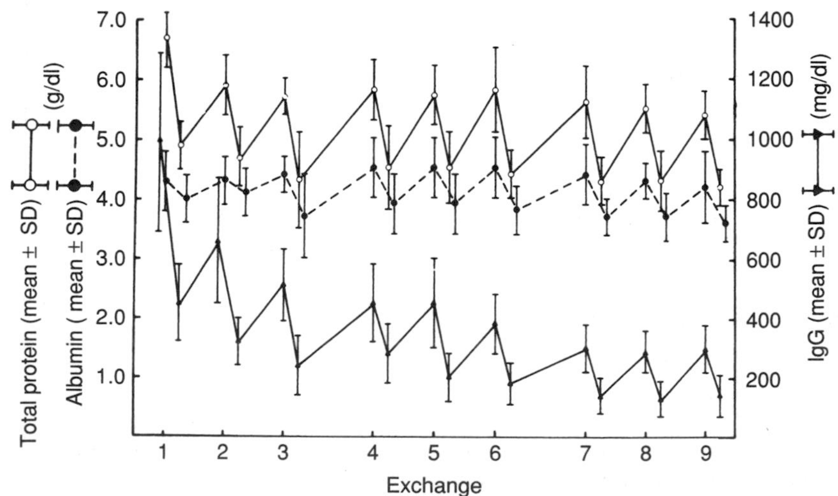

Figure 55–3 Total protein, albumin, and immunoglobulin G (IgG) levels before and after therapeutic plasma exchange with albumin/saline replacement. Exchanges were carried out 3 times per week for 3 weeks on seven patients. Points and ranges represent means and standard deviations. Note the disproportionate decrease in IgG levels. (From McLeod BC, Sassetti RJ, Stefoski D, Davis FA. Partial plasma protein replacement in therapeutic plasma exchange. J Clin Apheresis 1983;1:117.)

Table 55–2 Colloid Replacement Fluids for Therapeutic Plasma Exchange

Fluid	Advantages	Disadvantages
5% Albumin	Viral safety Convenience Reactions rare	High cost Most proteins not replaced
Single-donor plasma*	All proteins replaced	High cost Inconvenient† Citrate reactions Urticaria Infection possible
6% Hetastarch	Low cost Viral safety Convenience	No proteins replaced Hypotensive reactions Dosage limit Slow catabolism

*Fresh frozen plasma or cryoprecipitate-poor plasma.
†Must be thawed before use; must match patient's ABO type.

A meta-analysis published in 1998 suggested that critically ill patients resuscitated with albumin had a somewhat higher mortality than did those resuscitated exclusively with crystalloid.[29] A subsequent meta-analysis that included more patients did not confirm this finding,[30] and a recent prospectively randomized study comparing albumin with saline for fluid resuscitation in all patients admitted to intensive care units showed no survival disadvantage for albumin recipients.[31] Although further developments in this area will bear watching, no trend toward increased mortality has been apparent in decades of albumin use in TPE.

In a few circumstances, replacement with donor plasma is deemed preferable. Prominent among these is the treatment of thrombotic microangiopathies.[32] Affected patients are customarily exchanged with fresh frozen plasma (FFP) or cryoprecipitate-poor plasma because of abundant evidence that thrombotic thrombocytopenic purpura (TTP) responds better to plasma than to albumin. In addition, plasma is often given to patients with preexisting thrombocytopenia or humoral coagulopathy, who may have bleeding complications when the dilutional coagulopathy of an albumin exchange is superimposed. Use of plasma is associated with a higher incidence of immediate adverse effects, however, most notably urticarial and hypocalcemic reactions.[33]

One group has tried infusing a solution of hydroxyethyl starch (HES), a less costly volume expander, in the early part of an exchange. They reasoned that recommended dosage limitations for HES would not actually be exceeded because much of the infused HES would be removed in exchange for albumin infused later. This group has reported successes, albeit with a higher incidence of side effects.[34]

Selective Extraction of Plasma Components

Practitioners of TPE have long recognized the apparent wastefulness inherent in removing and discarding *all* plasma components in an effort to deplete just *one*. The concept of selective extraction of the pathogenic component from separated plasma, with recovery and reinfusion of the rest, was recognized early as an attractive goal. Experience with off-line separation of cryoglobulins[35] provided early evidence of practicality and efficacy; however, although a number of methods and applications for on-line separation have been explored,[36] commercial availability and widespread acceptance have been slow to be realized.

Prominent obstacles to commercially practical devices have included the high cost and limited capacity of sorbents that are biocompatible and truly selective, and the high extracorporeal volume associated with on-line sorbent modules that have a depletion capacity equivalent to that of TPE. In the past decade, several devices have become available that use pairs of small, low-capacity sorbent modules. Flow cycles are alternated, with one module absorbing material from patient's plasma, while the absorbent capacity of the other is regenerated by elution. This approach to selective extraction requires an additional instrument to manage the cycling-elution-regeneration process. A semiselective system of this type uses staphylococcal protein A to deplete IgG.[37] Other devices extract LDL selectively from the plasma of patients with familial hypercholesterolemia.[38,39]

Indication Categories

Subsequent sections of this chapter deal with specific indications for TPE. To help practitioners assess the potential utility of apheresis therapy in specific circumstances, two organizations, the American Society for Apheresis (ASFA) and AABB, have described indication categories for therapeutic apheresis.[40,41] The definitions used by the two organizations are similar and can be summarized as follows. Category I denotes diseases for which apheresis therapy is a standard and acceptable first-line therapy, although not always mandatory. Category II includes diseases in which it is a valuable second-line therapy, to be offered when first-line measures are contraindicated, fail, or are poorly tolerated. Category III indicates either uncertainty related to a paucity of data or controversy because of conflicting reports. Category IV implies negative data from controlled trials or anecdotal reports. The indication categories assigned by both organizations are given in tabular form for the diseases in each of the following sections.

THERAPEUTIC PLASMA EXCHANGE IN NEUROLOGIC DISORDERS

Immune processes, especially those that produce circulating antibody to structures in the nervous system, have been implicated in a number of neurologic diseases, and TPE has become an important therapeutic modality for many of them.[42] The diseases to be considered in this section are listed in Table 55–3, along with the indication categories assigned them by ASFA and AABB.[40,41]

Guillain-Barré Syndrome

Guillain-Barré syndrome (GBS) is a disease of the peripheral nervous system. It is the most common cause of acute paralysis with areflexia in the Western world, having an incidence of 1 to 2 cases per 100,000 population per year. It typically begins with symmetrical distal paresthesias, followed by leg and arm weakness. Symptoms progress proximally and reach a nadir by 14 to 30 days after onset. About one fourth of those affected have a mild illness and remain ambulatory throughout. The remaining patients are disabled by more serious paralysis and may have oropharyngeal and respiratory weakness as well. About one fourth require ventilatory

Table 55–3 ASFA/AABB Indication Categories for Therapeutic Plasma Exchange in Neurologic Disorders

Disorder	Indication Category*
Guillain-Barré syndrome	I
Chronic inflammatory demyelinating polyneuropathy	I
Peripheral neuropathy with monoclonal gammopathy	I/II
Myasthenia gravis	I
Lambert-Eaton myasthenic syndrome	II
Paraneoplastic neurologic syndromes	III
Stiff-person syndrome	III
Rasmussen encephalitis	III
Sydenham chorea	II
PANDAS	III
Multiple sclerosis	III

*I, standard first-line therapy; II, second-line therapy; III, controversial; IV, no efficacy.

PANDAS, pediatric autoimmune neuropsychiatric disorders associated with streptococcal infection.

assistance at some point, and the worst cases are marked by quadriplegia, ophthalmoplegia, and prolonged ventilator dependence. Variant presentations—with arm weakness predominating, with axonal degeneration instead of demyelination, or with symptoms limited to ophthalmoplegia, ataxia, and areflexia (Fisher syndrome)—are also possible. Spinal tap usually reveals few cells and only a moderately elevated protein concentration. A conduction block indicative of demyelination is usually found in electrophysiological studies, although inexcitability may be seen in the axonal form of GBS.[43–45]

Several lines of evidence suggest that the demyelination observed histopathologically is due to circulating antineuronal antibodies. Early experiments showed that sera from GBS patients produced demyelination in experimental animals.[46,47] Other studies have identified a variety of antimyelin antibodies in the sera of many patients with GBS.[48–50] A clinical association of GBS is found with a history of recent infection.[43] An association with *Campylobacter jejuni* infection[51–53] is especially strong, and studies have suggested a specific link to the Penner strain 19 of *C. jejuni* in 30% to 40% of GBS cases,[54] with antibodies formed to a strain-specific lipopolysaccharide that may be antigenically similar to the myelin ganglioside GM1.[55] Epidemic Chinese acute motor neuropathy, an illness of rural Chinese children, is clinically similar to GBS and is also associated with *C. jejuni* infection and anti-GM1 antibodies.[56] A number of other infectious agents, including cytomegalovirus, Epstein-Barr virus, *Mycoplasma pneumoniae,* and *Hemophilus influenzae* have also been associated with GBS.[57]

Spontaneous recovery is the rule in GBS and is perhaps associated with the decline in antibody levels expected after recovery from infection. Patients with mild illness require no therapy, but more severely affected patients need careful observation so that appropriate intervention with supportive therapies, such as mechanical ventilation, can be accomplished in a timely fashion.[43–45] Neither oral nor pulse intravenous steroids are beneficial in GBS.[58] Several small series and case reports suggested that TPE could favorably alter the course of the disease.[59–63] This evidence of benefit was confirmed by sizable randomized controlled trials that documented its effectiveness in shortening recovery time and reducing disability.[64–69]

The North American trial enrolled 245 disabled patients, 142 of whom received TPE.[66] At 4 weeks after entry, 59% of the treated patients had improved one clinical grade versus 39% of control subjects, with the mean improvements being 1.1 and 0.4 grades, respectively. The median time to improve one grade was only 19 days in treated patients versus 40 days in control patients, and median times to walk unassisted were 53 and 85 days, respectively. For ventilated patients, the median times to weaning were 24 and 48 days, respectively, and the median times to walk unassisted were 97 and 169 days. Similar hastening of recovery in severely affected patients was shown in the trial by the French Cooperative Group involving 220 patients.[67] In another study that enrolled 556 patients, the French group showed that benefit from TPE accrued even to mildly affected patients.[68] The typical treatment schedule in these trials included five or six exchanges of 1 to 1.5 plasma volumes over 7 to 14 days. Albumin replacement and FFP were specifically compared in the French trial. FFP caused more side effects[70] but offered no therapeutic advantage.[67] GBS patients may need careful monitoring, perhaps in an intensive care unit, because they may have autonomic neuropathy and are more likely to experience hemodynamic instability during TPE.[71]

Later evidence suggested that IVIG also is beneficial in GBS.[72] A large multi-institutional trial compared IVIG, TPE, and TPE followed by IVIG, with 121 to 130 patients in each treatment group.[73] The mean disability-grade improvements at 4 weeks were 0.8, 0.9, and 1.1, respectively, and the median times to walk unassisted were 51, 49, and 40 days, respectively. Although the trends favored TPE plus IVIG, none of the differences was statistically significant. TPE and IVIG are considered equivalent recommended therapies for GBS by the Quality Standards Subcommittee of the American Academy of Neurology.[74]

Chronic Inflammatory Demyelinating Polyneuropathy

Chronic inflammatory demyelinating polyneuropathy (CIDP) is an acquired neuropathy that has either a continuously progressive or an intermittent, relapsing course. Both sensory loss and weakness are typically present, with both proximal and distal sites usually affected. Proximal weakness helps to distinguish CIDP from other chronic neuropathies, and progression for more than 2 months differentiates it from GBS. Nerve-conduction studies should reveal evidence of demyelination, as should nerve biopsies. Nerve-root biopsies may show patchy inflammatory infiltrates. The cerebrospinal fluid protein is moderately elevated, but the cell count is usually less than 10 per microliter. Diagnostic criteria prepared by the American Academy of Neurology require lumbar puncture and nerve biopsy for a definitive diagnosis of CIDP; however, other diagnostic schemes require these tests only when clinical and/or nerve-conduction findings are inconclusive. Treatment is recommended for all CIDP patients, and responsiveness to treatment is expected in 60% to 80%. CIDP may be idiopathic or may arise in the context of an associated disease, such as inflammatory bowel disease, chronic active hepatitis, connective tissue disease, Hodgkin's disease, human immunodeficiency virus (HIV) infection, or monoclonal gammopathy.[75–77]

The etiology of CIDP remains unclear; however, the disease associations, the similarities to GBS, and the histopathology all support an immune process. The fact that some cases are associated with a monoclonal protein suggests an antibody-mediated disorder, as do the findings that experimental allergic neuritis, an animal model of CIDP, can be transferred with serum[78] and that antimyelin IgG from patient sera can cause electrophysiologic and pathologic features of CIDP in animals.[79] Later studies have shown antibody to myelin components such as GM1,[80] P_0 and P_2 proteins,[81] and β-tubulin[82] in the sera of patients with CIDP, although no cause-and-effect relation has been established. Abnormalities of cell-mediated immunity have also been identified.[77]

Most patients with CIDP respond to corticosteroids in moderately high doses. Standard therapy consists of a course of prednisone at perhaps 100 mg/day for an adult, followed by gradual tapering to alternate-day therapy when a functional plateau is reached.[75] The successful application of TPE in GBS, along with evidence for a circulating factor in CIDP, provided the rationale for early trials of TPE in CIDP patients who had not responded to steroids or were unable to tolerate them. A double-blind, sham-controlled crossover trial of 3 weeks of TPE reported by Dyck and colleagues[83] in 1986 showed improvement in 5 of 15 treated patients, with a similar proportion responding after crossover in the group randomly assigned to sham. Many patients worsened after TPE was stopped, however. A similar study was reported by Hahn and coworkers[84] in 1996 with 18 previously untreated patients. Twelve of 15 patients who completed the trial improved during the TPE portion. Improvement began after a shorter delay than is usually seen with steroid therapy, and its rate was more rapid. These patients were given prednisone for 6 months after completing TPE, and many maintained good function after recovery from a brief relapse when TPE was stopped.

An effect of IVIG on CIDP has also been sought.[85] Early controlled trials comparing IVIG with a control infusion of albumin were not conclusive but suggested a superior effect for IVIG.[86–89] Hahn and colleagues[90] published a double-blind, placebo-controlled trial with crossover in 30 patients. Study patients were permitted to take low stable doses of prednisone. Overall, 19 patients, or 63%, responded to IVIG, and 5 (17%) responded to placebo. Hughes and colleagues.[91] reported a randomized crossover trial in 32 patients comparing 6 weeks of oral prednisone with IVIG, 1.0 g/kg on 2 consecutive days. The responses were similar, supporting efficacy for IVIG. Two studies comparing IVIG with TPE in CIDP have been published. In an uncontrolled retrospective study by Choudhary and Hughes,[92] 21 (64%) of 33 patients had major improvement after TPE treatment while, at the same institution, 14 (67%) of 21 patients responded to IVIG. In a prospective observer-blinded crossover study of 20 patients at the Mayo Clinic, both therapies were adjudged to produce rapid and statistically significant improvement, and the authors concluded that either therapy was appropriate as a primary treatment.[93] TPE protocols in the preceding studies have tended to specify relatively long courses of treatment. A proposed schedule is three 1 plasma volume exchanges per week for 2 weeks, followed by two exchanges per week for another 4 weeks.[76]

Peripheral Neuropathy and Monoclonal Gammopathy

About 10% of patients with polyneuropathy have a circulating monoclonal immunoglobulin. The background incidence of such proteins is only 1% in adults older than 50 and increases to only 3% in adults older than 70.[94,95] Thus, the epidemiology suggests a causal relation. This idea has been strengthened by studies showing that antimyelin antibody activity is expressed by the monoclonal proteins of many patients with neuropathy. Antibody to a carbohydrate epitope on myelin-associated glycoprotein (MAG) is found in a majority of IgM-associated neuropathies.[96] The same epitope occurs in myelin glycoprotein P_0 and on other gangliosides in nerve cell membranes.[97,98] Anti-MAG injection is known to produce demyelination in experimental animals.[99] Other patients have antibodies to myelin sheath sulfatides, to membrane-associated chondroitin sulfate C moieties, or to the GM1 ganglioside.[97,98]

Clinical features of monoclonal gammopathy–associated neuropathy are mostly similar to those of CIDP[76]; however, sensory features tend to be more prominent, and although progression tends to be slower, it is also more relentless, and spontaneous improvement is uncommon.[100,101] Neuropathy is more prevalent in patients with IgM paraproteins than in those with IgG or IgA[102] except in osteosclerotic myeloma, in which the prevalence of neuropathy with IgG or IgA proteins is quite high, sometimes as a part of the POEMS syndrome (polyneuropathy, organomegaly, endocrinopathy, monoclonal protein, skin changes).[103] Nerve biopsies show demyelination, axonal degeneration, and fiber loss, and immunofluorescence may demonstrate IgM and complement in IgM-associated cases.[95]

Patients with B-cell malignancies such as myeloma or Waldenström macroglobulinemia should be treated with chemotherapy protocols appropriate for their diagnosis and may experience improvement in the neuropathy. Many patients have neuropathy in the context of a monoclonal gammopathy of undetermined significance (MGUS) and are treated with immunosuppressive regimens similar to those used in CIDP.[95]

TPE has been shown to be effective in MGUS-associated neuropathy. In a sham-controlled trial in 39 patients, twice-weekly exchange led to improvement in disability scores, weakness scores, and electrodiagnostic parameters in the blinded portion of the trial. Similar improvement occurred subsequently in sham-treated patients who received true TPE in an open follow-up.[104] Response was more frequent in patients with IgG and IgA paraproteins than in those with IgM. This trend was also noted in other studies.[105–107]

Myasthenia Gravis

Myasthenia gravis (MG) is a disease of the neuromuscular junction characterized by weakness or undue fatigability, or both, in skeletal muscle. Ocular myasthenia, with diplopia and ptosis, is a frequent presentation, but other muscles are eventually affected in most patients. Involvement of muscles innervated by other cranial nerves leads to the most serious symptoms, including inability to swallow secretions and respiratory insufficiency.[108,109]

Most patients with myasthenia have circulating antibodies to a portion of the α-subunit of the acetylcholine receptor molecule (AChR) on the muscle cell motor end plate.[108–110] At least three mechanisms exist by which such antibodies can cause weakness:

1. They can block receptors competitively so that acetylcholine released from the nerve ending cannot gain access.

2. They can increase turnover of receptors in a manner that requires crosslinking and leads to a decreased number of receptors available to receive signals.
3. They can mediate target-cell damage by complement or inflammatory cell attack, or both.[111]

The third mechanism probably leads to the most common histopathologic findings, which are simplification of the normally convoluted junctional folds that bear the receptors and occasional inflammatory cell infiltrates in these areas.[108]

Antibody to AChR is lacking in about half of patients with ocular myasthenia only and in about 10% of patients with typical generalized myasthenia. In the latter group, about half the patients have circulating antibody to MuSK, a tyrosine kinase in the motor end plate membrane. Antibodies to one of two intracellular proteins (titin and the ryanodine receptor) or the internal end plate protein rapsyn have been detected in some patients with myasthenia.[108,109]

Two approaches to drug therapy are available for myasthenia. Agents such as neostigmine and pyridostigmine inhibit degradation of acetylcholine at the neuromuscular junction and thereby enhance its action on remaining receptors. Immunosuppressive drugs, such as prednisone and azathioprine, are also used to reduce damage to receptors through either general anti-inflammatory properties or decreased antibody levels.[108,109]

Surgical treatment is also used. The incidence of malignant thymoma is increased among patients with myasthenia. Some of these patients improve after surgical resection of the thymus. This observation stimulated trials of thymectomy in patients not known to have tumors, and these patients may experience disease remission as well.[108,109]

Given the relation between circulating antibody, pathology, and symptoms in myasthenia, TPE has seemed a reasonable approach to therapy.[112] A controlled trial has never been published, but numerous open trials have suggested that the therapy can bring about rapid symptomatic improvement in concert with lower levels of circulating anti-AChR antibody. TPE has also been effective in patients who test negative for AChR antibody, perhaps suggesting that not all pathogenic antibodies are detected by this assay.[108,109]

As a result of this universally favorable experience, TPE is widely accepted as a therapy for myasthenia. It is not, however, recommended for all patients. Rather, it is reserved for those with severe disease and those who either do not respond to other therapies or cannot tolerate them. Patients whose respiration, deglutition, or locomotion is inadequate are good candidates for the rapid improvement brought by TPE, even at initial treatment.[113] TPE can also be useful to optimize muscle function before surgery, especially thymectomy.[114] Occasional patients do best with regular TPE at 2- to 4-week intervals in addition to maintenance drug therapy.[115] Semiselective adsorption of IgG with protein A-Sepharose has been tried in myasthenia, also with favorable results.[116–120]

Myasthenia may also respond to IVIG.[121] Although no randomized trials have been done to prove efficacy, a controlled study compared IVIG with TPE in 87 patients. Either three or five infusions of IVIG at 0.4 g/kg were found equivalent to three TPE treatments. A shorter median time to response for TPE-treated patients (9 days vs 15 days) did not achieve statistical significance ($P = 0.14$).[122] A multicenter retrospective chart review found significantly better ventilatory status at 2 weeks and functional status at 1 month in patients treated with TPE.[123]

Lambert-Eaton Myasthenic Syndrome

Lambert-Eaton myasthenic syndrome (LEMS) is characterized clinically by fatigue and weakness. It differs from MG in that oculomotor and bulbar symptoms are rarely prominent, but signs of dysautonomia, such as dry mucous membranes and orthostatic hypotension, are common. LEMS most often occurs as a paraneoplastic syndrome. About 60% of cases are associated with small cell lung cancer, and associations with other tumors are also known. In many cases, the neuromuscular symptoms antedate any other sign of tumor.[124–126]

LEMS also is a disease of the neuromuscular junction, but the defect is in the nerve cell ending instead of the muscle cell. LEMS is caused by circulating antibody directed against the voltage-gated calcium channels (VGCCs) in the nerve terminus that mediate electrical events in neuromuscular impulse transmission. The physiologic result is a reduction in the amount of acetylcholine released by depolarization events, with consequent weakness in affected skeletal muscles as well as dysfunction at some autonomic nerve endings.[127,128] The LEMS antibodies appear to be restricted to the P/Q subset of VGCCs.[127]

Curiously, cholinesterase inhibitors are less effective in LEMS than in MG. Agents that prolong nerve action potentials by blocking voltage-gated potassium channels may improve muscle strength in LEMS patients, presumably by enhancing acetylcholine release; 3,4-diaminopyridine is currently considered the most useful of these.[129,130] Immunosuppressive drugs such as cortisone and azathioprine may be helpful in LEMS, and paraneoplastic cases may respond to specific antitumor therapy.[130–132] TPE has been helpful in LEMS. Responses are often slower and more modest than those seen in MG, suggesting that more time is required to heal a damaged nerve ending.[129,132] IVIG has also been reported to be effective in trials in both the short and long term.[130]

Other Paraneoplastic Neurologic Syndromes

A number of distinct neurologic syndromes are associated with malignant tumors and are characterized by circulating antibody to structures in the nervous system. Paraneoplastic encephalomyelitis is characterized by seizures, mental changes, and cerebellar and autonomic dysfunction. It is often associated with anti-Hu (also called ANNA-1), an antibody to a 38- to 40-kDa antigen found in the nuclei of neurons and of small cell lung cancer cells. Paraneoplastic cerebellar degeneration produces ataxia, dysarthria, and downbeating nystagmus. It may arise in association with ovarian, breast, and small cell lung cancers as well as with Hodgkin's disease. About 40% of patients have circulating anti-Yo, an antibody to 34- and 62-kDa antigens in Purkinje cells. Paraneoplastic opsoclonus-myoclonus syndrome is characterized by both vertical and horizontal dysrhythmic conjugated eye movements. It may occur in children with neuroblastoma and in adults with lung, breast, or other tumors. Cases seen with breast or gynecologic cancers may have circulating anti-Ri (also called ANNA-2), an antibody to 55- and 80-kDa antigens in neuronal nuclei. Cancer-associated retinopathy causes photosensitivity and gradual visual loss. It is associated with anti-CAR, an antibody to antigens shared by retinal neurons and small cell lung cancer cells.[133–135]

Treatment of these syndromes is difficult. They seldom respond well to antitumor measures, even when these are otherwise effective, or to pharmacologic immunosuppression.

TPE has been used in a number of these cases, usually with disappointing results.[133,134]

Stiff-Person Syndrome

Stiff-person syndrome (SPS), originally known as stiff-man syndrome, is characterized by progressive rigidity or spasms of trunk and proximal limb muscles or both.[136,137] About 60% of patients have high titers of circulating antibody to glutamic acid decarboxylase (GAD), which is the rate-limiting enzyme in the synthesis of γ-aminobutyric acid (GABA), the neurotransmitter for the majority of inhibitory central nervous system (CNS) synapses.[137–139] When present, anti-GAD is believed to have a pathogenic role even though neuronal GAD, as a cytoplasmic enzyme, should be inaccessible to antibody. CNS histology is normal in SPS, suggesting that anti-GAD causes functional rather than structural changes. Pathogenesis is more uncertain in patients who lack antibody to GAD.[137–139]

About 5% of cases are associated with cancer, usually breast cancer. Instead of anti-GAD, most such patients have antibody to amphiphysine, a 128-kDa presynaptic vesicle protein.[138,140,141] A few have antibody to a postsynaptic protein called gephyrin that is associated with receptors for GABA and for glycine, another inhibitory neurotransmitter.[142]

Symptoms often respond to diazepam or other agents that increase CNS GABA levels. Immunomodulatory therapies such as prednisone, TPE, and IVIG have also seemed beneficial in individual cases, but no controlled trials have been performed.[143] In paraneoplastic cases, improvement may follow removal of the malignancy.

Other Non-neoplastic Disorders with Anti-CNS Antibodies

Rasmussen encephalitis is a rare, acquired disorder that may begin in childhood, adolescence, or adulthood, often after a viral infection. Seizures are a prominent clinical feature but, unlike patients with idiopathic epilepsy, patients with Rasmussen encephalitis develop progressive, usually unilateral neurologic deficits including hemiparesis and mental retardation. Histopathologic studies show inflammation and atrophy of brain tissue, usually confined to one hemisphere. Children progress faster and have more atrophy and more severe hemiparesis than do adolescents and adults.[144,145]

Studies have revealed circulating IgG antibody to the Glu R3 receptor for the CNS neurotransmitter glutamate,[146] as well as cytotoxic T cells reactive against neurons.[147] It is hypothesized that the autoantibodies arise in response to a crossreactive microbial antigen.[148] Treatment with either TPE,[149] IVIG,[150] and/or other immunosuppressive therapies[151] has been reported to bring temporary clinical improvement.

Sydenham chorea is an acquired movement disorder of children that follows group A streptococcal infection.[152] Many children with typical chorea also exhibit obsessive-compulsive symptoms,[153] and some children who have obsessive-compulsive disorder, tics, and other neurologic symptoms without chorea have evidence of streptococcal infection (pediatric autoimmune neuropsychiatric disorders associated with streptococcal infection [PANDAS]).[154]

Some evidence suggests that an antibody response to streptococcal antigens that crossreacts with antigens in the basal ganglia could mediate symptoms in some patients,[155–157] although this is not universally accepted.[158] Small controlled trials have indicated that TPE and IVIG may both be beneficial in Sydenham chorea[159] and in PANDAS.[160] More recent studies have linked a number of other movement and behavior disorders to antibodies against antigens in the basal ganglia that arise after a streptococcal infection.[161] Trials of TPE or other immunosuppressive therapies have not yet been reported in these conditions.

Multiple Sclerosis

Multiple sclerosis (MS) is a demyelinating disease of the CNS that results in localized neurologic dysfunction. Two clinical patterns can be distinguished. About 70% of patients have acute attacks that resolve partially or fully over time (relapsing-remitting). The other 30% have gradual but continual progression of disease (chronic progressive). Attack frequency in relapsing-remitting MS tends to decrease with disease duration, and some patients may change to a chronic progressive pattern.[162]

Discrete plaques of demyelination in white matter are the pathologic hallmarks of MS. These areas, which are easily visualized on magnetic resonance imaging (MRI), are initially inflammatory but progress to fibrosis.[162] The mechanism of their appearance remains a mystery, but most experts in the field suspect involvement of the immune system. An animal model of MS (experimental allergic encephalomyelitis [EAE]) can be induced by immunization with myelin basic protein (MBP) or other myelin proteins. EAE appears to be mediated by T cells and can be passively transferred with T cells from immunized animals.[163,164] Most evidence points to a disordered cellular immune response in MS as well.[165] Recent studies have demonstrated antibodies to MBP or myelin oligodendrocyte glycoprotein (MOG) or both in CNS lesions[166] and in serum of some MS patients.[167] Although they are predictive of progression to MS in patients with a clinically isolated demyelinating event,[168] such antibodies do not produce MS in experimental animals, and thus the role of circulating antibody in pathogenesis, if any, remains unclear.[165]

Treatment of MS is problematic. Observational studies are complicated by the natural tendencies for acute attacks to subside and for attack frequency to decline, as well as other spontaneous fluctuations in disease activity. Clinical measurement tools such as the Expanded Disability Status Scale have been devised to quantify improvement or progressive disability, or both. These bring some objectivity to clinical studies but are arithmetically arbitrary and subject to interrater variability.[162,169]

Immunosuppressive and immunomodulatory drugs have been the mainstay of pharmacologic treatment in MS. Resolution of acute attacks is thought to be promoted by short courses of either corticosteroids or adrenocorticotropic hormone. These agents may promote faster return of normal nerve conduction by lessening edema and inflammation around new plaques.[162] It is doubtful whether the relentless progression of disability is halted by these measures, although vigorous use of intravenous steroids for optic neuritis may delay the onset of frank MS that it often portends.[170,171] Cyclosporin, total lymphoid irradiation, and cytotoxic immunosuppressants such as azathioprine and cyclophosphamide provide only modest benefits that may not warrant their attendant risks.[171] Low-dose methotrexate[171] has also been tried. Mitoxantrone, interferon-β, and glatiramer acetate (a mixture of synthetic polypeptides that may modulate immune responses to myelin basic protein) are immunomodulatory agents that have been shown to reduce the frequency of acute attacks and the appearance of new lesions on MRI.[172,173]

IVIG has also been tried in MS. Prophylactic administration was reported to reduce the frequency of attacks in open trials. In three controlled trials, a decrease in the frequency of attacks was noted.[174–176] MRI was not monitored in one study[174]; in another, fewer gadolinium-enhancing lesions were found in IVIG-treated patients[175]; in the third, the number of lesions seen without enhancement was the same after 2 years in both treatment and control groups.[176] Recent guidelines state that IVIG is of little benefit in MS.[173]

The rationale for use of TPE in MS is unclear because so little evidence implicates any circulating factor in the etiology of acute attacks or chronic progression. TPE has been used, however, and uncontrolled studies have reported encouraging results.[177–179] In controlled studies, it has been more difficult to discern benefit, even with vigorous TPE regimens.[180,181] The first randomized double-blind sham-controlled study in chronic progressive MS was reported to show significant benefit for patients receiving TPE in addition to cyclophosphamide and prednisone.[182] The study was subsequently questioned because of anomalies in statistical analysis and because extraordinary recoveries in several of the TPE patients have not been reproduced in subsequent trials, suggesting that some patients with the relapsing-remitting form were inadvertently misclassified and entered into the trial.[183–185] Two later sham-controlled trials did not show convincing benefit.[186,187] Although TPE may yet be found useful in some subset of MS patients, such as previously nondisabled individuals with prolonged severe demyelination unresponsive to other therapies,[188,189] most neurologists view it as controversial at best. The Therapeutics and Technology Assessment subcommittee of the American Academy of Neurology and the MS Council for Clinical Practice Guidelines have classified TPE as "of little or no value" in progressive MS and of uncertain value in acute severe demyelination in previously nondisabled individuals.[173]

THERAPEUTIC PLASMA EXCHANGE IN HEMATOLOGIC AND ONCOLOGIC DISORDERS

Blood is the organ that can be most directly manipulated by therapeutic apheresis, and TPE has been tried in a variety of hematologic and oncologic conditions. These are listed in Table 55–4 along with the indication categories assigned by ASFA and AABB.[40,41]

Table 55–4 ASFA/AABB Indication Categories for Therapeutic Plasma Exchange in Hematologic-Oncologic Disorders

Disorder	Indication Category*
Myeloma/paraproteins/hyperviscosity	II
Myeloma/acute renal failure	II
Hemolytic disease of the newborn	III
ABO-incompatible marrow transplant	II
Platelet alloimmunization and refractoriness	III
Thrombotic thrombocytopenic purpura	I
Hemolytic-uremic syndrome	III
Post-transfusion purpura	I
Idiopathic thrombocytopenic purpura (IA)	II
Autoimmune hemolytic anemia	III
Aplastic anemia/pure red blood cell aplasia	III
Coagulation factor inhibitors	II

*I, standard first-line therapy; II, second-line therapy; III, controversial; IV, no efficacy.

IA, Protein A-silica immunoadsorption.

Monoclonal Proteins

In addition to peripheral neuropathy, four other syndromes associated with monoclonal immunoglobulins are regarded as clinical indications for TPE. All five are listed in Table 55–5. The three syndromes that almost always occur in the setting of a malignant B-cell disorder are discussed here, and cryoglobulinemia is discussed in a later section.

The hyperviscosity syndrome was the first condition to be treated successfully with manual plasmapheresis, the precursor to TPE.[2,3] The full-blown syndrome includes neurologic symptoms, a bleeding diathesis, a distinctive retinopathy characterized by alternating dilated and constricted segments in retinal veins (link-sausage veins), and hypervolemia related to an expanded plasma volume. Symptoms seldom occur if the relative serum viscosity is less than 4 and become more likely when it exceeds 6. The syndrome is most often seen in patients with IgM paraproteins in the context of Waldenström macroglobulinemia but may occur in multiple myeloma as well.[190–192]

At higher paraprotein levels, the relationship between viscosity and paraprotein concentration is nonlinear such that a relatively large change in viscosity may follow a relatively small change in paraprotein concentration. As a consequence, the two-unit manual plasmapheresis technique available in the 1950s could lower an elevated viscosity enough to relieve symptoms. When combined with the fact that most affected patients have IgM paraproteins that are roughly 80% intravascular, this nonlinear relation also predicts that a 1 plasma volume automated exchange will provide a wide margin of safety and can be done less often in the hyperviscosity syndrome than is necessary in many other conditions.[190,193] Viscosity measurements should guide therapy, of course, but treatment every 1 to 2 weeks is often adequate.

Interference by paraprotein molecules in platelet and clotting factor interactions may occur even in the absence of hyperviscosity. Coagulopathies are found in 60% of patients

Table 55–5 Paraprotein-Related Indications for Therapeutic Plasma Exchange

Indication	Implicated Ig classes
Hyperviscosity	IgM > IgG/IgA
Coagulopathy	IgM > IgA > IgG
Myeloma kidney	Light chains
Neuropathy	IgM > IgG/IgA
Cryoglobulinemia	
Type I	IgM/IgG/IgA
Type II	IgM >> IgG/IgA

Ig, immunoglobulin.

with macroglobulinemia, 40% of patients with IgA myeloma, and 15% of patients with IgG myeloma.[194] Should they prove clinically significant, TPE therapy can help to restore adequate hemostasis.

Renal failure occurs in 3% to 15% of myeloma patients and carries a poor prognosis. In many such cases, renal biopsy demonstrates accumulation of free light chains in renal tubules. With normal renal function, urinary excretion of light chains far exceeds the amounts that could be removed by TPE, but in renal failure, the reverse may be true.[195–198] Two controlled studies have shown higher rates of recovery of renal function in patients who received TPE therapy. In one study, three of seven dialysis-dependent patients who received TPE recovered renal function whereas none of five control patients did.[199] In the other, 13 of 15 patients in the treatment group recovered renal function compared with only 2 of 14 control subjects.[200] Thus TPE is recommended for such patients.[201]

Alloantibodies to Blood Cells

Alloantibodies to red blood cells and platelets may contribute to a disease process in a number of situations. Antibody removal has been used as a treatment in several of these pathologic states.

Hemolytic disease of the newborn was one of the first conditions to be approached with automated apheresis instruments.[8–10,202] Efforts were made to lower anti-D titers by TPE in sensitized D-negative mothers carrying a D-positive fetus in the hope of ameliorating fetal red blood cell destruction. The incidence of this condition has decreased dramatically as prophylaxis with Rh immune globulin has become more widespread, and intrauterine transfusion with D-negative red blood cells has proved to be a more effective treatment for an affected fetus.[203] TPE is seldom used in this circumstance now, but it may still be helpful in pregnancies with early evidence of fetal involvement because intrauterine transfusion is not feasible before about 18 weeks of gestation.[204,205] Early institution of TPE was associated with successful delivery after multiple prior abortions in compelling case reports involving anti-M[206] and anti-P.[207]

TPE has also been used to remove isoagglutinins in the context of transplantation. Allogeneic stem cell transplantation across a major ABO barrier (e.g., group A donor into group O recipient) is feasible if a hemolytic transfusion reaction to red blood cells in the transplant can be avoided. For bone marrow transplants, this was first accomplished by exhaustive pretransplantation TPE of the recipient to reduce the relevant isoagglutinin titer.[208] Immunoadsorption columns containing A or B substance have subsequently been used.[209] Ultimately, however, it has proved preferable simply to remove most of the red blood cells from the bone marrow graft before transplantation.[210] Peripheral blood stem cell grafts contain smaller quantities of red blood cells and can usually be infused safely without any manipulation. Red blood cell engraftment is sometimes delayed after ABO-incompatible transplantation, however, and TPE has been tried, both before transplantation to avoid delayed engraftment and after transplantation to correct it, with uncertain results in both cases.[211–213] Resolution of delayed engraftment after donor leukocyte infusions has also been reported.[214]

Solid-organ transplantation across a major ABO barrier can result in hyperacute rejection and is usually avoided for this reason. In desperate circumstances, however, considerations of organ availability have sometimes dictated use of an ABO-incompatible liver after pretransplantation TPE of the recipient, often with a satisfactory outcome.[215–217] More recently, the prolonged shortage of donor kidneys has been addressed by elective transplantation of kidneys from informed living donors across major ABO barriers.[218–220] Both A_2 and non-A_2 organs have been successfully engrafted. Pretransplant immunosuppressive regimens include TPE to lower isoagglutinin titers.[221]

Organ transplantation across a minor ABO barrier (e.g., group O donor into group A recipient) does not increase the risk of rejection; however, it is sometimes followed, within 1 to 3 weeks after transplantation, by a hemolytic anemia related to isoagglutinin secretion by B lymphocytes carried in the transplanted organ. Hemolysis mediated by these "passenger lymphocytes" is most often seen in heart-lung or liver transplantation, where the volume of lymphoid tissue transplanted is relatively high.[222] It may, however, be seen after renal transplantation and may involve anti-D.[223] Severe hemolysis in this setting may be partially ameliorated by TPE in combination with compatible red blood cell transfusion.[224]

Alloimmunization to platelets can cause clinical refractoriness to platelet transfusions.[225] Removal of antibody has been attempted, both with TPE[226] and with a protein A-silica column.[227,228] IVIG has also been tried.[229–231] However, the results have been inconclusive and transfusion of compatible platelets is still the best option.

Thrombotic Thrombocytopenic Purpura and Hemolytic-Uremic Syndrome

Thrombotic Thrombocytopenic Purpura

Thrombotic thrombocytopenic purpura (TTP) is characterized by microangiopathic hemolytic anemia and thrombocytopenia, often severe. Fever, CNS changes, and renal abnormalities may be seen in advanced cases, although frank renal failure is uncommon.[232] A rare relapsing form usually begins in childhood, but most cases are sporadic and occur in adults.[233] Women are predominantly affected, accounting for 70% of cases.[234] TTP is usually idiopathic, but the syndrome may be seen in association with other illnesses, such as SLE[235] and HIV infection.[236] Idiopathic TTP was formerly associated with a mortality rate of 95%, but empirical studies in the 1970s and 1980s demonstrated much better survival in patients who received TPE with plasma replacement. Some patients, including children with the relapsing form of the disease, respond to simple plasma infusion.[233]

A convincing account of the pathogenesis of TTP has been offered. It involves a plasma enzyme (a metalloproteinase designated ADAMTS 13) that cleaves the ultralarge von Willebrand factor (ULvWF) multimers secreted by endothelial cells, yielding the smaller polymers found in normal plasma. Children with relapsing TTP have an inherited deficiency of this enzyme,[237] whereas an acquired deficiency, related to the presence of an autoantibody that inhibits the enzyme, has been found in idiopathic adult cases[238,239] and some SLE[240] and HIV-associated[241] cases. In either instance, persistence of ULvWF in the circulation or on the surface of endothelial cells or both apparently promotes inappropriate adherence of platelets to endothelial cells and to each other, leading to consumptive thrombocytopenia and microvascular obstructions. The latter cause mechanical trauma to red blood cells and varying degrees of end-organ ischemia.[233] Periodic plasma infusion may abort or prevent attacks in congenitally deficient patients.[237] Idiopathic cases respond better to TPE (78% response rate vs 63% for plasma infusion in a Canadian study),[242] presumably because exchange removes inhibitory antibody as well as supplying the deficient enzyme. Exchanges are usually carried out daily until the platelet count and lactate dehydrogenase (as a marker of hemolysis) have normalized.

Various immunosuppressive measures, such as glucocorticoid therapy,[243] vincristine,[244] rituximab,[245] and splenectomy,[246] have been advocated as adjunctive treatments. Discovery of an autoimmune etiology provides support for their use in idiopathic but not in congenital cases. A syndrome similar to TTP has been identified in some patients taking the antiplatelet drug ticlopidine. Autoantibody-induced deficiency of the metalloproteinase has been demonstrated in patients with this syndrome,[247] and TPE has been reported to improve survival (76% survival vs 50% for patients without exchange in a retrospective study).[248]

Hemolytic-Uremic Syndrome

The hemolytic-uremic syndrome (HUS) is characterized by microangiopathic hemolysis, renal insufficiency, and mild to moderate thrombocytopenia.[249] In children, it may occur in a self-limited form that follows infection with a verotoxin-producing *Escherichia coli* (diarrhea + or D+); however, some pediatric cases lack this association (D–).[250,251] Familial and nonfamilial forms affect adults.[238] Nonfamilial cases may be idiopathic or may be associated with prior chemotherapy or stem cell transplantation.[252]

Because of overlapping manifestations that sometimes preclude distinction on clinical grounds alone, it has long been supposed that the pathogenesis of HUS was similar to that of TTP. Largely on this basis, TPE and protein A column therapy have been recommended for D-childhood HUS and for adult HUS. Although this is a prevalent standard of care, responses have generally been less favorable than in TTP, particularly in thrombotic microangiopathy associated with chemotherapy and transplantation.[233,253–255]

Levels of the vWF-cleaving metalloproteinase have now been studied in adult patients with both familial and nonfamilial forms of HUS. Neither severe deficiency nor inhibitory activity has been found.[238] Another study in patients with clinically uncategorized thrombotic microangiopathy compared 50 patients with severe ADAMTS 13 deficiency to 57 patients who were not severely deficient. The severely deficient patients had a lower median platelet count (13,000/μL vs 44,000/μL; $P < 0.001$), a lower median creatinine (1.3 mg/dL vs 2.7 mg/dL; $P < 0.001$), and a higher rate of relapse (16 of 46 vs 4 of 47 evaluable patients; $P < 0.01$).[256] Thus the prior supposition of a shared pathogenic mechanism for TTP and HUS would seem to be in error. Deficiency of complement factor H has been identified in some patients with familial HUS.[257–259] This might provide some rationale for plasma therapy; however, for most cases, the role of TPE is unclear at this time. Similar comments apply to the HELLP syndrome of hemolysis, elevated liver enzymes, and low platelets in pregnant women,[260] which shares clinical features with TTP, HUS, and preeclampsia.

ADAMTS 13 Assays

Several techniques have been devised to measure ADAMTS 13 activity in patient plasma and to detect inhibition of exogenous enzyme by patient plasma. End points after incubation of vWF with a putative enzyme or inhibitor source include electrophoretic assessment of vWF multimer size, extent of collagen binding by residual vWF, residual ristocetin cofactor activity, and immunoradiometric quantitation of cleavage sites.[261] Currently none of these assays is widely available to clinicians with a rapid turnaround time. This inaccessibility alone limits the value of such assays in clinical decision making. Furthermore, in multilaboratory comparative studies, the intra- and interlaboratory precision and accuracy of results obtained on replicate samples have been far from ideal (with coefficients of variation as high as 83%, even in the most respected laboratories), although most laboratories seem capable of recognizing severely deficient samples, variously defined as containing less than 5% or less than 10% of the ADAMTS 13 activity level in pooled normal plasma.[262,263] Interlaboratory variability in detection and quantitation of ADAMTS 13 inhibitors has been even more disappointing.[262]

Several retrospective surveys have questioned the value of ADAMTS 13 inhibitor assays in recognizing TTP, in differentiating TTP from HUS, and/or in predicting responsiveness to TPE.[264,265] Given the limitations of current assays and the disagreement about what degree of deficiency is "clinically significant," it is perhaps not surprising that their predictive value is suboptimal. Other confounding factors may also contribute to apparent discrepancies. These might include (1) alternative pathogenic mechanisms in some patients (for example, an antibody that blocks access of ADAMTS 13 to endothelial cell membranes could theoretically produce a TPE-responsive TTP syndrome with normal plasma enzyme levels[233]); (2) inability to eliminate very high titer inhibitors even with aggressive TPE, as is seen with some factor VIII inhibitors; and (3) spontaneous resolution of illness or response to concurrent therapies such as corticosteroids in patients with disease processes unrelated to ADAMTS 13 who nevertheless undergo TPE. Despite these reservations, it seems certain that the elucidation of ADAMTS 13 deficiency was a major advance in understanding the pathogeneses of TTP. It is likely that accurate assays for ADAMTS 13 activity and inhibitors that are widely available and have short turnaround times would be useful in evaluation of patients with thrombocytopenia and microangiopathic hemolysis.[240,265,266] However, prospective controlled studies and/or additional clinical experience will be necessary to assess fully the value of such assays.

Post-transfusion Purpura

Post-transfusion purpura (PTP) is a rare syndrome in which the platelet count decreases abruptly to dangerously low levels about 1 week after an allogeneic transfusion. Patients who develop the syndrome lack the common allele for one of the platelet-specific glycoprotein antigens, most often the human platelet-specific antigen 1a (HPA-1a) on glycoprotein IIIa. Most affected patients have had multiple pregnancies or prior transfusions and have been immunized thereby to the platelet-specific antigen coded by the prevalent allele. The transfusion that precipitates the illness appears to stimulate an anamnestic response with an increasing IgG antibody titer, most often anti–HPA-1a. PTP is self-limited and usually resolves without treatment in several weeks; however, bleeding complications, including fatal CNS hemorrhage, may occur.[267–269]

Although PTP is linked to a platelet-specific alloantibody response, the mechanism of extensive destruction of antigen-negative autologous platelets remains obscure. The following four possibilities have been proposed: (1) platelet antigen-antiplatelet antibody immune complexes bind to autologous platelets and mediate their destruction; (2) autologous platelets adsorb soluble alloantigen derived from the transfusion; (3) a simultaneous platelet autoantibody response occurs; and (4) a broad alloimmune response produces antibodies that crossreact with autologous platelets.[270]

Treatment of PTP is advisable because many patients have bleeding complications. High-dose corticosteroids are usually given empirically, and pulse methylprednisolone at 1 g/day has been reported effective. Platelet transfusions, even those from antigen-negative donors, do not increase the platelet count and may cause severe reactions. Daily TPE usually promotes an increase in platelet count within a few days and is considered an effective treatment for this reason, even though controlled trials have not been done.[271] Exchanges usually include FFP replacement to avoid a superimposed humoral coagulopathy. IVIG leads to similarly prompt increases in platelet count and has become the favored treatment modality for this group of patients.[272]

Idiopathic Thrombocytopenic Purpura

Idiopathic thrombocytopenic purpura (ITP) is an autoimmune illness affecting platelets. Most patients have an IgG autoantibody directed against a platelet membrane glycoprotein antigen. ITP sometimes accompanies warm autoimmune hemolytic anemia (Evans syndrome). A pediatric form of ITP is acute and self-limited; recovery is the rule with or without treatment. Adult cases, most of which occur in women, seldom remit without therapy, and most progress to the chronic form of the disease. An ITP-like syndrome also occurs in association with SLE and HIV.[273]

The goal of treatment in ITP is prevention of bleeding. Because most platelets circulating in ITP patients are relatively young and more hemostatically active, avoidance of hemorrhage can be accomplished without normalization of the platelet count. Corticosteroids, splenectomy, and IVIG are the mainstays of therapy.[273] Some favorable anecdotal reports of TPE in ITP appeared in the 1970s.[274,275] One small controlled trial suggested a lower rate of splenectomy in patients receiving exchange,[276] whereas a retrospective survey found little difference.[277] In the absence of confirmatory trials, however, enthusiasm for this approach has waned, and TPE is seldom used in ITP.

Favorable responses to protein A–silica column treatment have been reported, first in ITP associated with HIV infection[278] and later in patients with chronic ITP without HIV.[279] The mechanism of action of protein A in this disease is uncertain. A subtractive mechanism involving antiplatelet antibody is unlikely because responses have been reported with treatment of as little as 250 mL of plasma per week. Bearing this uncertainty in mind, the protein A–silica column remains an option for chronic ITP refractory to more standard therapies.

Autoimmune Hemolytic Anemia

Autoimmune hemolytic anemia (AHA) is caused by autoantibodies to red blood cells. Such antibodies are either cold or warm agglutinins. Cold agglutinins are usually IgM antibodies directed against the I/i antigens; they bind preferentially at low temperatures and produce the syndrome of complement-mediated intravascular hemolysis known as cold agglutinin disease (CAD). Warm agglutinins are usually IgG and are often directed against an antigen that is not expressed on Rh_{null} cells. They bind better at body temperature and produce a predominantly extravascular hemolytic syndrome (warm autoimmune hemolytic anemia [WAHA]). AHA can be idiopathic but may also be associated with an infection, a lymphoproliferative disorder, or another autoimmune disease.[280,281]

Most cases require treatment. Standard therapy is aimed at inhibiting antibody production or reducing destruction of sensitized cells, or both. Corticosteroids, IVIG, and splenectomy are often effective in WAHA, and other immunosuppressive drugs may be tried if these measures fail.[280] All approaches are less successful in CAD.[281]

TPE to deplete circulating antibody has been tried in both WAHA and CAD when conventional treatments have failed.[282–288] IgM antibodies in CAD are predominantly intravascular and only loosely bound to cells; thus their removal by TPE should be relatively efficient. Such therapy, when added to conventional drug treatment, has been reported to transiently reduce antibody titers and transfusion requirements in CAD. In WAHA much of the circulating antibody is bound to red blood cells; TPE has also been tried in this disorder, but it is less likely to be helpful.

Aplastic Anemia and Pure Red Blood Cell Aplasia

Aplastic anemia and pure red blood cell aplasia are bone marrow disorders. The former leads to pancytopenia, whereas in the latter, only reticulocytopenic anemia results. At least some cases of both conditions are likely to be immunologically mediated. Allogeneic bone marrow transplantation is the preferred treatment for aplastic anemia if a suitable donor is available, but immunosuppressive therapies, such as corticosteroids, cytotoxic drugs, cyclosporin, and antithymocyte globulin, are effective in some cases.[289–291]

In a minority of patients, it is possible to demonstrate a serum factor, probably antibody, that is inhibitory to the growth of relevant marrow-derived precursor cells in culture.[292] These observations provided an explicit rationale for TPE, and this therapy has been reported in a handful of cases in both disorders. Results in aplastic anemia have been mixed, with responses more likely in patients demonstrating serum inhibitory activity.[292–294] In pure red blood cell aplasia, all reported instances of TPE treatment have led to improvement, which is sometimes quite dramatic in patients with serum inhibitory activity.[295–298] Thus although TPE is not a primary therapy for either disorder, it is an option for patients who have not responded to more conventional treatment, especially those who have serum inhibitory factors.

Coagulation Factor Inhibitors

Coagulation factor inhibitors are IgG antibodies directed against components of the humoral clotting cascade. They inactivate the targeted factor and interfere with clotting. They may be autoantibodies that arise in individuals with no prior bleeding disorder. Alternatively, they may be alloantibodies arising in genetically deficient patients as a result of exposure to a "foreign protein" in the course of factor-replacement therapy.[299,300] Factor VIII is the clotting protein most often affected by antibodies of either type.

The goals of treatment for patients with inhibitors are, first, control of individual bleeding episodes and, eventually, suppression of inhibitor synthesis.[301,302] Depending on the inhibitor titer, the first goal can usually be achieved by infusion of high doses of human factor VIII, porcine factor VIII (which is usually only partially crossreactive with anti–human factor VIII antibodies),[303] or, for patients with the highest titers, factor VIII–bypassing products, including recombinant factor VIIa.[304] TPE with plasma replacement may be used during a bleeding episode to reduce inhibitor titers enough to allow infused human or porcine factor VIII to circulate and bring about hemostasis.[305–307] Immunoadsorption with protein A–Sepharose may also be effective for this purpose.[308] Suppression of inhibitor synthesis is approached with immunosuppressive measures, including high-dose corticosteroids, cytotoxic agents,[309] cyclosporin,[310] IVIG,[311] and rituximab.[312,313] Tolerance-inducing protocols have been devised for congenitally deficient patients with alloimmune inhibitors.[314,315] These involve regular infusion of exogenous factor VIII. In the so-called Malmö protocol, extensive TPE or IgG depletion with protein A–Sepharose column procedures is used to reduce the inhibitor titer at the onset of treatment so that infused factor can circulate.[316] Patients with inhibitors usually need frequent, large (two or three plasma volumes) exchanges with FFP replacement. Central venous access is frequently required; catheter placement in the context of a refractory bleeding disorder is challenging to all concerned and often mandates use of a factor VIII–bypassing product for wound hemostasis.[317]

TPE has also been reported for treatment of patients with antiphospholipid antibodies.[318] These may interfere with in vitro assays of coagulation, such as the partial thromboplastin time. However, unlike the inhibitory antibodies described earlier, they usually promote inappropriate coagulation in vivo and cause thrombotic events.

THERAPEUTIC PLASMA EXCHANGE IN OTHER IMMUNOLOGIC DISORDERS

TPE has been tried in a number of rheumatic diseases and other diseases that are considered to have an immune or autoimmune etiology. These are listed in Table 55–6 along with the indication categories assigned by ASFA and AABB.[40,41]

Table 55–6 ASFA/AABB Indication Categories for Therapeutic Plasma Exchange in Rheumatic and Other Immune Disorders

Disorder	Indication Category*
Cryoglobulinemia	II
Rheumatoid arthritis (IA)	II
Systemic lupus erythematosus	IV
Systemic vasculitis	III
Polymyositis and dermatomyositis	IV
Goodpasture syndrome	I
Rapidly progressive glomerulonephritis	II
Renal transplantation	
Rejection	IV
Presensitization	III
Recurrent focal glomerulosclerosis	III
Heart transplant rejection	III

*I, standard first-line therapy; II, second-line therapy; III, controversial; IV, no efficacy.

IA, protein A-silica immunoadsorption.

Cryoglobulinemia

Cryoglobulins are defined as serum proteins that precipitate reversibly at 4° C, although some precipitate at higher temperatures. The precipitates always contain immunoglobulins, and immunoelectrophoretic or immunofixation analysis allows distinction of three types.[319]

Type I cryoglobulins consist of a single species of monoclonal immunoglobulin. These are usually found in myeloma, Waldenström macroglobulinemia, or other lymphoproliferative disorders (see Table 55–5). Cryoglobulin levels are often quite high (>500 mg/dL) and may cause Raynaud phenomenon or acral necrosis related to microvascular obstruction, as well as other symptoms. Type II cryoglobulins have both a monoclonal and a polyclonal component. The former is usually an IgM*k* with anti-IgG activity that binds polyclonal IgG in an immune complex. These typically produce a lower-extremity cutaneous vasculitis and may cause other, more serious visceral manifestations of immune complex disease. Many cases occur in association with chronic hepatitis C infection.[320] Type III cryoglobulins are mixed polyclonal, often with IgM anti-IgG that binds IgG in immune complexes. These may arise in acute infections, such as hepatitis B, and in severe rheumatoid arthritis or other chronic inflammatory states. Clinical manifestations resemble those of serum sickness.[319,321]

If an associated condition is present, cryoglobulin levels and related symptoms may decrease with treatment of the primary disorder (for example, chemotherapy for myeloma or interferon for hepatitis C virus infection). For idiopathic and secondary cases of mixed cryoglobulinemia, prednisone therapy may be effective in relieving symptoms, and alkylating agents may be useful for patients with severe symptoms resistant to prednisone.[321]

TPE reduces cryoglobulin levels and controls symptoms.[322] It can do so even in the absence of other treatments,[35] but expense and inconvenience usually preclude such use. Plasma exchange therapy should be started promptly for patients with severe acral ischemia or visceral manifestations of vasculitis.[323] In such patients, it can help gain and maintain control of symptoms until aggressive drug therapy takes hold. Patients with chronic ulcers in the setting of cutaneous vasculitis may also benefit.[324] Care should be taken to warm replacement fluids to body temperature before reinfusion.

Rheumatoid Arthritis

Rheumatoid arthritis (RA) is a disease of unknown etiology that is more prevalent in women. It is the most common chronic inflammatory joint disease and a leading cause of disability. Most patients have rheumatoid factor, an IgM autoantibody to IgG; however, because this finding is absent in many otherwise typical cases and because it occurs in other patients who do not have arthritis, it is not thought to be directly involved in pathogenesis.[325]

Conservative treatment of RA includes nonsteroidal anti-inflammatory agents, low-dose oral corticosteroids, and intra-articular steroids. More severely affected patients eventually receive slow-acting antirheumatic agents that are probably immunomodulatory, such as antimalarials, gold compounds, and methotrexate.[326] Tumor necrosis factor inhibitors have been approved for use in RA, and other cytokine antagonists may be beneficial as well.[326,327]

TPE was tried in RA in the 1970s and 1980s, but controlled trials did not show benefit.[328,329] Subsequent reports of lymphapheresis were published, with or without TPE in addition. Some controlled trials showed significant but short-lived benefit,[330] whereas others did not.[331] In practice, the prospect of no more than a modest chance of only modest benefit from a costly and inconvenient therapy has discouraged treatment with therapeutic apheresis.

A sham-controlled trial of 12 weekly protein A–silica column treatments produced improvement in 33% of 48 treated patients versus only 9% of 43 control subjects. Benefit persisted for about 8 months on average, and a subsequent course was again beneficial in seven of nine initial responders.[332] Although its mechanism of action is unclear, this device has gained Food and Drug Administration (FDA) approval for use in RA, and postmarketing clinical experience is beginning to accumulate.

Systemic Lupus Erythematosus

SLE has been viewed as the prototypical autoimmune disease. The occurrence of antibodies to DNA, especially those specific for double-stranded DNA (anti-ds-DNA), identifies a group of patients who may have autoantibodies to a variety of other determinants. Their clinical syndromes compose a disparate mixture in which skin disease, joint disease, cytopenias, or nephritis may be the sole or dominant manifestation.[333,334]

Immunosuppressive measures are the cornerstone of therapy for SLE. Most patients receive prednisone in varying doses, and those with severe disease may also be given azathioprine or cyclophosphamide.[335,336] The plethora of autoantibodies that seem relevant to clinical signs made SLE an obvious target for plasma-exchange therapy, and it was one of the first illnesses to be treated with automated TPE in the early 1970s. A number of case reports and uncontrolled series suggested a favorable effect.[11,12,337,338]

Lupus nephritis is a particularly devastating expression of SLE in which glomerular deposition of anti-ds-DNA and immune complexes is believed to play a prominent pathogenic role. It thus seemed an attractive context for randomized trials. A controlled trial with only eight patients suggested benefit.[339] However, a multi-institutional randomized controlled trial comparing oral cyclophosphamide plus TPE with oral cyclophosphamide alone failed to show any advantage for the patients receiving TPE.[26] A later international trial included patients with a variety of severe manifestations. It was structured to take advantage of an enhanced sensitivity to a properly timed pulse dose of intravenous cyclophosphamide that was believed to follow removal of pathogenic antibody by TPE.[340] As mentioned earlier, subsequent work with knockout mice deficient for the FcRn receptor suggested that enhanced susceptibility would not occur.[24] In any case, this trial also failed to show any benefit associated with TPE, either in all patients[341] or in a subgroup with nephritis.[342] One group has also reported a higher incidence of infection in SLE patients treated with TPE.[343] Thus several large controlled studies have failed to reveal any worthwhile effect of TPE in SLE.

Systemic Vasculitis

Systemic vasculitis is an inclusive term applied to a group of disorders that cause inflammation in blood vessel walls with resultant ischemic tissue damage. Vasculitis syndromes are conveniently classified on the basis of the size of vessels typically involved, as shown in Table 55–7. Most are of unknown etiology. The presence of immune complexes in some syndromes and of autoantibodies in others, such as antineutrophil cytoplasmic antibodies (ANCAs) found in Wegener granulomatosis (c-ANCA) and polyarteritis (p-ANCA), has lent credence to the notion that humoral immune factors are somehow involved.[344]

Prednisone is the first-line therapy for most vasculitic syndromes. Cyclophosphamide or methotrexate is often added in more severe cases.[345] Randomized controlled trials in renal vasculitis,[346] as well as in a group of patients with polyarteritis or Churg-Strauss angiitis,[347] have shown little evidence that long-term benefit is conferred by addition of TPE to immunosuppressive drug therapy. Nevertheless, it may be requested for patients who are not responding to maximal drug therapy. A recent observational trial revealed good outcomes in patients with polyarteritis nodosa associated with hepatitis B who received TPE in conjunction with an antiviral drug.[348]

Polymyositis and Dermatomyositis

Polymyositis and dermatomyositis are inflammatory diseases of skeletal muscle. A characteristic dermatitis, typically involving the eyelids, knuckles, neck, and shoulders, is also found in the latter condition. Proximal weakness with biochemical evidence of muscle cell enzyme leakage is the usual presentation. The diagnosis is confirmed by characteristic inflammatory histology and immunopathology in a biopsy specimen from an affected muscle. The natural history is progressive fiber loss, eventually leading to profound, irreversible weakness. An autoimmune etiology is suspected, but an antibody specific for skeletal muscle has not yet been implicated in pathogenesis.[349]

Initial treatment is high-dose prednisone, which can often be tapered to levels that are tolerable in the long term. Resistant disease is treated with azathioprine, methotrexate, cyclosporine, or an alkylating agent, or a combination thereof.[349] Controlled trials have also shown that IVIG infusion reduces muscle enzyme levels and improves strength temporarily.[350]

Several uncontrolled series have been interpreted to show that TPE was beneficial, but these were confounded by concurrent

Table 55–7 Classification of Systemic Vasculitis

Large-vessel vasculitis
Giant cell (temporal) arteritis
Takayasu arteritis
Medium-sized vessel vasculitis
Polyarteritis nodosa
Kawasaki syndrome
Small-vessel vasculitis
Wegener granulomatosis
Churg-Strauss syndrome
Microscopic polyangiitis
Henoch-Schönlein purpura
Essential cryoglobulinemic vasculitis
Cutaneous leukocytoclastic angiitis

escalations in immunosuppressive drug therapy.[351–353] A randomized, controlled trial was reported in which 12 patients received TPE, 12 received lymphapheresis, and 12 received sham apheresis, with no changes in drug therapy.[354] No difference in the response rate was found among the three groups. Thus despite the successes with IVIG, no role for TPE appears obvious in the treatment of polymyositis.

Goodpasture Syndrome

Goodpasture syndrome (GPS) is an illness characterized clinically by rapidly progressive glomerulonephritis and in some cases by pulmonary hemorrhage. Renal biopsy shows crescent formation in many glomeruli on light microscopy and linear subendothelial immune deposits on immunofluorescence and electron microscopy. Lung biopsy may show similar subendothelial deposits. In 95% of cases, the syndrome is associated with circulating antibody that binds to glomerular basement membrane (anti-GBM). These antibodies are directed against a noncollagenous sequence (NC1) of the α-3 chain of a type of collagen (type IV) that is found in appreciable quantities only in renal and pulmonary basement membranes. Untreated GPS progresses quickly and relentlessly, and most patients die of uremia or of complications of lung hemorrhage.[355,356]

Since the classic report by Lockwood and colleagues in 1975,[357] the recommended treatment for GPS has been aggressive TPE combined with high-dose prednisone and cyclophosphamide.[358,359] TPE reduces anti-GBM levels quickly to minimize progression of tissue damage.[360] Exchanges are usually carried out daily and may be continued for 2 weeks. It is therefore prudent to give some FFP replacement in the latter part of each exchange to replete coagulation factors and avoid exacerbations of lung bleeding related to dilutional coagulopathy.[355,356]

The only controlled trial on record failed to show an advantage for GPS patients who received TPE; however, this study has been largely discounted because the TPE schedule (every 3 days) was not sufficiently aggressive and because, despite randomization, the extent of renal damage at entry was not comparable in the TPE and control groups.[361] Early treatment is preferred because it has been noted that patients with dialysis-dependent renal failure at the onset of treatment are not likely to recover renal function.[362,363] A corollary is that patients whose renal biopsies show an irreversible lesion and who do not have pulmonary hemorrhage are unlikely to benefit from TPE.

Other Rapidly Progressive Glomerulonephritis

In addition to GPS, two other categories of rapidly progressive glomerulonephritis (RPGN) exist, as shown in Table 55–8. In both of these, the light microscopic findings are similar to those in GPS with severe glomerular inflammation and crescent formation. Some cases may even have associated lung hemorrhage. The distinction among RPGN subcategories rests on immunofluorescence microscopy and electron microscopy, which show granular (vs linear in GPS) subendothelial immune deposits, usually taken to be immune complexes, in one group of patients and absence or relative scarcity of immune deposits in the other (pauci-immune RPGN). Patients in each group may have isolated, idiopathic renal disease or may have accompanying features that suggest a diagnosis of systemic vasculitis (for example, mixed cryoglobulinemia or Henoch-Schönlein purpura for granular-immune complex RPGN and microscopic polyangiitis or Wegener granulomatosis for patients with pauci-immune RPGN, many of whom test positive for ANCA).[364]

Table 55–8 Subtypes of Rapidly Progressive Glomerulonephritis (RPGN)

Nomenclature	Quality of Subendothelial Immune Deposits
Goodpasture syndrome	Linear
Immune complex RPGN	Granular
Pauci-immune RPGN	Scant or none

Because treatments for the two categories are similar, some trials and series have included patients with both types of RPGN.[365,366] Virtually all patients receive prednisone, and most receive cyclophosphamide, either orally or intravenously. TPE has been used extensively in patients with both types of disease, and early uncontrolled series tended to credit it with a beneficial effect. Two controlled trials, one published in 1988[367] and the other in 1992,[368] showed no advantage overall for patients who received TPE in addition to immunosuppressive drugs. However, a separate analysis of the small subgroup in the second study who had dialysis-dependent renal failure suggested that such patients have a better chance of recovering renal function if they receive TPE.[368] A comparable trend was not noticed in the trial conducted by Guillevin and colleagues.[369] A prospective, randomized trial by Stegmayr and coworkers[362] compared TPE with immunoadsorption. Among 38 patients with non-GPS RPGN, 87% of whom had ANCA, 70% avoided long-term dialysis. TPE and immunoadsorption were equally effective. In a more recent study of 22 patients with ANCA-positive RPGN, 12 patients who received prednisone, cyclophosphamide, and plasmapheresis had better outcomes than did 10 patients who received only drug therapy.[370] Criteria used for treatment-arm assignment were not specified. Thus TPE continues to be controversial in non-GPS RPGN. It is probably not justified as a first-line therapy, except (paradoxically) in patients who initially have dialysis dependence,[371] but it may be offered to patients who progress despite immunosuppressive drug therapy.

Solid Organ Transplantation

TPE has been used in the organ transplant setting both to treat and to prevent rejection as well as to treat recurrence of certain diseases in a transplanted organ. Photopheresis has also been tried for the same purposes, mostly in heart transplantation.

Rejection

Cellular immunity is thought to mediate rejection of most organ allografts; however, rapid antibody-mediated rejection may occur in patients who have preexisting antibodies to ABO or human leukocyte antigen (HLA) expressed by the graft.[372] Histologically, such hyperacute rejection is characterized by fibrin deposition, endothelial damage, and neutrophil infiltration in small blood vessels; damage to the graft parenchyma is mainly ischemic.[373] All treatments, including TPE, have been futile in hyperacute rejection. Vascular changes reminiscent of hyperacute rejection may be seen in later rejection episodes. These have sometimes been taken to indicate antibody-mediated rejection, even when immunofluorescence microscopy for immunoglobulin and tests for circulating antibody are negative.[373]

Prophylactic immunosuppression with corticosteroids and either cyclosporine or tacrolimus is standard post-transplantation management for kidney and liver transplantation. Heart recipients may also receive azathioprine or mycophenolate mofetil. Rejection episodes occurring in spite of these measures are treated with pulse steroids and/or therapeutic antibodies that deplete T cells, B cells, or both.[374,375]

TPE was used extensively in the late 1970s and early 1980s to treat renal transplant rejection after a number of case reports and uncontrolled series suggested it was beneficial.[376–381] In the middle and late 1980s, however, five controlled trials were reported. Four showed no significant benefit for patients receiving TPE in addition to standard drug therapy, even in the subgroups with vascular histology in transplant biopsies.[382–385] In the single study suggesting benefit, the mean time of treatment was 10 to 11 months after transplantation, when antibody-mediated rejection has been considered less likely.[386] The last and largest study was reported by Blake and colleagues,[385] who concluded that TPE therapy could no longer be recommended for this purpose. All of the aforementioned studies enrolled patients based on the timing of rejection (i.e., early rejection) and/or routine histologic criteria (i.e., acute rejection; vascular rejection). In none of them were patients assessed for the presence of donor-specific antibodies (DSAs). Despite this discouraging experience, use of TPE for renal transplant rejection continued to be reported.[387–389]

In the recent past, a new wave of enthusiasm for TPE has focused on patients with clinical and histologic evidence of acute rejection who also have DSAs and/or deposition of complement component C4d in transplant biopsy tissue.[390–394] DSAs can be shown by a positive crossmatch with donor cells or by flow-cytometric reactions with donor antigens. C4d deposition is demonstrated by immunofluorescence microscopy.[393]

Uncontrolled studies have been encouraging. Observations in the pretransplant period have shown that titers of donor specific HLA and/or ABO antibodies can be reduced by TPE.[219,395] Furthermore, in open trials, patients with refractory acute rejection who demonstrate DSAs and/or C4d have had relatively good long-term graft survival (>80%) after treatment regimens that include TPE and IVIG.[392,393] A recent conference on antibody-mediated rejection recommended that demonstration of circulating DSA be considered an essential criterion for diagnosis of humoral rejection and that the effectiveness of TPE and IVIG in this entity be studied in "rigorous prospective, multicenter" trials.[396]

Notwithstanding its ineffectiveness in controlled trials in renal transplantation, preliminary experience with TPE has also been reported in the context of cardiac allograft rejection. Favorable courses have been seen in individual patients who were also receiving other therapies, but no controlled trials have been reported.[397,398] The criteria for a diagnosis of humoral rejection in this setting remain controversial.[372] Vascular histology is more difficult to detect or exclude in the endomyocardial biopsies done to monitor cardiac allografts because few blood vessels are found in this part of the heart muscle. Immunofluorescence microscopy positive for IgG is the usual criterion for humoral rejection; however, it has been suggested that this diagnosis be made, and TPE used, in patients who have relatively normal biopsies in the context of deteriorating cardiac function.[399] Controlled data to support this assertion are lacking, as are any published data correlating this clinical syndrome with circulating DSAs.

TPE has been used before transplantation in patients presensitized to HLA antigens. Patients whose sera react with lymphocytes from a large proportion of the population have a diminished chance of a compatible crossmatch with an available donor and hence a low likelihood of receiving a transplant. Prospective immunosuppression, combined with removal of antibody by TPE or protein A–Sepharose immunoadsorption, has been tried as a means to obtain a compatible crossmatch and prevent hyperacute rejection. Several groups have reported that patients prepared in this way who receive cadaveric kidney transplants have quite respectable graft survival rates.[400–407] Similar protocols have facilitated successful transplantation of ABO-incompatible kidneys and livers.[217,408–412] In more recent studies, pretransplant TPE has facilitated elective living-donor transplantation of HLA-crossmatch positive as well as ABO-incompatible organs.[220,395,413,414]

In summary, the preponderance of evidence from controlled trials shows that TPE is not effective in reversing established rejection of renal allografts, except possibly in patients with circulating DSAs. Pretransplantation antibody removal can allow transplantation for otherwise ineligible candidates, especially those with high-titer antibodies to one or two HLA antigens whose titer-sensitive crossreactions can be suppressed. It can also facilitate transplantation of kidneys from living donors across ABO and donor-specific crossmatch barriers. The role of TPE in cardiac transplantation, if any, remains unclear.

Recurrence of Disease

Focal glomerulosclerosis (FGS) is a disease that causes nephrosis and renal failure, predominantly in children. It recurs after transplantation in at least 30% of patients who receive an allograft for FGS, suggesting that a humoral factor may play a role in pathogenesis.[415] Some evidence implicates a plasma factor having a molecular mass of 30 to 50 kDa that binds to protein A, is heat sensitive, and is soluble in 70% ammonium sulfate.[416,417] Other factors having estimated masses of 12 to 100 kDa have also been described in some patients.[418] All remain poorly characterized as to structure and half-life. Several reports describe reductions in proteinuria and improved renal function when recurrence of FGS is treated with stepped-up immunosuppression and TPE,[415,419–423] but no prospective randomized controlled studies have been reported.

GPS may occasionally recur in an allograft,[424] although this can usually be avoided by delaying renal transplantation until anti-GBM titers have decreased spontaneously. If it recurs, it should be treated promptly with TPE and cyclophosphamide.

A diffuse coronary artery disease, termed allograft vasculopathy, sometimes develops in transplanted hearts. It is a leading cause of morbidity and mortality in allograft recipients who survive beyond 1 year. It may be related to continuing hyperlipidemia as well as chronic immune injury.[425] Selective depletion of LDLs, discussed in more detail in the following section on hypercholesterolemia, has been thought to be helpful in a few transplant patients with persistent lipoprotein abnormalities.[426] Photopheresis has also been used as an antirejection measure in this setting (see chapter 56 on cytapheresis).[427]

THERAPEUTIC PLASMA EXCHANGE IN TOXIC AND METABOLIC DISORDERS

This section covers several conditions in which removal of nonantibody substances present in plasma has been deemed therapeutically attractive or advisable. These are listed in Table 55–9, along with the indication categories assigned to them by ASFA and AABB.[40,41]

Hypercholesterolemia

Familial hypercholesterolemia (FH) is an inherited disorder characterized by highly elevated levels of circulating LDL, cholesterol (650 to 1000 mg/dL), and lipoprotein (a) (Lpa). In homozygotes, cholesterol deposits in the form of skin xanthomas and coronary atheromas develop in the first decade of life, and death from myocardial infarction before age 20 years is common. Heterozygotes also have elevated LDL, cholesterol (350 to 500 mg/dL), and Lpa levels; xanthomas may develop by age 20 years, and coronary atherosclerosis, by age 30 years. A genetically determined deficiency of cell surface LDL receptors in these patients interferes with cholesterol off-loading from LDL into cells and with the normal negative-feedback regulation of LDL synthesis, leading to the elevations in LDL and cholesterol.[428,429]

Less severe forms of hypercholesterolemia can be influenced by dietary modifications and are amenable to therapy with several categories of drugs, including 3-hydroxy-3-methylglutaryl coenzyme A reductase inhibitors, bile acid–binding resins, nicotinic acid, and ezetimibe, a new agent that inhibits gut absorption of both dietary and biliary cholesterol.[429] However, FH homozygotes and some FH heterozygotes respond poorly to these measures and remain at high risk for premature death. For such patients, repeated physical removal of LDL and its associated cholesterol can be accomplished by various modalities of therapeutic apheresis.

A 1-plasma-volume TPE lowers LDL and cholesterol levels by 50% or more, and long-term treatment every 1 to 2 weeks can bring about shrinkage of cutaneous xanthomas and regression of coronary deposits.[430–433] TPE removes both LDL and Lpa, but it also depletes high-density lipoproteins (HDLs), which are thought to have a salutary antiatherogenic action. This apparent disadvantage has engendered efforts to remove LDL semiselectively and on-line from patient plasma separated by an apheresis device and then return the LDL-depleted plasma to the patient.

Several systems that have been designed to accomplish this goal are listed in Table 55–10. Secondary filtration systems use a plasma filter with a pore size that retains the very large LDL molecule while sieving smaller ones such as albumin[434]; however, these systems typically remove about half of plasma HDL.[435] In a heparin extracorporeal LDL precipitation (HELP) system, LDL precipitated by heparin at acid pH is removed by filtration from patient plasma that is then dialyzed on-line to restore a physiologic pH.[39,436] Lpa is also depleted, and HDL levels decline by 15%.[435] LDL immunoadsorption columns contain an LDL-specific antibody linked to Sepharose particles.[437,438] The need to reuse columns to achieve cost effectiveness is an awkward feature of this technology.[435] A final system, the Kaneka Liposorber, uses a pair of regenerable dextran sulfate columns that absorb LDL but not HDL or Lpa.[38,439] All these systems remove LDL effectively, but only the dextran sulfate and HELP systems are FDA approved and commercially available in the United States. FDA eligibility guidelines for these devices specify the following minimum LDL cholesterol levels on maximal drug therapy: more than 500 mg/dL for homozygous FH; more than 300 mg/dL for heterozygous FH; and more than 200 mg/dL for heterozygous FH with documented coronary artery disease.[440] Although these systems reduce HDL considerably less than TPE for a given decrement in LDL, they have no application other than the treatment of hypercholesterolemia. Consequently, a center acquiring one of them must use it regularly on multiple patients to make it economically feasible.

Table 55–9 ASFA/AABB Indication Categories for Therapeutic Plasma Exchange in Metabolic Disorders

Disease	Indication Category*
Homozygous familial hypercholesterolemia	II (I for LDL-P)
Refsum disease	I
Overdose or poisoning	III
Acute hepatic failure	III

*I, standard first-line therapy; II, second-line therapy; III, controversial; IV, no efficacy.
LDL-P, low-density lipoprotein apheresis (i.e., selective depletion of LDL).

Refsum Disease

Refsum disease is an inherited disorder caused by deficiency of the peroxisomal enzyme phytanoyl-CoA hydroxylase, which participates in the normal degradation of phytanic acid by α-oxidation. Symptoms usually begin in the third decade of life as a result of accumulation of diet-derived phytanic acid in plasma lipoproteins and in tissue lipid stores. Peripheral neuropathy, cerebellar ataxia, and retinitis pigmentosa are found in almost all cases. Anosmia, deafness, ichthyosis, renal failure, and arrhythmias may also occur. Slow progression is the usual course, but abrupt deterioration, including sudden death, may follow a marked increase in plasma phytanic acid levels.[441]

Early diagnosis is important so that dietary intake of phytanic acid through dairy products, meats, and ruminant fats can be curtailed. Diet is the mainstay of treatment, leading to gradual clearing of phytanate stores by slow ω-oxidation and gradual symptomatic improvement in most patients. Adequate nutrition must be maintained, however, because overly rapid

Table 55–10 Selective Extraction Methods for Lipoproteins

Immunoadsorption with anti-LDL antibody
Secondary membrane filtration
Heparin precipitation (HELP system)
Chemical adsorption to dextran sulfate

HELP, heparin extracorporeal low-density lipoprotein precipitation; LDL, low-density lipoprotein.

catabolism of endogenous fat can increase plasma phytanic acid levels acutely and cause clinical exacerbations.[441]

TPE has been reported in a number of cases of Refsum disease and removes large quantities of phytanic acid incorporated into plasma lipids.[442] Selective lipoprotein depletion is also effective.[443] Apheresis is probably most appropriate for patients who have very high plasma phytanate levels, particularly those with exacerbation of symptoms. Skin disease, neuropathic symptoms, and ataxia usually improve as plasma levels decrease. Cranial nerve defects usually do not.[441]

Drug Overdose and Poisoning

Toxic effects may arise from intentional or inadvertent exposure to excessive doses of pharmacologic agents as well as from harmful agents encountered in the environment. Management techniques are similar for both types of events and include attempts to remove toxin still in the gastrointestinal tract, efforts to promote or enhance renal elimination, and direct removal from the blood by hemodialysis, hemoperfusion (e.g., over charcoal columns), or TPE.[444] If available, specific antidotes may also be given.[445] Most patients are treated with more than one modality.

TPE has been tried in a number of patients with drug overdose or poisoning. It has been reported to be beneficial, when used along with other therapies, in cases involving substances that bind tightly to plasma proteins.[446,447] Examples include methylparathion,[448] vincristine,[449] vinblastine,[450] cisplatin,[451] carbamazipine,[452] and digoxin bound to antidigoxin Fab fragments.[453] It has also been reported for severe hyperthyroidism, either endogenous or exogenous, although its effectiveness is limited by extensive binding of L-thyroxine to tissue proteins.[454] TPE has been used in several cases of poisoning caused by ingestion of the *Amanita phalloides* mushroom[455,456]; however, diuresis has been shown to clear far more *Amanita* toxin.[457]

Most of the literature on this topic is older and all of it is anecdotal. Furthermore, TPE has always been used in combination with other, presumably effective therapies, making it difficult to formulate firm, rational guidelines. Nevertheless, it seems reasonable to offer TPE to severely affected patients with poisoning or overdose who have high blood levels of an agent known to bind to plasma proteins. Conversely, TPE has shown minimal or no beneficial effect in overdose of drugs known to bind to tissue proteins and lipids, including barbiturates,[458] chlordecone,[459] aluminum,[460] tricyclic antidepressauts,[461] benzodiazepines,[458] quinine,[462] phenytoin,[463] digoxin, digitoxin,[464] prednisone, prednisolone,[465] tobramycin,[466] and propranolol.[467]

Acute Hepatic Failure

Acute hepatic failure (AHF) is an uncommon condition that arises from a severe liver insult. Hepatitis B and acetaminophen overdosage are important causes. Additional cases are due to drug reactions, Wilson disease, vascular anomalies, acute fatty liver of pregnancy, and a variety of toxins. AHF results in myriad metabolic imbalances and synthetic defects. Clinical symptoms include jaundice, coagulopathy, renal failure, and encephalopathy. Liver transplantation is the treatment of choice, leading to 60% to 80% long-term survival versus greater than 60% mortality for patients without transplantation. Many fatal outcomes are due to complications of cerebral edema.[468–470]

Conservative therapy is essentially supportive. Fluid, electrolyte, and nutritional supplements are adjusted to correct metabolic abnormalities. Bowel sterilization with enteral antibiotics is recommended to minimize ammonia production by intestinal flora. Pressors are given as needed for hemodynamic support, and plasma products are infused to combat coagulopathy. Osmotic diuretics, sedatives, hyperventilation, and proper positioning are all used to reduce intracranial pressure.[468–470]

TPE with plasma replacement has inherent appeal as a strategy to restore metabolic homeostasis, remove toxic metabolites that may cause cerebral edema, and supply deficient plasma proteins, such as coagulation factors, in quantity without inducing volume overload. However, evaluations of the effectiveness of this approach have been mixed.[469] Some investigators have thought that TPE is helpful in stabilizing patients and maintaining them until an organ became available for transplantation.[471] Improvements in neurologic status, blood pressure, and cerebral blood flow were attributed to exchanges in one study[472]; however, intracranial pressure, which is a key prognostic indicator, did not decrease. Hemoperfusion over activated charcoal, which reduces plasma ammonia levels, has also shown no advantage over intensive supportive care alone.[470]

Potential problems with extensive TPE arise from the diminished ability of patients with AHF to metabolize the citrate in infused plasma. Citrate accumulation leads to ionized hypocalcemia and to alterations in arterial ketone body ratios that may interfere with regeneration of hepatocytes.[473] Thus although TPE can partially reverse coagulopathy and other synthetic deficits in these patients, a favorable net impact on outcome has been difficult to demonstrate, and it is seldom used for this indication in the United States.[474]

Other methods for extracorporeal support of patients with liver failure have been investigated. Several devices place patient plasma in "metabolic contact" with hepatocyte suspensions of either human or porcine origin. It is proposed that such devices could provide both detoxification and synthetic functions; however, evidence for the latter has been disappointing. Other devices aim to remove toxins via binding to extracorporeal albumin molecules. None of these approaches has yet been shown to improve outcomes for acute liver failure patients in a large controlled trial, but research is ongoing.[474,475]

CONCLUSION

It can be seen from the foregoing that TPE is an effective therapy for a number of disorders, especially those mediated by autoreactive antibodies or paraproteins. Refinements in instrumentation that are outside the scope of this chapter have made it a safe therapy as well; thus it should play an important role in the treatment of selected diseases for the foreseeable future.

REFERENCES

1. Abel JJ, Rowntree LG, Turner BB. Plasma removal with return of corpuscles (plasmapheresis). J Pharmacol Exp Ther 1914;5:625.
2. Skoog WA, Adams WS. Plasmapheresis in a case of Waldenström's macroglobulinemia. Clin Res 1959;7:96.
3. Schwab PJ, Fahey JL. Treatment of Waldenström's macroglobulinemia by plasmapheresis. N Engl J Med 1960;263:574.
4. Cohn EJ, Tullis JL, Surgenor DM, et al. Biochemistry and biomechanics of blood collection, processing and analysis: abstract of paper

presented at the National Academy of Science, New Haven, Conn., Nov 5–7, 1951. Science 1951;114:479.
5. Latham A. Early developments in blood cell separation technology. Vox Sang 1986;51:249.
6. De Laval CGP. U.S. Patent 247,804, 1881.
7. Freireich EJ, Judson G, Levin RH. Separation and collection of leukocytes. Cancer Res 1965;25:1516.
8. Powell L. Intense plasmapheresis in the pregnant Rh sensitized woman. Am J Obstet Gynecol 1968;101:153.
9. Bowman JM, Peddle LJ, Anderson C. Plasmapheresis in severe Rh isoimmunization. Vox Sang 1968;15:272.
10. Clarke CA, Elson CJ, Bradley J, et al. Intensive plasmapheresis as a therapeutic measure in Rhesus-immunised women. Lancet 1970;2:793.
11. Verrier Jones J, Cumming RH, Bucknall RC, et al. Plasmapheresis in the management of acute systemic lupus erythematosus. Lancet 1976;1:709.
12. Verrier Jones J, Cumming RH, Bacon PA, et al. Evidence for a therapeutic effect of plasmapheresis in patients with systemic lupus erythematosus. Q J Med 1979;448:555.
13. Chopek M, McCullough J. Protein and biochemical changes during plasma exchange. In Berkman EM, Umlas J (eds). Therapeutic Hemapheresis: A Technical Workshop. Washington, D.C., American Association of Blood Banks, 1980, p 13.
14. Kellogg RM, Hester JP. Kinetics modeling of plasma exchange: Intra- and post-plasma exchange. J Clin Apheresis 1988;4:183.
15. Orlin JB, Berkman EM. Partial plasma exchange using albumin replacement: removal and recovery of normal plasma constituents. Blood 1980;56:1055.
16. McLeod BC, Sassetti RJ, Stefoski D, Davis FA. Partial plasma protein replacement in therapeutic plasma exchange. J Clin Apheresis 1983;1:115.
17. Waldmann TA, Strober W. Metabolism of immunoglobulins. Prog Allergy 1969;13:1
18. Strober W, Wochner RD, Barlow MH, et al. Immunoglobulin metabolism in ataxia telangiectasia. J Clin Invest 1968;47:1905.
19. Wells JV, Fudenberg HH. Metabolism of radio-iodinated IgG in patients with abnormal serum IgG levels. 1: Hypergamma-globulinaemia. Clin Exp Immunol 1971;9:761.
20. Wells JV, Fudenberg HH. Metabolism of radio-iodinated IgG in patients with abnormal serum IgG levels. II. Hypogamma-globulinaemia. Clin Exp Immunol 1971;9:775.
21. Brambell FWR, Hemmings WA, Morris IG. A theoretical model of γ-globulin catabolism. Nature 1964;203:1352.
22. Junghans RP, Anderson CL. The protection receptor for IgG catabolism is the β_2-microglobulin-containing neonatal intestinal transport receptor. Proc Natl Acad Sci U S A 1996;93:5512.
23. Dau PC. Immunologic rebound. J Clin Apheresis 1995;10:210.
24. Junghans RP. IgG biosynthesis: No "immunoregulatory feedback." Blood 1997;90:3815.
25. Yu Z, Lennon VA. Mechanism of intravenous immune globulin therapy in antibody-mediated autoimmune diseases. N Engl J Med 1999;340:227.
26. Lewis EJ, Hunsicker LG, Lan SP, et al. A controlled trial of plasmapheresis therapy in severe lupus nephritis. N Engl J Med 1992;326:1371.
27. Pool M, McLeod BC. Pyrogen reactions to human serum albumin in plasma exchange. J Clin Apheresis 1995;10:81.
28. Keller AJ, Urbaniak SJ. Intensive plasma exchange on the cell separator: effects on serum immunoglobulins and complement components. Br J Haematol 1978;38:531.
29. Cochrane Injuries Group Albumin Reviewers. Human albumin administration in critically ill patients: Systematic review of randomized controlled trials. 1998;317:235.
30. Wilkes MM, Navickis RJ. Patient survival after human serum albumin administration: a meta-analysis of randomized, controlled trials. Ann Intern Med 2001;135:149–164.
31. Finfer S, Bellomo R, Boyce N, et al. A comparison of albumin and saline for fluid resuscitation in the intensive care unit. N Engl J Med 2004;350:2247–2256.
32. Rossi EC. Plasma exchange in the thrombotic microangiopathies. In Rossi EC, Simon TL, Moss GS, Gould SA (eds). Principles of Transfusion Medicine, 2nd ed. Baltimore, Williams & Wilkins, 1996, p 577.
33. McLeod BC, Price TH, Owen H, et al. Frequency of immediate adverse effects associated with therapeutic apheresis. Transfusion 1999;39:282.
34. Owen HG, Brecher ME. Partial colloid replacement for therapeutic plasma exchange. J Clin Apheresis 1997;12:146.
35. McLeod B, Sassetti R. Plasmapheresis with return of cryoglobulin depleted autologous plasma (cryoglobulinpheresis) in cryoglobulinemia. Blood 1980;55:866.
36. Vamvakas EC, Pineda AA. Selective extraction of plasma constituents. In McLeod BC, Price TH, Drew MJ (eds). Apheresis: Principles and Practice. Bethesda, Md., AABB Press, 1997, p 378.
37. Gjöstrup P, Watt RM. Therapeutic protein A immunoadsorption: A review. Transfus Sci 1990;11:281.
38. Gordon BR, Kelsy SF, Dau PC, et al. Long-term effects of low-density lipoprotein apheresis using an automated dextran sulfate cellulose adsorption system: Liposorber Study Group. Am J Cardiol 1998;81:407.
39. Jaeger BR. The HELP system for treatment of atherothrombotic disorders. Ther Apheresis Dial 2003;7:391–396.
40. McLeod BC. Introduction to the third special issue on clinical applications of therapeutic apheresis. J Clin Apheresis 2000;15:1.
41. Smith JW, Weinstein R, Hillyer KL for the AABB Hemapheresis Committee. Therapeutic apheresis: a summary of current indication categories endorsed by the AABB and the American Society for Apheresis. Transfusion 2003;43:820–822.
42. Consensus Conference. The utility of therapeutic plasmapheresis for neurological disorders. JAMA 1986;256:1333.
43. Ropper AH. The Guillain-Barré syndrome. N Engl J Med 1992;326:1130.
44. van der Meché FGA. The Guillain-Barré syndrome. Baillieres Clin Neurol 1994;3:73.
45. Hughes RA, Rees JH. Guillain-Barré syndrome. Curr Opin Neurol 1994;7:386.
46. Cook SD, Dowling PC, Murray MR, Whitaker JN. Circulating demyelinating factors in acute idiopathic polyneuropathy. Arch Neurol 1971;24:136.
47. Feasby TE, Hahn AF, Gilbert JJ. Passive transfer studies in Guillain-Barré polyneuropathy. Neurology 1982;32:1159.
48. Koski CI, Gratz E, Sutherland J, et al. Clinical correlation with anti-peripheral myelin antibodies in Guillain-Barré syndrome. Ann Neurol 1986;19:573.
49. McFarlin DE. Immunological parameters in Guillain-Barré syndrome. Ann Neurol 1990;27(Suppl 1):525.
50. Vriesendorp FJ, Mayer RF, Koski CL. Kinetics of anti-peripheral nerve myelin antibody in patients with Guillain-Barré syndrome treated and not treated with plasmapheresis. Arch Neurol 1991;48:858.
51. Vriesendorp FJ, Mishu B, Blaser MJ, Koski CL. Serum antibodies to GM1, GD16, peripheral nerve myelin, and *Campylobacter jejuni* in patients with Guillain-Barré syndrome and controls. Ann Neurol 1993;34:130.
52. Rees JH, Gregson NA, Hughes RA. Anti-ganglioside GM1 antibodies in Guillain-Barré syndrome and their relationship to *Campylobacter jejuni* infection. Ann Neurol 1995;38:809.
53. Rees JH, Soudain SE, Gregson NA, Hughes RAC. *Campylobacter jejuni* infection and Guillain-Barré syndrome. N Engl J Med 1995;333:1374.
54. Willison HJ, Kennedy PGE. Gangliosides and bacterial toxins in Guillain-Barré syndrome. J Neuroimmunol 1993;46:105.
55. Yuki N, Taki T, Inagaki F, et al. A bacterium lipopolysaccharide that elicits Guillain-Barré syndrome has a GM_1, ganglioside-like structure. J Exp Med 1993;178:1771.
56. McKhann GM, Cornblath DR, Griffen JW, et al. Acute motor axonal neuropathy: A frequent cause of flaccid paralysis in China. Ann Neurol 1993;33:333.
57. Jacobs BC, Rothbarth PH, van der Meche FG, et al. The spectrum of antecedent infections in Guillain-Barré syndrome: a case-control study. Neurology 1998;51:1110–1115.
58. Guillain-Barré Syndrome Steroid Trial Group. Double-blind trial of intravenous methylprednisone in Guillain-Barré syndrome. Lancet 1993;341:586.
59. Brettle RP, Gross MLP, Legg NJ, et al. Treatment of acute polyneuropathy by plasma exchange. Lancet 1978;2:1100.
60. Schooneman F, Janot C, Streiff F, et al. Plasma exchange in Guillain-Barré syndrome: ten cases. Plasma Ther 1981;2:117.
61. Valbonesi M, Garelli S, Mosconi L, et al. Plasma exchange as a therapy for Guillain-Barré syndrome with immune complexes. Vox Sang 1981;41:74.
62. de Jager AEJ, The TH, Smit Sibinga CTS, Das PC. Plasma exchange in the Guillain Barré syndrome. Br Med J 1981;283:794.
63. Rumpl E, Mayr U, Gerstenbrand F, et al. Treatment of Guillain-Barré syndrome by plasma exchange. J Neurol 1981;225:207.
64. Greenwood RJ, Newsom-Davis J, Hughes RA, et al. Controlled trial of plasma exchange in acute inflammatory polyradiculoneuropathy. Lancet 1984;1:877.
65. Osterman PG, Lundemo G, Pirskanen R, et al. Beneficial effects of plasma exchange in acute inflammatory polyradiculoneuropathy. Lancet 1984;2:1296.
66. The Guillain-Barré Syndrome Study Group. Plasmapheresis and acute Guillain-Barré syndrome. Neurology 1985;35:1096.

67. French Cooperative Group on Plasma Exchange and Guillain-Barré Syndrome. Efficiency of plasma exchange in Guillain-Barré syndrome: role of replacement fluids. Ann Neurol 1987;22:753.
68. French Cooperative Group on Plasma Exchange in Guillain-Barré Syndrome. Plasma exchange in Guillain-Barré syndrome: one-year follow-up. Ann Neurol 1992;32:94.
69. Jansen PW, Perkin RM, Ashwal S. The Guillain-Barré syndrome in childhood: natural course and efficacy of plasmapheresis. Pediatr Neurol 1993;9:16.
70. Bouget J, Chevret S, Chastang C, Raphael J-C, et al. Plasma exchange in Guillain-Barré syndrome: results from the French prospective, double-blind, randomized, multicenter study. Crit Care Med 1993;21:651.
71. McLeod BC. The technique of therapeutic apheresis. J Crit Illness 1991;6:487.
72. van der Meché FGA, Schmitz PIM, The Dutch Guillain-Barré Study Group. A randomized trial comparing intravenous immune globulin and plasma exchange in Guillain-Barré syndrome. N Engl J Med 1992;326:1123.
73. Plasma Exchange/Sandoglobulin Guillain-Barré Syndrome Trial Group. Randomised trial of plasma exchange, intravenous immunoglobulin, and combined treatments in Guillain-Barré syndrome. Lancet 1997;349:225.
74. Hughes RAC, Wijdicks EFM, Borohn R, et al. Practice parameter: immunotherapy for Guillain-Barré syndrome. Neurology 2003;61:736–740.
75. Mendell JR. Chronic inflammatory demyelinating polyradiculopathy. Annu Rev Med 1993;44:211.
76. Glass JD, Cornblath DR. Chronic inflammatory demyelinating polyneuropathy and paraproteinemic neuropathies. Curr Opin Neurol 1994;7:393.
77. Köller H, Kieseier BC, Jander S, Hartung H-P. Chronic inflammatory demyelinating polyneuropathy. N Engl J Med 2005;352:1343–1356.
78. Saida K, Sumner AJ, Saida T, et al. Antiserum-mediated demyelination: relationship between remyelination and functional recovery. Ann Neurol 1980;8:12.
79. Yan WX, Taylor J, Andrias-Kauba S, Pollard JD. Passive transfer of demyelination by serum or IgG from chronic inflammatory demyelinating polyneuropathy patients. Ann Neurol 2000;47:765–775.
80. Simone IL, Annunziata P, Maimone D, et al. Serum and CSF anti-GM1 antibodies in patients with Guillain-Barré syndrome and chronic inflammatory demyelinating polyneuropathy. J Neurol Sci 1993;114:49.
81. Khalili-Shirazi A, Atkinson P, Gregson N, Hughes RAC. Antibody response to P_0 and P_2 myelin proteins in Guillain-Barré syndrome and chronic inflammatory demyelinating polyradiculoneuropathy. J Neuroimmunol 1993;46:245.
82. Connolly AM, Pestronk A, Trotter JL, et al. High-titer selective anti-beta-tubulin antibodies in chronic demyelinating polyneuropathy. Neurology 1993;43:557.
83. Dyck PJ, Daube J, O'Brien P, et al. Plasma exchange in chronic inflammatory demyelinating polyradiculoneuropathy. N Engl J Med 1986;314:461.
84. Hahn AF, Bolton CF, Pillay N, et al. Plasma-exchange therapy in chronic inflammatory demyelinating polyneuropathy: a double-blind, sham-controlled, cross-over study. Brain 1996;119:1055.
85. Dalakas MC. Intravenous immunoglobulin in autoimmune neuromuscular diseases. JAMA 2004;291:2367–2375.
86. van Doom PA, Vermeulen M, Brand A, et al. Intravenous immunoglobulin treatment in patients with chronic inflammatory demyelinating polyneuropathy. Arch Neurol 1991;48:217.
87. Faed JM, Day B, Pollack M, et al. High-dose intravenous human immunoglobulin in chronic inflammatory demyelinating polyneuropathy. Neurology 1989;39:422.
88. van Doom PA, Brand A, Strengers PFW, et al. High-dose intravenous immunoglobulin treatment in chronic inflammatory demyelinating polyneuropathy. Neurology 1990;40:209.
89. Vermeulen M, van Doom PA, Brand A, et al. Intravenous immunoglobulin treatment in patients with chronic inflammatory demyelinating polyneuropathy: A double blind, placebo controlled study. J Neurol Neurosurg Psychiatry 1993;56:36.
90. Hahn AF, Bolton CF, Zochodne D, Feasby TE. Intravenous immunoglobulin treatment in chronic inflammatory demyelinating polyneuropathy: a double-blind, placebo-controlled, cross-over study. Brain 1996;119:1067.
91. Hughes R, Bensa S, Willison H, et al. Randomized controlled trial of intravenous immunoglobulin versus oral prednisone in chronic inflammatory demyelinating polyneuropathy. Ann Neurol 2001;50:195–201.
92. Choudhary PP, Hughes RAC. Long-term treatment of chronic inflammatory demyelinating polyradiculoneuropathy with plasma exchange or intravenous immunoglobulin. Q J Med 1995;88:493.
93. Dyck PJ, Litchy WJ, Kratz KM, et al. A plasma exchange versus immune globulin infusion trial in chronic inflammatory demyelinating polyradiculoneuropathy. Ann Neurol 1994;36:838.
94. Kyle RA. Monoclonal proteins in neuropathy. Neurol Clin 1992; 10:713.
95. Bosch EP, Smith BE. Peripheral neuropathies associated with monoclonal proteins. Med Clin North Am 1993;77:125.
96. Baldini L, Nobile-Orazio E, Guffanti A, et al. Peripheral neuropathy in IgM monoclonal gammopathy and Waldenström's macroglobulinemia: a frequent complication in elderly males with low MAG-reactive serum monoclonal component. Am J Hematol 1994;45:25.
97. Nemni R, Gerosa E, Piccolo G, Merlini G. Neuropathies associated with monoclonal gammopathies. Haematologica 1994;79:557.
98. Gabriel JM, Erne B, Miescher GC, et al. Expression patterns of human PNS myelin proteins in neuropathies associated with anti-myelin antibodies. Schweiz Arch Neurol Psychiatry 1994;145:22.
99. Tatum AH. Experimental paraprotein neuropathy: demyelination by passive transfer of human IgM anti-myelin-associated glycoprotein. Ann Neurol 1993;33:502.
100. Smith IS. The natural history of chronic demyelinating neuropathy associated with benign IgM paraproteinemia: a clinical and neurophysiological study. Brain 1994;117:949.
101. Simmons Z, Albers JW, Bromberg MB, Feldman EL. Long-term follow-up of patients with chronic inflammatory demyelinating polyradiculoneuropathy, without and with monoclonal gammopathy. Brain 1995;118:359.
102. Nobile-Orazio E, Barbieri S, Baldini L, et al. Peripheral neuropathy in monoclonal gammopathy of undetermined significance: prevalence and immunopathogenetic studies. Acta Neurol Scand 1992;85:383.
103. Miralles GD, O'Fallon JR, Talley NJ. Plasma-cell dyscrasia with polyneuropathy: The spectrum of POEMS syndrome. N Engl J Med 1992;327:1919.
104. Dyck PJ, Low PA, Windebank AJ, et al. Plasma exchange in polyneuropathy associated with monoclonal gammopathy of undetermined significance. N Engl J Med 1991;325:1482.
105. Siciliano G, Moriconi L, Gianni G, Richieri E. Selective techniques of apheresis in polyneuropathy associated with monoclonal gammopathy of undetermined significance. Acta Neurol Scand 1994;89:117.
106. Oksenhendler E, Chevret S, Leger JM, et al. Plasma exchange and chlorambucil in polyneuropathy associated with monoclonal IgM gammopathy. J Neurol Neurosurg Psychiatry 1995;59:243.
107. Bleasel AF, Hawke SH, Pollard JD, McLeod JG. IgG monoclonal paraproteinemia and peripheral neuropathy. J Neurol Neurosurg Psychiatry 1993;56:52.
108. Richman DP, Agius MA. Treatment of autoimmune myasthenia gravis. Neurology 2003;61:1652–1661.
109. Romi F, Gilhus NE, Aarli JA. Myasthenia gravis: clinical, immunological, and therapeutic advances. Acta Neurol Scand 2005;111:134–141.
110. Masselli, RA. Pathophysiology of myasthenia gravis and Lambert-Eaton syndrome. Neurol Clin 1994;12:285.
111. Richman DP, Wollman RL, Maselli RA, et al. Effector mechanisms of myasthenic antibodies. Ann N Y Acad Sci 1993;681:264.
112. Dau PC, Lindstrom JM, Cassel CK, et al. Plasmapheresis and immunosuppressive drug therapy in myasthenia gravis. N Engl J Med 1977; 297:1134.
113. Gajdos P, Chevret S, Toyka K. Plasma exchange for myasthenia gravis. Cochrane Database Sys Rev 2002;4:CD002275.
114. d'Empaire G, Hoaglin DC, Perlo VP, Pontoppidan H. Effect of prethymectomy plasma exchange on postoperative respiratory function in myasthenia gravis. J Thorac Cardiovasc Surg 1985;89:592.
115. Rodnitzy RL, Bosch EP. Chronic long-interval plasma exchange in myasthenia gravis. Arch Neurol 1984;41:715.
116. Splendiani G, Passlacqua S, Barbera G, et al. Semi-selective immunoadsorption treatment in myasthenia gravis. Biomater Artif Cells Immobilization Biotechnol 1992;20:1145.
117. Ichikawa M, Koh CS, Hata Y, et al. Immunoadsorption plasmapheresis for severe generalized myasthenia gravis. Arch Dis Child 1993;69:236.
118. Sawada K, Malchesky PS, Koo AP. Myasthenia gravis therapy: Immunoadsorbent may eliminate need for plasma products. Cleve Clin J Med 1993;60:60.
119. Berta E, Confalonieri P, Simoncini O, et al. Removal of antiacetylcholine receptor antibodies by protein-A immunoadsorption in myasthenia gravis. Int J Artif Organs 1994;17:603.
120. Benny WB, Sutton DMC, Oger J, et al. Clinical evaluation of a staphylococcal protein A immunoadsorption system in the treatment of myasthenia gravis patients. Transfusion 1999;39:682.
121. Gajdos P, Chevret S, Toyka K. Intravenous immunoglobulin for myasthenia gravis. Cochrane Database Sys Rev 2002;4:CD002277.

122. Gajdos P, Chevret S, Clair B, et al. Clinical trial of plasma exchange and high-dose intravenous immunoglobulin in myasthenia gravis. Ann Neurol 1997;41:789.
123. Al-Qureshi AI, Choudry MA, Akber MS, et al. Plasma exchange vs. intravenous immunoglobulin treatment in myasthenic crisis. Neurology 1999;52:629.
124. Newsom-Davis J. Lambert-Eaton myasthenic syndrome. Springer Semin Immunopathol 1985;8:129.
125. Jablecki C. Lambert-Eaton myasthenic syndrome. Muscle Nerve 1984;7:250.
126. O'Neill JH, Murray NM, Newsom-Davis J. The Lambert-Eaton myasthenic syndrome: A review of 50 cases. Brain 1988;11:577.
127. Takamori M. Lambert-Eaton myasthenic syndrome as an autoimmune calcium channelopathy. Biochem Biophys Res Commun 2004; 322:1347–1351.
128. Rosenfield MR, Wong E, Dalmace J, et al. Cloning and characterization of a Lambert-Eaton myasthenic syndrome antigen. Ann Neurol 1993;33:113.
129. Kokontis L, Gutmann L. Current treatment of neuromuscular diseases. Arch Neurol 2000;57:939–940.
130. Maddison P, Newsome-Davis J. Treatment for Lambert-Eaton myasthenic syndrome. Cochrane Database Syst Rev 2005;3:CD003279.
131. Chalk CH, Murray NM, Newsom-Davis J, et al. Response of the Lambert-Eaton myasthenic syndrome to treatment of associated small-cell lung carcinoma. Neurology 1990;40:1552.
132. Dau PC, Denys EH. Plasmapheresis and immunosuppressive drug therapy in the Eaton-Lambert syndrome. Ann Neurol 1982;11:570.
133. Moll JWB, Vecht CJ. Immune diagnoses of paraneoplastic neurological disease. Clin Neurol Neurosurg 1995;97:71.
134. Graus F, Rene R. Clinical and pathological advances on central nervous system paraneoplastic syndromes. Rev Neurol (Paris) 1992;148:496.
135. Sutton I, Winer JB. The immunopathogeneses of paraneoplastic neurological syndrome. Clin Sci 2002;102:475–486.
136. Lorish TR, Thorsteinsson G, Howard FM Jr. Stiff-man syndrome updated. Mayo Clin Proc 1986;64:629–636.
137. Levy LM, Dalakas MC, Floeter MK. The stiff-person syndrome: An autoimmune disorder affecting neurotransmission of γ-aminobutyric acid. Ann Intern Med 1999;131:522–530.
138. Helfgott SM. Stiff-man syndrome. Arthritis Rheum 1999;42: 1312–1320.
139. Dalakas MC, Fujii M, Li M, McElroy B. The clinical spectrum of anti-GAD antibody-positive patients with stiff-person syndrome. Neurology 2000;55:1531–1535.
140. Moll JWB, Vecht CJ. Immune diagnoses of paraneoplastic neurological disease. Clin Neurol Neurosurg 1995;97:71–81.
141. Graus F, Rene R. Clinical and pathological advances in central nervous system paraneoplastic syndromes. Rev Neurol (Paris) 1992;148: 496–501.
142. Butler MH, Hayashi A, Ohkoshi N, et al. Autoimmunity to gephyrin in stiff-man syndrome. Neuron 2000;26:307–312.
143. Hao W, Davis C, Hirsch IB, et al. Plasmapheresis and immunosuppression in stiff-man syndrome with type 1 diabetes: a 2-year study. J Neurol 1999;246:731–735.
144. Oguni H, Andermann F, Rasmussen TB. The natural history of the syndrome of chronic encephalitis and epilepsy: a study of the MNI series of forty-eight cases. In Andermann F (ed). Chronic Encephalitis and Epilepsy: Rasmussen's Syndrome. Boston, Butterworth-Heinemann, 1991, p 7.
145. Bien CG, Widman G, Urbach H, et al. The natural history of Rasmussen's encephalitis. Brain 2002;125:1751–1759.
146. Rodgers SW, Andrews PI, Gahring LC, et al. Autoantibodies to glutamate receptor Glu R3 in Rasmussen's encephalitis. Science 1994; 265:648.
147. Bien CG, Bauer J, Dechwerth TL, et al. Destruction of neurons by cytotoxic T cells: a new pathogenic mechanism in Rasmussen's encephalitis. Ann Neurol 2002;51:311–318.
148. Andrews PI, McNamara JO. Rasmussen's encephalitis: An autoimmune disorder? Curr Opin Neurobiol 1996;6:673.
149. Andrews PI, Dichter MA, Berkovic SF, et al. Plasmapheresis in Rasmussen's encephalitis. Neurology 1996;46:242.
150. Hart YM, Cortez M, Andermann F, et al. Medical treatment of Rasmussen's syndrome (chronic encephalitis and epilepsy): effect of high dose steroids or immunoglobulins in 19 patients. Neurology 1994;44:1030.
151. Gronata T, Fusco L, Gobbi G, et al. Experience with immunomodulatory treatments in Rasmussen's encephalitis. Neurology 2003;61:1807–1810.
152. Swedo SE, Leonard HL, Schapiro MB, et al. Sydenham's chorea: physical and psychological symptoms of St. Vitus' dance. Pediatrics 1993;91:706.
153. Swedo SE, Rapoport JL, Cheslow DL, et al. High prevalence of obsessive-compulsive symptoms in patients with Sydenham's chorea. Am J Psychiatry 1989;146:246.
154. Swedo SE, Leonard HL, Garvey M, et al. Pediatric autoimmune neuropsychiatric disorders associated with streptococcal infections: Clinical description of the first 50 cases. Am J Psychiatry 1998;155:264.
155. Husby G, van de Rijn I, Zabriskie JB, et al. Antibodies reacting with cytoplasm of subthalamic and caudate nuclei neurons in chorea and acute rheumatic fever. J Exp Med 1976;144:1094.
156. Zabriskie JB. Rheumatic fever: a model for the pathological consequences of microbial-host mimicry. Clin Exp Rheumatol 1986;4:65.
157. Snider LA, Swedo SE. Post-streptococcal autoimmune disorders of the central nervous system. Curr Opin Neurol 2003;16:359–365.
158. Singer HS. PANDAS and immunomodulatory therapy. Lancet 1999; 354:1137.
159. Garvey MA, Swedo SW, Shapiro MB, et al. Intravenous immunoglobulin and plasmapheresis as effective treatments in Sydenham's chorea. Neurology 1996;46:A147.
160. Perlmutter SJ, Leitman SF, Garvey MA, et al. Therapeutic plasma exchange and intravenous immunoglobulin for obsessive-compulsive disorder and tic disorders in childhood. Lancet 1999;354:1153.
161. Martino D, Giovannoni G. Antibasal ganglia antibodies and their relevance to movement disorders. Curr Opin Neurol 2004;17:425–432.
162. Weinshenker BG, Sibley WA. Natural history and treatment of multiple sclerosis. Curr Opin Neurol Neurosurg 1992;5:203.
163. Owens T, Sriram S. The immunology of multiple sclerosis and its animal model, experimental allergic encephalomyelitis. Neurol Clin 1995;13:51.
164. Hafler DA, Weiner HL. Immunologic mechanisms and therapy in multiple sclerosis. Immunol Rev 1995;144:75.
165. Weiner HL. Multiple sclerosis is on inflammatory T-cell-mediated autoimmune disease. Arch Neurol 2004;61:1613–1615.
166. Genain CP, Cannella B, Hauser SL, Raine CD. Identification of autoantibodies associated with myelin damage in multiple sclerosis. Nat Med 1999;5:170–175.
167. Egg R, Reindl M, Deisenhammer F, et al. Anti-MOG and anti-MBP antibody subclasses in multiple sclerosis. Mult Scler 2001;7:285–289.
168. Berger T, Rubner P, Schautzer F, et al. Antimyelin antibodies as a predictor of clinically definite multiple sclerosis after a first demyelinating event. N Engl J Med 2003;349:139–145.
169. Noseworthy JH, Ebers GC, Vandervoort MK, et al. The impact of blinding on the results of a randomized, placebo-controlled multiple sclerosis clinical trial. Neurology 1994;44:16.
170. Jacobs L, Goodkin DE, Rudick RA, Herndon R. Advances in specific therapy for multiple sclerosis. Curr Opin Neurol 1994;7:250.
171. Rizvi SA, Bashir K. Other therapy options and future strategies for treating patients with multiple sclerosis. Neurology 2004;63(Suppl 6): S47–S54.
172. Rizvi Sa, Bashir K. Current approved options for treating patients with multiple sclerosis. Neurology 2004;63(Suppl 6):S8–S14.
173. Goodin DS, Frohman EM, Garmany GP, et al. Disease modifying therapies in multiple sclerosis: report of the therapeutics and technology assessment subcommittee of the American Academy of Neurology and the MS Council for Clinical Practice Guidelines. Neurology 2002;58:169–178.
174. Fazekas F, Deisenhammer F, Strasser-Fuchs S, et al. Randomised placebo-controlled trial of monthly intravenous immunoglobulin therapy in relapsing-remitting multiple sclerosis. Austrian Immunoglobulin in Multiple Sclerosis Study Group. Lancet 1997;349:589.
175. Sorensen PS, Wanscher B, Jensen CV, et al. Intravenous immunoglobulin G reduces MRI activity in relapsing multiple sclerosis. Neurology 1998;50:1273.
176. Achiron A, Gabbay U, Gilad R, et al. Intravenous immunoglobulin treatment in multiple sclerosis: Effect on relapses. Neurology 1998;50:398.
177. Dau PC, Petajan JM, Johnson KP, et al. Plasmapheresis and immunosuppressive drug therapy in multiple sclerosis. Neurology 1980;30:1023.
178. Weiner HL, Dawson DM. Plasmapheresis in multiple sclerosis: preliminary study. Neurology 1980;30:1029.
179. Khatri BO, McQuillen MP, Hoffman RG, et al. Plasma exchange in chronic progressive multiple sclerosis: a long term study. Neurology 1991;41:409.
180. Hauser SL, Dawson DM, Lehrich JR, et al. Intensive immunosuppression in progressive multiple sclerosis: a randomized three-arm study of high dose intravenous cyclophosphamide, plasma exchange, and ACTH. N Engl J Med 1983;308:173.
181. Tindall RSA, Walker JE, Ehle AL, et al. Plasmapheresis in multiple sclerosis: prospective trial of pheresis and immunosuppression versus immunosuppression alone. Neurology 1982;32:739.

182. Khatri BO, McQuillen MP, Harrington GJ, et al. Chronic progressive multiple sclerosis: double-blind controlled study of plasmapheresis in patients taking immunosuppressive drugs. Neurology 1985;35:312.
183. Weiner HL. An assessment of plasma exchange in progressive multiple sclerosis. Neurology 1985;35:320.
184. Goodin DS. The use of immunosuppressive agents in the treatment of multiple sclerosis: a critical review. Neurology 1991;41:980.
185. Goodkin DE, Ransohoff RM, Rudick RA. Experimental therapies for multiple sclerosis: current status. Cleve Clin J Med 1992;59:63.
186. Weiner HL, Dau P, Khatri BO, et al. Double-blind study of true versus sham plasma exchange in patients being treated with immunosuppression for acute attacks of multiple sclerosis. Neurology 1989;39:1143.
187. The Canadian Cooperative Multiple Sclerosis Study Group. The Canadian cooperative trial of cyclophosphamide and plasma exchange in progressive multiple sclerosis. Lancet 1991;337:441.
188. Weinshenker B, O'Brien PC, Petterson TM, et al. A randomized trial of plasma exchange in acute central nervous system inflammatory demyelinating disease. Ann Neurol 1999;46:878–886.
189. Keegan M, Pineda AA, McClelland RL, et al. Plasma exchange for severe attacks of CNS demyelination: predictors of response. Neurology 2002;58:143–146.
190. McGrath MA, Penny R. Paraproteinemias: blood hyperviscosity and clinical manifestations. J Clin Invest 1996;58:1155.
191. Salmon SE, Cassady RJ. Plasma cell neoplasms. In DeVita VT, Hellman S, Rosenberg SA (eds). Cancer: Principles and Practice of Oncology. New York: Lippincott-Raven, 1997, p 2344.
192. Kipps TJ. Macroglobulinemia. In Lichtman MA, Beutler E, Kipps TJ, Seligsohn U, et al (eds). Williams Hematology, 7th ed. New York, McGraw-Hill, 2006, p 1549.
193. Gertz MA. Waldenström macroglobulinemia: a review of therapy. Am J Hematol 2005;79:147–157.
194. Glaspy JA. Hemostatic abnormalities in multiple myeloma and related disorders. Hematol Oncol Clin North Am 1992;6:1301.
195. Bear RA, Cole EH, Slang A, et al. Treatment of acute renal failure due to myeloma kidney. Can Med Assoc J 1980;123:750.
196. Knudsen LM, Hjorth M, Hippe E, for the Nordic Myeloma Study Group. Renal failure in multiple myeloma: Reversibility and impact on the prognosis. Eur J Hematol 2000;65:175–181.
197. Misiani R, Tiraboschi G, Mingardi G, Mecca G. Management of myeloma kidney: an anti-light chain approach. Am J Kidney Dis 1987; 10:28.
198. Solling K, Solling J. Clearance of Bence-Jones proteins during peritoneal dialysis or plasmapheresis in myelomatosis associated with renal failure. Contrib Nephrol 1988;68:259.
199. Johnson WJ, Kyle RA, Pineda AA, et al. Treatment of renal failure associated with multiple myeloma: plasmapheresis, hemodialysis, and chemotherapy. Arch Intern Med 1990;150:863.
200. Zucchelli P, Pasquali S, Cagnoli L, Ferrari G. Controlled plasma exchange trial in acute renal failure due to multiple myeloma. Kidney Int 1988;33:1175.
201. Kaplan AA. Therapeutic apheresis for the renal complications of multiple myeloma and the dysglobulinurias. Ther Apheresis 2001;5:171–175.
202. Fraser ID, Bothamley JE, Bennett MO, et al. Intensive antenatal plasmapheresis in severe Rhesus isoimmunisation. Lancet 1976;1:6.
203. Mollison PL, Engelfriet CP, Contreras M. Haemolytic disease of the fetus and newborn. In Blood Transfusion in Clinical Medicine. London: Blackwell Science, 1997, p 390.
204. Filbey D, Berseus O, Lindeberg S, Wesstrom G. A management programme for Rh alloimmunization during pregnancy. Early Hum Dev 1987;15:11.
205. Watson WJ, Katz VL, Bowes WA. Plasmapheresis during pregnancy. Obstet Gynecol 1990;76:451.
206. Furukawa K, Nakajima T, Kogure T, et al. Example of a woman with multiple intrauterine deaths due to anti-M who delivered a live child after plasmapheresis. Exp Clin Immunogenet 1993;10:161.
207. Shirey R, Ness P, Kickler T, et al. The association of anti-P and early abortion. Transfusion 1987;27:189.
208. Gale RP, Feig S, Ho W, et al. ABO blood group system and bone marrow transplantation. Blood 1977;50:185.
209. Bensinger WI, Baker DA, Buckner DD, et al. Immunoadsorption for removal of A and B blood group antibodies. N Engl J Med 1981; 301:160.
210. Braine HG, Sensenbrenner LL, Wright SK, et al. Bone marrow transplantation with major ABO incompatibility using erythrocyte depletion of marrow prior to infusion. Blood 1982;60:420.
211. Gmur JP, Burger J, Schaffner A, et al. Pure red cell aplasia of long duration complicating major ABO incompatible bone marrow transplantation. Blood 1990;75:290.
212. Benjamin RJ, Connors JM, McGurk S, et al. Prolonged erythroid aplasia after major ABO-mismatched transplantation for chronic myelogenous leukemia. Biol Blood Marrow Transplant 1998;4:151–156.
213. Üstün C, Celebi H, Arat M, et al. Treatment of aregeneratoric anemia following an ABO-incompatible allogeneic peripheral blood stem cell transplantation: a case report. Ther Apheresis 1999;3:275–277.
214. Verholen F, Stalder M, Helg C, Chalandon Y. Resistant pure red cell aplasia after allogeneic stem cell transplantation with major ABO mismatch treated by escalating dose donor leukocyte infusion. Eur J Hematol 2004;73:441–446.
215. Fischel RJ, Ascher NL, Payne WD, et al. Pediatric liver transplantation across ABO blood group barriers. Transplant Proc 1989;21:2221.
216. Renard TH, Shimaoka S, Le Bherz D, et al. ABO incompatible liver transplantation in children: a prospective approach. Transplant Proc 1993;25:1953.
217. Mor E, Skerrett D, Manzarbeitia C, et al. Successful use of an enhanced immunosuppressive protocol with plasmapheresis for ABO-incompatible mismatched grafts in liver transplant recipients. Transplantation 1995;59:986.
218. Gloor JM, Lager DJ, Moore B. ABO-incompatible kidney transplantation using both A_2 and non-A_2 living donors. Transplantation 2003; 75:971–977.
219. Warren DS, Zachary AA, Sonnenday CJ, et al. Successful renal transplantation across simultaneous ABO incompatible and positive crossmatch barriers. Am J Transplant 2004;4:561–568.
220. Sonnenday CJ, Warren DS, Cooper M, et al. Plasmapheresis, CMV hyperimmune globulin, and anti-CD20 allow ABO-incompatible renal transplantation without splenectomy. Am J Transplantation 2004; 4:1315–1322.
221. Winters JL, Gloor JM, Pineda AA, et al. Plasma exchange conditioning for ABO-incompatible renal transplantation. J Clin Apheresis 2004;19:79–85.
222. Ramsey G. Red cell antibodies arising from solid organ transplants. Transfusion 1991;31:76.
223. Ramsey G, Israel L, Lindsay GD, et al. Anti-rho(D) in two Rh-positive patients receiving kidney grafts from an Rh-immunized donor. Transplantation 1986;41:67–69.
224. Lundgren G, Asaba H, Bergstrom J, et al. Fulminating anti-A autoimmune hemolysis with anuria in a renal transplant recipient: a therapeutic role of plasma exchange. Clin Nephrol 1981;16:211.
225. Kickler TS. The challenge of platelet alloimmunization: Management and prevention. Transfusion 1990;30:8.
226. Bensinger WI, Buckner CD, Clift RA, et al. Plasma exchange for platelet alloimmunization. Transplantation 1986;41:602.
227. Christie DJ, Howe RB, Lennon SS, Sauro SC. Treatment of refractoriness to platelet transfusion by protein A column therapy. Transfusion 1993;33:234.
228. Lopez-Plaza I, Miller K, Leitman SF. Ineffectiveness of protein A adsorption in the treatment of platelet refractoriness. J Clin Apheresis 1992;7:33.
229. Lee EJ, Norris D, Schiffer CA. Intravenous immune globulin for patients alloimmunized to random donor platelet transfusions. Transfusion 1987;27:245.
230. Kickler T, Braine HG, Piantadosi S, et al. A randomized, placebo-controlled trial of intravenous gammaglobulin in alloimmunized thrombocytopenic patients. Blood 1987;70:313.
231. Ziegler ZR, Shadduck RK, Rosenfeld CS, et al. High-dose intravenous gamma globulin improves responses to single-donor platelets in patients refractory to platelet transfusion. Blood 1987;70:1433.
232. Amorosi EL, Ultmann JE. Thrombotic thrombocytopenic purpura: report of 16 cases and review of the literature. Medicine (Baltimore) 1966;45:139.
233. Moake JL. Thrombotic microangiopathies. N Engl J Med 2002;347: 589–600.
234. Torok TJ, Holman RC, Chorba TL. Increasing mortality from thrombotic thrombocytopenic purpura in the United States: analysis of national mortality data, 1968–1991. Am J Hematol 1995;50:84.
235. Porta C, Caporali R, Montecucco C. Thrombotic thrombocytopenic purpura and autoimmunity: a tale of shadows and suspects. Haematologia 1999;84:260.
236. Rarick MU, Espina B, Mocharnuk R, et al. Thrombotic thrombocytopenic purpura in patients with human immunodeficiency virus infection: a report of three cases and review of the literature. Am J Hematol 1992;40:103.
237. Furlan M, Robles R, Solenthaler M, et al. Deficient activity of von Willebrand factor-cleaving protease in chronic relapsing thrombotic thrombocytopenic purpura. Blood 1997;89:3097.
238. Furlan M, Robles R, Galbusera M, et al. Von Willebrand factor-cleaving protease in thrombotic thrombocytopenic purpura and the hemolytic-uremic syndrome. N Engl J Med 1998;339:1578.

239. Tsai H-M, Lian EC-Y. Antibodies to von Willebrand factor-cleaving protease in acute thrombotic thrombocytopenic purpura. N Engl J Med 1998;339:1585.
240. Rick ME, Austin H, Leitman SF, et al. Clinical usefulness of a functional assay for the von Willebrand factor cleaving protease (ADAMTS 13) and its inhibitor in a patient with thrombotic thrombocytopenic purpura. Am J Hematol 2004;75:96–100.
241. Sahud MA, Claster S, Liu L, et al. Von Willebrand factor-cleaving protease inhibitor in a patient with human-immunodeficiency syndrome-associated thrombotic thrombocytopenic purpura. Br J Haematol 2002;116:909–911.
242. Rock GA, Shumak KH, Buskard NA, et al. The Canadian Apheresis Study Group: comparison of plasma exchange with plasma infusion in the treatment of thrombotic thrombocytopenic purpura. N Engl J Med 1991;325:393.
243. Bell WR, Braine HG, Ness PM, Kickler TS. Improved survival in thrombotic thrombocytopenic purpura-hemolytic uremic syndrome: Clinical experience in 108 patients. N Engl J Med 1991;325:398.
244. O'Connor NTJ, Bruce-Jones P, Hill LF. Vincristine therapy for thrombotic thrombocytopenic purpura. Am J Hematol 1992;39:234.
245. Reddy PS, Deanna-Limayo D, Cook JD, et al. Rituximab in the treatment of relapsed thrombotic thrombocytopenic purpura. Ann Hematol 2005;84:232–235.
246. Onundarson PT, Rowe JM, Heal JM, Francis CW. Response to plasma exchange and splenectomy in thrombotic thrombocytopenic purpura. Arch Intern Med 1992;152:791.
247. Tsai H-M, Rue L, Sarode R, et al. Antibody inhibitors to von Willebrand factor metalloproteinase and increased binding of von Willebrand factor to platelets in ticlopidine associated thrombotic thrombocytopenic purpura. Ann Intern Med 2000;132:794.
248. Bennett CL, Weinberg PD, Rozenberg-Ben-Dor K, et al. Thrombotic thrombocytopenic purpura associated with ticlopidine: a review of 60 cases. Ann Intern Med 1998;128:541.
249. Gasser C, Gautier E, Steck A, et al. Hämolytisch-urämische Syndrome: Bilaterale Nierenrinden-nekrosen bei akuten erworbenen hämolytischen Anämien. Schweitz Med Wochenschr 1955;85:905.
250. Robson WL, Leung AKC, Kaplan BS. Hemolytic-uremic syndrome. Curr Probl Pediatr 1993;23:16.
251. Loirat C, Baudouin V, Sonsino E, et al. Hemolytic-uremic syndrome in the child. Adv Nephrol 1993;22:141.
252. George JN, Gilcher RO, Smith JW, et al. Thrombotic thrombocytopenic purpura-hemolytic uremic syndrome: diagnosis and management. J Clin Apheresis 1998;13:120.
253. Von Baeyer H. Plasmapheresis in thrombotic microangiopathy associated syndromes: review of outcome data derived from clinical trials and open studies. Ther Apheresis 2002;4:320–328.
254. George JN, Li X, McMinn JR. Thrombotic thrombocytopenic purpura-hemolytic uremic syndrome following allogeneic HPC transplantation: a diagnostic dilemma. Transfusion 2004;44:294–304.
255. Elliot MA, Nichols WL, Plumhoff EA, et al. Post transplantation thrombotic thrombocytopenic purpura: a single-center experience and a contemporary review. Mayo Clin Proc 2003;78:421–430.
256. Raife T, Atkinson B, Montgomery L, et al. Severe deficiency of VWF-cleaving protease (ADAMTS 13) activity defines a distinct population of thrombotic microangiopathy patients. Transfusion 2004;44:146–150.
257. Rougier N, Kazatchkine MD, Rougier J-P, et al. Human complement factor H deficiency associated with hemolytic uremic syndrome. J Am Soc Nephrol 1998;9:2318.
258. Warwicker P, Donne RL, Goalship JA, et al. Familial relapsing haemolytic uraemic syndrome and complement factor H deficiency. Nephrol Dial Transplant 1999;14:1229.
259. Zipfel PF, Hellwage J, Friese MA, et al. Factor H and disease: a complement regulator affects vital bodily functions. Mol Immunol 1999;36:241.
260. Martin JN, Files JC, Blake PG, et al. Plasma exchange for preeclampsia. I: Postpartum use for persistently severe preeclampsia-eclampsia with HELLP syndrome. Am J Obstet Gynecol 1990;162:126.
261. Veyradier A, Girma J-P. Assays of ADAMTS-13 activity. Semin Hematol 2004;41:41–47.
262. Studt JD, Böhm M, Budde U, et al. Measurement of von Willebrand-cleaving protease (ADAMTS-13) activity in plasma: a multicenter comparison of different assay methods. J Thromb Haemost 2003;1:1882–1887.
263. Tripodi A, Chantarangkul V, Böhm M, et al. Measurement of von Willebrand factor cleaving protease (ADAMTS-13): results of an international collaborative study involving 11 methods testing the same set of coded plasmas. J Thromb Haemost 2004;2:1601–1609.
264. Vesely SK, George JN, Lämmle B, et al. ADAMTS-13 activity in thrombotic thrombocytopenic purpura-hemolytic uremic syndrome: relation of presenting features and clinical outcomes in a prospective cohort of 142 patients. Blood 2003;102:60–68.
265. Zheng X, Majerus EM, Sadler JE. ADAMTS 13 and TTP. Curr Opin Hematol 2002;9:389–394.
266. Zheng X, Kaufman RM, Goodnough LT, Sadler JE: Effect of plasma exchange on plasma ADAMTS 13 metalloprotease activity, inhibitor level, and clinical outcome in patients with idiopathic and nonidiopathic thrombotic thrombocytopenic purpura. Blood 2004;103:4043–4049.
267. Mueller-Eckhardt C. Post-transfusion purpura. Br J Haematol 1986; 64:419.
268. Shulman NR, Reid DM: Platelet immunology. In Colman RW, Hirsh J, Marder VJ, Salzman EW (eds). Hemostasis and Thrombosis. Philadelphia: JB Lippincott, 1994, p 414.
269. McCrae KR, Herman JH. Posttransfusion purpura: two unusual cases and a literature review. Am J Hematol 1996;52:205.
270. Newman PJ, McFarland JG, Aster RH. Alloimmune thrombocytopenias. In Loscalzo J, Schafer AI (eds). Thrombosis and Hemorrhage. Boston: Blackwell Scientific, 1994, p 429.
271. Laursen B, Morling N, Rosenkvist J, et al. Post-transfusion purpura treated with plasma exchange by Haemonetics cell separator. Acta Med Scand 1978;203:539.
272. Mueller-Eckhardt C, Kiefel V. High dose IgG for post-transfusion purpura-revisited. Blut 1988;57:163.
273. Diz-Küçcükkaya R, Gushiken FC, Lopez JA. Thrombocytopenia. In Lichtman MA, Beutler E, Kipps TJ, Seligsohn U, et al (eds). Williams Hematology, 7th ed. New York, McGraw-Hill, 2006, p 1749.
274. Branda RF, Tate DY, McCullough JJ, et al. Plasma exchange in the treatment of fulminant idiopathic (autoimmune) thrombocytopenic purpura. Lancet 1978;1:688.
275. Isbister JP, Biggs JC, Penny R. Experience with large volume plasmapheresis in malignant paraproteinemia and immune disorders. Aust N Z J Med 1978;8:154.
276. Marder VJ, Nusbacher J, Anderson FW. One-year follow-up of plasma exchange therapy in 14 patients with idiopathic thrombocytopenic purpura. Transfusion 1981;21:291.
277. Buskard N, Rock G, Nair R. The Canadian experience using plasma exchange for immune thrombocytopenic purpura. Transfusion Sci 1998;19:295–300.
278. Mittelman A, Bertram J, Henry DH, et al. Treatment of patients with HIV thrombocytopenia and hemolytic uremic syndrome with protein A (proSorba) immunoadsorption. Semin Hematol 1989;26(Suppl 11):15.
279. Snyder HW Jr, Cochran SK, Balint JP, et al. Experience with protein A-immunoadsorption in treatment resistant immune thrombocytopenic purpura. Blood 1992;79:2237.
280. Packman CH. Hemolytic anemia resulting from immune injury. In Lichtman MA, Beutler E, Kipps TJ, Seligsohn U, et al (eds). Williams Hematology, 7th ed. New York, McGraw-Hill, 2006, p 729.
281. Packman CH. Cryopathic hemolytic syndromes. In Beutler E, Lichtman MA, Coller BS, Kipps TJ, Seligsohn U (eds). Williams Hematology, 6th ed. New York, McGraw-Hill, 2001, p 649.
282. Silberstein LE, Berkman EM. Plasma exchange in autoimmune hemolytic anemia (AIHA). J Clin Apheresis 1983;1:238.
283. Valbonesi M, Guzzini D, Zerbi D, et al. Successful plasma exchange for a patient with chronic demyelinating polyneuropathy and cold agglutinin disease due to anti-Pr_a. J Clin Apheresis 1986;3:109.
284. Kutti J, Wadenvik H, Safai-Kutti S, et al. Successful treatment of refractory autoimmune hemolytic anemia by plasmapheresis. Scand J Hematol 1984;32:149.
285. Andersen O, Taaning E, Rosenkvist J, et al. Autoimmune hemolytic anemia treated with multiple transfusions, immunosuppressive therapy, plasma exchange and desferrioxamine. Acta Paediatr Scand 1984;73:145.
286. McConnell ME, Atchison JA, Kohaut E, Castleberry RP. Successful use of plasma exchange in a child with refractory autoimmune hemolytic anemia. Am J Pediatr Hematol Oncol 1987;9:158.
287. von Keyserlingk H, Meyer-Sabellek W, Arntz R, Hiller H. Plasma exchange treatment in autoimmune hemolytic anemia of the wane antibody type with renal failure. Vox Sang 1982;52:298.
288. Geurs F, Ritter K, Mast A, Van Maele V. Successful plasmapheresis in corticosteroid-resistant hemolysis in infectious mononucleosis: Role of autoantibodies against triosephosphate isomerase. Acta Haematol 1992;88:142.
289. Segel GB, Lichtman MA. Aplastic anemia. In Lichtman MA, Beutler E, Kipps TJ, Seligsohn U, et al (eds). Williams Hematology, 7th ed. New York, McGraw-Hill, 2006, p 419.

290. Young NS. Pure red cell aplasia. In Lichtman MA, Beutler E, Kipps TJ, Seligsohn U, et al (eds). Williams Hematology, 7th ed. New York, McGraw-Hill, 2006, p 437.
291. Young NS, Barrett AJ. The treatment of severe acquired aplastic anemia. Blood 1995;85:3367.
292. Fitchen JJ, Cline MJ, Saxon A, et al. Serum inhibitors of hematopoiesis in a patient with aplastic anemia and systemic lupus erythematosus. Am J Med 1979;6:537.
293. Abdou NI. Plasma exchange in the treatment of aplastic anemia. In Tindall RSA (ed). Therapeutic Apheresis and Plasma Perfusion. New York: Alan R. Liss, 1982, p 337.
294. Young NS, Klein HG, Griffith P, et al. Therapeutic plasma exchange and lymphocyte depletion in aplastic anemia and pure red cell aplasia. In Nose Y, Malchesky PS, Smith JW, et al (eds). Plasmapheresis. New York, Raven Press, 1983, p 339.
295. Messner HA, Fause AA, Curtis JE, et al. Control of antibody-mediated pure red cell aplasia by plasmapheresis. N Engl J Med 1981;304:1334.
296. Freund LG, Hippe E, Strandgaard S, et al. Complete remission in pure red cell aplasia after plasmapheresis. Scand J Hematol 1985;35:351.
297. Khelif A, Van HV, Tremisi JP, et al. Remission of acquired pure red cell aplasia following plasma exchanges. Scand J Hematol 1985;35:13.
298. Berlin G, Lieden G. Long-term remission of pure red cell aplasia after plasma exchange and lymphocytapheresis. Scand J Haematol 1986;36:121.
299. Delgado J, Jimenez-Yuste V, Hernandez-Navarro F, Villar A. Acquired haemophilia: review and meta-analysis focused on therapy and prognostic factors. Br J Haematol 2003;121:21–35.
300. Ewenstein BM. Factor VIII and other coagulation factor inhibitors. In Loscalzo J, Schafer AI (eds). Thrombosis and Hemorrhage. Boston: Blackwell Scientific, 1994, p 729.
301. Garvey MB. Incidence and management of patients with acquired factor VIII inhibitors: the practical experience of a tertiary care hospital. In Kessler CM (ed). Acquired Hemophilia. Princeton, NJ, Excerpta Medica, 1995, p 91.
302. Kessler CM. Factor VIII inhibitors: an algorithmic approach to treatment. Semin Hematol 1994;31(Suppl 4):33.
303. Gribble J, Garvey MD. Porcine factor VIII provides clinical benefit to patients with high levels of inhibitors to human and porcine factor VIII. Haemophilia 2000;6:482–486.
304. Lusher J, Ingerslev S, Roberts H, Hedner U. Clinical experience with recombinant factor VIIa. Blood Coagul Fibrinol 1998;9:119.
305. Wensley RT, Stevens RF, Burn AM, et al. The role of intensive plasma exchange in the prevention and management of haemorrhage in patients with inhibitors to factor VIII. Br Med J 1980;281:1388.
306. Slocombe GW, Newland AC, Colvin MP, et al. The role of intensive plasma exchange in the management of hemophilia patients with inhibitors. Br J Haematol 1981;47:577.
307. Bona RD, Pasquale DN, Kalish RI, et al. Porcine factor VIII and plasmapheresis in the management of hemophilia patients with inhibitors. Am J Hematol 1986;21:201.
308. Freedman J, Garvey MB. Immunoadsorption of factor VIII inhibitors. Curr Opin Hematol 2004;11:327–333.
309. Lusher JM. Management of patients with factor VIII inhibitors. Transfus Med Rev 1987;1:123.
310. Pflieger G, Boda Z, H'arsfalvi J, et al. Cyclosporin treatment of a woman with acquired hemophilia due to factor VIII:C inhibitor. Postgrad Med J 1989;65:400.
311. Schwartz RS, Gabriel DA, Aledort LM, et al. A prospective study of treatment of acquired (autoimmune) factor VIII inhibitors with high-dose intravenous gammaglobulin. Blood 1995;86:797.
312. Mathias M, Khair K, Hann I, Liesner R. Rituximab in the treatment of alloimmune factor VIII and IX antibodies in two children with severe haemophilia. Br J Haematol 2004;125:366–368.
313. Stasi R, Brunetti M, Stipa E, Amadori S. Selective B-cell depletion with rituximab for the treatment of patients with acquired hemophilia. Blood 2004;103:4424–4428.
314. Ewing NP, Sanders NL, Dietrich SL, Kaspar CK. Induction of immune tolerance to factor VIII in hemophiliacs with inhibitors. JAMA 1988;259:65.
315. Gruppo RA, Valdez LP, Stout RD. Induction of immune tolerance in patients with hemophilia A and inhibitors. Am J Pediatr Hematol Oncol 1992;4:82.
316. Nilsson IM, Berntorp E, Zettervoll O. Induction of immune tolerance in patients with hemophilia and antibodies to factor VIII by combined treatment with intravenous IgG, cyclophosphamide, and factor VIII. N Engl J Med 1988;318:947.
317. Smith OP, Hann IM. Factor VIIa therapy to secure haemostasis during central line insertion in children with high-responding FVIII inhibitors. Br J Haematol 1992;92:1002.
318. Nakamura Y, Yoshida K, Itoh S, et al. Immunoadsorption plasmapheresis as a treatment for pregnancy complicated by systemic lupus erythematosus with positive antiphospholipid antibodies. Am J Reprod Immunol 1999;41:307.
319. Brouet JC, Clauvel JP, Danon F, et al. Biologic and clinical significance of cryoglobulins: a report of 86 cases. Am J Med 1974;57:775.
320. Bloch KJ. Cryoglobulinemia and hepatic C Virus. N Engl J Med 1992; 327:1521.
321. Ferri C, Zignego AL, Pileri SA. Cryoglobulins. J Clin Pathol 2002; 55:4–13.
322. Berkman EM, Orlin JB. Use of plasmapheresis and partial plasma exchange in the management of patients with cryoglobulinemia. Transfusion 1980;20:171.
323. Bombardieri S, Maggiore Q, L Abbate A, et al. Plasma exchange in essential mixed cryoglobulinemia. Plasma Ther Transfus Technol 1981; 2:101.
324. McGovern TW, Enzenauer RJ, Fitzpatrick JE. Treatment of recalcitrant leg ulcers in cryoglobulinemia types I and II with plasmapheresis. Arch Dermatol 1996;132:498.
325. Goronzy J, Weyland C. Rheumatoid arthritis. In Klippel R (ed). Primer on the Rheumatic Diseases. Atlanta, Arthritis Foundation, 1997, p 155.
326. O'Dell JR. Therapeutic strategies for rheumatoid arthritis. N Engl J Med 2004;350:2591–2602.
327. Weaver AL. The impact of new biologicals in the treatment of rheumatoid arthritis. Rheumatology 2004;43(Suppl 3):iii17–iii23.
328. Rothwell R, Davis P, Gordon P, et al. A controlled study of plasma exchange in the treatment of severe rheumatoid arthritis. Arthritis Rheum 1980;23:785.
329. Dwosh I, Giles A, Ford P. Plasmapheresis therapy in rheumatoid arthritis: A controlled, double-blind, crossover trial. N Engl J Med 1983; 308:1124.
330. Wallace D, Goldfinger D, Lowe C, et al. A double-blind, controlled study of lymphoplasmapheresis versus sham apheresis in rheumatoid arthritis. N Engl J Med 1982;306:1406.
331. Karch J, Klippel J, Plotz P, et al. Lymphapheresis in rheumatoid arthritis: A randomized trial. Arthritis Rheum 1981;24:867.
332. Hester J, Felson D, Gendreau M. Phase III trial of ProSorba column for severe rheumatoid arthritis. J Clin Apheresis 1998;13:90.
333. Pisesky D. Systemic lupus erythematosus. In Klippel J (cd). Primer on the Rheumatic Diseases. Atlanta, Arthritis Foundation, 1997, p 246.
334. Moc CC, Lau CS. Pathogenesis of systemic lupus erythematosus. J Clin Pathol 2003;56:481–490.
335. Klippel J. Systemic lupus erythematosus: treatment. In Klippel J (ed). Primer on the Rheumatic Diseases. Atlanta, Arthritis Foundation, 1997, p 258.
336. Ad Hoc Working Group. Criteria for steroid-sparing ability of interventions in systemic lupus erythematosus: report of a consensus meeting. Arthritis Rheum 2004;50:3427–3431.
337. Parry HF, Moran CJ, Snaith ML, et al. Plasma exchange in systemic lupus erythematosus. Ann Rheum Dis 1981;40:224.
338. Jones JV. Plasmapheresis in SLE. Clin Rheum Dis 1982;8:243.
339. Huston DP, White MJ, Maltiolo C, et al. A controlled trial of plasmapheresis and cyclophosphamide therapy of lupus nephritis. Arthritis Rheum 1983;26(Suppl):S33.
340. Euler HH, Schwab UM, Schroeder JO, Hasford J. The Lupus Plasmapheresis Study Group: Rationale and updated interim report. Artif Organs 1996;20:356.
341. Schroeder JO, Schwab U, Zennet R, et al. Plasmapheresis and subsequent pulse cyclophosphamide in severe systemic lupus erythematosus: preliminary results of the LPSG Trial. Arthritis Rheum 1997; 40:S325.
342. Wallace DJ, Goldfinger D, Pepkowitz S, et al. Randomized control of pulse/synchronization cyclophosphamide/apheresis for proliferative lupus nephritis. J Clin Apheresis 1998;13:163.
343. Aringer M, Smolen JS, Graninger WB. Severe infections in plasmapheresis-treated systemic lupus erythematosus. Arthritis Rheum 1998; 41:414–420.
344. Langford CA. Vasculitis. J Allergy Clin Immunol 2003;111:S602–S612.
345. Jayne D. Evidence-based treatment of systemic vasculitis. Rheumatol 2000;39:589–595.
346. Pusey CD, Rees AJ, Evans DJ, et al. Plasma exchange in focal necrotizing glomerulonephritis without anti-GBM antibodies. Kidney Int 1991;40:757.
347. Guillevin L, Fain O, Lhote F, et al. Lack of superiority of steroids plus plasma exchanges to steroids alone in the treatment of polyarteritis nodosa and Churg-Strauss syndrome: a prospective, randomized trial in 78 patients. Arthritis Rheum 1992;35:208.

348. Guillevin L, Mahr A, Cohen P, et al. Short-term corticosteroids then lamivudine and plasma exchanges to treat Hepatitis B virus-related polyarteritis nodosa. Arthritis Rheum 2004;51:482–487.
349. Dalakas MC. Polymyositis and dermatomyositis. Lancet 2003;362: 971–982.
350. Dalakas MC. Controlled studies with high-dose intravenous immunoglobulin in the treatment of dermatomyositis, inclusion body myositis and polymyositis. Neurology 1998;51:537.
351. Dau PC. Plasmapheresis in idiopathic inflammatory myopathy. Arch Neurol 1981;38:544.
352. Khatri BO, Luprecht G, Weiss SA. Plasmapheresis and immunosuppressive drug therapy in polymyositis. Muscle Nerve 1982;5:568.
353. Cecere FA, Spiva DA. Combination plasmapheresis/leukocytapheresis for the treatment of dermatomyositis/polymyositis. Plasma Ther Transfus Technol 1982;3:401.
354. Miller FW, Leitman SF, Cronin ME, et al. Controlled trial of plasma exchange and leukapheresis in polymyositis and dermatomyositis. N Engl J Med 1992;326:1380.
355. Salama AD, Levy JB, Lightstone L, Pusey CD. Goodpasture's disease. Lancet 2001;358:917–920.
356. Hudson BG, Tryggvason K, Sundaramoorthy M, Nelson EG. Alport's syndrome, Goodpasture's syndrome and type IV collagen. N Engl J Med 2003;348:2543–2556.
357. Lockwood CM, Boulton-Jones JM, Lowenthal RM, et al. Recovery from Goodpasture's syndrome after immunosuppressive treatment and plasmapheresis. Br Med J 1975;2:252.
358. Pusey CD, Lockwood CM, Peters DK. Plasma exchange and immunosuppressive drugs in the treatment of glomerulonephritis due to antibodies to the glomerular basement membrane. Int J Artif Organs 1983;6:15.
359. Glassock RJ. Intensive plasma exchange in crescentic glomerulonephritis: help or no help? Am J Kidney Dis 1992;20:270.
360. Madore F, Lazarus JM, Brady HR. Therapeutic plasma exchange in renal diseases. J Am Soc Nephrol 1997;7:367.
361. Johnson JP, Moore J, Austin HA, et al. Therapy of anti-glomerular basement membrane antibody disease: Analysis on the prognostic significance of clinical, pathologic, and treatment factors. Medicine (Baltimore) 1985;64:219.
362. Stegmayr BG, Almroth G, Berlin G, et al. Plasma exchange or immunoadsorption in patients with rapidly progressive glomerulonephritis: a Swedish multicenter study. Int J Artif Organs 1999;22:81.
363. Levy JB, Turner AN, Rees AJ, Pusey CD. Long-term outcome of anti-glomerular basement membrane antibody disease treated with plasma exchange and immunosuppression. Ann Intern Med 2001;134: 1033–1042.
364. Jennette JC. Rapidly progressive glomerulonephritis. Kidney Int 2003;63:1164–1177.
365. Burran WP, Avasthi P, Smith KJ, et al. Efficacy of plasma exchange in severe idiopathic rapidly progressive glomerulonephritis. Transfusion 1986;26:382.
366. Sakellariou G. Plasmapheresis as a therapy in specific forms of acute renal failure. Nephrol Dial Transplant 1994;9:210.
367. Glöckner WM, Sieberth HG, Wichmann HE, et al. Plasma exchange and immunosuppression in rapidly progressive glomerulonephritis: a controlled, multi-center study. Clin Nephrol 1988;29:1.
368. Cole E, Cattran D, Magil A, et al. A prospective randomized trial of plasma exchange as additive therapy in idiopathic crescentic glomerulonephritis. Am J Kidney Dis 1992;20:261.
369. Guillevin L, Fain O, Lhote F, et al. Lack of superiority of steroids plus plasma exchange to steroids alone in the treatment of polyarteritis nodosa and Churg-Strauss syndrome: a prospective, randomized trial in 78 patients. Arthritis Rheum 1992;35:208.
370. Nakamura T, Matsuda T, Kawagoe Y, et al. Plasmapheresis with immunosuppressive therapy vs. immunosuppressive therapy alone for rapidly progressive anti-neutrophil cytoplasmic autoantibody-associated glomerulonephritis. Nephrol Dial Transplant 2004;19:1935–1937.
371. Levy JB, Pusey CD. Still a role for plasma exchange in rapidly progressive glomerulonephritis? J Nephrol 1997;10:7.
372. Michaels PJ, Fishbein MC, Colvin RB. Humoral rejection of human organ transplants. Springer Semin Immunopathol 2003;25:119–40.
373. Croker BP, Ramos EL. Pathology of the renal allograft. In Tishler CC, Brenner BM (eds). Renal Pathology with Clinical and Functional Correlations. Philadelphia, JB Lippincott, 1994, p 1591.
374. Halloran PF. Immunosuppressive drugs for kidney transplantation. N Engl Med 2004;351:2115–2129.
375. Lindenfeld J, Miller GG, Shakar SF, et al. Drug therapy in the heart transplant recipient. Part I: Cardiac rejection and immunosuppressive drugs. Circulation 2004;110:3734–3740.
376. Cardella CJ, Sutton D, Uldall PR, de Veber GA. Intensive plasma exchange and renal transplant rejection. Lancet 1977;1:264.
377. Rifle G, Chalopin JM, Ture JM, et al. Plasmapheresis in the treatment of renal allograft rejections. Transplant Proc 1979;11:20.
378. Adams MB, Kauffman HM, Hussey CV, et al. Plasmapheresis in the treatment of refractory renal allograft rejection. Transplant Proc 1981; 13:491.
379. Vangelista A, Frasca GM, Nanni Costa A, et al. Value of plasma exchange in renal transplant rejection induced by specific HLA antibodies. Trans Am Soc Artif Intern Organs 1982;28:599.
380. Cardella CJ, Sutton D, Falk JA, et al. Effect of intense plasma exchange on renal transplant rejection and serum cytotoxic antibody. Transplant Proc 1978;10:617.
381. Bankowski LHW, Corteste J, Lutton JL, Saunders PH. Plasmapheresis: adjunctive treatment for steroid-resistant rejection in renal transplantation. J Urol 1984;131:14.
382. Soulillou JP, Guyot C, Guimbretiere J, et al. Plasma exchange in early kidney graft rejection associated with anti-donor antibodies. Nephron 1983;35:158.
383. Allen NH, Ayer P, Geoghegan T, et al. Plasma exchange in acute renal allograft rejection: a controlled trial. Transplantation 1983;35:425.
384. Kirubakaran MG, Disney APS, Norman J, et al. A controlled trial of plasmapheresis in the treatment of renal allograft rejection. Transplantation 1981;32:164.
385. Blake P, Sutton D, Cardella C. Plasma exchange in acute renal transplant rejection. Prog Clin Biol Res 1990;337:249.
386. Bonomini V, Vangelista A, Frasca GM, et al. Effects of plasmapheresis in renal transplant rejection: a controlled study. Trans Am Soc Artif Intern Organs 1985;31:698.
387. Grandtnerova B, Javorsky P, Kolacny J, et al. Treatment of acute humoral rejection in kidney transplantation with plasmapheresis. Transplant Proc 1995;27:934.
388. Loss GE Jr, Grewal HP, Siegel CT, et al. Reversal of delayed hyperacute renal allograft rejection with a tacrolimus-based therapeutic regimen. Transplant Proc 1998;30:1249.
389. Aichberger C, Nussbaumer W, Rosmanith P, et al. Plasmapheresis for the treatment of acute vascular reaction in renal transplantation. Transplant Proc 1997;29:169.
390. Gannedahl G, Ohlman S, Persson U, et al. Rejection associated with early appearance of donor-reactive antibodies after kidney transplantation treated with plasmapheresis and administration of 15-deoxyspergualin: a report of two cases. Transplant Int 1992;5:189.
391. Abe M, Sannomiya A, Koike T, et al. Removal of anti-donor antibody by double-filtration plasmapheresis to prevent chronic rejection in kidney transplantation. Transplant Proc 1998;30:3108.
392. Montgomery RA, Zachary AA, Racusen LC, et al. Plasmapheresis and intravenous immune globulin provides effective rescue therapy for refractory humoral rejection and allows kidneys to be successfully transplanted into cross-match-positive recipients. Transplantation 2000;70:887–895.
393. Crespo M, Pascual M, Tolkff-Rubin M, et al. Acute humoral rejection in renal allograft recipients. I: Incidence, serology and clinical characteristics. Transplantation 2001;71:652–658.
394. Jordan SC, Vo AA, Tyan D, et al. Current approaches to treatment of antibody-mediated rejection. Pediatr Transplant 2005;9:408–415.
395. Zachary AA, Montgomery RA, Ratner LE, et al. Specific and durable elimination of antibody to donor HLA antigens in renal-transplant patients. Transplantation 2003;76:1519–1525.
396. Takemoto SK, Zeevi A, Feng S, et al. National conference to assess antibody-mediated rejection in solid organ transplantation. Am J Transplantation 2004;4:1033–1041.
397. Partanen J, Nieminen MS, Krogerus L, et al. Heart transplant rejection treated with plasmapheresis. J Heart Lung Transplant 1992;11:301.
398. Malafa M, Mancini MC, Myles JL, et al. Successful treatment of acute humoral rejection in a heart transplant patient. J Heart Lung Transplant 1992;11:486.
399. Fishbein MC, Kobashigawa J. Biopsy-negative cardiac transplant rejection: etiology, diagnosis, and therapy. Curr Opin Cardiol 2004;19:166–169.
400. Taube D, Palmer A, Welsh K, et al. Removal of anti-HLA antibodies prior to transplantation: an effective and successful strategy for highly sensitized renal allograft recipients. Transplant Proc 1989;21:694.
401. Backman U, Fellstrom B, Frodin L, et al. Successful transplantation in highly sensitized patients. Transplant Proc 1989;21:762.
402. Alarabi A, Backman U, Wikstrom B, et al. Plasmapheresis in HLA-immunosensitized patients prior to kidney transplantation. Int J Artif Organs 1997;20:51.
403. Hodge EE, Klingman LL, Koo AP, et al. Pretransplant removal of anti-HLA antibodies by plasmapheresis and continued suppression on

cyclosporine-based therapy after heart-kidney transplant. Transplant Proc 1994;26:2750.
404. Hakim R, Milford E, Himmelfarb J, et al. Extracorporeal removal of anti-HLA antibodies in transplant candidates. Am J Kidney Dis 1990;16:423.
405. Kupin WL, Venkat KK, Hayashi H, et al. Removal of lymphocytotoxic antibodies by pretransplant immunoadsorption therapy in highly sensitized renal transplant recipients. Transplantation 1991;51:324.
406. Miura S, Okazaki H, Sato T, et al. Beneficial effects of double-filtration plasmapheresis on living related donor renal transplantation in presensitized recipients. Transplant Proc 1995;27:1040.
407. Miura S, Okazaki H, Sato T, et al. Successful renal transplantation in presensitized recipients with double-filtration plasmapheresis and 15-deoxyspergualin. Transplant Proc 1997;29:350.
408. Ishikawa A, Itoh M, Ushlyama T, et al. Experience of ABO-incompatible living kidney transplantation after double filtration plasmapheresis. Clin Transplant 1998;12:80.
409. Renard TH, Andrews WS. An approach to ABO-incompatible liver transplantation in children. Transplantation 1992;53:116.
410. Takahashi K, Yogisawa T, Sonda K, et al. ABO-incompatible kidney transplantation in a single center trial. Transplant Proc 1993;25:271.
411. Boudreaux JP, Hayes DH, Mizrahi S, et al. Successful liver/kidney transplantation across ABO incompatibility. Transplant Proc 1993;25:1874.
412. Aswad S, Mendez R, Mendez RG, et al. Crossing the ABO blood barrier in renal transplantation. Transplant Proc 1993;25:267.
413. Montgomery RA, Zachary AA. Transplanting patients with a positive donor-specific crossmatch: a single center's perspective. Pediatr Transplant 2004;8:535–542.
414. Sonnenday CJ, Ratner LE, Zachary AA, et al. Preemptive therapy with plasmapheresis/intravenous immunoglobulin allows successful live donor renal transplantation in patients with a positive cross-match. Transplant Proc 2002;34:1614–1616.
415. Vincenti F, Ghigger GM. New insights into the pathogenesis and the therapy of recurrent focal glomerulosclerosis. Transplantation 2005;5:1179–1185.
416. Artero ML, Sharma R, Savin VJ, Vincenti F. Plasmapheresis reduces proteinuria and serum capacity to injure glomeruli in patients with recurrent focal glomerulosclerosis. Am J Kidney Dis 1994;23:574.
417. Savin VJ, McCarthy ET, Sharma M. Permeability factors in focal segmental glomerulosclerosis. Semin Nephrol 2003;23:147–160.
418. Benchimal C. Focal segmental glomerulosclerosis: pathogenesis and treatment. Curr Opin Pediatr 2003;15:171–180.
419. Cochat P, Kassir A, Colon S, et al. Recurrent nephrotic syndrome after transplantation: early treatment with plasmapheresis and cyclophosphamide. Pediatr Nephrol 1993;7:50.
420. Oetliker OH, Zimmerman A, Bianchetti MG. Treatment of recurrent idiopathic nephrotic syndrome after transplantation using plasmapheresis and intensified immunosuppression over 2 months [Letter]. Pediatr Nephrol 1993;7:508.
421. Delucchi A, Cano F, Rodriguez E, Wolff E. Focal segmental glomerulosclerosis relapse after transplantation: treatment with high cyclosporine doses and a short plasmapheresis course [Letter]. Pediatr Nephrol 1994;8:786.
422. Davenport RD. Apheresis treatment of recurrent focal segmental glomerulosclerosis after kidney transplantation: reanalysis of published case-reports and case-series. J Clin Apheresis 2001;16:175–178.
423. Deegens JKJ, Andresdottir MB, Crookewit S, Wetzels JFM. Plasma exchange improves graft survival in patients with recurrent focal glomerulosclerosis after renal transplantation. Transplant Int 2004; 17:1511–1517.
424. Dixon FJ, McPhaul JJ, Lemer RA. The contribution of transplantation to the study of glomerulonephritis: the recurrence of glomerulonephritis in renal transplants. Transplant Proc 1969;1:194.
425. Ramzy D, Rao V, Brahm J, et al. Cardiac allograft vasculopathy. Can J Surg 2005;48:319–327.
426. Thiery J, Meiser B, Wenke K, et al. Heparin-induced extracorporeal low-density-lipoprotein plasmapheresis (HELP) and its use in heart transplant patients with severe hypercholesterolemia. Transplant Proc 1995;27:1950.
427. Barr ML, McLaughlin SN, Murphy MP, et al. Prophylactic photopheresis and effect on graft atherosclerosis in cardiac transplantation. Transplant Proc 1995;27:1993.
428. Goldstein JL, Hobbs HH, Brown MS. Familial hypercholesterolemia. In Scriver CR, Beuadet AL, Sly WS, Valle D (eds). The Metabolic and Molecular Basis of Inherited Disease. New York, McGraw-Hill, 2001, pp 1863–1913.
429. Rader DJ, Cohen J, Hobbs HH. Monogenic hypercholesterolemia: new insights in pathogenesis and treatment. J Clin Invest 2003;11:1795–1803.
430. Thompson GR, Miller JP, Breslow JL. Improved survival of patients with homozygous familial hypercholesterolaemia treated with plasma exchange. Br Med J 1985;291:1671.
431. Kamanabroo D, Ulrich K, Grobe H, Assman G. Plasma exchange in type II hypercholesterolemia. Prog Clin Biol Res 1988;255:347.
432. Leren TP, Fagerhol MK, Leren P. Sixteen years of plasma exchange in a homozygote for familial hypercholesterolemia. J Intern Med 1993; 233:195.
433. Beigel Y, Bar J, Cohen M, Hod M. Pregnancy outcome in familial homozygous hypercholesterolemic females treated with long-term plasma exchange. Acta Obstet Gynecol Scand 1998;77:603.
434. Leitman SF, Smith JW, Gregg RE. Homozygous familial hypercholesterolemia: selective removal of low-density lipoproteins by secondary membrane filtration. Transfusion 1989;9:341.
435. Matsuda Y, Malchesky PS, Nose Y. Assessment of currently available low-density lipoprotein apheresis systems. Artif Organs 1994;18:93.
436. Armstrong VW, Eisenhauer T, Noll D, et al, Extracorporeal plasma therapy: the HELP system for the treatment of hyperlipoproteinemia. In Widhalm K, Maito HK (eds). Recent Aspects of Diagnosis and Treatment of Lipoprotein Disorders: Impact on Prevention of Atherosclerotic Diseases. New York, Alan R. Liss, 1988, p 327.
437. Stoffel W, Borberg H, Greve V. Application of specific extracorporeal removal of low density lipoprotein in familial hypercholesterolaemia. Lancet 1981;2:1005.
438. Saal SD, Parker TS, Gordon BR, et al. Removal of low-density lipoproteins in patients by extracorporeal immunoadsorption. Am J Med 1986;80:583.
439. Yamamoto A, Kojima S, Shiba-Harada M, et al. Assessment of the biocompatibility and long-term effect of LDL-apheresis by dextran sulfate-cellulose column. Artif Organs 1992;16:177.
440. Vella A, Pineda AA, O'Brien T. Low-density lipoprotein apheresis for the treatment of refractory hyperlipidemia. Mayo Clin Proc 2003;76:1039–1046.
441. Wills AJ, Manning NJ, Reilly MM. Refsum's disease. Q J Med 2001; 94:403–406
442. Gibberd FB. Plasma exchange for Refsum's disease. Transfus Sci 1993;14:23.
443. Gutsche H-U, Siegmund JB, Hoppmann I. Lipapheresis: an immunoglobulin-sparing treatment for Refsum's disease. Acta Neurol Scand 1996;94:190.
444. Giorgi DF, Jagoda A. Poisoning and overdose. Mt Sinai J Med 1997; 64:283.
445. Trujillo MH, Guerrero J, Fragachan C, Fernandez MA. Pharmacologic antidotes in critical care medicine: a practical guide for drug administration. Crit Care Med 1998;26:377.
446. Jones JS, Dougherty J. Current status of plasmapheresis in toxicology. Ann Emerg Med 1986;15:474
447. Kale-Pradhan PB, Woo MH. A review of the effects of plasmapheresis on drug clearance. Pharmacology 1997;17:684–695.
448. Luzhnikov EA, Yaroslavsky AA, Molodenkov MN, et al. Plasma perfusion through charcoal in methylparathion poisoning. Lancet 1977;1:38.
449. Pierga JY, Beuzeboc P, Dorval T, et al. Favorable outcome after plasmapheresis for vincristine overdose. Lancet 1992;1:185.
450. Spiller M, Marson P, Perilongo G, et al. A case of vinblastine overdosage managed with plasma exchange. Pediatr Blood Cancer 2005;45:344–346.
451. Chu G, Mantin R, Shen YM, et al. Massive cisplatin overdose by accidental substitution for carboplatin: toxicity and management. Cancer 1993;72:3707.
452. Duzova A, Baskin E, Usta Y, Ozen S. Carbamazepine poisoning: treatment with plasma exchange. Hum Exp Toxicol 2001;20:175–177.
453. Chillet P, Korach JM, Petitpas JM, et al. Digoxin poisoning and acute anuric renal failure: efficiency of treatment associating digoxin-specific antibodies (Fab) and plasma exchanges. Int J Artif Organs 2002;25:538–541.
454. Ligtenberg J, Tulleken J, Zijlstra J. Plasmapheresis in thyrotoxicosis. Ann Intern Med 1999;131:71.
455. Mercuriali F, Sichia G. Plasma exchange for mushroom poisoning. Transfusion 1977;17:644.
456. Ponikvar R, Drinovec J, Kandus A, et al. Plasma exchange in management of severe acute poisoning with *Amanita phalloides*. In Rock G (ed). Apheresis. New York, Wiley-Liss, 1990, p 327.
457. Piqueras J, Duran-Suarez JR, Massuet L, Hernandez-Sanchez JM. Mushroom poisoning: therapeutic apheresis or forced diuresis. Transfusion 1987;27:116.
458. Seyffart G. Plasmapheresis in treatment of acute intoxications. Trans Am Soc Artif Organs 1982;28:673.
459. Guzelian PS. New approaches for treatment of humans exposed to a slowly excreted environmental chemical (chlordecone). Z Gastroenterol 1984;22:16.

460. Elliott HL, MacDougall AI, Haase G, et al. Plasmapheresis in the treatment of dialysis encephalopathy. Lancet 1978;2:940.
461. Tilz GP, Teubl I, Kopplhuber C, et al. Therapeutic plasmapheresis: A new form of adjuvant treatment. Med Klin 1976;71:1952.
462. Sabato JK, Pierce RM, West RH, Gurr FW. Hemodialysis, peritoneal dialysis, plasmapheresis and forced diuresis for the treatment of quinine overdose. Clin Nephrol 1981;16:264.
463. Larsen LS, Sterrett JR, Whitehead B, Marcus SM. Adjunctive therapy of phenytoin overdose: a case report using plasmapheresis. J Toxicol Clin Toxicol 1986;24:37.
464. Keller F, Hauff A, Schultze G, et al. Effect of repeated plasma exchange on steady state kinetics of digoxin and digitoxin. Arzneimittelforschung 1984;34:83.
465. Stigelman WH, Henry DH, Talbert RL, Townsend RJ. Removal of prednisone and prednisolone by plasma exchange. Clin Pharm 1984;3:402.
466. Appelgate R, Schwartz D, Bennett WM. Removal of tobramycin during plasma exchange therapy. Ann Intern Med 1981;94:820.
467. Talbert RL, Wong YY, Duncan DB. Propranolol plasma concentrations and plasmapheresis. Drug Intell Clin Pharm 1981;15:993.
468. Lee WM. Acute liver failure. Am J Med 1994;96(Suppl 1A):3S.
469. Lee WM. Acute liver failure. N Engl J Med 1993;329:1862.
470. Caraceni P, van Thiel DH. Acute liver failure. Lancet 1995;345:163.
471. Kondrup J, Almdal T, Vilstrup H, et al. High volume plasma exchange in fulminant hepatic failure. Int J Artif Organs 1992;15:669.
472. Larsen FS, Hansen BA, Ejlersen L, et al. Cerebral blood flow, oxygen metabolism and transcranial Doppler sonography during high-volume plasmapheresis in fulminant hepatic failure. Eur J Gastroenterol Hepatol 1995;8:261.
473. Saibara T, Maeda T, Onishi S, Yamamoto Y. Plasma exchange and the arterial blood ketone body ratio in patients with acute hepatic failure. J Hepatol 1994;20:617.
474. Barshes NR, Gay AN, Williams B, et al. Support for the acutely failing liver: a comprehensive review of historic and contemporary strategies. J Am Col Surgeons 2005;201:458–476.
475. Jalan R, Sen S, Williams R. Prospects for extracorporeal liver support. Gut 2004;53:890–898.

Chapter 56

Therapeutic Cytapheresis

Bruce C. McLeod

INTRODUCTION

This chapter will cover apheresis procedures performed on patients to modify or remove excess or abnormal formed elements. Because leukocytes and platelets occupy only a small fraction of total blood volume, they can generally be collected or depleted without a need for volume replacement. Red cells, by contrast, occupy a major fraction of total blood volume. In addition, their presence in the blood in adequate quantities is essential for respiratory gas transport. For these reasons, therapeutic manipulation of the red cell content of blood most often takes the form of an exchange procedure in which patient red cells are removed and simultaneously replaced with normal donor cells.

THERAPEUTIC CYTAPHERESIS

Cytapheresis procedures deplete or collect a component of the buffy coat having a density intermediate between red cells and plasma (Table 56–1). These procedures were the original goal for which centrifugal apheresis instruments were designed, which is why these instruments are sometimes called "blood cell separators."

It is possible for procedures to emphasize collection of either platelets or mononuclear white blood cells (MNCs) depending on centrifugal force, separation-chamber geometry, and, for intermittent collection techniques, the timing of collection events. Addition of an agent such as hydroxyethyl starch to blood entering the centrifuge will promote rouleaux formation, which will accelerate red cell sedimentation in the centrifuge. This enhances the separation between red cells and granulocytes (polymorphonuclear leukocytes; PMNs) (whose density is higher than that of MNCs and overlaps that of the youngest red cells) and thereby enables efficient collection of PMN by an apheresis instrument.[1,2]

Strictly speaking, the term *therapeutic cytapheresis* might be reserved for procedures designed to deplete an abnormal and/or overabundant buffy-coat component. This chapter will have a somewhat larger scope and will include other cytapheresis procedures performed on patients, even though some of them could equally well be considered autologous donations because the expected benefit is not realized until the collected cells are reinfused at a later time. Examples of the latter type of procedure would include collection and infusion of peripheral blood progenitor cells to restore hematopoiesis and collection and subsequent reinfusion of cells that have undergone ex vivo immunization or genetic alteration intended to enhance host immunity or correct a genetic defect.

The extent of reduction in the concentration of a targeted cell in blood by therapeutic cytapheresis is not easily predicted. Formulas based on blood volume, initial cell concentration, and volume of blood processed may give unreliable estimates for several reasons, including (1) the blood volume of patients with elevated cell counts is sometimes underestimated by standard nomograms, (2) more cells can be released into the circulation during a procedure from bone marrow or an enlarged spleen, and (3) the behavior of abnormal cells in a centrifugal field may differ from expectations[2] (Table 56–2) Therefore, rather than prescribe in advance a specific volume to be processed for a therapeutic cell-depletion procedure, it is more reasonable to monitor the cell count of interest during a procedure and, if possible, continue until a meaningful reduction (e.g., 30% to 50%) has been achieved.

Therapeutic Plateletpheresis

An elevated platelet count may be found in three settings: (1) rare familial cases may be due to excessive production of thrombopoietin; (2) a reactive thrombocytosis can occur after several types of inciting events including splenectomy, iron deficiency, malignancy, and chronic inflammation; and (3) finally, a supernormal platelet count may be seen in clonal myeloproliferative disorders such as chronic myelogenous leukemia. When a high platelet count is the only sign of an abnormal clone, the disorder is called essential thrombocythemia. Symptoms attributable to thrombocytosis are seen only in patients who have a myeloproliferative disorder.[3,4]

Rationale

Many patients with thrombocytosis remain asymptomatic indefinitely; however, both thrombosis and hemorrhage are noted with increased frequency in the context of a myeloproliferative disorder. Clotting may be venous (e.g., deep vein thrombosis, Budd-Chiari syndrome) or arterial (e.g., erythromelalgia, stroke). Hemorrhage may be caused by a platelet-function defect or by aspirin given to protect against thrombosis. An age exceeding 60 years, a preexisting cardiovascular disease, or a prior history of thrombosis (or a combination of these) all confer an increased risk for clinical events, the magnitude of which correlates roughly with platelet count (Table 56–3). In younger patients without cardiovascular disease, the risk of clinical events seems unrelated to platelet count (i.e., symptoms may develop with a platelet count of 500,000/μL in some patients, whereas others may remain problem free for years with platelet counts exceeding 1 million/μL).[3,4]

Table 56–1 Density of Plasma and Formed Elements

Component	Specific Gravity
Plasma	1.025–1.029
Platelets	1.040
Lymphocytes	1.050–1.061
Monocytes	1.065–1.070
Granulocytes	1.087–1.092
Erythrocytes	1.093–1.096

Clinical Studies

Little definitive evidence guides therapy for thrombocytosis. A single trial in high-risk patients revealed a reduced incidence of clinical events when the platelet count was kept below 600,000/μL,[5] but no comparable data exist for lower-risk patients. Drug therapy with hydroxyurea or anagrelide will reduce the platelet count of most patients. Therapeutic plateletpheresis is usually reserved for patients with acute, serious thrombotic or hemorrhagic events, or for higher-risk patients with very high platelet counts. When it occurs in such circumstances, thrombocytosis has been rated a category I (standard practice) indication for therapeutic plateletpheresis by the American Society for Apheresis (ASFA)[6] and AABB[7] (Table 56–4). An urgent plateletpheresis will reduce the platelet count promptly, and additional procedures can maintain a reduced level until drug therapy takes effect.[2,3]

Technique

Therapeutic plateletpheresis can be performed with any centrifugal apheresis instrument. Procedural variables such as anticoagulation, centrifuge speed, and separatory chamber configuration are usually the same as those used for a platelet donation; however, it may be desirable to maintain a higher flow rate in the component-removal line in an instrument so equipped.[2] As mentioned, the platelet count decrement for a single procedure cannot be reliably predicted on the basis of the volume of blood processed. Monitoring intraprocedural platelet counts is the best way to ensure that the desired decrement (e.g., a 50% decline) is obtained before a procedure is discontinued.

Therapeutic Leukapheresis

The great majority of therapeutic leukapheresis procedures are carried out to treat hyperleukocytosis occurring in association with leukemia, but a few other indications should be briefly mentioned. Depletion of nonmalignant lymphocytes by apheresis, with or without simultaneous therapeutic plasma exchange (TPE), has been reported in several autoimmune disorders. Rheumatoid arthritis,[8] progressive multiple sclerosis,[9] inclusion body myositis,[10] polymyositis, and dermatomyositis[11] have all been assigned indication categories by ASFA[6] and AABB[7] (see Table 56–4); however, leukapheresis to deplete nonmalignant lymphocytes has not become an accepted treatment for any autoimmune disorder. Leukapheresis has been used to remove malignant lymphocytes from patients who have Sézary syndrome in the context of cutaneous T-cell lymphoma (CTCL)[12,13]; this is also a category III indication (see Table 56–4).[6,7] However, it has been largely replaced by photopheresis, as discussed later.

Table 56–2 Sources of Error in Predicting the Extent of Cell Depletion by Leukapheresis

1. Blood volume exceeds predictions
2. Extravascular cells mobilized during procedure
3. Collection efficiency differs from expectations

Table 56–3 Risk Factors for Clinical Events in Myeloproliferative Disease with Thrombocytosis

1. Age older than 60 years
2. Cardiovascular disease
3. History of thrombosis

Rationale

The clinical manifestations associated with a highly elevated white blood cell (WBC) count (hyperleukocytosis) in leukemia patients include leukostasis, tumor lysis syndrome, and early mortality. These are not mutually exclusive, and it is therefore useful to keep all of them in mind when considering the potential for benefit from therapeutic leukapheresis.

Leukostasis is diagnosed when evidence is present of organ dysfunction due to microvascular obstruction and consequent patchy ischemia. Neurologic and pulmonary dysfunction are the most common examples in acute leukemia; priapism is another possible complication in patients with chronic myelogenous leukemia (CML).[14,15] The pathologic basis for these symptoms is believed to be small-vessel occlusion by masses of leukemic cells, possibly with thrombosis, and sometimes with hemorrhage distal to the occlusion.[16,17] Such obstructions have been attributed to rheologic consequences of an increased blood concentration of WBCs,

Table 56–4 ASFA/AABB Indication Categories for Therapeutic Cell Depletion

Disease	Procedure	Category
Thrombocytosis	Plateletpheresis	I
Hyperleukocytosis	Leukapheresis	I
Rheumatoid arthritis	Lymphoplasmapheresis	II
Progressive multiple sclerosis	Leukapheresis	III
Inclusion body myositis	Leukapheresis	IV
Polymyositis	Leukapheresis	IV
Dermatomyositis	Leukapheresis	IV
Heart transplant rejection	Photopheresis	III
Cutaneous T-cell lymphoma	Photopheresis	I
	Leukapheresis	III
Sickle cell disease	Red cell exchange	I
Severe malaria/ babesiosis	Red cell exchange	III

I, standard therapy; II, evidence suggests efficacy; III, inadequately tested; IV, ineffective in controlled trials.

especially increased viscosity.[18] However, concomitant anemia keeps the whole blood viscosity within the normal range in most patients with leukemia,[19,20] unless ill-advised red cell transfusions are given before the WBC count has been lowered.[21] More recent studies have identified reduced deformability, cytokine secretion, and altered adherence properties of blasts or other primitive cells as factors contributing to leukostasis.[2,22,23] These factors could explain not only why leukostasis correlates more closely with the circulating blast count than with total WBC count, but also why the absolute blast count at which symptoms occur can vary widely from patient to patient.[24,25]

Leukostasis occurs in about 5% of patients with acute myelogenous leukemia (AML).[14] Autopsy studies have shown microscopic evidence of leukostasis in most AML nonsurvivors whose WBC counts exceeded 200,000/μL.[17] The blast count exceeds 100,000/μL in most clinically evident instances of leukostasis; however, the syndrome is occasionally suspected in patients when the blast count is only in the 50,000 to 100,000/μL range.[26] Leukostasis is seldom seen in acute lymphocytic leukemia, and then only when the WBC count reaches the 250,000 to 300,000/μL range.[24] Higher cell counts, usually in the 300,000 to 500,000/μL range, are required before the more mature cells that circulate in CML can cause signs of leukostasis,[15] whereas counts above even this level may be tolerated without symptoms in chronic lymphocytic leukemia.[2]

Even in patients who do not have leukostasis, hyperleukocytosis is a marker for a poorer prognosis in both acute and chronic leukemias. Both short-term and long-term survival are inversely correlated with presenting WBC count, as are the complete remission rate and the mean duration of response to chemotherapy.[27] Finally, hyperleukocytosis is associated with a higher incidence of hyperuricemia and other manifestations of tumor lysis syndrome, all of which may be exacerbated by cytotoxic chemotherapy.[28]

Clinical Studies

It is widely accepted, based on accumulated clinical experience rather than controlled studies, that reducing the WBC count by leukapheresis can reverse symptoms of leukostasis, although it may not do so if tissue infarction as well as ischemia has occurred. This is the basis for the ASFA/AABB ranking of hyperleukocytosis as a category I indication for leukapheresis (see Table 56–4).[6,7] Leukapheresis should be carried out as an emergency in leukemia patients with symptomatic leukostasis, especially acute leukemia patients with blast counts exceeding 100,000/μL. Wide acceptance of this principle led to the question of whether urgent prophylactic leukapheresis might be prudent in acute leukemia patients with WBC or blast counts exceeding 100,000/μL, even if they do not have signs of leukostasis. Evidence for benefit from such prophylactic leukapheresis is limited, and this practice remains controversial; nevertheless, urgent leukapheresis may be requested routinely on this basis by individual physicians or as institutional policy, and requests for repeated leukapheresis may be made when acute leukemia patients' WBC counts remain high for several days before chemotherapy is instituted.[24,25] An extreme example of the latter was a pregnant patient who received only leukapheresis therapy for several weeks after a diagnosis of acute leukemia was made because she wished to delay chemotherapy until after delivery.[29]

It is still not clear that reducing the WBC count by leukapheresis before initiation of chemotherapy prevents or meaningfully reduces the severity of tumor lysis syndrome. A counter-argument to the prediction of such benefit is that the leukemic cells accessible for removal from the circulation represent only a small fraction of the total tumor burden and that a meaningful reduction in tumor load is not likely to be achieved in this way. Controlled studies that address this point have not been reported. It is also unclear whether prophylactic leukapheresis improves survival in patients with hyperleukocytosis, either by attenuating tumor lysis syndrome or in some other way.

Three observational studies of prophylactic leukapheresis have been published in the past decade. One group reported 48 consecutive AML patients who received leukapheresis if the presenting WBC count exceeded 100,000/μL. The extent of WBC count reduction was not significantly different between the 14 patients who died within 2 weeks and the remaining patients, suggesting that WBC count reduction was not an important predictor of mortality.[30] Another nonrandomized, retrospective study of 146 patients with AML and a WBC count exceeding 50,000/μL showed a higher 2-week survival (87% vs 77%) in patients who had leukapheresis; this was statistically significant only in a logistic regression analysis. Follow-up observation, however, showed no advantage in 4-week, 6-week, or overall survival. Paradoxically, long-term survival was significantly lower in the group that had leukapheresis.[31] A third study looked at outcomes in 53 patients with AML and WBC counts exceeding 100,000/μL, all of whom underwent daily leukapheresis (76 procedures total) until the WBC count dropped below 100,000/μL or the performance status improved. Only two patients died in the first week; however, despite the prophylactic WBC removal, 47% developed coagulopathy, 85% developed tumor lysis syndrome that was severe in 53%, and only 55% achieved a complete remission. Median survival among the responders was only 8 months.[32]

Taken as a whole, these reports provide little indication of benefit from routine prophylactic leukapheresis in hyperleukocytic AML patients. Indeed, the results might equally well imply that hyperleukocytosis is merely a marker for other risk factors, such as morphologic category, specific chromosomal abnormalities, and/or total tumor burden, that cannot be altered simply by leukapheresis. Prospective randomized controlled studies are needed before routine prophylactic leukapheresis can be recommended.

Technique

Therapeutic leukapheresis can be accomplished with most centrifugal apheresis instruments. Urgent treatment of patients with inadequate peripheral venous access may require equally urgent placement of a dual-lumen central venous catheter, which can be challenging in acutely ill patients with the low platelet counts that often occur in leukemia. When contemplating leukapheresis in a patient who does not have leukostasis, the unproven benefits of treatment should be balanced against the potential hazards of emergency central-line placement and delay in starting pharmacologic cytoreduction with hydroxyurea and definitive chemotherapy.[24,25]

Cell removal will be more efficient in most instances if hydroxyethyl starch or another sedimenting agent is added to patient blood before it enters the centrifuge. Also, removal of leukemic cells, even in a concentrate containing 500,000 to 750,000 leukocytes per microliter, may entail large plasma losses. The volume-expanding properties of a sedimenting agent can offset this to some extent, but additional colloid replacement is wise if the volume of leukocyte concentrate removed exceeds 1 L.[2]

The extent to which the WBC count must be reduced to prevent or reverse leukostasis cannot be known in advance for an individual patient with any degree of certainty. Nevertheless, it is reasonable to expect clinical improvement in a patient with leukostasis if the WBC count is promptly reduced by 30% to 50%, ideally to less than 100,000/μL in AML or less than 300,000/μL in CML. The extent of prophylactic leukocyte removal that might be needed to prevent tumor lysis syndrome or improve survival is even more uncertain. As mentioned previously, it is difficult to predict WBC count reduction merely on the basis of the volume of blood processed.[2] It is therefore worthwhile to monitor intraprocedural WBC counts to assure that a targeted reduction is reached.

Photopheresis

In an extracorporeal photochemotherapy (ECP or photopheresis) treatment, patient MNCs separated by leukapheresis are exposed to a standardized dose of ultraviolet A radiation (UVA) in the presence of 8-methoxypsoralen (8-MOP) at a concentration of 60 to 200 ng/μL. 8-MOP is a photoactive compound that will crosslink nuclear DNA in the treated cells by means of diadducts between proximate thymidine residues in complementary strands. Protein changes may occur as well. After a short incubation, the irradiated cells are returned to the patient. Although conceptually independent, the modules performing the apheresis and irradiation steps can be housed in a single instrument such as the UVAR XTS system (Therakos, Exton, Pa.). 8-MOP was originally given orally shortly before apheresis but is now available in a preparation suitable for intravenous administration that can be added to the MNC concentrate after collection but before UVA irradiation. This provides much better control of 8-MOP concentration during irradiation; in addition, it reduces the dose of 8-MOP given to the patient by a hundredfold, thereby reducing side effects such as photosensitivity. In most of the applications to be discussed, ECP has usually been performed on one or two consecutive days at 2- to 4-week intervals.[33]

Cutaneous T-Cell Lymphoma

ECP was devised in the 1980s as a therapy for CTCL, a disease in which malignant lymphocytes are typically abundant in the bloodstream as well as in skin infiltrates.[34] Certain cutaneous manifestations of CTCL were known to improve after depletion of malignant cells by leukapheresis[12,13] and also after UVA irradiation of skin after ingestion of 8-MOP (psoralen-UVA treatment; PUVA).[35] Collection, UVA irradiation and reinfusion of 5% to 10% of circulating MNCs on 2 consecutive days monthly led, after a delay of some months, to dramatic improvement in some patients. Responses of the magnitude observed cannot be accounted for simply by destruction of UVA-irradiated tumor cells, and this quantitative discrepancy suggested the possibility that ECP may elicit, enhance, or otherwise modulate a host immune response to the tumor.[23,24] This hypothesis provides a theoretical framework for trials of ECP in other diseases in which immunomodulation seems a reasonable approach to therapy.

Nine North American studies have reported 282 CTCL patients who received ECP.[34,36–43] Of these, 18% had a complete response, and another 38% had a partial response.[44] Long-term follow-up suggested better median survival than had been observed in historic controls. ECP seems most active in patients who have had relatively recent onset of diffuse skin disease (erythroderma) but still have relatively little of the immunosuppression that often accompanies advanced disease. Results are not as good in patients with localized skin plaques, long-standing disease, and/or involvement of lymph nodes and viscera.[44,45]

The FDA approved Therakos's original UVAR system for treatment of CTCL in 1987, and this use has been rated a category I indication for ECP by ASFA[6] and AABB[7] (see Table 56-4). Unfortunately, although its ability to produce regression of erythroderma is well established, the optimal role of ECP in CTCL remains uncertain because, unlike almost all drug therapies for malignant disease, it has never been subjected to controlled trials with uniform enrollment and response criteria comparing it with no treatment, sham ECP, or alternative therapies.[46]

Graft versus Host Disease (GVHD)

GVHD is most often encountered as a complication of allogeneic stem cell transplantation. It affects skin, liver, and gastrointestinal (GI) tract. Acute GVHD begins before day 100 after transplant and is mostly inflammatory, whereas chronic GVHD begins after day 100 and may include scleroderma-like skin thickening and other fibrotic changes. Both forms occur frequently in allograft recipients despite prophylaxis with corticosteroids and other immunosuppressive drugs. Each form has about a 30% incidence after HLA-matched sibling transplants; after partially mismatched related or matched unrelated transplants, the respective incidences are in the 50% to 80% range.[33,47]

Skin GVHD sometimes improves after PUVA therapy.[48] ECP was tried in hopes of addressing visceral involvement via a similar mechanism and has been reported to be beneficial in both acute and chronic GVHD. In both settings, the best responses are noted in skin manifestations.[33,49] Eleven reports on acute GVHD,[47,50–59] including observations of 76 patients, have been analyzed.[47] Of the patients with skin disease, 83% showed improvement after ECP, with a complete response recorded in 67%. Complete regression was also observed in 54% of cases with GI involvement and 38% of cases with liver disease. Twenty reports on chronic GVHD[47,52–54,56,59,60–72] also have been analyzed.[47] Of 160 patients with skin disease, 76% improved after ECP, with a complete response being noted in 35%. Improvement was also reported in 48% of 84 patients with liver involvement, 39% of 31 patients with lung disease, and 63% of 59 patients with oral manifestations. Responses in this context are said to be quicker than those seen in CTCL, with improvement evident in a matter of weeks. Survival is also thought to be improved.[47] Again, however, the precise contribution of ECP to treatment of GVHD must be regarded as uncertain because ECP-treated patients generally receive other therapies concomitantly, and no prospective controlled trials have been reported. GVHD has not been rated as an indication for ECP by either ASFA or AABB.

Solid Organ Transplant Rejection

Immunomodulation by means of ECP has also been undertaken in patients who are rejecting a solid organ transplant. A number of case studies and small series have described recipients of kidney[73–75] and lung[76–80] allografts who improved when ECP was added to a conventional antirejection regimen. The largest experience, however, has come from heart transplantation.

In considering the use of ECP in heart transplantation, it is important to point out that the term *rejection* has a subtle additional connotation in that context that does not apply to other organ allografts. Transplanted kidneys and lungs are seldom biopsied unless signs of organ dysfunction are present; however, the low risk and relative simplicity of endomyocardial biopsy (EMB) permits a cardiac allograft to be sampled routinely, often in the absence of cardiac dysfunction. It is also customary for patients who have mild histologic changes in such surveillance biopsies to be treated preemptively and aggressively for rejection in the absence of any signs of cardiac dysfunction.

The first reports of ECP in cardiac allograft recipients described cases with severe, hemodynamically significant rejection who improved after ECP was added to other antirejection therapies.[33,81] Subsequent studies have tended to focus on the more common patients with normal hemodynamics and mild histologic changes on EMB. A controlled trial with eight patients per arm found ECP to be equivalent to high-dose corticosteroids in reversing mild histologic changes on EMB.[82] The significance of this finding is open to question, however, because other studies have suggested that such changes usually resolve without adjustments to antirejection therapy.[83] A controlled trial of prophylactic ECP in 60 patients with cardiac transplants showed a lower incidence of mild histologic changes in patients who received ECP prophylaxis, but no difference in the rate of severe rejection with hemodynamic compromise.[84] Absent controlled trials in patients with severe rejection, the uncertainty about the prognostic significance of mild histologic changes contributes to uncertainty about the proper role for ECP in treatment of rejection of heart and other organ transplants. Heart transplant rejection has been rated as a category III indication for ECP by ASFA[6] and AABB[7] (see Table 56–4).

Autoimmune Diseases

Immunomodulation with ECP has been tried in a number of autoimmune diseases, including scleroderma,[85] systemic lupus erythematosus,[86] pemphigus vulgaris,[87] rheumatoid arthritis,[88] and psoriatic arthritis.[89] Favorable results have been reported in case studies and small series. More extensive experience in scleroderma has indicated limited benefit at most,[90] whereas data from controlled trials of ECP in other autoimmune disorders are still lacking.

Mechanism of Action

The mechanism of action of ECP is not known with certainty for any of the applications mentioned earlier. No doubt exists, however, that it leads to apoptosis in a majority of treated lymphocytes while leaving treated monocytes relatively intact and viable. UVA-induced DNA crosslinking by 8-MOP is probably an important contributor to this effect, although other mechanisms, such as protein damage, may operate as well.

In CTCL, it is supposed that apoptosis of malignant lymphocytes exposes or releases tumor-specific antigens in a more immunogenic fashion, thereby eliciting or enhancing host immune responsiveness to the tumor. Recent studies suggest that contact with plastic surfaces of the disposables in the apheresis instrument and the UVA irradiation apparatus induces collected monocytes to differentiate into dendritic cells. It is theorized that activated dendritic cells then ingest tumor antigens being released from apoptotic cells and facilitate antigen presentation, thus leading to enhanced immunity.[91,92]

A similar mechanism could be envisioned for ECP in other applications; that is, a downregulating response to a pathogenic though nonmalignant lymphocyte clone is enhanced through release of clone-specific antigens by apoptosis, followed by vigorous presentation of these antigens by abundant activated dendritic cells.[49,93] At present, however, this mechanism should be regarded as hypothetical. Circulating clonal lymphocytes have been found in scleroderma[94] and GVHD,[49] but thus far, neither pathogenicity nor downregulation by ECP has been shown for such clones.

The putative effects of ECP in GVHD have also been attributed to more general immunomodulatory effects. One hypothesis involves a shift from an inflammatory Th1 cytokine expression profile to a more inhibitory Th2 profile.[95] A second envisions a paradoxical decrease in dendritic cell function in this context.[96]

Peripheral Blood Progenitor Cell Collection

Autologous MNCs, collected by leukapheresis and cryopreserved, have all but replaced bone marrow as the preferred source of stem and progenitor cells for autologous hematopoietic rescue after myeloablative antitumor therapy for lymphomas, leukemias, myeloma, and other malignancies.[97] A similar approach is being tried in some autoimmune diseases.[98] Stem and progenitor cells do not circulate in the basal state in quantities sufficient for this purpose; however, they can be stimulated to enter the bloodstream in any of several ways. One is to give a "conventional" dose of an appropriate chemotherapeutic agent as "mobilizing chemotherapy" roughly 10 to 14 days before the planned date of collection. When the WBC count begins to increase after the expected interval of leukopenia, the blood concentration of CD34-positive cells, which is a marker for peripheral blood progenitor cell (PBPC) concentration, increases by as much as 25-fold and remains elevated for up to a week.[99,100] A second method is to give daily injections of a hematopoietic growth factor. Both granulocyte colony–stimulating factor (G-CSF; filgrastim; Neupogen)[101,102] and granulocyte-macrophage colony–stimulating factor (GM-CSF; sargramostim; Leukine)[103] injections will induce worthwhile levels of circulating CD34-positive cells in most individuals in 4 to 5 days; these levels will persist for up to a week with continued daily injections. In the autologous setting, G-CSF or GM-CSF or both can be given during recovery from mobilizing chemotherapy for maximal mobilization.[104–106] A number of other cytokines will also mobilize PBPCs, but none is commercially available at this time.[107]

Goals for total CD34-positive cell yield from autologous PBPC collections range from 2×10^6 to 5×10^6 CD34-positive cells per kilogram per transplant at different centers. Most patients will respond to mobilizing stimuli well enough to reach their goal after one to three daily leukapheresis procedures. A smaller proportion with suboptimal mobilization may require four to five daily collections. Perhaps 10% of patients, most of whom are older or have had extensive prior chemotherapy or both, will fail to have a useful response to conventional mobilization strategies. Their blood CD34-positive cell levels (expressed in cells per microliter) will not increase above the low single-digit range, levels at which daily leukapheresis procedures will seldom produce the target yield within the limited period of mobilization.[107]

PBPCs are preferred over cells from bone marrow harvests for two reasons. The first is that the collection procedure does not require hospitalization or general anesthesia. The second is that WBC and platelet counts recover about a week sooner after PBPC transplantation than after bone marrow transplantation. The resultant reduction in early morbidity and mortality from infection and bleeding more than offsets a somewhat higher incidence of GVHD with PBPC.[97]

Candidates for PBPC collection have unique vascular-access needs. They require a multilumen, tunneled central vein catheter for diagnostic blood draws, transfusion support, fluid maintenance, and chemotherapy infusions during both the pre- and post-transplant periods; however, catheters designed solely for these purposes are too flexible and have a diameter too small to support the flow rates required for efficient leukapheresis. Fortunately, tunneled dual- or triple-lumen apheresis catheters (e.g., Raaf catheter) that accommodate both PBPC collection and the full range of other intravenous-access requirements are now commercially available. Potential autologous PBPC transplant recipients will usually benefit from having such a catheter placed. A notable exception would be a patient having a precautionary collection that would only be used in the event of an unexpected or late relapse. Such "harvest and hold" patients should have leukapheresis via peripheral veins if possible.

PBPC collections are quite prolonged apheresis procedures. It is commonplace for 15 to 30 L of patient blood to be processed in a 4- to 6-hour period. Such extensive procedures may entail enough incidental platelet loss to warrant platelet transfusions for patients who are already somewhat thrombocytopenic. They also entail prolonged infusion of citrate anticoagulant and therefore a large cumulative citrate dose. Conflicting reports concerned the frequency of adverse effects during PBPC collection. A multicenter survey that included both autologous and allogeneic donors but did not track either mild paresthesias or calcium-replacement practices revealed only a 1.33% incidence of spontaneously reported adverse effects in 664 PBPC collections.[108] A later study at a single center found a 54% incidence of symptoms in carefully questioned donors during 71 allogeneic PBPC collections performed without intravenous calcium supplementation. Serum ionized calcium decreased by 20% to 35% during these procedures. Symptoms were especially prevalent in smaller female donors. The same investigators found a 20% incidence of symptoms among 244 donations performed with prophylactic intravenous calcium supplementation, with only a 10% to 15% decrease in ionized serum calcium.[109] Although the latter studies monitored allogeneic donations, they suggest that intravenous calcium supplementation might prevent mild paresthesias during autologous PBPC collections as well, especially those done on smaller female patients.

Autologous Mononuclear White Blood Cells Altered Ex Vivo

Autologous MNCs collected by leukapheresis provide the starting material for a number of established and experimental cellular therapy techniques.

Purification and Expansion

Purification of MNC subsets has been explored in autologous PBPC transplantation. This has been done primarily to address potential tumor cell contamination. In positive selection approaches, stem and progenitor cells are purified from all other MNC, including any contaminating tumor cells. The most prevalent techniques are immunologic ones that target the CD34 antigen. Several of these are commercially available. Stem cells thus purified also provide an attractive starting material for in vitro expansion techniques that could enhance the outcome of transplantation in other ways. An alternative approach to purification is negative selection to deplete tumor cells actively from an MNC concentrate. Sequential positive and negative selection approaches also are possible.[110] Gene-marking experiments identified tumor cells derived from autograft contamination in metastases developing after transplantation[111]; however, to date, no stem cell purification process has been shown to enhance survival after transplantation in any illness.

Immunization

A number of in vitro strategies have been proposed to induce and/or enhance antimicrobial or antitumor immunity expressed by autologous immunocytes present in MNC concentrates. Enhanced antigen presentation, release from inhibitory influences operative in vivo, and/or selective stimulation by supraphysiologic "cytokine cocktails" are potential mechanisms that could facilitate immune responses that could not be achieved in vivo and might result in desirable therapeutic effects after reinfusion of treated cells. Some approaches of this nature have shown promise in melanoma, renal cell carcinoma, and prostate cancer.[112]

Gene Insertion

Autologous hematopoietic stem and progenitor cells collected by leukapheresis are promising targets for therapeutic gene insertion. They can be obtained in abundance with relative ease, and they or their progeny can potentially survive indefinitely after genetic alteration and reinfusion. Encouraging early successes were achieved in correcting immunodeficiency due to adenosine deaminase deficiency, but gene therapy has subsequently proven to be a very challenging endeavor.[113]

RED CELL EXCHANGE

Description of Procedure

The most common manipulation of red cells by apheresis is red cell exchange (RCE), in which patient red cells separated by the instrument are removed while compatible donor red cells are added to patient plasma and reinfused. Two other manipulations are possible. Red cells can be depleted rapidly and isovolemically from patients with polycythemia by removing red cells and adding 5% human serum albumin (HSA) or fresh frozen plasma (FFP) at the same rate to the patient's plasma for reinfusion.[114,115] Alternatively, red cells can be transfused rapidly and isovolemically to anemic patients by removing patient plasma while adding compatible donor cells to the patient's red cells at the same rate to be reinfused.[116]

The kinetics of a "pure" RCE are similar to those of TPE, such that the equation and graph in the previous chapter (see Fig. 55–1) can be used to determine the fraction of patient red cells remaining (FCR) after exchange of a given number of patient red cell volumes. Some apheresis instruments include programming that accepts operator input for patient height, weight, hematocrit, the desired FCR, and the expected hematocrit of donor PRBCs, and then calculates the volume of packed red cells that should be exchanged.

Outcomes of RCE in some applications can be made more effective and efficient in ways not feasible for TPE. If the patient's baseline hematocrit is not too low (i.e., >24%), isovolemic removal of patient red cells with HSA replacement can be carried out at the beginning of the exchange to an extent that will reduce the hematocrit to the minimum safe level. Because no donor cells are infused, none can be subsequently withdrawn, and removal of patient cells during this preliminary phase is therefore 100% efficient. Similarly, if the hematocrit at the end of an exchange is not too high (i.e., <30%), additional donor red cells can be infused simultaneously with patient plasma removal to increase the hematocrit isovolemically to the desired or maximal safe level. Because no red cells are removed in this phase, provision of normal donor red cells is 100% efficient. A benefit similar to such postexchange red cell transfusion can be achieved during the exchange by withdrawing red cells at a hematocrit lower than that of infused PRBCs, thus raising the hematocrit gradually. Combining these two strategies (that is, pure patient cell removal at the beginning of a procedure and pure infusion of donor cells or gradual raising of hematocrit at the end of the procedure) can make a red cell "exchange" procedure more efficient (i.e., produce a lower FCR) than the formula in Figure 55-1 would predict for the volume of donor red cells used.[117]

Because red cell volume is less than plasma volume, especially in anemic patients, the total volume of blood processed in an RCE procedure tends to be less than that in TPE. Flow rates can also be lower. These factors predict a lower risk for citrate toxicity. Conversely, patients having RCE are at risk for both hemolytic and nonhemolytic reactions to red cell transfusions, and these risks are higher in patients who have had multiple RCE or are multitransfused for other reasons, because such patients have an increased likelihood of becoming alloimmunized to minor red cells antigens that could mediate a hemolytic reaction, as well as to HLA antigens that may be involved in febrile nonhemolytic transfusion reactions. In a multicenter study, the risk of an adverse reaction observed in 78 RCE procedures was 10.3%.[108]

Finally, many RCEs are performed on pediatric patients with sickle cell disease (SCD) whose small body size can make them more susceptible than adults to imprudent levels of hypovolemia or anemia during the procedure. The latter risk can be avoided in younger children by priming the apheresis instrument with 5% HSA and/or donor PRBCs as appropriate.

Sickle Cell Disease

The great majority of RCEs are done for complications of SCD in patients who are homozygous for hemoglobin S (HbS) or have another hemoglobinopathy. Briefly stated, the rationale for removing patient red cells and transfusing normal red cells containing hemoglobin A (HbA) in RCE is to create a hemoglobin mixture similar to that found in sickle trait cells, in which a majority of circulating hemoglobin is HbA. Because HbS-containing cells are less likely to sickle in such cell mixtures, RCE can interrupt the vicious cycle of sickling, stasis, and progressive hypoxia that occurs during sickle cell crisis.[118] The exact proportions of HbA and HbS needed to achieve this are not known with certainty; however, plans for RCE are usually formulated with a goal of increasing HbA above 70% of the total (i.e., FCR <30% in an untransfused patient) so that a HbA level above 50% will persist for several weeks. For some indications discussed later, it is desirable to maintain HbA above 70% for a prolonged interval. In appropriate circumstances, SCD is rated a category I indication for RCE by ASFA[6] and AABB[7] (see Table 56–4).

When transfusing SCD patients, it is important to avoid raising hematocrit much above 30% because at higher hematocrits, blood viscosity reaches levels that can exacerbate the microvascular ischemia that transfusion therapy is intended to combat. RCE is favored over simple transfusion in urgent circumstances because it can increase HbA quickly without a proportionate increase in hematocrit.[119] By contrast, long-term maintenance of a high HbA and low HbS can be achieved and sustained in SCD patients by repeated simple transfusion to a hematocrit of about 30% at 2- to 4-week intervals. Transfused cells survive longer than the patient's own cells and will tend to accumulate on that basis alone. In addition, suppression of erythropoietin synthesis by the higher post-transfusion hematocrit leads to reduced production of patient cells. In a comparison with RCE, the advantages cited for repeated simple transfusion are a lower cost and a reduced number of PRBC units needed per unit of time in a prolonged transfusion program. The advantages cited for RCE are (1) used as an emergency, it can raise HbA to 70% to 90% rapidly (in a few hours rather than a few weeks); (2) treatments are shorter and can be less frequent; and (3) less iron loading occurs with RCE because red cell removal is nearly equal to red cell transfusion.[119–121] This comparison is summarized in Table 56–5. In the present era, when the perceived risk of transfusion-transmitted infection is low, the reduction in iron loading with RCE is often deemed to outweigh the incremental infection risk associated with the greater number of units transfused. This leads many practitioners to favor RCE over simple transfusion as a means for long-term maintenance transfusion therapy.

If RCE is to be done, the number of units to be exchanged must be specified. This will depend on the patient's body size, the goal for post-treatment HbA and HbS levels, and the patient's recent transfusion history. The latter is important because a smaller exchange will suffice to reach a given post-treatment HbA goal if the patient already has some HbA circulating. A patient who has not been transfused for several months can be assumed to have no circulating HbA, whereas a patient in a regular maintenance exchange program might be expected, based on previous measurements,

Table 56–5 Comparison of Red Cell Exchange and Simple Transfusion for Long-Term Maintenance Transfusion in Hemoglobinopathies

	Simple Transfusion	Red Cell Exchange
Cost	Lower	Higher
PRBC units required	Fewer	More
Convenience of treatment	Worse	Better
Frequency of treatment	Higher	Lower
Iron overloading	More	LESS

PRBCs, packed red blood cells.

to have a 50% to 70% HbA level before the next exchange. In the absence of a recent hemoglobin electrophoresis, one must make a reasonable, preferably conservative estimate of pretreatment HbA.

Certain special requirements are appropriate for PRBCs to be transfused to SCD patients in either RCE or long-term simple transfusion regimens. Donors should be tested for and found negative for sickle trait, so that all transfused hemoglobin will be HbA. Leukocyte depletion is warranted to avoid febrile transfusion reactions; when these occur, the time required to rule out a hemolytic reaction is especially disruptive during RCE because the procedure must be halted for an hour or more. Some practitioners prefer to provide PRBCs that are phenotypically matched with the recipient to a greater or lesser extent to avoid alloantibody formation.[121] Others are content to deal with antibody workups as they arise and provide antigen-negative PRBCs only to the minority of patients who develop specific antibodies. Finally, some authors consider it important to provide relatively fresh PRBCs to certain patients, such as those with a new stroke or acute chest syndrome, who might have difficulty tolerating a temporary deficit in oxygen delivery associated with transfusion of older blood. None of these requirements should be regarded as absolute, and judgment must be exercised when adherence to any or all of them would delay a procedure in an emergency situation. Thus one might accept some units from donors with sickle trait if they are the only compatible cells available for a patient with a difficult constellation of alloantibodies. One might also waive prophylactic phenotypic matching for a patient with an uncommon phenotype or accept the freshest units available rather than insist on a predefined maximal age for PRBC units.

Stroke

Central nervous system (CNS) infarction is a common and potentially devastating complication of SCD that poses a particular threat to children with the disease.[122] In the United States, the prevalence of overt stroke is 11% by age 20 years in untreated SCD patients; another 17% will have evidence of clinically silent infarcts in CNS imaging studies.[123,124] Furthermore, children who have had one stroke are at high risk for subsequent CNS events. The recurrence rate was 67% in one study of patients with a history of overt stroke,[125] and a 14-fold increase in the risk of overt stroke was found in children with silent infarcts on CNS magnetic resonance imaging (MRI).[126]

Most childhood strokes are due to thrombosis at sites of previous narrowing in cerebral arteries. The presence of predisposing vascular lesions can be inferred from elevated blood-flow velocities detected by transcranial Doppler ultrasonography (TCD).[127] The incidence of stroke in children with abnormal TCDs is 10% to 13% per year versus the baseline risk of 0.5% to 1.0% per year.[128]

Long-term simple transfusion or maintenance RCE regimens designed to keep HbS below 30% have been used empirically to prevent recurrences in children who have had a stroke.[129,130] A randomized study of prophylactic transfusion to maintain HbS at less than 30% in children with abnormal TCDs showed a 90% reduction in the incidence of stroke in the transfused arm over a period of about 2 years. The incidence of new silent infarcts was similarly reduced. Most patients in that arm received simple transfusion. Iron overload requiring chelation therapy was a significant problem but was less severe in the minority of patients who received transfusions via RCE.[128] In another study of children with an abnormal TCD and a silent infarct on MRI, prolonged transfusion reduced the incidence of both overt stroke and new silent infarcts.[131]

Long-term simple transfusion or maintenance RCE to keep HbS less than 30% is recommended for SCD children with abnormal TCDs, overt strokes, or silent infarcts on MRI. Early cessation of transfusion after a primary stroke restores the baseline risk of recurrence.[132,133] In a randomized study performed in children who had received prophylactic transfusion for high-risk TCD findings for 30 to 91 months with correction of TCD velocities to low-risk values, discontinuation of transfusion was followed by reversion to high-risk TCD velocities or by clinical stroke within 4 to 9 months in 16 of 41 patients, versus no such events in patients who continued transfusion.[134] Transfusion becomes less onerous if the HbS goal is relaxed to less than 50% after several years without a CNS event,[135] but the risk of stroke after such an adjustment has not been established and may therefore be increased.[130] It may be reasonable to discontinue transfusion therapy when patients reach age 18 years because the baseline incidence of stroke is lower in young adults with SCD,[136–138] but this too remains unproven.

The incidence of a CNS event increases again in older SCD patients. These are usually hemorrhagic strokes. No conclusive evidence exists that urgent RCE improves short-term outcomes in children or adults with acute strokes, or that either long-term simple transfusion or maintenance RCE reduces the risk of recurrent stroke in adults.[139,140] Nevertheless, these are common practices in some institutions.

Acute Chest Syndrome

Acute chest syndrome (ACS) is an important cause of morbidity and mortality in SCD. It may be diagnosed in SCD patients who have a new infiltrate on a chest radiograph.[141] Such patients may also have fever, chest pain, tachypnea, wheezing, and/or cough. ACS is often precipitated or accompanied by lung infection or fat embolism. Hypoxemia is common, and 13% of patients in a recent series required mechanical ventilation.[142] ACS is more common in children but more severe in adults; thus mortality in one large series was 1.1% in patients younger than 20 versus 4.3% in adults. Furthermore, patients who have one episode of ACS are at increased risk (up to an 80% likelihood) of having a recurrence.[143,144]

Progressive sickling in the pulmonary microcirculation has long been thought to play a role in the pathogenesis of ACS. More recent studies point to excessive scavenging of nitric oxide (NO) by abundant free Hb,[145] along with release of other vasoactive mediators and enhanced expression of adhesion molecules, as additional factors favoring vascular obstruction, tissue ischemia, and the prolonged local hypoxia that leads to irreversible sickling.[146–149]

Management of ACS should include an aggressive search for a precipitating causal factors and appropriate measures (e.g., antibiotics for infection) to address such factors as they are identified. General supportive measures such as bronchodilators, supplemental oxygen, and adequate hydration are also appropriate. Transfusion therapy is generally given in more severe cases, including all those requiring mechanical ventilation.[141,150] Simple transfusion and RCE have never been systematically compared, but both have deemed helpful in series that lacked any comparison with untransfused controls. RCE seems particularly apt for patients with relatively high hematocrits who could not receive much HbA via simple transfusion without raising the hematocrit above recommended levels. In the randomized trial of prophylactic transfusion to prevent strokes, ACS was less frequent in the group receiving transfusions (2.2 vs 15.7 events per 100 patient years).[151]

Chronic progressive pulmonary hypertension is another important cause of pulmonary morbidity and mortality in SCD patients that is distinct from ACS.[152] It has been suggested that long-term RCE might, by reducing plasma Hb and increasing NO availability, be beneficial to SCD patients with early pulmonary hypertension recognized by echocardiographic screening.[152,153]

Priapism

Priapism is a prolonged, painful penile erection. Its pathogenesis in males with SCD presumably involves a self-perpetuating cycle of sickling and stasis in engorged penile vessels. In one survey, 27.5% of male SCD patients between the ages of 5 and 20 years reported at least one brief episode (median duration of 60 minutes) of priapism, and the actuarial probability of having at least one episode by age 20 years was estimated to be 89%.[154] More prolonged episodes are less frequent but can lead to penile fibrosis and impotence.[155,156]

Initial treatments for episodes lasting several hours may include hydration and analgesics. If detumescence is not achieved, penile aspiration and/or intrapenile injection of a dilute epinephrine solution may be tried. Surgical shunting may be performed as a last resort in prolonged, resistant episodes, although this can also lead to impotence.[157,158]

Transfusion therapy including RCE has been recommended for resistant episodes and is often tried.[159] Use of RCE has been reported with enthusiasm, although not all patients have responded.[160–164] In a recent series, however, only one of seven patients responded to RCE implemented 1 to 7 days into an episode of priapism when other measures had failed.[165]

Use of RCE for priapism is occasionally followed in a matter of days by neurologic events, including stroke (CVA; *a*ssociation of *p*riapism, *e*xchange transfusion and *n*eurologic events; ASPEN syndrome).[166] This has been attributed to an increase in an already relatively high post-transfusion hematocrit when intrapenile red cells are released during detumescence, and a consequent increase in blood viscosity, perhaps exacerbated by release of vasoactive mediators from the same source.

Use of RCE for refractory priapism must be regarded as problematic at this time. Its value in terminating episodes has not been established in controlled trials, although it is possible that earlier implementation might give better results than the "last ditch" implementation tried in some trials. Conversely, RCE has been linked to a potentially serious adverse event, albeit one that might be avoided by maintaining post-RCE hematocrit at less than 30%. The question of whether prophylactic RCE might prevent recurrent attacks, as it does with strokes and ACS, has also not been examined in a controlled trial.

Severe Pain Crisis and Multiorgan Failure

The uncomplicated pain crises that are the most frequent complication of SCD are usually self-limited and brief. They do not seem to be appreciably shortened by RCE.[161] Prolonged, severe pain crises, conversely, may entail considerable suffering and disability and may occasionally be followed by otherwise unexplained death.[167,168] In addition, a potentially fatal multiorgan failure syndrome has been described after severe painful crises in patients with historically mild SCD and relatively high baseline hematocrit levels.[169] Aggressive transfusion was associated with better outcomes in such patients, with the best outcomes seen in patients having RCE. Preemptive RCE might therefore be considered for a patient with an unusually prolonged severe crisis, especially if the hematocrit is high.

An occasional SCD patient has pain crises so frequently as to become almost continuously disabled. Anecdotal experience indicates that maintenance RCE can reduce or eliminate future crises in such patients and thereby improve quality of life.[118] This conclusion is supported by the reduced frequency of pain crises observed among patients in the transfusion arm in a randomized trial of maintenance transfusion for stroke prevention.[170]

Perioperative Management

SCD patients have long been considered to be at increased risk for morbidity and mortality after general anesthesia and surgery.[171,172] This has been attributed in part to perioperative development of metabolic circumstances that favor sickling, such as dehydration, hypoxia, and acidosis. Prophylactic preoperative transfusion strategies, including RCE to increase HbA to 70%, have been widely recommended and practiced.[173] Improvements in anesthetic technique, however, have decreased the likelihood that circumstances favoring sickling will occur during anesthesia, leading some to question whether routine perioperative transfusion is necessary for all SCD patients.[174]

Four large studies have furnished data that bear on this question. A prospective but nonrandomized multicenter survey of 1079 surgical procedures in SCD patients revealed no advantage for transfused patients homozygous for HbS in the overall postoperative complication rates for low-risk (17.3% vs 18.6%) or moderate-risk (23.9% vs 18.6%) surgeries. Transfused patients with hemoglobin SC disease had a lower complication rate for moderate-risk surgeries (24.5% vs 42.9%). All patients having high-risk surgeries received perioperative transfusions.[175] A randomized study in 604 low- or moderate-risk surgeries compared an aggressive preoperative transfusion strategy (to increase HbA to ≥70%) to a more conservative strategy (to increase Hb to ≥10 g/dL).[176] No difference was found in the postoperative complication rates between the two groups except that complications of transfusion were more frequent in the aggressively transfused patients.

Two other studies followed up patients having similar surgeries who were either randomized preoperatively to the aggressive or conservative transfusion regimens previously described, or "registered" as preoperatively nontransfused or transfused. A study of 364 cholecystectomies (moderate-risk procedures) included 234 randomized patients and 134 registered patients, 37 of whom were nontransfused. The overall complication rate was 39%. Sickle cell–related events such as pain crisis and ACS were more frequent in the nontransfused group, but no other differences in outcome were apparent between the two randomized arms.[177] A study of 138 low- and moderate-risk orthopedic procedures included 74 randomized procedures and 64 "registered" procedures, 24 of which were done without preoperative transfusion. The overall rate of serious complications was 67%. The only significant difference in complication rate across the four groups was that ACS was more common in both the untransfused (21%) and aggressively transfused (21%) groups.[178]

These studies do not permit a definitive conclusion regarding the necessity of preoperative transfusion in low- and moderate-risk surgeries, but they do suggest that RCE to increase HbA to ≥70% is not warranted. For high-risk (intrathoracic or intracranial) surgeries, however, perioperative transfusion or RCE continues to be the standard of practice.

Pregnancy

Although most pregnancies in women with SCD have a satisfactory outcome, certain complications are more frequent. A recent survey comparing SCD and control pregnancies confirmed increased risks for spontaneous abortion, prematurity, low-birth-weight infants, and postpartum infection. The risks of hypertension and preeclampsia are not increased above controls, and the incidence of pain crisis is not increased above patient-specific baselines.[179–181]

The possibility that prophylactic transfusion, particularly in the third trimester, might improve the outcome of SCD pregnancies has been the subject of a number of uncontrolled surveys. Some of these have concluded that transfusion has a favorable effect.[182–185] One has recommended third-trimester prophylactic transfusion for all SCD pregnancies despite finding that this practice did not improve obstetric outcomes.[186]

A single prospective controlled trial has addressed this question. Seventy-two pregnant women with SCD were randomly assigned before week 28 of gestation to receive either prophylactic transfusion to increase Hb to 10 to 11 g/dL or selective transfusion only if Hb was less than 6 g/dL. The incidence of pain crisis was decreased in the prophylactic transfusion group, but no difference between the two arms was found for any other outcome.[187] Mindful of adverse effects of transfusion, these authors recommended it only for treatment of SCD-related complications, such as ACS, that had actually arisen in association with pregnancy.[188]

The precise role of RCE as a method of delivering transfusion therapy in this context has not been directly examined; however, several reports indicate that it can be carried out safely during pregnancy, even in the outpatient setting.[182,184,185,189,190]

Hepatopathy

A variety of liver problems can develop in patients with SCD, several of which arise as complications of transfusion. Iron overload is almost inevitable with long-term transfusion therapy; however, as mentioned earlier, its onset can be delayed by using RCE instead of simple transfusion. Acute and chronic viral hepatitis are other potential hazards that are theoretically more common with RCE because it requires more donor exposures than simple transfusion. Currently, however, the risk of viral hepatitis is quite low with either approach.[191]

Acute liver disease that is deemed to be a consequence of intrahepatic sickling may also occur. In some cases, it may be further complicated by intrahepatic cholestasis, leading to very high bilirubin levels, or by sequestration of a large volume of red cells in an engorged liver; both of these syndromes are potentially fatal.[191] Scattered case reports have suggested that exchange transfusion (ET) can reverse intrahepatic sickling.[192,193] RCE has been recommended for hepatic as well as splenic sequestration crisis on the theoretic grounds that it can increase HbA without increasing the hematocrit to a level that could become dangerously high if sequestered red cells were to be rapidly released back into the bloodstream.[191,194]

Malaria and Babesiosis

Malaria

Malaria is a mosquito-borne illness caused by several protozoal species of the genus *Plasmodium* that can parasitize red cells. The most severe infections are due to *P. falciparum*, which can infect circulating red cells of any age and therefore causes higher levels of parasitemia than other species that can infect only reticulocytes. Severe malaria with parasitemia greater than 5% can include cerebral, renal, and/or lung dysfunction as well as profound anemia and disseminated intravascular coagulation. Parasitized red cells swell and develop increased adherence to vascular endothelium; they may therefore contribute directly to organ failure via microvascular obstruction and ischemia. An alternative mechanism for tissue damage has been proposed that implicates high levels of cytokines, especially tumor necrosis factor-α (TNF-α) and interferon-γ (IFN-γ); however, these two mechanisms are not necessarily mutually exclusive.[195]

Most patients with malaria can be cured by antimicrobials such as chloroquine. Even *P. falciparum*, which is often chloroquine resistant, is usually sensitive to quinine, quinidine, or artemisinins.[196] In patients with severe or resistant disease and high levels of parasitemia, some form of ET has been used as a means to remove both the infectious agent and potentially obstructive red cells. The literature contains many case reports and small series describing patients who had a prompt decrease in parasitemia and concomitant clinical improvement after ET.[197–203] The only randomized study unfortunately had insufficient power to be meaningful.[204] In contrast, a meta-analysis of eight case-control studies encompassing 279 patients found no survival advantage for patients who received ET. However, the meta-analysis also concluded that exchanged patients were sicker than controls.[205]

Most patients in the aforementioned reports received manual whole-blood ET rather than automated RCE. Some authors contend that removal of TNF-α, IFN-γ, and/or other pro-inflammatory mediators in plasma may contribute to a beneficial effect from ET. If this is the case, it would be important because, although RCE will reduce parasitemia faster with less hemodynamic alteration, it would not be expected to deplete mediators of inflammation. Few data support these contentions, however,[206] and I deem it unlikely that low-molecular-weight cytokines with relatively short half-lives could be meaningfully depleted by the exchange of plasma inherent in ET. Additional treatment with TPE has been reported for this purpose[207] but is again deemed unlikely to produce therapeutically meaningful depletion.

Further studies of ET in malaria are clearly needed but are likely to be problematic. ET and RCE are reported most frequently from developed countries where safe donor blood is readily available and where most patients with malaria are travelers who have no underlying immunity. In contrast, the vast bulk of malaria occurs in underdeveloped areas where safe donor blood is often not available and where many individuals have partial immunity that influences disease outcome. Thus randomized studies in endemic areas would be challenging both to conduct and to interpret.[194] Nevertheless, based on current information, the World Health Organization recommends that ET be done for malaria, if safe blood is available, in patients with severe disease and parasitemia greater than 10%, and in any patient with more than 30% parasitemia.[208] Severe malaria has been rated a category III indication for RCE by ASFA[6] and AABB[7] (see Table 56–4).

Babesiosis

Babesiosis also is a protozoal red cell infection. It is endemic in wild and domesticated mammals in many parts of the world. *Babesia microti* infection occurs in deer, mice, and other animals in the northeastern and upper midwestern United States and can be transmitted to humans by tick bites.[209] Most cases in immunocompetent individuals are mild, and the incidence of immunity in endemic areas exceeds that of clinical disease, suggesting that subclinical cases are common. Severe disease with high fever, profound anemia, cardiorespiratory and/or renal failure, and coma may occur, however, and is more likely in immunodeficient or asplenic patients.[209]

Babesiosis usually responds to antimicrobials; however, reduction in parasitemia accompanied by clinical improvement has been reported after ET or RCE in several patients with severe, resistant disease.[210–213] Here also the question of mediator depletion as an extra therapeutic benefit of whole-blood ET has been raised in the absence of supporting data.[209] Controlled trials are lacking, but some authorities recommend ET or RCE for severe cases of babesiosis with more than 5% parasitemia.[209] Severe babesiosis is rated as a category III indication for RCE by ASFA[6] and AABB[7] (see Table 56–4).

REFERENCES

1. Burgstaler EA. Current apheresis instrumentation. In McLeod BC, Price TH, Weinstein R (eds). Apheresis: Principles and Practice, 2nd ed. Bethesda, Md., AABB Press, 2003, pp 95–130.
2. Hester J. Therapeutic cell depletion. In McLeod BC, Price TA, Weinstein R (eds). Apheresis: Principles and Practice, 2nd ed. Bethesda, Md., AABB Press, 2003, pp 183–194.
3. Schafer AI. Essential thrombocythemia and thrombocytosis. In Lichtman MA, Beutler E, Kipps TJ, Seligsohn U, et al (eds). Williams Hematology, 7th ed. New York, McGraw-Hill. 2006, pp1785–1794.
4. Greist A. The role of blood component removal in essential and reactive thrombocytosis. Ther Apheresis 2002;6:36–44.
5. Cortelazzo S, Finazzi G, Ruggieri M, et al. Hydroxyurea for patients with essential thrombocythemia and a high risk of thrombosis. N Engl J Med 1995;332:1132–1136.
6. McLeod BC. Clinical applications of therapeutic apheresis. J Clin Apheresis 2000;15:1–5.
7. Smith JW, Weinstein R, Hillyer KL for the AABB Hemapheresis Committee. Therapeutic apheresis: a summary of current indication categories endorsed by the AABB and the American Society for Apheresis. Transfusion 2003;43:820–822.
8. Karch J, Klippel J, Plotz O, et al. Lymphapheresis in rheumatoid arthritis: a randomized trial. Arthritis Rheumatism 1981;24:867–873.
9. Rose J, Klein H, Greenstein J, et al. Lymphocytapheresis in chronic progressive multiple sclerosis: results of a preliminary trial. Ann Neurol 1983;14:593–594.
10. Dau PC. Leukocytapheresis in inclusion body myositis. J Clin Apheresis 1987;3:167–170.
11. Miller FW, Leitman SF, Cronin ME, et al. Controlled trial of plasma exchange and leukapheresis in polymyositis and dermatomyositis. N Engl J Med 1992;326:1380–1384.
12. Bongiovanni MB, Katz RS, Tomaszewski JE, et al. Cytapheresis in a patient with Sezary syndrome. Transfusion 1981;21:332–334.
13. Decaro JH, Novoa FE, de Anda G, et al. Leukapheresis in a patient with Sézary syndrome. Vox Sang 1984;47:276–279.
14. Liesveld JL, Litchman MA, Acute myelogenous leukemia. In Lichtman MA, Beutler E, Kipps TJ, Seligsohn U, et al (eds). Williams Hematology, 7th ed. New York, McGraw-Hill. 2006, pp 1183–1236.
15. Lichtman MA, Liesveld JL. Chronic myelogenous leukemia and related disorders. In Lichtman MA, Beutler E, Kipps TJ, Seligsohn U, et al (eds). Williams Hematology, 7th ed. New York, McGraw-Hill, 2006, pp 1237–1294.
16. Freireich EJ, Thomas LB, Frei E III, et al. A distinctive type of intracerebral hemorrhage associated with blast crisis in patients with leukemia. Cancer 1960;13:146–150.
17. McKee C, Collins R. Intravascular leukocyte thrombi and aggregates as a cause of morbidity and mortality in leukemia. Medicine 1974;53:463–478.
18. Litchmann MA, Heal J, Rowe JM. Hyperleukocytic leukemia: rheological and clinical features and management. Baillieres Clin Hematol 1987;1:725–742.
19. Litchmann MA. Rheology of leukocytes, leukocyte suspensions and blood in leukemia. J Clin Invest 1973;52:350–358.
20. Steinberg MH, Charm SE. Effect of high concentration of leukocytes on whole blood viscosity. Blood 1971;38:299–301.
21. Harris AL. Leukostasis associated with blood transfusion in acute myeloid leukemia. Br Med J 1978;1:1169–1171.
22. Stucki A, Rivier AS, Gikic M, et al. Endothelial cell activation by myeloblasts: molecular mechanisms of leukostasis and leukemic cell dissemination. Blood 2001;97:2121–2129.
23. Reuss-Borst MA, Klein G, Waller HD, Muller CA. Differential expression of adhesion molecules in acute leukemia. Leukemia 1995;9:869–874.
24. Porcu P, Cripe LD, Ng EW, et al. Hyperleukocytic leukemias: a review of pathophysiology, clinical presentation and management. Leuk Lymphoma 2000;39:1–18.
25. Porcu P, Farag S, Marcucci G, et al. Leukocytoreduction for acute leukemia. Ther Apheresis 2002;6:15–23.
26. Soares FA, Magnani-Landell GA, de Miranda Cardoso MC. Pulmonary leukostasis without hyperleukocytosis: a clinicopathologic study of 16 cases. Am J Hematol 1992;40:28–32.
27. Dutcher JP, Schiffer CA, Wiernik PH. Hyperleukocytosis in adult acute non-lymphocytic leukemia: impact on remission rate and duration and survival. J Clin Oncol 1987;9:1364–1372.
28. Davidson MB, Thakkar S, Hix JK, et al. Pathophysiology, clinical consequences and treatment of tumor lysis syndrome. Am J Med 2004; 116:546–554.
29. Caplan SN, Coco FV, Berkman EM. Management of chronic myelocytic leukemia in pregnancy by cell pheresis. Transfusion 1978;18:120–124.
30. Porcu P, Danielson CF, Orazi A, et al. Therapeutic leukapheresis in hyperleucocytic leukaemias: lack of correlation between degree of cytoreduction and early mortality rate. Br J Haematol 1997;98:433–436.
31. Giles FJ, Shen Y, Kantarjian HM, et al. Leukapheresis reduces early mortality in patients with acute myeloid leukemia with high white cell counts but does not improve long-term survival. Leuk Lymphoma 2001;42:67–73.
32. Thiébaut A, Thomas X, Belhabri A, et al. Impact of pre-induction therapy leukapheresis on treatment outcome in adult acute myelogenous leukemia presenting with hyperleukocytosis. Ann Hematol 2000;79:501–506.
33. Foss FM. Photopheresis. In McLeod BC, Price TH, Weinstein R (eds). Apheresis: Principles and Practice, 2nd ed. Bethesda, Md., AABB Press, 2003, pp 623–642.
34. Edelson R, Berger C, Gasparro F, et al. Treatment of cutaneous T-cell lymphoma by extracorporeal photochemotherapy: preliminary results. N Engl J Med 1987;316:297–303.
35. Thomsen K, Hammer H, Molin L, Volden G. Retinoids plus PUVA (RePUVA) and PUVA in mycosis fungoides, plaque stage: a report from the Scandinavian mycosis fungoides group. Acta Derm Venereol 1989;20:416–428.
36. Heald PW, Perez MI, Christensen I, et al. Photopheresis therapy of cutaneous T-cell lymphoma: the Yale-New Haven hospital experience. Yale J Biol Med 1989;62:629–638.
37. Koh HK, et al: Extracorporeal photopheresis for the treatment of 34 patients with cutaneous T-cell lymphoma (CTCL). Soc Invest Dermatol 1994;43:54–60.
38. Zic JA, Stricklin GP, Greer JP, et al. Longterm follow-up of patients with cutaneous T-cell lymphoma treated with extra-corporeal photochemotherapy. J Am Acad Dermatol 1996;35:935–945.
39. Gottlieb SL, Wolfe JT, Fox FE, et al. Treatment of cutaneous T-cell lymphomas with extracorporeal photopheresis monotherapy and in combination with recombinant interferon alfa: a 10-year experience at a single institution. J Am Acad Dermatol 1996;35:946–957.
40. Duvic M, Hester JP, Lemak NA. Photopheresis therapy for cutaneous T-cell lymphoma. J Am Acad Dermatol 1996;35:573–579.
41. Vonderheid EC, Zhang Q, Lessin SR, et al. Use of serum soluble interleukin-2 receptor levels to monitor the progression of cutaneous T-cell lymphoma. J Am Acad Dermatol 1998;38:207–220.

42. Jiang SB, Dietz SB, Kim M, Lim HW. Extra-corporeal photochemotherapy for cutaneous T-cell lymphoma: a 9.7 year experience. Photoimmunol Photomed 1999;15:161–165.
43. Bisaccia E, Gonzalez J, Palangio M, et al. Extracorporeal photochemotherapy alone or with adjuvant therapy in the treatment of cutaneous T-cell lymphoma: a 9-year retrospective study at a single institution. J Am Acad Dermatol 2000;43:263–271.
44. Knobler R, Girardi M. Extracorporeal photochemoimmunotherapy in cutaneous T cell lymphoma. Ann N Y Acad Sci 2001;941:123–138.
45. Zic JA. The treatment of cutaneous T-cell lymphoma with photopheresis. Dermatol Ther 2003;16:337–346.
46. Bunn PA, Hoffman SJ, Norris D, et al. Systemic therapy of cutaneous T-cell lymphomas (mycosis fungoides and the Sézary syndrome). Ann Intern Med 1994;121:592–602.
47. Dall'Amico R, Messina C. Extracorporeal photochemotherapy for the treatment of graft-versus-host disease. Ther Apheresis 2002;6:296–304.
48. Kapoor N, Pellegrini AE, Copelan EA, et al. Psoralen plus ultraviolet A (PUVA) in the treatment of chronic graft-versus-host disease: preliminary experience in standard treatment resistant patients. Semin Hematol 1992;29:108–112.
49. Foss FM, Gorgun G, Miller KB. Extracorporeal photopheresis in chronic graft-versus-host disease. Bone Marrow Transplant 2002;29:719–725.
50. Girardi M, McNiff JM, Heald PW. Extracorporeal photochemotherapy in human and murine graft-versus-host disease. J Dermatol Science 1999;9:106–113.
51. Looks A, Fuchs D, Rulke D, et al. Successful treatment of acute graft versus host disease after bone marrow transplantation in a 16-year-old girl with extracorporeal photopheresis. Onkologie 1997;20:340–342.
52. Smith EP, Sniecinski I, Dagis AC, et al. Extracorporeal photochemotherapy for the treatment of drug-resistant graft-vs.-host disease. Biol Blood Marrow Transplant 1998;4:27–37.
53. Miller JL, Goodman SA, Stricklin GP, Lloyd EK. Extracorporeal photochemotherapy in the treatment of graft-versus-host disease: Abstract Book IBMTR/ABMTR Meeting Keystone Resort Colorado 1998:7a.
54. Besnier DP, Chabannes D, Mahe B, et al. Treatment of graft-versus-host disease by extracorporeal photochemotherapy. Transplantation 1997;64:49–54.
55. Richter HI, Stege H, Ruzicka T, et al. Extracorporeal photopheresis in the treatment of acute graft-versus-host disease. J Am Acad Dermatol 1997;36:787–789.
56. Salvaneschi L, Perotti C, Zecca M, et al. Extra-corporeal photochemotherapy for treatment of acute and chronic graft-versus-host disease in childhood. Transfusion 2001;41:1299–1305.
57. Greinix HT, Volc-Platzer B, Rabitsch W, et al. Successful use of extracorporeal photochemotherapy in the treatment of severe acute and chronic graft-versus-host disease. Blood 1998;92:3098–3104.
58. Greinix HT, Volc-Platzer B, Kalhs P, et al. Extracorporeal photochemotherapy in the treatment of severe steroid-refractory acute graft-versus-host disease: a pilot study. Blood 2000;96:2426–2431.
59. Sniecinski I, Smith B, Parker PM, Dagis A. Extracorporeal photochemotherapy for treatment of drug resistant chronic graft-versus-host disease. J Clin Aphresis 1995;10:51.
60. Balda BR, Kostantinow A, Starz H, et al. Extracorporeal photochemotherapy as an effective treatment modality in chronic graft-versus-host disease. J Eur Acad Dermatol Venereol 1996;7:155–162.
61. Owsianowski M, Gollnick H, Siegert W, et al. Successful treatment of chronic graft-versus-host disease with extracorporeal photopheresis. Bone Marrow Transplant 1994;14:845–848.
62. Child FJ, Ratnavel R, Watkins P, et al. Extracorporeal photopheresis (ECP) in the treatment of chronic graft-versus-host disease (GVHD). Bone Marrow Transplant 1999;23:881–887.
63. Dippel E, Goerdt S, Orfanos CE. Long-term extracorporeal photoimmunotherapy for treatment of chronic cutaneous graft-versus-host disease: observations in four patients. Dermatology 1999;198:370–374.
64. Schooneman F, Claise C. Treatment of graft-versus-host disease by photopheresis. Transfus Sci 1996;17:527–536.
65. Abhvankar S, Godder K, Chiang KY, et al. Extracorporeal photopheresis (ECP) with UVADEX for the treatment of chronic graft-versus-host disease (cGVHD). J Exp Hematol 1998;26:8.
66. Bolwell B, Fisleder A, Lichtin A, et al. Photopheresis in the treatment of chronic graft-versus-host disease (cGVHD). Blood 1990;76:529a.
67. Crovetti G, Carabelli A, Bertani E. Case report: Chronic graft-versus-host disease (cGVHD) treated with extracorporeal photochemotherapy (ECP). Florence, Italy: Sixth World Apheresis Association Meeting 137a, 1996.
68. Biagi E, Perseghin P, Buscemi F, et al. Effectiveness of extracorporeal photochemotherapy in treating refractory chronic graft-versus-host disease. Haematologica 2000;85:329–330.
69. Bloom EJ, Telang GH, Jegosothy BV. Extracorporeal photochemotherapy in the treatment of chronic graft-versus-host disease after allogenic bone marrow transplantation. American Society Clinical Oncology Annual Meeting 19–21, 1991.
70. Sniecinski I, Parker P, Dagis A, Smith B. Extracorporeal photopheresis (EP) is effective treatment for chronic refractory graft-versus-host disease. J Am Soc Hematol 1998;92:454.
71. Zic JA, Miller JL, Stricklin GP, King LE Jr. The North American experience with photopheresis. Ther Apheresis 1990;3:50–62.
72. Apisarnthanarax N, Duvic M, Donato M. Extracorporeal photopheresis in the management of steroid refractory or steroid dependent extensive cutaneous chronic graft-versus-host disease after allogenic stem cell transplantation: feasibility and results. Blood 1998;92:398a.
73. Horina JH, Mullegger RR, Horn S, et al. Photopheresis for renal allograft rejection [Letter]. Lancet 1995;346:61.
74. Sunder-Plassman G, Druml W, Steininger R, et al. Renal allograft rejection controlled by photopheresis [Letter]. Lancet 1995;346:506.
75. Dall'Amico R, Murer L, Montini G, et al. Successful treatment of recurrent rejection in renal transplant patients with photopheresis. J Am Soc Nephrol 1998;9:121–127.
76. Salerno CT, Park SJ, Kreykes NS, et al. Adjuvant treatment of refractory lung transplant rejection with extracorporeal photopheresis. J Thorac Cardiovasc Surg 1999;117:1063–1069.
77. Slovis BS, Loyd JE, King LE Jr. Photopheresis for chronic rejection of lung allografts. N Engl J Med 1995;332:962.
78. Villanueva J, Bhorade SM, Robinson JA, et al. Extracorporeal photopheresis for the treatment of lung allograft rejection. Ann Transplant 2000;5:44–47.
79. O'Hagan AR, Stillwell PC, Arroliga A, Koo A. Photopheresis in the treatment of refractory bronchiolitis obliterans complicating lung transplantation. Chest 1999;115:1459–1462.
80. Andreu G, Achkar A, Couetil JP, et al. Extracorporeal photochemotherapy treatment for acute lung rejection episode. J Heart Lung Transplant 1995;14:793–796.
81. Constanzo-Nordin MR, McManus BM, Wilson JE, et al. Efficacy of photopheresis in the rescue therapy of acute cellular rejection in human heart allografts: a preliminary clinical and immunopathologic report. Transplant Proc 1993;25:881–883.
82. Costanzo-Nordin MR, Hubbell EA, O'Sullivan EJ, et al. Photopheresis versus corticosteroids in the therapy of heart transplant rejection: preliminary clinical report. Circulation 1992;86:242–250.
83. Lloveras JJ, Escourrou G, Delisle MB, et al. Evolution of untreated mild rejection in heart transplant recipients. J Heart Lung Transplant 1992;11:751–756.
84. Barr ML, Meiser BM, Eisen HJ, et al. Photopheresis for the prevention of rejection in cardiac transplantation: photopheresis Transplantation Study Group. N Engl J Med 1998;339:1744–1751.
85. Di Spaltro FX, Cottrill C, Cahill C, et al. Extra-corporeal photochemotherapy in progressive systemic sclerosis. Int J Dermatol 1993;32: 417–421.
86. Knobler RM, Graninger W, Lindmaier A, et al. Extracorporeal photochemotherapy for the treatment of systemic lupus erythematosus: a pilot study. Arthritis Rheum 1992;35:319–324.
87. Rook AH, Jegasothy BV, Heald P, et al. Extracorporeal photochemotherapy for drug-resistant pemphigus vulgaris. Ann Intern Med 1990;112:303–305.
88. Malawista SE, Trock D, Edelson RL. Photopheresis for rheumatoid arthritis. Ann N Y Acad Sci 1991;636:217–226.
89. Wilfert H, Honigsmann H, Steiner G, et al. Treatment of psoriatic arthritis by extracorporeal photochemotherapy. Br J Dermatol 1990;122:225–232.
90. Fries JF, Seibold JR, Medsger TA Jr. Photopheresis for scleroderma? No! J Rheumatol 1992;19:1011–1013.
91. Edelson RL. Cutaneous T-cell lymphoma: the helping hand of dendritic cells. Ann N Y Acad Sci 2001;941:1–11.
92. Rook AH, Suchin KR, Kao DM, et al. Photopheresis: Clinical applications and mechanism of action. J Invest Dermatol Symp Proc 1999; 4:85–90.
93. Fimiani M, Di Renzo M, Rubegni P. Mechanism of action of extracorporeal photochemotherapy in chronic graft-versus-host disease. Br J Dermatol 2004;150:1055–1060.
94. French LE, Lessin SR, Kathakali A, et al. Identification of clonal T cells in the blood of patients with systemic sclerosis. Arch Dermatol 2001;137:1309–1313.
95. Tokura Y, Seo N, Yagi H, et al. Treatment of T lymphocytes with 8-methoxypsoralen plus ultraviolet A induces transient but biologically active Th1-skewing cytokine production. J Invest Dermatol 1999;113:202–208.

96. Alcindor T, Gorgun G, Miller KB, et al. Immunomodulatory effects of extracorporeal photochemotherapy in patients with extensive chronic graft-versus-host disease. Blood 2001;98:1622–1625.
97. Kessinger A. Clinical features of autologous and allogeneic peripheral blood progenitor cell transplantation. In McLeod BC, Price TH, Weinstein R (eds). Apheresis: Principles and practice, 2nd ed. Bethesda, Md., AABB Press, 2003, pp 493–502.
98. Burt RK, Slavin S, Burns WH, Marmont AM. Induction of tolerance in autoimmune diseases by hematopoietic stem cell transplantation: getting closer to a cure? Int J Hematol 2002;76(Suppl 1):226–247.
99. Richman CM, Weiner RS, Yankee RS. Increase in circulating stem cells following chemotherapy in man. Blood 1976;47:1031–1039.
100. To LB, Haylock DN, Kimber RJ, Juttner CAL. High levels of circulating haematopoietic stem cells in very early remission from acute non-lymphoblastic leukaemia and their collection and cryopreservation. Br J Haematol 1984;58:399–410.
101. Duhren U, Villeval J-L, Boyd J, et al. Effects of recombinant human granulocyte colony-stimulating factor on hematopoietic progenitor cells in cancer patients. Blood 1988;72:2074–2081.
102. Tjonnfjord GE, Steen R, Evensen SA, et al. Characterization of CD34+ peripheral blood cells from healthy adults mobilized by recombinant human granulocyte colony-stimulating factor. Blood 1994;84:2795–2801.
103. Haas R, Ho AD, Bredthauer U, et al. Successful autologous transplantation of blood stem cells mobilized with recombinant human granulocyte-macrophage colony-stimulating factor. Exp Hematol 1990;18:94–98.
104. Herrman F, Brugger W, Kanz L, Mertelsmann R. In-vivo biology and therapeutic potential of hematopoietic growth factors and circulating progenitor cells. Semin Oncol 1992;19:422–431.
105. Antman K, Griffin J, Elias A, et al. Effect of recombinant human granulocyte-macrophage colony-stimulating factor on chemotherapy-induced myelosuppression. N Engl J Med 1988;319:593–598.
106. Ravagnani F, Siena S, Bregni M, et al. Large-scale collection of circulating hematopoietic progenitors in cancer patients treated with high-dose cyclophosphamide and recombinant human GM-CSF. Eur J Cancer 1990;26:562–564.
107. Mechanic SA, Krause D, Proytcheva MA, Snyder EL. Mobilization and collection of peripheral blood progenitor cells. In McLeod BC, Price TH, Weinstein R (eds). Apheresis: Principles and Practice, 2nd ed. Bethesda, Md., AABB Press, 2003, pp 503–530.
108. McLeod BC, Price TH, Owen H, et al. Frequency of immediate adverse effects associated with therapeutic apheresis. Transfusion 1999;39: 282–288.
109. Bolan CD, Cecco SA, Wesley RA, et al. Controlled study of citrate effects and response to IV calcium administration during allogeneic peripheral blood progenitor cell donation. Transfusion 2002;42:935–946.
110. Meagher RC. Peripheral blood progenitor cell graft engineering. In McLeod BC, Price TH, Weinstein R (eds). Apheresis:Principles and Practice, 2nd ed. Bethesda, Md., AABB Press, 2003, pp 545–563.
111. Brenner MK, Rill DR, Moen RC, et al. Gene marking and autologous bone marrow transplantation. Ann NY Acad Sci 1994;716:204–214.
112. Ribas A, Butterfield LH, Glaspy JA, Economou JS. Current developments in cancer vaccines and cellular immunotherapy. J Clin Oncol 2003;21:2415–2432.
113. Klein HG. Cellular gene therapy. In McLeod BC, Price TH, Weinstein R (eds). Apheresis: Principles and Practice, 2nd ed. Bethesda, Md., AABB Press, 2003, pp 643–656.
114. Cesana M, Mandelli C, Tiribelli C, et al. Concomitant primary hemochromatosis and B-thalassemia trait: iron depletion by erythrocytapheresis and desferrioxamine. Am J Gastroenterol 1989;84:150–152.
115. Kaboth U, Rumph KW, Liersch T, et al. Advantages of isovolemic large-volume erythrocytapheresis as a rapidly effective and long-lasting treatment modality for red blood cell depletion in patients with polycythemia vera. Ther Apheresis 1997;1:131–134.
116. McLeod BC, Reed SR, Viernes AV, Valentino L. Rapid red cell transfusion by apheresis. J Clin Apheresis 1994;9:142–146.
117. Myers L, Paranjape G, Anderson C, et al. Isovolemic hemodilution-red blood cell exchange is superior to red blood cell exchange in the management of sickle cell disease in patients on hypertransfusion programs following cerebrovascular accident. Blood 2002;102:764a.
118. Kleinman SH, Goldfinger D. Erythrocytapheresis in sickle cell disease. In MacPherson JL, Kasprisin DO (eds). Therapeutic Hemapheresis, Vol 2. Boca Raton, Fla., CRC Press, 1985, pp 129–142.
119. Danielson CFM. The role of red blood cell exchange transfusion in the treatment and prevention of complications of sickle cell disease. Ther Apheresis 2002;6:24–31.
120. Kim HC, Dugan NP, Silber JH, et al. Erythrocytapheresis therapy to reduce iron overload in chronically transfused patients with sickle cell disease. Blood 1994;83:1136–1142.
121. Adams DM, Schultz WH, Ware RE, Kinney TR. Erythrocytapheresis can reduce iron overload and prevent the need for chelation therapy in chronically transfused pediatric patients. J Pediatr Hematol Oncol 1996;18:46–50.
122. Hoppe C. Defining stroke risk in children with sickle cell anemia. Br J Haematol 2004;128:751–766.
123. Sarnaik SA, Lusher JM. Neurological complications of sickle cell anemia. Am J Pediatr Hematol/Oncol 1982;4:386–394.
124. Balkaran B, Char G, Morris JS, et al. Stroke in a cohort of patients with sickle cell disease. J Pediatr 1992;120:360–366.
125. Powars D, Wilson B, Imbus C, et al. The natural history of stroke in sickle cell disease. Am J Med 1978;65:461–471.
126. Miller ST, Macklin EA, Pegelow CH, et al. Silent infarction as a risk factor for overt stroke in children with sickle cell anemia: a report from the Cooperative Study of Sickle Cell Disease. J Pediatr 2001;139:385–390.
127. Adams R, McKie V, Nichols F, et al. The use of transcranial ultrasonography to predict stroke in sickle cell disease. N Engl J Med 1992; 326:605–610.
128. Adams RJ, McKie VC, Hsu L, et al. Prevention of a first stroke by transfusions in children with sickle cell anemia and abnormal results on transcranial Doppler ultrasonography. N Engl J Med 1998;339:5–11.
129. Russell MO, Goldberg HI, Hodson A, et al. Effect of transfusion therapy on arteriographic abnormalities and on recurrence of stroke in sickle cell disease. Blood 1984;63:162–169.
130. Pegelow CH, Adams RJ, McKie V, et al. Risk of recurrent stroke in patients with sickle cell disease treated with erythrocyte transfusions. J Pediatr 1995;126:896–899.
131. Pegelow CH, Wang W, Granger S, et al. Silent infarcts in children with sickle cell anemia and abnormal cerebral artery velocity. Arch Neurol 2001;58:2017–2021.
132. Wilimas J, Goff JR, Anderson HR, et al. Efficacy of transfusion therapy for one to two years in patients with sickle cell disease and cerebrovascular accidents. J Pediatr 1980;96:205–208.
133. Wang W, Kovnar EH, Tonkin IL, et al. High risk of recurrent stroke after discontinuance of five to twelve years of transfusion therapy in patients with sickle cell disease. J Pediatr 1991;118:377–382.
134. http://nhlbi.nih.gov/health/prof/blood/sickle/clinical-alert-scd.htm.
135. Cohen AR, Martin MB, Silber JH, et al. A modified program for prevention of stroke in sickle cell disease. Blood 1992;79:1657–1661.
136. Charache S, Lubin B, Reid CD. Management and Therapy of Sickle Cell Disease. Washington, D.C., Public Health Service, US Dept of Health and Human Services, 1992, p 22. NIH publication 92–2117.
137. Rana S, Houston PE, Surana N, et al. Discontinuation of long-term transfusion therapy in patients with sickle cell disease and stroke. J Pediatr 1997;131:757–760.
138. Powars DR. Management of cerebral vasculopathy in children with sickle cell anemia. Br J Haematol 2000;108:666–678.
139. Adams RJ. Stroke prevention and treatment in sickle cell disease. Arch Neurol 2001;58:565–568.
140. Riddington C, Wang W. Blood transfusion for preventing stroke in people with sickle cell disease. Cochrane Library/Database of Systematic Reviews 2005;2:CD003146.
141. Vichinsky EP, Styles LA, Colangelo LH, et al. Acute chest syndrome in sickle cell disease: clinical presentation and course: The Cooperative Study of Sickle Cell Disease. Blood 1997;89:1787–1792.
142. Vichinsky EP, Neumayr LD, Earles AN, et al. Causes and outcomes of the acute chest syndrome in sickle cell disease. N Engl J Med 2000; 342:1855–1865.
143. Castro O. Systemic fat embolism and pulmonary hypertension in sickle cell disease. Hematol Oncol Clin North Am 1996;10:1289–1303.
144. Vichinsky E, Styles L. Sickle cell disease: pulmonary complications. Hematol Oncol Clin North Am 1997;10:1275–1287.
145. Gladwin MT, Schechter AN, Shelhamer JH, et al. The acute chest syndrome in sickle cell disease: possible role of nitric oxide in its pathophysiology and treatment. Am J Respir Crit Care Med 1999; 159:1368–1376.
146. Hassell KL, Deutsch JC, Kolhouse JF, et al. Elevated serum levels of free fatty acid in sickle cell patients with acute chest syndrome and multi-organ failure syndrome. Blood 1994;84:1633A.
147. Platt OS. Sickle cell anemia as an inflammatory disease. J Clin Invest 2000;106:337–338.
148. Hebbel RP. Adhesive interactions of sickle erythrocytes with endothelium. J Clin Invest 1997;100:83–86.
149. Setty BN, Stuart MJ. Vascular cell adhesion molecule-1 is involved in mediating hypoxia-induced sickle red cell adherence to endothelium: Potential role in sickle cell disease. Blood 1996;88:2311–2320.
150. Siddique AK, Ahmed S. Pulmonary manifestations of sickle cell disease. Postgrad Med J 2003;79:384–390.

151. Miller ST, Wright E, Abboud M, et al. Impact of chronic transfusion on incidence of pain and acute chest syndrome during the stroke prevention trial (STOP) in sickle-cell anemia. J Pediatr 2001;139:785–789.
152. Vichinsky EP. Pulmonary hypertension in sickle cell disease. N Engl J Med 2004;350:857–859.
153. Gladwin MT, Sachdev V, Jison ML. Pulmonary hypertension as a risk factor for death in patients with sickle cell disease. N Engl J Med 2004;350:886–895.
154. Mantadakis E, Cavender JD, Rogers ZR, et al. Prevalence of priapism in children and adolescents with sickle cell anemia. J Pediatr Hematol/Oncol 1999;21:518–522.
155. Mykulak DJ, Glassberg KI. Impotence following childhood priapism. J Urol 1990;144:134–135.
156. Chakrabarty A, Upadhyay J, Dhabuwala CB, et al. Priapism associated with sickle cell hemoglobinopathy in children: long-term effects on potency. J Urol 1995;155:1419–1423.
157. Hamre MR, Harmon EP, Kirkpatrick DV, et al. Priapism as a complication of sickle cell disease. J Urol 1991;145:1–5.
158. Cavender JD, Ewalt D, Rogers Z, et al. Treatment of severe priapism in young patients with sickle cell disease with oral or intrapenile adrenergic agonists, abstracted. Proceedings of the 20th Annual Meeting of the National Sickle Cell Disease program 1995:147.
159. Powars DR, Johnson CS. Priapism. Hematol/Oncol Clinic N Am 1996;10:1363–1372.
160. Rifkind S, Waisman J, Thompson R, Goldfinger D. RBC exchange for priapism. JAMA 1979;242:2317–2318.
161. Kleinman SH, Hurvitz CG, Goldfinger D. Use of erythrocytapheresis in the treatment of patients with sickle cell anemia. J Clin Apheresis 1984;2:170–176.
162. Walker EM, Mitchum EN, Rous SN, et al. Automated erythrocytapheresis for relief of priapism in sickle cell hemoglobinopathies. J Urol 1983;130:912–916.
163. Talacki CA, Ballas SK. Modified method of exchange transfusion in sickle cell disease. J Clin Apheresis 1990;5:183–187.
164. Kevy S, Fosburg M. Therapeutic apheresis in childhood. J Clin Apheresis 1990;5:87–90.
165. McCarthy LJ, Vattuone J, Weidner J, et al. Do automated red cell exchanges relieve priapism in patients with sickle cell anemia? Ther Apheresis 2000;4:256–258.
166. Siegel JR, Rich MA, Brock WA. Association of sickle cell disease, priapism, exchange transfusion and neurological events: ASPEN syndrome. J Urol 1993;150:1480–1482.
167. Platt OS, Brambilla DJ, Rosse WF, et al. Mortality in sickle cell disease: Life expectancy and risk factors for early death. N Engl J Med 1994;330:1639–1644.
168. Parfrey NA, Moore W, Hutchins GM. Is pain crisis a cause of death in sickle cell disease? Am J Clin Pathol 1985;84:209–212.
169. Hassell KL, Eckman JR, Lane PA. Acute multiorgan failure syndrome: a potentially catastrophic complication of severe sickle cell pain episodes. Am J Med 1994;96:155–162.
170. Styles LA, Vichinsky E. Effects of a long-term transfusion regimen on sickle cell-related illnesses. J Pediatr 1994;125:909–911.
171. Holzmann L, Finn H, Lichtman HC, Harmel MH. Anesthesia in patients with sickle cell disease: a review of 112 cases. Anesth Analg 1969;48:566–572.
172. Spigelman A, Warden MJ. Surgery in patients with sickle cell disease. Arch Surg 1972;104:761–764.
173. U.S. Department of Health and Human Services. Management and Therapy of Sickle Cell Disease. NIH Publication No. 84–2117. Washington, D.C., National Institutes of Health, September 1984.
174. Griffin TC, Buchanan GR. Elective surgery in children with sickle cell disease without preoperative blood transfusion. J Pediatr Surg 1993; 28:681–685.
175. Koshy M, Weiner SJ, Miller ST, et al. Surgery and anesthesia in sickle cell disease. Blood 1995;86:3676–3684.
176. Vichinsky EP, Haberkern CM, Neumayr L, et al. A comparison of conservative and aggressive transfusion regimens in the perioperative management of sickle cell disease. N Engl J Med 1995;333:206–213.
177. Haberkern CM, Neumayr L, Orringer EP, et al. Cholecystectomy in sickle cell anemia patients: Perioperative outcome in 364 cases from the National Perioperative Transfusion Study. Blood 1997;89:1533–1542.
178. Vichinsky EP, Neumayr LD, Haberkern C, et al. The perioperative complication rate of orthopedic surgery in sickle cell disease: report of the National Sickle Cell Surgery Study Group. Am J Hematol 1999;62:129–138.
179. Serjeant GR, Loy LL, Crowther M, et al. Outcome of pregnancy in homozygous sickle cell disease. Obstet Gynecol 2004;103:1278–1285.
180. Sun PM, Wilburn W, Raynor D, Jamieson D. Sickle cell disease in pregnancy: twenty years of experience at Grady Memorial Hospital, Atlanta, Georgia. Am J Obstet Gynecol 2001;184:1127–1130.
181. Smith JA, Espeland M, Bellvue R, et al. Pregnancy in sickle cell disease: experience of the cooperative study of sickle cell disease. Obstet Gynecol 1996;87:199–204.
182. Cunningham G, Pritchard JA, Mason R. Pregnancy and sickle cell hemoglobinopathies: results with and without prophylactic transfusions. Obstet Gynecol 1983;62:419–424.
183. Tuck SM, James CE, Brewster EM, et al. Prophylactic blood transfusion in maternal sickle cell syndromes. Br J Obstet Gynecol 1987;94: 121–125.
184. Morrison JC, Schneider JM, Whybrew WD, et al. Prophylactic transfusions in pregnant patients with sickle hemoglobinopathies: benefit versus risk. Obstet Gynecol 1980;56:274–280.
185. Morrison JC, Douvas SG, Martin JM, et al. Erythrocytapheresis in pregnant patients with sickle hemoglobinopathies. Am J Obstet Gynecol 1984;149:912–914.
186. Howard RJ, Tuck SM, Pearson TC. Pregnancy in sickle cell disease in the UK: results of a multicenter survey of the effect of prophylactic blood transfusion on maternal and fetal outcome. Br J Obstet Gynecol 1995;102:947–951.
187. Koshy M, Burd L, Wallace D, et al. Prophylactic red-cell transfusions in pregnant patients with sickle cell disease. N Engl J Med 1988;319: 1447–1452.
188. Koshy M, Chisum D, Burd L, et al. Management of sickle cell anemia and pregnancy. J Clin Apheresis 1991;6:230–233.
189. Janes SL, Pocock M, Bishop E, Bevan D. Automated red cell exchange in sickle cell disease. Br J Haematol 1997;97:256–258.
190. Morrison JC, Morrison FS, Floyd RC, et al. Use of continuous flow erythrocytapheresis in pregnant patients with sickle cell disease. J Clin Apheresis 1991;6:224–229.
191. Banerjee S, Owen C, Chopra S. Sickle cell hepatopathy. Hepatology 2001;33:1021–1028.
192. Sheehy TW, Low DE, Wade BH. Exchange transfusion for sickle cell intrahepatic cholestasis. Arch Intern Med 1980;140:1364–1365.
193. Rossof AH, McLeod BC, Holmes AW, Fried W. Intrahepatic sickling crises in hemoglobin SC disease; management by partial exchange transfusion. Plasma Ther 1981;2:7–12.
194. Pepkowitz S. Red cell exchange and other therapeutic alterations of red cell mass. In McLeod BC, Price TH, Weinstein R (eds). Apheresis: Principles and Practice, 2nd ed. Bethesda, Md., AABB Press, 2003, pp 411–435.
195. Powell VI, Grima K. Exchange transfusion for malaria and Babesia infection. Transfus Med Rev 2002;16:239–250.
196. Singhal T. Management of severe malaria. Indian J Pediatr 2004;71: 81–88.
197. Gyr K, Speck B, Ritz R, et al. Cerebral tropical malaria with blackwater fever: a current diagnostic and therapeutic problem. Schweiz Med Wochenschr 1974;104:1628–1630.
198. Alfandari S, Dixmier G, Guery B, et al. Exchange transfusion for severe malaria, Infection 2001;29:96–97.
299. Phillips P, Nantel S, Benny WB. Exchange transfusion as an adjunct to the treatment of severe falciparum malaria: case report and review. Rev Infect Dis 1990;12:1100–1108.
200. Macallan DC, Pocock M, Robinson GT, et al. Red cell exchange, erythrocytapheresis, in the treatment of malaria with high parasitaemia in returning travelers. Trans R Soc Trop Med Hyg 2000;94:353–356.
201. Mordmüller B, Kremsner PG. Hyperparasitemia and blood exchange transfusion for treatment of children with falciparum malaria. Clin Infect Dis 1998;26:850–852.
202. Vachon F, Wolff M, Lebras J. Exchange transfusion as an adjunct to the treatment of severe falciparum malaria. Clin Infect Dis 1992;14: 1269–1270.
203. Weir EG, King KE, Ness PM, et al. Automated RBC exchange transfusion: Treatment for cerebral malaria. Transfusion 2000;40:702–707.
204. Saddler M, Barry M, Ternouth I, et al. Treatment of severe malaria by exchange transfusion [Letter]. N Engl J Med 1990;322:58.
205. Riddle MS, Jackson JL, Sanders JW, Blazes DL. Exchange transfusion as an adjunct therapy in severe Plasmodium falciparum malaria: a meta-analysis. Clin Infect Dis 2002;34:1192–1198.
206. Kumar S, Karnad D, Vaingankar J, et al. Serum tumor necrosis factor and levels in severe malaria: effect of partial exchange transfusion. Intensive Care Med 2003;29:1857–1858.
207. Lercari G, Paganini G, Malfanti L, et al. Apheresis for severe malaria complicated by cerebral malaria, acute respiratory distress syndrome, acute renal failure and disseminated intravascular coagulation. J Clin Apheresis 1992;7:93–96.

208. World Health Organization, Communicable Diseases Cluster. Severe falciparum malaria. Trans R Soc Trop Med Hyg 2000;94(Suppl 1):S1–S90.
209. Krause PJ. Babesiosis diagnosis and treatment. Vector Borne Zoonotic Dis 2003;3:45–51.
210. Cahill KM, Benach JL, Reich LM, et al. Red cell exchange: treatment of babesiosis in a splenectomized patient. Transfusion 1981;21:193–198.
211. Machtinger L, Telford SR III, Inducil C, et al. Treatment of babesiosis by red blood cell exchange in an HIV-positive, splenectomized patient. J Clin Apheresis 1993;8:78–81.
212. Bonoan JT, Johnson DH, Cunha BA. Life-threatening babesiosis in an asplenic patient: treatment with exchange transfusion, azithromycin, and atovaquone. Heart Lung 1998;27:424–428.
213. Dorman ME, Cannon SR, Telford SR III, et al. Fulminant babesiosis treated with clindamycin, quinine, and whole blood exchange transfusion. Transfusion 2000;40:375–380.

D. Cellular Therapies and Tissue Banking

Chapter 57

The Role of Transfusion Medicine in Cellular Therapies

Simon Mantha • Edward L. Snyder

Over the past 2 decades, blood bank and transfusion medicine specialists and practitioners have been called on to expand their traditional roles of collection, processing, storing, and administering blood components derived from human whole blood or via apheresis, to the manipulation, processing, storage, and administration of other human cell and plasma-based therapeutic elements, and to assisting the scientists and clinicians involved with these concepts or procedures. Thus the field of "blood banking" has evolved into "transfusion medicine and cellular therapies." Perhaps an even broader application of transfusion medicine and requiring expertise in collection, manufacture, processing, storage, and administration, along with its increasing regulation, is the addition of the hospital tissue-banking function described in the final chapter of this text. Thus, what has only recently come to be called "transfusion medicine and cellular therapies" is now undergoing additional definition and falling under the abbreviation "HCT/P" for "Human Cellular and Tissue-Based Products." Indeed, those framing the mission statement for the American Association of Blood Banks (AABB) adopted the terminology of "transfusion medicine and cellular and related biological therapies" to cover the continually evolving arena in which the transfusion medicine practitioner is found. It is the cellular and related biologic therapies and the HCT/Ps that are the subject of this section of this textbook. This chapter provides an overview of the role of transfusion medicine in cellular therapies, with subsequent chapters providing more detail on peripheral blood, bone marrow, umbilical cord blood progenitor cells, mononuclear cell and related preparations, and tissue banking in the hospital setting.

ORIGINS OF "BLOOD BANKING"

Blood banks, initially and traditionally, have been involved in the collection, storage, and use of blood products containing mature, end-stage cellular blood elements with no potential for further mitosis or expansion, including red blood cells, platelets, and granulocytes. Red blood cells were the first cellular constituent of human blood for which standardized, reliable methods of collection, storage, and administration were established. Instrumental to the ability to transfuse red blood cells safely was the discovery of the ABO system by Landsteiner in 1901.[1] Then, the use of sodium citrate as an anticoagulant, pioneered by Albert Hustin in 1914, and the development of refrigerated storage by Richard Weil allowed the creation of a "blood depot" by Oswald Hope Robertson in Great Britain during World War I.[2] By 1940, the first Blood Bank had been established in the United States by Bernard Fantus in Chicago.[3] Eventually procedures were developed to separate whole blood into its different components, so that red blood cells, platelets, plasma, and its various fractions could be stored and administered individually.

BONE MARROW TRANSPLANTATION

The First Years of Bone Marrow Transplantation

Bone marrow transplantation (BMT) inaugurated the era of modern cellular therapy, in which the cells transferred to the recipient engraft and divide in vivo, thus generating long-term therapeutic effects.[4] Initially, the role of transfusion medicine in BMT was basically to support the transplant procedure by providing the patient with appropriate red blood cells and platelets via transfusion. Minimal if any manipulation of the stem cell products was done by the Blood Bank, as was seen in E.E. Osgood's report of an attempt to treat aplastic anemia with injections of crude marrow extracts.[5]

By 1960, Dr. E. Donnall Thomas[6] initiated trials on dogs before attempting bone marrow transplantation in humans, by using intravenous infusion of allogeneic donor bone marrow aspirated from the iliac crest and filtered to remove aggregates and fat. In many instances, the preparative regimen was minimal, especially in patients treated for aplastic anemia. Initial procedures almost always resulted in death, either from lack of engraftment or "secondary disease," the entity that would be later referred to as graft-versus-host disease (GVHD).[7] The only successful procedures were those in which the donor and the recipient were identical twins. In those syngeneic transplants, the two individuals shared the same cellular antigens, and histoincompatibility was not an issue. Consequently, clinical interest in bone marrow transplantation decreased after 1962, when it became clear that a better understanding of the immune processes involved would be necessary before its more widespread application.

Such advances would come in the early 1970s, with elucidation of the physiologic role of the human leukocyte antigen (HLA) system.[8–11] Initial demonstration of inherited determinants that affected the tolerance of transplanted allogeneic tumors in mice dates back to 1916.[12] Twenty years later, Gorer[13,14] identified the murine major histocompatibility complex (MHC). The human equivalent to the mouse MHC was discovered independently in the form of the HLA system, when it was found that the sera of some multiparous women and blood donors contained agglutinating antibodies against allogeneic leukocytes.[15–17] This led to the identification of type I HLA antigens. Discovery of the type II HLA allelic group occurred with the advent of the mixed lymphocyte culture (MLC) technique. Advances in molecular biology in the 1980s allowed localization of the genomic sequences involved and provided a detailed knowledge of the amino acid sequences they encode.[18] This would prove instrumental in improving the quality of matches for patients undergoing allogeneic stem cell transplant, thus helping to decrease the morbidity and mortality associated with GVHD.[19]

The immune attack mounted by the immunocompetent donor lymphocytes against the recipient's cells was eventually found to be a significant contributor to the long-term remissions observed in some hematologic malignancies, and this phenomenon was named the graft versus leukemia/lymphoma effect (GVL). However, to date, induction of GVL often occurs in parallel with the untoward effects of GVHD. Whereas immunosuppressive agents have been administered to patients to control acute GVHD,[20] chronic GVHD is less responsive, and still no effective treatment exists for this devastating complication.[21]

Refining the Transplantation Process

The stage for the involvement of transfusion medicine in the collection of hematopoietic stem cells (HSCs) was set by the coming together of three events: the development of apheresis technology, the identification of the CD34 antigen as a marker of early progenitors, and the identification and synthesis of granulocyte colony–stimulating factor (G-CSF) and granulocyte-macrophage CSF (GM-CSF).

Leukapheresis

Leukapheresis had initially been designed as a palliative treatment for leukemia by decreasing the disease burden, with only limited efficacy.[22] In the beginning, patients with chronic myelogenous leukemia were treated with leukapheresis. Later, this technique was used as a treatment modality for hyperleukocytic acute myeloid leukemia, with published reports confirming the beneficial effects of cytoreduction on cerebral leukostasis.[23] In the latter condition, the efficiency of cell removal is higher because of cell-density considerations. Finally, leukapheresis has been used to collect granulocytes to transfuse into neutropenic patients with bacterial or fungal infections. Such colonization by opportunistic infections is a common and often lethal complication of myeloablative chemotherapy. Unfortunately, to this date, no documentation of a survival benefit is attributable to granulocyte transfusion, probably because of the low cell doses used in most published studies. This might change with new clinical trials using G-CSF–mobilized neutrophils.[24]

Because it had been shown that humans have small amounts of circulating hematopoietic progenitors at any one time, the idea of processing large volumes of peripheral blood for isolation of the mononuclear cell fraction emerged as an alternative to bone marrow aspiration in the operating room.[25] Early efforts at peripheral blood stem cell harvest from an unstimulated allogeneic donor yielded products that failed to engraft, probably because of an insufficient number of cells collected.[26] Later attempts by Dr. Ann Kessinger[27,28] at the University of Nebraska, using multiple apheresis sessions in steady-state donors, were more successful. It had been observed, however, that 2 weeks after chemotherapy, the number of hematopoietic progenitors in the peripheral blood more than doubled.[29] The exact mechanism by which this occurred was not well understood, and the term *mobilization* was used to describe the exit of cells from the marrow and into the blood stream. This had the potential to allow completion of the collection process in a shorter time.

An unexpected benefit, however, was that for the same amount of early progenitor cells infused, peripheral blood–derived products elicited a faster engraftment of neutrophils and platelets.[30] A possible explanation for that effect is that a significant increase in more committed progenitors is observed in the peripheral blood of patients immediately after chemotherapy.[31] Those cells, once transplanted, are thought to take less time to generate mature neutrophils than do the pluripotent stem cells in the bone marrow, which are less differentiated and take longer to mature. Shortening the duration of the nadir for both granulocytes and platelets is a major concern in HSC transplant, as most early complications occur in the vulnerable period when the absolute neutrophil count is less than 500 cells/μL and the platelet count is less than 20,000 cells/μL. Of note, apheresis products contain more lymphocytes than do those derived from marrow. However, they do not seem to cause significantly more GVHD, and their use in hematologic malignancies might be associated with a better disease-free survival.[32]

The transfusion medicine service performs apheresis in most United States medical centers where this therapeutic modality is available. It follows stringent regulations that determine how the procedures are done and who can perform them (i.e., level of training and supervision). The blood bank is therefore well suited to be in charge of the peripheral blood stem all harvest process, as it is basically a variant of leukapheresis. Additionally, because processing and storage of the product is usually also performed in the blood bank, the whole sequence from harvest to delivery can be kept under the supervision of one entity, which greatly facilitates quality control.

Refinements in the apheresis techniques also opened the door to donor lymphocyte infusions (DLIs), a new application designed to harness the therapeutic effects of GVL without going through conditioning of the patient and aspiration of marrow from the donor. Individuals who had donated stem cells were asked to provide lymphocytes to the recipient whose disease had relapsed. This proved to be of particular benefit in chronic myeloid leukemia, in which responses were observed in most patients.[33] Infused donor lymphocytes were also shown to be useful in fighting infection by cytomegalovirus (CMV) and Epstein-Barr virus (EBV). Such a transfer of active immunity to the immunosuppressed recipient can help control a potentially lethal condition. Even though the doses of cells used to treat a viral infection are lower than those for relapsed leukemia, the potential to induce GVHD is present in both settings. The blood bank is accordingly very involved in the collection and storage of lymphocytes, as this procedure requires leukapheresis and, often, cryopreservation of a white blood cell fraction.

CD34+ Cell Identification

The science of transplantation passed another milestone when Dr. Curt Civin[34,35] at Johns Hopkins Medical School created a monoclonal antibody against an antigen present on hematopoietic progenitor cells capable of long-term engraftment. Mice were immunized against poorly differentiated human myeloid cells from the KG-1a line, by intraperitoneal and intravenous injection. The mouse spleen cells were fused with murine plasmacytoma cells. Hybridomas were then screened for production of an antibody that would bind KG-1a cells but not human granulocytes. The corresponding antigen was initially called My-10, but its designation would eventually be changed to CD34. This seminal discovery would allow a better assessment of the graft and its potential to reconstitute hematopoiesis in a particular donor, thereby improving standardization of the transplantation process. Additionally, use of such an antibody would permit positive selection of HSCs before transplant as a way to deplete the graft of undesired cellular elements.[36–39]

This technique is still used today to decrease the number of lymphocytes in the graft, to reduce the incidence of GVHD.[40] The procedure is usually performed with a commercial immunomagnetic selection apparatus, operated under strict aseptic conditions or within a closed system.[41] Paramagnetic beads are covered with a monoclonal antibody directed against the CD34 antigen. When put in contact with the stem cell product, the early progenitors expressing CD34 are bound to the beads. Exposure of the cell suspension to a strong magnetic field results in separation of the CD34-positive cell fraction from the remaining of the product. Some systems use a releasing agent to free the isolated cells from the paramagnetic beads before storage or infusion into the patient.

To ensure quality at all steps of this complex process and ultimately the safety of the patient, it should be undertaken only by thoroughly trained staff working under expert supervision. The product must be sampled for assessment of leukocyte populations by flow cytometry, and critical calculations must be done to ensure that the adequate amounts of reagents are mixed with the cells. The selection process itself is now essentially automated, but often the device will require intervention by the operator. The blood bank is the ideal setting to accomplish this, given its long history of processing cellular products and ensuring quality control. Blood bank quality systems also provide for strict adherence to current good manufacturing practices (cGMP) during the entire CD34+ selection process.

Hematopoietic Growth Factors

The growth of HSC transplantation accelerated with the development and commercialization of G-CSF and GM-CSF. Both of these cytokines improved the efficiency of peripheral blood stem cell collection via apheresis. The existence of these cytokines and their effects on committed progenitors were well known in the early 1980s,[42] but industrial production by means of recombinant DNA technology became feasible only after the genes were cloned.[43,44] It was soon demonstrated that when used as single agents, G-CSF and GM-CSF mobilized HSCs into the peripheral blood.[45,46] This effect is further improved by combination of any one cytokine with chemotherapy, but not much when only the two cytokines are combined together.[47] The physiology of cytokine-induced mobilization is being studied intensely, and researchers understand the mechanism(s) of mobilization much more clearly than they had previously. It is thought that on exposure to pharmacologic doses of the agent, progenitors already present in the marrow release their attachments to osteoblastic stromal cells and enter the peripheral circulation. For example, it is thought that G-CSF acts by promoting release of proteolytic enzymes from granulocytes, which cleave the bond between progenitor cells and the marrow stromal cells.

An interesting investigational drug that works through a different mechanism is AMD-3100. It selectively blocks the binding of CXCR4 receptor present on leukocytes with CXCL12 present on osteoblasts. This bond mediates adhesion of hematopoietic progenitors to marrow stromal cells. Blockade of the receptor results in a shift of those progenitors to the peripheral blood. Use of this drug is now being evaluated in clinical trials for patients who do not mobilize enough stem cells with current modalities.[48] Cytokines other than G-CSF and GM-CSF have been used to achieve mobilization, including stem cell factor (SCF), erythropoietin (EPO), interleukin 3 (IL-3), interleukin 6 (IL-6), and FLT3 ligand.[49–53] Single-agent G-CSF or GM-CSF, however, remains the standard regimen for healthy donors, with tolerable acute toxicity and no evidence of long-term effects on hematopoiesis.[54] Patients often experience bone pain and headache. Thrombocytopenia is often noticed but usually is not severe. Splenomegaly is common, but splenic rupture is a very rare event.

As the use of HSC transplantation became widespread, blood banks and their staff became more involved clinically. They were instrumental in streamlining the collection process, which is often logistically complex, as it involves careful timing between start of mobilization (cytokine with or without chemotherapy), assessment of peripheral blood CD34+ cell counts, central-line placement, and start of apheresis. The kinetics of mobilization vary from one patient to another, and the experience of the transfusionist in that matter is crucial in ensuring that the collection goal is met.

Emergence of a Body of Regulations

As HSC transplantation continued to grow, it became clear that programs for practices, standards, and accreditation needed to be firmly in place. The AABB (formerly the American Association of Blood Banks) developed a series of standards for cellular therapy (starting in 1991, addressing hematopoietic cellular therapy and more recently relating to cellular therapy, in general), as well as an accreditation program designed to support the adherence to these standards. The Food and Drug Administration (FDA) originally determined that bone marrow would be considered within the practice of medicine and therefore would not be regulated. However, when peripheral blood stem cell collections were being developed, the FDA mandated that these biologics would need to be regulated, as was the blood industry. Other organizations, such as the Foundation for Accreditation of Cellular Therapies (FACT), also developed standards for the laboratory and clinical aspects of stem cell transplantation. Strict adherence to these standards is critical to ensure that the process of HSC transplantation is performed under conditions of maximal safety and quality. The opportunity for the blood bank or hospital transfusion service to play a role in this process is clear.

The National Marrow Donor Program

The requirement for a compatible family member has often limited the use of allogeneic stem cell transplantation, creating the need for a large, nationwide stem cell donor bank. Early proponents of such an organization were Robert and Sherry Graves from Colorado. Their 10-year-old girl Laura had developed acute leukemia and needed a bone marrow transplant. After a search involving platelet donors, an HLA-matched individual was found. Realizing that other families shared the same struggle, Robert Graves became an advocate for the creation of a national marrow donor registry. In 1984, Congress passed the National Organ Transplant Act, which among other things evaluated the feasibility of a national marrow donor registry. Thanks to the support of Congressman Bill Young (R-FL), the National Bone Marrow Donor Registry (NBMDR) began operating in 1986. Its goal was to provide matched unrelated transplants for anyone in need of a stem cell or bone marrow transplant. By the end of that year, 39 donor centers were already affiliated with the organization. The Registry was originally supported by the AABB, the Council of Community Blood Centers (now America's Blood Center), and the American Red Cross (which administered the program), in addition to funds from Health Resources and Services Administrations (HRSA) and the Navy. In 1988, its name was changed to National Marrow Donor Program (NMDP).

In 1990 the organization took charge of its administration and became a nonprofit entity separate from the Red Cross. The Transplant Amendments Act of 1990 further codified its functions. As this program continued to grow, peripheral blood stem cells as the source for transplants caught up with and exceeded the percentage of BMTs. In current practice, the majority of grafts are collected from peripheral blood, mainly because of their faster engraftment and ease of collection.

UMBILICAL CORD BLOOD

Another major source of HSCs was evaluated and established by Dr. Harold Broxmeyer[55] when he identified umbilical cord blood as being rich in these cells. Benefits already obvious at that time were availability of the resource, ease of collection, and absence of risk to the donor. One major inconvenience, however, was the limited amount of hematopoietic progenitors available in one sample, making it difficult to use in adult recipients. The first case of a patient receiving an umbilical cord blood progenitor cell transplant from a sibling donor was reported in 1989.[56] Applicability of this treatment in the unrelated allogeneic setting was evaluated, and it became obvious that a cord blood bank would be necessary to ensure availability of adequately matched products for potential recipients.[57] Dr. Pablo Rubinstein[58] established the first umbilical cord blood bank at the New York Blood Center in 1992. The NHLBI fostered the development of this program with the establishment of the Cord Blood Transplantation Program (COBLT). This effort resulted in the large-scale collection and storage of umbilical and placental stem cells in both public and private umbilical cord blood banks.[59] Now umbilical cord blood is considered a good alternative to marrow for pediatric HSC transplant, especially given the lower risk of acute and chronic GVHD with cord blood.[60]

Again, because the technology was similar to that of peripheral blood stem cell collection and manipulation, the FDA chose to regulate the cord blood field as a manufacturing process rather than within the practice of medicine. This was done to ensure the quality of the product, its appropriate storage, and that the highest levels of cGMP and current good tissue practices (cGTP) were being followed. As illustrated by the experience of the New York Blood Center, the blood bank was involved from the beginning in cord blood storage. Its familiarity with cryopreservation of cells but also its ability to keep a large registry of products were instrumental in the success of this enterprise. Today, cord blood banking is being monitored and regulated by Congress (HR 2520) with the responsibility for administrative oversight being assigned to HRSA (Health Resources Service Administration). This Bill will help to ensure that cord blood is available to patients of all ethnic backgrounds and that the stem cells will be of the highest quality. Blood banks and hospital transfusion services will clearly have an opportunity to play a major role in this process.

OTHER STEM CELLS

The field of stem cells expanded yet again when researchers showed that bone marrow–derived cells (BMCs) are able to become epithelial cells specific to various organs and tissues such as the liver, pancreas, kidney, central nervous system, gastrointestinal tract, skin, cardiac muscle, and skeletal muscle.[61–70] A debate is going on as to whether this really is transdifferentiation (supporting the hypothesis of stem cell plasticity) or, alternatively, a fusion process.[71–74] It is possible that both processes are occurring. The exact nature of BMCs involved is still largely unknown, and if fusion is the underlying mechanism, then they are likely hematopoietic cells. At this point, only two distinct marrow populations capable of self-renewal and multilineage differentiation have been well characterized: HSCs and mesenchymal stem cells (MSCs). MSCs can give rise to adipocytes, chondrocytes, and osteoblasts.[75,76] Attempts at clinical applications in humans have yielded encouraging results, notably in the treatment of osteogenesis imperfecta, a congenital disease characterized by defective synthesis of type I collagen, which causes brittle bones.[77] Other potential uses include repair of bone and cartilage at sites of trauma.[78] The blood bank will likely be involved in the storage and manipulation of MSCs, given its existing record with HSCs. Blood banks could also be involved in the harvesting process, depending on the anatomic site of origin.

REPAIRING THE HUMAN BODY (REGENERATIVE MEDICINE)

Regenerative medicine is the new name for the field previously referred to as tissue engineering. The potential for using stem cells of various types to replace human tissues and even organs appears limitless at this time.

Pancreatic Islet Cells

Pancreatic islet cell transplantation is one emerging application that is used for the treatment of type I diabetes. Efficient processing of the pancreas to obtain a highly purified preparation was first described by Dr. Camillo Ricordi in 1988.[79] However, attempts at transplantation in the 1990s usually gave short-lived results, as the allogeneic cells were quickly destroyed by the host's immune system. Graft survival improved with the introduction of a new, glucocorticoid-free immunosuppressive regimen in 2000.[80] Research is ongoing to better prevent rejection, if possible without the use of immunosuppression, which is a significant cause of complications for this procedure.[81,82] Although blood banks are not as involved in retrieval of the cells, they could participate in the processing.

Cell Therapies in Myocardial Infarction

Acute treatment of myocardial infarction aims at early reperfusion, but patients who survive the initial event often develop cardiac failure due to ventricular remodeling. This process is characterized by replacement of the dead myocardium by fibrous tissue, which eventually undergoes expansion, with secondary dilation of the ventricular cavity.[83] Animal studies suggested that stem cells could differentiate into myocardial cells and regenerate infarcted tissue.[84] Early trials in humans revealed the safety and feasibility of this approach.[85] Some randomized studies have been completed, with variable initial results.[86–88] More time is needed to appreciate fully the impact of such a treatment on the natural history of those patients.

IN VITRO AND IN VIVO REGENERATION

Although scientists have become better at handling and administering single-cell suspensions, as illustrated in the previous examples, much more must be learned for the field of regenerative medicine to proceed to the next step: the in vitro or even in vivo generation of functional tissue elements of adequate size, possessing the necessary physical, electrical, and metabolic properties to support normal function.[89–93] Such engineered tissues would be able to replace abnormal or diseased human structures (for example, skin, bone, muscle, tendons, blood vessels, or corneas). Ideally, autologous cells would be used to avoid the transmission of viruses and prions. In this process, the starter cells are expanded in vitro and used to seed a support structure (mandril). These structures can be made of either permanent materials such as ceramic or bone or biodegradable materials such as seaweed or alginates. Once the cells have grown in vitro, the mold is ready to be implanted in a human host to replace a damaged body tissue or eventually even an organ. After the cells and the mold are implanted, over a period of time, the implanted cells grow and differentiate so that they are able to replace the damaged tissue and restore normal function. Ceramic molds, for example, are used to repair bony abnormalities, whereas degradable molds are used for blood vessel repair.

Expansion of these cells and creation of an artificial tissue or even organ would probably occur in a designated facility, as the process will certainly require very specialized staff and equipment. The experience of the blood bank with maintenance of an inventory of cellular products and all the related quality-control issues will make transfusion services the best candidate for the collection, storage, processing, and distribution of these biologics in the hospital setting.

GOVERNMENTAL OVERSIGHT

The FDA has exercised oversight of blood and blood components for almost 4 decades. In the 1990s, they started developing regulations for other human cells, tissues, and cellular and tissue-based products, including peripheral blood stem cells. The FDA derives its regulatory power from the Public Health Service Act, Sections 351 and 361. Title 21 CFR Part 1270, under Section 351, governs the collection, storage, and manipulation of human cells and tissues from unrelated donors. Title 21 CFR Part 1271, under Section 361, covers minimally manipulated autologous and allogeneic cellular products of first- and second-degree relatives and includes the most recent regulations on cellular therapies. The first Final Rule of 21 CFR Part 1271, published on January 19, 2001, and effective January 19, 2002, addresses establishment registration and listing of human cells, tissues, and cellular and tissue-based products (Subparts A and B). Published on May 25, 2004, the second Final Rule of 1271 covers eligibility determinations for donors (Subpart C). The third Final Rule (Subpart D) establishes standards for current Good Tissue Practices (cGTPs) and was published on November 24, 2004, to become effective at the same time as the Donor Eligibility Final Rule (Subpart C), May 25, 2005. The FDA inspects registered facilities on a regular basis to ensure compliance. Importantly, many aspects of the new field of regenerative medicine does not clearly fall under the current regulatory guidelines. Some techniques, for example, may involve collection of bone marrow from the autologous donor for use in the operating room. Regulations will likely be developed to address these areas. Here, too, specialists in transfusion medicine will likely play an advisory and consultative role to the FDA.

THE NEW BLOOD BANK

The term *transfusion medicine* was coined in the 1980s by the late Dr. Tibor Greenwalt and by Dr. Fann Harding, then of the NHLBI. The efforts of those and other visionaries led to the NHLBI-sponsored Transfusion Medicine Academic Awards (TMAAs), which were awarded to about 40 medical schools during the 1980s and 1990s. This federal program provided enormous impetus for researchers to study the science of transfusion, and this resulted in the attraction of many of the current transfusion leaders into the field. Although blood banking started with collecting, processing, and storing end-stage blood cells, the TMAA program and other factors led, in part, to the field's current involvement with hematopoietic and other types of stem cells. Indeed, at this point, the field of transfusion medicine is deeply involved in the collection, processing, storage, and distribution of HSCs whether the HSCs are from bone marrow, peripheral blood, or cord blood. These core competencies will be built on in the future to ensure the role of the blood bank in the field of regenerative medicine. As other aspects of blood banking will become more automated, the amount of time devoted to traditional blood products and practices by blood banks will likely decrease, with the activities of the transfusion service of tomorrow becoming more oriented toward cell processing in any number of its many facets (Fig. 57–1). The transfusionist will manage an increasingly more complex inventory of products, many of them likely to be standardized cellular suspensions or tissues produced in specialized bio-factories. This will be an exciting era with myriad challenges. However, the central and overriding consideration

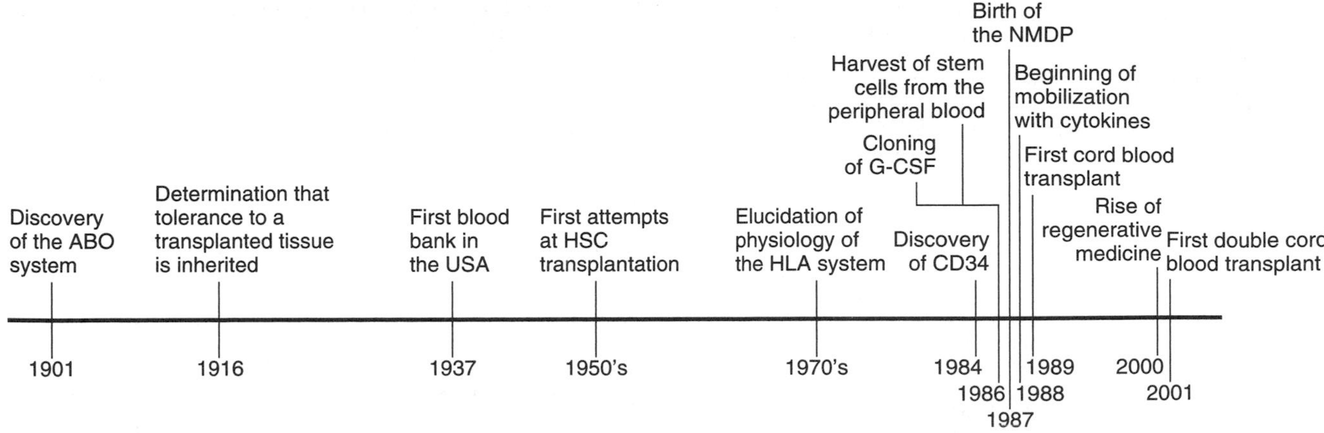

Figure 57–1 Chronology of some major advances in cell therapies.

will always be quality and quality controls designed to ensure that the patient will receive the safest and most efficacious blood-borne material possible, just as it was when transfusion medicine first began in the 19th century.

REFERENCES

1. Landsteiner K. Uber Agglutinationserscheinungen normalen menschlichen Blutes. Wien Klin Wochenschr 1991;46:1132–1134.
2. Robertson O. A method of citrated blood transfusion. Br Med J 1918; 1:477–479.
3. Fantus B. Landmark article July 10, 1937: The therapy of the Cook County Hospital, by Bernard Fantus. JAMA 1984;251:647–649.
4. Thomas ED. Landmarks in the development of hematopoietic cell transplantation. World J Surg 2000;24:815–818.
5. Osgood EE, Riddle MC, Mathews TJ. Aplastic anaemia treated with daily transfusions and intravenous marrow. Ann Intern Med 1939;13:357–360.
6. Thomas ED, Lochte HL Jr, Lu WC, Ferrebee JW. Intravenous infusion of bone marrow in patients receiving radiation and chemotherapy. N Engl J Med 1957;257:491–496.
7. Bortin MM. A compendium of reported human bone marrow transplants. Transplantation 1970;9:571–587.
8. McDevitt HO, Chinitz A. Genetic control of the antibody response: relationship between immune response and histocompatibility (H-2) type. Science 1969;163:1207–1208.
9. Shevach EM, Paul WE, Green I. Histocompatibility-linked immune response gene function in guinea pigs: specific inhibition of antigen-induced lymphocyte proliferation by alloantisera. J Exp Med 1972;136:1207–1221.
10. Rosenthal AS, Shevach EM. Function of macrophages in antigen recognition by guinea pig T lymphocytes. I: Requirement for histocompatible macrophages and lymphocytes. J Exp Med 1973;138:1194–1212.
11. Zinkernagel RM, Doherty PC. Restriction of in vitro T cell-mediated cytotoxicity in lymphocytic choriomeningitis within a syngeneic or semiallogeneic system. Nature 1974;248:701–702.
12. Little CC, Tyzzer EE. Further experimental studies on the inheritance of susceptibility to a transplantable tumor, carcinoma (JWA) of the Japanese waltzing mouse. J Med Res 1961;33:393–453.
13. Gorer PA. The detection of antigenic differences in mouse erythrocytes by the employment of immune sera. Br J Exp Pathol 1936;17:42–50.
14. Gorer PA. The genetic and antigenic basis for tumor transplantation. J Pathol Bacteriol 1937;44:691–697.
15. Dausset J. [Iso-leuko-antibodies.] Acta Haematol 1958;20:156–166.
16. Payne R, Rolfs MR. Fetomaternal leukocyte incompatibility. J Clin Invest 1958;37:1756–1763.
17. Van Rood JJ, Eernisse JG, Van Leeuwen A. Leucocyte antibodies in sera from pregnant women. Nature 1958;181:1735–1736.
18. Wake CT, Long EO, Mach B. Allelic polymorphism and complexity of the genes for HLA-DR beta-chains: direct analysis by DNA-DNA hybridization. Nature 1982;300:372–374.
19. Flomenberg N, Baxter-Lowe LA, Confer D, et al. Impact of HLA class I and class II high-resolution matching on outcomes of unrelated donor bone marrow transplantation: HLA-C mismatching is associated with a strong adverse effect on transplantation outcome. Blood 2004;104:1923–1930.
20. Storb R, Deeg HJ, Whitehead J, et al. Methotrexate and cyclosporine compared with cyclosporine alone for prophylaxis of acute graft versus host disease after marrow transplantation for leukemia. N Engl J Med 1986;314:729–735.
21. Weisdorf DJ. Chronic graft-versus-host disease: where is promise for the future? Leukemia 2005;19:1532–1535.
22. Freireich EJ, Judson G, Levin RH. Separation and collection of leukocytes. Cancer Res 1965;25:1516–1520.
23. Giles FJ, Kantarjian H, O'Brien SM. Leukapheresis reduces early risk of mortality in AML patients with high white cell counts receiving first induction therapy. Blood 1998;92(Suppl):237a.
24. Oza A, Hallemeier C, Goodnough L, et al. Granulocyte-colony-stimulating factor-mobilized prophylactic granulocyte transfusions given after allogeneic peripheral blood progenitor cell transplantation result in a modest reduction of febrile days and intravenous antibiotic usage. Transfusion 2006;46:14–23.
25. McCredie KB, Hersh EM, Freireich EJ. Cells capable of colony formation in the peripheral blood of man. Science 1971;171:293–294.
26. Hershko C, Gale RP, Ho WG, Cline MJ. Cure of aplastic anaemia in paroxysmal nocturnal haemoglobinuria by marrow transfusion from identical twin: failure of peripheral-leucocyte transfusion to correct marrow aplasia. Lancet 1979;1:945–947.
27. Kessinger A, Armitage JO, Landmark JD, Weisenburger DD. Reconstitution of human hematopoietic function with autologous cryopreserved circulating stem cells. Exp Hematol 1986;14:192–196.
28. Kessinger A, Vose JM, Bierman PJ, Armitage JO. High-dose therapy and autologous peripheral stem cell transplantation for patients with bone marrow metastases and relapsed lymphoma: an alternative to bone marrow purging. Exp Hematol 1996;19:1013–1016.
29. Richman CM, Weiner RS, Yankee RA. Increase in circulating stem cells following chemotherapy in man. Blood 1976;47:1031–1039.
30. Le Corroller AG, Faucher C, Auperin A, et al. Autologous peripheral blood progenitor-cell transplantation versus autologous bone marrow transplantation for adults and children with non-leukaemic malignant disease: a randomised economic study. Pharmacoeconomics 1997;11:454–463.
31. To LB, Haylock DN, Kimber RJ, Juttner CA. High levels of circulating haemopoietic stem cells in very early remission from acute non-lymphoblastic leukaemia and their collection and cryopreservation. Br J Haematol 1984;58:399–410.
32. Bensinger WI, Martin PJ, Storer B, et al. Transplantation of bone marrow as compared with peripheral-blood cells from HLA-identical relatives in patients with hematologic cancers. N Engl J Med 2001;344:175–181.
33. Kolb HJ, Mittermuller J, Clemm C, et al. Donor leukocyte transfusions for treatment of recurrent chronic myelogenous leukemia in marrow transplant patients. Blood 1990;76:2462–2465.
34. Civin CI, Strauss LC, Brovall C, et al. Antigenic analysis of hematopoiesis. III: A hematopoietic progenitor cell surface antigen defined by a monoclonal antibody raised against KG-1a cells. J Immunol 1984;133:157–165.
35. Civin CI, Trischmann T, Kadan NS, et al. Highly purified CD34-positive cells reconstitute hematopoiesis. J Clin Oncol 1996;14:2224–2233.
36. Civin CI, Strauss LC, Fackler MJ, et al. Positive stem cell selection: basic science. Prog Clin Biol Res 1990;333:387–401, discussion 2.
37. Brugger W, Henschler R, Heimfeld S, et al. Positively selected autologous blood CD34+ cells and unseparated peripheral blood progenitor cells mediate identical hematopoietic engraftment after high-dose VP16, ifosfamide, carboplatin, and epirubicin. Blood 1994;84:1421–1416.

38. Fruehauf S, Haas R, Zeller WJ, Hunstein W. CD34 selection for purging in multiple myeloma and analysis of CD34+ B cell precursors. Stem Cells 1994;12:95–102.
39. Shpall EJ, Jones RB, Bearman SI, et al. Transplantation of enriched CD34-positive autologous marrow into breast cancer patients following high-dose chemotherapy: influence of CD34-positive peripheral-blood progenitors and growth factors on engraftment. J Clin Oncol 1994;12:28–36.
40. Waldmann H, Polliak A, Hale G, et al. Elimination of graft-versus-host disease by in-vitro depletion of alloreactive lymphocytes with a monoclonal rat anti-human lymphocyte antibody (CAMPATH-1). Lancet 1984;2:483–486.
41. Miltenyi S, Muller W, Weichel W, Radbruch A. High gradient magnetic cell separation with MACS. Cytometry 1990;11:231–238.
42. Metcalf D. The granulocyte-macrophage colony-stimulating factors. Science 1985;229:16–22.
43. Wong GG, Witek JS, Temple PA, et al. Human GM-CSF: molecular cloning of the complementary DNA and purification of the natural and recombinant proteins. Science 1985;228:810–815.
44. Nagata S, Tsuchiya M, Asano S, et al. Molecular cloning and expression of cDNA for human granulocyte colony-stimulating factor. Nature 1986;319:415–418.
45. Socinski MA, Cannistra SA, Elias A, et al. Granulocyte-macrophage colony stimulating factor expands the circulating haemopoietic progenitor cell compartment in man. Lancet 1988;1:1194–1198.
46. Duhrsen U, Villeval JL, Boyd J, et al. Effects of recombinant human granulocyte colony-stimulating factor on hematopoietic progenitor cells in cancer patients. Blood 1988;72:2074–2081.
47. Koc ON, Gerson SL, Cooper BW, et al. Randomized cross-over trial of progenitor-cell mobilization: high-dose cyclophosphamide plus granulocyte colony-stimulating factor (G-CSF) versus granulocyte-macrophage colony-stimulating factor plus G-CSF. J Clin Oncol 2000;18:1824–1830.
48. Flomenberg N, Devine SM, Dipersio JF, et al. The use of AMD3100 plus G-CSF for autologous hematopoietic progenitor cell mobilization is superior to G-CSF alone. Blood 2005;106:1867–1874.
49. Shpall EJ, Wheeler CA, Turner SA, et al. A randomized phase 3 study of peripheral blood progenitor cell mobilization with stem cell factor and filgrastim in high-risk breast cancer patients. Blood 1999;93:2491–2501.
50. Kessinger A, Bishop MR, Jackson JD, et al. Erythropoietin for mobilization of circulating progenitor cells in patients with previously treated relapsed malignancies. Exp Hematol 1995;23:609–612.
51. Vose JM KA, Bierman PJ. The use of rhIL-3 for mobilization of peripheral blood stem cells in previously treated patients with lymphoid malignancies. Int J Cell Cloning 1992;10(Suppl 1):62–64.
52. Pettengell R, Luft T, de Wynter E, et al. Effects of interleukin-6 on mobilization of primitive haemopoietic cells into the circulation. Br J Haematol 1995;89:237–242.
53. Lebsack ME, McKenna HJ, Hoek JH, et al. Safety of FLT3 ligand in healthy volunteers. Blood 1997;90(Suppl 1):170a.
54. Pulsipher MA, Nagler A, Iannone R, Nelson RM. Weighing the risks of G-CSF administration, leukopheresis, and standard marrow harvest: Ethical and safety considerations for normal pediatric hematopoietic cell donors. Pediatr Blood Cancer 2006;46:422–433.
55. Broxmeyer HE, Douglas GW, Hangoc G, et al. Human umbilical cord blood as a potential source of transplantable hematopoietic stem/progenitor cells. Proc Natl Acad Sci USA 1989;86:3828–3832.
56. Gluckman E, Broxmeyer HA, Auerbach AD, et al. Hematopoietic reconstitution in a patient with Fanconi's anemia by means of umbilical-cord blood from an HLA-identical sibling. N Engl J Med 1989;321:1174–1178.
57. Dunn PM. Banking umbilical cord blood. Lancet 1992;340:309.
58. Rubinstein P, Carrier C, Scaradavou A, et al. Outcomes among 562 recipients of placental-blood transplants from unrelated donors. N Engl J Med 1998;339:1565–1577.
59. Fraser JK, Cairo MS, Wagner EL, et al. Cord Blood Transplantation Study (COBLT): Cord blood bank standard operating procedures. J Hematother 1998;7:521–561.
60. Rocha V, Wagner JE Jr, Sobocinski KA, et al. Graft-versus-host disease in children who have received a cord-blood or bone marrow transplant from an HLA-identical sibling: Eurocord and International Bone Marrow Transplant Registry Working Committee on Alternative Donor and Stem Cell Sources. N Engl J Med 2000;342:1846–1854.
61. Poulsom R, Forbes SJ, Hodivala-Dilke K, et al. Bone marrow contributes to renal parenchymal turnover and regeneration. J Pathol 2001;195:229–235.
62. Tomita S, Li RK, Weisel RD, et al. Autologous transplantation of bone marrow cells improves damaged heart function. Circulation 1999;100(19 Suppl):II247–II256.
63. Petersen BE, Bowen WC, Patrene KD, et al. Bone marrow as a potential source of hepatic oval cells. Science 1999;284:1168–1170.
64. Krause DS, Theise ND, Collector MI, et al. Multi-organ, multi-lineage engraftment by a single bone marrow-derived stem cell. Cell 2001;105:369–377.
65. Theise ND, Badve S, Saxena R, et al. Derivation of hepatocytes from bone marrow cells in mice after radiation-induced myeloablation. Hepatology 2000;31:235–240.
66. Alison MR, Poulsom R, Jeffery R, et al. Hepatocytes from non-hepatic adult stem cells. Nature 2000;406:257.
67. Eglitis MA, Mezey E. Hematopoietic cells differentiate into both microglia and macroglia in the brains of adult mice. Proc Natl Acad Sci USA 1997;94:4080–4085.
68. Ferrari G, Cusella-De Angelis G, Coletta M, et al. Muscle regeneration by bone marrow-derived myogenic progenitors. Science 1998;279:1528–1530.
69. Ianus A, Holz GG, Theise ND, Hussain MA. In vivo derivation of glucose-competent pancreatic endocrine cells from bone marrow without evidence of cell fusion. J Clin Invest 2003;111:843–850.
70. Mezey E, Chandross KJ, Harta G, et al. Turning blood into brain: cells bearing neuronal antigens generated in vivo from bone marrow. Science 2000;290:1779–1782.
71. Ying QL, Nichols J, Evans EP, Smith AG. Changing potency by spontaneous fusion. Nature 2002;416:545–548.
72. Terada N, Hamazaki T, Oka M, et al. Bone marrow cells adopt the phenotype of other cells by spontaneous cell fusion. Nature 2002;416:542–545.
73. Wang X, Willenbring H, Akkari Y, et al. Cell fusion is the principal source of bone-marrow-derived hepatocytes. Nature 2003;422:897–901.
74. Vassilopoulos G, Wang PR, Russell DW. Transplanted bone marrow regenerates liver by cell fusion. Nature 2003;422:901–904.
75. Prockop DJ. Marrow stromal cells as stem cells for nonhematopoietic tissues. Science 1997;276:71–74.
76. Pittenger MF, Mackay AM, Beck SC, et al. Multilineage potential of adult human mesenchymal stem cells. Science 1999;284:143–147.
77. Horwitz EM, Prockop DJ, Fitzpatrick LA, et al. Transplantability and therapeutic effects of bone marrow-derived mesenchymal cells in children with osteogenesis imperfecta. Nat Med 1999;5:309–313.
78. Caplan AI. Review: Mesenchymal stem cells: cell-based reconstructive therapy in orthopedics. Tissue Eng 2005;11:1198–1211.
79. Ricordi C, Lacy PE, Finke EH, et al. Automated method for isolation of human pancreatic islets. Diabetes 1988;37:413–420.
80. Shapiro AM, Lakey JR, Ryan EA, et al. Islet transplantation in seven patients with type 1 diabetes mellitus using a glucocorticoid-free immunosuppressive regimen. N Engl J Med 2000;343:230–238.
81. Bretzel RG, Eckhard M, Brendel MD. Pancreatic islet and stem cell transplantation: new strategies in cell therapy of diabetes mellitus. Panminerva Med 2004;46:25–42.
82. Hirshberg B, Rother KI, Digon BJ 3rd, et al. Benefits and risks of solitary islet transplantation for type 1 diabetes using steroid-sparing immunosuppression: the National Institutes of Health experience. Diabetes Care 2003;26:3288–3295.
83. Sutton MG, Sharpe N. Left ventricular remodeling after myocardial infarction: pathophysiology and therapy. Circulation 2000;101:2981–2988.
84. Orlic D, Kajstura J, Chimenti S, et al. Bone marrow cells regenerate infarcted myocardium. Nature 2001;410:701–705.
85. Assmus B, Schachinger V, Teupe C, et al. Transplantation of progenitor cells and regeneration enhancement in acute myocardial infarction (TOPCARE-AMI). Circulation 2002;106:3009–3017.
86. Chen SL, Fang WW, Ye F, et al. Effect on left ventricular function of intracoronary transplantation of autologous bone marrow mesenchymal stem cell in patients with acute myocardial infarction. Am J Cardiol 2004;94:92–95.
87. Wollert KC, Meyer GP, Lotz J, et al. Intracoronary autologous bone-marrow cell transfer after myocardial infarction: the BOOST randomised controlled clinical trial. Lancet 2004;364:141–148.
88. Janssens S, Dubois C, Bogaert J, et al. Autologous bone marrow-derived stem-cell transfer in patients with ST-segment elevation myocardial infarction: double-blind, randomised controlled trial. Lancet 2006;367:113–121.
89. Nishida K, Yamato M, Hayashida Y, et al. Corneal reconstruction with tissue-engineered cell sheets composed of autologous oral mucosal epithelium. N Engl J Med 2004;351:1187–1196.
90. Shin'oka T, Imai Y, Ikada Y. Transplantation of a tissue-engineered pulmonary artery. N Engl J Med 2001;344:532–533.
91. Vunjak-Novakovic G, Altman G, Horan R, et al. Tissue engineering of ligaments. Annu Rev Biomed Eng 2004;6:131–156.
92. Joraku A, Sullivan CA, Yoo JJ, Atala A. Tissue engineering of functional salivary gland tissue. Laryngoscope 2005;115:244–248.
93. Jain RK, Au P, Tam J, et al. Engineering vascularized tissue. Nat Biotechnol 2005;23:821–823.

Chapter 58

Bone Marrow and Peripheral Blood Stem Cell Transplantation

Howard Benn • Scott D. Rowley

INTRODUCTION

The intent of hematopoietic stem cell (HSC) transplantation, regardless of the type of HSC component infused, any modifications of the component performed, and the disease being treated, is to achieve long-term engraftment of the cells infused. HSC transplantation was initially developed to correct the consequences of bone marrow (BM) failure, whether this failure was the result of a disease such as severe aplastic anemia or iatrogenic, resulting from the treatment of disease with administration of dose-intense chemoradiotherapy regimens. Restoration of hematopoietic function after administration of an intensive conditioning regimen in the treatment of those malignant diseases that show a dose-response effect, such as leukemia, continues to be the most common use of HSC transplantation. However, the ability to establish a different immune system in a properly prepared recipient with the resulting graft-versus-disease effect extends the utility of HSC transplantation to treatment of diseases that are not sensitive to escalation of chemotherapy dosage. Furthermore, the ability to establish a lymphohematopoietic chimera with allogeneic HSC transplantation opens the possibility of using HSC transplantation as a foundation for other treatments such as cell-based immunotherapy or solid organ transplantation.

Several thousands of patients undergo HSC transplantation each year, a testament to the facility with which this particular stem cell therapy can be used. Advancements in supportive care including newer antibiotics and the development of pretransplant conditioning regimens with lower nonhematologic toxicities widen the diagnoses and age range of patients who can be treated successfully. The availability of alternate stem cell sources such as umbilical cord blood (Chapter 59) and unrelated volunteer donors extends allogeneic transplantation to patients lacking an appropriate related donor.

TRANSPLANTATION TECHNIQUES

Selection of Patients

Careful patient selection and timing of treatment are critical to the success of HSC transplantation (Table 58–1). For example, in the treatment of cancer, patients with bulky tumor masses or chemotherapy-resistant diseases are much less likely to achieve durable responses, even with the use of dose-intense regimens. The immune suppression required with allogeneic transplantation also may exacerbate underlying infections such as mold infections, viral hepatitis, or tuberculosis. The early introduction of dose-intense therapy in the treatment of a patient, before chemotherapy resistance and excessive chemotherapy-induced organ toxicity develop, is paramount. Therefore, treatment algorithms incorporating HSC-transplant salvage strategies must be part of the initial therapeutic decisions for each patient with a disease possibly treatable by high-dose therapy. Patients being prepared for HSC transplantation will frequently undergo several cycles of chemotherapy, intended to demonstrate the sensitivity of the disease to chemotherapy, reduce the bulk of the disease before transplantation, and facilitate the collection of peripheral blood stem cells (PBSCs).[1] Radiotherapy can be used to debulk large tumor masses but is, in general, reserved for administration after recovery from transplantation because of the deleterious effects of this treatment modality on the collection of PBSCs and the increase in organ toxicity within the treatment field with subsequent administration of chemotherapy.[2] Radiotherapy used as consolidation therapy after autologous transplantation may require the infusion of additional HSCs to offset the marrow-suppressive effects of this therapy, again illustrating the need for comprehensive planning of the patient undergoing HSC transplantation, including possible collection of reserve quantities of HSCs.

Many patients eligible for HSC transplantation using marrow-ablative or reduced-intensity regimens also have comorbidities that can affect the tolerance of the patient to this treatment, possibly increasing the risk of nonhematologic complications. Patients undergo a detailed evaluation to uncover any organ dysfunction that may preclude the safe administration of this therapy. Although HSC infusion rescues the patient from the hematologic toxicity of the conditioning regimen, the nonhematologic (organ) toxicity of dose-intense therapies may be formidable, particularly if a dose-intense conditioning regimen is administered. The presence of single-organ comorbidity or abnormal laboratory values predicts regimen-related nonhematologic toxicities.[3,4] A retrospective review of 383 consecutive transplants noted individual factors predictive of early transplant-related mortality to include a forced expiratory volume $(FEV)_1$ less than 78% of predicted, serum creatinine greater than 1.1 mg/dL, and serum bilirubin greater than 1.1 mg/dL.[4] Unfortunately, many patients, especially older patients, initially have more than a single comorbidity. Investigators in Seattle applied the multiparameter Charlson Comobidity Index to patients undergoing unrelated or related donor HSC transplantation and reported a direct correlation between patient score and

Table 58–1 Factors Influencing Transplant Decision

Disease-Related Issues	Patient-Related Issues	Availability of Donor
Diagnosis IPSS score Previous treatment Response to treatment Current extent (bulk) of disease Current chemotherapy sensitivity of disease	Age Performance status Other medical conditions	Autologous Family member Unrelated donor Umbilical cord blood

nonrelapse mortality.[5] (These investigators subsequently published a modified HSC transplant–specific comorbidity index developed from data from 1055 patients that showed better predictive value for nonrelapse mortality and post-transplant survival).[6] For these reasons, the timing of transplantation is critical, and efforts should be made both to reduce tumor bulk and to correct comorbid conditions before initiation of transplant conditioning.

Selection of Donors

A variety of sources of HSCs for transplantation are available, and details regarding the collection, processing, and infusion of marrow, peripheral blood, and umbilical cord blood products are described in Chapters 57–60. All patients storing cells for autologous HSC transplantation and donors for allogeneic (or syngeneic) transplantation must be evaluated for risks involved with the collection of HSCs and the risks to the recipient from diseases of the donor that may be transmitted into an immunoincompetent recipient. Patients undergoing autologous transplantation are not at risk for transmission of infectious diseases but must be evaluated for the risks of the collection procedure (and subsequent treatment). As a broad consideration, donors can be evaluated by using the same criteria currently applied to blood donors, although the United States Food and Drug Administration (FDA) has enacted specific regulations for the handling of certain tissues including PBSCs obtained from allogeneic donors. However, numerous infectious diseases that would not exclude the donor from blood donation, such as cytomegalovirus, may be transmitted with the allograft.[7] Donors who would otherwise be excluded for health reasons from donating blood for transfusion (e.g., history of hepatitis) may still be eligible to donate BM if the needs of the recipient outweigh the risks of disease transmission. Hematopoietic disorders of the donor, such as hemoglobinopathies, will be transmitted to the recipient. Cancer can be transmitted to a conditioned host, as illustrated by the transmission of donor leukemia not detected during initial evaluation of the donor.[8] Standards are now published that describe the evaluation of the donor both for the risk of the donation process and for the risk of transmission of disease to the recipient.[9,10]

Anesthesia and blood loss present the greatest risks of serious complications for marrow collection. Marrow harvesting has the luxury of the intensive support capability of the operating room, allowing collection of patients and donors with significant comorbid conditions. Most marrow harvesting is performed under general anesthesia, which requires intubation for control of the airway for a surgical procedure performed on a prone patient. Regional (spinal or epidural) anesthesia is acceptable for the donor who is not at risk for the hypotension that frequently occurs with this form of anesthesia. Regional anesthesia occasionally fails, so patients and donors who express a preference for this anesthesia must also be counseled about the potential need for general anesthesia. The health assessment of the marrow donor must include questioning about a history of joint disease of the cervical spine and mandible and examination of the mouth if general anesthesia requiring intubation is chosen. Patients and donors with comorbid conditions, such as aortic stenosis or sensitivity to changes in blood volume and blood pressure, may require anesthesia consultation and plans for invasive monitoring during the surgical procedure. A history of marrow fibrosis, previous pelvic irradiation, or pelvic tumor involvement will exclude a patient from marrow harvesting.

In contrast, collection of PBSCs is generally an outpatient procedure conducted in the clinic setting. For this reason, PBSC collection should never be viewed as a safer alternative to marrow harvesting for the donor with underlying health problems. PBSC donation presents its own unique risks resulting from the logistics of cytokine administration and the extracorporeal circulation of blood. The risks of cytokine administration are presented in Chapter 60. Adverse events that have been associated, at least temporally, with the collection procedure include myocardial infarction, cerebral vascular accident, and rupture of the spleen.[11–14] Most donations can be obtained by using a vein-to-vein procedure. Some donors, especially pediatric donors, may require the placement of a temporary central venous catheter. The risks of catheter placement are well known and are not repeated here.

Allogeneic Donors

HLA MATCHING

Human leukocyte antigen (HLA) compatibility is the primary consideration in selection of a donor for allogeneic transplantation. Both major and minor histocompatibility-locus antigens may contribute to host-versus-graft (HVG; with HSC rejection) and graft-versus-host reactions (GVH; resulting in graft-versus-host disease [GVHD]), as shown by the increased risks of engraftment failure and GVHD after HLA-matched allogeneic compared with syngeneic transplantation. HLA antigens are classified as class I (HLA-A, -B, -C) and class II (HLA-DR, -DQ, -DP); typing of donors and patients can be performed by using low- or high-resolution techniques. The low-resolution techniques will discriminate, generally, between antigens (e.g., A02 vs A03, phenotypic matching), whereas high-resolution molecular techniques will identify allelic differences (e.g., A0201 vs A0202, genotypic matching). Various reports describe deleterious effects of mismatching at each of these loci on transplant outcomes, although the effect may not be clinically evident in all patient populations, demonstrating an influence of nongenetic factors on the tolerability of HLA mismatching.[15–19]

Transplantation of HSCs from HLA-disparate donors increases the risk of GVHD and transplant-related mortality, with greater numbers of mismatches increasing these risks of transplantation. Ideally, genotypically matched unrelated donors (URDs) will be available for patients lacking an HLA-identical sibling donor. However, not all ethnic groups are well represented in the various donor registries, and genotypically matched donors are not available for all patients who are candidates for allogeneic transplantation. What is not known is whether certain allelic mismatches are more permissive than others, allowing the use of mismatched donors without increased risk of adverse outcomes. A large series involving 1874 donor-recipient pairs for whom retrospective high-resolution typing was performed found increased risks of mortality for recipients of HSCs from donors mismatched at a single HLA-A, -B, -C, and -DRB1 locus, with much higher risks for patients with multiple mismatches.[20] The risk of mortality was increased for patients mismatched at either the antigen (low-resolution) or allelic level, although the relative risk was greater for the former. Importantly, 56% of patients matched at HLA-A, -B, and -DR by using low-resolution techniques were found to have one or more mismatches when high-resolution typing for these antigens and HLA-C was performed. These investigators found no additional contribution of mismatching at either HLA-DQ or HLA-DP loci, suggesting that mismatches at these loci can be ignored in the algorithm used for the selection of a URD. Similar findings regarding the importance of HLA-DR, but not HLA-DQ or -DP matching was reported in another large (831 patients) registry data study from the National Marrow Donor Program.[21]

The large study by Flomenberg and colleagues[20] did not detect a difference in engraftment success for patients undergoing mismatched transplants, although another single-center study reported higher risks of engraftment failure for patients receiving transplants mismatched at class I loci at the antigen (low-resolution) level.[22] The risk of rejection was increased, in particular, for recipients homozygous at the mismatched class I locus and for recipients mismatched at more than one locus. A large study of 1298 patients from the Japan Marrow Donor Program found a deleterious effect of class I allelic mismatching on success of engraftment.[23] Single disparities of the HLA-A, -B, -C, or -DRB1 allele were independent risk factors for acute GVHD, and HLA-A and/or HLA-B allele mismatch was found to be a significant factor for the occurrence of chronic GVHD. However, this study did not find an adverse effect of mismatching at the HLA-DR locus on transplant outcomes in contrast to the other studies cited earlier.

DONOR AGE/GENDER

The effects of donor/patient age and gender are primarily on the logistics of the collection procedure, such as the possible need for central venous catheterization for pediatric donors, the presence of comorbid conditions for older donors and patients, and the generally smaller blood volumes of pediatric and female donors. Gender mismatches, especially female donors for male recipients, and older donors increase the risk of GVHD.[24] Donor-selection algorithms will incorporate age and gender into selection criteria.

DONOR HEALTH

Infectious and malignant diseases can be transmitted to the allogeneic/syngeneic transplant recipient, and donors must undergo a comprehensive evaluation before the recipient is conditioned for transplantation.[7,8] Currently, most HSC transplant procedures are performed in the treatment of patients with fatal malignancies who lack other treatment options. In these situations, the recipient, with appropriate informed consent (the donor must first consent to the release of confidential medical information to the recipient), may opt to accept the risk of disease transmission. If time allows, donors with hepatitis may be treated to reduce the risk of disease transmission. Human immunodeficiency virus (HIV) infection is an absolute contraindication to HSC donation. Cytomegalovirus (CMV) is the most common infection likely to be transmitted because of the high incidence of infection in the general population. Fortunately, with current post-transplant monitoring of patients and the availability of effective antiviral drugs, CMV infection has little effect on transplant outcomes. A large retrospective review of 7018 patients seropositive for CMV reported to the European Group for Blood and Marrow Transplantation (EBMT) who received related (5910 patients) or unrelated (1108 patients) found that patients receiving grafts from CMV-seropositive HLA-identical sibling donors had the same survival as patients grafted from seronegative donors.[25] Interestingly, URD recipients receiving grafts from CMV-seropositive donors had an improved 5-year survival (35% vs 27%, an improved event-free survival (EFS; 30% vs 22%), and a reduced transplant-related mortality (49% vs 62%). In patients with chronic myelogenous leukemia (CML), T-cell depletion abrogated the beneficial effect of donor status, suggesting that the effect is mediated through transfer of donor immunity and that for a CMV-seropositive patient, a seropositive donor might be preferable.

RELATIONSHIP

Most patients who are candidates for allogeneic transplantation will lack an appropriate related donor. URD transplantation is facilitated by the large donor registries now totaling more than 10 million potential worldwide donors. However, paradoxically, the advances in high-resolution HLA typing that now can often detect single amino acid differences complicate the search for the ideal HLA-compatible donor. No randomized studies comparing the use of related or URDs are reported. In general, recipients of URD products face higher risks of graft failure, acute and chronic GVHD, and transplant-related mortality.[26]

BLOOD-GROUP MATCHING

The major histocompatibility antigens are located on chromosome 6, and red cells antigens are located on a number of other chromosomes. For this reason, HLA-compatible donors may differ for red cell antigens including ABO, Rh, and other potentially hemolytic antigens. Red cell antigens are not major histocompatibility antigens, and red cell incompatibility does not appear to increase the risk of GVH or HVG reactions. Depletion of red cell and/or plasma from the HSC product will reduce the risks of hemolytic transfusion reactions during HSC infusion, but careful transfusion practices are required to avoid acute or delayed hemolytic transfusion reactions from the infusion of incompatible red blood cells or immunocompetent B lymphocytes. Eventually, recipient red cells and isoagglutinins are replaced by donor type. Red cell incompatibility may be classified into three categories, one in which the recipient has antibodies directed against donor red cells with the potential of acute hemolysis on infusion of the component (major incompatibility), one in which the donor has antibodies against the recipient (minor incompatibility), and one in which both major and minor incompatibility exist (bidirectional incompatibility). Although minor incompatibility rarely causes difficulty during infusion of incompatible plasma, B lymphocytes carried in the component can form increasing titers of isoagglutinins, resulting in a delayed transfusion reaction 7 to

12 days after transplantation. Apheresis devices are commonly used to remove red cells from marrow component for major or bidirectional red cell incompatibility.[27] Red blood cell quantities of 10 mL or less appear, generally, to be tolerable, although no lower limit of red cells exists below which clinical reactions will not occur. Secondary processing of a PBSC component collected by the same technology used for the depletion of red cells from marrow grafts and already containing low quantities of red cells is not required. The persistence of donor isoagglutinins directed against donor red cell antigens will prolong the time to red-cell transfusion independence, and individual patients requiring several years of red-cell support have been reported. Administration of erythropoietin or attempts to remove donor isoagglutinins by plasmapheresis are usually ineffective. Elimination of donor B cells by administration of rituximab or donor lymphocytes (resulting in GVHD) are more likely effective. Minor ABO incompatibility can result in delayed transfusion reactions that may be fatal if appropriate blood-transfusion support (avoiding the infusion of donor-type red cells) is not initiated before the transplant. Two case reports of severe red cell hemolysis after allogeneic PBSC transplantation have been reported. In the first, transfusion support before the event was not described.[28] The second patient received recipient-type red cells on day 7 after transplantation,[29] which is the point at which donor-derived isoagglutinins will be increasing in the recipient. Although both authors discussed the much greater numbers of B cells in PBSCs compared with BM products as a possible factor in these events, it is not clear from these reports that delayed-type transfusion reactions will be more likely or of greater severity in PBSC recipients. The risk of delayed-type reaction may be ameliorated by the use of combination post-transplant immunosuppressive regimens. The Seattle transplant program, for example, found no delayed transfusion reactions in a large retrospective review of patients undergoing PBSC transplantation and who received the two-drug immunosuppressive regimen of cyclosporine and methotrexate.[30]

Syngeneic Donors

Syngeneic HSC transplantation avoids the risk of tumor reinfusion that may complicate autologous transplantation and also avoids the immunologic complications (and benefits) of allogeneic transplantation. Few reports exist of syngeneic transplantation for the treatment of malignant diseases, but the published series, in general, describe a lower risk of relapse compared with autologous transplantation. One review of large transplant databases identified 89 NHL patients who received syngeneic transplants and compared these patients with NHL patients who received allogeneic (T-cell depleted and T-cell replete) or autologous (purged and unpurged) transplants. No significant differences in relapse rates were observed when results of allogeneic transplantation were compared with those of syngeneic transplantation for any histology. However, patients who received unpurged autografts for low-grade NHL had a fivefold ($P = .008$) greater risk of relapse than did recipients of syngeneic transplants, and recipients of unpurged autografts had a twofold ($p = .0009$) greater relapse risk than did patients who received purged autografts.[31] A comparable retrospective study that compared 25 patients with multiple myeloma who received BM grafts ($n = 24$) or PBSCs ($n = 1$) from twin donors to 125 patients who underwent autologous transplantation, and 125 who underwent allogeneic transplantation described no difference in achieving complete remission, but a trend to better overall survival (OS; 73 vs 44 months) and significantly better progression-free survival (72 vs 25 months) for the syngeneic recipients.[32] Syngeneic transplantation requires the administration of dose-intense conditioning and is not appropriate in the setting in which an immunologic response to the underlying disease is required for optimal transplant outcome.

Pediatric Donors

PBSCs and marrow can be collected from pediatric donors, including infants. The special challenges of the pediatric donor arise from the smaller blood volume of the donor, the need for venous catheters for blood access if apheresis is to be used, and the management of a patient who may be unwilling or unable to rest quietly for the period of collection. It is especially important in management of the pediatric PBSC donor (or patient) that timing of apheresis be optimal to minimize the number of procedures required to achieve the desired quantity of PBSCs. Virtually all pediatric patients undergo insertion of a venous catheter adequate for the flow rates expected, although older (older than 12 years) patients may tolerate vein-to-vein procedures.

Selection of Product

PBSCs have virtually replaced BM as the HSC source for autologous transplantation and are widely used for allogeneic transplantation. The ease of collection and the rapid engraftment kinetics of PBSCs compared with BM are widely recognized. Median times to achieve an absolute neutrophil count (ANC) greater than 500 per microliter are typically about 11 to 14 days, and platelet recovery is even faster.[33–35] The more rapid engraftment kinetics for recipients of PBSCs have been confirmed in a number of phase III studies involving either autologous or allogeneic HSC transplantation (Table 58–2). This effect is not limited to HSCs collected from the peripheral blood, because cytokine administration to the patient or donor before marrow harvesting will also increase the number of HSCs collected and result in quicker hematologic recovery.[36–40]

Disadvantages to the use of PBSC components as a source of HSCs for autologous or allogeneic transplantation include the usual need for multiple days of collection (especially for autologous transplantation), the current need for sophisticated flow-cytometric analysis of the components (or hematopoietic cell cultures) to ensure adequacy of HSC content, the inability to collect adequate components from all patients and donors, the risks associated with administration of hematopoietic cytokines and the apheresis procedures, the risks of infusion if the components are cryopreserved, and a possibly higher risk of GVHD or the occurrence of GVHD that is more difficult to control (see Table 58–2).[41–43]

Although GVHD prophylaxis with post-transplant administration of methotrexate will slow engraftment, the kinetics of engraftment for the allogeneic PBSC recipient is similar to that experienced by the autologous PBSC recipient. After multiple phase I and II studies of allogeneic (or syngeneic) PBSC transplantation confirmed the feasibility of this technique,[44–51] at least 11 phase III studies comparing PBSC and marrow transplantation in the related donor setting were published.[52–58] A meta-analysis of 9 of these trials described a lower relapse rate and improvements in overall and disease-free survivals (DFSs) after PBSC transplantation for patients with advanced hematologic malignancies,

Table 58–2 Phase III Studies of PBSC versus Marrow

	No. of Patients		CD34+ Cell Dose		ANC > 500/μL			PLT > 20,000/μL			Acute GVHD		
	BM	PBSC	BM	PBSC	BM	PBSC	*P*	BM	PBSC	*P*	BM	PBSC	*P*
Allogeneic													
BM vs. PBSC													
Blaise et al[52]	52	48	2.4	6.6	21	15	10^{-5}	21	13	10^{-4}	42%	44%	NS
Bensinger et al[56]	91	81	2.4	7.3	21	16	<0.001	19	13	<0.001	57%	64%	0.35
Couban et al[53]	118	109	2.4	6.7	23	19	<0.001	22	16	<0.001	44%	44%	>0.9
Schmitz et al[54]	116	163	2.7	5.8	15	12	<0.001	20	15	<0.001	39%	52%	0.013
G-BM vs. PBSC#													
Morton et al[37]	28	29	2.6	7.2	16	14	<0.1	14	12	<0.1	52%	54%	<0.6
Autologous													
BM vs. PBSC													
Beyer et al[33]	23	24	ND	ND	11	10	<0.01	17	10	<0.01			
Schmitz et al[34]	31	27	ND	ND	14	11	0.005	23	16	0.02			
Hartmann et al[35]	65	64	ND	ND	12	8	<0.001	29	9	<0.001			
G-BM vs. PBSC													
Damiani et al[39]	36	19	0.6	3.3	12	11	0.22	13	11	0.24			
Weisdorf et al[40]	17	15	ND	ND	14	13	ND	25	17	ND			

BM, bone marrow; PBSCs, peripheral blood stem cells; G-BM, G-CSF–stimulated bone marrow; ND, not done.

although at the cost of a significant risk of extensive chronic GVHD.[59] Multiple studies suggest that chronic GVHD may be more common after PBSC transplantation or may be more difficult to control.[41–43,57] However, treatment-related mortality (TRM) rates may also be lower and leukemia-free survival rates higher with blood stem cell transplants in patients with advanced leukemia (acute leukemia in second remission or CML in accelerated phase) but not in early leukemia (acute leukemia in first remission or CML in chronic phase).[44] The reports of improved survival for patients who undergo PBSC transplantation may, similarly, be particular to transplant regimens or patient selection.

Umbilical cord blood (UCB) is a rich source of HSCs, leading to use as a source of stem cells for transplantation in both adults and children. The major limitation of UCB is the small quantity of cells collected. Advantages are the immediate availability of units, a lower risk of GVHD, and the ability to use mismatched units without a prohibitory increase in transplant complications. Multiple large series of both pediatric and adult transplants using UCB have been reported. In general, as with other sources of HSCs, outcomes of transplantation reflect patient characteristics, with lower survival probabilities for patients with advanced diseases or poorer performance status at time of transplantation. The easy availability and the lack of risk to a donor of an already collected UCB unit promote the treatment of patients who may not be able to wait for identification of an unrelated or related marrow donor or who appear for transplantation with advanced diseases and significant comorbidities. In the multicenter Cord Blood Transplantation (COBLT) study of 34 adult patients, 94% of patients were classified as poor risk according to National Marrow Donor Program criteria, and 4 died before transplantation. The probability of survival to 180 days after transplantation, the primary end point of the study, was 30%, and only two patients survived over the long term.[60] In contrast, a case-controlled series comparing the outcome of adult patients receiving UCB products matched at five of six (34 patients) or four of six (116 patients) loci to recipients of marrow with no (367 patients) or one antigen mismatch (83 patients) treated at multiple centers described 2-year survival probabilities of 20% for recipients of mismatched marrow, 26% for recipients of UCB, and 35% for recipients of HLA-matched marrow ($P < .001$).[61] In this study, however, the survival probability did not differ for recipients of mismatched marrow or UCB products. A similar case-controlled study of 98 adult UCB recipients (6 receiving 6/6 matched products) and 584 HLA-compatible marrow recipients reported 2-year survivals probabilities of 36% and 42%, respectively ($P = .08$) with nonsignificant differences in subgroups classified by diagnosis or stage of disease at the time of transplantation.[62] These data regarding the differing outcomes for different stem cell sources require that transplant programs establish algorithms for selection of an HSC source depending on patient characteristics and treatment plan.

Cell Dose

Cell dose is an important predictor of transplant outcome for both autologous and allogeneic transplantation. An early study of patients undergoing allogeneic transplantation reported higher risks of engraftment failure for patients receiving less than 3×10^8 nucleated BM cells per kilogram, but this was a study of patients with aplastic anemia who received only methotrexate for postgrafting immunosuppression.[63] It is now recognized that successful establishment of donor cell chimerism is a complex interplay of pre- and post-transplant suppression of the host immune system, the dose of HSCs and accessory cells (including donor lymphocytes) contained in the graft, and HLA compatibility between donor and host. HLA-mismatching, T-cell depletion, and less-intensive (less-immunosuppressive) conditioning regimens all increase the risk of graft failure. Autologous transplantation does not present a likely risk of engraftment failure if HSC product viability is maintained during postcollection processing and storage. Instead, the speed of hematologic recovery is related to the quantity of HSCs reinfused, with initial studies demonstrating an exponential relation between cell dose and engraftment speed.[64] Lower doses of CD34+ cells appear satisfactory for nonablative regimens.[65,66] For example, Bokemeyer and colleagues.[65] infused 0.9×10^6 CD34+

cells per cycle for patients treated with high-dose ifosfamide and doxorubicin. Despite an overall doubling of the ifosfamide dose in this phase I study, the median times between cycles did not progressively increase, indicating that adequate marrow stores were maintained. For marrow-ablative regimens, increasingly higher CD34+ doses results in greater likelihood of rapid recovery of peripheral blood counts.[67] Patients who receive a dose of CD34+ cells above an undefined threshold will engraft. At lower doses of CD34+ cells, considerable heterogeneity in engraftment speed is found, especially for platelet recovery, with some patients experiencing quick engraftment despite low doses of PBSCs. As the dose of CD34+ cells increases, the engraftment speed becomes more consistent for the population studied, although the median days of cytopenia are minimally affected in the dose ranges usually administered.[68,69] Several investigators showed more consistently rapid granulocyte and platelet engraftment for recipients of products containing a quantity of CD34+ cells above a dose of about 2–3 $\times$ 10^6 per kilogram recipient weight.[67,69–71] Importantly, the duration of aplasia predicts the incidence of peritransplant mortality after autologous or allogeneic transplantation.[72]

Similarly, the cell dose is a predictor of outcome for patients undergoing allogeneic (or syngeneic) transplantation.[72–76] A study of 905 patients undergoing BM transplantation from related ($n = 770$) or unrelated ($n = 135$) donors stratified patients in three groups ranging from fewer than 2.4 to more than 5 $\times$ 10^8 nucleated cells/kg and reported that the recipients in the highest group had significantly higher platelet and higher white blood cell (WBC) counts both early and late after transplantation as compared with other patients.[76] The actuarial 5-year transplant-related mortality, OS, and DFS significantly favored patients receiving grafts with higher cell doses. The cell-dose effect was more pronounced in patients older than 30 years, with advanced disease, with a diagnosis of CML, and with alternative donors (other than HLA-compatible siblings). Nucleated cell count is a poor surrogate for HSC content, and similar studies reported an association between CD34+ cell dose and outcome of allogeneic transplantation with either marrow or PBSCs.[77]

Accessory cells contained in the graft also appear to affect the outcome of transplantation in both autologous and allogeneic transplantation. The dose of lymphocytes and the kinetics of lymphocyte recovery after autologous transplantation predicts the probability of disease relapse.[79,80] The quantities of natural killer cells (NK cells), T-lymphocyte subsets, and dendritic cells have been correlated with the risks of GVHD and disease relapse after allogeneic transplantation.[80,81] The ability to manipulate the quantities or function of various cell populations in the HSC graft to improve the outcome of transplantation remains an area of active research.[82] For example, various studies suggest that G-CSF priming changes the cytokine response of lymphocytes contained in the PBSC product,[83] may decrease the risk of acute GVHD,[84] and may increase the graft-versus-leukemia effect.[85] The potential influence of these changes in outcome of allogeneic (or autologous) transplantation is not clear.

Selection of Transplant-Conditioning Regimen

The infusion of HSCs allows the administration of a dose-intense, myeloablative regimen without concern for the effects on hematopoiesis. The efficacy of dose intensity is demonstrated by randomized trials of autologous transplantation for diseases such as multiple myeloma,[86] Hodgkin's disease (HD),[87] and NHL[88]—these trials illustrate that dose-intense therapy is more effective than available nontransplant regimens delivered in multiple cycles over time.

Autologous (and syngeneic) HSC transplantation lacks the immunologic graft-versus-disease (GVD) effect of allogeneic transplantation and cures diseases through the administration of dose-intensive regimens. Therefore, the conditioning regimen used should include drugs that are effective in the treatment of the particular malignancy and, ideally, induce minimal nonhematopoietic organ damage at the myeloablative doses used for transplantation. Immunosuppression is not required for engraftment of autologous HSCs. Some regimens, such as high-dose melphalan for the treatment of patients with multiple myeloma and carmustine (BCNU)-based regimens for the treatment of lymphoma, are commonly used based on the results of multicenter phase III studies showing the tolerability of these regimens. However, the relative efficacy of different conditioning regimens in the treatment of a particular disease has not been studied in large randomized studies. Relapse is the major cause of failure of autologous HSC transplantation and novel techniques to deliver yet more intensive conditioning regimens continue to be explored. One example of this is the addition of radiolabeled antibodies to a chemotherapy or total-body irradiation (TBI)-based regimen to target specifically areas of tumor while sparing radiation-sensitive organs such as the liver, lung, and kidney.[89] Press and colleagues.[89] added 20 to 27 Gy of ^{131}I-labeled anti-CD20 antibody to a conditioning regimen of etoposide (20 mg/kg) and cyclophosphamide (CY; 100 mg/kg) and reported a 77% CR rate and a 68% 2-year probability of progression-free survival (PFS) for patients with relapsed NHL. The two-year PFS was almost double that previously experienced (36%) by similar patients treated with chemotherapy alone. Similar attempts to target therapy to the tumor and increase the intensity of the conditioning are being investigated in allogeneic transplantation.[90]

Allogeneic transplantation differs in the need to achieve adequate immunosuppression of the patient to permit the establishment of donor-cell chimerism, but also in the beneficial effect of the immunologic GVD effect that occurs. The regimen-related (nonhematologic) toxicity is greater after allogeneic transplantation, possibly because of the need for immunosuppressive regimens but also because of GVHD and opportunistic infections. The GVD effect of allogeneic transplantation, however, also allows the use of lower-intensity conditioning regimens for older patients or patients with comorbid conditions that would otherwise preclude transplant-based therapy.

Dose-Intense Regimens

TBI became the primary component of myeloablative conditioning regimens because of its efficacy in the treatment of hematologic malignancies, its ability to treat sanctuary sites of disease such as the central nervous system (CNS), and (for allogeneic transplantation) its immunosuppressive effects. TBI is usually combined in sequence with chemotherapy agents such as CY. The nonhematopoietic toxicities of TBI are reduced by fractioning the dose over several days, allowing higher treatment doses. Increasing the total dose of TBI decreases the risk of relapse but increases the risk of transplant-related complications[91]; often, these effects are offsetting, and event-free survival remains the same.[92–94] The primary dose-limiting toxicities of TBI include pneumonitis, veno-occlusive disease of the liver, renal impairment, and mucositis. Other attempts to develop regimens with greater tumoricidal effects included the addition of a third agent such as busulfan or etoposide, but again with increased regimen-related toxicities.[95,96]

Busulfan-based regimens were developed as alternatives to TBI-based regimens for the treatment of patients who had received prior dose-limiting radiotherapy, to avoid the effects of TBI on growth and development in children, and to eliminate the difficulty in scheduling patients to the limited number of radiation machines available. Initially, one of the limitations in the use of busulfan was the lack of an intravenous preparation, and wide variation in plasma levels with consequent effects on regimen-related toxicities such as hepatic veno-occlusive disease, failure of engraftment, and relapse of disease.[97–100] Close monitoring of plasma busulfan levels with adjustment of dose reduces the risks of treatment failure, as does the recent availability of an intravenous formulation of this drug.

A number of retrospective analyses and prospective phase III studies compared the outcomes of transplantation using busulfan or TBI-based regimens in allogeneic transplantation.[101–104] One review of four such studies conducted in the treatment of patients with CML or acute myelogenous leukemia (AML) found no statistically significant difference in survival or DFS for patients with CML, with a nonsignificant improvement in survival for patients with AML treated with the TBI regimen.[104] CML patients who received the TBI-based regimen had an increased risk of cataract formation, and patients treated with the busulfan-based regimen had an increased risk of irreversible alopecia. Other late complications occurred equally after both conditioning regimens. Chronic GVHD was the primary risk factor associated with late pulmonary disease and avascular osteonecrosis.

A number of studies explored the addition of agents to protect against nonhematopoietic toxicities of the dose-intense conditioning regimens. This can be as simple as having a patient "chew" ice during the infusion of a single dose of melphalan, which is effective in protecting against oral mucositis because of the quick elimination of this drug from the plasma. Amifostine has been used as a cytoprotective agent in a number of studies, with conflicting results.[105,106] Kerotinocyte growth factor was recently approved for prophylaxis of patients undergoing autologous HSC transplantation based on the results of a phase III study showing a reduction in mucositis.[107]

Reduced-Dose Regimens

Allogeneic transplant recipients benefit from the immunologic GVD effect that develops with establishment of hematopoietic chimerism. Thus control of disease does not result only from the administration of a dose-intense regimen, and nonmyeloablative regimens have been developed for patients ineligible for myeloablative conditioning because of age or comorbid conditions. The primary requirement in developing a reduced-intensity regimen is the need to achieve adequate immunosuppression to permit the development of hematopoietic chimerism. Storb and others[108–111] proposed that the HVG reaction leading to HSC rejection and the GVH reaction could both be modified by an appropriate immunosuppressive regimen administered after transplantation, allowing a reduction in the intensity of the pretransplant conditioning regimen. In a series of canine followed by human trials, this group demonstrated the ability to achieve durable donor cell engraftment with low levels of TBI (2 Gy given in a single fraction) if high concentrations of cyclosporine and mycophenylate mofetil were maintained after transplantation. Engraftment success was improved subsequently with the addition of the purine analog, fludarabine. Again, a variety of regimens are available, including combinations of fludarabine with melphalan and fludarabine with busulfan.[112–114] These regimens can pose less immediate risk of regimen-related toxicities[115,116] and open the option of combining in tandem dose-intense regimens with autologous support (for optimal cytoreduction of the tumor) followed by allogeneic transplantation by using a reduced-intensity regimen (to induce a GVD effect).[115,117,118] For example, a study of tandem autologous transplantation using dose-intense melphalan conditioning followed several months later by allogeneic transplantation using conditioning with a single fraction of TBI reported median days of neutropenia, thrombocytopenia, and hospitalization of none.[117] Comparative studies of myeloablative and reduced-intensity regimens have not been reported, but patients with advanced malignancies may require the increased cytoreduction of the dose-intense regimens for optimal results.[119]

HEMATOLOGIC RECOVERY AFTER HEMATOPOIETIC STEM CELL TRANSPLANTATION

HSC engraftment encompasses two concepts: recovery of hematopoietic and immunologic function of the BM (e.g., yes or no), and the rate at which this recovery occurs (e.g., time to achieve a particular milestone of engraftment). Delay in or failure of sustained engraftment after administration of a myeloablative-conditioning regimen greatly increases the morbidity and cost of the treatment and may result in the death of the patient.[72] Engraftment is a complex interplay of donor, host, and HSC-component characteristics. Engraftment failure can occur as a result of inadequate HSC quantity from poor collection or loss in postcollection processing, or because of inadequate host support of the infused cells,[120] post-transplant events or medications, or the immunologically mediated rejection of the allogeneic donor's cells. Failure of engraftment is a very rare complication of autologous or syngeneic HSC transplantation and is likely only with poor preservation of HSCs after collection. For allogeneic transplants, the risk of engraftment failure is proportional to the disparity between donor and recipient for HLA and minor transplant antigens, occurring more commonly in URD transplantation than in sibling donor transplantation, and for mismatched in comparison with HLA-matched transplants. The risk of engraftment failure is also increased by the removal of T lymphocytes from the marrow inoculum because of the loss of the GVH effect mediated by donor immunoreactive cells.[121] This risk of immunologically mediated rejection can be reduced by increasing the intensity of the pretransplant conditioning regimen to suppress the HVG reaction,[122] such as with increased doses of TBI, but with increased regimen-related toxicity as well. The HVG reaction can also be overcome by increasing the quantity of HSCs in the inoculum, a technique made feasible for human transplantation by the availability of PBSCs that can be used in conjunction with marrow cells.[122] Studies in dogs and humans demonstrated the feasibility of increasing the intensity of the post-transplant immunosuppression to offset a weaker conditioning regimen.[108]

Delayed engraftment has a deleterious effect on transplant outcomes after either autologous or allogeneic transplantation. In an analysis of duration of severe neutropenia and risk of death in 2276 patients after marrow transplantation, the risk ratio for patients still neutropenic between days 10 and 14 remained close to 1.0, indicating that the risk of death before day 100 for patients with an ANC less than 100 per microliter was similar to that for patients who achieved an ANC ≥100/μL during this time.[73] However, between day 15, when 38% of patients had an ANC less than 100 per microliter, and day 26, when 3.8% of patients had an ANC less than 100 per microliter, the risk ratio showed an overall upward trend, indicating that patients with an ANC less than 100 per microliter had a higher risk of death before day 100 than did those with an ANC ≥100/μL. Similar studies described an adverse correlation between persistent thrombocytopenia and outcomes of allogeneic transplantation.[26,123]

Administration of hematopoietic growth factors may speed engraftment after allogeneic or autologous transplantation. Randomized studies of sargramostim or filgrastim administration after autologous transplantation demonstrated that these hematopoietic cytokines speed granulocyte recovery, may decrease the morbidity of the transplant procedure, and may be associated with a smaller probability of relapse.[124–126] Hematologic recovery after allogeneic transplantation is similarly hastened,[127] but this fact has not consistently translated into earlier hospital discharge or reduced transplant cost because mucositis and other complications of transplantation, not blood cell recovery, are often the primary reasons for continued hospitalization. Assessment of chimerism is important in evaluating poor marrow function after allogeneic HSC transplantation. A decrease in peripheral blood counts could indicate HVG-mediated rejection of the graft or early relapse after transplantation or could be a result of post-transplant events such as GVHD or viral infection. Documentation of stable persistence of donor cells will help discriminate between these possibilities. It is also important that sustained chimerism be demonstrated if infusion of donor T cells is to be used in the treatment of disease relapse after transplantation.[128] The level of donor-host chimerism after allogeneic transplantation is currently demonstrated through the detection of sex chromosomes by using fluorescent in situ hybridization (FISH) techniques or, for same-gender donor-patient pairs, through evaluation of single-nucleotide tandem repeats (STRs) by using molecular analysis techniques. Obviously, these studies are of no value in assessing engraftment after autologous or syngeneic transplantation.

Much of the emphasis in transplantation has been on myeloid engraftment, because initial patient survival depends on recovery of phagocytes and, to a lesser extent, platelets. However, severe immunosuppression is also a consequence of both allogeneic and autologous BM transplantation, resulting from damage to normal barriers such as skin and mucosal linings, loss of phagocytic cells, loss of lymphoid function, and the use of immunosuppressive regimens to prevent or treat GVHD. Lymphoid reconstitution may take months, and even longer, if GVHD occurs. Recoveries of both B- and T-lymphoid function appear to recapitulate ontogeny, with lymphoid subpopulations recovering at different rates.[129,130] Recovery of lymphoid populations (in the absence of GVHD) is similar in allogeneic, syngeneic, and autologous transplantation, although ex vivo purging of T or B cells can delay recovery of specific subpopulations removed by the purge procedure.[131–133] Opportunistic infections occur commonly until host immunity is recovered. Infections are an especially common cause of both morbidity and mortality for transplants complicated by GVHD because of the delay in recovery of immune function caused by this disease and its treatment. Fungal and viral infections commonly occur in association with acute GVHD and its treatment; sinusitis, otitis, and pneumonia are common complications of chronic GVHD.[134] Administration of immunoglobulin (Ig) supplementation to patients with low IgG levels can prevent some of these infectious complications.[135] Reconstitution of dendritic cell function may also predict post-transplant outcomes.[136]

COMPLICATIONS OF HEMATOPOIETIC STEM CELL TRANSPLANTATION

Patients who undergo HSC transplantation face a series of complications arising from the underlying disease, previous treatments that may have been administered, the conditioning regimen used for transplantation, the supportive procedures including antibiotic administration and blood-component transfusions, and (for recipients of allogeneic cells) the immunologic complications of transplantation. Transplantation is given, usually, with curative intent, and the proper management of the transplant recipient includes lifelong monitoring for such complications. The early complications associated with the treatment regimen ("regimen-related toxicities") usually occur within the first 3 months after transplantation. Long-term complications such as the osseus or ocular complications of transplantation may not be detected until several years after treatment. Although patients may achieve a cure of the underlying disease with HSC transplantation, these patients face a higher mortality rate than the general population. One study evaluated the mortality rate of 6691 patients listed in the International Bone Marrow Transplant Registry who were alive and free of their original disease 2 years after allogeneic BMT.[137] Mortality rates in this cohort were compared with those of an age-, sex-, and nationality-matched general population. For these patients, the probability of living for 5 more years was 89%. For patients with a diagnosis of aplastic anemia, the risk of death by the sixth year after transplantation did not differ significantly from that of a normal population. However, mortality remained significantly higher than normal among patients who underwent transplantation for acute lymphoblastic leukemia or CML and through the ninth year among those who underwent transplantation for AML. Recurrent leukemia was the chief cause of death among patients who received a transplant for leukemia, whereas chronic GVHD was the chief cause among those who received a transplant for aplastic anemia. However, most patients who undergo allogeneic transplantation enjoy good health after transplantation. One study evaluated 798 recipients of BM transplants (477 adults, 321 children) from 43 European centers who were alive more than 5 years after transplantation.[138] Fifty-five of these patients died more than 5 years after transplantation, and the actuarial mortality was 8% at 10 years and 14% at 15 years. The leading causes of death were disease recurrence (21 patients), chronic GVHD with complicating infections and lung disease (11 patients), secondary cancer

(8 patients), and the acquired immunodeficiency syndrome (AIDS) (5 patients). The clinical performance was normal (Karnofsky score, 100%) or minimally reduced (Karnofsky score, 90%) in 93% of patients; 89% of patients resumed full-time work or school. Factors associated with poorer quality of life include older age at time of transplantation, presence of long-term sequelae of the treatment, and presence of chronic GVHD.

Infectious Complications of Hematopoietic Stem Cell Transplantation

HSC transplantation predisposes to a unique spectrum of infectious complications as a result chemotherapy damage to host defenses and the immunologic consequences of this treatment. The risk of and type of infection vary over time after transplantation and also for donor type (autologous vs allogeneic). Bacterial infections predominate in the early post-transplant period when the absolute neutrophil count is less than 100 per microliter, and the mucosal and skin barriers are most compromised. The duration and depth of neutropenia independently predict the risk of infection in this the early recovery phase.[139] The majority (70%) of the bacterial pathogens are gram-positive species, with the gram-negative incidence decreasing significantly within the past 20 years. In the mid-recovery phase beginning immediately after engraftment when profound depression of cellular and humoral immunity occurs, viral pathogens, especially CMV, are the major causes of infections. Invasive fungal infections (IFIs)—*Aspergillus*, *Candida* spp.—are increasingly recognized as the major causes of death in allogeneic SCT (ASCT) with an overall incidence of 8% to 15%. This incidence has been correlated with T cell–depleted or CD34-selected HSC products, acute and chronic GVHD, treatment with corticosteroids, secondary neutropenia, CMV infection, and respiratory virus infection.[139]

Pretransplant diagnosis does not appear to predict different risks of bacterial infections after transplantation. Auner and colleagues[140] analyzed data from 114 patients who had undergone high-dose chemotherapy and autologous HSC transplantation in the treatment of AML, NHL/HD, and MM, and found no differences with respect to the type or incidence of infections despite a longer median duration of neutropenia in the leukemia and lymphoma populations. In contrast, the choice of preparative regimen may independently influence the risk of infection. In a study published by Ketterer and associates[141] of 277 patients, fludarabine or TBI-based preparative regimens were associated with a higher risk (26%) of late infections, with viral infections, mainly varicella zoster virus (VZV) and pneumonia the main etiologies. Junghanss and coworkers[142] compared the infectious complications of allogeneic transplantation by using either myeloablative or reduced-intensity conditioning (RIC) regimens. Patients undergoing a reduced-intensity regimen experienced a shorter duration of neutropenia and fewer episodes of bacteremia during the initial 30- and 100-day periods (9% vs 27%, P = .01; and 27% vs 41%, P = .07, respectively) after transplantation. However, the rates of invasive aspergillosis during the first year after transplantation were the same for both groups, illustrating the effects of GVHD and its treatment on the risk of infection after allogeneic transplantation. Multivariate analysis identified neutropenia and CMV disease as the major factors associated with bacteremia and aspergillus infection.

Although transplant-related mortality continues to decrease as a result of improved transplant techniques, supportive care, and judicious patient selection, infective death rates continue to be significant. In a landmark special report by Gratwohl and colleagues[143] of the EBMT, data from 14,403 patients with a diagnosis of leukemia undergoing transplantation with reduced-intensity conditioning regimens were retrospectively analyzed to determine the causes of post-transplant death. They reported an 11% infective death rate. Of the 597 deaths from infection, 36%, 31%, 28%, and 5% were attributed to bacteria, viruses, fungi, and parasites, respectively. Remarkably, even though the cumulative incidence of death from infection decreased over time, the relative contributions remained stable. Bacterial infections predominated during the initial 3 months after transplantation, with approximately 50% of all infections occurring in this period. The risk of infectious death diminished with time after transplantation, with 25% of infectious deaths occurring in the first 2 months, 25% after 7 months, and 10% beyond 1 year, and the majority of deaths occurring after initial hematologic recovery. They reiterated that the pretransplant factors associated with infectious death were advancing age and T-cell depletion. An advantage was noted for patients undergoing PBSC transplantation with respect to all infectious etiologies. Inexplicably, they reported a higher incidence of death from viral infections among female patients. They postulated that this phenomenon may be as a result of transmission of respiratory syncytial virus (RSV) and VZV from children. The conclusion was that delayed immune reconstitution is probably more important than marrow hypoplasia as a factor contributing to infectious death.

Reports have also been published detailing the infectious complications and mortality after unrelated donor cord blood transplant (UCBT). Because of the different kinetics of myeloid and lymphoid recovery after UCBT, there was a higher rate of early bacterial blood stream infections. Absence of grade II-IV GVHD was associated with higher incidence of *VZV* reactivation but lower incidence of CMV antigenemia and disease. However, the major cause of infectious mortality was multiresistant *Acinetobacter* spp.[144,145]

The incidence of postengraftment invasive aspergillosis is increasing. A large single-institution study of 1682 patients undergoing allogeneic transplantation identified older patient age and diagnosis as risk factors for early infection.[146] Transplantation of PBSCs conferred protection against early (<40 days) infection compared with the use of BM. Factors that increased risks for later (beyond 40 days) infection included receipt of T cell–depleted or CD34-selected stem cell products, receipt of corticosteroids, neutropenia, lymphopenia, GVHD, CMV disease, and respiratory virus infections. Very late infection (>6 months after transplantation) was associated with chronic GVHD and CMV disease.

Regimen-Related Toxicities

Early Complications

The patient undergoing dose-intense therapy with autologous HSC transplantation experiences a period of marrow hypoplasia that can persist for days or weeks. During this time, the patient will require antibiotic and blood component support, but death from infection or hemorrhage is uncommon. Nonhematopoietic toxicity that is common but not life threatening may include alopecia and varying degrees of mucositis with concomitant mouth pain, inanition, and diarrhea. Rarely, mucositis compromises the safety of the airway, and intubation of the patient is temporarily required for airway protection. Serious organ toxicity includes hepatic venocclusive disease (from high-dose regimens in general), interstitial pneumonitis (e.g., BCNU induced), cardiomyopathy (e.g., CY induced), and hemorrhagic cystitis (e.g., CY induced). The risk of nonhematopoietic toxicity increases for older patients and for patients who previously received intensive chemotherapy regimens. For these patients, reduction of dose of the transplant conditioning regimen may be appropriate, but at possibly increased risk of relapse of disease.

Mucositis and gastrointestinal toxicity are the most prevalent early nonhematologic complications of dose-intense therapy, usually occurring within the first 10 to 14 days after transplantation. In one study of 202 recipients of high-dose therapy and autologous or allogeneic stem-cell rescue, a diagnosis of leukemia, use of TBI, allogeneic transplantation, and delayed neutrophil recovery were associated with increased oral mucositis and longer parenteral nutritional support.[147] Administration of keratinocyte growth factor may reduce the incidence and severity of mucositis. A randomized, placebo-controlled study of palifermin in patients undergoing dose-intense therapy with autologous HSC support reported that the incidence of oral mucositis of World Health Organization (WHO) grade 3 or 4 was 63% in the palifermin group and 98% in the placebo group ($P < .001$). Furthermore, among patients with this degree of mucositis, the median duration of mucositis was 6 days (range, 1 to 22 days) in the palifermin group and 9 days (range, 1 to 27 days) in the placebo group. As compared with placebo, palifermin was also associated with significant reductions in the use of opioid analgesics and the incidence of use of total parenteral nutrition.[148]

The incidence of hepatic venocclusive disease (VOD) ranges from 5% to 50%. It is defined as a conditioning regimen-related and dose-limiting toxicity and is significantly more prevalent after allogeneic SCT compared with autologous SCT, and with the use of dose-intense compared with reduced-intensity conditioning regimens. The factors predisposing to its incidence are the transplant procedure itself, use of TBI as part of the conditioning regimen, use of methotrexate for post-transplant immunosuppression, and pre-existing or antecedent hepatic dysfunction. Clinical signs suggestive of VOD are tender hepatomegaly, noncardiogenic weight gain, and hyperbilirubinemia, which usually occur within the first 3 weeks after transplantation. Overall mortality ranges from 20% to 50% in various series, reaching 98% for patients with severe disease.[149] Oral busulfan has been the standard in many myeloablative regimens since the 1970s. However, its use is productive of increased VOD secondary to the hepatic first-pass effect, unpredictable absorption kinetics, and variable bioavailability, with sinusoidal obstruction as the terminal event.[150] With the formulation of intravenous busulfan, the incidence of VOD significantly decreased with no loss of myeloablative efficacy.[151–153] Treatment of VOD is usually best supportive care, although defribotide may be effective.[154]

Late Complications

Avascular necrosis (AVN) of bone is an uncommon but not rare complication of HSC transplantation, with an average time of onset of about 2 years after transplantation. The cause of this complication is not defined, although vasculitis involving intraosseous blood vessels induced by GVHD has been proposed for patients undergoing allogeneic HSC transplantation.[155] Two large retrospective studies have defined risk factors associated with this complication. A multicenter study of 4388 patients, recorded in the Societe Francaise de Greffe de Moelle (SFGM) database, who had undergone a single allogeneic BMT, described 77 patients who developed avascular necrosis, leading to a 4.3% projected incidence at 5 years. Symptoms developed 2 to 132 months after transplantation. A mean of 1.87 joints per patient were affected (range, 1–7 joints), with the hip joint being the most often affected (88% of patients) and 48% of the patients required joint replacement. In univariate analysis, six risk factors were shown to be linked to an increased risk: older age, diagnosis of aplastic anemia or acute leukemia, an irradiation-based conditioning regimen, type of GVHD prophylaxis regimens, and occurrence of acute and chronic GVHD. In multivariate logistic regression analysis, five factors remained significantly associated with an increased risk for developing avascular necrosis: chronic GVHD (odds ratio [OR], 3.52), acute GvHD (OR, 3.73), age older than 16 years (OR, 5.81), aplastic anemia (OR, 3.90), and acute leukemia (OR, 1.72).[156] A case-control study of 1939 long-term survivors who underwent BMT at a single center found 88 who developed AVN after transplantation (an addition eight patients developed AVN before transplant) at a mean of 26.3 months. Post-transplant steroid use was a risk factor for the occurrence of AVN (adjusted OR, 14.4; 95% confidence interval [CI], 2.8–73.2), with the greatest risk associated with those receiving steroids at the time of diagnosis of AVN (adjusted OR, 31.9; 95% CI, 4.4–248.9). No further increasing risk was associated with increasing duration of steroid use. Conditioning with TBI was also associated with the occurrence of AVN (adjusted OR, 3.2).[157]

Cataract formation is a frequent long-term complication of HSC transplantation and is associated with administration of TBI and corticosteroids. A retrospective analysis of 1063 patients from the EBMT registry who were evaluable for survival and ophthalmologic status after transplant for acute leukemia reported an overall 10-year estimated cataract incidence of 50%. In this analysis, factors independently associated with an increased risk of cataract were older age, higher radiation dose rate (>0.04 Gy/min), allogeneic HSC transplantation, and longer-term steroid administration (>100 days).[158]

Bronchiolitis obliterans is a late complication of BMT associated with chronic GVHD and is frequently fatal. One retrospective analysis of 2859 HSC transplantation recipients found no cases of among 1070 autologous transplant recipients.[159] Among the 1789 allogeneic recipients, 47 patients with this pulmonary complication were found, and older ages of recipients and donors and the development of acute GVHD were significantly associated with the development of bronchiolitis obliterans. Among patients with this complication, the 5-year survival from the time of transplantation was only 10% compared with 40% among allogeneic recipients without. Pulmonary failure was the leading cause of death.

The majority of dose-intense conditioning regimens invariably cause gonadal failure, with only a minority of patients able to regain gonadal function after HSCT. Therefore, puberty and menarche are delayed or abrogated completely. For women, ovarian failure is guaranteed in the face of busulfan and or TBI conditioning. Indeed, fertility will already have been seriously compromised by induction and consolidation chemotherapeutic and radiotherapeutic strategies. Despite this, more than 50% of women younger than 26 years will regain ovarian functioning if CY only is used and approximately 10% in patients conditioned with TBI. Clinically recognized pregnancies among women who have received a marrow transplant incorporating TBI are likely to be accompanied by an increased risk of spontaneous abortion. Pregnancies among all women who received a marrow transplant are likely to be accompanied by preterm labor and delivery of low-birth-weight (LBW) or very LBW (VLBW) babies who do not seem to be at an increased risk of congenital anomalies.[160] However, determination of possible adverse effects of parental exposure to high-dose alkylating agents with or without TBI on children born after transplant requires longer, additional follow-up.

The need for hormone-replacement therapy (HRT) should be investigated for both men and women after HSC transplantation. For female patients unopposed estrogen predisposes to endometrial cancer, whereas combined estrogen receptor (ER) + progesterone receptor (PR) increases the risk of cardiovascular events and invasive breast cancer beginning 2 to 5 years after HSCT. In view of the foregoing management of menopausal symptoms, loss of bone mineral density becomes more important. Individualization of management with informed consent before systemic or topical HRT is recommended. The importance of screening mammography, breast self-exams, and pap smears cannot be overstated.[161] For men, decreased libido, low testosterone levels, and osteopenia mandate the use of HRT, but, as is the case with their female counterparts, scrupulous informed consent and preventive screening for prostate cancer, liver-function test monitoring, and detection of lipid abnormalities are necessary.[162]

Second Cancers after Hematopoietic Stem Cell Transplantation

The development of second cancers, including myelodysplasia or secondary leukemia, is a well-described complication of allogeneic or autologous HSC transplantation.[163–167] Possible explanations include administration of chemotherapy or radiotherapy, prolonged administration of immunosuppressive agents, and chronic irritation of tissues (e.g., lining of mouth) that are target organs of GVHD. A prevalence of myelodysplasia or secondary leukemia appears to exist after autologous transplantation, and this risk may be increased with certain pretransplant agents such as etoposide or TBI.[163] Studies of second cancers after allogeneic transplantation report a variety of nonhematologic malignancies. One series of 1036 patients enrolled into cooperative group transplant trials reported second cancers in 53 patients, with an actuarial incidence of 3.5% at 10 years and 12.8% at 15 years.[168] The rate of new malignant disease was 3.8-fold higher than that in an age-matched control population, with the most frequent malignant diseases being neoplasms of the skin (14 patients), oral cavity (7 patients), uterus (5 patients), thyroid gland (5 patients), breast (4 patients), and glial tissue (3 patients). Malignant neoplasms were more frequent in older patients and in patients with chronic GVHD. A very large study of more than 19,000 patients who underwent allogeneic or syngeneic transplantation also found a higher risk of cancer compared with that in the general population, with the risk increasing to 8.3 times that expected among those who survived 10 years or longer after transplantation.[169] The risk was significantly elevated for malignant melanoma (ratio of observed-to-expected cases, 5.0) and cancers of the buccal cavity (11.1), liver (7.5), brain or other parts of the central nervous system (7.6), thyroid (6.6), bone (13.4), and connective tissue (8.0). The cumulative incidence rate was 2.2% at 10 years and 6.7% at 15 years. In this study, the risk was higher for recipients who were younger at the time of transplantation than for those who were older. Multivariate analyses found an association between higher doses of TBI and a higher risk of solid cancers, and chronic GVHD and male gender were strongly linked with an excess risk of squamous cell cancers of the buccal cavity and skin. An increased risk of solid tumors was also reported by one center after autologous transplantation in the treatment of patients with NHL.[170] In this series of 605 patients, the risk of a nonhematologic malignancy was 10%, with the risk continuing to increase with continued follow-up. The risk of any second cancer was 29%, and a second malignancy was the cause of death for 10% of patients treated. Again, older age was the primary factor associated with the development of a second cancer.

Relapse of Disease after Hematopoietic Stem Cell Transplantation

Relapse of disease is the most frequent cause of treatment failure after autologous or allogeneic HSC transplantation. Factors associated with higher risk of relapse include transplantation at a more-advanced stage of disease, autologous transplantation, absence of GVHD, T-cell depletion of the allograft, and less-intensive conditioning regimen. A small proportion of patients can undergo a second transplant, although the peritransplant mortality is greatly increased with use of a second dose-intense regimen.[171,172] The probability of successful outcome is greater for patients with longer disease-free intervals between transplants. Manipulation of the donor-derived immune system in the allogeneic recipient (cf., GVL effects, described later) may achieve control of disease in a minority of patients.

IMMUNOLOGIC CONSEQUENCES OF HEMATOPOIETIC STEM CELL TRANSPLANTATION

Establishment of hematopoietic chimerism with its attendant GVH reaction has both advantageous and deleterious consequences for the patient undergoing allogeneic HSC transplantation. Acute and chronic GVHD (the clinical sequelae of this reaction) are major causes of both early and late mortality and may result in considerable morbidity if not adequately controlled. However, the GVD benefit of allografting is the justification for the development of reduced-intensity transplant-conditioning regimens and is the primary reason for the lower relapse rate observed after allogeneic compared with autologous transplantation. The mechanisms involved in the development of GVHD and GVD continue to be dissected in both human and animal studies. Similarly, studies are being conducted in an attempt to separate the beneficial GVD from the detrimental GVHD to improve the outcome of allogeneic transplantation. In 1966, Billingham[173] postulated that three requirements must be met for GVHD to occur: the transplanted graft must contain immunocompetent cells, the host must be incapable of rejecting the transplanted cells, and the host must express tissue antigens that are not present in the transplant donor and can be recognized as foreign. GVHD is a much more complex phenomenon, involving cytokine networks as well as a variety of cellular mediators including antigen-presenting cells.

Graft-versus-Host Disease

Acute Graft-versus-Host Disease

The form of GVHD occurring early after transplantation, usually within the first 100 days, is referred to as acute

GVHD. Organs involved include skin, gastrointestinal tract, and liver; involvement of skin is most common, but any organ may be involved either alone or in combination with other tissue targets of immunologic attack. GVHD is a clinical diagnosis with laboratory confirmation. No laboratory studies, including tissue biopsies, are available to confirm or exclude this diagnosis. Skin rash, which is the most common presenting manifestation of GVHD, may also result from an allergic reaction to medication or toxicity from the conditioning regimen. Nausea, anorexia, and diarrhea may result from the conditioning regimen or infectious consequences of transplantation as well as from GVHD. Each of these complications of transplantation more commonly occurs at distinct times after transplantation, simplifying the diagnosis.

In contrast to the simple concepts proposed by Bellingham, the results of murine and human studies now show that acute GVHD (aGVHD) can be considered a three-step process: (1) damage to host tissues from chemotherapy/radiotherapy inducing the secretion of inflammatory cytokines; (2) activation and amplification of donor T cells interacting with host antigen-presenting cells along with increased expression of major histocompatibility complex (MHC) antigens; and (3) target cell apoptosis via both cellular and inflammatory mediators.[174,175]

The risk of developing aGVHD increases primarily with HLA disparity between donor and recipient,[176] but also with increasing age of donor and recipient, gender disparity, and infusion of T cell–replete HSC products. Conditioning with reduced-intensity regimens, with lower regimen-related toxicities to nonhematologic tissues, also results in a lower risk of aGVHD (but not chronic GVHD [cGVHD]), but may also shift the time to initial manifestations of GVHD.[177]

Pharmacologic agents are the mainstay of prophylaxis of aGVHD. Most patients receive a combination of a calcineurin inhibitor (tacrolimus or cyclosporine) along with an antimetabolite such as methotrexate or mycophenylate mofetil (MMF). Randomized studies in related donor and URD transplantation of tacrolimus and cyclosporine showed a lower incidence of aGVHD for recipients of tacrolimus, but no differences in event-free survival, at least for patients with less-advanced diseases.[178,179] Methotrexate is associated with delayed engraftment, mucositis, idiopathic pneumonia syndrome, and other transplant-related complications, prompting the development of other combination regimens such as a calcineurin inhibitor in combination with sirolimus or MMF. In these studies, mucositis was modest, engraftment was prompt, and transplant-related toxicity was modest.[180–182] Other centers reported possible success of reduced doses of methotrexate, although randomized studies have not been conducted.[183] The addition of antithymocyte globulin (ATG) to the conditioning regimen lowers the GVH and HVG reactions because of the persistence of this agent for several days after HSC infusion.[111,186] However, patients treated with ATG may face higher risks of infectious complications including Epstein-Barr virus (EBV)-associated post-transplant lymphoproliferative disorder as a result of the greater immunosuppression achieved.

T lymphocytes are primary mediators of the GVH reaction, and multiple studies have demonstrated lower risks of aGVHD for recipients of T cell–depleted grafts, including large randomized studies.[185] Unfortunately, T-cell depletion increases the risks of engraftment failure and relapse after disease, as a result of the loss of the beneficial effects of the GVH reaction, and long-term event-free survivals are similar for patients receiving T cell–depleted or T cell–replete grafts. Several transplant groups explored depletion of T-cell subsets in attempts to discriminate between the beneficial and deleterious effects of the GVH reaction.[186] To date, no specific technique has shown superiority in clinical studies in humans.

Glucocorticoids remain the standard approach to initial systemic management of clinically significant aGVHD. Patients who fail to respond to initial therapy have a poor prognosis, as additional agents added for control increase the risk of opportunistic infections and other complications. The use of higher doses of corticosteroids, concomitant addition of ATG, for example, have not proven to improve the outcomes of patients who develop aGVHD and should be reserved for patients who are refractory to initial therapy.[187,188] A number of drugs including ATG, pentastatin, switching to tacrolimus from cyclosporine, and newer monoclonal antibodies have shown (limited) activity in the salvage treatment of patients with steroid-refractory aGVHD.[189–191] Extracorporeal exposure of peripheral blood mononuclear cells to the photosensitizing agent 8-methoxypsoralen and UVA radiation (photopheresis) has been shown to be effective in the treatment of selected diseases mediated by T cells, including both aGVHD and cGVHD and is a novel approach to the treatment of patients with steroid-refractory GVHD.[192]

Chronic Graft-versus-Host Disease

Chronic GVHD is the leading cause of late treatment-related deaths among recipients of allogeneic BM and blood transplants. cGVHD resembles autoimmune disorders such as scleroderma, Sjögren syndrome, and primary biliary cirrhosis. Diagnosis is, as with acute GVHD, based on clinical observations with secondary laboratory confirmation (Table 58–3) A falling performance status, progression weight loss, or recurrent infections are usually signs of clinical extensive cGVHD. About 50% of long-term survivors will develop this complication of transplantation at a median of 9 months, and patients must be monitored closely for at least 2 years after transplantation so that appropriate treatment can be initiated before extensive tissue damage develops.

Factors predicting the development of cGVHD again include degree of HLA disparity but also include source of HSCs (PBSC transplantation conveys a higher risk compared with marrow or cord blood transplantation). Patients who develop cGVHD have a higher risk of TRM but a lower risk of relapse as a result of the immunologic GVD effect.[193] T cell depletion may decrease the risk of cGVHD, although this has not been demonstrated in all studies. A randomized study of 404 patients undergoing marrow transplantation from URDs reported similar incidences of cGVHD for recipients of T cell–depleted or T cell–replete grafts; the duration of post-transplant immunosuppression and OS were also similar for the two arms of this study.[196]

Most patients require at least two drugs for treatment of cGVHD. Again, glucocorticoids along with a calcineurin inhibitor are the standard initial treatment. About half of the patients with cGVHD do not achieve a complete remission with first-line therapy. No clear recommendations exist regarding second-line treatments, and a variety of pharmacologic and immunologic techniques have been used. Retransplantation is ineffective, but a single-center report of low-dose thoracoabdominal irradiation described an 82% response rate, with the best responses observed for patients

Table 58–3 Manifestations of Chronic Graft-versus-Host Disease

Target Organ	Physical Manifestation	Target Organ	Physical Manifestation
Skin	Erythema Dryness Exfoliation Macular-papular or urticarial rash Pigmentary changes (hyperpigmentation, vitiligo, mottling) Papulosquamous or lichenoid plaques Keratosis Nodules Scleroderma Morphea	Vagina/vulva	Dryness Dyspareunia Strictures or stenosis Erythema Atrophy or lichenoid changes not attributed to ovarian failure
Nails	Ridging Onychodystrophy Onycholysis	Liver	Elevated bilirubin or liver-function tests not resulting from other cause
Hair	Premature graying Thinning scalp hair Alopecia Decreased body hair	Lung	Bronchiolitis obliterans Cough Wheezing Dyspnea on exertion History of recurrent bronchitis or sinusitis
Mouth	Burning Gingivitis Mucositis Ulcers Erythema Striae Dryness Atrophy Lichenoid changes Labial atrophy or pigmentary changes Tightness around the mouth Sensitivity to acidity, strong flavors, heat or cold Tooth decay	GI	Anorexia Nausea Vomiting Diarrhea Malabsorption Weight loss Dysphagia Odynophagia
Eyes	Dryness Burning Blurring Gritty eyes Photophobia Pain		

with fasciitis or oral involvement.[195] Photopheresis has an overall response rate of 50% to 60%, with many patients achieving complete control of this complication of transplantation.[196]

Graft-versus-Leukemia Effect

The chemoradiotherapy regimen used for the treatment of patients is intended to cure the underlying disease, with the HSCs infused merely to rescue the patient from the marrow-lethal toxicity of the regimen. However, it became evident very early that patients who experienced acute or chronic GVHD had a much lower risk of relapse after transplantation than did those without these complications. The potential of the GVD effect is demonstrated by the infusion of unmodified peripheral blood mononuclear cells from the marrow donor for the treatment of relapse after allogeneic BMT. Kolb and colleagues[128] reported the administration of donor lymphocytes to 135 patients with chronic and acute leukemias who relapsed after allogeneic transplantation. Complete remissions were achieved in 73% of patients with CML, but only 29% of patients with AML. None of the patients treated for acute lymphoblastic leukemia (ALL) responded to this treatment, suggesting that this approach is most practical for more indolent diseases. Complications of this therapy include the development of GVHD (41%) and myelosuppression (34%). The number of lymphocytes infused is important in achieving this effect, and it may be possible to induce GVD by using doses of lymphocytes that are less likely to result in GVHD.[197] However, a distinction between the cells responsible for inducing GVD and those causing GVHD has not been found. The delay in response between lymphocyte infusion and the development of a GVD effect suggests that only a minority of the cells infused recognize the tumor cell antigens and must undergo in vivo expansion before a therapeutic effect is achieved. It may be possible to develop cytotoxic lymphocytes in the laboratory, decreasing the delay in effect and possibly increasing the effect in the more rapidly proliferative acute leukemias.[198]

Peripheral blood mononuclear cell components (donor-cell lymphocytes infusion, DLI) collected from donors either with or without treatment with granulocyte colony–stimulating factor (G-CSF) are also effective in the immunotherapy of patients with progressive disease after allogeneic transplantation.[199–201] Patients with low-grade lymphoid malignancies such as CLL or indolent NHL, mantle cell

NHL, and CML have the highest likelihood of response. The results of a survey of 25 transplant programs identified 140 patients who received DLI and reported a CR rate of 60% in patients with CML; response rates were higher in patients with cytogenetic and chronic-phase relapse (75.7%) than in patients with accelerated-phase (33.3%) or blastic-phase (16.7%) relapse, and almost 90% of these patients remained in remission at 2 years after treatment.[202] Complete remission rates in AML and ALL patients who had not received pre-DLI chemotherapy were 15.4% and 18.2%, respectively. Complications of DLI included aGVHD (60%), cGVHD (60.7%), and pancytopenia (18.6%). The development of GVHD after DLI was highly correlated with disease response ($P < .00001$).

Donor immunity can be transferred at least transiently to the host, as demonstrated by delayed-type transfusion reactions to host red blood cells mediated by donor lymphocytes transfused along with the marrow.[203] Adoptive transfer of donor immunity against specific targets can be achieved, but its persistence requires immunization of both the donor and the recipient.[204,205] A clinical utility for such manipulation of the immune system has not yet been demonstrated but is clearly of interest as a technique to prevent post-transplant infections or, possibly, relapse.

DISEASES TREATED

Acute Myelogenous Leukemia

Induction chemotherapy yields complete remission for most patients with AML, but these patients will rapidly relapse if postinduction consolidation therapy is not administered. Randomized studies of consolidation regimens of varying intensity demonstrate that more-intensive regimens will achieve a higher probability of durable remissions. Despite this, even with the administration of several cycles of consolidation therapy, the probability of cure is only on the order of 35%. Cytogenetic status remains the single most important prognostic factor, although other factors can also help in risk stratification.[206]

Because chemotherapy-only regimens achieve disease control for a minority of patients, transplant strategies were investigated to evaluate their relative efficacy. To date no fewer than 16 studies have failed to demonstrate conclusively the superiority of allogenic stem cell transplantation (SCT) over autologous and nontransplant modalities in the consolidative treatment of AML. Indeed, these published reports have been conflicting about the true relative merits of the three modalities. This seems in no small part to be due to the widely disparate treatment regimens used and the number and intensity of consolidation cycles before SCT.

The selection of a postremission treatment plan hinges on multiple factors: the age and performance status of the patient, the number of cycles of treatment required to achieve remission, the pretreatment cytogenetics, and the minimal residual disease (MRD) status.[207,208] Assessment of these prognostic factors and the fact that AML represents an intermediate disease sensitivity to a graft-versus-malignancy effect provides a risk-stratification basis for the implementation of autologous versus allogenic SCT and the timing (CR1 vs CR2) of further consolidation.

In general, autologous BMT has not proven to be more effective than nontransplant intensive consolidation chemotherapy (Table 58–4), although studies reported by Burnett and colleagues[209] and Zittoun and colleagues[210] demonstrated significantly better DFS for recipients of autologous (54% vs 41%) and allogeneic (48% vs 30%) transplantation compared with recipients of chemotherapy, respectively. Therefore, the timing and patient selection are critical because the best results for allogenic SCT have been noted in younger patients in CR1. If a patient in CR1 relapses, then early preemptive allogenic SCT should be undertaken, as opposed to reinduction to CR2. The rationale is that even though CR2 may be achieved by reinduction chemotherapy, the DFS is short with probable early relapse and relentlessly difficult-to-control disease due to increased tumor cell resistance and disease burden.[211]

Table 58–4 Multicenter Randomized Studies Comparing Autologous Marrow Transplantation to Intensive Consolidation Chemotherapy

	Probability of Event-Free Survival (%)		
Investigator	Allogeneic	Autologous	Chemotherapy
Zittoun et al[210]	55*	48	30 (4 yr)‡
Cassileth et al[394]	43	35	35 (4 yr)
Burnett et al[209]	ND†	53*	40 (7 yr)
Harousseau et al[395]	44	44	40 (4 yr)
Ravindranath et al[396]	ND†	38	36 (3 yr)

*Significantly different compared with chemotherapy treatment arm.
†ND: Allogeneic transplantation was not performed as part of this trial.
‡Shown is the median duration of follow-up at time of analysis.

Publication of CALGB 8461 has been instrumental in classifying AML patients into low-, intermediate-, or high-risk groups based on the pretreatment cytogenetic status. The t(15;17), t(8;21), inv16, and t(16;16) are the favorable cytogenetic abnormalities, and based on cytogenetic stratification, this good-risk group of patients in CR1 would benefit most from high-dose consolidation chemotherapy as the risks of an SCT outweigh the benefit.[210,213] Indeed the remarkable advances in the treatment of APL with t(15;17) have minimized the role of transplantation in first remission in this subtype.[214,215] Therefore, patients with these abnormalities should be offered ASCT only on relapse or if identified to have molecular abnormalities that predict relapse despite overt good-risk karyotype. To this end, Acute Leukemia French Association (ALFA) centers carried out two consecutive trials considering allogeneic sibling SCT in 92 young AML patients with t(8;21)/inv(16) (core-binding factor [CBF] group) or a normal karyotype (NN group). Sixty-six (66%) achieved CR2. Donor availability was an independent prognostic factor for survival in the patient population as a whole as well as in the CBF subset, but not in NN patients, further supporting this strategy for CBF-AML. The presence of an FLT3 internal tandem duplication (ITD) was found to be the main poor prognostic factor for attaining second CR and survival, mandating earlier consideration of SCT, especially in NN patients.[216] Additionally, Kim and associates[217] published their investigation of AML patients with normal cytogenetics in which a multiple drug resistance (MDR) phenotype was found to be an independent prognostic factor for EFS and OS.

Allogenic SCT has the lowest risk of relapse with the highest TRM. In the unfavorable-risk group, an allogeneic sibling SCT in CR1 would be acceptable, as the outcomes with chemotherapy alone or with an autologous SCT are dismal.[218] Patients with poor-risk cytogenetics such as trisomy 8, monosomy 5 or 7, and complex cytogenetics merit early ASCT in CR1. Additionally, chromosome 5 and/or 7 abnormalities are indicative of a poor prognosis and the only potential cure for such patients is allogeneic SCT, although data in this context are limited. In a retrospective study between 1983 and 2001 recorded by the Netherlands Stem Cell Transplant Registry (Typhon), OS was 25%. Factors that predicted lower relapse rate and better OS were age younger than 40 years, unrelated grafts, and chromosome 5 or chromosome 7 abnormalities, but not both. The development of GVHD grades II to IV was independently associated with significantly higher TRM albeit similar to patients with a secondary AML and normal cytogenetics. Therefore, although patients with AML with chromosome 5 and/or 7 abnormalities do rather poorly after ASCT, this is the only approach that can achieve a substantial long-term survival and cure in patients with high-risk acute leukemia.[219]

Controversy still centers around the suitability of early matched sibling SCT in CR1 versus at relapse. Approximately 25% of patients in CR1 may indeed be cured, and to subject them to an unnecessarily toxic procedure must be weighed against the specter of relapsed disease with compromised performance status, resistant disease, and increased disease burden. This therefore confirms the importance of pre-treatment cytogenetic assessment and post-treatment MRD assays.

For intermediate-risk patients ABMT/ASCT is an appropriate treatment choice and seems to improve outcomes compared with conventional chemotherapy.[220] Autologous SCT has an intermediate risk of relapse and TRM, although its role in CR1 is not obvious, and questions remain about the selection of HSC source, value of ex vivo purging, and timing of transplantation relative to other cycles of postinduction consolidation. Autologous SCT appears to be effective therapy for the patient with AML in second CR, as reported in a number of phase II studies where the survival probabilities of ≥35% are significantly superior to standard chemotherapy regimens.[221]

AML is a disease in which purging of tumor cells may be beneficial because the presence of MRD predisposes to earlier and higher relapse rates. In nonrandomized studies, patients who received marrow cells treated with chemotherapy agents were less likely to relapse after transplantation. Indeed, Osborne and colleagues[222] recently published a study using the WT1 transcript, as a marker of MRD in BM harvests of 24 patients slated for autologous SCT. At median follow-up of 92 months, they reported an relapse-free survival (RFS) of 10.4 months for patients with WTI more than 2000 (high risk) and an as-yet-reached RFS for patients with scores less than 2000 (low risk) ($P < .05$). Similarly, indirect laboratory assessments of purging efficacy suggest a benefit for patients who are treated with an aggressive purging technique. Despite the foregoing, the role of purging has not been proven in randomized studies, nor has it been shown to be of benefit in PBSCT.

However, the change that may have the greatest impact on AML treatment is the advent of reduced intensity or NST.[223] Reduced-intensity hematopoietic cell transplantation (HCT) relies on the GVL effect of the allograft rather than the direct tumoricidal activity of the conditioning regimen. Because of the paucity of any direct antileukemic effect of the conditioning regimens, the truly nonmyeloablative regimens can be used only in patients with low volumes of disease, whereas the reduced-intensity conditioning regimens, which usually contain fludarabine and some alkylating agent, do have direct antileukemia activity and can be used with more-extensive disease.[224] The shortened duration of cytopenias and the minimal mucosal toxicity of the newer reduced-intensity conditioning regimens provide a reasonably safe transplant option for patients 2 decades older than the population that was treated with traditional fully ablative high-dose chemoradiotherapy regimens.[225]

A lack of consensus is found in the literature about the true definition of primary refractory disease with respect to the morphologic criteria and the number of induction regimens required before it is deemed refractory. Nevertheless, TRM occurs and risk of relapse with a 5-year EFS of only 10% to 20%. Factors to consider before implementing allogeneic transplantation for primary refractory AML are those that are critically predictive of outcome, such as BM blast cell count, karyotype, degree of pretreatment, age, performance status, and availability of a related donor.[226] Those patients with many favorable prognostic factors and an HLA-matched related donor available would be the best candidates; whereas those with many poor prognostic factors and only an URD available should be offered enrollment in investigational studies or palliation.

Acute Lymphoblastic Leukemia

In contrast to treatment of the pediatric patient with ALL, only a small minority of adults with ALL are currently cured with available induction and consolidation regimens.[227,228] Results have improved modestly with more intensive postremission chemotherapy and with tailoring of protocols to specific subsets of ALL.[229] Multicenter trials have demonstrated CR rates of 75% to 89% and leukemia-free survival rates of 33% mainly due to the intensified chemotherapy regimens.[230] ALL patients have traditionally been categorized as either standard risk or high risk. High-risk factors are older age, high white cell count, CNS involvement, B-cell phenotype, T-cell phenotype, cytogenetic abnormalities such as t(4;11), t(8;14), t(1;19), 11q23 abnormalities, Ph^+, and longer time to achieve CR.[231] In view of the poor response rates and OS of adult ALL, SCT continues to be explored and refined in an effort to bridge the gap.

The questions to be answered in adult ALL are: (1) does SCT improve outcomes over chemotherapy, (2) what is the optimal timing of SCT in standard-risk and high-risk subgroups, (3) what is the value of purging in autologous SCT, (4) is ASCT superior to auto- and nontransplant modalities, (5) is related donor superior to URD, (6) what is the appropriate treatment for relapsed ALL, and (7) what is the role of targeted therapy?

SCT has been recommended in first remission for patients with risk factors for relapse, and for standard-risk patients only after relapse. The international ALL trial E2993 clearly established the favorable results of ASCT in CR1 for standard-risk patients.[232] However, the optimal treatment of postremission high-risk adult ALL has still not been clearly elucidated. The GOELAMS trial concurred that early intent-to-treat allogeneic BMT was productive of significantly better outcomes than consolidation chemotherapy followed by delayed unpurged autologous SCT (6-year OS, 75% vs 41%; 6-year DFS, 72% vs 33%). Also they determined that after autologous SCT, interferon-α maintenance did not confer any advantage with respect to relapse or survival.[233]

For relapsed or high-risk disease, Thiebaut and colleagues[234] demonstrated a DFS benefit (43% vs 31%) for patients allografted versus controls, with an even more pronounced benefit noted in the high-risk cohort (DFS, 44% vs 11%, respectively). Additionally, a subsequent study demonstrated similar outcomes in the URD versus related-donor setting and for BM versus PBSC grafts. Significantly though, improved survival was noted in B-lineage ALL versus their T-lineage ALL and that DFS for younger patients was superior.[235]

After relapse, should all patients without exception be allografted? Data from the IBMTR reported a DFS of 42% in CR2. However, beyond CR2 or in primary refractory disease, the DFS is a precipitately dismal 5% to 15%. To confirm these data, two U.S. centers evaluated the relative efficacy of allogeneic BMT in CR1 ($n = 41$), complete response (CR) ≥2 ($n = 46$), or relapse ($n = 95$) and demonstrated a significantly better 5-year DFS for the early SCT group (CR1 [43%] vs CR ≥2 (23%) vs relapsed, 9%; $P < .001$) and an overall 5-year DFS of 21%. These data underscore the contention that early ASCT improves outcomes.[236] In another study of standard-risk patients in CR1 or 1(st) relapse, DFS was similar between autologous, related, and unrelated cohorts. Again, DFS was superior for transplantation in CR1. In the Ph^+ subset, 5-year DFS was clearly superior for allogeneic versus autologous SCT (30% vs 0; $P = .04$) and was further augmented by the occurrence of limited cGVHD (53% vs 22%).[237]

For patients with high-risk or relapsed ALL lacking a related histocompatible donor, autologous and URD transplantation are available options.[238] Comparatively, both URD and auto-SCT extend survival, but URD offers better protection against leukemia relapse. To confirm this assertion, an analysis of 712 patients in CR1 revealed that URD predisposed to a higher TRM in both CR1 and CR2. Conversely, relapses were more frequent in the auto-SCT arm irrespective of CR status. Although 3-year DFSs were similar for both CR1 and CR2, an advantage in initial 6-month DFS was recorded in the URD group for younger patients, patients in CR2 with initial CR1 more than 1 year, WBC fewer than 50×10^9/L), performance status ≥90%, and in those who have undergone transplantation since 1995. Of note, more URD recipients were high risk. Further analysis revealed that ex vivo purging delayed but did not abrogate engraftment. In conclusion, improvements in allo-SCT safety and refinements in patient selection are required the better to aid treatment decision making for optimal OS.[239]

For Ph^+ ALL, the greatest improvements in DFS and OS are a consequence of in vivo purging of *BCR/ABL*$^+$ transcripts by the incorporation of imatinib mesylate into pre-/post-SCT treatment regimens. This factor becomes more important when viewed in the context of quantification of MRD by reverse transcription–polymerase chain reaction (RT-PCR) to predict pre-SCT risk of relapse and therefore necessary therapy adjustment. Second, MRD quantification is used in conjunction with chimerism studies not only to predict relapse but also to modulate the GVL effect mediated by GVHD. MRD quantification therefore more precisely defines remission, prognosis, responsiveness to therapy, and expected long-term survival.[240,241]

Chronic Myelogenous Leukemia

Allogeneic HSC transplantation is an appropriate treatment for CML, with long-term survival rates exceeding 80% in some series.[242,243] However, newly developed inhibitors of the tyrosine kinase encoded by the Philadelphia chromosome has relegated transplantation to the treatment of patients with advanced disease or the rare patient with CML not responsive to that targeted therapy. Unfortunately, the probability of long-term survival decreases for patients who undergo allogeneic transplantation more than 1 year after diagnosis and for patients with more-advanced diseases, and the effect of prior therapy with a tyrosine kinase inhibitor on the outcome of transplantation is not known. CML is highly responsive to the immunologic GVD effect, and many patients in relapse after transplantation can be salvaged by the administration of donor lymphocytes.

Limited numbers of patients with CML in chronic phase or with more-advanced disease have been treated with autologous HSC transplantation.[244] In a large, single-center study of 73 patients, the survival of patients with chronic-phase disease who underwent transplantation did not differ from that of patients treated with interferon: 58% of patients with more-advanced disease achieved a complete hematologic remission, but only 10% achieved a complete cytogenetic response, and the median survival for this group of patients was only 5 months. Of speculative interest is the collection of autologous cells after cytogenetic remission is achieved by using one of the new tyrosine kinase inhibitors for subsequent use at the time of disease relapse.[245]

Chronic Lymphocytic Leukemia

To date, the factors that have limited the implementation of HSC transplantation in CLL have been the long natural history of the disease and the advanced age of most patients at diagnosis. Although traditionally considered a disease of the elderly, up to 40% and 12% of CLL patients are younger than 60 and 50 years, respectively. These younger patients invariably will die of their disease or its complications. The understanding of the pathophysiology of CLL is rapidly advancing, and risk stratification of patients is now possible through examination for chromosome 17p and 11q deletions and detection of ZAP-70 and CD38 expression.[246]

Allogeneic transplantation is very effective in the control of CLL.[247,248] In the study from Dana-Farber Cancer Institute of 162 patients with high-risk CLL who had undergone full myeloablative SCT from 1989 through 1999, 25 patients underwent related donor T cell–depleted HSC transplantation, and 137 patients without sibling donors underwent autologous SCT.[247] The 100-day mortality was similar in both groups at 4%. OSs were also similar—58% and 55% in the allogeneic and autologous cohorts, respectively. The probability of relapse after allogeneic HSC transplantation was 68%, possibly as a result of the T-cell depletion and resultant loss of the GVD effect. The exquisite sensitivity of CLL cells to the GVD effect allows the use of reduced-intensity regimens with lower risks of regimen-related mortality in these, generally, older patients.[249,250] The Seattle program described 64 patients with advanced CLL treated with a nonmyeloablative regimen of a single fraction of TBI with or without fludarabine and either related ($n = 44$) or unrelated ($n = 20$) HSC transplantation.[249] The probability of relapse was 26%, but the probability of relapse-free survival was 52%.

The extensive infiltration of BM by malignant lymphocytes complicates autologous transplantation. Investigators from the M.D. Anderson Cancer Institute reported that 6 of 11 patients treated with autologous marrow cells (7 purged ex vivo) surviving in remission up to 29 months after transplantation.[251] Investigators at the Dana-Farber reported a high CR rate for 137 patients who received autologous BM that had been purged with multiple monoclonal antibodies.[247] However, disease relapse and a high incidence (19%) of secondary malignancies were frequent sources of late mortality in that large series. As with autologous transplantation for CML, autologous HSC transplantation for this disease is, in general, limited to clinical research protocols and cannot be generally advocated for any group of these patients.

Myeloma

Newly diagnosed multiple myeloma (MM) has become one of the most common indications for transplantation as a result of multiple randomized studies showing improved outcomes after dose-intense therapy with autologous HSC support. In 1983, McElwain and Powles[252] used melphalan, 140 mg/m^2, without stem cell support as a salvage therapy in nine patients with refractory myeloma and noted that all patients responded to treatment, with five patients achieving complete biochemical and BM responses. Further dose escalation was precluded by the hematopoietic toxicity of this drug. After multiple phase I and II studies of high-dose melphalan therapy with autologous marrow or PBSC support confirmed the feasibility of this technique,[253–255] at least 6 phase III studies comparing dose-intense with standard-dose therapy in the autologous transplant setting were published (Table 58–5).[86,256–260] The French Myeloma Intergroup reported a large-scale randomized trial (IFM 90) that randomized 200 patients to either conventional dose VMCP/VBAP or autologous BMT with melphalan and TBI after four cycles of induction treatment.[86] The findings were strikingly in favor of the dose-intense approach with improvements in CR rates (22% vs 5%) and median probabilities of event-free (27 months vs 18 months) and OSs (60+ months vs 37 months). The Medical Research Council Myeloma VII trial of 407 patients reported similar results[256]; the French group Myelome Autogreffe (MAG) achieved results comparable to the IFM 90 trial, but no significant difference in OSs was found as a result of unexpected prolonged survivals in the chemotherapy arm.[257] The Spanish PETHEMA group did not find a statistically significant difference in EFS and OS between chemotherapy and dose-intensive therapy.[258] However, only patients who responded to conventional-dose chemotherapy were randomized, and patients in the chemotherapy arm were allowed to cross over into the dose-intensive therapy group. The MRC trial comparing dose-intense with conventional therapy deserves special consideration, in that it is the most recent of the randomized trials and was carried out in the era of more-advanced supportive care and with the availability of newer therapeutic agents.[256] It still showed a statistically significant advantage for dose intensity in terms of CR, EFS, and OS. These randomized trials, all of which showed a trend to, or significantly improved results for patients treated with dose-intense therapy, with the support of numerous phase II trials, clearly indicate that dose-intense therapy with autologous HSCT should be offered to appropriate patients as part of their initial treatment. The median EFS is remarkably constant in all these trials (25–31 months). It is more difficult to analyze OS results because OS partly depends on salvage therapy. However, median OS was significantly longer in the three studies in which differences in EFS were more marked. In all studies, procedure-related death rate was less than 5% and not greater than that observed with conventional chemotherapy. Factors associated with long-term EFS included initial transplantation within 1 year of diagnosis, absence of chromosome 11 or 13 abnormalities, and a lower β_2 microglobulin at initial diagnosis.[261] About one fourth of the patients will enjoy EFSs of ≥5 years, with few additional relapses seen after 7 years.

Tandem cycles of dose-intense therapy appear to improve further the outcomes of autologous HSC transplantation. The Arkansas transplant program described 42 patients who received two consecutive autologous PBSC transplants by using melphalan, 200 mg/m^2.[262] In patients that were capable of receiving two transplants, the CR rate increased from 24% after the first transplant to 43% after two transplants. This experience has now been extended in more than 1000 patients with overall CR rates of 40% and projected 5-year EFS and OSs of 25% and 40%, respectively.[263] The French Intergroup randomized 399 newly diagnosed myeloma patients younger than 60 years to single versus tandem transplants.[264] They found similar CR rates between the two groups (42% single transplant vs 50% tandem transplant), but superior 7-year EFSs (10% vs 20%; $P = .03$) and OSs (21% vs 42%, $P = .01$) for the tandem transplant group. For patients w ho did not achieve a very good partial response (<90% reduction in serum or urine paraprotein) after one transplant, the improvement in 7-year OS was even more dramatic (11% vs 43%; $P < .01$). These results support tandem autologous transplants for patients with a diagnosis of MM who do not show disease progression after the first transplant.

Table 58–5 Randomized Trials Comparing Conventional Chemotherapy with High-Dose Therapy in Multiple Myeloma

				CR Rate (%)			Median EFS (mo)			Median OS (m)		
	N	Age (yr)	Median F/U	CC	HDT	*P*	CC	HDT	*P*	CC	HDT	P
IFM 90[86]	200	<65	7 yr	5	22	<.001	18	28	.01	44	57	.03
MAG91[256]	190	55–65	56 mo	NE	NE		19	25	.05	45	42	NS
PETHEMA[258]	164	≤65	42 mo	11	30	.002	34	42	NS	67	65	NS
Italian MMSG[259]	195	50–70	2 yr	7	26	<.001	16	28	.0036	43	58+	.0008
USIG[260]	50			15	17	NS	21	25	.05	53	58	NS
MRC7[255]	407	<65	42 mo	8	44	<.001	19.6	31.6	<.0001	42	54	<.001

CC, conventional chemotherapy; CR, complete remission; EFS, event-free survival; HDT, high-dose therapy; OS, overall survival; NE, not evaluated; NS, difference not statistically significant; F/U, follow-up; mo, months.

The incidence of myeloma increases with increasing age, and many patients with plasma cell dyscrasias have renal impairment as a result of their disease; early studies of dose-intense therapy tended to exclude these patients. However, the favorable characteristics of melphalan permit transplant therapy to be extended to patients with renal impairment, including patients with end-stage renal failure (ESRF). Pharmacokinetic studies of melphalan show comparable clearance rates regardless of renal function.[265] The Arkansas group compared 42 patients with renal failure (including 19 requiring dialysis) with 84 patients matched for other prognostic features. Regimen-related mortality was 7% for the group with renal impairment compared with 6% for those with normal renal function. Engraftment kinetics and probabilities of EFSs and OSs were also similar. This group reported a subsequent series involving 81 patients with renal insufficiency that showed no difference in quality of stem cell collection and engraftment, even for patients on dialysis.[266] This transplant group also demonstrated the tolerability of dose-intense therapy in the older patient, reporting a slight increase in 60-day mortality for patients older than 65 years (8% vs 2%). However, median EFSs (1.5 vs 2.8 years) and OSs (3.3 vs 4.8 years) were statistically similar for the older and younger patients.[267]

The EBMTR performed a case-matched study comparing 25 patients receiving syngeneic transplants with 125 patients receiving autologous transplants and 125 patients receiving allogeneic transplants.[268] They reported a CR rate of 68%, which was not significantly different from autologous (48%) or allogeneic (58%) transplants. Median OS was better for syngeneic compared with autologous (73 vs 44 months) transplants, and the progression-free survival was significantly better (72 vs 25 months). From this study, the EBMTR recommends a syngeneic transplant if an identical twin donor is available.

Allogeneic transplantation after dose-intense therapy in the treatment of myeloma is characterized by unacceptable transplant-related morbidity, approaching 40% by day 100.[269] Use of a reduced-intensity conditioning regimen decreases the risk of regimen-related mortality to less than 20%, but patients with advanced disease are unlikely to respond to this treatment.[270] The lower risk of complications with non-myeloablative conditioning regimens has led to studies of tandem autologous transplantation (to achieve dose-intense tumor debulking) followed by allogeneic transplantation (to achieve immunotherapy). In a study of tandem autologous followed by allogeneic transplantation published by Maloney and associates[271] the median days of neutropenia and hospitalization and the median number of platelet transfusions after allogeneic transplantation with a conditioning regimen of 2-Gy TBI were each 0. However, a similar study of patients with adverse risk features including chromosome 13 abnormalities did not demonstrate a benefit of tandem autologous followed by allogeneic transplantation in comparison to tandem cycles with autologous HSC support.[272]

The Amyloidoses

Primary amyloidosis, recognized as plasma cell dyscrasia in 1931, is a protein-conformation disorder caused by a clonal plasma cell disorder. The plasma cells in the BM produce a monoclonal immunoglobulin protein. The M protein light chains or light-chain fragments form insoluble fibrils from β-pleated sheet aggregates that are deposited into the extracellular matrix in kidney, heart, liver, gut, peripheral nervous system, and other tissues. The deposits disrupt organ function and ultimately lead to death. The two most common forms, amyloid light chain (AL) and reactive, may be primary, secondary, or familial, with 21 causative proteins identified to date. The prognosis of systemic AL amyloidosis is poor; fewer than 5% of all patients survive 10 years or longer. With conventional chemotherapy, such as vincristine, doxorubicin (Adriamycin), and dexamethasone (VAD), the median survival could be prolonged by 4 months.

In a study from MSKCC, Comenzo and colleagues[273] concluded that all patients with systemic amyloid syndromes (more than two organ systems) should be considered for PBSCT because no other modality of therapy is as effective in achieving complete hematologic responses and reversal of amyloid-related organ dysfunction in 66% of surviving patients. Autologous SCT is the treatment of choice because AL deposits in BM do not obviously impair stem cell mobilization. G-CSF mobilization is the standard recommended approach. The CD34+ optimal recommended dose is 5E+06/kg. More importantly, CD34+ selected cells require the same time to myeloid engraftment as unselected cells but have delayed lymphoid recovery with increased incidence of opportunistic infections. This procedure, however, remains controversial because TRM in AL amyloidosis is substantially higher (15%–40%) than in MM (<5%). The same study also explored the role of cytoreduction before autologous SCT. They found that reducing clonotypic cells yielded no benefit in DFS or OS in MM studies and hence questionable utility in AL.

In another study by DiSpenzieri and coworkers[274] 63 PBSCT case and 63 control subjects were strictly matched. OS at 1, 2, and 4 years from diagnosis were 89% and 71%, 81% and 55%, and 71% and 41% ($P < .001$) in favor of the SCT cohort. Additionally, the OS rates at 1, 2, and 4 years from start of therapy were 82% and 68%, 81% and 53%, and 70% and 40% ($P < .001$) for the PBSCT and conventional therapy cohorts, respectively. Randomized studies have shown that treatment with high-dose melphalan (HDM) and autologous stem cell transplantation (ASCT) of selected patients has been effective in arresting and even reversing the disease course with induction of CRs. Responders who achieve a complete disappearance of light-chain secretion are more likely to achieve reversal of underlying organ dysfunction.[275] Multiorgan disease, and cardiac dysfunction in particular, predicts poor transplant outcome. AL invariably has multisystem involvement and, indeed, one of the major criteria for post-transplant survival is intact organ function, specifically renal and cardiac function. (In one study, the EFS was 60% for patients with cardiac involvement but 100% for patients with renal involvement and no evidence of cardiac dysfunction.[278])

To this end, recent reports by Gillmore and colleagues[277] and Leung and colleagues[278] have detailed their individual successes with tandem cardiac and tandem living donor renal autologous SCT, respectively. However, genetic testing to document the presence of the *VλV1IGL6VS1* and *DPL2* mutations seen in cardiac and renal AL involvement, respectively, is still not widely used.[279]

Waldenström's Macroglobulinemia

Waldenström's macroglobulinemia (WM) is a rare monoclonal gammopathy associated with lymphoplasmacytic lymphoma.[280] It has been a hitherto incurable lymphoproliferative disorder characterized by the production of IgM paraprotein.[281] Asymptomatic WM patients who are diagnosed by chance need not be treated, and initiation of treatment should not be based on level of serum monoclonal protein per se but rather on the presence of cytopenia, significant adenopathy or organomegaly, symptomatic hyperviscosity, severe neuropathy, or cryoglobulinemia.[282]

The need for rapid disease control may favor the use of nucleoside analogs, although it may be prudent to avoid these agents in patients who are candidates for high-dose therapy because of the deleterious effects on subsequent HSC collection.[283,284] The presence of significant cytopenias may favor rituximab.[285] Despite the lack of randomized trials, a rational approach to the treatment of patients with WM is possible. Several factors, including the presence of cytopenias and need for rapid disease control, imply candidacy for high-dose therapy with autologous HSCT, which may induce responses even in patients with resistance to all three classes of agents (Table 58–6).[286]

Desikan and associates[287] reported a study of six patients conditioned with melphalan and TBI followed by autologous stem cell rescue. Five patients achieved a PR with EFS ranging from 2 to 52 months, and one patient achieved a durable CR. In this study, the importance of restriction of excessive purine analog use to the post–stem cell–collection period was stressed. This B-cell disorder appears to be sensitive to a GVL effect, and allogeneic transplantation may be effective in the treatment of patients with WM. Martino and colleagues[288] reported on two patients who had undergone ASCT after multiple relapses and have EFSs of 3 and 9 years. More studies need to be performed to elucidate the GVL effect of the allograft.

Non-Hodgkin's Lymphoma

The lymphomas represent a diverse group of malignancies. The incidence has doubled within the past 3 decades with 55,000 to 60,000 new cases diagnosed annually in the United States. These statistics represent a 3% annual increase within this period.[289,290] These malignancies have been reclassified by the WHO into B-cell and T-cell neoplasms.[291] Increasingly an association with chronic inflammatory disorders (Sjögren syndrome), chronic infection (*Helicobacter pylori*, EBV) and immune suppression (solid organ transplant) has been noted in the pathogenesis of the NHLs.[292] As a group, the lymphomas are highly responsive to chemotherapy, radiation, radioimmunotherapy (RIT), and increasingly biologic therapies such as monoclonal antibodies (anti-CD20, rituximab; anti-CD52, alemtuzumab) and a variety of vaccine-based therapies. Importantly, prognostic indices (IPI, FLIPI) and genetic and molecular markers in combination with the histology and extent of disease are increasingly being used to aid and refine treatment decisions.[293,294] Despite these advances, the majority of patients experience some initial responses, but only a minority are cured.

These tumors exhibit a strong dose-response relation, and the benefit of high-dose treatment with autologous stem cell rescue is well established for some categories of this disease. Several high-dose chemotherapy regimens have been developed for the treatment of the lymphomas. Radiation-based regimens, including CY with TBI and etoposide plus TBI, have significant activity but frequently are difficult to administer in that many patients have already been exposed to radiotherapy. Popular chemotherapy regimens include CY, BCNU, and etoposide (CBV) and BCNU, etoposide, Ara-C, and melphelan (BEAM). However, no single chemotherapeutic regimen has emerged as a superior treatment.

Autologous HSCT is a standard of care for many patients with NHL either in the treatment of relapse or as consolidation therapy for patients with aggressive disease. The success of this therapy reflects the extent and the responsiveness of the disease to chemotherapy at the time of transplantation. Relapse is the major cause of failure of autologous transplantation.

Indolent Non-Hodgkin's Lymphoma

In low-grade NHL, conventional chemotherapy has increased PFS, but OS has not been improved. Low-grade NHL, in general, exhibits a variable and prolonged natural course, with many patients not requiring treatment until symptoms or organ toxicity appear. Therefore, most of the experience with HSC transplantation has been in patients after initial relapse rather than at initial diagnosis, avoiding the potential for the morbidity and mortality of dose-intense therapy. The optimal timing of HSC transplantation (consolidation vs salvage) remains to be determined by prospective randomized trials, such as the ongoing multicenter trial of the German Low-grade Lymphoma Study Group, which indicates that up-front transplant after CHOP/MCP (mitoxantrone, chlorambucil, and prednisone) induction produces significant prolongation of PFS versus maintenance in patients attaining CR/PR.[295]

Clearly, HSC0 transplantation aims to eradicate residual tumor cells and prolongs OS, although it certainly does not guarantee cure, with the majority of patients eventually

Table 58–6 Autologous Stem-Cell Transplantation in Waldenström Macroglobulinemia

Reference	No. of Patients	Median age (yr)	Disease Status	Response (%)	CR (%)
Desikan et al[287]	8	58	Relapse	100	13
Anagnostopoulos et al[286]	4	49	Refractory	75	0
Tournilhac et al[393]	18	55	Chemosensitive, $n = 14$; chemoresistant, $n = 4$	95	11
Dreger et al[392]	10	51	First response or primary refractory	100	14

CR, complete response; WM, Waldenström macroglobulinemia.

relapsing.[296] Current data suggest that noncontaminated grafting (obtained with stem cell purging) does improve OS. As an example, up-front purged autograft (TBI, etoposide, CY) has proven to be valuable in patients with advanced follicular lymphoma, providing 10-year disease-specific survival of 97% with an RR of 30%.[297] However, data from prospective randomized trials comparing purged versus unpurged autografts are pending. A number of phase II and registry data have been published. Although response rates are high, a continuing pattern of relapse has been observed with autologous transplant. Bierman and colleagues[298] reported a 68% CR rate for a single-center series of 100 patients with relapsed disease but, at a median of 4 years, a probability of failure-free survival of 44% with no plateau to the curve depicting probability of relapse. The Dana-Farber transplant program reported a series of 86 patients with advanced follicular lymphoma who underwent autologous marrow transplantation as part of initial therapy in a publication that raised the question about the necessity for and efficacy of tumor cell purging.[299] Patients who received marrow products that were free of disease (based on a sensitive PCR detection technique for the t(14;18) abnormality commonly found in follicular NHL) experienced a much lower rate of relapse than did similar patients whose products contained detectable tumor after purging. However, again, no plateau to the curve depicting probability of relapse was reported.

The indolent lymphomas exhibit a strong response to the GVL effect of allogeneic transplantation and appears to provide the best chances for cure, providing a noncontaminated graft along with a graft versus lymphoma (GVL) effect.[300,301] Reduced intensity SCT may therefore be a reasonable approach in patients with advanced disease, allowing a GVL effect with less toxicity compared with conventional allograft. However, data are still limited, and follow-up in the majority of studies is relatively short, highlighting the need for longer follow-up to establish the role of reduced-intensity SCT in low-grade lymphoma.[302] Patients who undergo allogeneic transplantation will experience a higher probability of transplant-related mortality, but a lower risk of relapse after transplantation.[303] The difference in relapse rates could result from reintroduction of lymphoma cells in the HSC product or from the lack of a GVD effect of autologous transplantation.

Small numbers of patients have undergone autologous HSC transplantation for indolent NHL after transformation to aggressive NHL.[304] A large proportion of these patients achieved durable remissions, suggesting that this is effective therapy and should be considered for older patients or for those lacking an allogeneic donor. For patients with refractory or recurrent indolent NHL, allogeneic has returned superior DFS and OS as compared with autologous SCT, although the high TRM continues to indicate that nonmyeloablative allogeneic SCT (NST) should be explored in controlled trials.[305]

Aggressive Non-Hodgkin's Lymphoma

The role of high-dose chemotherapy with stem cell rescue in patients with chemotherapy-sensitive aggressive (intermediate or high-grade) lymphomas in relapse has become well established. The PARMA trial clearly demonstrated superior 5-year EFS treatment (46% vs 12%; $P = .001$) and OS (53% vs 32%; $P = .038$) in favor of HDT/autologous SCT versus conventional dose treatment for patients in first chemosensitive relapse. They also found that no patients assigned to the conventional-dose salvage therapy could be rescued at the time of second relapse with a delayed transplant. Therefore, excessive pretransplant "debulking" therapy and/or delays in transplant timing should be avoided. This randomized trial, which confirmed the findings of previous phase II studies, conclusively demonstrated that transplantation therapy represents the treatment of choice for first-relapse chemosensitive aggressive NHL.[306]

The International Prognostic Index (IPI) identifies patients with aggressive NHL who have a high likelihood of relapse and poor OS with conventional first-line therapy.[307] The French LNH-87 trial examined the role of consolidation transplantation for patients in first CR after standard-dose treatment.[308] The initial analysis of this trial demonstrated no advantage gained by the addition of intensive consolidation. However, subsequent analysis, which included only those patients with high intermediate or high risk by the more restrictive criteria of the IPI, revealed a superior DFS for those patients undergoing high-dose transplant. Similarly, the Italian Non-Hodgkin's Lymphoma Study Group showed no benefit to high-dose therapy with stem cell rescue in patients judged to be at high risk by virtue of tumor bulk or advanced-stage disease.[309,310] However, a striking advantage in DFS was noted when the 70 patients who qualified as high-intermediate or high risk based on the IPI were analyzed. In this subgroup, transplantation yielded a superior 6-year DFS rate (87% vs 48%; $P = .008$). In total, these studies suggest that for patients with high-risk disease by virtue of the IPI, the use of autologous transplantation therapy may be beneficial as part of the overall initial therapeutic strategy.

In other circumstances, HSCT may be indicated, such as for the patient who responds slowly to initial therapy, has high-risk disease or disease resistant to initial therapy, and relapse with chemotherapy-insensitive disease.[311] The appropriate approach for patients who achieve less than a CR or who exhibit a slow response to conventional induction therapy is not yet clear. In one small trial of 69 slow responders to CHOP chemotherapy, the use of early transplant compared with five additional cycles of CHOP was not associated with an overall improvement in survival or EFS ($P < .10$).[312]

Analysis of the ABMTR data showed that among 184 patients who had never achieved a CR with conventional therapy (primarily induction failures), 44% could achieve a CR after autologous BM or PBSC transplantation. The probability of PFS at 5 years after transplantation was 31%. Variables predictive of poor outcome in the multivariate analysis were chemotherapy resistance, administration of multiple cycles of chemotherapy before transplantation, poor performance status at time of transplantation, older age, and the lack of use of consolidative radiotherapy before or after transplantation.[313]

Patients with diffuse large cell lymphoma (DLCL) in chemosensitive first relapse have a 40% to 50% chance of long-term DFS after autologous transplantation.[314] This approach may also confer a survival advantage for high-risk patients in first CR. Patients relapsing after an autograft have a particularly poor prognosis, with a median survival of less than 12 months.[315] Comparatively, an earlier EBMT analysis failed to demonstrate superiority for allogenic SCT versus auto-SCT, but an updated analysis by Peniket and colleagues[324] confirmed better outcomes for the allogeneic cohort despite a higher proportion of chemoresistance in this subgroup. Given the reasonable outcomes and limited toxicity of salvage high-dose therapy and autologous stem cell rescue in DLCL, allogeneic transplantation should be considered only after autograft failure unless outcome is predicted to be particularly poor.

Mantle cell lymphoma is known for its unremitting clinical course when treated conventionally and has proven relatively resistant to high-dose treatment, especially when used as a salvage therapy.[316] Incorporating high-dose therapy into the initial overall treatment plan, however, may be more likely to provide durable remissions. At M.D. Anderson, the results of using an intensive induction regimen followed by autologous transplantation have been encouraging.[317] Among previously untreated patients, the EFS rate at 3 years was 72%. Despite this, relapse remains a problem after autologous SCT, and ASCT currently appears to provide more durable remissions. The role of high-dose therapy and autologous rescue remains unclear. Use early in the disease may improve OS, but little evidence indicates that the procedure is curative.[318] Given the lack of long-term DFS with autologous approaches, the role of allogeneic transplantation in newly diagnosed patients must be addressed in appropriate extended phase II studies.

Burkitt's lymphoma, Burkitt-like lymphomas, and lymphoblastic lymphomas are high-grade NHLs associated with relatively poor long-term survival rates. The role of both autologous and allogeneic transplantation in these disorders remains unclear. No convincing risk models identify clear indications for transplantation in CR1. Allogeneic transplantation should probably therefore be restricted to chemosensitive relapsed patients. The lack of a clear contributory benefit of GVL in these disorders suggests that for patients without BM involvement in whom a sibling is not available, autologous transplantation may provide a reasonable alternative to URD transplantation, particularly if the potential delay incurred by the donor search is likely to be considerable. Data from the EBMTR suggest that disease status at the time of transplant is the most important predictor of outcome in patients with high-grade disease.[319] For Burkitt's and Burkitt-like lymphoma, the 3-year actuarial OS rate was 72% for patients transplanted during first CR, compared with 37% in those with chemotherapy-sensitive relapse, and 7% in patients with disease that is unresponsive to chemotherapy. For patients with lymphoblastic lymphoma, the 6-year actuarial survival rate ranged from 63% in patients who were in first CR to 15% in those who had resistant disease. Patients in second CR had an intermediate survival rate of 31% at 6 years. These results with transplantation appear to be superior to those with conventional-dose salvage therapy.

T-cell lymphomas are less common entities, classified by the WHO into leukemic, nodal, and extranodal variants.[283] These lymphomas may first be seen with numerous unusual clinical syndromes (hemophagocytic syndrome, sinus tumors with angiocentric T-cell proliferation).[292] No well-defined management strategy exists for these disorders, and treatment is based on the disease stage and immunopathologic grade. Few comparative trials have been performed, and hence little evidence exists that any one combination regimen is superior to another. The relative chemotherapy sensitivity to common B cell–type treatment regimens is lower, corresponding to the inferior CR rates noted in these diseases. Some entities remain localized, such as the nasal T/NK cell lymphoma, requiring only CHOP-like chemotherapy followed by involved field radiotherapy (IFRT) and are generally associated with good prognosis. Conversely, visceral involvement such as hepatosplenic T-cell lymphoma, intestinal T-cell lymphomas, and the leukemic variants are aggressive with poor prognoses and are generally treated with high-dose chemotherapy and autologous stem cell rescue.[320] Currently, numerous novel targeted therapies are being explored for the treatment of the T-cell lymphomas.[321]

Autologous HSCT continues to be associated with a high risk of relapse because of the presence of MRD in the harvested, reinfused stem cells, or remaining in the patient after chemotherapy. As a result, monitoring and eradicating MRD has become a major focus of many studies in NHL. Rearrangement and gene expression of the bcl-1 and bcl-2 genes are the hallmarks of mantle-cell and follicular lymphoma, respectively, and evidence suggests that they are promising surrogate markers of MRD. Clearance of bcl-1/JH- and bcl-2/JH-positive cells after treatment is associated with a significant improvement in outcome.[322,323]

Allogenic HSCT continues to be investigated to improve outcomes. Allogenic HSCT has several potential advantages over autologous transplantation for NHL, including procurement of an uncontaminated stem-cell graft, GVL effects, and the elimination of HSC damage and consequent secondary leukemia. However, because of a 1-year TRM of 30% to 40% and complications caused by GVHD, conventional, myeloablative, allogeneic transplantation is a high-risk option for low-grade lymphoproliferative disorders.[326] Even though the ideal application of allogeneic transplantation in aggressive and high-grade lymphomas is still unclear, the high rates of CR and the lower relapse rates demonstrated in several comparisons of the two approaches make this an exciting area to pursue. Allo-SCT also induces complete remission in advanced lymphoma patients, even when the tumor had relapsed after autologous HSCT. Freytes and associates[325] investigated conventional myeloablative allogenic SCT in 114 relapsed patients after auto-SCT. They demonstrated higher rates of disease progression (52%), TRM (22%), 3-year OS and PFS (33% and 25%), respectively. Despite the foregoing, this approach is usually not curative. In conclusion, allo-SCT should be considered earlier as a therapeutic option in poor-risk patients to avoid the high nonrelapse mortality associated with extensive pretreatment.

Nonmyeloablative (NST) or reduced-intensity SCT broadens the applicability of allogeneic transplantation by lowering regimen-related mortality while capitalizing on the GVL effect.[326] For aggressive disease, NST is indicated only for patients with minimal disease burden, as the nonmyeloablative regimens lack the ability to control rapidly proliferating disease before the generation of a GVT effect, a major limiting factor with this modality.

Results for patients with truly chemotherapy-refractory disease are poor. Patients with disease that is unresponsive to chemotherapy at the time of relapse have a low (about 15%–20%) chance of achieving a long-term remission with high-dose therapy and stem cell rescue (Table 58–7).

Hodgkin's Disease

Many patients will achieve durable remissions with nontransplant chemotherapy and/or radiation therapy, and algorithms for staging and treatment of this disease are well defined. For patients who have a relapse, the prognosis with conventional salvage therapy is directly related to the duration of the initial remission. The outcome for patients whose remission lasted less than 1 year is dismal, and most experts concur that approximately 40% to 50% of patients with HD who have a relapse within 1 year will achieve durable remissions after autologous HSCT.[327,328]

Table 58–7 **Outcomes of Transplantation of Low-Grade Non-Hodgkin's Lymphoma**

Study	Total Points/ LG-NHL Points	Median FU/mo (range)	Median age/yr (range)	Median Prior Treatments (range)	Conditioning regimen	Post transplant IS	Donors	GVHD: acute (II–IV)/ chronic (%)	Graft failure	Outcome
Khouri et al[397]	15 (CLL 6, FL 4, MCL 1, Richt 2, Tf FL 2)	6	55 (45–71)	3 (2–7)	Cyclo+Flu or Cisplat+ Flu+ Cytarabine	Tacro±MTX	All MSD	5 acute (4 gd 1 skin; 1 gd 2 liver)+2 postDLI	4	8 CR (2 with aGVHD, 4 with cGVHD)
Nagler et al[398]	23	22.5	41 (13–63)	3 (2–6)	Flu+Bu+ATG	CSA	22 MSD 1 MUD	8 aGVHD 2 CL	0	37 mo DFS 40% 6 died PD 7 died TRM
Kottaridis et al[399]	44 (including 5 FL, 4 Tf FL, 3 MCL, 1 CLL)	9 (3–29)	41 (18–56)	3 (0–6)	Flu+Mel+Al emtuzumab	CSA±MTX	36 MSD 8 MUD	3 gd 1 skin; 2 gd 2 GI; 1 CE	1 (+1 N/E)	22 CR, 4 PR, 7 stable PR, 3 progression
Khouri et al[400]	20 (all FL or small lymphocytic lymphoma)	21 (5–46)	51 (31–68)	2 (1–5)	Cyclo+Flu± Rituximab	Tacro+MTX	All MSD	20% gd II-IV aGVHD 64% cGVHD	0	20 CR, 2 died TRM 84% DFS at 2 yrs
Chakraverty et al[401]	47 (including 4 FL, 1 T-PLL, 3 MCL)	11 (3–27)	44 (18–62)	29 prior autografts	Flu+Mel+ Alemtuzumab	CSA	All MUD	7 gd 1; 7 gd 2; 3 gd 3; 3 CL (+9 N/E for cGVHD)	2	1 yr OS 75.5% 1 yr PFS 61.5%
Robinson et al[402]	188 (including 52 LGNHL, 22 MCL)	9 (range not given)	40 (2–61)	3 (x–x) 48% prior autografts	Various (EBMT Registry data)	Various	167 MSD 16 MUD	37% aGVHD (12% gd 1, 24% gd II-IV) 7% CL, 9% CE	3	LGNHL: OS at 2 yr 65% PFS at 2 yr 54% TRM at 2 yr 30.9%
Faulkner et al[406]	65 (including 13 CLL/PLL, 28 FL, 5 MCL)	17 (1–67)	46 (19–60)	2 (1–6) 11% prior autograft	BEAM+ Alemtuzumab	CSA+MTX	57 MSD 8 MUD	17% gd 1–2 17% CL (38% post DLI gd 1–3)	3	EFS at 2 yr 69% (LGNHL) TRM at 1 yr 8% (if no prior autograft)
Dreger et al[403]	77 (all CLL)	18 (1–44)	54 (30–66)	3 (0–8)	Various (EBMT Registry data)	CSA±MTX ±MMF	62 MSD 15 MUD	34% gd 2–4 (of which 16% gd 3–4) 58% CL or CE	0	1 yr TRM 18%, 2 yr EFS 56%, 2 year OS 72%
Khouri et al[404]	17 (all CLL)	21	54, (44–73)	3, (1–8)	Flu+Cyclo± Rituximab	Tacro+MTX	All MSD	29/60	0	7 CR, 2 PR (8 of the 9 responders received rituximab at conditioning)
Morris et al[405]	88 (including 29 FL, 9 CLL, LPC 3, MCL 10)	36 (18–60)	48 (18–73)	4 (2–6) HG NHL; 3 (1–6) LG NHL 42% prior autograft	Flu+Mel+ Alemtuzumab	CSA	63 MSD 23 MUD 2 MM related	15% gd 1 15% gd 2–4 (of which, 4% gd 3–4)	4	LG-NHL only: 3 yr OS 73% 3 yr PFS 65% 3 yr TRM 11%

aGVHD, acute graft-versus-host disease; ATG, anti-thymocyte globulin; BEAM, BCNU etoposide cytarabine melphalan; Bu, busulphan; CE, chronic extensive; cGVHD, chronic graft-versus-host disease; Cisplat, cisplatin; CL, chronic limited; CLL, chronic lymphocytic leukemia; CR, complete remission; CSA, cyclosporin A; Cyclo, cyclophosphamide; DFS, disease-free survival; DLI, donor lymphocyte infusion; EBMT, European Bone Marrow Transplant; EFS, event-free survival; FL, follicular lymphoma; Flu, fludarabine; gd, grade; GI, gastrointestinal; GVHD, graft-versus-host disease; LPC, lymphoplasmacytoid; MCL, mantle cell lymphoma; Mel, melphalan; MM, mismatched; MMF, mycophenylate mofetil; MSD, matched sibling donor; MTX, methotrexate; MUD, matched unrelated donor; N/E, not evaluable; PD, progressive disease; PFS, progression-free survival; PR, partial remission; OS, overall survival; Richt, Richter's transformation; Tacro, tacrolimus; TBI, total body irradiation; Tf FL, transformed follicular lymphoma; T-PLL, T-cell prolymphocytic leukaemia; TRM, transplant-related mortality.

For patients whose first remission lasts more than 1 year, two randomized trials comparing HDT/autologous SCT with conventional salvage treatment suggested similar overall long-term survival rates but possibly a greater DFS rate for the transplant arms.[329,330] Also, patients with refractory HD may achieve durable CRs with HDT/SCT. ABMTR and EBMTR analyses demonstrated that HDT can overcome drug resistance in HD. After autologous transplantation, the probability of 3-year PFS was 38% and 30%, with an OS rate of 50% and 34%, respectively.[331]

Previous reports from Seattle and Baltimore strongly suggested that allografting resulted in a lower relapse rate with evidence of a GVL effect in relapsed refractory HD. In two large registry-based randomized retrospective analyses published in 1996, Gajewski and colleagues[332] analyzed the results of 100 HD patients with advanced resistant disease, who had undergone matched-sibling SCT. The 3-year OS, DFS, and probability of relapse were 21%, 15%, and 65%, respectively. A lower relapse rate was noted in patients who developed GVHD but at the risk of higher TRM. The second analysis by Milipied and coworkers[333] of 45 autografted and 45 allografted case-matched patients revealed no significant difference in OS, PFS, relapse and nonrelapse mortality. The pattern of decreased relapse rate in 17 allografted patients with GVHD grade ≥2 was repeated compared with 17 matched autografted patients.

With the TRM from conventional myeloablative ASCTs approaching 60% in some reports, nonmyeloablative SCT (NST) is being actively studied as an alternative to classic SCT, although the question of whether the relatively low doses of cytotoxic drugs in the preparative regimens will suffice to debulk the tumor burden to a level at which the allografted T cells can expand and control residual tumor to permit lifelong remission still must be answered.

The EBMT collected data on 94 heavily pretreated patients who underwent NST.[334] Of these, 50% had failed a prior autograft, and 31% were deemed primary progressive or refractory to conventional salvage regimens. The majority of the patients received HLA-identical family donor grafts. Among the 80 evaluable patients, the OS patterns in 35 chemosensitive- and 23 chemoresistant-disease patients revealed that none of the chemoresistant patients were surviving at 1.4 years, whereas fully 78% of the chemosensitive cohort was alive at 4.3-year follow-up. Univariate and multivariate analyses confirmed that the only factor negatively influencing both OS and DFS was chemoresistant compared with chemosensitive disease ($P = .025$ and $P = .015$, respectively). This therefore underscores the importance of early selection of appropriate chemosensitive patients for NST. To this end, the EBMT has launched two new studies to better understand and exploit the true potential of NST.

HDT followed by tandem autoallogeneic transplants is being explored as a more effective approach in the relapsed refractory setting. As a prelude to this, Ahmed and associates[335] recently reported their experience with HDT combined with tandem auto-SCT. They reported a 32.14% long-term survival in their resistant/refractory group. Multivariate analysis identified age younger than 35 years and no B symptoms as predictors of superior outcome.

Marrow Failure States

The inherited BM failure syndromes are becoming less enigmatic as their genetic and molecular bases are further elucidated. These rare disorders may present only with tricytopenia, and interestingly enough, children and young adults may not display all the classically described physical characteristics. It is therefore imperative to make an early diagnosis, as it affects therapeutic approaches and management strategies. Currently the only option for reestablishing normal hematopoiesis in this patient population is HSCT.[336,337] T-cell depletion of BM or PBSC or use of UCB are frequently used to decrease GVHD, early post-transplant toxicity, and therefore promote promising early survival.[338]

Fanconi anemia is an autosomal recessive disease with a median survival of 30 years. This disorder should be suspected in any child, adolescent, or adult with BM failure, MDS, or early-onset epithelial malignancies. The only option for reestablishing normal hematopoiesis in otherwise normal patients with tricytopenia (ANC < 1000/mm^3; HgB, 8 g/dL; or platelet count, 40–50,000/mm^3) and a suitable HLA-matched sibling is HSCT. NST avoids the pitfalls of the exquisite chemotherapy and radiotherapy sensitivities unique to this patient population, thereby preventing fatal toxicity. It is recommended that all siblings be HLA typed and have their cord blood stored, as 5-year survival figures for sibling HSCT approach 75%. The 5-year OS for matched URD SCT is 58% at some centers.[339]

For dyskeratosis congenita, HSCT is not an optimal option, as there have been reports of multiple unexplained post-transplant morbidities with the development of fatal lung toxicities and secondary cancers. Currently HSCT is recommended only in the context of clinical trials.

In the Schwachman-Diamond syndrome, exocrine pancreatic insufficiency, and clonal evolution to MDS and AML are the consistent features of this chromosome 7 autosomal recessive disorder.[340] Hypoplastic granulopoiesis is the most reliable hematologic abnormality with more than 90% of patients demonstrating neutropenia; 40%, anemia; 28%, thrombocytopenia; but only 20% with tricytopenia.[341] However, the rarity of this disorder limits large-scale trials with no consensus recommendations. Therefore, each case is managed on an individual basis with a distinctive trend toward management by SCT after preparation with attenuated conditioning regimens.

The Diamond-Blackfan syndrome occurs with pure red cell aplasia, elevated HB F and RBC adenosine deaminase (ADA), and is also classified as a cancer-predisposition syndrome. Sibling-matched HSCT confers an actuarial survival of approximately 80, although reserved for steroid-refractory cases. As previously noted for the other BM failure states, early typing of the proband and siblings and also preservation of UCB samples are strongly advocated.

Aplastic anemia (AA) is a disorder characterized by tricytopenia with concomitant hypocellular BM. This disorder preferentially affects adolescents and individuals older than 60 years. Diverse etiologies are proposed with the current focus on an autoimmune origin. It is critical to differentiate AA from hypoplastic MDS, hairy cell leukemia (HCL), and the HCL variant because of the differing treatment strategies used. Immunosuppressive therapy (IST) is the current frontline option with a remission rate close to 70%, an 80% to 90% 5-year EFS in responding patients, and a relapse rate of 10%. For the 30% of patients who have an HLA-matched sibling donor, BM or PBSCT has yielded cure rates of approximately 90% and graft failure/rejection rates of 5% to 10%.[342] The decision-making process for selection of patients must take into account the fact that younger patients tolerate SCT significantly better and have fewer long-term issues with GVHD than their older counterparts.[343] Even though in one retrospective study, the OS for BMT and IST were no different (63% vs 61%) for all comers, the preponderance of evidence significantly favored the choice of BMT for younger patients (64% vs 38%). As a corollary to the foregoing, because some patients may require IST for up to 6 months to achieve resolution of neutropenia, therefore even middle-aged patients with an HLA-matched sibling donor and few comorbid conditions must be seriously considered for early HSCT because the risk of mortality from infectious complications increases exponentially with the increased duration of neutropenia.

Sickle cell disease (SCD) is a single-nucleotide genetic disorder with protean manifestations contributing to relentlessly omnipresent morbidity. Currently, HSCT is the only curative modality of treatment for this disorder. The two cardinal concepts of SCT in SCD are that (1) engraftment of normal donor cells ameliorates ongoing pathologic effects, and (2) mixed chimerism was sufficient to achieve this diminution of progressive chronic organ damage. Wu and colleagues[344] reported that after SCT, ineffective native erythropoiesis of Hbss provides a growth advantage for HbA or heterozygous Hbs/HbA donor-derived erythroid precursors, resulting in improvement of clinical disease. By virtue of the nature of inheritance of the genetic mutation responsible for this disorder and other factors, significant difficulty exists in finding appropriate matched sibling donors, with only 20% having suitable donors available, therefore requiring wider employment of matched URD SCT with the attendant undesirable complication of GVHD, which typically is worse in adults.[340] Results of HSCT in 200 patients who had undergone myeloablative SCT from matched-sibling donors demonstrated an 85% DFS, 7% TRM, and 9% graft failure rate with recrudescence of the SCD genotype.[346] To combat this, and as previously stated, because at worst only a minority fraction of donor-derived stem cells was necessary to achieve mixed chimerism, NST appears to be a much more attractive modality of treatment. This principle was initially established by Krishnamurthi and others[344] and further elucidated by Chakrabarti and Beresford[347] who commented on a multicenter study in which the U.S. arm donor chimerism ranged from 11% with representative Hbs of only 7%, to 99% with all patients experiencing stable mixed chimerism and resolution of SCD symptoms.

Myeloproliferative Disorders

The myeloproliferative disorders (MPDs) are clonal stem cell diseases. Based on the WHO classification, they comprise Philadelphia (Ph) chromosome/BCR-ABL–positive CML, polycythemia vera (PV), idiopathic myelofibrosis (IF), essential thrombocytosis (ET), and, more recently, chronic myelomonocytic leukemia (CMML) and atypical CML(Ph/BCR-ABL negative).[348] These disorders display overlapping clinical features but exhibit different natural histories and different therapeutic requirements. Phenotypic mimicry among these disorders, between them and nonclonal hematopoietic disorders, lack of clonal diagnostic markers, lack of understanding of their molecular bases and paucity of controlled, prospective therapeutic trials have made the diagnosis and management of these disorders problematically difficult. A potentially curative approach is allogeneic HSCT, although limited data exist on the impact of HSCT on the natural history of these disorders.[349] The preparative regimens used in fully ablative techniques rule out older patients for consideration, and many younger patients with good prognostic criteria may do sufficiently well on medical treatment or observation to avoid transplantation.[350] Indeed, some[351] have suggested that specific inhibitory molecules analogous to imatinib may be designed for each disease or disease subtype, and future trends may be identification and exploitation of the basic mechanism underlying the GVL effect for eradication of minimal residual disease without the need for allografting. Older patients may have the option to undergo an HLA-identical sibling NST to minimize peritransplant toxicity and mortality. Thus, a prerequisite to the broad use of transplantation is objective determination of candidacy. Several evaluation methods agree that anemia, age, and cytogenetic abnormalities all predict poor survival in IF, suggesting that patients with anemia and an abnormal karyotype undergo allogenic HSCT. Ample scope remains for improving the clinical results of allogenic HSCT, which in theory should "cure" most patients with MPD. The median survival for patients with myelofibrosis ranges from 13 to 93 months and myeloablative allogeneic transplantation results in high rates of durable engraftment and cure in approximately 50% of patients.

Three studies by Mittal and associates,[349] Przepiorka and associates,[352] and Anderson and associates[353] have demonstrated the effectiveness of SCT in these disorders challenging the previously held belief that this procedure resulted in delayed hematopoietic recovery.[352,353] TRM, associated with more-advanced disease and age rather than disease recurrence, accounts for the majority of treatment failures. In the Mittal study, four of six atypical CML patients died, underscoring the worse prognosis of this disorder. More recently, reduced-intensity conditioning regimens have been shown to induce encouraging rates of engraftment and prolonged survival by exploiting the GVT effect mediated by donor immunocompetent cells.[354]

Rondelli and colleagues published their small study of 21 patients in support of the use and efficacy of NST in IF. Eighty percent of the cohort displayed grades III to IV myelofibrosis. The patients all underwent fludarabine-based conditioning. Post-transplantation chimerism analysis showed more than 95% donor cells in 18 patients. Acute GVHD, grades II to IV, was observed in 7 patients, grades III to IV in 2, and extensive chronic GVHD in 8. Eighteen patients were surviving at 12 to 122 months (median, 31 months) after transplantation with 17 in remission (1 after a second transplantation). They concluded that the use of RIC regimens in allogenic SCT results in prolonged survival in intermediate/high-risk IF patients.[355] With regard to CMML, Zang and associates[356] reported on 12 patients who had undergone myeloablative allogenic SCT. They noted that early HSCT recipients (disease duration <12 months) enjoyed better survival than did those with disease duration ≥12months.

Myelodyplasia

The myelodysplastic syndrome (MDS) comprises a heterogeneous group of hematologic disorders. They are characterized by a clonal HSC abnormality engendering variable degrees of cytopenias, lineage dysplasias, and frequent evolution to AML. Currently, HSCT is the only modality of treatment that can accomplish palliation of anemia, trilineage response, cytogenetic response, delay to transformation to AML, improve survival, and, most importantly, achieve a cure. HSCT for MDS is characterized by high TRM, especially in older patients and those with more-advanced disease and secondary MDS. Outcomes after PBSCT may be superior to earlier results with BMT.[357,358] In a report from the NMDP by Castro-Malaspina on 510 patients treated with URD BMT, the TRM ranged from 40% to 50%. Martino and coworkers[288] reported on 43 patients (aged 12–73 years; median, 49 years) who had received an HLA-identical sibling donor PBSCT. Twenty-three patients aged 55 years or older without prohibitive comorbidity received myeloablative TBI-based conditioning, followed by a T cell–depleted PBSCT and delayed DLI. Older patients or those with comorbidities (n = 20) received reduced-intensity conditioning and an unmanipulated PBSCT. Thirty-seven (86%) had advanced disease. The median follow-up was 18 months. Actuarial probabilities of 3-year OS, DFS, relapse, and TRM were 64%, 59%, 26%, and 23%, respectively, for 34 primary MDS patients. The best results were seen in 19 patients 50 years of age or older undergoing myeloablative PBSCT. Outcomes for all stages of primary MDS were improved over the data for marrow SCT, confirming a GVL effect for RIST. However, results for therapy-related MDS remained dismal, with a high relapse rate (89%).

Nakai and colleagues[359] evaluated the impact of chemotherapy before allo-SCT. In an analysis of the data of 283 patients who underwent allo-SCT from an HLA-identical sibling donor for MDS that were reported to the Japan Society for Hematopoietic Cell Transplantation, multivariate analyses identified karyotype, FAB classification, and the history of chemotherapy before allo-SCT as significant predictors for OS. OS at 5 years was 57% for patients who underwent allo-SCT as a primary treatment for refractory anemia with excess blasts in transformation (RAEB-t) or secondary acute myeloid leukemia (AML) and 54% for those who underwent allo-SCT in remission after induction chemotherapy (P = .81). These results do not support the administration of induction chemotherapy for patients with RAEB-t or secondary AML before allo-SCT. As a corollary to the foregoing, Kebriaei and associates[360] investigated the impact of disease burden at the time of myeloablative or RIST ASCT in a cohort of 68 patients (60 AML, 8 MDS). After multivariate analysis, they concluded that the factors predicting a worse outcome were increased blast count in the BM at HSCT, presence of GVHD, mismatched donor, Zubrod performance of ≥2, age 45 years or older, and residual cytogenetic abnormalities. These data support an association between pre-SCT disease burden and quality of outcome.

Solid Tumors

Autologous transplantation for the treatment of solid tumors is less established, primarily because most malignancies do not exhibit the strong dose response to myelosuppressive chemotherapeutic agents. Exceptions to this are germ cell tumors and some pediatric malignancies, such as neuroblastoma. Breast cancer, which at one point was the most frequent indication for autologous transplantation,[134] is still a subject of controversy pending the final analysis of randomized trials. Small-cell lung cancer and ovarian carcinoma are still being studied in clinical trials of autologous transplantation.

Breast Cancer

Approximately 180,000 women in the United States will develop this cancer each year, and nearly 40,000 will die. Although disease confined to the breasts and the lymph nodes is curable with multimodality therapy including surgery, radiation, chemotherapy, and hormone manipulation, once breast cancer has spread to distant organs, cure may not be possible. Therefore, all efforts to treat patients in an aggressive fashion in hopes of preventing distant spread are typically undertaken. The use of adjuvant chemotherapy became commonplace in the treatment of patients with breast cancer involving axillary lymph nodes as a result of clinical trials showing improved EFS for patients at high risk of developing metastatic disease.

To date, 18 randomized trials of high-dose therapy in breast cancer have been published.[361] Overall the consensus has been that with stage II (or above) disease, inflammatory or metastatic breast cancer prognosis is poor. Inflammatory breast cancer represents a unique clinical entity with a high propensity for both local and distant metastatic spread. Given the rarity of inflammatory breast carcinoma, no formal randomized trials have been performed in this disease. Metastatic breast cancer rarely is curable, although some women will benefit from a more-indolent course lasting years, with responses to a variety of different regimens. A role of dose-intense therapy is not clear for this stage of this disease. Currently combinations of chemotherapy and subsequently, tamoxifen or an aromatase inhibitor, have improved survival.[362,363] Trastuzumab is an encouraging example of the exploitation of a newer mechanism of action, monoclonal antibody–based immunotherapy, to produce antitumor effects in patients with metastatic tumor.

Demonstration of the efficacy of conventional adjuvant therapy with and without auto-SCT was published by Tallman and colleagues[364] who were able to achieve superior results in the combined chemotherapy transplant arm. Studies of autologous transplant as adjuvant consolidation in high-risk breast cancer have varied in the chemotherapy regimen. Because of the historic trials detailing improved outcomes with high-dose chemotherapy in high-risk patients,[365] German investigators first studied double high-dose doxorubicin (Adriamycin), paclitaxel, CY, and thiotepa as a four-drug regimen preparatory to autologous-PBS transplantation. Of the 21 evaluable patients, 8 were able to achieve CR, and 10 achieved PR. At 3 years, 4 patients remained in CR.[366] Sayer et al.[367] then studied the feasibility of intensive tandem high-dose chemotherapy consisting of epirubicin, CY, and thiotepa versus epirubicin and cyclophosphamide followed by accelerated CY, methotrexate, and fluorouracil. They demonstrated no TRM, and the intent-to-treat analysis showed a 4-year EFS of 60% versus 40% in the control arm, with an OS of 75% versus 70% (P = .02.) These findings are in contrast to other studies but reflect a difference in the design of the chemotherapy regimens.

Although statistically significant evidence indicates that high-dose chemotherapy and auto-SCT improve EFS compared with conventional chemotherapy, no consensus exists that an OS benefit results from this approach.[367]

Full myeloablative allogeneic transplantation for breast cancer has been explored by several investigators; these studies have produced preliminary and indirect evidence for a graft-versus–breast cancer effect.[368,369] Allogeneic lymphocytes can induce regression of advanced metastatic breast cancer. These results indicate that an immunological GVT effect from allogeneic lymphocytes exists against metastatic breast cancer and provide rationale for further development of allogeneic cellular therapy.[370] Currently, reduced-intensity or nonmyeloablative regimens that have less TRM but preserve the T cell–mediated GVT effects led to increased investigation of allo-HSCT in MBC.[371] To distinguish an immunologic GVT effect from any antitumor effect of cytotoxic chemotherapy in the transplant-conditioning regimen, allogeneic T lymphocytes were removed from the stem-cell graft and were subsequently administered late after allo-HSCT. The responses, observed in 20% to 40% of patients, appear to be associated with the development of complete donor lymphoid chimerism and may be delayed with objective tumor regressions occurring after day +28 after allo-HSCT. These results indicate that an immunologic GVT effect from allogeneic lymphocytes exists against metastatic breast cancer and provide a rationale for further development of allogeneic cellular therapy for this largely incurable disease.[372]

Germ Cell Tumors

Germ cell cancers are relatively uncommon diseases accounting for about 1% of all malignancies in (primarily, adolescent and young) men. Germ cell tumors, highly curable with nontransplant therapies, are classified as seminomatous or nonseminomatous tumors.

Despite a propensity for metastatic spread, germ cell cancers remain one of the most highly curable human malignancies. For example, more than 60% of patients with high-risk disseminated disease will achieve durable responses after treatment with four cycles of cis-platinum, etoposide, and bleomycin. Patients with refractory disease or who relapse after initial treatment can be effectively rescued with one or two cycles of dose-intense therapy.

Forty cis-platinum–refractory patients were entered into a large multi-institutional phase II (ECOG-sponsored) trial of carboplatinum and etoposide, of whom 58% (22 patients) were able to proceed to a second cycle.[373] Toxicity included five (13%) patients dying of treatment-related causes, including infection, hemorrhage, and hepatic veno-occlusive disease. All treatment-related deaths occurred during the first course of therapy. Nine (24%) patients achieved a CR (including two patients after surgical resection of residual disease). Another eight patients achieved a PR for an overall response rate of 45%. Three of the CRs occurred after the first BMT, and for four patients, the PR converted to CR after the second BMT. Five of the 9 patients were alive and free of disease at a minimum follow-up of 18 months. A striking finding of this study was the poor outcome in patients with nonseminomatous primary mediastinal germ cell tumors. Eleven patients with this diagnosis were enrolled in this study, and none obtained a durable CR.

The initial ECOG experience with multiple cycles of high-dose therapy has been replicated at single centers. The Memorial Sloan Kettering group treated 58 patients with refractory germ cell tumors with two cycles of high-dose carboplatin, etoposide, and cisplatin; 40% achieved a CR, with a 2-year survival rate of 31%. Patients having pretreatment β-human chorionic gonadotropin (HCG) values less than 100 and those without retroperitoneal masses fared better.[374]

The Indiana University group reported 25 patients who had relapsed after cis-platinum–based regimens.[375] Patients received one to two cycles of conventional-dose salvage, followed by two cycles of high-dose carboplatin and etoposide with stem cell support. At a median of 26 months of follow-up, 13 (52%) patients remain progression free. This very aggressive schedule resulted in one of the highest response rates noted to date. Based on this and other reports from this program, two cycles of dose-intense therapy with autologous transplantation is now considered to be standard for patients for whom initial therapy fails.

Ovarian Carcinoma

Autologous transplantation for the treatment of ovarian carcinoma remains under active investigation, but promising results have been reported for some groups of women.[376–378] A randomized study of high-dose chemotherapy for women with low amounts of residual tumor demonstrated a prolongation of DFS for women who received the dose-intense regimen.[375] The median survival for these women was 22 months, compared with 11 months for women who received standard-dose chemotherapy (P = .03). Bengala and colleagues[380] recently published the EBMT retrospective analysis on the utility of high-dose chemotherapy with autologous stem cell rescue for 91 advanced ovarian cancer patients in first remission. No subgroup of patients likely to benefit in particular from dose-intense therapy could be identified, but the median duration of remission had not been reached for patients who had no residual disease. These studies indicate that remission status at time of transplantation and the ability to achieve a CR after transplantation are determining factors for long-term responses. Preliminary studies of allogeneic transplantation demonstrate a potential GVD effect in this patient population, and studies involving allogeneic transplantation are ongoing.[381]

Renal Cell Carcinoma

Renal cell carcinoma has a response rate to most chemotherapeutic agents of only about 5%. In contrast, immunotherapy with agents such as interleukin-2 have response rates as high as 15% to 20%, justifying attempts to achieve disease control through allogeneic transplantation. Investigators at the National Institutes of Health reported a seminal trial of 45 patients who were conditioned with a reduced-intensity regimen of fludarabine and CY.[382] Twenty of the patients achieved PR and CR, with four patients experiencing complete regression of all metastatic disease. The response was delayed, at a median of 5 months, and observed only for patients who developed clinically evident GVHD. Other investigators also reported GVD effect in their cohorts despite differing preparative regimens. Others have reported similar experiences, although only a minority of patients benefit from this therapy.[383] These studies, however, demonstrate the feasibility of using the GVD effect in the treatment of solid tumors.

Autoimmune Disorders

The improved safety of autologous PBSC transplantation encourages studies of dose-intense therapy in the treatment of nonmalignant diseases, including autoimmune disorders such as multiple sclerosis, scleroderma, systemic lupus erythematosus (SLE), and refractory rheumatoid arthritis. The hypothesis of currently ongoing studies is that dose-intense lymphoablative conditioning regimens will achieve prolonged remission or cure of these diseases by destruction of the clone of cells responsible for the disease. This hypothesis is supported by reports of remission of autoimmune diseases (e.g., rheumatoid arthritis, SLE) that existed as a comorbid condition for patients undergoing autologous or allogeneic transplantation,[384,385] although this has not been a universal finding.[386] The use of intensive chemoradiotherapy with HSC rescue offers an opportunity to deliver maximally tolerated immunosuppression. Factors that may influence the relative efficacy of this approach include the number and relative resistance to ablation of the responsible lymphoid effector populations and the nature and persistence of the relevant antigen against which the immune response is raised. Although the pathogenesis of these disorders is not fully understood and lymphoid effectors are not well defined for these diseases, evidence points to the involvement of T and B lymphocytes. High-dose therapy followed by autologous HSC transplantation may allow the immune system to "reset" with control of the autoreactive lymphocytes. As with the treatment of malignant diseases, depletion of the unwanted lymphoid cell population from the HSC inoculum (purging) may be necessary for optimal clinical outcome. These diseases, although nonmalignant, can be equally debilitating, and appropriate patient selection is necessary so that the risks (morbidity and mortality) are appropriately balanced against the benefits (possibly, lack of progression instead of reversal of damage already incurred) of this therapy.

Some preliminary data on autologous transplantation carried out specifically for the treatment of autoimmune diseases have now been reported. Fassas and coworkers[387] reported stabilization or improvement for patients undergoing autologous transplantation for multiple sclerosis. In a recent publication, Traynor and colleagues[388] reported seven patients with SLE treated with autologous PBSC transplantation. All patients had severe active SLE refractory to conventional intensive immunosuppressive therapy, and two patients had a creatinine clearance of less than 30 mL/min. Treatment involved mobilization of PBSCs with CY, 2 g/m^2, followed by filgrastim; the PBSCs were depleted of lymphocytes by enrichment of CD34+ cells. The dose-intense immunoablative regimen consisted of cyclophosphamide, 50 mg/kg × 4, and antithymocyte globulin, 90 mg/kg. At a median of 25 (range, 12–40) months, all patients were free of clinical signs of active SLE. A larger series of patients confirms these findings, but also reported considerable regimen-related mortality.[389] Similar studies have been reported in other autoimmune disorders including rheumatoid arthritis and Crohn disease.[390,391]

REFERENCES

1. Moskovitz CH, Nimer SD, Zelenetz AD, et al. A 2-step comprehensive high-dose chemoradiotherapy second-line program for relapsed and refractory Hodgkin disease: analysis by intent to treat and development of a prognostic model. Blood 2001;97:616–623.
2. Bensinger W, Appelbaum F, Rowley S, et al. Factors that influence collection and engraftment of autologous peripheral-blood stem cells. J Clin Oncol 1995;13:2547–2555.
3. Parimon T, Madtes DK, Au DH, et al. Pretransplant lung function, respiratory failure, and mortality after stem cell transplantation. Am J Respir Crit Care Med 2005;172:384–390.
4. Goldberg SL, Klumpp TR, Magdalinski AJ, et al. Value of the pretransplant evaluation in predicting toxic day 100 mortality among blood stem cell and bone marrow recipients. J Clin Oncol 1998;16:3796–3802.
5. Diaconescu R, Flowers CR, Storer B, et al. Morbidity and mortality with nonmyeloablative compared with myeloablative conditioning before hematopoietic cell transplantation from HLA-matched related donors. Blood 2004;104:1550–1558.
6. Sorror ML, Maris MB, Storb R, et al. Hematopoietic cell transplantation (HCT)-specific comorbidity index: a new tool for risk assessment before allogeneic HCT. Blood 2005;106:2912–2919.
7. Gottesdiener KM. Transplanted infections: donor to host transmission with the allograft. Ann Intern Med 1989;110:1001–1016.
8. Niederwieser DW, Appelbaum FR, Gastl G, et al. Inadvertent transmission of a donor's acute myeloid leukemia in bone marrow transplantation for chronic myelocytic leukemia. N Engl J Med 1990; 25:1794–1796.
9. Foundation for the Accreditation of Hematopoietic Cell Therapy. Standards for blood and marrow progenitor cell collection, processing & transplantation. Omaha, NE: FAHCT, 2002.
10. AABB. Standards for hematopoietic progenitor cells. Bethesda, Md., American Association of Blood Banks, 1996.
11. Anderlini P, Korbling M, Dale D, et al. Allogeneic blood stem cell transplantation: considerations for donors. Blood 1997;90:903–908.
12. Becker PS, Wagle M, Matous S, et al. Spontaneous splenic rupture following administration of granulocyte colony-stimulating factor (G-CSF): occurrence in an allogeneic donor of peripheral blood stem cells. Biol Blood Marrow Transplant 1997;3:45–49.
13. Platzbecker U, Prange-Krex G, Bornhauser M, et al. Spleen enlargement in healthy donors during G-CSF mobilization of PBPCs. Transfusion 2001;41:184–189.
14. LeBlanc R, Roy J, Demers C, et al. A prospective study of G-CSF effects on hemostasis in allogeneic blood stem cell donors. Bone Marrow Transplant 1999;23:991–996.
15. Petersdorf EW, Malkki M. Human leukocyte antigen matching in unrelated donor hematopoietic cell transplantation. Semin Hematol 2005;42:76–84.
16. Petersdorf EW, Anasetti C, Martin PJ, et al. Limits of HLA mismatching in unrelated hematopoietic cell transplantation. Blood 2004;104:2976–2980.
17. Speiser DE, Tiercy JM, Rufer N, et al. High resolution HLA matching associated with decreased mortality after unrelated bone marrow transplantation. Blood 1996;87:4455–4462.
18. Szydlo R, Goldman JM, Klein JP, et al. Results of allogeneic bone marrow transplants for leukemia using donors other than HLA-identical siblings. J Clin Oncol 1997;15:1767–1777.
19. Drobyski WR, Klein J, Flomenberg N, et al. Superior survival associated with transplantation of matched unrelated versus one-antigen-mismatched unrelated or highly human leukocyte antigen-disparate haploidentical family donor marrow grafts for the treatment of hematologic malignancies: establishing a treatment algorithm for recipients of alternative donor grafts. Blood 2002;99:806–814.
20. Flomenberg N, Baxter-Lowe LA, Confer D, et al. Impact of HLA class I and class II high-resolution matching on outcomes of unrelated donor bone marrow transplantation: HLA-C mismatching is associated with a strong adverse effect on transplantation outcome. Blood 2004;104:1923–1930.
21. Petersdorf EW, Kollman C, Hurley CK, et al. Effect of HLA class II gene disparity on clinical outcome in unrelated donor hematopoietic cell transplantation for chronic myeloid leukemia: the U.S. National Marrow Donor Program Experience. Blood 2001;98:2922–2929.
22. Petersdorf EW, Hansen JA, Martin PJ, et al. Major-histocompatibility-complex class I alleles and antigens in hematopoietic-cell transplantation. N Engl J Med 2001;345:1794–1800.
23. Morishima Y, Sasazuki T, Inoko H, et al. The clinical significance of human leukocyte antigen (HLA) allele compatibility in patients receiving a marrow transplant from serologically HLA-A, HLA-B, and HLA-DR matched unrelated donors. Blood 2002;99:4200–4206.
24. Randolph SS, Gooley TA, Warren EH, et al. Female donors contribute to a selective graft-versus-leukemia effect in male recipients of HLA-matched, related hematopoietic stem cell transplants. Blood 2004;103:347–352.
25. Ljungman P, Brand R, Einsele H, et al. Donor CMV serologic status and outcome of CMV-seropositive recipients after unrelated donor stem cell transplantation: an EBMT megafile analysis. Blood 2003;102:13255–13260.
26. Davies SM, Kollman C, Anasetti C, et al. Engraftment and survival after unrelated-donor bone marrow transplantation: a report from the national marrow donor program. Blood 2000;96:4096–4102.
27. Braine HG, Sensenbrenner LL, Wright SK, et al. Bone marrow transplantation with major ABO blood group incompatibility using erythrocyte depletion of marrow prior to infusion. Blood 1982;60:420–425.
28. Toren A, Dacosta Y, Manny N, et al. Passenger B-lymphocyte-induced severe hemolytic disease after allogeneic peripheral blood stem cell transplantation [Letter]. Blood 1996;87:843–844.
29. Oziel-Taieb S, Faucher-Barbey C, Chabannon C, et al. Early and fatal immune haemolysis after so-called "minor" ABO-incompatible peripheral blood stem cell allotransplantation. Bone Marrow Transplant 1997;19:1155–1156.
30. Rowley SD, Liang, PS, Ulz L. Transplantation of ABO-incompatible bone marrow and peripheral blood stem cell components. Bone Marrow. Transplant 2000;26:749–757.
31. Bierman PJ, Sweetenham JW, Loberiza FR Jr, et al. Syngeneic hematopoietic stem-cell transplantation for non-Hodgkin's lymphoma: a comparison with allogeneic and autologous transplantation: The

Lymphoma Working Committee of the International Bone Marrow Transplant Registry and the European Group for Blood and Marrow Transplantation. J Clin Oncol 2003;21:3744–3753.
32. Gahrton G, Svensson H, Bjorkstrand B, et al. Syngeneic transplantation in multiple myeloma: a case-matched comparison with autologous and allogeneic transplantation: European Group for Blood and Marrow Transplantation. Bone Marrow Transplant 1999;24:741–745.
33. Beyer J, Schwella N, Zingsem J, et al. Hematopoietic rescue after high-dose chemotherapy using autologous peripheral-blood progenitor cells or bone marrow: a randomized comparison. J Clin Oncol 1995;13:1328–1335.
34. Schmitz N, Linch DC, Dreger P, Goldstone, et al. Randomised trial of filgrastim-mobilised peripheral blood progenitor cell transplantation versus autologous bone-marrow transplantation in lymphoma patients. Lancet 1996;347:353–357.
35. Hartmann O, Le Corroller AG, Blaise D, et al. Peripheral blood stem cell and bone marrow transplantation for solid tumors and lymphomas: hematologic recovery and costs: A randomized, controlled trial. Ann Intern Med 1997;126:600–607.
36. Serody JS, Sparks SD, Lin Y, et al. Comparison of granulocyte colony-stimulating factor (G-CSF)–mobilized peripheral blood progenitor cells and G-CSF–stimulated bone marrow as a source of stem cells in HLA-matched sibling transplantation. Biol Blood Marrow Transplant 2000;6:434–440.
37. Morton J, Hutchins C, Durrant S. Granulocyte-colony-stimulating factor (G-CSF)-primed allogeneic bone marrow: significantly less graft-versus-host disease and comparable engraftment to G-CSF-mobilized peripheral blood stem cells. Blood 2001;98:3186–3191.
38. Couban S, Messner HA, Andreou P, et al. Bone marrow mobilized with granulocyte colony-stimulating factor in related allogeneic transplant recipients: a study of 29 patients. Biol Blood Marrow Transplant 2000;6:422–427.
39. Damiani D, Fanin R, Silvestri F, et al. Randomized trial of autologous filgrastim-primed bone marrow transplantation versus filgrastim-mobilized peripheral blood stem cell transplantation in lymphoma patients. Blood 1997;90:36–42.
40. Weisdorf D, Miller J, Verfaillie C, et al. Cytokine-primed bone marrow stem cells vs. peripheral blood stem cells for autologous transplantation: a randomized comparison of GM-CSF vs. G-CSF. Biol Blood Marrow Transplant 1997;3:217–223.
41. Storek J, Gooley T, Siadak M, et al. Allogeneic peripheral blood stem cell transplantation may be associated with a high risk of chronic graft-versus-host disease. Blood 1997;90:4705–4709.
42. Mohty M, Kuentz M, Michallet M, et al. Chronic graft-versus-host disease after allogeneic blood stem cell transplantation: long-term results of a randomized study. Blood 2002;100:3128–3134.
43. Flowers ME, Parker PM, Johnston LJ, et al. Comparison of chronic graft-versus-host disease after transplantation of peripheral blood stem cells versus bone marrow in allogeneic recipients: long-term follow-up of a randomized trial. Blood 2002;100:415–419.
44. Körbling M, Przepiorka D, Huh Y, et al. Allogeneic blood stem cell transplantation for refractory leukemia and lymphoma: potential advantages of blood over marrow allografts. Blood 1995;85:1659–1665.
45. Bensinger WI, Clift R, Martin P, et al. Allogeneic peripheral blood stem cell transplantation in patients with advanced hematologic malignancies: A retrospective comparison with marrow transplantation. Blood 1996;88:2794–2800.
46. Schmitz N, Dreger P, Suttorp M, et al. Primary transplantation of allogeneic peripheral blood progenitor cells mobilized by filgrastim (granulocyte colony-stimulating factor). Blood 1995;85:1666–1672.
47. Rosenfeld C, Collins R, Piñeiro L, et al. Allogeneic blood cell transplantation without posttransplant colony-stimulating factors in patients with hematopoietic neoplasm: a phase II study. J Clin Oncol 1996;14:1314–1319.
48. Bacigalupo A, Van Lint MT, Valbonesi M, et al. Thiotepa cyclophosphamide followed by granulocyte colony-stimulating factor mobilized allogeneic peripheral blood stem cells in adults with advanced leukemia. Blood 1996;88:353–357.
49. Brown RA, Adkins D, Goodnough LT, et al. Factors that influence the collection and engraftment of allogeneic peripheral-blood stem cells in patients with hematologic malignancies. J Clin Oncol 1997;15:3067–3074.
50. Champlin RE, Schmitz N, Horowitz MM, et al. Blood stem cells compared with bone marrow as a source of hematopoietic cells for allogeneic transplantation: IBMTR Histocompatibility and Stem Cell Sources Working Committee and the European Group for Blood and Marrow Transplantation (EBMT). Blood 2000;95:3702–3709.
51. Pavletic ZS, Bishop MR, Tarantolo SR, et al. Hematopoietic recovery after allogeneic blood stem-cell transplantation compared with bone marrow transplantation in patients with hematologic malignancies. J Clin Oncol 1997;15:1608–1616.
52. Blaise D, Kuentz M, Fortanier C, et al. Randomized trial of bone marrow versus lenograstim-primed blood cell allogeneic transplantation in patients with early-stage leukemia: a report from the Societe Francaise de Greffe de Moelle. J Clin Oncol 2000;18:537–546.
53. Couban S, Simpson DR, Barnett MJ, et al. A randomized multicenter comparison of bone marrow and peripheral blood in recipients of matched sibling allogeneic transplants for myeloid malignancies. Blood 2002;100:1525–1531.
54. Schmitz N, Beksac M, Hasenclever D, et al. Transplantation of mobilized peripheral blood cells to HLA-identical siblings with standard-risk leukemia. Blood 2002;100:761–767.
55. Weaver CH, Buckner CD, Longin K, et al. Syngeneic transplantation with peripheral blood mononuclear cells collected after the administration of recombinant human granulocyte colony-stimulating factor. Blood 1993;82:1981–1984.
56. Bensinger WI, Martin PJ, Storer B, et al. Transplantation of bone marrow as compared with peripheral-blood cells from HLA-identical relatives in patients with hematologic cancers. N Engl J Med 2001; 344:175–181.
57. Ustun C, Arslan O, Beksac M, et al: A retrospective comparison of allogeneic peripheral blood stem cell and bone marrow transplantation results from a single center: a focus on the incidence of graft-vs.-host disease and relapse. Biol Blood Marrow Transplant 1999;5:28–35.
58. Oehler VG, Radich JP, Storer B, et al. Randomized trial of allogeneic related bone marrow transplantation versus peripheral blood stem cell transplantation for chronic myeloid leukemia. Biol Blood Marrow Transplant 2005;11:85–92.
59. Stell Cell Trialists Collaborative Group. Allogeneic peripheral blood stem-cell compared with bone marrow transplantation in the management of hematologic malignancies: an individual patient data meta-analysis of nine randomized trials. J Clin Oncol 2005;23:5074–5087.
60. Cornetta K, Laughlin M, Carter S, et al. Umbilical cord blood transplantation in adults: results of the prospective Cord Blood Transplantation (COBLT). Biol Blood Marrow Transplant 2005;11:149–160.
61. Laughlin MJ, Eapen M, Rubinstein P, et al. Outcomes after transplantation of cord blood or bone marrow from unrelated donors in adults with leukemia. N Engl J Med 2004;351:22265–22275.
62. Rocha V, Labopin M, Sanz G, et al. Transplants of umbilical-cord blood or bone marrow from unrelated donors in adults with acute leukemia. N Engl J Med 2004;351:22276–22285.
63. Storb R, Prentice RL, Thomas ED. Marrow transplantation for treatment of aplastic anemia. N Engl J Med 1977;296:61–66.
64. Rowley SD, Zuehlsdorf M, Braine HG, et al. CFU-GM content of bone marrow graft correlates with time to hematologic reconstitution following autologous bone marrow transplantation with 4-hydroperoxycyclophosphamide purged bone marrow. Blood 1987;70:271–275.
65. Bokemeyer C, Franzke A, Hartmann JT, et al. A phase I/II study of sequential, dose-escalated, high dose ifosfamide plus doxorubicin with peripheral blood stem cell support for the treatment of patients with advanced soft tissue sarcomas. Cancer 1997;80:1221–1227.
66. Pettengell R, Woll PJ, Thatcher N, et al. Multicyclic, dose-intensive chemotherapy supported by sequential reinfusion of hematopoietic progenitors in whole blood. J Clin Oncol 1995;13:148–156.
67. Weaver CH, Hazelton B, Birch R, et al. An analysis of engraftment kinetics as a function of the CD34 content of peripheral blood progenitor cell collections in 692 patients after the administration of myeloablative chemotherapy. Blood 1995;86:3961–3969.
68. Bensinger W, Appelbaum F, Rowley S, et al. Factors that influence collection and engraftment of autologous peripheral-blood stem cells. J Clin Oncol 1995;13:2547–2555.
69. Haas R, Möhle R, Frühauf S, et al. Patient characteristics associated with successful mobilizing and autografting of peripheral blood progenitor cells in malignant lymphoma. Blood 1994;83:3787–3794.
70. Tricot G, Jagannath S, Vesole D, et al. Peripheral blood stem cell transplants for multiple myeloma: identification of favorable variables for rapid engraftment in 225 patients. Blood 1995;85:588–596.
71. Schwella N, Beyer J, Schwaner I, et al. Impact of preleukapheresis cell counts on collection results and correlation of progenitor-cell dose with engraftment after high-dose chemotherapy in patients with germ cell cancer. J Clin Oncol 1996;14:1114–1121.
72. Offner F, Schoch G, Fisher LD, et al. Mortality hazard functions as related to neutropenia at different times after marrow transplantation. Blood 1996;88:4058–4062.

73. Singhal S, Powles R, Treleaven J, et al. A low CD34+ cell dose results in higher mortality and poorer survival after blood or marrow stem cell transplantation from HLA-identical siblings: should 2×10^6 CD34+ cells/kg be considered the minimum threshold? Bone Marrow Transplant 2000;26:489–496.
74. Sierra J, Storer B, Hansen JA, et al. Transplantation of marrow cells from unrelated donors for treatment of high-risk acute leukemia: the effect of leukemic burden, donor HLA-matching, and marrow cell dose. Blood 1997;89:426–435.
75. Barrett AJ, Ringden O, Zhang MJ, et al. Effect of nucleated marrow cell dose on relapse and survival in identical twin bone marrow transplants for leukemia. Blood 2000;95:3323–3327.
76. Dominietto A, Lamparelli T, Raiola AM, et al. Transplant-related mortality and long-term graft function are significantly influenced by cell dose in patients undergoing allogeneic marrow transplantation. Blood 2002;100:3930–3934.
77. Ringden O, Barrett AJ, Zhang MJ, et al. Decreased treatment failure in recipients of HLA-identical bone marrow or peripheral blood stem cell transplants with high CD34 cell doses. Br J Haematol 2003;121:874–885.
78. Porrata LF, Gertz MA, Inwards DJ, et al. Early lymphocyte recovery predicts superior survival after autologous hematopoietic stem cell transplantation in multiple myeloma or non-Hodgkin lymphoma. Blood 2001;98:579–585.
79. Porrata LF, Litzow MR, Inwards DJ, et al. Infused peripheral blood autograft absolute lymphocyte count correlates with day 15 absolute lymphocyte count and clinical outcome after autologous peripheral hematopoietic stem cell transplantation in non-Hodgkin's lymphoma. Bone Marrow Transplant 2004;33:291–298.
80. Panse JP, Heimfeld S, Guthrie KA, et al. Allogeneic peripheral blood stem cell graft composition affects early T-cell chimaerism and later clinical outcomes after non-myeloablative conditioning. Br J Haematol 2005;128:659–667.
81. Kim DH, Sohn SK, Lee NY, et al. Transplantation with higher dose of natural killer cells associated with better outcomes in terms of non-relapse mortality and infectious events after allogeneic peripheral blood stem cell transplantation from HLA-matched sibling donors. Eur J Haematol 2005;75:299–308.
82. Solomon SR, Mielke S, Savani BN, et al. Selective depletion of alloreactive donor lymphocytes: a novel method to reduce the severity of graft-versus-host disease in older patients undergoing matched sibling donor stem cell transplantation. Blood 2005;106:1123–1129.
83. Pan L, Delmonte J, Jalonen CK, Ferrara JL. Pretreatment of donors with granulocyte colony-stimulating factor polarizes donor T lymphocytes toward type 2 cytokine production and reduces severity of experimental graft versus host disease. Blood 1995;86:4422.
84. Feng D, Dejbakhsh-Jones S, Strober S. Granulocyte colony-stimulating factor reduces the capacity of blood mononuclear cells to induce graft-versus-host disease: Impact on blood progenitor cell transplantation. Blood 1997;90:453.
85. Glass B, Uharek L, Zeis M, et al. Allogeneic peripheral blood progenitor cell transplantation in a murine model: evidence for an improved graft-versus-leukemia effect. Blood 1997;90:1694.
86. Attal M, Harousseau J-L, Stoppa A-M, et al. A prospective, randomized trial of autologous bone marrow transplantation and chemotherapy in multiple myeloma. N Engl J Med 1996;335:91–97.
87. Linch DC, Winfield D, Goldstone AH, et al. Dose intensification with autologous bone-marrow transplantation in relapsed and resistant Hodgkin's disease: results of a BNLI randomized trial. Lancet 1993;341:1051–1054.
88. Philip T, Guglielmi C, Hagenbeek A, et al. Autologous bone marrow transplantation as compared with salvage chemotherapy in relapses of chemotherapy-sensitive non-Hodgkin's lymphoma. N Engl J Med 1995;333:1540–1545.
89. Press O, Eary JF, Gooley T, et al. A phase I/II trial of iodine-131-tositumomab (anti-CD20), etoposide, cyclophosphamide, and autologous stem cell transplantation for relapsed B-cell lymphomas. Blood 2000;96:2934–2942.
90. Pagel JM, Appelbaum FR, Eary JF, et al. ^{131}I-ANTI-CD45 antibody plus busulfan and cyclophosphamide before allogeneic hematopoietic cell transplantation for treatment of acute myeloid leukemia in first remission. Blood 2005;107:2184–2191.
91. Petersen FB, Deeg HJ, Buckner CD, et al: Marrow transplantation following escalating doses of fractionated total body irradiation and cyclophosphamide: a phase I trial. Int J Radiat Oncol Biol Phys 1992;23:1027–1032.
92. Clift RA, Buckner CD, Appelbaum FR, et al. Allogeneic marrow transplantation in patients with acute myeloid leukemia in first remission: a randomized trial of two irradiation regimens. Blood 1990;76:1867–1871.
93. Clift RA, Buckner CD, Appelbaum FR, et al. Allogeneic marrow transplantation in patients with chronic myeloid leukemia in the chronic phase: a randomized trial of two irradiation regimens. Blood 1991;77:1660–1665.
94. Clift RA, Buckner CD, Appelbaum FR, et al. Long-term follow-up of a randomized trail of two irradiation regimens for patients receiving allogeneic marrow transplants during first remission of acute myeloid leukemia. Blood 1998;92:1455–1456.
95. Petersen FB, Buckner CD, Appelbaum FR, et al. Busulfan, cyclophosphamide and fractionated total body irradiation as a preparatory regimen for marrow transplantation in patients with advanced hematological malignancies: a phase I study. Bone Marrow Transplant 1989;4:617–623.
96. Petersen FB, Buckner CD, Appelbaum FR, et al. Etoposide, cyclophosphamide and fractionated total body irradiation as a preparative regimen for marrow transplantation in patients with advanced hematological malignancies: a phase I study. Bone Marrow Transplant 1992;10:83–88.
97. Groshow LB. Busulfan disposition: The role of therapeutic monitoring in bone marrow transplantation induction regimens. Semin Oncol 1993;20:18–25.
98. Slattery JT, Sanders JE, Buckner CD, et al. Graft-rejection and toxicity following bone marrow transplantation in relation to busulfan pharmacokinetics. Bone Marrow Transplant 1995;16:31–42.
99. Grochow LB, Jones RJ, Brundrett RB, et al. Pharmacokinetics of busulfan: correlation with veno-occlusive disease in patients undergoing bone marrow transplantation. Cancer Chemother Pharmacol 1989;25:55–61.
100. Slattery JT, Clift RA, Buckner CD, et al. Marrow transplantation for chronic myeloid leukemia: the influence of plasma busulfan levels on the outcome of transplantation. Blood 1997;89:3055–3060.
101. Ringden O, Labopin M, Tura S, et al. A comparison of busulphan versus total body irradiation combined with cyclophosphamide as conditioning for autograft or allograft bone marrow transplantation in patients with acute leukaemia: Acute Leukaemia Working Party of the European Group for Blood and Marrow Transplantation (EBMT). Br J Haematol 1996;93:637–645.
102. Blume KG, Kopecky KJ, Henslee-Downey JP, et al. A prospective randomized comparison of total body irradiation-etoposide versus busulfan-cyclophosphamide as preparatory regimens for bone marrow transplantation in patients with leukemia who were not in first remission: a Southwest Oncology Group study. Blood 1993;81:2187–2193.
103. Devergie A, Blaise D, Attal M, et al. Allogeneic bone marrow transplantation for chronic myeloid leukemia in first chronic phase: a randomized trial of busulfan-cytoxan versus cytoxan-total body irradiation as preparative regimen: a report from the French Society of Bone Marrow Graft (SFGM). Blood 1995;85:2263–2268.
104. Socie G, Clift RA, Blaise D, et al. Busulfan plus cyclophosphamide compared with total-body irradiation plus cyclophosphamide before marrow transplantation for myeloid leukemia: long-term follow up of 4 randomized studies. Blood 2001;98:3569–3574.
105. Spencer A, Horvath N, Gibson J, et al. Prospective randomised trial of amifostine cytoprotection in myeloma patients undergoing high-dose melphalan conditioned autologous stem cell transplantation. Bone Marrow Transplant 2005;35:971–977.
106. Benesch M, McDonald GB, Schubert M, et al. Lack of cytoprotective effect of amifostine following HLA-identical sibling transplantation for advanced myelodysplastic syndrome (MDS): a pilot study. Bone Marrow Transplant 2003;32:1071–1075.
107. Spielberger R, Stiff P, Bensinger W, et al. Palifermin for oral mucositis after intensive therapy for hematologic cancers. N Engl J Med 2004;351:2590–2598.
108. Storb R, Yu C, Wagner JL, Deeg JH, et al. Stable mixed hematopoietic chimerism in DLA-identical littermate dogs given sublethal total body irradiation before and pharmacological immunosuppression after marrow transplantation. Blood 1997;89:3048–3054.
109. McSweeney PA, Niederwieser D, Shizuru JA, et al. Hematopoietic cell transplantation in older patients with hematologic malignancies: Replacing high-dose cytotoxic therapy with graft-versus-tumor effects. Blood 2001;97:3390–3400.
110. Maris MB, Niederwieser D, Sandmaier BM, et al. HLA-matched unrelated donor hematopoietic cell transplantation after nonmyeloablative conditioning for patients with hematologic malignancies. Blood 2003;102:2021–2030.

111. Rowley SD, Goldberg SL, Pecora AL, et al. Unrelated donor hematopoietic stem cell transplantation for patients with hematological malignancies using a non-myeloablative conditioning regimen of fludarabine, low-dose total body irradiation, and rabbit anti-thymocyte globulin. Biol Blood Marrow Transplant 2004;10:784–793.
112. Giralt S, Aleman A, Anagnostopoulos A, et al. Fludarabine/melphalan conditioning for allogeneic transplantation in patients with multiple myeloma. Bone Marrow Transplant 2002;30:367–373.
113. Russell JA, Tran HT, Quinlan D, et al. Once-daily intravenous busulfan given with fludarabine as conditioning for allogeneic stem cell transplantation: study of pharmacokinetics and early clinical outcomes. Biol Blood Marrow Transplant 2002;8:468–476.
114. Kroger N, Schwerdtfeger R, Kiehl M, et al. Autologous stem cell transplantation followed by a dose-reduced allograft induces high complete remission rate in multiple myeloma. Blood 2002;100:755–760.
115. Diaconescu R, Flowers CR, Storer B, et al. Morbidity and mortality with nonmyeloablative compared with myeloablative conditioning before hematopoietic cell transplantation from HLA-matched related donors. Blood 2004;104:1550–1558.
116. Alyea EP, Kim HT, Ho V, et al. Comparative outcome of nonmyeloablative and myeloablative allogeneic hematopoietic cell transplantation for patients older than 50 years of age. Blood 2005;105:1810–1814.
117. Carella AM, Cavaliere M, Lerma E, et al. Autografting followed by nonmyeloablative immunosuppressive chemotherapy and allogeneic peripheral-blood hematopoietic stem-cell transplantation as treatment of resistant Hodgkin's disease and non-Hodgkin's lymphoma. J Clin Oncol 2000;18:3918–3924.
118. Maloney DG., Graft-vs-lymphoma effect on various histologies of non-Hodgkin lymphoma. Leuk Lymphoma 2003;44(Suppl 3):S99–105. Review
119. Robinson SP, Goldstone AH, Mackinnon S, et al. Chemoresistant or aggressive lymphoma predicts for a poor outcome following reduced-intensity allogeneic progenitor cell transplantation: an analysis from the Lymphoma Working Party of the European Group for Blood and Bone Marrow Transplantation. Blood 2002;100:4310–4316.
120. Migliaccia AR, Migliaccio G, Johnson G, et al. Comparative analysis of hematopoietic growth factors released by stromal cells from normal donors or transplanted patients. Blood 1990;75:305–312.
121. Martin PJ, Hansen JA, Buckner CD, et al. Effects of in vitro depletion of T cells in HLA-identical allogeneic marrow grafts. Blood 1985;66:664–672.
122. Aversa F, Tabilio A, Terenzi A, et al. Successful engraftment of T-cell-depleted haploidentical "three-loci" incompatible transplants in leukemia patients by addition of recombinant human granulocyte colony-stimulating factor-mobilized peripheral blood progenitor cells to bone marrow inoculum. Blood 1994;84:3948–3955.
123. Dominietto A, Raiola AM, van Lint MT, et al. Factors influencing haematological recovery after allogeneic haemopoietic stem cell transplants: graft-versus-host disease, donor type, cytomegalovirus infections and cell dose. Br J Haematol 2001;112:219–227.
124. Nemunaitis J, Rabinowe SN, Singer JW, et al. Recombinant granulocyte-macrophage colony-stimulating factor after autologous bone marrow transplantation for lymphoid cancer. N Engl J Med 1991; 324:1773–1778.
125. Gulati SC, Bennett CL. Granulocyte-macrophage colony-stimulating factor (GM-CSF) as adjunct therapy in relapsed Hodgkin disease. Ann Intern Med 1992;116:177–182.
126. Advani R, Chao NJ, Horning SJ, et al. Granulocyte-macrophage colony-stimulating factor (GM-CSF) as an adjunct to autologous hemopoietic stem cell transplantation for lymphoma. Ann Intern Med 1992;116:183–189.
127. De Witte T, Gratwohl A, Van der Lely N, et al. Recombinant human granulocyte-macrophage colony-stimulating factor accelerates neutrophil and monocyte recovery after allogeneic T-cell-depleted bone marrow transplantation. Blood 1992;79:1359–1365.
128. Kolb H-J, Schattenberg A, Goldman JM, et al. Graft-versus-leukemia effect of donor lymphocyte transfusions in marrow grafted patients. Blood 1995;86:2041–2050.
129. Lum LG. The kinetics of immune reconstitution after human marrow transplantation. Blood 1987;69:369–380.
130. Atkinson K. Reconstruction of the haemopoietic and immune systems after marrow transplantation. Bone Marrow Transplant 1990;5:209–226.
131. Anderson KC, Soiffer R, DeLage R, et al. T-cell-depleted autologous bone marrow transplantation therapy: analysis of immune deficiency and late complications. Blood 1990;76:235–244.
132. Pedrazzini A, Freedman AS, Andersen J, et al. Anti-B-cell monoclonal antibody-purged autologous bone marrow transplantation for B-cell non-Hodgkin's lymphoma: phenotypic reconstitution and B-cell function. Blood 1989;74:2203–2211.
133. Daley JP, Rozans MK, Smith BR, et al. Retarded recovery of functional T cell frequencies in T cell-depleted bone marrow transplant recipients. Blood 1987;70:960–964.
134. Ferrara JLM, Deeg HJ. Graft-versus-host disease. N Engl J Med 1991; 324:667–674.
135. Sullivan KM, Kopecky KJ, Jocom J, et al. Immunomodulatory and antimicrobial efficacy of intravenous immunoglobulin in bone marrow transplantation. N Engl J Med 1990;323:705–712.
136. Reddy V, Iturraspe JA, Tzolas AC, et al. Low dendritic cell count after allogeneic hematopoietic stem cell transplantation predicts relapse, death, and acute graft-versus-host disease. Blood 2004;103: 4330–4335.
137. Socie G, Stone JV, Wingard JR, et al. Long-term survival and late deaths after allogeneic bone marrow transplantation: Late Effects Working Committee of the International Bone Marrow Transplant Registry. N Engl J Med 1999;341:14–21.
138. Duell T, van Lint MT, Ljungman P, et al. Health and functional status of long-term survivors of bone marrow transplantation: EBMT Working Party on Late Effects and EULEP Study Group on Late Effects: European Group for Blood and Marrow Transplantation. Ann Intern Med 1997;126:184–192.
139. Leather HL, Wingard JR. Infection following hematopoietic stem cell transplantation. Infect Dis Clin North Am 2001;15:483–520.
140. Auner HW, Sill H, Mulabecirovic A, et al. Infection complication after autologous hematopoietic stem cell transplantation: comparison of patients with acute myeloid leukemia, malignant lymphoma and multiple myeloma. Ann Hematol 2002;81:374–377.
141. Ketterer N, Espinouse D, Chomerat M, et al. Infections following peripheral blood progenitor cell transplantation for lymphoproliferative malignancies: etiology and potential risk factors. Am J Med 1999;106:191–197.
142. Junghanss C, Marr KA, Carter RA, et al. Incidence and outcome of bacterial and fungal infections after nonmyeloablative compared with myeloablative allogeneic stem cell transplantation: a matched control study. Biol Blood Marrow Transplant 2002;8:512–520.
143. Gratwohl A, Brand R, Frassoni F, et al. Cause of death after allogeneic haematopoietic stem cell transplantation in early Leukaemias: an EBMT analysis of lethal infectious complications and changes over relative time. Bone Marrow Transplant 2005;36:757–769.
144. Saavedra S, Sanz GF, Jarque I, et al. Early infections and adults patients undergoing unrelated donor cord blood transplantation. Bone Marrow Transplant 2002;30:937–943.
145. Hamza NS, Lisgaris M, Yadavalli G, et al. Kinetics of myeloid and lymphocyte recovery and infectious complications after unrelated umbilical cord blood vs HLA matched unrelated donor allogeneic transplantation in adults. Br J Haematol 2004;124:488.
146. Marr KA, Carter RA, Boeckh M, et al. Invasive aspergillosis in allogeneic stem cell transplant recipients: changes in epidemiology and risk factors. Blood 2000;100:4358–4366.
147. Rapoport AP, Miller Watelet LF, et al. Analysis of factors that correlate with mucositis in recipients of autologous and allogeneic stem-cell transplants. J Clin Oncol 1999;17:2446–2453.
148. Spielberger R, Stiff P, Bensinger W, et al. Palifermin for oral mucositis after intensive therapy for hematologic cancers. N Engl J Med 2004;351:2590–2598.
149. Kumar S, DeLeve LD, Kamath PS, Tefferi A. Hepatic veno-occlusive disease (sinusoidal obstruction syndrome) after hematopoietic stem cell transplantation. Mayo Clin Proc 2003;78:589–598.
150. Kashyap A, Wingard J, Cagnoni P, et al. Intravenous versus oral busulfan as part of a busulfan/cyclophosphamide preparative regimen for allogeneic hematopoietic stem cell transplantation: decreased incidence of hepatic venoocclusive disease (HVOD), HVOD-related mortality, and overall 100-day mortality. Biol Blood Marrow Transplant 2002;8:493–500.
151. Williams CB, Day SD, Reed MD, et al. Dose modification protocol using intravenous busulfan (Busulfex) and cyclophosphamide followed by autologous or allogeneic peripheral blood stem cell transplantation in patients with hematologic malignancies. Biol Blood Marrow Transpl 2004;10:614–623.
152. Fernandez HF, Tran HT, Albrecht F, et al. Evaluation of safety and pharmacokinetics of administering intravenous busulfan in a twice-daily or daily schedule to patients with advanced hematologic malignant disease undergoing stem cell transplantation. Biol Blood Marrow Transplant 2002;8:486–492.
153. Russell JA, Tran HT, Quinlan D, et al. Once-daily intravenous busulfan given with fludarabine as conditioning for allogeneic stem cell transplantation: study of pharmacokinetics and early clinical outcomes. Biol Blood Marrow Transplant 2002;8:468–476.

154. Richardson PG, Murakami C, Jin Z, et al. Multi-institutional use of defibrotide in 88 patients after stem cell transplantation with severe veno-occlusive disease and multisystem organ failure: response without significant toxicity in a high-risk population and factors predictive of outcome. Blood 2002;100:4337–4343.
155. Sixou L, Lassoued S, Attal M, et al. Symptomatic osteonecrosis in recipients of nonautologous bone marrow transplants. Rev Rheum Engl Ed 1995;62:359–363.
156. Socie G, Cahn JY, Carmelo J, et al. Avascular necrosis of bone after allogeneic bone marrow transplantation: analysis of risk factors for 4388 patients by the Societe Francaise de Greffe de Moelle (SFGM). Br J Haematol 1997;97:865–870.
157. Fink JC, Leisenring WM, Sullivan KM, et al. Avascular necrosis following bone marrow transplantation: a case-control study. Bone 1998;22:67–71.
158. Belkacemi Y, Labopin M, Vernant JP, et al. Cataracts after total body irradiation and bone marrow transplantation in patients with acute leukemia in complete remission: a study of the European Group for Blood and Marrow Transplantation. Int J Radiat Oncol Biol Phys 1998;41:659–668.
159. Dudek AZ, Mahaseth H, DeFor TE, Weisdorf DJ. Bronchiolitis obliterans in chronic graft-versus-host disease: analysis of risk factors and treatment outcomes. Biol Blood Marrow Transplant 2003;9:657–666.
160. Sanders JE, Hawley J, Levy W, et al. Pregnancies following high-dose cyclophosphamide with or without high-dose busulfan or total-body irradiation and bone marrow transplantation. Blood 1996;87:3045–3052.
161. Tauchmanova L, De Simone G, Musella T, et al. Effects of various antireabsorptive treatments on bone mineral density in hypogonadal young women after allogeneic stem cell transplantation. Bone Marrow Transplant 2006;37:81–88.
162. Harris E, Mahendra P, McGarrigle HH, et al. Gynaecomastia with hypergonadotrophic hypogonadism and Leydig cell insufficiency in recipients of high-dose chemotherapy or chemo-radiotherapy. Bone Marrow Transplant 2001;28:1141–1144.
163. Krishnan A, Bhatia S, Slovak ML et al. Predictors of therapy-related leukemia and myelodysplasia following autologous transplantation for lymphoma: an assessment of risk factors. Blood 2000;95:1588–1593.
164. Micallef IN, Lillington DM, Apostolidis J, et al. Therapy-related myelodysplasia and secondary acute myelogenous leukemia after high-dose therapy with autologous hematopoietic progenitor-cell support for lymphoid malignancies. J Clin Oncol 2000;18:947–955.
165. Sobecks RM, Le Beau MM, Anastasi J, et al. Myelodysplasia and acute leukemia following high-dose chemotherapy and autologous bone marrow or peripheral blood stem cell transplantation. Bone Marrow Transplant 1999;23:1161–1165.
166. Lowsky R, Lipton J, Fyles G, Minden M, et al. Secondary malignancies after bone marrow transplantation in adults. J Clin Oncol 1994;12:2187–2192.
167. Hasegawa W, Pond GR, Rifkind JT, et al. Long-term follow-up of secondary malignancies in adults after allogeneic bone marrow transplantation. Bone Marrow Transplant 2005;35:51–55.
168. Kolb HJ, Socie G, Duell T, et al. Malignant neoplasms in long-term survivors of bone marrow transplantation: Late Effects Working Party of the European Cooperative Group for Blood and Marrow Transplantation and the European Late Effect Project Group. Ann Intern Med 1999;131:738–744.
169. Curtis RE, Rowlings PA, Deeg HJ, et al. Solid cancers after bone marrow transplantation. N Engl J Med 1997;336:897–904.
170. Brown JR, Yeckes H, Friedberg JW, et al. Increasing incidence of late second malignancies after conditioning with cyclophosphamide and total-body irradiation and autologous bone marrow transplantation for non-Hodgkin's lymphoma. J Clin Oncol 2005;23:2208–2214.
171. Radich JP, Sanders JE, Buckner CD, et al. Second allogeneic marrow transplantation for patients with recurrent leukemia after initial transplant with total-body irradiation-containing regimens. J Clin Oncol 1993;11:304–313.
172. Bosi A, Laszlo D, Labopin M, et al. Second allogeneic bone marrow transplantation in acute leukemia: results of a survey by the European Cooperative Group for Blood and Marrow Transplantation. J Clin Oncol 2001;19:3675–3684.
173. Billingham RE. The biology of graft-versus-host reactions. Harvey Lec 1996;62:21–78.
174. Ferrara JL, Yanik G. Acute graft versus host disease: Pathophysiology, risk factors, and prevention strategies. Clin Adv Hematol Oncol 2005;3:415–419.
175. Reddy P. Pathophysiology of acute graft-versus-host disease. Hematol Oncol 2003;21:149–161.
176. Ottinger HD, Ferencik S, Beelen DW, et al. Hematopoietic stem cell transplantation: contrasting the outcome of transplantations from HLA-identical siblings, partially HLA-mismatched related donors, and HLA-matched unrelated donors. Blood 2003;102:1131–1137.
177. Mielcarek M, Martin PJ, Leisenring W, et al. Graft-versus-host disease after nonmyeloablative versus conventional hematopoietic stem cell transplantation. Blood 2003;102:756–762.
178. Ratanatharathorn V, Nash RA, Przepiorka D, et al. Phase III study comparing methotrexate and tacrolimus (prograf, FK506) with methotrexate and cyclosporine for graft-versus-host disease prophylaxis after HLA-identical sibling bone marrow transplantation. Blood 1998;92:2303–2314.
179. Nash RA, Antin JH, Karanes C, et al. Phase 3 study comparing methotrexate and tacrolimus with methotrexate and cyclosporine for prophylaxis of acute graft-versus-host disease after marrow transplantation from unrelated donors. Blood 2000;96:2062–2068.
180. Cutler C, Kim HT, Hochberg E, et al. Sirolimus and tacrolimus without methotrexate as graft-versus-host disease prophylaxis after matched related donor peripheral blood stem cell transplantation. Biol Blood Marrow Transplant 2004;10:328–336.
181. Bolwell B, Sobecks R, Pohlman B, et al. A prospective randomized trial comparing cyclosporine and short course methotrexate with cyclosporine and mycophenolate mofetil for GVHD prophylaxis in myeloablative allogeneic bone marrow transplantation. Bone Marrow Transplant 2004;34:621–625.
182. Nash RA, Johnston L, Parker P, et al. A phase I/II study of mycophenolate mofetil in combination with cyclosporine for prophylaxis of acute graft-versus-host disease after myeloablative conditioning and allogeneic hematopoietic cell transplantation. Biol Blood Marrow Transplant 2005;11:495–505.
183. Przepiorka D, Ippoliti C, Khouri I, et al. Tacrolimus and minidose methotrexate for prevention of acute graft-versus-host disease after matched unrelated donor marrow transplantation. Blood 1996;88:4383–4389.
184. Bacigalupo A, Lamparelli T, Bruzzi P, et al. Antithymocyte globulin for graft-versus-host disease prophylaxis in transplants from unrelated donors: 2 randomized studies from Gruppo Italiano Trapianti Midollo Osseo (GITMO). Blood 2001;98:2942–2947.
185. Wagner JE, Thompson JS, Carter SL, et al. Effect of graft-versus-host disease prophylaxis on 3-year disease-free survival in recipients of unrelated donor bone marrow (T-cell Depletion Trial): a multi-centre, randomised phase II-III trial. Lancet 2005;366:733–741.
186. Ho VT, Kim HT, Li S, et al. Partial CD8+ T-cell depletion of allogeneic peripheral blood stem cell transplantation is insufficient to prevent graft-versus-host disease. Bone Marrow Transplant 2004;34:987–994.
187. Van Lint MT, Uderzo C, Locasciulli A, et al. Early treatment of acute graft-versus-host disease with high- or low-dose 6-methylprednisolone: a multicenter randomized trial from the Italian Group for Bone Marrow Transplantation. Blood 1998;92:2288–2293.
188. Cragg L, Blazar BR, Defor T, et al. A randomized trial comparing prednisone with antithymocyte globulin/prednisone as an initial systemic therapy for moderately severe acute graft-versus-host disease. Biol Blood Marrow Transplant 2000;6:441–447.
189. MacMillan ML, Weisdorf DJ, Davies SM, et al. Early antithymocyte globulin therapy improves survival in patients with steroid-resistant acute graft-versus-host disease. Biol Blood Marrow Transplant 2002;8:40–46.
190. Bolanos-Meade J, Jacobsohn DA, Margolis J, et al. Pentostatin in steroid-refractory acute graft-versus-host disease. J Clin Oncol 2005;23:2661–2668.
191. Kobbe G, Schneider P, Rohr U, et al. Treatment of severe steroid refractory acute graft-versus-host disease with infliximab, a chimeric human/mouse anti-TNF-alpha antibody. Bone Marrow Transplant 2001;28:47–49.
192. Greinix HT, Volc-Platzer B, Kalhs P, et al. Extracorporeal photochemotherapy in the treatment of severe steroid-refractory acute graft-versus-host disease: A pilot study. Blood 2000;96:2426–2431.
193. Lee SJ, Klein JP, Barrett AJ, et al. Severity of chronic graft-versus-host disease: Association with treatment-related mortality and relapse. Blood 2002;100:406–414.
194. Pavletic SZ, Carter SL, Kernan NA, et al. Influence of T-cell depletion on chronic graft-versus-host disease: results of a multicenter randomized trial in unrelated marrow donor transplantation. Blood 2005;106:3308–3313.
195. Robin M, Guardiola P, Girinsky T, et al. Low-dose thoracoabdominal irradiation for the treatment of refractory chronic graft-versus-host disease. Transplantation 2005;80:634–642.
196. Apisarnthanarax N, Donato M, Korbling M, et al. Extracorporeal photopheresis therapy in the management of steroid-refractory or steroid-dependent cutaneous chronic graft-versus-host disease after allo-

geneic stem cell transplantation: feasibility and results. Bone Marrow Transplant 2003;31:459–465.
197. Mackinnon S, Papadopoulos EB, Carabasi MH, et al. Adoptive immunotherapy evaluating escalating doses of donor leukocytes for relapse of chronic myeloid leukemia after bone marrow transplantation: Separation of graft-versus-leukemia responses from graft-versus-host disease. Blood 1995;86:1261–1268.
198. Choudhury A, Gajewski JL, Liang JC, et al. Use of leukemic dendritic cells for the generation of antileukemic cellular cytotoxicity against Philadelphia chromosome-positive chronic myelogenous leukemia. Blood 1997;89:1133–1142,
199. Kolb HJ, Mittermüller J, Clemm CH, et al. Donor leukocyte transfusions for treatment of recurrent chronic myelogenous leukemia in marrow transplant patients. Blood 1990;76:2462–2465.
200. Szer J, Grigg AP, Phillips GL, Sheridan WP. Donor leucocyte infusions after chemotherapy for patients relapsing with acute leukaemia following allogeneic BMT. Bone Marrow Transplant 1993;11:109.
201. Drobyski WR, Keever CA, Roth MS, et al. Salvage immunotherapy using donor leukocyte infusions as treatment for relapsed chronic myelogenous leukemia after allogeneic bone marrow transplantation: Efficacy and toxicity of a defined T-cell dose. Blood 1993;82:2310.
202. Collins RH Jr, Shpilberg O, Drobyski WR, et al. Donor leukocyte infusions in 140 patients with relapsed malignancy after allogeneic bone marrow transplantation. J Clin Oncol 1997;15:433–44.
203. Hows J, Beddow K, Gordon-Smith E, et al. Donor-derived red blood cell antibodies and immune hemolysis after allogeneic bone marrow transplantation. Blood 1986;67:177–181.
204. Gottlieb DJ, Cryz SJ, Furer E, et al. Immunity against *Pseudomonas aeruginosa* adoptively transferred to bone marrow transplant recipients. Blood 1990;76:2470–2475.
205. Donnenberg AD, Hess AD, Duff SC, et al. Regeneration of genetically restricted immune functions after human bone marrow transplantation: influence of four different strategies for graft-v-host disease prophylaxis. Transplant Proc 1987;19(Suppl 7):144–152.
206. Linker CA. Autologous stem cell transplantation for acute myeloid leukemia. Bone Marrow Transplantation 2003;31:731–738.
207. Wallen H, Gooley TA, Deeg HJ, et al. Ablative allogeneic hematopoietic cell transplantation in adults 60 years of age and older. Clin Oncol 2005;23:439–446. Epub 2005.
208. Kebriaei P, Kline J, Stock W, et al. Impact of disease burden at the time of allogeneic stem cell transplantation in adults with acute myeloid leukemia and myelodysplastic syndromes. BMT 2005;35:965–970.
209. Burnett AK, Wheatley K, Rees JH, et al. The value of allogeneic bone marrow transplant in patients with acute myeloid leukemia at differing risk of relapse: Results of the UK MRC AML 10 trial. Br J Haematol 2002;118:385–400.
210. Zittoun RA, Mandelli F, Willemenze R, et al. Autologous or allogeneic bone marrow transplantation compared with intensive chemotherapy in acute myelogenous leukemia: European Organization for Research and Treatment of Cancer (EORTC) and the Gruppo Italiano Malaitte Ematologiche Maligne dell'Adulto (GINEMA) Leukemia cooperative groups. N Engl J Med 1995;332:217–223.
211. Suciu S, Mandelli F, de Witte T, et al. Allogeneic compared with autologous stem cell transplantation in the treatment of patients younger than 46 years with acute myeloid leukemia in first complete remission: an intention to treat analysis of the EORTC/GINEMA AML10 trial. Blood 2003;102:1232–1240.
212. Byrd JC, Mrozek K, Dodge RK, et al. Pretreatment cytogenetic abnormalities are predictive of induction success, cumulative incidence of relapse, and overall survival in adult patients with de novo acute myeloid leukemia: results from Cancer and Leukemia Group B (CALGB 8461). Blood 2002;100:325–336.
213. Slovak MI, Kopecky KJ, Cassileth PA, et al. Karyotype analysis predicts preremission and post remission therapy in adult acute myeloid leukemia. Blood 2000;96:4075–4083.
214. Au WY, Lie AK, Chim CS, et al. Arsenic trioxide in comparison with chemotherapy and bone marrow transplantation for the treatment of relapsed acute promyelocytic leukemia Ann Oncol 2003;14:752–757.
215. de Botton S, Fawaz A, Chevret S, et al. Autologous and allogeneic stem-cell transplantation as salvage treatment of acute promyelocytic leukemia initially treated with all-*trans*-retinoic acid: a retrospective analysis of the European Acute Promyelocytic Leukemia group. J Clin Oncol 2005;23(a):120–126. Epub 2004 Nov 8.
216. deLabarthe A, Pautas C, Thomas X, et al. French Association. Allogeneic stem cell transplantation in second rather than first complete remission in selected patients with good-risk acute myeloid leukemia. Bone Marrow Transplant 2005;35:767–773.
217. Kim DH, Lee NY, Sung WJ, et al. Multidrug resistance as a potential prognostic indicator in acute myeloid leukemia with normal karyotypes. Acta Haematol 2006;114;78–83.
218. Stone RM, O'Donnell MR, Sekeres MA. Acute myeloid leukemia. Hematology, Am Soc Hematol Ed 2004:98–117.
219. Van der Straaten HM, Van Biezen A, Brand R, et al. Allogeneic stem transplantation for patients with acute myeloid leukemia or myelodysplastic syndrome who have chromosome 5 and or 7 abnormalities. Haematologica 2005;90:1339–1345.
220. C A Linkerl Autologous stem cell transplantation for acute myeloid leukemia. Bone Marrow Transplant 2003;31:731–738.
221. Breems DA, Lowenberg B. Autologous stem cell transplantation in the treatment of adults with acute myeloid leukaemia. Br J Haematol 2005;130:825–833.
222. Osborne D, Frost L, Tobal K, et al. Elevated levels of WT1 transcripts in bone marrow harvests are associated with a high relapse risk in patients autografted for acute myeloid leukaemia. Bone Marrow Transplant 2005;36:17–70.
223. Mohty M, de Lavallade H, Ladaique P, et al. The role of reduced intensity conditioning allogeneic stem cell transplantation in patients with acute myeloid leukemia: a donor vs. no donor domparsion. Leukemia 2005;19:916–920.
224. Schmid C, Schleuning M, Ledderose G, et al. Sequential regimen of chemotherapy, reduced intensity conditioning for allogeneic stem cell transplantation, and prophylactic donor lymphocyte transfusion in high risk acute myeloid leukemia and myelodysplastic syndrome. J Clin Oncol 2005;23:5675–5687.
225. Cornillon J, Fawaz A, Depil S, et al. Outcome of patients less than 55 years of age with high-risk acute leukemia who did not have a human leukocyte antigen-identical related donor: a long-term study of 97 consecutive patients. Leuk Lymphoma 2005;46:641–649.
226. Song KW, Lipton J. Is it appropriate to offer allogeneic hematopoietic stem cell transplantation to patients with primary refractory acute myeloid leukemia? Bone Marrow Transplant 2005;36: 183–191.
227. Ribera JM, Oriol A, Bethencourt C, et al. Comparison of intensive chemotherapy, allogeneic or autologous stem cell transplantation as post-remission treatment for adult patients with high-risk acute lymphoblastic leukemia: results of the PETHEMA ALL-93 trial. Haematologica 2005;90:1346–1356.
228. Pui CH, Relling MV, Downing JR. Acute lymphoblastic leukemia. N Engl J Med 2004;350:1535–1538.
229. Redaelli A, Laskin BL, Stephens JM, et al. A systematic literature review of the clinical and epidemiological burden of acute lymphoblastic leukaemia (ALL). Eur J Cancer Care (Engl) 2004;14:53–62.
230. Durrant IJ, Prentice HG, Richards SM. Intensification of treatment of adults with acute lymphoblastic leukemia: results of the UK -MRC randomized trial UKALLXA: Medical research council working party on leukemia in adults. Br J Haematol 1997;99:84–92.
231. Copelan EA, McGuire EA. The biology and treatment of all in adults. Blood 1995;85:1151–1168.
232. Durrant IJ, Prentice HG, Richards SM. Intensification of treatment of adults with acute lymphoblastic leukemia: results of the UK MRC ALLXA. Medical research council working party on leukemia in adults. Br J Haematol 1997;99:84–92.
233. Hunault M, Harousseau JL, Delain M, et al. Better outcome of adult acute lymphoblastic leukemia after early genoicentical allogeneic bone marrow transplantation (BMT) than after late high-dose therapy and autologous BMT: a GOELAMS trial. Blood 2004;104:28–37. Epub.
234. Thiebaut A, Vernant JP, Degos L. Adult ALL study testing chemotherapy and autologous and allogenewneic transplantation: a follow up to report of the French LALA 87 protocol. Hematol Oncol Clin North Am 2000;14:1353–1366.
235. Kiehl MG, Kraut L, Schwerdfeger R, et al. Outcomes of allogeneic hematopoietic stem cell transplantation in adult patients with acute ALL: no difference in related compared with unrelated transplant in first complete remission. J Clin Oncol 2004;22:2816–2825.
236. Doney K, Hägglund H, Leisenring W, et al. Predictive factors for outcome of allogeneic hematopoietic cell transplantation for adult acute lymphoblastic leukemia. Biol Blood Marrow Transplant 2003;9: 472–481.
237. Hallbook H, Hasglund H, Stockelberg D, et al. Autologous and allogeneic stem cell transplantation in adult ALL: The Swedish Adult All Group experience. Bone Marrow Transplant 2005;35:141–148.
238. Dahlke J, Kroger Nzabelina T, et al. Comparable results in patients with ALL after related and unrelated stem cell transplantation. Bone Marrow Transplant 2006;37:155–163.

239. Weisdorf D, Bishop M, Dharan B, et al. Autologous versus allogeneic unrelated donor transplantation for acute lymphoblastic leukemia: comparative toxicity and outcomes. Biol Blood Marrow Transplant 2002;8:213–220.
240. Schilham MW, Balduzzi A, Bader P. PD-WP of the EBMT: Is there a role for minimal residual disease levels in the treatment of ALL patients who receive allogenic stem cells? Bone Marrow Transplant 2005;35(Suppl 1):S49–S52.
241. Radaelli A, Laskin BL, Stephens JM, et al. A systematic literature review of the clinical and epidemiological burden of acute lymphoblastic leukemia. Eur J Cancer Care 2005;14:53–62.
242. Radich JP, Gooley T, Bensinger W, et al. HLA-matched related hematopoietic cell transplantation for chronic-phase CML using a targeted busulfan and cyclophosphamide preparative regimen. Blood 2003;102:31–105.
243. Hansen JA, Gooley TA, Martin PJ, et al. Bone marrow transplants from unrelated donors for patients with chronic myeloid leukemia. N Engl J Med 1998;338:962–968.
244. Khouri IF, Kantarjian HM, Talpaz M, et al. Results with high-dose chemotherapy and unpurged autologous stem cell transplantation in 73 patients with chronic myelogenous leukemia: the MD Anderson experience. Bone Marrow Transplant 1996;17:775–779.
245. Hui CH, Goh KY, White D, et al. Successful peripheral blood stem cell mobilisation with filgrastim in patients with chronic myeloid leukaemia achieving complete cytogenetic response with imatinib, without increasing disease burden as measured by quantitative real-time PCR. Leukemia 2003;17:821–828.
246. Calin GA, Ferracin M, Cimmino A, et al. A MicroRNA signature associated with prognosis and progression in chronic lymphocytic leukemia. N Engl J Med 2005;353:1793–1801.
247. Gribben JG, Zahrieh D, Stephans K, et al. Autologous and allogeneic stem cell transplantations for poor-risk chronic lymphocytic leukemia. Blood 2005;106:4389–4396.
248. Pavletic SZ, Khouri IF, Haagenson M, et al. Unrelated donor marrow transplantation for B-cell chronic lymphocytic leukemia after using myeloablative conditioning: results from the Center for International Blood and Marrow Transplant research. J Clin Oncol 2005;23: 5788–5794.
249. Schetelig J, Thiede C, Bornhauser M, et al. Evidence of a graft-versus-leukemia effect in chronic lymphocytic leukemia after reduced-intensity conditioning and allogeneic stem-cell transplantation: the Cooperative German Transplant Study Group. J Clin Oncol 2003;21:2747–2753.
250. Sorror ML, Maris MB, Sandmaier BM, et al. Hematopoietic cell transplantation after nonmyeloablative conditioning for advanced chronic lymphocytic leukemia. J Clin Oncol 2005;23:3819–3829.
251. Khouri IF, Keating MJ, Vriesendorp HM, et al. Autologous and allogeneic bone marrow transplantation for chronic lymphocytic leukemia: Preliminary results. J Clin Oncol 1994;12:748–758.
252. McElwain TJ, Powles RL. High-dose intravenous melphalan for plasma-cell leukaemia and myeloma. Lancet 1983;2:22–24.
253. Attal M, Huguet F, Schlaifer D, et al. Intensive combination therapy for previously untreated aggressive myeloma. Blood 1992;79:1130–1136.
254. Harousseau JL, Attal M, Divine M, et al. Autologous stem cell transplantation after first remission induction treatment in multiple myeloma: a report of the French Registry on autologous transplantation in multiple myeloma. Blood 1995;85:3077–3085.
255. Barlogie B, Jagannath S, Vesole DH, et al. Superiority of tandem autologous transplantation over standard therapy for previously untreated multiple myeloma. Blood 1997;189:789–793.
256. Child JA, Morgan GJ, Davies FE, et al. High-dose chemotherapy with hematopoietic stem-cell rescue for multiple myeloma. N Engl J Med 2003;348:1875–1883.
257. Fermand JP, Ravaud P, Katsahian S, et al. High dose therapy and autologous blood stem cell transplantation versus conventional treatment in multiple myeloma results of a randomized trial in 190 patients 55 to 65 years of age. Blood 1999;94(Suppl 1):396a.
258. Blade J, Rosinol L, Sureda A, et al. High-dose therapy intensification compared with continued standard chemotherapy in multiple myeloma in patients responding to initial treatment chemotherapy: long-term results from a prospective randomized trial from the Spanish cooperative group PETHEMA. Blood 2005;106:3755–3759.
259. Palumbo A, Bringhen S, Rus C, et al. A prospective randomized trial of intermediate dose melphalan (100 mg/m^2) vs. oral melphalan/prednisone. Blood 2003;102(Suppl 1):984a.
260. Barlogie G, Kyle R, Anderson K, et al. Comparable survival in multiple myeloma with high dose therapy employing Mel 140 mg/m^2 + TBI 12 Gy autotransplants versus standard dose therapy with VBMCP and no benefit from interferon maintenance: results of Intergroup trial S9321. Blood 2003;102(Suppl 1):42a.
261. Tricot G, Spencer T, Sawyer J, et al. Predicting long-term (≥5 years) event-free survival in multiple myeloma patients following planned tandem autotransplants. Br J Haematol 2002;116:211–217.
262. Vesole D, Barlogie B, Jagannath S, et al. High dose chemotherapy for refractory multiple myeloma: improved prognosis with better supportive care and double transplants. Blood 1994;84:950–956.
263. Desikan R, Barlogie B, Sawyer J, et al. Results of high dose therapy for 1000 patients with multiple myeloma: durable complete remission and superior survival in the absence of chromosome 13 abnormalities. Blood 2000;95:4008–4010.
264. Attal M, Harousseau JL, Facon T, et al. Single versus double autologous stem-cell transplantation for multiple myeloma. N Engl J Med 2003;349:2495–2502.
265. Tricot G, Alberts DS, Johnson C, et al. Safety of autotransplants with high-dose melphalan in renal failure: a pharmacokinetic and toxicity study. Clin Ca Res 1996;2:947–952.
266. Badros A, Barlogie B, Siegel E, et al. Results of autologous stem cell transplant in multiple myeloma patients with renal failure. Br J Haematol 2001;114:822–829.
267. Siegel DS, Desikan KR, Mehta J, et al. Age is not a prognostic variable with autotransplants for multiple myeloma. Blood 1999;93:51–54.
268. Gharton G, Svensson H, Bjorkstrand B, et al. Syngeneic transplantation in multiple myeloma: a case-matched comparison with autologous and allogeneic transplantation: European Group for Blood and Marrow Transplantation. Bone Marrow Transplant 1999;24: 741–745.
269. Bensinger WI, Buckner CD, Anasetti C, et al. Allogeneic marrow transplantation for multiple myeloma: An analysis of risk factors on outcome. Blood 1996;88:2787–2793.
270. Crawley C, Lalancette M, Szydlo R, et al. Outcomes for reduced-intensity allogeneic transplantation for multiple myeloma: an analysis of prognostic factors from the Chronic Leukaemia Working Party of the EBMT. Blood 2005;105:4532–4539.
271. Maloney DG, Molina AJ, Sahebi F, et al. Allografting with nonmyeloablative conditioning following cytoreductive autografts for the treatment of patients with multiple myeloma. Blood 2003;102: 3447–3454.
272. Garban F, Attal M, Michallet M, et al. Prospective comparison of autologous stem cell transplantation followed by a dose-reduced allograft (IFM99-03 trial) with tandem autologous stem cell transplantation (IFM99-04 trial) in high-risk de novo multiple myeloma. Blood 2006 [Epub ahead of print].
273. Comenzo RL, Gertz MA. Autologous stem cell transplantation for primary systemic amyloidosis. Blood 2002;99;12:4276–4282.
274. Dispenzieri A, Kyle RA, Lacy MQ, et al. Superior survival in primary systemic amyloidosis patients undergoing peripheral blood stem cell transplantation: a case-control study. Blood 2004;103:3960–3963.
275. Dember LM, Sanchorawala V, Seldin DC, et al. Effect of dose-intensive intravenous melphalan and autologous blood stem-cell transplantation on AL amyloidosis-associated renal disease. Ann Intern Med 2001;134:746–753.
276. Comenzo RL, Vosburgh E, Simms RW, et al. Dose-intensive melphalan with blood stem-cell support for the treatment of AL (amyloid light-chain) amyloidosis: survival and responses in 25 patients. Blood 2998;91:3662–3670.
277. Gillmore J, Apperley J, Craddock C, et al. High-dose melphalan and stem cell rescue for AL amylodosis. VIII International Symposium on Amyloidosis; August 7–11, 1998; Rochester, Minn.
278. Leung M, Park JW, Ray-Chowdury R. Heart transplantation for restrictive cardiomyopathy: development of cardiac amyloidosis in pre-existing monoclonal gammopathy. J Heart Lung Transplant 1992;11:139.
279. Merlini et al. Molecular mechanisms of amyloidosis. N Engl J Med. 2003;349:583–596.
280. Jaffe ES, Harris NL, Stein H (eds). WHO Classification of Tumors of Hematopoietic and Lymphoid Tissue. Lyon, France, IARC Press, 2001.
281. Owens RG, Treon SP, Al-Katib AL, et al. Clinicopathological definition of Waldenstrom's macroglobulinemia: consensus panel recommendations from the 2nd International workshop on Waldenstrom's macroglobulinemia. Semin Oncol 2003;30:110–115.
282. Kyle RA, Treon SP, Alexanian R, et al. Prognostic markers and criteria to initiate therapy in Waldenstrom's macroglobulinemia: Consensus panel recommendations from the 2nd International workshop on Waldenstrom's macroglobulinemia. Semin Oncol 2003;30:16–120.

283. Gertz MA, Anagnostopoulos A, Anderson K, et al. Treatment recommendations in Waldenstrom's macroglobulinemia: consensus panel recommendations from the 2nd International workshop on Waldenstrom's macroglobulinemia. Semin Oncol 2003;30:121–126.
284. Munshi NC, Barlogie B. Role of high dose therapy with autologous hematopoietic stem cell support in Waldenstrom's macroglobulinemia. Semin Oncol 2003;30:243–247.
285. Treon SP, Agus DB, Link B, et al. CD20 directed antibody mediated immunotherapy induces responses and facilitates hematologic recovery patients with Waldenstrom's macroglobulinemia. J Immunother 2001;24:272–279.
286. Anagnostopoulos A, Dinopoulos MA, Aleman A, et al. High dose chemotherapy followed by stem cell transplantation inpatients with resistant Waldenstrom's macroglobulinemia. Bone Marrow Transplant 2001;27:1027–1029.
287. Desikan R, Dhodapkar M, Siegel D, et al. High dose therapy with autologous hematopoietic stem cell support for Waldenstrom's macroglobulinemia. Br J Haematol 1999;105:993–996.
288. Martino R, Shah A, Romero P, et al. Alogeneic bone marrow transplantation for advanced Waldenstrom's macroglobulinemia. Bone Marrow Transplant 1999;3:747–749.
289. American Cancer Society. Cancer Facts and Figures 2002. Atlanta, Ga., ACS, 2002.
290. Howe HL, Wingo PA, Thun MJ, et al. Annual reports to the nation on the status of cancer 1973–1998. J Natl Cancer Inst 2001;92: 824–842.
291. Jaffe ES, Harris NL, Stein H, Vardiman JW, et al (eds). World Health Organization Classification of Tumors: Pathology and Genetics of Tumors of Hematopoietic and Lymphoid Tissues. Geneva, World Health Organisation, 2001.
292. Ansell SM, Armitage J. Non-Hodgkin lymphoma: Diagnosis and treatment. Mayo Clin Proc 2005;80:1087–1097.
293. International Non-Hodgkin Lymphoma Prognostic Factors project. A predictive model for aggressive NHL. N Engl J Med 1993;329: 987–994.
294. Cameron DA, Leonard RCF, Mao JH, et al. Identification of prognostic groups in follicular lymphoma. Leuk Lymphoma 1993;10:89–99.
295. Lenz G, Dreyling M, Schiegnitz E, et al. Myeloablative radiochemotherapy followed by autologous stem cell transplantation on first remission prolongs progression-free survival in follicular lymphoma: results of a prospective, randomized trial of the German Low-Grade Lymphoma Study Group. Blood 2004;104:2667–2674.
296. Schouten HC, Qian W, Kvaloy S, et al. High dose therapy improved progression free survival and overall survival in relapsed follicular non Hodgkin's lymphoma: results from the randomized European CUP trial. J Clin Oncol 2003;19:4014–4022.
297. Horning SJ, Negrin RS, Hoppe RT, et al. High-dose therapy and autologous bone marrow transplantation for follicular lymphoma in first complete or partial remission: results of a phase II clinical trial. Blood 2002;97:404–409.
298. Bierman PJ, Vose JM, Anderson JR, et al. High-dose therapy with autologous hematopoietic rescue for follicular low-grade non-Hodgkin's lymphoma. J Clin Oncol 1997;15:445–450.
299. Freedman AS, Gribben JG, Neuberg D, et al. High-dose therapy and autologous bone marrow transplantation in patients with follicular lymphoma during first remission. Blood 1996;88:2780–2786.
300. Toze CL, Shepherd JD, Connors JM, et al. Allogeneic bone marrow transplantation for low-grade lymphoma and chronic lymphocytic leukemia. Bone Marrow Transplant 2000;25:605–612.
301. van Besien K, Sobocinski KA, Rowlings PA, et al. Allogeneic bone marrow transplantation for low-grade lymphoma. Blood 1998;92:1832–1836.
302. Avivi I, Goldstone A. Conventional allograft and autograft in low grade lymphoma: Best practice and research. Clin Hematol 2005;18:113–128.
303. van Besien K, Sobocinski KA, Rowlings PA, et al. Allogeneic bone marrow transplantation for low-grade lymphoma. Blood 1998;92:1832–1836.
304. Williams CD, Harrison CN, Lister TA, et al. High-dose therapy and autologous stem-cell support for chemosensitive transformed low-grade follicular non-Hodgkin's lymphoma: a case-matched study from the European Bone Marrow Transplant Lymphoma Working Party-European Bone Marrow Transplant Registry. J Clin Oncol 2000;19:727–735.
305. Hosing C, Saliba RM, McLaughlin P, et al. Long term results favor allogeneic over autologous hematopoietic stem cell transplantation in patients with refractory or recurrent indolent non-Hodgkin's lymphoma. Ann Oncol 2003;14:737–744.
306. Blay JY, Gomez F, Sebban C, et al. The IPI correlates to survival in patients with aggressive lymphoma in relapse: an analysis of the PARMA trial. Blood 1998;92:3562–3568.
307. The International Non-Hodgkin's lymphoma prognostic factors project. A predictive model for aggressive non-Hodgkin's lymphoma. N Engl J Med 1993;329:987–992.
308. Haioun C, Lepage E, Gisselbrecht C, et al. Benefit of autologous bone marrow transplant over sequential chemotherapy in poor risk aggressive non-Hodgkin's lymphoma: updated results of the prospective study LNH 87–2. J Clin Oncol 1997;15:1131–1136.
309. Martelli M, Gherlinzoni F, Zinzani PL, et al. Early autologous stem cell transplantation as first line therapy in poor prognosis non-Hodgkin's lymphoma: an Italian randomized trial. Ann Oncol 1999;10(Suppl):594a.
310. Santini G, Salvagno L, Leoni P, et al. VACOP-B versus VACOP-B plus autologous bone marrow transplantation for advanced diffuse non-Hodgkin's lymphoma: results of a prospective randomized trial by the non-Hodgkin's Lymphoma Cooperative Study Group. J Clin Oncol 1998;16:2796–2802.
311. Verdonck LF, van Putten WL, Hagenbeek A, et al. Comparison of CHOP chemotherapy with autologous bone marrow transplantation for slowly responding patients with aggressive non-Hodgkin's lymphoma. N Engl J Med 1995;332:1045–1051.
312. Verdonck LF, van Putten WL, Hagenbeek A, et al. Comparison of CHOP chemotherapy with autologous bone marrow transplantation for slowly responding patients with aggressive non-Hodgkin's lymphoma. N Engl J Med 1995;332:1045–1051.
313. Vose JM, Zhang MJ, Rowlings PA, et al. Autologous transplantation for diffuse aggressive non-Hodgkin's lymphoma in patients never achieving remission: a report from the Autologous Blood and Marrow Transplant Registry. J Clin Oncol 2001;19:406–413.
314. Philip T, Gugliemi C, Somers R, et al. Autologous bone marrow transplantation as compared with salvage chemotherapy in relapses with chemotherapy sensitive non-Hodgkin's lymphoma. N Engl J Med 1995;333:1540–1545.
315. Paltiel O, Rubinstein C, Or R, et al. Factors associated with survival in patients with progressive disease following autologous transplant for lymphoma. Bone Marrow Transplant 2003;31:565–569.
316. Freedman AS, Neuberg D, Gribben JG, et al. High-dose chemoradiotherapy and anti-B-cell monoclonal antibody-purged autologous bone marrow transplantation in mantle-cell lymphoma: no evidence for long-term remission. J Clin Oncol 1998;16:13–18.
317. Khouri IF, Romaguera J, Kantarjian H, et al. Hyper-CVAD and high-dose methotrexate/cytarabine followed by stem-cell transplantation: An active regimen for aggressive mantle-cell lymphoma. J Clin Oncol 1998;16:3803–3809.
318. Jacobsen A, Freedman A. An update on the role of high dose therapy with autologous or allogeneic stem cell transplantation in mantle cell lymphoma. Curr Opin Oncol 2004;16:106–113.
319. Sweetenham JW, Pearce R, Taghipour G, et al. Adult Burkitt's and Burkitt-like non-Hodgkin's lymphoma: Outcome for patients treated with high-dose therapy and autologous stem-cell transplantation in first remission or at relapse: Results from the European Group for Blood and Marrow Transplantation. J Clin Oncol 1996;14: 2465–2472.
320. Blystad AK, Enblad G, Kvaloy S, et al. High-dose therapy with autologous stem cell transplantation in patients with peripheral T-cell lymphomas. Bone Marrow Transplant 2001;27:711–716.
321. Savage KJ. Aggressive peripheral T-cell lymphomas. Am Soc Hematol Ed Program book. 2005;267–277.
322. McGregor DK, Keever-Taylor CA, Bredeson C, et al. The implication of follicular lymphoma patients receiving allogeneic stem cell transplantation from donors carrying t(14;18)-positive cells. Bone Marrow Transplant 2005;35:1049–1054.
323. Brugger W, Hirsch J, Grunebach F, et al. Rituximab consolidation after high-dose chemotherapy and autologous blood stem cell transplantation in follicular and mantle cell lymphoma: a prospective, multicenter phase II study. Ann Oncol 2004;15:1691–1698.
324. Peniket AJ, Ruiz de Elvira MC, Taghipour G, et al. EBMT Lymphoma registry. Bone Marrow Transplant 2003;31:667–678.
325. Feytes CO, Lodrriza FR, Rizzo JD, et al. Lymphoma working committee of the IBMTR. Blood 2004;104:3797–3803.
326. Peggs KS, Hunter A, Chopra R, et al. Clinical evidence of a graft-versus-Hodgkin's-lymphoma effect after reduced-intensity allogeneic transplantation. Lancet 2005;365:1906–1908.
327. Chopra R, McMillan AK, Linch DC, et al. The place of high-dose BEAM therapy and autologous bone marrow transplantation in poor-risk Hodgkin's disease: a single-center eight-year study of 155 patients. Blood 1993;81:1137–1145.
328. Yuen AR, Rosenberg SA, Hoppe RT, et al. Comparison between conventional salvage therapy and high-dose therapy with autografting for recurrent or refractory Hodgkin's disease. Blood 1997;89:814–822.

329. Linch DC, Winfield D, Goldstone AH, et al. Dose intensification with autologous bone-marrow transplantation in relapsed and resistant Hodgkin's disease: results of a BNLI randomized trial. Lancet 1993;341:1051–1054.
330. Schmitz N, Sextro M, Pfistner D, et al. High-dose therapy (HDT) followed by hematopoietic stem cell transplantation (HSCT) for relapsed chemosensitive Hodgkin's disease (HD): final results of a randomized GHSG and EBMT trial (HD-R1). Proc Am Soc Clin Oncol 1999;18:2a.
331. Lazarus HM, Rowlings PA, Zhang MJ, et al. Autotransplants for Hodgkin's disease in patients never achieving remission: a report from the Autologous Blood and Marrow Transplant Registry. J Clin Oncol 1999;17:534–545.
332. Gajewski JL, Phillips GL, Sobocinski KA, et al. Bone marrow transplantation from HLA-matched siblings in advanced Hodgkin's disease. J Clin Oncol 1996;14:572–578.
333. Milpied N, Fielding AK, Pierce RM, et al. Allogeneic bone marrow transplant is better than autologous transplant for patients with relapsed Hodgkin's disease. J Clin Oncol 1996;14:1291–1296.
334. Schmitz N, Sureda A, Robinson S. Allogeneic transplantation of hematopoietic stem cells after nonmyeloablative conditioning for Hodgkin's disease. Indications and results. Semin Oncol 2004;31:27–32.
335. Ahmed T, Rashid K, Waheed F, et al. Long-term survival of patients with resistant lymphoma treated with tandem stem cell transplant. Leuk Lymph 2005;46:405–414.
336. MacMillan ML, Wagner JE. Hematopoietic cell transplantation for congenital bone marrow failure. Curr Opin Oncol 2005;17:106–113.
337. Evilla J, Fernandez-Plaza S, Diaz MA, Madero L. Paediatric disease working party of the EBMT: Haematopoietic transplantation for bone marrow failure syndromes and thalassemia. Bone Marrow Transplant 352005;(Suppl 1):S17–S21.
338. Bagby GC, Lipton JM, Sloand EM, Schiffer CA. Marrow Failure. Hematology (Am Soc Hematol Educ Program) 2004;318–336.
339. Ferry C, Ouachee M, Leblanc T, et al. Hematopoietic stem cell transplantation in severe congenital neutropenia: Experience of the French SCN register. Bone Marrow Transplant 2005;35:45–50.
340. Dokal I, Rule S, Chen F, et al. Adult onset of AML(M6) in patients with the Shwachman-Diamond syndrome. Br J Haematol 1997;99: 171–173.
341. Dror Y, Freedman MH. Shwachman-Diamond syndrome. Br J Haematol 2002;118:701–713.
342. Vibhakar R, Radhi M, Rumelhart S, et al. Successful unrelated umbilical cord blood transplantation in children with Shwachman-Diamond syndrome. Bone Marrow Transplant 2005;36:855–861.
343. Jaime-Perez JC, Ruiz-Arguelles GJ, Gomez-Almauger D. Haematopoietic stem cell transplantation to treat aplastic anaemia. Expert Opin Biol Ther 2005;5:617–626.
344. Wu CJ, Krishnamurthi L, Kutok JL, et al. Evidence for ineffective erythropoiesis in severe sickle cell disease. Blood 2005;106:3639–3645.
345. Brachet C, Azzi N, Demulder A, et al. Hydroxyurea treatment for sickle cell disease: impact on haematopoietic stem cell transplantations's outcome. Bone Marrow Transplant 2004;33:799–803.
346. Woodard P, Helton KJ, Khan RB, et al. Brain parenchymal damage after hematopoietic stem cell transplantation for severe sickle cell disease. Br J Haematol 2005;129:550–552.
347. Chakrabarthi S, Beresford D. Will developments in allogeneic transplantation influence treatment of adult patients with sickle cell disease? Biol Blood Marrow Transplant 2004;10:23–31.
348. Harris NL, Jaffe ES, Diebold J, et al. World Health Organization classification of neoplastic diseases of the hematopoietic and lymphoid tissues: Report of the clinical advisory committee meeting. Airlie house, Virginia, November 1997. J Clin Oncol 1999;17:3835–3849.
349. Mittal P, Salibe RM, Giralt SA, et al. Allogeneic transplantation: A therapeutic option for myelofibrosis, chronic myelomonocytic leukemia and Philadelphia-negative/BCR-ABL-negative chronic myelogenous leukemia. Bone Marrow Transplant 2004;33:1005–1009.
350. Fruchtman SM. Transplant decision-making strategies n the myeloproliferative disorders. Semin Hematol 2003;40(Suppl 1):30–33.
351. Champlin R, Khouri I, Shimoni A, et al. Harnessing graft versus malignancy: non-myeloablative preparative regimens for allogeneic hematopoietic transplantation, an evolving strategy for adoptive immunotherapy. Br J Haematol 2000;111:19–29.
352. Przepiorka D, Giralt S, Khouri I, et al. Allogeneic marrow transplantation for myeloproliferative disorders other than CML: review of 40 cases. Am J Hematol 1998;57:24–28.
353. Anderson JE, Sale G, Appelbaum FR, et al. Allogeneic marrow transplantation for primary myelofibrosis secondary to polycythemia vera or essential thrombocytosis. Br J Haematol 1997;98:1010–1016.
354. Mittal P, Saliba RM, Giralt SA, et al. Allogeneic transplantation: a therapeutic option for myelofibrosis, chronic myelomonocytic leukemia and Philadelphia-negative/BCR-ABL-negative chronic myelogenous leukemia. Bone Marrow Transplant 2004;33:1005–1009.
355. Rondelli D, Barosi C, Bacigalupo A, et al. Allogeneic hematopoietic stem-cell transplantation with reduced-intensity conditioning in intermediate- or high-risk patients with myelofibrosis with myeloid metaplasia. Blood 2005;105:4115–4119.
356. Zand DY, Deeg HJ, Gooley T, et al. Treatment of CMML by allogeneic transplantation. Br J Haematol 2000;110:217–222.
357. Giralt S. Bone Marrow transplant in myelodysplastic syndromes: new technologies, same questions. Curr Hematol Rep 2005;413:200–207.
358. Solomon S, Savani B, Childs R, et al. Improved outcome for peripheral blood stem cell transplantation for advanced primary myelodysplastic syndrome. Biol Blood Marrow Transplant 2005;11:619–626.
359. Nakai K, Kanda Y, Fukuhara S, et al. Value of chemotherapy before allogeneic hematopoietic stem cell transplantation from an HLA-identical sibling donor for myelodysplastic syndrome. Leukemia 2005;19:396–364.
360. Kebriae P, Kline J, Stock W, et al. Impact of disease burden at time of allogeneic stem cell transplantation in adults with acute myeloid leukemia and myelodysplastic syndromes. Bone Marrow Transplant 2005;35:965–970.
361. Antman KH. Hematopoietic cell transplantation for breast cancer. In Blume KG, Forman SJ, Applebaum FR (eds), Thomas' Hematopoietic Cell Transplantation, 3rd ed. Malden, Mass., Blackwell, 2004, pp1298–1307.
362. Bonadonna G, Valagusa P, Molitermi A, et al. Adjuvant cyclophosphamide, methotrexate and fluorouracil in node-positive breast cancer: the results of 20 years of follow-up. N Engl J Med 1995;332:901–906.
363. Fisher B, Dignan J, Bryant J, et al. Five versus more than five years of tamoxifen for lymph node-negative breast cancer: updated findings from the national surgical adjuvant breast and bowel project B-14. randomized trial. J Natl Cancer Inst 2001;93:684–690.
364. Tallman MS, Gray R, Robert NJ, et al. Conventional adjuvant chemotherapy with or without high-dose chemotherapy and autologous stem-cell transplantation in high-risk breast cancer. N Engl J Med 2003;349:17–26.
365. Damon LE, Hu WW, Stockerl-Goldstein KE, et al. High-dose chemotherapy and hematopoietic stem cell rescue for breast cancer: experience in California. Biol Blood Marrow Transplant 2000;6:496–505.
366. Sayer HG, Schilling K, Vogt T, et al. Double high dose chemotherapy with Adriamycin, paclitaxel, cyclophosphamide and thiotepa followed by autologous peripheral blood stem cell transplantation in women with metastatic breast cancer. J Cancer Res Clin Oncol 2003;129:361–366.
367. Farquhar C, Marjoribanks J, Basser R, et al. High dose chemotherapy and autologous bone marrow or stem cell transplantation versus conventional chemotherapy for women with metastatic breast cancer. Cochrane database system review 2003;cd003142.
368. Eibl B, Schwaighofer H, Nachbaur D, et al. Evidence for a graft-versus-tumor effect in a patient treated with marrow ablative chemotherapy and allogeneic bone marrow transplantation for breast cancer. Blood 1996;88:1501–1508.
369. Ueno NT, Rondon G, Mirza NQ, et al. Allogeneic peripheral blood progenitor cell transplantation for poor-risk patients with metastatic breast cancer. J Clin Oncol 1998;16:986–993.
370. Bishop MR, Fowler DH, Marchigiani D, et al. Allogeneic lymphocytes induce tumor regression of advanced metastatic breast cancer. J Clin Oncol 2004;22:3886–3892.
371. Bishop MR. Allogeneic hematopoietic stem cell transplantation for metastatic breast cancer. Haematologica 2004;89:599–605.
372. Bishop MR, Fowler DH, Marchigiani D, et al. Allogeneic lymphocytes induce tumor regression of advanced metastatic breast cancer. J Clin Oncol 2004;22:3846–3847.
373. Nichols CR, Andersen J, Lazarus HM, et al. High-dose carboplatin and etoposide with autologous bone marrow transplantation in refractory germ cell cancer: An Eastern Cooperative Oncology Group protocol. J Clin Oncol 1992;10:558–563.
374. Motzer RJ, Mazumdar M, Bosl GJ, et al. High-dose carboplatin, etoposide, and cyclophosphamide for patients with refractory germ cell tumors: treatment results and prognostic factors for survival and toxicity. J Clin Oncol 1996;14:1098–1105.
375. Broun ER, Nichols CR, Gize G, et al. Tandem high dose chemotherapy with autologous bone marrow transplantation for initial relapse of testicular germ cell cancer. Cancer 1997;79:1605–1610.
376. Bertucci F, Viens P, Gravis G, et al. High-dose chemotherapy with hematopoietic stem cell support in patients with advanced epithelial ovarian cancer: analysis of 67 patients treated in a single institution. Anticancer Res 1999;19:1455–1461.

377. Stiff PJ, Veum-Stone J, Lazarus HM, et al. High-dose chemotherapy and autologous stem-cell transplantation for ovarian cancer: an autologous blood and marrow transplant registry report. Ann Intern Med 2000;133:504–515.
378. Stiff PJ, Shpall EJ, Liu PY, et al. Randomized phase II trial of two high-dose chemotherapy regimens with stem cell transplantation for the treatment of advanced ovarian cancer in first remission or chemosensitive relapse: a Southwest Oncology Group study. Gynecol Oncol 2004;94:98–106.
379. Cure H, Battista C, Guastalia J, et al. Phase III randomized trial of high-dose chemotherapy (HDC) and peripheral blood stem cell (PBSC) support as consolidation in patients (pts) with responsive low-burden advanced ovarian cancer (AOC): preliminary results of a GINECO/FNCLCC/SFGM-TC study. Proc Am Soc Clin Oncol 2001;204a.
380. Bengala C, Guarneri V, Ledermann J, et al. High-dose chemotherapy with autologous haemopoietic support for advanced ovarian cancer in first complete remission: Retrospective analysis from the Solid Tumour Registry of the European Group for Blood and Marrow Transplantation (EBMT). Bone Marrow Transplant 2005;36:25–31.
381. Bay JO, Fleury J, Choufi B, et al. Allogeneic hematopoietic stem cell transplantation in ovarian carcinoma: results of five patients. Bone Marrow Transplant 2002;30:95–102.
382. Childs R, Chernoff A, Contentin N, et al. Regression of metastatic renal-cell carcinoma after nonmyeloablative allogeneic peripheral-blood stem-cell transplantation. N Engl J Med 2000;343:750–758.
383. Artz AS, Van Besien K, Zimmerman T, et al. Long-term follow-up of nonmyeloablative allogeneic stem cell transplantation for renal cell carcinoma: The University of Chicago experience. Bone Marrow Transplant 2005;35:253–260.
384. Schachna L, Ryan PF, Schwarer AP. Malignancy-associated remission of systemic lupus erythematosus maintained by autologous peripheral blood stem cell transplantation. Arthritis Rheum 1998;41:2271–2272.
385. Snowden JA, Kearney P, Kearney A, et al. Long-term outcome of autoimmune disease following allogeneic bone marrow transplantation. Arthritis Rheum 1998;41:453–459.
386. Euler HH, Marmont AM, Bacigalupo A, et al. Early recurrence or persistence of autoimmune diseases after unmanipulated autologous stem cell transplantation. Blood 1996;88:3621–3625.
387. Fassas A, Anagnostopoulos A, Kazis A, et al. Peripheral blood stem cell transplantation in the treatment of progressive multiple sclerosis: first results of a pilot study. Bone Marrow Transplant 1997;20:631–638.
388. Traynor AE, Schroeder J, Rosa RM, et al. Treatment of severe systemic lupus erythematosus with high-dose chemotherapy and haemopoietic stem-cell transplantation: a phase I study. Lancet 2000;356:701–707.
389. Jayne D, Passweg J, Marmont A, et al. Autologous stem cell transplantation for systemic lupus erythematosus. Lupus 2004;13:168–176.
390. Snowden JA, Passweg J, Moore JJ, et al. Autologous hemopoietic stem cell transplantation in severe rheumatoid arthritis: a report from the EBMT and ABMTR. J Rheumatol 2004;31:482–488.
391. Burt RK, Traynor A, Oyama Y, Craig R. High-dose immune suppression and autologous hematopoietic stem cell transplantation in refractory Crohn disease. Blood 2003;101:2064–2066.
392. Dreger P, Glass B, Kuse R, et al. Myeloablative radiochemotherapy followed by reinfusion of purged autologous stem cells for Waldenstrom's macroglobulinaemia. Br J Haematol 1999;106:115–118.
393. Tournilhac O, Leblond V, Tabrizi R, et al. Transplantation in Waldenstrom's macroglobulinemia—the French experience. Semin Oncol 2003;30:291–296.
394. Cassileth PA, Harrington DP, Appelbaum FR, et al. Chemotherapy compared with autologous or allogeneic bone marrow transplantation in the management of acute myeloid leukemia in first remission. N Engl J Med. 1998;339:1649–1656.
395. Harousseau JL, Cahn JY, Pignon B, et al. Comparison of autologous bone marrow transplantation and intensive chemotherapy as post-remission therapy in adult acute myeloid leukemia. The Groupe Ouest Est Leucemies Aigues Myeloblastiques (GOELAM). Blood 1997; 90:2978–2986.
396. Ravindranath Y, Yeager AM, Chang MN, et al. Autologous bone marrow transplantation versus intensive consolidation chemotherapy for acute myeloid leukemia in childhood. Pediatric Oncology Group. N Engl J Med 1996;334:1428–1434.
397. Khouri IF, Keating M, Korbling M, et al. Transplant-lite: induction of graft-versus-malignancy using fludarabine-based nonablative chemotherapy and allogeneic blood progenitor-cell transplantation as treatment for lymphoid malignancies. J Clin Oncol 1998;16: 2817–2824.
398. Nagler A, Slavin S, Varadi G, et al. Allogeneic peripheral blood stem cell transplantation using a fludarabine-based low intensity conditioning for malignant lymphoma. Bone Marrow Transplant 2000;25: 1021–1028.
399. Kottaridis PD, Milligan DW, Chopra R, et al. In vivo CAMPATH-1H prevents graft-versus-host disease following nonmyeloablative stem cell transplantation. Blood 2000;96:2419–2425.
400. Khouri IF, Saliba RM, Giralt SA, et al. Nonablative allogeneic hematopoietic transplantation as adoptive immunotherapy for indolent lymphoma: low incidence of toxicity, acute graft-versus-host disease, and treatment-related mortality. Blood 2001;98:3595–3599.
401. Chakraverty R, Peggs K, Chopra R, et al. Limiting transplantation-related mortality following unrelated donor stem cell transplantation by using a nonmyeloablative conditioning regimen. Blood 2002;99:1071–1078.
402. Robinson SP, Goldstone AH, Mackinnon S, et al. Chemoresistant or aggressive lymphoma predicts for a poor outcome following reduced-intensity allogeneic progenitor cell transplantation: an analysis from the Lymphoma Working Party of the European Group for Blood and Bone Marrow Transplantation. Blood 2002;100:4310–4316.
403. Dreger P, Brand R, Hansz J, et al. Treatment-related mortality and graft-versus-leukemia activity after allogeneic stem cell transplantation for chronic lymphocytic leukemia using intensity-reduced conditioning. Leukemia 2003;17:841–848.
404. Khouri IF, Lee MS, Saliba RM, et al. Nonabilitive allogeneic stem cell transplantation for chronic lymphocytic leukemia: impact of rituximab on immunomodulation and survival. Exp Hematol 2004;32: 28–35.
405. Morris EC, Mackinnon S. Reduced intensity allogeneic stem cell transplantation for low grade non-Hodgkin's lymphoma. Best Pract Res Clin Haematol 2005;18:129–142.
406. Faulkner RD, Craddock C, Byrne JL, et al. BEAM-alemtuzumab reduced-intensity allogeneic stem cell transplantation for lymphoproliferarative diseases: GVHD, toxicity, and survival in 65 patients. Blood 2004;103:428–434.

Chapter 59

Umbilical Cord Blood Stem Cells: Collection, Processing, and Transplantation

Hal E. Broxmeyer

INTRODUCTION

The first cord blood transplantation was performed successfully in October 1988.[1] This clinical effort was initiated based on a basic science study coordinated by the author's laboratory that suggested umbilical cord blood as a potential source of transplantable hematopoietic stem and progenitor cells.[2] The clinical study, which demonstrated hematopoietic reconstitution in a patient with Fanconi anemia by using human leukocyte antigen (HLA)-identical sibling cells, served as the first proof-of-principal for the initiating scientific study,[2] and as a precursor to the more than 6000 umbilical/placental cord blood transplants performed to the present for a wide variety of malignant and nonmalignant disorders that required a hematopoietic stem cell transplant for treatment and cure. Similarly, the author's laboratory served as the first cord blood bank that stored the cord bloods used for the first five cord blood transplants performed as well as for two of the second five done.[2–5]

Both the laboratory[2] and clinical[1] studies were the result of a multi-institutional national study in the United States,[2] which then opened up into a multi-institutional international study between investigators in the United States and in Paris, France.[1] The background leading to both efforts has been reviewed in a number of articles.[3–6] At first, the clinical cord blood transplants were limited to HLA-matched sibling donor cord bloods, with the recipients being children.[7] These encouraging results led to the use of HLA-partially matched transplants in children and then the use of unrelated cord blood transplants that were completely and then subsequently partially matched for HLA.[8–13] However, because of the limiting number of cells that one can collect from the cord blood at the birth of the baby and the need for greater numbers of cells the larger the recipient's body weight, relatively fewer cord blood transplants have been performed in adults than in children and lower-weight individuals.[11,14–17] This is changing as transplanters have become more comfortable with the use of cord blood as a source of transplantable cells and as clinical understanding and efforts have better developed.[18–24]

CORD BLOOD TRANSPLANTS IN ADULTS

Although the number of cord blood transplants in adults is still relatively low compared with that for children, these numbers are increasing.[11,14–24] The recent article by Laughlin and colleagues[19] compared results of 150 patients being transplanted with cord blood mismatched for one or two antigens, in comparison to 367 matched and 83 one-antigen-mismatched bone marrow transplants. Overall, the recipients of the cord blood transplants were younger, and they were more likely to manifest advanced leukemia than were the recipients of bone marrow transplantation. Moreover, because of the limiting numbers of cells in cord blood compared with bone marrow collections, the recipients of cord blood transplants received a lower dose of nucleated cells. For as yet unknown reasons, which may not entirely relate to the dose of nucleated cells infused, neutrophil and platelet recovery was slower with transplantation of mismatched bone marrow and cord blood, than with matched marrow transplantation. This delayed engraftment with cord blood has been noted since the first cord blood transplant[1] and may relate to the relatively immature nature of cord blood cells. Interestingly, acute graft-versus-host disease (GVHD) was more likely to occur after mismatched marrow transplantation, but chronic GVHD was more evident after cord-blood transplantation. Recipients of mismatched bone marrow or cord blood transplants were similar in treatment-related mortality, treatment failure, and overall mortality, with no differences in the rate of relapse of leukemia. Although the authors noted infections being more prevalent with cord blood, the types of infections did not differ among the three comparison groups. An article by Rocha and associates[20] in the same issue of the *New England Journal of Medicine* as that of Laughlin and colleagues[19] evaluated outcomes in 682 adults with acute leukemia. Ninety-eight were recipients of cord blood transplantation, and 584 received bone marrow. This effort was confined to those transplants performed from 1998 to 2002.[20] The cord blood transplant recipients were younger, weighed less, and had more-advanced disease than bone marrow recipients at the time of transplantation. The authors reported lower risks of grade 2 to 4 acute GVHD, but significant delays in neutrophil recovery with cord blood. However, incidence of chronic GVHD, transplant-related mortality, relapse, and leukemia-free survival were not significantly different in the two groups. Attempts to reconcile the data[25] in these two articles[19,20] pointed to several possibilities in the two studies that might explain some of the differences noted. The article by Laughlin and colleagues[19] encompassed patients given transplants over a longer period than that of Rocha and associates[20] when the relevance of nucleated cell dose and HLA matching had not yet been fully appreciated. By restricting their analysis to after 1998, Roche and associates[20] likely had better patient and cord blood unit selectivity based on identification of potential reasons for better patient outcomes.[22] A prospective study published by the Cord Blood Transplantation (COBLT) study group, supported in part by the U.S. National Institutes of Health, reported somewhat less-favorable results for cord blood transplantation in adults.[23] The primary end point of this study[23] was survival at 6 months, with secondary end points analyzing engraftment, GVHD, relapse, and longer-term survival. Enrollment into the program required a cord blood collection that contained more than 10^7 nucleated cells per kilogram recipient body weight with equal to or greater than four HLA-A and -B (low or intermediate resolution) and -DRB1 (high resolution) matches. Patients included those with acute and chronic myelogenous leukemia and acute lymphoblastic leukemia, as well as myelodysplastic syndrome, paroxysmal nocturnal hemoglobinuria, and non-Hodgkin's lymphoma. Of these patients, 94% were considered poor-risk candidates by criteria put forth by the National Marrow Donor Program (NMDP). The overall conclusion of the COBLT study[23] was that cord blood transplantation should continue to be performed in specialized centers with a research focus on cord blood cells because of the high treatment-related mortality and slow engraftment kinetics they noted. The less-favorable results noted by the COBLT study,[23] compared with that of the results of the articles reported earlier,[19,20] may in part reflect the much greater poor-risk patients studied in the COBLT study, even though the study was open to both good- and poor-risk patients, as defined by the NMDP. A comparative analysis of the major clinical studies for cord blood transplantation for adults was reviewed by Chao.[26]

Most cord blood transplants have been performed by using myeloablative conditioning regimens for the recipients, however, some patients have undergone nonmyeloablative conditioning,[27,28] and these have also been summarized by Chao.[26]

CURRENT AND FUTURE EFFORTS TO EXTEND THE REACH OF CORD BLOOD TRANSPLANTATION TO MORE PATIENTS

Although many unanswered questions remain regarding how to best broaden the applicability of cord blood transplantation, a major effort has gone into trying to adapt cord blood for more-efficient use in adults and high-weight individuals. Limits in the numbers of cord blood cells available in the individual collections of cord blood at the births of babies are clearly a major limiting factor in successful transplantation into adults and high-weight individuals. Current clinical practice uses in the range of greater than or equal to about 2×10^7 nucleated cells per kilogram recipient body weight. Whereas this is about a log lower than that recommended for bone marrow transplantation, this is compensated for in part by the increased frequency and quality of hematopoietic stem and progenitor cells found in the cord blood compared with bone marrow.[2,29–38] However, even being able to generate equal to or greater than 2×10^7 nucleated cells per kilogram body weight from single cord blood collections to use in adults is problematic on a routine basis. Attempts to compensate for limiting numbers of nucleated cells in single cord blood collections include (1) use of multiple cord blood units for transplantation into single recipients, (2) ex vivo expansion of single cord blood units, and (3) enhanced quality of the hematopoietic stem and progenitor cells for homing to and engraftment in the appropriate microenvironment niches of recipient bone marrow.

Use of Multiple Cord Blood Units for Transplantation into Single Recipients

This mode of using multiple cord blood units for potential transplantation is not new in concept[39] but has only recently demonstrated possible efficacy.[40] Barker and coworkers[40] evaluated the safety of combining two partially HLA cord blood units for transplantation after myeloablative conditioning in 23 patients manifesting high-risk hematologic malignancy. Of the 21 evaluable patients, all engrafted at 15 to 41 days, with a median time to engraftment of 23 days. Of interest, and not yet fully understood, engraftment was seen at 21 days for 24% of the patients with both cord bloods, and with only one cord blood in the rest of the recipients. However, only one unit predominated at 100 days in all the patients. The mystery is not only why only one cord blood unit eventually predominated, but also how to predict which of 2 units will predominate. This information would be of great interest, especially in the context of a number of clinical trials evaluating an ex vivo expanded cord blood unit in combination with an unmanipulated unit. If only one unit predominates, and it is not clear which unit will "win out," combining a manipulated cord blood unit (e.g., one that is "expanded" ex vivo) with an unmanipulated cord blood unit may make it extremely difficult to interpret the results. Thus far, neither nucleated nor CD34+ cell doses nor HLA-type of the cord blood collections is predictive of predominance in the host, and CD3+ T-cell dose, which was originally suggested as a possible criterion for predominance,[40] has not been substantiated. Many centers are currently using two or more cord blood units for transplantation, although a controlled clinical trial has not yet been performed to prove definitively that the transplantation of more than one cord blood unit is any more efficacious than that of a single unit.

Ex Vivo Expansion of Single Cord Blood Units

Hematopoietic stem cells are defined by their capacity to self-renew. Being able to harness the self-renewal capacity of these stem cells ex vivo would likely open up the possibility for more-consistent use of cord blood transplantation for adults. Also, it is possible that a single collection of cord blood, if effectively expanded in the context of functional stem cells, could be used for engraftment and repopulation of the blood cell system for multiple recipients. Harnessing self-renewal capacity for production/expansion of stem cells is clear for murine stem cells. Unfortunately, it is not apparent that anyone has been able truly ex vivo to expand human hematopoietic stem cells. Without question, ex vivo expansion of hematopoietic progenitor cells is possible, but progenitors do not have the capacity to provide the long-term engraftment needed for successful transplantation. Progenitors may to some extent provide short-term engraftment, and it is possible that this may be of some value when expanded progenitors or short-term repopulating stem cells are combined with unmanipulated cord blood units that themselves do not have a high enough nucleated cell content to guarantee long-term engraftment. The expanded progenitors may allow the long-term repopulating cells in the unmanipulated cord blood unit the opportunity to "take hold" and repopulate over the long term in the recipient.

Several clinical attempts to use ex vivo expanded cells[41,42] have not provided encouraging results, although efforts in this area are ongoing at a number of centers. Hematopoietic stem and progenitor cells are controlled by both stromal cell interactions and soluble cytokines. Although many such key players have been identified to act on hematopoietic progenitor cells,[43] far less is known about the factors influencing stem cell self-renewal and other functions of stem cells. Players implicated in stem cell proliferation and self-renewal are Notch ligands and their receptor, Notch,[44–47] Wnt3a/Frizzled,[48–51] Hox B4/PBX1,[52–58] and Bmi-1.[59–61] Whether Notch ligands effect the long-term repopulating or short-term hematopoietic stem cell is not clear,[62,63] and no clinical reports are available yet on use of Wnt3a/Frizzled, Hox B4/PBX1, and Bmi-1 manipulation for enhancement of clinical transplantation efficiency. Other intracellular factors implicated in hematopoietic stem cell function include C/EBPα,[64] Gfi-1,[65,66] Stat5,[67,68] and possibly Stat3,[69] although a role for Stat3 in hematopoietic stem cell activity is not yet clear.[68] What is clear is that self-renewal of mouse embryonic stem cells is mediated by activation of Stat3,[70] and the author's group has preliminary evidence, from using mice in which Stat3 is conditionally deleted in hematopoietic cells, that Stat3 is involved in mouse hematopoietic cell engraftment (unpublished observations). Interestingly, mouse embryonic stem cells produce a number of factors that provide functional support for themselves as well as for hematopoietic progenitor cells.[71,72] It is possible that factors produced by embryonic stem cells may have functional activity on hematopoietic stem cells. The study of both hematopoietic stem cells and embryonic stem cells could shed light on the capacity of hematopoietic stem cells for self-renewal and engrafting capability.

Stromal cell–derived factor-1 (SDF-1/CXCL12) and its receptor, CXCR4, have been implicated in a number of functions on hematopoietic stem and progenitor cells, including directed movement, as well as the survival of these cells.[43] SDF-1/CXCL12, a stromal cell–derived factor, is also produced by mouse embryonic stem cells.[71] The author's laboratory is also investigating a potential role for SDF-1/CXCL12 in hematopoietic stem cell proliferation, self-renewal, and engrafting activity. SDF-1/CXCL12 enhances the replating capacity in vitro of multipotential and macrophage progenitor cells (unpublished observations). Because replating capacity in vitro is a measure of self-renewal of these progenitors,[33,34] it is possible that SDF-1/CXCL12 may enhance the self-renewal capacity of hematopoietic stem cells.

It is probably only a matter of time before investigators uncover the factors and mechanisms of action responsible for stem cell self-renewal. When this occurs, it is likely that ex vivo expansion of stem cells will become a reality for clinical transplantation efforts. In the meantime, another option is to enhance the capacity of hematopoietic stem cells efficiently to home to their microenvironment niches in the bone marrow, and in this way, to increase the engrafting capability of these cells.

Enhanced Homing of Hematopoietic Stem Cells for More Efficacious Engraftment of Limiting Numbers of Cells

Homing of hematopoietic stem cells is a poorly understood event but is believed to involve a coordinated series of steps involving SDF-1/CXCL12, stem cell factor, lymphocyte function-associated antigen 1 (LFA-1), the integrins VLA-4 and VLA-5, CD44, metalloproteinases, and additional players.[73,74] It is believed that not all hematopoietic stem cells, when infused into recipients, reach their microenvironmental niches where these stem cells can be nourished for optimal proliferation, self-renewal, and differentiation. Thus being able to enhance homing to the appropriate niches in the bone marrow could enhance the engrafting capability of these cells. This may be of special interest for situations such as cord blood, where sometimes only limiting numbers of cells are available for transplantation.

One possible means to enhance the stem cell homing process is to increase the efficiency of the SDF-1/CXCL12-CXCR4 axis for chemotaxis/migration/homing.[73] CD26, a cell surface component, manifests dipeptidylpeptidase IV activity. This peptidase activity truncates SDF-1/CXCL12; truncated SDF-1/CXCL12 is not active as a chemotactic activity but does block the chemotactic activity of full-length CXCL12 for hematopoietic stem/progenitor cells.[75] Thus it was reasoned by us that inhibiting or deleting the CD26 expressed on hematopoietic stem and progenitor, as well as other cell types (e.g., T cells), which could enhance the chemotactic effectiveness of SDF-1/CXCL12 by blocking truncation of SDF-1/CXCL12, might enhance homing of these cells after infusion. To test this hypothesis, mouse bone marrow cells were pretreated with either Diprotin A or Val-Pyr, both inhibitors of the peptidase activity of CD26, or bone marrow cells from CD26-/- mice were used. The cells were transplanted into lethally irradiated mice congenic for CD45 in either a competitive or noncompetitive in vivo hematopoietic stem cell–engrafting assay.[76] Inhibition or deletion of CD26 on hematopoietic stem cells greatly enhanced the homing capacity of the stem cells and led to enhanced stem cell engraftment, effects most apparent when limiting numbers of stem cells were used for engraftment. Preliminary experiments suggest that Diprotin A inhibition of CD26 on CD34+ human cord blood cells enhances the engraftment of these cells in sublethally irradiated NOD/SCID mice,[77] an assay used to evaluate human hematopoietic stem cells functionally.[35–37,78] Whether inhibition of CD26 on human stem cells, or other means to enhance homing of these cells will be of clinical efficacy to increase engraftment by using limiting numbers of cells, or will enhance the time to engraftment, a problem with cord blood stem cell transplantation, remains to be determined.

CORD BLOOD BANKING

Cord blood transplantation is dependent on being able to bank the cord blood cells, which in turn requires that these cells can be cryopreserved.

Cryopreservation of Cord Blood Stem and Progenitor Cells

The first recipient of a cord blood transplant[1] is still alive and well 17 years after the transplant. He received cord blood from his HLA-matched sister that had been cryopreserved by and stored frozen for a number of months in the author's laboratory before the actual transplant.[1,3] The longest time a cord blood has been stored in cyropreserved form before actual transplantation is not clear but is likely in the time frame of at least 5 years. Theoretically, once cord blood is appropriately frozen, the cells should remain cryopreserved for at least a lifetime, assuming of course that problems did not exist with the freezing process, the storage, and the defrosting protocol. In actual experimental terms, cord blood cells have been stored at least up to 15 years without loss of functional hematopoietic stem and progenitor cell activity.[2,29,79,80] In the most recent study from the author's laboratory to evaluate cord blood cryopreservation,[80] highly efficient recovery was noted for granulocyte-macrophage (CFU-GM), erythroid (BFU-E), and multipotential (CFU-GEMM) progenitor cells in terms of numbers and proliferative capacity of these progenitor cells in vitro after 15 years of storage. Moreover, the recovered CD34+ population of stem/progenitor cells showed more than 250-fold ex vivo expansion of progenitor cells, and the CD34+ cells isolated after defrosting of the cord blood were able to engraft sublethally irradiated NOD/SCID mice with a frequency that was equivalent to that of freshly isolated cord blood CD34+ cells. The author's laboratory, as of the date of this writing, has cord blood cells frozen for as long as 18 to 19 years and will be able to continue to evaluate the efficacy of recovery of cryopreserved cord blood stem/progenitor cells stored over the long term. However, others continue to define more-effective cryopreservation methods for cord blood stem/progenitor cells.[81]

Cord Blood Banking

In general terms, currently two types of cord blood banks are available. There are those that store cord blood for autologous or related use. These are termed "Private" banks and usually charge an upfront fee as well as a continuing maintenance fee. Once entered into a contractual agreement with the cord blood banking company, the individual that signed the contract and/or the donor of the cord blood essentially own the blood. The other type of cord blood bank is generally called a "Public Bank." Once donated to a "Public Bank," the cord blood is no longer owned by the donor or family of the donor and is available for use, for a fee, by one who is in need of a cord blood stem cell transplant. Cord blood banking has a number of benefits,[82] which include (1) rapid availability of cord blood when needed, as the blood is stored in banks and has been HLA-typed and assessed for the possibility of infectious agents; (2) no donor risk or attrition, as collection of the cord blood is essentially an easy and safe process in the hands of experienced personnel, and can theoretically be replenished from the multitude of births every day. In contrast to registries such as the National Marrow Donor Program (NMDP) for bone marrow, the cord blood is already present, whereas when the bone marrow is needed, those who signed up to donate the marrow have to be tracked down to see if they can be found and are still willing to donate the marrow, which is obtained through an invasive although relatively safe procedure; and (3) the potential for increasing the pool of donor stem cells for ethnic and racial minorities. In addition, cord blood use opens up the probability for a lower risk of transmitting infectious diseases and appears to manifest a reduced risk of GVHD, as mismatched cord blood appears to elicit less GVHD than does mismatched bone marrow. The first operational "Public" cord blood banks were established in 1993 in New York, Milan, and Dusseldorf.[82] In 2001, a number of selected organizations were available to ensure quality and standards in cord blood banking,[82] and these included in alphabetical order: American Association of Blood Banks, American Red Cross, Bone Marrow Donors World, Cord Blood Transplantation Study, European Blood and Marrow Transplant Group (EBMT), Eurocord, Foundation for the Accreditation of Hematopoietic Cell Therapy, Group for the Collection and Expansion of Hematopoietic Cells, International Society for Hemotherapy and Graft Engineering (ISHAGE), Joint Accreditation Committee of ISHAGE-Europe and EBMT, Netcord, and National Marrow Donor Program. Many of these organizations are still available today.

Techniques have been developed and continue to be refined efficiently and safely to select donors and to collect, store, process, and distribute cord blood units to areas of need throughout the world.[82]

A recent review on new trends in umbilical cord blood transplantation,[83] cited a 2003 reference that listed about 150,000 available cord bloods from 35 different cord blood banks in 21 countries, almost all of which were typed for HLA-A, -B, and -DR, with 76% of the units typed by molecular analysis for major histocompatibility complex (MHC) class II antigens, and 49% molecularly typed for MHC class I antigens. These numbers of stored cord blood are now likely an underestimate of those cord blood units available. It was noted that most Cord Blood Banks in the United States operate under an Investigational New Drug (IND) application from the Food and Drug Administration (FDA), as well as an Institutional Review Board (IRB)-approved research consent.[83] Efforts are also still needed to define the best application of cord blood transplantation in the transplant donor-choice algorithm,[83] which currently involves a decision between use of mobilized peripheral blood, bone marrow, and cord blood as sources of transplantable and long-term engrafting stem cells.

Report from the Institute of Medicine of the National Academies of Science, U.S.A.

It was noted that the increase in numbers of cord blood banks in the United States raised a number of important questions,[84] including adequacy of cord blood inventories, standardization of collecting cord bloods, as well as their processing, storage, documentation, and quality control. Moreover, the lack of a single outcomes database has been thought to block the ability of the scientific community to determine best-practice guidelines. Because of these concerns, the U.S. Congress provided money, under a 2004 appropriations bill of the U.S. Department of Health and Human Services, to establish a U.S. National Cord Blood Bank Program under the leadership of the Health Resources and Services Administration.

The Institute of Medicine report was broken down into questions and recommendations.[84] Among the questions considered, the most specific were (1) What is the role of cord blood in hematopoietic progenitor cell (Author's note: this should have read hematopoietic stem cell) transplantation in the context of other sources of progenitor cells? (2)What is the current status of cord blood banks? (3) What is the optimal structure for the cord blood program? (4) What is the current use and utility of cord blood collections for stem cell transplants? (5) What standards should be set for storage, collection, information sharing, distribution, and outcome measures? (6) What is the best way to make cord blood units available for research? (7) What consent procedures are needed for both the research and transplantation use of cord blood? and (8) Should the cord blood program set practice guidelines for both "Public" and "Private" banks? It was recommended that a national program should have as its primary mission the goal of maximizing access to high-quality cord blood units for patient care and research in the most efficient, cost-effective, and ethical manner.[84] This program needed to avoid duplication of efforts in services provided and the steps necessary for a transplant center to access appropriate sources of grafts, with promotion of the best possible chance for patient recovery through the establishment of high-quality, HLA-diverse cord blood units, and an integral part of the program should be support and education for all individuals involved. It was emphasized that a barrier to the goal of unimpeded access to treatment was the lack of sufficient ethnic and racial diversity in existing stored cord blood units.

Specific recommendations for banks and banking included[84] (1) identify a cord blood accrediting organization; (2) establish uniform standards for cord blood collection; (3) establish uniform quality-assurance systems; (4) establish FDA licensure of cord blood units; and (5) apply quality standards to all banks.

Specific recommendations for ethical and legal issues included[84] (1) cord blood centers need policies regarding who must provide consent; (2) informed consent should be obtained before the labor and delivery; (3) donors must be provided with clear information about their options (Author's note: This of course is not possible for cord blood donors but would likely fall up front to the parents of the baby); (4) promote the security of medical information; (5) cord blood donors must understand the limits of their rights (Author's note: Again, this is not possible for the baby).

The key functions of a National Cord Blood Program were[84] governance, database, unit selections, source of transplanted material, finances, cord blood bank selection, standards, and outcomes data.

Although the Institute of Medicine report[84] is clearly a step in the right direction, it may be some time before the differing groups in cord blood banking come to any consensus and the recommendations of the report are implemented.

CORD BLOOD CHARACTERISTICS

Cord blood contains, among a number of cell types, hematopoietic stem and progenitor cells, which are very rare in the total population; and more mature blood cells including B and T lymphocytes, natural killer cells, dendritic cells, monocytes, and granulocytes. It also contains endothelial progenitor cells and mesenchymal stem cells, the latter giving rise to a number of different cell types other than blood cells. Recent reviews are available on cord blood immune cells.[85–88] This chapter covers hematopoietic stem and progenitor cells, endothelial progenitor cells, and mesenchymal stem cells. Table 59–1 lists a brief description of these cells, but this table is not meant to be an all-encompassing assessment of knowledge about these cells. Information on many of these cells, especially those that are not hematopoietic stem and progenitor cells, is still lacking but we hope will emerge soon. Because the author is not clear how these different cells, other than those of hematopoietic stem and progenitor cells, relate to each other in terms of ontogeny and parent-progeny relations, no effort has been made to describe the ontogeny and relations of these apparently different cells to each other.

Hematopoietic Stem and Progenitor Cells

In this group of cells, most is known about hematopoietic progenitor cells in terms of their frequency and proliferative characteristics. Overall, these cells in cord blood appear to have a high quality in terms of their capacity to give rise to progeny and replate in vitro.[2,29–34] These cells are found in the CD34+ and mainly in the subset of CD34+ CD38+ cells. They can be highly enriched in the CD34+++ population, those CD34+ cells expressing the highest-density distribution of cell surface CD34 antigens. Given the right separation procedure, functional hematopoietic progenitors, as determined by in vitro colony assessment in the presence of combinations of colony-stimulating factors (CSF), such as granulocyte-macrophage CSF, interleukin-3, and erythropoietin, and potent costimulating factors such as stem cell factor and Flt3-ligand, can be found at a frequency of up to 80% in the CD34+++ preparations of sorted cells. Hematopoietic stem cells are functionally assessed by their capacity to repopulate the bone marrow of sublethally irradiated NOD/SCID mice[35–37,78] and are highly enriched in the CD34+ CD38− population of cells, but only 1 in about 700 CD34+CD38− cord blood cells is a NOD/SC1D repopulating cell (SRC). This frequency is much greater than that for SRC in bone marrow or mobilized peripheral blood.

Genomic[89–93] and proteomic[94] profiling of hematopoietic stem and progenitor cells has been reported, and future studies could shed light on profiles of stem cells and progenitor cells. However, current genomic and proteomic analysis of hematopoietic stem and progenitor cells is only as good as the methods used and the cell populations analyzed. As noted earlier, even phenotypically isolated human cord blood hematopoietic progenitor cell populations are not pure, and the best separations for human cord blood SRC only yield a preparation in which the hematopoietic stem cell population is present in rare frequency. Thus information obtained on the genomics and proteomics of human hematopoietic stem and progenitor cells has to be interpreted with caution.

Endothelial Progenitor Cells

Progenitors for endothelial cells are present in human cord blood,[95–105] and an hierarchy of cells within the endothelial progenitor cell population has been identified,[103] based on their clonogenicity and proliferative potential. The high-proliferative-potential endothelial progenitor cell achieved at least 100 population doublings and could be replated to form colonies in secondary and tertiary dishes with maintenance of high telomerase activity. Of interest, endothelial progenitor cells from cord blood had much greater proliferative potential than those found in adults.[103]

Cells with Differentiating Capacity for More than Blood Cells

Stem cells in various organs do not always meet the same definition rigor. This was especially apparent in recent discussions on the topic.[106,107] The most rigorous definition of stem cells is that for hematopoietic stem cells, which should serve as the paradigm for stem cells of all organs, but agreement on this is far from unanimous.[106]

Mesenchymal stem cells are reported to produce bone, fat, and cartilage, and this multipotentiality may be the best reason for considering a mesenchmyal stem cell to be a stem

Table 59–1 **Description of Progeny of Stem and Progenitor Cells Identified in Human Cord Blood***

Cell (Abbreviations)	Progeny	Functional Identification	Cell Surface Phenotype	Engrafting Capability in vivo	Proven Therapeutically Useful in Humans	Selected References
Hematopoietic Stem Cell (HPC)	All blood cell lineages including erythroid cells, granulocytes, monocytes/macrophages, platelets, lymphocytes, natural killer cells (NK), dendritic cells, etc.	Repopulates bone marrow of sublethally irradiated NOD/SCID mice and bone marrow and blood of myeloablated human recipients	CD34+ CD38– CD45+ lineage–. HSC are rare within this phenotype. About 1 SCID repopulating cells is present in 700 CD34+ CD38– cells.	Yes	Yes	13, 35–38, 78
Hematopoietic Progenitor Cells (HPC):		Form colonies in vitro stimulated by cytokines. The cytokines used to stimulate colony formation determine the progenitor detected.	CD34+ CD38+ CD45+ lineage–	Yes	Not clear	2, 29–34, 38,
(i) Multipotential (CFU-GEMM: Colony Forming Unit—erythroid, granulocyte, macrophage, megakaryocyte; also termed (CFU-MIX)	Erythroid cells, granulocytes, macrophages, and megakaryocytes					
(ii) Erythroid (BFU-E: Burst Forming Unit—erythroid)	Erythroid cells					
(iii) Granulocyte Macrophage (CFU-GM) Colony-Forming unit—granulocyte, macrophage	Granulocytes, macrophages					
(iv) Granulocyte (CFU-G)	Granulocytes					
(v) Macrophage (CFU-M)	Macrophages					
(vi) Megakaryocyte (CFU-MK)	Megakaryocyte					
(vii) Lymphoid	T-lymphocyte, B-lymphocyte, NK, etc.	In vitro analysis	?	Yes	Not clear	
Endothelial Progenitor Cells (EPC)	Endothelial Cells	In vitro analysis	?	Not clear	Not clear	95–105
Mesenchymal Stem Cells (MSC)	Bone, fat, cartilage	In vitro analysis; stemness not proven and until it is proven these cells may more accurately be termed progenitor cells	CD45–; poorly characterized which leaves open the possibility that the varying differentiation capacities attributed to these cells may not be due to a single cell	Yes	Not clear	108–118
Unrestricted somatic stem cell (USSC)	Osteoblasts, chondroblasts, adipocytes, hematopoietic cells, neural cells (including astrocytes and neurons)	In vitro analysis mainly; this cell type and its differentiation capacity requires verification by other groups.	CD45–, MHC class II–	Yes (?)	Not clear	126

*Multipotential Adult Progenitor Cells (MAPC)[120–124] are not listed above as they have not yet been identified in cord blood.[125] This cell type and its differentiation capabilities still remain to be verified by other investigators.

cell. However, in most cases, these cells are poorly defined by both phenotypic markers and functional activity as actually being stem cells, at least as assessed by single isolated cells giving rise to all different tissue types.[108] Lack of evidence exists for self-renewal capacity, although their proliferative potential is not in question.

Mesenchymal stem cells are found in a number of tissues, including cord blood.[108–115] However, not all reports have shown these cells to be present in cord blood, and great variability is found in detection of the frequency of these cells in different cord blood collections, even when they are found.[116–118] This could be a technical problem of detection or may truly reflect variability in presence of mesenchymal stem cells in cord blood. Such variability and their low frequency in some cord bloods may dampen the potential therapeutic usefulness of these cells, making it difficult to translate the use of these cells into clinical application. Cryopreservation of mesenchymal stem cells has been reported.[119]

Multipotent adult progenitor cells (MAPCs), which are reported to differentiate into endothelial, epithelial, and mesenchymal cells, have been detected in bone marrow,[120–124] but not in cord blood.[125] However, an unrestricted somatic stem cell (USSC) population has been reported to be present in cord blood.[126] USSCs are CD45− and MHC class II antigen− cells, which are found in only 40% of cord blood collections (94 of 233) analyzed, and even when found, are extremely rare. In contrast to mesenchymal stem cells, the USSCs were purported to be able to differentiate into osteoblasts, chondroblasts, adipocytes, and hematopoietic and neural cells, including astrocytes and neurons.[126] They were reported to differentiate along mesodermal and endodermal pathways in vivo.[126] More information on USSCs will need to be forthcoming from the group that published the original article on this cell,[126] as well as verification from the other groups, before the true value and ramifications of its clinical relevance are appreciated.

Plasticity of stem cells, the ability of one cell to give rise to numerous cells of different tissues, is still a controversial issue, in no small part due to the lack of rigor described for the experiments performed. Moreover, other potential possibilities exist for the purported plasticity, including cell fusions and the presence of separate progenitor cells in the population, rather than one stem cell population giving rise to the different tissue types. Recent reviews and original scientific papers have discussed the issue of plasticity.[127–129] Because of the ill-defined surface characteristics of mesenchymal stem cells, it is also unclear how multipotential these cells are, and if indeed attributes associated with these cells are actually due to one cell or to a number of different cells in the population.

CONCLUDING REMARKS

Ongoing studies will delineate which cell in cord blood has what functional property and differentiation capacity and should allow us to determine whether cord blood cells can be used in cellular therapy and regenerative medicine for more than replenishment and correction of the blood cell system. It is clear that more rigorous information on the properties of the cells present in cord blood will help not only to define their ontogeny, but also further to broaden therapeutic applications of these cells.

REFERENCES

1. Gluckman E, Broxmeyer HE, Auerbach AD, et al. Hematopoietic reconstitution in a patient with Fanconi anemia by means of umbilical-cord blood from an HLA-identical sibling. N Engl J Med 1989;321:1174–1178.
2. Broxmeyer HE, Douglas GW, Hangoc G, et al. Human umbilical cord blood as a potential source of transplantable hematopoietic stem/progenitor cells. Proc Natl Acad Sci USA 1989;86:3828–3832.
3. Broxmeyer HE, Gluckman E, Auerbach A, et al. Human umbilical cord blood: a clinically useful source of transplantable hematopoietic stem/progenitor cells. Int J Cell Cloning 1990;8:76–91.
4. Broxmeyer HE. Introduction: The past, present, and future of cord blood transplantation. In Broxmeyer HE (ed). Cellular Characteristics of Cord Blood and Cord Blood Transplantation. Bethesda, Md., American Association of Blood Banks Press, 1998, pp 1–9.
5. Broxmeyer HE. Introduction: Cord blood transplantation: looking back and to the future. In Cohen SBA, Gluckman E, Rubinstein P, et al. (eds). Cord Blood Characteristics: Role in Stem Cell Transplantation. London, Martin Dunitz, 2000, pp 1–12.
6. Gluckman E, Rocha V. History of the clinical use of umbilical cord blood hematopoietic cells. Cytotherapy 2005;7:219–227.
7. Wagner JE, Kernan NA, Steinbuch M, et al. Allogeneic sibling umbilical cord blood transplantation in forty-four children with malignant and non-malignant disease. Lancet 1995;346:214–219.
8. Kurtzberg J, Laughlin M, Graham ML, et al. Placental blood as a source of hematopoietic stem cells for transplantation into unrelated donors. N Engl J Med 1996;335:157–166.
9. Wagner JE, Rosenthal J, Sweetman R, et al. Successful transplantation of HLA-matched and HLA-mismatched umbilical cord blood from unrelated donors: analysis of engraftment and acute graft-versus-host disease. Blood 1996;88:795–802.
10. Gluckman E, Rocha V, Boyer-Chammard A, et al. Outcome of cord blood transplantation from related and unrelated donors: Eurocord Transplant Group and the European Blood and Marrow Transplantation Group. N Engl J Med 1997;337:373–381.
11. Rubinstein P, Carrier C, Scaradavou A, et al. Outcomes among 562 recipients of placental-blood transplants from unrelated donors. N Engl J Med 1998;339:1565–1577.
12. Wagner JE, Barker JN, DeFor TE, et al. Transplantation of unrelated donor umbilical cord blood in 102 patients with malignant and non-malignant diseases: influence of CD34 cell dose and HLA disparity on treatment-related mortality and survival. Blood 2002;100:1611–1618.
13. Broxmeyer HE, Smith FO. Cord blood hematopoietic cell transplantation. In Blume KG, Forman SJ, Appelbaum FR (eds). Thomas' Hematopoietic Cell Transplantation, 3rd ed. Cambridge, Mass., Blackwell Scientific Publications, 2004, pp 550–564.
14. Laughlin MJ, Barker J, Bambach B, et al. Hematopoietic engraftment and survival in adult recipients of umbilical-cord blood from unrelated donors. N Engl J Med 2001;344:1815–1822.
15. Sanz GF, Saavedra S, Jimenez C, et al. Unrelated donor cord blood transplantation in adults with chronic myelogenous leukemia: results in nine patients from a single institution. Bone Marrow Transplant 2001;27:693–701,
16. Ooi J, Iseki T, Takahashi S, et al. A clinical comparison of unrelated cord blood transplantation and unrelated bone marrow transplantation for adult patients with acute leukaemia in complete remission. Br J Haematol 2002;118:140–143.
17. Sanz GF, Saavedra S, Planelles D, et al. Standardized, unrelated donor cord blood transplantation in adults with hematologic malignancies. Blood 2001;98:2332–2338.
18. Long GD, Laughlin M, Madan B, et al. Unrelated umbilical cord blood transplantation in adult patients. Biol Blood Marrow Transplant 2003;9:772–780.
19. Laughlin MJ, Eapen M, Rubinstein P, et al. Outcomes after transplantation of cord blood or bone marrow from unrelated donors in adults with leukemia. N Engl J Med 2004;351:2265–2275.
20. Rocha V, Labopin M, Sanz G, et al. Transplants of umbilical-cord blood or bone marrow from unrelated donors in adults with acute leukemia. N Engl J Med 2004;351:2276–2285.
21. Takahashi S, Iseki T, Ooi J, et al. Single-institute comparative analysis of unrelated bone marrow transplantation and cord blood transplantation for adult patients with hematologic malignancies. Blood 2004;104:3813–3820.
22. Gluckman E, Rocha V, Arcese W, et al. Factors associated with outcomes of unrelated cord blood transplant: guidelines for donor choice. Exp Hematol 2004;32:397–407.
23. Cornetta K, Laughlin M, Carter S, et al. Umbilical cord blood transplantation in adults: results of the prospective cord blood transplantation (COBLT). Biol Blood Marrow Transplant 2005;11:149–160.

24. Tse W, Laughlin MJ. Cord blood transplantation in adult patients. Cytotherapy 2005;7:228–242.
25. Sanz MA. Cord blood transplantation in patients with leukemia: a real alternative for adults. N Engl J Med 2004;351:2328–2330.
26. Chao NJ. Stem cell transplantation (cord blood transplants): how close are we to using this in adults? In Broudy VC, Berliner N, Larson RA, et al (eds). Hematology. Washington, D.C., American Society of Hematology, 2004, pp 355–359.
27. Chao NJ, Liu CX, Rooney B, et al. Non myeloablative regimen preserves "niches" allowing for peripheral expansion of donor T cells. Biol Blood Marrow Transplant 2002;8:249–256.
28. Barker JN, Weisdorf DJ, DeFor TE, et al. Rapid and complete donor chimerism in adult recipients of unrelated donor umbilical cord blood transplantation after reduced intensity conditioning. Blood 2003;102:1915–1919.
29. Broxmeyer HE, Hangoc G, Cooper S, et al. Growth characteristics and expansion of human umbilical cord blood and estimation of its potential for transplantation of adults. Proc Natl Acad Sci USA 1992;89:4109–4113.
30. Lu L, Xiao M, Shen RN, et al. Enrichment, characterization and responsiveness of single primitive $CD34^{+++}$ human umbilical cord blood hematopoietic progenitor cells with high proliferative and replating potential. Blood 1993;81:41–48.
31. Lansdorp PM, Dragowska W, Mayani H. Ontogeny-related changes in proliferative potential of human hematopoietic cells. J Exp Med 1993;178:787–791.
32. Cardoso AA, Li ML, Batard P, et al. Release from quiescence of $CD34^{+}CD38^{-}$ human umbilical cord blood cells reveals their potentiality to engraft adults. Proc Natl Acad Sci USA 1993;90:8707–8711.
33. Carow C, Hangoc G, Cooper S, et al. Mast cell growth factor (c-kit ligand) supports the growth of human multipotential (CFU-GEMM) progenitor cells with a high replating potential. Blood 1991;78:2216–2221.
34. Carow CE, Hangoc G, Broxmeyer HE. Human multipotential progenitor cells (CFU-GEMM) have extensive replating capacity for secondary CFU-GEMM: an effect enhanced by cord blood plasma. Blood 1993;81:942–949.
35. Vormoor J, Lapidot T, Pflumio F, et al. Immature human cord blood progenitors engraft and proliferate to high levels in immune-deficient SCID mice. Blood 1994;83:2489–2497.
36. Orazi A, Braun SE, Broxmeyer HE. Immunohistochemistry represents a useful tool to study human cell engraftment in SCID mice transplantation models. Blood Cells 1994;20:323–330.
37. Bock TA, Orlic D, Dunbar CE, et al. Improved engraftment of human hematopoietic cells in severe combined immunodeficient (SCID) mice carrying human cytokine transgenes. J Exp Med 1995;182:2037–2043.
38. Broxmeyer HE. Proliferation, self-renewal, and survival characteristics of cord blood hematopoietic stem and progenitor cells. In Broxmeyer HE (ed). Cord Blood: Biology, Immunology, Banking, and Clinical Transplantation. Bethesda, Md., American Association of Blood Banking, 2004, pp 1–21.
39. Shen BJ, Hou HS, Zhang HQ, et al. Unrelated, HLA-mismatched multiple human umbilical cord blood transfusion in four cases with advanced solid tumors: Initial studies. Blood Cells 1994;2/3:285–292.
40. Barker JN, Weisdorf DJ, DeFor TE, et al. Transplantation of 2 partially HLA-matched umbilical cord blood units to enhance engraftment in adults with hematologic malignancy. Blood 2005;105:1343–1347.
41. Shpall EJ, Quinones R, Giller R, et al. Transplantation of ex vivo expanded cord blood. Biol Bone Marrow Transplant 2002;8:368–376.
42. Jaroscak J, Goltry K, Smith A, et al. Augmentation of umbilical cord blood (UCB) transplantation with ex-vivo-expanded UCB cells: results of a phase I trial using the AstromReplicell system. Blood 2003;101:5061–5067.
43. Shaheen M, Broxmeyer HE. The humoral regulation of hematopoiesis. In Hoffman R, Benz E, Shattil S, et al (eds). Hematology: Basic Principles and Practice, Philadelphia, Elsevier/Churchill Livingstone, 4th ed. 2005, pp 233–265.
44. Milner LA, Kopan R, Martin DIK, et al. A human homologue of the Drosophila developmental gene, notch, is expressed in $CD34^{+}$ hematopoietic precursors. Blood 1994;83:2057–2062.
45. Varnum-Finney B, Purton LE, Yu M, et al. The notch ligand, jagged-1, influences the development of primitive hematopoietic precursor cells. Blood 1998;91:4084–4091.
46. Varnum-Finney B, Brashem-Stein C, Bernstein ID. Combined effects of Notch signaling and cytokines induce a multiple log increase in precursors with lymphoid and myeloid reconstituting ability. Blood 2003;101:1784–1789.
47. Suzuki T, Chiba S. Notch signaling in hematopoietic stem cells. Int J Hematol 2005;82:285–294.
48. Austin TW, Solar GP, Ziegler FC, et al. A role for Wnt gene family in hematopoiesis: Expression of multilineage progenitor cells. Blood 1997;89:3624–3635.
49. Van DerBerg DJ, Sharma AK, Bruno E, et al. Role of members of the Wnt gene family in human hematopoiesis. Blood 1998;92:3189–3202.
50. Reya T, Duncan AW, Ailles L, et al. A role for Wnt signaling in self-renewal of haematopoietic stem cells. Nature 2003;423:409–414.
51. Willert K, Brown JD, Danenberg E, et al. Wnt proteins are lipid-modified and can act as stem cell growth factors. Nature 2003;423:448–452.
52. Antonchuk J, Sauvageau G, Humphries RK. HOXB4 overexpression mediates very rapid stem cell regulation and competitive hematopoietic repopulation. Exp Hematol 2001;29:1125–1134.
53. Buske C, Feuring-Buske M, Abramovich C, et al. Deregulated expression of HOXB4 enhances the primitive growth activity of human hematopoietic cells. Blood 2002;100:862–868.
54. Antonchuk J, Sauvageau G, Humphries RK. HOXB4-induced expansion of adult hematopoietic stem cells ex vivo. Cell 2002;109:39–45.
55. Kyba M, Perlingeiro RCR, Daley GQ. HoxB4 confers definitive lymphoid-myeloid engraftment potential on embryonic stem cell and yolk sac hematopoietic progenitors. Cell 2002;109:29–37.
56. Krosi J, Beslu N, Mayotte N, et al. The competitive nature of HOXB4-transduced HSC is limited by PBX1: the generation of ultra-competitive stem cells retaining full differentiation potential. Immunity 2003;18:561–571.
57. Krosl J, Austin P, Beslu N, et al. In vitro expansion of hematopoietic stem cells by recombinant TAT-HOXB4 protein. Nat Med 2003;9: 1428–1432.
58. Amsellem S, Pflumio F, Bardinet D, et al. Ex vivo expansion of human hematopoietic stem cells by direct delivery of the HOXB4 homeoprotein. Nat Med 2003;9:1423–1427.
59. Park I-K, Qian D, Kiel M, et al. Bmi-1 is required for maintenance of adult self-renewing haematopoietic stem cells. Nature 2003;423:302–305.
60. Lessard J, Sauvageau G. Bmi-1 determines the proliferative capacity of normal and leukaemic stem cells. Nature 2003;423:255–260.
61. Iwama A, Oguro H, Negishi M, et al. Enhanced self-renewal of hematopoietic stem cells mediated by the polycomb gene product Bmi-1. Immunity 2004;21:843–851.
62. Delaney C, Varnum-Finney B, Aoyama K, et al. Dose-dependent effects of the Notch ligand Delta1 on ex vivo differentiation and in vivo marrow repopulating ability of cord blood cells. Blood 2005;106:2693–2699.
63. Duncan AW, Rattis FM, DiMascio LN, et al. Integration of Notch and Wnt signaling in hematopoietic stem cell maintenance. Nat Immunol 2005;6:314–322.
64. Zhang P, Iwasaki-Arai J, Iwasaki H, et al. Enhancement of hematopoietic stem cell repopulating capacity and self-renewal in the absence of the transcription factor C/EBPα. Immunity 2004;21:853–863.
65. Hock H, Hamblen MJ, Rooke HM, et al. Gfi-1 restricts proliferation and preserves functional integrity of haematopoietic stem cells. Nature 2004;431:1002–1007.
66. Zeng H, Yücel R, Kosan C, et al. Transcription factor Gfi1 regulates self-renewal and engraftment of hematopoietic stem cells. EMBO J 2004;23:4116–4125.
67. Schuringa JJ, Chung KY, Morrone G, et al. Constitutive activation of STAT5A promotes human hematopoietic stem cell self-renewal and erythroid differentiation. J Exp Med 2004;200:623–635.
68. Kato Y, Iwama A, Tadokoro Y, et al. Selective activation of STAT5 unveils its role in stem cell self-renewal in normal and leukemic hematopoiesis. J Exp Med 2005;202:169–179.
69. Oh IH, Eaves CJ. Overexpression of a dominant negative form of STAT3 selectively impairs hematopoietic stem cell activity. Oncogene 2002;21:4778–4787.
70. Niwa H, Burdon T, Chambers I, et al. Self-renewal of pluripotent embryonic stem cells is mediated via activation of STAT3. Genes Dev 1998;12:2048–2060.
71. Guo Y, Hangoc G, Bian H, et al. SDF-1/CXCL12 enhances survival and chemotaxis of murine embryonic stem cells and production of primitive and definitive hematopoietic progenitor cells. Stem Cells 2005;23:1324–1332.
72. Guo Y, Graham-Evans B, Broxmeyer HE. Murine embryonic stem cells secrete cytokines/growth modulators that enhance cell survival/anti-apoptosis and stimulate colony formation of murine hematopoietic progenitor cells. Stem Cells 2005 (in press).
73. Christopherson KW II, Broxmeyer HE. Hematopoietic stem and progenitor cell homing, engraftment, and mobilization in the context of the CXCL12/SDF-1 - CXCR4 Axis. In Broxmeyer HE (ed). Cord Blood: Biology, Immunology, and Clinical Transplantation. Bethesda, Md., American Association of Blood Banks Press, 2004, pp 65–86.

74. Lapidot T, Dar A, Kollet O. How do stem cells find their way home? Blood 2005;106:1901–1910.
75. Christopheron KW, Hangoc G, Broxmeyer HE. Cell surface peptidase CD26/DPPIV regulates CXCL12/SDF-1α mediated chemotaxis of human CD34+ progenitor cells. J Immunol 2002;169:7000–7008.
76. Christopherson KW II, Hangoc G, Mantel C, et al. Modulation of hematopoietic stem cell homing and engraftment by CD26. Science 2004;305:1000–1003.
77. Campbell T, Hangoc G, Broxmeyer HE. The role of CD26 in human umbilical cord blood CD34+ cell engraftment of NOD/SCID mice. Blood 2005;106(Pt 1):487a (Abstract 1708).
78. Bodine DM. Animal models for the engraftment and differentiation of human hematopoietic stem and progenitor cells. In Broxmeyer HE (ed.). Cord Blood: Biology, Immunology, and Clinical Transplantation. Bethesda, Md., American Association of Blood Banks Press, 2004, pp 47–64.
79. Broxmeyer HE, Cooper S. High efficiency recovery of immature hematopoietic progenitor cells with extensive proliferative capacity from human cord blood cryopreserved for ten years. Clin Exp Immunol 1997;107:45–53.
80. Broxmeyer HE, Srour EF, Hangoc G, et al. High efficiency recovery of hematopoietic progenitor cells with extensive proliferative and ex-vivo expansion activity and of hematopoietic stem cells with NOD/SCID mouse repopulation ability from human cord blood stored frozen for 15 years. Proc Natl Acad Sci USA 2002;100:645–650.
81. Wood EJ, Liu J, Pollok K, et al. A theoretically optimized method for cord blood stem cell cryopreservation. J Hematother Stem Cell Res 2003;12:341–350.
82. Ballen K, Broxmeyer HE, McCulloch J, et al. Current status of cord blood banking and transplantation in the United States and Europe. Biol Blood Marrow Transplant 2001;7:635–645.
83. Ballen KK. New trends in umbilical cord blood transplantation. Blood 2005;105:3786–3792.
84. Meyer EA, Hanna K, Gebbre K (eds). Cord Blood: Establishing a National Hematopoietic Stem Cell Bank Program. Washington, D.C., The National Academies Press, 2005.
85. Smith FO. Immune reconstitution following umbilical cord blood transplantation. In Broxmeyer HE (ed). Cord Blood: Biology, Immunology, and Clinical Transplantation. Bethesda, Md., AABB Press, 2004, pp 151–162.
86. Gluckman JC, Canque B. Dendritic cell and lymphoid progenitors in cord blood. In Broxmeyer HE (ed). Cord Blood: Biology, Immunology, and Clinical Transplantation. Bethesda, Md., AABB Press, 2004, pp 163–185.
87. Navarrete CV, Gomez J, Borras FE. Cord blood dendritic cells. In Broxmeyer HE (ed). Cord Blood: Biology, Immunology, and Clinical Transplantation. Bethesda, Md., AABB, 2004, pp 187–198.
88. Kim Y-J, Broxmeyer HE. Cytotoxic T lymphocytes in the context of cord blood transplantation. In Broxmeyer HE (ed). Cord Blood: Biology, Immunology, and Clinical Transplantation. Bethesda, Md., AABB, 2004, pp 199–217.
89. Phillips RL, Ernst RE, Brunk B, et al. The genetic program of hematopoietic stem cells. Science 2000;288:1635–1640.
90. Ramalho-Santos M, Yoon S, Matsuzaki Y, et al. "Stemness": Transcriptional profiling of embryonic and adult stem cells. Science 2002;298:597–600.
91. Ivanova NB, Dimos JT, Schaniel C, et al. A stem cell molecular signature. Science 2002;298:601–604.
92. Tao W, Hangoc G, Hawes JW, et al. Profiling of differentially expressed apoptosis-related genes by cDNA arrays in human cord blood CD34+ cells treated with VP-16 etoposide. Exp Hematol 2003;31:251–260.
93. Tao W, Broxmeyer HE. Toward a molecular understanding of hematopoietic stem and progenitor cells. In Broxmeyer HE (ed). Cord Blood: Biology, Immunology, and Clinical Transplantation. Bethesda, Md., AABB Press, 2004, pp 87–123.
94. Tao W, Wang M, Voss ED, et al. Comparative proteomic analysis of human CD34+ stem/progenitor cells and mature CD15+ myeloid cells. Stem Cells 2004;22:1003–1014.
95. Crisa L, Cirulli V, Smith K, et al. Human cord blood progenitors sustain thymic T-cell development and a novel form of angiogenesis. Blood 1999;94:3928–3940.
96. Peichev M, Naiyer A, Pereira D, et al. Expression of VEGFR-2 and AC133 by circulating human CD34+ cells identifies a population of functional endothelial precursors. Blood 2000;95:952–958.
97. Kang HJ, Kim SC, Kim YJ, et al. Short-term phytohaemagglutinin-activated mononuclear cells induce endothelial progenitor cells from cord blood CD34+ cells. Br J Haematol 2001;113:962–969.
98. Pesce M, Orlandi A, Iachininoto MG, et al. Myoendothelial differentiation of human umbilical cord blood-derived stem cells in ischemic limb tissues. Circ Res 2003;93:e51–e62.
99. Eggermann J, Kliche S, Jarmy G, et al. Endothelial progenitor cell culture and differentiation in vitro: a methodological comparison using human umbilical cord blood. Cardiovasc Res 2003;58:478–486.
100. Fan C-L, Li Y, Gao P-J, et al. Differentiation of endothelial progenitor cells from human umbilical cord blood CD34+ cells in vitro. Acta Pharmacol Sin 2003;24:212–218.
101. Murga M, Yao L, Tosato G. Derivation of endothelial cells from CD34– umbilical cord blood. Stem Cells 2004;22:385–395.
102. Hildbrand P, Cirulli V, Prinsen RC, et al. The role of angiopoietins in the development of endothelial cells from cord blood CD34+ progenitors. Blood 2004;107:2010–2019.
103. Ingram D, Mead L, Tanaka H, et al. Identification of a novel hierarchy of endothelial progenitor cells using human peripheral and umbilical cord blood. Blood 2004;104:2752–2760.
104. Aoki M, Yasutake M, Murohara T. Derivation of functional endothelial progenitor cells from human umbilical card blood mononuclear cells isolated by a novel cell filtration device. Stem Cells 2004;22: 994–1002.
105. Bompais H, Chagraoui J, Canron X, et al. Human endothelial cells derived from circulating progenitors display specific functional properties compared with mature vessel wall endothelial cells. Blood 2004;107:25777–25784.
106. Parker GC, Anastassova-Kristeva M, Broxmeyer HE, et al. Stem cells: Shibboleths of development. Stem Cell Dev 2004;13:579–584.
107. Parker GC, Anastassova-Kristeva M, Eisenberg LM, et al. Stem cells: Shibboleths of development. Part II: Toward a functional definition. Stem Cell Dev 2005;14:463–469.
108. Javazon EH, Beggs KJ, Flake AW. Mesenchymal stem cells: Paradoxes of passaging. Exp Hematol 2004;32:414–425.
109. Erices A, Conget P, Minguell JJ. Mesenchymal progenitor cells in human umbilical cord blood. Br J Haematol 2000;109:235–242.
110. Goodwin HS, Bicknese AR, Chien SN, et al. Multilineage differentiation activity by cells isolated from umbilical cord blood: expression of bone, fat and neural markers. Biol Blood Marrow Transplant 2001;7:581–588.
111. Bieback K, Kern S, Kluter H, et al. Critical parameters for the isolation of mesenchymal stem cells from umbilical cord blood. Stem Cell 2004;22:625–634.
112. Yang S-E, Ha C-W, Jung MH, et al. Mesenchymal stem/progenitor cells developed in cultures from UC blood. Cytotherapy 2004;6:476–486.
113. Lee OK, Kuo TK, Chen W-M, et al. Isolation of multipotent mesenchymal stem cells from umbilical cord blood. Blood 2004;103: 1669–1675.
114. Rosada C, Justesen J, Melsvik D, et al. The human umbilical cord blood: A potential source for osteoblast progenitor cells. Calcif Tissue Int 2003;72:135–142.
115. Bonanno G, Perillo A, Rutella S, et al. Clinical isolation and functional characterization of cord blood CD133+ hematopoietic progenitor cells. Transfusion 2004;44:1087–1097.
116. Gutierrez-Rodriguez M, Reyes-Maldonado E, Mayani H. Characterization of the adherent cells developed in Dextertype long-term cultures from human umbilical cord blood. Stem Cell 2000;18:45–52.
117. Mareschi K, Biasin E, Piacibello W, et al. Isolation of human mesenchymal stem cells: bone marrow versus umbilical cord blood. Haematologica 2001;86:1099–1100.
118. Wexler S, Donaldson C, Denning-Kendall P, et al. Adult bone marrow is a rich source of human mesenchymal "stem" cells but umbilical cord and mobilized adult blood are not. Br J Haematol 2003;121:368–374.
119. Lee MW, Choi J, Yang MS, et al. Mesenchymal stem cells from cryopreserved human umbilical cord blood. Biochem Biophys Res Commun 2004;320:273–278.
120. Reyes M, Lund T, Lenvik T, et al. Purification and ex-vivo expansion of postnatal human marrow mesodermal progenitor cells. Blood 2001;98:2615–2625.
121. Jiang Y, Jahagirdar BN, Reinhardt RL, et al. Pluripotency of mesenchymal stem cells derived from adult marrow. Nature 2002;418:41–49.
122. Schwartz RE, Reyes M, Koodie L, et al. Multipotent adult progenitor cells from bone marrow differentiate into functional hepatocyte-like cells. J Clin Invest 2002;109:1291–1302.
123. Jiang Y, Vaessen B, Lenvik T, et al. Multipotent progenitor cells can be isolated from postnatal murine bone marrow, muscle, and brain. Exp Hematol 2002;30:896–904.
124. Reyes M, Dudek A, Jahagirdar B, et al. Origin of endothelial progenitors in human postnatal bone marrow. J Clin Invest 2002;109:337–346.

125. Adassi A, Verfaille CM. Multipotent adult progenitor cells. In Lanza R, Blau H, Melton D, et al (eds). Handbook of Stem Cells, Vol 2: Adult and Fetal Cells. Amsterdam, Elsevier Academic Press, 2004, pp 293–297.
126. Kogler G, Sensken S, Airey J, et al. A new human somatic stem cell from placental cord blood with intrinsic pluripotent differentiation potential. J Exp Med 2004;200:123–135.
127. Wagers A, Weissman I. Plasticity of adult stem cells. Cell 2004;116: 639–648.
128. Verfaillie C. "Adult" stem cells: Tissue specific or not? In Lanza R, Blau H, Melton D, et al (eds.) Handbook of Stem Cells, Vol 2: Adult and Fetal Cells. Amsterdam, Elsevier Academic Press, 2004, pp 13–20.
129. Goodell MA. Potential nonhematopoietic uses for stem cells in cord blood. In Meyer EA, Hanna K, Gebbre K (eds). Cord Blood, Establishing a National Hematopoietic Stem Cell Bank Program. Washington, D.C., Institute of Medicine of the National Academies, 2005, pp 208–220.

Chapter 60

Collection and Processing of Peripheral Blood Stem Cells and Bone Marrow

Scott D. Rowley • Howard Benn

INTRODUCTION

Hematopoietic stem cell (HSC) transplantation, by definition, requires the collection and processing of HSCs from the bone marrow or peripheral circulation of the patient or a volunteer donor. Most bone marrow products are collected from the posterior iliac crests by using the techniques originally described more than 30 years ago by Thomas and Storb.[1] Bone marrow HSCs can be collected for autologous transplantation from almost all patients who are eligible for dose-intense therapy, and bone marrow harvesting from healthy donors presents little risk of serious morbidity, permitting the ethical recruitment of allogeneic donors including unrelated and pediatric bone marrow donors.[2,3] The advent of cytokine mobilization simplified the use of this cell source for transplantation. The presence of HSCs in the peripheral circulation was suggested by animal studies as early as 1951.[4] Although the nature of the survival agent was not recognized at that time, parabiosis experiments demonstrated that a factor in the blood of a healthy animal was able to rescue another animal from the effects of lethal irradiation. Subsequently, the presence of HSCs in the peripheral blood and the use of these cells to rescue animals from the marrow-lethal effects of radiation were demonstrated in a number of animal models.[5,6] Peripheral blood stem cells (PBSCs) now have virtually replaced bone marrow as the HSC component for autologous transplantation and are widely used for allogeneic transplantation. The clinical advantages and disadvantages of each cell source are described in Chapter 57.

COLLECTION OF BONE MARROW

Bone Marrow–Collection Techniques

Bone marrow is typically harvested from the posterior iliac crests.[1] Multiple aspirations are performed, with collection of about 5 mL of marrow from each puncture site to avoid dilution of the marrow sample with blood. If properly spaced, no more than two to three skin-puncture sites per side are usually required. Other harvest sites, such as the anterior iliac crests or sternum, may be used, but at increased risk of complications from accidental laceration or perforation of contiguous anatomic structures. Extending the harvest to the anterior crests or sternum is more likely to be done in patients with poor marrow function as a result of prior treatments, but is unusual, required for less than 10% of patients undergoing autologous collections.[7] For patients with a history of radiation or tumor involvement of one pelvic crest, adequate cells can be harvested from the anterior and posterior crests of the other side.

Marrow is collected in the day-surgery suite by using either general or regional anesthesia.[7] With proper fluid and blood replacement, overnight hospitalization should not be required. For the healthy donor, the risks of serious complications of either general or regional anesthesia are about the same, and choice of anesthesia can be left to the donor. Spinal or epidural anesthesia avoids the nausea that may occur with general anesthesia, especially for younger women, but hypotension from loss of vascular tone in the lower extremities often occurs as the volume of marrow is collected. General anesthesia is preferable for the donor with comorbid disorders such as cardiovascular or cerebral vascular disease because of the better control of donor airway and lower risk of hypotension. Local anesthesia is acceptable only if a limited harvest is being performed; large quantities of lidocaine used for local anesthesia are cardiotoxic, and local anesthesia does not achieve anesthesia of the interior marrow space. The operating theater is an intensive care unit, which is preferable to blood stem cell harvesting in an outpatient apheresis unit for the patient with serious comorbid illnesses.

Evaluation of Bone Marrow Donors

Anesthesia and blood loss present the greatest risks of serious complications, and patients and donors must undergo a thorough medical examination. Most marrow harvesting is performed under general anesthesia, which requires intubation for control of the airway for this surgical procedure that is performed on a prone patient. Regional (spinal or epidural) anesthesia may not be effective, so patients and donors who express a preference for this form of anesthesia must also be counseled about the potential need for general anesthesia. The health assessment must include questioning about a history of joint disease of the cervical spine and mandible and examination of the mouth if general anesthesia requiring intubation is chosen. Arthritis of the cervical spine and poor dentition may greatly increase the risk of intubation. Patients and donors with comorbid conditions such as aortic stenosis sensitive to changes in blood volume and blood pressure may require anesthesia consultation and plans for invasive monitoring during the surgical procedure. A history of marrow fibrosis, previous pelvic irradiation, or pelvic tumor involvement may exclude a patient from marrow harvesting.

All allogeneic donors must be evaluated by using the criteria currently applied to blood donors, including a targeted history regarding behaviors exposing the donor to virus infection, recent and concurrent illnesses, and medication use.[8–11] Some groups advocate age-specific screening, possibly including marrow examination, because of the higher risk of malignant diseases in older donors.[12,13] Donors with concurrent acute illnesses should be delayed, if at all possible, because of the risk of virus transmission such as West Nile virus.[14] Numerous infectious diseases that would not exclude the donor from blood donation, such as cytomegalovirus (CMV), may be transmitted with the allograft.[15] However, donors who would otherwise be excluded for health reasons from donating blood for transfusion (e.g., history of hepatitis) may still be eligible to donate bone marrow if the needs of the recipient outweigh the risks of disease transmission. Guidance regarding the management of patients and donors with hepatitis virus infection has been published.[16] Hematopoietic disorders, such as hemoglobinopathies, will be transmitted to the recipient. Cancer can be transmitted, as illustrated by the transmission of donor leukemia not detected during initial evaluation of the donor,[17] and donors with a history of malignancy, even if in a current complete remission, should not be used if an alternate source of HSCs is available.

Complications of Bone Marrow Collection

Anesthesia complications present the major health risk to the donor or patient undergoing bone marrow collection. The actual marrow aspirations are generally well tolerated. Major complications occur in about 0.27% of healthy allogeneic donors[18] and up to 0.97% of autograft patients.[19] Complications include hemorrhage and infections at the skin-puncture sites. Severe hematomas and neuralgias rarely occur, but accidental perforation of both sides of the bone may occur, with risk of damage to vessels and nerves lying under or adjacent to the iliac crest harvest sites. Irritation of the sacral nerves, possibly requiring several months of physical therapy, may result from needle penetration through the pelvic bone into the sacral plexus or from blood tracking into the regions of the nerve roots. All donors and patients will experience localized pain at the harvest sites, which may last for several days, and may require a brief period of opioid medications.[20] Topical application of ice after collection of bone marrow may help alleviate these symptoms, and donors should be counseled to avoid strenuous exercise until after the pain has resolved. In a survey of almost 500 donors for unrelated marrow transplantation, the average time for recovery (resolution of all symptoms) was 15.8 days, although 10% of the donors required more than 30 days for complete recovery.[2] Most donors are able to return to routine activities 1 or 2 days after harvesting.

The usual volume harvested from healthy donors is about 10 to 15 mL of marrow per kilogram of recipient body weight, resulting in an average blood loss of 800 to 1000 mL. The quantity of marrow harvested from autologous patients may be greater, reflecting the previous chemotherapy given to these patients. Most donors receive blood transfusions to alleviate symptoms of volume depletion and to lessen the probability that overnight hospitalization for control of hypotension will be required. With proper preharvest autologous blood storage, the use of homologous blood for allogeneic donors should be extremely rare. For blood loss of less than 10 mL/kg, crystalloid (salt) solutions are acceptable replacement. Colloid solutions such as hydroxyethylstarch may also be used to avoid homologous blood transfusion. Blood transfusions for both autologous patients and healthy donors must be irradiated to prevent transfusion-associated graft-versus-host disease in the recipient. Donors undergoing a second harvest shortly after the first are more likely to require homologous blood.[21] Oral iron supplements should be considered for healthy donors.

Quantity of Bone Marrow Cells Harvested

Cell dose is a surrogate for the stem cell content of the marrow product. For autologous transplantation, cell doses of 1×10^8 nucleated cells/kg are adequate. Most centers target 3×10^8 nucleated cells/kg of recipient weight for allogeneic transplantation, based on early reports that smaller quantities increased the risk of engraftment failure.[22] Those reports, however, were of patients being treated for aplastic anemia, in which engraftment failure is a more common event. A study of 100 patients who received allogeneic transplantation for the treatment of acute leukemia found that cell dose per kilogram of recipient body weight (over the range of 0.5 to 13.0×10^8) did not predict the likelihood of successful engraftment.[23] A review of unrelated donor transplantation found that recipients of higher cell doses experienced faster neutrophil and platelet engraftment as well as better leukemia-free survival.[24] The pretreatment of the marrow donor with either sargramostim (GM-CSF) or filgrastim (G-CSF) may increase the number of myeloid progenitor cells harvested, especially more mature committed progenitor cells, and decrease the period of post-transplant aplasia.[25–27]

Postcollection Processing

Bone marrow is packaged in blood-transfer packs, usually after filtration to remove fat, blood clots, and bone spicules. Commercial collection kits with disposable filters are available and simplify the process of product packaging. Additional bone marrow–processing procedures including frozen or nonfrozen storage, removal or enrichment of various cell populations, and transportation are discussed later and apply to both marrow and PBSC sources.

COLLECTION OF PERIPHERAL BLOOD STEM CELLS

The ease of collection and the rapid engraftment kinetics of PBSCs compared with bone marrow, leading to shorter hospital stays and reduced costs of (autologous) transplantation, are widely recognized (Table 60–1).[28–31] Median times to achieve an absolute neutrophil count (ANC) greater than 500 per microliter are typically about 11 to 14 days, and platelet recovery is even faster.[32–37] Although graft-versus-host disease (GVHD) prophylaxis with methotrexate will slow engraftment, the kinetics of engraftment for the allogeneic PBSC recipient is similar to that experienced by the autologous PBSC recipient.[38–44] The more-rapid engraftment kinetics for recipients of PBSCs have been confirmed in a number of phase III studies involving either autologous or allogeneic HSC transplantation.[45–50] This effect is not limited to HSCs collected from the peripheral blood because cytokine administration to the patient or donor before marrow harvesting will also increase the number of HSCs collected and result in quicker hematologic recov-

Table 60–1 Engraftment Outcomes and Costs of Transplantation for Autologous Marrow or PBSC Transplantation

Study	Patient Number	Time to Engraftment: ANC >500/µL	Time to Engraftment: Platelet >20,000/µL	Hospital Stay (days)	Costs
Hartmann[28]	BM 65	12	36.5*	31	$28,429
	PBSC 64	8	17.5	24	$23,591
Smith[29]	BM 31	14	23	23	$59,314
	PBSC 27	11	16	17	$45,792
Vellenga[30]	BM 42	26	18	34	$17,668
	PBSC 76	15	13	27	$13,954
Van Agthoven[31]	BM 29	15	18	34	$ 39,610
	PBSC 62	10	13	27	$ 38,742

* Platelet ≥ 50,000/µL.
BM, bone marrow; PBSC, peripheral blood stem cell.

ery.[51–55] The disadvantages to the use of PBSC components are the usual need for multiple days of collection (especially for autologous donors with poor marrow function), the current need for sophisticated flow-cytometric analysis of the components to ensure adequacy of HSC content, the inability to collect adequate components from all patients and donors, the risks associated with administration of hematopoietic cytokines and the apheresis procedures, and a possibly higher risk of GVHD, or the occurrence of GVHD that is more difficult to control.[56–58] The clinical uses of bone marrow and PBSCs are discussed in Chapter 58.

The concentration of HSCs in the peripheral blood is normally very low. Thus, very large quantities of blood must be processed to collect a quantity of HSCs equivalent to what could be collected in a single bone marrow harvest. For this reason, PBSC transplantation was limited initially to a few centers that explored this source of HSCs for patients who were otherwise ineligible for marrow harvesting. The availability of cytokines (and chemokines) with the effective mobilization of HSCs into the peripheral blood is the direct reason for the rapid and widespread adoption of PBSCs as a source of HSCs for transplantation.

Peripheral Blood Stem Cell Collection Techniques

A variety of mobilization schemes have been developed for both patients and donors. Before the availability of hematopoietic cytokines, it was noted that marrow hypoplasia–producing chemotherapy, such as that used as induction therapy for acute leukemia or the salvage therapy for non-Hodgkin's lymphoma, results in a transient increase in the number of HSCs circulating in the peripheral blood.[59–61] It was subsequently discovered that the administration of GM-CSF or G-CSF during the recovery from chemotherapy increased the numbers of circulating progenitor cells, leading to the exploration of efficacious mobilization regimens using hematopoietic cytokines, cytokine combinations, chemotherapy plus cytokines, or chemokines alone or in combination with cytokines.

Cytokine Mobilization with Granulocyte–Colony-Stimulating Factor

At present, G-CSF is the cytokine most commonly used because of its higher efficacy compared with other cytokines and its relatively benign toxicity profile. r-metHuG-CSF (filgrastim) and rHuG-CSF (lenograstim) are the two forms of this cytokine available for clinical use.[62] Slight, if any, difference between these two cytokines is found in the ability to mobilize PBSCs. Watts and colleagues[63] studied 20 healthy volunteers and found that the peak levels of colony-forming units–granulocyte macrophage (CFU-GM) in the peripheral blood were 28% higher after treatment with the glycosylated molecule (lenograstim). Hoglund and colleagues[64] found a similar comparative effect in 32 healthy male donors with an average of 104 versus 82 CD34– cells per microliter of blood ($p < .0010$) on the fifth day of administration of either drug at a dose of 10 µg/kg/day. The glycosylated molecule has a higher specific activity that may account for this difference, although some authors also suggest a gender specificity for this difference.[65] De Arriba and associates[66] treated 30 women with breast cancer in a randomized study of these two drugs by using dosages containing bioequivalent units of activity and found no difference in the mobilization of CD34+ cells. The two forms have otherwise similar biologic activity and are not further distinguished in this discussion. A pegylated form of filgrastim is now available, avoiding the need for daily injections, and may also be effective in the mobilization of PBSCs, as demonstrated in a study involving healthy donors given a single injection of 12 mg.[67]

G-CSF is the most potent cytokine currently available for the mobilization of HSCs. In a randomized study of healthy volunteers comparing G-CSF, GM-CSF, and the combination of both, Lane and colleagues[68] reported an average 0.99% CD34+ cells in the peripheral blood of healthy donors treated with 10 µg/kg/day of G-CSF compared with 0.25% for donors treated with the same dose of GM-CSF. The quantity of CD34+ cells in the peripheral blood before treatment averaged 1.6 per microliter. After GM-CSF treatment, this increased to 3 per microliter, but with G-CSF, the level increased to 61 per microliter. Each group underwent one leukapheresis on the fifth day of treatment, and the collections from donors treated with G-CSF averaged 119 × 10^6 CD34+ cells compared with 12.6 × 10^6 for the GM-CSF–treated donors. Similar results are seen in autologous transplant candidates given either cytokine after mobilization chemotherapy.[69]

A distinct time course of appearance of CD34+ cells occurs during the administration of G-CSF, with the maximal level of CD34+ cells occurring on day 5 after 4 days of G-CSF administration.[70,71] Smaller numbers of CD34+ are present on days 4 and 6, and the level decreases rapidly on subsequent days, despite a continual increase in white blood cells (WBCs).

The number of CD34+ cells collected after G-CSF treatment is proportional to the number of these cells in the peripheral blood before the initiation of this cytokine.[43] Although doses as low as 5 μg/kg/day have been used for allogeneic PBSC transplantation,[72] a dose response to G-CSF occurs, with higher average levels of CD34+ cells being achieved with 10 μg/kg/day compared with 5 μg/kg/day.[73] The average collection from one group of healthy donors treated with 10 μg/kg/day averaged 4×10^8 CD34+ cells.[73] With this dose of G-CSF and appropriate apheresis technique, adequate numbers of CD34+ cells can be collected in one procedure for transplantation of most patients. A similar dose response is observed in autologous patients and may extend to doses as high as 40 μg/kg/day.[74] Waller and colleagues[75] studied twice-daily administration of G-CSF to healthy donors and found greater yields of CD34+ cells in the apheresis component. However, the total amount of G-CSF administered was also doubled, so it is not clear if the twice-daily administration or the higher dose is responsible for this observation. Anderlini and associates[76] compared administration of 6 μg/kg given twice daily with 12 μg/kg given once daily and found no differences in CD34+ cells/L of blood processed or the yield of CD34+ cells/kg collected. A similar study, however, found a benefit to twice-daily dosing,[77] and a third trial enrolling primarily pediatric subjects noted better results with a twice-daily schedule.[78] A retrospective study of allogeneic donors reported that single daily dosing of G-CSF predicted a lower yield of HSCs.[79] Patients, especially those previously treated with chemotherapy or radiotherapy (see later) will generally have lower quantities of CD34+ cells mobilized. However, previous treatment with chemotherapy does not preclude the use of G-CSF. De Luca and colleagues[80] noted a median 76-fold increase in CFU-GM for a population of 30 patients who were previously extensively treated for B-cell malignancies. Older donors will also have lower levels of CD34+ cells mobilized into the peripheral blood after G-CSF administration.[81]

Lymphocytes are also increased in the peripheral blood, and G-CSF priming may change the cytokine response of these cells,[82,83] possibly decreasing the risk of acute GVHD,[84] and augmenting the graft-versus-leukemia effect.[85] The potential influence of these changes in outcome of allogeneic (or autologous) transplantation is not clear.

The toxicity of G-CSF has been most clearly defined in studies of allogeneic donors.[72,73,86,87] The autologous patient will experience a similar toxicity profile, but with the added complications of the underlying malignancy and its treatment. Virtually all recipients of G-CSF will develop somatic complaints, of which skeletal pain is most prominent (Table 60–2). Few serious complications of the mobilization regimen and donation process have been reported.[88,89] Splenic rupture that occurred for a healthy donor appeared to be temporally related to the donation process, and a small study of normal donors showed an average increase in spleen size of 1.1 cm.[90] Filgrastim induces a hypercoagulable state, possibly increasing the risk of vascular events in some patients or donors.[91,92] Patients with autoimmune disorders may experience a flare of their disease during administration of filgrastim.[93] A variety of case reports of ophthalmologic and other adverse events have been reported for healthy donors or patients treated with filgrastim.[94–97] No clinical evidence exists that these agents will induce abnormalities in the hematopoietic cell, and no reports exist of an increased risk of myelodysplasia or hematologic malignancies in either healthy donors or patients who have been treated with short courses of G-CSF.

Table 60–2 Incidence of Somatic Complaints for Healthy Donors Treated with Filgrastim

	Anderlini[86]	Stroncek[73]	Bishop[72]
Number of donors	43	85	41
G-CSF dose	6 μg/kg/d	2–10 μg/kg/d	5 μg/kg/d
Symptom			
Malaise	82	86	83
Headache	70	28	44
Fatigue	20	14	NR
Fever	0	NR	27
Chills	NR	NR	22
Nausea	10	11	22

The reported proportion of donors experiencing the somatic complaint is shown. NR means this particular complaint was not reported in the series.

G-CSF administration results in a number of changes in blood counts and chemistries in addition to the coagulation factor changes noted earlier.[73,86] Alanine aminotransferase (ALT), lactate dehydrogenase (LDH), and alkaline phosphatase levels will increase, and the levels of blood urea nitrogen and bilirubin may decrease. These abnormalities of serum chemistries will resolve within 2 weeks after discontinuation of this medication. G-CSF administration will also result in a decrease in platelet count, especially if the cytokine is administered over many days.[73,87] WBC counts decrease rapidly after discontinuation of G-CSF. In about 10% of donors, the WBC may decrease to abnormal levels (but generally remain >1000 per microliter), reaching a nadir at 10 to 14 days after discontinuation of the cytokine before stabilizing at normal levels.

Cytokine Mobilization with GM-CSF

Much of the early experience with the use of hematopoietic cytokines for the mobilization of HSCs involved GM-CSF and chemotherapy.[32,98,99] The increase in CFU-GM in the peripheral blood can increase by as much as 1000-fold in this setting.[32] Moreover, at least for some patients, the combination of cyclophosphamide and GM-CSF is more effective than mobilization with G-CSF alone.[100] GM-CSF is not as potent as G-CSF, as discussed earlier. Haas and colleagues[101] treated 12 patients with 250 μg/m²/day of GM-CSF and observed only an 8.5-fold increase in the number of CFU-GM in the peripheral blood (to a median of 1347 CFU-GM/mL). As with G-CSF, a dose response also occurs in mobilization of PBSCs with GM-CSF over a range of 0.3 to 20 μg/kg/day without a plateau being observed.[102] In this latter study, however, the average increase in CFU-GM in the blood at this highest dose level was again only 8.4-fold. In a randomized study comparing GM-CSF with G-CSF or both drugs used in sequence after chemotherapy administration, patients recovered counts faster, required less supportive care including transfusions, and achieved greater collections of CD34+ cells if given one of the G-CSF–containing regimens.[103] However, administration of GM-CSF (alone or in combination with G-CSF) to healthy donors may result in a lower risk of acute GVHD.[104]

Administration of GM-CSF results in similar somatic complaints and liver-function abnormalities reported after G-CSF administration.[105] In addition, 44% to 80% of patients will experience fever, sometimes after each dose, and generalized or local skin reactions. Lieschke and Burgess[106] noted that doses greater than 20 μg/kg/day are poorly tolerated because of fluid retention, pleural and pericardial inflammation, and venous thrombosis. A "first-dose reaction" characterized by hypoxia and hypotension occurring within 3 hours after administration has been described for some recipients, especially after intravenous (IV) administration.[107]

Mobilization with Other Hematopoietic Cytokines

Recognition of the mobilization potential of G-CSF led many investigators to study other hematopoietic cytokines for their capacity to mobilize HSCs into the peripheral blood, including M-CSF, interleukin 3 (IL-3), IL-3 and GM-CSF fusion protein, erythropoietin, and stem cell factor (SCF).[108–118] Used as single agents, these cytokines resulted in only about a 5- to 10-fold increase in circulating CFU-GM or CD34+ cells. Moreover, many of these cytokines also caused unique toxicities, and most of these products are not commercially available.

Mobilization with Combinations of Cytokines

G-CSF + GM-CSF: The addition of G-CSF to GM-CSF greatly increases the number of HSCs mobilized. The converse is not true. Winter and others[119] treated patients with a variety of malignancies to regimens of GM-CSF or G-CSF (both at 5 μg/kg/day) to which the other cytokine was added at day 7 of treatment and both continued through day 12. The addition of GM-CSF on day 7 resulted in greater numbers of CFU-GM being collected in subsequent apheresis procedures than were collected on day 5, although the effect was not very great. In contrast, the addition of G-CSF on day 7 to patients treated with GM-CSF resulted in a strong release of CFU-GM 4 days later. Ho and coworkers[120] similarly studied the administration of GM-CSF or G-CSF at doses of 10 μg/kg/day, or both cytokines together at doses of 5 μg/kg/day each and found that G-CSF alone achieved greater mobilization than GM-CSF or both drugs given in combination at a lower dose. Among healthy allogeneic donors, the sequential combination of GM-CSF followed by G-CSF yielded superior CD34+ cell collections compared with GM-CSF at the same dose or concurrent G/GM-CSF.[121] Of interest, however, is the observation that the addition of GM-CSF to G-CSF in the treatment of healthy donors will affect the dendritic cell profile in the collected product, possibly leading to an enhanced antitumor effect and reduced risk of relapse after transplantation.[122]

Other Combinations: The combination of G-CSF with other cytokines such as SCF and IL-3 has also been the subject of clinical studies with additive or synergistic effects being described.[123–131] The combination of erythropoietin with G-CSF has been found to enhance HSC collection in two autologous transplant studies,[132,133] but to be antagonistic in another study involving allogeneic donors.[134] Again, the use of these agents in combination is precluded by the lack of commercial availability.

Mobilization with Chemotherapy Plus Cytokine

Chemotherapy plus cytokine will generally mobilize greater numbers of PBSCs than either alone.[100,135–137] No differences in the degree of tumor cell contamination of PBSC components, engraftment kinetics, or survival were found. A wide variety of different chemotherapy regimens have been used successfully for the mobilization of HSCs into the blood. The primary consideration is that the choice of chemotherapy used must meet the treatment needs of the patient. However, evidence also exists that the choice of chemotherapy regimens will affect the mobilization of HSCs. Schwartzberg and colleagues[138] reported an average daily apheresis yield of 4.0×10^7 CD34+ cells in 395 apheresis components collected from 61 patients treated with cyclophosphamide (CY) and average yields of 8.3×10^7 CD34+ cells in 218 collections from 33 patients treated with both CY and etoposide. (Another group of 24 patients were treated with this latter chemotherapy regimen, but also received 6 μg/kg/day of G-CSF. The average CD34+ cell contents for 122 collections from these patients were significantly higher at 38.8×10^7.) The average quantities of CFU-GM paralleled the numbers of CD34+ cells collected. Similarly, Demirer and coworkers[139] studied the effect of different chemotherapy regimens for the mobilization of HSCs for patients with breast cancer. Four regimens were used, all involving CY, but including etoposide with or without cisplatin, or paclitaxel. All patients also received G-CSF. The median quantity of CD34+ cells collected on the first day of apheresis after CY mobilization was 0.9×10^6 per kilogram of patient weight. The addition of etoposide, and then etoposide and cisplatin increased this to 8.1×10^6 and 3.5×10^6 CD34+ cells/kg, respectively. The median number of CD34+ cells harvested on the first day of apheresis after CY plus paclitaxel was 11.1×10^6 per kilogram. More than 50% of the women mobilized with this last regimen achieved the target dose of CD34+ cells in one apheresis procedure. Of the 100 women studied, 94 achieved the target dose of more than 5×10^6 CD34+ cells per kilogram. Only 4 patients failed to reach a lower but acceptable dose of 2.5×10^6 CD34+ cells per kilogram.

Mobilization with Chemokines

The chemokines are a superfamily of small peptide molecules instrumental in the regulation of leukocyte migration and trafficking. They may be subdivided into four families (CXC, CC, CX3C, and C), with important developmental immunologic and hematopoietic functions, and play a critical role in host defense.[140,141] They mediate their function through specific receptor proteins on the cell surface. Therefore, the interaction of the chemokine with its specific receptor forms an axis that may be manipulated to enhance stem cell mobilization from the bone marrow to the peripheral blood to optimize PBSC harvesting.[142]

Recently the role of the stromal cell–derived factor (SDF-1α) has been intensely investigated in hematopoietic progenitor and stem cells with long-term repopulating capability homing to the bone marrow in humans. Reports suggest that this mobilization effect relies on both the interaction with CCXR4 and its plasma concentration.[143,144] These findings also suggest that functional interaction between SDF-1α, CCXR4, and hematopoietic growth factors is implicated in cell migration. To exploit this effect, antagonists to CCXR4 (CTCE-0021 and AMD3100) have been studied alone and in combination with G-CSF in both murine and human systems to assess mobilizing capacity.[145–147] CTCE-0021 demonstrated both polymorphonuclear leukocyte (PMN) and hematopoietic progenitor cell (HPC) mobilization with a strong dose-effect differential in the two populations; multiday administration favored augmented PMN but not HPC mobilization. Strong synergism with G-CSF existed in the mobilization of both populations, but no alteration of plasma or marrow proteases was noted, and the primary end point of downmodulation of

CCXR4 and disruption of the SDF-1α/CCXR4 axis to induce mobilization was reached. The role of AMD3100 in mobilization of autografts for patients with NHL and MM was recently explored and published. This trial demonstrated that AMD3100 in combination with G-CSF produced a median 2.9-fold increase in circulating CD34+ cells 6 hours after initial dose with higher daily harvest totals, fewer apheresis procedures, early neutrophil recovery after transplantation, and minimal toxicity during mobilization.[148] The precise mode of action of AMD3100 remains to be elucidated. Because of the rapid mobilization engendered by the combination of the AMD31000 and G-CSF, studies are under way to ascertain whether AMD3100 alone may be sufficient to mobilize patients for autologous or allogeneic transplantation.[149]

In a primate study, the administration to rhesus monkeys of a modified CXC chemokine GROβ after 4 days of G-CSF resulted in a fivefold increase in the number of circulating stem and progenitor cells compared with G-CSF alone within a time course measured in hours.[150] The studies with GROβ have been translated to human volunteers where a variant GROβ-T, even though it lacks intrinsic colony stimulating activity, in combination with colony-stimulating factors has been proven to augment synergistically CFU-GM to levels far greater than either agent alone, as well as mobilization of early high-proliferative-potential progenitor cells into the peripheral blood.[151] This phenomenon may be explained by the codependence of the GROβ-T receptor CXCR2 and G-CSF receptors. IL-8 mobilizes stem cells within 15 to 30 minutes of injection into mice, an effect too rapid to result from an increase in the numbers of HSCs in the marrow compartment.[152] IL-8 also exerts its effects via the CCXR2 receptor, and an association between IL-8 levels in the blood and the numbers of CD34+ cells in normal donors undergoing G-CSF mobilization of PBSCs was found by Watanabe and others.[153] Studies are also under way to elucidate the precise role of the Flt3 ligand and its Flt3 receptor on the SDF-1α/CXCR4 axis and its effects on the kinetics of mobilization of both normal CD34+ cells and leukemic clone proliferation.[154]

These studies indicate that chemokines play a definitive role in the enhanced migration (mobilization) of HSCs into the peripheral blood preparatory to initiation of the apheresis procedure. These molecules do not expand the number of HSCs but increase the number available for collection, thereby reducing the volume of blood necessary to be processed to achieve the desired quantity of HSCs.

Management of Mobilization Failure

Most patients achieve the targeted dose of CD34+ cells after the processing of 20 to 30 L of blood in one to three apheresis procedures. However, about 5% to as many as 30% of patients in various series will have inadequate collections because only small numbers of HSCs are present in the peripheral blood despite the administration of hematopoietic cytokines. As discussed earlier, different chemotherapy and cytokine regimens will affect the mobilization of HSCs. Patient-specific factors predictive for poor mobilization include older age, marrow disease, prior radiotherapy, and prior chemotherapy.[29,155–158] The previous administration of marrow-toxic drugs suppresses the subsequent mobilization of HSCs.[159–162] About 50% of patients who fail to achieve the targeted dose of CD34+ cells will achieve this goal on a second attempt,[163] and a second-line harvest of PBSCs may be more efficacious than bone marrow harvesting.[164] High-dose (15 mg/kg BID) G-CSF after a 2- to 4-week drug holiday to allow marrow recovery is one strategy. Combination cytokine therapy is also of potential value in this situation but not adequately explored in clinical trials. An interesting report describes the administration of human growth hormone in combination with G-CSF in a series of 16 hard-to-mobilize patients.[165] Repetition of a chemotherapy-plus-cytokine regimen will also work, but may be associated with increased toxicity.[158] Bone marrow can be harvested, but the poor mobilization of PBSC predicts for a poor marrow harvest.[166] Consideration should also be given to infusing a lower dose of CD34+ cells (as low as 1×10^6 CD34+ cells/kg) because, although the risk of delayed engraftment is incurred,[181,182] failure of engraftment has not been reported.[158,167]

Consideration should also be given to collection of PBSCs early in the course of treatment for patients who may later be candidates for autologous HSC transplantation but who are advised to receive multiple courses of therapy or therapy involving alkylating agents or radiation therapy. HSCs may be collected and cryopreserved before extensive therapy while the patient has good marrow function and stored for years without obvious progressive loss of engraftment potential.[168]

Large-Volume Leukapheresis

The apheresis device has a uniform and fairly reproducible efficiency of collection. Thus, for a consistent quantity of blood processed through the machine, the quantity of CD34+ cells collected is directly related to the number present in the peripheral blood. Greater quantities of CD34+ cells can be collected by increasing the number of these cells in the peripheral circulation or by increasing the volume of blood processed by the device. For those patients with lower CD34+ cell levels, multiple apheresis procedures will be required to achieve the target dose of CD34+ cells needed for transplantation. An alternate approach is to process the same total quantity of blood, but in fewer, longer procedures. Large-volume leukapheresis (LVL) is not standardly defined, but in general use refers to the processing of more than 2 or 3 times the patient's blood volume.[169–178] Typically, the quantity of blood processed is 6 or more times the patient's blood volume, often 25 to 36 L of blood. The advantage of LVL is that this reduces the number of days of cytokine administration and apheresis with associated reduced costs of laboratory processing and testing. The apheresis techniques are the same as used for the processing of smaller volumes of blood, although blood flow rates may be increased to reduce the time required. The risks of LVL are the increased time required and the higher risk of citrate (or other anticoagulant) toxicity. Patients will also incur a proportional decrease in platelet counts and may become profoundly thrombocytopenic.

Most reports of LVL describe the collection of more CD34+ cells than are calculated to be present in the peripheral blood at the initiation of the apheresis procedure. Obviously, release of cells from the marrow replaces those removed by apheresis. Apheresis of CD34+ cells is a three-compartment system consisting of the extracorporeal circuit of the apheresis device (including the collection bag), the peripheral blood, and the marrow. However, it is not obvious that the apheresis technique itself consistently "mobilizes" CD34+ cells. The experience with patients and donors treated with cytokines or chemotherapy-plus-cytokine is variable, with reports describing an increase,[171–175] no change,[169,177,178] or even an exhaustion of CD34+ cells from the peripheral blood.[177,179] An increase also may not be evident in patients with poor marrow function.[176]

Clinically, most important is the possibility of exhaustion of HSCs such that the processing of the large blood volumes exposes the patient to the risks of anticoagulant toxicity and thrombocytopenia without achieving an increased collection of HSCs. However, studies at the Fred Hutchinson Cancer Research Center demonstrated a continuous release of CD34+ cells from the marrow (and, presumably, return to the marrow space).[180] Patients having higher levels of CD34+ cells in the peripheral blood appeared to have a greater number of these cells circulating between the marrow and peripheral blood compartments. In this model, the apheresis device merely serves as a siphon, removing these cells from the blood as they are released from the marrow. If this is an appropriate description of CD34+ cell kinetics, it may be possible to deplete these cells from the blood and marrow by prolonged processing, but probably only if limited numbers of these cells are in the marrow compartment. Also, the model suggests that higher blood flow rates used to shorten the apheresis procedure may be counterproductive for the patient with low CD34+ cell levels in the blood because of the slower rate of release of CD34+ cells for these patients.

LVL is appropriate management for the patient or donor who needs to complete apheresis in a limited number of procedures. The quality of the component collected by LVL does not differ from that collected by the processing of smaller volumes of blood, and patients experience the same rapid kinetics of engraftment after infusion of these components.[174]

Definition of Adequate Component(s)

The quantity of CD34+ cells in a PBSC component varies greatly and is dependent on the number in the peripheral blood at the time of collection and the volume of blood processed. Therefore, any definition of an adequate component cannot include a set number of CD34+ cells in a single apheresis component. Instead, one or more components will be collected to meet the appropriate dose of these cells for transplantation. What dose of CD34+ cells is required for infusion depends on the intended treatment regimen. For marrow-ablative regimens, increasingly higher CD34+ doses results in greater likelihood of rapid engraftment.[181,182] Although most transplant centers will probably accept components containing at least 1×10^6 to 2×10^6 CD34+ cells per kilogram of recipient weight, cell doses of 2.5×10^6 to 5×10^6 CD34+ cells per kilogram are desirable, and quicker engraftment will even be observed with higher doses.[181,182] Administration of G-CSF after transplantation will further speed the recovery of granulocytes[183–185] but may have a detrimental affect on platelet engraftment for patients receiving components containing low numbers of CD34+ cells.[181]

At lower doses of CD34+ cells, considerable heterogeneity is found in engraftment speed, especially for platelet engraftment. It is not known why this heterogeneity exists, but it may reflect a weakness in the correlation between CD34+ cells and the cells responsible for engraftment, or more simply, a greater degree of error in the measurement of CD34+ cells at the lower cell concentrations. As the dose of CD34+ cells increases, the engraftment speed becomes more consistent for the population studied.[181,182] Several investigators showed more rapid granulocyte and platelet engraftment for recipients of products containing a quantity of CD34+ cells above a dose of about 2 to 3×10^6 per kilogram recipient weight.[156,157,186] Investigators at the Fred Hutchinson Cancer Research Center found a threshold of 5×10^6 CD34+ cells per kilogram to achieve reliably prompt platelet engraftment,[187] and studies that include large patient populations found that higher doses of CD34+ cells will result in even higher proportions of patients achieving quick engraftment.[182] Investigators at the Hutchinson Center noted that the dose of CD34+ cells infused was more important than the type of mobilization therapy. In a study of allogeneic transplant recipients, Singhal and colleagues[188] reported a higher transplant-related mortality for patients who received a CD34+ cell dose less than 2×10^6 per kilogram, regardless of source of HSCs.

A major problem with chemotherapy-based mobilization regimens is the difficulty in determining the optimal time to commence HSC collection. Although many protocols call for the initiation of apheresis when the WBC count has recovered to greater than 1000 per microliter, a poor, if any, correlation exists between the peripheral blood WBC counts and the CD34+ cells in the peripheral blood. Characteristics that suggest a higher CD34+ cell level are rapidly increasing WBC count, a shift in differential to immature myeloid cells, circulating nucleated red cells, and platelet transfusion independence. These features may be more valuable in a homogeneous patient population receiving a uniform mobilization regimen.[189] However, it may be cost effective to obtain an actual measurement of CD34+ cells in the blood for the timing of apheresis collection. The published experience from many transplant centers describes a correlation between the CD34+ cells in the peripheral blood and in the harvested component.[156,186,190,191]

At what level of CD34+ cells in the peripheral blood to start apheresis is a clinical decision. Although levels in the range of 50 to 100/μL or greater will reduce the number of apheresis procedures necessary to achieve a target goal of CD34+ cells, each day's delay in initiating apheresis also incurs the costs of additional cytokine administration and blood testing. For some patients who have been extensively treated, it may be necessary to accept multiple apheresis procedures to achieve the target goal. Certainly, no patient should undergo apheresis if the peripheral blood count is less than 5 per microliter. For patients with CD34+ cell counts in the range of 10 to 20 per microliter, it is possible to process more blood per day by using LVL techniques. Most patients will have an increasing CD34+ cell count in the peripheral blood, so it is generally feasible to start apheresis the day after the patient has achieved a desirable CD34+ level.[191]

The timing of apheresis after G-CSF mobilization differs from the timing after chemotherapy and cytokine mobilization. For both patients and healthy donors, the peak concentration of CD34+ cells occurs on the fifth day of G-CSF administration (after four daily doses).[70,71] Lower levels are present on day 4, and the concentration continues to decrease after day 6 even if cytokine administration is continued and despite a continued increase in the WBC count. Thus, PBSC collection should be initiated on day 4 or 5 of G-CSF administration. The kinetics of CD34+ cells in the peripheral blood for patients and donors mobilized with G-CSF alone are so reliable that it is not necessary to monitor peripheral blood levels unless concern is felt that the patient has failed to mobilize cells and it is practical to obtain the cell count rapidly enough to initiate apheresis on the same day.

Evaluation of the Peripheral Blood Stem Cell Donor

The PBSC donor must meet the same donor health criteria applied to the bone marrow donor. The unique considerations for the PBSC donor are the need for adequate venous access and the risks of cytokine administration. The risks of cytokine administration are unique to each drug and are described earlier in this chapter. Anderlini and coworkers[88] suggested that G-CSF specifically not be administered to patients with a history of inflammatory ocular disorders, venous thrombosis, autoimmune disorders, or malignancy treated with chemoradiotherapy. Beelen and colleagues[192] reported in an interim analysis of an ongoing study of healthy donors receiving one of two different doses of G-CSF that 478 acute adverse events were noted in the first 150 donors enrolled. Most (80%) of these adverse events were transient bone pain or headache, and no persistent hematologic or nonhematologic events were recorded.

Older donors will have more underlying medical conditions, and the risks to the donor with underlying health problems must be fully considered before subjecting the donor to mobilization and apheresis.[193] The special challenges of the pediatric patient arise from the fixed extracorporeal blood volume of the apheresis device, the need for venous catheters for blood access, and the management of a patient who may be unwilling or unable to rest quietly for the period of apheresis. Virtually all pediatric patients undergo insertion of a venous catheter adequate for the flow rates expected, although older (older than 12 years) patients may tolerate vein-to-vein procedures. The whole blood flow rate for the pediatric patient is much reduced compared with that in adult patients, and catheters as small as 5F be adequate.[205]

Appropriate management of fluid balance during the apheresis procedure is critical for the smaller patient. The volume of red blood cells contained in the extracorporeal circuit of continuous flow apheresis device could represent 30% to 50% of the red cell mass of a pediatric donor. The obvious solution to this problem is to prime the apheresis device with ABO-compatible, irradiated, red blood cells (leukocyte depleted and CMV-negative blood may also be desirable) when the blood in the extracorporeal circuit is expected to exceed 15% of the patient's blood volume.

Complications of Peripheral Blood Stem Cell Collection

Apheresis technology is widely used for the collection of platelets from healthy donors and is considered to be without major risk to the donor. The important safety considerations for PBSC collection are the same as for platelet collection and include the venous access to be used for the procedure, the extracorporeal volume of blood during the procedure, and the solutions administered to the donor. However, it must also be acknowledged that PBSC collection for autologous transplantation involves patients with underlying medical conditions who may require considerable nursing care during the procedure. In a retrospective review of more than 5000 patient plasmapheresis procedures for the treatment of a variety of diseases, complications of apheresis were observed in 12% of procedures, and 40% of patients experienced at least one complication during a course of therapy.[194] Most of these were mild and transient, such as fever, chills, urticaria, hypotension, and reactions to citrate anticoagulants. In contrast, patients and donors undergoing PBSC collection do not require the replacement fluids used during plasmapheresis and will not experience the toxicities associated with plasma protein infusions. However, rare anaphylactic reactions may occur for the pediatric patient who requires blood priming of the extracorporeal circuit, patients treated with angiotensin-converting enzyme (ACE) inhibitors,[195] or those allergic to ethylene oxide used to sterilize the apheresis disposable set.[196] Goldberg and colleagues[197] studied the complications occurring during 554 PBSC collections from 75 consecutive patients. Patient diagnoses were varied, as were the mobilization treatment regimens. All but one patient had subclavian or jugular venous system catheters placed for apheresis. A median of 9 collections per patient was performed by using a discontinuous-flow apheresis device. The most common problems were related to the venous catheters, with 50% of the patients developing at least one occlusion. Hypocalcaemia occurred in 14.6% of patients and hypotension in 13.3%. Sixteen percent of patients experienced infectious complications during the PBSC collection period.

The discomfort, pain, and high levels of anxiety produced by PBSC donation has been rated as equivalent to that experienced by marrow donors enrolled in two randomized trials comparing marrow with PBSC transplantation. However, the PBSC donors reported more-rapid resolution of symptoms.[198,199] To the contrary, Switzer and associates[200] conducted a National Marrow Donor Program (NMDP) retrospective analysis of donor experiences that underwent PBSC donation after a prior bone marrow donation. These donors found the marrow harvest procedure physically more difficult, time consuming, and inconvenient. The comparative risks attendant to the allogeneic PBSC donor and platelet donor should not differ greatly if the apheresis techniques are similar, even though the PBSC donor may undergo larger volume and repetitive exchanges with different anticoagulants compared with the platelet donor. Although platelets can be separated from the component for infusion back to the donor, LVL and repetitive exchanges will result in platelet depletion.[73,86] The platelet count may reach its nadir several days after the completion of the apheresis collections and discontinuation of G-CSF, and donors should be counseled in this regard.[73,87]

Venous Access

Adequate venous access is required for optimal apheresis technique. Therefore, consultation with apheresis unit staff about the suitability of a particular type of venous access for an individual patient/donor is appropriate before commencement of treatment. Continuous-flow apheresis devices require dual-lumen access with a stable blood-flow capacity in the range of 60 to 100 mL/min.[201] Approximately 90% of adult allogeneic PBSC donors have adequate antecubital venous access for the procedure to be conducted "vein-to-vein." Consecutive day procedures may be performed, with scrupulous phlebotomy technique. Autologous transplant patients will have received previous chemotherapy or are proceeding directly to transplantation with tunneled access commonly placed. Often, this venous access can be appropriate both for the apheresis procedures and the subsequent transplant. A short, stiff, tunneled catheter or a temporary percutaneous dialysis/apheresis catheter is an appropriate choice.[202–204] Catheters of 10F or larger size are appropriate for adult patients. Pediatric patients whose blood flow rates are considerably slower may use catheters of 5F to 7F size.[205]

Venous-access complications account for a considerable amount of the toxicity associated with PBSC collection. Mobilization with either G-CSF or GM-CSF is associated with an increase in the incidence of catheter occlusion.[206,207] Goldberg and colleagues[197] reported this complication in 50% of patients. In contrast, Alegre and associates[203] reported only a 1.8% incidence of thrombosis or clotting of catheters, possibly because of differences in cytokine or catheter type and care. Catheter thromboses are easily managed with streptokinase, urokinase, or recombinant tissue plasminogen activator (rt-PA) instillation by the apheresis unit staff. One randomized study reported that low doses of warfarin decreased the incidence of venous thrombosis associated with indwelling catheters, but this study did not address catheter patency, nor were the patients enrolled in this study treated with hematopoietic cytokines.[208] Because of the rare but serious complication of heparin-induced thrombocytopenia (HIT), some centers avoid the use of heparin in favor of saline flushes. A study by Stephens and coworkers[209] demonstrated that the rate of catheter occlusion by thrombosis was similar, irrespective of the use of heparin or saline.

Anticoagulation

Anticoagulants are added to the blood during apheresis to prevent clotting of the extracorporeal circuit and clumping of cells in the component. Citrate (ACD-A) is the most widely used anticoagulant in apheresis procedures for the collection of PBSCs. The major drawback is the risk of a symptomatic hypocalcemia ("citrate toxicity"), especially during LVL.[210,211] ACD-A chelates calcium and magnesium, lowering the serum levels by as much as 35% and 56%, respectively, in inverse proportion to serum citrate levels, thus rendering them unavailable for Ca^{2+}-dependent metabolic reactions. Citrate redistribution throughout the circulation combined with metabolism by liver, kidney, and muscle is instrumental in preventing citrate toxicity.[212] Alterations in electrolytes, plasma protein levels, muscle mass, or renal or hepatic function that may occur for patients receiving chemotherapy may predispose patients to citrate toxicity. The initial signs include circumoral or acral paresthesias and may progress to nausea, vomiting, loss of consciousness, tetany, and seizures. Rarely, fatal cardiac dysrhythmias have been reported for patients undergoing plasmapheresis.[213] Citrate infusions may depress myocardial function, and this may be exacerbated by the concomitant use of calcium channel blockers, although reports of such complications for patients or donors undergoing apheresis have not been published.[210] Pediatric patients may not be able to relate the initial symptoms of citrate toxicity, and this should be considered for any change of behavior such as crying for these patients during the apheresis procedure. Prevention of citrate toxicity is by limiting the quantity of citrate infused either by decreasing the blood flow rate through the apheresis device or changing the blood-to-citrate ratio. The processing of blood of patients experiencing the initial symptoms of citrate toxicity should be temporarily halted until the symptoms abate and then resumed at a slower rate. Heparin may be used as a replacement for some or all of the citrate, although additional citrate is added to the component bag to prevent clumping of platelets.[33,214] Some centers using citrate anticoagulants will also administer intermittent or continuous infusions of calcium gluconate during the procedure, especially if large volumes of blood are being processed.[169] Buchta and colleagues[215] have suggested that female donors with total blood volume of less than 4.5 L may be ideal candidates for calcium administration. However, excessive calcium replacement can also induce cardiac dysfunction.[210]

PROCESSING OF HEMATOPOIETIC STEM CELLS

Management of Red Blood Cell Incompatibility

Management of red blood cell incompatibility is the same for PBSCs and bone marrow transplantation.[216] The infusion of incompatible red blood cells or immunocompetent B lymphocytes may provoke acute or delayed hemolytic transfusion reactions; therefore, red cell and/or plasma depletion may be required, and careful transfusion practices are critical. Red cell incompatibility may be classified into two major categories. First, major incompatibility is the situation in which host antibodies directed against infused donor red cells may produce acute hemolysis. Red blood cell quantities of 10 mL or less appear to be tolerable, although no safe level can be defined. Most PBSC components will contain small amounts of red blood cells, and apheresis devices are commonly used to remove red cells from marrow products.[217] Second, minor incompatibility is the situation in which donor-derived antibodies exist or may develop against the recipient. Although the latter rarely causes immediate infusion reactions, B lymphocytes within the component can form isoagglutinins, resulting in a delayed transfusion reaction 7 to 12 days after transplantation. Minor ABO incompatibility can result in delayed transfusion reactions that are potentially fatal if appropriate blood-transfusion support (avoiding the infusion of donor-type red cells) is not initiated before the transplant. Some authors suggest that the much greater numbers of B cells in PBSC products increase the risk of delayed hemolysis in the setting of minor ABO incompatibility.[218] However, the risk of delayed-type reaction may be reduced by the use of multiple post-transplant immunosuppressive medications, and the Seattle transplant program reported no delayed transfusion reactions in a large retrospective review of patients undergoing PBSC transplantation with cyclosporine and methotrexate immunosuppression.[219] Some patient/donor pairs may be incompatible with each other (bidirectional incompatibility) and must be managed by using the strategies for both major and minor red blood cell incompatibility.

Red cell depletion of bone marrow products is usually accomplished by centrifugation with or without the addition of hydroxyethylstarch,[220,221] or by processing of the product through an apheresis device.[222,223] The goal of processing is maximal recovery of HSCs with maximal depletion of red blood cells. At least 80% of nucleated cells should be recoverable through centrifugation; processing using an apheresis device may result in a relative enrichment of mononuclear cell fraction including HSCs and lymphocytes. PBSCs collected through apheresis technology already contain a small quantity of red blood cells, and further processing is more likely to result in cell losses without benefit. Plasma depletion is often performed for minor red cell incompatibility and is achieved through simple centrifugation of the product.

Tumor Cell Purging of Hematopoietic Stem Cell Components for Autologous Transplantation

The probability that tumor cell contamination of the component could contribute to relapse was demonstrated by Brenner and others[224–226] in studies involving the transplantation of genetically marked marrow cells. As a corollary to this, van Besien and colleagues[227] and Bierman and colleagues[228] suggested that tumor-free grafts may improve outcomes. Sensitive immunocytostaining techniques, clonal assays, flow-cytometric analysis, and polymerase chain reaction (PCR) amplification of malignant genetic material detect tumor cells in the PBSC components of many patients with a variety of malignancies.[229–232] In general, the incidence of contamination and the level of contamination is much less for PBSCs than for marrow components,[229] although this has not been a consistent finding in all studies.[230] In light of the clinical advantages of autologous PBSC transplantation, a phase III study to assess the relative relapse rates of PBSC versus bone marrow transplantation is unlikely to be conducted without preliminary evidence justifying the randomization of patients to the bone marrow transplant control arm. In a retrospective study, Sharp and associates[233] demonstrated similar probabilities of relapse-free survival for recipients of PBSC or marrow components if the HSC products were free of lymphoma cells. In that study, patients with marrow involvement by lymphoma were assigned to transplantation with PBSCs, suggesting that PBSC collection is a sensible approach to the patient with overt marrow involvement. Brugger and coworkers[234] however, demonstrated that patients with breast cancer involvement of the marrow at the time of chemotherapy mobilization were just as likely to mobilize tumor cells as CD34+ cells into the blood. Similarly, Pecora and colleagues[235] found a relation between the ability to detect tumor in PBSC components and in bone marrow samples, but also found a higher incidence of positive PBSC components for patients who required greater numbers of apheresis procedures to achieve the target dose of CD34+ cells. Investigators at The Johns Hopkins Oncology Center found no difference in the incidence of tumor contamination of PBSC components between patients mobilized with chemotherapy plus cytokines versus cytokines alone.[236] Because the probability of tumor contamination of PBSC components decreases after induction chemotherapy,[237] patients with marrow involvement should benefit from several cycles of debulking (in vivo purging) chemotherapy before collection of PBSCs with the caveat that extensive chemotherapy will decrease the subsequent yield of PBSCs. This concept was demonstrated in a randomized study comparing precollection treatment of patients with non-Hodgkin's lymphoma with rituximab to postcollection purging of the PBSC product.[238] The PBSC products for both patient groups were equally likely to be tumor cell positive and to achieve similar event-free survivals, but the products that were purged contained fewer CD34+ cells, and patients receiving the purged components experienced delayed hematologic recovery.

Considerable effort has been devoted to the development of purging techniques based on physical characteristics, immunologic differences, or relative sensitivities of normal and malignant cells to chemotherapeutic agents. PBSC components can be purged of tumor cells by using the same techniques originally developed for marrow, although the larger cell quantities collected and the multiple days of collection will increase the cost of this processing. The commercial availability of devices that enrich CD34+ cells has served to focus recent purging studies on this technology. The presence of this marker on hematopoietic stem and progenitor cells enables the enrichment of these cells from the HSC product. The enriched populations can then be used for transplantation or for further manufacturing, such as gene therapy or cell expansion. Numerically, simple enrichment of CD34+ cells from less than 1% to levels of 70% to 95% results in a greater than 90% to 99% depletion of CD34− cells, leading many investigators to explore CD34+ cell enrichment as a technique of T-cell depletion to prevent GVHD in allogeneic cell recipients,[239–242] or tumor depletion to decrease the risk of relapse for autologous component recipients.[243–246] Engraftment does not appear to be affected by the CD34+ cell enrichment unless low quantities of CD34+ cells are infused.[243]

Positive enrichment of HSCs achieves nonspecific tumor cell depletion as CD34+ cells are separated from the antigen-negative cells. Because this depletion is nonspecific, the degree of purging achieved will equal the depletion of other CD34− cells such as lymphocytes. Typically, this will range from 99.0% to 99.99% depletion. By itself, CD34+ cell enrichment will reduce the number of tumor cells below the level of detection of some assay systems. For example, Shiller and colleagues[243] reported that five of eight components were negative for myeloma cells after processing, but Lemoli and associates[246] found the persistence of detectable disease in five of six patients tested. The median purity of the CD34+ cells was actually greater in the latter study (77% vs 89.5%). Phase III studies of CD34 enrichment for patients undergoing treatment for myeloma show the feasibility of CD34+ cell enrichment of PBSC components, although these studies were not powered to demonstrate efficacy in control of disease.[247] In an effort to improve the specificity of purging, some investigators have used a double-purging technique. Altes and coworkers[248] used a positive CD34 and negative CD19 double-selection method to improve the efficacy of single purging in 26 patients with a poor prognosis in lymphoproliferative disorders with minimal residual disease (MRD) detected by PCR and flow cytometry. Half of the patients mobilized an adequate number of CD34+ cells and proceeded into the double-purge arm. Twelve harvests became PCR negative after double selection, and 10 patients were autografted. At a median follow-up of 30 months, only 2 patients had molecular relapse. However, a high frequency of life-threatening infections was found in this study, underscoring the risks associated with this double-enrichment modality. A recent study of double-enrichment technique (based on CD34 and CD133 expression) reported a 50% improvement in tumor cell depletion, but clinical studies have not yet been reported.[249] No benefit for survival has been shown in any randomized study of ex vivo purging (Table 60–3).[238,247,250,251]

T-Cell Purging of Hematopoietic Stem Cell Components for Allogeneic Transplantation

Effective removal of mature T lymphocytes from the stem cell inoculum can reduce both the incidence and the severity of acute and chronic GVHD. A number of depletion techniques have been developed, including physical techniques such as elutriation or agglutination; and antibody-based techniques involving complement-mediated killing, solid-phase separation, or the more recently developed CD34+ cell-enrichment techniques that nonspecifically separate T

Table 60–3 **Randomized Studies of Autologous HSC Transplantation Using Tumor Cell–Depleted Grafts**

Study	Diagnosis Purging Technique	Time to ANC >500/μL	Survival Probability	
			Progression Free	Overall
Stewart[250]	Multiple myeloma CD34 enrichment	Purged 12 Unpurged 12	71 67	64 66
Schouten[257]	Follicular NHL Antibody depletion	Purged NS Unpurged NS	55 58	77 71
Van Heeckeren[238]	Large cell and follicular NHL CD34 enrichment vs. rituximab	Purged (CD34) 11 Unpurged 10	76 81	70 79

NS, not stated.

*Initial data published in Vescio, R, Schiller G, Stewart AK, et al. Multicenter phase III trial to evaluate CD34+ selected versus unselected autologous peripheral blood progenitor cell transplantation in multiple myeloma. Blood 1999;93:1858–1868.

lymphocytes and other CD34– cell populations from the CD34+ stem cell population. The intent of these procedures is to deplete mature T lymphocytes from the stem cell inoculum. The occurrence of GVHD decreases as T-cell quantities are reduced below 10^5 per kilogram of recipient weight.[252]

The major risks of T-cell depletion are widely recognized and include loss of the graft-versus-tumor (GVL) effect with increased risk of disease relapse, increased risk of infections if delayed immunologic reconstitution results from the depletion method used, and failure of engraftment or graft rejection. Higher doses of HSCs, which can be achieved by combining marrow and PBSC components, will reduce the risk of graft failure.[253] Fixed doses of lymphocytes, as opposed to maximal T-cell depletion, may also reduce the risk of graft failure.[254] The clinical benefit of reduced GVHD may be offset by the complications of T-cell depletion. A large, multicenter, randomized trial that enrolled more than 400 patients found more rapid engraftment for the recipients of T-depleted grafts (who did not receive post-transplant methotrexate), fewer grade III to IV nonhematopoietic toxicities, shorter hospitalization, and a lower risk of severe acute GVHD.[255] However, the recipients of the T-depleted grafts experienced higher likelihood of infectious complications and relapse, and overall survival at 3 years after transplantation did not differ statistically (27% for T-depleted recipients; 34% for control group). This study also found no difference in the risk of chronic GVHD,[256] and economic analysis found no difference in the costs of transplantation with the reduced costs from not treating acute GVHD offset by the increased costs of treating serious infections.[257]

QUALITY CONTROL OF HEMATOPOIETIC STEM CELL PRODUCTS

Microbial Contamination of Hematopoietic Stem Cell Components

Bone marrow harvesting, by virtue of the procedural techniques, has a risk of contamination of the product by bacterial skin flora. However, this contamination is, generally, not a cause of clinically significant infections in the recipient, although some serious infections have been reported from contamination of products during postharvesting processing.[258–264] Any decision regarding the disposition of culture-positive HSCs must be made by the patient's transplant physician after considering the type of contamination, the anticipated risks from use of the component, and the ability to replace the culture-positive component(s) in a timely manner. As a consequence of the different collection modality, the incidence of contamination of PBSC products is considerably less than that for marrow.[262–264] Attarian and colleagues[168] reported only 3 products with bacterial contamination in a prospective study of 1263 PBSC collections from 376 sequential patients, even though 50% of the patients were receiving antibiotics for the treatment of neutropenic fever on the day of apheresis. Clinically stable but febrile patients may safely have PBSCs harvested based on the kinetics of mobilization of CD34+ cells into the peripheral blood. Bone marrow harvesting, the timing of which is not determined by cytokine administration, should be delayed for the comfort and safety of the donor.

Quantitation of CD34+ Cells

Quantification of CD34 antigen-positive cells by flow cytometry has become the standard of care for the management of the PBSC donor because it provides a rapid and clinically relevant assessment of HSC content in the peripheral blood or the PBSC component. Cell viability using propidium iodide (PI) or 7-aminoactinomycin D (7-AAD) exclusion can simultaneously be determined if the cells are analyzed while still fresh.[265] Many centers are finding strong correlations between the numbers of CD34+ cells and CFU-GM in the sample, but with a ratio of about 520:1.[190,266] Thus, CD34 analysis will provide data similar to those obtainable with cell cultures, with the exception that the growth of cells in the laboratory demonstrates the viability of the progenitor cells.

The major difficulty with the analysis of CD34+ cells is the low frequency of these cells. This enumeration is possible because of the multidimensional measurements possible with the flow cytometer, which can measure at least five characteristics of each cell including size, granularity, and the presence of up to three different fluorochromes. Thus the cells of interest can be separated in five-dimensional space, achieving discrimination of cells as rare as 1 in 10,000. The difficulties arise from developing an adequate technique that makes optimal use of the cytometer to measure these rare cells. Sources of errors include (1) sampling of the component, (2) cell counting, (3) cytometer calibration and operation, (4) choice of antibody and fluorochrome, (5) lysis technique, and (6) gating strategy. The steps involved in preparing a specimen for cytometry may alter the proportion of cells in the sample, and this error will be translated into an error in the absolute number.[267] Serke and colleagues[268] found a coefficient of variation of 30% in counting of CFU-GM colonies and of 10% in flow-cytometric counting of CD34+ cells. The coefficient of variation in CD34+ cell enumeration could be as high as 65% for specimens containing few cells, and this variation was decreased by the analysis of larger cell samples. A variety of different cytometry techniques are used in measuring CD34+ cells.[269–271] Considerable variation is found in results even between laboratories using the same cytometry technique, and no cytometer-based technique has proven to have a lower interlaboratory variability.[270]

Subset analysis will provide additional information but does not appear to be clinically useful at this time. Pecora and associates[272] reported that the quantity of CD34+CD33− cells infused was identified as an independent factor predictive of engraftment kinetics. Derksen and coworkers[273] reported better correlation between the number of CD34+CD33− cells and time to granulocyte engraftment and between the number of CD34+CD41+ cells and time to platelet engraftment than found with the overall number of CD34+ cells. This group reported a similar finding for the number of CD34+ L-selectin+ cells infused and platelet engraftment.[274] Given the limited range in recovery times when adequate numbers of CD34+ cells are collected and infused, however, this additional information is of limited clinical value.

Progenitor Cell Cultures

Unlike other measures of component quality, progenitor cell cultures also demonstrate the functional capacity of the cells. These techniques require expertise and equipment not available in many clinical laboratories, and have other drawbacks that may limit their utility as routine quality control. Other than availability of equipment and expertise, the major limitation is that progenitor cell assays require 10 to 14 days of culture before the results are available. Thus, progenitor cell cultures cannot be used in the day-to-day management of the PBSC donor. No standard culture technique has been adopted by all laboratories. The clinical relevance of the culture technique to the transplant population must be determined if the data obtained are to be used in the management of individual patients. Progenitor cell cultures are the only currently available relevant assay of HSC viability other than actual engraftment of the recipient, and should be available at the PBSC processing facility for use in quality control or if questions about the viability of a particular component are raised.

STORAGE OF HEMATOPOIETIC STEM CELL PRODUCTS

Cryopreservation

HSCs harvested from the peripheral blood, bone marrow, or umbilical cord blood are frozen and stored by using the same techniques. The general parameters include cryopreservation in dimethylsulfoxide (DMSO) and a source of plasma protein with or without hydroxyethylstarch (HES), cooling at 1° C to 3°C per minute, and storage at −80°C or colder.[275] Variations on this technique include the concentration at which the cells are frozen, the amount and source of the plasma protein, and the cooling techniques used.[276,277] Most of these variations probably have little effect on the survival of the HSCs, but cryopreservation results in the loss of an undefined but potentially substantial proportion of HSCs. Delay in engraftment can occur if the component being frozen has borderline quantities of HSCs.[278,279] A considerable incidence of generally minor toxicity is associated with the infusion of cryopreserved cells.[280]

PBSCs differ from marrow components because of their much larger cell quantity, frequently exceeding 4×10^{10} cells. Cryopreservation of these cells at a set cell concentration, especially if multiple days of collection are performed, may result in large volumes of cryopreserved material to be infused. DMSO itself has a variety of pharmacologic effects,[281] which may be compounded by the presence of lysed blood cells, foreign proteins from tumor-cell purging procedures, or contaminants from nonpharmaceutical grades of reagents used in the processing. The acute toxic dose of DMSO for humans has not been determined. One report cited two instances of encephalopathy after the infusion of cryopreserved PBSC products, possibly containing more than 2 g DMSO per kilogram patient weight.[282] For these reasons, the volume of DMSO infused should be limited to 1 g/kg/day. Patients with larger volumes can receive the cells over more than 1 day.

To minimize the volume infused, PBSCs and bone marrow may be concentrated before cryopreservation. In one series, the average cell concentration of cryopreserved PBSCs was 5.59×10^8 nucleated cells per milliliter.[283] No detrimental effect of cryopreservation at these high cell concentrations on the recovery of nucleated cells, mononuclear cells, or CD34+ cells was found. No clinical studies have addressed the effect of cell concentration during cryopreservation of bone marrow or PBSCs on engraftment speed. Of concern, however, is that several patients infused at that center developed alterations in mental status, including seizures, after infusion of PBSCs concentrated before cryopreservation.[284] It is very unlikely that these events were related to the small volumes of DMSO infused but may be related to the concentration of cells frozen.

HSCs can be frozen in solutions using reduced concentrations of DMSO. A large (294 patients) randomized phase III study comparing engraftment after autologous transplantation of PBSCs frozen using either 10% DMSO or 5% DMSO with 6% HES showed faster granulocyte recovery for patients receiving cells frozen by using the combination cryoprotectant solution.[285] No difference in platelet-recovery speeds was found, suggesting a lineage-specific benefit. These investigators did not report on infusion-related toxicity, although others have suggested that infusion-related toxicities are, in general, proportional to the quantity of DMSO infused.[286]

Alternately, the cells can be washed after thawing, with removal of most of the DMSO.[287] The risk is again one of cell loss, and it is preferable, if possible, that a strategy be adopted to ensure that not all cells are at risk during a single processing. An effect of post-thaw washing on the speed or success of engraftment after infusion of marrow or PBSC components has not been published.

Nonfrozen storage

HSCs may be kept in nonfrozen conditions for transportation or before infusion or subsequent processing. Nonfrozen storage is a less costly alternative to cryopreservation and allows greater flexibility in timing of transplantation relative to HSC collection, including the ability to modify or postpone a transplant-conditioning regimen already started.

A progressive loss of HSCs occurs during nonfrozen storage. One author reported a 61% loss of myeloid colony-forming progenitor cells (CFU-GM) from marrow after 72 hours of storage at 4°C.[288] Yet another found only a 3% loss of CFU-GM from marrow stored for 96 hours, but a 95% loss if the source of the cells was peripheral blood.[289] Preti and colleagues[290] compared the survival of mature hematopoietic progenitor cells isolated from marrow during frozen or nonfrozen storage, and reported an immediate loss of myeloid (CFU-GM) progenitors of 33% during cryopreservation and thawing. In contrast, cells stored at 4°C showed a progressive, linear loss of total nucleated cells, cell viability, and HSCs cloned in vitro. The quantity of erythroid colony-forming progenitor cells (BFU-E) in these nonfrozen samples became significantly less than those in cryopreserved samples only after 5 days of storage. The difference for myeloid progenitor cells (CFU-GM) was not yet significant even after 9 days of storage. These differing reports demonstrate that storage conditions such as concentration of cells, chemicals added, product volume, storage bag, and temperature of storage will affect the survival of cells kept in nonfrozen storage.[291]

Most published reports of noncryopreserved storage describe storage at 4° C, which provides a stable temperature compared with storage at ambient temperatures. The optimal storage temperature is unknown and will probably depend on such concerns as the prestorage processing, the quantity and concentration of mature blood cells, the buffering capacity of the solution, and the gas-diffusion capacity of the storage container. Beaujean and associates[292] for example, reported a greater acidity for PBSC products stored overnight at room temperature compared with storage at 4° C, although they did not find a difference in the recovery of progenitor cells. Storage conditions for nonfrozen storage have not been tested in an engraftment model, so proper storage conditions are not adequately defined. For laboratories intending to store stem cell products, particularly PBSC components, for prolonged periods without freezing, rigorous validation of the storage conditions must be performed.

REGULATORY ASPECTS OF STEM CELL COLLECTION AND PROCESSING

The regulation of the wide range of cellular- and tissue-based products being developed requires either an extensive number of focused regulations specific for each possible product or an adaptable regulatory strategy that can encompass a broad and expanding range of products and manufacturing techniques. The Food and Drug Administration (FDA) proposed in 1997 a new approach for the regulation of cellular- and tissue-based products by using a continuum of regulation that is intended to enable the FDA to meet its task of protecting public health without being unfair to specific practitioners of this field of medicine or stifling to the development of novel uses of these products. These regulations were implemented in May 2005.[9] The intended rigor of control is proportional to the extent of risk involved with use of the tissue or cellular product, with the level of regulation dictated by the following five considerations: prevention of disease transmission, processing controls to prevent contamination and maintain product integrity and function, clinical safety and efficacy, labeling and promotion of the products, and communication with and monitoring of the tissue industry. The regulatory approach taken by the FDA addresses facility registration, selection and evaluation of the tissue donor, and manufacturing of the product. The FDA views cell processing to be a manufacturing activity. Therefore, the FDA expects that the collection, processing, and distribution of HSC-derived components will comply, at least, to current Good Tissue Practices (cGTPs) with the much more detailed current good manufacturing practices (cGMPs) required for extensively manipulated products. cGMPs and cGTPs differ in the level of control over the manufacturing pathway required to prevent contamination or loss of potency of the final product. The FDA developed part 1271 of chapter 21 of the CFR for these regulations. Part 1271 does not replace cGMP regulations for drugs and medical devices found elsewhere in Chapter 21 of the Code of Federal Regulations (CFR); cell-therapy products that combine cell products with devices or drugs must comply with part 1271 and with the applicable cGMP regulations.

The regulations described in part 1271 are designed to prevent the introduction, transmission, and spread of communicable diseases. For example, compliance with cGTPs would require such precautions as cleaning of facilities and equipment, storage procedures designed to prevent product mix-ups, and controls over processing to prevent product contamination and impairment to function or integrity. cGTPs include, at a minimum, requirements for the appropriate collection, processing, labeling, storage, and distribution of cellular products to ensure maintenance of the product's function and integrity but do not require the rigorous environmental and manufacturing controls inherent in cGMPs.

In the final rule enacting establishment registration, the FDA defined products regulated solely under this section (lowest level of regulation) if they are (1) minimally manipulated; (2) intended for homologous use only (e.g., serves same basic function as cells being replaced); (3) not combined with a drug or a device, except for a sterilizing, preserving, or storage agent; and (4) either without a systemic effect and not dependent on the metabolic activity of living cells or have a systemic effect or are dependent on the metabolic activity of living cells for their primary function and are for autologous use or for allogeneic use in a first-degree or second-degree blood relative.[293] This includes most HSC transplantation. Products not meeting this description are still subject to these core requirements found in part 1271, but are also subject to more stringent requirements, including the requirement for premarketing approval (gained through submission of data from preclinical and clinical studies demonstrating safety and efficacy for the use being requested) and cGMP manufacturing requirements, as described in the regulatory approach for somatic cell therapy products.[294]

REFERENCES

1. Thomas ED, Storb R. Technique for human marrow grafting. Blood 1970;36:507–515.
2. Stroncek DF, Holland PV, Bartch G, et al. Experiences of the first 493 unrelated marrow donors in the National Marrow Donor Program. Blood 1993;81:1940–1946.
3. Sanders J, Buckner CD, Bensinger WI, et al. Experience with marrow harvesting from donors less than two years of age. Bone Marrow Transplant 1987;2:45–50.
4. Brecher G, Cronkite RP. Postradiation parabiosis and survival in rats. Proc Soc Exp Biol Med 1951;77:292–294.
5. Goodman JW, Hodgson GS. Evidence for stem cells in the peripheral blood of mice. Blood 1962;19:702–714.

6. Storb R, Graham TC, Epstein RB, et al. Demonstration of hemopoietic stem cells in the peripheral blood of baboons by cross circulation. Blood 1977;50:537–542.
7. Brandwein JM, Callum J, Rubinger M, et al. An evaluation of outpatient bone marrow harvesting. J Clin Oncol 1989;7:648–650.
8. CDC, Infectious Disease Society of America, and the American Society of Blood and Marrow Transplantation. Guidelines for preventing opportunistic infections among hematopoietic stem cell transplant recipients: Recommendations of CDC, the Infectious Disease Society of America, and the American Society of Blood and Marrow Transplantation. Biol Blood Marrow Transplant 2000;6:659–713, 715, 717–727.
9. Chapter 21, Code of Federal Regulations, part 1271.
10. Foundation for the Accreditation of Cellular Therapy. Standards for Hematopoietic Progenitor Cell Collection, Processing and Transplantation, 2nd ed. Omaha, Neb., Foundation for the Accreditation of Cellular Therapy, 2002.
11. American Association of Blood Banks. Standards for Hematopoietic Progenitor Cells. Bethesda, Md., American Association of Blood Banks, 1996.
12. Niederwieser D, Gentilini C, Hegenbart U, et al. Transmission of donor illness by stem cell transplantation: should screening be different in older donors? Bone Marrow Transplant 2004;34:657–665.
13. Kiss TL, Chang H, Daly A, et al. Bone marrow aspirates as part of routine donor assessment for allogeneic blood and marrow transplantation can reveal presence of occult hematological malignancies in otherwise asymptomatic individuals. Bone Marrow Transplant 2004;33:855–858.
14. Iwamoto M, Jernigan DB, Guasch A, et al. Transmission of West Nile virus from an organ donor to four transplant recipients. N Engl J Med 2003;348:2196–2203.
15. Gottesdiener KM. Transplanted infections: donor to host transmission with the allograft. Ann Intern Med 1989;110:1001–1016.
16. Strasser SI, McDonald GB. Hepatitis viruses and hematopoietic cell transplantation: a guide to patient and donor management. Blood 1999;93:1127–1136.
17. Niederwieser DW, Appelbaum FR, Gastl G, et al. Inadvertent transmission of a donor's acute myeloid leukemia in bone marrow transplantation for chronic myelocytic leukemia. N Engl J Med 1990; 25:1794–1796.
18. Buckner CD, Clift RA, Sanders JE, et al. Marrow harvesting from normal donors. Blood 1984;64:630–634.
19. Jin NR, Hill RS, Petersen FB, et al. Marrow harvesting for autologous marrow transplantation. Exp Hematol 1985;13:879–884.
20. Hill HF, Chapman CR, Jackson TI, Sullivan KM. Assessment and management of donor pain following marrow harvest for allogeneic bone marrow transplantation. Bone Marrow Transplant 1989;4: 157–161.
21. Stroncek DF, McGlave P, Ramsay N, McCullogh J. Effects on donors of second bone marrow collections. Transfusion 1991;31:819–822.
22. Storb R, Prentice RL, Thomas ED. Marrow transplantation for treatment of aplastic anemia. N Engl J Med 1977;296:61–66.
23. Thomas ED, Buckner CD, Benaji M, et al. One hundred patients with acute leukemia treated by chemotherapy, total body irradiation, and allogeneic marrow transplantation. Blood 1977;49:511–533.
24. Sierra J, Storer B, Hansen JA, et al. Transplantation of marrow cells from unrelated donors for treatment of high-risk acute leukemia: the effect of leukemic burden, donor HLA-matching, and marrow cell dose. Blood 1997;89:4226–4235.
25. Zaucha JM, Knopinska-Posluszny W, Bieniaszewska M, et al. The effect of short G-CSF administration on the numbers and clonogenic efficiency of hematopoietic progenitor cells in bone marrow and peripheral blood of normal donors. Ann Transplant 2000;5:20–26.
26. Weisdorf D, Jiller J, Verfaillie C, et al. Cytokine-primed bone marrow stem cells vs. peripheral blood stem cells for autologous transplantation: a randomized comparison of GM-CSF vs. G-CSF. Biol Blood Marrow Transplant 1997;3:217–223.
27. Dicke KA, Hood DL, Arneson M, et al. Effects of short-term in vivo administration of G-CSF on bone marrow prior to harvesting. Exp Hematol 1997;25:34–38.
28. Hartmann O, Le Corroller AG, Blaise D, et al. Peripheral blood stem cell and bone marrow transplantation for solid tumors and lymphomas: Hematologic recovery and costs: a randomized, controlled trial. Ann Intern Med 1997;126:600–607.
29. Smith TJ, Hillner BE, Schmitz N, et al. Economic analysis of a randomized clinical trial to compare filgrastim-mobilized peripheral-blood progenitor-cell transplantation and autologous bone marrow transplantation in patients with Hodgkin's and non-Hodgkin's lymphoma. J Clin Oncol 1997;15:5–10.
30. Vellenga E, van Agthoven M, Croockewit AJ, et al. Autologous peripheral blood stem cell transplantation in patients with relapsed lymphoma results in accelerated haematopoietic reconstitution, improved quality of life and cost reduction compared with bone marrow transplantation: The Hovon 22 study. Br J Haematol 2001;114:319–326.
31. van Agthoven M, Vellenga E, Fibbe WE, et al. Cost analysis and quality of life assessment comparing patients undergoing autologous peripheral blood stem cell transplantation or autologous bone marrow transplantation for refractory or relapsed non-Hodgkin's lymphoma or Hodgkin's disease: A prospective randomised trial. Eur J Cancer 2001;37:781–789.
32. Gianni AM, Siena S, Bregni M, et al. Granulocyte-macrophage colony-stimulating factor to harvest circulating haemopoietic stem cells for autotransplantation. Lancet 1989;2:580–585.
33. Bensinger W, Singer J, Appelbaum F, et al. Autologous transplantation with peripheral blood mononuclear cells collected after administration of recombinant granulocyte stimulating factor. Blood 1993;81:31–58.
34. Elias AD, Ayash L, Anderson KC, et al. Mobilization of peripheral blood progenitor cells by chemotherapy and granulocyte-macrophage colony-stimulating factor for hematologic support after high-dose intensification for breast cancer. Blood 1992;79:30–36.
35. Sheridan WP, Begley CG, To, LB et al. Phase II study of autologous filgrastim (G-CSF): mobilized peripheral blood progenitor cells to restore hemopoiesis after high-dose chemotherapy for lymphoid malignancies. Bone Marrow Transplant 1994;14:105–111.
36. To LB, Roberts MM, Haylock DN, et al. Comparison of haematological recovery times and supportive care requirements of autologous recovery phase peripheral blood stem cell transplants, autologous bone marrow transplants and allogeneic bone marrow transplants. Bone Marrow Transplant 1992;9:277–284.
37. Sheridan WP, Begley CG, Juttner CA, et al. Effect of peripheral-blood progenitor cells mobilised by filgrastim (G-CSF) on platelet recovery after high-dose chemotherapy. Lancet 1992;339:640–644.
38. Körbling M, Przepiorka D, Huh Y, et al. Allogeneic blood stem cell transplantation for refractory leukemia and lymphoma: potential advantages of blood over marrow allografts. Blood 1995;85:1659–1665.
39. Bensinger WI, Clift R, Martin P, et al. Allogeneic peripheral blood stem cell transplantation in patients with advanced hematologic malignancies: a retrospective comparison with marrow transplantation. Blood 1996;88:2794–2800.
40. Schmitz N, Dreger P, Suttorp M, et al. Primary transplantation of allogeneic peripheral blood progenitor cells mobilized by filgrastim (granulocyte colony-stimulating factor) Blood 1995;85:1666–1672.
41. Rosenfeld C, Collins R, Piñeiro L, et al. Allogeneic blood cell transplantation without post transplant colony-stimulating factors in patients with hematopoietic neoplasm: a phase II study. J Clin Oncol 1996;14:1314–1319.
42. Bacigalupo A, Van Lint MT, Valbonesi M, et al. Thiotepa cyclophosphamide followed by granulocyte colony-stimulating factor mobilized allogeneic peripheral blood stem cells in adults with advanced leukemia. Blood 1996;88:353–357.
43. Brown RA, Adkins D, Goodnough LT, et al. Factors that influence the collection and engraftment of allogeneic peripheral-blood stem cells in patients with hematologic malignancies. J Clin Oncol 1997;15:3067–3074.
44. Pavletic ZS, Bishop MR, Tarantolo SR, et al. Hematopoietic recovery after allogeneic blood stem-cell transplantation compared with bone marrow transplantation in patients with hematologic malignancies. J Clin Oncol 1997;15:1608–1616.
45. Blaise D, Kuentz M, Fortanier C, et al. Randomized trial of bone marrow versus lenograstim-primed blood cell allogeneic transplantation in patients with early-stage leukemia: a report from the Societe Francaise de Greffe de Moelle. J Clin Oncol 2000;18:537–546.
46. Bensinger WI, Martin PJ, Storer B, et al: Transplantation of bone marrow as compared with peripheral-blood cells from HLA-identical relatives in patients with hematologic cancers. N Engl J Med 2001;344:175–181.
47. Couban S, Simpson DR, Barnett MJ, et al. A randomized multicenter comparison of bone marrow and peripheral blood in recipients of matched sibling allogeneic transplants for myeloid malignancies. Blood 2002;100:1525–1531.
48. Schmitz N, Beksac M, Hasenclever D, et al. Transplantation of mobilized peripheral blood cells to HLA-identical siblings with standard-risk leukemia. Blood 2002;100:761–767.
49. Beyer J, Schwella N, Zingsem J, et al. Hematopoietic rescue after high-dose chemotherapy using autologous peripheral-blood progenitor cells or bone marrow: A randomized comparison. J Clin Oncol 1995;13:1328–1335.

50. Schmitz N, Linch DC, Dreger P, et al. Randomised trial of filgrastim-mobilised peripheral blood progenitor cell transplantation versus autologous bone-marrow transplantation in lymphoma patients. Lancet 1996;347:353–357.
51. Serody JS, Sparks SD, Lin Y, et al. Comparison of granulocyte colony-stimulating factor (G-CSF)–mobilized peripheral blood progenitor cells and G-CSF–stimulated bone marrow as a source of stem cells in HLA-matched sibling transplantation. Biol Blood Marrow Transplant 2000;6:434–440.
52. Morton J, Hutchins C, Durrant S. Granulocyte-colony-stimulating factor (G-CSF)-primed allogeneic bone marrow: significantly less graft-versus-host disease and comparable engraftment to G-CSF-mobilized peripheral blood stem cells. Blood 2001;98:3186–3191.
53. Couban S, Messner HA, Andreou P, et al: Bone marrow mobilized with granulocyte colony-stimulating factor in related allogeneic transplant recipients: a study of 29 patients. Biol Blood Marrow Transplant 2000;6:422–427.
54. Damiani D, Fanin R, Silvestri F, et al. Randomized trial of autologous filgrastim-primed bone marrow transplantation versus filgrastim-mobilized peripheral blood stem cell transplantation in lymphoma patients. Blood 1997;90:36–42.
55. Weisdorf D, Miller J, Verfaillie C, et al. Cytokine-primed bone marrow stem cells vs. peripheral blood stem cells for autologous transplantation: a randomized comparison of GM-CSF vs. G-CSF. Biol Blood Marrow Transplant 1997;3:217–223.
56. Storek J, Gooley T, Siadak M, et al. Allogeneic peripheral blood stem cell transplantation may be associated with a high risk of chronic graft-versus-host disease. Blood 1997;90:4705–4709.
57. Mohty M, Kuentz M, Michallet M, et al. Chronic graft-versus-host disease after allogeneic blood stem cell transplantation: long-term results of a randomized study. Blood 2002;100:3128–3134.
58. Flowers ME, Parker PM, Johnston LJ, et al. Comparison of chronic graft-versus-host disease after transplantation of peripheral blood stem cells versus bone marrow in allogeneic recipients: long-term follow-up of a randomized trial. Blood 2002;100:415–419.
59. Juttner CA, To LB, Ho JQK, et al. Early lympho-hemopoietic recovery after autografting using peripheral blood stem cells in acute non-lymphoblastic leukemia. Transplant Proc 1988;20:40–42.
60. Fermand J-P, Levy Y, Gerota J, et al. Treatment of aggressive multiple myeloma by high-dose chemotherapy and total body irradiation followed by blood stem cells autologous graft. Blood 1989;73:20–23.
61. Brice P, Marolleau JP, Dombret H, et al. Autologous peripheral blood stem cell transplantation after high dose therapy in patients with advanced lymphomas. Bone Marrow Transplant 1992;9:337–342.
62. Welte K, Gabrilove J, Bronchud MH, et al, Filgrastim (r-metHuG-CSF): the first 10 years. Blood 1996;88:1907–1929.
63. Watts MJ, Addison I, Long SG, et al. Crossover study of the haematological effects and pharmacokinetics of glycosylated and non-glycosylated G-CSF in healthy volunteers. Br J Haematol 1997;98:474–479.
64. Hoglund M, Smedmyr B, Bengtsson M, et al. Mobilization of CD34+ cells by glycosylated and nonglycosylated G-CSF in healthy volunteers: A comparison study. Eur J Haematol 1997;59:177–183.
65. Fischer JC, Frick M, Wassmoth R, et al. Superior mobilization of haematopoietic progenitor cells with glycosylated G-CSF in male but not female unrelated stem cell donors. Br J Haematol 2005;130:740–746.
66. De Arriba F, Lozano ML, Ortuño F, et al. Prospective randomized study comparing the efficacy of bioequivalent doses of glycosylated and nonglycosylated rG-CSF for mobilizing peripheral blood progenitor cells. Br J Haematol 1997;96:418–420.
67. Kroschinsky F, Holig K, Poppe-Thiede K, et al. Single-dose pegfilgrastim for the mobilization of allogeneic CD34+ peripheral blood progenitor cells in healthy family and unrelated donors. Haematologica 2005;90:1665–1671.
68. Lane TA, Law P, Maruyama M, et al. Harvesting and enrichment of hematopoietic progenitor cells mobilized into the peripheral blood of normal donors by granulocyte-macrophage colony-stimulating factor (GM-CSF) or G-CSF: Potential role in allogeneic marrow transplantation. Blood 1995;85:275–282.
69. Weaver CH, Schulman KA, Buckner CD. Mobilization of peripheral blood stem cells following myelosuppressive chemotherapy: A randomized comparison of filgrastim, sargramostim, or sequential sargramostim and filgrastim. Bone Marrow Transplant 2001;27(Suppl 2):S23–S29.
70. Tjønnfjord GE, Steen R, Evensen SA, et al. Characterization of CD34+ peripheral blood cells from healthy adults mobilized by recombinant human granulocyte colony-stimulating factor. Blood 1994;84:2795–2801.
71. Grigg AP, Roberts AW, Raunow H, et al. Optimizing dose and scheduling of filgrastim (granulocyte colony-stimulating factor) for mobilization and collection of peripheral blood progenitor cells in normal volunteers. Blood 1995;86:4437–4445.
72. Bishop MR, Tarantolo SR, Jackson JD, et al. Allogeneic-blood stem-cell collection following mobilization with low-dose granulocyte colony-stimulating factor. J Clin Oncol 1997;15:1601–1607.
73. Stroncek DF, Clay ME, Petzoldt ML, et al. Treatment of normal individuals with granulocyte-colony stimulating factor: donor experiences and the effects on peripheral blood CD34+ cell counts and on the collection of peripheral blood stem cells. Transfusion 1996;36:601–610.
74. Weaver CH, Birch R, Greco FA, et al. Mobilization and harvesting of peripheral blood stem cells: randomized evaluations of different doses of filgrastim. Br J Haematol 1998;100:338–347.
75. Waller CF, Bertz H, Wenger MK, et al. Mobilization of peripheral blood progenitor cells for allogeneic transplantation: efficacy and toxicity of a high-dose rhG-CSF regimen. Bone Marrow Transplant 1996;18:279–283.
76. Anderlini P, Donato M, Lauppe MJ, et al. A comparative study of once-daily versus twice-daily filgrastim administration for the mobilization and collection of CD34 peripheral blood progenitor cells in normal donors. Br J Haematol 2000;109:770–772.
77. Kroger N, Renges H, Kruger W, et al. A randomized comparison of once versus twice daily recombinant human granulocyte colony-stimulating factor (filgrastim) for stem cell mobilization in healthy donors for allogeneic transplantation. Br J Haematol 2000;111:761–765.
78. Lee V, Li CK, Shing MM, et al. Single vs. twice daily G-CSF dose for peripheral blood stem cells harvest in normal donors and children with non-malignant diseases. Bone Marrow Transplant 2000;25:931.
79. de la Rubia, Arbone C, de Arriba F, et al. Analysis of factors associated with low peripheral blood progenitor cell collection in normal donors. Transfusion 2002;42:4–9.
80. DeLuca E, Sheridan WP, Watson D, et al. Prior chemotherapy does not prevent effective mobilisation by G-CSF of peripheral blood progenitor cells. Br J Cancer 1992;66:893–899.
81. Anderlini P, Przepiorka D, Seong C, et al. Factors affecting mobilization of CD34+ cells in normal donors treated with filgrastim. Transfusion 1997;37:507–512.
82. Weaver CH, Longin K, Buckner CD, Bensinger W. Lymphocyte content in peripheral blood mononuclear cells collected after the administration of recombinant human granulocyte colony-stimulating factor. Bone Marrow Transplant 1994;13:411–415.
83. Pan L, Delmonte J, Jalonen CK, Ferrara JL. Pretreatment of donors with granulocyte colony-stimulating factor polarizes donor T lymphocytes toward type 2 cytokine production and reduces severity of experimental graft versus host disease. Blood 1995;86:4422–4429.
84. Zeng D, Dejbakhsh-Jones S, Strober S. Granulocyte colony-stimulating factor reduces the capacity of blood mononuclear cells to induce graft-versus-host disease: Impact on blood progenitor cell transplantation. Blood 1997;90:453–463.
85. Glass B, Uharek L, Zeis M, et al. Allogeneic peripheral blood progenitor cell transplantation in a murine model: evidence for an improved graft-versus-leukemia effect. Blood 1997;90:1694–1700.
86. Anderlini P, Przepiorka D, Seong D, et al. Clinical toxicity and laboratory effects of granulocyte-colony-stimulating factor (filgrastim) mobilization and blood stem cell apheresis from normal donors, and analysis of charges for the procedure. Transfusion 1996;36:590–595.
87. Akizuki S, Mizorogi F, Inoue T, et al. Pharmacokinetics and adverse events following 5-day repeated administration of lenograstim, a recombinant human granulocyte colony-stimulating factor, in healthy subjects. Bone Marrow Transplant 2000;26:939–946.
88. Anderlini P, Korbling M, Dale D, et al. Allogeneic blood stem cell transplantation: considerations for donors. Blood 1997;90:903–908.
89. Becker PS, Wagle M, Matous S, et al. Spontaneous splenic rupture following administration of granulocyte colony-stimulating factor (G-CSF): occurrence in an allogeneic donor of peripheral blood stem cells. Biol Blood Marrow Transplant 1997;3:45–49.
90. Platzbecker U, Prange-Krex G, Bornhauser M, et al. Spleen enlargement in healthy donors during G-CSF mobilization of PBPCs. Transfusion 2001;41:184–189.
91. Sohngen D, Wienen S, Siebler, et al. Analysis of rhG-CSF on platelets by in vitro bleeding test and transcranial Doppler ultrasound examination. Bond Marrow Transplant 1998;22:1087–1090.
92. LeBlanc R, Roy J, Demers C, et al. A prospective study of G-CSF effects on hemostasis in allogeneic blood stem cell donors. Bone Marrow Transplant 1999;23:991–996.
93. Snowden JA, Biggs JC, Milliken ST, et al. A randomize, blinded, placebo-controlled, dose escalation study of the tolerability and efficacy of filgrastim for haemopoietic stem cell mobilization in patients with severe active rheumatoid arthritis. Bone Marrow Transplant 1998;22:1035–1041.
94. Parkkali T, Volin L, Siren MJ, et al. Acute iritis induced by granulocyte colony-stimulating factor used for mobilization in a volunteer

unrelated peripheral blood progenitor cell donor. Bone Marrow Transplant 1996;1:433–434.
95. Huhn RD, Yurkow EJ, Tushinski R, et al. Recombinant human interleukin-3 (rhIL-3) enhances the mobilization of peripheral blood progenitor cells by recombinant granulocyte colony-stimulating factor (rhG-CSF) in normal volunteers. Exp Hematol 1996;24:839–847.
96. Salloum E, Stoessel KM, Cooper DL. Hyperleukocytosis and retinal hemorrhages after chemotherapy and filgrastim administration for peripheral blood progenitor cell mobilization. Bone Marrow Transplant 1998;21:835–837.
97. Esmaeli B, Ahmadi M, Kim S, et al. Marginal keratitis associated with administration of filgrastim and sargramostim in a healthy peripheral blood progenitor cell donor. Cornea 2002;21:621–622.
98. Siena S, Bregni M, Brando B, et al. Circulation of CD34+ hematopoietic stem cells in the peripheral blood of high-dose cyclophosphamide-treated patients: enhancement by intravenous recombinant granulocyte-macrophage colony-stimulating factor. Blood 1989;74:1905–1914.
99. Socinski MA, Cannistra SA, Elias A, et al. Granulocyte-macrophage colony stimulating factor expands the circulating haemopoietic progenitor cell compartment in man. Lancet 1988;1:1194–1198.
100. Alegre A, Tomás JF, Martínez-Chamorro C, et al. Comparison of peripheral blood progenitor cell mobilization in patients with multiple myeloma: high-dose cyclophosphamide plus GM-CSF vs. G-CSF alone. Bone Marrow Transplant 1997;20:211–217.
101. Haas R, Ho AD, Bredthauer U, et al. Successful autologous transplantation of blood stem cells mobilized with recombinant human granulocyte-macrophage colony-stimulating factor. Exp Hematol 1990;18:94–98.
102. Villeval J-L, Dührsen U, Morstyn G, Metcalf D. Effect of recombinant human granulocyte-macrophage colony stimulating factor on progenitor cells in patients with advanced malignancies. Br J Haematol 1990;74:36–44.
103. Weaver CH, Schulman KA, Wilson-Relyea G, et al. Randomized trial of filgrastim, sargramostim, or sequential sargramostim and filgrastim after myelosuppressive chemotherapy for the harvesting of peripheral-blood stem cells. J Clin Oncol 2000;18:43–53.
104. Devine SM, Brown RA, Mathews V, et al. Reduced risk of acute GvHD following mobilization of HLA-identical sibling donors with GM-CSF alone. Bone Marrow Transplant 2005;36:531–538.
105. Lieschke GJ, Maher D, Cebon J, et al. Effects of bacterially synthesized recombinant human granulocyte-macrophage colony-stimulating factor in patients with advanced malignancy. Ann Intern Med 1989;110:357–364.
106. Lieschke GJ, Burgess AW. Granulocyte colony-stimulating factor and granulocyte-macrophage colony-stimulating factor (first of two parts). N Engl J Med 1992;327:28–35.
107. Lieschke GJ, Maher D, O'Connor M, et al. Phase I study of intravenously administered bacterially synthesized granulocyte-macrophage colony-stimulating factor and comparison with subcutaneous administration. Cancer Res 1990;50:606–614.
108. Eto T, Takamatasu Y, Harada M, et al. Effects of macrophage colony-stimulating factor (M-CSF) on the mobilization of peripheral blood stem cells. Bone Marrow Transplant 1994;13:125–129.
109. Pettengell R, Woll PJ, Chang J, et al. Effects of erythropoietin on mobilisation of haemopoietic progenitor cells. Bone Marrow Transplant 1994;14:125–130.
110. Ganser A, Lindemann A, Ottmann OG, et al. Sequential in vivo treatment with two recombinant human hematopoietic growth factors (interleukin-3 and granulocyte-macrophage colony-stimulating factor) as a new therapeutic modality to stimulate hematopoiesis: Results of a phase I study. Blood 1992;79:2583–2591.
111. Brugger W, Bross K, Frisch J, et al. Mobilization of peripheral blood progenitor cells by sequential administration of interleukin-3 and granulocyte-macrophage colony-stimulating factor following polychemotherapy with etoposide, ifosfamide, and cisplatin. Blood 1992; 79:1193–1200.
112. Geissler K, Peschel C, Niederwieser D, et al. Potentiation of granulocyte colony-stimulating factor-induced mobilization of circulating progenitor cells by seven-day pretreatment with interleukin-3. Blood 1996;87:27–32.
113. Geissler K, Valent P, Mayer P, et al. Recombinant human interleukin-3 expands the pool of circulating hematopoietic progenitor cells in primates-synergism with recombinant human granulocyte/macrophage colony-stimulating factor. Blood 1990;75:2305–2310.
114. Bishop MR, Jackson JD, O'Kane-Murphy B, et al. Phase I trial of recombinant fusion protein PIXY 321 for mobilization of peripheral-blood stem cells. J Clin Oncol 1996;14:2521–2526.
115. Demetri GD, Gordon M, Horrman R, et al. Effects of recombinant methionyl human stem cell factor on hematopoietic progenitor cells in vivo: Preliminary results from a phase I trial [Abstract]. Proc Am Assoc Cancer Res 1993;34:217.
116. Kurtzberg J, Meyers F, McGuire B, Crawford J. Mobilization of peripheral blood progenitor cells in patients given recombinant methionyl human stem cell factor [Abstract]. Proc Am Assoc Cancer Res 1993;34:211.
117. Crawford J, Lau D, Erwin R, et al. A phase I trial of recombinant human stem cell factor (SCF) in patients with advanced non-small cell carcinoma [Abstract]. Proc Am Soc Clin Oncol 1993;12:135.
118. Demetri G, Costa J, Hayes D, et al. A phase I trial of recombinant methionyl human stem cell factor (SCF) in patients with advanced breast carcinoma pre- and post-chemotherapy (chemo) with cyclophosphamide (C) and doxorubicin (A) [Abstract]. Proc Am Soc Clin Oncol 1993;12:142.
119. Winter JN, Lazarus HM, Rademaker A, et al. Phase I/II study of combined granulocyte colony-stimulating factor and granulocyte-macrophage colony-stimulating factor administration for the mobilization of hematopoietic progenitor cells. J Clin Oncol 1996;14:277–286.
120. Ho AD, Young D, Maruyama M, et al. Pluripotent and lineage-committed CD34+ subsets in leukapheresis products mobilized by G-CSF, GM-CSF vs. a combination of both. Exp Hematol 1996;24:1460–1468.
121. Sohn SK, Kim JG, Seo KW, et al. GM-CSF based mobilization effect in normal healthy donors for allogeneic peripheral blood stem cell transplantation. Bone Marrow Transplant 2002;30:81–86.
122. Lonial S, Hicks M, Rosenthal H, et al. A randomized trial comparing the combination of granulocyte-macrophage colony-stimulating factor plus granulocyte colony-stimulating factor versus granulocyte colony-stimulating factor for mobilization of dendritic cell subsets in hematopoietic progenitor cell products. Biol Blood Marrow Transplant 2004;10:848–857.
123. Ganser A, Lindemann A, Ottmann OG, et al. Sequential in vivo treatment with two recombinant human hematopoietic growth factors (interleukin-3 and granulocyte-macrophage colony-stimulating factor) as a new therapeutic modality to stimulate hematopoiesis: Results of a phase I study. Blood 1992;79:2583–2591.
124. de Revel T, Appelbaum FR, Storb R, et al. Effects of granulocyte colony-stimulating factor and stem cell factor, alone and in combination, on the mobilization of peripheral blood cells that engraft lethally irradiated dogs. Blood 1994;83:3795–3799.
125. Andrews RG, Briddell RA, Knitter GH, et al. In vivo synergy between recombinant human stem cell factor and recombinant human granulocyte colony-stimulating factor in baboons: Enhanced circulation of progenitor cells. Blood 1994;84:800–810.
126. Moskowitz CH, Stiff P, Gordon MS, et al. Recombinant methionyl human stem cell factor and filgrastim for peripheral blood progenitor cell mobilization and transplantation in non-Hodgkin's lymphoma patients: Results of a phase I/II trial. Blood 1997;89:3136–3147.
127. Begley CG, Basser R, Mansfield R, et al. Enhanced levels and enhanced clonogenic capacity of blood progenitor cells following administration of stem cell factor plus granulocyte colony-stimulating factor to humans. Blood 1997;90:3378–3389.
128. Dipersio JF, Schuster MW, Abboud CN, et al. Mobilization of peripheral blood stem cells by concurrent administration of daniplestin and granulocyte colony-stimulating factor in patients with breast cancer or lymphoma. J Clin Oncol 2000;18:2761–2771.
129. Weaver A, Ryder D, Crowther D, et al. Increased numbers of long-term culture-initiating cells in the apheresis product of patients randomized to receive increasing doses of stem cell factor administered in combination with chemotherapy and a standard dose of granulocyte colony-stimulating factor. Blood 1996;88:3323–3328.
130. Somlo G, Sniecinski I, ter Veer A, et al. Recombinant human thrombopoietin in combination with granulocyte colony-stimulating factor enhances mobilization of peripheral blood progenitor cells, increases peripheral blood platelet concentration, and accelerates hematopoietic recovery following high-dose chemotherapy. Blood 1999;93:2798–2806.
131. Goldman SC, Bracho F, Davenport V, et al. Feasibility study of IL-11 and granulocyte colony-stimulating factor after myelosuppressive chemotherapy to mobilize peripheral blood stem cells from heavily pretreated patients J Pediatr Hematol/Oncol 2001;23:300–305.
132. Olivieri A, Offidani M, Ciniero L, et al. Addition of erythropoietin to granulocyte colony-stimulating factor after priming chemotherapy enhances hemopoietic progenitor mobilization. Bone Marrow Transplant 1995;16:765–770.
133. Pierilli L, Perillo A, Greggi S, et al. Erythropoietin addition to granulocyte colony-stimulating factor abrogates life-threatening neutropenia and increases peripheral blood progenitor cell mobilization after epirubicin, paclitaxel, and cisplatin combination chemotherapy: results of a randomized comparison. J Clin Oncol 1999;17:1288.

134. Sautois B, Baudoux E, Salmon JP, et al. Administration of erythropoietin and granulocyte colony-stimulating factor in donor/recipient pairs to collect peripheral blood progenitor cells (PBSC) and red cell units for use in the recipient after allogeneic PBSC transplantation. Haematologica 2001;86:1209–1218.
135. Demirer T, Buckner CD, Gooley T, et al. Factors influencing collection of peripheral blood stem cells in patients with multiple myeloma. Bone Marrow Transplant 1996;17:937–941.
136. Narayanasami U, Kanteti R, Morelli J, et al. Randomized trial of filgrastim versus chemotherapy and filgrastim mobilization of hematopoietic progenitor cells for rescue in autologous transplantation. Blood 2001;98:2059–2064.
137. Koc ON, Gerson SL, Cooper BW, et al. Randomized cross-over trial of progenitor-cell mobilization: High-dose cyclophosphamide plus granulocyte-colony stimulating factor 9G-CSF) vs. granulocyte-macrophage colony-stimulating factor plus G-CSF. J Clin Oncol 2000;18:1824–1830.
138. Schwartzberg LS, Birch R, Hazelton B, et al. Peripheral blood stem cell mobilization by chemotherapy with and without recombinant human granulocyte colony-stimulating factor. J Hematother 1992;1:317–327.
139. Demirer T, Buckner CD, Storer B, et al. Effect of different chemotherapy regimens on peripheral-blood stem-cell collections in patients with breast cancer receiving granulocyte colony-stimulating factor. J Clin Oncol 1997;15:684–690.
140. Zlotnik A, Yoshie O. Chemokines: A new classification system and their role in immunity. Immunity 2000;12:121–127.
141. Murphy PM. Chemokine receptors: structure, function and role in microbial pathogenesis. Cytokines Growth Factor Rev 1996;7:47–64.
142. Pelus LM, Horowitz D, Cooper SC, King AG. Peripheral blood stem cell mobilization: a role for CXC chemokines. Crit Rev Oncol/Hematol 2002;43:257–275.
143. Auiuti A, Web IJ, Bleul C, et al. The chemokine SDF-1 is a chemoattractant for human CD 34+ hematopoietic progenitor cells and provides a new mechanism to explain the mobilization of CD 34+ progenitors to peripheral blood. J Exp Med 1997;185:111–120
144. Ratajczak MZ, Kucia M, Recca R, et al. Stem cell plasticity revisited: CCXR4-positive cell expressing mRNA for muscle, liver and neural cells "hide out" in the bone marrow. Leukemia 2004;18:29–40.
145. Pelus LM, Bian H, Fukuda S, et al. The CCXR4 agonist peptide, CTCE-0021 rapidly mobilizes polymorphonuclear neutrophils and hematopoietic progenitor cells into peripheral blood and synergizes with granulocyte colony stimulating factor. Exp Hematol 2005;33:295–307.
146. Brxmeyer HE, Orschell CM, Clapp DW, et al. Rapid mobilization of murine and human hematopoietic stem cells with AMD3100, a CXCR4 antagonist. J Exp Med 2005;201:1307–1318.
147. Flomenberg N, DiPersio J Calandra G. Role of CCXR4 chemokine receptor blockade using AMD3100 for mobilization of autologous hematopoietic progenitor cells. Acta Haematol 2005;114:198–205.
148. Flomenberg N, Devine SM, DiPersoio JF, et al. The use of AMD3100 plus G-CSF for autologous hematopoietic progenitor cell mobilization is superior to G-CSF alone. Blood 2005;106:1867–1874.
149. Devine SM, Bonde J, Hess DA, et al. A pilot study evaluating the safety and efficacy of AMD1300 for the mobilization and transplantation of HLA-matched sibling donor hematopoietic stem cells in patients with advanced hematological malignancies [Abstract]. Blood 2004;104:913a.
150. King AG, Horowitz D, Dillon SB, et al. Rapid mobilization of murine hematopoietic stem cells with enhanced engraftment properties and evaluation of hematopoietic progenitor cell mobilization in rhesus monkeys by a single injection of SB-251353, a specific truncated form of the human CXC chemokine GRObeta. Blood 2001;97:1534.
151. King AG, Johanson K, Frey CA, et al. Identification of unique truncated KC/GROβ chemokines with potent hematopoietic and anti-infective activities. J Immunol 2000;164:3774–3782.
152. Pruijt JF, van Kooyk Y, Figdor CG, et al. Anti-LFA-1 blocking antibodies prevent mobilization of hematopoietic progenitor cells induced by interleukin-8. Blood 1998;91:4099–4105.
153. Watanabe T, Kawano Y, Kanamaru S, et al. Endogenous interleukini-8 (IL-8) surge in granulocyte colony-stimulating factor-induced peripheral blood stem cell mobilization. Blood 1999;93:1157–1163.
154. Fukuda S, Broxmeyer HE, Pelus LM. Flt3 ligand and the Flt3 receptor regulate hematopoietic cell migration by modulating the SDF-1α(CXCL 12)/CXCR4 axis. Blood 2005;105:3227–3126–831.
155. Bensinger WI, Longin K, Appelbaum F, et al. Peripheral blood stem cells (PBSCs) collected after recombinant granulocyte colony stimulating factor (rhG-CSF): an analysis of factors correlating with the tempo of engraftment after transplantation. Br J Haematol 1994;87:825–831.
156. Haas R, Möhle R, Frühauf S, et al. Patient characteristics associated with successful mobilizing and autografting of peripheral blood progenitor cells in malignant lymphoma. Blood 1994;83:3787–3794.
157. Tricot G, Jagannath S, Vesole D, et al. Peripheral blood stem cell transplants for multiple myeloma: Identification of favorable variables for rapid engraftment in 225 patients. Blood 1995;85:588–596.
158. Weaver CH, Schwartzberg LS, Birch R, et al. Collection of peripheral blood progenitor cells after the administration of cyclophosphamide, etoposide, and granulocyte-colony-stimulating factor: an analysis of 497 patients. Transfusion 1997;37:896–903.
159. Dreger P, Klöss M, Petersen B, et al. Autologous progenitor cell transplantation: Prior exposure to stem cell-toxic drugs determines yield and engraftment of peripheral blood progenitor cell but not of bone marrow grafts. Blood 1995;86:3970–3978.
160. Singhal S, Mehta J, Desikan K, et al. Collection of peripheral blood stem cells after a preceding autograft: unfavorable effect of prior interferon-alpha therapy. Bone Marrow Transplant 1999;24:13–17.
161. Visani G, Lemoli RM, Tosi CL, et al. Fludarabine-containing regimens severely impair peripheral blood stem cell mobilization and collection in acute myeloid leukemia patients. Br J Haematol 1999;105:775–779.
162. Boccadoro M, Palumbo A, Bringhen S, et al. Oral melphalan at diagnosis hampers adequate collection of peripheral blood progenitor cells in multiple myeloma. Haematologica 2002;87:846–850.
163. Fraipont V, Sautois B, Baadoux E, et al: Successful mobilization of peripheral blood HPCs with G-CSF alone in patients failing to achieve sufficient numbers of CD34 cells and/or CFU-GM with chemotherapy and G-CSF. Transfusion 2000;40:339–347.
164. Goterris R, Hernandez-Boluda JC, Teruel A, et al. Impact of different strategies of second-line stem cell harvest on the outcome of autologous transplantation in poor peripheral blood stem cell mobilizers. Bone Marrow Transplant 2005;36:847–853.
165. Carlo-Stella C, Di Nicola M, Limani R, et al. Use of recombinant human growth hormone (rhGH) plus recombinant human granulocyte colony-stimulating factor (rhG-CSF) for the mobilization and collection of CD34+ cells in poor mobilizers. Blood 2004;103:3287–3295.
166. Watts MJ, Sullivan AM, Leverett D, et al. Back-up bone marrow is frequently ineffective in patients with poor peripheral-blood stem-cell mobilization. J Clin Oncol 1998;16:1554–1560.
167. Weaver CH, Potz J, Redmond J, et al. Engraftment and outcomes of patients receiving myeloablative therapy followed by autologous peripheral blood stem cells with a low CD34+ cell content. Bone Marrow Transplant 1997;19:1103–1110.
168. Attarian H, Feng Z, Buckner CD, et al. Long-term cryopreservation of bone marrow for autologous transplantation. Bone Marrow Transplant 1996;17:425–430.
169. Passos-Coelho JL, Braine HG, Wright SK, et al. Large-volume leukapheresis using regional citrate anticoagulation to collect peripheral blood progenitor cells. J Hematother 1995;4:11–19.
170. Comenzo RL, Malachowski ME, Miller KB, et al. Large-volume leukapheresis for collection of mononuclear cells for hematopoietic rescue in Hodgkin's disease. Transfusion 1995;35:42–45.
171. Hillyer CD, Tiegerman KO, Berkman EM. Increase in circulating colony-forming units-granulocyte-macrophage during large-volume leukapheresis: Evaluation of a new cell separator. Transfusion 1991;31:327–332.
172. Malachowski ME, Comenzo RL, Hillyer CD, et al. Large-volume leukapheresis for peripheral blood stem cell collection in patients with hematologic malignancies. Transfusion 1992;32:732–735.
173. Comenzo RL, Vosburgh E, Weintraub LR, et al. Collection of mobilized blood progenitor cells for hematopoietic rescue by large-volume leukapheresis. Transfusion 1995;35:493–497.
174. Murea S, Goldschmidt H, Hahn U, et al. Successful collection and transplantation of peripheral blood stem cells in cancer patients using large-volume leukaphereses. J Clin Apheresis 1996;11:185–194.
175. Hillyer CD, Lackey DA, Hart KK, et al. CD34+ progenitors and colony-forming units-granulocyte macrophage are recruited during large-volume leukapheresis and concentrated by counterflow centrifugal elutriation. Transfusion 1993;33:316–321.
176. Passos-Coelho JL, Braine HG, Davis JM, et al. Predictive factors for peripheral-blood progenitor-cell collections using a single large-volume leukapheresis after cyclophosphamide and granulocyte-macrophage colony-stimulating factor mobilization. J Clin Oncol 1995;13:705–714.
177. Kobbe G, Soehngen D, Heyll A, et al. Large volume leukapheresis maximizes the progenitor cell yield for allogeneic peripheral blood progenitor donation. J Hematother 1997;6:125–131.
178. Cull G, Ivey J, Chase P, et al. Collection and recruitment of CD34+ cells during large-volume leukapheresis. J Hematother 1997;6:309–314.
179. Gorlin JB, Vamvakas EC, Cooke E, et al. Large-volume leukapheresis in pediatric patients: processing more blood diminished the apparent magnitude of intra-apheresis recruitment. Transfusion 1996;36:879–885.

180. Rowley SD, Yu J, Heimfeld S, et al. Trafficking of CD34+ cells into the peripheral circulation during collection of peripheral blood stem cells by apheresis. Bone Marrow Transplant 2001;28:649–656.
181. Bensinger W, Appelbaum F, Rowley S, et al. Factors that influence collection and engraftment of autologous peripheral-blood stem cells. J Clin Oncol 1995;13:2547–2555.
182. Weaver CH, Hazelton B, Birch R, et al. An analysis of engraftment kinetics as a function of the CD34 content of peripheral blood progenitor cell collections in 692 patients after the administration of myeloablative chemotherapy. Blood 1995;86:3961–3969.
183. Spitzer G, Adkins DR, Spencer V, et al. Randomized study of growth factors post-peripheral-blood stem-cell transplant: neutrophil recovery is improved with modest clinical benefit. J Clin Oncol 1994;12:661–670.
184. Shimazaki C, Oku N, Uchiyama H, et al. Effect of granulocyte colony-stimulating factor on hematopoietic recovery after peripheral blood progenitor cell transplantation. Bone Marrow Transplant 1994; 13:271–275.
185. Klumpp TR, Mangan KF, Goldberg SL, et al. Granulocyte colony-stimulating factor accelerates neutrophil engraftment following peripheral-blood stem-cell transplantation: a prospective randomized trial. J Clin Oncol 1995;13:1323–1327.
186. Schwella N, Beyer J, Schwaner I, et al. Impact of preleukapheresis cell counts on collection results and correlation of progenitor-cell dose with engraftment after high-dose chemotherapy in patients with germ cell cancer. J Clin Oncol 1996;14:1114–1121.
187. Bensinger W, Rowley S, Longin K, et al. Peripheral blood mononuclear cells (PBMCs) collected after recombinant granulocyte colony stimulating factor (rhG-CSF): Number of CD34+ cells infused correlate with platelet recovery after transplantation. Exp Hematol 1993;21:1149.
188. Singhal S, Powles R, Treleaven J, et al. A low CD34+ cell dose results in higher mortality and poorer survival after blood or marrow stem cell transplantation from HLA-identical siblings: should 2×10^6 CD34+ cells/kg be considered the minimum threshold? Bone Marrow Transplant 2000;26:489–496.
189. Krieger MS, Schiller G, Berenson JR, et al. Collection of peripheral blood progenitor cells based on a rising WBC and platelet count significantly increases the number of CD34 cells. Bone Marrow Transplant 1999;24:25–28.
190. Schots R, Van Riet I, Damiaens S, et al. The absolute number of circulating CD34+ cells predicts the number of hematopoietic stem cells that can be collected by apheresis. Bone Marrow Transplant 1996;17:509–515.
191. Elliott C, Samson DM, Armitage S, et al. When to harvest peripheral-blood stem cells after mobilization therapy: prediction of CD34-postive cell yield by preceding day CD34-positive concentration in peripheral blood. J Clin Oncol 1996;14:970–973.
192. Beelen DW, Ottinger H, Kolbe K, et al. Filgrastim mobilization and collection of allogeneic blood progenitor cells from adult family donors: first interim report of a prospective German multicenter study. Ann Hematol 2002;81:701–709.
193. Anderlini P, Przepiorka D, Lauppe J, et al. Collection of peripheral blood stem cells from normal donors 60 years of age or older. Br J Haematol 1997;97:485–487.
194. Sutton DMC, Nair RC, Rock G. The Canadian Apheresis Study Group: complications of plasma exchange. Transfusion 1989;29:124–127.
195. Owen HG, Brecher ME. Atypical reactions associated with use of angiotensin-converting enzyme inhibitors and apheresis. Transfusion 1994;34:891–894.
196. Leitman SF, Boltansky H, Alter JH, et al. Allergic reactions in healthy plateletpheresis donors caused by sensitization to ethylene oxide gas. N Engl J Med 1986;315:1192–1196.
197. Goldberg SL, Mangan KF, Klumpp TR, et al. Complications of peripheral blood stem cell harvesting: review of 554 PBSC leukaphereses. J Hematother 1995;4:85–90.
198. Rowley SD, Donaldson G, Lilleby K, et al. Experiences of donors enrolled in a randomized study of allogeneic bone marrow or peripheral blood stem cell transplantation. Blood 2001;97:2541–2548.
199. Fortanier C, Kuentz M, Sutton L, et al. Healthy sibling donor anxiety and pain during bone marrow or peripheral blood stem cell harvesting for allogeneic transplantation: results of a randomised study. Bone Marrow Transplant 2002;29:145–149.
200. Switzer GE, Goycoolea JM, Dew MA, et al. Donating stimulated peripheral blood stem cells vs bone marrow: do donors experience the procedures differently? Bone Marrow Transplant 2001;27:917–923.
201. Reddy RL. Mobilization and collection of peripheral blood progenitor cells for transplantation. Trans Apheresis Sci 2005;32:63–72.
202. Grishaber JE, Cunningham MC, Rohret PA, Strauss RG. Analysis of venous access for therapeutic plasma exchange in patients with neurological disease. J Clin Apheresis 1992;7:119–123.
203. Alegre A, Requena MJ, Fernández-Villalta MJ, et al. Quinton-mahurkar catheter as short-term central venous access for PBSC collection: single-center experience of 370 aphereses in 110 patients. Bone Marrow Transplant 1996;18:865-869.
204. Lazarus HM, Trehan S, Miller R, et al. Multi-purpose Silastic dual-lumen central venous catheters for both collection and transplantation of hematopoietic progenitor cells. Bone Marrow Transplant 2000;25:779–785.
205. Madero L, Diaz MA, Benito A, et al. Non-tunneled catheters for the collection and transplantation of peripheral blood stem cells in children. Bone Marrow Transplant 1997;20:53–56.
206. Stephans LC, Haire WD, Schmit-Pokorny K, et al. Granulocyte macrophage colony stimulating factor: high incidence of apheresis catheter thrombosis during peripheral stem cell collection. Bone Marrow Transplant 1993;11:51–54.
207. Canales MA, Arrieta R, Gomez-Rioja R, et al. Induction of a hypercoagulability state and endothelial cell activation by granulocyte colony-stimulating factor in peripheral blood stem cell donors. J Hematother Stem Cell Res 2002;11:675–681.
208. Bern MM, Lokich JJ, Wallach SR, et al. Very low doses of warfarin can prevent thrombosis in central venous catheters: a randomized prospective trial. Ann Intern Med 1990;112:423–428.
209. Stephens L, Haire W, Tarantolo S, et al. Normal saline versus heparin flush for maintaining central venous catheter patency during apheresis collection of peripheral blood stem cells. Transfus Sci 1997;18:187–193.
210. Dzik WH, Kirkley SA. Citrate toxicity during massive blood transfusion. Transfus Med Rev 1988;2:76–94.
211. Strauss RG. Mechanisms of adverse effects during hemapheresis. J Clin Apheresis 1996;11:160–164.
212. Bolan C, Cecco S, Wesley R, et al. Controlled study of citrate effects and response to IV calcium administration during allogeneic peripheral blood progenitor cell donation. Transfusion 2002;42:935–946.
213. Huestis DW. Risks and safety practices in hemapheresis procedures. Arch Pathol Lab Med 1989;113:273–278.
214. Gorlin JB, Humphreys D, Kent P, et al. Pediatric large volume peripheral blood progenitor cell collections from patients under 25 kg: A primer. J Clin Apheresis 1996;11:195–203.
215. Buchta C, Macher M, Bieglmeyer C, et al. Reduction of adverse reactions during autologous large volume PBPC apheresis by continuous infusion of calcium gluconate. Transfusion 2003;43:1615–1621.
216. O'Donnell MR. Blood group incompatibilities and hemolytic complications of hematopoietic cell transplantation. In Forman SJ, Blume KG, Thomas ED (eds). Thomas' Hematopoietic Cell Transplantation, 3rd ed. Malden, Blackwell Publishing, 2004, pp 824–832.
217. Braine HG, Sensenbrenner LL, Wright SK, et al. Bone marrow transplantation with major ABO blood group incompatibility using erythrocyte depletion of marrow prior to infusion. Blood 1982;60:420–425.
218. Bolan CD, Childs RW, Procter JL, et al. Massive immune haemolysis after allogeneic peripheral blood stem cell transplantation with minor ABO incompatibility. Br J Haematol 2001;112:787–795.
219. Rowley SD, Liang PS, Ulz L. Transplantation of ABO-incompatible bone marrow and peripheral blood stem cell components. Bone Marrow Transplant 2000;26:749–757.
220. Buckhalter R, Watkins K, Ericson SG. Inverted spin method for removing RBCs from BM buffy coat products. Cytotherapy 2003;5:553–557.
221. Montuoro A, De Rosa L, Del Monte C, et al. A technique for isolation of bone marrow cells using hydroxyethyl starch (HES) sedimentation agent. Haematologica 1991;76(Suppl 1):7–9.
222. Hester JP, Rondon G, Huh YO, et al. Principles of bone marrow processing and progenitor cell/mononuclear cell concentrate collection in a continuous flow blood cell separation system. J Hematother 1995;4:299–306.
223. Cassens U, Ostkamp-Ostermann P, Garritsen H, et al. Efficacy and kinetics of bone marrow processing and enrichment of haematopoietic progenitor cells (HPC) by a large-volume apheresis procedure. Bone Marrow Transplant 1997;19:835–840.
224. Brenner MK, Rill DR, Moen RC, et al. Gene-marking to trace origin of relapse after autologous bone-marrow transplantation. Lancet 1993; 341:85–86.
225. Rill DR, Santana VM, Roberts WM, et al. Direct demonstration that autologous bone marrow transplantation for solid tumors can return a multiplicity of tumorigenic cells. Blood 1994;84:380–383.
226. Deisseroth AB, Zu Zhifei, Claxton D, et al. Genetic marking shows that Ph+ cells present in autologous transplants of chronic myelogenous leukemia (CML) contribute to relapse after autologous bone marrow in CML. Blood 1994;83:30–68.
227. van Besien K, Loberiza F, Balorunaite R, et al. Comparison of autologous and allogeneic hematopoietic stem cell transplantation for follicular lymphoma. Blood 2003;102:3521–3529.

228. Bierman P, Sweeten ham J, Loberiza F, et al, Lymphoma Working committee of the International Bone marrow Transplant Registry and the European Group for Blood and Marrow Transplantation. Syngeneic hematopoietic stem cell transplantation for non-Hodgkin's lymphoma: A comparison with allogeneic and autologous transplantation. J Clin Oncol 2003;21:3744–3753.
229. Ross AA, Cooper BW, Lazarus HM, et al. Detection and viability of tumor cells in peripheral blood stem cell collections from breast cancer patients using immunocytochemical and clonogenic assay techniques. Blood 1993;82:2605–2610.
230. Moss TJ, Cairo M, Santana VM, et al. Clonogenicity of circulating neuroblastoma cells: implications regarding peripheral blood stem cell transplantation. Blood 1994;83:3085–3089.
231. Mariette X, Fermand J.-P, Brouet J-C. Myeloma cell contamination of peripheral blood stem cell grafts in patients with multiple myeloma treated by high-dose therapy. Bone Marrow Transplant 1994;14:47–50.
232. Gertz JA, Witzig TE, Pineda AA, et al. Monoclonal plasma cells in the blood stem cell harvest from patients with multiple myeloma are associated with shortened relapse-free survival after transplantation. Bone Marrow Transplant 1997;19:337–342.
233. Sharp JG, Kessinger A, Mann S, et al. Outcome of high-dose therapy and autologous transplantation in non-Hodgkin's lymphoma based on the presence of tumor in the marrow or infused hematopoietic harvest. J Clin Oncol 1996;14:214–219.
234. Brugger W, Bross KJ, Glatt M, et al. Mobilization of tumor cells and hematopoietic progenitor cells into peripheral blood of patients with solid tumors. Blood 1994;83:636–640.
235. Pecora AL, Lazarus HM, Jennis AA, et al. Breast cancer cell contamination of blood stem cell products in patients with metastatic breast cancer: predictors and clinical relevance. Biol Blood Marrow Transplant 2002;8:536–543.
236. Passos-Coelho JL, Ross AA, Kahn DJ, et al. Similar breast cancer cell contamination of single-day peripheral-blood progenitor-cell collections obtained after priming with hematopoietic growth factor alone or after cyclophosphamide followed by growth factor. J Clin Oncol 1996;14:2569–2575.
237. Moss TJ, Sanders DG, Lasky LC, Bostrom B. Contamination of peripheral blood stem cell harvests by circulating neuroblastoma cells. Blood 1990;76:1879–1883.
238. van Heeckeren WJ, Vollweiler J, Fu P, et al. Randomised comparison of two B-cell purging protocols for patients with B-cell non-Hodgkin lymphoma: in vivo purging with rituximab versus ex vivo purging with CliniMACS CD34+ cell enrichment device. Br J Haematol 2005;132:42–55.
239. Link H, Aseniev L, Bahre O, et al. Transplantation of allogeneic CD34+ blood cells. Blood 1996;87:4903–4909.
240. Bensinger WI, Buckner CD, Shannon-Dorcy K, et al. Transplantation of allogeneic CD34+ peripheral blood stem cells in patients with advanced hematologic malignancy. Blood 1996;88:4132–4138.
241. Finke J, Brugger W, Bertz H, et al. Allogeneic transplantation of positively selected peripheral blood CD34+ progenitor cells form matched related donors. Bone Marrow Transplant 1996;18:1081–1086.
242. Urbano-Ispizua A, Roxman C, Martinez C, et al. Rapid engraftment without significant graft-versus-host disease after allogeneic transplantation of CD34+ selected cells from peripheral blood. Blood 1997;89:3967–3973.
243. Schiller G, Vescio R, Freytes C, et al. Transplantation of CD34+ peripheral blood progenitor cells after high-dose chemotherapy for patients with advanced multiple myeloma. Blood 1995;86:390–397.
244. Shpall EJ, Jones RB, Bearman SI, et al. Transplantation of enriched CD34-positive autologous marrow into breast cancer patients following high-dose chemotherapy: influence of CD34-positive peripheral-blood progenitors and growth factors on engraftment. J Clin Oncol 1994;12:28–36.
245. McQuaker IG, Haynes AP, Anderson S, et al. Engraftment and molecular monitoring of CD34+ peripheral-blood stem-cell transplants for follicular lymphoma: a pilot study. J Clin Oncol 1997;15:2288–2295.
246. Lemoli RM, Fortuna A, Motta MR, et al. Concomitant mobilization of plasma cells and hematopoietic progenitors into peripheral blood of multiple myeloma patients: Positive selection and transplantation of enriched CD34+ cells to remove circulating tumor cells. Blood 1996;87:1625–1634.
247. Vescio R, Schiller G, Stewart AK, et al. Multicenter phase III trial to evaluate CD34+ selected versus unselected autologous peripheral blood progenitor cell transplantation in multiple myeloma. Blood 1999;93:1858–1868.
248. Altes A, Sierra J, Esteve J, et al. CD34+ enriched CD19 depleted autologous peripheral blood stem cell transplantation for chronic lymphoproliferative disorders: high purging efficacy but increased risk of severe infections. Exp Hematol 2002;30:824–830.
249. Feller N, van der Pol MA, Waaijman T, et al. Immunological purging of autologous peripheral blood stem cell products based on CD34 and CD133 expression can be effectively and safely applied in half of the acute myeloid leukemia patients. Clin Cancer Res 2005;11:4793–4801.
250. Stewart AK, Vescio R, Schiller G, et al. Purging of autologous peripheral-blood stem cells using CD34 selection does not improve overall or progression-free survival after high-dose chemotherapy for multiple myeloma: results of a multicenter randomized controlled trial. J Clin Oncol 2001;19:3771–3779.
251. Schouten HC, Qian W, Kvaloy S, et al. High-dose therapy improves progression-free survival and survival in relapsed follicular non-Hodgkin's lymphoma: results from the randomized European CUP trial. J Clin Oncol 2003;21:3918–3927.
252. Kernan NA, Collings NH, Juliano L, et al. Clonable T lymphocytes in T cell-depleted bone marrow transplants correlate with development of graft versus host disease. Blood 1986;68:770–773.
253. Aversa F, Tabilio A, Terenzi A, et al. Successful engraftment of T-cell-depleted haploidentical "three-loci" incompatible transplants in leukemia patients by addition of recombinant human granulocyte colony-stimulating factor-mobilized peripheral blood progenitor cells to bone marrow inoculum. Blood 1994;84:3948–3955.
254. Verdonck LF, Dekker AW, de Gast GC, et al. Allogeneic bone marrow transplantation with a fixed low number of T cells in the marrow graft. Blood 1994;83:3090–3096.
255. Wagner JE, Thompson JS, Carter SL, et al. Effect of graft-versus-host disease prophylaxis on 3-year disease-free survival in recipients of unrelated donor bone marrow (T-cell Depletion Trial): a multi-centre, randomised phase II-III trial. Lancet 2005;366:733–741.
256. Pavletic SZ, Carter SL, Kernan NA, et al. Influence of T-cell depletion on chronic graft-versus-host disease: results of a multicenter randomized trial in unrelated marrow donor transplantation. Blood 2005;106:3308–3313.
257. de Lissovoy G, Hurd D, Carter S, et al. Economic analysis of unrelated allogeneic bone marrow transplantation: results from the randomized clinical trial of T-cell depletion vs unmanipulated grafts for the prevention of graft-versus-host disease. Bone Marrow Transplant 2005;36:539–546.
258. Henslee J, Kenyon P, Ferrieri P, et al. Prevention of early gram positive (gm+) septicemia in autologous bone marrow transplant (ABMT) patients (PTS). Proc Am Soc Clin Oncol 1984;3:100.
259. Lazarus HM, Magalhaes-Silverman M, Fox RM, et al. Contamination during in vitro processing of bone marrow for transplantation: clinical significance. Bone Marrow Transplant 1991;7:241–246.
260. Morbidity and Mortality Weekly Report. Reported contamination of heparin sodium with *Pseudomonas putida*. MMWR Morb Mortal Wkly Rep 1986;35:123.
261. Schwella N, Rick O, Heuft HG, et al. Bacterial contamination of autologous bone marrow: reinfusion of culture-positive grafts does not result in clinical sequelae during the posttransplantation course. Vox Sang 1998;74:88–94.
262. Attarian H, Bensinger WE, Buckner CD, et al. Microbial contamination of peripheral blood stem cell collections. Bone Marrow Transplant 1996;17:699–702.
263. Schwella N, Rick O, Zimmermann R, et al. Microbiologic contamination of peripheral blood stem cell autografts. Vox Sang 1994;67:32–35.
264. Prince HM, Page SR, Keating A, et al. Microbial contamination of harvested bone marrow and peripheral blood. Bone Marrow Transplant 1995;15:87–91.
265. Schmid I, Krall WJ, Uittenbogaart CH, et al. Dead cell discrimination with 7-amino-actinomycin D in combination with dual color immunofluorescence in single laser flow cytometry. Cytometry 1992; 13:204–208.
266. Bender JG, Lum L, Unverzagt KL, et al. Correlation of colony-forming cells, long-term culture initiating cells and CD34+ cells in apheresis products from patients mobilized for peripheral blood progenitors with different regimens. Bone Marrow Transplant 1994;13:479–485.
267. Fritsch G, Printz D, Stimpfl M, et al. Quantification of CD34+ cells: Comparison of methods. Transfusion 1997;37:775–784.
268. Serke S, Arseniev L, Watts M, et al. Imprecision of counting CFU-GM colonies and CD34-expressing cells. Bone Marrow Transplant 1997;20:57–61.
269. Johnsen HE. Report from a Nordic workshop on CD34+ cell analysis: technical recommendations for progenitor cell enumeration in leukapheresis from multiple myeloma patients. J Hematother 1995;4:21–28.
270. Brecher ME, Sims L, Schmitz J, et al. North American multicenter study on flow cytometric enumeration of CD34+ hematopoietic stem cells. J Hematother 1996;5:227–236.

271. Sutherland DR, Anderson L, Keeney M, et al. The ISHAGE guidelines for CD34+ cell determination by flow cytometry. J Hematother 1996;5:213–226.
272. Pecora AL, Preti RA, Gleim GW, et al. CD34+CD33– cells influence days to engraftment and transfusion requirements in autologous blood stem-cell recipients. J Clin Oncol 1998;16:2093–2104.
273. Dercksen MW, Rodenhuis S, Dirkson MKA, et al. Subsets of CD34+ cells and rapid hematopoietic recovery after peripheral-blood stem-cell transplantation. J Clin Oncol 1995;13:1922–1932.
274. Dercksen MW, Gerritsen WR, Rodenhuis S, et al. Expression of adhesion molecules on CD34+ cells: CD34+L-selectin+ cells predict a rapid platelet recovery after peripheral blood stem cell transplantation. Blood 1995;85:3313–3319.
275. Rowley SD. Hematopoietic stem cell cryopreservation: A review of current techniques. J Hematother 1992;1:233-250.
276. Areman EM, Sacher RA, Deeg HJ. Processing and storage of human bone marrow: a survey of current practices in North America. Bone Marrow Transplant 1990;6:203–209.
277. Elliot C, McCarthy D. A survey of methods of processing and storage of bone marrow and blood stem cells in the EBMT. Bone Marrow Transplant 1994;14:419–423.
278. Gorin NC. Collection, manipulation and freezing of haemopoietic stem cells. In Goldstone AH (ed). Clinics in Haematology. London, Saunders, 1986, pp 19–48.
279. Rowley SD, Piantadosi S, Santos GW. Correlation of hematologic recovery with CFU-GM content of autologous bone marrow grafts treated with 4-hydroperoxycyclophosphamide culture after cryopreservation. Bone Marrow Transplant 1989;4:553–558.
280. Davis JM, Rowley SD, Braine HG, et al. Clinical toxicity of cryopreserved bone marrow graft infusion. Blood 1990;75:781–786.
281. David NA. The pharmacology of dimethyl sulfoxide 6544. Annu Rev Pharm 1972;12:353–374.
282. Dhodapkar M, Goldberg SL, Tefferi A, Gertz MA. Reversible encephalopathy after cryopreserved peripheral blood stem cell infusion. Am J Hematol 1994;45:187–188.
283. Rowley SD, Bensinger WI, Gooley TA, Buckner CD. The effect of cell concentration on bone marrow and peripheral blood stem cell cryopreservation. Blood 1994;83:2731–2736.
284. Rowley SD, MacLeod B, Heimfeld S, et al. Severe central nervous system toxicity associated with the infusion of cryopreserved PBSC components. Cytotherapy 1999;1:311–317.
285. Rowley SD, Feng Z, Chen L, et al. A randomized phase III clinical trial of autologous blood stem cell transplantation comparing cryopreservation using dimethylsulfoxide versus dimethylsulfoxide with hydroxyethylstarch. Bone Marrow Transplant 2003;31:1043–1051.
286. Davis JM, Rowley SD, Braine HG, et al. Clinical toxicity of cryopreserved bone marrow graft infusion. Blood 1990;75:781–786.
287. Beaujean F, Hartmann O, Kuentz M, et al. A simple, efficient washing procedure for cryopreserved human hematopoietic stem cells prior to reinfusion. Bone Marrow Transplant 1991;8:291–294.
288. Burnett AK, Tansey P, Hills C, et al. Haematological reconstitution following high dose and supralethal chemo-radiotherapy using stored, non-cryopreserved autologous bone marrow. Br J Haematol 1983;54:309–316.
289. Delforge A, Ronge-Collard E, Stryckmans P, et al. Granulocyte-macrophage progenitor cell preservation at 4° C. Br J Haematol 1983;53:49–54.
290. Preti RA, Razis E, Ciavarella D, et al. Clinical and laboratory comparison study of refrigerated and cryopreserved bone marrow for transplantation. Bone Marrow Transplant 1994;13:253–260.
291. Kohsake M, Yanes B, Ungerleider JS, Murphy MJ. Non-frozen preservation of committed hematopoietic stem cells from normal human bone marrow. Stem Cell 1981;1:111–123.
292. Beaujean F, Pico J, Norol F, et al. Characteristics of peripheral blood progenitor cells frozen after 24 hours of storage. J Hematother 1996;5:681–686.
293. Human cells, tissues, and cellular and tissue-based products; establishment registration and listing (Final Rule). 66 FR 5447, 2001.
294. Kessler DA, Siegel JP, Noguchi PD, et al. Regulation of somatic-cell therapy and gene therapy by the Food and Drug Administration. N Engl J Med 1993;329:1169–1173.

Chapter 61
Tissue Banking in the Hospital Setting

A. Bradley Eisenbrey • D. Michael Strong

INTRODUCTION

Tissue for transplantation belongs in the hospital blood bank. No other service in the hospital has the experience with the regulatory environment and compliance, Good Manufacturing Practices (GMPs), diverse storage requirements, inventory and record management, and tracking and tracing of human products. Like blood products, tissues have transmitted infectious diseases to recipients[1–10] and have required look-backs and recalls.[11] Application of the skills honed with blood components to "banking" tissue is a logical and conceptually simple expansion of services for the hospital blood bank.

Most hospital blood bankers were unaware of the volume and extent of human tissue use within their institutions until the Joint Commission on Healthcare Organization (JCAHO) published updated Standards in 2005, effective in July 2005.[12] The updated Standards require JCAHO-accredited institutions to name a single authority for oversight of tissue acquisition, storage, and tracking, and to create storage and tracking procedures and protocols consistent with the GMP standards followed in the transfusion medicine community. The new JCAHO Standards were a direct response to new federal regulations that brought United States Food and Drug Administration (FDA) oversight of nonmedical device human hematopoietic stem cell and tissue use in the United States and establishment of Good Tissue Practices (GTPs).[12,13]

Bone, tendon, skin, heart valves, corneas, sclera, fascia, and other tissues from deceased donors are transplanted every day in hospitals throughout the United States.[14–16] These tissues are recovered by registered eye and tissue banks, which screen the donors, perform disease-marker testing, process, package, and distribute the tissues to the physicians and dentists who implant the tissues. Tissues are recovered under aseptic conditions and undergo processing, which may vary from simple packaging to extensive computer-controlled milling, freezing, lyophilization, irradiation, or complicated washing processes. Some vendors report that their process produces sterile tissues.[15]

Most hospital blood banks have had little contact with these tissues other than informal arrangements for temporary storage of frozen tissue in a blood bank freezer or for holding a cornea in the blood bank refrigerator because of a delay in an operation. Although some hospitals are registered tissue banks and participate in the whole manufacturing process, "hospital tissue banking," for the purpose of this chapter, will refer to acting as a "consignee" or storage and distribution point for tissues within the hospital setting.

HOSPITAL TISSUE BANKING MODELS

Two models exist for handling tissues within the hospital setting. The most common model is the "decentralized" or "distributed" model, in which tissue is ordered, received, stored, and used within each of the separate hospital service areas. The decentralized model is exemplified by an ophthalmologist who places a direct order for a cornea from an eye bank, takes receipt of the cornea in the surgical suite, performs the transplant, and records the tissue information in the patient record. Similarly, an orthopedic surgeon may obtain a milled piece of lyophilized bone, or a vascular surgeon may obtain a frozen venous graft directly from a vendor and take delivery in the operating room. In each of these examples, the transplanting surgeon, and/or the surgical service, takes responsibility for ensuring the proper handling of the tissues from receipt to implantation. There may or may not be a log in which the receipt of the tissue at the hospital is recorded.

Alternatively, tissue "banking" in the hospital can be centralized in the department that runs the operating rooms, the hospital central supply, the pharmacy, or the blood bank. The knowledge, skills, and experience of hospital blood bankers make the blood bank the optimal choice.

The business of the hospital blood bank has been to provide patients with the appropriate blood products for their needs and to ensure that an adequate inventory of those blood products is maintained to prevent harmful delays in patient care. As technology advanced, the menu of blood products has expanded from the humble beginnings in whole blood kept in a refrigerator to a complex selection of packed red cells in the refrigerator, frozen plasma products in the freezers, and platelets maintained at room temperature. All of these are monitored. Add irradiation, leukocyte reduction, and screening for specific antibody or antigen negativity, and the inventory of most large hospital blood banks rivals other centralized services in complexity. The variety of monitored storage conditions resulted in the blood bank's becoming a useful intermediate storage place for human tissues foreign to most blood bankers. Bone, skin, vascular tissues, and other tissues such as corneas found their way onto the shelves of many blood banks, most often with informal agreements, if any.

Until 2005, the retrieval, processing, and distribution of bone, ocular, vascular, and connective tissue were virtually unregulated, with the exception of a few state laws and voluntary standards. Unless the tissues were substantially altered, federal regulations did not apply. It was routine in most hospitals for business transactions between the surgeon implanting the tissue and the vendor to occur without oversight by the institution in which the tissue was used.

Changes in federal regulations and voluntary standards of organizations like JCAHO and American Association of Blood Banks (AABB) have resulted in substantial changes in the way tissues are handled in hospitals.[13,17]

Ocular, vascular, and connective tissue and fresh and frozen bone have all been implicated in the transmission of bacterial, fungal, and viral diseases to transplant recipients, occasionally resulting in death. Retrieval of unused (stored) tissue after the identification of infectious cases has been complicated by the lack of formal tracking mechanisms. In some cases, the disposition of tissues was never known. The principle of being able to track a human tissue from the donor to the recipient (or backward) has, only recently, been applied to tissue banking, although the voluntary Standards of the American Association of Tissue Banks (AATB) and Eye Bank Association of America (EBAA) have incorporated the principle for years.[18,19] The tracking and traceability Standards of AATB and EBAA were enforceable only with their member tissue and eye banks. No enforcement existed for the end-user. AABB and JCAHO Standards require tracking and traceability to the patient.[12,20]

PROCESSES AND PROTOCOLS

Hospital tissue banking requires certain processes. A system must exist for a surgeon to select and order tissues appropriate for the types of surgery he or she performs and which meet the special anatomic and medical needs of the patient. The tissue must be ordered from the vendor (manufacturer). This requires establishment of purchasing and contractual arrangements. The tissue must be delivered to the hospital, and someone must take responsibility for acceptance of the tissue. The tissue may need to be stored before use, particularly if surgery is delayed or the tissue is found to be unsuitable for the particular patient. Informed consent for the use of allogeneic tissue must be obtained and documented. The tissue must be properly handled in the operating room, including careful final inspection to verify its type, suitability, and condition. The tissue must be properly reconstituted, if applicable. The use of the tissue must be appropriately documented in the patient's permanent medical record. The vendor must be notified of the disposition of the tissue to allow tracking in the event of a recall, usually by return of preaddressed reporting forms. Finally, a mechanism must exist for recognition and reporting of complications due to the tissue implanted.

A decentralized system for tissue handling places responsibility for ordering, receipt, storage, and tracking in the hands of the surgeon or service in which the tissue is used. This has been efficient for the surgeon because it eliminates administrative layers and allows ordering tissue on a highly individualized basis, when needed. If the salesperson for the tissue manufacturer is responsible, the support staff for the surgeon is appropriately trained to ensure proper storage and handling of the tissue, and the surgeon or operating room staff ensures proper documentation of the use of the tissue, including reporting to the vendor, this process can be effective. Tracking and traceability can be augmented in this system by the use of a tissue log in the surgical suite (tissue-accession register or record). In many cases, the salesperson for the vendor delivers the tissue and takes responsibility for ensuring proper handling and storage, up to and including the operating room.

JCAHO recognized the lack of standardization of tissue handling in hospitals and the difficulties that had been reported for tracking tissues that had been delivered to hospitals and established new Standards for member hospitals, beginning July 1, 2005.[12] The new JCAHO Standards incorporated many of the voluntary standards of the AATB, EBAA, and AABB (formerly American Association of Blood Banks). A Standard "unique" to JCAHO is a single individual responsible for the oversight of tissue in the hospital. JCAHO has created a responsible party for all tissue delivered to each member hospital.[12]

The JCAHO Standards do not preclude decentralized tissue handling in a hospital, but do modify the process and require a single person to keep track of each of the individual practices within the institution. Creation of a standardized protocol with uniform documentation will simplify the work of the tissue monitor.

Tissue banking at the author's organization, William Beaumont Hospital, Royal Oak, Michigan, evolved over a decade from a casual arrangement of holding tissues in the Blood Bank refrigerator or freezer to a formal process mandated by the hospital Blood Transfusion and Tissue Committee. Initial resistance to an ordered and centralized process is contrasted, today, with ready acceptance, high praise for the quality of the services provided, and swift rejection of a proposal to move responsibility to the operating room service.

The transition from casual to fully controlled was facilitated by four critical components: (1) an existing blood bank computer system that was readily adapted to manage tissue products like blood products, (2) an existing working relationship with the operating room team for specialized products that were already being stored in the blood bank, (3) a team of outstanding medical technologists with excellent supervision, and (4) a dedicated senior medical technologist (Hospital Tissue Coordinator) who had a good working knowledge of the tissue requirements and was able to communicate effectively with surgeons as problems arose. The process does not happen overnight, is unlikely to work as a "turn-key" operation, and continues to evolve as the product mix and size of the inventory changes.

The tissue banking process used at William Beaumont Hospital (WBH), Royal Oak, is a logical extension of the existing processes used for receipt, acceptance, storage, inventory, issuing, and tracking of blood products. The process is built with consideration of the published Standards of the AABB for handling and storage of tissues. Although most tissue products were not regulated by the federal government when the procedures and protocols used at WBH were established, all the tissue products were treated in the same manner as blood products. Experience as a registered blood establishment and a well-established quality assurance program helped in developing the procedures and processes for handling fresh, frozen, and lyophilized tissues.

Product Selection

Tissues for transplantation can be recovered from deceased donors (skin, cornea, sclera, cartilage), frozen (bones, vessels, valves) after initial aseptic recovery and processing, or further processed (bone, connective tissue) through lyophilization, patented washing/sterilization methods (Allowash; LifeNet, Virginia Beach, Va.; Bio-cleanse; Bio-cleanse Technologies, Bellingham, Wash.). Bone, in particular, can be milled and

Hospital

TISSUE BANK REQUEST

Frozen Bone

Quantity	Description and size
	Achilles Tendon (>19.5 cm)
	Anterior Tibialis Tendon (Call Blood Bank for dimensions)
	Distal Femur (See Frozen Allograft Bone Book for aailable sizes)
	Femoral Cortical Strut (20 cm, half of a femur)
	Femoral Head
	Femoral Shaft (15 cm)
	Femoral Trap—Anterior (10.75) *Depuy Bullets*
	Femoral Trap—Anterior Lateral(10.75) *Depuy Bullets*
	Femoral Trap—Anterior (12.75) *Depuy Bullets*
	Femoral Trap—Anterior Lateral(12.75) *Depuy Bullets*
	Femoral Trap—Anterior (14.75) *Depuy Bullets*
	Femoral Trap—Anterior Lateral(14.75) *Depuy Bullets*
	Femoral Trap—Anterior (16.74) *Depuy Bullets*
	Femoral Trap—Anterior Lateral(16.74) *Depuy Bullets*
	Fibula Shaft (18 cm)
	Fibula Shaft (12 cm)
	Gracilis Tendon (Call Blood Bank for dimensions)
	Patella-tibial Tendon (Hemi)
	Patella-tibial Tendon (Whole/special order)
	PLIF (9 x 9, W:9)
	PLIF (11 x 11, W:9)
	PLIF (13 x 13, W:9)
	Proximal Femur (See Frozen Allograft Bone Book for available sizes)
	Tibia Shaft (10 cm)
	Tibia Shaft (20 cm)

Lyophilized Bone *stored at room temperature*

Quantity	Description and Size
	Cervical Spacer (6 mm) (*Graftech™*)
	Cervical Spacer (7 mm) (*Graftech™*)
	Cervical Spacer (8 mm) (*Graftech™*)
	Cervical Spacer (9 mm) (*Graftech™*)
	Chips, Cancellous (15 cc)
	Chips, Cancellous (30 cc)
	Chips, Cancellous (60 cc)
	Cortical Cancellous Struts (1 x 10 cm, 1 per bottle)
	Cortical Cancellous Struts (6 cm x 8 mm, 6 per bottle)
	Cortical Cancellous Struts (6 cm x 3–6 cm, Matchsticks/4 per bottle)
	Crushed, Cancellous (30 cc)
	Dowel (12 mm)
	Dowel (14 mm)
	Fibula Shaft (8 cm)
	Fibula Wedge (8 mm)
	Flex (2.5 x 10 cm)
	Gel (10 cc) Circle Brand Preferred: *Graftech™* *Optium™*
	Gel (5.0 cc) *Optium™*
	Iliac Wedge (10–12 mm)
	Iliac Wedge (9 mm)
	Ilium Tricortical Strip (5 cm)
	Ilium Tricortical Strip (5.5 cm)
	Ilium Tricortical Strip (6.0 cm, Special order)
	Patella Wedge (13–15 mm)
	Putty (10 cc) Circle Brand Preferred: *DBX®* *Optium™*
	Putty (1 cc) Circle Brand Preferred: *DBX®*

ORA Runner ID#: ________________

Patient's information

SoftTissues

Quantity	Description and Size	*Storage*
	Amniotic Membrane (4 x 4 cm)	RT
	Cornea (Special order)	4°C
	Fascia Lata (2 x 12 cm)	RT
	Heart Valve	−190°C
	Pericardium (1.5 x 1.5 cm) *Tutoplast®*	RT
	Pericardium (5 x 10 cm) *Graft Jacket™*	4°C
	Saphenous Vein—group A	−190°C
	Saphenous Vein—group B	−190°C
	Saphenous Vein—group O	−190°C
	Sclera (0.5 x 8 cm) *Tutoplast®*	RT
	Sclera (Special order)	RT
	Skin product (2 x 4 cm) *Alloderm®*	4°C
	Skin product (2 x 7 cm) *Repliform™*	4°C
	Skin product (3 x 7 cm) *Alloderm®*	4°C
	Skin product (4 x 12 cm) *Alloderm®*	4°C
	Skin product (4 x 16 cm) *Alloderm®*	4°C

SPECIAL ORDER Indicate

Product:

Size:

Quantity:

Date reserved:

Figure 61–1 Tissue request form.

tooled to obtain unique shapes and structural characteristics unavailable in the native tissue.[15,21]

Product selection is driven by the transplanting surgeon. The surgeon contacts the Hospital Tissue Coordinator (HTC) with a request for a particular tissue product by using the Request Form (Fig. 61–1). If the product is from a vendor that has already been evaluated and qualified, the product is ordered and placed into the inventory on receipt. If a similar product is already in the inventory or is available from a qualified vendor, the HTC will contact the surgeon with that information and will attempt to persuade the surgeon to accept the existing product as a substitute. If the vendor has not been qualified, the surgeon is notified that the request cannot be filled as requested until the vendor qualification is complete and a site visit is arranged. Tissues from nonqualified vendors are not allowed into the hospital. This is enforced through the inability of the vendor to bill for any products not authorized by the HTC.

A key component of a successful centralized hospital tissue bank is the support of the hospital Purchasing Department. Vendors are not allowed to deliver tissues to the operating rooms, and payments are not authorized for tissues that are not ordered by the HTC. These practices keep unauthorized tissues from being brought into the hospital and ensure compliance with tracking requirements.

Vendor Qualification

Vendor qualification includes documentation of certification by AATB, all necessary licensure (i.e., Florida and New York) and/or registrations, and evaluation of the processes used in donor acceptance, prevention of cross-contamination, tissue processing, storage, tracking, quality assurance, and staff training and competency evaluation. Vendor qualification has required site visits by the Medical Director or Associate Medical Director, HTC and/or Blood Bank Quality Assurance Officer. A template can be used for evaluation to ensure completeness. The supporting documents are requested before the site visit.

Inventory Control

Inventory control is dynamic and similar to management of the blood product inventory. The turnover rate of each product is carefully monitored so that enough tissue is maintained in the inventory to prevent having to postpone surgery. If a particular tissue is nearing outdate, the HTC works closely with surgeons and operating room staff so that the tissue will not be discarded. The most significant problem with tissue is the unusual special-order bone or cardiovascular tissue that is obtained (usually frozen) for a particular patient. Outdates happen and can be significant financial events as well as an unfortunate waste of donated cadaveric tissue.

Inventory is communicated to the surgeons through continuously updated catalogs of available tissues. The catalogs are kept in the operating room cores. Telephone calls are placed to the surgeons' offices when special-order tissue arrives. The inventory is available to all of the blood bank staff through the blood bank computer system as a look-up function so that availability can be confirmed. A copy of the catalog is kept in the blood bank.

In 2005, no uniform labeling or nomenclature exists for tissue products. As a result, unique product codes are generated by the HTC to allow tracking of the inventory. In some cases, the product codes of the manufacturer can be directly incorporated; however, unique identifiers are not standardized across vendors, so some creativity is necessary until standardization develops. The result is an unusual mixture of product codes that may defy logic in the naming because of the complexity of the inventory and the number of different product codes required. A movement to adopt ISBT code 128 labeling standards by European Tissue Bank organizations would greatly simplify inventory management and tracking.[22]

Because of the lack of a uniform national labeling standard, each product brought into the inventory is given a unique tracking number generated by the blood bank. These can be referenced to the individual product for recalls. The unique tracking number can be referenced from the patient back to the product and the vendor in the event of an adverse outcome from the transplant.

The challenges of inventory control include the large number of highly specialized, milled bone products, many designed solely for a single surgical-instrument manufacturer's tools. This boutique approach to inventory can result in expensive duplication and waste if a surgical tool goes out of fashion. Although tissue invoices will not be paid if the tissue was not ordered by the blood bank HTC, and all tissue must be delivered to the blood bank to be accessioned, vendors and salespeople continue to approach the surgeons directly and enter the operating room to pitch their wares, occasionally under the guise of demonstrating new products.

ECONOMIC CONSIDERATIONS

Tissue products are expensive. The vendor charges for tissues range from approximately \$360 for a 30-mL volume of cancellous chips to \$2900 for complex milled products (femoral trapezoid ring) and \$3700 for special-order frozen bone products (whole femur) (W. Frizzo, MT [ASCP], personal communication). Cryopreserved heart valves can exceed \$7500 (D. Michael Strong, PhD, personal communication). A centralized inventory and bank in the hospital allows close tracking of the inventory to ensure that "short-dated" products get used rather than being discarded. Improper handling resulting in wastage can be identified and corrective actions put in place. For example, a circulating nurse, who opens multiple tissue packages in the operating room instead of waiting for the surgeon to select the appropriate product, can be educated on the expense and the impact of wasting the products.

An additional benefit of a centralized program is the ability to negotiate better pricing from the vendors because of better knowledge of the competing products and the ability to do volume purchasing and standing orders. The cost of "drop-shipping" or hand delivery of individual tissue products is always greater than the scheduled purchasing arrangement. Even products with short "shelf life" can be scheduled into an inventory with careful management.

Another benefit of centralized purchasing and inventory is the ability to encourage competition between vendors for quality improvements, improvements in supply, and customer service. The direct sales model, preferred by the vendors because of the loyalty factor created by the interaction of the salesperson and the surgeon, restricts any cost comparisons.

ACCESSIONING TISSUES

Accessioning tissues follows the template of the receipt of blood products. The packaging is inspected for damage, labels are checked, and the temperature of the shipped product is evaluated to ensure that the product stayed within the acceptable range determined by the manufacturer. If these are in order, the tissue is accessioned into the inventory and assigned unique product and tracking numbers for the computer system. The process is facilitated by vendors that barcode products. Barcode labels are printed with the unique product identification/tracking numbers for the products that are not barcoded (or when barcoding is unusable) by the manufacturer. The accessioning process includes the storage location to ease finding the tissue when it is requested.

Storage and Handling

Storage and handling requirements are set by the vendor (manufacturer) for each tissue product. AABB and JCAHO Standards require continuous temperature monitoring and documentation of the temperatures of refrigerators and freezers.[12,20] In addition, storage equipment must have functional alarms and emergency backup. AABB Standards require monitoring and recording of the room temperature.[20] The importance of this is not immediately apparent without recognition of the number of products that are stored at "room temperature." Most manufacturers are becoming more explicit in the definition of room temperature.

Packaging

Packaging is not generally an issue for the end user or consignee unless the product is damaged in handling. For those institutions that store autologous tissues, however, packaging becomes an important step in the manufacturing process. The ideal packaging is built of sealable clear plastic pharmaceutical grade bags that will remain flexible at freezer temperatures and will tolerate gamma or x-ray irradiation. Clear packaging allows inspection of the contents without opening the package and immediate recognition that the correct tissue product has been selected (e.g., Rollprint Packaging Products, Inc., Addison, Ill., and Kimberly-Clark, Roswell, Ga.). Opaque overwraps may ease handling within the operating room by allowing traditional opening procedures for the nurse assisting the surgeon, but the contents are collected aseptically and should not be considered sterile unless sterility is proven.

Barcoding

Barcodes are not standardized between vendors. When barcoding is present on the tissue product packaging, the information encoded can vary dramatically from vendor to vendor, ranging from simple product identification to embedded coding allowing traceability to the individual donor. In many cases, the coded information is not sufficient to allow an individual tissue product to be uniquely identified. In these circumstances, the addition of a locally produced barcode label may improve inventory control, tracking, and the ability to trace from the patient back to a specific tissue-product vendor when complications occur.

Issuing

Issuing tissues requires a request form for each tissue (see Fig. 61–1). The request forms are patient specific, and the tissues are issued to a specific patient rather than to a surgeon or operating room. The unique identifier is used to link the specific tissue product permanently to the specific patient. When the tissue product is issued, it is accompanied by a multiple-part form for tracking similar to the "transfusion tag" used in most blood banks (Fig. 61–2). The first page of the multipart form is placed in the patient record, and the duplicate page is returned to the blood bank. Reporting forms (frequently a postcard format) for the manufacturer can be returned directly by the surgeon or the HTC.

Tracking

Tracking is performed on multiple levels. Because all tissue comes to the blood bank in the centralized model, the location of all unused tissue is known, virtually immediately. In the author's experience, a major vendor recall was completed in less than 15 minutes, with all tissues accounted for. Because tissue is issued for a specific patient, the assurance that it is used for the specified patient is very high (chart record audits have been consistent for the final disposition) but will be improved when electronic records allow a direct link between the barcoded product and a specific patient's record. Untoward events can be linked to the specific tissue because surgical complications (e.g., wound infections) reported to the hospital epidemiologists are crosschecked against the daily tissue-use listing.

Traceability

Traceability is maintained by the direct one-to-one link of a patient to a specific tissue issued from the blood bank, which is linked to the unique identifiers of the tissue and for the manufacturer. Some manufacturers embed the donor information that can be recovered to allow tracing back from the recipient to the donor. The blood bank computer database is archived on a continuous basis with routine backups and results in a stable platform for future look-backs, if needed. Appropriately completed, vendor supplied transplant report forms can also improve traceability by documenting the link between the recipient and the donor.

Autologous Tissues

Calvaria (skull bone flaps),[23,24] bone,[25,26] skin,[27–29] and parathyroids[30,31] are frequently stored for various amounts of time for reimplantation in the original anatomic position (skull bone flap) or new location (iliac crest bone for spinal fusion, skin autografts for burn or plastic surgery, limb site for parathyroid reimplantation). The role of the hospital tissue bank can range from processing the tissue for long-term storage (see Packaging) to holding a tissue in culture media overnight. In most cases of autologous tissue transplants in the hospital setting, the tissue is removed, minimally manipulated, and reimplanted during the same surgical procedure. Careful records must be kept because autologous tissue can be forgotten by the surgeon and never used, thus becoming the blood bank's problem. Some limits must be placed on length of storage to avoid this situation.

Stem Cells and Reproductive Tissues

Stem cells and reproductive tissues are beyond the scope of this chapter. Stem cell and reproductive tissue collection, processing, storage, handling, and transplantation are regulated under 21CFR1271.[13] Stem cell laboratories and transplant centers are

Section 1—Allograft Information and Receipt

Type of Allograft	Product Name	Description	Volume
			OC

Blood Product Code	Identification Number	Expiration Date	ABO/Rh	Source Code

Shipping Method	Graft Transport Temperature OK?	Graft Storage
□ Frozen □ Refrigerated □ Room Temp	□ Yes □ No	□ Blood Bank □ Other (specify)

Graft Packaging Intact?	ID on Graft Match Invoices?	If either answer is NO, notify Tissue Coordinator:	Tissue Coordinator Notified:
□ Yes □ No	□ Yes □ No		Date: Tech:

Processing Tech Initials	Receipt Date:	Receipt Time:	

Section 2—Product Tracking and Disposition
(**Surgical nursing** complete shaded areas)

Product Issue	**Product Preparation—Nursing**	**Product Return to Blood Bank**
Transplant Surgeon:	Packing intact prior to use? □ Yes □ No* **If NO, return product to Blood Bank*	Tech receiving product return:
Issued to:	Expiration date verified as: □ In-date □ Expired* **If expired, return product to Blood Bank*	**Return Transport Condition** □ On dry ice □ Room temperature □ On liquid N_2 □ On wet ice □ Lacking transport coolant (*explain below*)
Issuing Tech	Graft Prepared by:	*(observations of inappropriate transport conditions)*
Issue Date & Time	**Graft Disposition** □ Implanted □ Discarded □ Returned	Return Date & Time

Figure 61–2 Tissue tracking form.

accredited by the AABB, Foundation for the Accreditation of Cellular Therapy (FACT, Omaha, Nebr.), American Society for Blood and Marrow Transplantation (ASBMT, Arlington Heights, Ill.), National Marrow Donor Program (NMDP, Minneapolis, Minn.), and other organizations. Reproductive tissue laboratories and transplant centers are accredited by the AABB, AATB (McLean, Va.), and the American Society for Reproductive Medicine (ASRM, Birmingham, Ala.).[32]

TRANSFER OF TISSUES BETWEEN INSTITUTIONS

Current regulations consider hospitals and surgical centers as "consignees" or end users for tissues for transplantation.[13] If tissue for transplantation is stored at a hospital but transferred to another hospital for use, the hospital storing the tissue must meet GTP requirements and may be considered a vendor if the practice is routine. In May 2006, the Health Resources and Services Administration (HRSA) revised the definition of "organ" to include blood vessels (usually segments of iliac arteries and veins) recovered from an organ donor during the same recovery procedure such as organ(s) and intended for use in organ transplantation. This excluded blood vessels intended for use in organ transplantation from the definition of human cells, tissues, and cellular and tissue-based products (HCT/Ps).

Because of this revision, blood vessels labeled and intended solely for use in organ transplantation became subject to HRSA requirements in 42 CFR part 121 and any enforceable organ procurement and transplantation network (OPTN) policies established under 42 CFR part 121.[34]

ORGANS AND THE HOSPITAL TISSUE BANK

The solid organ (renal, heart, lung, liver, pancreas, small bowel) transplant community has always understood the critical nature of ABO compatibility in transplant. Untoward events involving unintended ABO-incompatible transplants of organs resulted in revisions to the Standards of the United Network for Organ Sharing in 2005 (Standard 3.1.4.2; UNOS, Richmond, Va.). Many transplant centers changed internal procedures before the revision of the Standards to confirm the ABO group of the donor and recipient and to improve the documentation of the checks during the organ acceptance and transplant process.

Although time is critical and delays do result in poorer graft and recipient outcomes, ABO-incompatibility may be fatal and certainly can result in immediate graft loss. Accessioning solid organs through the hospital blood bank, confirming the ABO of the recipient (from review of repeated testing of blood group typing), and confirming the ABO of the donor organ by using a sample tube included with the organ gives the surgeon and transplant team a final opportunity to check for ABO-compatibility and to document the acceptance of the organ for transplant. The greater the sensitivity of the organ to cold ischemia time, the more urgent the process. However, assumptions about prior testing and the inherent sense of urgency have contributed to fatal mistakes.[33]

Organs can be triaged in the hospital blood bank with the same efficiency that is present when handling a trauma or massive transfusion case. Well-defined procedures, carefully constructed tracking forms, and clear documentation facilitate the process and result in minimal delays. The author has seen the system work when two kidneys from deceased donors were accepted for two patients on the hospital transplant service within a couple of hours, and the second kidney arrived first. The blood bank check of the records stopped a fairly rapid process in which the first transplant team assumed that the kidney that was sent by the Organ Procurement Organization was for their patient and began prepping the operating room and preparing the patient. The chain of assumptions was broken, and the second transplant team was called in to proceed with the appropriate organ and recipient. Admittedly, this is highly unusual, and even less likely for other organs, but it demonstrated that the system worked.

CONCLUSIONS

The use of tissue will continue to increase until cultured or synthetic replacements are found for these highly successful, but potentially dangerous, transplants. Changes in federal regulations and JCAHO Standards have resulted in increased scrutiny and controls on the handling of these human products. The transfusion medicine community, particularly blood bankers, has had more experience than any other hospital organization with operating in the GMP environment and dealing with federal and state regulators and voluntary accreditation organizations. Tissues (and organs) are amenable to the processes, procedures, and protocols used by the hospital blood bank to order, accession, store, track, issue, and trace blood products.

REFERENCES

1. Zou S, Dodd RY, Stramer SL, Strong DM, for the Tissue Safety Study Group. Probability of viremia with HBV, HCV, HIV, and HTLV among tissue donors in the United States. N Engl J Med 2004;351:751–759.
2. CDC. Epidemiologic notes and reports transmission of HIV through bone transplantation: case report and public health recommendations. MMWR Morb Mortal Wkly Rep. 1988;37:597–599.
3. Henkel J. Safeguarding human tissue transplants. FDA Consumer, September 1994. Available at http://www.fda.gov/bbs/ topics/CONSUMER/ CON0289c.html.
4. CDC. *Candida albicans* endocarditis associated with a contaminated aortic valve allograft: California, 1996. MMWR Morb Mortal Wkly Rep. 1997;46:261–263.
5. CDC. Septic arthritis following anterior cruciate ligament reconstruction using tendon allografts: Florida and Louisiana, 2000. MMWR Morb Mortal Wkly Rep. 2001;50:1081–1083.
6. CDC. Update: Allograft-associated bacterial infections: United States, 2002. MMWR Morb Mortal Wkly Rep. 2002;51:207–210.
7. CDC. Hepatitis C virus transmission from an antibody-negative organ and tissue donor: United States, 2000–2002. MMWR Morb Mortal Wkly Rep. 2003;52:273–276.
8. CDC. Invasive *Streptococcus pyogenes* after allograft implantation: Colorado, 2003. MMWR Morb Mortal Wkly Rep. 2003;52:1173–1176.
9. CDC. Clostridial endophthalmitis after cornea transplantation: Florida, 2003. MMWR Morb Mortal Wkly Rep. 2003;52:1176–1179.
10. CDC. Update: Investigation of rabies infections in organ donor and transplant recipients: Alabama, Arkansas, Oklahoma, and Texas, 2004. MMWR Morb Mortal Wkly Rep. 2004;53:615–616.
11. FDA Public Health Web Notification. Human Tissue Processed by Cryolife, Inc., 21 August 2002. Available at http://www.fda.gov/cdrh/ safety/humantissue.html.
12. Joint Commission on Accreditation of Healthcare Organizations. Overcoming challenges: Tissue standards: Joint Commission. The Source 2005;Feb;3(2):5–12(8).
13. Code of Federal Regulations, Title 21, Part 1271, Human cells, tissues, and cellular and tissue-based products (21CFR1271).
14. Strong DM, Eastlund T, Mowe J. Tissue bank activity in the United States: 1992 survey of AATB-inspected tissue banks. Tissue Cell Rep 1992;3:15–18.
15. Woll J. Tissue banking overview. Clin Lab Med 2005;25(3):473–486.
16. Gandhi M, Strong DM. Cardiovascular tissues for transplantation. Clin Lab Med 2005;25(3):571–585.
17. Eisenbrey AB, Frizzo W. Tissue banking regulations and oversight. Clin Lab Med 2005;25(3):487–498.
18. American Association of Tissue Banks. Standards for Tissue Banking, 10th ed. McLean, Va., AATB, 2002.
19. EBAA. EBAA Medical Standards. Washington, D.C., EBAA, June 2004.
20. AABB. Standards for Blood Banks and Transfusion Services, 23rd ed. Bethesda, Md., AABB, 2004.
21. Woll J, Smith D. Bone and connective tissue. Clin Lab Med 2005;25(3):499–518.
22. Fehily D, Ashford P, Poniatowski S. Traceability of human tissues for transplantation: the development and implementation of a coding system using ISBT 128. Organs Tissues 2004;2:83–88.
23. Crotti F, Mangiagalli E. Cranial defects repair by replacing bone flaps. J Neurosurg Sci 1979;23:289–294.
24. Iwama T, Yamada J, Imai S, et al. The use of frozen autogenous bone flaps in delayed cranioplasty revisited. Neurosurgery 2003;52:591–596.
25. Ahlmann E, Patzakis M, Roidis N, et al. Comparison of anterior and posterior iliac crest bone grafts in terms of harvest-site morbidity and functional outcomes. J Bone Joint Surg Am 2002;84:716–720.
26. Roselli R, Muscatello L, Valdatta L, et al. Mandibular reconstruction with frozen autologous mandibular bone and radial periosteal fasciocutaneous free flap: preliminary report. Ann Otol Rhinol Laryngol 2004;113:956–960.
27. Bannasch H, Fohn M, Unterberg T, et al. Skin tissue engineering. Clin Plast Surg 2003;30:573–579.
28. Carsin H, Ainaud P, Le Bever H, et al. Cultured epithelial autografts in extensive burn coverage of severely traumatized patients: A five year single-center experience with 30 patients. Burns 2000;26:379–387.
29. Hierner R, Degreef H, Vranckx JJ, et al. Skin grafting and wound healing-the "dermato-plastic team approach." Clin Dermatol 2005;23: 343–352.
30. Lo C. Parathyroid autotransplantation during thyroidectomy. Aust NZ J Surg 2002;72:902–907.
31. Gauger P, Reeve T, Wilkinson M, Delbridge L. Routine parathyroid autotransplantation during total thyroidectomy: the influence of technique. Eur J Surg 2000;166:605–609.
32. Shah T, Keye W. Fertility: tissue and cell banking overview. Clin Lab Med 2005;25(3):557–569.
33. Campion E. A death at Duke. N Engl J Med 2003;348:1083–1084.
34. Health Resources and Services Administration. Blood vessels recovered with organs intended for use in organ transplantation; companion document to direct final rule. Federal Register 21CFR121 Proposed Rules 2006 May;71(92):27649–27651.

Index

Note: Page numbers followed by f indicate figures; those followed by t indicate tables; those followed by b indicate boxes.

C

D

M

N

O

P

Q

R

X

Y

Z

eye: Hole in the axe head where the handle is inserted

ferrite: Structural designation for irons with cubic body-centered crystal lattice

field forge: Transportable forge that can be set up outdoors

flame cutting: Cutting method using a gas flame to cut the metals

flash layer: Gap between upper and lower die parts; in drop forging, this results in working with excess material.

flattening: Forging technique to increase the length and decrease the thickness of the workpiece

flux: Agent for soldering

forge: Apparatus for heating forged pieces. Most are powered by gas or coal.

forge welding: Historical welding process using the smithy fire

forging temperature: Favorable temperature for forging

free-form forging: Forging process in which the blacksmith uses a hammer and an anvil to make the forged piece

fullering: The workpiece diameter is reduced at one place.

gas forge: Forge that primarily burns gas with ceramic chips to evenly heat the workpieces better

gas furnace: Liquid-gas-fueled gas firing

grooving hammer: Hammer to make round or pointed grooves

hammer face: Square side of the hammer used to strike the blows

hammer peen: Half-rounded side of a hammer

harden by quenching: Steel hardness can be significantly increased by quenching in cold water.

hardening: Process to increase the hardness of a material

hardening the welding point: If steel with a carbon content of more than 0.4 percent is welded, the rapid cooling of the welding point in the air causes a hardening process at the welding point.

hatchet (*Beil* in German): Axe without an eye to insert the handle (such as a stone axe)

heat: Term for heating to forging temperature (such as first heat for first heating)

honing: Hammering out small indentations in the scythe blade

ingot: Preform cut from flat steel for forging a scythe

iron: Chemical element from the group of metals with a melting point of 2,797°F (1,536°C)

iron-carbon diagram: A graph showing the connections of the iron and carbon systems in an idealized form

locking pliers: Self-locking pliers

logging staples: U-shaped curved and pointed staple for wood

manipulator: Device to hold and move large forged pieces

material number: System for identifying metals

neutral axis: An imaginary line that is neither compressed nor subject to tension when a workpiece is bent

normal annealing: Annealing process to produce the initial state for a steel

oxyfuel welding system: System for gas welding

perlite: A structural area made of cementite (Fe_3C) and ferrite.

prerequisite: Carbon content of at least 0.4 percent.

puddling furnace: Historical furnace for making pig iron fired with hard coal. Product = puddled steel.

punch: Noncutting method to make an opening in a workpiece

pure iron: Chemically pure iron

refining: Burning unwanted metalloids out of pig iron, which creates steel

residual heat: Workpiece is not completely quenched during hardening

residual stresses: There may be internal stresses in a workpiece from outside without any external force effect. This can occur due to uneven cooling, for example.

sappie: Tool used by woodsmen to move round logs

scale: Oxide layer on steel surface, caused by oxygen in the air

sledgehammer: Heavy hammer for powerful blows; can be replaced by a power hammer

spark test: Simple method to roughly determine steel composition

spectral analysis: Modern method for determining a steel grade

splitting: Forging technique using a splitting hammer or splitting chisel to separate a forged piece lengthwise

spreading: Forging process used to increase the width of the workpiece

star washer: Grinding wheel with several fan-shaped grinding disks made of cardboard

steel: Alloy of iron with carbon

stress cracks: Cracks in the hardened area caused by rapid cooling

striker: Blacksmith's helper who does the "striking"

tang: Connecting piece between the scythe snath and the blade portion

tempering: Heat treatment of steel that increases the workpiece's toughness by reducing hardness

tempering color: Steel shows various colors when heated, depending on temperature.

tensile strength: (Resistance to) stress on a material that leads to breakage

tilt hammer: Heavy-duty forging hammers driven by waterpower; the hammer is raised and dropped by cams on the drive shaft. They are no longer used.

TTT diagram: Indicates how structural changes occur depending on time and temperature

ultimate strain: Expansion until the sample piece breaks

upsetting: Forging technique to decrease the length and increase the thickness of the workpiece

volute: Term for a decorative curved piece

weldability: Welding capacity of steel. High-alloy steels cannot be welded well without additional processes.

whetting: Cold forging of the worn cutting edge of a scythe

wrought iron: Steel made by forging for forging work (historical)

yield strength: Maximum load for a material where no permanent deformation occurs

Sources and Notes

Feiner Sappel–Manufaktur Feiner GmbH
Industriepark 8 A-8682 Hönigsberg
www.feiner.at

Höhere Technische Bundeslehranstalt Kapfenberg
Viktor-Kaplan-Straße 1 A-8605 Kapfenberg
www.htl-kapfenberg.ac.at

Krenhof Schmiedetechnik
Judenburger Straße 188 A-8580 Köfach
www.krenhof.at

Loidolt Johann, proprietor Maria Dirnbacher
Smithy Untertal 1 8611 St. Kathrein an der Laming

Himmelberger Zeughammerwerk Leonhard Müller & Söhne GmbH
Zellach 4 A-9413 St. Gertraud
www.mueller-hammerwerk.at

Franz de Paul Schröckenfux GmbH
Sensenwerk ("scythe factory") Roßleithen 7 A-4575 Roßleithen
www.schroeckenfux.at

Literature

Bergland, Håvard. ***Die Kunst des Schmiedens*** ("The art of forging"). 4th ed. Bruckmühl, Germany: Wieland Verlag, 2013.

Domke, Wilhelm. ***Werkstoffkunde und Werkstoffprüfung*** ("Materials science and materials testing"). 10th ed. Essen, Germany: Verlag Girardet, 1986.

Enander, Lars, and Karl-Gunnar Noren. ***Schmieden lernen*** ("Learn to forge"). 3rd ed. Hannover, Germany: Verlag Th. Schäfer, 2008.

Gissing, Karl. ***Einfach schmieden alle Grundtechniken*** ("Simple forging: All basic techniques"). 2nd ed. Stuttgart: Leopold Stocker Verlag Graz, 2013.

Guichard d' Arenc, Jean-Paul. ***Die Herrscher über den Stahl: Eine illustrierte Geschichte des Schmiedens*** ("The conquerors of steel: An illustrated history of forging"). 2nd ed. Reinstetten-Ochsenhausen, Germany: Angele-Verlag, 2009.

Hundeshagen, Herrmann. ***Der Schmied am Amboß: Eine praktisches Lehrbuch für all Schmiede*** ("The blacksmith at the anvil: A practical textbook for all blacksmiths"). 8th ed. Hannover, Germany: Vincentz Network, 2010.

Kopp, Reiner, and Herbert Wiegels. ***Einführung in die Umformtechnik*** ("Introduction to forming technique"). 2nd ed. Aachen, Germany: Verlag Mainz, 1999.

Lamp, Ingo. ***Werkzeugkunde für die Waldarbeit im Gebirge*** ("Tool design for mountain forestry"). 3rd ed. Graz, Austria: Steiermärkischer Forstverein, 1952.

Sims, Lorelei. T***he Complete Blacksmith: Traditional Techniques for the Modern Smith***. Gloucester, MA: Quarry Books, 2006.

Weißbach, Wolfgang. ***Aufgabensammlung Werkstoffkunde und Werkstoffprüfung*** ("Materials science and materials testing"). 11th ed. Wiesbaden, Germany: Verlag Vieweg, 1993.

OTHER SCHIFFER BOOKS ON RELATED SUBJECTS

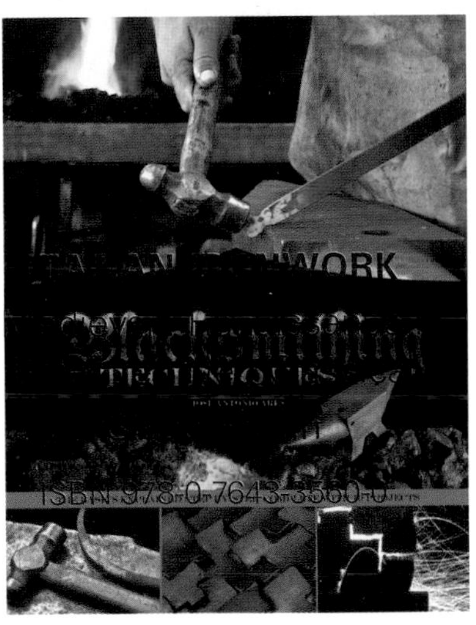

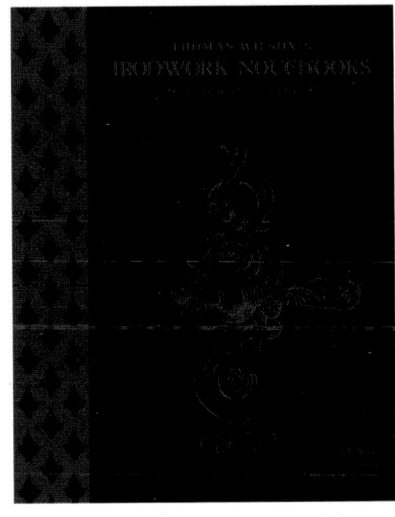

BLACKSMITHING TECHNIQUES

The Basics Explained Step by Step, Complete with 10 Projects

José Antonio Ares

ISBN 978-0-7643-4935-5

THOMAS WILSON'S IRONWORK NOTEBOOKS

Inspiration from a Master

Sally Adam
Foreword by
H. Russell Zimmermann

ISBN 978-0-7643-5180-8

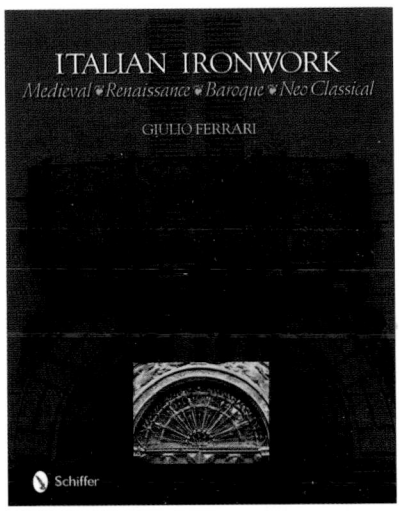

ITALIAN IRONWORK

Medieval : Renaissance : Baroque : Neo Classical

Giulio Ferrari

ISBN 978-0-7643-3560-0

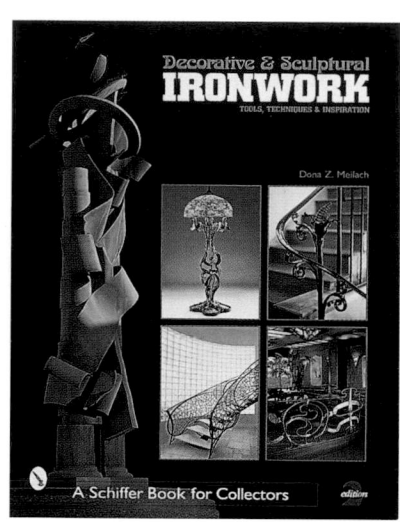

DECORATIVE & SCULPTURAL IRONWORK

Tools, Techniques & Inspiration

Dona Z. Meilach

ISBN 978-0-7643-0790-4

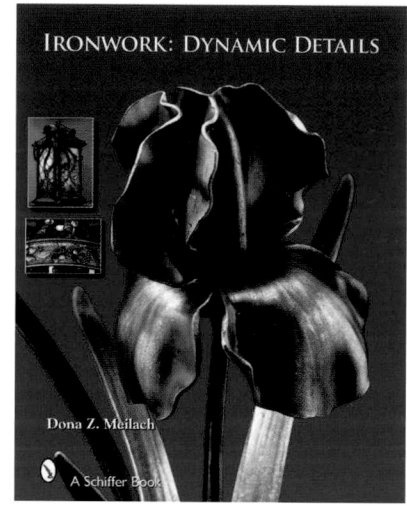

IRONWORK

Dynamic Details

Dona Z. Meilach

ISBN 978-0-7643-2549-6

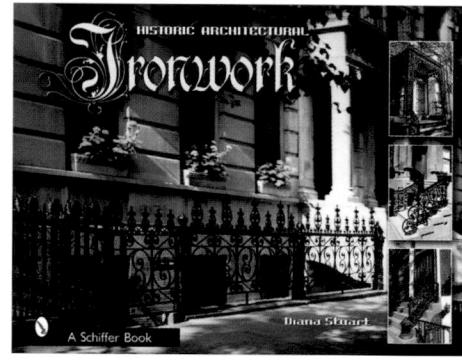

DECORATIVE ARCHITECTURAL IRONWORK

Featuring Wrought & Cast Designs

Diana Stuart

ISBN 978-0-7643-2192-4